Foundations for Osteopathic Medicine

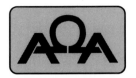

Bureau of Research

AMERICAN
OSTEOPATHIC
ASSOCIATION

Foundations for Osteopathic Medicine

Published under the auspices of the American Osteopathic Association and the Bureau of Research and carries their seal of approval

EXECUTIVE EDITOR

ROBERT C. WARD

SECTION EDITORS

JOHN A. JEROME

JOHN M. JONES III

ROBERT E. KAPPLER

ALBERT F. KELSO

MICHAEL L. KUCHERA

WILLIAM A. KUCHERA

MICHAEL M. PATTERSON

BARBARA A. PETERSON

FELIX J. ROGERS

MICHAEL A. SEFFINGER

SARAH A. SPRAFKA

RICHARD L. VAN BUSKIRK

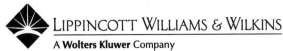

LIPPINCOTT WILLIAMS & WILKINS
A **Wolters Kluwer** Company
Philadelphia · Baltimore · New York · London
Buenos Aires · Hong Kong · Sydney · Tokyo

Editor: John P. Butler
Managing Editor: Linda S. Napora
Development Editor: Tom Lochhaas
Production Coordinators: Carol Eckhart, Kim Nawrozki
Copy Editors: Klemie Bryte, Karen Ruppert
Designer: Dan Pfisterer
Illustration Planner: Ray Lowman
Typesetter: University Graphics, Inc.
Printer & Binder: R.R. Donnelley & Sons

Copyright © 1997 Williams & Wilkins

351 West Camden Street
Baltimore, Maryland 21201-2436 USA

Rose Tree Corporate Center
1400 North Providence Road
Building II, Suite 5025
Media, Pennsylvania 19063-2043 USA

Accurate indications, adverse reactions and dosage schedules for drugs are provided in this book, but it is possible that they may change. The reader is urged to review the package information data of the manufacturers of the medications mentioned.

Printed in the United States of America

Library of Congress Cataloging-in-Publication Data

Foundations for osteopathic medicine / executive editor, Robert C. Ward ; section editors, John
  A. Jerome . . . [et al.] ; AOA.
        p.   cm.
    Includes index.
    ISBN 0-683-08792-4
    1. Osteopathic medicine.   2. Osteopathic medicine—Philosophy.
  I. Ward, Robert C., DO.   II. Jerome, John A.   III. American Osteopathic Association.
    [DNLM: 1. Osteopathic Medicine—methods.   WB 940 F771 1997]
    RZ342.F68   1997
    615.5′33—dc20
    DNLM/DLC
    for Library of Congress   96-16610
                                                                            CIP

The publishers have made every effort to trace the copyright holders for borrowed material. If they have inadvertently overlooked any, they will be pleased to make the necessary arrangements at the first opportunity.

To purchase additional copies of this book, call our customer service department at **(800) 638-0672** or fax orders to **(800) 447-8438.** For other book services, including chapter reprints and large quantity sales, ask for the special sales department.

Canadian customers should call **(800) 268-4178,** or fax **(905) 470-6780.** For all other calls originating outside of the United States, please call **(410) 528-4223** or fax us at **(410) 528-8550.**

99 00
4 5 6 7 8 9 10

ISBN 0-683-08792-4

90000

9 780683 087925

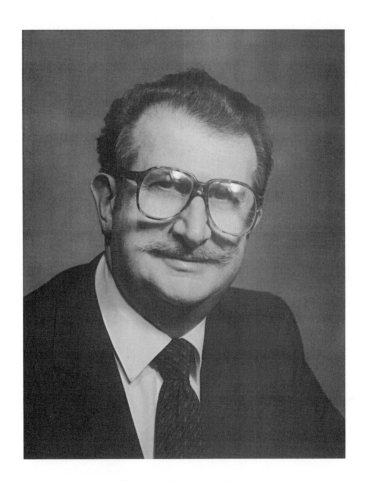

Howard M. Levine, D.O.

To Howard,
whose vision, support, determination, persistence,
and political skills have been invaluable

Foreword

It is my privilege to be an osteopathic physician. It has also been my great privilege to be involved with this textbook and its authors. For many years, students and osteopathic physicians alike have expressed concern that there was no major text dealing with the broad aspects of osteopathic medicine. *Foundations for Osteopathic Medicine* is our attempt to deal with this need. What follows reflects current understanding and knowledge of over 100 osteopathic physicians, basic science and behavioral science authors who have special wisdom in the field. Working closely with individuals of this caliber for the last five years has been my reward.

Our goal has been to create an authoritative publication that will help physicians to understand the rationale behind applications of osteopathic principles and the appropriate role of palpatory diagnosis and manipulative treatment. Admittedly, this process is increasingly difficult in an era of high technology/impersonal medical practice.

There are many fine reference books on osteopathic principles and practice and osteopathic manipulative treatment (OPP and OMT). However, this is the first comprehensive textbook written primarily for osteopathic medical students and practitioners. The education of an osteopathic physician includes the mission that students learn to "think osteopathically." The processes for achieving this end are not uniformly conceived, taught, or practiced. This book provides a practical source for students to grasp the scope of such thinking and practice, and uniformly provides information on the application of OPP and OMT in all clinical settings.

In the late 1980s the American Osteopathic Association (AOA) Board of Trustees and House of Delegates provided financial support for the development of this textbook. After several proposals were reviewed, this project was launched in July 1990 under the supervision of the AOA Bureau of Research. The venture, under the title "Osteopathic Principles Textbook Project," has culled endless ideas and suggestions from hundreds of sources in the basic, behavioral, and clinical sciences. *Foundations for Osteopathic Medicine* has been inspired by the dreams of numerous osteopathic physicians, educators, and scientists who have supported the growth and development of osteopathic medicine in every part of the country, every college of osteopathic medicine, and every arm of the AOA. It is through their determination and tenacity that the source materials in this book have been reviewed, compiled, edited, and published. All of those involved in the preparation of this text take great pride in its publication.

We commend this book to you and charge students with the task of believing in themselves as osteopathic physicians. Most importantly, we ask that you become a physician who "thinks osteopathically."

HOWARD M. LEVINE, D.O., F.A.C.G.P., D.OSTEO.SCI. (HON.)
CHAIRMAN, BUREAU OF RESEARCH, AMERICAN OSTEOPATHIC ASSOCIATION

Mission Statement

Osteopathic medicine (historically, osteopathy) is a philosophy, a science, and an art. Its philosophy embraces the concept of the unity of the living organism's structure and function in health and disease. Its science includes the biological, behavioral, chemical, physical, and spiritual knowledge related to the maintenance and restoration of health as well as identification, prevention, cure, and alleviation of disease. Its art is the application of the philosophy in the practice of medicine and surgery in all its branches and specialties.

EDITORIAL BOARD
FIRST MEETING, JULY 1990
CHICAGO, ILLINOIS

Preface

Osteopathic medical students and physicians alike have expressed the need for a major text dealing with the broad aspects of osteopathic medicine. For this and many other reasons, the American Osteopathic Association concluded that a wide variety of venues would benefit from a straightforward and practical explanation of osteopathic philosophy and its principles as practiced in a modern context. *Foundations for Osteopathic Medicine* reflects the current understanding and knowledge of osteopathic philosophy and principles as reflected by more than 70 osteopathically oriented authors and even greater number of peer reviewers from a variety of basic science, behavioral, and clinical disciplines.

This text provides an up-to-date multidisciplinary overview of osteopathic philosophy and principles with examples of clinical perspectives gleaned from a variety of disciplines. The book has been organized in ten sections, many of which are introduced with an editorial overview from the section editor. A brief overview of the ten sections follows.

I. Osteopathic Philosophy

This consensus statement comes from the Editors of *Foundations for Osteopathic Medicine* after an extensive peer-review process. The reader will note that many other philosophy references are scattered throughout the text, including the Mission Statement.

II. History

No text of this sort gives proper perspective to its essential ideas and practices without discussing its ancestry and evolution. In the United States, accelerating reorganization of health care services of all types emphasizes the importance of this profession's historical memory. Sometimes forgotten are the many individual and collective struggles for full medical licensure in all 50 states; general ostracism, then acceptance into military and public sector positions; moves from within sectors of the profession to restrict osteopathic physician licensure for their own short-term gain; and, most recently, the substantial growth of osteopathic education and training programs in universities, colleges, and schools, while at the same time there is a merging/closure and downsizing of hospitals in response to economic pressures.

III. Basic Sciences

From its earliest beginnings, osteopathic medicine emphasized the scientific basis for applications of its fundamental ideas. In the 19th century, there was little to go on other than clinical instincts and intuition. On the other hand, formal scientific investigation was exploding in many areas. Now, a century later, research and evidence-based clinical practices are becoming rules rather than exceptions. With this in mind, the section editors recognized the need for presentation of current osteopathic perspectives among the basic science disciplines. To this end, authors from a variety of basic science disciplines have skillfully crafted creative, pertinent, and current perspectives representing their fields of inquiry. A number of clinically applicable discussions relating the particular disciplines to neuromusculoskeletal structure and function perspectives are of particular interest.

IV. Behavioral Sciences

This offering is a first effort from within osteopathic medicine to highlight some of the important and complex behavioral, psychosocial, and cultural issues in a context that uses osteopathic philosophy and its principles as a frame of reference. Patients and physicians alike behave and are affected by their genetic endowments, cultural values, belief systems, gender, age, family background, education, and working environments. Health, impairment, and disease/illness outcomes are often determined by individual, family, and social group responses and choices deriving from these background elements. Authors highlight some of these important issues, such as life stages, stress, and depression.

V. Clinical Problem Solving

Like the Behavioral Science Section, this too is an osteopathic textbook first. Written by one of the pioneers in the field, the offering lays out both general and specific problem-solving strategies that enhance comprehensive clinical evaluations in a context that highlights osteopathic philosophy and principles. Emphasis is placed on integrative thinking processes in the clinical setting.

VI. Family Practice and Primary Care

Family practice and primary care form the backbone of osteopathic medicine. When these chapters were written, approximately 60% of graduates nationwide were entering the fields of family practice, general pediatrics, and general internal medicine. If general obstetrics and gynecology is added, the figures are higher. The authors have given general overviews of their disciplines, with an emphasis on osteopathic philosophy and principles.

VII. Clinical Specialties

In our complex, high technology, medically oriented society, applications of osteopathic medicine principles may, at times, be difficult to articulate. One outcome has been the inaccurate notion that osteopathic philosophy and its principles reflect alternative or complementary medicine rather than mainstream practices. Among many complex reasons for this view is the reality that some specialties and subspecialties seem less holistic than others, often inappropriately so.

VIII. Palpatory Diagnosis and Manipulative Treatment

Approximately half of this text presents a perspective on aspects of osteopathic palpatory diagnosis and manipulative treatment processes. Survey chapters cover the major curriculum content areas taught in American colleges of osteopathic medicine. Contributions have been peer reviewed by members of the Educational Council on Osteopathic Principles, an osteopathic manipulative skills teaching arm of the American Association of Colleges of Osteopathic Medicine.

IX. Health Restoration

Osteopathic palpatory diagnosis, manipulative treatment, and rehabilitative procedures are essential components of an osteopathic medical treatment program. These survey chapters address some of the pertinent issues.

X. Applications of Basic and Clinical Research for Osteopathic Theory and Practice

This section discusses appropriate research methods and opportunities confronting osteopathic medical practice. Particular emphasis is placed on appropriate research planning, data acquisition and documentation, basic science perspectives, clinical trials, epidemiologic considerations, and outcomes research in relation to somatic dysfunction.

In addition, the Glossary of Osteopathic Terminology, prepared by the Educational Council on Osteopathic Principles of the American Association of Colleges of Osteopathic Medicine, endorsed by the American Osteopathic Association, is included. The text concludes with a comprehensive Index.

The time for this text has been long in coming. One idea for such a textbook was informally discussed during the 1970s as part of a longitudinal osteopathic principles curriculum effort by the Educational Council on Osteopathic Principles. Other such forums had discussed additional alternatives over the years. However, the concept and plan for this text was developed within the Bureau of Research of the AOA. The Bureau officially termed the development activity the "Osteopathic Principles Textbook Project." Our goal has been to introduce both future and present osteopathic physicians to the rationale behind applications of osteopathic principles and the appropriate use of palpatory diagnosis and manipulative treatment in a wide range of disciplines. After years of soul-searching and peer review, our efforts are in your hands. We have given our best. We hope you agree.

Acknowledgments

The development of *Foundations for Osteopathic Medicine* has been accomplished through the vision, determination, and tenacity of the academic, administrative, and clinical leaders of the osteopathic profession. Support, both financial and intellectual, has been provided by the House of Delegates, Board of Trustees, Bureau of Research, and the members of the American Osteopathic Association (AOA).

We especially recognize the contributions of Frank J. McDevitt, D.O., and Eugene L. Sikorski, D.O., past presidents of the AOA, who demonstrated their courage, foresight, trust, and encouragement by donating their SmithKline & French presidential grants toward this publication, when it was only a dream.

Special appreciation and thanks is expressed to Robert C. Ward, D.O., Executive Editor, who with vision and leadership successfully completed a complex and difficult task. His effort required masterful diplomacy and was accomplished with tact and wisdom. Dr. Ward's knowledge of research and osteopathic medicine is encyclopedic. Throughout this project, he kept a diverse group of 100 authors moving toward agreed-upon goals.

A special thanks is also-extended to staff members of the AOA Department of Education: Douglas Ward, Ph.D., whose guidance and encouragement assisted in launching and gathering support for the project; Konrad C. Retz, Ph.D., who steadfastly assisted in managing the project through the Bureau of Research; and Andrea L. Change of the Division of Research for her secretarial assistance and handling of the daily details with dispatch.

Felix J. Rogers, D.O., has my deepest admiration. He adeptly coped with the most sensitive part of the book—that of ensuring that the clinical section was "osteopathic."

I wish to thank personally the AOA leadership, the House of Delegates, and the general membership of the AOA for their steadfast and patient support. We think the result has been well worth the investment and the effort.

The enthusiasm and help given by the staff of Williams & Wilkins was exceeded only by their understanding when we needed it the most.

Most importantly, we congratulate the section editors of *Foundations for Osteopathic Medicine* and all authors and contributors. Because of their efforts, this textbook has evolved and matured. Their wisdom, insight, and understanding have resulted in a book that describes the state of the art in osteopathic medical education, research, and OPP and OMT. This text ensures the future role of osteopathic medicine by highlighting its contributions and distinctiveness.

HOWARD M. LEVINE, D.O., F.A.C.G.P., D.OSTEO.SCI. (HON.)
CHAIRMAN, BUREAU OF RESEARCH, AMERICAN OSTEOPATHIC ASSOCIATION

In July 1990, the American Osteopathic Association (AOA) Board of Trustees and House of Delegates decided to sponsor the development and publication of an osteopathic medical textbook dealing with osteopathic principles and practice under the supervision of the AOA Bureau of Research. The first meeting was chaired by Tom Miller, an organizational development consultant from Madison, Wisconsin. As with any long-term project, the Board of Editors had some turnover. Unfortunately, one of our members, John Harakal, D.O., F.A.A.O., passed away after much work on his section. He was replaced by Michael A.

Seffinger, D.O. I am particularly grateful to Dr. Barbara A. Peterson, who took the risk of helping initially to organize the Project prior to the entry of our publisher Williams & Wilkins. Her considerable diplomatic skills and in-depth knowledge of the profession gained through her years as managing editor for AOA publications were invaluable. Special thanks also go to Ward Perrin, D.O., F.A.C.O.I., and Jill Hendra, D.O., who organized and delivered early Clinical and Behavior Science Sections, respectively.

I wish to personally thank all the associate editors both past and present, the leadership of the American Osteopathic Association, and its general membership for their generous and steadfast support through the seven-year development process. As time passed, countless ideas and content suggestions from hundreds of sources in the basic, behavioral, and clinical sciences have been collated, peer reviewed, and edited by this group.

Special thanks go to John Butler, Linda Napora, and Tom Lochhaas of Williams & Wilkins. John is the executive editor who took the risk of selling this project to his colleagues; Linda has served ably as general managing editor, cajoling laggards to finish. Tom carried out the editor's job with precision and swiftness. His ability to turn work around on a tight schedule has been truly remarkable. Much gratitude is extended to Richard Fritzler of DesignPointe for enhancing the book with illustrations and then more illustrations. Finally, the major glue for all of the administrative detail has been provided by Jane Walsh, who, by education and training, is a research histologist in the Department of Biomechanics at Michigan State University. She readily and cheerfully accepted the "detail person" role and has done a masterful job. Now the text is reality. We hope you think our efforts have been worthwhile.

Special recognition goes to the following individuals for their dedication, persistence, and, above all, patience in dealing with the myriad and commonly frustrating problems and details that go with a project of this magnitude.

Section Editors past and present
    John Harakal, D.O., F.A.A.O. (deceased)
    Jill Hendra, D.O.
    John A. Jerome, Ph.D.
    John M. Jones III, D.O.
    Robert E. Kappler, D.O., F.A.A.O
    Albert F. Kelso, Ph.D., D.Sci. (Hon.)
    Michael L. Kuchera, D.O., F.A.A.O.
    William A. Kuchera, D.O., F.A.A.O.
    Michael M. Patterson, Ph.D.
    Ward Perrin, D.O., F.A.C.O.I.
    Barbara A. Peterson, D.Litt.
    Felix J. Rogers, D.O., F.A.C.O.I., F.A.C.C.
    Michael A. Seffinger, D.O.
    Sarah A. Sprafka, Ph.D.
    Richard L. Van Buskirk, D.O., Ph.D.

Project Managers
    For the Osteopathic Principles Textbook Project
        Jane A. Walsh
    For Williams & Wilkins
        John P. Butler, Executive Editor
        Linda S. Napora, Managing Editor
        Tom Lochhaas, Development Editor
        Carol Eckhart and Kim Nawrozki, Production Coordinators

Klemie Bryte and Karen Ruppert, Copy Editors
Dan Pfisterer, Designer
Ray Lowman, Illustration Planner
For the American Osteopathic Association
Andrea Change, Bureau of Research
Konrad Retz, Ph.D., Secretary, Bureau of Research

Peer Reviewers

Myron Beal, D.O., F.A.A.O.
David Beatty, D.O.
Daniel Belsky, D.O., F.A.C.O.O.G.
Wesley Boudette, D.O., F.A.C.O.R.
Boyd R. Buser, D.O., C.S.P.-O.M.M.
Mark Cantieri, D.O., C.S.P.-O.M.M.
Constance Cashen, D.O., F.A.C.O.S.
Anthony G. Chila, D.O., F.A.A.O.
Gerald Cooper, D.O., F.A.A.O.
Eileen L. DiGiovanna, D.O., F.A.A.O.
Chester DeGroat, Ph.D.
Jerry Dickey, D.O., F.A.A.O.
Walter C. Ehrenfeuchter, D.O., F.A.A.O.
Mitchell L. Elkiss, D.O., F.A.C.N.
Wayne English, D.O., F.A.O.C.R.M.
Richard Feely, D.O., F.A.A.O.
Robert Foreman, Ph.D.
Bruce Flagg, D.O.
Harry D. Friedman, D.O., C.S.P.-O.M.M.
Melvin Friedman, D.O., C.S.P.-O.M.M.
Patrick Galvas, D.O.
Kenneth Glinter, D.O., F.A.C.O.O.G.
John P. Goodridge, D.O., F.A.A.O.
Philip E. Greenman, D.O., F.A.A.O.
Roger Grimes, D.O., F.A.O.A.O., F.A.C.O.S.
Ann Habenicht, D.O., C.S.P.-O.M.M.
Bruce Halas, D.O.
Shirley Harding, D.O.
Jane Harris, D.O., C.S.P.-O.M.M.
David Heilig, D.O., F.A.A.O.
Susan Hendrix, D.O.
E. Carlisle Holland, D.O., C.S.P.-O.M.M.
Raymond J. Hruby, D.O., F.A.A.O.
Robert Jackson, D.O.
John A. Jerome, Ph.D., B.C.F.E.
William L. Johnston, D.O., F.A.A.O.
Charles Kaluza, D.O., F.O.C.O.O.
Robert E. Kappler, D.O., F.A.A.O.

Albert F. Kelso, Ph.D.
Hollis King, D.O., C.S.P.-O.M.M.
George Kleiber, D.O., F.A.C.O.I.
Bradley Klock, D.O., C.S.P.-O.M.M.
Irvin M. Korr, Ph.D.
Michael L. Kuchera, D.O., F.A.A.O.
William A. Kuchera, D.O., F.A.A.O.
Edna M. Lay, D.O., F.A.A.O.
Howard M. Levine, D.O., F.A.C.O.F.P.
Michael Lockwood, D.O., C.S.P.-O.M.M.
Ronald Marino, D.O., F.A.C.O.P.
Alexander Nicholas, D.O., F.A.A.O.
William Nickey, D.O., F.A.C.O.I.
Judith O'Connell, D.O., C.S.P.-O.M.M.
Gerald G. Osborn, D.O., M.Phil., F.A.C.N.
Wendy Page-Echols, D.O., C.S.P.-O.M.M.
David A. Patriquin, D.O., F.A.A.O.
Michael M. Patterson, Ph.D.
Dennis Paulson, Ph.D.
Donald Pelino, D.O., F.A.C.O.P.
Ward Perrin, D.O., F.A.C.O.I.
Scott Ransom, D.O.
Eric Rentz, D.O., C.S.P.-O.M.M.
Felix J. Rogers, D.O., F.A.C.O.I., F.A.C.C.
Lisa Rogers, D.O.
Bernard R. Rubin, D.O., F.A.C.O.I.
John Schairer, D.O., F.A.C.O.I.
Michael A. Seffinger, D.O.
Frederic N. Schwartz, D.O., F.A.C.O.F.P.
Donald Stanton, D.O., F.A.O.A.P.M.R.
Karen M. Steele, D.O., F.A.A.O.
Edward Stiles, D.O., F.A.A.O.
James Stookey, D.O., F.A.A.O.
Benjamin Sucher, D.O., F.A.A.P.M.R.
Bernard TePoorten, D.O., F.A.A.O.
Richard Theriault, D.O., F.A.C.O.I.
Richard L. Van Buskirk, D.O., Ph.D.
Colleen Vallad-Hix, D.O.
David Vick, D.O., C.S.P.-O.M.M.
Elaine Wallace, D.O., C.S.P.-O.M.M.
Frank Walton, D.O., F.A.A.O.
Robert C. Ward III, D.O.

Lawrence Wickless, D.O.
Leon Wince, D.O.
Douglas Wood, D.O., Ph.D.,
    F.A.C.O.I.

Robert D. Wurster, Ph.D.
Gerald Zackey, D.O.

Osteopathic Student Reviewers
    Kevin Batterbee (D.O.–1997)
    David Hoffman (D.O.–1997)
    Karlin Sevensma (D.O.–1997)
    Troy Silvernale (D.O.–1997)

Donations of SmithKline & French Presidential Grants
    Frank J. McDevitt, D.O., F.A.C.F.P.
    Eugene L. Sikorski, D.O., F.A.C.F.P.

Another major project contributor
    Sharon Husch, Executive Secretary, Department of Biomechanics, Michigan State University College of Osteopathic Medicine

                                                    ROBERT C. WARD, D.O., F.A.A.O.
                                                              EXECUTIVE EDITOR

Contributors

JOSEPH A. ALDRICH, D.O., F.A.C.O.P.
Chairman
Department of Pediatric and Adolescent
Medicine
Department of Pediatrics
Kirksville College of Osteopathic Medicine
Kirksville, Missouri

THOMAS WESLEY ALLEN, D.O.
Dean and Professor of Medicine
Oklahoma State University College of
Osteopathic Medicine
Tulsa, Oklahoma

DAVID A. BARON, M.S.Ed., D.O., F.A.C.N.
Clinical Professor
Department of Psychiatry
Temple University School of Medicine
Philadelphia, Pennsylvania
Associate Clinical Professor
Department of Pharmacology
College of Osteopathic Medicine
New York Institute of Technology
Old Westbury, New York

BOYD R. BUSER, D.O., C.S.P.-O.M.M.
Chairman
Department of Osteopathic Manipulative
Medicine
University of New England College of
Osteopathic Medicine
Biddeford, Maine

RICHARD M. BUTLER, D.O.
Clinical Associate Professor
Department of Medicine
College of Osteopathic Medicine
Michigan State University
East Lansing, Michigan
Director of Medical Education
Oakland General Hospital
Madison Heights, Michigan

THOMAS A. CAVALIERI, D.O.
Professor of Clinical Medicine
Chairman, Department of Medicine
School of Osteopathic Medicine
University of Medicine and Dentistry
Stratford, New Jersey

ANTHONY G. CHILA, D.O., F.A.A.O.
Professor
Department of Family Medicine
College of Osteopathic Medicine
Ohio University
Athens, Ohio

CARMELLA D'ADDEZIO, D.O., F.A.C.O.I.
Director of Medical Education
Graduate Medical Education
Bay Medical Center
Bay City, Michigan

GILBERT E. D'ALONZO, Jr., D.O., F.A.C.O.I.
Professor of Medicine
Division of Pulmonary and Critical Care
Medicine
Temple University School of Medicine
Philadelphia, Pennsylvania

EILEEN L. DiGIOVANNA, D.O., F.A.A.O.
Chairperson and Professor
Stanley Schiowitz Department of Osteopathic
Manipulative Medicine
Assistant Dean of Student Affairs
New York College of Osteopathic Medicine
Old Westbury, New York

DENNIS J. DOWLING, D.O., C.S.P.-O.M.M.
Associate Chairman
Academic Health Care Center
Department of Osteopathic Manipulative
Medicine
New York College of Osteopathic Medicine
Old Westbury, New York
Director of Manipulation
Department of Physical Medicine and
Rehabilitation
Nassau County Medical Center
East Meadow, New York

MARK E. EFRUSY, D.O., F.A.C.G.
Director of Gastroenterology
Professor of Medicine
Department of Internal Medicine
Chicago College of Osteopathic Medicine
Midwestern University
Chicago, Illinois

WALTER C. EHRENFEUCHTER, D.O.,
    F.A.A.O.
Professor and Vice Chairman
Department of Osteopathic Manipulative
    Medicine
Philadelphia College of Osteopathic Medicine
Philadelphia, Pennsylvania

MITCHELL L. ELKISS, D.O., F.A.C.N.,
    C.S.P.-O.M.M.
Clinical Professor, Neurology
Department of Internal Medicine
College of Osteopathic Medicine
Michigan State University
East Lansing, Michigan
Associate Director
Gertrude Levin Pain Clinic
Southfield, Michigan

WILLIAM M. FALLS, PH.D.
Professor
Department of Anatomy
College of Osteopathic Medicine
Michigan State University
East Lansing, Michigan

HARRY D. FRIEDMAN, D.O.,
    C.S.P.-O.M.M.
Clinical Assistant Professor
Department of Family Practice
College of Osteopathic Medicine
Michigan State University
East Lansing, Michigan
Staff Physician
St. Mary's Spine Center
Cofounder
San Francisco Manual Medicine Society
San Francisco, California

JEREL H. GLASSMAN, M.P.H., D.O.,
    C.S.P.-O.M.M.
Clinical Assistant Professor
Department of Physical Medicine and
    Rehabilitation
Michigan State University
East Lansing, Michigan
Staff Physician
St. Mary's Spine Center
St. Mary's Medical Center
San Francisco, California

JOHN C. GLOVER, D.O.
Chair and Associate Professor
Department of Osteopathic Principles and
    Practice
University of Health Sciences
College of Osteopathic Medicine
Kansas City, Missouri

JOHN P. GOODRIDGE, D.O., F.A.A.O.,
    C.S.P.-O.M.M.
Professor Emeritus
Department of Family and Community
    Medicine
College of Osteopathic Medicine
Michigan State University
East Lansing, Michigan

PHILIP E. GREENMAN, D.O., F.A.A.O.
Professor
Department of Osteopathic Manipulative
    Medicine
Department of Physical Medicine and
    Rehabilitation
College of Osteopathic Medicine
Michigan State University
East Lansing, Michigan

DEBORAH M. HEATH, D.O., C.S.P.-O.M.M.
Private Practice
Arizona Center for Health and Medicine
Phoenix, Arizona

DAVID HEILIG, D.O., FAAO
Emeritus Professor
Department of Osteopathic Manipulative
    Medicine
Philadelphia College of Osteopathic Medicine
Philadelphia, Pennsylvania

KURT HEINKING
Family Medicine Resident
Department of Family Medicine
Chicago College of Osteopathic Medicine
Midwestern University
Chicago, Illinois

RAYMOND J. HRUBY, D.O., F.A.A.O.
Professor and Chairperson
Department of Osteopathic Manipulative
*   Medicine*
College of Osteopathic Medicine
Michigan State University
East Lansing, Michigan

ALLEN W. JACOBS, D.O., PH.D.
Acting Dean
College of Osteopathic Medicine
Associate Professor and Team Physician
Department of Osteopathic Manipulative
*   Medicine*
Michigan State University
East Lansing, Michigan

JOHN A. JEROME, PH.D., B.C.F.E.
Psychologist
Department of Osteopathic Manipulative
*   Medicine*
Michigan State University
Clinical Director
Sparrow Pain Center
Sparrow Hospital
Lansing, Michigan

JOYCE M. JOHNSON, D.O., M.A.
Psychiatrist
Chevy Chase, Maryland

WILLIAM L. JOHNSTON, D.O., F.A.A.O.
Professor Emeritus
Department of Family Medicine
College of Osteopathic Medicine
Michigan State University
East Lansing, Michigan

JOHN M. JONES III, D.O.
Chair, Department of Osteopathic Manipulative
*   Medicine*
College of Osteopathic Medicine of the Pacific
Western University of Health Sciences
Pomona, California

ROBERT E. KAPPLER, D.O., F.A.A.O.
Director, Center for Osteopathic Research and
*   Education Development (C.O.R.E.D.)*
Professor, Family Medicine
Department of Family Medicine
Chicago College of Osteopathic Medicine
Midwestern University
Chicago, Illinois

ALBERT F. KELSO, PH.D., D.SCI. (HON.)
Professor Emeritus
Center for Osteopathic Education and Research
University Health Sciences
Chicago College of Osteopathy
Chicago, Illinois

IRVIN M. KORR, B.H., M.A., PH.D.
Professor Emeritus (1975)
Department of Physiology
Kirksville College of Osteopathic Medicine
Kirksville, Missouri
Professor Emeritus, Medical Education (1990)
College of Osteopathic Medicine
University of North Texas
Fort Worth, Texas

SAMUEL L. KRACHMAN, D.O.
Assistant Professor of Medicine
Department of Pulmonary Medicine and
*   Critical Care*
Temple University
Philadelphia, Pennsylvania

MICHAEL L. KUCHERA, D.O., F.A.A.O.
Professor and Chairperson
Department of Osteopathic Manipulative
*   Medicine*
Kirksville College of Osteopathic Medicine
Kirksville, Missouri

WILLIAM A. KUCHERA, D.O., F.A.A.O.
Professor Emeritus
Department of Osteopathic Manipulative
*   Medicine*
Kirksville College of Osteopathic Medicine
Kirksville, Missouri

EDNA M. LAY, D.O., F.A.A.O.
Associate Professor Emeritus
Department of Osteopathic Manipulative
*   Medicine*
Kirksville College of Osteopathic Medicine
Kirksville, Missouri

JED G. MAGEN, D.O.
Assistant Professor
Department of Psychiatry
Michigan State University
Residency Education Director
Colleges of Osteopathic and Human Medicine
East Lansing, Michigan

JOHN M. McPARTLAND, D.O., M.S.
Director
Vermont Alternative Medicine/AMRITA
Middlebury, Vermont
Adjunct Assistant Professor
Department of Osteopathic Manipulative
  Medicine
Michigan State University
East Lansing, Michigan

EUGENE MOCHAN, PH.D., D.O.
Professor and Chairman
Department of Biochemistry/Molecular Biology
Professor of Family Medicine
Philadelphia College of Osteopathic Medicine
Philadelphia, Pennsylvania

DAVID J. MOKLER, PH.D.
Associate Professor
Department of Pharmacology
University of New England
Biddeford, Maine

P. J. MORGANE, PH.D.
Professor of Pharmacology
Department of Pharmacology
University of New England
Biddeford, Maine

REGINA C. MOROZ, D.O.
Chairman and Clinical Assistant Professor of
  Internal Medicine
Department of Internal Medicine
University of Health Sciences
College of Osteopathic Medicine
Kansas City, Missouri

ALEXANDER S. NICHOLAS, D.O., FAAO
Professor
Department of Osteopathic Manipulative
  Medicine
Philadelphia College of Osteopathic Medicine
Philadelphia, Pennsylvania

MICHAEL I. OPIPARI, D.O.
Vice President and Chief Medical Officer
Horizon Health System/Henry Ford Health
  System
Southfield, Michigan
Attending Physician
Department of Internal Medicine
Bi-County Community Hospital
Warren, Michigan

GERALD G. OSBORN, D.O., M.PHIL.,
  F.A.C.N.
Professor
Departments of Psychiatry, Medicine, and
  History
College of Osteopathic Medicine
Michigan State University
East Lansing, Michigan

DAVID A. PATRIQUIN, D.O., F.A.A.O.
Professor Emeritus of Family Medicine
Department of Family Medicine
College of Osteopathic Medicine
Ohio University
Athens, Ohio

MICHAEL M. PATTERSON, PH.D.
Professor of Osteopathic Principles and Practice
  and of Physiology
Department of Osteopathic Principles and
  Practice
Director of Basic Science Research
University of Health Sciences
College of Osteopathic Medicine
Kansas City, Missouri

BARBARA A. PETERSON, D.LITT.
Evanston, Illinois

DAVID A. PLUNDO, D.O.
Director
Osteopathic Family Practice Residency Program
St Vincent Medical Center
Toledo, Ohio

RONALD PORTANOVA, PH.D.
Associate Professor
Department of Basic Sciences
College of Osteopathic Medicine
Ohio University
Athens, Ohio

KENNETH A. RAMEY, D.O.
Family Medicine Resident
Department of Family Medicine
Olympia Fields Osteopathic Hospital and
*   Medical Center*
Olympia Fields, Illinois

LOUIS E. RENTZ, D.O.
Clinical Professor of Neurology
Wayne State University
Chairman, Department of Neuroscience
Oakland General Hospital
Detroit, Michigan

FELIX J. ROGERS, D.O., F.A.C.O.I., F.A.C.C.
Clinical Professor
Department of Internal Medicine
College of Osteopathic Medicine
Michigan State University
Downriver Cardiology Consultants
Trenton, Michigan

SYDNEY P. ROSS, D.O., F.A.C.O.S.
Vice President for Academic Affairs and Dean
Kirksville College of Osteopathic Medicine
Kirksville, Missouri

RICHARD M. ROTNICKI, D.O.
Attending Physician
Department of Gastroenterology
Morris Hospital
Morris, Illinois
Attending Physician
Department of Gastroenterology
St. Joseph Medical Center
Joliet, Illinois

BERNARD R. RUBIN, D.O., F.A.C.O.I.
Professor of Medicine
Chief, Division of Rheumatology
Department of Medicine
University of North Texas Health Science Center
Fort Worth, Texas

STANLEY SCHIOWITZ, D.O., F.A.A.O.
Dean, New York College of Osteopathic
*   Medicine*
Old Westbury, New York

FREDERIC N. SCHWARTZ, D.O., F.A.C.F.P.
Professor of Family Medicine
Director, Division of Family Medicine
Arizona College of Osteopathic Medicine
Medical Director
East Valley Center for Primary Care
Tempe, Arizona

RICHARD A. SCOTT, D.O.
Associate Clinical Professor
College of Osteopathic Medicine
Michigan State University
East Lansing, Michigan
Private Physician
Department of Orthopaedics
Bi-County Hospital
Warren, Michigan

MICHAEL A. SEFFINGER, D.O.
Family Physician
Department of Family Medicine
Health Care Partners Medical Group
Gardena, California

HARRIET H. SHAW, D.O.
Associate Professor
Department of Osteopathic Family Medicine
College of Osteopathic Medicine
Oklahoma State University
Tulsa, Oklahoma

MICHAEL B. SHAW, D.O.
Clinical Lecturer
Department of Surgery
College of Osteopathic Medicine
Oklahoma State University
Tulsa, Oklahoma

STEPHEN H. SHELDON, D.O.
Director, Sleep Disorders Center
Division of Pulmonary and Critical Care
*   Medicine*
Children's Memorial Hospital
Assistant Professor of Pediatrics
Northwestern University Medical School
Chicago, Illinois

GARY L. SLICK, D.O.
Professor and Chairman
Department of Internal Medicine
Chicago College of Osteopathic Medicine
Chicago, Illinois

NEIL SPIEGEL, D.O.
Private Physician
Center for Physical Medicine and Rehabilitation
Rockville, Maryland

SARAH A. SPRAFKA, PH.D.
Director, Predoctoral Education
College of Osteopathic Medicine
University of New England
Biddeford, Maine

KAREN M. STEELE, D.O., F.A.A.O.
Associate Professor
Department of Osteopathic Principles and
*   Practices*
West Virginia School of Osteopathic Medicine
Lewisburg, West Virginia

BARBARA SWARTZLANDER
Public Services Coordinator
Library
University of New England
Biddeford, Maine

MELICIEN A. TETTAMBEL, D.O., F.A.A.O.,
**   F.A.C.O.O.G.**
Adjunct Clinical Instructor
Department of Family Medicine
Chicago College of Osteopathic Medicine
Chicago, Illinois

ROBERT J. THEOBALD, JR., PH.D.
Professor and Chairman
Department of Pharmacology
Kirksville College of Osteopathic Medicine
Kirksville, Missouri

LEX C. TOWNS, PH.D.
Professor and Chairman
Department of Anatomy
Kirksville College of Osteopathic Medicine
Kirksville, Missouri

RICHARD L. VAN BUSKIRK, D.O., PH.D
Private Practice
Sarasota, Florida

ELAINE WALLACE, D.O.
Associate Dean of Academics
Associate Professor of Family Medicine
Associate Professor of Osteopathic Principles and
*   Practices*
University of Health Sciences
Kansas City, Missouri

ROBERT C. WARD, D.O., F.A.A.O.
Professor
Departments of Osteopathic Manipulative
*   Medicine and Family Medicine*
College of Osteopathic Medicine
Michigan State University
East Lansing, Michigan

FRANK H. WILLARD, PH.D.
Associate Professor
Department of Anatomy
University of New England
Biddeford, Maine

MICHAEL K. WILLMAN, D.O., F.A.O.C.R.
Professor
Department of Radiology
Kirksville College of Osteopathic Medicine
Kirksville, Missouri

ROBERT D. WURSTER, PH.D.
Professor
Departments of Physiology and Neurosurgery
Loyola University Medical Center
Maywood, Illinois

HERBERT A. YATES, D.O., F.A.A.O., H.L.M.
Clinical Professor of Family Medicine
Department of Osteopathic Family Medicine
College of Osteopathic Medicine
Oklahoma State University
Tulsa, Oklahoma

Contents

Foreword / HOWARD M. LEVINE.. *vii*

Mission Statement... *ix*

Preface.. *xi*

Acknowledgments.. *xv*

Contributors... *xix*

SECTION I

OSTEOPATHIC PHILOSOPHY

  1. Osteopathic Philosophy / MICHAEL A. SEFFINGER, IRVIN M. KORR 3

SECTION II

OSTEOPATHIC HISTORY

  2. Major Events in Osteopathic History / BARBARA A. PETERSON....................... 15

SECTION III

OSTEOPATHIC CONSIDERATIONS IN THE BASIC SCIENCES

Introduction / MICHAEL M. PATTERSON 24

  3. Anatomy / ALLEN W. JACOBS, WILLIAM M. FALLS.................................... 27

  4. Rules of Anatomy / LEX C. TOWNS 45

  5. Autonomic Nervous System / FRANK H. WILLARD 53

  6. Endocrine System and Body Unity: Osteopathic Principles at a Chemical Level /
       RONALD PORTANOVA 83

  7. Pharmacologic and Osteopathic Basic Principles / ROBERT J. THEOBALD, JR.......... 93

  8. Human Regulatory Adaptations in Health and Disease: A Molecular Perspective /
       EUGENE MOCHAN 99

  9. Neuroendocrine-Immune System and Homeostasis / FRANK H. WILLARD,
       DAVID J. MOKLER, P.J. MORGANE.. 107

 10. Neurophysiologic System: Integration and Disintegration / MICHAEL M. PATTERSON,
       ROBERT D. WURSTER 137

SECTION IV

OSTEOPATHIC CONSIDERATIONS IN THE BEHAVIORAL SCIENCES

Introduction / JOHN A. JEROME 154

 11. Lifestyles and Health Habits / GERALD G. OSBORN 157

 12. Psychoneuroimmunology / DAVID A. BARON 167

 13. Osteopathic Management of Pain / JOHN A. JEROME 171

 14. Health Maintenance / JOYCE M. JOHNSON... 187

 15. Life Phases and Health / JED G. MAGEN.. 191

 16. Exercise, Fitness, and Health / RICHARD M. BUTLER, FELIX J. ROGERS 197

 17. Stress Management in Primary Care / JOHN A. JEROME 205

SECTION V

OSTEOPATHIC CONSIDERATIONS IN CLINICAL PROBLEM SOLVING

18. Clinical Problem Solving / SARAH A. SPRAFKA 217

SECTION VI

OSTEOPATHIC CONSIDERATIONS IN FAMILY PRACTICE AND PRIMARY CARE

Introduction / RICHARD L. VAN BUSKIRK 244
19. Family Practice / RICHARD L. VAN BUSKIRK, DAVID A. PLUNDO 249
20. General Internal Medicine / REGINA C. MOROZ 257
21. Primary Care Pediatrics / JOSEPH A. ALDRICH 261

SECTION VII

OSTEOPATHIC CONSIDERATIONS IN THE CLINICAL SPECIALTIES

Introduction / FELIX J. ROGERS 264
22. Pediatrics / STEPHEN H. SHELDON 267
23. Geriatrics / THOMAS A. CAVALIERI 273
24. Sports Medicine / THOMAS WESLEY ALLEN 285
25. Ear, Nose, and Throat / HARRIET H. SHAW, MICHAEL B. SHAW 289
26. Cardiology / FELIX J. ROGERS 299
27. Hypertension / GARY L. SLICK 319
28. Orthopaedics / RICHARD A. SCOTT 329
29. Obstetrics / MELICIEN A. TETTAMBEL 349
30. Gynecology / MELICIEN A. TETTAMBEL 363
31. Gastroenterology / MARK E. EFRUSY, RICHARD M. ROTNICKI 375
32. General Surgery / SYDNEY P. ROSS 387
33. Nephrology / CARMELLA D'ADDEZIO 393
34. Neurology / MITCHELL L. ELKISS, LOUIS E. RENTZ 401
35. Oncology / MICHAEL I. OPIPARI 417
36. Physical Medicine and Rehabilitation / NEIL SPIEGEL 431
37. Respiratory System / GILBERT E. D'ALONZO, JR., SAMUEL L. KRACHMAN 441
38. Rheumatology / BERNARD R. RUBIN 459

SECTION VIII

**OSTEOPATHIC CONSIDERATIONS IN PALPATORY DIAGNOSIS AND
MANIPULATIVE TREATMENT**

Introduction / JOHN M. JONES III, ROBERT E. KAPPLER 468

Part A. Overview: Evaluation and Management 473

39. Palpatory Skills: An Introduction / ROBERT E. KAPPLER 473
40. Progressive Exercises for Developing the Sense of Touch / ROBERT E. KAPPLER 479
41. Diagnosis and Plan for Manual Treatment: A Prescription / ROBERT E. KAPPLER,
    JOHN M. JONES III, WILLIAM A. KUCHERA 483
42. Musculoskeletal Examination for Somatic Dysfunction / WILLIAM A. KUCHERA,
    JOHN M. JONES III, ROBERT E. KAPPLER, JOHN P. GOODRIDGE 489

Part B. Regional Examination and Treatment 511

43. Examination and Diagnosis: An Introduction / MICHAEL L. KUCHERA 511
44. Head: Diagnosis and Treatment / ROBERT E. KAPPLER, KENNETH A. RAMEY 515

45. Cervical Spine / ROBERT E. KAPPLER 541
46. Upper Extremities / ROBERT E. KAPPLER, KENNETH A. RAMEY 547
47. Thoracic Region and Rib Cage / RAYMOND J. HRUBY, JOHN P. GOODRIDGE,
    JOHN M. JONES III 563
48. Lumbar and Abdominal Region / WILLIAM A. KUCHERA 581
49. Pelvis and Sacrum / KURT HEINKING, JOHN M. JONES III, ROBERT E. KAPPLER 601
50. Lower Extremities / MICHAEL L. KUCHERA, JOHN P. GOODRIDGE 623

Part C. Palpatory Diagnosis and Manipulative Treatment 661

51. Thrust Techniques: An Introduction / ROBERT E. KAPPLER 661
52. High-Velocity Low-Amplitude Thrust Techniques / ROBERT E. KAPPLER,
    JOHN M. JONES III 667
53. Muscle Energy Technique Procedures / JOHN P. GOODRIDGE 691
54. Muscle Energy Treatment Techniques for Specific Areas / JOHN P. GOODRIDGE,
    WILLIAM A. KUCHERA 697
55. Articulatory Techniques / DAVID A. PATRIQUIN, JOHN M. JONES III 763
56. Soft Tissue Techniques / WALTER C. EHRENFEUCHTER, DAVID HEILIG,
    ALEXANDER S. NICHOLAS 781
57. Functional Technique: An Indirect Method / WILLIAM L. JOHNSTON 795
58. Strain and Counterstrain Techniques / JOHN C. GLOVER, HERBERT A. YATES 809
59. Fascial-Ligamentous Release: Indirect Approach / ANTHONY G. CHILA 819
60. Facilitated Positional Release / STANLEY SCHIOWITZ 831
61. Facilitated Positional Release Techniques / EILEEN L. DiGIOVANNA,
    DENNIS J. DOWLING 833
62. Integrated Neuromusculoskeletal Release and Myofascial Release: An Introduction
    to Diagnosis and Treatment / ROBERT C. WARD 843
63. Integrated Neuromusculoskeletal Techniques for Specific Areas / ROBERT C. WARD .. 851
64. Cranial Field / EDNA M. LAY 901
65. Myofascial Trigger Points: An Introduction / MICHAEL L. KUCHERA,
    JOHN M. McPARTLAND 915
66. Travell and Simons' Myofascial Trigger Points / MICHAEL L. KUCHERA 919
67. Chapman's Reflexes / DAVID A. PATRIQUIN 935
68. Lymphatic System: Lymphatic Manipulative Techniques / ELAINE WALLACE,
    JOHN M. McPARTLAND, JOHN M. JONES III, WILLIAM A. KUCHERA, BOYD R. BUSER...... 941

Part D. Goals and Expectations 969

69. General Postural Considerations / MICHAEL L. KUCHERA, WILLIAM A. KUCHERA........ 969
70. Management of Group Curves / ROBERT E. KAPPLER 979
71. Postural Considerations in Coronal and Horizontal Planes / MICHAEL L. KUCHERA,
    WILLIAM A. KUCHERA 983
72. Postural Considerations in the Sagittal Plane / MICHAEL L. KUCHERA 999
73. Efficacy and Complications / EILEEN L. DiGIOVANNA, MICHAEL L. KUCHERA,
    PHILIP E. GREENMAN 1015
74. Radiographic Technical Aspects of the Postural Study / MICHAEL K. WILLMAN,
    MICHAEL L. KUCHERA, WILLIAM A. KUCHERA..................... 1025

SECTION IX
OSTEOPATHIC CONSIDERATIONS IN HEALTH RESTORATION

75. Treatment of the Acutely Ill Hospitalized Patient / KAREN M. STEELE................ 1037
76. Exercises and Recovery / ROBERT E. KAPPLER 1049

SECTION X

APPLICATIONS OF BASIC AND CLINICAL RESEARCH FOR OSTEOPATHIC THEORY AND PRACTICE

Introduction / ALBERT F. KELSO 1058

77. Somatic Dysfunction: Effects of Manipulative Treatment and Impact on Health Status / DEBORAH M. HEATH 1067

78. Medical Records in Clinical Research / HARRY D. FRIEDMAN 1077

79. Use of Data on Osteopathic Aspects of Health Care / JEREL H. GLASSMAN 1087

80. Clinical Research and Clinical Trials / STEPHEN H. SHELDON 1091

81. Epidemiology: Application to Clinical Research / ALBERT F. KELSO, FREDERIC N. SCHWARTZ 1095

82. Planning Research on Health Care: Access to Safe, Quality Health Care / ALBERT F. KELSO, DEBORAH M. HEATH 1101

83. Basic Research and Osteopathic Medicine / FRANK H. WILLARD, BARBARA SWARTZLANDER 1107

84. Osteopathic Research: The Future / MICHAEL M. PATTERSON 1115

GLOSSARY

Introduction / WILLIAM A. KUCHERA 1126

Glossary of Osteopathic Terminology / EDUCATIONAL COUNCIL ON OSTEOPATHIC PRINCIPLES 1127

Index *1141*

Osteopathic Philosophy

I. Osteopathic Philosophy

Key Concepts

- Evolution of the osteopathic philosophy from A.T. Still to present

- Principle of body unity

- Principle of the body's self-regulation, self-healing, and health maintenance

- Principle that structure and function are complexly interdependent

- Osteopathic treatment is based on body unity, self-regulation, and interrelationship of structure and function

Development of Osteopathic Philosophy

MICHAEL A. SEFFINGER[a]

Osteopathic medicine, as a profession, is predicated on a philosophy of health and health care. Deceptively simple in its presentation, the osteopathic philosophy sets osteopathic medicine apart from other approaches to health care. Osteopathic medicine is distinctive in the very fact that it has been and continues to be practiced according to an articulated philosophy. Osteopathic medicine, including its philosophy and interpretation, has evolved with time. While American osteopathic physicians are educated and practice in all aspects and disciplines of medicine and surgery, an integral component of their education highlights the osteopathic philosophy, including its basic concepts and problem-solving perspectives.

Because thinking and philosophical orientation are not always obvious, what an osteopathically oriented physician does in particular clinical situations may appear similar to what others do in comparable circumstances.

How did osteopathy, as conceived by Andrew Taylor Still, come to have a philosophical foundation? A major influence may have been the philosophy of pragmatism, which was a popular contemporary school of thought. Charles S. Pierce was a philosopher of science, among other things, and as a 1859 graduate of Harvard University, he was a contemporary of Andrew Taylor Still. Pierce was known to many thinkers of his time as the father of pragmatism. Pierce addressed the following major themes in his discussions of the philosophy of science:[1]

1. Concepts are fundamental to any philosophy.
2. Philosophical analyses of key concepts provide a systematic description of a philosophy.
3. Reasoning or inquiry is a knowledge-seeking activity that seeks stable beliefs.
4. A belief is a readiness or disposition to respond in certain ways to certain situations, i.e., it reflects complex habits of behaving and expecting.
5. Beliefs may be stable or unstable.
6. To be scientific is to subject beliefs to the tests of experience.
7. If a belief is judged to be true, it will not be eliminated by the test of experience.
8. Scientific reasoning tends to self-correct, both the conclusions and the premises.

The osteopathic philosophy arises from the teachings and writings of Andrew Taylor Still, MD (1828–1917). Still was a forward-thinking iconoclast who was convinced that 19th and early 20th century patient care was severely inadequate. Completely rejected by the medical establishment, he chose to establish a parallel medical educational system that he called "osteopathy." Osteopathy, as conceived by Still represented several of the themes articulated by Pierce in his writings. In addition to being a reaction to what he saw as a dysfunctional approach by mainstream (heroic) medicine, Still's beliefs were based in his conceptualization of humankind as self-sustaining, and they were strengthened by successful outcomes of his efforts at testing those beliefs with patients. Although we have

[a]Note: This statement of osteopathic philosophy was developed, peer-reviewed, and approved by the Osteopathic Principles Textbook Project Board of Editors under the direction of Michael A. Seffinger.

no direct evidence from his writings, Still may have been familiar with Charles Pierce's work and may have fashioned his science of osteopathy after the ideas of Pierce and his pragmatist colleagues.

We do know that, as a young man, Still was immersed in a culture that supported alternative, at times radical, thinking. The mid-19th century in America was a period when spiritualism was challenging mainstream Christianity for religious adherents, when Herbert Spencer's interpretations of Darwin's theories of natural selection and evolution where having their influence, and when American society was enjoying a fascination with technology in the form of machines. These positive influences were coupled with that of Still's disillusionment with mainstream medicine. By the time Still was 40 years old, three of his children and his father had died from infectious diseases, against which mainstream medicine of the time was powerless.

Drawing on several sources of enlightenment, Still came to see humans as marvelous machines, created and sustained by laws of nature and ultimately capable of achieving perfection here on earth. On June 22, 1874, Still was "shot," as he described it, by the revelation of God as the embodiment of perfection and with the mandate for the physician to use reason and an understanding of Nature's laws as the keys to health and disease. It was at that point that Still divorced himself from traditional medicine.[2]

Blessed with a vivid imagination and a practical clinical background, Still was adept with descriptive metaphors and aphorisms. Some, by today's standards, are quaintly arcane. On the other hand, many are incisive and witty, making them easy to remember. The best and most insightful of them remain pertinent a century later and have formed the foundation for the osteopathic philosophy as we know it today. The *Autobiography of A.T. Still*[3] and *The Philosophy and Mechanical Principles of Osteopathy*[4] highlight his observations.

EVOLUTION OF THE OSTEOPATHIC PHILOSOPHY

As interpretation of Still's ideas evolved into a cogent set of tenets, it became possible to define and codify the concepts into more precise statements that could be understood by those other than members of the profession, most particularly by students of osteopathic medicine. This occurred in 1953 with publication of the Kirksville consensus declaration.[5] We offer here a verbatim quotation of the introduction to that document, followed by a brief statement of four key principles. Together they comprise a concise statement of the osteopathic philosophy.

Osteopathy, or Osteopathic Medicine is a philosophy, a science and an art. Its philosophy embraces the concept of the unity of body structure and function in health and disease. Its science includes the chemical, physical and biological sciences related to the maintenance of health and the prevention, cure, and alleviation of disease. Its art is the application of the philosophy and the science in the practice of osteopathic medicine and surgery in all its branches and specialties.

Health is based on the natural capacity of the human organism to resist and combat noxious influences in the environment and to compensate for their effects; to meet, with adequate reserve, the usual stresses of daily life and the occasional severe stresses imposed by extremes of environment and activity.

Disease begins when this natural capacity is reduced, or when it is exceeded or overcome by noxious influences.

Osteopathic medicine recognizes that many factors impair this capacity and the natural tendency towards recovery, and that among the most important of these factors are the local disturbances or lesions of the musculoskeletal system. Osteopathic medicine is therefore concerned with liberating and developing all the resources that constitute the capacity for resistance and recovery, thus recognizing the validity of the ancient observation that the physician deals with a patient as well as a disease.

THE FOUR PRINCIPLES

The four key principles of osteopathic philosophy are as follows:

I. The body is a unit; the person is a unit of body, mind, and spirit.
II. The body is capable of self-regulation, self-healing, and health maintenance.
III. Structure and function are reciprocally interrelated.
IV. Rational treatment is based upon an understanding of the basic principles of body unity, self-regulation, and the interrelationship of structure and function.

Following is an interpretation of those principles as they apply to the contemporary practice of osteopathic medicine.

Body Unity

This first principle clearly refers to unity of person. As humans, each of us is an expression of the unity of body, mind, and spirit. The person is regulated, coordinated, and integrated through the interdependent functions of multiply associated anatomical, physiological, and psychosocial systems. Any separation for purposes of diagnosis, treatment, teaching, or discussion is always artificial.

Anatomically, all body structures are enveloped in connective tissue or fascia, making them contiguous and mechanically interdependent. Physiologically, synergy of body function is facilitated by the nervous and circulatory systems, which enable communication and interaction among the various body systems. Furthermore, we know the nervous, endocrine, immune, and musculoskeletal systems interact, reflect, and respond to internal and external environments and events as an integrated unit.

IMPLICATIONS OF BODY UNITY PRINCIPLE

A basic premise of osteopathic medicine is the principle of health, wellness, and body unity and their many applications in clinical medicine. Applied clinically, the concepts suggest that both healthy states and physiologic breakdowns are intimately linked with physical, mental, emotional, and spiritual factors. When one component is stressed or altered, other components are affected and respond accordingly. Insult or imbalance in one area alters structure and function throughout the organism. It is through appreciation of this basic principle of unity that the osteopathic physician is able to evaluate and treat the whole patient in his or her life context. Far from perceiving the patient as a host for disease, the osteopathic physician seeks to understand how the condition of the patient as a whole has deviated from health and how disease may have ensued.

Self-regulation, Self-healing, and Health Maintenance

The human organism is inherently self-regulating. Under optimum conditions, the body, mind, and spirit work to maintain health and heal to the extent possible. This principle embodies several important ideas found in traditional osteopathy: homeostatic regulation, *vis medicatrix naturae* (the healing power of nature), proper circulation (the rule of the artery is supreme), good nutrition, and a healthy psychological and spiritual life.

IMPLICATIONS OF SELF-REGULATION PRINCIPLE

Still suggests, "*Within man's body there is a capacity for health. If this capacity is recognized and normalized, disease can be both prevented and treated.*"[6]

Health is the adaptive and optimal attainment of physical, mental, emotional, and spiritual well-being. It is based on our natural capacity to meet, with adequate reserves, the usual stresses of daily life and the occasional severe stresses imposed by extremes of environment and activity. It includes our ability to resist and combat noxious influences in our environment and to compensate for their effects. One's health at any given time depends on many factors including his or her polygenetic inheritance, environmental influences, and adaptive response to stressors.

Students and investigators in medicine and the life sciences have long understood the basic homeostatic mechanisms of the immune system, the body's system of thermal control, the body's capacity for healing wounds, and other regulatory processes that we often take for granted until something goes wrong with them or their ability to cope with stressors is overwhelmed.

Andrew Taylor Still promulgated his ideas during a period in which research in medicine and the life sciences was very active. New learning and new theories were emerging left and right, Still's among them. This was the era when the invasive approaches of heroic medicine coexisted with the minimalist theory of homeopathy. It was also an era when the mechanisms of pharmacotherapeutics were poorly understood, and the pharmacopoeia was limited. Still believed that the body produced substances that would help remove poisons, dissolve lumps or thickened places, and perform numerous other poorly understood functions. In his words: "... *nature at will, can*

and does produce solvents, necessary to melt down deposits of fiber, bone, or any fluid or solid found in the human body."[3(p207)] And "*osteopathy believes that all parts of the human body do work on chemical compounds, and from the general supply manufacture for local wants....*"[7] And "*... the brain of man was God's drug store, and had in it all liquids, drugs, lubricating oils, opiates, acids, and antacids, and every quality of drugs that the wisdom of God thought necessary for human happiness and health.*"[8] Modern medicine, of course, knows these "solvents" and "chemicals" as endorphins, enkephalins, prostaglandins, and the numerous other entities produced by the human body that affect our well-being.

Proper circulation was of paramount importance to Still. One of his most quoted aphorisms is: "*The rule of the artery must be absolute, universal and unobstructed, or disease will be the result.*"[9] Furthermore, although Still acknowledged that lymph and its function were poorly understood, he believed that one accomplishment of manipulating the musculoskeletal system was "*turning on the lymph, giving it time to do its work of atomizing all crudities.*"[3(p209)] Since then, modern medicine has come to appreciate the role of circulation in health maintenance and management of chronic illness. Obvious examples are wound healing, congestive heart failure and related accumulation of fluid in the lungs and edema of the extremities, kidney failure, and other end organ damage resulting from decreased circulation.

The most visible current expression of the medical profession's appreciation of the person's capacity for self-regulation, self-healing, and self-maintenance comes through our ever-increasing understanding of the importance of health maintenance and illness prevention as a key to the health care process. In recent years we have seen an evolution in the role of the physician, especially in primary care and in the managed care movement, away from intervention following the occurrence of illness or disease, toward emphasis on prevention. Osteopathic medicine has had this principle as a foundation of practice since its inception.

Structure and Function Complexly Interdependent

A.T. Still, typically astute, saw altered structure–function relationships in situations that others had yet to consider. Some were neuromusculoskeletal; many were not. At one point he boldly suggested that all diseases are effects of altered structure–function relationships: "*Disease is the result of anatomical abnormalities followed by physiologic discord.*"[9(p36)]

IMPLICATIONS OF INTERDEPENDENT STRUCTURE AND FUNCTION

In modern medicine and the life sciences, we are daily becoming more and more aware of the artificiality of separating the study of structure from that of function. Clinically, our understanding of such abnormalities as sickle cell disease is just one manifestation of our application of the structure–function relationship, at the cellular level. Furthermore, our structuring of the knowledge base for understanding normal biologic structure and function has undergone a revolution in the last 10 years, as we have come to the realization that separating fields of knowledge into the traditional disciplines such as anatomy, biochemistry, and physiology, for example, is artificial. The evolution of teaching and research in the basic sciences from separate disciplines with clear boundaries to the integrated conceptualizations of cell biology is a highly visible acknowledgment of our realization that, beginning at the cellular level and moving to the level of the total being, there is an interdependent relationship of structure and function.

Closer to home for osteopathic medicine, Northup writes:

Where does an idea start? As an original idea in the mind of one person? Hardly so. The origin of an idea is rarely certain, and too much energy often is expended in fixing the credit, which more often than not goes to the one to first put the idea to good use. Therefore, the idea of the interdependent relationship between structure and function has been attributed to . . . the founder of osteopathy, because he was one of the first to make practical application of this fundamental concept in the diagnostics and therapeutics of medicine. Whether Dr. Still has received more or less credit for the structure–function concept than he deserves is of minor importance. It is, however, of major importance that he recognized the validity of the concept and applied it in diagnosis and therapy.[6(p33)]

Because the neuromusculoskeletal system interacts interdependently with all aspects of structure and function, osteopathic physicians commonly use palpatory diagnosis and osteopathic manipulative treatment to identify and treat related somatic components, i.e., areas of somatic dysfunction. These skills and applied philosophical concepts serve to distinguish the osteopathic profession.

Rational Treatment Based on Body Unity, Self-regulation, and Interrelationship of Structure and Function

Along with standard medical, behavioral, and surgical care, osteopathically oriented problem-solving and treatment plans commonly incorporate basic osteopathic principles. Patient evaluation by the osteopathic physician includes application of the principles to gain an understanding of the patient's health or illness status. Management planning for the osteopathic physician invokes these principles in the development of an approach that will optimize the patient's function and/or restore him or her to health if ill.

The key to effective application of the principles for the osteopathic physician is the understanding that what we identify and call disease is not the invasion of a host by some etiologic entity that can then be labeled but rather a breakdown in the body's capacity for self-maintenance. Still repeatedly reminded us that disease was an effect rather than a cause of dysfunction or illness. For example, one of his most colorful assertions:

It appears perfectly reasonable to any person born above the condition of an idiot, who has familiarized himself with anatomy

and its working with the machinery of life, that all diseases are mere effects, the cause being a partial or complete failure of the nerves to properly conduct the fluids of life.

On this stone I have builded and sustained Osteopathy for twenty-five years. Day by day the evidences grow stronger and stronger that this philosophy is correct.[3(p94)]

Peppered throughout Still's writings we find similar reminders:

Sickness is an effect caused by the stoppage of some supply of fluid or quality of life.[3(p252)]

When all parts of the human body are in line we have perfect health. When they are not, the effect is disease. When the parts are readjusted disease gives place to health.[9(p33)]

All diseases are only effects.[9(p34)]

Still's perspective was principally mechanical, as that was his level of understanding, and the analogies to physics and mechanics worked well for him. In more modern times, we have come to appreciate a broader conceptualization of illness or disease as an effect or consequence of compromise in the body's ability to sustain health, as expressed in the introduction to the Kirksville consensus declaration quoted earlier.

IMPLICATIONS OF RATIONAL TREATMENT PRINCIPLE

The osteopathic physician realizes that the neuromusculoskeletal system, through its interdependent structure–function relationships, can positively or negatively influence inherent healing and health maintenance mechanisms. Abnormal structure leads to abnormal function, and vice versa. In many instances, palpably evident somatic dysfunction is commonly associated with a range of medically identifiable somatic and visceral problems, and thus differential diagnosis becomes more accurate.

One of Still's more famous aphorisms states: "*To find health should be the object of the doctor. Anyone can find disease.*"[7(p28)] This emphasis on health and a healthy lifestyle is a long-standing osteopathic tradition. From a clinical point of view, it also suggests that diagnostic and treatment plans emphasize enhancements of normal physiologic functions as methods for coping with pathophysiologic processes.

Among important osteopathically oriented considerations are changes in the neuromusculoskeletal system. In some cases, palpatory diagnosis is used to help identify preclinical states. Still notes viscerosomatic and somaticovisceral responses in the following way: "*The body's musculoskeletal system . . . forms a structure which, when disordered, may effect changes in the function of other parts of the body. This effect may be created through irritation and abnormal response of the nerve and blood supply to other organs.*"[6(p15)] He also states his views very well at another point:

. . . When a patient comes to me for examination and begins to talk to me about symptoms . . . while listening, I am seeing in my mind's eye the combinations of systems which go to make up the whole of that body structure. I am concentrating on her story,

trying to determine through the description given to me the structural alterations which have occurred to produce the symptoms described. I am seeing first the bony framework and the joints which hold it together as one system, the foundation upon which all other structures in the human body are built. I am seeing, especially, the positions of those bony parts and their relationships, one with the other. Then I see the ligaments . . . the muscles . . . the nervous system in all its relationships, in every function of the body . . . controlling the functions of the internal organs, the circulation of body fluids, and nutrition of the various body parts. . . . I further see the arterial system . . . the venous system . . . the lymphatic system (and their functions) . . . and last but not least I see the glandular system of the body and wonder how it brings about its effect in each particular case.[10]

In a more general sense, the evolution of American health care practices from the more interventionist approach to that of emphasizing health maintenance and illness prevention is eloquent testimony to our understanding of the origins of illness. Modern interpretations of the concept of disease as an effect are more refined and are able to take into consideration exceptions such as congenital and heritable disease processes as well as other less well-understood infectious diseases (such as AIDS) and certain cancers. However, our ability to stave off infectious diseases through immunization; our understanding of the relationship between exposure to noxious substances such as tobacco smoke and the development of lung diseases; and, perhaps most importantly, our ability to forestall and even avoid degenerative processes such as coronary artery disease through pursuit of a healthy lifestyle all derive from our understanding (albeit implicit in some cases) that much disease and illness is not the cause of, but is caused by, a deterioration in health.

Along with this understanding comes the evolution of the role of the physician from one who treated the patient who came to him or her with a problem, to a partner in health maintenance and disease prevention.

DRUGS, SURGERY, AND OTHER CONSIDERATIONS

The roles of surgery, drugs, and applied pharmacology in Still's system have been a source of confusion for some. Notably, his observations and experiences occurred prior to the control of infections and infectious diseases. They also were before adequate vaccinations were available. Still often referred to the dangers of contemporary medical and surgical practices. On the other hand, he established an obstetrical hospital and lived to see the establishment of the first osteopathic hospitals in such cities as Chicago, Philadelphia, and Detroit. He notes the importance of surgery for cancers: *"Cancer begins long before recognized symptoms can be detected. When positively diagnosed, it may have spread its seeds in other parts of the body like a brush pile on fire. It will burst forth its sparks to other areas producing more fire. Cancer is first a local disease when it can be cured by surgery. When it becomes general, it is beyond human efforts. . . ."*[9(p26)]

During his lifetime, Still remained adamantly opposed to so-called "materia medica" and did not permit its teaching in his school. On the other hand, he said, *"To be able to intelligently prescribe any and all drugs, one must first learn the fundamental principles that govern their administration. Namely: There must exist within the body the physiologic wrong for which the drug is given. Otherwise, it becomes a poison instead of a remedial agency."*[9(p37)]

An Explication of Osteopathic Principles

IRVIN M. KORR

At this stage of your medical training, you have become familiar with osteopathic principles and can recite them in their usual brief, maxim form. The purpose of this section is to explore more fully the meaning, biological foundations, and clinical implications of the founding principles of osteopathic medicine.

Remember that these principles began to evolve centuries ago, even before the time of Hippocrates. However, their basis in animal and, more specifically, human biology did not begin to become evident through research until late in the 19th century. The origin of these principles, therefore, was largely empirical; that is, they were the product of thoughtful and widely shared observations of ill and injured people. For example, it could hardly escape notice, even in primitive societies, that people (and animals) recovered from illness and wounds healed without intervention and, therefore, some natural indwelling healing power must be at work.

Even at the time of the founding of the osteopathic profession in 1892, the available knowledge in the sciences of physiology, biochemistry, microbiology, immunology, and pathology was meager. Indeed, immunology, biochemistry, and various other neurosciences and biomedical sciences had yet to appear as distinct disciplines. Therefore, these principles could only be expressed as aphorisms, embellished perhaps with conjectures about their biological basis. It is to the credit and honor of the osteopathic profession that it contributed cogent elaboration of the principles, developed effective methods for their implementation, built a system of practice upon those principles, and disclosed much about their basis in biological mechanisms through research.

In view of the enormous burgeoning of biomedical knowledge during this century, it is timely to examine the principles that guide osteopathic practice in the light of that vast and growing body of knowledge and to explore their relevance to clinical practice and to current and future health problems. What follows is an effort in that direction, without detailed reference to individual research.

THE PERSON AS A WHOLE

The Body

The principle of the unity of the body, so central to osteopathic practice, states that every part of the body depends on other parts for maintenance of its optimal function and even of its integrity. This interdependence of body components is mediated by the communication systems of the body: exchange of substances via circulating blood and other body fluids and exchange of nerve impulses and neurotransmitters through the nervous system.

The circulatory and nervous systems also mediate the regulation and coordination of cellular, tissue, and organ functions and thus the maintenance of the integrity of the body as a whole. The organized and integrated collaboration of the body components is reflected in the concept of homeostasis, the maintenance of the relative constancy of the internal environment in which all the cells live and function.

In view of this interdependence and exchange of influences, it is inevitable that dysfunction or failure of a major body component will adversely affect the competence of other organs and tissues and, therefore, one's health.

The Person

Important and valid as is the concept of body unity, it is incomplete in that it is, by implication, limited to the physical realm. Physicians minister not to bodies but to individuals, each of whom is unique by virtue of his or her genetic endowment, personal history, and the variety of environments in which that history has been lived.

The person, obviously, is more than a body, for the person has a mind, also the product of heredity and biography. Separation of body and mind, whether conceptually or in practice, is an anachronistic remnant of such dualistic thinking as that of the 17th century philosopher-scientist, René Descartes. It was his belief that body and mind are separate domains, one publicly visible and palpable, the other invisible, impalpable, and private. This dualistic concept is anachronistic because, while it is almost universally rejected as a concept, it is still acted out in much of clinical practice and in biomedical research.

Clinical and biomedical research (as well as everyday experience) has irrefutably shown that body and mind are so inseparable, so pervasive to each other, that they can be regarded—and treated—as a single entity. It is now widely recognized (whether or not it is demonstrated in practice) that what goes on (or goes wrong) in either body or mind has repercussions in the other. It is for reasons such as these that I prefer "unity of the person" to "unity of the body," conveying totally integrated humanity and individuality.

The Person as Context

Phenomena assigned to mind (consciousness, thought, feelings, beliefs, attitudes, etc.) have their physiological and behavioral counterparts; conversely, bodily and behavioral changes have psychological concomitants, such as altered feelings and perceptions. It must be noted, however, that it is the *person* who is feeling, perceiving, and responding—not the body or the mind. It is you who feels well, ill, happy, or sad, and not your body or mind. What goes on in body and mind is conditioned by who the person is and his or her entire history.

In short, the person is far more than the union of body and mind, in the same sense that water is more than the union of hydrogen and oxygen. Nothing that we know about either oxygen or hydrogen accounts for the three states of water (liquid, solid, and gas), their respective properties, the boiling and freezing points, viscosity, and so forth. Water incorporates yet transcends oxygen and hydrogen. To understand water we must study water and not only its components. In the same way, at an enormously more complex level, the person comprises yet transcends body and mind.

Moreover, once hydrogen and oxygen are joined to form water, they become subject to the laws that govern water. In the same but infinitely more complex sense, it is you who makes up your mind, changes your mind, trains and enriches your mind, and puts it to work. It is you who determines from moment to moment whether and in what way you will express, through your body, what is in or on your mind.

Thus the person is the context, the environment, in which all the body parts live and function and in which the mind finds expression. Everything about the person—genetics, history from conception to the present moment, nutrition, use and abuse of body and mind, parental and school conditioning, physical and sociocultural environments, and so on—enters into determining the quality of physical and mental function. The better the quality of the "environment" provided by the person for the mental and bodily components, the better they will function. For example, someone who has a peptic ulcer is not ill because of the ulcer. The ulcer exists because of an unfavorable internal environment.

In conclusion, just as "*the proper study of mankind is man*" (Alexander Pope), so is the study of human health and illness also man. As will become evident, the principle of the unity of the person leads us naturally to the next principle.

THE PLACE OF THE MUSCULOSKELETAL SYSTEM IN HUMAN LIFE

The Means of Expression of Our Humanity and Individuality

"Structure determines function," "structure and function are reciprocally interrelated," and similar aphorisms have traditionally represented another osteopathic principle. That principle recognizes the special place of the musculoskeletal system among the body systems and its relation to the health of the person. We examine now the basis for the osteopathic emphasis on the musculoskeletal system in total health care.

Human life is expressed in human behavior, in humans doing the things that humans do. And whatever humans do, they do with the musculoskeletal system. That system is the ultimate instrument for carrying out human action and behavior. It is the means through which we manifest our human qualities and our personal uniqueness—personality, intellect, imagination, creativity, perceptions, love, compassion, values, and philosophies. The most noble ethical, moral, or religious principle has value only insofar as it can be overtly expressed through behavior.

That expression is made possible by the coordinated contractions and relaxations of striated muscles, most of them acting upon bones and joints. The musculoskeletal system is the means through which we communicate with each other, whether it be by written, spoken, or "signed" language, or by gesture or facial expression. Agriculture, industry, technology, literature, the arts and sciences—our very civilization—are the products of human action, interaction, communication, and behavior, that is, by the orchestrated contractions and relaxations of the body's musculature.

Relation to the Body Economy

The musculoskeletal system is the most massive system in the community of body systems. Its muscular components are collectively the largest consumer in the body economy. This is true not only because of their mass, but because of their high energy requirements. Furthermore, those requirements may vary widely from moment to moment according to what the *person* is doing, with what feelings and in what environments.

The high and varying metabolic requirements of the musculoskeletal system are met by the cardiovascular, respiratory, digestive, renal, and other visceral systems. Together, they supply the required fuels and nutrients, remove the products of metabolism, and control the composition and physical properties of the internal environment. In "servicing" the musculoskeletal system in this manner, these organ systems are at the same time servicing each other (and, of course, the nervous system).

The nervous system is also, to a great degree, occupied with the musculoskeletal system, that is, with behavior and motor control. Indeed, most of the fibers in the spinal nerves are those converging impulses to and from the muscles and other components of the musculoskeletal system. In addition, the nervous system, its autonomic components, and the circulatory system mediate communication and exchange of signals and substances between the soma and the viscera. In this way, visceral, metabolic, and endocrine activity is continually tuned to moment-to-moment requirements of the musculoskeletal system, that is, to what the person is doing from moment to moment.

Consequences of Visceral Dysfunction

Impairment or failure of some visceral function or of communication between the musculoskeletal system and the viscera is reflected in the musculoskeletal system. When the resulting dysfunction is severe and diffuse, motor activity and even maintenance of posture are difficult or impossible and automatically imposed.

The Musculoskeletal System as Source of Adverse Influences on Other Systems

In view of the rich afferent input of the musculoskeletal system into the central nervous system and its rich interchange of substances with other systems through the body fluids, it is inevitable that structural and functional disturbances in the musculoskeletal system will have repercussions elsewhere in the body.

Such structural and functional disturbances may be of postural, traumatic, or behavioral origin (neglect, misuse, or abuse by the person). Further, it must be appreciated that the human framework is, compared with other (quadruped) mammals, uniquely unstable and vulnerable to compressive, torsional, and shearing forces, because of the vertical configuration, higher center of gravity, and the comparatively small, bipedal base.

The human musculoskeletal system, therefore, is the frequent source of aberrant afferent input to the central nervous system and its autonomic distribution, with at least potential consequences to visceral function. Which organs, blood vessels, etc. are at risk is determined by the site of the musculoskeletal dysfunction and the part(s) of the central nervous system, (e.g., spinal segments) into which it discharges its sensory impulses.

When a dysfunction or pathology has developed in a visceral organ, that disturbance is reflected in segmentally related somatic tissues. Viscus and soma become linked in a vicious circle of afferent and efferent impulses, which sustain and exacerbate the disturbance. Appropriate treatment of the somatic component reduces its input to the vicious circle and may even interrupt that circle with therapeutic effect.

Importance of the Personal Context

Whether or not visceral or vasomotor consequences of somatic dysfunction occur, and with what consequences to the person, depends on other factors in the person's life, such as the genetic, nutritional, psychological, behavioral, sociocultural, and environmental. As research has shown, however, the presence of somatic dysfunction and the accompanying reflex and neurotrophic effects exaggerate the impact of other detrimental factors on the person's health. *Effective treatment of the musculoskeletal dysfunction shields the patient by reducing the deleterious effects of the other factors. Such treatment, therefore, has preventive as well as therapeutic benefits.*

Such treatment directed to the musculoskeletal system assumes even greater and often crucial significance when it is recognized that the other kinds of harmful factors, such as those enumerated above, are not readily subject to change and may even require social or governmental intervention. The musculoskeletal system, however, is readily accessible and responsive to osteopathic manipulative treatment. I view these considerations as the rationale for osteopathic manipulative treatment and its strategic role in total health care.

Finally, the osteopathic philosophy and the unity of the person concept enjoins the physician to treat the patient as a whole and not merely the affected parts. Hence, appropriate corrective attention should also be given by both patient and physician to other significant risk factors that are subject to change.

OUR PERSONAL HEALTH CARE SYSTEMS

The Natural Healing Power

Appreciation, even in ancient times, of our inherent recuperative, restorative, and rehabilitative powers is reflected in the Latin phrase, *vis medicatrix naturae* (nature's healing force). We recover from illnesses, fevers drop, blood clots and wounds heal, broken bones reunite, infections are overcome, skin eruptions clear up, and even cancers are known to occasionally undergo "spontaneous remission." But miraculous as is the healing power (and appreciated as it was until we became more impressed by human-made "miracles" and "breakthroughs"), the other, more recently revealed components of the health care system with which each of us is endowed are no less marvelous.

The Component System That Defends against Threats from Without

This component includes, among others, immune mechanisms that defend us against the enormous variety and potency of foreign organisms that invade our bodies, wreaking damage and even bringing death. These same immune mechanisms guard us against those of our own cells that *become* foreign and malignant as the result of mutation. Included also are the mechanisms that defend against foreign and poisonous substances that we may take in with our food and drink or that enter through the skin and lungs, by disarming them, converting them to innocuous substances, and eliminating them from the body. They defend us (until overwhelmed) even against the toxic substances that we ourselves introduce into the atmosphere, soil, water, or more directly into our own bodies.

MECHANISMS THAT DEFEND AGAINST CHANGES IN THE INTERNAL ENVIRONMENT

We humans are exposed to, and adapt to, wide variations in physical and chemical properties of our environment (e.g., temperature, barometric pressure, oxygen, and carbon dioxide concentrations) and sustain ourselves with chemically diverse food and drink. But the cells of our body can function and survive only in—the internal environment of interstitial fluids

which maintain body functions within relatively narrow limits as regards variations in chemical composition, temperature, tissue, osmotic pressure, pH, etc.

This phenomenon, called homeostasis, is based on thousands of simultaneously occurring dynamic equilibria throughout the body. Examples are: rates of energy consumption and replenishment by the cells. Homeostasis—constancy and quick restoration of constancy—must be accomplished regardless of the variations in the external environment, composition of food and drink, and the moment-to-moment activities of the person. It is accomplished by an enormously complex array of regulatory mechanisms that continually monitor and control respiratory, circulatory, digestive, renal, metabolic, and countless other functions and processes. Maintenance of optimal environments for cellular function is essential to health. The homeostatic mechanisms may, therefore, be viewed as the health-maintenance system of the body.

Commentary

These, then are the three major components of our indwelling health care system, each comprising numerous component systems. In the order in which humans became aware of them, they are (a) the healing (remedial, curative, palliative, recuperative, rehabilitative) component; (b) the component that defends against threats from the external environment; and (c) the homeostatic, health-maintaining component. These major component systems, of course, share subcomponents and mechanisms.

When the internal health care system is permitted to operate optimally, without impediment, its product is what we call "health." Its natural tendency is always toward health and the recovery of health. Indeed, the personal health care system is the very *source* of health, upon which all externally applied measures depend for their beneficial effects. The internal health care system, in effect, makes its own diagnoses, issues its own prescriptions, draws upon its own vast pharmacy, and in most situations, administers each dose—without side effects.

Health and healing, therefore, come from within. It is the patient who *gets* well, and not the practitioner or the treatment that *makes* them well.

THE THREE PRINCIPLES AS GUIDES TO MEDICAL PRACTICE

The Unity of the Person

In caring for the whole person, the well-grounded osteopathic physician goes beyond the presenting complaint, beyond relief of symptoms, beyond identification of the disease and treatment of the impaired organ, malfunction, or pathology, important as they are to total care. The osteopathic physician also explores those factors in the person and the person's life that may have contributed to the illness and that, appropriately modified, compensated, or eliminated, would favor recovery, prevent recurrence, and improve health in general.

The physician then selects that factor or combination of

factors that are readily subject to change and that would be of sufficient impact to shift the balance toward recovery and enhancement of health. The possible factors include such categories as the biological (e.g., genetic, nutritional), psychological, behavioral (use, neglect, or abuse of body and mind; interpersonal relationships; habits; etc.), sociocultural, occupational, and environmental. Some of these factors, especially some of the biological, are responsive to appropriate clinical intervention, some are responsive only to social or governmental action, and still others require changes by patients themselves. Osteopathic whole-person care, therefore, is a collaborative relationship between patient and physician.

The Place of the Musculoskeletal System in Human Biology and Behavior: The Strategic Role of Osteopathic Manipulative Treatment

It is obvious that some of the most deleterious factors are difficult or impossible for patient and physician to change or eliminate. These include (at least at present) genetic factors (although some inherited predispositions can be mitigated by lifestyle change). They include also such items as social convention, lifelong habits (e.g., dietary and behavioral), widely shared beliefs, prejudices, misconceptions and cultural doctrines, attitudes, and values. Others, such as the quality of the physical or socioeconomic environments, may require concerted community, national, and even international action.

Focus falls, therefore, upon those deleterious factors that *are* favorably modifiable by personal and professional action, and that, when appropriately modified or eliminated, mitigate the health-impairing effects of the less changeable factors. Improvement of body mechanics by osteopathic manipulative treatment is a major consideration when dealing with these complex interactions.

Our Personal Health Care Systems

This principle has important implications for the respective responsibilities of patient and physician and for their relationship. Since each person is the owner and hence the guardian of his or her own personal health care system, the ultimate source of health and healing, the *primary* responsibility for one's health is each individual's. That responsibility is met by the way the person lives, thinks, behaves, nourishes himself or herself, uses body and mind, relates to others, and the other factor usually called "lifestyle." Each person must be taught and enabled to assume that responsibility.

It is the physician's responsibility, while giving palliative and remedial attention to the patient's immediate problem, to support each patient's internal health care system, to remove impediments to its competence, and above all, to do it no harm. It is also the responsibility of physicians to instruct patients on how to do the same for themselves and to strive to motivate them to do so, especially by their own example.

The relationship between patient and osteopathic physician is therefore a collaborative one, a partnership, in maintaining and enhancing the competence of the patient's personal health care system. The maintenance and enhancement of health is the most effective and comprehensive form of preventive medicine, for "health is the best defense against disease." As stated by A.T. Still, *"To find health should be the object of the doctor. Anyone can find disease."*

Relevance to the Current and Future Health of the Nation

The preventive strategy of health maintenance and health enhancement, intrinsic to the osteopathic philosophy, is urgently needed by our society today. One of the greatest burdens on the nation's health care system and on the national economy is in the care of victims of the chronic degenerative diseases, such as heart disease, cancer, stroke, and arthritis, which require long-term care.

The incidence of these diseases has increased and will continue to increase well into the next century as the average age of our population continues to increase. The widely accepted (but usually unspoken) assumption that guides current practice (and national policy) is that the chronic degenerative diseases are an inevitable aspect of the aging process, that is, that aging is itself pathological. It is now increasingly apparent, however, that the increase of their incidence with age is because the longer one lives, the greater the toll taken by minor, seemingly inconsequential, inconspicuous, treatable impairments and modifiable contributing factors in and around the person. They are, therefore, largely the natural culmination of less-than-favorable lifestyles, and, hence, they are largely preventable.

The great national strategy is that, while the nation's health care system is so extensively and expensively absorbed in the care of millions of elderly victims of chronic disease (at per capita cost 3.5 times that of persons under the age of 65 years), tens of millions of younger people and children are living on and embarking on life paths that culminate in the same diseases. The health care system simply must move upstream to move people from pathogenic to salutary paths. And the osteopathic profession can show the way.

The osteopathic profession has a historic opportunity to make an enormous contribution to the enhancement of the health of our nation. It can do this by giving leadership in addressing this great tragedy by bringing its basic strategy of whole-person, *health-oriented* care to bear on the problem and demonstrating its effectiveness in practice.

Having reviewed and enlarged on the principles of osteopathic medicine, their meaning, biological foundations, and clinical implications, it seems appropriate to propose a definition of osteopathic medicine. The author offers the following: Osteopathic medicine is a system of medicine that is based on the continually deepening and expanding understanding of (a) human nature; (b) those components of human biology that are centrally relevant to health, namely the inherent regulatory, protective, regenerative, and recuperative biological mechanisms, whose combined effect is consistently in the direction of the maintenance, enhancement, and recovery of health; and (c) the factors in and around the person that both favorably and unfavorably affect those mechanisms.

The *practice* of osteopathic medicine is, essentially, the potentiation of the intrinsic health-maintaining and health-restoring resources of the individual. The methods and agents employed are those that are effective in enhancing the favorable factors and diminishing or eliminating the unfavorable factors affecting each individual. Osteopathic medical practice necessarily includes the application of palliative and remedial measures, but always on the condition that they do no harm to the patient's own health-maintaining and health-restoring resources. This stipulation governing the choice of methods and agents is based on the recognition that *all* therapeutic methods depend on the patient's own recuperative power for their effectiveness and are valueless without it and that health and the recovery of health come from within.

The *art and science* of osteopathic medicine are expressed in the identification and selection of those factors in each individual that are accessible and amenable to change and that, when changed, would most decisively potentate the person on health-supporting resources.

Osteopathic physicians give special emphasis to factors originating in the musculoskeletal system, for the following reasons:

1. The vertical human framework (a) is highly vulnerable to compressive (gravitational), torsional, and shearing forces, and (b) encases the entire central nervous system.
2. Since the massive, energy-demanding system has rich two-way (communication with all other body systems, it is, because of its vulnerability, a common and frequent source of impediments to the functions of other systems.
3. These impediments exaggerate the physiological impact of other detrimental factors in the person's life, and, through the central nervous system, focus it on specific organs and tissues.

4. The musculoskeletal impediments (somatic dysfunctions) are readily accessible to the hands and responsive to the manipulative and other methods developed and refined by the osteopathic medical profession.

REFERENCES

1. Pierce, Charles S. (1839–1914). *Essays in the Philosophy of Science.* In: Thomas V, ed. Brown University, Liberal Arts Press, American Heritage Series. New York, NY: Bobbs-Merrill Co; 1957.
2. Trowbridge C. *Andrew Taylor Still.* Kirksville, Mo: Thomas Jefferson University Press, Northeast Missouri State University; 1991:122–125.
3. Still AT. *Autobiography of Andrew T. Still.* rev ed. Kirksville, Mo; 1908. Published by the author. Distributed, Indianapolis, Ind; American Academy of Osteopathy.
4. Still AT. *The Philosophy and Mechanical Principles of Osteopathy.* Kansas City; 1902. Reprinted, Kirksville, Mo: Osteopathic Enterprises; 1986.
5. Special Committee on Osteopathic Principles and Osteopathic Technic, Kirksville College of Osteopathy and Surgery. An interpretation of the osteopathic concept. Tentative formulation of a teaching guide for faculty, hospital staff and student body. *J Osteop.* 1953; 60(Oct):8–10.
6. Northup GW. *Osteopathic Medicine, An American Reformation.* Chicago, Ill: American Osteopathic Association; 1966:15.
7. Still AT. *Philosophy of Osteopathy.* Kirksville, Mo; 1899. Reprinted, Academy of Applied Osteopathy; January, 1946:40.
8. Still AT. *Autobiography of Andrew T. Still.* 1st ed. p 219. Quoted by: Booth ER. *History of Osteopathy and Twentieth Century Medical Practice.* Cincinnati: Jennings and Graham; 1905:53.
9. Truhlar RE. *Doctor AT Still in the Living.* Privately published, Cleveland, Ohio; 1950. Distributed, Indianapoils, Ind: American Academy of Osteopathy; p 13.
10. Hildreth AG. *The Lengthening Shadow of Dr. Andrew Taylor Still.* Privately published, Macon, Mo; 1942. Reprinted and distributed, Kirksville, Mo: Osteopathic Enterprises, Inc; pp 181–183.

Osteopathic History

2. Major Events in Osteopathic History

BARBARA A. PETERSON

Key Concepts

- **Beginnings of osteopathic medicine**
- **Growth of the osteopathic profession**
- **Educational issues**
- **Areas of conflict and agreement with allopathic medicine**
- **Osteopathic professional organizations**
- **Recognition by state and federal governments**
- **Role in specialties, hospitals, and primary care**

The founder of the osteopathic profession was Andrew Taylor Still (1828–1917), a frontier physician in Kansas and Missouri.[1,2] Like most American physicians of his time, he learned medicine by apprenticeship, reading, and his own anatomic dissections, probably with a course of lectures from a long-defunct Kansas City medical school.[3] In addition to practicing medicine, he farmed, fought in the Civil War[a] on the side of the Union,[4] and served briefly in the Kansas Free-State Legislature.[5]

After losing members of his own family to spinal meningitis in 1864,[1] his longtime dissatisfaction with the "heroic" methods of orthodox medicine[6] intensified his search for a better way. He searched by studying, thinking, and examining the anatomy of cadavers obtained from Indian burial grounds.

After a decade of study, in 1874 Still "*flung to the breeze the banner of osteopathy.*"[1] He did not say precisely what that meant, but it was followed by attempts to present his findings at Baker University, an institution he had helped to found. He could not get a hearing. Further, he was ejected from the church on the basis that only Christ was allowed to heal by laying on of hands. His description of that experience makes it clear that the "*laying on of hands*" was therapeutic manipulation.[1]

During 1875 Still spent some time with his brother, who had become addicted to morphine through medical treatment. This experience, added to the uselessness of medication in sav-

ing his family, roused in Still a new hatred for the drugs of the day. This enmity later became absolute, even when the armamentarium of drugs began to move from harmful toward helpful.

Late in 1875 Still moved from Kansas to Kirksville, Missouri, where he spent the rest of his life. For several years he used Kirksville as a base to conduct a marginal itinerant practice.[7] By 1887 there finally were enough patients so that Still could stay in Kirksville. When a little recognition came, a lot soon followed, and the burden of practice quickly became heavy. Still began to think about teaching others his methods; unlike many alternative practitioners of his day, he never intended to keep therapeutic secrets to himself or to grow rich from his methods. There were abortive attempts first to train apprentices and then to teach a class of "operators" to assist in the practice of osteopathy. The attempts were unsuccessful largely because the students lacked Still's detailed knowledge of anatomy and bodily function.

The term osteopathy was coined by Still in about 1889. The story is told[8] that, when challenged because this word was not in the dictionary, Still replied "*We are going to put it there.*" The word became for Still and his followers a symbol for medical reform, for a science that would refocus medicine on "*the perfect works of the Creator.*" Osteopathy worked with and facilitated the natural machinery of the body for normal and reparative function and did not work against it, as seemed to be the case with purgatives, emetics, bloodletting, and addictive drugs.

PROFESSIONAL EDUCATION AND GROWTH

First School

The first successful school, the American School of Osteopathy, was chartered in May 1892 and opened that Fall with a class of about 21 men and women, including members of Still's family and other local people.[9] The faculty consisted of Still and Dr. William Smith, an Edinburgh-trained physician who taught anatomy in exchange for learning osteopathy. The goal, as stated in the revised (1894) charter for the school,[9] was "*to improve our present system of surgery, obstetrics, and treatment of diseases generally, and to place the same on a more rational and scientific basis, and to impart information to the medical profession. . . .*" The charter would have permitted granting of the MD degree, but Still insisted on a distinctive recognition for graduates, DO, for Diplomate in Osteopathy (later Doctor of Osteopathy).

The first course was just a few months long; most of the students voluntarily returned for a second year of additional

---

[a]Still wrote in 1877 that he did the duties of a surgeon although he was placed on the roll as a hospital steward.

training. By 1894 the course was 2 years long, two terms of 5 months each. In addition to their study of anatomy, students worked in the clinic under experienced operators, at first only under Still but later under other graduates as well.

During the last 5 years of the century the growth of both clinic and school were spectacular. Patients came from near and distant places, having heard by either word of mouth or printed accounts of near-miraculous cures. There were enough of such "miracles" that the osteopathic profession was widely promoted by grateful patients. A significant number of early DOs were either former patients or family members of patients who came to their studies with a kind of evangelical fervor. The town of Kirksville prospered and came to regard Still, who once was ridiculed, as a citizen of immense importance. His statue even stands in the town square.[10]

Data on the number of enrolled students illustrate the school's growth. In October 1895 there were 28 students. By the following summer there were 102. By 1900, there were over 700 students, with a faculty of 18.[9] There were by the turn of the century more than a dozen daughter schools founded by graduates of the original school.

Conflict with the American Medical Association

Medical education at the time was not well regulated. Many schools, both medical and osteopathic, had virtually no entrance requirements except tuition payments, and many schools were for-profit institutions. Licensing laws had not yet reached a stage where they were effective in setting educational standards. The American Medical Association (AMA), later a powerful influence for the raising of educational standards, was then weak and about to reorganize itself.

The new AMA, observing that there were too many doctors, made its first order of business under a revised constitution the regulation of medical education. Its Council on Medical Education was formed in 1904, with a charge (among others) to improve the academic requirements for medical schools. This charge was fulfilled by rating as Class A (approved), B (probation), or C (unapproved) all medical schools and making the findings available to state licensing boards.[11]

Even before the AMA formed its Council on Medical Education, the young American Osteopathic Association (AOA) had adopted standards for approval of osteopathic colleges (1902) and begun inspections (1903).[12] This had the effect of causing many small osteopathic colleges to close or merge with larger institutions.

Osteopathic schools were not included in the first AMA survey, but they were included in the influential Flexner Report, published in 1910.[13] The sequelae of this report, which harshly condemned osteopathic schools along with many medical schools, was major reform. Marginal schools closed, and the surviving ones converted to a not-for-profit status. State licensing boards began to enforce stricter requirements.

Curriculum

Many medical schools formed affiliations with universities and by doing so gained additional funding. This was not an option for osteopathic institutions at that time, and they faced a difficult dilemma: raise entry standards and lose major portions of tuition payments, which were at that time their only income, or adopt a "go slow" attitude. They chose the latter, which meant that they were perhaps two decades behind in the educational reforms that many agreed were desirable.[14] AOA standards did increase the required length of osteopathic curricula, to 3 years in 1905 and to 4 years in 1915.[14]

The profession officially responded to external criticism by pointing out the differences between osteopathic and orthodox medical education. However, when there was an opportunity to raise general standards, as came beginning in the 1930s, the profession did so. By the mid-1930s, osteopathic colleges were requiring at least 2 years of college before matriculation; in 1954, 3 years were required; by 1960, over 70% had either baccalaureate or advanced degrees.[14] At present, virtually all osteopathic students enter with at least baccalaureate degrees; many have advanced degrees as well. Curriculum content similarly grew and changed with the times. An 1899–1900 Kirksville catalog describes the course as follows:[15]

The course of study extends over two years, and is divided into four terms of five months each.

The first term is devoted to Descriptive Anatomy, including Osteology, Syndesmology and Myology; lectures on Histology illustrated by micro-stereopticon; the principles of General Inorganic Chemistry, Physics and Toxicology.

The second term includes Descriptive and Regional Anatomy with demonstrations; didactic and laboratory work in Histology; Physiology and physiological demonstrations; Physiological Chemistry and Urinalysis; Principles of Osteopathy; Clinical Demonstrations in Osteopathy.

The third term includes Demonstrations in Regional Anatomy; Physiology and physiological Demonstrations; lectures on Pathology illustrated by micro-stereopticon; Symptomatology; Bacteriology; Physiological Psychology; Clinical Demonstrations in Osteopathy and Osteopathic diagnosis and therapeutics.

The fourth term includes Symptomatology; Surgery; didactic and laboratory work in Pathology; Psycho-Pathology and Psycho-Therapeutics; Gynaecology; Obstetrics; Hygiene and Public Health; Venereal diseases; Medical Jurisprudence; Dietetics; Clinical Demonstrations; Osteopathic and operative clinics.

A major difference between this curriculum and that of an allopathic medical school, in addition to the distinctive osteopathic content, was the exclusion of materia medica, now known as pharmacology.

Early in osteopathic history a difference appeared between so-called lesion osteopaths and broad osteopaths, those who limited their therapeutic practice essentially to manipulation and those who used all the tools available to medicine, including materia medica.

Andrew Taylor Still practiced midwifery and surgery; both were taught under his guidance. Indeed, when the issue of surgery became controversial among later DOs, Still's son provided an affidavit concerning his father's practice.[16] However, to the end of his life Still was adamantly opposed to teaching about or using any form of pharmaceuticals.

Still's opposition to drugs did not prevent some early DOs from using them for treatment. Quite a few had been trained as MDs before they came to osteopathic schools; others went on to earn MDs after they became DOs; still others simply decided to use all the adjunctive treatments available. The most direct early confrontation came in 1897 when a DO–MD opened a short-lived Columbian School of Osteopathy in Kirksville, with the announced intention of offering DO and MD degrees upon graduation from a course in manipulation, surgery, and materia medica. The competitive and personal issues in this case extended beyond the academic questions, and the school closed after graduating only three classes.[9] The issue was professionally divisive for many years after.

Adjunctive treatments became a major subject of debate within the AOA and the Associated Colleges of Osteopathy (now the American Association of Colleges of Osteopathic Medicine) for many years. The question finally was resolved in favor of the broad osteopaths, not by consensus over the idea but by recognizing that state licensing laws required fuller training. In 1916, against the direct protest of Still,[17] the trustees revoked a previous year's action condemning individuals and colleges who taught drug therapy, effectively opening the way for the colleges to form their own curricula. The profession's great success in using manipulative treatment during the 1918 influenza epidemic probably slowed the integration of materia medica into the osteopathic curriculum. However, by the late 1920s it became officially permissible to institute courses in supplementary therapeutics, of which pharmacology was one subheading.[14] By the mid-1930s the integration was complete. The change was further validated, of course, as drugs improved, making it possible to offer pharmaceutical treatment without doing harm.

STATE LICENSURE

Closely related to the issue of educational standards was licensure under increasingly strict state laws.

The first legislative recognition of osteopathic practice came from Vermont in 1896,[18] where graduates of the American School of Osteopathy, Kirksville, were accorded the right to practice in that state. Missouri had a successful bill as early as 1895, but it was vetoed by the governor; what was hailed as a better bill was passed and signed into law in March 1897.[19,20]

Such laws as these, greeted with much rejoicing in the profession, made tremendous growth possible in the osteopathic profession in states where legislation provided a friendly welcome. Osteopathic history includes numerous stories about legal action against DOs for practicing without a valid license, David-and-Goliath encounters of DOs with MD-dominated legislatures, and testimony or influence offered by prominent people who were osteopathic patients. These colorful tales were the war stories of an energetic first generation of DOs, who managed to secure legislative rights to at least limited practice in a majority of states.

Registration and licensure were related but often different matters. Some states provided for formation of separate osteopathic licensing boards; some permitted the addition of an osteopathic representative to an existing or composite board; and a few permitted DOs to apply through a medical board without osteopathic representation.

The roles of these boards were not immediately clear at the time of their formation. There was opposition on ideological grounds even to the idea of licensure. Some populists said that medical licensure was discriminatory. Others said that licensing would interfere with freedom of medical research. Some social Darwinists went so far as to say that, if the poor died of their own foolishness in choosing bad medical practitioners, the species would improve.[21]

By 1901, however, every state had some form of legislation: at least registration, with a diploma from an accepted school, or a state examination of some type. When the Missouri board began to function in 1903, the first certificate it issued was to A.T. Still.[22]

Licensure to practice a full scope of medicine was another matter, and in most places it was related first to the content of the osteopathic curriculum and later to the results of examinations. Again using Missouri as an example, by 1897 the subjects taught had expanded to include:

Anatomy
Physiology
Surgery
Midwifery
Histology
Chemistry
Urinalysis
Toxicology
Pathology
Symptomatology

Everything was included except materia medica; academic consciences were satisfied temporarily. By 1937, however, only 26 states had any provision to provide unlimited licenses to DOs.

In some states DOs were ineligible to apply because their education did not meet specific criteria. As late as 1937, in 16 states osteopathic standards did not meet preprofessional college requirements; in 8, a year's internship was needed. DOs who took examinations under medical or composite boards showed a much lower pass rate. Whether, as it was argued, this was a difference in osteopathic curricula rather than an educational deficiency, in due course the curricula were altered and the pass rates increased. The major changes were addition of more basic science courses and faculty and larger clinical facilities.[14]

After World War II, a major effort was made to reverse the old discriminatory laws. These efforts, along with major changes in osteopathic education, enabled the enactment of new practice laws for all 50 states.[23]

A final dramatic chapter in the American licensing story came when the California Osteopathic Association agreed in 1961 to merge with the California Medical Association, and the College of Osteopathic Physicians and Surgeons, Los Angeles, became the California College of Medicine. Consenting DOs were given MD degrees as a preparation for a referendum approved by voters in 1962, which discontinued licensure of DOs in that state.[14]

A new state osteopathic group, Osteopathic Physicians and Surgeons of California, was chartered by the American Osteopathic Association. This group fought against the referendum but lost; then they began a long legal battle that culminated in a 1974 decision by the California Supreme Court that licensure of DOs must be resumed.[24] A new college was chartered in that state, and professional continuity was restored.

By the end of the 20th century, state licensure could be attained in various ways: through the standard national osteopathic licensing examination and/or through the standard national medical licensing examination, depending on state requirements. Some states maintained separate osteopathic and allopathic licensing boards; many were composite boards. Graduate education required for new licenses still varied state by state. In every state, however, as well as in a number of foreign countries, it was possible to be licensed for unlimited practice.

OSTEOPATHIC ORGANIZATION

The AOA was formed at Kirksville under the name "American Association for the Advancement of Osteopathy" in 1897. Its present name was adopted in 1901. The second national association was the Associated Colleges of Osteopathy (now American Association of Colleges of Osteopathic Medicine), formed in 1898. Both groups sought to protect and raise standards for education and practice of DOs. The AOA became the regulatory group; the Associated Colleges became a discussion and consensus group.

State (divisional) and local (district) osteopathic organizations grew up to serve physicians in their own localities. When the AOA grew too large for general membership meetings, state societies began (in 1920) to name representatives to serve in the AOA House of Delegates. That body thereafter became the chief policy-making group for the osteopathic profession; the Board of Trustees, elected by the house, oversaw the implementation of those policies, a role it still fills.

Students were involved in the early organization of the AOA. They now participate as voting members of the delegations from the states in which their schools are located, and they have a number of organizations[b] of their own.

A major early effort of the AOA was to produce a code of ethics, accomplished in 1904. A participant in those deliberations observed that the problem *"was not because anyone really wished to practice unethically, but rather that on some points it was difficult to agree upon what was ethical."*[25] To put this in perspective: the issue of advertising was a hard-fought question among all professionals at that time. The question was resolved by declaring advertising unethical except for brief professional card listings. By the 1990s advertising by professionals again became considered ethical.

In 1907 the first organization devoted to osteopathic research began, though the first recorded osteopathic research was done almost a decade earlier.[26,27] The role of the AOA in encouraging and supporting osteopathic research was vital. Study of the scientific questions raised by osteopathic practice has never been easy. For example, taking only an obvious aspect of manipulative treatment: What is a manipulative placebo? Research money has never been plentiful; a major portion of the support for osteopathic research, especially in earlier days, has come from financial contributions by DOs themselves. However, a number of significant accomplishments have been recorded.[27]

Over time many osteopathic organizations grew, from starting points as various as special tasks, geographic or school affinity, and practice interest. A current guide to osteopathic organization is the annual *AOA Yearbook and Directory of Osteopathic Physicians.*[28]

The AOA was and remains the umbrella group that recognizes and coordinates their efforts on behalf of the profession. The AOA itself has many important functions. Through its bureaus, councils, and committees, it is the osteopathic accrediting organization for undergraduate, graduate, and continuing medical education and for health care facilities. It certifies specialists in all fields, through a network of specialty boards and a its own central bureau. Research grants and related projects, as well as educational meetings, are arranged through AOA bureaus and councils.

Staff, directed by elected officers and trustees, provide professional services, including:

Maintenance of central records on all DOs
Public and legislative education
Ombudsman services
Procurement and administration of member services
Educational activities including publications and conventions
Maintenance of a central office facility

Special committees deal with such categories as:

Student affairs
Young physicians' interests
Small states' concerns
Ethics
Fund raising
Awards
Basic documents

Position papers on various topics are approved by the House of Delegates and presented as the profession's position on questions of public health and professional interest.

In addition to activities of the AOA itself, a network of divisional and affiliate societies is recognized by the AOA. Certain major subumbrella organizations have networks of their own: the associations of osteopathic colleges, health care organizations, licensing groups, and foundations.

Specialty colleges, distinct from the certifying boards, conduct educational affairs and recognize their own members'

---

[b]For a current list of component or affiliate osteopathic organizations, see the annual *AOA Yearbook and Directory of Osteopathic Physicians.*

achievements through fellowships and other awards. State (divisional) and local (district) societies typically deal with state legislative and regulatory affairs, conduct educational programs, and provide a variety of member services.

Colleges typically have student and alumni groups, student chapters of certain specialty organizations, fraternities and sororities, and a variety of special interest groups.

Many of the physicians' and students' organizations have auxiliaries for spouses.

All organizations recognized by the AOA accept such ongoing controls as approval of any changes in basic documents and designation of how many representatives (if any) are sent to the AOA House of Delegates for voice and vote in professional policy affairs.

FEDERAL GOVERNMENTAL RECOGNITION

The first major attempt by the AOA to obtain federal governmental recognition was during World War I, when it tried to gain commissions for DOs as military physicians. This effort was unsuccessful, in spite of active support by such prominent advocates as former President Theodore Roosevelt.[29]

At that time, an examination was set, and it was understood that if DOs (along with MDs) took this and passed it, they could be commissioned as medical officers. About 25 DOs took the examination and were recommended for commissions. The Surgeon General unilaterally ruled that only MDs were eligible. Bills were then introduced (1917) in both the House of Representatives and the Senate to correct this inequity. The bills were referred to the Military Affairs Committees, and hearings were held. The committee then referred the issue to the Surgeon General, who in his statement of opposition claimed that regular physicians would withhold their services if DOs were allowed to serve. The bills remained in committee without resolution until the end of the war. Meanwhile, DOs served as regular soldiers, unable to use their medical training.

The situation remained uncorrected when World War II began. Again there were efforts to obtain commissions for DOs, this time emphasizing regulatory rather than legislative barriers.[30] DOs were deferred rather than drafted, waiting for the possibility that never came. Ironically, the DOs left behind became family physicians to thousands of the patients left by the MDs in military service, with the effect of enhancing the public's view of DOs as full-service physicians.

The pressure for federal recognition continued after World War II ended, and in 1956 a new law specifically provided for the appointment of DOs as commissioned officers in the Medical Corps. However, implementation of that law was blocked for another 10 years, until the Vietnam conflict created another special need for military physicians. The first DO finally was commissioned in May 1966. The next year the AMA withdrew its long-standing opposition, and DOs were included in the doctor draft. It was another 20 years, in 1983, until the first DO was promoted to be a flag officer in the military Medical Corps.[12]

Acceptance of DOs as medical officers under the Civil Service was accomplished 3 years earlier, in 1963. Careers in this field became possible after that date.

Nearly every federal recognition came after a long and difficult fight. Among the important federal recognitions were the following:[14]

1951: The U.S. Public Health Service first awarded renewable teaching grants to each of the six osteopathic colleges.

1957: The AOA was recognized by the U.S. Office of Education, Department of Health, Education and Welfare (DHEW), as the accrediting body for osteopathic education.

1963: The Health Professions Educational Assistance Act included a provision for matching construction grants for osteopathic colleges and loans to osteopathic students.

1966: The AOA was designated by DHEW (now Department of Health and Human Services (DHHS)) as official accrediting body for hospitals under Medicare.

1967: The AOA was recognized by the National Commission on Accrediting as accrediting agency for all facets of osteopathic education.

The AOA continues to maintain a presence in Washington, where it directs efforts to include DOs and osteopathic institutions as a separate but equal partner in all legislative and regulatory initiatives.

SPECIALTIES

Perhaps the first osteopathic activity in what now is called a medical specialty began only 3 years after Wilhelm Roentgen announced discovery of x-rays. The second x-ray machine west of the Mississippi was installed in Kirksville in 1898. With it, Dr. William Smith formulated a method to inject a radiopaque substance in cadaveric veins and arteries to demonstrate the normal pattern of circulation. Two articles were published late that year, one in the *Journal of Osteopathy*, a Kirksville journal associated with the American School of Osteopathy, and the other in the fledgling *American X-Ray Journal*. These were reprinted for modern reference in AOA publications in 1974.[31] When formal certifying boards for osteopathic specialties were organized, radiology was first (1939).[12]

Among those events came the long story of the development of:

Osteopathic hospitals
Internships
Residencies
Specialty organizations
Standards
Examinations
Recognitions for those standards

By the 1990s a full complement of specialties, training programs, and certifying boards were well established in the osteopathic profession, including a board recognizing special proficiency in osteopathic manipulative medicine. At the same time, the profession was unknowingly developing what would come to be the most needed type of practice for the 1990s: primary care.

Throughout its history, osteopathic clinical education has taken place in primary care settings: community hospitals and clinics. The profession has supported very few academic medical centers. This disadvantage, by the 1990s, became an advantage because of the profession's success in producing primary care physicians, including many willing to work in underserved communities.

Many factors have been cited as influential in the choice of practice type and venue, but the chief ones seem to be undergraduate experiences and role models.[32] Whereas students trained in academic medical centers tend to have as role models only subspecialists, and clinical contacts tend to be the types of cases referred to a tertiary medical center, osteopathic students have continued to have regular contact with community clinics and hospitals and to have many faculty role models among primary care physicians.

For example, rural clinics, long a mainstay of clinical education for the Kirksville college and later for other osteopathic schools, have become a model for primary care education.[33] In the last decade of the 20th century, the osteopathic profession has found itself in the enviable role of advisor on how to replicate its educational processes in other places.

HOSPITALS

As with medicine in general, hospitals had their share of problems in the 19th century. Inadequate facilities and staff, infection, disagreement over who should get patient fees, social stigma, and hospital ownership all entered the picture. By about 1900, however, with the growth of an educated nursing profession and a new sense of sanitation, hospitals began to be at least safe. Many small institutions were privately owned by surgeons who furnished hotel services and nursing for their own patients. New general hospitals began to appeal to patients other than the poor, and patient fees began to help with hospital developments.[21]

There were osteopathic hospitals early in the 20th century; at the time of Flexner's inspection, Kirksville had the largest, with 54 beds. Chicago had 20 beds; the Pacific College, 15; Boston, 10; and Philadelphia, 3. No others were listed in that report.[14]

Eventually the numbers and size of osteopathic hospitals grew, but few reached the size and diversity of specialties that characterized the academic medical centers associated with university medical schools. However, the osteopathic profession did set hospital standards, first for training of interns and residents and then for accreditation of the institutions themselves.

The growth of osteopathic hospitals was especially marked in the period during and after World War II, when MD hospitals did not permit DOs to join their medical staffs. When U.S. government programs were approved to help with construction of hospitals, osteopathic institutions participated along with medical institutions; many community teaching hospitals were constructed during that period.

In 1954, a landmark court decision in Audrain County, Missouri, made it illegal for public hospitals to deny staff membership and admitting privileges to qualified DOs. This initiated a series of changes in areas outside California, where for many years DOs had been in charge of half the Los Angeles County Hospital. By the 1960s, most public hospitals were open to DOs; by the 1980s most private hospitals were open as well.

By the 1990s, with medical residencies open to both MDs and DOs, the need for a network of osteopathic hospitals for training purposes was much reduced. Mechanisms were adopted to recognize training that took place in allopathic institutions as acceptable for osteopathic board certification. This is now possible either by affiliation of the MD institution with an accredited osteopathic college or by direct AOA accreditation of the training institution.

Reorganization of the health care system itself made these changes necessary. Payment mechanisms led to the formation of large networks of health care providers, including hospitals, outpatient facilities, home care, extended and long-term care, and multiple independent contractors and physician organizations. Community hospitals, including many osteopathic institutions, were merged with larger groups or simply closed. The lines between osteopathic and allopathic hospitals blurred, as both came under the umbrella of for-profit managed care organizations.

In a case of history repeating itself, economic factors control health care delivery, and the profit motive is once again a respectable part of the medical scene. Against a call for serious reform of medical education and better distribution of primary care physicians is a majority voice, seeking through corporate management to find ways to survive in a competitive environment.

CONCLUSION

As the 20th century moves toward its close, the separate but equal osteopathic profession is respected in many quarters for a variety of reasons. First is the osteopathic emphasis on primary care. This arose not only from the earlier circumstances of training opportunities and role models but also from the traditional whole person philosophy.

There has been a rebirth of interest in manual medicine and other osteopathic methods. In most osteopathic colleges and graduate education programs, there is increased emphasis on historic tenets and clinical skills. A mechanism has been established for an osteopathic board to certify both MDs and DOs in proficiency in osteopathic manual medicine. The process assumes additional studies by MDs not educated in osteopathic institutions.

Throughout the profession, there is a continued emphasis on preventive care and health maintenance. This reemerging trend is also in line with traditional osteopathic values.

Osteopathic physicians have had a positive voice in public affairs. In the public arena, DOs are regarded as a *"separate but equal"* profession in regulatory and legislative affairs, and the profession is consulted on most matters of public health policy.

For all these reasons, the mood of the profession in the last decade of the 20th century is one of optimism. As an AOA president repeatedly said, "*Osteopathic medicine is an idea whose time has come.*"[c]

REFERENCES

1. Still AT. *Autobiography of Andrew T. Still,* with a history of the discovery and development of the science of osteopathy. rev ed. Published by the author, Kirksville, Mo; 1908:28.

2. Trowbridge C. *Andrew Taylor Still, 1828–1917.* Kirksville, Mo: Thomas Jefferson University Press, Northeast Missouri State University; 1991.

3. Laughlin GM. Asks if A.T. Still was ever a doctor. *Osteopathic Physician.* 1909;15(Jan):8.

4. A.T. Still Pension File, Still National Osteopathic Museum, Kirksville, Mo. Cited by: Trowbridge C. *Andrew Taylor Still, 1828–1917.* Kirksville, Mo: Thomas Jefferson University Press, Northeast Missouri State University; 1991.

5. Andrew Taylor Still: the Kansas years. In: From the Archives. *The DO.* 1974;June:31–41.

6. Magner LN. *A History of Medicine.* New York, NY: Marcel Dekker; 1992:203–207; 223; 341.

7. Still CE. A.T. Still: the itinerant years. In: From the Archives. *The DO.* 1975;(Mar)27–30.

8. Riley GW. Following osteopathic principles. In: Hildreth AG, ed. *The Lengthening Shadow of Dr. Andrew Taylor Still.* Published by the author, Macon, Mo; 1938:412.

9. Walter GW. *The First School of Osteopathic Medicine; A Chronicle, 1892–1992.* Kirksville, Mo: Thomas Jefferson University Press, Northeast Missouri State University; 1992.

10. Violette EM. *History of Adair County.* Kirksville, Mo: Denslow History Co, 1911:253.

11. Johnson V, Weiskotten HG. *A History of the Council on Medical Education and Hospitals of the American Medical Association.* Chicago, Ill: American Medical Association; 1960.

12. Important dates in osteopathic history. In: Allen TW, ed. *AOA Yearbook and Directory of Osteopathic Physicians.* Chicago, Ill: American Osteopathic Association; 1995:554–556. (This feature is published annually.)

13. Flexner A. *Medical Education in the United States and Canada; A Report to the Carnegie Foundation for the Advancement of Teaching.* Boston, Mass: The Merrymount Press; 1910.

14. Gevitz N. *The D.O.s: Osteopathic Medicine in America.* Baltimore: Johns Hopkins University Press; 1982:75–87.

15. *Catalogue of the American School of Osteopathy, Session of 1899–1900.* Kirksville, Mo; seventh annual announcement.

16. The memoirs of Dr. Charles Still; IV. a postscript. In: From the Archives. *The DO.* 1975;(Jun):25–26.

17. Booth ER. *History of Osteopathy and Twentieth-Century Medical Practice.* Printed for the author, Cincinnati, Ohio: Caxton Press; 1924:442.

18. "A Vermont story" and "Contacts with the law." In: From the Archives. *The DO.* 1972;(Nov):46–50.

19. Hildreth AG. *The Lengthening Shadow of Dr Andrew Taylor Still.* 1938: Published by the author, Macon, Mo; 1938:94–98.

20. Schnucker RV, ed. *Early Osteopathy in the Words of A.T. Still.* Kirksville, Mo: Thomas Jefferson University Press, Northeast Missouri State University; 1991:87–88.

21. Starr P. *The Social Transformation of American Medicine.* New York, NY: Basic Books; 1982:104–105.

22. The Old Doctor gets first certificate. *J Osteopathy* 1904;11(Jan):28.

23. Year of passing unlimited practice laws. In: Allen TW, ed. *AOA Yearbook and Directory of Osteopathic Physicians.* Chicago, Ill: American Osteopathic Association; 1995:556. (This chart is published in each issue.)

24. Alexander Tobin, 1921–1992. In: *The Collected Papers of Viola M. Frymann, DO.* Indianapolis, Ind: American Academy of Osteopathy; 1996. In press. (Includes information on the legal battle.)

25. Evans AL. The beginnings of the AOA (1928 manuscript). In: From the Archives. *The DO.* 1972;(Sep)34–38.

26. Peterson B. How old is osteopathic research? In: Time Capsule. *The D.O.* 1978;(Dec)24–26.

27. Cole WV. Historical basis for osteopathic theory and practice. In: Northup GW, ed. *Osteopathic Research: Growth and Development.* Chicago: American Osteopathic Association; 1987:5–7.

28. *AOA Yearbook and Directory of Osteopathic Physicians.* Chicago, Ill: American Osteopathic Association. (Published annually.)

29. They passed the exam, but they could not serve: the DO doughboys. In: From the Archives. *The D.O.* 1975;(Aug)39–46. (Part of this material was excerpted from Booth ER, *History of Osteopathy and Twentieth Century Medicine.* Cincinnati, Ohio: Caxton Press; 1905:790–823, which also contains an account of attempts at national legislation hostile to the osteopathic profession which preceded the action governing military physicians.)

30. How DOs gained commissions. In: Time Capsule. *The D.O.* 1980; (Apr)25–32.

31. 1898: Radiology in Kirksville. In: Time Capsule. *JAOA* 1974; 74(Oct):167–172.

32. Rodos JJ, Peterson B. *Proposed Strategies for Fulfilling Primary Care Manpower Needs; A White Paper Prepared for the National Advisory Council, National Health Service Corps, U.S. Public Health Service.* Rockville, Md: National Health Service Corps; 1990.

33. Blondell RD, Smith IJ, Byrne ME, Higgins CW. Rural health, family practice, and area health education centers: a national study. *Fam Med* 1989;3(May–Jun):183–186.

---

[c]William G. Anderson, DO, AOA president in 1994–1995, often included this statement in his presidential addresses.

Osteopathic Considerations in the Basic Sciences

INTRODUCTION

Michael M. Patterson

Osteopathic medical practice is built on the foundation of both scientific knowledge and a medical philosophy that guides the application of facts within the art of treatment. Too often, in the practice of medicine, we overlook the fact that medical knowledge must be delivered in the context of a philosophy of how life, health, and disease processes function, with treatment stemming from that understanding.

OSTEOPATHIC PHILOSOPHY

The philosophy of the osteopathic profession was put forward by A.T. Still and the early members of the profession, and this formulation in turn had its roots in the earliest of medical thought and practice. To these earlier views, Still added important insights and understandings gained from his own experience and knowledge. The philosophy of the profession has been refined and expanded over the years as increasing knowledge has led to greater understanding of osteopathy's basic tenets. This philosophy is meant to guide osteopathic physicians to the best use of scientific knowledge in optimizing health and diminishing disease processes in their patients.

Within osteopathic philosophy, one of the most important tenets is that for optimal function there must be integration of the various functions of the body, from the subcellular to systems to psychological levels. When a breakdown in the integration of these functions develops, the individual can no longer maintain the best level of health, and disease can appear. This leads to another of the tenets of the profession, that the underlying cause of disease is disturbance of function; homeostatic mechanisms can no longer ward off invasions of bacteria or viruses or contain the degeneration of aging or use. Osteopathic philosophy suggests that one of the most important things for the osteopathic physician to understand is how body functions are integrated, how that integration can be broken, and how it can be restored.

The amount of knowledge available to the student of human function is now almost beyond the wildest dreams of those in the field only a few years ago. Information is increasing at an astounding rate, and all indications are that it will continue to compound even more rapidly in the years ahead. It is becoming increasingly difficult for any one person to have even a basic understanding of most of the fields of biomedical knowledge, not to mention a mastery of them. Rather than decreasing the need for having a philosophical base for the practice of medicine, the increasing knowledge base makes it even more important to have a philosophy as a means of organizing the vast numbers of facts and theories and to allow that knowledge to be put into practice.

It is the purpose of this section to present ways to look at various areas of knowledge in the light of an important part of osteopathic philosophy, that of integration of function. It is not possible for one or even a series of books to present all the knowledge of the various scientific areas underlying biomedical science. Some physiology texts alone are longer than this entire book, and the same holds for most of the other basic science areas. Chapters in this section provide information and knowledge in these areas in terms of integration of function and, in some cases, in terms of the ways in which lack of integration, or disintegration, can occur. These chapters do not attempt to cover all areas of basic science or even to summarize the current knowledge in an area, but rather provide a way of looking at that area with an osteopathic understanding of health and loss of health.

Anatomy

In the first chapter, Jacobs and Falls provide an overview of the concepts of anatomy, one of the most basic areas of knowledge for the osteopathic physician. They point out that a thorough understanding not only of anatomical structures but of how they function and interrelate is key to understanding the basis of health. They discuss the often-overlooked, all-encompassing fascial tissues as important contributors to continuity throughout the body. The authors show that disturbance in one muscle has consequences for function in many other structures. They emphasize the importance of myofascial continuity throughout the body as a means to understanding the disparate effects of disturbances in an often distant structure.

In the companion chapter on the rules of anatomy, Towns uses his years of experience in teaching anatomy to draw attention to some of the important means of viewing the structures of the body and the principles that combine these structures with their function. He points out that it is important for the physician to be able to visualize the true relationships between structures not only to understand their function but also to know when they are not functioning correctly, and how to use the best manipulative techniques to improve functional capacity. How fluids move into and out of an area is vital to understanding normal and abnormal function. This includes not only arterial and venous supply but also lymph movement and drainage. Improper fluid movement is a vital and primary cause of loss of integration. A knowledge of what connects to what and how pain can be used or misunderstood is a vital part of an anatomical understanding. It contributes to a physician's ability to help the patient; these topics are treated here as well. The reader gains a renewed appreciation for the importance of a deep understanding of structure and relationships between structures from these two chapters.

Autonomic Nervous System

The autonomic nervous system is one of the most important and poorly understood systems of the body. Usually thought of as a rather dull and even uninteresting system of the body, it is actually one of the most important of integrating systems. Willard, in his chapter on the autonomic nervous system, provides a picture of the vast complexity of this system as it influences all areas of the body. Within the chapter, Willard not only examines the structure of the system but outlines the neurochemical aspects of this great communicating system and gives a flavor of the complexity of the processes involved in the ongoing control of various body functions. He emphasizes the vital importance of this system in coordinating the activities of the visceral systems to meet the demands imposed by the musculoskeletal system. This system is a singularly important part of the osteopathic physician's understanding of the integration of total body function.

Endocrine System

The endocrine system is treated in a unique way in Portanova's chapter. As with all the other systems treated here, this author has room only to provide an overview of the system as it applies to the concept of integration of function. Portanova uses the complexity and ubiquity of endocrine function to illustrate the beauty of interactions at every level of function. He points out that, while the level of knowledge in Still's time was very rudimentary (will our great grandchildren say that of our understanding now relative to theirs?), the concepts of functional integration held by Still are beautifully shown by the control loops and feedback pathways within the endocrine system. Indeed, Portanova uses several of the basic tenets of the osteopathic philosophy as tenets of endocrine function. This allows the reader to see the application of these concepts at a systems level; the author points out that the osteopathic philosophy is so *deeply rooted in the fabric of life*" that even knowledge gained in the future will be embraced by this philosophy. Certainly, the reader will gain a new and deeper appreciation for the endocrine system from this chapter.

Pharmacology

In the early days of the osteopathic profession, drug use was looked upon with great suspicion. In retrospect, it is easy to see why Still took this attitude. Most if not all common drugs of the time either were detrimental to function and health or were used in harmful ways. Now the use of the pharmacopoeia is common and viewed as a necessary adjunct for proper treatment. There is the remaining suspicion that in many cases drugs are still often misused, overused, or abused. In his chapter on pharmacology and osteopathy, Theobald presents parallels between the concepts of osteopathy and the uses of pharmacologic agents. He points out that the rational use of any pharmacologic agent necessitates understanding that each individual is unique. Chemical agents used properly can help the body regain control of improperly functioning systems and help redress balance of function. His description of the treatment of hypertension with pharmacologic agents using the principles of integration is a wonderful example of how endogenous agents can help the body restore properly integrated function.

Musculoskeletal System

The means by which the body regulates its responses and goes about healing itself after insult is determined by the smooth function of all body systems. Even the musculoskeletal system must be involved in this effort. In the next two chapters, Mochan and Willard, Mokler, and Morgane discuss how what were previously thought to be rather separate systems with only incidental or hierarchical interactions actually function more as one great system to produce the miracles of homeostasis and healing. In his chapter, Mochan looks at the adaptive capacity of the body from the biochemical level up to the level of the musculoskeletal system in their activities as regulators that act to achieve stability in the face of stressors and injury. The importance of processes such as inflammation in the regulation of function is viewed here in the context of an integrated response to external threats. This chapter shows the importance of viewing what seem to be bothersome side effects of injury as necessary steps in the restoration of normal functional integration.

Neuro-Endocrine-Immune System

In their chapter on the neuro-endocrine-immune system, Willard and coauthors present a fascinating view of the complexity apparent in the finely honed interactions of these great communicating systems of the body. They present a picture of our growing understanding of the delicate interactions between the neural, endocrine, and immune systems. These interactions allow responses to demands on the body in a well-orchestrated, coordinated fashion. The authors show that psychological factors can alter the functions of the immune system. They detail the evidence for innervation by the sympathetic system of much of the immune tissue and discuss the detrimental influence of somatic dysfunction on the function of this finely tuned network.

Neurophysiology

In the final chapter of the section, Patterson and Wurster provide an overview of the neural basis for interactions between the somatic and autonomic systems in the spinal cord. They discuss how inputs from one system directly influence the activity of the other system. The heart is used as an example of the complexity of innervation and control in the context of an integrating system. The authors then discuss the factors that cause disintegration of normal neural function in terms of alterations in neural excitability and how these alterations of function can become long-lasting and even permanent, as a part of somatic dysfunction.

CONCLUSION

The chapters of this section show the levels of integration within and between various body systems and units. They provide a basis for understanding the ways in which structure and function are interrelated. The interrelationship produces the smooth integration that is the hallmark of health. They show some of the ways in which this integration and function can become compromised to produce the first and necessary cause of disease. Osteopathic philosophy is admirably demonstrated in these chapters; the authors show the fit between the emerging scientific understanding of human function and osteopathic philosophy. Thus, these chapters provide a deeper understanding of the application of osteopathic philosophy to the optimization of human health.

3. Anatomy

ALLEN W. JACOBS AND WILLIAM M. FALLS

Key Concepts

- **How the fully developed human body's segmental nervous system is directly related to embryological growth patterns**

- **Differences among major types of connective tissue, the constituents of each, and their functional significance**

- **Differences between synovial and nonsynovial joints; joint play and its significance in the diagnosis of joint-related dysfunctions**

- **Structures in synovial joints and their functional basis**

- **Examples of nonsynovial joints and the differences between fibrous and cartilaginous types**

- **Anatomy of the muscle–tendon complex and its functional significance**

- **How the innervation from spinal segments is distributed throughout the body and how the limbs are supplied from this source**

- **Structural implications of myofascial continuity and its impact on the osteopathic diagnosis and treatment of musculoskeletal dysfunction**

A fundamental understanding of basic human anatomy is the foundation of osteopathic medicine. The embryologic development of the neuromusculoskeletal system is the basis for understanding the segmental dermatomal representation of the nervous system as well as the distribution of somatic and visceral nerve supply to the entire body.

The microscopic structure of connective tissue is a key element in the myofascial continuity of the body. The gross structure of the musculoskeletal system is based on the microscopic structural and functional components of connective tissue and their interrelationship with skeletal muscle. The ability of the tissues of the musculoskeletal system to heal and repair following injury is directly related to their cellular content and microscopic structure. At the macroscopic level, the arrangement of neurovascular bundles that supply somatic tissue is intimately related to connective tissue spaces and fascial planes.

The functional units of the musculoskeletal system include the synovial joint, the muscle–tendon complex, and the fascial elements that support skeletal muscles and their neurovascular supply.

At the macroscopic level, the embryologic segmental organization of the body is represented in the axial skeleton. The arrangement of nerve and arterial supply, as well as venous and lymphatic drainage, is repeated segmentally throughout the axial skeleton. It is modified to serve the upper and lower limbs. An understanding of this segmental organization is essential for diagnosis and treatment of neuromusculoskeletal system dysfunction and disorders.

The functional adaptation of the limbs is best understood through the concept of myofascial continuity. Posture, balance, and stability during dynamic activity are directly related to the functional capacity and adaptability of the myofascial elements of the body.

Understanding embryologic development, microscopic anatomy, functional units, and segmental organization of the neuromusculoskeletal system depends on understanding anatomy, which is presented in detail in major anatomical textbooks.[1-8] The application of this knowledge and an understanding of myofascial continuity are the foundations of osteopathic medicine used in the diagnosis and treatment of neuromusculoskeletal dysfunctions and disorders.

NEUROMUSCULOSKELETAL EMBRYOLOGY

The embryologic development of the neuromusculoskeletal system exemplifies the segmental organization of the body. The formation of somites in the developing embryo, composed of embryonic mesoderm (mesenchyme), is specifically related to the segmentation of the neural tube. Each somite differentiates into two parts: a sclerotome and a dermatomyotome (Fig. 3.1). As the mesenchyme migrates from these parts of the somites during development to form the segmental elements of the axial skeleton (e.g., vertebral column and ribs from the sclerotome, and intercostal muscles from the myotome), the segmental nerve supply from the developing neural tube (spinal cord) is maintained (Figs. 3.2 and 3.3). This segmentation in the axial skeleton is sustained in the adult.

With the development of the upper and lower limbs, the mesenchyme, which forms bone, muscle, and connective tissue, maintains segmental connections with the developing spinal cord through nerves growing into the developing limbs (Fig. 3.4). However, through differential limb growth and development, the initial segmental representation of the embryo is modified in the adult.

Figure 3.1. **A** and **B**. Transverse sections showing differentiation of a somite in relation to development of neural tube. (Reprinted with permission from Sadler TW. *Langman's Medical Embryology*. 7th ed. Baltimore, Md: Williams & Wilkins; 1995:148.)

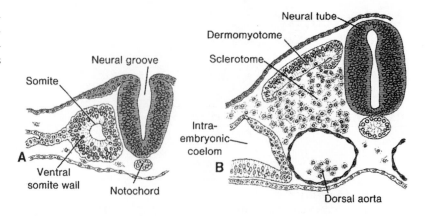

Figure 3.2. **A** and **B**. Transverse sections showing migration of cells from sclerotome and myotome during development. (Reprinted with permission from Sadler TW. *Langman's Medical Embryology*. 7th ed. Baltimore, Md: Williams & Wilkins; 1995:167.)

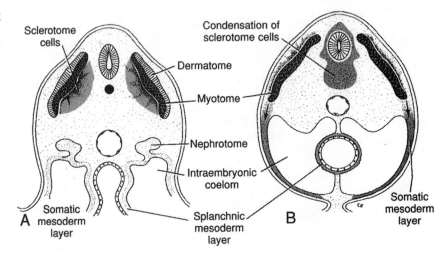

Figure 3.3. **A** and **B**. Transverse sections showing segmental nerve from developing spinal cord innervating developing musculature of thorax and abdomen. (Reprinted with permission from Sadler TW. *Langman's Medical Embryology*. 7th ed. Baltimore, Md: Williams & Wilkins; 1995:167.)

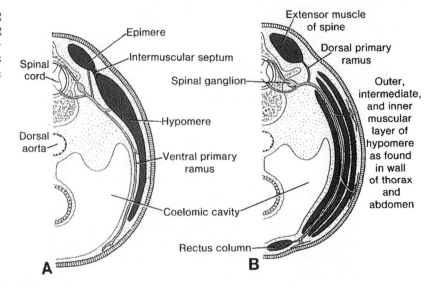

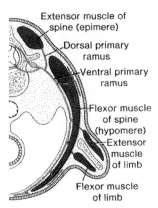

Figure 3.4. Transverse section showing that muscles (as well as bone and connective tissues) of developing limbs maintain segmental innervation from developing spinal cord. (Reprinted with permission from Sadler TW. *Langman's Medical Embryology.* 7th ed. Baltimore, Md: Williams & Wilkins; 1995:169.)

The segmentally organized nervous system provides the link between the somatic tissue and the viscera that develop internally in a similar segmental manner. Through the segmental organization of the nervous system there is a structural relationship between the nerve supply to the somatic tissue and the autonomic visceral nerve supply of each segment of the developing embryo.

MUSCULOSKELETAL MICROSCOPIC ANATOMY

The connective tissues of the body are derived from mesenchyme and include connective tissue, bone, and cartilage.

These developing tissues contain cells that produce a matrix of ground substance and fibers that surround the cells. The cells are of these types:

Fibroblasts
Osteoblasts
Chondroblasts

Each type of connective tissue has a unique arrangement of cell types within a specific matrix of ground substance and fibers. Changing these three elements—cells, ground substance, and fibers—produces the variable composition and consistency of each type of connective tissue in the musculoskeletal system. Connective tissue is classified on the basis of the arrangement of these three elements.

Connective Tissue

Loose connective tissue forms an open meshwork of cells (fibrocytes, fibroblasts) and fibers (collagen, elastic, reticular), with a large amount of fat cells and ground substance in between. Loose connective tissue also surrounds neurovascular bundles and fills the spaces between individual muscles and fascial planes (Fig. 3.5).

Dense fibrous connective tissue is classified on the basis of the dense, regular arrangement of the predominant collagen fiber bundles that run in the same direction. This tissue forms the substance of:

Periosteum
Tendons
Ligaments
Deep fascia

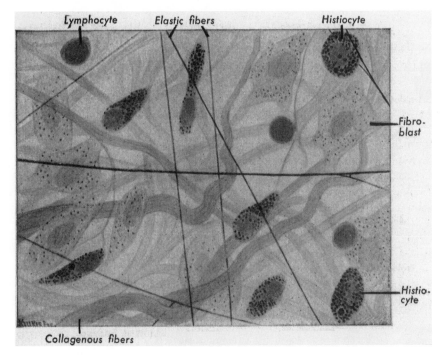

Figure 3.5. Cellular elements of loose connective tissue. (Reprinted with permission from Copenhaver WM, Bunge RP, Bunge MB. *Bailey's Textbook of Histology.* 16th ed. Baltimore, Md: Williams & Wilkins; 1971.)

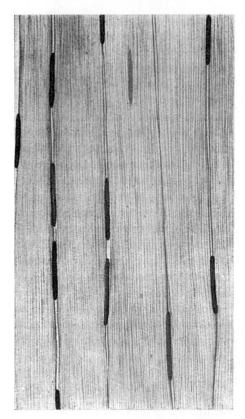

Figure 3.6. Cellular elements of dense regular fibrous tissue. Dark fibroblast nuclei lie between bundles of regularly arranged collagen fibers. (Reprinted with permission from Copenhaver WM, Bunge RP, Bunge MB. *Bailey's Textbook of Histology.* 16th ed. Baltimore, Md: Williams & Wilkins; 1971.)

This tissue is commonly described as regular or irregular depending upon the arrangement of the closely packed collagen fiber bundles (Fig. 3.6).

Cartilage and Bone

Cartilage and bone are highly specialized connective tissues in which the ground substance of the matrix is predominant over the cellular and fibrous elements.

The chondroblast is responsible for producing the ground substance and fibers of the three types of cartilage:

Hyaline (articular)
Elastic
Fibrous

These three cartilage types vary in histological makeup on the basis of their ground substance and predominant fiber type (collagen or elastin) (Figs. 3.7–3.9).

The osteocytes of bone are maintained in a rigid matrix that is calcified and reinforced by connective tissue fibers that are produced by the osteoblasts. The structural unit of bone, the osteon (haversian system), is formed by concentric lamellae of bone surrounding a microscopic neurovascular bundle in the haversian canal. The osteocytes are located within microscopic spaces (lacunae) between the concentric bone matrix lamellae and extend processes into the matrix (Fig. 3.10).

Skeletal Muscle

Skeletal muscle tissue is also derived from mesenchyme and is modified for the specific function of contraction. The individual skeletal muscle cells (fibers) are arranged in a regular sys-

Figure 3.7. Cellular elements of hyaline (articular) cartilage. (Reprinted with permission from Copenhaver WM, Bunge RP, Bunge MB. *Bailey's Textbook of Histology.* 16th ed. Baltimore, Md: Williams & Wilkins; 1971.)

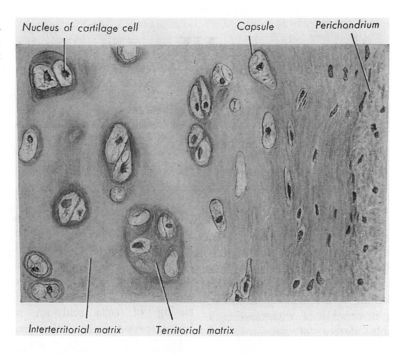

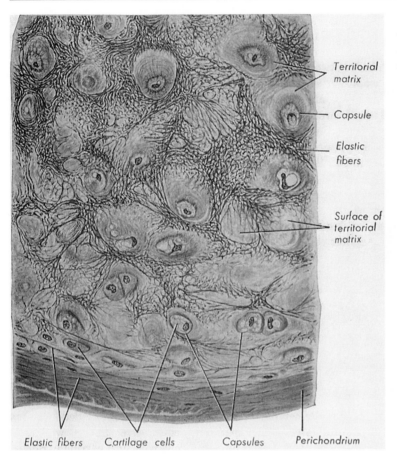

Figure 3.8. Cellular elements of elastic cartilage. (Reprinted with permission from Copenhaver WM, Bunge RP, Bunge MB. *Bailey's Textbook of Histology.* 16th ed. Baltimore, Md: Williams & Wilkins; 1971.)

tematic manner to facilitate contraction when stimulated by a nerve impulse. The microscopic appearance of skeletal muscle presents a classic banding pattern that represents the internal organization of the protein contractile elements in each muscle fiber (Fig. 3.11).

Response to Injury

The inherent capacity of the musculoskeletal system to heal and repair itself following injury is a direct reflection of the histological organization of connective tissue. At the macroscopic level, connective tissue invests the neurovascular bundles that supply specific parts of the body. At the microscopic level, the capillary beds are located within the open meshwork of loose connective tissue and nourish the cellular elements of the tissue. These cells in turn produce the ground substance and fibers of the connective tissue. Following injury, a complex biochemical reaction results in stimulating the inherent capacity of healing and repair.

FUNCTIONAL MUSCULOSKELETAL CONCEPTS

Synovial and Nonsynovial Joints

All synovial joints of the body are freely movable and similar in structure. The "typical" synovial joint is exemplified in Fig-

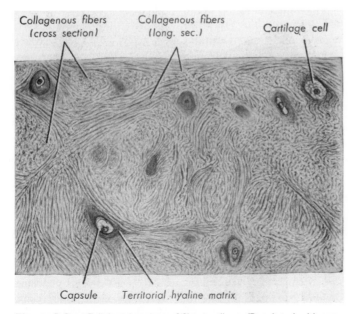

Figure 3.9. Cellular elements of fibrocartilage. (Reprinted with permission from Copenhaver WM, Bunge RP, Bunge MB. *Bailey's Textbook of Histology.* 16th ed. Baltimore, Md: Williams & Wilkins; 1971.)

Figure 3.10. Transverse section showing cellular elements of compact bone. (Reprinted with permission from Copenhaver WM, Bunge RP, Bunge MB. *Bailey's Textbook of Histology.* 16th ed. Baltimore, Md: Williams & Wilkins; 1971.)

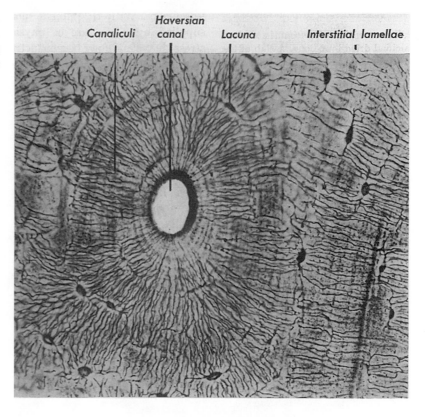

Canaliculi   Haversian canal   Lacuna   Interstitial lamellae

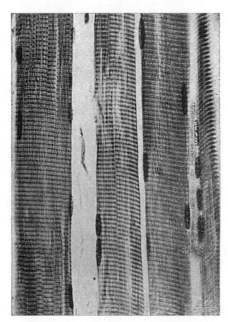

Figure 3.11. Longitudinal section of skeletal muscle showing classic banding pattern found in individual fibers. (Reprinted with permission from Copenhaver WM, Bunge RP, Bunge MB. *Bailey's Textbook of Histology.* 16th ed. Baltimore, Md: Williams & Wilkins; 1971.)

ure 3.12. The articular surfaces of the two bones that form the joint are covered by hyaline (articular) cartilage that is specifically modified for the function of articular motion. The two articular surfaces are separated by a monolayer of synovial fluid in the joint cavity. The joint capsule is composed of two layers. The fibrous outer layer is in continuity with the periosteum of the proximal and distal bones that form the synovial joint. It is classified as dense irregular fibrous connective tissue.

At the point where the articular hyaline cartilage ends, the bone tissue is covered by the periosteum. The fibrous outer layer of the joint capsule could be described as the free periosteum that envelops the freely movable joint and connects the proximal and distal bones at the articulation. The unique inner layer is the synovial membrane that lines the fibrous outer layer. This membrane secretes the synovial fluid that lubricates the internal joint surfaces and the articular hyaline cartilage. The uniqueness of this membrane is that it is derived from mesenchyme. However, microscopically and functionally, this tissue is similar to epithelial tissue, which is an ectodermal derivative.

Each synovial joint is stabilized by specific ligaments. Ligaments may be classified as capsular or accessory. A capsular ligament is a part of the fibrous outer layer of the joint capsule, while accessory ligaments are either located within the joint cavity (intracapsular) or outside the joint capsule, separated from the fibrous outer layer (extracapsular). All ligaments are histologically composed of dense regular fibrous connective tissue and have microscopic, structural, and functional continuity with the periosteum of adjacent bone.

There are several highly specialized types of synovial joints:

Temporomandibular
Sternoclavicular
Ulnomeniscotriquetral
Knee

These joints have the unique feature of either a disk or meniscus (incomplete disk) within the joint cavity (Fig. 3.13). The fibrocartilaginous disk provides for additional support and stability as it separates the two hyaline cartilage articular surfaces. Peripherally, disks are connected to the fibrous outer layer of the joint capsule. A disk extends across a synovial joint, dividing it structurally and functionally into two synovial cavities. The disk, derived from mesoderm, represents a highly specialized form of connective tissue that is distinct, in that the fibrous element of the matrix predominates. A synovial joint with a fibrocartilaginous disk displays a structure that is similar to the embryologically developing synovial joint. This type of synovial joint maintains the fibrocartilaginous element that is developmentally lost in the "typical" synovial joint.

Synovial joints are commonly classified according to the shape of the articular surfaces and/or the movements permitted. None of the articular surfaces are truly flat. Biomechanically, these joint surfaces permit motion that is described as spin, roll, or slide (Fig. 3.14). Spin represents rotation about the longitudinal axis of a bone. Roll is the result of decreasing and increasing the angle between the two bones at an articulation. Slide is the result of a translatory motion of one bone gliding or sliding on the other at the joint. Specific details regarding the classification system and individual synovial joints can be found in anatomy textbooks.[1,2,4,5,7,8]

Nonsynovial joints consist of fibrous and cartilaginous types. These joints, where the articulating bones are directly connected by either fibrous tissue or cartilage, have no free surface for movement but provide for strength and stability between adjacent bones. The fibrous joints include:

Sutures of the skull (Fig. 3.15)
Teeth in the mandible and maxilla
Distal tibiofibular joint

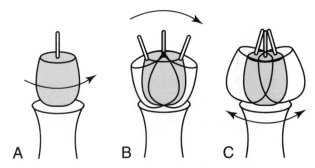

Figure 3.14. Motion at a synovial joint. **A.** Spin. **B.** Roll. **C.** Slide. (Modified from DiGiovanna EL, Schlowitz S. *An Osteopathic Approach to Diagnosis and Treatment*. Philadelphia, Pa: JB Lippincott; 1991.)

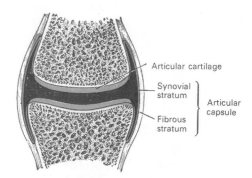

Figure 3.12. Typical synovial joint. (Reprinted with permission from Clemente CD. *Gray's Anatomy of the Human Body*. American 3rd ed. Philadelphia, Pa: Lea & Febiger, 1985:333.)

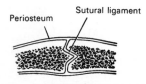

Figure 3.15. A suture is an example of a fibrous joint. (Reprinted with permission from Clemente CD. *Gray's Anatomy of the Human Body*. American 3rd ed. Philadelphia, Pa: Lea & Febiger; 1985:332.)

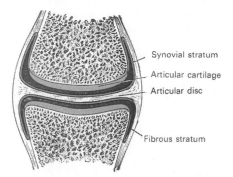

Figure 3.13. Synovial joint with an articular disk. (Reprinted with permission from Clemente CD. *Gray's Anatomy of the Human Body*. American 3rd ed. Philadelphia, Pa: Lea & Febiger; 1985.)

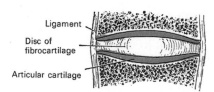

Figure 3.16. A symphysis is an example of a cartilaginous joint. (Reprinted with permission from Clemente CD. *Gray's Anatomy of the Human Body*. American 3rd ed. Philadelphia, Pa: Lea & Febiger; 1985:333.)

The fibrocartilaginous intervertebral disk between adjacent vertebral bodies and the pubic symphysis (Fig. 3.16) are examples of cartilaginous joints.

The sutures of the skull are a classic example of the interrelationship between structure and function. Each suture (joint) between adjacent cranial bones uniquely provides support and mobility. Unlike the freely movable synovial joints, the sutures are highly restricted to slight gliding motion. However, motion loss or restriction is the clinically significant factor in somatic dysfunction of the joint.

Cranial bone motion is also influenced by the tension of the cranial dura mater that covers the brain and forms the internal lining of the skull. Cranial dura mater consists of two layers: periosteal and meningeal. The periosteal layer is the periosteal lining of the cranium. There is histological continuity of this layer with the fibrous tissue (sutural ligament) at each cranial suture. The meningeal layer of cranial dura mater has continuity with the spinal dura mater (thecal sac) at the foramen magnum of the occipital bone (Fig. 3.17). The direct effect of these connective tissues on cranial bone motion has been described by Sutherland[9] as the reciprocal tension membrane.

Synovial and nonsynovial joints exemplify the osteopathic concept of the interrelationship between structure and function. Synovial joints that are freely movable allow for the body to have mobility and greater range of motion. The nonsynovial joints (fibrous and cartilaginous) provide strength and stability within a limited range of motion.

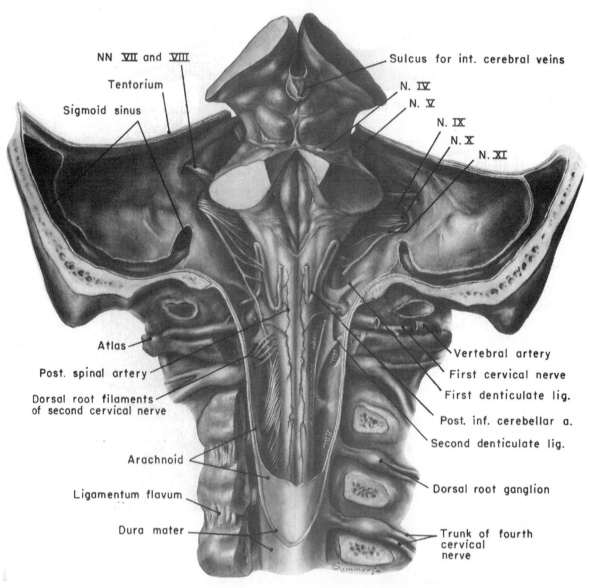

Figure 3.17.   Area of foramen magnum. Cranial dura mater lines internal surface of cranium, is continuous with fibrous tissue of sutures, and is continuous with spinal dura mater at foramen magnum. (Reprinted with permission from Carpenter MB. *Core Text of Neuroanatomy.* 4th ed. Baltimore, Md: Williams & Wilkins; 1991:5.)

Joint Play

The voluntary movement of synovial joints is accommodated by joint play as described by Mennell.[10] Joint play is defined as a small but precise amount of movement (less than ⅛ inch) that is independent of the action of voluntary muscle function. The normal, easy, voluntary range of active motion at a synovial joint depends on the integrity of joint play. Joint play is present only in the living synovial joint. The movement of joint play can only be demonstrated by passive examination. Each synovial joint has one or more joint play movements.

Joint dysfunction is defined as the loss of joint play and therefore a limitation of the voluntary range of motion at a synovial joint. Joint dysfunction is a component of somatic dysfunction (acute or chronic) that is diagnosed in the evaluation of the neuromusculoskeletal system. The restoration of joint play appears to be the basis for the success of synovial joint mobilization using direct or indirect action treatment techniques in osteopathic manipulation.

Muscle–Tendon Complex

Individual skeletal muscle fibers are surrounded by a delicate network of fine connective tissue. At each end of the muscle, this connective tissue forms a tendon composed of dense regular fibrous connective tissue. The tendon is attached to bone through a microscopic interlacing of its connective tissue with the periosteal connective tissue covering of the bone (Fig. 3.18). Each muscle has two parts: a predominant connective tissue at its ends that are attached to bones and a predominance of muscle tissue in its functional contractile belly. The change to connective tissue at its ends provides the muscle a firm attachment to bone. The musculotendinous junction represents the point at which there is a significant change in the histological composition of skeletal muscle from predominantly muscle fibers to predominantly collagen fibers. Muscle contraction exerts force on the musculotendinous junction and the tendon that moves a bone at a joint.

Fascia and Neurovascular Bundle

Fascia is a derivative of mesoderm. Throughout the body there is a subcutaneous layer of loose connective tissue called the superficial fascia (Figs. 3.5 and 3.19). It contains collagen fibers as well as variable amounts of fat. Superficial fascia increases skin mobility, acts as a thermal insulator, and stores energy for metabolic use. The dense connective tissue envelope that invests and separates individual muscles of the limbs and trunk is deep fascia. It is also composed primarily of collagen fibers.

Between individual muscles there is a fascial plane that represents the separation of the connective tissue investment (wrapper) of the individual muscles. In the limbs and neck deep fascia pass over and between muscle groups and connect to bone periosteum. The deep fascia passing between muscle groups are called intermuscular septa. Together with the deep fascia passing over muscle groups, they serve to compartmentalize muscle groups of similar functions and innervations (Figs. 3.19 and 3.20). Deep fascia between individual muscles that move extensively are loose connective tissue, which facilitate movement. As connective tissue, fascia provide for mobility and stability of the musculoskeletal system. There is a myofascial continuity throughout the body.

Peripheral nerves, blood, and lymph vessels lie in the loose connective tissue fascia between muscles. This fascia binds together these nerves and vessels, and collectively these components form the neurovascular bundle (Fig. 3.20).

Muscle Action

A muscle contracts because it is stimulated by a motor nerve. A single motor nerve fiber innervates more than one skeletal muscle fiber. The nerve fiber and all the muscle fibers it innervates are called the motor unit (Fig. 3.21). In general, small muscles that react quickly, such as extraocular muscles, have 10 or fewer muscle fibers innervated by a single nerve fiber. In contrast, large muscles that do not require fine central nervous system control, for example, deep back muscles, may have up

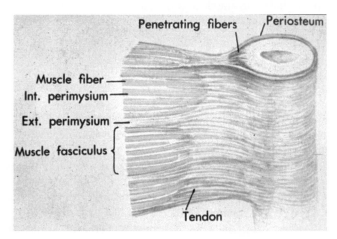

Figure 3.18. Diagrammatic representation of how muscle attaches to bone. (Source unknown.)

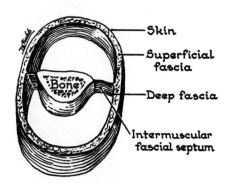

Figure 3.19. Diagrammatic representation of a transverse section through arm illustrating organization of superficial and deep fascia. Deep fascia divides arm into compartments by way of intermuscular septa. (Reprinted with permission from Basmajian JV, Slonecker CE. *Grant's Method of Anatomy.* 11th ed. Baltimore, Md: Williams & Wilkins; 1989:388.)

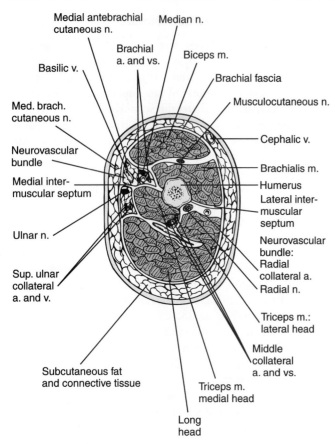

Figure 3.20. Transverse section through arm. Neurovascular bundles are found between skeletal muscles in anterior and posterior compartments. (Modified from Woodbourne RT, Burkel WE. *Essentials of Human Anatomy*. 9th ed. New York, NY: Oxford University Press; 1994.)

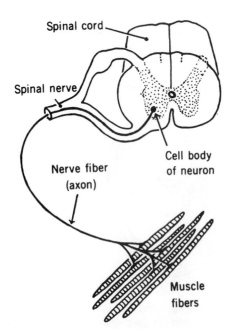

Figure 3.21. A motor unit. (Reprinted with permission from Basmajian JV, Slonecker CE. *Grant's Method of Anatomy*. 11th ed. Baltimore, Md: Williams & Wilkins; 1989:22.)

to 1000 muscle fibers in a motor unit. When a muscle is resting, some motor units are always discharging. It may not be the same motor units at each instance in time. This type of motor activity is the background for muscular contraction in the performance of a purposeful movement.

When most muscles contract, their fibers act through tendons on movable bones to cause the desired action (Fig. 3.18). Movements result in the activation of motor units in some muscles and the simultaneous relaxation of motor units in other muscles. Movement from muscle contraction causes the muscles to change in length. When this occurs, tension created within the muscle remains constant, and the contraction is called isotonic. If movement does not occur as a result of muscle contraction and muscle length stays constant with elevated tension generated within the muscles, the contraction is called isometric, as occurs with posterior compartment muscles of the leg when standing. Isotonic contractions may be concentric (shortening of the muscle) or eccentric (lengthening of the muscle).

Most movements require the combined action of several muscles. The term "prime mover" is used for those muscles that act directly to bring about the desired movement. Every muscle that acts on a joint is paired with another muscle that has the opposite action on the same joint. These muscles are antagonists of each other, for example, the biceps brachi-flexor and triceps-extensor. An antagonist does not significantly block the action of the prime mover. Its primary effect only occurs at the initiation of the movement after which it relaxes until the movement is finished. There are times when prime movers and antagonists contract together and are called fixators. This occurs to stabilize a joint or hold a part of the body in an appropriate position.

Muscles that contract at the same time as prime movers are called synergists. These can be either muscles that aid the prime movers in the performance of the desired action or antagonist muscles that contract at the same time as a prime mover and thereby prevent unwanted movement that would be counterproductive to the desired action. Individual muscles should not always be considered as units with a single function. Different parts of the same muscle may have different, even antagonistic, actions, such as occur with the deltoid muscle.

SEGMENTAL ORGANIZATION OF THE NEUROMUSCULOSKELETAL AND VASCULAR SYSTEMS

A typical transverse section through the thoracic region demonstrates the basic organization of the axial skeleton (Figs. 3.3 and 3.22). Throughout the thoracic region each vertebral level is organized symmetrically about a central axis composed of the vertebra, spinal cord, and aorta. The distribution of a typical spinal nerve and posterior intercostal artery are repeated at each segmental level of the thoracic spine (T_1 through T_{12}).

The typical spinal nerve is formed by the union of the anterior and posterior roots just lateral to the intervertebral foramen. Within a short distance, the spinal nerve divides to

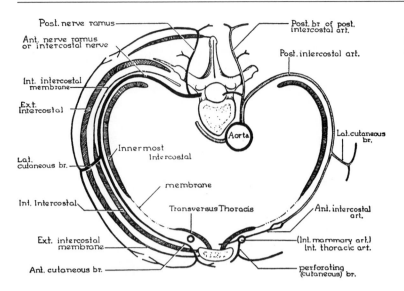

Figure 3.22. Transverse section illustrating contents of a segmental level through thorax. (Reprinted with permission from Basmajian JV, Slonecker CE. *Grant's Method of Anatomy*. 11th ed. Baltimore, Md: Williams & Wilkins; 1989:74.)

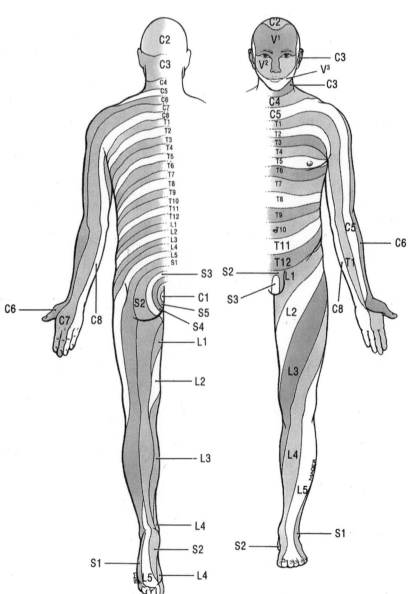

Figure 3.23. Dermatomal maps of body. (Reprinted with permission from Agur AMR. *Grant's Atlas of Anatomy*. 9th ed. Baltimore, Md: Williams & Wilkins; 1991:252.)

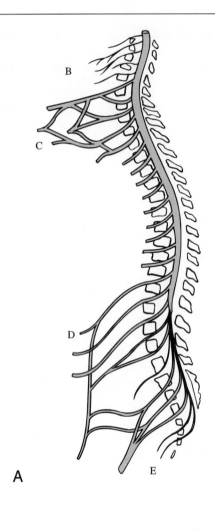

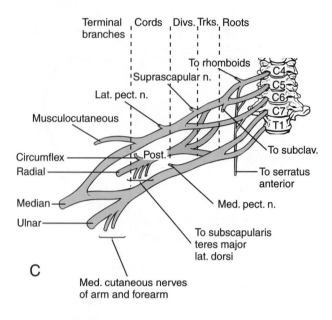

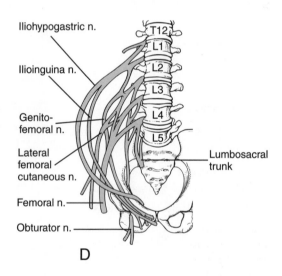

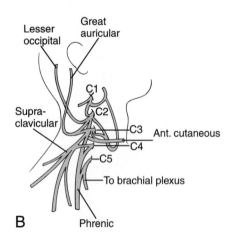

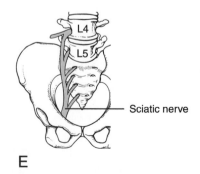

Figure 3.24.   Spinal cord and plexuses. **A.** Sagittal view of spinal cord and plexuses. **B.** Cervical plexus.
C. Brachial plexus. **D.** Lumbar plexus. **E.** Sacral plexus. (Modified from Romero-Sierra C. *Neuroanatomy: A Con-*
ceptual Approach. New York, NY: Churchill Livingstone; 1986.)

form a posterior primary ramus and an anterior primary ramus (Fig. 3.22). The posterior primary ramus is distributed to the deep ("true") back muscles, the skin over these muscles, and the joints that the muscles functionally move. Posterior primary rami distribute segmentally from the base of the skull to the coccyx. The anterior primary ramus in the thoracic region (intercostal nerve) passes between the muscle layers of the intercostal space and distributes laterally and anteriorly to supply the muscles and skin of the thorax and abdomen.

The pattern of thoracic and abdominal distribution is clinically demonstrated as dermatomal bands from the base of the neck to the pubis (Fig. 3.23). The anterior primary rami are distributed in a more complex manner above and below the thoracic region (Fig. 3.24). The anterior primary rami of $C_{1,2,3}$ and C_4 form the cervical plexus. The anterior primary rami of $C_{5,6,7,8}$ and T_1 form the brachial plexus, which supplies the upper limb. Lumbar and sacral anterior primary rami ($L_{1,2,3,4}$ and L_5, $S_{1,2,3}$) form the lumbosacral plexus, which is distributed to the pelvis, perineum, and lower limb.

In the thoracic region the abdominal aorta gives rise to right and left posterior intercostal arteries that supply the thoracic and abdominal walls segmentally (Fig. 3.22). This area of supply includes the:

Skin
Superficial and deep fascia
Intercostal and abdominal musculature
Ribs
Vertebrae
Paravertebral musculature

The costal groove on the internal inferior surface of each rib contains a segmental neurovascular bundle that includes the:

Intercostal nerve and artery
Venae comitans of the intercostal artery (intercostal veins)
Segmental intercostal lymphatics (Fig. 3.22)

These structures supply and drain the muscle, connective tissue, and skin within and over the thorax and abdomen.

The segmental pattern of neurovascular distribution in the thorax and abdomen is an example of developmental segmentation that the body maintains in the adult. However, this segmental pattern is modified in the limbs by differential growth and development.

LIMB ANATOMY

Upper and Lower Limbs

The anatomy of the upper and lower limbs is comparable. If one is to understand this basic anatomy, as well as how the limbs function, then one must understand limb development. The limbs are divided into four major parts. The upper limb is divided into the shoulder (shoulder girdle), arm, forearm, and hand. The lower limb consists of the pelvic girdle, thigh, leg, and foot. The bones of the upper and lower limbs form the appendicular skeleton. These bones form in situ in the developing limb buds. They begin as mesenchyme that con-

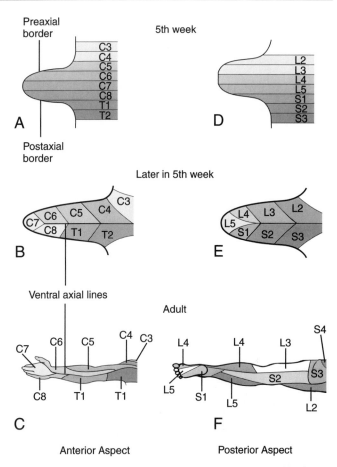

Figure 3.25. Developing dermatomal patterns in upper (**A–C**) and lower (**D–F**) limbs. **A–C.** anterior view upper limb. **D** and **F.** posterior view lower limb. **A, B, D,** and **E.** Limb buds in embryo. **C** and **F.** Adult limbs. (Modified from Moore KL. *The Developing Human.* 3rd ed. Philadelphia, Pa: WB Saunders Co; 1982.)

denses and differentiates into hyaline cartilage bone models. These cartilaginous models eventually ossify through endochondral ossification.

Limb musculature is also derived from mesenchyme, but muscle mesenchyme, unlike that which form the bones, is derived from somites adjacent to the developing neural tube. It migrates into the limb bud where it condenses adjacent to the developing bones (Fig. 3.4). As the limb elongates, the muscular tissue splits into flexor (anterior) and extensor (posterior) components. Initially the muscles of the limbs are segmental in character, but in time they fuse and are composed of muscle tissue from several segments. Upper limb buds are opposite neural tube (spinal cord) segments $C_{5,6,7,8}$ and T_1, while lower limb buds lie opposite segments $L_{2,3,4,5}$ and S_1 and S_2.

As the limbs grow, posterior and anterior branches derived from anterior primary rami of spinal nerves penetrate into the developing muscles (Fig. 3.4). Posterior branches enter extensor musculature; anterior branches enter flexor musculature. With development, the segmental posterior and anterior branches from each anterior primary ramus unite to form large

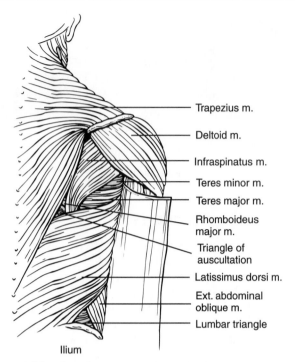

Figure 3.26. Superficial muscles of upper limb located on back. Notice extensive broad attachment of latissimus dorsi muscle as it covers posterior and lateral trunk. (Modified from Woodbourne RT, Burkel WE. *Essentials of Human Anatomy.* 9th ed. New York, NY: Oxford University Press; 1994.)

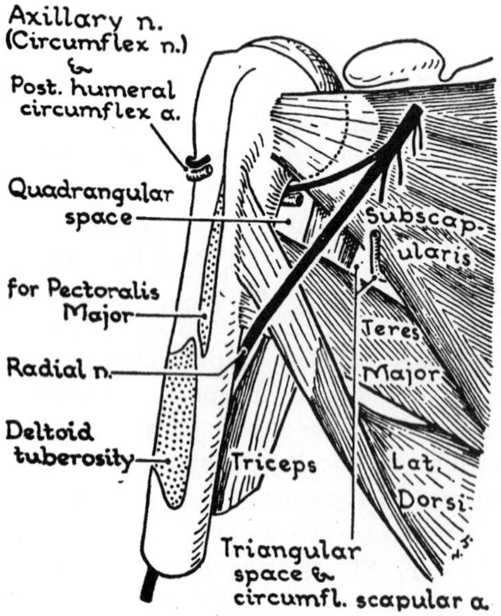

posterior and anterior nerves. This union of the original segmental posterior and anterior branches from each anterior primary ramus is the basis for the formation of the brachial and lumbosacral plexuses (Fig. 3.24). It comes about with the fusion of segmental muscles.

The large posterior and anterior nerves are represented in the adult upper limb as the radial nerve, supplying extensor musculature, and the median and ulnar nerves, innervating flexor musculature, respectively (Fig. 3.24). In the adult lower limb, the large posterior and anterior nerves are represented as the femoral and common peroneal nerves, supplying extensor musculature, and the tibial nerve, supplying flexor musculature, respectively (Fig. 3.24). Contact between nerves and differentiating muscle cells is a prerequisite for complete func-

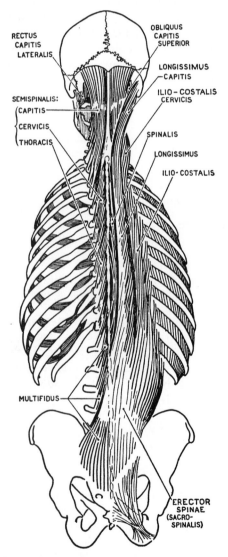

Figure 3.27. Posterior wall of axilla showing attachment of latissimus dorsi muscle into intertubercular groove of humerus. (Reprinted with permission from Basmajian JV, Slonecker CE. *Grant's Method of Anatomy.* 11th ed. Baltimore, Md: Williams & Wilkins; 1989:358.)

Figure 3.28. Deep muscles of back provide myofascial continuity from cranium through vertebral column to pelvis. (Reprinted with permission from Basmajian JV, Slonecker CE. *Grant's Method of Anatomy.* 11th ed. Baltimore, Md: Williams & Wilkins; 1989:349.)

tional muscle differentiation. The segmental spinal nerves also provide sensory innervation of the limb dermatomes. The original segmental dermatomal pattern is modified with growth of the limbs, but an orderly sequence is present in the adult (Fig. 3.25).

The development of the upper and lower limbs is similar. However, there are two differences. First, the lower limb develops later than the upper limb. Second, the limbs rotate in opposite directions. The upper limb rotates 90° laterally so that the elbow points posteriorly. The extensor musculature lies on lateral and posterior surfaces, while the flexor musculature lies on anterior and medial surfaces, and the thumb lies laterally on the anterior facing palm. The lower limb rotates 90° medially so that the knee points anteriorly, and the extensor muscles are on the anterior surface. The flexor muscles are on the posterior surface, and the big toe is medial. These rotations are necessary based on the functions that the limbs will be asked to perform. In the limbs, deep fascia and intermuscular septa connecting with bone separate or compartmentalize groups of muscles. The muscles in each compartment share the following:

Similar functions
Developmental histories
Nerve and arterial supply
Venous and lymphatic drainage

Functional Adaption

Through their development, the upper and lower limbs have adapted anatomically to perform different functions. The upper limb is involved in manual activity. It moves freely, especially the hand, which is adapted for manipulating and grasping. The stability of the upper limb has been sacrificed for mobility. The digits are the most mobile parts of the upper limb. The lower limb is involved in locomotion, weight bearing, and maintaining equilibrium. Because of its weight-bearing function, some movement has been sacrificed in order to achieve stability.

MYOFASCIAL CONTINUITY

The concept of myofascial continuity is best understood by examining the attachment of a tendon to a bone. The dense fibrous connective tissue is anchored to the compact cortical substance of bone by microscopic connective tissue penetrating fibers, Sharpey's fibers. The connective tissue that then forms the mass of the tendon becomes feathered to interdigitate with the skeletal muscle fibers that will form the substance of the muscle. The same architecture is duplicated at the proximal and distal muscle attachments to bone (Fig. 3.18).

Through the attachment of the dense regular fibrous tissue of tendon and ligament to bone there is microscopic fiber continuity with the periosteum covering the substance of each

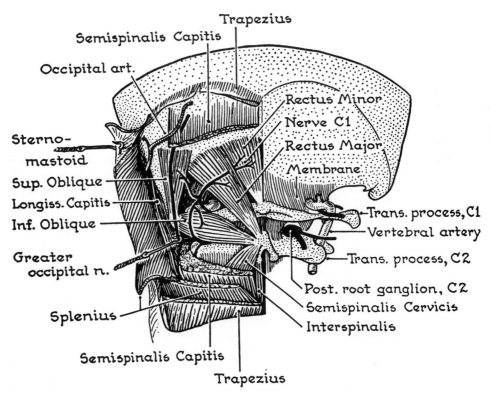

Figure 3.29. Suboccipital region. Suboccipital muscles (obliques capitus superior and rectus capitis posterior minor) provide myofascial continuity between cranium and C$_1$/atlas. (Reprinted with permission from Basmajian JV, Slonecker CE. *Grant's Method of Anatomy.* 11th ed. Baltimore, Md: Williams & Wilkins; 1989:496.)

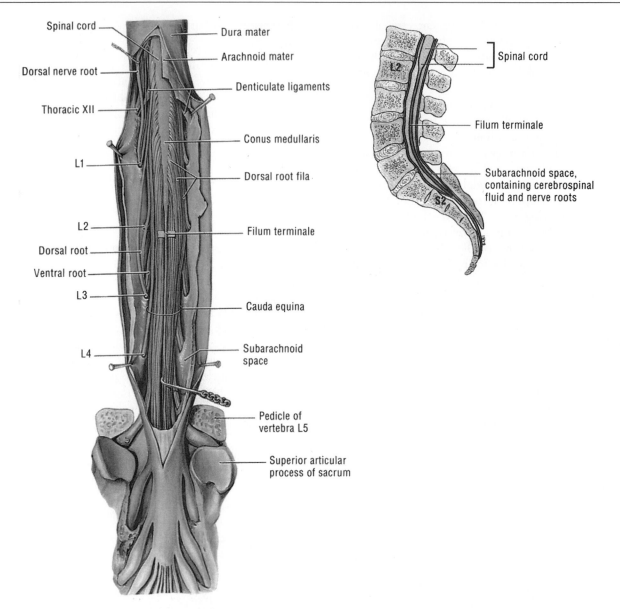

Figure 3.30. Lower end of spinal cord, including cauda equina, and its coverings. Inferior end of dura mater at S₂ is attached to coccyx by coccygeal ligament. Dura mater provides a direct connection from internal surface of cranium to coccyx. (Reprinted with permission from Agur AMR. *Grant's Atlas of Anatomy*. 9th ed. Baltimore, Md: Williams & Wilkins; 1991:249.)

bone. The tendon attachment provides direct continuity of a muscle at its origin and insertion to bone. The connection of tendon to bone provides functional integrity of each part of the body across each synovial joint by way of the muscle tendon complex. This can best be described as myofascial continuity (Fig. 3.18).

The latissimus dorsi muscle exemplifies myofascial continuity. Through attachment to the lumbar spine and iliac crest by way of the lumbodorsal (thoracolumbar) fascia, the latissimus dorsi tendon/aponeurosis has continuity with the flat sheet of skeletal muscle that covers the posterior and lateral trunk. The latissimus dorsi muscle then converges to a narrow

flat tendon that crosses the posterior axilla and inserts into the floor of the intertubercular groove on the anterior aspect of the humerus (Figs. 3.26 and 3.27). The latissimus dorsi muscle provides functional and structural continuity among the upper limb, spine (thoracic, lumbar, and sacral), ribs, and pelvis. It does so through an attachment to the crest of the ilium and pelvis. Dysfunction of the latissimus dorsi muscle can therefore have a direct effect on all these joints:

Glenohumeral joint
Scapulothoracic articulation
Acromioclavicular joint
Thoracic facet joints

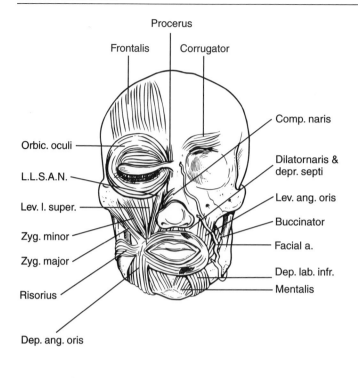

Procerus
Frontalis   Corrugator

Comp. naris

Orbic. oculi

L.L.S.A.N.

Lev. l. super.

Zyg. minor

Zyg. major

Risorius

Dep. ang. oris

Dilatornaris & depr. septi

Lev. ang. oris

Buccinator

Facial a.

Dep. lab. infr.

Mentalis

Superficial   Deeper

Figure 3.31. Muscles of facial expression. Periosteum covering bones of viscerocranium provides attachment for these muscles inserting into skin. (Modified from Basmajian JV, Slonecker CE. *Grant's Method of Anatomy.* 11th ed. Baltimore, Md: Williams & Wilkins; 1989.)

Costovertebral joints
Lumbar facet joints
Stability of the pelvis at the sacroiliac joint

Myofascial continuity from one region of the body to another can best be understood through consideration of the regional structure of the body, which includes the:

Cranium
Cervical spine and upper limb
Thoracic spine and trunk
Lumbosacral spine
Pelvis and lower limb (Fig. 3.28)

The myofascial continuity of the cranium is best understood by studying the internal and external structure of the skull as

it articulates with the first cervical vertebra (C_1/atlas). Suboccipital muscles (obliquis capitis superior and rectus capitis posterior minor) provide for this continuity (Fig. 3.29).

The meningeal layer of cranial dura mater is continuous with the spinal dura at the occipital foramen magnum (Fig. 3.17). The spinal dura surrounding and supporting the spinal cord is free within the vertebral canal. The inferior aspect of the spinal dura mater at S_2 is attached to the coccyx by the coccygeal ligament (Fig. 3.30). Through the dura mater there is a direct connection between the internal aspect of the cranium and the inferior aspect of the vertebral column.

Externally, the bones of the face (viscerocranium) and the cranial vault (neurocranium) are covered by a thin layer of connective tissue periosteum. This periosteum provides a protective covering of each bone and a mechanism for attachment of specific muscles (e.g., muscles of facial expression Fig. 3.31).

CONCLUSION

An understanding of basic human anatomy and myofascial continuity enables the osteopathic physician to use the basic principles of osteopathic medicine in the diagnosis and treatment of neuromusculoskeletal dysfunctions and disorders.

REFERENCES

1. Basmajian JV, Slonecker CE. *Grant's Method of Anatomy.* 11th ed. Baltimore, Md: Williams & Wilkins; 1989.
2. Clemente CD. *Gray's Anatomy of the Human Body.* American 30th ed. Philadelphia, Pa: Lea & Febiger; 1985.
3. Copenhaver WM, Bunge RP, Bunge MB. *Bailey's Textbook of Histology.* 16th ed. Baltimore, Md: Williams & Wilkins; 1971.
4. Hollinshead WH, Rosse C. *Textbook of Anatomy.* 4th ed. Philadelphia, Pa: Harper & Row; 1985.
5. Moore KL. *Clinically Oriented Anatomy.* 3rd ed. Baltimore, Md: Williams & Wilkins; 1992.
6. Sadler TW. *Langman's Medical Embryology.* 7th ed. Baltimore, Md: Williams & Wilkins; 1995.
7. Williams PL, Warwick R, Dyson M, Bannister LH. British 37th ed. *Gray's Anatomy.* London, Churchill Livingstone; 1989.
8. Woodburne RT, Burkel WE. *Essentials of Human Anatomy.* 9th ed. New York, NY: Oxford University Press; 1994.
9. Magoun HI. *Osteopathy in the Cranial Field.* 3rd ed. Kirksville, Mo: The Journal Printing Company; 1976.
10. Mennell J. *Joint Pain.* Boston, Mass: Little, Brown & Co; 1964.

4. Rules of Anatomy

LEX C. TOWNS

Key Concepts

- **Seven "rules" of anatomy**

- **Rule of proximity**

- **Rule of function including special relevance of function of musculoskeletal system to practice of osteopathic medicine**

- **Two anatomical entities that provide supply**

- **Two anatomical entities that provide drainage**

- **Reasons pain is the most anatomical of all symptoms; similarities and differences between direct and referred pain**

- **Structures and functional systems that connect the body into a unified whole**

- **Fascia and examples of how fascia separates areas of the body and unites different areas and structures**

- **Two reasons for variation in human form with examples of each that illustrate disease process or normal variation in structure**

An understanding of anatomy is fundamental to the practice of medicine. To assess health and disease, physicians must have a detailed knowledge of the structures of the body with which they deal. Yet the anatomical knowledge of many physicians is often restricted to a particular body area or functional system with which they deal in a specialized practice. Effective physicians, even those in very specialized practices, need and use a working knowledge of the reciprocal, interactive nature of the body's structure and function. Osteopathic physicians need sufficient knowledge of body structure and function to understand how focal destructive causes may lead not only to localized effects but also to more subtle widespread or distant degenerative morbid events. The payoff for mastering anatomy is the ability to practice osteopathic medicine in a more rational, predictable, and effective manner.

This chapter does not attempt to thoroughly review anatomy. Numerous excellent books and programs are available on human anatomy. The purpose of this chapter is to provide some conceptual bases to guide the study of anatomy and

thereby maximize the positive impact of anatomical knowledge on osteopathic medical practice. These concepts are sketched here as a series of "rules." These rules illustrate that effective osteopathic medical treatment proceeds from a fundamental, accurate understanding of structure.

RULE 1: RULE OF PROXIMITY

Understanding spatial relationships forms the essence of the use of anatomy in medical practice. The most usable admonition is also the most obvious: in any particular part of the body, you must know the spatial arrangement of all the organs and tissues. Knowledge of spatial relations, gained from lectures, readings, and dissections, allows one to reconstruct mentally the entire anatomy of an area when only limited cues are available. For example, when palpating the abdomen, the physician must be able to visualize accurately the entire abdominal contents based on a few large organs or bony landmarks that can be seen or felt manually. When casting a limb, the physician must be able to visualize the placement of important arteries, veins, and nerves to avoid the disastrous consequences of compromise to these important structures. Their locations may be inferable only from bony or muscular surface landmarks.

A necessary first step is often to memorize basic facts of anatomy, such as these examples:

What is the attachment of the biceps humerus?
What are the branches of the femoral artery?
How is the brachial plexus formed and what are its branches?

The more important task is to place those memorized facts into a larger morphological context. For example, one must initially memorize the layout of the brachial plexus, but the brachial plexus bears important spatial relations to other components in the arm, axilla, and root of the neck. Without this subsequent understanding, the memorization is largely wasted effort.

With the advent of powerful new imaging technologies, some might assume that the eventual task of the practicing physician would be greatly simplified, that the study of anatomy would become unnecessary. In fact, a new level of complexity is added by the ready availability of computerized tomography (CT), magnetic resonance imaging (MRI), and other modern imaging technologies. Recognizing and reconstructing whole anatomical structures on the basis of their sectional representation is not an inconsequential mental task. Most teaching programs of anatomy now emphasize how the three-dimensional morphology seen in dissection and represented in textbooks and atlases appears when imaged via various technologies. Physicians must now be conversant with the contemporary images of structure, and they must also become facile at translating these static or dynamic images into complete, inclusive, three-dimensional living patients. Realistically, the advent of modern imaging technology has replaced the need to infer deep anatomy from subtle surface landmarks. However, the clarity with which previously unviewable structures can now be seen is offset by the necessity to reconstruct three-dimensionally whole regions of the body from slices.

Also, despite the power of these remarkable new tools, many important small structures are not visualized. Physicians must still rely on detailed relational anatomy and must be able to place small nerves and vessels into the context of CT or MRI images.

The rule of proximity is applied with the visualization of spatial relations as the osteopathic physician uses the most distinctive features of his or her practice: palpatory diagnosis and musculoskeletal manipulative therapy. The physician must have a clear comprehension of the localized relationships of muscles, muscle attachments, and bones to each other and to vessels, nerves, lymphatics, fascia, and organs. This is prerequisite to most osteopathic diagnostic and therapeutic strategies. Together, palpation and manipulation can be thought of as anatomy in practice. This mental reconstruction of the anatomical structure of a region proceeds from only a few palpable or visible superficial landmarks.

The accurate diagnosis and treatment of many conditions and diseases proceeds from knowing where things are located. Virtually all the utilization of anatomy in a clinical setting, and all of the other rules described below, is based on the rule of proximity.

RULE 2: RULE OF FUNCTION

Like the first rule, the rule of function is obvious. The companion goal of knowing where things are is knowing what they do.

For many of the structures, organs, or organ systems, most gross anatomy courses appropriately limit the discussion of function, as, for example:

The function of the lung is to provide gas exchange in the blood
The function of the kidneys is to filter the blood and make urine
The function of the gastrointestinal tract is to digest and absorb nutrients and water

Details of these functions are left to the other basic sciences, which in turn assume an understanding of gross structure. It remains important to grasp the intimate relationship of structure and function. The human organism is a complex, unified organism; relating structure and function is one basic and necessary strategy to understand the functioning, integrated, whole human being.

The musculoskeletal system is approximately 75% of the body mass; this vast system can give stability in health, provide

clues to dysfunction and disease, and offer a mode of treatment to support the patient who is diseased or stressed. Osteopathic physicians must understand well the function of the individual components of the musculoskeletal system.

This function is seen from two fundamental complementary perspectives:

What action does a muscle (joint, bone, ligament, etc.) produce?
Which muscle (joint, bone, ligament, etc.) produces a specific action or function?

For example, the deltoid muscle is a large, easily identified muscle with well-defined bony attachments. Its functions are complex; it participates in:

Abduction
Flexion
Extension
Medial and lateral rotation of the arm

In a clinical situation, however, the physician is simply presented with a patient who has, among other symptoms, a weakness in abducting the arm. Working from that complaint, the physician must recall which muscle produces that action and then assess the strength of the deltoid in its various movements.

These two related questions of function are the beginning of a series of questions predicated on an understanding of a more complex structural and functional interrelationship:

How might dysfunction of the muscle (or other musculoskeletal component) affect total body efficiency and health?
How might dysfunction of some visceral element degrade the structural or functional integrity of the musculoskeletal system?

In the previous example, if there is a deltoid weakness, the physician must then recall the innervation of the muscle (the axillary nerve) and assess the strength of other muscles (teres minor) innervated by that nerve. Working backward, the physician checks the function of muscles that, like the deltoid, receive their motor supply from bunches of the posterior cord of the brachial plexus. The innervation of the deltoid muscle is principally from the fifth cervical spinal nerve. The thoracic diaphragm also receives part of its innervation from that same cervical segment. The physician looks for answers to the following questions:

Is there any compromise in respiratory function?
What postural or functional compensation has the patient made for weakness of the deltoid?
Is weakness of abduction unrelated to the deltoid and simply a function of pain in the shoulder; that is, does the patient not raise the arm because it hurts to do so?
Is the pain in the joint itself or does it result from disease of some internal organ?

These questions can be fully answered only with an understanding of the structure and function of the musculoskeletal system.

RULE 3: RULE OF SUPPLY

Two structural entities, arteries and nerves, are important for the health and maintenance of any organ or area. Arteries supply nutrients, oxygen, and a variety of hormonal regulatory substances to the area of their distribution. Nerves provide ongoing neural control of skeletal and smooth muscle and glandular tissue and deliver trophic or regulatory factors to the muscles or organs that they innervate. The rule of supply illustrates a major source for maintenance of health or, conversely, origin of pathology when disrupted.

Few statements are more cogent than A.T. Still's insightful dictum, "*The rule of the artery is supreme.*"[1] An adequate blood supply during varying physiological conditions is a prerequisite for health of an organ or region. Conversely, compromise to the blood supply often leads to diminished functional capacity, cascading, in turn, toward disease. The osteopathic physician must work to ensure continued blood supply in the healthy state and, when treating injury or disease, should attempt to enhance arterial supply to affected regions. One important condition of compromise is bleeding due to trauma or disease. The physician must be able to halt the hemorrhage quickly and restore adequate blood flow to ischemic areas. But the physician must also be able to recognize the clinical signs of ischemia due to blockage of arterial supply and work to relieve the blockage.

To optimize strategies that continue arterial supply (and health) in the healthy state, and to use appropriate therapeutic interventions in disease or injury to restore adequate blood supply, a physician must have an accurate knowledge of the arterial supply to an area. Consistent with rule 1 above, it is not sufficient simply to know the name of the artery that provides supply; rather, the passage of the arterial supply must be placed in the context of surrounding muscles, bones, organs, lymphatics, fascia, etc.

One of the goals of an osteopathic approach to medical treatment is, first, to recognize which piece of surrounding tissue might be compressing an artery and, having visualized the mechanical impediment to blood flow, adopt appropriate therapies to relieve the compression and thereby restore normal flow. Similarly, the osteopathic physician works to recognize in the healthy individual those areas or organs that might be at risk for reduced blood flow caused by lifestyle, activities, posture, obesity, etc., and adopt a treatment plan to maintain health in risk zones.

As do arteries, nerves supply vital components to every portion of the body. Nerves supply control; they are a major component of the body's homeostatic mechanisms. Nerve cell bodies in the central nervous system (CNS) send nerve fibers to control contraction of smooth (involuntary) muscles and skeletal (voluntary) muscles and to control secretion of glands. Nerves also supply sensory input; they convey either exteroceptive input concerning physical forces that impinge on the body or interoceptive stimuli about the status of the internal milieu. Nerve fibers also supply chemical materials from the CNS to the periphery and vice versa. Through the mechanism of axoplasmic transport, trophic (growth promoting) chemicals are manufactured in the neuron cell body and carried to target muscles or organs where, after release into the synaptic space, they are taken into the target tissue and there promote healthy function. In the opposite direction, chemicals from the muscle or organ can cross the synapse, be taken up, and be transported retrogradely to the neuron cell bodies where the chemicals can then alter basic neuron function.

Individual nerves have their origins in the spinal cord (for spinal nerves) or brainstem (for cranial nerves); the segmental origins of specific nerves are important. The segmental origin of nerves is pertinent to three general targets of innervation: skin, muscles, and internal organs. The dermatomal (skin) innervation pattern is relatively straightforward. Pain or sensory loss over some specific dermatomal zone leads to inferences about the integrity of restricted areas of the central nervous system or nerves near their origin.

The innervation pattern of muscles is particularly pertinent to osteopathic medicine because changes in the tone, texture, or function of a muscle are related to the segmental source of nerve supply to that muscle. The innervation of muscles of the trunk is relatively simple and follows a pattern similar to that of the dermatomes. Nerve fibers to the muscles of the limbs, on the other hand, arise from the spinal cord and are woven through complex networks (the brachial plexus and lumbosacral plexus) which combine fibers from several spinal cord segments into motor nerves that typically serve functional groups of muscles. A physician must understand innervation of limb muscles well enough to reconstruct those nerve fibers from their termination through the plexus to their spinal cord origin.

The internal viscera receive abundant autonomic nerve supply. The pattern by which this nerve supply arises from the spinal cord or brainstem and passes to target tissue is schematically simple but anatomically complex. The sensory innervation to the internal viscera that signals functional status, distention, and pain typically accompanies the autonomic innervation to the target organ.

Because of developmental and maturational events, the origin of autonomic and sensory innervation of a specific organ may be relatively distant from that particular viscus. As a result, changes in a particular visceral organ may appear as pain or changes in muscle texture some distance from the organ. On the other hand, localized musculoskeletal misalignment may produce alteration in autonomic outflow from the related segmental zone of the spinal cord and may disturb function in an internal organ some distance away from that segment. The physician must understand both the general segmental origin and anatomical pathway by which autonomic nerve fibers and the accompanying sensory nerve fibers pass to the various internal organs.

Nerves supply important functional and trophic control to all parts of the body. An important aspect of osteopathic medical practice is to recognize and treat conditions that alter nerve supply to a region or organ. The success of palpation and treatments in recognizing and relieving compression or irritation to nerves and the effectiveness of maintenance of nerve traffic by healthy lifestyles depend directly on how well the physician understands the route that nerves take from their origin to their destination.

RULE 4: RULE OF DRAINAGE

While the arterial supply is the only means by which fluid and blood cellular components are taken to an area, two pathways remove fluids and blood cells from a region. The venous network collects the deoxygenated blood from the capillary bed; the lymphatic channels drain the relatively cell-free extracellular fluid. Compromise to either of these return channels leads to edema in the affected area: more fluid goes in than comes out.

To alleviate edema, the osteopathic physician may choose to use protocols to enhance venous and/or lymphatic return. That strategy depends on a thorough knowledge of the anatomy of the venous and lymphatic systems. As with the arterial system, the knowledge of anatomy places venous and lymphatic channels into the context of surrounding organs, muscles, bones, fascia, etc., usually by visualizing those structures on the basis of subtle palpable or surface landmarks.

Peripheral venous channels tend to be somewhat idiosyncratic, with considerable anastomoses. For general medical application, it is acceptable to understand the overall pattern of peripheral venous drainage and concentrate one's effort on the larger, more predictable central veins. Anastomoses of peripheral venous channels, however, are useful in treatment of the venous system. For example, venous anastomoses offer therapeutic strategies for the physician as alternate routes of venous drainage are established. Significant venous blood flow through some anastomoses is unusual and may indicate a pathological condition. Most venous blood from the gastrointestinal system, for example, is drained through the portal system to the liver. Internal hemorrhoids or esophageal varices indicate shunting of blood from the portal to the vena caval system (which drains the lower body) and may, thus, indicate blockage of venous drainage to the liver, or so-called portal hypertension.

The rule of venous drainage is to know by which veins an area is typically drained of blood, by what routes blood drains if the typical route is blocked, and where the veins lie relative to the surrounding structures.

Lymphatic channels are typically even more idiosyncratic than veins in their gross morphology; knowing general patterns and spatial relations of lymph drainage is usually sufficient. Although they are less well defined anatomically, they are important to understand. As with venous return, selecting osteopathic approaches to treatment of edema assumes a working knowledge of the location of lymph channels and how to augment lymphatic flow. Lymph collects into blind-ended endothelial tubes in the periphery. These channels throughout the body merge into ever larger channels, are filtered at predictable intervals by lymph nodes, and finally converge on two large lymphatic ducts in the thorax.

These two lymphatic ducts then empty into the venous system near the heart. As the lymphatic system has no intrinsic pump, fluid is moved from peripheral to central regions by osmotic pressure, muscular contractions, external pressure, and pressure differences between the thorax and the abdomen. There are various techniques to increase lymphatic return. When using techniques of muscle contraction or applying local pressure or lymphatic pump mechanisms, one needs prerequisite knowledge of the anatomy of lymphatic flow.

In addition to lymph flow, the lymphatic system and the lymph nodes are often indicators of disease. The lymphoid system houses important cells of the immune system. As a result of infection, lymphocytes proliferate and are sequestered in lymph nodes, where they attack pathogens (bacteria, viruses, etc.) in the lymph. Because of this important immune function, lymph nodes draining an infected area are often swollen and palpable.

Cancer in an organ will often metastasize to adjacent lymph nodes; the examining physician must understand the potential significance of enlarged nodes. For example, breast cancer may metastasize to the lymph nodes on the lateral thoracic wall or in the axilla that drain lymph from the breast. Or, illustrating a less obvious anatomical relationship, an enlarged node above the clavicle in the root of the neck may indicate cancer of the stomach. Knowledge of the pattern by which lymph drains from one zone to another can be used by the examining physician to infer the source of a disease process.

RULE 5: RULE OF PAIN

Pain brings more people to the physician than any other single complaint. Because of the prevalence of pain as a symptom, it is important to understand the anatomy of pain. Pain is almost always a symptom, not the disease or disturbance itself.

Pain as a symptom, whether sharp or dull, constant or intermittent, recent or long-standing, can usually be localized by the patient. Where the pain is easily attributed to an identifiable injury or lesion, the physician's use of anatomy is somewhat simplified; the pain is generally alleviated by healing the wound and administering systemic analgesics. Even in these cases, however, a working knowledge of the anatomy of the damaged area is a useful tool in the treatment of pain resulting from injury. The structural and functional integrity of the arterial supply, venous and lymphatic drainage, and nerve supply to the wounded area must be optimized to treat pain caused by a superficial wound.

A common medical scenario is of a patient who has a symptom of localized pain, yet no superficial tissue damage is visible. Swelling or redness may help direct the examination, but often the complaint is without an obvious external physical manifestation. Whether local signs are present or not, the physician must be able to visualize the deep anatomy of the affected area and understand the structures in that area and what their spatial relationships are. Using this mental map of the area, and guided by the history, the physician gently palpates in an effort to more clearly identify the source of the pain. Such palpatory examinations are of limited use without an understanding of anatomy.

The task of inferring anatomy from surface palpation is somewhat more simple in the limbs. These areas are not intrinsically easier (some of the most complex spatial relationships of structure are associated with the limbs), but a proportionally greater amount of the limbs are available for direct visual inspection and palpation. Similarly, much of the superficial neck anatomy can be assessed with palpation, but deep prevertebral structures are inaccessible to palpation. The walls of the thorax, abdomen, or pelvis are readily palpated; superficial pain in these walls can often be assessed with limited necessity to recall deep anatomy. However, to address a patient's pain inside the thorax, abdomen, or pelvis, one must know the normal anatomy of the affected region. Preliminary judgments of the size, integrity, and health of the viscera are based on superficial cues.

In most medical environments, the initial visual or palpatory inference of anatomy may be rapidly checked with one or more medical imaging modalities, such as plane radiographic films, CT, MRI, or ultrasound. The task for the physician is anatomically more concrete but requires in some cases an even more sophisticated level of anatomical knowledge. The examining physician must call on a detailed mental image of the anatomy of an area during initial examination. Reconstructing to dimensional spatial relations from CT or MRI sections, inferring placement of structures from shades of gray in a radiograph, or visualizing unseen structures in the shadows of an ultrasound sector also requires a detailed knowledge of anatomy. It is difficult to localize and interpret the source of that most common symptom, pain, without an accurate understanding of the anatomy of a region.

Be alert to referred pain, as well, when an organ or structure is damaged but the pain is felt somewhere else. The most coherent hypothesis of referred pain postulates that individual pain transmission neurons in the spinal cord receive afferents from both somatic pain fibers and visceral pain fibers. Individual pain transmission cells are almost always stimulated by somatic pain affects; higher somatosensory centers interpret that cell's firing as localized to a somatic site. In the rare circumstance that a pain transmission cell in the spinal cord is stimulated by visceral pain afferents, the pain is interpreted by higher centers as originating at the somatic site.

Referred pain is often difficult to localize and may move as the disease state progresses. Initially, pain may be vague and gnawing, felt in the midline of the body. Later the pain may become paravertebral and then follow a segmental or dermatomal pattern. Examples of referred pain are numerous. The following are two examples:

Damage to heart tissue invokes a sensation of pain in the left arm, shoulder, neck, and jaw
Gall bladder irritation causes referred pain in the right flank

Physicians by experience recognize referred pain and further understand its significance in a patient. The osteopathic physician should be particularly attentive to pathways of sensory innervation and pain innervation. The somatic innervation to the body wall and limbs is via spinal nerves, while the pain innervation of thoracic, abdominal, and pelvic viscera is via peripheral processes of dorsal root ganglia cells that generally accompany the distribution of autonomic fibers.

Pain is the most anatomical of symptoms. The proper localization and identification of the source of pain, whether superficial or deep, direct or referred, is essential to understanding the significance of the pain and a necessary prerequisite to holistic treatment of the underlying condition.

RULE 6: RULE OF CONNECTEDNESS

It has not been customary in modern medicine to point out that the human is a complex, unified organism made up of many overlapping, interconnected systems. Recently, conventional medicine has attempted to reassemble its various specialties and subspecialties, each focused on a body region or functional system, into a holistic understanding of health and disease. Nevertheless, the structure of medicine retains much of its compartmentalization; it is difficult for even the most thoughtful physician, particularly those in a demanding specialty practice, to step back routinely and holistically assess a patient.

One's understanding of body unity and the propensity to view the patient holistically is heightened by remembering a basic unifying principle: although the body is made up of many structurally and functionally discrete elements, the elements are linked together by a number of connectors. These connectors, or the connectedness of the body, make up a significant portion of the study of medicine in general and the study of anatomy in particular.

Some of the connectors are easily listed. Among the major connectors are the nervous systems:

Central
Peripheral
Autonomic
Enteric

The nervous system constantly receives external and internal stimuli filters, sorts and integrates those stimuli, and then causes the coordinated contraction of muscles and/or secretion of glands in response to those stimuli. The nervous system can even impel muscular contraction and/or glandular secretion independent of stimulation.

The endocrine and immune systems, interconnected to each other and to the nervous systems, are also major connectors, serving to bring tissues distant from each other under unified, coordinated control. Medical practice requires attention to the connected nature of the unified human organism. Typically, one disturbing force (a localized injury, lesion, or infection) causes a cascade of altered structural and functional changes in other areas or systems. Similarly, the treatment of localized disease or injury must be not only localized but must also attempt to bring the whole organism into healthy equilibrium. Planned treatments must account for not only the effect of the treatment protocol on the target site or organ system, but also the so-called side effect alterations brought about in distant, relatively healthy systems by the treatment.

Observe the obvious examples of body unity. Take time to appreciate the connected nature of the body. For didactic reasons the body is traditionally disassembled into component parts or regions such as these:

Bones
Muscles
Vessels
Nerves
Thorax
Abdomen
Upper limb

Yet it is important to be able mentally to reconstruct the intact specimen. The fundamental idea of holistic medicine is predicated on this.

One class of connectors is connective tissue in general, and fascia in particular. Connective tissue binds organ to organ, muscle to bone, and bone to bone and literally is the fundamental connector that allows structural and functional systems to be physically grouped into a unified package. Without connective tissue, the body is a dissociated mass of dying cells. It is the connective tissue, most of it a proteinaceous extracellular matrix, that enforces form and thereby permits function. Connective tissue plays a critical role in body health and disease, but ironically it is so pervasive it is easily overlooked in the study of anatomy, in the maintenance of health, and in the diagnosis and treatment of disease.

Fascia is one readily identifiable component of body connective tissue. It is particularly pertinent to osteopathic medical practice. Fascia are sheets of connective tissue that envelop specific structures and segregate one area from another. For example, each individual muscle is wrapped in a layer of tightly investing connective fascia. Groups of muscle of similar location and function are further ensheathed in an enveloping fascia.

At a basic anatomical level, these fascia define the individual muscles and muscle groups. For example, each of the muscles in the anterior compartment of the leg has its own investing fascia. The entire group is bounded laterally by a wall of fascia, the anterior crural septum, medially by fascia that is continuous with the periosteum of the tibia, and anteriorly by the encasing deep fascia of the leg. As is typical, the blood and nervous supply to these muscles, as well as venous and lymphatic return, is principally contained within this fascial compartment. These fascia collectively define the anterior compartment. More importantly, they enhance the extensor functions of the muscles, while simultaneously providing protection, support, and separation from other muscle groups. The fascia define the normal, healthy limit of the group; they tend to constrain destruc-

tive states and prevent the spread of bleeding, infection, tumor growth, etc., into adjacent compartments.

Fascial compartments also separate muscles of the trunk. The muscles of the anterior abdominal wall, for example, are easily divided into planes and groups by tough enveloping fascia. The external oblique, internal oblique, transverses abdominis, and rectus abdominis are delineable as a group and from one another not only by their attachments and orientations but by the tight-fitting sheets of fascia that enclose them. Planes of fascia are also found in the subcutaneous space, external to the deep fascia that bounds the surfaces of the muscles. Understanding the placement of these fascia is important in a variety of medical and surgical settings.

Many of the layers of fascia, whether subcutaneous or investing, merge together and/or have common points of attachment. The fascia that separate and ensheathe the external and internal abdominal obliques merge posteriorly. They also merge with the thick connective tissue thoracolumbar fascia; they are continuous upward, encasing and separating the erector spinae muscle groups. Anteriorly the fascia of the abdominal muscles merge, split, and are reflected to contribute to the inguinal anatomy and abdominal aponeurosis. These fascia are continuous with connective tissue sheets flowing over the crest of the pelvis and becoming the fascia lata of the thigh. They are continuous, in turn, with the crural fascia of the leg. As a consequence of the widespread continuity of fascia, distortion or damage to fascia in one area can have effects in a distant, seemingly unrelated area.

The subcutaneous fascia are also continuous from one body region to another. The deep layer of superficial fascia of the abdomen (Scarpa's fascia) defines a space that is more or less continuous from the flank onto the abdominal wall. It continues inferiorly into the perineum, where it is the superficial perineal space (bounded by Colles' and dartos fascia, continuations of Scarpa's fascia). Fluid or infection in the abdominal subcutaneous space can, thus, spread to the lumbar area or into the perineum.

The importance of the two-faceted aspect of fascia, that it at once not only separates and segregates but is also continuous structure-to-structure and area-to-area, should not be overlooked. This pervasive connector (along with muscle and bone) helps to regionalize the body and also connects region to region. Such a dualism is apparent in many physical manifestations of both health and disease.

The body, so often represented as a group of discrete regions or functional systems, is in reality an integrated whole. The integration of the body region to region and system to system is accomplished by a series of connectors. Some of these connectors, the endocrine and immune systems, are more commonly included in the context of physiology, biochemistry, or immunology. The nervous system, the vascular system, and the lymphatics are also important connectors, the structural components of which are part of anatomical disciplines. Finally, the visible connective tissues of the body, and particularly the fascia, are great physical connectors that bind organs or muscles into larger groups.

RULE 7: RULE OF DIFFERENCE

Things are not always built the way they are supposed to be: they do not look like the atlas. The important lesson is again the most obvious: the structure of each human body is different from all others. There are two reasons for variation of human form: developmental and historical. Variation in structure may be based on either or both.

During development and maturation of the human form, each person's genetic pool, along with extrinsic intrauterine and environmental signals, determines his or her ultimate form. Developmental deviations of structure are so common that descriptions of normal anatomy can more usefully be translated as usual anatomy, with variations assumed. For example, the pattern of venous drainage of surface structures (the limbs and neck are all good examples) is so variable that only a general plan can be described, and even with the propensity of anatomists to name everything, only the larger elements can typically be identified. Similar normal variation is common in arterial supply. The branching of the celiac trunk to supply the stomach, liver, pancreas, spleen, and duodenum follows a general pattern, but there are numerous deviations. There are often variations in normal anatomy; deviation of structure from the norm does not necessarily imply a pathological condition.

There are also instances where structures have been altered by injury or disease. Virtually every cadaver has localized and/ or widespread, visible, pathological alteration of structure, caused by examples such as these:

Ravages of atherosclerotic disease
Metastatic carcinoma
Prolapsed rectum or uterus
Arthritic changes

The structural outcome of systemic disorders, be they cardiovascular, pulmonary, gastrointestinal, musculoskeletal, etc., are often visible in the morphological condition of those organs. There are morphological manifestations of many of the diseases that currently drive disease-oriented medicine in the United States.

The cadavers available for teaching anatomy are usually of aged individuals and, in addition to the types of systemic pathology outlined above, these bodies also show the structural changes caused by the wear and tear of seven or eight decades. One can find arthritic joints, muscles withered by disuse, worn or infected teeth, or resorbed bones of the jaw when teeth are missing. The list of the normal alterations of anatomy that accompany aging is lengthy; these are important consequences of each person's life history. Many patients show morphological evidence of age-related deterioration, and the physician can benefit from recollecting the texture and appearance of those changes first seen in cadaver dissection.

CONCLUSION

The rules that have been outlined here are, for the most part, self-evident. Anatomy is the study of structure and general function. Learn where things are, what they do, how they are connected, how they influence each other, and how they change with time and life's experience.

REFERENCES

1. Still AT. *Autobiography of A.T. Still.* Published by the author, Kirksville, Mo, 1897:219.

5. Autonomic Nervous System

FRANK H. WILLARD

Key Concepts

- **Two components of peripheral nervous system: somatic and autonomic**

- **Somatic component innervation of skeletal muscle; influence of autonomic portion, representing predominant component, on almost all other tissues in body**

- **Organization of autonomic nervous system similar to the somatic nervous system, including following roles: receiving afferent fibers, processing information in central circuits, and forming output to connective tissue cells, smooth muscle cells, secretory cells, and immune cells**

- **Distinctive feature of autonomic nervous system: two-step output pathway involving centrally located preganglionic neurons and peripherally located ganglionic neurons**

- **Two anatomically, biochemically, and functionally distinct divisions: sympathetic and parasympathetic, with dual effects on organ systems**

- **Innervation of the visceral organs through great autonomic plexus extending from base of neck, through thorax, diaphragm, and abdomen to terminate in pelvis. Plexus supplied with parasympathetic fibers from vagus nerve and pelvic splanchnic nerves and sympathetic fibers from thoracic, lumbar, and sacral splanchnic nerves**

- **Central origin of sympathetic and parasympathetic innervation for organ systems in head, neck, thorax, abdomen, and pelvis, and their importance**

- **Origin of sympathetic innervation for peripheral vasculature, and its importance.**

- **Primary afferent innervation of organ systems instrumental in controlling output of autonomic nervous system**

- **Neuropeptide markers in afferent nerve fibers; small caliber, primary afferent fibers involved with detection of nociceptive stimuli**

Our daily existence depends on the coordinated activities of our internal organ systems. A major factor in orchestrating the diverse functions of these internal structures is the autonomic nervous system. Through an extensive network of connections, the autonomic nervous system helps maintain the normal rhythm of activity in the visceral organs as well as adjust their output to accommodate any external challenge. The limbic structures of the brain control the autonomic nervous system through the hypothalamus. The hypothalamus itself is closely integrated into a complex network involving the endocrine and immune systems. This conglomerate of interlocking systems, with its pervasive influence on our physiology and psychology, is called the neuroendocrine-immune network. This neuroendocrine-immune network is described in Chapter 9.

The terminology used to describe the part of the nervous system usually not under voluntary control varies widely. Since the 18th century, different terms have been used by researchers in different countries. None of these terms refers to the same group of structures or functions. Examples include:

Vegitive Nervensystem
Grand symapathique
Ganglionic nervous system
Visceral nervous system

The two most commonly used terms today are vegetative and autonomic nervous system. For a thorough discussion of the history of terminology concerning this system, see Clarke and Jacyna.[1] This chapter uses the term "autonomic nervous system" to refer to all components of the nervous system using preganglionic and ganglionic neurons as an efferent pathway. This definition excludes only the neuromuscular junctions between the ventral horn of the spinal cord (and a few cranial nuclei) and skeletal muscle.

The clinical importance of understanding the circuits of the autonomic nervous system cannot be overstated. Almost all communication between neurons in these circuits occurs via synaptic transmission. This process depends on the production, distribution, and recognition of specific neurochemicals.

These metabolic and stereological events are affected by most pharmaceutical agents, either as a desired first action or as an undesired side effect. A knowledge of nervous system structure, function, and chemistry is a necessity for the educated use of these substances and the intelligent approach to the maintenance of health.

The autonomic nervous system is sensitive to events occurring in somatic tissue such as cutaneous and musculoskeletal systems. The autonomic and somatic nervous systems are interlocked through numerous somatovisceral and viscerosomatic reflexes. Visceral symptoms may be the primary manifestations of somatic dysfunction and vice versa. This chapter examines the organization of the autonomic nervous system and its afferent component and emphasizes the pattern of innervation reaching the major organs of the thoracoabdominopelvic viscera and segmental representation of these organs in the spinal cord.

ORGANIZATION OF AUTONOMIC NERVOUS SYSTEM

The autonomic nervous system has components in both the central and peripheral nervous systems (Fig. 5.1). The major autonomic components of the central nervous system (CNS) include:

Limbic forebrain
Hypothalamus
Several brainstem nuclei
Intermediolateral cell column of the spinal cord

The autonomic components of the peripheral nervous system (PNS) include numerous ganglia (collections of neuron cell bodies located outside of the central nervous system) and a network of fibers distributed to all tissues of the body with the exception of the hyaline cartilages, the centers of the intervertebral disks, and the parenchymal tissues of the central nervous system. This review focuses on the peripheral distribution of the autonomic nervous system.

Peripheral Nervous Systems

The axons from neurons located in the CNS enter the periphery through spinal and cranial nerves. The peripheral portion of the nervous system can be divided into two fundamental parts based on the target structures of efferent fibers. Axons derived from the somatic component of the peripheral nervous system innervate skeletal muscle. Axons derived from the autonomic component of the peripheral nervous system enter the periphery and form complex interwoven plexuses containing clusters of cell bodies called ganglia. Neurons in these ganglia innervate all other targets, including:

Smooth muscle
Cardiac muscle
Glands
Connective tissue
Cells in the immune system

This fundamental division in the peripheral nervous system also reflects differential methods in cellular communication.

Figure 5.1. General organization of the autonomic nervous system. *CNS*, central nervous system; *PNS*, peripheral nervous system.

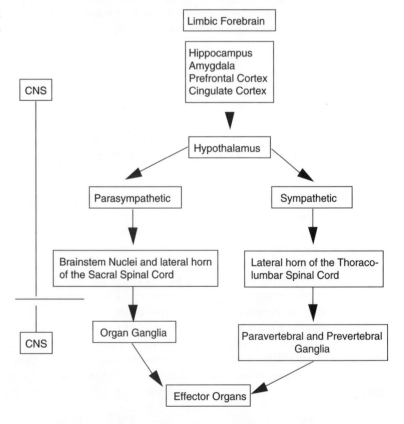

The mechanism of transmission in the neuromuscular junction of the somatic system involves ionotrophic principles.[2] The mechanism uses the ion-gated channels to quickly depolarize the cell membrane, a process referred to as fast transmission. Conversely, chemical signaling in the autonomic peripheral nervous system chiefly uses metabotrophic principles and volume transmission,[3] the diffusion of transmitter substance away from axonal vesicles. These latter methods of signaling usually involve a neuromodulator that activates a second-messenger pathway within the target cell. These methods are also called slow transmission. To further understand the distinction between somatic and visceral peripheral nervous systems, compare the typical neural circuitry present in reflex arcs.

SOMATIC REFLEX ARC

Input and output for the peripheral somatic nervous system occur through spinal and cranial nerves. Figure 5.2 diagrams a typical spinal nerve illustrating the basic circuitry of the somatic reflex arc. In its simplest form, the reflex arc contains a primary afferent neuron in a ganglion and a centrally located motoneuron connected by a synaptic junction. Since only one synapse separates the input from the output, this circuit is called a monosynaptic reflex. The cell body of the primary sensory neuron is located in the dorsal root ganglia or in the peripheral ganglia of a cranial nerve. The peripheral process of the sensory neuron is directed outward along a spinal or cranial nerve to reach its target in the peripheral tissue. This process either acts as a receptor end organ itself or is attached to one located in skin, muscle, or connective tissue. Each sensory neuron also has a central process (axon) that extends into the dorsal horn of the spinal cord or into the brainstem.

Two fundamental types of primary afferent neurons are present in sensory ganglia. One class of sensory neuron features a large cell body with a myelinated process; this kind of cell forms the A-afferent system and is involved in proprioception or discriminative mechanoreception.[4] Conversely, other sensory neurons have small cell bodies, with lightly myelinated or unmyelinated processes. These cells form the B-afferent system and are involved in crude touch and nociception.[4]

The second component of the monosynaptic reflex arc, the motor neuron, has a cell body in the ventral horn of the spinal cord or a brainstem nucleus with long dendrites that ramify in the surrounding gray matter and receive synapses from the central processes of primary afferent neurons. Motor neuron axons leave the central nervous system in the ventral root of a spinal nerve or in a cranial nerve, eventually innervating its effector organ, skeletal muscle, through a neuromuscular synaptic junction. These monosynaptic reflex connections occur between the largest sensory neurons (the A-afferent system) and ventral horn motoneurons innervating skeletal muscle.

All other somatic reflexes involve the presence of interneurons situated between the central processes of the sensory neuron and the motoneurons; several synaptic connections must be traversed to complete the arc. Such circuits are called disynaptic or polysynaptic reflex arcs. The polysynaptic reflexes involve input from both A-afferent and B-afferent systems. Although the addition of interneurons into the circuit slows the conduction of information through these reflex arcs, it greatly facilitates the construction of more complex circuits and, consequently, more complicated behavior patterns in response to sensory information.

AUTONOMIC REFLEX ARC

Input and output for the peripheral autonomic nervous system occurs via spinal, cranial, and splanchnic (visceral) nerves. Figure 5.3 is a diagram of a typical spinal nerve and its connections with a splanchnic nerve. The afferent neuron has a peripheral process ending in a visceral organ, a cell body located in the dorsal root ganglia, and a central process that terminates in the dorsal horn of spinal cord. This central process terminates on interneurons that, in turn, innervate the effector (motor or pseudomotor) neurons in the gray matter of the spinal cord or brainstem. The effector or preganglionic neurons are found in the lateral horn of the spinal cord or in specific brainstem nuclei; their myelinated preganglionic axons terminate on ganglionic neurons located outside of the central nervous system. These peripheral neurons are found either in encapsulated ganglia in the fascia of the body wall or in ganglia embedded in the fascia surrounding a specific organ. Unmyelinated, postganglionic axons travel from these ganglia to cellular targets in visceral organs. The presence of two sequential neurons in its output pathway is a critical feature distinguishing the autonomic from somatic peripheral nervous systems. The sensory neurons of these two systems are otherwise very similar in morphology and function.

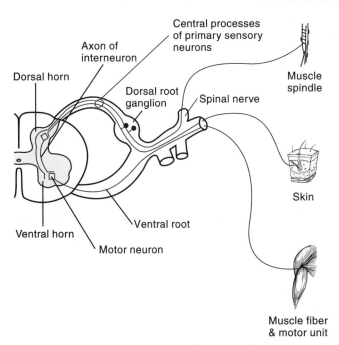

Figure 5.2. Components of somatic reflex arc.

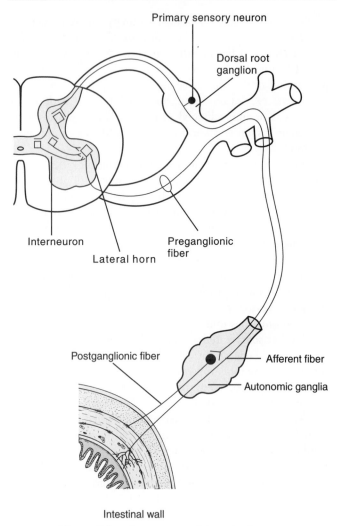

Figure 5.3. Components of visceral reflex arc.

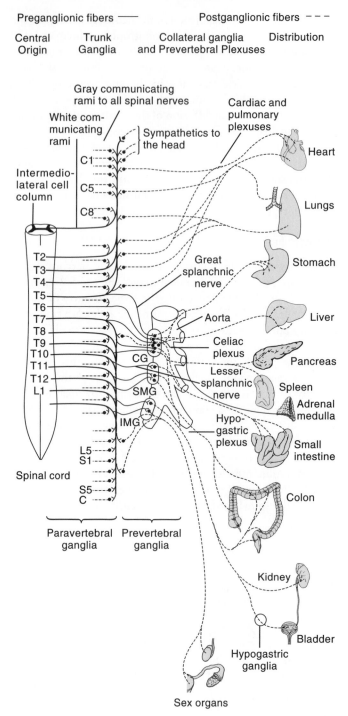

Figure 5.4. Sympathetic division of peripheral autonomic system. *CG*, celiac ganglion; *SMG*, superior mesenteric ganglion; *IMG*, inferior mesenteric ganglion. (Modified from Chusid JG. *Correlative Neuroanatomy and Functional Neurology*. Los Altos, Calif: Lange Medical Publishers; 1985.)

Ganglionic neurons of the autonomic system are found primarily in three locations (Fig. 5.4):

1. The paravertebral ganglia or sympathetic trunk lying along the side of the spinal cord
2. The prevertebral ganglia or collateral ganglia scattered in several clusters associated with the large vessels of the abdominal cavity
3. In isolated ganglia or hypogastric ganglia embedded in the adventitial tissue of specific visceral organs of the pelvis

These ganglia contain a variety of chemically differentiated neurons producing numerous neuroregulators. Preganglionic axons innervate multiple neurons within each ganglia. Values of 1:15 to 1:20 are the ratio between preganglionic and postganglionic axons; this suggests a very divergent system. One study has even found a ratio of 1:196 in the human superior cervical ganglion.[5] This arrangement of a few central neurons influencing effector organs through a large battery of chemically distinct, postganglionic neurons allows for a limited number of input channels to initiate numerous, complex motor and secretomotor responses.

Many of the ganglia in the output channels also contain sensory neurons that do not communicate with the central nervous system; instead, their axons terminate on ganglionic efferent cells. Local reflex arcs are established that do not communicate with the central nervous system. In this respect, the visceral autonomic ganglia act as small brains; in fact, some visceral organ function can be maintained by the ganglia even when all communication with the central nervous system is severed. In such cases, even though the organ responds to changing internal stimuli, it is not able to respond to changes in external stimuli. Autonomic ganglia are capable of managing their specific organ systems in isolation but rely on input from the central nervous system for signals concerning the conditions in the external environment.

Divisions of Autonomic Nervous System

The peripheral autonomic nervous system can be separated into two major divisions based on structure, chemistry, and function: sympathetic and parasympathetic. In general, each organ receives innervation from both divisions, one acting to enhance or accelerate the activity of the organ and the other division acting as an inhibitor or de-accelerator. The major exception to this rule is the innervation of the peripheral vasculature, hair follicles, and sweat glands of the trunk and extremities. These latter structures are serviced solely by the sympathetic system. Two chemically distinct components of the sympathetic system are involved, catecholaminergic and cholinergic, thereby providing a dual innervation. The distribution of the sympathetic nervous system is illustrated in Figure 5.4 and that of the parasympathetic nervous system in Figure 5.5.

A morphological distinction between sympathetic and parasympathetic systems is seen in the arrangement of their ganglia. In general, the ganglionic neurons of the sympathetic nervous system are located in the paravertebral and prevertebral ganglia with the exception of a few scattered neurons found in the hypogastric plexus of the pelvis. Those of the parasympathetic nervous system are found in ganglia located on organ walls. The preganglionic axons of the sympathetic system tend to be short, reaching only to the paravertebral and prevertebral ganglia, while the postganglionic axons, which reach to the visceral organs, are longer. The situation is reversed in the parasympathetic system where the preganglionic axons tend to be long, extending all the way to the ganglia in the organ wall, and the postganglionic axons short, being confined to a distribution along the organ wall (Fig. 5.6).

This distinction between the major divisions of the autonomic nervous system is further reflected in their chemistry. The sympathetic system arises from cholinergic preganglionic neurons located in the lateral horn of the thoracic and lumbar spinal cord; it is also called the thoracolumbar system. In general, the postganglionic neurons of the sympathetic system secrete norepinephrine. However, there are important exceptions. For example, some cholinergic ganglionic neurons contribute to the innervation of the peripheral vasculature and sweat glands. The parasympathetic system arises from cholin-

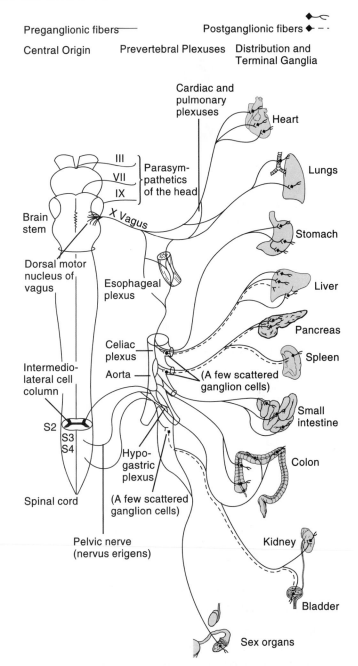

Figure 5.5. Parasympathetic division of peripheral autonomic system. (Modified from Chusid JG. *Correlative Neuroanatomy and Functional Neurology.* Los Altos, Calif: Lange Medical Publishers; 1985.)

ergic preganglionic neurons located in either cranial nerve nuclei of the brainstem or the lateral horn of the sacral spinal cord and is called the craniosacral system. The postganglionic neurons of the parasympathetic system secrete acetylcholine and a wide variety of other neuron modulators such as the neuropeptides. Given that these two divisions of the autonomic nervous system can be differentiated on the basis of their anatomy and chemistry, it is not surprising that they have differing influences on their target organs.

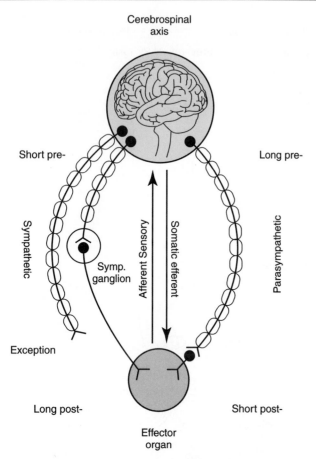

Figure 5.6. Major anatomical differences between sympathetic and parasympathetic divisions of autonomic system. (Modified from Harati Y. Anatomy of the spinal and peripheral autonomic nervous system. In: Low P, ed. *Clinical Autonomic Disorders.* Boston, Mass: Little, Brown & Co; 1993.)

SYMPATHETIC AUTONOMIC NERVOUS SYSTEM

The sympathetic autonomic nervous system has two distinct components: vascular and visceral. The vascular component is associated with the spinal nerves and innervates:

Fascia
Smooth muscle of vasculature
Smooth muscle of hair follicles
Secretory cells in the sweat glands of the skin

The visceral component innervates:

Smooth muscle
Cardiac muscle
Nodal tissue
Glandular organs of the thoracic, abdominal, pelvic, and perineal viscera

Also, portions of the sympathetic visceral component provide an innervation to the neurons of the parasympathetic ganglia in the walls of the visceral organs.

The ganglionic neurons of the sympathetic autonomic nervous system are located in two types of ganglia: paravertebral and prevertebral (Fig. 5.4). The paravertebral ganglia form two long chains, the sympathetic trunks, located on either side of the vertebral column (Fig. 5.7). Each sympathetic trunk extends from the upper cervical vertebrae, along the heads of the ribs in the thorax, on the sides of the lumbar vertebral bodies in the abdomen, and along the ventromedial aspect of the sacroiliac joint in the pelvis. Inferiorly, the two trunks terminate by uniting to form the ganglion impar, a small neural structure on the ventral aspect of the coccygeal vertebrae. The three major prevertebral ganglia are found in clusters, embedded in the abdominal plexuses that surround the anterior branches of

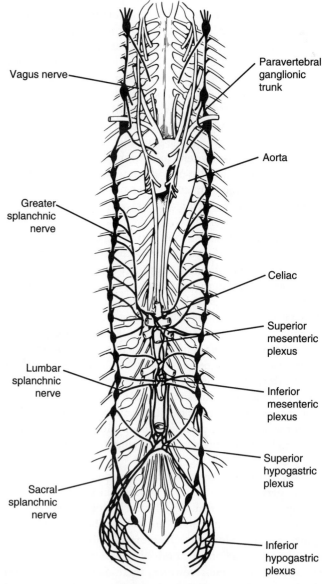

Figure 5.7. Paravertebral ganglia (sympathetic trunk) lying along median axis of body. (Modified from Rohen JW, Yokochi C. *Color Atlas of Anatomy.* New York, NY: Igaku-Shoin; 1983.)

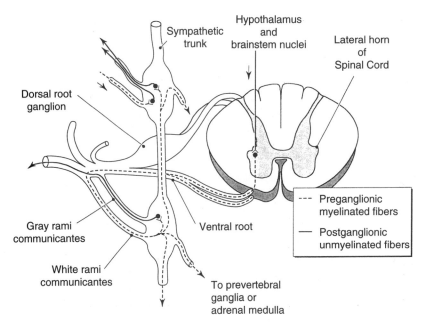

Figure 5.8. Neuronal circuitry present in typical peripheral thoracic spinal segment. (Modified from Harati Y. Anatomy of the spinal and peripheral autonomic nervous system. In: Low P, ed. *Clinical Autonomic Disorders.* Boston, Mass: Little, Brown & Co; 1993.)

the aorta. Additional small clusters of prevertebral ganglia are found scattered in the autonomic plexus of the pelvic basin.

The detailed organization of the sympathetic system is illustrated in Figure 5.4. The following features are critical:

1. All preganglionic cell bodies are located in the lateral horn of spinal cord segments mainly between T1 and L2; however, this can extend as high as C7 and as low as L3. Their axons leave the spinal cord through ventral roots T1-L2 and course along the corresponding spinal nerves to reach white communicating rami (Fig. 5.8). The white rami carry the myelinated, preganglionic fibers from the spinal nerve directly into the paravertebral ganglia. They also carry sensory processes from the vasculature and viscera back to the spinal nerve.

2. The paravertebral ganglia are present on both sides of the spinal cord at:

    3 cervical segments (superior, middle, and stellate)
    11 thoracic segments
    4 lumbar segments
    At least 3 or 4 sacral segments

    Often the upper thoracic and lower cervical ganglia are fused to form the stellate ganglion. Only the ganglia between T1 and L2 receive white rami since preganglionic fibers arise from only these segments.

3. Neurons in paravertebral ganglia located either above T1 or below L2 receive their innervation from preganglionic fibers arising in spinal segments T1-L2. These preganglionic axons enter the sympathetic trunk at their segmental level of origin and ascend or descend through the trunk to reach ganglia positioned above or below T1-L2.

4. Ganglionic neurons, destined to innervate blood vessels, smooth muscles, and glands of the skin, are found in all the paravertebral ganglia. Their postganglionic axons gain access to spinal nerves by passing over gray rami (Fig. 5.8). All para-

vertebral ganglia give rise to gray rami; each spinal nerve receives at least one gray ramus. The postganglionic axons follow the spinal nerves distally before shifting to assume a position in the fascia along the wall of a blood vessel.

5. Ganglionic neurons with axons innervating thoracic, abdominal, and pelvic viscera are found in the three cervical ganglia, the upper five thoracic paravertebral ganglia, and the prevertebral ganglia. These are the celiac and the superior and inferior mesenteric ganglia, as well as small scattered ganglia in the pelvic plexus. These prevertebral ganglia receive their preganglionic axons through thoracic, lumbar, and sacral splanchnic nerves. The term splanchnic refers to the viscera; splanchnic nerves are simply visceral nerves. Thoracic, lumbar, and sacral splanchnic nerves carry sympathetic fibers and pelvic splanchnic nerves carry parasympathetic fibers.

The sympathetic ganglia receive information from the central nervous system through the axons of the preganglionic neurons. A preganglionic axon of the sympathetic system, after passing through a white ramus between T1 and L2 to enter a paravertebral ganglion, has a number of options:

1. It can innervate a ganglionic neuron in the paravertebral ganglion at its spinal cord level of entry.

2. It can pass either up or down in the sympathetic trunk to innervate ganglionic neurons located at levels not serviced by white rami.

3. It can proceed through the paravertebral ganglia without forming synaptic contacts, join a thoracic, lumbar, or sacral splanchnic nerve, and subsequently innervate a neuron in one of the retroperitoneal prevertebral ganglia.

These options are diagrammed in Figure 5.8, which illustrates a typical thoracic spinal segment and its accompanying spinal nerve and paravertebral ganglia. The significance of these innervation patterns are considered further as the innervation of specific organs are examined.

PARASYMPATHETIC AUTONOMIC NERVOUS SYSTEM

The parasympathetic autonomic nervous system, unlike its sympathetic counterpart, innervates only visceral organs and blood vessels in the:

Head and neck
Thorax
Abdomen
Pelvis

The parasympathetic nervous system lacks a division innervating the peripheral vasculature of the extremities and trunk. The parasympathetic system is divided into two portions: cranial and sacral. These are based on the location of its preganglionic neurons (Figs. 5.5 and 5.9). The cranial portion consists of several brainstem nuclei and their preganglionic nerves. Cranial

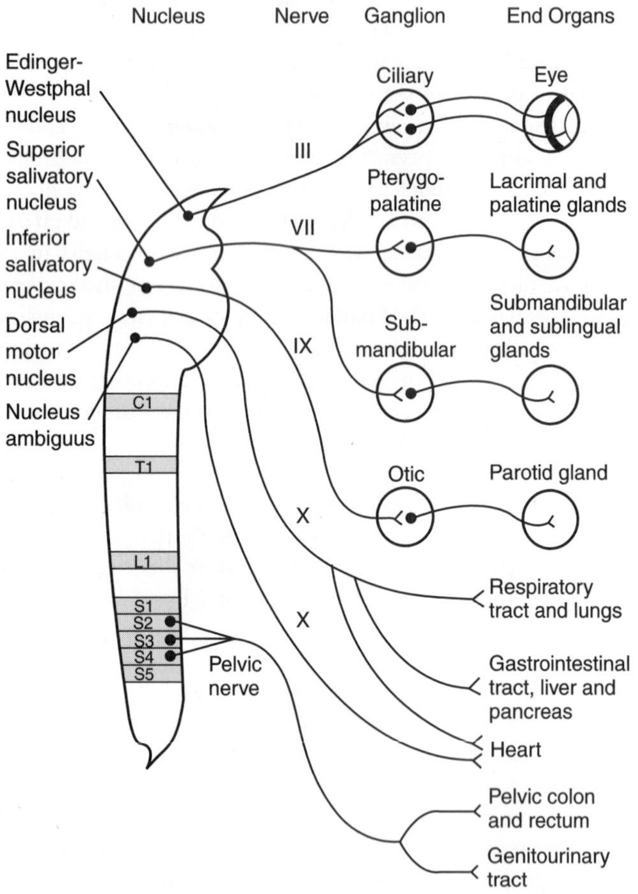

Figure 5.9. Summary of parasympathetic nervous system emphasizing distribution of cranial nerves III, VII, IX, and X. (Modified from Barron KD, Chokroverty S. Anatomy of the autonomic nervous system: brain and brainstem. In: Low P, ed. *Clinical Autonomic Disorders*. Boston, Mass: Little, Brown & Co; 1993.)

nerves III, VII, and IX give rise to parasympathetic preganglionic fibers that innervate ganglia located in the:

Orbit (ciliary ganglion)
Sphenopalatine fossa (sphenopalatine ganglion)
Inferior temporal fossa (otic ganglion)
Floor of the mouth (submandibular and sublingual ganglia)

Cranial nerve X, the vagus, innervates ganglia in the organs of the cervical, thoracic, and superior portions of the abdominal viscera.

The vagus nerve is a significant source of parasympathetic innervation to the thoracic and upper abdominal viscera. It enters the thoracic cavity along the upper portion of the mediastinal wall and passes posterior to the root of the lung to gain a position on the walls of the esophagus. Vagal branches are given off to the cardiac and pulmonary plexuses and to the esophageal plexus. Through the vagus, the nucleus ambiguus contributes innervation to the pharynx, larynx, and skeletal muscle portion of the upper esophagus. Preganglionic vagal fibers from the dorsal motor nucleus in the medulla terminate in ganglia on the walls of each organ beginning in the upper esophagus. From these ganglia the postganglionic fibers arise and course in and around the smooth muscle layers and glands of the organ. The left and right trunks of the vagus rotate around the esophagus (due to the fetal rotation of the gut), forming the anterior and posterior trunks of the vagus, respectively. At the distal end of the esophagus, these two trunks slip through the esophageal hiatus of the diaphragm riding in the fatty adventitial fascia of the esophageal walls. The identity of the vagus nerve is lost as its axons join the celiac plexus. These vagal preganglionic fibers continue in the celiac and superior mesenteric plexus to reach the full extent of these two corresponding neurovascular territories. The vagal preganglionic axons reach only as far inferiorly as the splenic flexure of the colon.

The lower portion of the gastrointestinal tract, distal to the splenic flexure, as well as the pelvic viscera receive their parasympathetic innervation from the pelvic splanchnic nerves. These latter nerves form the sacral component of the parasympathetic nervous system. The preganglionic neurons are located in the lateral horn of spinal cord segments S2-4. Their axons exit the spinal cord by traveling in the sacral nerve roots. As these roots pass through the endopelvic fascia, small pelvic splanchnic nerves branch off. These branches quickly join the inferior hypogastric plexus (pelvic plexus) also located in the endopelvic fascia. Through this plexus, the preganglionic axons can reach the visceral organs of the pelvic basin such as the urinary bladder, the internal reproductive organs, and the rectum. By ascending along the hypogastric plexus, these axons also enter the inferior mesenteric plexus of the abdomen.

From this point the preganglionic axons follow the vascular branches of the inferior mesenteric artery to service its structures such as the descending and sigmoid colon. The preganglionic axons of the vagus and of the pelvic splanchnic nerves terminate in ganglia located in the walls of the abdominopelvic viscera. Short, postganglionic axons invade the organ to terminate in layers of smooth muscle and in surrounding glands. The pattern of parasympathetic innervation of the visceral organs continues in an uninterrupted manner through the abdominopelvic cavity even though the source of this innervation shifts from cranial origins to sacral origins at the splenic flexure of the large bowel.

The autonomic nervous system provides input to the:

Vasculature and fascias
Organs of the head
Organs of the neck
Organs of the thoracoabdominopelvic cavity
Spleen
Thymus
Bone marrow
Lymph modes

The remainder of the chapter focuses on the innervation of the vasculature, fascia, and major organs. The innervation of the immune glands are examined in the chapter on the neuroendocrine-immune network (Chapter 9).

Primary Afferent Fibers

The autonomic nervous system is not strictly an efferent system.[6] All nerves containing autonomic efferent axons also carry primary afferent fibers. The principal targets of these primary afferent fibers are the:

Dorsal horn of the spinal cord from approximately T1-L2 and S2-S4
Solitary nucleus of the vagal complex in the medulla

Although the majority of primary afferent fibers in autonomic nerves are of the small caliber variety (B-afferent system), some larger, myelinated fibers are also present (A-afferent system). In general, the input over visceral afferent fibers to the medullary brainstem involves the nonnoxious regulation of organ function. Conversely, many of the primary afferent fibers targeting the spinal cord have the characteristics of nociceptive fibers. They produce neuropeptides such as substance-P and calcitonin gene-related polypeptide and respond to nociceptive stimuli. In addition, some are capable of eliciting a neurogenic inflammatory response in the surrounding tissue.[7,8] Nociceptive input from these fibers to the spinal cord can facilitate spinal segments. This initiates vasomotor changes and alters the output to somatic musculature (viscerosomatic reflexes) as well as refers pain to the somatic structures.[9,10]

REGIONAL DISTRIBUTION OF THE AUTONOMIC NERVOUS SYSTEM

Peripheral Vasculature

The vascular tree is divided into four different types of vessels based on their distinctive functions:[11]

1. Conduit vessels comprise the arterial system prior to arterioles.
2. Resistance vessels represent arterioles.

3. Exchange vessels are capillaries.
4. Capacitance vessels consist of veins.

Most aspects of the vascular tree receive an efferent innervation that controls the resistance of these vessels to blood flow.[11-13] Different types of axons in these vascular nerves can be identified by their neurochemistry. Sensory fibers, coursing in the vascular nerves, typically contain neuropeptides such as substance-P and calcitonin gene-related polypeptide. Efferent axons in the peripheral autonomic nerves can be:[11]

Adrenergic
Cholinergic
Histaminergic
Purinergic

In general, the adrenergic fibers function as constrictors, contracting smooth muscle in the tunica media and increasing the resistance in the peripheral vasculature. These norepinephrine-containing fibers arise from the paravertebral ganglia of the sympathetic nervous system and innervate all vasculature of the body. Cholinergic fibers are much fewer in number in most tissue and are vasodilating in nature. These nerves are of mixed origin, some arising from parasympathetic ganglia and some from sympathetic origin (the sympathetic–cholinergic system). Cholinergic axons from ganglia of the parasympathetic nervous system participate in the innervation of vasculature in the head and neck and in the visceral organs of the thorax, abdomen, and pelvis. A few cholinergic axons from the sympathetic ganglia also reach visceral vasculature, but they are far more numerous in the vasculature in the trunk of the body. They provide exclusive cholinergic innervation of resistance vessels in the extremities. Purinergic and histaminergic axons also mediate relaxation of vascular wall smooth muscle, but their origin and role in vasodilation are not clear.[11]

The sympathetic innervation of blood vessels in muscle and skin is accomplished by preganglionic neurons located in the lateral horn of spinal segments T2 through L2-3. Their axons leave the spinal cord in the ventral roots and pass through white rami to innervate neurons located in the paravertebral ganglia (Fig. 5.8). Vasomotor neurons present in the paravertebral ganglia give rise to axons that leave the ganglia over the gray rami to rejoin the spinal nerves. In this way they reach the somatic peripheral tissue where they innervate blood vessels, sweat glands, and hair follicles. As such, these axons are called vasomotor or sudorisecretory fibers. A topographic map of the vasculature in the body is contained within paravertebral ganglia such that:[14,15]

1. The vasomotor fibers to the head and neck come from spinal segments T1-4. Their axons travel up the sympathetic trunk to reach the cervical ganglia. Postganglionic axons follow the carotid vascular tree to reach the head and neck. Segments T1-T2 provide innervation for the brain and meninges; T2-T4 provides innervation to the vasculature of the face and neck.[14]
2. The vasomotor fibers to the upper extremity come from spinal segments T5-7. Their axons course rostrally in the sympathetic

trunk to reach the upper thoracic and lower cervical ganglia. Postganglionic axons join the spinal nerves of the brachial plexus to reach the vasculature of the upper extremity.

3. The vasomotor fibers to the lower extremity come from spinal segments T10 through L2-3. Their axons descend in the sympathetic trunk to reach the lower lumbar and sacral ganglia. Postganglionic axons join the spinal nerves of the lumbosacral plexus to reach the vasculature of the lower extremity.

Sympathetic fibers course along the outer border of the tunica media of the artery and secrete their neuroregulators into the extracellular fluids surrounding the vascular smooth muscle. Most sympathetic fibers release norepinephrine from small swellings along the terminal distribution of the axon. This neuromodulator interacts with its specific receptors on the vascular smooth muscle cell membranes. Both α- and β-adrenergic receptors are present on these plasma membranes. Activation of α-adrenoceptors leads to contraction of the smooth muscle cells and vasoconstriction, while activation of the β-adrenoceptors mediates relaxation of the muscle cell, resulting in vasodilatation. In general, the α-adrenoceptors predominate on the smooth muscle of resistance vessels; adrenergic stimulation yields vasoconstriction in skeletal muscle.

Additional control of skeletal muscle resistance arteries is accomplished through numerous endothelium-derived substances such as the vasodilator nitric oxide or the vasoconstrictors prostacyclin, endothelin, and angiotensin.[16] The tone in the vessel wall is the product of a complex interaction of these vasoactive substances.[17] In certain skeletal muscle vascular beds there are sympathetic axons that also secrete acetylcholine and vasoactive intestinal polypeptide, two neuroregulators usually associated with the ganglionic neurons of the parasympathetic system. These substances act on vascular smooth muscle to facilitate dilation of the vessel and as such represent a sympathetic vasodilator system. The cholinergic fibers do not appear to innervate the cutaneous vascular tree; instead, a nonadrenergic, noncholinergic vasodilatory mechanism exists for these vessels.[18]

Along with the output to the vascular tree, afferent or sensory fibers also course in the walls of the blood vessels. Little is known of the sensory feedback to the spinal cord provided by these fibers. The nomenclature of these afferent fibers is confusing since it is not clear whether they are somatic or visceral afferent fibers. Jinkins et al.[19] have called the vascular afferent fibers found in somatic tissue somatosympathetic fibers since they course through somatic tissue but are related to the autonomic nervous system. However, since these afferent fibers are generally of small caliber and contain an array of neuropeptides such as substance-P, much of the information they carry is most likely related to nociceptive stimuli. The normal, baseline release of such neuropeptides as substance-P from these fibers may play an important role in maintaining vascular tone.[20] The small caliber, primary afferent fibers appear to have additional homeostatic functions in the peripheral tissue beyond that of nociception.

When irritated, some of these small caliber, sensory axons can secrete quantities of substance-P, a proinflammatory, vasodilatory neuropeptide, into the surrounding tissue. This release of an inflammatory agent from a peripheral nerve terminal is involved in initiating the processes of neurogenic inflammation and edema.[21] Neurogenic inflammation is a critical component in inflammatory joint disease; this suggests an important role for the small caliber, primary afferent fibers in these diseases.[22]

An interaction between sensory axons and sympathetic neurons appears to occur in the peripheral tissues. Sympathetic adrenergic terminals often end in close association with the peripheral processes of sensory neurons. Secretion of norepinephrine can increase the levels of prostaglandins E_2 and I_2 in the tissue.[23] Prostaglandins are irritating to many small caliber, primary afferent fibers. Sufficient sympathetic discharge can result in a nociceptive input to the spinal cord. In addition, evidence strongly suggests that small caliber, primary afferent fibers can become sensitized to sympathetic nervous system activity.[23] This interaction between sympathetic efferent axons and primary afferent neurons is a possible mechanism for sympathetically dependent hyperalgesia such as is present in reflex sympathetic dystrophy.[24]

Sweat Glands and Connective Tissue

Along with innervating the vasculature, the autonomic fibers also provide an innervation to sweat glands and fascia. Sweat glands receive an exclusively cholinergic innervation from the sympathetic trunk ganglia, through the sympathetic–cholinergic system.[12] These cholinergic fibers stimulate secretory activity in the gland.

The connective tissues of the body are innervated by small caliber, primary afferent fibers. These fibers, many containing neuropeptides, along with adrenergic sympathetic axons are found coursing throughout the fascias of the body. The relationship between these fibers and the connective tissue components of the fascia is seen in such tissue as the:

Cranial dura[25,26]
Gastrointestinal tract[27]
Synovium of diarthrodial joints[28]

In several locations, such as joints, these fibers have been demonstrated to play a role in modulating the cellular components (mast cells) of the connective tissue and to contribute to the maintenance of tissue integrity.[28,29] Finally, the interaction of these two fiber types appears to play an important role in the maintenance of normal vascular tone in connective tissue.[20]

Head and Neck

The autonomic innervation of the head and neck arises from two general sources: sympathetic and parasympathetic. The sympathetic innervation originates in the intermediolateral nucleus of the upper thoracic segments (T1-T4) of the spinal cord, and their ganglionic neurons are located in the cervical sympathetic ganglia of the neck. Postganglionic fibers from the superior cervical ganglion gain access to the head by following the course of the carotid and vertebral arteries and the jugular vein. The parasympathetic innervation originates from several nuclei in the brainstem; the ganglionic neurons are located in these ganglia (Fig. 5.9):

Ciliary sphenopalatine
Otic
Geniculate

Recently, additional parasympathetic ganglia located on the walls of the internal carotid artery have been described.[30–32] The autonomic innervation of the cranial viscera, the function of these nerves, and the neurology of their dysfunctioning are amply described elsewhere.[14,33–36]

The third cranial nerve contains parasympathetic axons that arise in the Edinger-Westphal nucleus of the midbrain and innervate the ciliary ganglion of the eye (Fig. 5.9). They are responsible for constricting the pupil through the pupillary sphincter muscles and contracting the ciliary body to thicken the lens in the accommodation reflex. The facial (VII) cranial nerve carries parasympathetic preganglionic axons from the superior salivatory and lacrimal nuclei in the pontine region of the brainstem. These secretomotor and vasomotor axons course along the superficial petrosal nerve to reach sphenopalatine ganglion. Postganglionic axons follow branches of the trigeminal nerve to reach the lacrimal gland and mucosal glands of the nasal and oral cavities. Preganglionic axons from the superior salivatory nucleus also follow the chorda tympani, a branch of the facial nerve, to reach the submandibular and sublingual ganglia. Postganglionic axons from these ganglia supply the salivatory glands on the floor of the mouth. The glossopharyngeal nerve carries secretomotor and vasomotor axons from the inferior salivatory nucleus located at the pontomedullary border to the otic ganglion. These latter axons pass over the lesser petrosal nerve. Postganglionic axons from the otic ganglion extend to the parotid gland over branches of the third division of the trigeminal nerve.

Cranial nerve X, the vagus, is the largest of the parasympathetic nerves. It supplies preganglionic parasympathetic innervation of the viscera in the thorax and abdomen to the level of the transverse colon. Efferent vagal axons arise in the dorsal motor nucleus and nucleus ambiguus of the medulla. The vagus is largely a sensory nerve; afferent fibers outnumber efferent fibers in the mammalian vagus by more than 10:1.[37] These sensory fibers include the afferent innervation of the thoracoabdominal viscera and the general sensory innervation of the:

Pharynx
Larynx
Skin of the ear
External auditory meatus
External surface of the tympanic membrane

The cell bodies for these afferent fibers are located in the two nuclei of the vagus: the superior (jugular) ganglion and the inferior ganglion. Their central brainstem targets include the nucleus solitarius, nucleus ambiguus, and spinal trigeminal nucleus.

An area of much recent interest is the autonomic innervation of the vascular and dural systems in the head. Preganglionic sympathetic input to the cranial vasculature and dura arises in the upper thoracic spinal segments. Those controlling the vasculature of the brain and meninges are located in segments T1-T2, and those involved with the vasculature of the face and neck are located in T2-T4.[14] Ganglionic neurons are located in the superior cervical sympathetic ganglion and in small ganglia embedded in the fibers of the internal carotid nerve.[15] Their axons course along the carotid arteries; those going to the cerebral vessels and dura form the well-developed internal carotid nerve. Within the dura, the adrenergic fibers diverge away from the vasculature to form a dense plexus within the connective tissue substrate of the dura itself.[26] The extensive autonomic innervation may play a role in regulating the metabolic activity of the dural tissue. The sympathetic innervation of the dura and associated vasculature is of interest due to its possible role in the cause of migraine headache.[38]

Parasympathetic axons innervating the cerebral vasculature arise in these ganglia: sphenopalatine, otic, and internal carotid.[39–42] Axons from the ganglia contain acetylcholine and neuropeptides such as vasoactive intestinal polypeptide and neuropeptide-Y, among others.[31,43] The axons form a delicate plexus wrapped around cerebral arteries as they travel through the subarachnoid space. Also present in the plexus surrounding the cerebral vessels are primary afferent fibers containing neuropeptides such as substance-P and calcitonin gene-related polypeptide. These fibers arise in the ophthalmic and maxillary divisions of the trigeminal ganglion.[44] Similar primary afferent fibers containing substance-P and calcitonin gene-related polypeptide have been described in the dura mater.[26] Some of these fibers form free-endings and are postulated to form trophic relationships with the connective tissue cells in the dura such as the fibroblast and mast cells. Release of these proinflammatory peptides has been indicated in the pathogenesis of certain inflammatory headaches such as the migraine and cluster varieties.[45,46]

Thorax

A great autonomic plexus of fibers extends from the superior mediastinum downward through the posterior mediastinum and, using the esophageal hiatus of the diaphragm as a conduit, continues into the abdominopelvic cavity (Fig. 5.10). The thoracic component of this conjoint plexus is derived from the vagus nerve and its branches and from splanchnic branches from the paravertebral ganglia. Superiorly, this complex arrangement of fibers contains the cardiac and pulmonary plexuses; inferiorly in the thorax it contains the esophageal plexus.

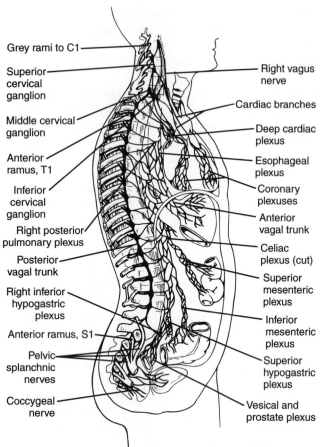

Figure 5.10. Great autonomic plexus extending from lower cervical region, through thorax and abdomen to reach pelvis. (Modified from Bannister LH, Berry MM, Collins P, Dyson M, Dussek JE, Ferguson MWJ, eds. *Gray's Anatomy*. New York, NY: Churchill Livingstone; 1995.)

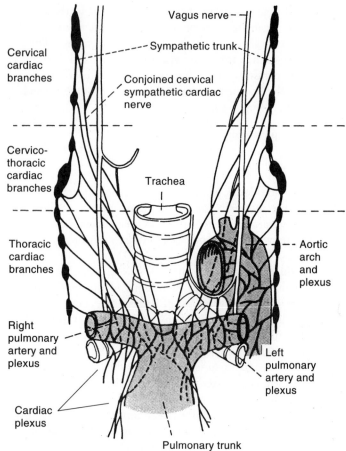

Figure 5.11. Nerve supply of heart. (Modified from Bonica JJ. General considerations of pain in the chest. In: Bonica JJ. *The Management of Pain*. Philadelphia, Pa: Lea & Febiger; 1990.)

Branches from the great autonomic plexus supply the following with afferent and efferent nerves:

Heart
Trachea
Bronchi
Lungs
Esophagus
Thoracic duct

The thoracic viscera receive sympathetic preganglionic axons arising in spinal cord segments T1 through T5 or T6. These axons synapse with ganglionic neurons in the superior, middle, and inferior cervical ganglia and in the sympathetic trunk ganglia T1 to T5-T6. Sympathetic postganglionic axons from the paravertebral ganglia join the conjoint plexus of the thorax via a series of small, delicate cardiac, pulmonary, and esophageal nerves. Within the thoracic portion of the great autonomic plexus, sympathetic cardiac and pulmonary nerves descend through the superior mediastinum joining with similarly named parasympathetic branches from the vagus and recurrent

laryngeal nerves. They form the complex cardiopulmonary plexus of fibers surrounding the great vessels of the heart (Fig. 5.11) and the vasculature and airway structures of the lungs (Fig. 5.12). The individual superior, middle, and inferior cardiac nerves of the sympathetic trunk and vagus are extremely inconsistent in actual form.[47] The esophageal sympathetic nerves arise from the thoracic paravertebral ganglia and course diagonally downward across the thoracic vertebral bodies to reach the adventitial fascia surround the esophagus in the posterior mediastinum. Here they join with the main trunks of the vagus nerve (parasympathetic) to form the esophageal plexus.

The mixing of parasympathetic and sympathetic axons begins in the most superior aspect of the great autonomic plexus, as it extends upward into the cervical region. Scattered communicating branches unite the vagus and recurrent laryngeal nerves with the sympathetic trunk. Therefore, even at the most superior aspect of the plexus there are no pure sympathetic or parasympathetic nerves. All fibers in the plexus contain a mixture of afferent and efferent axons, so the plexus cannot be considered a purely efferent structure.

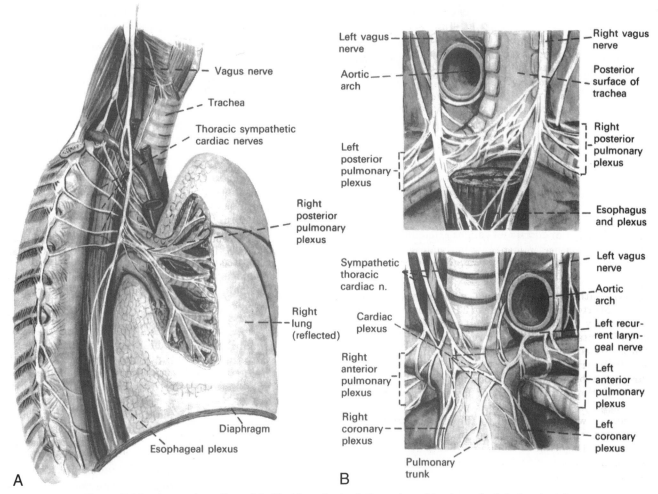

Figure 5.12.   Innervation of lung. (Modified from Bonica JJ. General considerations of pain in the chest. In:
Bonica JJ. *The Management of Pain.* Philadelphia, Pa: Lea & Febiger; 1990:981.)

Cardiovascular

The cardiac plexus consists of a mixture of sympathetic and parasympathetic fibers, as well as afferent fibers, surrounding the great vessels of the heart (Fig. 5.11). Preganglionic sympathetic cardiac fibers arise in the nucleus intermediolateralis of the lateral horn of spinal cord segments T1-5. The ventricular innervation is represented in the higher thoracic segments, while the atrial representation is found in the lower segments.[48] The preganglionic axons of these neurons enter the sympathetic trunk over upper thoracic white rami. Most of these fibers ascend in the trunk to reach their ganglionic neurons primarily in the cervical ganglia. Variable numbers of cervical and thoracic sympathetic cardiac nerves leave the cervical and upper thoracic ganglia, course through the fascia of the mediastinum, and join the cardiac branches of the vagus to form the cardiac plexus. This plexus is primarily located on the walls of the pulmonary arterial tree.[49] Adrenergic, postganglionic fibers from this plexus form a rich network of fibers distributed along the coronary vasculature, coursing throughout the myo-

cardium of the atria and ventricles, as well as reaching the sinoatrial and atrioventricular nodes.[50]

Preganglionic parasympathetic fibers arise in the dorsal motor nucleus of the vagus and the nucleus ambiguus located in the medulla.[51,52] These preganglionic axons leave the vagus nerve over its variable (one to three) cardiac branches beginning in the neck and extending into the superior mediastinum. The axons target parasympathetic ganglia embedded in the cardiac plexuses. Short cholinergic axons from these ganglia reach the sinoatrial and atrioventricular nodes, and course in the myocardium of the ventricles. The parasympathetic innervation of the ventricular wall is much less dense than that of the sympathetic fibers.[50]

Stimulation of the sympathetic fibers on the left side accelerates cardiac output and is arrhythmogenic. A similar reaction is obtained by cooling the right sympathetic fibers, indicating that cardiac activity is influenced by the balance of activity between the two sympathetic inputs.[53] Stimulation of the parasympathetic vagal fibers tends to stabilize the heart rate. It appears that heart rate and volume output are influenced, in part, by the balance of tonic neural activity occurring in the vagus and sympathetic systems.

Cardiac afferent nerves are an important consideration in understanding reflex control of the heart, patterns of referred cardiac pain, and patterns of cardiac facilitated segments. Small caliber, primary afferent fibers are distributed throughout the:[54–56]

Myocardium
Coronary vasculature
Roots of its great vessel
Parietal pericardium

There are at least two different pathways for these sensory fibers. Those coursing with the sympathetic nerves have their cell bodies located in dorsal root ganglia extending from C_6 to T_7; their central processes terminate in the dorsal horn of the spinal cord.[57,58] Sensory axons coursing with the parasympathetic nerves have cell bodies located in the nodose ganglion of the vagus nerve and central processes that terminate in the solitary nucleus of the medulla. In addition to the autonomic nerves supplying an afferent innervation of the pericardium, afferent fibers reach this structure over the phrenic nerve as well. These fibers enter the spinal cord over segments C3-5.

Along with the dual origin of sensory nerves, there is a differential distribution of these two sensory pathways in the cardiovascular system. The afferent fibers of the vagus nerve terminate in the:

Ascending aorta
Aortic arch
Pulmonary trunk
Arterial walls
Atrial walls
Atrioventricular valve
Ventricular walls

The afferent fibers from the sympathetic nerves reach the:[55]

Atrial walls
Pulmonary arteries
Atrioventricular and aortic valves
Parietal peritoneum

Afferent fibers from both systems reach the coronary arteries. Those from the vagus extend to a more distal level of the vasculature closer to the apex of the heart than do afferent fibers associated with the sympathetic nervous system. Both Aδ and C afferent fibers are present in the heart;[59] many of these fibers contain neuropeptides such as substance-P or calcitonin gene-related polypeptide that are typical of small caliber, primary afferent fibers. At least one population of these cardiac C-fibers has the physiological properties of nociceptive axons.

In general, the afferent fibers coursing with the sympathetic nerves are involved with cardiac nociception; those following the parasympathetic nerves are mainly involved in reflexogenic regulation of heart functions through their brainstem connection.[57] Section of the sympathetic nerves to the heart can relieve cardiac pain in the chest, arms, and neck.[60] These cardiac afferent fibers reach the spinal cord over a range of segments from C6 to T7; the influence of these nerves can extend at least two segments below T7.[61] The signs of segmental facilitation due to cardiac disease can present in the vicinity of the cervicothoracic junction and extend downward through at least T9.[62] Importantly, the nociceptive afferent fibers reaching the dorsal horn of the spinal cord influence neurons with concomitant somatic receptive fields. This viscerosomatic convergence of nociceptive information provides an explanation for the referral of pain from cardiac structures to the body wall and extremity.[63]

Respiratory

The respiratory system receives its innervation through the large pulmonary plexus that surrounds the pulmonary artery and extends onto the posterior surface of the trachea and bronchi (Fig. 5.12). Sympathetic preganglionic neurons that contribute to this plexus are located in the lateral horn of spinal segments T2-7; their ganglionic neurons are located in the cervical and first four thoracic ganglia. Postganglionic axons from these ganglia course through cardiac and esophageal nerves from the sympathetic trunk to reach the pulmonary plexus. These adrenergic axons primarily target the glandular tissue surrounding the bronchi and bronchioles; little direct adrenergic innervation of the bronchial musculature has been noted. β-Adrenergic receptors are present on the glandular cells and on bronchial smooth muscle cells. Stimulation of the β-adrenergic, sympathetic nervous system leads to bronchial dilation and the release of a more viscous secretion.[64]

The vagus nerve is the source of parasympathetic innervation for the respiratory airways. After entering the thorax, the vagus shifts posteriorly in the mediastinum to pass around the root of the lung. Anterior and posterior pulmonary branches are given off that contribute to the pulmonary plexus. Parasympathetic ganglia in the walls of the airways receive preganglionic fibers from these vagal branches. Postganglionic parasympathetic fibers course in the arteriobronchial tree to terminate around bronchial smooth musculature, mucosal glands, and blood vessels. Stimulation of these cholinergic fibers causes:[64]

Bronchoconstriction
Hypersecretion of a serous secretion
Vasodilation

The pulmonary plexus and ganglia contain intrinsic neurons, that is, cells whose processes remain in the peripheral tissue and do not innervate the central nervous system. Such cells are called interneurons. Some of these cells produce a variety of neuropeptides, among which is vasoactive intestinal polypeptide, a potent bronchodilator.[65] In addition, several neuropeptides co-release with norepinephrine from sympathetic terminals and with acetylcholine from parasympathetic terminals. These ubiquitous neuropeptides have gained considerable interest recently due to their role in controlling the diameter of the bronchial lumen.

Small caliber, primary afferent fibers are also present in the pulmonary plexus. These fibers provide sensory information to the brainstem via the vagus and to the spinal cord via the sympathetic trunk. This information is involved in reflex arcs related to:

Sneezing
Coughing
Bronchospasms
Pulmonary congestion

Many of these fibers, and particularly the smallest of them, contain neuropeptides such as substance-P and calcitonin gene-related polypeptide, among others. Irritation of these sensory fibers results in the release of these proinflammatory substances, leading to neurogenic edema and inflammation in the lung. Substance-P, released from these sensory axons into the pulmonary parenchyma, is a potent bronchoconstrictor, vasodilator, and secretagogue.[66]

Activation of these primary afferent nociceptors can also facilitate segments in the spinal cord extending from the cervical region into the low thoracic cord.[62] The extended range of activation most likely relates to the wide distribution of the central processes of these primary afferent fibers. Changes in spinal cord activity are seen in response to pulmonary afferent stimulation; electrical stimulation of inflamed tracheobronchial mucosa produces a decrease in electrical skin resistance in the T2 to T5 dermatomes followed hours later by cutaneous hyperalgesia.[60] Unlike the heart, pain from the lungs and bronchial tree is carried in the vagal fibers as well as in the spinal afferent fibers. Lung tumors can refer pain to the skin around the ear.[67] Electrical stimulation of the laryngeal and tracheal mucosa refers pain to the neck; similar irritation of the bronchial tree refers pain to the anterior chest wall. Section of the vagus below the recurrent laryngeal branch ameliorates the pain,[68] suggesting that the vagus nerve is the conduit for this referred pain.

The costal parietal pleura surrounding the plural cavity receives an afferent in innervation derived from the intercostal nerves of the thorax; the mediastinal pleura is innervated by sensory fibers from the phrenic nerve. The plural membrane is sensitive to noxious stimuli. The visceral pleura in the lungs receives sympathetic and sensory fibers from the autonomic plexuses surrounding the bronchi but is insensitive to pain.[60]

Esophageal

The esophagus is surrounded by a plexus of autonomic nerves derived from the vagus and branches of the sympathetic trunk.[69] The preganglionic parasympathetic innervation to the rostral portion of the esophagus (skeletal muscle portion) is derived from the nucleus ambiguus; the smooth muscle of the esophagus is derived primarily from the dorsal motor nucleus of the vagus.[70] The left and right vagal trunks approach the esophagus at the root of the lung and form an elaborate plexus, which follows this structure through the esophageal hiatus in the diaphragm. The postganglionic parasympathetic neurons

are contained in two intrinsic ganglia in the walls of the esophagus: Auerbach's, or the myenteric plexus, and Meissner's, or the submucosal plexus. Preganglionic sympathetic neurons are located in the intermediolateral nucleus of spinal cord segments ranging from T2 to T8:[71]

Cervical esophageal portion
T2-T4
Thoracic esophageal portion
T3-T6
Abdominal portion
T5-T8

They synapse in the cervical and upper thoracic sympathetic ganglia. Small esophageal branches, derived from the cervical to fourth and fifth thoracic ganglia and carrying postganglionic sympathetic fibers, join the vagal plexus along the walls of the esophagus.[72]

Afferent fibers from the esophageal walls follow the vagus back to the solitary nucleus of the medulla. They also follow the sympathetic fibers back to the dorsal horn of the upper segment of the spinal cord.[73] Vagal afferent fibers ending in the solitary nucleus of the medulla contribute to a viscerovisceral reflex arc by synapsing on premotor neurons of the nucleus ambiguus. These premotor neurons subsequently innervate the motor neurons of the nucleus ambiguus. The premotor neurons form the central pattern generator for organized movements of the esophagus such as swallowing.[74] The spinal afferent fibers from the esophagus contribute to the referral of pain. These afferent fibers innervate spinal segments that also receive afferent information from the:

Heart
Pulmonary tree
Chest
Back

Esophageal pain can refer substernally (heartburn) or posteriorly through the back into the area of the scapula.[75]

Thoracic Aorta

The thoracic aorta has an intimate relationship with both divisions of the autonomic nervous system. Sympathetic input and sensory fibers reach the superior thoracic aorta through cardiac and pulmonary nerves as well as by following direct branches from the sympathetic trunk. The inferior thoracic aorta receives branches of the thoracic splanchnic nerves. The preganglionic sympathetic axons arise in the upper five thoracic spinal segments and the postganglionic fibers arise from the upper five thoracic paravertebral ganglia. Once on the wall of the aorta, these fibers form an adrenergic plexus in the adventitial tissue. Afferent fibers from this large elastic artery follow the sympathetic nerves back to the upper five thoracic spinal segments.[71] This observation accounts for the referral of pain from the thoracic aorta to the thoracic spinal segments, resulting in their subsequent facilitation. Vagal cardiac nerves traverse the walls of the aorta as they descend toward their targets.

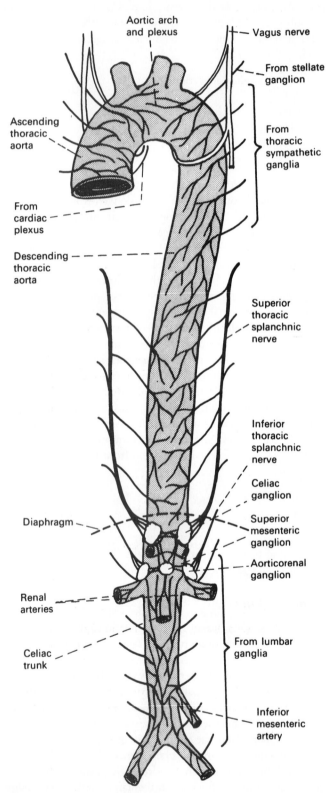

Figure 5.13. Innervation of thoracic and abdominal aorta. (Modified from Bonica JJ. General considerations of pain in the chest. In: Bonica JJ, ed. *The Management of Pain.* Philadelphia, Pa: Lea & Febiger; 1990:979.)

Small twigs from these branches provide afferent as well as parasympathetic efferent innervation (Fig. 5.13).

Thoracic Duct

The thoracic duct, located in the posterior mediastinum near the esophagus, receives a innervation similar to the vasculature of the body. Its muscular walls receive cholinergic innervation from the vagus and adrenergic innervation from branches of the intercostal nerves in a segmental pattern. The cisterna chyli, the origin of the thoracic duct, is innervated by the eleventh thoracic ganglion and the left splanchnic nerve.[76]

Abdominopelvic Region

The great autonomic plexus of the thorax passes through the diaphragm to continue inferiorly in the abdominopelvic cavity. At the level of the diaphragm, the plexus has two major components: parasympathetic and sympathetic. The two vagal trunks and their associated branches, representing the parasympathetic component, enter the abdomen on the walls of the esophagus. The sympathetic component, or thoracic splanchnic nerves, pass directly through the crura of the diaphragm to enter the abdomen. Once in the abdominal cavity, the vagal trunks and thoracic splanchnic nerves unite around the aortic prevertebral ganglia. The resultant abdominopelvic plexus of fibers follows the abdominal aorta to the pelvic brim and bifurcates slightly above the sacral promontory; the two divisions descend into the pelvic basin (Fig. 5.14). Throughout the abdomen, the plexus contains both sympathetic and parasympathetic axons and has numerous afferent fibers as well. Toward the inferior end of the abdominopelvic plexus, additional sympathetic contributions arise in the lumbar and sacral splanchnic nerves, while additional parasympathetic contributions come from the pelvic splanchnic nerves.

The abdominopelvic plexus can be divided into several geographical regions. Along the abdominal aorta, differing territories are marked out by the major prevertebral ganglia:

Celiac
Superior mesenteric
Inferior mesenteric

Between the inferior mesenteric plexus and the sacral promontory lies the superior hypogastric plexus. Below the sacral promontory, the plexus splits to pass laterally around the pelvic organs; this region is called the inferior hypogastric plexus or simply the pelvic plexus. Frequently, the fibers of the superior hypogastric plexus unite into a few large cords in the region directly over the sacral promontory and just prior to bifurcation into the two inferior hypogastric plexuses. These cords are often referred to in the surgical literature as the presacral nerve.[77] Although the abdominal autonomic nervous system has regional names, in reality the components blend together to form one great abdominopelvic plexus. The abdominal portion of this great plexus supplies efferent and afferent nerves to the organs of the abdominal cavity including the gastrointes-

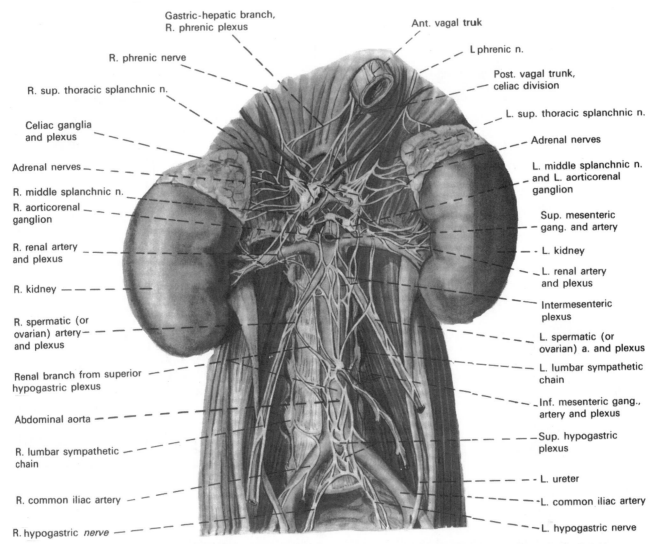

Figure 5.14. Position of major prevertebral sympathetic ganglia in great autonomic plexus of abdomen. (Modified from Bonica JJ. General considerations of pain in the chest. In: Bonica JJ, ed. *The Management of Pain*. Philadelphia, Pa: Lea & Febiger; 1990:1157.)

tinal organs, spleen, and kidneys. The pelvic portion of this plexus supplies the rectum, urinary organs, and reproductive organs. In addition to the organs, the abdominopelvic plexus also provides innervation of the vasculature of the abdominopelvic cavity.

Gastrointestinal Tract

The gastrointestinal system receives a complex pattern of innervation involving splanchnic nerves derived from the thoracolumbar and sacral portions of the spinal cord and the terminal portion of the vagus (Figs. 5.4 and 5.5). This innervation, like its visceral blood supply, can be divided into three zones based on embryological partitions of the gastrointestinal system:

1. Celiac (foregut)
2. Superior mesenteric (midgut)
3. Inferior mesenteric (hindgut)

Within the walls of the gut is an elaborate and ubiquitous network of fibers and neurons called the enteric nervous system. The enteric or intrinsic neural system controls the activity of gut smooth muscle and glands. It in turn is modulated by input from the central nervous system via the sympathetic and parasympathetic nerves. Numerous sensory feedback loops exist in the gastrointestinal system. Afferent fibers within the luminal surface and gut wall form short loops with the enteric nervous system. Longer feedback loops connect the gut to the prevertebral ganglia, and still longer loops connect the gut with the spinal cord and brainstem.[10,78–81]

The gastrointestinal tract has a special pattern of sympathetic innervation that differs significantly from that of the thoracic viscera. Preganglionic fibers arise in the lateral horn of spinal segments T9-L2 but they do not terminate in the paravertebral ganglia. Instead they pass through a series of thoracic, lumbar, and sacral splanchnic nerves (branches off of the sympathetic truck) to reach the prevertebral sympathetic gan-

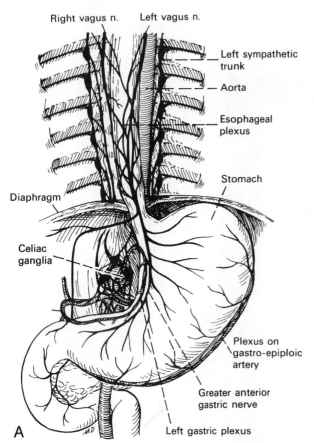

Figure 5.15. Connections of celiac ganglion and innervation of stomach. (Modified from Kimmey MB, Silverstein FE. Diseases of the gastrointestinal tract. In: Bonica JJ, ed. *The Management of Pain*. Philadelphia, Pa: Lea & Febiger; 1990:1189.)

glia on the anterior wall of the abdominal aorta (Fig. 5.15). The major prevertebral ganglia are distributed around the three abdominal arteries:

Celiac
Superior mesenteric
Inferior mesenteric

Anatomical authorities subdivide the celiac ganglia into numerous parts based on its location about the celiac artery and aorta; however, from a clinical perspective, it is simpler to treat it as one anatomical unit. Additional clusters of sympathetic ganglia neurons are scattered in the hypogastric plexus as it enters the pelvic basin.

Neurons in each prevertebral ganglia give rise to postganglionic fibers that innervate abdominal and pelvic viscera. These axons travel to their target organs by hitchhiking on abdominal and pelvic arteries. Each ganglia innervates different regions of the viscera.

CELIAC GANGLION

This large ganglionic mass surrounds the celiac trunk. It receives afferent fibers from the thoracic splanchnic nerves; and in turn it supplies postganglionic sympathetic axons to the vas-

cular territory of the celiac artery including the (Figs. 5.15 and 5.16):

Stomach
Liver
Gall bladder
Spleen
Portions of the pancreas and duodenum

SUPERIOR MESENTERIC GANGLION

This ganglion is found wrapped around the superior mesenteric artery. It receives preganglionic axons from the thoracic splanchnic nerves and supplies postganglionic axons to the territory supplied by the superior mesenteric artery (Fig. 5.17):

Portions of the pancreas and duodenum
Jejunum
Ilium
Ascending colon
Proximal two-thirds of the transverse colon

INFERIOR MESENTERIC GANGLION

The most ventral of the three prevertebral ganglia, the inferior mesenteric ganglia, surrounds the abdominal artery of the same

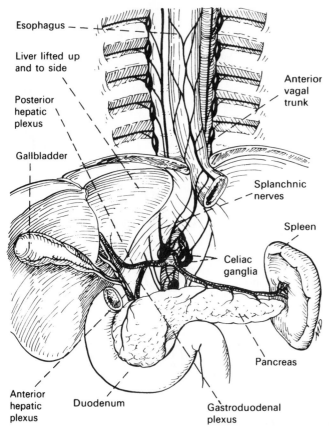

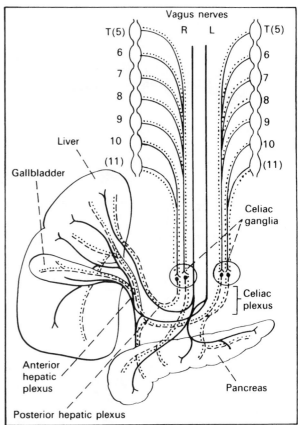

Figure 5.16.　Connections of celiac ganglia and innervation of liver and biliary tree. (Modified from Mulholland MW, Debas HT. Diseases of the liver, biliary system, and pancrease. In: Bonica JJ, ed. *The Management of Pain.* Philadelphia, Pa: Lea & Febiger; 1990:1215.)

name. It receives axons from the three lumbar splanchnic nerves and supplies postganglionic axons to the vascular territory of the inferior mesenteric vessels, namely the (Fig. 5.18):

Distal third of the transverse colon
Descending colon
Sigmoid colon
Rectum

Postganglionic fibers from the prevertebral ganglia follow their specific blood supplies through the mesenteric ligaments to reach the specific organs. The termination of these noradrenergic fibers is primarily on the neurons in the enteric ganglia.[82] Sympathetic fibers also terminate in the muscular coat of blood vessels, and an abundance of these fibers reaches the sphincteral musculature of the enteric wall. Only scattered sympathetic fibers are present in the muscularis externa and submucosa of the gastrointestinal tract.[83] There are almost no adrenergic cell bodies in the enteric plexus; most enteric adrenergic fibers are of external origin. In general, stimulation of these sympathetic fibers inhibits the activity of cholinergic neurons of the parasympathetic system.

The parasympathetic innervation of the organs located below the thoracoabdominal diaphragm has a dual origin, which also segregates along vascular and embryological divisions. The organs of the foregut and midgut, serviced by the celiac and superior mesenteric arteries, receive parasympathetic preganglionic fibers from the vagus (Figs. 5.15–5.17). The vagus follows the esophagus through the diaphragm to enter the abdominal cavity on the walls of the stomach. The esophageal hiatus of the diaphragm is the last place the vagus can be identified as a distinct nerve. Vagal axons, however, continue into the abdominal cavity, joining those of the sympathetic system in the celiac and superior mesenteric ganglia and forming mixed nerves, which pass along celiac and superior mesenteric blood vessels eventually to reach the abdominal viscera. Vagal fibers are plentiful in the walls of the stomach and small bowel; a few reach as far distally in the enteric plexus as the splenic flexure of the large colon. The preganglionic vagal axons terminate on neurons in enteric ganglia. Short postganglionic fibers from these neurons innervate the glands and course within the layers of smooth muscle of the alimentary canal. Cholinergic stimulation increases glandular secretions and peristaltic activity.

The organs of hindgut origin (transverse colon to anus), serviced by the inferior mesenteric artery, receive parasympathetic preganglionic innervation from the pelvic splanchnic nerves (Fig. 5.18). These nerves arise in the lateral horn of the S2-3 spinal cord segments and exit the spinal canal with the sacral nerve roots. As the roots pass along the pelvic wall on

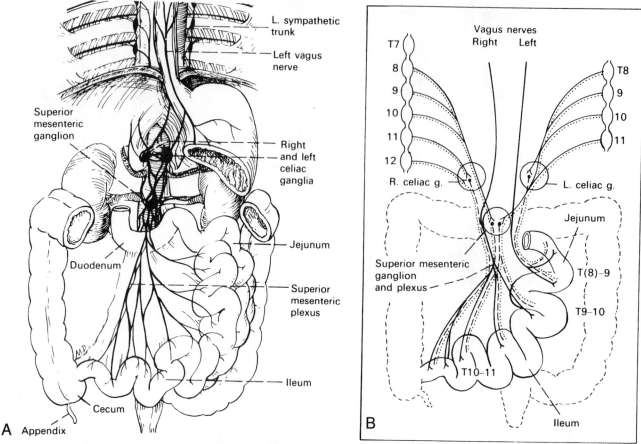

Figure 5.17. Connections of superior mesenteric ganglion and innervation of small bowel. (Modified from Kimmey MB, Silverstein FE. Diseases of the gastrointestinal tract. In: Bonica JJ, ed. *The Management of Pain.* Philadelphia, Pa: Lea & Febiger; 1990:1198.)

their way to the greater sciatic foramen, the delicate pelvic splanchnic nerves are given off. These thin nerves course through the endopelvic fascia to reach the inferior hypogastric plexus surrounding the walls of the rectum. Once in the hypogastric plexus, these parasympathetic preganglionic fibers can ascend to the origin of the inferior mesenteric artery. By hitchhiking along its branches they reach upward to the splenic flexure of the large colon. Not all parasympathetic axons from the pelvis follow this route to reach the inferior abdominal organs. Some preganglionic fibers in the inferior hypogastric plexus gain access to the enteric plexus in the wall of the rectum and ascend along the colon to reach more proximal levels of the gastrointestinal system. The preganglionic axons of the pelvic splanchnic nerves eventually terminate on the neurons of the enteric nervous system.

The enteric ganglia and plexus within the walls of the gut form a highly complex and elaborate network, often referred to as the third division of the autonomic nervous system. It exerts a major influence over all activities in the gut.[84] The enteric nervous system is estimated to possess as many neurons as are found in the entire spinal cord.[85] The enteric system is divided into two layers: the external layer is the myenteric plexus (Auerbach's), and the internal layer is the submucosal

(Meissner's). A full understanding of these structures requires a knowledge of the gastrointestinal histology and is beyond the scope of this review.[86,87]

Numerous neurotransmitters and neuromodulators are found within enteric neurons, for example:

Acetylcholine
Serotonin
Purines
γ-Amino butyric acid
Histamine

There are also many peptides such as:

Substance-P
Somatostatin
Vasoactive intestinal polypeptide
Enkephalins

Recently, nitric oxide has been described as a significant noncholinergic, nonadrenergic mechanism of neurotransmission in the enteric nervous system as well as elsewhere.[88,89] Nitric oxide is synthesized from the amino acid arginine by neurons in the myenteric plexus and is a potent smooth muscle relaxing factor.

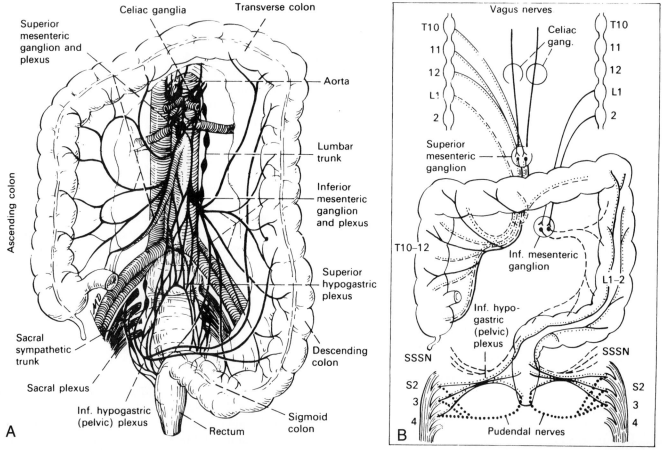

Figure 5.18. Connections of inferior mesenteric ganglion and innervation of large bowel and rectum. *SSSN*, sacral sympathetic splanchnic nerve. (Modified from Kimmey MB, Silverstein FE. Diseases of the gas-trointestinal tract. In: Bonica JJ, ed. *The Management of Pain*. Philadelphia, Pa: Lea & Febiger; 1990:1199.)

For this reason it is postulated to be important in dilation of the alimentary canal.

Three levels of sensory information processing are necessary for the proper regulation of gastrointestinal tract function.[78] The first level features afferent neurons that form a short loop interconnecting the gut mucosa, submucosa, or muscle to the enteric ganglia only. These neurons are responsible for local reflexes along the gut wall. The second level of sensory information processing involved is arranged in a longer loop involving afferent neurons from the mucosa that project to the prevertebral ganglia along the aorta. These sensory neurons participate in intraabdominal reflex arcs coordinating various regions of the gastrointestinal system. Finally, the third level of sensory feedback loops involves afferent neurons that project from the gut wall to the brainstem via the vagus nerve or to the spinal cord via the thoracic, lumbar, and pelvic splanchnic nerves. These visceral afferent neurons assist the central nervous system in integrating the activity of the alimentary canal with that of external environmental conditions.

There are some significant differences in distribution and neurochemistry between the visceral afferent fibers associated with sympathetic nerves and those coursing with the parasympathetic nerves. There are a few large encapsulated nerve end-

ings in the gut wall, most of which are related to axons from the parasympathetic vagus nerve. However, the majority of afferent terminals in the gut are small caliber, naked nerve endings.[78] In the vagus nerve, mechanoreceptive, chemoreceptive, and polymodal fibers have been described with their receptive fields in the mucosa and submucosa of the gut wall. At least in the stomach, very few of these vagal fibers contain calcitonin gene-related polypeptide, a neuropeptide typically related in nociceptive afferent fibers of the somatic tissue. However, some nociceptive information is carried in the vagus because pain from a hiatal hernia can be referred to the face.[90] Little is known of nociceptive function in vagal fibers below the level of the diaphragm.

The visceral afferent fibers that follow the sympathetic nerves to the spinal cord are mechanoreceptive and chemoreceptive; they tend to be distributed to the mesenteries and peritoneal ligaments of the gut and along its vascular system. In contrast to the vagal fibers, those projecting to the spinal cord are mostly of small caliber and are rich in calcitonin gene-related polypeptide, suggesting that they have a role in nociception. Their endings are commonly distributed within the mesentery and supporting ligaments of the abdominal organs.[79] Frequently these nerve endings are present near the branch points for the vasculature in the peritoneal lining. Few small-caliber nerve endings are present within the visceral organs themselves.

Physiological[63] as well as clinical studies support the general separation of regulatory information into the vagal system and nociceptive information into the spinal cord. Stimulating the greater thoracic splanchnic nerve at surgery elicits severe pain; blockade of the splanchnic nerve relieves pain.[91] In addition, applying local anesthetic to the greater thoracic splanchnic nerve following abdominal surgery prevents the endocrine–metabolic responses, such as increased plasma cortisol and urinary adrenaline levels, usually present in the early stages of recovery.[92] The projection of the viscera afferent through the sympathetic system creates a nociceptive map of the abdominopelvic organs on the dorsal horn of the spinal cord. This map has been demonstrated in humans by sectioning the white rami commicans during the surgical treatment of visceral pain (White and Sweet, as cited in Janig and Morrison[79]). A summary of the organotopic map of the human viscera is presented in Table 5.1. The position of a specific organ in the visceral afferent organotopic map of the spinal cord coincides approximately with the origin of the sympathetic efferent system to that specific organ. The nociceptive input to the spinal cord over these visceral afferent fibers is not precisely mapped; instead, input from any one organ overlaps considerably with that from surrounding organs.[79]

Hepatobiliary Tree and Pancreas

The vasculature and parenchyma of the liver and pancreas, as well as their associated ducts, receive innervation from both divisions of the autonomic nervous system (Fig. 5.16). In addition, these organs have an abundant supply of visceral afferent fibers that course in the vagus and thoracic splanchnic nerves. Preganglionic sympathetic innervation to these organs arises in thoracic segments T6 to T9-11 and approaches the abdomen through the thoracic splanchnic nerves. Sympathetic ganglionic neurons are located in the celiac ganglia; their post-

ganglionic axons reach the liver and pancreas by hitchhiking on the hepatic and pancreatic branches of the celiac trunk. Preganglionic parasympathetic axons, derived from the vagus nerve, pass through the fascia of the celiac region and follow the vasculature to the target organs.

A significant percentage of the axons in the vagus and thoracic splanchnic nerves traveling to the liver and pancreas are sensory in nature. Approximately 90% of the vagal axons and 50% of the splanchnic axons to the liver are visceral afferent fibers.[93] These two afferent systems perform different functions.[10] Those afferent axons traveling with the vagus respond to such stimuli as plasma glucose concentration, portal venous blood osmotic pressure, and temperature changes. The visceral afferent associated with the splanchnic nerves are high-threshold mechanoreceptors and chemoreceptors located in the walls of the biliary system, among other places, and are responsive to stretch and bradykinin concentration. The evidence available to date suggests that all pain sensation from the liver and biliary tree is transmitted via the splanchnic nerves and not the vagus.

Kidney and Urinary Tract

KIDNEY

Although the kidney is primarily controlled by endocrine mechanisms, it does receive significant innervation from the sympathetic (adrenergic) system that regulates, in part, the retention of sodium (Table 5.1).[94–97] Alterations in the neural activity in sympathetic fibers are involved in the generation of certain forms of hypertension.[98] Very little vagal parasympathetic (cholinergic) input to the kidney has been reported. This organ does, however, receive neuropeptide-containing, primary afferent fibers that course along with the adrenergic fibers (Fig. 5.19).

The kidney receives most of its innervation from the thoracolumbar spinal cord. Preganglionic sympathetic neurons regulating the kidney are located in the lateral horn of the spinal cord extending from approximately segments T11 to L1; their axons travel to the great autonomic plexus of the abdomen over the lower thoracic and first lumbar splanchnic nerves (Table 5.1). The postganglionic sympathetic (adrenergic) fibers are derived from laterally positioned ganglia (sometimes called renal ganglia) in the celiac and superior mesenteric plexuses and course into the hilus kidney along the renal vasculature.

The adrenergic axons of the mammalian kidney terminate on the:[99]

Afferent and efferent glomerular arterioles
Proximal and distal renal tubules
Ascending limb of Henle's loop
Juxtaglomerular apparatus

All portions of the cortical tubular nephron are under neural influence; the relative density of adrenergic fibers is greatest around the ascending limb of the loop of Henle, followed in decreasing relative density by the distal convoluted tubule and the proximal convoluted tubule.[100,101] α-Adrenoceptors have

Table 5.1
Visceral Organs and Their Approximate Spinal Cord Level for the Origin of Their Preganglionic Neurons[a]

Heart	T1-T5	
Stomach	T5-T9	
Liver and gall bladder	T6-T9	
Pancreas	T5-T11	
Small intestine	T9-T11	
Colon and rectum	T8-L2	S2-S4
Kidney and ureters	T10-L1	
Urinary bladder	T10-L1	S2-S4
Ovary and fallopian tube	T9-T10	
Testicle and epididymus	T9-T10, L1-L2	S2-S4
Uterus	T10-L1	
Cervix		S2-S4
Prostate	L1-L2	

[a]These levels create a viscerotopic map in the lateral horns of the spinal cord.

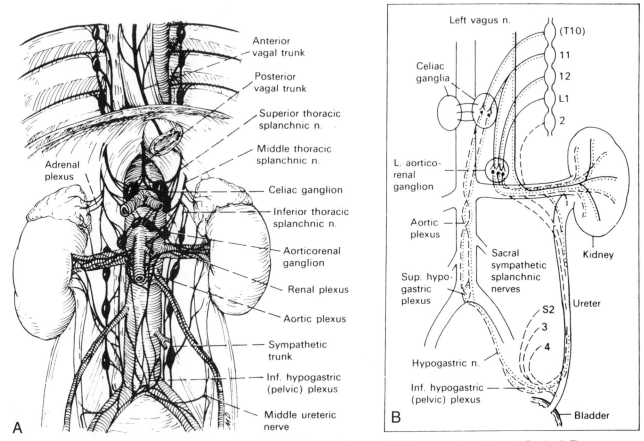

Figure 5.19. Innervation of kidney. (Modified from Ansell JS, Gee WF. Diseases of the kidney. In: Bonica JJ. *The Management of Pain*. Philadelphia, Pa: Lea & Febiger; 1990:1233.)

been located on the proximal convoluted tubule[102] as well as on the smooth muscle of the vasculature. Sympathetic innervation of the kidney is involved in the normal regulation of sodium retention, both by increasing the transport of sodium across the tubule walls and by directly increasing the release of renin from the juxtaglomerular apparatus.[99,103] Studies have shown that there is an increased activity in the renal sympathetic nervous system in essential hypertension in humans.[98]

A dual sensory innervation of the kidney exists: afferent fibers follow the thoracic splanchnic nerves back to the spinal cord and the vagus nerve back to the brainstem. Within the kidney, peripheral endings of both mechanoreceptors and chemoreceptors are found in close association with blood vessels (arteries and veins) and in the walls of the pelvis of the ureter.[104] Their cell bodies are in the dorsal root ganglia located mainly in segments at the thoracolumbar junction (T10-L3); their central processes terminate in the dorsal horn of the spinal cord. These afferent axons are classified as Aδ and C-fibers. Vagal afferent fibers, both mechanoreceptors and chemoreceptors, play a role in renorenal reflexes; the mechanoreceptors are also involved in modulating cardiovascular reflexes, thus regulating blood pressure.[104] Pain is the only detectable sensory perception that can be elicited from the kidney;[10] this modality is carried in the visceral afferent nerves of the thoracic splanchnic nerves to reach the spinal cord and the spinothalamic tracts.

In a study of the sympathetic renal afferent fibers in the primate, all spinothalamic tract cells excited by renal afferent fibers were also excited by somatic afferent fibers, indicating a powerful somatovisceral convergence on these cells.[105] This convergence has been suggested as a mechanism to explain the referral of pain from the kidney out to somatic structures such as the flank of the body.[105] In addition, this relationship may explain the changes in the tone of muscle innervated by the segments T10-L1 that accompany renal infection or inflammation.

URETER

The ureter is the conduit for urine from the kidney to the bladder. Its course is retroperitoneal, lying along the posterior abdominal body wall. The walls of the ureter consist of interlacing bundles of smooth muscle fibers woven into a theca muscularis. Individual smooth muscle cells interconnect via numerous gap junctions, making the muscularis a functional syncytium.[106] Modified smooth muscle cells within the muscular layer serve as pacemakers initiating peristaltic contractions.[107] Wrapped around the muscularis is a plexus of efferent and afferent nerve fibers, capable of regulating the pacemaker cells.[106]

The ureter receives its innervation in a segmental fashion.

The upper portion is innervated by the lower thoracic and upper lumbar segments (T10-L1) and by the vagus nerve. The lower portion of the ureter is innervated by the upper lumbar segments (L1-L2) and the pelvic splanchnic nerves (Table 5.1). The sympathetic innervation reaches the upper ureter through the lesser splanchnic nerves, and celiac and associated renal and gonadal (testicular or ovarian) ganglia. The lower ureter receives its sympathetic innervation from lumbar and sacral splanchnic nerves that contribute to ganglia located in the superior and inferior hypogastric plexus.[108]

Fibers containing tyrosine hydroxylase and neuropeptide-Y, markers for sympathetic axons, are in the outer muscle layers and the surrounding adventitia of the human ureter.[109–111] Activation of α-adrenergic receptors increases ureteral peristalsis and elevates luminal pressures; activation of β-adrenergic receptors decreases ureteral peristaltic frequency and lowers intraureteral pressures.[112]

Parasympathetic innervation for the upper portion of the ureter arises in the vagus nerve and reaches the ureter through the celiac and superior mesenteric plexus. The lower portion receives its cholinergic innervation from spinal segments S2-4. These pelvic splanchnic nerves communicate with the ureter via the inferior hypogastric plexus. Acetylcholine-containing neurons are present in the mural ganglia of the ureter; fibers containing acetylcholine are present in the mammalian ureter. These fibers are of greatest density as the ureter enters the vesical wall. Stimulation of ureteral wall with acetylcholine results in an increased contractile activity and an increased basal tone of the mural smooth muscle.[112,113] Acetylcholine also relaxes the ureteral resistance arteries using a mechanism involving endothelium-derived nitric oxide.[112]

Afferent fibers to the ureter are derived from dorsal root ganglia ranging from L2-3 to S1-2 (in guinea pigs).[114] Two classes of mechanoreceptors have been described in the ureteral walls.[115] One class has low thresholds and is responsive to peristaltic type contractions of the ureteric smooth muscle. The other class of mechanoreceptor has higher thresholds of activation and is most likely related to nociception. Many of these primary afferent fibers contain neuropeptides such as substance-P and calcitonin gene-related polypeptide, thereby suggesting that they are involved in nociceptive activities.

Pain, presumably from these nociceptors, is the only sensory perception obtainable from the human ureter.[10] In the thoracolumbar dorsal horn of the spinal cord, input from the ureter converges with somatic input from thoracolumbar spinal segments. Pain from distention of the ureter is often referred to the somatic body wall over a range of body segments. From the upper ureter, pain refers to the area from the anterior superior spine of the ilium anteriorly to the border of the rectus abdominis muscle (T11-T12). From the middle ureter, pain refers to the area from the inguinal ligament anteriorly to the rectus abdominis muscle (T12-L1). From the lower ureter, pain refers to the suprapubic area (L1) and below into the scrotum or labia (L2).[108] This descending segmental pattern of primary afferent fibers from the ureter is responsible for the descending movement of facilitated segments as any obstructing material moves through the ureteric lumen.

URINARY BLADDER

The muscular components of the urinary bladder can be divided into two anatomical and functional parts: the body or detrusor muscle and the base or the trigonal muscle. The detrusor muscle is the largest of the two parts and is active during expulsion of urine from the bladder. The trigone muscle surrounds the openings of the ureter in the base and the opening of the urethra in the neck of the bladder. It acts as an internal sphincter and, when contracted, helps to prevent the flow of urine from the bladder. The detrusor and the trigone tend to oppose each other in activity. Both detrusor and trigone muscles comprise multiple layers of smooth muscle fibers and receive an efferent innervation from the large autonomic pelvic plexus. A third muscle, related to bladder function, is located inferior to the trigone in the layers of the perineum. It is the deep transverse perineal muscle; the portion of this muscle that surrounds the urethra is called the sphincter urethra. Unlike the detrusor and trigone, this component of the perineal diaphragm is composed of skeletal muscle and innervated by branches of the pudendal, a somatic nerve.

The autonomic innervation of the urinary bladder is accomplished through the hypogastric plexus that is embedded in endopelvic fascia (Fig. 5.20). Parasympathetic preganglionic (cholinergic) fibers from the intermediolateral nucleus of spinal segments S2-4 enter the hypogastric plexus via the pelvic splanchnic nerves. These axons continue anteriorly into the vesicle plexus to terminate on ganglionic neurons located in the walls of the bladder. Their postganglionic (cholinergic and purinergic) axons supply motor innervation to all portions of the bladder wall. Stimulation of the parasympathetic system, which occurs during voiding, is excitatory to the detrusor muscle and inhibitory to the trigone muscle.

Sympathetic preganglionic fibers arise in the intermediolateral nucleus of spinal segments T11-L2 (Fig. 5.20). They leave the sympathetic trunk coursing on lumbar and sacral splanchnic nerves to enter the inferior hypogastric plexus, eventually targeting prevertebral ganglia.[116] Sympathetic postganglionic (adrenergic) axons pass anteriorly through the inferior hypogastric plexus and ultimately contribute to the vesicle plexus in the bladder adventitia. Their major target is the smooth muscle cells of the trigone muscle with a much smaller contribution to the smooth muscle of the detrusor. Sympathetic tone facilitates contraction of the trigone muscles and relaxation of the detrusor muscle, necessary to allow filling of the bladder.

The vesicle plexus contains many ganglionic neurons traditionally associated with the parasympathetic system. However, it is now clear that these neurons also receive input from adrenergic axons from the sympathetic system. Thus, the sympathetic system can influence the activity of the parasympathetic system by modulating the activity of the ganglion cells. The ganglion cells innervating the trigone muscle have α-adrenoceptors on their membranes and respond to sympathetic stimulation with contraction. Conversely, ganglion cells innervating the detrusor muscle have β-adrenoceptors on their membranes and respond to sympathetic stimulation with relaxation. It is through this differential distribution of adreno-

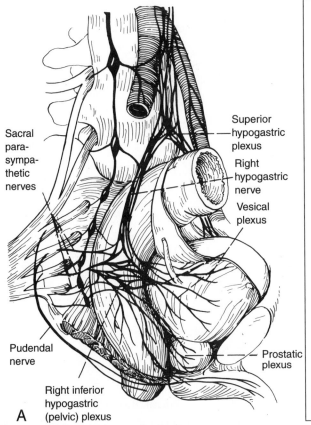

Figure 5.20. **A.** Inferior hypogastric plexus as it innervates viscera of pelvic basin. **B.** Somatic innervation of urinary bladder and its external sphincter. (Modified from Gee WF, Ansell JS. Pelvic and perineal pain of urologic origin. In: Bonica JJ. *The Management of Pain*. Philadelphia, Pa: Lea & Febiger; 1990:1369.)

ceptors that the sympathetic nervous system is capable of increasing the tone in the trigone while simultaneously relaxing the detrusor.[116]

The sphincter urethrae muscle, or external urethral sphincter, at the base of the bladder is skeletal muscle; it receives its innervation from the peroneal branches of the pudendal nerve (Fig. 5.20). This is a somatic nerve containing axons from motoneurons located in the ventral horn of the spinal cord (S2-4). The release of urine from the bladder requires an integrated viscerosomatic reflex involving:

1. Excitation of the parasympathetic system to activate the detrusor
2. Inhibition of the sympathetic system to relax the trigone and internal sphincteral muscles
3. Subsequent inhibition of the pudendal nerve to relax the external sphincteral muscles

Vesicle afferent fibers arise from mechanoreceptor endings in the connective tissue and epithelium of the vesicle mucosa and travel over the lumbar and pelvic splanchnic nerves as well as pudendal nerves to reach the cord at the L1-2 and S2-4 levels. Cell bodies for these nerves are present in the associated dorsal root ganglia. Many of these fibers contain neuropeptides such as those represented in the small caliber, primary afferent

fibers system.[116] The afferent fibers reach only to the dorsal horn of the spinal cord near their segmental level of entry; a small number of these fibers enter the spinal cord and follow the ascending tracts rostrally to terminate in the lower regions of the medulla.

Sensory information from distension of the bladder initiates reflexes involved in voiding.[116] Initial filling of the bladder triggers low-level afferent volleys that increase the tone in the trigone muscle and external sphincter muscles and inhibit the tone in the detrusor, allowing the bladder to serve as a reservoir for urine. After a certain level of filling is reached, a higher intensity of afferent volleys from the bladder wall reverse these reflexes such that the detrusor muscle tone is enhanced and the tone of the trigone and external sphincter is inhibited. This reversal of reflexes prepares the bladder for voiding. The last step, relaxation of the external sphincter, requires cooperation of the suprasegmental control of the bladder musculature, allowing volitional control of voiding.

Reproductive Tract

The pelvic and perineal organs of the male and female reproductive systems receive both sympathetic and parasympathetic innervation through the complex abdominopelvic plexus (Fig. 5.21). This innervation targets the glandular cells and smooth

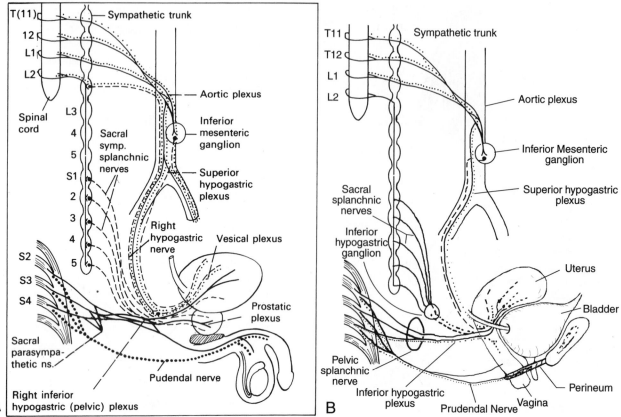

Figure 5.21. **A.** Innervation of male reproductive organs. **B.** Innervation of female reproductive organs. (Modified from Gee WF, Ansell

JS. Pelvic and perineal pain of urologic origin. In: Bonica JJ. *The Management of Pain.* Philadelphia, Pa: Lea & Febiger; 1990:1369.)

muscle of the vasculature as well as the mural smooth muscle present in the tubular portions of these organs. The origin of this innervation varies according to the embryonic origin of the specific organs. The testis and ovary, which arise in the gonadal ridge of the posterior abdominal wall, receive their afferent and efferent supply from the abdominal portions of the abdominopelvic plexus; the remaining pelvic organs of reproduction are innervated from the pelvic portion of the plexus. Afferent fibers are present in each of these organs, and their input to the spinal cord is a key feature in the presentation of pelvic pain.

TESTIS AND OVARY

Gonadal tissue receives sympathetic innervation from preganglionic neurons located in spinal segments T10 and T11 (Fig. 5.21). These preganglionic axons target neurons in the celiac and superior mesenteric ganglia. The gonadal (spermatic or ovarian) plexus of fibers arises from these ganglia and follows the course of the gonadal arteries. Additional sympathetic postganglionic axons join the gonadal plexus from the superior hypogastric plexus in the lower abdomen. In females, the gonadal (ovarian) plexus innervates the ovary and extends on to reach the uterine tubes. In males, the gonadal (spermatic) plexus joins the spermatic cord with the vas deferens and proceeds through the inguinal canal to reach the scrotum. Adren-

ergic fibers in the testis are present around blood vessels and interstitial cells of the seminiferous tubules and in the tubules of the epididymis.[112] Stimulation of the sympathetic nervous system initiates strong peristaltic waves in the vas deferens responsible for the propulsion of sperm. Parasympathetic innervation of the gonadal tissue is less dense than that of the sympathetic fibers. Cholinergic fibers arise from the vesical plexus and join the gonadal plexus as it passes though the pelvis. These fibers primarily target the vas deferens and the seminal vesicles.

Afferent fibers from the testis, epididymis, and vas deferens course through the gonadal plexus to reach the thoracolumbar spinal cord. Fibers arising in the testis target segment T10, those from the epididymis enter the spinal cord at T11 and T12, and those from the vas deferens enter at T10-L1.[117] Afferent fibers from the ovary also ascend in the gonadal plexus to enter the spinal cord at the T10 level. The return of afferent axons from the gonadal tissue to the lower thoracic level of the spinal cord is responsible for the referral of pain to the thoracolumbar junction and the facilitation of segments in this area consequent to irritation of the gonadal tissue.

UTERUS, UTERINE TUBE, CERVIX, AND VAGINA

The distal portion of the abdominopelvic plexus bifurcates as it descends over the sacral promontory to enter the pelvic basin. The pelvic portion of this complex neural structure is called the inferior hypogastric or pelvic plexus. This plexus sweeps laterally along the pelvic walls to surround the midline organs of the female pelvis. As this plexus crosses over the transverse cervical ligament, its fibrous network thickens to form the elaborate plexus of Frankenhäuser (a regional subset of the inferior hypogastric plexus). From here, autonomic axons accompany the uterine vessels medially along the transverse cervical ligament to gain access to the uterus, cervix, and vagina. The remainder of the inferior hypogastric plexus extends anteriorly to surround the bladder (this collection of fibers is often referred to as the vesical plexus).

Sympathetic preganglionic neurons capable of influencing the uterus and cervix are located in the T10-L2 spinal segments (Fig. 21). Their axons target neurons in the celiac ganglia and other prevertebral ganglia. Postganglionic fibers from these ganglia descend into the pelvic basin coursing in the superior and inferior hypogastric plexus to eventually reach the uterus. For the most part, these adrenergic fibers end on the vasculature of the uterus. Some axons terminate in the smooth muscle of the myometrium, particularly in the longitudinal layer[118] and among the glands of the endometrium. The parasympathetic input to the uterus and cervix arises in the intermediolateral nucleus of spinal segments S2-4. These axons target ganglia located in the plexus of Frankenhäuser; postganglionic (cholinergic) axons extend into the uterus following the uterine artery. Most of the cholinergic input to the uterus is confined to the vascular supply with a small amount reaching the glands of the endometrium and a few fibers in the circular muscle layer of the myometrium.[118] The function of this elaborate autonomic innervation of the uterus, beyond regulation of the vasculature, is not well known. Evidence suggests that stimulation of the adrenergic and cholinergic inputs can enhance the contraction of mammalian uterine myometrium.[119] The number and size of adrenergic nerves appears to increase in the uterus during pregnancy,[120] further suggesting a role for these fibers in the uterine contractions of birth.

The uterus, cervix, and vagina receive a complex afferent innervation that influences the referral of pain during birth.[121] Experimental studies in cats demonstrate that afferent fibers from the uterus and cervix enter the spinal cord over a range of levels (T12-S3).[122] The majority of fibers from the fallopian tubes have cell bodies in the dorsal root ganglia of the lumbar segments while the majority of fibers from the cervix have cell bodies in the dorsal root ganglia of the sacral segments. Clinical studies suggest that the afferent fibers from the human uterus project to even higher levels of the spinal cord (T10)[121] and that the majority of pain fibers from the uterus enter the thoracolumbar spinal cord.[123,124] Nociceptive fibers from the uterus pass upward through the superior hypogastric plexus and lumbar splanchnic nerves to enter the spinal cord over the white rami of the lower thoracic and lumbar segments. For this reason, the white ramus at L1 can be particularly large. The pathways handling sensory information from the female reproductive tract are split. Input from above the cervix ascends through the superior hypogastric plexus to the thoracolumbar junction while afferent fibers from the cervix and below descend into the sacral spinal cord.[63] This arrangement of primary afferent fibers is responsible, in part, for the presentation of low back pain late in pregnancy as well as accompanying facilitation of spinal segments around the thoracolumbar junction.

ERECTILE TISSUE OF PENIS AND CLITORIS

The sympathetic innervation of the vasculature and erectile tissue in the penis and clitoris has its origin in the intermediolateral cell column of spinal cord segments T11-L2 (Fig. 5.21). At least two routes exist through which these fibers reach the penis. One route involves preganglionic axons that arise in the thoracolumbar spinal cord and synapse in the associated paravertebral ganglia. From these ganglia, adrenergic postganglionic fibers join the hypogastric plexus to pass into the pelvic basin, eventually entering the penis at its root on the perineal diaphragm. The second route comprises sympathetic preganglionic axons from thoracolumbar segments that pass by the paravertebral ganglia to terminate in pelvic ganglia located deep in the pelvic plexus. Postganglionic adrenergic axons from these ganglia reach the root of the penis or clitoris by following the associated peroneal vasculature.

Parasympathetic innervation of the vasculature and erectile tissue arises in the sacral (S2-4) spinal cord. Postganglionic axons from neurons in the scattered ganglia of the pelvic plexus join the sympathetic axons entering the penis or clitoris over its root. Nonadrenergic, noncholinergic axons, presumably from cells located in the pelvic ganglia, also innervate the erectile tissue. Somatic motor innervation of the clitoris and penis arises in Onuf's nucleus of the ventral horn of spinal cord segments S2-4. Their axons travel the course of the pudendal to the perineum where they innervate the following structures, all of which are composed of skeletal muscle:

Bulbocavernosus muscles
Ischiocavernosus muscles
Superficial and deep perineal muscles
External urethral sphincters
Anal sphincters

The sex act requires coordinated viscerosomatic reflexes involving the organs and musculature of the pelvic and perineal region.[116] Initially, somatic and/or emotional stimuli activate parasympathetic outflow from the sacral cord to the vasculature of the erectile tissue. The cholinergic fibers activate the release of nitric oxide from endothelial cells; this relaxes the vessel walls, resulting in increased perfusion of the tissue. Once the erectile tissue is engorged, additional stimuli initiate a sympathetic barrage from the thoracolumbar junction of the cord. This output results in contraction of smooth muscle in the vas deferens in the male and in the walls of the vagina in the female. Subsequently, coordinated reflex activation of the peroneal nerve results in contraction of the bulbospongiosus, ischiocavernosus, and transverse peroneal muscles. The rhythmic contraction of these muscles assists in forcing the ejaculum along the urethra in the male and constricts the vestibule of the vagina in the female. Integration of these three efferent pathways, parasympathetic, sympathetic, and somatic, occurs in the circuitry of the sacral spinal cord segments and is necessary for successful completion of the sex act.

CONCLUSION

A major factor in orchestrating the diverse functions of internal structures is the autonomic nervous system. Through an extensive network of connections, the autonomic nervous system helps maintain the normal rhythm of activity in the visceral organs as well as adjust their output to accommodate any external challenge. This conglomerate of interlocking systems, with its pervasive influence on our physiology and psychology, is called the neuroendocrine-immune network, which is described in more detail in Chapter 9.

REFERENCES

1. Clarke E, Jacyna LS. *Nineteenth-Century Origins of Neuroscientific Concepts*. Berkeley, Calif: University of California Press; 1987.
2. McGeer PL, Eccles JC, McGeer EG. *Molecular Neurobiology of the Mammalian Brain*. New York, NY: Plenum Press; 1987.
3. Agnati LF, Bjelke B, Fuxe K. Volume transmission in the brain. *Am Sci*. 1992;80:362–373.
4. Prechtl JC, Powley TL. β-Afferents: a fundamental division of the nervous system mediating homeostasis? *Behav Brain Sci*. 1990; 13:289–331.
5. Ebbesson SOE. Quantitative studies of superior cervical sympathetic ganglia in a variety of primates including man, II: Neuronal packing density. *J Morphol*. 1968;124:181–186.
6. Freire-Maia L, Azevedo AD. The autonomic nervous system is not a purely efferent system. *Med Hypotheses*. 1990;32:91–99.
7. Dockray GJ, Sharkey KA. Neurochemistry of visceral afferent neurones. *Prog Brain Res*. 1986;67:133–148.
8. Schott GD. Visceral afferents: their contribution to "sympathetic dependent" pain. *Brain*. 1994;117:397–413.
9. Cervero F. Mechanisms of acute visceral pain. *Br Med Bull*. 1991; 47:549–560.
10. Cervero F. Sensory innervation of the viscera: peripheral basis of visceral pain. *Physiol Rev*. 1994;74:95–138.
11. Vanhoutte PM, Shepherd JT. Autonomic nerves of the systemic blood vessels. In: Dyck PJ, Thomas PK, eds. *Peripheral Neuropathy*. Philadelphia, Pa: WB Saunders Co; 1993:208–227.
12. Burnstock G. Cholinergic and purinergic regulation of blood vessels. *Handbook of Physiology*. Sect. 2. Vol. II. 1980:567–612.
13. Renkin EM. Control of microcirculation and blood-tissue exchange. *Handbook of Physiology*. Sect. 2. Vol. IV. 1984:627–687.
14. Bonica JJ. General considerations of pain in the head. In: Bonica JJ, ed. *The Management of Pain*. Philadelphia, Pa: Lea & Febiger; 1990:651–675.
15. Mitchell GAG. The cranial extremities of the sympathetic trunks. *Acta Anat (Basel)*. 1953;18:195–201.
16. Shepherd RFJ, Shepherd JT. Control of blood pressure and the circulation in man. In: Bannister R, Mathias CJ, eds. *Autonomic Failure*. Vol. 3. Oxford: Oxford Medical Publications; 1992:78–93.
17. Joyner MJ, Shepherd JT. Autonomic control of circulation. In: Low PA, ed. *Clinical Autonomic Disorders*. Boston, Mass: Little, Brown & Co; 1993:55–67.
18. Kawarai M, Koss MC. Neurogenic cutaneous vasodilation in the cat forepaw. *J Auton Nerv Syst*. 1992;37:39–46.

19. Jinkins JR, Whittemore AR, Bradley WG. The anatomic basis of vertebrogenic pain and the autonomic syndrome associated with lumbar disk extrusion. *Am J Radiol*. 1989;152:1277–1289.
20. Yonehara N, Chen J-Q, Imai Y, Inoki R. Involvement of substance P present in primary afferent neurons in modulation of cutaneous blood flow in the instep of the rat hind paw. *Br J Pharmacol*. 1992; 106:256–262.
21. Basbaum AI, Levine JD. The contributions of the nervous system to inflammation and inflammatory disease. *Can J Physiol Pharmacol*. 1991;69:647–651.
22. Kidd BL, Gibson SJ, O'Higgins F, Mapp PI, Polak JM, Buckland-Wright JC, et al. A neurogenic mechanism for symmetrical arthritis. *Lancet*. 1989;1128–1131.
23. Gonzales R, Sherbourne CD, Goldyne ME, Levine JD. Noradrenaline-induced prostaglandin production by sympathetic postganglionic neurons is mediated by 2-adrenergic receptors. *J Neurochem*. 1991;57:1145–1150.
24. Levine JD, Fields HL, Basbaum AI. Peptides and the primary afferent nociceptor. *J Neurosci*. 1993;13:2273–2286.
25. Keller JT, Marfurt CF, Dimlich RVW, Tierney BE. Sympathetic innervation of the supratentorial dura mater of the rat. *J Comp Neurol*. 1989;290:310–321.
26. Keller JT, Marfurt CF. Peptidergic and serotonergic innervation of the rat dura mater. *J Comp Neurol*. 1991;309:515–534.
27. Stead RH, Dixon MF, Bramwell NH, Riddell RH, Bienenstock J. Mast cells are closely apposed to nerves in the human gastrointestinal mucosa. *Gastroenterology*. 1989;97:575–585.
28. Levine JD, Coderre TJ, Covinsky K, Basbaum AI. Neural influences on synovial mast cell density in rat. *J Neurosci Res*. 1990; 26:301–307.
29. Levine JD, Dardick SJ, Roizen MF, Helms C, Basbaum AI. Contribution of sensory afferents and sympathetic efferents to joint injury in experimental arthritis. *J Neurosci*. 1986;6:3423–3429.
30. Hardebo J-E. Activation of pain fibers to the internal carotid artery intercranially may cause the pain and local signs of reduced sympathetic and enhanced parasympathetic activity in cluster headache. *Headache*. 1991;31:314–320.
31. Suzuki N, Hardebo J-E. The cerebrovascular parasympathetic innervation. *Cerebrovasc Brain Metab Rev*. 1993;5:33–46.
32. Suzuki N, Hardebo J-E. Anatomical basis for a parasympathetic and sensory innervation of the intracranial segment of the internal carotid artery in man. Possible implication for vascular headache. *J Neurol Sci*. 1991;104:19–31.
33. Spalding JMK, Nelson E. The autonomic nervous system. In: Joynt RJ, ed. *Clinical Neurology*. Philadelphia, Pa: JB Lippincott; 1986:1–58.
34. Williams PL, Warwick R, Dyson M, Bannister LH. *Grays's Anatomy*. 37th ed. Edinburgh: Churchill Livingstone; 1989.
35. Wilson-Pauwels L, Akesson E, Stewart P. *Cranial Nerves: Anatomy and Clinical Comments*. Toronto: BC Decker, Inc; 1988.
36. Haerer AF. *DeJong's The Neurologic Examination*. Philadelphia, Pa: JB Lippincott; 1992.
37. Grundy D. Speculations on the structure/function relationship for vagal and splanchnic afferent endings supplying the gastrointestinal tract. *J Auton Nerv Syst*. 1988;22:175–180.
38. Lance JW. Current concepts of migraine. *Neurology*. 1993;43:S11–S15.
39. Ruskell GL. The orbital branches of the pterygopalatine ganglion and their relationship with internal carotid nerve branches in primates. *J Anat*. 1970;106:323–339.
40. Suzuki N, Hardebo J-E, Skagerberg G, Owman C. Central origins

of preganglionic fibers to the sphenopalatine ganglion in the rat. A fluorescent retrograde tracer study with special reference to its relation to central catecholaminergic systems. *J Auton Nerv Syst.* 1990;30:101–109.

41. Walters BB, Gillespie SA, Moskowitz MA. Cerebrovascular projections from the sphenopalatine and otic ganglia to the middle cerebral artery of the cat. *Stroke.* 1986;17:488–494.

42. Suzuki N, Hardebo J-E. Anatomical basis for a parasympathetic and sensory innervation of the intracranial segment of the internal carotid artery in man. Possible implication for vascular headache. *J Neural Sci.* 1991;104:19–31.

43. Hardebo J-E, Suzuki N, Ekblad E, Owman C. Vasoactive intestinal polypeptide and acetylcholine coexist with neuropeptide Y, dopamine-beta-hydroxylase, tyrosine hydroxylase, substance P or calcitonin gene-related peptide in neuronal subpopulations in cranial parasympathetic ganglia of rat. *Cell Tissue Res.* 1992;267:291–300.

44. Suzuki N, Hardebo J-E, Owman C. Origins and pathways of cerebrovascular nerves storing substance P and calcitonin gene-related peptide in rat. *Neuroscience.* 1989;31:427–438.

45. Diamond S. Head pain. *Clin Symp.* 1994;46:1–34.

46. Moskowitz MA. Basic mechanisms in vascular headache. *Neurol Clin North Am.* 1990;8:801–815.

47. Pick J. *The Autonomic Nervous System.* Philadelphia, Pa: JB Lippincott; 1970.

48. Mitchell GAG. *Cardiovascular Innervation.* London: ES Livingstone; 1956.

49. Mizeres NJ. The cardiac plexus of nerves. *Am J Anat.* 1963; 112:141.

50. Levy M, Martin PJ. Neural control of the heart. *Handbook of Physiology.* Sect. 2. The Nervous System, Vol. 1. Bethesda, Md: American Physiological Society; 1979:581–620.

51. Standish A, Enquist LW, Schwaber JS. Innervation of the heart and its central medullary origin defined by viral tracing. *Science.* 1994; 263:232–234.

52. Standish A, Enquist LW, Escardo JA, Schwaber JS. Central neuronal circuit innervating the rat heart defined by transneuronal transport of pseudorabies virus. *J Neurosci.* 1995;15:1998–2012.

53. Talman WT. The central nervous system and cardiovascular control in health and disease. In: Low PA, ed. *Clinical Autonomic Disorders.* Boston, Mass: Little, Brown & Co; 1993:39–53.

54. Baluk P, Gabella G. Some intrinsic neurons of the guinea-pig heart contain substance-P. *Neurosci Lett.* 1989;104:269–273.

55. Quigg M, Elfvin L-G, Aldskogius H. Distribution of cardiac sympathetic afferent fibers in the guinea pig heart labeled by anterograde transport of wheat germ agglutinin-horseradish peroxidase. *J Auton Nerv Syst.* 1988;25:107–118.

56. Quigg M. Distribution of vagal afferent fibers of the guinea pig heart labeled by anterograde transport of conjugated horseradish peroxidase. *J Auton Nerv Syst.* 1991;36:13–24.

57. Hopkins DA, Armour JA. Ganglionic distribution of afferent neurons innervating the canine heart and cardiopulmonary nerves. *J Auton Nerv Syst.* 1989;26:213–222.

58. Malliani A, Lombardi F, Pagni M. Sensory innervation of the heart. *Prog Brain Res.* 1986;67:39–48.

59. Foreman RD, Blair RW, Ammons WS. Neural mechanisms of cardiac pain. *Prog Brain Res.* 1986;67:227–243.

60. Bonica JJ. General considerations of pain in the chest. In: Bonica JJ, ed. *The Management of Pain.* Philadelphia, Pa: Lea & Febiger; 1990:959–1000.

61. Ammons WS. Cardiopulmonary sympathetic afferent excitation of lower thoracic spinoreticular and spinothalamic neurons. *J Neurophysiol.* 1990;64:1907–1916.

62. Beal MC. Viscerosomatic reflexes: a review. *JAOA.* 1985;85:786–801.

63. Ruch TC. Pathophysiology of pain. In: Ruch TC, Patton HD, eds. *Physiology and Biophysics.* 19th ed. Philadelphia, Pa: WB Saunders Co; 1965:345–363.

64. Thurlbeck WM, Miller RR. The respiratory system. In: Rubin E, Farber JL, eds. *Pathology.* Philadelphia, Pa: JB Lippincott; 1988:542–627.

65. Barnes PJ, Baraniuk JN, Belvisi MG. Neuropeptides in the respiratory tract. *Am Rev Respir Dis.* 1991;144:1187–1198.

66. Drazen JM, Gaston B, Shore SA. Chemical regulation of pulmonary airway tone. *Ann Rev Physiol.* 1995;57:151–170.

67. Bindoff LA, Heseltine D. Unilateral facial pain in patients with lung cancer: a referred pain via the vagus? *Lancet.* 1988;1:812–815.

68. Morton DR, Klassen KP, Curtis GM. Clinical physiology of the human bronchi, I: Pain of tracheobronchial origin. *Surgery.* 1950; 28:669.

69. Richards WG, Sugarbaker DJ. Neuronal control of esophageal function. *Chest Surg Clin North Am.* 1995;5:157–171.

70. Collman PI, Tremblay L, Diamant NE. The central vagal efferent supply to the esophagus and lower esophageal sphincter of the cat. *Gastroenterology.* 1993;104:1430–1438.

71. Bonica JJ. Applied anatomy relevant to pain. In: Bonica JJ, ed. *The Management of Pain.* Philadelphia, Pa: Lea & Febiger; 1990:133–158.

72. Hightower NC. Applied anatomy and physiology of the esophagus. In: Bockus HL, ed. *Gastroenterology.* Philadelphia, Pa: WB Saunders Co; 1974:127–142.

73. Collman PI, Tremblay L, Diamant NE. The distribution of spinal and vagal sensory neurons that innervate the esophagus of the cat. *Gastroenterology.* 1992;103:817–822.

74. Barrett RT, Bao X, Miselis RR, Altschuler SM. Brain stem localization of rodent esophageal premotor neurons revealed by transneuronal passage of pseudorabies virus [see comments]. *Gastroenterology.* 1994;107:728–737.

75. Pope CE. Heartburn, dysphagia, and chest pain of esophageal origin. In: Sleisenger MH, Fordtran JS, eds. *Gastrointestinal Disease: Pathophysiology, Diagnosis, Management.* Philadelphia, Pa: WB Saunders Co; 1983:145–148.

76. Bulloch K. Neuroanatomy of lymphoid tissue: a review. In: Guillemin R, Cohn M, Melnechuk T, eds. *Neural Modulation of Immunity.* New York, NY: Raven Press; 1985:111–141.

77. Elaut L. The surgical anatomy of the so-called presacral nerve. *Surg Gynecol Obstet.* 1932;55:581–589.

78. Mayer EA, Raybould HE. Role of visceral afferent mechanisms in functional bowel disorders. *Gastroenterology.* 1990;99:1688–1704.

79. Janig W, Morrison JFB. Functional properties of spinal visceral afferents supplying abdominal and pelvic organs, with special emphasis on visceral nociception. *Prog Brain Res.* 1986;67:87–114.

80. Paintal AS. The visceral sensations—some basic mechanisms. *Prog Brain Res.* 1986;67:3–19.

81. Cervero F, Tattersall JEH. Somatic and visceral sensory integration in the thoracic spinal cord. *Prog Brain Res.* 1986;67:189–204.

82. Wood JD. Physiology of the enteric nervous system. In: Johnson LR, ed. *Physiology of the Gastrointestinal Tract.* Vol. 1. New York, NY: Raven Press; 1981:1–37.

83. Gabella G. Structure of muscles and nerves in the gastrointestinal tract. In: Johnson LR, ed. *Physiology of the Gastrointestinal Tract.* New York, NY: Raven Press; 1981:197–241.

84. Goyal RK, Crist JR. Neurology of the gut. In: Sleisenger MH, Fordtran JS, eds. *Gastrointestinal Disease*. Philadelphia, Pa: WB Saunders Co; 1989:21–52.

85. Ottaway CA. Neuroimmunomodulation in the intestinal mucosa. *Gastroenterol Clin North Am*. 1991;20:511–529.

86. Schofield GC. Anatomy of muscular and neural tissues in the alimentary canal. In: Code C, ed. *Handbook of Physiology*. Sect. 6, Alimentary Canal: Vol. IV. Motility. Bethesda, Md: American Physiology Society; 1968:1579–1627.

87. Fawcett D. *A Textbook of Histology*. Philadelphia, Pa: WB Saunders Co; 1986:619–678.

88. Stark ME, Szurszewski JH. Role of nitric oxide in gastrointestinal and hepatic function and disease. *Gastroenterology*. 1992;103:1928–1949.

89. Sanders KM, Ward SM. Nitric oxide as a mediator of nonadrenergic noncholinergic neurotransmission. *Am J Physiol*. 1992;262:G379–G392.

90. Blau JN, MacGregor EA. Migraine and the neck. *Headache*. 1994;34:88–90.

91. Cervero F. Neurophysiology of gastrointestinal pain. *Bailliere's Clin Gastroenterol*. 1988;2:183–199.

92. Shirasaka C, Tsuji H, Asoh T, Takeuchi Y. Role of the splanchnic nerves in the endocrine and metabolic response to abdominal surgery. *Br J Surg*. 1986;73:142–145.

93. Mulholland MW, Debas HT. Diseases of the liver, biliary system, and pancreas. In: Bonica JJ, ed. *The Management of Pain*. Philadelphia, Pa: Lea & Febiger; 1990:1214–1231.

94. Osborn JL. Relation between sodium intake, renal function, and the regulation of arterial pressure. *Hypertension*. 1991;17:191–196.

95. DiBona GF, Wilcox CS. The kidney and the sympathetic nervous system. In: Bannister R, Mathias CJ, eds. *Autonomic Failure*. Vol. 3. Oxford: Oxford Medical Publications; 1992:178–196.

96. DiBona GF. Sympathetic neural control of the kidney in hypertension. *Hypertension*. 1992;19:I28–35.

97. DiBona GF, Jones SY. Analysis of renal sympathetic nerve responses to stress. *Hypertension*. 1995;25:531–538.

98. Hollenbreg NK. Renal vascular tone in essential and secondary hypertension. *Medicine*. 1975;54:29–44.

99. DiBona GF. Neural control of renal function: cardiovascular implications. *Hypertension*. 1989;13:539–548.

100. Barajas L, Powers K. Innervation of the renal proximal convoluted tubule of the rat. *Am J Anat*. 1989;186:378–388.

101. Barajas L, Powers K, Wang P. Innervation of the renal cortical tubules: a quantitative study. *Am J Physiol*. 1984;247:F50–F60.

102. Insel PA, Snavely MD, Healy DPM, Munzel PA, Potenza CL, Nord EP. Radioligand binding and functional assays demonstrate postsynaptic alpha2-receptors on proximal tubules of rat and rabbit kidney. *J Cardiovasc Pharmacol*. 1985;7:S9–S17.

103. Gottschalk CW. Renal nerves and sodium excretion. *Annu Rev Physiol*. 1979;41:229–240.

104. Ammons WS. Renal afferent inputs to the ascending spinal pathways. *Am J Physiol*. 1992;262:R165–R176.

105. Ammons WS. Electrophysiological characteristics of primate spinothalamic neurons with renal and somatic inputs. *J Neurophysiol*. 1989;61:1121–1130.

106. Tahara H. The three-dimensional structure of the musculature and the nerve elements in the rabbit ureter. *J Anat*. 1990;170:183–191.

107. Weiss RM. Physiology and pharmacology of the renal pelvis and

ureter. In: Walsh PC, Gittes RF, Perlmutter AD, Stamey TA, eds. *Campbell's Urology*. Philadelphia, Pa: WB Saunders Co; 1986:94–128.

108. Ansell JS, Gee WF. Diseases of the kidney and ureter. In: Bonica JJ, ed. *The Management of Pain*. Philadelphia, Pa: Lea & Febiger; 1990:1232–1249.

109. Edyvane KA, Smet PJ, Trussell DC, Jonavicius J, Marshall VR. Patterns of neuronal colocalisation of tyrosine hydroxylase, neuropeptide Y, vasoactive intestinal polypeptide, calcitonin gene-related peptide and substance P in human ureter. *J Auton Nerv Syst*. 1994; 48:241–255.

110. Smet PJ, Edyvane KA, Jonavicius J, Marshall VR. Colocalization of nitric oxide synthase with vasoactive intestinal peptide, neuropeptide Y, and tyrosine hydroxylase in nerves supplying the human ureter. *J Urol*. 1994;152:1292–1296.

111. Edyvane KA, Trussell DC, Jonavicius J, Henwood A, Marshall VR. Presence and regional variation in peptide-containing nerves in the human ureter. *J Auton Nerv Syst*. 1992;39:127–137.

112. Stewart JD. Autonomic regulation of sexual function. In: Low PA, ed. *Clinical Autonomic Disorders*. Boston, Mass: Little, Brown and Co; 1993:117–123.

113. Prieto D, Simonsen U, Martin J, Hernandez M, Rivera L, Lema L, et al. Histochemical and functional evidence for a cholinergic innervation of the equine ureter. *J Auton Nerv Syst*. 1994;47:159–170.

114. Semenenko FM, Cervero F. Afferent fibres from the guinea-pig ureter: size and peptide content of the dorsal root ganglion cells of origin. *Neuroscience*. 1992;47:197–201.

115. Cervero F, Sann H. Mechanically evoked responses of afferent fibres innervating the guinea-pig's ureter: an in vitro study. *J Physiol (Lond)*. 1989;412:245–266.

116. De Groat WC, Booth AM. Autonomic systems to the urinary bladder and sexual organs. In: Dyck PJ, Thomas PK, eds. *Peripheral Neuropathy*. Philadelphia, Pa: WB Saunders Co; 1993:149–165.

117. Gee WF, Ansell JS. Pelvic and perineal pain of urologic origin. In: Bonica JJ, ed. *The Management of Pain*. Philadelphia, Pa: Lea & Febiger; 1990:1368–1394.

118. Taneike T, Miyazaki H, Nakamura H, Ohga A. Autonomic innervation of the circular and longitudinal layers in swine myometrium. *Biol Reprod*. 1991;45:831–340.

119. Bulat R, Kannan MS, Garfield RE. Studies of the innervation of rabbit myometrium and cervix. *Can J Physiol Pharmacol*. 1989; 67:837–844.

120. Thilander G. Adrenergic and cholinergic nerve supply in the porcine myometrium and cervix. A histochemical investigation during pregnancy and parturition. *Zentralbl Veterinarmed A*. 1989; 36:585–595.

121. Bonica JJ. The nature of pain in parturition. *Clin Obstet Gynecol*. 1975;2:499.

122. Kawatani M, Takeshige C, De Groat WC. Central distribution of afferent pathways from the uterus of the cat. *J Comp Neurol*. 1990; 302:294–304.

123. Bonica JJ, McDonald JS. The pain of childbirth. In: Bonica JJ, ed. *The Management of Pain*. Philadelphia, Pa: Lea & Febiger; 1990:1313–1343.

124. Bonica JJ, Chadwick HS. Labor pain. In: Wall PD, Melzack R, eds. *Textbook of Pain*. Edinburgh: Churchill Livingstone; 1989:482–499.

6. Endocrine System and Body Unity

OSTEOPATHIC PRINCIPLES AT A CHEMICAL LEVEL

RONALD PORTANOVA

Key Concepts

- **General chemical types of hormones (amines, peptide/protein, and steroid) and for each chemical type of hormone the:**
  - **—Biosynthesis, storage, and release**
  - **—Characteristics of transport in the blood**
  - **—Mechanism of action (receptor, signal transduction, and effector mechanisms)**
  - **—Metabolism/degradation**

- **"Classic" endocrine glands, the hormone(s) secreted, the mechanisms that control the rate of hormone secretion, including feedback (positive, negative) mechanisms, and the principal biologic action(s) of the hormone(s).**

- **Integration of hormone action with regard to the regulation of:**
  - **—Reproduction**
  - **—Growth and development**
  - **—Energy management**
  - **—Preservation and stabilization of the internal environment**

- **Intimate relationship between the principles that underlie endocrinology and the principles that guide the study and practice of osteopathic medicine**

The endocrine system is a whole-body communications system. Endocrine information is transmitted in the form of structurally specific chemical messengers, the hormones, and received by equally specific chemical structures, the cell receptors. The endocrine system participates in the control and integration of bodily processes that are fundamental to human life:

Reproduction, growth, and development
Energy management
Preservation and stabilization of the internal environment

ENDOCRINOLOGY

Terms and Definitions

The traditional view of hormones and endocrine glands dates from the work of Baylis and Starling in the early part of this century. Accordingly, a hormone is an information-carrying molecule, secreted in small amounts by a specific gland and transported in the blood to a distant site, where it exerts its biologic effect. These ideas pertain to what might be called the traditional or classic hormones and endocrine glands. It is now clear that certain hormones and hormonelike substances (e.g., prostaglandins, various growth factors) do not fit this description. These nonclassic hormones have two key characteristics:

1. They are produced in organs that are not normally thought of as endocrine glands; for example, the atrial natriuretic peptide is secreted by the heart. The kidney produces renin, erythropoietin, and the hormonally active metabolite of vitamin D $(1,25\text{-}(OH)_2\text{-}D_3)$.
2. They may act locally, without transport in the blood, on contiguous cells or even on the cells that produce them, functions that are referred to, respectively, as paracrine and autocrine.

Chemical Structure of Hormones

Endocrine information is encoded in specific chemical structure. Every hormone is structurally unique; seemingly minor differences in chemical structure can dramatically affect the activity of the molecule. Nevertheless, chemically, all of the hormones fall into one of three broad structural categories (Table 6.1):

1. Amino acid derivatives
2. Peptides and proteins
3. Steroids

These structural categories are associated with typical physical and chemical characteristics that have important functional implications.

ENDOCRINOLOGY AND OSTEOPATHY

This chapter discusses the basic elements of endocrine physiology. The information is presented in summary form and is meant to serve as a guide for further study. The information is organized with reference to principles that guide the study and practice of osteopathic medicine. This arrangement is didactic *and* natural since body unity is the focus of endocrinology and osteopathy.

Table 6.1
Classical Endocrine Glands and Hormones Based on Structure[a]

Chemical Structure	Gland	Hormone	Major Target and/or Function
Amines	Adrenal medulla	Epinephrine, norepinephrine	Whole-body adaptation to stress, including regulation of CVS and energy flux
	Thyroid	Thyroxine (T_4), triiodothyronine (T_3)	Whole-body including CNS; growth and development, organ system performance, energy metabolism
Peptides and proteins	Neurohypophysis	Vasopressin (AVP, antidiuretic h., ADH)	Nephron, water metabolism; CVS, regulation of blood flow/pressure
		Oxytocin	Smooth muscle; milk let down, uterine motility
	Hypophysis, pars intermedia	Melanocyte-stimulating h. (MSH)	Melanocytes in lower vertebrates; however, role in humans unknown
	Adenohypophysis	Adrenocorticotrophic h. (ACTH, corticotropin)	Adrenal cortex; regulation of growth and functional status (especially steroidogenesis)
		Prolactin (PRL)	Mammary; growth of gland and milk synthesis
		Growth h. (GH) (somatotropin, STH)	Whole-body; growth and development, organic metabolism
		Thyroid-stimulating h. (TSH, thyrotropin)[b]	Thyroid; regulation of growth and functional status (especially thyroid h. secretion)
		Follicle-stimulating h. (FSH)[b] Luteinizing h. (LH)[b]	Gonads; regulation of reproduction including gamete production and development and gonadal steroidogenesis
	Hypothalamus	Corticotropin-releasing h. (CRH) Thyrotropin-releasing h. (TRH) Gonadotropin-releasing h. (GnRH, LHRH) Growth h.-releasing h. (GHRH, somatocrinin) Growth h. inhibiting h. (somatostatin)	Adenohypophysis, regulation of adenohypophysial h. secretion; also found at other sites (extrahypothalamic regions of CNS, pancreas, others) and may serve neurotransmitter, neuromodulation, or other local (paracrine) functions
	Blood (via hepatic precursor), CNS	Angiotensin	Adrenal cortex; regulation of steroidogenesis (aldosterone) CNS, neurotransmission/modulation
	Parathyroids	Parathyroid h. (PTH, parathormone)	Bone/kidney; regulation of calcium and phosphate metabolism
	Pancreatic islets, β-cells	Insulin	Liver, adipocyte, muscle, other; regulation of energy metabolism, plasma levels of glucose and other metabolites; widespread anabolic actions
	Pancreatic islets, α-cells	Glucagon	Liver, adipocyte, regulation of energy metabolism, mobilizes glucose and other oxidative substrates
	Thyroid, C cells	Calcitonin	Bone; calcium metabolism
Steroids	Adrenal cortex, zona fasciculata	Cortisol	Liver, adipocyte, muscle, other; energy metabolism, widespread catabolic actions; adaptations to a wide variety of whole-body noxious insults (stresses)
	Adrenal cortex, zona glomerulosa	Aldosterone	Nephron, sweat glands, salivary glands, other; promotes sodium retention and potassium loss
	Ovary	Estrogens (E_2, E_3)	Reproductive tract, mammary; regulation of growth, development, function; tissue-specific anabolic effects
		Progesterone	Reproductive tract, mammary; regulation of reproduction, lactation
	Testes	Testosterone (T)	Reproductive tract; regulation of growth, development, function; tissue-specific and general somatic anabolic effects
	T-sensitive tissues (via T as precursor)[c]	Dihydrotestosterone (DHT)	

[a]The information contained in this table is not intended to be all-inclusive. A given hormone may be produced at multiple sites and may be known by additional synonyms. Certainly, with regard to hormone-responsive targets and function, the information summarized here is grossly incomplete; many targets and biologic actions, indeed important biologic actions, are not included. It must also be stressed that only those glands and substances "classically" recognized as primarily endocrine in nature are included. Indeed, a comprehensive tabulation of the large and growing list of hormones (or hormonelike substances) would include, at least, the following: the pituitary endorphins and lipotropins, the placental hormones (human chorionic gonadotropin (hCG) and human placental lactogen (hPL)), additional pancreatic and gastrointestinal hormones (gastrin, vasoactive intestinal peptide (VIP), pancreatic polypeptide, cholecystokinin (CCK), gastric inhibitory peptide (GIP), and secretin), as well as a number of hormones produced in organs traditionally considered to be nonendocrine, such as heart (atrial natriuretic peptides (ANP), kidney (cholecalciferol metabolites, erythropoeitin (ESF), renin), lymphocytes (interleukins), liver (insulinlike growth peptides (IGFs, somatomedins)), platelets (growth or transforming factors, including PDGF and TGF-β), and other sites (various growth and/or transforming factors, including EGF and TGF-α)].

[b]TSH, FSH, and LH contain a carbohydrate moiety attached to the protein component and are thus glycoproteins.

[c]Testosterone is converted to dihydrotestosterone (DHT) in various peripheral tissues; both metabolites, T and DHT, are biologically active.

Structure and Function

I. Structure and function are not only interrelated but are inseparably linked at all levels of the biologic spectrum.

The interdependence of structure and function, a basic principle of osteopathic medicine, is also a fundamental principle of endocrinology. Indeed, the specific biologic activity of a hormone originates in the structural characteristics of the molecule. Endocrine physiology is most usefully studied and understood in terms of molecular structure. In the following discussion the interrelation of hormone structure and function is considered in relation to endocrine processes that underlie the actions of all hormones. In this regard, it is useful to view the hormone as part of a simple endocrine system (Fig. 6.1), consisting of the following:

1. An endocrine gland and the hormone it produces
2. A transport system to deliver the hormone from its site of production to its site(s) of action
3. An effector organ (target) that undergoes a biologic change in response to the hormone

The biochemical events that occur in the endocrine gland are referred to as cellular processing. They include the biosynthesis, storage, and release of the hormone. Transport of the hormone in the plasma depends on the physical and chemical characteristics of the hormone. The nature of the transport process is an important determinant of the metabolism of the hormone and its rate of removal from the plasma, that is, the metabolic clearance rate (MCR) of the hormone. The biochemical events that account for the biologic change in the target are referred to as the mechanism of action of the hormone. These three fundamental components of an endocrine system—cellular processing, transport, and mechanism of action—are considered in the following sections with reference to the inexorable link between structure and function.

CELLULAR PROCESSING

The cellular and subcellular events involved in the biosynthesis, storage, and release of hormones are generally differentiated and grouped on the basis of the chemical structure of the hormone (peptide/protein, steroid, and amine).

Peptides and Proteins

The biosynthesis of peptide and protein hormones is basically consistent with the typical pattern of eucaryotic protein synthesis. That is, specific messenger RNAs are transcribed in the nucleus on DNA and carry the genetic message to the cytoplasm, where it is translated into the specific sequence of amino acids that constitute the hormone. In the case of proteins destined to be exported from the cell, including hormones, peptide bond formation occurs on membrane-bound ribosomes, that is, the rough endoplasmic reticulum (RER). As peptide bond formation occurs, the polypeptide is extruded through the lipid membrane of the endoplasmic reticulum, sequestered within the lumen of the RER, and transported to the Golgi apparatus, where it is packaged into secretory vesicles. During this entire process, the polypeptide is effectively segregated from other cellular proteins and constituents of the cell cytosol. This feature has the advantage of simultaneously protecting and concentrating the nascent polypeptide.

The molecule that is initially synthesized on the RER is not the hormone per se, but rather one of two larger precursor molecules, referred to as a prohormone or a preprohormone. The authentic (mature) hormone is formed by sequential proteolytic cleavages of the precursor as it is transported through the RER and packaged into secretory vesicles in the Golgi apparatus. In response to an adequate stimulus, the secretory vesicles fuse with the cell membrane and release their contents, including the hormone, into the extracellular perivascular space. This "*bulk*" transport process is known as exocytosis, or reverse pinocytosis, and characteristically involves these processes:

Expenditure of energy (ATP)
Mobilization of calcium ion
Participation of the contractile microtubular system

In most cases, polypeptide hormone-secreting cells store ample amounts of hormone-filled secretory vesicles as a means of rapidly responding to demands for increased hormone secretion. That is, the hormone has been presynthesized and prepackaged and is held in the cell in a form ready for release.

Steroids

Just as polypeptide hormone-secreting cells are able to respond rapidly to circumstances that require increased secretion of the hormone, so too are cells that secrete steroid hormones. The strategy employed by these cells is different from that described above. The cells that secrete steroid hormones (adrenocortical, ovarian, testicular) all originate from a common embryologic site, the primitive urogenital ridge. As such, it is not surprising that these functionally distinct cells are not only structurally similar but also employ basically similar pathways for steroid hormone biosynthesis (steroidogenesis).

In all cases, steroid hormones are produced from a common precursor, cholesterol, via sequential enzymatic modifications of the steroid nucleus. The steroid-secreting cells store large amounts of esterified-cholesterol (in the form of fat droplets). The intracellular pool of the precursor is maintained by cholesterol biosynthesis in the cell and also by taking up preformed

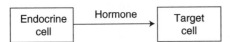

Figure 6.1. A simple endocrine system consisting of endocrine cell and hormone it produces, transport system to deliver hormone from its site of production to its site of action, and target (effector) cell that undergoes a biologic change in response to hormone.

cholesterol from the blood. Ring modifications to the steroid nucleus are catalyzed by enzymes that are associated with specific subcellular structures (e.g., mitochondria, endoplasmic reticulum). The enzyme profile of the cell determines the nature and location of the ring modifications. In so doing, it determines whether the final steroid product is cortisol, aldosterone, androgen, or estrogen. Steroid hormones are highly lipid-soluble and are released from the cell by simple diffusion across the plasma membrane. Unlike peptide and protein hormones, the steroids are not packaged into secretory vesicles and are not stored within the cells in significant amounts. Increasing the rate of steroid synthesis meets demands for increased secretion of the hormones.

Amino Acid Derivatives

The amine type hormones are secreted by the adrenal medulla (catecholamines, including epinephrine and norepinephrine) and the thyroid gland (triiodothyronine and thyroxine). In both glands, the active hormones are derived from a precursor, the amino acid tyrosine, supplied via the blood. Once formed, the catecholamines are packaged into secretory granules and stored within the cell. Release of the hormones occurs by means of an exocytotic process similar to that described for peptide and protein hormones.

The biosynthesis and release of the thyroid hormones is closely tied to the metabolism of a large glycoprotein, thyroglobulin. Thyroid hormones are derived from the iodination and linkage of two residues of the amino acid tyrosine. During the entire biosynthetic sequence, however, the tyrosine molecules are not free within the cell but instead are incorporated into thyroglobulin via peptide bonds. After the thyroid hormones are formed, they remain covalently linked to thyroglobulin. This macromolecule, thyroglobulin with its attached hormones, comprises the major constituent of a gelatinous material known as the thyroid colloid. Large amounts of the colloid are stored in the lumen of the thyroid follicle, that is, outside of the thyroid follicular cell.

Release of the thyroid hormones involves the exquisite interplay of several subcellular organelles. In brief, follicular cells take up droplets of colloid (by endocytosis). In the cell, lysosomes (containing hydrolytic enzymes) merge with the colloid droplets, and proteolysis of the thyroglobulin molecule frees the active thyroid hormones that then diffuse across the cell membrane and enter the bloodstream. It is difficult to imagine that A.T. Still would not consider the subcellular ballet involved in production and release of the thyroid hormones to be graphic representation of the interrelationship of structure and function.

TRANSPORT AND METABOLISM

Once the hormone is released at its site of production, it is transported in the blood to a distant target site, where it produces a biologic change. The magnitude of the change in the target, the biologic response, is proportional to the concentration of the hormone in the blood. This, in turn, is a function not only of the rate at which the hormone enters the blood (rate of secretion), but also of the rate at which it is removed from the blood, that is, the MCR. The characteristics of a particular hormone's transport process have a significant effect on the MCR and therefore on the biologic action of the hormone.

In general, hormones circulate in the blood in one of two ways, depending on the chemical structure and solubility characteristics of the molecule. Amine and polypeptide hormones are readily soluble in the aqueous phase of the plasma and circulate in a free, unbound form. In contrast, steroid and thyroid hormones are hydrophobic and travel in the blood in association with carrier proteins. The carrier, or transport, protein may be a specific plasma globulin with high-affinity binding sites for a particular hormone, for example, testosterone-binding globulin (TeBG). It can also be a nonspecific plasma protein, for example albumin, that associates loosely with a number of hormones.

Several aspects of the binding of hormones to carrier proteins are of particular importance and again underscore the notion that form indeed gives rise to function. First, only the free, unbound fraction of the hormone is biologically active. Functionally, the transport protein-hormone complex serves as a circulating hormone reservoir that can be used to augment or replenish the free, biologically active, hormone pool.

Second, changes in plasma levels of binding proteins occur both physiologically (for example, cortisol-binding globulin levels increase during pregnancy) and pathologically (for example, liver disease). Such changes are reflected in the total (bound plus free) hormone concentration, but not necessarily in the concentration of free, biologically active hormone. This is of practical importance to the osteopathic physician, since diagnostic procedures may measure total plasma hormone, an unreliable index of the actual activity of the hormone.

Third, the MCR of a circulating hormone is directly related to its binding characteristics. Hormones that are tightly bound to carrier proteins have a longer lifetime in the plasma than hormones that circulate in a free or loosely bound form (for example, respectively, thyroxine, days, versus vasopressin, minutes).

MECHANISM OF ACTION

The mechanism of action of a hormone refers to the sequence of chemical and morphological events that mediate the specific biologic action of the molecule on a particular target tissue. At minimum, these intermediary processes must account for certain general characteristics of hormone action. That is, hormones are distributed (via the blood) indiscriminately throughout the body, but only certain tissues (targets) respond to the hormone. A particular tissue may respond to only one hormone or to several different hormones. Some hormones act on only a single tissue or tissue type, whereas other hormones act at numerous, distinct sites. Finally, a particular hormone may elicit widely differing responses in different target tissues.

HYDROPHILIC HORMONES

Peptide hormones and catecholamines act on target cells through a four-stage process.

Hormone Receptor Interaction; Signal Generation

Stage 1 occurs when the interaction of the hormone with a specific, high-affinity receptor on the cell membrane "*signals*" the initiation of the response sequence. It is the presence or absence of the receptor that determines whether the cell responds to the hormone. A particular cell may have receptors for one or more hormones. Fasciculata cells in the adrenal cortex respond selectively to adrenocorticotropic hormone (ACTH), whereas adipose cells respond to several hormones, including glucagon, epinephrine, ACTH, and vasopressin. Both the number of receptors and the affinity of the receptors are physiologically regulated and significantly affect the biologic response. Moreover, abnormal receptor structure and/or function is an important component of the pathophysiology of endocrine disorders (e.g., diabetes mellitus).

Signal Transduction

Stage 2 is signal transduction. Hormone receptor interaction influences guanine nucleotide-sensitive components of the cell membrane, G-proteins, which, in turn, regulate (increase or decrease) the generation of substances referred to as second messengers.

Second Messengers

Stage 3 is that of the second messengers. The biologic response is initiated by the hormone (first messenger), but it is mediated by intracellular second messengers. Cyclic AMP was the first of the intracellular mediators to be recognized, but it is now clear that other substances also fill this role, including, for example, cyclic GMP, calcium ion, and phospholipid metabolites such as diacylglycerol and inositol triphosphate.

Biologic Response

Stage 4 occurs when the second messenger interacts with the chemical machinery of the cell to produce the biologic response. The interaction normally involves a change in the activity of a protein, often an enzyme. It is this protein (enzyme) that determines the characteristics of the biologic response. For instance, in the hepatocyte, cyclic AMP generated in response to glucagon stimulates the phosphorylase enzymes and glycogen breakdown. In the adipocyte, glucagon increases the production of cyclic AMP, activation of an enzyme known as hormone-sensitive lipase, and the hydrolysis of triglyceride.

One characteristic feature of peptide and protein hormones requires further discussion. A particular hormone may elicit widely differing responses in different target tissues. For example, the same posterior pituitary hormone that produces antidiuresis in the nephron produces vasoconstriction in the vasculature and thus is known, respectively, as antidiuretic hormone (ADH) and vasopressin. In the case of the parathyroid hormone (PTH), even a partial list of biologic actions and respective targets would include:

Phosphaturia and bicarbonaturia in renal proximal tubules
Increased calcium reabsorption in renal distal tubules
Bone resorption in osteoblasts
Increased thymidine incorporation in osteocytes

The presence of multiple distinct biologic actions within a single molecule gives rise to the notion that some hormones may contain multiple distinct structural features (amino acid sequences), that is, that some hormones are in fact "*polyhormones.*"[1]

LIPOPHILIC HORMONES

Steroid hormones and thyroid hormones enter the target cell and bind to specific receptor proteins, localized primarily within the nucleus. The hormone-receptor complex regulates the transcription of specific genetic segments in DNA and ultimately the synthesis of specific messenger RNAs and cellular proteins. In contrast to the hydrophilic hormones that regulate the activity of existing cellular proteins (enzymes), the response to lipophilic hormones is mediated by changes in the amount of "*new*" protein (e.g., enzyme). The final biologic response is characterized by the chemical activity (function) of the protein(s) synthesized in response to the hormone. It can range from the increased synthesis of a particular enzyme or functionally related group of enzymes, such as increased hepatic synthesis of gluconeogenic enzymes in response to cortisol, to cellular differentiation and tissue growth, such as prostate hypertrophy in response to androgens.

Body Functions as a Whole

II. The body functions as a whole. It is regulated, coordinated, and integrated through multiple interactive systems.

Hormones play a major role in the orchestration of body unity. In this endeavor, the endocrine system does not operate in isolation but is interdependent with other body systems. The following discussion deals with the interrelation of endocrine, cardiovascular, and neural function.

CARDIOVASCULAR SYSTEM

Endocrine function is dependent on cardiovascular function. This is most obvious in that hormones rely on the cardiovascular system (CVS) as a means of transport to distant sites. The transport function of the CVS usually involves the systemic circulation, but other specialized vascular networks are also employed to great advantage (see below). The circulatory system also participates in controlling the secretion of hormones and in determining the magnitude of their effect at the site of action (target). That is, alterations in blood flow to the endocrine gland contribute to alterations in secretion rate. For example, hyperemia often accompanies increased secretion, and changes in blood flow to the target affect the rate of delivery and the effect of the hormone. Commensurate with the role of the CVS in endocrine function, endocrine glands are typically highly vascularized. For example, throughout the mammalian kingdom, blood supply to the pituitary (milliliter per milligram of tissue weight) is greater than that of any other tissue. In the adrenal gland, cells of the zona fasciculata are arranged in bicellular columns separated by capillaries; that is, each cell is in direct contact with a capillary.

While the endocrine system clearly depends on cardiovascular function, hormones have a major influence on the CVS:

Catecholamines have well-known actions on the heart and vasculature.

Adrenergic cardiac fibers influence myocardial contractility and rhythm.

Adrenergic vasoconstrictor fibers are a dominant influence on systemic vascular resistance.

Catecholamines of adrenal medullary origin and a number of other hormones also influence the cardiovascular system:

Vasopressin and angiotensin are vasoconstrictors.

Thyroid hormones affect heart rate.

Thyroid hormones and aldosterone increase the force of ventricular contraction.

In addition to these "*direct*" actions, endocrine mechanisms (the renin-angiotensin-aldosterone system, antidiuretic hormone, atrial natriuretic peptides) are an important component in the regulation of whole-body fluid and electrolyte metabolism, the extracellular fluid (ECF) and blood volume and, indirectly, cardiovascular function. The endocrine mechanisms serve to maintain fluid homeostasis and cardiovascular function under normal conditions and to "*protect*" cardiovascular function against the consequences of challenges such as water deprivation or hemorrhage.

NERVOUS SYSTEM

A wide variety of external stimuli, or changes in the external environment, alter the activity of the endocrine system by means of multisynaptic neural pathways. For example, auditory stimuli activate the hypothalamic-pituitary axis and increase cortisol secretion. Light cycles influence endocrine rhythms, and groups of females living together may develop synchronous periods of gonadotropin secretion and ovarian function. Changes in the internal environment, such as the chemical composition of the blood, directly affect hormone secretion without the necessity of neural intervention (discussed below). Nevertheless, even in cases like this, neural influences may play a role. Insulin secretion is a typical example: Although glucose and other metabolites stimulate release of the polypeptide, β-cell innervation (sympathetic and parasympathetic) modulates the secretory response.

Just as the nervous system influences endocrine activity, hormones have significant effects on neural activity. The endocrine effects can range from actions on single neurons to alterations of complex mental activity and behavior.

PEPTIDES

A number of peptide hormones have been found to alter CNS activity. For example, vasopressin acts in the CNS to decrease body temperature and to improve memory. In some cases, peptide hormones have been found not only to act in the CNS but also to be produced in the CNS. Examples of these hormones include the atrial natriuretic peptides (ANPs) and angiotensin, which, respectively, inhibit and stimulate the sensation of thirst.

STEROIDS

Gonadal and adrenocortical steroids affect the activity of the hypothalamic neurons that control the anterior pituitary. They thus play a major role in regulating pituitary-gonadal and pituitary-adrenocortical activity. Moreover, both types of steroids influence complex patterns of neural activity; for example, androgens stimulate libido (sex drive) in both males and females. Cortisol deficiency (adrenal insufficiency, Addison's disease) is accompanied by an abnormal electroencephalographic pattern and behavioral and emotional disturbances including anxiety and depression. The cortisol deficiency is corrected by administering the steroid, but caution must be exercised since cortisol excesses also lead to behavioral disorders.

AMINES

The actions of the thyroid amines on the development and function of the CNS are especially profound. Thus, infantile hypothyroidism (cretinism) is associated with retarded mental development. The earlier the condition appears and the longer it goes untreated, the more severe the effects, culminating in irreversible damage to the brain. Congenital hypothyroidism is a current leading cause of preventable mental deficiency. Even after the developmental period, thyroid hormones influence neural activity. In the adult, thyroid status is related to gross behavior such as alertness, mental acuity, and irritability.

In some cases the interaction of endocrine and neural function is so complete that the distinction between the two systems is in fact blurred. Nowhere is this more true than in the hypothalamic-pituitary complex, where neural and endocrine activity are combined in the same neuroendocrine cell. The peptide hormones oxytocin and vasopressin are secreted by neurons having their cell bodies located in the hypothalamus and sending their axons into the neurohypophysis (posterior pituitary). Instead of ending on another nerve or effector, such as a muscle, the neuroendocrine cells terminate on pituitary capillaries and release their hormones into the systemic circulation. Another group of hypothalamic neuroendocrine cells deliver their hormones not to the systemic circulation, but rather to a specialized (portal) vascular system that supplies blood to the adenohypophysis (anterior pituitary). These cells, referred to as hypophysiotropic neurons, regulate the secretory activity of the anterior pituitary.

"FINAL COMMON PATH"

Neural influences predominate in the regulation of anterior pituitary hormone secretion. It is well known that ACTH secretion is related to photoperiod. Growth hormone (GH) secretion is associated with sleep stages. Not only light, odor, auditory, and tactile stimuli but also emotional disturbances influence gonadotropin secretion and reproductive function. For a time, the relationship between anterior pituitary and CNS function presented a conceptual difficulty, since the adenohypophyseal secretory cells are not innervated. (The anterior pituitary is innervated by vasomotor fibers.) Indeed, the (older) endocrine literature refers to the anterior pituitary as *"a gland under neural control, but lacking a nerve supply."*

The physical link between the CNS and the anterior pituitary is not neural but vascular, consisting of a specialized arrangement of vessels, alternatively known as the pituitary portal vessels or the hypothalamo-hypophyseal portal vessels. In brief, the anterior pituitary is regulated by neurohormones that are produced in the hypothalamus and transported to the pituitary in the portal venous blood. The portal vessels originate in a capillary network (primary plexus) located in the hypothalamus. The capillaries coalesce to form the pituitary portal veins, which enter the anterior pituitary and give rise to a secondary capillary plexus. The hypothalamic neurohormones, hypophysiotropic hormones, are produced by neurons that terminate in the hypothalamus in close contact with the primary capillary plexus. The neurohormones enter the portal venous blood and are delivered to the anterior pituitary. This exquisite interrelationship of neural, vascular, and endocrine function is sometimes referred to as *"the final common path."*

The functional significance of the pituitary portal vessels was postulated by Sir Geoffrey Harris about 40 years ago. It is a credit to A.T. Still that he recognized the importance of such relationships almost half a century earlier.

Self-regulating, Self-healing

III. The body is inherently self-regulating and self-healing. Responses to internal and external events are modulated through feedback mechanisms with homeostasis of the internal environment, the internal milieu, as a major goal.

Homeostasis of the internal environment is a primary goal of endocrine physiology. To accomplish this goal, the rate of hormone secretion is modulated according to changes in the internal environment. The relationship between hormones and the internal environment is completely interactive: Changes in the internal environment affect hormone secretion, and changes in hormone concentration influence the composition of the internal environment.

REGULATION OF HORMONE SECRETION

The rate of hormone secretion is controlled by specific chemical signals that increase or decrease the rate of hormone biosynthesis and release. The chemical signals include neural transmitters (e.g., acetylcholine, norepinephrine), supplied at a synaptic junction, and numerous constituents of the blood and extracellular fluid, such as:

Various substrates, such as glucose, amino acids
Ions, such as sodium, potassium, calcium
Other hormones

Regardless of the chemical nature of the signal(s), in all cases the rate of hormone secretion is tightly coupled to demands for the hormone. This is in response to changes in the internal environment, which in turn are, of course, responsive to changes in the external environment. The control mechanisms are designed to ensure that the rate of hormone secretion is, in fact, *appropriate* to environmental conditions. When these mechanisms succeed, as they usually do, the hormone plays a vital role in the self-regulating and self-healing aspects of the body. On the other hand, failure of these mechanisms leads to hormone imbalances and the creation of an internal environment hostile to the health, well-being, and even the very survival of the individual.

CONTROL MECHANISMS

The secretion of a hormone is typically controlled by a self-regulating servomechanism designed to match circulating concentrations of the hormone to the momentary needs of the individual. Two essential features of the control scheme are readily apparent. First, the systemic concentration of the hormone, or of some variable related to the hormone, such as a metabolite, must be monitored. Second, this information must be returned or fed back to the endocrine organ. The secretion of the hormone is adjusted up or down according to the nature of the information returned: inhibitory, negative feedback or stimulatory, positive feedback.

Negative feedback mechanisms are more common than positive feedback mechanisms throughout the endocrine system. Negative feedback mechanisms are inherently self-limiting. In their most basic form they operate as follows:

1. The hormone produces a response in a target cell.
2. Some feature of that response acts back on the cell that produces the hormone to decrease (limit) its secretion.

For example, the adenohypophysis secretes ACTH, which then acts on fasciculata cells in the adrenal cortex to stimulate the production of cortisol. Cortisol has widespread effects throughout the body. One important action of the steroid is to act back on the adenohypophysis to inhibit ACTH secretion.

This closed-loop information pathway is diagrammed in Figure 6.2 as one component of a multifaceted control scheme that regulates the hypothalamo-pituitary-adrenocortical axis. This complex control scheme includes several hormones and multiple negative feedback loops. The first hormone, corticotropin-releasing hormone (CRH), is produced in the hypothalamus and delivered to the pituitary in the portal venous

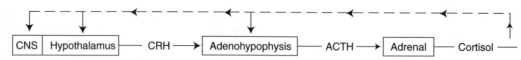

Figure 6.2. Cortisol feeds back at several sites to "dampen" activity of hypothalmic-pituitary-adrenal axis and ultimately to limit own secretion. *CNS*, central nervous system; *CRH*, corticotropin-releasing hormone; *ACTH*, adrenocorticotropic hormone; *solid arrow*, stimulates; *dashed arrow*, inhibits.

blood. The hypothalamic peptide stimulates the secretion of a second hormone, ACTH, that enters the systemic circulation, and activates the adrenocortical secretion of still another hormone, cortisol. The adrenal steroid feeds back on the anterior pituitary, the hypothalamus, and on other sites in the CNS. Negative feedback effects at these several loci all contribute to "dampen" the activity of the hypothalamic-pituitary-adrenal axis and ultimately to limit the secretion of cortisol. Since negative feedback mechanisms are inherently self-limiting in nature, it is perhaps not apparent that this mechanism is equally important as a means of increasing hormone secretion. For example, inadequate circulating levels of cortisol are accompanied by decreased negative feedback that leads to activation of the hypothalamic-pituitary-adrenal axis and increased secretion of the steroid.

As noted above, positive feedback mechanisms are also employed to control endocrine systems. Here, two hormones (or other variables) change in the same direction, so that an initial increase in the activity of the system leads to further increased activity. This type of mechanism does not limit but rather amplifies the magnitude of the effect and produces an abrupt, "explosive" change in the activity of the system.

Although positive feedback mechanisms are rather uncommon, they nevertheless play a vital role in regulating certain aspects of endocrine function. A particularly noteworthy example is the role of positive feedback in regulating reproductive function. The pituitary gonadotropins, follicle-stimulating hormone and luteinizing hormone (FSH and LH, respectively), stimulate the production of estrogen. The steroid acts back on the ovary to promote growth and development of the ovarian follicle and additional estrogen secretion. As a consequence, plasma concentrations of estrogen rise dramatically. Near the midpoint of the menstrual cycle, the high circulating levels of steroid trigger a sudden, marked increase in LH secretion, which, in turn, induces ovulation. Ovulation depends on the preovulatory LH surge, and LH secretion is driven by the positive feedback effects of estrogen at at least two sites, the ovary and the pituitary. The importance of these events to normal reproductive function is underscored by the fact that contraceptive steroid regimens are expressly designed to create steroid imbalances that prevent the preovulatory LH surge.

TEMPORAL PATTERNS

As described above, the rate of hormone secretion is tightly controlled and responsive to physiological demands. Although it is clear that secretion rate (the amount of hormone delivered to the blood per unit time) influences the circulating concentration and activity of the hormone, hormone activity is not a simple function of concentration. That is, the temporal pattern of changes in secretory rate and circulating concentration of the hormone also influence hormone activity. Many, perhaps all, endocrine glands secrete hormones in a repetitious "stop and go" fashion, a quiescent period followed by a burst of secretory activity. This leads to small but physiologically significant oscillations in plasma hormone concentrations. This secretory pattern, referred to as pulsatile or episodic secretion, has two important characteristics:

1. The rate of hormone secretion (amount/time) is the product of the frequency (episodes/time) and amplitude (amount/episode) of the secretory episodes.
2. Changes in secretory rate are produced by corresponding changes in both parameters; for example, negative feedback signals decrease both the frequency and amplitude of the secretory episodes.

Episodic secretion is characteristically associated with high-frequency oscillations in secretory activity: Release episodes are separated by only brief intervals of time (minutes). In some cases the high-frequency secretory episodes are superimposed upon other lower-frequency temporal patterns or rhythms having periodicities of hours, days, or even months. For example, ACTH and the pituitary gonadotropins are secreted episodically and display high-frequency oscillations in plasma concentration. At the same time, plasma levels of ACTH (and also cortisol) are well known to cycle on a daily basis, in the classic diurnal rhythm. In reproductively competent females, pituitary gonadotropins (and also the gonadal steroids) cycle rhythmically with a period of approximately a month.

The cellular and molecular mechanisms that generate patterned or rhythmic hormone secretion are not well understood. The implication of phasic hormone release also requires further study. Nevertheless, it is clear in a few cases that the oscillations are physiologically significant. For example, inadequate secretion of hypothalamic luteinizing hormone-releasing hormone (LH-RH) leads to reproductive failure. This condition is corrected by administration of the peptide, but only if the LH-RH is given in a pulsatile fashion that approximates normal endogenous secretion.

PROCESSES REGULATED BY HORMONES

Hormones are involved in regulating the most fundamental aspects of human life. Indeed, hormones play a vital role with regard to the survival of the species. That role includes:

Reproduction
Growth
Development to reproductive maturity

Hormones also play a vital role with regard to the survival of the individual:

Maintenance of the internal environment
Energy metabolism

Reproduction

Hormones produced by the hypothalamus (gonadotropin-releasing hormone (GnRH)), the pituitary (FSH, LH, prolactin (PRL), GH), and the gonads (androgens, estrogens, progestogens) interact to regulate reproductive function. Reproductive competence requires the ability to produce gametes (ova, sperm) and the ability to unite the gametes by attracting and mating with members of the opposite sex. There are several aspects of this process:

Gamete formation, that is, spermatogenesis, oogenesis
Mating ability, that is, growth, development, and maintenance of the reproductive tract
Mutual attractiveness, that is, male and female phenotype, and pattern of sexual behavior

All are influenced by or totally depend on the reproductive hormones. After conception, maternal support for the developing fetus (pregnancy) is hormone-dependent, and in mammals, even after birth, hormones continue to play a role in nurturing the infant during lactation.

Growth and Development

The regulation of intrauterine growth is poorly understood. Surprisingly, hormones having dramatic effects on the neonate (growth hormone, thyroid hormone) appear to have little influence on fetal growth. Somatomedins and other growth factors undoubtedly play a role in prenatal growth, but much research must be done to clarify that role.

The regulation of postnatal growth is better understood. In addition to a number of nonhormonal factors, such as nutrition, hygiene, and general health, normal growth and development depend on the interplay of several hormones, including:

GH and the somatomedins
Thyroid hormone
Insulin
Cortisol
Gonadal steroids

Imbalances in the secretion of these hormones, excesses as well as deficiencies, dramatically affect growth, especially if the imbalance occurs during the normal growing period. For example, hyposecretion of GH produces dwarfism. Hypersecretion of the hormone leads to giantism. Thyroid hormone deficit impairs growth of the body and also has devastating effects on the development of the CNS and mental capacity. Cortisol or

the gonadal steroids in excess slow or even arrest growth and lead to short adult stature.

Internal Environment

Many, and in a broad sense all, hormones participate in the "defense" of the internal environment. Although no aspect of the internal environment is unimportant to health and well being, certain features are regulated and "guarded" especially closely by functional groups of hormones. These include the:

1. Ionic composition (Na^+, K^+, and H^+) of the body fluids, most notably the blood and cerebrospinal fluid (the renin-angiotensin-aldosterone system, ANP, insulin, and other hormones)
2. Volume of the body fluids, especially the ECF volume and the blood volume (ADH, the renin-angiotensin-aldosterone system, ANP, cortisol, and others)
3. Plasma level of calcium and phosphate ions (PTH, 1,25-dihydroxycholecalciferol ($1,25\text{-}(OH)_2\text{-}D_3$), calcitonin, and others)
4. Structural integrity and function of body tissues, including bone, muscle, and adipose tissue (GH and the somatomedins, PTH, $1,25\text{-}(OH)_2\text{-}D_3$, gonadal steroids, insulin, glucagon, cortisol, and others)
5. Direction and rate of flow of metabolic energy

Energy Metabolism

The hormonal regulation of energy metabolism allows the body to meet its need for a constant supply of energy in spite of the intermittent intake of food. Even at rest, vital bodily processes must be maintained. There is a significant metabolic "cost of living"—the basal metabolic rate. On the other hand, the intake of energy (calories contained in food) is sporadic; the consumption of excess food (caloric intake exceeds momentary needs) is interspersed with periods of fasting. To resolve this problem, excess energy is stored in a form that is readily mobilized and available for use when necessary. The metabolic flow in both directions, storage and retrieval, is directed and controlled by hormones.

During the period when exogenous fuels are available, insulin is of primary importance. The polypeptide stimulates the uptake and metabolism of glucose (glycolysis) and promotes the storage of small metabolites in their respective macromolecular forms, that is, glucose as glycogen, amino acids as protein, and free fatty acids as triglyceride. When exogenous fuels are not available, several hormones, most notably glucagon and cortisol, collaborate to mobilize energy from endogenous storage sites. Glucagon stimulates the hydrolysis of glycogen (glycogenolysis) and triglyceride (lipolysis). It increases the formation of new glucose from noncarbohydrate sources (gluconeogenesis). Cortisol stimulates gluconeogenesis and mobilizes amino acids (gluconeogenic precursors) from protein depots.

The importance of the hormonal controls is dramatically illustrated in clinical conditions such as diabetes mellitus and Addison's disease (cortisol deficiency). The absence of insulin leads to a metabolic profile that in many respects resembles that seen in long-term food deprivation (starvation) and, if left untreated, death. In the absence of cortisol, gluconeogenesis is so seriously impaired that short periods of food deprivation, even an overnight fast, pose a serious threat to life.

CONCLUSION

This chapter reviews the endocrine system with reference to osteopathic philosophy and concepts. The picture that emerges is that osteopathy embraces endocrine physiology. The principles that direct the study and practice of osteopathic medicine might well have been formulated on the basis of a through understanding of endocrine physiology. Yet A.T. Still never studied endocrinology, for this is a new science, evolving entirely during this century. Almost all of the endocrine information presented here is a product of the last few years and virtually *none* of this information was available at the time osteopathy came into being. The future surely holds still more, and even unexpected, information concerning not only endocrinology but all body systems. However, the conclusion is inescapable: Osteopathic philosophy is so deep-rooted in an understanding of the fabric of life that this new information too will be embraced.

REFERENCES

1. Mallette LE. The parathyroid polyhormones: new concepts in the spectrum of peptide hormone action. *Endocr Rev.* 1991;12:110–117.

SUGGESTED READINGS

Clark JH, Schrader WT, O'Malley BW. Mechanism of steroid hormone action. In: Wilson JD, Foster DW, eds. *Textbook of Endocrinology*. Philadelphia, Pa: WB Saunders Co; 1985:33–75.

Daughaday W. Prolactin and growth hormone in health and disease. In: Ingbar SH, ed. *Contemporary Endocrinology*. vol 2. New York, NY: Plenum Publishing Co; 1985:27–86.

Griffin JE, Ojeda SR, eds. *Textbook of Endocrine Physiology*. New York, NY: Oxford University Press, 1988.

Kelly RB. Pathways of protein secretion in eukaryotes. *Science.* 1985;230:25–28.

Nunez J. Effects of thyroid hormones during brain differentiation. *Mol Cell Endocrinol.* 1984;37:125.

Roth J, Grunfeld C. Mechanism of action of peptide hormones and catecholamines. In: Wilson JD, Foster DW, eds. *Textbook of Endocrinology*. Philadelphia, Pa: WB Saunders Co; 1985:76–122.

Sayers G, Portanova R. Regulation of the secretory activity of the adrenal cortex: cortisol and corticosterone. In: Greep RO, Astwood EB, eds. *Handbook of Physiology*, Section 7: Endocrinology, vol 2. Baltimore: Williams & Wilkins; 1975:41–53.

Schrier RW. *Vasopressin*. New York, NY: Raven Press, 1985.

Shupnik MA. Effects of gonadotropin-releasing hormone on rat gonadotropin gene transcription in vitro: requirement for pulsatile administration for luteinizing hormone gene stimulation. *Mol Endocrinol.* 1990;4(10):1444–1450.

Wilson SK, Lynch DR, Ladenson PW. Angiotensin II and atrial natriuretic factor-binding sites in various tissues in hypertension: comparative receptor localization and changes in different hypertension models in the rat. *Endocrinology.* 1989;124:2799–2808.

Wise PM, Scarbrough K, Weiland NG, et al. Diurnal pattern of proopiomelanocortin gene expression in the arcuate nucleus of proestrous, ovariectomized, and steroid-treated rats: a possible role in cyclic luteinizing hormone secretion. *Mol Endocrinol.* 1990;4(6):886–892.

7. Pharmacologic and Osteopathic Basic Principles

ROBERT J. THEOBALD, JR.

Key Concepts

- **Similarities between basic pharmacologic concepts and the basic tenets of osteopathic medicine**

- **Differences between a reductionist view and a holistic view of biomedical science**

- **Several intrinsic and extrinsic factors that influence drug responses of an individual**

- **Pharmacologic phases of drug responses**

The goal of this chapter is to help the reader appreciate the relationship between the biomedical science of pharmacology and the basic tenets of osteopathic medicine. The fundamental concepts of biomedical science are the foundation of all medicine. The basic osteopathic concepts include:

Structure–function relationship
Homeostasis
Unity

The concepts of pharmacology and the concepts of osteopathy are similar. They complement each other and other medical modalities. The principles of osteopathy are crucial to practicing good medicine, to making sound clinical decisions, and to integrating basic science and clinical science in the treatment of patients.

Korr[1] emphasizes the need to redirect basic biomedical research away from a reductionist view to a view more suited to investigation of the body as a whole unit. He states, *"the reductionist paradigm is not unproductive, but it is incomplete"* and *"reductionist, mechanistic medical research fails to see that when illness occurs, whatever the affected part, it is illness of the person."*[1] The logical corollary to this is the need for clinical medicine to treat the whole person, not just the diseased part. Korr further states that this *"mechanistic biomedical philosophy"* espouses *"that the way to understand anything, including humans, their illnesses, and the origins of their vulnerability, is to take them apart; that is, to reduce them to their components, and to study these and their interactions as minutely as possible."*[1] The major problem with this view is that it fails to appreciate the effect of illness and treatment of illness on the whole organism, the total human body. The reductionist view, held by many practicing clinicians, is contrary to basic tenets of both pharmacology and osteopathy. Korr's paper implies that whatever the

physician does to any part of the patient the physician also does to the whole body because the body is a unit whose parts respond to anything done to any part.

The osteopathic principles—body unity, homeostasis, and the relationship of structure and function—are mutually supportive of the basic principles of pharmacokinetics and pharmacodynamics. These pharmacokinetic and pharmacodynamic principles provide the foundation for our understanding of how the body deals with these drugs and how drugs work in the body. The principles complement osteopathy and the role of osteopathic manipulative techniques (OMT) similarly to the way they complement other medical modalities. Use of drugs to treat an illness does not, and should not, preclude the use of OMT anymore than it should preclude the use of other modalities, such as surgery. The role of the physician is to orchestrate the use of all appropriate interventions to the best advantage of the patient, always basing decisions on fundamental principles of osteopathy and of all good medicine.

This chapter focuses on the principles of pharmacology, providing a basis for the understanding of the similarities of pharmacology and osteopathy. It shows how pharmacology, OMT, and other medical modalities are complementary. This chapter also discusses the interaction of these principles, showing that they are intertwined and must be considered together in any decision-making process.

PHARMACOLOGIC PRINCIPLES

Individualization of Therapy

The most important pharmacologic concept to remember when considering the use of drugs is that of individualization of therapy. Physicians treat people, whole people, and whatever they do to any part of a person, they also do to the whole person. The body, as a unit, is comprised of many components and factors. Some are intrinsic and some extrinsic. They all affect responses to drugs and other medical interventions. To individualize drug therapy, one must be fully aware of both intrinsic and extrinsic factors that are part of each person and may influence any response to drugs. The intrinsic factors include characteristics such as:

Age
Sex
Genetics
Health
Race
Other factors inherent in a person's makeup

The extrinsic factors include characteristics such as:

Occupation
Smoking
Alcohol consumption
Physical activity
Diet
Home environment
Other factors that may be altered if necessary

These factors, found in Table 7.1, determine in part who the patient is and influence how the patient will respond to any drug prescribed. These are the aspects a physician must consider when choosing medication for any patient, because that person is the composite of the extrinsic and intrinsic factors. In other words, the body is a unit (one osteopathic principle) made up of these factors, each of which will be affected by whatever the physician does to the patient.

Homeostasis

A second osteopathic principle states that the body has inherent self-regulatory, defensive, and recuperative powers. This principle is very similar to the phenomenon called homeostasis. Homeostatic mechanisms are a system of control mechanisms that use feedback loops to maintain stability of bodily functions. These mechanisms help the body self-regulate, provide defense against anything that triggers an untoward response, and help maintain a stable internal environment in which injured tissues can use the natural recuperative powers inherent in the body, described so well by Still.[2] Many diseases, in fact probably all diseases, may be considered disruptions of homeostasis. They are disruptions of the stability of activity or function of some system in the body. Discussion of homeostatic mechanisms is vital to understanding the effects of many drugs on the systems of the body. Drugs produce many effects throughout the body, changing levels of activity in organ systems, changes that stimulate reflex responses in the body, or sometimes blunt these responses. Drugs also alter the environment in which an organ functions, such that the body's reflex mechanisms, homeostatic mechanisms, can reclaim control of a malfunctioning system. This reinforces the concept of body unity.

Structure Activity

The third osteopathic principle states that structure and function are reciprocally related. This principle is analogous to the structure–activity relationship described for many drugs. In the mid-19th century an English physician, James Blake, established the principle that the chemical structure of drugs determines their effect on the body.[3] The relationship between functional groups of drugs and the characteristics of the drugs was defined further by Fraser, another English physician, and Brown, a chemist.[3] The concept of structure–activity relationships for drugs and their effects is important to the understanding of the pharmacokinetics and pharmacodynamics of a drug, including:

Administration
Distribution
Biotransformation
Excretion
Effect at specific receptor sites

PHARMACOLOGIC PROCESSES

The processes occurring with the administration of a drug and the production of effects in a living system can be divided into three phases:

1. Pharmaceutic
2. Pharmacokinetic
3. Pharmacodynamic

These phases are described in Table 7.2.

Pharmaceutics

The pharmaceutic phase is the study of the relationship between the nature and intensity of the biological effects observed, and the different factors related to the nature of the drugs, such as the physical state, particle size, which salt is used, etc. These factors are important and affect the dissolution and disintegration of a drug after oral administration. To be ab-

Table 7.1
Factors That Influence Drug Responses

Intrinsic Factors	Extrinsic Factors
Body weight and size	Diet
Age	Smoking
Sex	Occupation
Body composition	Lifestyle
Genetic factors	Physical activity level
Somatovisceral factors	Home environment
Physical health	
Psychological health	

Table 7.2
Three Pharmacologic Phases

Administration of drug ↓ Disintegration and dissolution of drug	]—Pharmaceutical
↓	
Absorption Distribution Biotransformation Elimination	]—Pharmacokinetic
↓	
Drug receptor interaction ↓ Drug effects	]—Pharmacodynamic

sorbed into the body from the gastrointestinal tract, a drug must be dissolved in the aqueous contents of the stomach. For this to occur, it must disintegrate from the tablet or capsule form. The importance of this for pharmacology involves the assumption that drugs dissolve completely in the gastrointestinal tract upon oral administration. The validity of this assumption involves consideration of differences in various commercial preparations. Consider this factor when choosing preparations for administration to patients. It is important to determine bioavailability of drugs, which can be critical in certain clinical situations.

Pharmacokinetics

Pharmacokinetics is the study of factors that determine the amount of drug at sites of biologic effect at various times after application of the drug to a biologic system. These factors deal with the concentration of drugs in the body as a function of time. Pharmacokinetics considers what the body does to the drug, that is, the phenomena of:

Absorption
Distribution
Biotransformation (metabolism)
Elimination

To have any effect on the body, a drug must reach the appropriate sites of action within the body, usually receptors. It must be absorbed in sufficient amounts to produce effective concentrations at the sites of action. Some of the factors influencing absorption include:

Age
Diet
Blood flow through the site of administration
pH of body fluids at the site of administration

Distribution of the drug from the site of administration to the site of action is influenced by factors such as:

Structure of the drug
Binding of the drug to plasma proteins
pK_a
Other factors

Only the portion of drug that is free (not bound to plasma proteins) is active and capable of producing an effect, of distributing and equilibrating in the body, of being biotransformed and excreted.

Termination of drug effects in the body occurs several ways:

Through redistribution to nonsites of action
Biotransformation
Excretion

Just because the effects of a drug are no longer apparent, the drug is not necessarily excreted from the body. The clinical manifestation of effects that are expected are not the only effects of the drug.

Pharmacodynamics

Pharmacodynamics is the study of biochemical and physiological effects of drugs as they interact with the body at various levels of organization and systems in the body. The focus is on the characteristics of drugs, what a drug does to the body. The effects of a drug are the consequence of the interaction of the drug with structures in the body called receptors. This interaction occurs through the attachment of the drug to the receptor via some type of chemical binding, such as hydrogen or ionic or covalent binding. The interaction can occur because the structure of any given drug determines if it will bind to a specific receptor and, if it binds, what type of effect, agonistic or antagonistic, it will have. An agonist is a drug whose structure allows it to bind to its receptor and produce some action or effect. An agonist is said to possess intrinsic activity. An antagonist is a drug whose structure allows it to bind to its receptor without producing an action or effect; it possesses no intrinsic activity.

This phenomenon of drug–receptor interaction exemplifies the osteopathic principle of structure–function relationships. The structures of the drugs and receptors determine their function. Many drugs are structural analogs of endogenous substances that have been isolated from the body and identified. Still strongly encouraged this when he said in his autobiography, *"Man should study and use the drugs compounded in his own body."*[4] In effect, that is what has been done. Structural analogs of endogenous substances have been synthesized and altered to have agonist or antagonist effects on specific receptors. Alteration of structure, for example, addition of an OH group or a methyl group, can produce an altered function. This exemplifies the basic osteopathic principle that structure and function are intimately related. Recent examples of this include immunologic agents, such as the interferon analogs, and the prostaglandin-based antisecretory/cytoprotective agent, misoprostol.

Most drug effects, but not all, are mediated through receptors. Receptors are proteins or protein-related structures in membranes that link drugs to intracellular functional systems through signal transduction mechanisms. The interaction of receptors and signal transduction mechanisms are varied and include:

Receptors coupled to ion channels
Receptors coupled to G-proteins
Receptors linked to tyrosine kinase
Intracellular steroid receptors interacting with specific target DNA elements

Non–receptor-mediated drug actions include mechanisms such as drug interaction with small molecules (e.g., chelation, or gastric acid neutralization) and inhibition of enzymes (e.g., inhibitors of angiotensin-converting enzyme). Although drugs are classified by a major mechanism of action, such as α-adrenergic receptor antagonists, drugs may have other mechanisms of action; all drugs have multiple effects.

OSTEOPATHIC AND PHARMACOLOGIC INTERACTIONS

There are different ways osteopathic and pharmacologic principles may interact. For example, when considering treatment for a patient with a CNS disorder that requires medication that will enter the CNS, the physician must consider the structure–function relationship of the tissues involved, as well as the structure–activity relationship of any drug being considered.

Structure–Function Relationship

The blood–brain barrier, a barrier that restricts the entry of polar molecules from entering the brain readily, protects the brain from severe toxic effects of drugs like penicillins or tubocurarine. The cerebral capillaries have an essentially continuous layer of endothelial cells with tight gap junctions that form the barrier. The blood–brain barrier is neither absolute nor invariable. Very large doses of drugs, such as penicillin, will cross the barrier. In addition, inflammation of the barrier lessens its effectiveness.

Knowing that the barrier allows small molecules and lipid-soluble molecules to enter the CNS much more readily, the physician could choose a drug with those characteristics. A drug like succinylcholine is a neuromuscular blocking agent that is used as an adjuvant in surgery. It possesses a charged ion in its structure, is not very lipid-soluble, and therefore does not readily cross the blood–brain barrier. However, a drug like thiopental, a barbiturate that is highly lipid-soluble, so rapidly enters the CNS that it produces effects within seconds after an intravenous administration of sufficient dose. Subsequently, because of its lipid solubility, thiopental rapidly leaves the CNS and sequesters in other lipid tissues that are not sites of action, such as adipose tissue. This termination of effects is due to redistribution of the drug to a nonsite of action.

Structure–Activity Relationship

Structure–activity relationships are also important when considering drugs that readily sequester in certain tissues for clinical effect. In treating a patient with a lower urinary tract infection, for example, consider several factors when choosing an appropriate antimicrobial agent. First, the antimicrobial agent must be effective against the infecting organism. Second, any pharmacologic agent used must concentrate in the urine in large enough levels to provide adequate antimicrobial activity. Structural characteristics of pharmacologic agents influence mechanisms of termination of effects and clearance of the drug from the plasma. Agents such as sulfonamides and trimethoprim are rapidly cleared into the urine, providing ample concentrations in the urine for antimicrobial activity. Drugs such as minocycline and doxycycline do not concentrate in the urine and therefore would not be appropriate choices for treatment of lower urinary tract infections.

Considering the interactions of osteopathic and pharmacologic principles in this manner should aid an understanding of the interrelationship. The physician needs to integrate these principles so that he or she can provide a comprehensive approach to caring for each individual patient.

Interaction of Principles and Hypertension

ETIOLOGY

The cause of primary hypertension, although not clearly understood, apparently involves an initial increase in cardiac output.[5] This increase in cardiac output increases blood flow to tissues, which in turn causes a compensatory autoregulation at the tissue level. The autoregulation involves a twofold action. First, a functional autoregulation produces a vasoconstriction that decreases flow to the tissue. Second, a structural autoregulation causes hypertrophy of the vessel wall that amplifies any vasoconstrictor activity or stimulus, such as sympathetic nerve stimulation.

The structural change, hypertrophy, contributes and amplifies the functional change, vasoconstriction, producing an even greater elevation of blood pressure.[6] This interaction of structure as an amplification of the functional change provides support for the osteopathic tenet involving structure and function relationships.

The structural change, vascular hypertrophy, is not solely responsible for the elevation of blood pressure, but it is an important contributor and, in fact, may be the autoregulatory component responsible for the chronic elevation of blood pressure seen in hypertension.[5] To understand this chronic role of hypertrophy, consider the concept of down-regulation of receptors that are under chronic neurotransmitter stimulation. The basic concept is that some trigger, unknown perhaps, creates a change that produces a structural/functional alteration in vascular smooth muscle that results in an abnormal homeostatic level of blood pressure.

PHARMACOLOGIC TREATMENT

Treatment of hypertension with pharmacologic agents alters this abnormal state and attempts to return blood pressure to a "normal" level, that level which would be maintained by the body's own homeostatic mechanisms if they were functioning properly. The pharmacologic intervention provides several benefits. During the time of pharmacologic maintenance of blood pressure, there is some evidence that the hypertrophy of vascular smooth muscle regresses, leading to a decrease in blood pressure.[6] This supports the osteopathic tenet that structure and function are related. A decrease in muscle mass leads to a decrease in muscle tension and a decrease in blood pressure. There is also evidence emerging that, after some period of time, pharmacologic intervention may be decreased or ceased completely because the patient's own homeostatic mechanisms are then capable of normal regulatory control of blood pressure, eliminating the need for pharmacologic intervention.

Treating hypertension with pharmacologic agents is not inconsistent with the osteopathic tenet of the body's self-healing potential. It actually supports this and may provide benefit similar to OMT, where a treatment regimen, in addition to other benefits, provides an opportunity for the body to heal itself. In this instance, the body's homeostatic mechanisms are allowed to regain proper control of blood pressure. The pharmacologic agents maintain blood pressure at the appropriate level while the self-healing actions of the body occur, the decrease in vascular smooth muscle mass in this instance. Additionally, OMT has been shown to decrease hypersympathetic tone, decrease total peripheral resistance, and affect the renin-angiotensin-aldosterone system.[7] Therefore, appropriate OMT in conjunction with pharmacologic therapy could hasten the return of normal function of the body's autoregulatory systems.

Before starting pharmacologic treatment of hypertension, consider several points in light of the principles of viewing the body as a unit and individualization of therapy. First, fully investigate the cause of the hypertension to determine if the hypertension is primary or secondary. If any factors are present that tend to raise blood pressure, such as smoking, eliminate them, or at least modify them to lessen their influence. Second, when treating very high blood pressure, begin treatment without delay. Overaggressive treatment may be risky, however; carry it out with extreme care. It is important in treating patients with very high blood pressure to lower blood pressure gradually so that hypotension does not result. Third, treatment of hypertension requires a long-term, perhaps lifelong, relationship between the patient and the physician. Reassess patients periodically to determine if pharmacotherapy is still necessary, and, if so, is still effective. The reassessment should be an evaluation of the total patient. The aim is to find a therapeutic regimen, including a drug or combination of drugs, that lowers blood pressure effectively, is not contraindicated in any way, and may be positively helpful in other ways. These are Simpson's key points on the treatment of hypertensive disease.[8]

Drugs used to treat hypertension fall into several classes, including:

Diuretics
β-Adrenergic receptor blocking drugs
α-Adrenergic receptor blocking drugs
Adrenergic neuron blocking drugs
Centrally acting α-adrenergic agonists
Calcium channel blocking drugs
Direct acting vasodilators
Angiotensin-converting enzyme inhibitors
Ganglionic blocking agents

The choice of which agent to use depends upon fully evaluating the patient, including all factors listed above. For example, use of a β-adrenergic receptor blocking drug, such as propranolol, would be effective in lowering blood pressure. However, consideration must be given to other factors such as concurrent diseases. Blockade of β-adrenergic receptors can exacerbate symptoms of other diseases, such as congestive heart failure, peripheral vascular disease, bronchial asthma, or chronic obstructive pulmonary disease (COPD). Some of these agents could also interfere with the control of diabetes because of blockade of β_2-adrenergic receptors. Other agents with intrinsic sympathomimetic activity (ISA) could aggravate anginal symptoms or increase risk for patients with a previous myocardial infarction. These agents are also known to cause sexual dysfunction in some men. Counseling may be necessary before and during use of these agents in male patients, indicating the need to consider sex and age factors in clinical decisions.

Other antihypertensive agents, such as the adrenergic neuron-depleting agent reserpine, cross the blood–brain barrier and can cause central nervous system side effects like depression and sedation. Consider the patient's lifestyle when agents such as these are part of the clinical options. If a patient lives alone and must be self-sufficient, as many elderly patients do, then agents that cause depression and sedation may produce very detrimental side effects. Other agents with no or fewer CNS effects would be a better choice.

In making pharmacologic decisions, consider the total patient including physical, mental, and spiritual aspects. The physician does *not* treat just the hypertension; the physician treats the whole patient. The intrinsic and extrinsic factors listed in Table 7.1 are just a checklist, a beginning for total patient evaluation.

CONCLUSION

Pharmacologic therapy does not preclude therapy with other modalities, especially osteopathic modalities, and can be effectively integrated into an osteopathic approach for the treatment of disease and dysfunction. The principles of osteopathy and pharmacology are mutually supportive, and are very similar. Individualization of therapy, based on an understanding of body unity, should be the framework of all clinical decisions. Do what is best for the patient, the whole patient, remembering that whatever drug you give, or treatment you apply to any part of the body, you do to the whole body.

REFERENCES

1. Korr IM. Osteopathic research: The Needed Paradigm Shift. *JAOA.* 1991;91(2):156–171.
2. Still AT. In: Schmucker RV, ed. *Early Osteopathy in the Words of A.T. Still.* Kirksville, Mo: The Thomas Jefferson University Press, Northeast Missouri State University; 1991:36.
3. Levine RR. *Pharmacology: Drug Actions and Reactions.* 4th ed. Boston, Mass: Little, Brown and Co; 1990:12.
4. Still AT. *Autobiography of Andrew T. Still.* 1908:89. Reprinted Indianapolis, Ind: American Academy of Osteopathy; 1981.
5. Onrot J, Rangno RE. Treatment of cardiac disorders: hypertension. In: Melmon KL, Morrelli HF, Hoffman BB, Nierenberg DW, eds. *Melmon and Morrelli's Clinical Pharmacology: Basic Principles in Therapeutics.* 3rd ed. New York, NY: McGraw-Hill, Inc, 1992:52–83.
6. Folkow B. Early structural changes. Brief historical background and principle nature of process. *Hypertension.* 1984;6(suppl 3):1–3.
7. Mannino JR. The application of neurologic reflexes to the treatment of hypertension. *JAOA.* 1979;79(10):225–231.
8. Simpson FO. Hypertensive disease: In: Speight TM, ed. *Avery's Drug Treatment.* 3rd ed. New York, NY: Churchill-Livingston; 1987:676–731.

8. Human Regulatory Adaptations in Health and Disease

A MOLECULAR PERSPECTIVE

EUGENE MOCHAN

Key Concepts

- **Importance of regulatory phenomena in health and disease**

- **Interacting molecular events that lead to homeostasis**

- **Molecular defenses, repair mechanisms, and adaptive responses that serve to protect individuals from internal and external stressors**

- **Potential role of the musculoskeletal system in the ability of the body to be self-regulating and self-healing**

Osteopathic philosophy embraces the concept of the unity of body structure and function in health and disease.[1,2] From the physiological point of view, the body contains the necessary units and regulatory devices to maintain the following:

Structural integrity
Functional capabilities
Growth
Development
Reproduction

The human body also has a tremendous capacity to maintain and heal itself.

At the molecular level,[3] health is the natural capacity of the human organism, through a complex set of metabolic regulatory devices, to achieve a biological steady state, referred to as homeostasis. This enables the individual to resist both internal and external stressors experienced during daily life. Healthy individuals use numerous molecular regulatory adaptations to compensate for these perturbations. Disease leading to illness results when this natural capacity to maintain homeostasis becomes overwhelmed. In addition, a person's adaptive responses to stressors themselves may become a source for producing pathologic changes.

This chapter presents an overview of the nature of perturbing stressors and the resulting human metabolic responses that lead to metabolic and physiologic homeostasis. Particular emphasis is placed on the molecular basis of human adaptive responses that protect individuals from internal and external disturbances, and their osteopathic significance.

OVERVIEW OF STRESSORS AND HUMAN DEFENSE SYSTEMS

Organisms have developed selective survival advantages by acquiring molecular regulatory devices that neutralize threatening stressors.[3] These stressors may be physical, chemical, and/or psychological in nature (Fig. 8.1).

Physical/chemical stressors include environmental pollutants such as these:

Radiation
Carcinogens
Teratogens
Mutagens

They also include environmental pressures, such as temperature extremes, and other physiological stressors:

Hypoxia
Hypoglycemia
Infectious agents
Trauma
Blood loss

Psychological stressors result from internal reactions to one's own personal thoughts and/or feelings regarding perceived threats. When the stressors result from social interactions, they are often referred to as psychosocial stressors.

The major categories of human protective adaptive responses to stressors (Fig. 8.1) include:

Physical barriers (e.g., skin, mucous membranes)
Phagocytes of the reticuloendothelial system
Chemical detoxification systems
Inflammatory reaction
Coagulation system
Complement system
Immune system
Stress response

HUMAN STRESS RESPONSE

Endocrine and Metabolic Factors

The adaptive responses can be specific to the stressor or can be generalized and nonspecific.[3] Responses of the latter type ap-

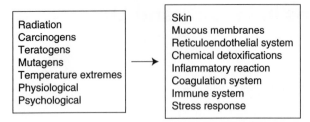

Figure 8.1. Major categories of stressors (*left*) and human protective/adaptive responses (*right*).

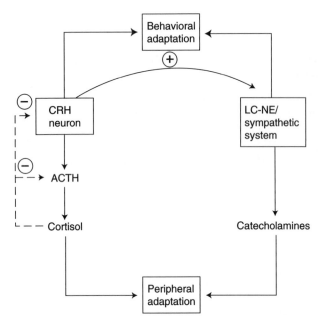

Figure 8.2. Neuroendocrine factors in human stress response. Stimulation of hypothalamic corticotropin-releasing hormone (*CRH*) neurons stimulate both pituitary adrenocorticotropic hormone (*ACTH*) and central autonomic-arousal systems (locus ceruleus-norepinephrine system (*LC-NE*)), leading, respectively, to glucocorticoid and catecholamine (norepinephrine (*NE*)) secretion.

pear to occur only if the magnitude of the stressor to homeostasis exceeds a certain threshold. In humans and other mammals, this response is referred to as the "stress response" or "general adaptation response." It includes a series of interactive molecular, cellular, physiologic, and behavioral responses that function to restore physiological homeostasis. The hypothalamic peptide hormone, corticotropin-releasing hormone (CRH), and the locus ceruleus-norepinephrine (LC-NE) systems are major effectors of the stress response.[4,5] Physiological effects (Fig. 8.2) mediated by CRH include:

Pituitary–adrenal activation
Sympathetic nervous system activation
Anorexia
Diminished sexual behavior
Increased arousal
Changes in motor activity
Other signs of peripheral and autonomic nervous system activation

CRH stimulation of the anterior pituitary results in the release of adrenocorticotropic hormone (ACTH), which in turn stimulates adrenal cortex production of the glucocorticoid cortisol. Cortisol produced in high levels during stress states inhibits CRH and ACTH production in a negative feedback loop commonly referred to as the hypothalamic–pituitary–adrenal (HPA) axis. The major function of cortisol in stress states is to prevent unrestrained activation of the stress response mechanisms.[5,6]

Acting together, the CRH and LC-NE systems produce a stress response that may be viewed as consisting of two categories of changes. Changes in behavior (behavioral adaptation) consist primarily of:

Improved alertness
Decrease in reflex time
Suppression of feeding
Suppression of sexual behavior

Peripheral adaptive changes include mainly an adaptive redirection of energy resulting in oxygen and nutrients being shunted toward organs that require additional energy to function under stress.

Increased catecholamine (epinephrine/norepinephrine) and cortisol production results in mobilization of energy stores via activation of glycogenolysis, gluconeogenesis, and lipolysis. In addition, increased glucagon and growth hormone secretion occurs, accompanied by inhibition of insulin release and increased peripheral resistance. All of these events are geared toward maximal energy utilization (Fig. 8.3). These four hormones oppose the major anabolic function of insulin, stimulating the synthesis of energy storage molecules. They have been referred to as counterregulatory hormones. As noted in Figure 8.2, an additional role for cortisol is apparently to contain the magnitude of the stress response (that is, counterregulate it) by feedback inhibition of CRH and ACTH production.

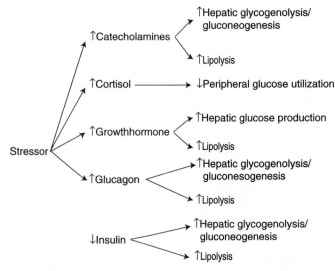

Figure 8.3. Stressor-induced hormone response.

Inflammatory Mediators

Inflammation is one of the fundamental defense reactions.[7,8] It is basically nonspecific. Cell or tissue injury evokes an acute reaction frequently referred to as the acute phase response. If no complications occur, homeostasis is usually restored within a week. If the process continues, chronic inflammation occurs, a characteristic of many diseases. Over the years, evidence has accumulated that most, if not all, features of inflammation are directly caused by the action of host-derived substances, rather than the accompanying environmental perturbation. Local and systemic inflammatory mediators are involved.

Locally, at the site of the tissue injury, inflammation is characterized by:

Vasodilation
Increased vascular permeability
Increased heat production
Increased tenderness
Swelling

A number of inflammatory mediators have been identified that are responsible for these properties (Table 8.1). The fact that there are many different types of mediators points to the complexity and coordinated activity involved with the localized inflammatory process.

Cytokines play a central role in the systemic effects of inflammation.[9–12] Cytokines are groups of polypeptide cell regulators produced primarily by monocytes and macrophages, although they can originate in a wide variety of cell types. They have been variously called lymphokines, interleukins, interferons, and colony-stimulating factors. Collectively, cytokines play an important role in many physiological responses. In particular, they are critical in the immune response. They reg-

Table 8.1
Inflammatory Mediators and Biological Role

Major Inflammatory Effect	Mediator
Vasodilation	Prostaglandins
Increased vascular permeability	Vasoactive amines
	C3a and C5a (through liberating amines)
	Bradykinin
	Leukotriene C_4, D_4, E_4, platelet-aggregating factor (PAF)
Chemotaxis	C5a
	Leukotriene B_4
	Other chemotactic lipids
	Bacterial products
Fever	IL-1, TNF
	Prostaglandins
Pain	Prostaglandins
	Bradykinin
Tissue damage	Neutrophil and macrophage lysosomal enzymes
	Oxygen metabolites

Table 8.2
Classes of Cytokines

I. Interleukins (IL)
    IL-1→IL-17
II. Interferons (IFN)
III. Colony-stimulating factors (CSF)
    Granulocyte (G-CSF)
    Granulocyte/monocyte (GM-CSF)
    Monocyte (M-CSF)
IV. Tumor necrosis factor (TNF)
V. Chemokines
VI. Growth factors

Table 8.3
Common Characteristics of Cytokines

Low molecular mass (<80kDa) secreted proteins, often glycosylated, involved in immunity and inflammation
Regulate amplitude and duration of response
Usually produced transiently and locally, acting in paracrine or autocrine manner
Extremely potent at picomolar concentrations
Interact with high affinity cell surface receptors specific for each cytokine or cytokine group
Receptors are expressed at relatively low number (10–10,000 per cell)
Cell surface binding ultimately leads to a change in the pattern of cellular RNA and protein synthesis and altered cell behavior
Individual cytokines have multiple overlapping cell regulatory actions
Interact in a network by:
    Inducing each other
    Transmodulating cytokine cell surface receptors
    Synergistic, additive, or antagonist interactions on cell function

ulate activation, growth, and functional activities of all immune cellular components. In addition, they are involved in the pathophysiology of many diseases and are currently used therapeutically. Table 8.2 summarizes the classes of cytokines.

At the cellular level, this heterogeneous group of proteins has a number of common characteristics (Table 8.3). Individual cytokines have multiple overlapping cell regulatory actions. Current evidence suggests that the response of a cell to a given cytokine depends on the local concentration of the cytokine and other cell modulators as well as the cell type. Cytokines appear to interact in a network by inducing each other, transmodulating cytokine cell surface receptors, and by synergistic, additive, or antagonistic interactions on cell function.

During physiological stresses, the genes for nearly all cytokines are expressed. Based on the observed biological activities, the cytokines may be grouped as being primarily proinflammatory or antiinflammatory molecules. Prominent proinflammatory cytokines include:

Interleukin-1 (IL-1)
IL-6
IL-8
Tumor necrosis factor (TNF)

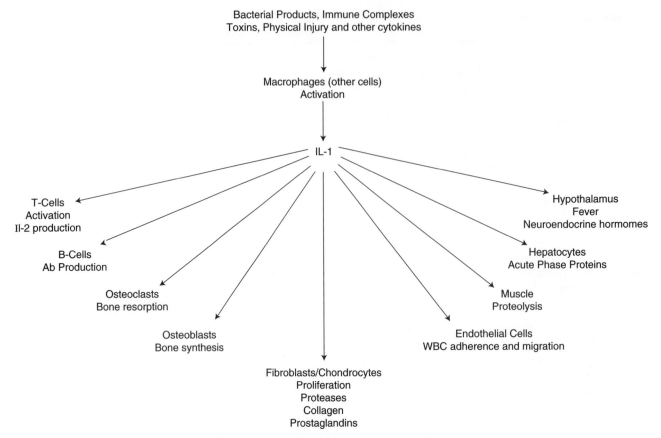

Figure 8.4. Multiple biological activation by IL-1.

The major antiinflammatory cytokines include:

IL-4
IL-10
Transforming growth factor-β (TGF-β)
Interferons

INTERLEUKIN-1: A KEY BIOLOGICAL MODULATOR

Although many interleukins interact in their functional roles, IL-1 appears to play a particularly important role.[8,9] IL-1 is a protein of molecular mass 17,500 kDa that exists in two molecularly distinct forms. Both forms appear to have similar biological activities. IL-1 is produced primarily by monocytes and macrophages but has been reported to be synthesized by a wide variety of cell types in response to infectious, toxic, and inflammatory stimuli. Once formed, IL-1 induces several metabolic and immunological changes that guard against excessive tissue damage and enhance the repair process. The multiple biological activities of IL-1 and the physiological consequences of these pleiotropic effects are summarized in Figure 8.4 and Table 8.4.

TISSUE REPAIR

The body's attempts to heal damage induced by local injury involve a series of coordinated activities.[13] The final successful

Table 8.4
Biological Effects of IL-1

Metabolic	Physiologic	Hematologic	Immunologic
↑ ACTH	Fever	Neutrophilia	T-cell activation
↑ Corticosteroids	Sleep	↑ CSFs	B-cell activation
↓ ↑ Insulin	↓ Appetite	Interferon	↑ Natural killer (NK) cell binding
↓ Plasma zinc and iron	Hypotension	↑ Endothelial procoagulant	Adjuvant
↑ Hepatic protein	↑ Sodium excretion	↑ Resistance to infection	↑ Lymphokines
↓ Albumin		Radioprotection	
↓ Cytochrome P-450			
↓ Lipoprotein lipase			
Weight loss			

outcome involves repair and replacement of damaged or dead cells by healthy cells. Once this process is complete, restoration to the normal homeostasis state is feasible.

Although the mechanistic details of this important process are poorly understood, four stages appear to be necessary:

1. New capillary growth
2. Fibroblast growth and proliferation

3. Collagen deposition
4. Scar tissue formation

Several growth factors (e.g., platelet-derived growth factor, IL-1, TNF, fibroblast growth factor) appear to be involved in these various steps.

CYTOKINE INTERACTION WITH IMMUNE AND CENTRAL NERVOUS SYSTEMS

The stress response, inflammation, and the neuroendocrine system are mechanistically linked.[4–6,14–20] The interrelationship between these systems is bidirectional. IL-1 produced by the peripheral immune system not only exerts proinflammatory and immunostimulatory effects at the inflammatory site, but also acts at the level of the hypothalamus to stimulate CRH production. Therefore, IL-1 appears to participate in a negative feedback loop that ultimately leads to the production of cortisol, which in turn depresses peripheral IL-1 production as well as other inflammatory mediators. These relationships are summarized in Figure 8.5.

HUMAN DEFENSE SYSTEMS[3]

Human beings are constantly being threatened with bodily injury from biological, chemical, and physical agents in the environment. Through the process of natural selection, humans have evolved elaborate mechanisms by which they are able to survive and function in a hostile world. The major categories of human protective mechanisms include:

Physical barriers (e.g., skin)
Stress reactions
Immune responses

Inflammation
Coagulation
Chemical detoxification
A widespread network of phagocytic cells in the reticuloendothelial system

The host, rather than using these modalities independently, responds to all injuries at the molecular level with a concerted constellation of host responses referred to collectively as the stress response. This response is most commonly seen in people following a number of inflammatory stimuli including:

Infection
Trauma
Burns
Tissue infarction
Immune-related diseases
Surgery

Characteristic changes occur involving the following functions:

Metabolic
Endocrinologic
Neurologic
Immunologic

Most of these changes are observed within hours or days after the onset of injury. They represent a series of local and systemic responses designed to aid survival by neutralizing the offending agent and restoring normal tissue functioning (Fig. 8.6). These responses represent a major adaptive phenomenon whereby homeostasis is maintained in an altered steady state. Complete recovery occurs by a return to the normal steady state.

In general, the magnitude of the stress response is related to the severity of the injured state. In cases of major injury, survival occurs only if these interactive defense responses are sufficient to compensate for the imposed stresses. Host factors are important in determining individual survival. These include:

Nutritional status
Immune status

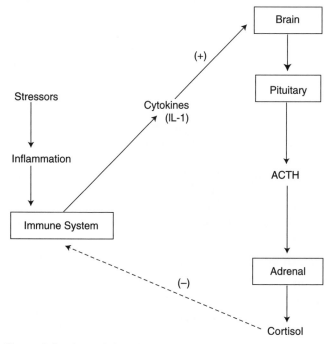

Figure 8.5. Interrelationships between neuroendocrine and immune systems.

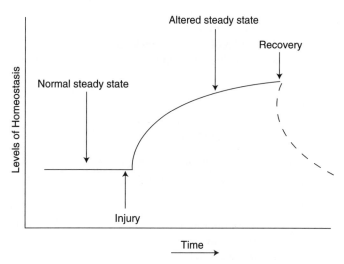

Figure 8.6. Effects of internal and external stressors on homeostasis.

Age
Gender
Concomitant disease

In addition, in many cases the return to the normal steady state can be unsuccessful, in that normal homeostasis is not achieved. Stress response changes can persist that themselves cause damage (e.g., chronic inflammatory disease such as rheumatoid arthritis).

Molecular Basis[3,14–20]

The host responds to injury with several common metabolic and physiological alterations collectively referred to as the stress response. Many metabolic changes can be measured within the first few hours to the first day after the tissue injury (Fig. 8.6). These responses are seen most dramatically in clinical settings involving rapidly progressive infections. They also follow the inflammatory reaction to local injury or chronic disease states like rheumatoid arthritis and connective tissue diseases. Whether the disease is chronic or acute, the host's response is similar and includes most, if not all, components of the stress response. However, there are additional host physiological changes that may occur secondarily to extended stress responses. These responses are usually measured in weeks following the resolution of the illness and include:

Hypergammaglobulinemia
Changes in T-lymphocyte function
Anemia

There is a molecular basis for the stress response. A number of stressors lead to the activation of monocytes or macrophages via stimulation of cytokines (IL-1, IL-6, TNF). These stressors include tissue injury, infection, and inflammation. Depending on the extent of injury, these mediators evoke responses either locally or systemically. Prominent effects include those biological activities summarized in Table 8.4. In addition, other blood-borne substances produced by the activated immune and clotting systems play an important role in inducing metabolic modulators.

When a cytokine enters the circulation, it affects many organs and tissues. Circulating cytokines reach the hypothalamus via the arterial blood supply and initiate the following:

Fever
Altered appetite
Altered sleep
Release of corticotropin-releasing hormone (CRH)

CRH also stimulates anterior pituitary release of adrenocorticotropic hormone (ACTH), which in turn stimulates adrenal production and release of cortisol. Cortisol and related corticosteroids suppress CRH and ACTH release and are potent inhibitors of the immune and inflammatory systems. A primary function of cortisol may be to prevent uncontrolled activation of the stress response.

Another important aspect of the varied metabolic changes

is known as the acute phase protein response. It involves increased production of hepatic protein synthesis that includes:

Serum amyloid A
C-reactive protein
Haptoglobin
Protease inhibitors
Complement components
Ceruloplasmin
Fibrinogen

Other aspects of this response include:

Decrease in albumin synthesis
Leukocytosis
Hypergammaglobulinemia

The roles that these proteins play in host defense systems are not completely understood. Since some acute phase proteins bind to lipids or directly to bacterial surfaces, it has been speculated that they may function as nonspecific opsonins. It also has been speculated that other acute phase proteins function as oxygen scavengers. The antiproteinases could function to neutralize destructive effects of proteolytic enzymes from tissue damage and/or bacterial infection. Induced metalloproteins that bind and remove iron and zinc from tissue fluids may inhibit bacterial or tumor cell replication.

Probably no function of the cytokine IL-1 has greater defensive significance than its ability to activate the immune system. Lymphocyte activation by IL-1 enhances immunoglobulin synthesis during the acute phase response. IL-1 activates helper T cells to produce IL-2 and γ-interferon, and macrophages to produce IL-6, all of which influence B-cell stimulation.

Recently, it has also been shown that IL-1 and TNF act as potent chemoattractants for neutrophils and T cells. This appears to occur via the ability of these cytokines to stimulate the synthesis of chemokines. Increased levels of chemokines at sites of tissue injury probably contribute to infiltration of neutrophils, monocytes, and T cells.

One of the most important nonleukocyte targets of IL-1 and TNF is the endothelial cell. Activation of endothelial cells by these cytokines leads to the vascular changes associated with tissue injury and inflammation. Important events include release of the vasodilators, prostacyclin I_2 (PGI_2) and prostaglandin E_2 (PGE_2), and alterations in endothelial surface adhesion molecules to enhance adherence of neutrophils, monocytes, and lymphocytes. The combination of these events initiates vascular congestion, clot formation, and cellular infiltration.

Health and Disease: Osteopathic Approach[1–2]

Health reflects a state of equilibrium between a person and his or her physical, emotional, and social environment that is compatible with full functional activity of the person (Fig. 8.7). Health can be described as a dynamic state that includes various aspects of both wellness and illness. At one end of the spectrum is a high level of wellness—the optimal state of well-

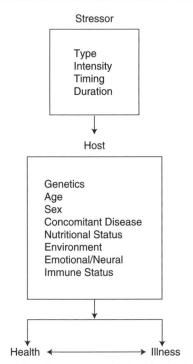

Stressor

Type
Intensity
Timing
Duration

Host

Genetics
Age
Sex
Concomitant Disease
Nutritional Status
Environment
Emotional/Neural
Immune Status

Health ⟷ Illness

Figure 8.7. Stress response in health and disease.

being of a person. At the other extreme is complete disabling illness.

Disease is a condition of impaired body function that is manifested by a characteristic set of symptoms and signs whose etiology, pathology, and prognosis may be known or unknown. Although disease usually includes alterations in body structure or in the composition of body fluids, it is the manifestations of these bodily changes that impair function and lead to an awareness of illness. Likewise, it is the return of normal function that usually marks recovery from illness.

Osteopathic medicine has long recognized the importance of the musculoskeletal system, as well as the body's ability to be self-regulating and self-healing. Since muscle comprises the greatest mass in the body and is responsible for body movements, it is clear how an extended stress response, leading to muscle tension, could have enormous impact on physiological functions. Likewise, it is easily seen how muscle relaxation from osteopathic manipulative therapy and other forms of manual medicine could be effective therapeutic modalities.

Since its inception, osteopathic medicine has emphasized that a patient be considered individually as a whole person belonging to a family living in a unique community environment. Therapies have been developed based on established physiological concepts of interrelationships between the various physiological regulatory mechanisms within the human body. Most recently, we have realized that integrative physiology must be viewed not only in terms of the interrelationships of the physiological regulatory mechanisms that occur within the organism, but must also incorporate the understanding that these mechanisms appear to be influenced by mental and emotional stimuli. Therefore, osteopathic physi-

cians have been especially well-trained to appreciate that physiological, emotional, and environmental factors affect health and must all be given specific consideration in the prevention, diagnosis, and treatment of illness.

CONCLUSION

In the last decade, the study of the human stress response has gained considerable attention in human health and disease. Suggestions have been made that a significant percentage of diseases prevalent in Western society today is related to abnormalities in this response.

Remember that we are just beginning to understand the mechanisms by which the human body maintains health and recovers from illness. It is important for the osteopathic physician to be actively involved in helping to define and promote use of these concepts in practice. The implications for the profession, and most importantly for health care, are potentially immense.

REFERENCES

1. Still AT. *Osteopathy, Research and Practice*. St. Paul, Minn: The Pioneer Co; 1910.
2. Greenman PE. *Principles of Manual Medicine*. Baltimore, Md: Williams & Wilkins; 1989.
3. Seyle H. *Stress in Health and Disease*. Reading, Mass: Butterworths; 1976.
4. Chrousos G, Loriax DL, Gold PW. *Mechanisms of Physical and Emotional Stress*. New York, NY: Plenum Press; 1988.
5. Munck A, Guyre PM, Holbrook NJ. Physiological functions of glucocorticoids in stress and their relation to pharmacological actions. *Endocr Rev.* 1984;5:25–44.
6. Wilder RL, Steinberg EM. Neuroendocrine hormonal factors in rheumatoid arthritis and related conditions. *Curr Opin Rheumatol.* 1990;2:436–440.
7. Zurier RB. Prostaglandins leukotrienes and related compounds. In: Kelley WN, Harris ED Jr, Ruddy S, Sledge CB, eds. *Textbook of Rheumatology*. 4th ed. Philadelphia, Pa: WB Saunders Co; 1993:201–210.
8. Pruzanski W, Vadas P. Phospholipase A_2—a mediator between proximal and distal effectors of inflammation. *Immunol Today.* 1991; 12:143–146.
9. Dinarello CA. The endogenous pyrogens in host–defense interactions. *Hosp Pract.* Nov. 15, 1989;24(11):111–128.
10. Dinarello CA. Interleukin-1 in disease. *N Engl J Med.* 1993; 328(2):106–113.
11. Larrick JW, Kunkel SL. The role of tumor necrosis factor and interleukin-1 in the immunoinflammatory response. *Pharm Res.* 1988; 5:129–139.
12. Tracey KJ, Cerami A. Tumor necrosis factor, other cytokines and disease. *Ann Rev Cell Biol.* 1993;9:317–343.
13. Kushner I. Regulation of the acute phase response by cytokines. *Perspect Biol Med.* 1993;36(4):611–622.
14. Bellinger DL, Lorton D, Romano TD, et al. Neuropeptide innervation of lymphoid organs. *Ann NY Acad Sci.* 1990;594:17–33.
15. Karalis K, Sono H, Redwine J, et al. Autocrine or paracrine proinflammatory actions of corticotropin releasing hormone in vivo. *Science.* 1991;254:421–423.

16. Smith HR, Steinberg AD. Autoimmunity—a perspective. *Ann Int Med.* 1986;105:37–44.

17. Johnston M. Basic concepts of immunity. In: Torrence P, ed. *Biological Response Modifiers.* New York, NY: Academic Press, 1985.

18. Gelfand RA, Matthews DE, Bier DM, et al. Role of counterregulatory hormones in the catabolic response to stress. *J Clin Invest.* 1984;74:2238–2248.

19. Ganong WF. The stress response—a dynamic overview. *Hosp Pract.* June 15, 1988;23(6):155–171.

20. Peterson PK, Chao CC, Molitor T, et al. Stress and pathogenesis of infectious disease. *Rev Infect Dis.* 1991;13:710–720.

9. Neuroendocrine-Immune System and Homeostasis

FRANK H. WILLARD, DAVID J. MOKLER, AND P.J. MORGANE

Key Concepts

- **Reciprocal interdependence of human structure, function, and mind**

- **Complex homeostatic equilibrium; self-regulatory and self-healing with respect to disease processes**

- **Homeostatic equilibrium represented by integrated network of messenger molecules produced by cells in the neural, endocrine, and immune systems**

- **Signal coding: messenger molecules communicating through receptor complexes located on cell membranes**

- **Critical role of neural system, especially limbic forebrain and hypothalamus, in influencing output of endocrine and immune systems**

- **Neural control of endocrine system via hypothalamic-pituitary axis; neural control over immune system via hypothalamus and peripheral autonomic nervous system, the latter of which innervates every immune gland in the body**

- **Modulatory effect on immune and neural systems of hormones produced by endocrine cells; critical role of feedback systems in controlling intensity of inflammatory processes**

- **Effect of external and internal stressors on normal homeostatic rhythms of neuroendocrine-immune system**

- **Role of general adaptive response in handling acute stressful stimuli by controlling immune system and initiating repair of body**

- **Requirements for return of normal homeostatic rhythms**

- **Effect on body function of prolonged exposure to altered homeostatic chemistry of general adaptive response**

- **Role of osteopathic physician to control stressful external or internal stimuli and assist patient in regaining normal complement of homeostatic rhythms**

Human beings are faced with protecting their bodies against extremely varied and often harsh external environmental conditions. Simultaneously, we also have to maintain a relatively constant internal environment, conducive to the complex chemistry of our metabolism. To accomplish this protection we have developed a sophisticated network of extracellular messenger molecules composed of the secretory products of many cells, chief of which are those in the neural, endocrine, and immune systems.

The protective mechanisms begin at the molecular and cellular levels with the release into the local microenvironment of a complex array of proinflammatory chemicals from nerve terminals as well as from various immune cells. Many of these same messengers also enter the systemic circulation and serve as complex signal codes, engaging the central nervous system and endocrine system to alter physiology and behavior (Fig. 9.1). These defensive alterations in homeostatic function are referred to as the general adaptive response; the events that initiate them are called stressors.[1] The resultant output of messengers from the autonomic pathways and hormones from the pituitary gland seeks to reestablish homeostatic balance as well

as provide feedback to the peripheral tissue, ultimately regulating the immune response. This extracellular chemical network represents the primary compensatory mechanism of the body, functioning to combat any threat to its homeostatic mechanisms.

The finely tuned balance present in the neuroendocrine-immune network is critical to the general health and function of the body and mind.[2] Understanding the neuroendocrine-immune network is of considerable significance to the practicing osteopathic physician. This network orchestrates the varied responses of the body to the presence of somatic dysfunction, an event defined in large part by the hyperalgesia and surrounding edema accompanying inflammation.[3] The three primary drives or stressors initiating the cascade of chemical messengers in the general adaptive response are somatic, visceral, or emotional dysfunction.

Examples of somatic origins of stress are the chronic inflammation or the inescapable nociception that can accompany somatic dysfunctions.[3] Numerous studies have demonstrated that a general demise of health occurs following chronic exposure to the stress-related chemical messengers.[4–6] This decline in health, typified by suppressed immune functions and increased susceptibility to infection diseases, is related to profound alterations in the activity of the neuroendocrine-immune network.[7–8]

In this chapter we discuss the:

Complex extracellular chemical network, elaborated by neural, endocrine, and immune cells (Fig. 9.1)

Various chemical equilibria that serve to maintain homeostasis

Disruption in the network that plays a significant role in the disease process

We first consider the regulatory molecules and their membrane receptors involved in signal coding among neural, endocrine, and immune systems. This is followed by discussion of the brain's ability to regulate the immune response via the autonomic nervous system (see Chapter 5, Autonomic Nervous System) and hypothalamic-endocrine output. The influences of external stimuli on the neuroendocrine-immune network as well as on the feedback of its neuroregulators, immunoregulators, and hormones are described. The major emphasis is on understanding the interactions between the various components of this network and the implications of these homeostatic regulations for the practice of osteopathic medicine.

SIGNAL CODING IN NEUROENDOCRINE-IMMUNE NETWORK

The cells of the neural, endocrine, and immune systems act in concert to produce numerous molecules that are released into the extracellular spaces (Fig. 9.2). These molecules represent the signals that encode information regulating homeostatic mechanisms both at the local microenvironmental level and systemically.[9] Traditionally, these three systems have been distinguished based on the distance between the cell producing the messenger and its site of activity, as well as the mode of transit used by the messenger. The immune system was typified by autocrine (self-stimulating) and paracrine (stimulating local tissues) methods of communication (Fig. 9.3). The endocrine system was described as using bloodborne messengers operating over longer distances by humoral transport. The neural system was described as using chemical transmitters released into a narrow synaptic cleft separating the presynaptic and

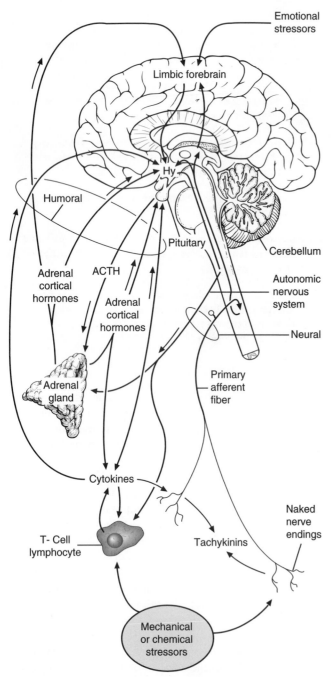

Figure 9.1. Some interactions among components of the neuroendocrine-immune network. ACTH, adrenocorticotropic hormone; Hy, hypothalamus.

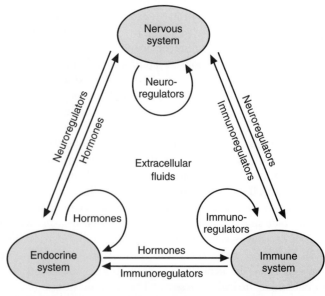

Figure 9.2. Complex neural, endocrine, and immune communication network in extracellular spaces.

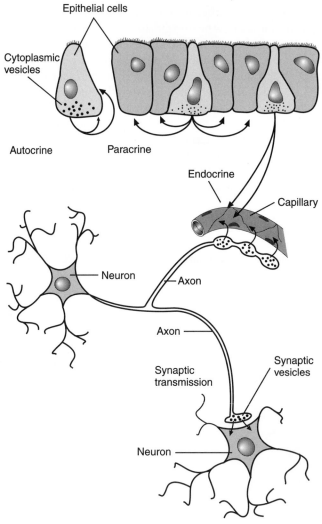

Figure 9.3. Four major forms of communication among cells in neuroendocrine-immune network.

postsynaptic specializations of nerve cells. However, it is now well-established that these four methods of communication are used to some extent in each of the three major systems.[a]

Substances long considered to be involved in one system are now recognized as playing integral roles in multiple other systems as well. In addition, a cross-distribution of receptor complexes for these messenger molecules exists.[8,10] Common cellular mechanisms of bidirectional communication[9] and the similar molecular structure of many of the messengers and their receptors are combined to transcend the traditional borders between neural, endocrine, and immune systems. This creates the concept of a shared communications network functioning in an integrated manner to maintain homeostatic balance.[11–12]

---

[a]We have extracted the salient features of the neuroregulators and immunoregulators without citing the many publications supporting this field of research. A review citation is included at the end of each section to assist in accessing the primary literature.

Neuroregulators

Neural communication in mammals is accomplished mainly by chemical transmission at synaptic endings. Messenger substances are released from the presynaptic terminal into the extracellular space of the synaptic cleft; they interact with specific receptors located on both presynaptic and postsynaptic neural membranes. Many different types of substances act as neuroregulators; a partial list of these substances is included in Table 9.1. To act on a given cell, each type of neuroregulator requires a specific receptor complex located on the surface membrane of that target cell. Identifying the location of specific receptor complexes is critical to this field of study. There are numerous reviews of neuroregulators and the distribution of their receptors.[13–17] Three major classes of neuroregulators are described here:

> Amino acids
> Biogenic amines
> Neuropeptides

As examples, one substance for each class is discussed below. In selecting a specific substance, we chose those most directly related to the general adaptive response to stressors.

GLUTAMATE

The amino acid glutamate is an extremely common excitatory transmitter in the central nervous system.[18] It is produced by

Table 9.1
Selected Neuroregulators

Catecholamines	dopamine
	norepinephrine
	epinephrine
Cholines	acetylcholine
Indolamines	serotonin
Peptides	substance P
	neuropeptide Y
	calcitonin gene-related polypeptide
	enkephalins
	endorphins
	neurotensin
	cholecystokinin
	angiotensin II
	vasoactive intestinal polypeptide
	bombesin
	adrenocorticotropin
	somatostatin
	corticotropin
	dynorphin
Amino acids	glutamate
	aspartate
	GABA
	glycine
Purines	adenosine
Diamines	histamine

neurons through the brain and spinal cord and is involved in most activities of the nervous system, such as:

Cognition and memory
Sensory system processing,[19] especially spinal cord activity in response to nociception[20]
Motor systems activity[21]
Neuroendocrine regulation[22]
As a trophic factor in neurodevelopmental mechanisms[23]

Multiple receptor complexes for glutamate have been described and are found on almost all cells of the nervous system.[24–25] Two basic classes of glutamate receptors are described: ligand-gated and voltage-gated ion channels. Ligand-gated ion channel glutamate receptors are involved in fast synaptic transmission. Voltage-gated ion channels are normally blocked by a cation. However, when activated by prolonged changes in membrane potential, these channels eject the cation and transmit calcium. This subsequently initiates metabolic changes in the cell's membrane.[26] These changes often result in facilitation of the cell's activities, called long-term potentiation.[27] The voltage-gated ion channels are involved in the memory process in the hippocampus[26] and in facilitation of spinal cord segments as a result of excessive small-caliber primary afferent fiber input.[28] Excessive production of glutamate has been associated with neurotoxicity[29] and the neuronal death occurring in many neurologic diseases.[8,30–31]

NOREPINEPHRINE

Norepinephrine, a catecholamine, is a biogenic amine used as a neuroregulator in the central and peripheral nervous systems. In the central nervous system, it is produced by a small number of neurons located in the reticular formation of the medulla, pons, and midbrain. Although the number of noradrenergic cells is limited, their axons are diverse, innervating:

Spinal cord
Brainstem
Cerebellum
Thalamus
Hypothalamus
Hippocampus
Portions of the cerebral cortex

In the peripheral nervous system, noradrenergic neurons represent the majority of ganglionic neurons in the sympathetic system. Their postganglionic sympathetic axons innervate smooth muscle in:

Organs throughout the body
Glandular cells
Cardiac cells
Parasympathetic ganglionic neurons
Immune cells

The extensive innervation of the primary and secondary lymphatic organs by noradrenergic axons (NA axons) has been well-documented.[32] Many cells express adrenergic

receptors; several different adrenoreceptors are known. Norepinephrine is a slow neuroregulator; adrenoreceptors alter cells by working through second messenger systems such as the G-proteins.[17,33] Activation of the central and peripheral noradrenergic system is accomplished by stressors such as tissue injury and inflammation. The proinflammatory cytokines, such as interleukin-1 (IL-1) and interleukin-6 (IL-6), are also potent stimuli for increased output of norepinephrine. In general, norepinephrine acts to suppress immune cell division and immune cell growth in the lymphoid organs.[32] On this basis it is postulated that the sympathetic system is acting as a long feedback loop to suppress excessive activity in the immune system.

SUBSTANCE P

The small-caliber, primary afferent fibers produce a wide range of neuropeptides of which substance P, an 11-amino acid polypeptide, is the best characterized. Stimuli resulting in the release of substance P include, among others (Fig. 9.4):

Noxious events
Antigenetic substances
Cytokines of immune cells
Histamine from mast cells

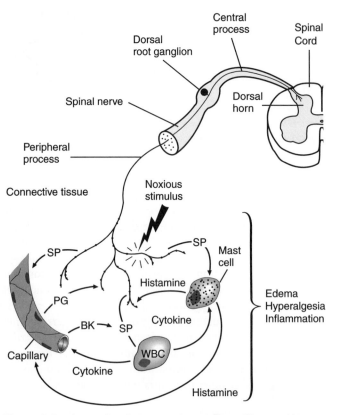

Figure 9.4. Interactions between primary afferent fibers and immune system. Noxious stimulus initiates secretion of neuropeptides such as substance P from primary afferent fiber. Result is feed-forward cascade of inflammatory events producing edema and hyperalgesia. PG, prostaglandins; SP, substance P; BK, bradykinin; WBC, white blood cells.

Bradykinin (BK)
Prostaglandin

Substance P is released from both the central and peripheral terminals of the primary afferent fibers. Although these peptides have been traditionally associated with the synaptic endings in the spinal cord, it is now understood that they are also secreted from the peripheral process of the sensory fiber.[34] The release of neuroregulators from the peripheral process of a dorsal root ganglion cell challenges the traditional concept of sensory neuron organization. The existence of neuroregulators was predicted from experiments on the classic axon reflex by Lewis in 1927.[35] Recent studies indicate that up to 90% of the substance P produced by sensory neurons is stored and released from its terminal branches; it thereby functions as a paracrine gland in peripheral tissue.[36]

In the periphery, this neuropeptide is proinflammatory, attracting lymphocytes and granulocytes, degranulating mast cells, and dilating capillaries (Fig. 9.4).[34,37–38] In the dorsal horn of the spinal cord, substance P is co-released with a fast-acting neurotransmitter such as the excitatory amino acid glutamate.[39] Substance P is a slow-acting neuromodulator; its release in the dorsal horn is responsible for the slow evoked potentials following noxious primary afferent stimulus.[40] Substance P induces slow potentials on dorsal horn cells; this appears to involve unmasking of voltage-gated calcium channels, such as the NMDA channel. Increasing intracellular calcium levels initiates second messenger systems and immediate early gene products in the dorsal horn cells, resulting in facilitation of spinal reflexes and ascending pathways.[41] In response to somatic dysfunctions, substance P plays an important role in the propagation of the local inflammatory response and, in concert with the excitatory amino acids, influences the plasticity of the dorsal horn. This leads to spinal facilitation and the shift from acute to chronic pain syndromes.

Immunoregulators

A host of regulatory substances called immunoregulators (cytokines, lymphokines, monokines) are produced by lymphoid (Table 9.2) and mononuclear cell lines (Table 9.3) as well as these others (Table 9.4):

Smooth muscle
Fibroblasts
Endothelial cells
Synoviocytes
Osteoblasts
Osteocytes
Mesangial cells
Glial cells
Neural cells

Immunoregulators are pleiotropic, glycoprotein messenger molecules, serving both as intercellular communicators and as growth factors regulating the proliferation and differentiation of many types of cells throughout the body. The production of immunoregulators by cells of the immune system can be initiated under many different circumstances, particularly those involving stimuli damaging to tissue. Cytokine expression is seen in most tissue throughout the body, including the nervous system. Cytokine induction consequent to injury and its contribution to fever and the inflammatory process is an important feature of neurodegenerative diseases.[42–43]

The immunoregulators, unlike the immunoglobulins, are not specific to a given stimulus. In essence, these messengers serve to multiply the variety and extent of the immune response. Initially, a specific antigen interacts with a limited number of lymphoid cells. The immunoregulators subsequently released by activated lymphoid cells then engage many other cells, both lymphoid and nonlymphoid. The result of this progression of events is a substantially increased response to the initial antigen. Many mammalian immunoregulators have been described, a partial list of which is presented in Table 9.5. Some of the interactions of the best known immunoregulators with the neuroendocrine system are summarized below.

Table 9.2
Cell Types in the Immune System

	Lymphoid Cells
Thymocytes	Lymphoid cells of the thymus
T cells	Lymphoid cells that mature in the thymus and express the T cell receptor (TCR)
Helper T cells	Lymphoid cells responding to cell surface antigens by secreting cytokines
Cytotoxic T Cells	Lymphoid cells responding to cell surface antigens by lysing cell producing the antigen
B cells	Lymphoid cells that, when activated, are capable of producing immunoglobulins
Natural killer cells	Lymphoid cells capable of killing tumor cells and virus-infected cells
Neutrophils	Major lymphoid cell of the acute inflammatory response and effector cells of humoral immunity
Basophils	Effector cell of IgE-mediated immunity that secrete histamine granules in response to IgE activation
Eosinophils	Lymphoid cell containing lysosomal granules that can destroy parasites

Table 9.3
Mononuclear Cells and Their Functions

Monocytes	Circulating immune cells whose primary function is phagocytosis
Macrophages	Tissue-based immune cells whose primary function is phagocytosis
Microglia	Macrophages found in the central nervous system
Kupffer cell	Macrophages found along the sinusoids of the liver
Alveolar macrophage	Macrophages found in the pulmonary alveoli
Type A synoviocytes	Macrophages found in the synovial membrane of joints
Mast cell	Tissue-based, histamine-containing cells similar to basophils

Table 9.4
Non-Lymphoid Cell Types

Fibroblast	Connective tissue cell capable of secreting and maintaining the collagenous fiber matrix
Endothelial cell	Squamous cell lining the inner aspect of the vascular system
Mesangial cells	Specialized mesenchymal cell found in the renal glomerulus
Chromaffin cell	Neuropeptide secreting cell found in the adrenal medulla
Enterochromaffin cell	Neuropeptide secreting cell found in the lining of the gastrointestinal system
Hepatocyte	Liver cell capable of secreting the acute phase proteins
Endometrial cell	Epithelial cell lining the internal surface of the uterus
Astrocyte	Neuroglial cell found in the central nervous system involved in forming the blood-brain barrier
Oligodendrocyte	Neuroglial cell forming myelin sheaths around axons in the central nervous system
Osteoblast	Specialized mesenchymal cells capable of secreting the osteoid matrix for the formation of bone
Osteocyte	Connective tissue cell found in bone representing a mature form of the osteoblast
Reticular cell	Endodermal cell creating a three-dimensional network for lymphocytes in the thymus, spleen, and lymph nodes

INTERLEUKIN-I

In response to challenge by foreign antigens, a family of IL-1 glycoproteins are produced by activated macrophage/monocytes, as well as by (Table 9.3):

Lymphocytes
Fibroblasts
Endothelial cells
Renal mesangial cells
Adrenal chromaffin cells

IL-1 acts as a bridge, coordinating the cells of the immune system with those of the neural and endocrine systems to bring into play the various components of the inflammatory reaction.[44] The influence of IL-1 is pleiotropic in the body. Receptors for IL-1 are widespread and are present on many cell types in the nervous and immune systems, as well as on connective tissue cells in the fascia.[45–46] The systemic effects of IL-1 on the body include[47]:

Shift into negative nitrogen balance
Decrease in the threshold of pain (hyperalgesia)
Fever
Sleep
Anorexia
Hypotension

Circulating IL-1 gains access to the cerebrospinal fluid of the third ventricle.[48] Through axonal connections with the hypo-

Table 9.5
Immunoregulators

Interleukins (1–7)
Interferons (alpha, beta, and gamma)
Tumor necrosis factor (beta)
Colony-stimulating factors
    granulocyte-stimulating factor
    macrophage-stimulating factor
    granulocyte-macrophage stimulating factor
    interleukin-3
Leukemia inhibiting factor or neuroleukin
Transforming growth factor (beta)

thalamus, IL-1 can influence the activity of the hypothalamic-pituitary adrenal axis, resulting in increased output of adrenal cortical steroid. It can also activate the release of norepinephrine from the sympathetic nervous system.[49] The adrenal cortical hormones and the catecholamines serve in a long feedback loop to depress the activity of the immune system (Figs. 9.1 and 9.5) and control the immune response.[50] Hypothalamic IL-1 also is a stimulus for thermogenesis as seen in fever,[42] possibly by regulating hypothalamic output to the thyroid (Fig. 9.5).[48] Based on its plethora of interactions both at the local level and systemically, IL-1 is a significant proinflammatory substance. It has been called "the hormone of the acute phase response."[51]

The effects of IL-1 in appropriate amounts are beneficial to the body. Injection of this immunoregulator in laboratory animals prior to challenge with various noxious or infectious agents offers significant protective effects.[52] Production of excessive amounts of IL-1 is also associated with numerous pathologies such as[47]:

Destruction of beta cells in the pancreas
Growth of myelogenous leukemia cells
Inflammation associated with arthritis and colitis
Growth of atherosclerotic plaques

Elevated levels of IL-1 are associated with sickness behavior as defined and described in numerous experimental paradigms.[53]

INTERLEUKIN-2

Interleukin-2 (IL-2) is best known for its function as an obligatory growth factor for thymocytes and as a major T cell cytokine for coordinating the immune response. This cytokine is produced by activated T-helper cells when they are exposed to antigens that are presented along with membrane proteins derived from the major histocompatibility genes and IL-1. Using an autocrine mechanism of communication (Fig. 9.3), IL-2 stimulates its T cells of origin to increase their production of more IL-2 and to induce the expression of its receptors on their surface membranes.[54] IL-2 multiplies the initial immune reaction, augmenting its own production as it recruits B cells into the response. In the absence of IL-2 or its receptor, the T-cell immune response fails. This immunoregulator occupies a pivotal position in the immune system.[54]

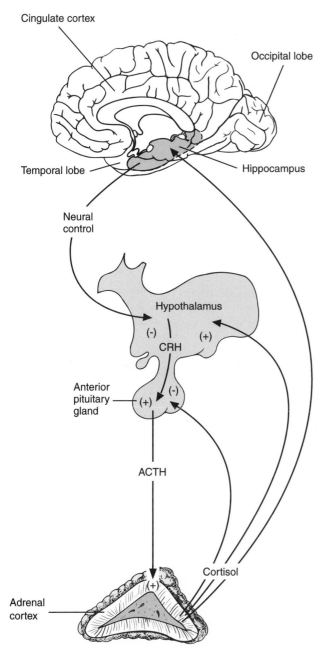

Figure 9.5. Major components of hypothalamic-pituitary-adrenal axis. CRH, corticotropin-releasing hormone.

IL-2 receptors have a wide distribution in the body. They are found on cells of the monocyte/macrophage and lymphoid cell lines, including natural killer cells. Nonlymphoid cell types expressing these receptors are, among others[55]:

Oligodendrocytes
Kupffer cells
Mast cells

Receptors for IL-2 are present on neurons in the hippocampal formation and cerebellum. Additionally, IL-2 receptors have been identified on a cultured line of pituitary cells.[56]
Production of IL-2 has been detected in microglia and mac-

rophages of the central nervous system, suggesting that this immunoregulator can be produced inside the blood-brain barrier. When released into the brain, IL-2 stimulates regions of the hypothalamus, resulting in increased output of β-endorphin and adrenocorticotrophic hormone (ACTH) from pituicytes,[57] both of which are involved in the general adaptive response. IL-2, acting through neural, endocrine, and immune structures, augments the activities of IL-1 in regulating the many cellular responses to external challenge.

INTERLEUKIN-6

Interleukin-6 (IL-6) is a proinflammatory substance, generally similar to IL-1 in its properties. It is produced in response to inflammatory stimuli by:

Lymphoid cells
Connective tissue
Endothelial cells
Glial and neuronal cells in the hypothalamus and pituitary

IL-6 receptors, of which there are several types, have a wide distribution in the body.[58] They are present on immune cells and macrophages, fibroblasts, and cells of hematopoietic and neural origin. Within the nervous system, receptors for IL-6 have also been found on hypothalamic neurons, suggesting direct hypothalamic activation by this proinflammatory immunoregulator.[59]

IL-6 is a mediator of the inflammatory response and is best known for stimulating the release of the acute phase proteins from hepatocytes. It also influences the growth and differentiation of numerous cell types in the neuroendocrine-immune and fascial tissues of the body.[60] It stimulates the production of immunoglobulins from activated B cells and stimulates the secretion of several hormones from the anterior pituitary, including ACTH.[57] When IL-6 is injected in the cerebral ventricular system, it produces a sustained elevation in temperature.[61] IL-6 is a pleiotropic immunoregulatory agent with many properties similar to IL-1. It acts in concert with the other immunoregulators to mediate the acute phase response, initiate fever, and prepare the neuroendocrine-immune network for defense of the body.[62]

Abnormal production of IL-6 is found in association with numerous pathologic states.[60] Excessive production of this immunoregulator is related to:

Polyclonal B-cell activation
Autoantibody production
Hypergammaglobulinemia accompanying cardiac myxoma
Proliferation of mesangial cells in certain forms of proliferative
    glomerulonephritis

Production of IL-6 has been demonstrated in synoviocytes; elevated levels of this immunoregulator have been reported in synovial fluid and serum of patients with rheumatoid arthritis.[63] IL-6 is also found in elevated levels in the cerebrospinal fluid in response to various tumors and bacterial and viral infections.

TUMOR NECROSIS FACTOR

This protein factor (originally called cachexin) is synthesized by activated[64]:

Macrophages
Monocytes
Lymphoid cells
Mast cells
Keratinocytes
Astrocytes
Microglia
Smooth muscle cells
Intestinal cells

Stimulation of tumor necrosis production can come from tissue injury or from the presence of bacterial endotoxins. Its receptors are ubiquitous, with almost all mammalian cells expressing them at one point or another in their life cycle. Release of this cytokine activates many tissue repair and remodeling processes involving blood cells, bone, and the cells in fascia. Slow release of tumor necrosis factor leads to granulomas and wound repair, whereas larger amounts can be lethal. Induction of this factor by bacterial endotoxins is responsible for initiating the toxic shock reaction leading to cachexia and, eventually, to death.[64–65]

Tumor necrosis factor is also a strong proinflammatory agent, inducing the release of other immunoregulators and attracting lymphoid cells, especially neutrophils, that become more adherent to vessel walls under its influence. Similar to IL-1 and IL-6, tumor necrosis factor also:

Stimulates the release of acute phase proteins from hepatocytes[65]
Initiates thermogenesis in the hypothalamus
Has some analgesic properties
Stimulates the release of corticotropin-releasing factor (CRF) from the hypothalamus

This last function initiates the release of ACTH from the anterior pituitary gland and the adrenal cortical hormones from the adrenal gland.[57] Tumor necrosis factor augments the response of the body to IL-1 and IL-6 and participates in the induction of the acute phase response.

INTERFERONS

The interferons represent a family of regulatory molecules consisting of more than 20 different proteins.[66] They were initially recognized based on their ability to interfere with viral replication. There are at least three major types of interferons, each with a slightly different functional profile.[67] In peripheral tissue they are produced by T cells, fibroblasts, and macrophages. In the central nervous system they are produced by astrocytes and also possibly by neurons.[57] Receptors for interferons are widespread, found on cells in all tissues of the body, including those of the nervous system.[57] Interferons also mimic ACTH in the adrenal gland, stimulating steroidogenesis and the release of the adrenal cortical hormones.[68] Interferons represent another link between the immune system and the hypothalamic-pituitary-adrenal axis in the coordination of the adaptive response.

The interferons are best known for antiviral, antibacterial, and antiprotozoal activities. In general circulation they also[66]:

Stimulate the synthesis of immunoglobulins from B cells
Enhance the cytotoxicity of natural killer lymphocytes
Increase the phagocytic properties of macrophages
Induce the production of numerous proteins including the class I and II antigens of the major histocompatibility complex

Within the central nervous system, interferons participate directly in the inflammatory response. Stimulation of hypothalamic neurons by interferons initiates thermogenesis.[69] There are elevated levels of interferons, as well as other immunoregulators, in the cerebrospinal fluid of patients with psychiatric disorders subsequent to viral infections such as measles and herpes simplex virus. This suggests a role for these immunoregulators and the inflammatory process in the cause of certain mental disorders.[70] Elevated levels of interferons can also be detected in the cerebrospinal fluid of individuals with bacterial and viral infections,[71–73] including the AIDS virus and its associated infections.[74–75] In the cerebrospinal fluid, these immunoregulators are also increased in autoimmune disorders such as lupus psychosis[76] and multiple sclerosis.[77] Finally, the effects of interferons on the body are seen in iatrogenic administration. Individuals injected with interferons respond with[57]:

Fever
Fatigue
Anorexia
Dizziness
Impaired cognition
Mood alteration
Depression

There are many immunoregulators. These pleiotropic molecules evolved out of a process of gene duplication and selection; many isoforms exist for both the specific messenger molecule and its receptors.[8] Production of these regulatory molecules is accomplished by:

Immune cells
Neural cells
Glial cells
Mast cells
Fibroblast
Smooth muscle cells
Endothelial cells

The stimuli initiating the production of cytokines involve noxious or potentially injurious events. Besides augmenting the inflammatory response, cytokines play an important role in preparing the body for defense and orchestrating the repair of tissue. When produced in inappropriate amounts or for excessive periods of time, these molecules can be destructive to the homeostatic mechanism both at the tissue level and systemically. Their importance in somatic dysfunction and the conversion of acute injury to a chronic state is just being realized.

Endocrine Regulators

Hormones related to the hypothalamic-pituitary-adrenal axis have wide-ranging effects on neural and immune cells and their endocrine targets (Table 9.5). In addition, they influence the cellular component of the fascia. The hypothalamic-pituitary-adrenal axis plays a major role in the maintenance of homeostasis and the general adaptive response of the body to challenge. These substances are listed in Table 9.6 and illustrated in Figure 9.5. Their role in the general adaptive response to stressful stimuli is considered in more detail below.

CORTICOTROPIN-RELEASING FACTOR

Control of the release of adrenal cortical hormones is exercised by neural substances called hypophysiotrophic factors. These are produced in the hypothalamus and secreted into the blood supply of the anterior pituitary (Fig. 9.5). Neurons in the paraventricular nuclei and adjacent areas of the hypothalamus synthesize CRF. Following its synthesis, CRF is trans-

Table 9.6
Endocrine Substances Known to Interact with the Neural and Immune Systems

Pituitary
    adrenocorticotrophin (ACTH)
    thyrotrophin (TSH)
    growth hormone-releasing factor (GRH)
    somatostatin (SS)
    prolactin
Adrenal medullary hormones
    epinephrine
    norepinephrine
Adrenal cortical hormones
    cortisol
    corticosterone
    aldosterone
Thyroid hormones
    thyroxine (T_4)
    triiodothyronine (T_3)
Growth hormones
    somatotropin (pituitary growth hormone)
    somatomammotropin (placental growth hormone)
    somatomedin
Thymus
    thymulin
    thymosin
    thymopoietin
    thymolymphotropin
    thymic factor X
Others
    estrogen
    testosterone
    insulin

ported by the axons of cells in the paraventricular nucleus to the median eminence at the base of the hypothalamus, where it is released in the hypothalamic-pituitary portal vascular system to act on cells in the anterior pituitary. Production of this hypothalamic hormone is elicited by somatic and visceral nociceptive neural pathways from the spinal cord and brainstem and by forebrain limbic pathways involving the hippocampus.[78] Production and release of CRF are regulated by the neurotransmitters[79–81]:

    Norepinephrine
    Serotonin
    Acetylcholine
    The opioid peptides

CRF is also regulated by the immunoregulators such as IL-1 and IL-6.[80] Many stimuli elicit the release of CRF including:

    Cold exposure
    Emotions
    Hemorrhage
    Exercise hypoglycemia
    Infection
    Inflammation
    Trauma
    Pain

ADRENOCORTICOTROPHIC HORMONE

ACTH is produced by basophilic cells in the anterior pituitary gland in response to stimulation by CRF (Fig. 9.5). Once released into the general circulation, ACTH induces the production of the adrenal cortical hormones. These hormones are major factors in the stress response because they stimulate catabolic metabolism and increase the overall activity of the sympathetic autonomic nervous system. ACTH is also produced by immunocytes in certain conditions. Stimulation of monocyte/macrophages and T cells with bacterial endotoxin (lipopolysaccharidase), exposure to certain tumor cells, or exposure to CRF initiates the production of an ectopic ACTH.[68] Using a mechanism similar to pituitary cells, lymphocytes produce ACTH molecules from the larger pro-opiomelanocortin polypeptide. Endorphins, the other cleavage product of pro-opiomelanocortin, are also released in this process. This lymphocyte production of ACTH and endorphin has been postulated as one underlying mechanism for the induction of pathologic manifestations experienced in endotoxic shock.[11]

ADRENAL CORTICAL HORMONES

Glucocorticoid steroid hormones, such as cortisol, are produced in the adrenal cortex in response to circulating ACTH (Fig. 9.5). These adrenal hormones initiate catabolic metabolism in the tissues of the body, converting stored forms of energy into those more rapidly available forms in the process of gluconeogenesis. The release of adrenal cortical hormones also acts as a stimulant to the sympathetic nervous system and is generally a suppressant to the parasympathetic nervous system. When present in sufficient quantities, the adrenal cortical hormones act as a buffer on immune system functions.[82] Taken together, all of these responses to the adrenal hormones assist the body in initiating and controlling the general adaptive response to physical and emotional stressors.

THYMIC HORMONES

The thymus gland is known for its role in the genesis of immunocytes involved in cell-mediated immunity. It also secretes a number of peptide hormones that play a role in the regulation of the immune and endocrine systems and thereby modulate the adaptive response.[83] The best-characterized of these proteins are thymulin and the thymosins. Thymulin is secreted by separate cell populations located in the subcapsular/perivascular cortex and in the medulla of the gland. Thymulin is released into both the gland itself and systemic circulation. In the immune system, this hormone promotes the differentiation of surface markers on T cells and modulates the movements of these cells as they migrate through peripheral tissue. It also influences the expression of other immunoregulators by mononuclear cells. Production and release of thymulin is stimulated by circulating hormones, particularly:

Prolactin
ACTH
Thyroid hormones
Growth hormone

All of these are factors known to be involved in the general adaptive response to stress. Finally, the thymic hormones, along with IL-1, act to stimulate the hypothalamic-pituitary-adrenal axis. The result of this is a diminution of the output of IL-1 and control of the immune response. The thymus is involved in the genesis and regulation of cell-mediated immunity. In addition, its thymic hormones play a role in modulation of the immune response through a long feedback control loop involving the hypothalamic-pituitary-adrenal axis.

The neuroregulators, endocrine regulators, and immunoregulators are multifunctional molecules making up an integrated extracellular signal network. An outstanding feature of these substances is their diverse pleiotropism, such that each molecule has a wide range of influence in multiple areas of the body. Ultimately this network of regulators controls the proliferation, differentiation, and molecular expression of all cells. The production of these regulators is influenced by external and internal noxious stimuli and psychological stimuli such as emotional stress. Locally these regulators become mediators of the inflammatory process. Once in the systemic circulation, these regulators interact with cells in the nervous, immune, and endocrine systems to facilitate a general adaptive response. Many of the events that are seen consequent to the inflammatory process are also the outward signs of the tissue changes accompanying a palpable somatic dysfunction. One underlying tenet of osteopathic manipulative treatment is the restoration of normal vascular dynamics in an effort to assist in the removal of proinflammatory mediators to return the tissue to its normal state.

CENTRAL NERVOUS SYSTEM MODULATION OF ENDOCRINE AND IMMUNE SYSTEMS

The central nervous system modulates the activity of cells in the immune system. The most convincing evidence for this is found in the altered lymphocyte functions consequent to lesions in the:

Cerebral cortex[84]
Hypothalamus[85]
Peripheral autonomic fibers[86]

The concept of neural-immune system linkage is further reinforced by the observations that some higher levels of neural processing, such as conditioned learning, also influence the production of immunoglobulins.[87] Two pathways mediate neural influences over the immune system: the hypothalamic-pituitary-endocrine outflow and the autonomic nervous system outflow (Fig. 9.1). Both routes employ a host of chemical messengers to modulate cell function in the immune system. How the central nervous system affects immunocyte functions and the neural and endocrine pathways involved represent the main themes of this section.

The interactions among neural, endocrine, and immune systems are bidirectional and extremely complex (Figs. 9.1 and 9.2). When an organism is invaded by microbes, exposed to microbial byproducts or toxins, or subjected to trauma, lymphocytes at the point of attack produce a variety of proinflammatory, polypeptide immunoregulators called cytokines. This immune response is phasic and involves a sequence of different steps. It is through these differing phases of cytokine release that the brain detects and monitors the various steps of the immune response. These immune signals are instrumental in closely coordinating the combined response of brain, peripheral autonomic, and endocrine systems to stressful stimuli. Within the brain, the hypothalamus is the nodal point for receiving these signals and functions to integrate the responses governing all these systems (Figs. 9.1 and 9.5). For this reason, hypothalamic circuits are critical for proper maintenance of the immune response.

The hypothalamus is positioned at the base of the brain and is composed of several nuclei and important nerve fiber pathways that link the forebrain with hindbrain regions (Figs. 9.1, 9.5, and 9.6). For a more detailed description of the location and internal structure of the hypothalamus, see Morgane[88] and Willard.[89] Situated immediately superior to the pituitary gland, the hypothalamus receives projections from the spinal cord and brainstem, which carry somatic and visceral sensory information. The hypothalamus also receives connections from the limbic forebrain-limbic midbrain circuitry, known to play a major role in various integrative behaviors (Fig. 9.6). The efferent connections of the hypothalamus have a major function in regulating the endocrine system through the hypothalamic-pituitary portal system to the anterior pituitary and through direct innervation of the posterior pituitary. This control of pituitary output allows the hypothalamus to influence all other endocrine activities in the body. In addition, descending pathways from the hypothalamus regulate the activity of many

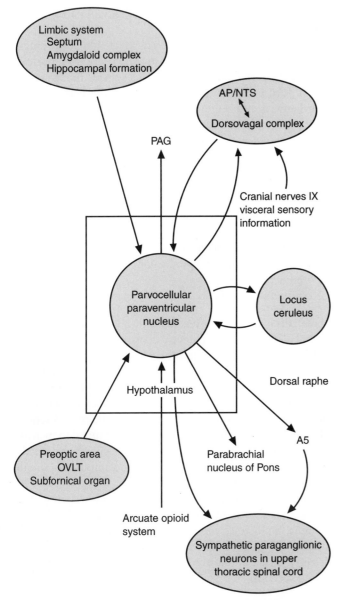

Figure 9.6. Schematic of paraventricular nucleus of hypothalamus and interconnected brain structures. OVLT, organum vasculosum of lamina terminalis; PAG, periaqueductal gray; AP/NTS, area postrema/nucleus tractus solitarii.

lower brainstem regions, especially those related to the origin of the autonomic nervous system. Its various nuclear structures are involved in regulating, among other functions:

Electrolyte balance
Feeding behavior
Body weight
Body temperature
Sexual activity
Aggressive behavior

The neurons of the hypothalamus can be classified in two major categories based on their size: magnocellular and parvicellular. Magnocellular neurons are the largest neurons of the

hypothalamus and are located primarily in two regions called the supraoptic and paraventricular nuclei. Axons from these nuclei directly innervate the posterior pituitary gland. Magnocellular neurons produce the peptides oxytocin and vasopressin for systemic release through the posterior pituitary vasculature. In addition, collateral axons from these same neurons have been demonstrated to descend into the brainstem and innervate many nuclei, including the solitary nucleus that is the primary viscerosensory nucleus of the vagus nerve. The more numerous and smaller parvicellular neurons largely compose the remaining nuclei of the hypothalamus. Many of these neurons are involved in local circuit activity; they also form projections to brainstem and forebrain. Certain groups of these cells located in the paraventricular nucleus, the arcuate nucleus, and the preoptic nucleus produce peptide regulators, called hypophysiotrophic factors, that control the production and release of anterior pituitary hormones.

The paraventricular nucleus has both magnocellular and parvicellular components. It has emerged as a key example of neuroendocrine-immune integration (Figs. 9.5 and 9.6). Stimuli converge on this nucleus from the limbic forebrain, brainstem, and spinal cord.[90] Among the neurons of this nucleus are those producing CRF. Their axons project to the neural-hemal contact zone in the median eminence,[91] a highly vascular type of circumventricular organ. The circumventricular organs are found in several localities along the walls of the third and fourth ventricles, and including the pineal gland. They represent highly vascularized zones of specialized ependymal cells that are capable of sampling the vascular and cerebrospinal fluids. Within these zones the blood-brain barrier becomes porous, and substances can pass from blood to cerebrospinal fluids of the ventricles or cerebral extracellular fluids of the surrounding tissue. These organs play a role in detecting changes in fluid ion concentration and the presence of such hormones as angiotensin and IL-1. Neurons contained within the circumventricular organs project axons to various regions of the hypothalamus.

The vasculature of the median eminence gives rise to a portal system that communicates with capillary beds in the anterior pituitary gland. Peptide regulators, such as CRF, are secreted from axon terminals into the neural-hemal contact zone to gain access to the portal blood supply. Once released into the portal blood, the regulators, called hypophysiotrophic hormones (Table 9.7), pass into a second capillary bed located in the anterior pituitary gland. In general, these hypophysiotrophic factors control the production and release of the six anterior pituitary hormones:

Follicle-stimulating hormone
Luteinizing hormone
ACTH
Thyroid stimulating hormone
Prolactin
Growth hormone

The consequences of elevated CRF secretion are multiple. There is an increased release of ACTH from the anterior pituitary gland and a related increase in the release of the adrenal

Table 9.7
Hypophyseotrophic Factors Produced in the Hypothalamus

Hypophyseotrophic Factor	Function
Corticotropin-releasing hormone	stimulates the release of ACTH
Thyrotropin-releasing hormone	stimulates the release of TSH
Growth hormone-releasing hormone	stimulates the release of GH
Somatostatin	inhibits the release of GH
Gonadotropin hormone-releasing hormone	stimulates the release of FSH
Prolactin-releasing hormone	stimulates the release of prolactin
Prolactin-inhibiting hormone	inhibits the release of prolactin

cortical hormones from the adrenal gland (Fig. 9.5). CRF also stimulates increased activity of neurons in the locus ceruleus and thus increases norepinephrine production and release, an event that activates the sympathetic autonomic nervous system. The increase in circulating adrenal cortical hormones and catecholamines acts to suppress immune system activities.

The hypothalamus also plays a significant role in controlling the central and peripheral autonomic nervous system. Again, the paraventricular nucleus is an example of how this regulatory circuitry is arranged. Descending projections from the paraventricular nucleus have recently been shown to project to extensive areas of the brainstem and spinal cord, including the sympathetic preganglionic neurons in the nucleus incallediolateralis of the upper thoracic spinal cord.[92–93] The incallediolateral nucleus is the origin of the preganglionic sympathetic axons that innervate the paravertebral and prevertebral ganglia of the body. The peripheral sympathetic system innervates the immune organs; norepinephrine from these axons acts as a self-regulating, long feedback loop to control immune system function.

Critical to the maintenance of homeostasis is the interface in the hypothalamus between the ascending monoamine systems of the brain and the adaptive response pathways of the neuroendocrine system. These ascending brainstem aminergic pathways project heavily onto hypothalamic nuclei and are major regulators of hypothalamic neuronal activity influencing the release of the hypophysiotrophic factors.[94–95] For example, noradrenergic fibers arising in the locus ceruleus of the midbrain innervate the hypothalamus, in particular the paraventricular nucleus, a major source of CRF. Recent studies suggest that this monoamine facilitates the secretion of CRF.[95] The positive influence of norepinephrine on the production and release of thyrotropin-releasing factor (TRF) has also been demonstrated.[94] The response of the locus ceruleus to external and internal stimuli, including the reticular activating system, immunoregulators, and hyperalgesia, is considered instrumental in increasing awareness and arousal, particularly when related to protective or defensive behaviors.[96] Similar activating or arousal behaviors have been obtained by injecting CRF into the ventricular cerebrospinal fluids.[79] The locus ceruleus-hypothalamic axis is a major component in translating feelings of

awareness and arousal into the altered body physiology of the adaptive response.

Through its pituitary-adrenal axis regulation of the adrenal cortical hormones and its brainstem regulation of the catecholamines in the autonomic nervous system, the hypothalamus influences immunocytes throughout the body. The hypothalamus is also responsive to immune system activity, as it is the primary site for interaction between circulating IL-1, also called the hormone of the acute phase response,[51] and the central nervous system.[97] Stimulation of the hypothalamus by administration of IL-1, either intravenously or intraperitoneally, results in:

Increased neural activity in the paraventricular nucleus[98]
Rising fever
Increased ACTH production
Increased corticosterone production
Decreased appetite
Increased slow-wave sleep[99–101]

These effects of IL-1 are mediated through increased production of CRF from the paraventricular nucleus of the hypothalamus.[97] The mechanism through which IL-1 accomplishes this feat is not well-known but might involve activation of circumventricular organs surrounding the third ventricle[48] or activation of IL-1 responsive cells in the solitary nucleus of the medulla.[97] The hypothalamus is the nodal point in a series of self-regulating, long feedback loops. They respond to increased output of immunoregulators such as IL-1 with the production of adrenal cortical hormones and catecholamines that are immunosuppressive in their activity.

Finally, the hypothalamus, through its connections with the limbic system, acts to integrate emotional behavior into the immune, endocrine, and autonomic nervous system circuits. Emotions, which are thought to be represented in the complex circuitry of the limbic system of the brain, relate to states of feeling such as:

Joy
Happiness
Mental pain
Grief
Anxiety
Depression

The hypothalamus acts as a bridge between the limbic forebrain-limbic midbrain system and the autonomic nervous system and endocrine system (Figs. 9.5 and 9.6).[90,102] A considerable body of evidence indicates that mood and emotional states influence disease susceptibility. Recent studies have begun to elucidate how these parts of the nervous system communicate with the immune system.[7] The limbic forebrain regions are involved in responses to various emotional stressors in several affective states (such as depression) and in emotional responses to sensory inputs. Stimulation or destruction of these forebrain areas alters immune activity; these same areas are responsive to circulating levels of the immunoregulators.[103] In particular, these limbic forebrain areas possess the highest concentration of glucocorticoid receptors[104–105] and link the endocrine system with neuronal outflows to autonomic and neuroendocrine systems. The limbic-hypothalamic-brainstem circuitry is the major component of the central nervous system responding to psychological, nociceptive, and immune signals and, in turn, regulating neuroendocrine outflow to the immune system.

AUTONOMIC NERVOUS SYSTEM MODULATION OF IMMUNE SYSTEM

The once well-defined boundary between the neural and immune systems is now indistinguishable. Cells in both systems produce similar intercellular messenger substances and contain cross-reacting receptors. In turn, these neuroregulators and immunoregulators modulate the activity of components of either systems. Distinctions between these two systems have become even less evident with the finding that axons from the autonomic nervous system are present within the parenchyma of immune organs (Fig. 9.7).[103,106] Many of these axons are involved in controlling the internal vasculature of the organ. These fibers also directly influence the proliferation, migration,

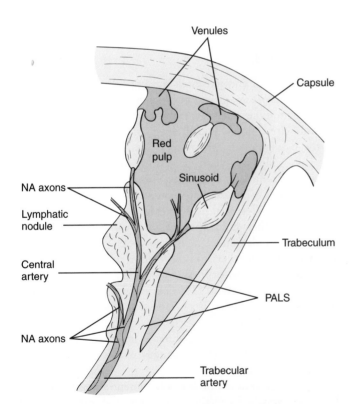

Figure 9.7. General pattern of immune gland innervation. Branch of splenic artery shown covered with small fibers marked by tyrosine hydroxylase, a marker for sympathetic postganglionic axons. Although many fibers follow the artery, others are seen in white pulp of spleen. PALS, periarteriolar lymphatic sheaths; NA axons, noradrenergic axons. (Modified from Felten SY, Felten DL. Innervation of lymphoid tissue. In: Ader R, Felten DL, Cohen N, eds. *Psychoneuroimmunology.* 2nd ed. San Diego, Calif: Academic Press; 1991.)

and maturation of immune cells.[103] Terminal endings of nerve fibers can occur in close juxtaposition to immune cells[106–107]; many immune cells have receptors for the neuroregulators of the autonomic nervous system.[10,57]

Not all axons present in lymphoid organs are efferent in nature. Some contain polypeptide neuroregulators, such as the tachykinins (substance P), that are commonly associated with the axons of unmyelinated primary afferent neurons. These sensory fibers respond to events in the immune tissue and thereby provide direct neural communication with the central nervous system.[106] In some lymphoid tissue, such as the submucosal plexus of the gastrointestinal system, interneurons containing tachykinin peptides have processes that remain entirely within the lymphatic tissue,[103] suggesting the presence of local reflex arcs.

There are several important issues concerning the function of this complex neural-immune interaction:

1. What specific properties of the immune system can be regulated by neural input?
2. Can altered output from the spinal cord, such as arises from a facilitated segment, affect neural input to specific immune glands and thereby alter function of the gland?
3. Can sensory information from somatic sources, such as muscles, joints, or connective tissue, affect the output of the autonomic nervous system to the immune organs?

These questions raise issues of considerable significance to the osteopathic physician, particularly with respect to manipulative treatment, and are promising areas for further basic and clinical research. In this section we review the innervation of the major immune organs and consider the functional aspects of this neural-immune communication.

Efferent Innervation of Immune Glands

THYMUS

The thymus is critical to the development of a specific class of lymphocytes called thymocytes or T-lymphocytes that are involved in orchestrating the cell-mediated immune responses. The thymus also plays an important role in subsequently programming the antigen-recognizing abilities of these T-lymphocytes. The thymus is divided into lobes, each containing a cortex densely populated with lymphocytes and an inner, less densely populated medulla. The thymus receives sympathetic innervation from the cervical and upper thoracic ganglia of the paravertebral ganglionic trunk.[108] These adrenergic fibers enter the cortex of the gland with the vasculature but have terminal branches that leave the vessels and can be seen distributed among the cortical immunocytes. Autonomic fibers also follow the vasculature into the medulla of the gland, but few adrenergic fibers are present in the parenchymal tissue of the medulla. It remains questionable whether any parasympathetic fibers innervate the thymus.[108]

The relationship between the sympathetic axons and thymocytes has also been examined. There are close contacts between adrenergic nerve fibers and lymphocytes of the thymus, and release of norepinephrine near thymocytes. Both immature and adult thymocytes possess β-adrenergic receptors on their external membranes.[86,106,109] β-Adrenergic stimulation of thymocytes tends to inhibit proliferation and stimulate differentiation of immunocytes.[108] The autonomic nervous system can[103,106]:

1. Control proliferation and differentiation of immune cells
2. Regulate cell metabolism in separate populations of thymocytes and T-lymphocytes
3. Control the integrity of the blood-thymus barrier
4. Modulate the secretion of thymic hormones that regulate the hypothalamus-pituitary axis

SPLEEN

The spleen is essentially a complex filter designed to maximize contact, through its specialized vasculature, of elements circulating in the blood with parenchymal macrophages and lymphocytes. Splenic macrophages participate in removing effete erythrocytes from circulation, converting their hemoglobin to bilirubin, and recycling their iron. The large splenic lymphocyte population traps circulating antigens and represents the prime source for initiation of the immune response to circulating pathogenic material.

Sympathetic innervation of the spleen arises from the thoracic spinal cord segments (T5-T9). Its preganglionic axons course via the thoracic splanchnic nerves to the celiac ganglion, from which postganglionic axons follow the splenic artery to reach the organ. Parasympathetic innervation stems from the vagus nerve that, after passing through the celiac ganglion, also follows the splenic artery. Once in the hilus, the vasculature and its mixed neural plexus courses along connective tissue septa deep into the organ (Fig. 9.7). Branches of the arterial tree leave the septi and acquire a coat of lymphocytes forming the periarteriolar lymphatic sheaths or white pulp. Subsequently, branches of these arteries lose their white pulp coats and terminate as sinusoids in the red pulp, an area rich in sinusoids.[106]

Acetylcholine-containing (parasympathetic) axons tend to remain in the extrasplenic tissue surrounding the splenic artery. Conversely, catecholamine-containing (sympathetic) axons leave the neurovascular network and enter the splenic parenchyma, terminating mainly in the white pulp. The catecholamine content of the spleen is high, suggesting that this organ might act as a catecholamine reservoir. This elevated concentration of norepinephrine has been postulated as being necessary to control both the proliferation and differentiation of B cells.[110] Depletion of norepinephrine in the adult animal by sympathectomy increases the rate of proliferation and differentiation of B cells. Although not well-understood, this excessive nonspecific or spontaneous proliferation of B cells appears disruptive to normal antigen-specific responses by the splenic immunocytes.[110] High levels of norepinephrine in the spleen

appear necessary to control B-cell proliferation and to maintain the ability of the organ to mount a specific immune response.

BONE MARROW

Hematopoiesis in adults occurs in the marrow cavities of long bones and in certain spongy bones such as the sternum and the squamous bones of the cranium. These marrow cavities are richly supplied with vasculature by nutrient canals passing through in the surrounding compact bone. Nerves enter the marrow by coursing in the perivascular sheaths of the nutrient vessels. The spinal cord segmental origins of these efferent nerves are related to the position of the bone in the body. Once inside the bone, these axons innervate the vasculature and parenchyma of the marrow cavity. Various neuroregulators have been identified in the bone marrow plexus, including catecholamines, acetylcholine, and various neuropeptides such as calcitonin gene-related polypeptide and neuropeptide Y.[106–107] These efferent nerves might modulate the proliferation kinetics of bone marrow lymphatic cells. This is suggested by the observation that catecholamine agonists increase, while stimulation by cholinergic agonists inhibits, the proliferative capabilities of these immunocytes. Also, myelination of the nerves in bone marrow coincides with the onset of hemopoiesis, suggesting a developmental relationship between these events.[106]

LYMPHATIC VESSELS

Lymphatic fluid and its vessels are important components of the immune system, providing a conduit through which extravascular immune cells and extracellular fluids can return to systemic circulation. Fluid drainage of tissue is accomplished by the passage of lymph from the extracellular tissue spaces into thin-walled lymphatic vessels that course along with neurovascular bundles. Lymphatic vessels contain numerous strong, one-way valves that facilitate directed movement of lymph using differential tissue pressures. Lymphatic vessels actively propel their fluids through these valves using peristaltic contraction under direct neural control.[111] Both cholinergic and adrenergic fibers exist in the walls of the lymphatic plexus; electrical stimulation of these nerves increases the effusion of material from the vessels. Electrical activity within the walls of the lymphatic vessel consists of one action potential preceding each peristaltic contraction.[112] Although little is known concerning the function of the cholinergic innervation, stimulating the sympathetic paravertebral ganglia results in a reflexive increase in lymph flow.[113]

A plexus of autonomic fibers is present along the walls of lymphatic vessels. The spinal cord segmental origin of the innervation of specific lymphatic vessels is correlated with the location of the vessel in the body. The largest lymphatic vessel, the thoracic duct, receives its parasympathetic innervation from the vagus and its sympathetic innervation from branches of the intercostal nerves. The cisterna chyli, the origin of the thoracic duct, is innervated by the eleventh thoracic ganglion and the left splanchnic nerve.[106] There is a distinct topographic pattern in lymphatic vessel innervation.

LYMPH NODES

Peripheral lymph nodes are specialized clusters of lymphatic tissue interposed in the lymphatic drainage routes of the body. Each node sits in a dense connective tissue capsule that is indented on one side to form a hilus. Neurovascular bundles gain access to the node by passing through the hilus. Internally, each node contains an outer cortical layer of nodules or follicles separated from the capsule by a subcapsular space. Each nodule is rich in B-lymphocytes and is surrounded by a zone of pericortical lymphatic tissue rich in T-lymphocytes. Inside the cortex is a highly vascular medulla containing venous sinuses separated by cords of lymphatic tissue. Lymph enters the node through afferent vessels that penetrate the nonhilar portion of the capsule. Lymph passes through the cortex and medulla, coming in contact with numerous lymphocytes. Filtered lymph is removed by efferent vessels that leave from the hilus. The lymph node is organized to screen lymph and trap any associated antigens.

A differential distribution of autonomic fibers is present in lymph nodes. Cholinergic fibers remain in the subcapsular area of the node while norepinephrine-containing fibers follow the vasculature into the subcapsular spaces, paracortex, and medullary cords. These latter areas are rich in T-lymphocytes as opposed to the centers of the nodules that contain primarily B-lymphocytes.[103,106,114] Neuropeptidergic fibers are also concentrated under the capsule and along the vasculature of the lymph node, but as in the case of the sympathetic innervation, few penetrate into the germinal centers of the nodules. Neuronal contacts between peptide-containing fibers and mast cells and macrophages are seen within the lymph node.[107] Autonomic fibers in the lymph node appear to control vascular size and blood flow as well as the movement of lymphocytes out of the node, a process called trafficking.[103,115] These observations suggest that the autonomic nervous system plays an instrumental role in modulating cell movement through the lymphatic system both at the level of the lymph node itself and in the lymph vessels.

The differential and complex innervation of the various immune glands underscores the powerful influence of the autonomic nervous system on their functions. There are significant changes in lymphocyte functions subsequent to lesions in the cerebral cortex,[84] hypothalamus,[85] or peripheral sympathetic fibers.[85,106] Bilateral lesions in portions of the hypothalamus (anterior hypothalamic area or ventromedial hypothalamic nucleus) decrease the number of thymocytes and splenocytes responding to activation by the mitogen concanavalin-A, whereas similar lesions in the hippocampal formation, amygdala, and frontal cortex increase the number of these immune cells activated by exposure to this mitogen.[85] Multiple areas of the central nervous system, such as the limbic forebrain and hypothalamus, acting through their peripheral connections

with immune glands modulate the proliferation kinetics and trafficking of immune cells. In addition, the hypothalamus, through the hypothalamic-pituitary-adrenal axis and the production of adrenal cortical hormones, also exerts control over the general reactivity of the immune system.

Primary Afferent Innervation of Immune Glands

Along with the autonomic or efferent innervation, the endings of afferent or sensory fibers carrying information to the central nervous system have also been found in the[106–107,116]:

Thymus
Spleen
Lymph nodes
Bone marrow
Lymphatic vessels

These afferent fibers contain neuropeptides typically present in sensory nerves such as the tachykinins (substance P) and calcitonin gene-related polypeptide, among others. Immunocytes in these glands have been demonstrated to contain receptors for these neuropeptides on their cell membranes.[103] Although the effects of neuropeptides on immunocyte activity is not well-understood, data suggest that the peptide-containing fibers can be paracrine in nature and, consequently, play a role in controlling such immunocyte activities as:

Mitosis
Differentiation
Migration
Maturation

The presence of sensory nerves in all immune glands might be one method for detecting what has been called noncognitive stimuli.[12,107] Examples of noncognitive stimuli are bacteria, foreign protein, or other allergenic molecules that gain access to the extracellular fluids. Because the immune system is capable of recognizing both self-antigens and foreign antigens, it has in effect constructed within its network an internal image or antigenic map of the body.[117] Distortions of this antigenic body image, by the presence of foreign substances, trigger the release of immunoregulators into the extracellular matrix. These immunoregulators, such as IL-1 and interferon, are potent stimulants of the small-caliber, primary afferent fibers as well as of hypothalamic neurons via the circumventricular organs of the ventricles. As immune cells begin to communicate with each other in response to the presence of foreign substances and initiate cellular and humoral-based immune responses, they also engage the afferent limb of the nervous system. The cells inform the brain of distortions in the antigenic body map and the current phase of the immune response in handling this potentially injurious situation. In the central nervous system this information is used to trigger a series of autonomic and neuroendocrine reflexes that, if of sufficient intensity, culminate in a general adaptive response. Ultimately, this response functions to control various components of the immune system.

ENDOCRINE MODULATION OF IMMUNE SYSTEM

Stressors interact with the hypothalamus through its many neural and humoral connections. Stressors initiate major adjustments in secretion of extracellular messengers within the neuroendocrine-immune network, forming the basis of the general adaptive response. An elaborate complex of feedback control pathways among neural, endocrine, and immune organs provides a series of buffering mechanisms to prevent overcompensation in the production and release of these extracellular messengers. Many of the pathways involve interactions between components of the endocrine and immune systems (Table 9.5). The scope of this section is limited to a summary of the specific endocrine-immune interactions related to the general adaptive response. Tables 9.2 and 9.3 list the types and functions of the immune cells germane to this summary. The focus is on hormones of the hypothalamic-pituitary-adrenal axis, as well as thyroid hormones, pineal hormones, and those factors related to growth hormone, called the somatomammotrophs.

Hormones of Hypothalamic-Pituitary-Adrenal Axis

The adrenal cortical hormones affect most metabolic processes in the body, enhancing those that are capable of deriving energy from the tissues of the body and repressing growth processes that require energy. The activity of this pituitary-adrenal axis is controlled through two peptides, ACTH, produced in the anterior pituitary gland, and CRF, produced in the paraventricular nucleus of the hypothalamus (Fig. 9.5). Neural control of the hypophyseotropic hormone is achieved through the limbic system as well as through ascending projections from brainstem and spinal cord. Emotional stimuli, acting through the limbic forebrain, as well as nociception from somatic and visceral dysfunctions, increase the hypothalamic output of CRF and consequently increase the production and release of adrenal cortical hormones.[78,118–119]

Circulating levels of adrenal cortical hormones provide a feedback signal to the hypothalamic-pituitary axis, thereby regulating the production of both CRF and ACTH. At least two control pathways are known in this neuroendocrine circuit; a long-term loop involving the central nervous system and a short-term loop involving the pituitary gland directly (Fig. 9.5). In the short-term or fast-acting loop, the release of ACTH by the anterior pituitary is directly inhibited by feedback of adrenal cortical hormones. Conversely, in the long-term feedback loop, involving minutes to hours, the glucocorticoids influence neural activity in the limbic system and hypothalamus to decrease the production of CRF. These neural control mechanisms involve receptors for the adrenal cortical hormones located on neurons in the paraventricular nucleus of the (Fig. 9.6)[104]:

Hypothalamus
Septal nuclei
Hippocampal formation
Frontal cerebral cortex

Circulating adrenal cortical hormones give feedback to the pituitary gland and multiple areas of the central nervous system, thereby diminishing the further release of CRF by the hypothalamus and ACTH by the anterior pituitary gland.

The relationship between adrenal cortical hormones and the immune system was one of the first endocrine-immune interactions to be studied. One of the best known functions of the adrenal cortical hormones is the inhibition of arachidonic acid release from cell membranes through blockage of the enzyme phospholipase A_2. The inhibition of arachidonic acid diminishes the formation of prostaglandins and leukotrienes, two proinflammatory compounds, from arachidonic acid.[120] Consequent to traumatic injury, arachidonic acid, a fatty acid component of most cell membranes, is released into the extracellular fluids. Its metabolic byproducts, the prostaglandins and leukotrienes, are primary mediators of the inflammatory response. They:

Induce edema
Sensitize sensory nerve endings (hyperalgesia)
Stimulate the central nervous system to initiate fever

The first two of these responses constitute the palpable signs of a somatic dysfunction.[3]

Adrenal cortical hormones also function to curb the cell-mediated aspects of the inflammatory process. These hormones suppress T-cell and B-cell secretions and natural killer cell activity.[120] Additionally, circulating glucocorticoids decrease the production and release of the proinflammatory immunoregulators such as[120]:

Interleukins -1, -2, and -3
Interferon
Tumor necrosis factor

The overall effect of the corticosteroids on the immune system is to suppress the cascading network of responses that lead to inflammation and tissue destruction. Glucocorticoid suppression of the immune response is suggested by Munck and colleagues[82] to be an important mechanism in the overall limiting of inflammation and of the general adaptive response.

These findings are derived primarily from experiments assessing immune function following administration of exogenous adrenal cortical hormones at pharmaceutical concentrations. The role of these steroids at physiologic concentrations is more complex and less clear. Although concentrations in the higher physiologic levels are generally inhibitory, especially to antibody formation, several studies have demonstrated enhanced immune functions when the physiologic levels of circulating adrenal cortical hormones have been repressed by antagonists or are reduced by genetic factors.[120] Conversely, low physiologic levels of the adrenal cortical hormones might have no effect on, or even tend to stimulate, immune functions such as monocyte and macrophage activity. In this regard, the daily output of the adrenal cortical steroids appears to establish a window of optimal function in which the activities of immunocytes are positioned. The boundaries of this window are flexible and can be influenced by the output of immunoregulators.

This is supported by the observation that IL-1 and other immunoregulators stimulate the release of CRF and ACTH.[103] The resulting increased levels of serum adrenal cortical hormones then limit feedback on immune cell function. These observations demonstrate the critical role of the hypothalamic-pituitary-adrenal axis in stabilizing the functions of the immune system (Fig. 9.6).

The interactions between the hypothalamic-pituitary-adrenal axis and the immune system are bidirectional. Cells of the immune system are capable of producing substances that regulate this major neuroendocrine axis[11,119]:

Proinflammatory cytokines
ACTH
β-endorphins
Tissue corticotropin-releasing hormone (CRH)

The proinflammatory cytokines are IL-1, IL-6, and tumor necrosis factor, which can synergistically stimulate the neuroendocrine axis. Although these cytokines influence hypothalamic function, it is not yet understood how they cross the blood-brain barrier. Several possibilities exist involving transfer to glial cells or interaction with the circumventricular organs.[119] The ACTH produced by immunocytes is derived from expression of the pro-opiomelanocortin gene and is identical to that produced in the anterior pituitary gland.[56] While the circulating ACTH influences the adrenal gland, the production and release of β-endorphin by mononuclear cells in peripheral tissue and the interaction of this opioid compound with the terminal processes of small-caliber, primary afferent fibers has been suggested as a key to the peripheral antinociceptive mechanisms.[121] The ectopic source of the stress-related hormones such as ACTH and CRH from the immunocytes stimulates the production of adrenal cortical steroid hormones and down-regulates the immune system response, thus helping to stabilize the homeostatic mechanism. This tissue release of neuroendocrine messengers can be severely damaging to body functions if excessive. For example, excessive production of pro-opiomelanocortin by lymphocytes that results in the excess formation and release of ACTH and endorphins has been implicated as the source of the pathologic processes in the endotoxic shock syndrome following exposure to bacterial endotoxins.[11]

A critical balance of activities in the hypothalamic-pituitary-adrenal axis is essential to the normal physiology and psychology of the body. Disruption of this axis results in a number of complex neuroendocrinologic syndromes.[119] Primary adrenal hyperactivity is seen in Cushing's disease; primary adrenal insufficiency is the underlying pathology in Addison's disease. Elevation in the activity of the hypothalamic-pituitary-adrenal axis as a result of stress does not necessarily present with these disease conditions. Long-term, stress-induced activation of this system, sufficient to result in hypercortisolism, has been linked to major psychiatric disorders such as melancholic depression and also with chronic immunosuppression.[122] Conversely, lowered levels of hypothalamic activity in this axis, resulting in hypocortisolism, has been demonstrated in some patients with chronic fatigue syndrome and in diseases featuring excessive

activity of the immune system, such as the inflammatory arthropathies.[123] Disruption of the hypothalamic-pituitary-adrenal axis is also suspected to occur in posttraumatic stress disorder.[124]

Hormones of Hypothalamic-Pituitary-Thyroid Axis

Thyroid gland hormones that act to increase the metabolic activity of cells in most organs of the body are also responsive to stressful stimuli. Hypothalamic control over the thyroid gland is exercised through the production of thyrotropin-releasing hormone (TRH). It acts through the hypothalamic-pituitary portal system and induces production and release of thyrotropin (thyroid-stimulating hormone) from the cells in the anterior pituitary gland. Thyrotropin, in turn, stimulates the synthesis and release of thyroxine and triiodothyronine from the thyroid gland. Throughout the body, these thyroid hormones influence the cellular consumption of oxygen and regulate the metabolism of lipids and carbohydrates. The thyroid hormones play a significant role in growth and development as well as in maintenance of adult tissue. Development of the musculoskeletal system is greatly affected by alterations in the hypothalamic-pituitary-thyroid axis.

Environmental factors, acting through the hypothalamic-pituitary-thyroid axis, influence the production of the thyroid hormones.[125] The thyroid responds positively to prolonged exposure to cold or even to moderately diminishing temperature. This response to decreasing temperature depends on an intact hypothalamic-pituitary axis; lesions of the preoptic area in the hypothalamus interrupt the reflex. Increased thyroid hormone output accelerates cellular metabolism and elevates the production of body heat. Conversely, emotional and physical stressors impact thyroid function negatively by acting through the hypothalamus and limbic system. In experimental situations, certain stressors result in suppression of thyroid output[125]:

Starvation
Somatic pain
Visceral pain
Restraint
Toxins
Infection

Stress-related sympathetic activation suppresses thyroid functions as detected by a decrease in thyroid size despite the presence of thyroid-stimulating factor.[126] In response to adrenal and sympathetic activation in stressful situations such as painful somatic dysfunction, several routes exist whereby thyroid gland activity can be depressed.

Pituitary thyrotropin and the thyroxins have effects on immune cell function. In systemic circulation, thyrotropin enhances the stimulation of natural killer cell activity by IL-2. Thyroxin, on the other hand, induces the production of T cells. Both of these events facilitate activation of the immune response. The communication between the hypothalamic-pituitary-thyroid axis and the immune system is bidirectional. Thyrotropin is also produced by activated lymphocytes, suggesting one route whereby the immune system can modulate body metabolism.[127] The lymphocyte-derived thyrotrophin enhances antigen-stimulated antibody production by immunocytes.[128] The thyroid gland and its associated regulatory factors modify the function of a number of immune cells and, in turn, these cells synthesize thyrotropin that could facilitate thyroid functions.

Somatomammotrophs

Several other anterior pituitary hormones, responsive to stressful stimuli, serve as potent regulators of immune functions. Two of these substances are collectively called the somatomammotrophs: growth hormone (somatotropin) and prolactin. They are closely related hormones.

GROWTH HORMONE

Growth hormone is the quintessential pleiotropic hormone. It is released from the somatotrophic cells in the anterior pituitary gland and regulates a wealth of cellular metabolic and growth activities throughout the body. Its release from the pituitary gland is closely regulated by two hypothalamic factors, somatostatin and growth hormone-releasing factor.[125] Regulation of growth hormone secretion is accomplished by two hypothalamic peptides acting through the hypothalamic-pituitary portal system. Growth hormone-releasing factor stimulates growth hormone secretion; conversely, somatostatin inhibits growth hormone secretion.

At the tissue level, growth hormone acts through an additional class of hormones, the somatomedins, that are produced in the liver and exist in general circulation. The growth hormone-somatomedin interaction enhances nucleic acids and protein synthesis at the cellular level, ultimately promoting growth. The entire growth hormone-somatomedin mechanism is regulated by the hypothalamus and is responsive to limbic system inputs. In experimental situations, increases in activity of the growth hormone-somatomedin axis has been demonstrated by stimulation of the:

Hippocampus
Amygdala
Locus ceruleus
Raphe nuclei

These are all areas of the brain known to be activated by stressful or noxious stimuli.

Somatostatin is found not only in the hypothalamus but also throughout the body. Like substance P, this polypeptide is produced and secreted from small-caliber, primary afferent fibers (C fibers or nociceptive fibers) involved in the transmission of painful stimuli.[34,38] Somatostatin is inhibitory to the secretion of substance P from the endings of the small-caliber, primary afferent fibers and might be antagonistic to other proinflammatory messengers as well. Because both of these neuropeptides are released from nociceptive afferent fibers when they are irritated by noxious stimuli, the ratio of the two should determine the overall proinflammatory activities occur-

ring in the tissue. The factors influencing the amounts of somatostatin and substance P release from nerve endings for a given stimulus have not yet been determined.

The messengers of the hypothalamic-pituitary-growth hormone axis also exert influence on the immune system. Growth hormone has several effects. It[129]:

Stimulates antibody synthesis by macrophages
Increases cytotoxic T-cell activity
Activates natural killer cells
Increases macrophage metabolism and T-cell proliferation

Somatostatin generally suppresses immune cell functions as evidenced by decreases in[129]:

Natural killer cell activity
T-cell response
Lymphocyte proliferation
Leukocyte migration

Splenocyte proliferation is also decreased by somatostatin, as is the synthesis of the immunoglobulins IgA and IgM.[130–131] Growth hormone production is stimulated by immunoregulators such as IL-1.[53] The immune system seeks to establish a growth-enhancing environment as it initiates an adaptive response to antigenic stimulation. Such a condition is of considerable benefit in the process of wound repair and healing.

PROLACTIN

Prolactin, another hormone of the family of somatomammotrophs, is produced and released from the anterior pituitary under control of the hypothalamus. Several inhibiting factors have been described, among which is dopamine, a catecholamine. Although releasing factors for prolactin are not as well-documented, numerous substances in the hypothalamus have been suggested for this function, among them being:

Vasoactive intestinal polypeptide
Oxytocin
TRF
Opioid peptides

Steroid hormones also have an influence on the production and release of prolactin. Estrogens are strong stimulants of prolactin release, whereas the glucocorticoids inhibit prolactin release.[132] In circulation, prolactin plays an important role in breast maturation and lactation.

Prolactin also has a major stimulatory impact on the immune response. Factors that inhibit the release of prolactin, such as dopamine, depress T-cell proliferative response to mitogen and increase susceptibility to infection[132]; these events can be reversed by administering prolactin. Conversely, stimulating the production of endogenous prolactin by administering antagonists for dopamine (disinhibiting prolactin secretion) increases the proliferative response of T cell to mitogen.[132] Hypoprolactinemia, such as seen following antipsychotic drug therapy, is associated with impaired lymphocyte proliferation and decreased production of macrophage-activating factor by T cells.[133] For these reasons, prolactin has been described as being immunopermissive; that is, its presence is necessary for the normal activity of the immune system.[132] Recently the immunopermissive actions of prolactin have been demonstrated to be antagonistic to the immunosuppressive activities of the adrenal cortical hormones, suggesting that prolactin functions as a counterregulatory stress hormone for the adrenal cortical hormones.[132]

External stimuli trigger the release of prolactin from the hypothalamus. These stimuli include a spinal reflex pathway arising from tissue around the nipple and uterine cervix as well as physical and emotional stressors. There is a rapid and significant increase in prolactin secretion initially in acute stress, but this response returns to baseline with prolonged stress.[132] This biphasic response of prolactin to stressors suggests that prolactin is initially acting as a stress hormone to increase immune system activity, but that in prolonged exposure to stressors prolactin diminishes, possibly preventing excessive proliferative activity in the immune system.

Opioid Peptides

The natural opioid peptides metenkephalin, leuenkephalin, and the endorphins (alpha, beta, and gamma) are central factors in the stress response, particularly the response to nociceptive events, such as somatic dysfunction. These opioids arise from three large precursor peptides[13]:

Pro-opiomelanocortin
Proenkephalin
Prodynorphin

The factors determining which of these opioid peptides are produced from the precursor molecule and in what concentrations in vivo are not well-established.

Opioid peptides are synthesized by neurons in numerous regions of the central nervous system, including the[134]:

Arcuate area of the hypothalamus
Solitary nucleus of the medullary brainstem
Dorsal horn of the spinal cord

Axonal projections from these sites provide a rich opioid-containing innervation of the following areas:

Cerebral cortex
Corpus striatum
Hippocampal formation
Amygdala
Periventricular thalamic
Hypothalamic
Many sensory and nociceptive areas of the brainstem

These peptides are also produced and released into systemic circulation from the pituitary and adrenal glands. Receptors for the opioid peptides are found in the numerous regions of the central nervous system receiving opioid projections and on many immune cells, including[11]:

Lymphocytes
T cells
B cells
Macrophages

As neuroregulators, the opioid peptides play important roles in modulating the perception of painful stimuli and regulating the production of hypophyseotropic hormones. In the central nervous system, opioid-induced analgesia is mediated through a neural circuit extending from the hypothalamus through the periaqueductal region of the midbrain and raphe of the medulla, to the dorsal horn of the spinal cord.[135] In addition to the central pathways for antinociception, recent studies have demonstrated that the peripheral processes of small-caliber, primary afferent neurons also have receptors for the opioids. Stimulation of these peripheral receptors by opioids released from local immunocytes has an analgesic effect and represents a primary level of pain control.[121,136–137] This peripheral-level analgesia can be blocked by the opioid antagonist naloxone, demonstrating the dependence of the analgesia on functioning opioid receptors. Clinical application of the peripheral antinociception pathways has been accomplished by injecting morphine into knee joints following arthroscopic surgery.[138]

Beyond their role in the antinociceptive response, opioid peptides influence the activity of cells in the endocrine and immune systems. Hypothalamic opioid pathways stimulate the production of CRF and inhibit the production of gonadotropin-releasing factor. This latter event is suggested as a source of the stress-induced amenorrhea seen in women who achieve excessive levels of physical exercise.

CRH, in the presence of mononuclear cells, induces β-endorphin production in peripheral B-lymphocytes.[139] It appears that the CRF interacts with the monocyte, which then releases IL-1, stimulating B cells to secrete β-endorphin into the peripheral tissue. These opioids assist in the generation of peripheral-level analgesia by interacting with opioid receptors on the terminals of the primary afferent fibers.[137] Opioid compounds have a major role in modulation of the immune system generally by enhancing cell-mediated immune functions.[9,139] All of the following increase the cytotoxic activity of natural killer cells:

Metenkephalin
Leuenkephalin
α-endorphin
β-endorphin
γ-endorphin

These effects are inhibited by naloxone,[140] an antagonist of the opioid compounds that blocks opioid receptors. The endorphins also stimulate the production of IL-1 from immunocytes.

The effects of the opioid peptides on the humoral immune system are subtle and depend on the current level of activity in the immune system. α-Endorphin and ACTH are inhibitory to the primary antibody response. δ-Endorphin either enhances or suppresses the secondary antibody response; the critical factor is the magnitude of the antibody response. High levels of response tend to favor an inhibitory action of δ-endorphin and low levels of response tend to result in a facilitatory action.[139] The opioids, especially the endorphins, act to fine-tune the antibody response and represent another example of the overall effort of the neuroendocrine-immune network to maintain homeostasis in the face of stressful stimuli.

Pineal Gland and Melatonin

The pineal gland is located at the posterior and superior corner of the third ventricle and is considered one of the circumventricular organs. This gland and its major hormone, melatonin, play an important role in the circadian control of immune function.[141] Melatonin is produced from serotonin in the gland and released in a circadian rhythm. Circadian control of the pineal gland is established by a pathway involving axons from retinal ganglion cells that project to the superchiasmatic nucleus of the hypothalamus. The pineal gland innervation arises in the hypothalamus from which it takes an indirect route involving the upper thoracic spinal cord and the cervical and thoracic sympathetic ganglia. From there, postganglionic axons follow the cervical and cerebral vasculature, eventually arriving at the pineal gland. Sympathetic nervous system regulation of the circadian clock is obtained by the light-related, β-adrenergic stimulation of the serotonin-converting enzyme serotonin-N-acetyltransferase. Under normal circumstances, melatonin is released during the dark phase and inhibited during the light phase of the day–night cycle. This gland is described as a sensory transducing organ, converting a light/dark sensorineural signal carried in the autonomic nervous system into a hormonal pulse.[141]

Modulation of the melatonin circadian cycle has effects on immune function. Eliminating the darkness cycle by exposing animals to continuous light decreases the amount of melatonin produced by the pineal gland and reveals a concomitant impairment in immune system function. The ability to mount a humoral response to challenge by T-dependent antigens is depressed, and there is cellular depletion of the thymic cortex and atrophy of the red and white pulp of the spleen. Replacement of the melatonin, using a circadian rhythm, significantly enhances the ability of the animals to mount a primary antibody response. This enhancement does not carry over to cellular immunity, suggesting that melatonin's immunoenhancement properties are focused on the humoral responses.

Melatonin counteracts the immunosuppressive functions of the hypothalamic-pituitary-adrenal axis during exposure to stressors. Restraining an animal creates a stressful condition featuring elevated output of adrenal cortical hormones from the hypothalamic-pituitary-adrenal axis. The result of this increase in circulating adrenal cortical hormones is immunosuppression characterized by involution of the immune organs and depressed response to antigenic challenge. Melatonin injection into restraint-stressed animals prevents some of the immunosuppressive properties of the stressor. Although the effects of the corticosteroids are still seen in the atrophy of the immune organs, the humoral antibody response is significantly increased. Melatonin appears to assist in the recovery of the immune system from the stress-induced suppression without negating the general systemic effects of the adrenal cortical hormones.[141]

The effects of melatonin as an anti-stress hormone on the hypothalamic-pituitary-adrenal axis are not direct. Melatonin stimulates the endogenous opioid system. It, in turn, counteracts some of the immunosuppressive effects of the adrenal cortical hormones. The endogenous opioids, dynorphin and β-endorphin, have an immunoenhancing effect that is more pronounced when they are administered in a circadian rhythm, particularly if they are injected during the evening. Melatonin stimulates T helper cells to release opioid agonists that, in turn, enhance the immune responses in an autocrine or paracrine fashion. This melatonin-induced stimulation of the immune system can be blocked by naltrexone, an opioid antagonist, further emphasizing its dependence on the natural opioid compounds. Based on its immunoenhancing effects, melatonin has been regarded as an anti-stress immunoregulator.

This section has demonstrated the complex hormonal response to stressors such as the pain involved in somatic or visceral dysfunction or in emotional distress. In response to proinflammatory cytokines or emotional stimuli, the hypothalamus releases CRF, stimulating the pituitary-adrenal axis, initiating a sympathetic response, and suppressing activity in other neuroendocrine axes such as that involving the pituitary and thyroid gland. Initially the hypothalamic-growth hormone axis is activated but can be repressed in the chronic state. In a situation of acute stress, the adrenal cortical hormones, although immunosuppressive in elevated amounts, shift body tissues to an energy-scavenging state. Growth hormone and the thyroid hormones enhance cellular metabolism and growth as well as possibly being immunostimulatory or immunopermissive in the early phases of the response. These stress hormones are counterbalanced by anti-stress hormones such as prolactin and melatonin. The combined action of these messenger molecules creates a tissue environment that is rich in available energy and promotes growth and metabolism, thereby facilitating the immune response and the overall healing process. In this regard, the adrenal cortical hormones can establish an upper limit or cap on the extent of the immune response because they become immunosuppressive at high levels of concentration. Under these conditions, the interplay of the nervous, endocrine, and immune systems allows for a highly integrated, multisystem response to external threats. This facilitates the major function of the network: to respond to external challenges and then to restore the body to its normal homeostatic condition.

FACTORS MODULATING NEUROENDOCRINE-IMMUNE NETWORK

The neuroendocrine-immune network is responsive to stimuli from both external and internal sources. External factors capable of altering the function of this network include:

Invasion by foreign substances or infectious diseases
Musculoskeletal injury such as somatic dysfunction
Predatory threat

Internal stressors influencing the neuroendocrine-immune network are represented by noxious mechanical or chemical sources in the visceral organs and associated vasculature. Finally, psychological or emotional states also serve as factors affecting the balance of activities in the neuroendocrine-immune network. Regardless of the type of noxious stimulus, the shift in homeostatic mechanisms can have similar features, suggesting common pathways of function. In this section, three major categories of stressful factors—somatic, visceral, and emotional—are examined for the effect they exert on the patient's compensatory mechanisms (Fig. 9.8).

Somatic Factors

Noxious somatic stimuli, in addition to initiating protective reflexes and providing the central nervous system with warning signs,[142–144] influence the release of extracellular messengers from the endocrine-immune axis (Fig. 9.8).[118] When activated by noxious stimuli such as arises in somatic dysfunction, small-caliber primary afferent fibers (called A-γ and C fibers, or collectively referred to as the B-afferent system) from peripheral nociceptive endings release neuropeptides such as substance P into the surrounding tissue, thereby initiating a neurogenic inflammation (Fig. 9.4).[38] The B-afferent fiber system represents a subset of small-caliber, primary afferent fibers with high threshold for activation that are present in both somatic and visceral tissue. These fibers form a system for detecting stimuli pertinent to homeostasis; for that reason they are referred to as the homeostatic fiber system. For a description of the B-afferent fiber see Prechtl and Powley[145] and Chapter 5, Autonomic Nervous System.

The central processes of these fibers stimulate cells in the dorsal horn of the spinal cord. Within the dorsal horn (Fig. 9.4), cells responding to the nociceptive input initiate signals carried to the motor nuclei of the ventral horn to alter the tone of muscles innervated by that particular spinal segment[142,144–146] and, through the anterolateral tract of the spinal cord, communicate with the brainstem and hypothalamus.[147]

A significant result of nociceptive input is increased activity in the hypothalamic-pituitary-adrenal axis, culminating in increased output of adrenal cortical hormones and increased output of norepinephrine from the sympathetic nervous system (Fig. 9.8). This reflex can be blocked by selectively eliminating the small-caliber, primary afferent fibers. Animals treated with capsaicin, which reduces levels of substance P in the peripheral nervous system by destroying the small-caliber, primary afferent fibers, show a blunted ACTH response to stress induced by a nociceptive stimulus such as foot shock.[118] Suppression of nociceptive input from the periphery, by removing small-caliber fibers, diminishes the hypothalamic response and reduces the pituitary-adrenal and autonomic responses to somatic stressors. In addition, capsaicin-treated animals, lacking the ability to release substance P, also accumulate fewer neutrophils at the site of injury, suggesting a blunted inflammatory response. The neuroendocrine-immune network is affected by the output of signals from a somatic dysfunction; it responds by initiating a compensatory shift in extracellular messengers that then alters the functions of the immune system.[148] Parts of this model for somatic dysfunction have been presented in Willard[149] and VanBuskirk.[150]

Visceral Factors

The cervical, thoracic, abdominal, and pelvic viscera as well as peripheral blood vessels communicate with the brainstem and spinal cord through an extensive complement of afferent fibers, also considered a portion of the B-afferent system.[147] These visceral afferent fibers reach their target organs by coursing in the same nerves as the efferent autonomic fibers; they follow the routes of the vascular system. The visceral sensory fibers, typically of small-caliber and having little or no myelin, have cell bodies located in the thoracolumbar dorsal root ganglia and in ganglia of the several cranial nerves. The central processes of these neurons terminate in:

Superficial and deep regions of the dorsal horn of the spinal cord
Spinal trigeminal nucleus
Solitary nucleus of the vagus

Thoracoabdominal and pelvic organs receive an extensive sensory innervation. These afferent fibers travel to the central ner-

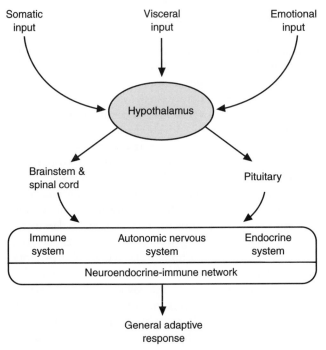

Figure 9.8. Response of neuroendocrine-immune network to signals emanating from somatic, visceral, or emotional dysfunction. (Reprinted with permission from Willard FH. Neuroendocrine-immune network, nociceptive stress, and the general adaptive response. In Everett T, Dennis M, Ricketts E, eds. *Physiotherapy in Mental Health: A Practical Approach.* Oxford, Boston: Butterworth/Heinemann; 1995.)

vous system in company with the efferent autonomic fibers. In general, those sensory fibers traveling in the parasympathetic nerves, such as the vagus, carry non-noxious information for reflex control of the organ. Those traveling with the sympathetic nerves, such as the greater splanchnic, carry noxious information.[151] Neurons of the deeper portions of the dorsal horn receive extensive convergence of information from the small-caliber sensory axons arising in both visceral and somatic sources.[152–154] A similar convergence of somatic and visceral input is seen in the solitary nucleus of the vagus.[155]

Neurons responsive to both visceral and somatic nociceptive stimuli are located in the spinal cord,[156] brainstem,[155] hypothalamus, and thalamus.[157] These dually responsive neurons provide an explanation for the phenomena of referred pain between visceral and somatic sources. Visceral sensory information is conducted through the same ascending spinal tracts to the brainstem and hypothalamus as somatic nociceptive information.[158] This suggests that nociception from visceral dysfunction is capable of eliciting similar changes in the output of the neuroendocrine-immune network as that derived from somatic dysfunction (Fig. 9.8). Support for this contention is seen in the observation that using an analgesic to block activity in the thoracic splanchnic nerves at the conclusion of abdominal surgery blunts the postoperative release of cortisol.[159]

Emotional Factors

Psychological input to the neuroendocrine-immune network arises largely from the limbic forebrain system and hypothalamus. The major components of the limbic forebrain include large portions of the association neocortex such as the:

Prefrontal area
Cingulate cortex
Insula cortex
Inferior medial aspect of the temporal lobe

The limbic forebrain also includes older portions of the forebrain such as the hippocampal formation and amygdala. The hippocampal formation and amygdala receive extensive connections from the frontal, parietal, and cingulate associational areas of neocortex and, in turn, project to the hypothalamus through the fornix and stria terminalis. By influencing the hypophyseotropic hormones of the hypothalamic nuclei, these limbic forebrain areas exert considerable modulation over the pituitary gland as well as the autonomic nervous system (Fig. 9.8). Under a state of excessive emotion the limbic system mediates from the pituitary gland, via the hypothalamus, the release of:

Growth hormone
ACTH
Prolactin
Somatostatin

The limbic system also increases the sympathetic output from the spinal cord. These alterations in neuroendocrine activity affect the metabolic processes of the body, shifting peripheral tissues to a catabolic form of metabolism and leading to marked changes in the function of the immune system, including stress-induced suppression of immune function. These conditions characterize the general adaptive response.

Highly stressful circumstances in life can initiate a general adaptive response and significantly alter the status of the immune system. These circumstances include:

Death of a loved one
Caring for a family member with a chronic, progressive disease
Change in lifestyle such as a divorce or beginning a new job
Summer vacation

These factors do not operate in isolation; instead they are interactive and combine in intensity to heighten the extent of any general adaptive response. As the body mounts this response, further compensations develop that then limit the ability to respond to additional potentially harmful stimuli.

General Adaptive Response

The word "stress" has been given many meanings specific to the type of causal factors such as cardiac stress, emotional stress, and mental stress, among others. This plethora of terms makes it difficult to present a generic definition for the word. For consistency in this chapter, we have used the phrase "general adaptive response" to indicate any event resulting in a change in homeostasis of the individual and aiming toward a state of compensated body function. The causal factors of the adaptive response are then called stressors.[1] The neuroendocrine-immune network, as described in this chapter, represents the device for detecting stressors, both external and internal, and the mechanism for orchestrating the adaptive response in the physiology and psychology of the body (Fig. 9.8). As this network of extracellular messenger molecules adapts to the stressor, it becomes increasingly compensated.

Detection of stressors can involve cognitive awareness, such as occurs with some nociceptive somatic or visceral stimuli and painful emotional circumstances. It can involve noncognitive warnings derived from detection of abnormal distortions in the distribution of antigens in the body, or antigenic map, as viewed through the immune system.[117] An important concept for osteopathic medicine is that the outward manifestations of a somatic dysfunction, namely hyperalgesia and inflammation,[3] represent stressors. Acting through the neuroendocrine-immune network, they can initiate the release of a plethora of neuroregulators, hormones, and immunoregulators into the extracellular fluids of the body, thereby altering homeostasis.

One of the primary events in initiating a response to stress is the activation of the hypothalamus either directly through its neural connections with the spinal cord and limbic forebrain or indirectly through its window on the extracellular fluids, the circumventricular organs of the third and fourth ventricles. In either case, neuroregulators and immunoregulators, initiated by stressors, activate adaptive limbic and hypothalamic neural circuits. Through these circuits significant alterations occur in autonomic nervous system function, and a common pathway is accessed into the endocrine system via the pituitary gland. There are changes in adrenal and thyroid gland output, mediated through the pituitary tropic hormones. When these changes are coupled to the increased activity in the sympathetic autonomic nervous system, they bring the organ systems of the body into metabolic preparation for defense of homeostasis. In analogy to the convergence of input onto spinal motoneurons before its relay to muscles, the hypothalamus and its connections have been referred to as representing the final common pathway in the adaptive response.

Suppression of the immune system represents part of the general adaptive mechanism to conserve energy for the immediate fight-or-flight response during conditions of acute stress. Studies show that many stressors ranging from chronic illness to the acute anxiety associated with medical school examinations leads to suppression of immune system function.[6,160] Importantly, immune system parameters continue to remain compensated in the face of chronic stressful stimuli.[6] Continued compromise of the immune system under conditions of chronic exposure to stressors lead to long-term imbalance in body homeostasis, and ultimately to illness. These changes induced by long-term stressful factors are the result of chronic modulation of the immune system by the endocrine and autonomic nervous systems.

Alteration in the output of the hypothalamic-pituitary-adrenal axis affects psychological as well as physiologic processes. For example, elevated blood cortisol levels represent a common feature of a cohort of individuals diagnosed with melancholic depression, a disease characterized by such disturbances in personality as[122]:

Increased anxiety
Vigilance
Obsessionalism
Hyperarousal
Aggressiveness
Feelings of worthlessness

Physiologic profiles of patients with melancholic depression reveal increased production of cortisol and norepinephrine and a breakdown in the regulation of these adaptive pathways with consequent immunosuppression. This disease represents a malfunction in the neural regulation of the hypothalamic-pituitary-adrenal axis, possibly involving the increased activity in the locus ceruleus.[122] Interestingly, the major depressions such as melancholia appear to develop through a kindling process similar to that which leads to seizure in the cerebral cortex. In this paradigm, episodes of melancholia occur at progressively shorter intervals and with progressively greater intensity in the natural history of the disease. To extrapolate from this observation, initial exposure to a stressor does not push the person's regulatory mechanisms irretrievably out of balance. However, repeated exposure to a given stressor or simultaneous exposure to multiple stressors can, in certain circumstances, contribute to a breakdown in the feedback control pathways leading to chronic dysregulation of the hypothalamic-pituitary-adrenal axis.[161]

A delicate feedback mechanism exists among the messenger molecules of the endocrine, immune, and nervous systems. One aspect of this feedback mechanism involves receptors for extracellular messengers, such as cortisol on neurons in the hypothalamus, and in portions of the brain capable of regulating neural activity in the hypothalamus, such as the hippocampal formation. Pyramidal cells in the CA1 region of the hippocampal formation, a specific portion of the hippocampus proper, project axons to the hypothalamus and contain receptors for adrenal cortical hormones. When activated by rising levels of blood cortisol, these neurons are capable of diminishing the output of CRF from neurons in the paraventricular nucleus of the hypothalamus.

Prolonged exposure to stress, especially unavoidable stress, manifests itself by disruption of this feedback control system. Chronic high levels of adrenal cortical hormones in the general circulation decrease the number of cortisol receptors as well as the number of pyramidal cells in a portion of the hippocampal formation (CA1 region). Inducing hypercortisolism in experimental paradigms potentiates these neurotoxic events, while adrenalectomy is protective of neuronal populations in the hippocampus exposed to certain neurotoxins.[162–163] These high levels of adrenal cortical hormones result in decreased suppression of the adaptive response via the hypothalamic-pituitary-adrenal axis; the once helpful adaptive response now becomes pathologic in nature. It is ironic that chronic exposure to unavoidable stress manifests in the destruction of the very feedback mechanisms designed to buffer the harmful effects of the adaptive response.

The initial response of the body to stressful factors is adaptive, allowing the patient to compensate for these conditions. However, under chronic exposure to stressful factors, the general adaptive response becomes pathologic, and the long-term suppression of immune function ultimately reduces the capacity of the body to resist additional attacks of infectious or noxious agents. The effects of somatic (and visceral) illness and psychological factors are cumulative. The addition of further stressful factors such as nascent infections or noxious agents, coupled with growing psychological concern with the illness, leads to a further suppression of immune function and a downward spiral of declining health as the patient slips further into dysregulation of compensatory mechanisms. Accordingly, the holistic treatment of the patient, with balanced attention to the psychological stress of illness as well as to its somatic and visceral components, can help to keep homeostatic mechanisms from becoming compromised to a greater extent than the effects from the causal disease process alone.

AGING AND NEUROENDOCRINE-IMMUNE SYSTEM

Aging of the organism has often been described in terms of altered functions in the neuroendocrine-immune network. As summarized above, the components of this network are tightly interactive; a breakdown in the mechanisms could represent a significant feature of the aging process.[164] Degeneration of any point in a network could initiate a progressive loss of function.

Any progressive disruption of homeostatic mechanisms results in a decrease in the ability of the body to compensate when exposed to stressful stimuli.

The hypothalamus is a key component in the control of the pituitary gland and consequently of the entire endocrine system. Major regressive changes in neuronal cytology and histochemistry occur in the aging hypothalamus. These changes involve cell degeneration and death and the loss of catecholamine-containing fibers.[164] Accompanying this cell death and the concomitant changes in neuronal circuitry is a decrease in the hypothalamic output of:

Gonadotropin-releasing factor
Growth hormone-releasing factor
Thyrotropin-releasing factor

This loss results in[164]:

Diminution in reproductive behavior
Decrease in protein synthesis and basal metabolic rate
Compromise of function in the immune system

The decline in immune functions can be directly related to the diminishing systemic levels of growth hormone and the thyroid hormones. A salient indicator of this decline in immune function is the well-known fatty involution of the thymic gland and the concomitant decrease of the circulating thymic hormone levels.[165] Each of these declining functions can be reversed by introducing the appropriate hypophysiotrophic factor, suggesting that a significant aspect of the aging process lies in failure of hypothalamic mechanisms and not in the pituitary or its target glands. Most notable is the recovery of histologic features in the thymus consequent to treatment with thyroid hormones. Since these same aging-related functional losses can be mimicked in young animals by prolonged blocking of the catecholamine pathways, it is also strongly suggested that disruption of these hypothalamic pathways plays a key role in the aging process (reviewed in Fabris[165]).

One possible origin for the age-related disruption of homeostatic mechanisms is the loss of specific forebrain mechanisms involved in the feedback control pathways for regulation of the adrenal cortical hormones in the hypothalamic-pituitary-adrenal axis. Cell death is a prominent feature in the normal ontogenic process of the vertebrate nervous system.[166] This event, responsive to both genetic programming and environmental cues, plays an integral role in shaping the morphology of the central and peripheral nervous systems.[167] Although cell death continues through adult life, the rate of cell death diminishes significantly after early development ceases. Recent studies have shown that the rate of this process can be accelerated by factors such as alcohol or other environmental toxins, as well as psychological factors such as stressful stimuli. Both an age-related and a stress-related loss of neurons in the hippocampal formation contributes to diminishing control of the hypothalamic-pituitary-adrenal axis. The altered control of the neural and endocrine systems could represent contributing factors for the overall decrease in functional properties of the immune system experienced in geriatric populations.[164] The significance of these observations lies in the progressive loss of stress management systems occurring in the elderly. The increased susceptibility to stressors in this population underscores the necessity on the part of the physician to identify and alter as many of the stress-related drives as possible on the homeostatic mechanism.

CONCLUSION

Traditionally, the immune and nervous systems were considered separate and independent, each with its own cell types, cell functions, and intercellular regulators. Altered function in each system also was related to diseases considered reasonably specific for that system. However, in the light of research done in the past 30 years, the illusion of independence of these systems has evaporated. We now recognize not only their interdependence and interlocking molecular organization but also their extensive integration with the endocrine system. The conceptual separations between the neuroendocrine-immune systems concerning structure, function, and communication have been discarded. In their stead is a combined multidimensional network contributing to the functional unity of the body (Fig. 9.2).

Today, we also recognize the multifactorial nature of practically all diseases as the result of interactions among the following components:

Genetic
Endocrine
Nervous
Immune
Behavioral-emotional

A relatively new field called psychoneuroimmunology[7] is concerned with the complex bidirectional interactions occurring in the neuroendocrine-immune network. This network forms the prime bulwark against disease and is responsible for resistance to infectious diseases and cancer. Sensory information from external and internal sources is tightly integrated with cognitive and emotional processes to influence the neuroendocrine-immune network through the hypothalamic-pituitary-adrenal axis. This chapter summarizes many of the pathways and mechanisms through which this integration is accomplished (Fig. 9.1).

The basis for communication in the neuroendocrine-immune system is the numerous messenger molecules that are released into the extracellular fluids. These messengers form the signal codes of the neuroendocrine-immune network:

Small peptides
Glycoproteins
Amines
Steroids

They express their activity through these mechanisms:

Autocrine
Paracrine
Synaptic
Hormonal

Receptors for these messengers are found on numerous cell types throughout the body. By monitoring the concentration of many of these extracellular messengers, the central nervous system, particularly the limbic system and hypothalamus, directly modulates the activity of the autonomic nervous system and the endocrine system. Both of these systems have extensive communication with the immune system, thereby bringing it under neural modulation as well. The combined action of this multidimensional network creates a compensatory reserve that enables the body to mount an adaptive response to stressful conditions regardless of their origin, whether somatic, visceral, or psychogenic.

Dysregulation of the neuroendocrine-immune network increases susceptibility to various disease states. Overproduction or underproduction of the extracellular messengers, in response to either external or internal stimuli or as a secondary response to another disease process, results in dysfunction of the many aspects of the network. For example, at the local tissue level, cellular damage and destruction can result when proinflammatory messengers are released into the central nervous system. At the systemic level, physiologic and psychological dysfunctions are expressed consequent to dysregulation of this network. The aging process also alters the regulation of this network and, as such, is associated in many instances with various disease states. The concept of a dysfunctional integrative network involving neural, endocrine, and immune components allows us to join together seemingly disparate disease presentations such as[168]:

Joint and artery pathology
Congenital anomalies
Autoimmune disorders
Cancers
Viral and bacterial infections
Cerebral dysfunctions (such as the dyslexias) as well as various psychiatric disorders

Somatic, visceral, and emotional stimuli act as the drivers capable of influencing activity in this axis (Fig. 9.8). Complex feedback loops, involving extracellular messengers, monitor the conditions in the peripheral tissue and adjust the output of the axis accordingly. This natural tendency toward recovery or reestablishing homeostasis, instituted by these control devices, can be altered by excessive driving stimuli or by dysfunction of the feedback circuits themselves. Abnormal regulation of the neuroendocrine-immune network results in a decrease in the compensatory reserve, rendering the body less tolerant of stressful stimuli. It is to the concept of body homeostasis described in this chapter that A.T. Still (1908)[169] spoke when he noted:

If this machine [the body] is self-propelling, self-sustaining, having all the machinery of strength, all the thrones of reason established, and all working to perfection, is it not reasonable to suppose that the amount of wisdom thus far shown in the complete forms and workings of the chemical department, the motor department, the nutritive [and] sensory [departments, and in] the compounding of the elements, provides the avenues and power to deliver these compounds to any part of the body, to make [in] the newly com- *pounded fluids, any change in the quality that is necessary for renovation and restoration to health.*

The osteopathic physician's role in this process is to assist the body in maintaining homeostasis by recognizing and modifying any or all of the driving stimuli (stressors).

ACKNOWLEDGMENT

The authors wish to thank Richard Van Buskirk, DO, PhD, for a helpful and constructive critical reading of this chapter.

REFERENCES

Note: A synthesis article of this scope covers a large range of material. The number of appropriate primary references is enormous. For this reason we have chosen to use mainly secondary (review) sources. The citations appearing in the body of the text do not necessarily represent the original source of the work but serve as a reference through which the reader can gain access to the primary literature.

1. Selye H. The general adaptive syndrome and the diseases of adaptation. *J Clin Endocrinol & Metab.* 1946;6:117–173.
2. Dubos R. *Man Adapting.* New Haven, Conn: Yale University Press; 1965.
3. Denslow JS. Pathophysiologic evidence for the osteopathic lesion: the known, unknown, and controversial. *JAOA.* 1975;74:415–421.
4. Stein M. Bereavement, depression, stress, and immunity. In: Guillemin R, Cohn M, Melnechuk T, eds. *Neural Modulation of Immunity.* New York, NY: Raven Press; 1985:29–44.
5. Kennedy S, Kiecolt-Glaser JK, Glaser R. Neuroimmunology of normal human behavior. In: Goetzl EJ, Spector NH, eds. *Neuroimmune Networks: Physiology and Diseases.* New York, NY: Alan R Liss Inc; 1989.
6. Kiecolt-Glaser JK, Glaser R. Stress and immune function in humans. In: Ader R, Felten DL, Cohen N, eds. *Psychoneuroimmunology.* 2nd ed. San Diego, Calif: Academic Press Inc; 1991:849–895.
7. Solomon GF. Psychoneuroimmunology: interactions between central nervous system and immune system. *J Neurosci Res.* 1987;18:1–9.
8. Merrill JE, Jonakait GM. Interactions of the nervous and immune systems in development, normal brain homeostasis, and disease. *Fed Am Soc Exp Biol J.* 1995;9:611–618.
9. Blalock JE. A molecular basis for bidirectional communication between the immune and neuroendocrine systems. *Physiol Rev.* 1989; 69:1–32.
10. Roszman TL, Brooks WH. Signal pathways of the neurotransmitter-immune network. In Freier S, ed. *The Neuroendocrine-Immune Network.* Boca Raton, Fla: CRC Press Inc; 1990:53–67.
11. Carr DJJ, Blalock JE. Neuropeptide hormones and receptors common to the immune and neuroendocrine systems: Bidirectional pathways of intersystem communication. In: Ader R, Felten DL, Cohen N, eds. *Psychoneuroimmunology.* San Diego, Calif: Academic Press Inc; 1991:573–558.
12. Weigent DA, Carr DJJ, Blalock JE. Bidirectional communication between the neuroendocrine and immune systems: common hormones and hormone receptors. *Ann NY Acad Sci.* 1990;579:17–27.

13. Bradford HF. *Chemical Neurobiology.* New York, NY: WH Freeman and Company; 1986.

14. Siegel GJ, Agranoff BW, Albers RW, Molinoff PB. *Basic Neurochemistry: Molecular, Cellular, and Medical Aspects.* New York, NY: Raven Press; 1989.

15. Cooper JR, Bloom FE, Roth RH. *The Biochemical Basis of Neuropharmacology: An Introduction to Molecular Neurobiology.* New York, NY: Oxford University Press; 1991.

16. Hall ZW. *An Introduction to Molecular Neurobiology.* Sunderland, Mass: Sinauer Associates Inc; 1992.

17. Hille B. *Ionic Channels of Excitable Membranes.* Sunderland, Mass: Sinauer Associates Inc; 1992.

18. Greenamyre JT, Porter RHP. Anatomy and physiology of glutamate in the CNS. *Neurology.* 1994;44(suppl 8):S7–S13.

19. Bunch ST, Fawcett JW. NMDA receptor blockade alters the topography of naturally occurring ganglion cell death in the rat retina. *Dev Biol.* 1993;160:434–442.

20. Davies SN, Lodge D. Evidence for involvement of N-methylaspartate receptors in "wind-up" of class 2 neurones in the dorsal horn of the rat. *Brain Res.* 1987;424:402–406.

21. Kashiwabuchi N, Ikeda K, Araki K, Hirano T, Shibuki K, Takayama C, Inoue Y, Kutsuwada T, Yagi T, Kang Y, Aizawa S, Mishina M. Impairment of motor coordination, Purkinje cell synapse formation, and cerebellar long-term depression in GluRγ2 mutant mice. *Cell.* 1995;81:245–252.

22. Brann DW. Glutamate: a major excitatory transmitter in neuroendocrine regulation. *Neuroendocrinology.* 1995;61:213–225.

23. Haydon PG, Drapeau P. From contact to connection: early events during synaptogenesis. *Trends Neurosci.* 1995;18:196–201.

24. Gasic GP, Hollman M. Molecular neurobiology of glutamate receptors. *Ann Rev Physiol.* 1992;54:507–536.

25. Petralia RS, Yokotani N, Wenthold RJ. Light and electron microscope distribution of the NMDA receptor subunit NMDAR1 in the rat nervous system using a selective anti-peptide antibody. *J Neurosci.* 1994;14:667–696.

26. Collingridge GL, Bliss TVP. Memories of NMDA receptors and LTP. *Trends Neurosci.* 1995;18:54–56.

27. Izquierdo I, Medina JH, Bianchin M, Walz R, Zanatta MS, Da Silva RC, Silva MBE, Ruschel AC, Paczko N. Memory processing by the limbic system: role of specific neurotransmitter systems. *Behav Brain Res.* 1993;58:91–98.

28. Dougherty PM, Palecek J, Paleckova V, Sorkin LS, Willis WD. The role of NMDA and non-NMDA excitatory amino acid receptors in the excitation of primate spinothalamic tract neurons by mechanical, chemical, thermal and electrical stimuli. *J Neurosci.* 1992;12:3025–3041.

29. Rothman SM, Olney JW. Excitotoxicity and the NMDA receptor—still lethal after eight years. *Trends Neurosci.* 1995;18:57–58.

30. Lu CZ, Fredrikson S, Xiao BG, Link H. Interleukin-2 secreting cells in multiple sclerosis and controls. *J Neurol Sci.* 1993;120:99–106.

31. Meinl E, Aloisi F, Ertl B, Weber F, De Waal Malefyt R, Wekerle H, Hohlfeld R. Multiple sclerosis: immunomodulatory effects of human astrocytes on T cells. *Brain.* 1994;117:1323–1332.

32. Madden KS, Felten DL. Experimental basis for neural-immune interactions. *Physiol Rev.* 1995;75:77–106.

33. Ross EM. Signal sorting and amplification through G-protein-coupled receptors. *Neuron.* 1989;3:141–152.

34. Payan DG, Levine JD, Goetzl EJ. Modulation of immunity and hypersensitivity by sensory neuropeptides. *J Immunol.* 1984; 132:1601–1604.

35. Lewis T. *The Blood Vessels of the Human Skin and Their Responses.* London, England: Shaw; 1927.

36. Pernow B. Substance P. *Pharmacol Rev.* 1983;35:85–141.

37. Payan DG. Substance P: a neuroendocrine-immune modulator. *Hosp Pract.* 1989;24(2):67–80.

38. Payan D. The role of neuropeptides in inflammation. In: Gallin JI, Goldstein IM, Snyderman R, eds. *Inflammation: Basic Principles and Clinical Correlations.* New York, NY: Raven Press; 1992.

39. Battaglia G, Rustioni A. Coexistence of glutamate and substance P in dorsal root ganglion neurons of the rat and monkey. *J Comp Neurol.* 1988;227:302–312.

40. Fisher ND, Baranauskas G, Nistri A. Multiple types of tachykinin receptor mediate a slow excitation of rat spinal motoneurones in vitro. *Neurosci Lett.* 1994;165:84–88.

41. Coderre TJ, Katz J, Vaccarina AL, Melzack R. Contribution of central neuroplasticity to pathological pain: review of clinical and experimental evidence. *Pain.* 1993;52:259–285.

42. Hopkins SJ, Rothwell NJ. Cytokines and the nervous system, I: expression and recognition. *Trends Neurosci.* 1995;18:83–88.

43. Rothwell NJ, Hopkins SJ. Cytokines and the nervous system, II: actions and mechanisms of action. *Trends Neurosci.* 1995;18:130–136.

44. Pober JS, Cotran RS. Cytokines and endothelial cell biology. *Physiol Rev.* 1990;70:427–451.

45. Le J, Vilcek J. Tumor necrosis factor and interleukin 1: cytokines with multiple overlapping biological activities. *Lab Invest.* 1987; 56:234–248.

46. Cunningham ET, Wada E, Carter DB, Tracey DE, Battey JF, De Souza EB. In situ histochemical localization of type I interleukin-1 receptor messenger RNA in the central nervous system, pituitary, and adrenal gland of the mouse. *J Neurosci.* 1992;12:1101–1114.

47. Dinarello CA, Wolff SM. The role of interleukin-1 in disease. *New Engl J Med.* 1993;328:106–113.

48. Breder CD, Dinarello CA, Saper CB. Interleukin-1 immunoreactive innervation of the human hypothalamus. *Science.* 1988; 240:321–323.

49. Lumpkin MD. The regulation of ACTH secretion by IL-1. *Science.* 1987;238:452–454.

50. Sundar SK, Cierpial MA, Kilts C, Ritchie JC, Weiss JM. Brain IL-1 induced immunosuppression occurs through activation of both pituitary-adrenal axis and sympathetic nervous system by corticotropin releasing factor. *J Neurosci.* 1990;10:3701–3706.

51. Dinarello CA. The biology of interleukin-1. *Res Staff Phys.* 1985; 31(7):25–29.

52. Dinarello CA. Role of interleukin-1 in infectious diseases. *Immunol Rev.* 1992;127:119–146.

53. Dantzer R, Bluthe RM, Kent S, Kelley KW. Cytokines and sickness behavior. In: Husband AJ, ed. *Psychoimmunology: CNS-Immune Interactions.* Boca Raton, Fla: CRC Press; 1993:1–16.

54. Waldmann TA. The structure, function, and expression of interleukin-2 receptors on normal and malignant lymphocytes. *Science.* 1986;232:727–732.

55. Kroemer G, Andreu JL, Gonzalo JA, Gutierrez-Ramos JC, Martinez AA. Interleukin-2, autotolerance, and autoimmunity. *Adv Immunol.* 1991;50:147–235.

56. Weigent DA, Blalock JE. Interactions between the neuroendocrine and immune systems: common hormones and receptors. *Immunol Rev.* 1987;100:79–108.

57. Plata-Salaman CR. Immunoregulators in the nervous system. *Neurosci Biobehav Rev.* 1991;15:185–215.

58. Van Snick J. Interleukin-6: an overview. *Ann Rev Immunol.* 1990; 8:253–278.

59. Cornfield LJ, Sills MA. High affinity interleukin-6 binding sites in bovine hypothalamus. *Eur J Pharmacol.* 1991;202:113–115.

60. Hirano T. Interleukin-6 and its relation to inflammation and disease. *Clin Immunol Immunopathol.* 1992;62:S60–S65.

61. Sakata Y, Morimoto A, Long NC, Murakami N. Fever and acute-phase response induced in rabbits by intravenous and intracerebroventricular injection of interleukin-6. *Cytokines.* 1991;3:199–203.

62. Heinrich PC, Castell JV, Andus T. Interleukin-6 and the acute phase response. *Biochem J.* 1990;265:51–66.

63. Houssiau F, Devogelaer JD, Van Damme J, de Deuxchaisnes CN, Van Snick J. Interleukin-6 in synovial fluid and serum of patients with rheumatoid arthritis and other inflammatory arthritides. *Arthritis Rheum.* 1988;31:784–788.

64. Vassalli P. The pathophysiology of tumor necrosis factors. *Ann Rev Immunol.* 1992;10:411–452.

65. Sherry B, Cerami A. Cachectin/tumor necrosis factor exerts endocrine, paracrine and autocrine control of inflammatory responses. *J Cell Biol.* 1988;107:1269–1277.

66. Borden EC. Interferons: pleiotropic cellular modulators. *Clin Immunol Immunopathol.* 1992;62:s18–s24.

67. Friedman RM. Interferons. In: Oppenheim JJ, Shevach EM, eds. *Immunophysiology: The Role of Cells and Cytokines in Immunity and Inflammation.* New York, NY: Oxford University Press; 1990:194–209.

68. Blalock JE, Harbour-McMenamin D, Smith ER. Peptide hormones shared by neuroendocrine and immunologic systems. *J Immunol.* 1985;135:858S–861S.

69. Shibata M, Blatteis CM. Differential effects of cytokines on thermosensitive neurons in guinea pig preoptic area slices. *Am J Physiol.* 1991;261:R1096–R1103.

70. Ahokas A, Rimon R, Koskiniemi M, Vaheri A, Julkunen I, Sarna S. Viral antibodies and interferon in acute psychiatric disorders. *J Clin Psychiatry.* 1987;48:194–196.

71. Frei K, Leist TP, Meager A, Gallo P, Leppert D, Zinkernagel RM, Fontana A. Production of B cell stimulatory factor-2 and interferon gamma in the central nervous system during viral meningitis and encephalitis. *J Exp Med.* 1988;168:449–453.

72. Chonmaitree T, Baron S. Bacteria and viruses induce production of interferon in the cerebrospinal fluid of children with acute meningitis: a study of 57 cases and review. *Rev Infect Dis.* 1991;13:1061–1065.

73. Griffin DE, Ward BJ, Jauregui E, Johnson RT, Vaisberg A. Immune activation during measles: interferon-gamma and neopterin in plasma and cerebrospinal fluid in complicated and uncomplicated disease. *J Infect Dis.* 1990;161:449–453.

74. Tyor WR, Glass JD, Griffin JW, Becker PS, McArthur JC, Bezman L, Griffin DE. Cytokine expression in the brain during the acquired immunodeficiency syndrome. *Ann Neurol.* 1992;31:349–360.

75. Griffin DE, McArthur JC, Cornblath DR. Neopterin and interferon-gamma in serum and cerebrospinal fluid of patients with HIV-associated neurologic disease. *Neurology.* 1991;41:69–74.

76. Shiozawa S, Kuroki Y, Kim M, Hirohata S, Ogino T. Interferon-alpha in lupus psychosis. *Arthritis Rheum.* 1992;35:417–422.

77. Traugott U, Lebon P. Multiple sclerosis: involvement of interferons in lesion pathogenesis. *Ann Neurol.* 1988;24:243–251.

78. Ganong W. The stress response—a dynamic overview. *Hosp Pract.* 1988;23(6):155–190.

79. Owens MJ, Nemeroff CB. Physiology and pharmacology of corticotrophin-releasing factor. *Pharmacol Rev.* 1991;43:425–473.

80. Navarra P, Tsagarakis S, Faria MS, Rees LH, Besser GM, Grossman AB. Interleukins-1 and -6 stimulate the release of corticotropin-releasing hormone-41 from rat hypothalamus in vitro via the eicosanoid cyclooxygenase pathway. *Endocrinology.* 1991;128:37–44.

81. Morgane PJ. Hypothalamic connections with brainstem, limbic and endocrine systems. In: Willard FH, Patterson MM, eds. *Nociception and the Neuroendocrine-Immune Connection.* Athena, Ohio: University Classics, Ltd; 1994:155–178.

82. Munck A, Guyre PM, Holbrook NJ. Physiological functions of glucocorticoids in stress and their relationship to pharmacological actions. *Endocr Rev.* 1984;5:25–44.

83. Millington G, Buckingham JC. Thymic peptides and neuroendocrine-immune communication. *J Endocrinol.* 1992;133:163–168.

84. Biziere K, Guillaumin JM, Degenne D, Bardos P, Renoux M, Renoux G. Lateralized neocortical modulation of the T-cell lineage. In: Guillemin R, Cohn M, Melnechuk T, eds. *Neural Modulation of Immunity.* New York, NY: Raven Press; 1985:73–79.

85. Brooks WH, Cross RJ, Roszman TL, Markesbery WR. Neuroimmunomodulation: neural anatomical basis for impairment and facilitation. *Ann Neurol.* 1982;12:56–61.

86. Felten DL, Felten SY, Bellinger DL, Carlson SL, Ackerman KD, Madden KS, Olschowki JA, Livnat S. Noradrenergic sympathetic neural interactions with the immune system: structure and function. *Immunol Rev.* 1987;100:225–260.

87. Ader R. Behaviorally conditioned modulation of immunity. In: Guillemin R, Cohn M, Melnechuk T, eds. *Neural Modulation of Immunity.* New York, NY: Raven Press; 1985:55–66.

88. Morgane P. Historical and modern concepts of hypothalamic organization and function. In: Morgane PJ, Panksepp J, eds. *Handbook of the Hypothalamus, Vol. 1: Anatomy of the Hypothalamus.* New York, NY: Marcel Dekker Inc; 1979:1–64.

89. Willard FH. *Medical Neuroanatomy.* Philadelphia, Penn: JB Lippincott; 1993.

90. Nauta WJH. Hippocampal projections and related neural pathways to the midbrain in the cat. *Brain.* 1958;81:319–340.

91. Palkovits M. Anatomy of neural pathways affecting CRH secretion. *Ann NY Acad Sci.* 1987;512:139–147.

92. Hosoya Y, Sugiura Y, Ito R, Kohno K. Descending projections from the hypothalamic paraventricular nucleus to the A5 area, including the superior salivatory nucleus in the rat. *Exp Brain Res.* 1990;82:513–518.

93. Hosoya Y, Sugiura Y, Okado N, Loewy AD, Kohno K. Descending input from the hypothalamic paraventricular nucleus to sympathetic preganglionic neurons in the rat. *Exp Brain Res.* 1991;85:10–20.

94. Engler D, Chad D, Jackson IMD. Thyrotropin-releasing hormone in the pancreas and brain of the rat is regulated by central noradrenergic and dopaminergic pathways. *J Clin Invest.* 1982;69:1310–1320.

95. Calogero AE, Gallucci WT, Chrousos GP, Gold PW. Catecholamine effects upon rat hypothalamic corticotropin-releasing hormone secretion in vitro. *J Clin Invest.* 1988;82:839–846.

96. Aston-Jones G, Foote S, Bloom FE. Anatomy and physiology of locus coeruleus neurons: Functional implications. In: Ziegler MG, Lake CR, eds. *Norepinephrine.* Baltimore, Md: Williams & Wilkins; 1984:92–116.

97. Ericsson A, Kovács KJ, Sawchenko PE. A functional anatomical analysis of central pathways subserving the effects of interleukin-1 on stress-related neuroendocrine neurons. *J Neurosci.* 1994;14:897–913.

98. Saphier D, Ovadia H, Abramsky O. Neural responses to antigenic challenges and immunomodulatory factors. *Yale J Biol Med.* 1990;63:109–119.

99. Berkenbosch F, van Oers J, del Rey A, Tilders F, Besedovsky HO.

Corticotropin-releasing factor producing neurons in the rat activated by interleukin-1. *Science.* 1987;238:524–528.

100. Besedovsky HO, del Rey A, Sorkin E, Dinarello CA. Immunoregulatory feedback between interleukin-1 and glucocorticoids hormone. *Science.* 1986;233:652–654.

101. Dinarello CA. The endogenous pyrogens in host-defense interactions. *Hosp Pract.* 1989;24(11):111–128.

102. Nauta WJH, Domesick VB. Ramifications of the limbic system. In: Matthyse S, ed. *Psychiatry and the Biology of the Human Brain.* Amsterdam, Holland: Elsevier; 1981;165–188.

103. Ader R, Felten D, Cohen N. Interactions between the brain and the immune system. *Annu Rev Pharmacol Toxicol.* 1990;30:561–602.

104. McEwen BS, De Kloet ER, Rostene W. Adrenal steroid receptors and actions in the nervous system. *Physiol Rev.* 1986;66:1121–1188.

105. McEwen BS. Glucocorticoid receptors in the brain. *Hosp Pract.* 1988;23(8):107–121.

106. Bulloch K. Neuroanatomy of lymphoid tissue: A review. In: Guillemin R, Cohn M, Melnechuk T, eds. *Neural Modulation of Immunity.* New York, NY: Raven Press; 1985:111–141.

107. Weihe E, Nohr D, Michel S, Muller S, Zentel HJ, Fink T, Krekel J. Molecular anatomy of the neuro-immune connection. *Intern J Neurosci.* 1991;59:1–23.

108. Felten SY, Felten DL. Innervation of lymphoid tissue. In: Ader R, Felten DL, Cohen N, eds. *Psychoneuroimmunology.* 2nd ed. San Diego, Calif: Academic Press; 1991:27–69.

109. Ackerman KD, Bellinger DL, Felten SY, Felten DL: Ontogeny and senescence of noradrenergic innervation of the rodent thymus and spleen. In: Ader R, Felten DL, Cohen N, eds. *Psychoneuroimmunology.* 2nd ed. San Diego, Calif: Academic Press; 1991:71–125.

110. Madden K, Ackerman KD, Livnat S, Felten S, Felten DL. Patterns of noradrenergic innervation of lymphoid organs and immunological consequences of denervation. In: Goetzl EJ, Spector NH, eds. *Neuroimmune Networks: Physiology and Diseases.* New York, NY: Alan R Liss; 1989:1–8.

111. Adair TH, Guyton AC. Introduction to lymphatic system. In: Johnston MG, ed. *Experimental Biology of Lymphatic Circulation.* Amsterdam, Holland: Elsevier; 1985:1–44.

112. McHale NG. Innervation of the lymphatic circulation. In: Johnston MG, ed. *Experimental Biology of the Lymphatic Circulation.* Amsterdam, Holland: Elsevier; 1985:121–140.

113. McHale NG. Lymphatic innervation. *Blood Vessels.* 1990;27:127–136.

114. Felten DL, Livnat S, Felten SY, Carlson SL, Lorton D, Bellinger DL, Yeh P. Sympathetic innervation of lymph nodes in mice. *Brain Res Bull.* 1984;13:693–699.

115. Giron LT, Crutcher K, Davis JN. Lymph nodes—a possible site for sympathetic neuronal regulation of immune responses. *Ann Neurol.* 1980;8:520–525.

116. Magni F, Bruschi F, Kasti M. The afferent innervation of the thymus gland in the cat. *Brain Res.* 1987;424:379–385.

117. Besedovsky HO, del Rey A. Immune-neuroendocrine circuits: integrative role of cytokines. *Front Neuroendocrinol.* 1992;13:61–94.

118. Donnerer J, Eglezos A, Helme RD. Neuroendocrine and immune function in the capsaicin-treated rat: Evidence for afferent neural modulation *in vivo.* In Freier S, ed. *The Neuroendocrine-Immune Network.* Boca Raton, Fla: CRC Press Inc; 1990:69–83.

119. Chrousos GP. The hypothalamic-pituitary-adrenal axis and immune-mediated inflammation. *N Engl J Med.* 1995;332:1351–1362.

120. Munck A, Guyre PM. Glucocorticoids and immune function. In: Ader R, Felten DL, Cohen N, eds. *Psychneuroimmunology.* 2nd ed. San Diego, Calif: Academic Press; 1991:447–474.

121. Stein C. Peripheral mechanisms of opioid analgesia. *Anesth Analg.* 1993;76:182–191.

122. Gold PW, Pigott TA, Kling MA, Kalogeras K, Chrousos GP. Basic and clinical studies with corticotropin-releasing hormone. *Psychol Clin North Am.* 1988;11:327–334.

123. Demitrack MA, Dale JK, Straus SE, Laue L, Listwak SJ, Kruesi MJP, Chrousos GP, Gold PW. Evidence for impaired activation of the hypothalamic-pituitary-adrenal axis in patients with chronic fatigue syndrome. *J Clin Endocrinol Metab.* 1991;73:1224–1234.

124. Lemieux AM, Coe CL. Abuse-related postraumatic stress disorder: evidence for chronic neuroendocrine activation in women. *Psychosom Med.* 1995;57:105–115.

125. Martin JB, Reichlin S. *Clinical Neuroendocrinology.* Philadelphia, Penn: FA Davis; 1987.

126. Maayan ML, Volpert EM, Debons AF. Neurotransmitter regulation of thyroid activity. *Endocr Res.* 1987;13:199–212.

127. Blalock JE. The immune system as a sensory organ. *J Immunol.* 1984;132:1067–1070.

128. Kruger TE, Smith LR, Harbour DV, Blalock JE. Thyrotropin: an endogenous regulator of the in vitro immune response. *J Immunol.* 1989;142:744–747.

129. Krueger E, Krueger GRF. How does the subjective experience of stress relate to the breakdown of the human immune system. *In Vivo.* 1991;5:207–216.

130. Stanisz AM, Scicchitano R, Payan DG, Bienenstock J. In vitro studies of immunoregulation by substance P and somatostatin. *Ann NY Acad Sci.* 1987;496:217–225.

131. Pawlikowski M, Stepien H, Kunert-Radek J, Zelazowski P, Schally AV. Immunomodulatory action of somatostatin. *Ann NY Acad Sci.* 1987;496:233–239.

132. Bernton EW, Bryant HU, Holaday JW. Prolactin and immune function. In: Ader R, Felten DL, Cohen N, eds. *Psychoneuroimmunology.* 2nd ed. San Diego, Calif: Academic Press; 1991:403–428.

133. Khansari D, Murgo AJ, Faith RE. Effects of stress on the immune system. *Immunol Today.* 1990;11:170–175.

134. Khachaturian H, Lewis ME, Schäfer MKH, Watson SJ. Anatomy of the CNS opioid systems. *Trends Neurosci.* 1985;8:111–119.

135. Basbaum AI, Fields HL. Endogenous pain control mechanisms: review and hypothesis. *Ann Neurol.* 1978;4:451–462.

136. Stein C, Gramsch C, Herz A. Intrinsic mechanisms of antinociception in inflammation: local opioid receptors and β-endorphin. *J Neurosci.* 1990a;10:1292–1298.

137. Stein C, Hassan AHS, Przewlocki R, Gramsch C, Peter K, Herz A. Opioids from immunocytes interact with receptors on sensory nerves to inhibit nociception in inflammation. *Proc Natl Acad Sci.* 1990b;87:5935–5939.

138. Stein C, Comisal K, Haimerl E, Yassouridis A, Lehrberger K, Herz A, Peter K. Analgesic effect of intraarticular morphine after arthroscopic knee surgery. *New Engl J Med.* 1991;325:1123–1126.

139. Heijnen CJ, Kavelaars A, Ballieux RE. β-Endorphin: cytokine and neuropeptide. *Immunol Rev.* 1991;119:41–63.

140. Teschemacher H, Koch G, Scheffler H, Hildebrand A, Brantl V. Opioid peptined: immunological significance. *Ann NY Acad Sci.* 1990;94:66–77.

141. Maestroni GJM, Conti A. Role of the pineal neurohormone melatonin in the psycho-neuroendocrine-immune network. In Ader R,

Felten DL, Cohen N, eds. *Psychoneuroimmunology*. 2nd ed. San Diego, Calif: Academic Press; 1991:495–513.

142. Mense S. Nociception from skeletal muscle in relation to clinical muscle pain. *Pain*. 1993;54:241–289.

143. Sato A. The reflex effects of spinal somatic nerve stimulation on visceral function. *J Manipulative Physiol Ther*. 1992;15:57–61.

144. Schaible H-G, Grubb BD. Afferent and spinal mechanisms of joint pain. *Pain*. 1993;55:5–54.

145. Prechtl JC, Powley TL. B-afferents: a fundamental division of the nervous system mediating homeostasis? *Behav Brain Sci*. 1990; 13:289–331.

146. He X, Proske U, Schaible H-G, Schmidt RF. Acute inflammation of the knee joint in the cat alters responses of flexor motoneurons to leg movements. *J Neurophysiol*. 1988;59:326–340.

147. Bonica JJ. Neurophysiologic and pathologic aspects of acute and chronic pain. *Arch Surg*. 1977;112:750–761.

148. Willard FH. Neuroendocrine-immune network, nociceptive stress, and the general adaptive response. In: Everett T, Dennis M, Ricketts E, eds. *Physiotherapy in Mental Health: A Practical Approach*. Oxford, Boston: Butterworth/Heinemann; 1995:102–126.

149. Willard FH. Nociception and the neuroendocrine immune network. Phoenix, Ariz: Presented at the American Academy of Osteopathy Convocation; 1989.

150. VanBuskirk RL. Nociceptive reflexes and the somatic dysfunction: a model. *JAOA*. 1990;90:792–809.

151. Cervero F. Neurophysiology of gastrointestinal pain. *Bailliere's Clin Gastroenterol*. 1988;2:183–199.

152. Selzer M, Spencer WA. Convergence of visceral and cutaneous afferent pathways in the lumbar spinal cord. *Brain Res*. 1969a; 14:331–348.

153. Selzer M, Spencer WA. Interactions between visceral and cutaneous afferents in the spinal cord: reciprocal primary afferent fiber depolarization. *Brain Res*. 1969b;14:349–366.

154. Sugiura Y, Terui N, Hosoya Y. Difference in distribution of central terminals between visceral and somatic unmyelinated (C) primary afferent fibers. *J Neurophysiol*. 1989;62:834–840.

155. Person RJ. Somatic and vagal afferent convergence on solitary tract neurons in cat: electrophysiological characteristics. *Neuroscience*. 1989;30:283–295.

156. Cervero F, Tattersall JEH. Somatic and visceral sensory integration in the thoracic spinal cord. *Prog Brain Res*. 1986;67:189–204.

157. McLeod JG. The representation of the splanchnic afferent pathways in the thalamus of the cat. *J Physiol*. 1958;140:462–478.

158. Willis WD. Visceral inputs to sensory pathways in the spinal cord. *Prog Brain Res*. 1986;67:207–225.

159. Shirasaka C, Tsuji H, Asoh T, Takeuchi Y. Role of the splanchnic nerves in the endocrine and metabolic response to abdominal surgery. *Br J Surg*. 1986;73:142–145.

160. Ader R, Cohen N. The influence of conditioning on immune responses. In: Adar R, Felten DL, Cohen N, eds. *Psychoneuroimmunology*. 2nd ed. New York, NY: Academic Press, Inc; 1991:611–646.

161. Johnson EO, Kamilaris TC, Chorusos GP, Gold PW. Mechanisms of stress: a dynamic overview of hormonal and behavioral homeostasis. *Neurosci Biobehav Rev*. 1992;16:115–130.

162. Sapolsky RM. A mechanism for glucocorticoid toxicity in the hippocampus: increased neuronal vulnerability to metabolic insults. *J Neurosci*. 1985;5:1228–1232.

163. Sapolsky RM, Uno H, Rebert CS, Finch CE. Hippocampal damage associated with prolonged glucocorticoid exposure in primates. *J Neurosci*. 1990;10:2897–2902.

164. Meites J. Aging: hypothalamic catecholamines, neuroendocrine-immune interactions, and dietary restriction. *Proc Soc Exp Biol Med*. 1990;195:304–311.

165. Fabris N. Immune system and aging: neuroimmunological implications. *Int J Immunol Pharmacol*. 1992;5:93–102.

166. Purves D, Lichtman JW. *Principles of Neural Development*. Sunderland, Mass: Sinauer Associates Inc; 1985:433.

167. Steward O. *Principles of Cellular, Molecular, and Developmental Neuroscience*. New York, NY: Springer-Verlag; 1989.

168. Behan PO, Geschwind N. Hemispheric laterality and immunity. In Guillemin R, Cohn M, Melnechuk T, eds. *Neural Modulation of Immunity*. New York, NY: Raven Press; 1985:73–79.

169. Still AT. *Autobiography of Andrew T. Still*. Kirksville, Mo; 1908.

10. Neurophysiologic System: Integration and Disintegration

MICHAEL M. PATTERSON AND ROBERT D. WURSTER

"The human body is a machine run by the unseen force called life, and that it may be run harmoniously it is necessary that there be liberty of blood, nerves, and arteries from the generating point to destination."[1]

Key Concepts

- **Reflex and the interactions affecting reflex activity**

- **Types of reflex interactions and the importance of reflexes in body function**

- **Neural basis of reflex interaction and integration and how reflex integration is exhibited in cardiac control**

- **How spinal and higher nervous areas interact in reflex control**

- **Concept of the "facilitated area" or "segment" of the spinal cord and how it affects function**

- **Effects of nociception on peripheral tissues and how nerve fibers transmit materials to and from peripheral structures**

- **Central excitation changes and four stages of alteration of spinal neuron excitability**

- **What causes the changes of spinal neuron excitability and the time course of each**

- **Importance of trophic factors for normal function**

- **The implications of alterations in neural integrative function for health**

- **Importance of manipulative treatment in maintaining optimal function and health**

The foundations of the osteopathic profession laid by its founder, A.T. Still, recognize that the state of health is a continuum from complete breakdown to perfect function. One of Still's basic beliefs about function was that the body was a totally integrated unit, its structures working together harmoniously to produce a state of health. Lacking that harmonious function, the body produced conditions promoting loss of health, or disease. Implicit in these assumptions is the idea that the various parts of the body are functionally interconnected, allowing for necessary adaptations when demands on the body change. This view necessitates that the supply and maintenance organs, mainly the visceral structures, be functionally connected with the primary energy consumer of the body, the musculoskeletal system. This interrelationship has long been neglected in medical practice. The communicating systems of the body, including the immune, endocrine, and neural systems, provide this interconnectedness. When a problem develops in the integrating systems of the body, function cannot help but be compromised, and the stage is set for a lowered state of health, and eventually disease, to occur.

The field of neurophysiology is important to the physician. A thorough knowledge of anatomy and the structural relationships within the body are vital. The physician must also know how these structures function and relate to each other. He or she needs a basis for providing the patient with a rational course of treatment, especially manipulative treatment. The physician must be aware of what palpatory diagnosis is telling him or her about the underlying state of the body, and therefore of the person. Many excellent neurophysiology texts are available that lay out the basics of the field.

This chapter does not attempt to give an overview of the entire field or all the areas of special interest to the osteopathic physician. It focuses on the integration of somatic and visceral function through the reflex pathways and relates these interactions to their specific neural basis. Functional alterations in reflex pathways that can disrupt integration are reviewed, along with the non–impulse-based or trophic function of the nervous system, and how this provides a means of two-way communication within the body not dependent on the better understood neural impulse-based communication. These aspects of the integrative activity of the nervous system are important in the osteopathic clinical experience and the role of manipulative treatment in health care. As Still recognized before the turn of the century, proper function necessitates the free interaction and integration of all body systems. Rational treatment of functional problems likewise requires an understanding of how these interactions occur and what can alter their function.

THE REFLEX

In 1906, Charles Sherrington published *The Integrative Action of the Nervous System.*[2] This classic text represented current knowledge about the fundamental aspects of how the nervous system handled and integrated information. Over the ensuing years, considerably more has been learned about the function of the nervous system and how it integrates the many functions of the body. A great deal is known about how the basic structural unit of the nervous system, the neuron, interacts with other cells through synaptic structures and release of neurotransmitters and neuromodulators. The billions of neurons and glial cells that make up the nervous system are organized into functional groups, often with widely differing structural and functional characteristics. Many of the neurons are involved in networks that respond to stimuli impinging on or even originating in the body. This results in commands to muscles and glands that produce activity or secretions. These networks, the reflexes, have been more fully analyzed in recent years. What were previously considered to be almost autonomous units of function are actually complex and interactive aspects of an organizational whole. The reflex has been found to be anything but a static unit of input–output relationships, but rather an active and ever-changing mosaic. The characteristics of reflex function are modulated by messages from other areas of the nervous system and by activity of the endocrine and immune systems.

Structure

The common concept of the reflex is basically one of a relationship between an input stimulus to the body and an output action to either a muscle or a secretory organ. Sherrington viewed the reflex as an input–output relationship between information coming into the body and a response to that information. He viewed a reflex as *"always inherited and innately given."*[2] The concept of a reflex includes an afferent or incoming limb from a sensory receptor, a central component in the spinal cord or brain. It also includes an output (efferent) limb that is usually a motor component to either somatic (musculoskeletal) or visceral structures terminating in synaptic connections that may either activate or inhibit activity in these structures (Fig. 10.1).

The usual concept of the reflex suggests that the reflex limbs are fairly well defined and limited primarily to one input and one output channel, with little interaction with other reflex networks (Figs. 10.2 and 10.3). Almost all reflex networks can be influenced by a wide variety of other excitatory and inhibitory signals, including those coming from higher or lower levels of the central nervous system. The picture of a reflex as a simple message pathway from the patellar tendon that causes the quadriceps femoris muscle to contract, resulting in a knee jerk, is a vast oversimplification of the interactions that occur

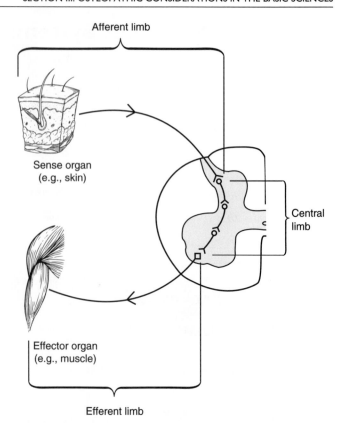

Figure 10.1. Schematic of "reflex" as it is usually envisioned, with afferent, central, and efferent limbs.

when a stimulus causes a response. The tendon tap reflex, exemplified by the patellar tap–knee jerk reflex activation, is, however, a prime example of the simplest reflex structure.

The tendon tap, or myotatic reflex, is a monosynaptic reflex. It is the only monosynaptic reflex present in the human. The stimulus of a tap to a tendon stretches the muscle attached to the tendon, which in turn stretches the muscle spindle organs in the muscle. Neural signals, or action potentials, are sent from the spindle organs to the spinal cord on the incoming, or afferent, limb of the reflex. In this case, the signals travel through the spinal cord on the axons from the spindles directly to the motoneurons that innervate the muscle that was stretched. They make synaptic contact with the motoneurons, causing the motoneurons to generate action potentials that travel over the efferent, or outgoing, limb of the reflex network back to the muscle, causing it to contract.

If this were all that happened, it would be a simple picture. However, the incoming axons send off branches that go to other neurons in the spinal cord that in turn send axons to the motoneurons of the antagonist of the stretched muscle. These axons provide signals that inhibit the motoneurons innervating the antagonist muscle. When the stretched muscle contracts, the antagonist muscle is inhibited, allowing a smooth movement to occur. In addition, other branches from the incoming axons go up the spinal cord to other spinal areas (for example, to the arms, if the patellar reflex was stimulated), and to the brainstem, as well as down the spinal cord to lower spinal cen-

Dorsal

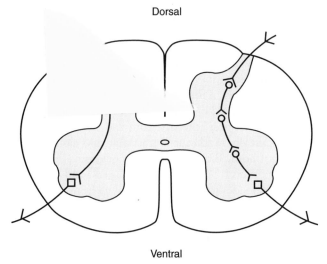

Ventral

Figure 10.2. A common, mistaken concept of how a reflex is constructed. Afferent limb simply connects with central limb, which activates efferent limb. *Left*, monosynaptic reflex; *right*, polysynaptic reflex. Actual complexity is better represented in Figure 10.3.

Dorsal

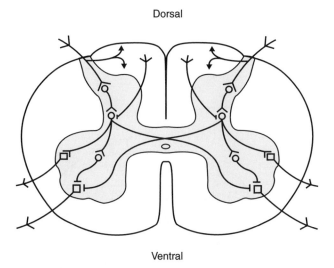

Ventral

Figure 10.3. Schematic of neural interactions at spinal level, indicating complexity of even simple "reflexes." An input to the spinal cord sends collaterals up and down cord and is acted upon by ascending and descending influences, as well as inputs from opposite side of cord. Input courses through several synapses and interneurons before acting (in thoracolumbar cord) on both somatic and sympathetic motoneurons. In cervical and sacral cord areas, parasympathetic pathways are involved.

ters. What appeared to be a simple reflex network has become a complex set of pathways within the spinal cord and brainstem. In addition, pathways from both above and below the level of the input axons can directly influence the basic excitability of the motoneurons involved and hence alter the reflex activity observed when the tendon is tapped. Indeed, when elicited clinically, the tendon tap reflex is used as a porthole into the nervous system to see how it is functioning, and the

clinician is not usually interested in that reflex per se. In fact, the main purpose of using the tendon tap reflex clinically is to test the excitability of the motoneurons, as a function of both local and distant influences.

SOMATO-SOMATIC

While the tendon tap reflex is used a great deal clinically, the most familiar of the spinal reflexes are the defensive reflexes, such as the withdrawal movements of a limb to a noxious stimulus. These somato-somatic reflexes occur when some stimulus is applied to a somatic structure. This initiates a volley of neural activity (often nociceptive) through the afferent limb of the reflex into the spinal cord. The afferent input activity flows through synapses into the interneurons of the spinal cord central gray, and finally into the ventral horn motoneurons. These motoneurons then cause somatic muscle contraction. The reflexes have at least one interneuron interposed between the sensory input in the dorsal horn of the cord and the motoneurons of the ventral horn (Fig. 10.3). They are named from the origin of the information and the locus of action, both somatic.

Many somato-somatic reflexes have been documented and studied. The simple somato-somatic reflexes are exemplified by defensive withdrawal actions such as when a person touches a hot object accidentally, and the arm jerks back. There are also very complex activities, such as the righting reflexes that occur, for example, when a cat is dropped upside down and lands on its feet. Even these reflexes do not occur in isolation but are accompanied by a spread of activity throughout the nervous system, just as are the myotatic reflexes.

VISCERO-VISCERAL

A second type of reflex is the viscero-visceral reflex, in which sensory inputs from a visceral structure cause activity in a visceral organ. These reflexes are involved, for example, in distention of the gut, that results in increased contraction of the gut muscle. Viscero-visceral reflexes involve afferent activity flowing from the receptors into the spinal cord, through interneurons, to produce efferent or outflow activity within the sympathetic and/or parasympathetic motoneurons.

REFLEX INTERACTIONS

We might expect to find that afferent inputs from somatic structures have some influence on visceral organs and that inputs from visceral structures have some effect on somatic organs. Somato-visceral and viscero-somatic reflexes have been known for many years but until recently have received little attention from the research and medical community. However, these types of reflex interactions are very important for the practice and understanding of osteopathic palpatory diagnosis and treatment, and for the integration of body function.

A familiar example of a viscero-somatic reflex is of a person feeling a pain and experiencing muscle tightness in the left shoulder with onset of a myocardial infarction (MI). The nociceptive inputs from the compromised myocardium (a visceral structure) are exciting not only the pathways that are interpreted as pain of the shoulder (a somatic structure), but are causing the motoneurons supplying the shoulder muscles to become active. In a classic study, Eble[3] showed several such reflexes by stimulating visceral structures and recording somatic muscle activity. He demonstrated that stimulation of various visceral structures would produce somatic muscle activity.

Conversely, activity in a somatic structure can alter visceral function. In a number of studies over the past several years, Sato[4] has demonstrated clearly the effect of somatic stimulation on various visceral functions, ranging from heart rate to adrenal output. These studies have also shown that some of these reflex interactions occur directly in the spinal cord. With others, the afferent activity from the somatic stimulation travels up the spinal cord to the brainstem, resulting in a cascade of activity from the brainstem back down to the spinal autonomic motoneurons.

In both viscero-somatic and somato-visceral reflex networks, the activity resulting from the stimulation of a structure can be either an excitatory or inhibitory influence on the motoneurons involved. For example, stimulation of the belly skin usually results in inhibition of gut activity (a somato-visceral reflex), but increased heart rate.

In an individual's daily life, the body's somatic system is active. The skeletal muscles are the machines that carry out the activities of the individual. The visceral organs are the means by which the energy demands and maintenance of the muscles are met and waste is disposed of. Without a continuous and highly integrated communication between these two systems, the body could not continue to achieve a balance among:

Its energy needs and supply
The amount of blood necessary to carry nutrients and waste and the demands of the muscles and bones
Supply and demand in general

The neural connections represented by these reflex systems is one of the primary ways this integration is carried out.

For the osteopathic physician, the viscero-somatic and somato-visceral reflexes are of extreme importance. When using palpatory diagnosis to detect subtle problems in function, whether it be tissue texture changes, motion characteristics, or temperature variations of the body, the physician is sensing clues from the musculoskeletal system—the skin, muscles, and fascias. These clues reflect not only aspects of these tissues but also functional characteristics of the underlying visceral organs and tissues through the viscero-somatic reflex networks. When the physician uses manipulative treatment to correct somatic dysfunctions, underlying visceral function is affected through the somato-visceral reflex networks. Thus, for both palpation and treatment, an understanding of reflex function is necessary.

Neural Basis for Reflex Interactions

Evidence is accumulating about the neural basis of viscerosomatic and somato-visceral interactions. When a stimulus is applied, afferent inputs from either visceral or somatic structures flow into the spinal cord along the dorsal roots and enter the upper areas of the spinal gray matter. The spinal gray is commonly divided into ten layers, first documented on cytoarchitectural evidence by Rexed (Fig. 10.4).[5] Large-diameter cutaneous afferent inputs that signal nonnociceptive stimuli enter the spinal gray of the dorsal horn and terminate primarily in layers III and IV. Nociceptive afferents from both somatic and visceral structures enter the cord and send branches rostrally and caudally in Lissauer's tract that runs along the apex of the dorsal horn. Branches of these nociceptive inputs then terminate in layers I, II, V, VII, and X. Layers I and V especially display a tremendous overlap of the inputs from somatic and visceral nociceptors.[6]

It now appears that in most areas of the spinal cord practically every interneuron that receives inputs from a visceral nociceptor also receives inputs from a somatic source. It also appears that almost 80% of interneurons that receive inputs from somatic structures also receive visceral inputs. There is at present no evidence for any ascending pathway that transmits only visceral sensory signals from the spinal cord to the brain. This raises the question of how an individual can distinguish visceral from somatic pain or sensation at all. In many cases, visceral pain is felt as a diffuse and poorly localized sensation and is referred to somatic structures. The overlap of somatic and visceral inputs explains the referral of visceral pain to somatic structures that is designated as "referred pain."

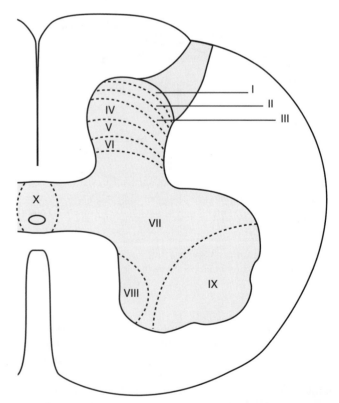

Figure 10.4. Rexed layers. Laminae at L-7 segment of cat spinal cord. (After Rexed B. The cytoarchitectonic organization of the spinal cord in the cat. *J Comp Neurol.* 1952;96:415–495.)

Impulses arriving from visceral structures and converging onto interneurons also receiving somatic afferents activate ascending pathways to the brain that result in the perception of pain in the somatic structure. In addition, there are many more somatic inputs than visceral, since the viscera are much more sparsely innervated with sensory receptors. This suggests that the visceral inputs have much more diffuse functional effects than do the corresponding somatic afferents. For example, it appears that many of the somatic C fiber inputs terminate primarily in focal areas of layer II of the cord. Visceral C fibers extend for several segments and give off collaterals at regular intervals. Only about 10% of the inflow into the thoracolumbar spinal cord comes from visceral structures.[7] This sparse innervation but wide distribution of visceral afferents may be the basis for the diffuse nature of most visceral pain. The evidence indicates that the widespread effects of visceral inputs are due more to functional (spread of activity through networks) than anatomical (many collateral branches) divergence.[8] Figure 10.5 shows the afferent terminations of somatic and visceral afferents in the various levels of the spinal cord.

The overlap of inputs onto common interneurons within the gray matter of the spinal cord is also the basis for the activation of somatic muscle activity seen with visceral disturbances. The excitatory drive provided onto common interneurons by visceral inputs activates not only sympathetic outflows back to visceral structures, but also motoneurons (both alpha and gamma) that innervate skeletal musculature. The result is a tonic activation of skeletal muscles in the referral area of visceral inputs. This is the viscero-somatic reflex manifestation, or "splinting," that is often seen, for example, in appendicitis.

These relationships also underlie the reverse phenomenon, that of the somato-visceral reflex, in which somatic inputs alter sympathetic and parasympathetic outflows. The data on the convergence of somatic and visceral inputs are beginning to explain the interrelations between visceral and somatic structures, especially when nociceptive inputs are activated.

There are descending influences on the activity of both somatic and visceral reflex pathways. In many of the reflex loops driven by both visceral and somatic inputs, there is a strong effect of descending pathways on the long-lasting excitability of the reflex outflows. These descending influences can maintain the excitability of the reflex for extended periods. They may account for some of the long-term increases in sensitivity, muscle contractions, and hyperexcitable sympathetic outputs seen especially with visceral disturbances. Likewise, the long-lasting descending influences can be inhibitory, resulting in lowered somatic or autonomic outflows. For example, the effects of rib-raising techniques (a somatic stimulation) on sympathetic outflows seem to be primarily inhibitory, resulting in decreased vasoconstriction and better fluid flow in the thoracic area.[9]

CARDIAC CONTROL

Neural input from somatic structures may affect neural activity to both somatic and visceral structures. A good example of this

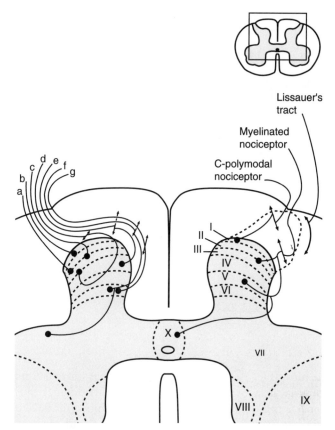

Figure 10.5. Terminal patterns of primary afferent collaterals in transverse plane of spinal cord. *Left*, primary afferent terminations of axons not associated with nociception. *a*, C-low threshold mechanoreceptor; *b*, innocuous cooling receptor; *c*, Aδ hair afferent; *d*, G-1 and G-2 hair receptors; *e*, slowly adapting type I and II afferents; *f*, primary and secondary muscle spindle afferents; *g*, Golgi tendon organ. *Arrow* indicates that parent axon bifurcates and ascends and descends spinal cord for 1–7 segments and gives off collaterals along this course. *Right*, nociceptor afferents from both somatic and visceral structures. Both visceral and somatic Aδ and c fiber nociceptor afferents terminate in Rexed lamina I, II, V, and to some extent in VII and X. Lamina are indicated on *right* and outlined by *dotted lines*. (From Light AR. *The Initial Processing of Pain and Its Descending Control: Spinal and Trigeminal Systems*. Basel: Karger; 1992:88.)

interaction between somatic afferents and autonomic outflows is the control of the heart. As with most visceral structures, the heart receives its autonomic innervation from both sympathetic and parasympathetic nerves.

SYMPATHETIC INNERVATION OF THE HEART

Excitation of the cardiac sympathetic nerves causes (Fig. 10.6) these effects:

Increased heart rate
Increased atrial and ventricular contractility
Decreased conduction time from the atrium to the ventricle

The heart's spinal innervation is associated with spinal cord levels from T1 to about T5, with T2 probably contributing

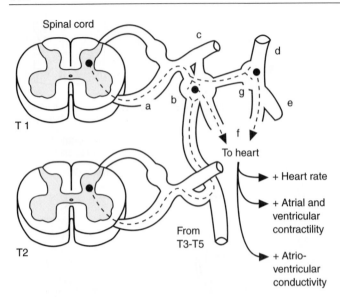

Figure 10.6. Sympathetic innervation of heart. *a*, ventral root; *b*, stellate ganglion; *c*, spinal nerve; *d*, vagosympathetic trunk; *e*, vagus nerve; *f*, cardiac nerves; *g*, middle cervical ganglion.

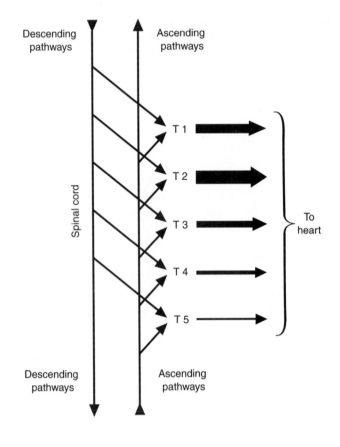

Figure 10.7. Spinal sympathetic innervation of heart and related ascending and descending pathways. Heart receives spinal cord control via T1 to T5 spinal cord levels with T2 making largest functional contribution. Lesions above T1 and below T5 block brain control of cardiac sympathetic activity and reflex responses to ascending afferent activation, respectively.

the most (Fig. 10.7). The preganglionic fibers leave the spinal cord via the ventral roots and course a short distance in the spinal nerves (Fig. 10.6). The preganglionic fibers then exit the spinal nerves to enter the adjoining sympathetic chain ganglia. Most preganglionic sympathetic fibers controlling the heart course though the stellate ganglion to the middle cervical ganglion. There they excite ganglion cells that send their axons, the postganglionic fibers, via the cardiac nerves to innervate:

Pacemaker cells
Myocardium
Conductile system
Coronary arteries

The first paravertebral ganglion associated with the heart is the stellate ganglion, where some preganglionic axons excite ganglion cells whose axons also run directly to the heart.[10]

Segmental-like innervation to different portions of the heart does not seem to occur.[11] In other words, a particular spinal level (e.g., T4), sends its sympathetic influences to most areas of the heart, not to one area. One should be cautious in relating problems in one portion of the heart to problems associated with one spinal level. However, different spinal segmental levels innervate different organs, for example, heart versus lungs. Some degree of segmental-like innervation does occur.

Understanding the spinal cord levels that control the heart is helpful to understand responses of spinal cord-injured patients (Fig. 10.7).[12,13] With spinal cord lesions above T1, the brain has no control of the heart via the spinal cord and sympathetic nerves, but can still activate the parasympathetic pathways. However, marked cardiac alterations may occur via reflexes mediated by sensory inputs that enter the spinal cord below the C8 level. For example, inputs from the urinary bladder may cause markedly increased sympathetic activity to the

heart. Patients with spinal lesions below T1 have some brain control of the heart via descending spinal pathways. Patients with lesions below T5 rarely show any spinal reflexes influencing the heart from the spinal afferents entering the cord below the lesion level. Specific levels of the spinal cord innervate specific visceral organs.

Sympathetic motoneurons located in both sides of the spinal cord and their corresponding sympathetic nerves innervate the heart. There are some quantitative differences in the regions of the heart that are innervated.[11] For example, stimulation of sympathetic preganglionic nerves from both sides of the spinal cord causes increases in heart rate. The right side has a greater influence on heart rate and the sinoatrial node function. Both sides innervate the atrioventricular node, both ventricles, and atria. However, sympathetic output from the left spinal cord has a greater effect on cardiac output and myocardial contractility.[11,13] Visceral organs receive asymmetrical autonomic control from the left and right sides of the spinal cord.

Several different descending spinal pathways can affect autonomic outflow from the spinal cord. Many of these pathways are located in the lateral funiculus of the spinal cord. Both anatomical[14] and physiological[15] evidence suggests that the descending spinal pathways are organized according to a viscerotopic pattern. Localized lesions of the spinal cord, or portions of the descending spinal pathways, may result in loss of brain control of one particular visceral organ. This also suggests that the brain has the potential to separately control different visceral organs (Fig. 10.8).

PARASYMPATHETIC INNERVATION OF THE HEART

Parasympathetic innervation of the heart is via the vagus nerves that cause the following (Fig. 10.9):

Decreased heart rate
Slowed atrioventricular conduction
Decreased atrial contraction
Limited decrease of ventricular contractility

The cardiac vagal fibers travel in the cervical vagus nerve (vagosympathetic trunk) into the thorax where they separate from the vagus nerve to form the cardiac nerves. These cardiac vagal nerves have their cell bodies in the medulla, that is, the nucleus ambiguus and the dorsomotor nucleus.[16–20]

These two medullary regions may subserve different cardiac functions. For example, the nucleus ambiguus may mediate heart rate, and the dorsomotor nucleus, ventricular contractility.[17] Not only are there regions of the brainstem controlling cardiac function that seem to be distinct from those controlling gastrointestinal function and other visceral organs, but different brainstem regions may control separate cardiac functions.

VISCERAL FUNCTION CONTROL

Cardiovascular function can be reflexively controlled by somatic afferents via the somatosympathetic reflexes. These reflexes may be mediated at the spinal cord level or via suprasegmental connections. The spinal somatosympathetic reflexes demonstrate dependency on segmental organization. These sympathetic reflex responses at one segmental level are larger if the somatic afferent activity enters at the same spinal level than at adjoining levels.[21–23] These reflexes also demonstrate

laterality, because they are larger for ipsilateral reflexes than for contralateral reflexes (Fig. 10.10).

Visceral afferents can also influence somatic reflexes, and muscle tone may be altered by visceral inputs. Many of these reflex possibilities are very important for osteopathic palpatory diagnosis and treatment. They provide mechanisms for the use of muscle tone as an indicator of visceral disturbances. The work by Eble[3] showed activation of skeletal muscles with stimulation of visceral structures, while Schoen and Finn[24] reported electromyographic (EMG) activity in shoulder muscles of the cat following experimental myocardial infarction. The cardiac viscero-somatic reflex has an influence on somatic musculature.

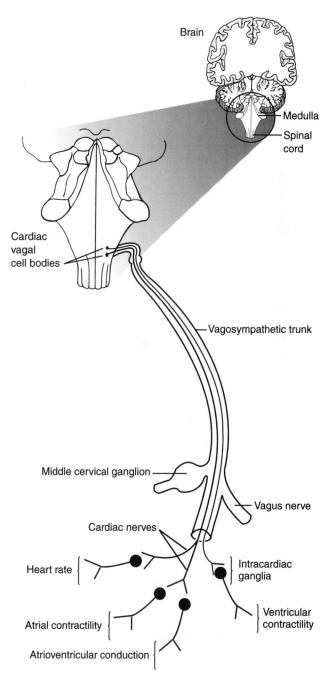

Figure 10.9. Parasympathetic innervation of heart.

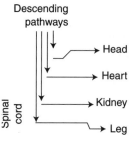

Figure 10.8. Viscerotopic organization of descending spinal pathways controlling autonomic outflow.

Not only can there be activity from somatic or visceral structures that influences the opposite structures, but another type of activity, independent of the brain or spinal cord, may occur. Recently, neural activity has been recorded from in vitro sympathetic ganglion cells and intracardiac ganglion cells, demonstrating considerable action potential activity even when the neuronal connections to the central nervous system are severed.[17–20] These observations suggest that the autonomic ganglia may function as "little brains" within peripheral ganglia and the heart. These ganglia may have the neural circuitry to act almost independently and have the ability to integrate intrinsic cardiocardiac reflexes as well as information from the central nervous system. However, the functional roles of these peripheral nervous system interactions are not known at present (Fig. 10.11).

The possibility of "little brains" within the autonomic ganglia present many possibilities. If visceral afferents have reflexes within the autonomic ganglia, somatic afferents could have reflex connections within the autonomic ganglia. Some somatic afferent fibers pass through the autonomic ganglia. It is possible that somatic afferents influence sympathetic activity not only to the somatic structure but also to visceral structures such as the heart. Activation of somatic afferents might cause reflex alteration of cardiac function via direct ganglionic reflexes as well as via the central nervous system-mediated reflexes. Likewise, visceral afferents might activate sympathetic ganglion cells with axons supplying somatic structures.[25–28] The therapeutic implications of reflexes within autonomic ganglia may be important.

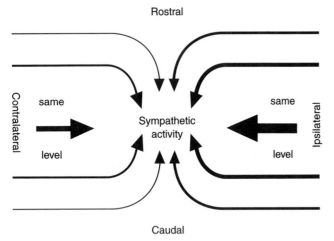

Figure 10.10. Laterality of cardiac sympathetic control and segmental organization of spinal sympathetic reflexes.

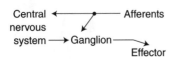

Figure 10.11. Afferent reflex control of autonomic effectors may be mediated via reflexes within peripheral autonomic ganglia as well as via central nervous system connections.

INTERACTIONS OF SOMATIC AFFERENTS AND BARORECEPTOR CONTROL OF AUTONOMIC ACTIVITY

Blood pressure and cardiac function are reflexively controlled through alteration of autonomic activity mediated by arterial blood pressure receptors, the baroreceptor afferents. Increased arterial blood pressure excites baroreceptor activity that is carried to the brainstem via the glossopharyngeal and vagus nerves. In the brainstem, the baroreceptor afferent activity eventually leads to excitation of the medullary cardiac vagal cell bodies. It also leads to inhibition of the sympathetic activity to the cardiovascular system via descending brainstem–spinal pathways.[29] Baroreflexes involving the cardiac vagus nerves have parallel inhibitory effects on the sinoatrial node (slowing heart rate) and atrioventricular node (slowing atrioventricular conduction).[30]

Although these baroreceptor reflexes have powerful influences on cardiovascular function, they also interact with other spinal reflexes, especially from small, high-threshold afferent fibers. With activation of these spinal afferents, reflex changes in sympathetic activity (somatosympathetic reflexes) occur at the spinal cord level and through suprasegmental reflexes involving ascending and then descending pathways to and from the brainstem.[31,32]

Baroreflexes inhibit both spinal and supraspinally mediated somatosympathetic reflexes.[33] Presumably, other visceral afferents that also mediate sympathetic reflexes are also inhibited by these powerful baroreceptor reflexes.

Somatic afferent activity can modulate baroreceptor reflex vagal control of the heart.[19,29,34,35] Baroreceptor activation excites the cardiac vagus nerve activity. However, somatic afferent stimulation attenuates or blocks the baroreceptor influence of vagal cardiac nerves. Somatic afferents and baroreceptors compete for control of autonomic activity. The ascending and descending pathways for these reflexes have been localized in the dorsal portion of the lateral funiculus of the spinal cord.[35–37]

Summation Characteristics of Somato-Visceral Reflexes

Somato-visceral reflexes demonstrate temporal and spatial summation as indicated by the "wind-up" phenomenon and the effects of multiple inputs from different parts of the body. These somato-visceral reflexes do not reach their maximal activity immediately.[38] Rather, when stimulated at a slow repetition rate, these reflexes exhibit wind-up. With each repetition of the stimulation up to about 20 times, the autonomic response increases in size (Fig. 10.12).

The wind-up, or as it has also been termed, sensitization, phenomenon suggests that maximal effectiveness of therapeutic procedures involving somatic afferent influences on autonomic control may require frequent repetitions of the procedure to allow the response to build to its maximum. Furthermore, afferent inputs from different portions of the body can summate together to activate autonomic responses.[39] Accordingly, one would expect that a subliminal or noneffective stimulus to one

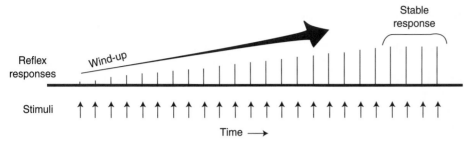

Figure 10.12. Wind-up or sensitization. When a stimulus is repeated at a rate of once every second or two, response to stimulus may continue to grow for 20 seconds or more. Finally, a stable response level is reached that can continue at increased level as long as stimulus is continued.

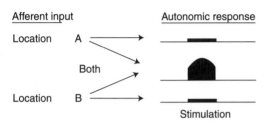

Figure 10.13. Summation of autonomic responses. Inputs from two different locations add together to produce a larger autonomic response than either input produces when it occurs alone.

portion of the body might actually have an effect if combined with stimulation to another area of the body (Fig. 10.13).

The reflex system is truly a complex integrating network. Perhaps most important for the osteopath is the fact that somatic inputs can and do influence visceral function, just as inputs from the viscera cause changes in the outputs to the somatic structures. This can often be felt as altered tissue tensions or changes in motion characteristics of joints. Maps have even been published listing somatic areas that become abnormal to palpation with various visceral disturbances.[40]

A corollary of this is that manipulation of the somatic structures can alter the function of visceral structures through the same pathways. The reflexes are not simple systems with only local influences, but interconnected networks that receive inputs from many sources and process that information for distribution to both local and distant areas of the body.

ALTERATION OF INTEGRATIVE FUNCTION

Inputs from each area of the body and from descending brain areas interact on a highly overlapping and integrated neural network in the spinal interneurons. Afferent inputs from any source influence both visceral or somatic structures. For normal functioning of organs, muscles, fluid motion, and other body activities, these complex and interacting networks within the nervous system must act in concert. Should one area of the neural network respond either more or less than normal, the finely tuned balance necessary for normal and optimal physiological function will be disturbed. Not only must the control mechanisms from the brain be normal for proper reflex function, but the networks of neurons that make up the reflexes

must also be acting normally. Unfortunately, these networks themselves can be altered, resulting in a loss of proper function.

While Sherrington postulated that reflexes are innately given, more and more evidence is accumulating that the function of reflex networks can be influenced by many factors. They are subject to both short-term and long-term changes that can have consequences for the health of the individual.

Among the first to show the results of changes in the integrative function of reflex networks in humans were Denslow and his colleagues in the early and mid-1940s. They performed a series of studies on normal young adult volunteers to determine whether the reflex excitabilities at various spinal levels of the body were stable and comparable.[41–43] They measured how much stimulation it took to evoke muscle activity (EMG) in the paraspinal muscles of the back at several levels of the thoracic spine.

They found that, on the average, reflex excitability to pressure on the spinous processes was highest in the upper thoracic area and lowest in the midlumbar area. While decreased excitability from the upper thoracic to the lower lumbar areas was seen overall in the subjects studied, practically all individuals studied had areas that were very highly excitable, responding to small amounts of pressure on the spinous process at that spinal level. In normal areas, in contrast, even a fairly heavy pressure in the spinous processes did not produce any muscle activity in the associated muscles. The highly excitable areas were characterized by not only the increased muscle activity to pressure on the spinous process but also often by pain and tenderness in the area. The areas of increased sensitivity to stimulation were not uniform from individual to individual and were long-lasting (some cases remaining almost the same for years). In most cases, the individual did not realize that any change was present.

These long-lasting, low-threshold areas to afferent inputs could be activated not only by stimulating tissues at the same level of the spinal cord but also by stimulating other areas of the back or even by providing a psychological stress to the individual. With remote inputs, such as pressure on a spinous process four vertebrae away from the level of the low-threshold area, the muscles at the level of the input remained silent, while those at the level of the low threshold became active. The same pattern would occur with psychological stressors. The normal areas remained silent, but the low-threshold areas showed muscle activity.

In later studies, Denslow and his coworkers found that not only was muscle activity affected but so were the activities of visceral organs through altered sympathetic outputs. Here again, the interrelatedness of the somatic and visceral portions of the body were shown.

While many otherwise normal subjects had low-threshold or high-excitability areas, it became evident from subject-to-subject variability, and from further data showing that the excitability increases often accompanied injury and disease, that the excitability changes were not a normal state. They represented areas of neural function that were operating out of synchrony with other areas of the neural system, causing the organs served by those neural supplies also to be out of synchrony with the total body function.

Korr[44] suggested that these low-threshold spinal reflexes represented pathways that were being held in a hyperexcited state, perhaps by a continued bombardment of inputs. He termed these areas "facilitated." He pointed out that they acted to magnify inputs to the area from any source and to cause a magnified outflow to the organs innervated by that level of the spinal cord. Thermographic studies were carried out.[45,46] Not only did the skeletal muscles respond in an exaggerated fashion in the low threshold areas, but also the sympathetic outflows increased. Such areas of abnormally increased excitability or decreased threshold within the otherwise normal areas of the spinal cord must act to decrease the overall integration of body function. No matter what the source of inputs to a facilitated spinal area, the neural outflows would be exaggerated relative to the same response at other spinal levels. Such a situation lasting over time can have only undesirable consequences for total body function.

Beginning and Maintenance of Reflex Facilitation

The finding that facilitated or low-threshold areas could continue for long periods of time and the fact that these areas were not the same from individual to individual suggested that some process could occur that would set up these chronically hyperactive areas. There was initial speculation that the hyperexcitability was maintained by tonic afferent inputs. Most inputs from either somatic or visceral structures, however, decrease dramatically with such activities as sleep and other forms of relaxation. Why should the hyperexcitability continue even with the loss of afferent activity? What is the nature of the neural processing within the reflex pathways to afferent stimuli that might explain the appearance of regions of hyperexcitability? More recent studies have provided some answers that have a bearing on how changes in reflex excitability can at times be an adaptive process and at times a detrimental one.

ALTERATION OF REFLEX EXCITABILITY

The concept of the reflex as basically a simple, unchanging, static input–output relationship is oversimplified. Although he characterized reflex function as "innately given," even Sherrington recognized that reflex excitability could be momentarily altered by such influences as signals from higher brain struc-

tures, or by rapid and repeated use, that he noted caused "reflex fatigue." The notion that reflexes are fundamentally unchanging, static input–output relationships is still widespread, despite the fact that it is now clear that the excitability of spinal reflex pathways can be altered by many influences. These changes can range from short-lasting, fleeting changes to very long-lasting ones that may even become permanent. These long-lasting alterations may well be the basis for the changes shown by Denslow in his studies of human motoneuron excitability, and for the facilitated state hypothesized by Korr. These threats to functional integration of the body may be related to the effects of nociceptive stimuli at the periphery.

ALTERATIONS OF NOCICEPTIVE STIMULI

Inflammation from strong stimulation of the skin or other peripheral somatic or visceral structures produces a set of changes in the sensory receptors of the organ that dramatically alters the amount of neural activity sent to the spinal cord.[47] Most tissues are innervated by various sensory receptors, such as these:

Touch
Temperature
Stretch
Nociceptors

The nociceptors are composed primarily of "naked" (unmyelinated) nerve endings that respond to potentially tissue-damaging stimuli. In the hollow visceral organs, they respond to stretch or dilation of the organ, for example. These receptors send impulses through thin myelinated (group III or Aδ) or unmyelinated (group IV or C) fibers into the spinal gray matter, where they synapse primarily in Rexed layers I and V. When activity occurs in these pathways, the resulting sensation is usually discomfort or pain, although the inputs may be blocked by other neural activity from reaching the areas of the brainstem where they are appreciated as pain. However, even though a nociceptive input to the spinal cord does not reach the conscious level, it may affect the dynamics of the spinal pathways.[48]

Once a stimulus sufficiently strong to activate nociceptive inputs begins, impulses travel into the spinal cord via the dorsal roots. At the branches of the peripheral neurons, the afferent impulses invade the afferent branches and are conveyed back out to the nerve terminals, where they cause release of various peptides into the surrounding tissues. The sites of peptide release may be some distance from the original stimulus. The result of this release is the start of a cascade of events that leads to involvement of the sympathetic postganglionic nerve terminals and to the release of serum from the surrounding capillaries. Prostaglandins released from the sympathetic nerve terminals continue the serum release that leads to local inflammation.

This process begins the healing process, although it may be sufficiently severe that the healing process is retarded.[49] The inflammation also produces dramatic changes in the characteristics of the local nociceptors in the area. Schmidt[47] demonstrated that in the cat knee joint after inflammation the number of nociceptors responding to a stretch stimulation may be between 3000 and 4000. In contrast, even severe stretch of the normal joint may cause only 400 nociceptors to fire. Also, the receptive fields of the active nociceptors enlarge dramatically in the inflamed area, and the threshold to activation goes down significantly. The result of an inflammatory process, or of a strong stimulus that produces tissue damage, will be to lower nociceptor thresholds and dramatically increase the number of inputs to the spinal cord. Peripheral events can lead to dramatic changes in the amount of stimulus input caused by changes in the peripheral receptors.

What happens to spinal reflex networks when stimulus inputs change? In the normal reflex pathway, repeated activation of the pathway by a weak afferent input results in a temporary decrease in the output of the network. Sherrington described this short-term decrease in reflex pathway excitability as reflex fatigue. This process, now termed "habituation," has been studied extensively and is a characteristic of polysynaptic reflex pathways in the spinal cord and brainstem.

Habituation is characterized by a decrease in output from a neural pathway with repeated stimulus input of a mild to moderate intensity. A stimulus may initially produce a response of a certain magnitude, but if the stimulus is repeated several times, the response decreases. If the stimulus is then terminated, the response returns to its initial level in a matter of seconds to minutes.[50] The process of habituation is a ubiquitous phenomenon, occurring in almost all animals and in all mammalian reflex pathways except the monosynaptic myotatic reflex. It is a necessary part of the neural integration, since it allows nonessential stimuli to be muted in their effects on the nervous system.

The opposite of habituation is an increase in reflex excitability. We described earlier the phenomenon of wind-up, in which a stimulus repeated several times causes an increased number of neural firings. Wind-up has also been called "sensitization" in earlier studies (Fig. 10.12). In this process, a repetitive stimulus can cause an increase in output rather than a decrease. A stimulus causing habituation can cause sensitization simply by increasing its intensity. This causes more nociceptors to become active, or the same nociceptors to produce more impulses. Like habituation, sensitization can occur within a matter of seconds, and it can also dissipate in a matter of seconds when the stimulus is terminated.[50]

Both habituation and sensitization have been extensively studied at the cellular level. In the mammal, both occur within the spinal central gray matter in the interneuron pathways. They are probably subserved by two different sets of interneurons, which then synapse on the motoneurons of both the sympathetic and somatic systems. Both sensitization and habituation are apparently presynaptic processes, which either inhibit (habituation) or enhance (sensitization) the release of neurotransmitter with each activation of the presynaptic terminal.[51] They are independent of descending influences from higher nervous centers. Both processes can be demonstrated in humans with spinal cord transections.

Habituation and sensitization are different processes but occur at the synaptic level and can occur over a few seconds of sensory input. While the process of sensitization may not be a unitary one, since there may be more than one form of sensitization, both processes do appear to dissipate in a fairly short time when the initiating stimulus is terminated.

Habituation allows the organism to damp the response to nonthreatening stimuli, while sensitization allows the individual to respond more forcefully to a stimulus that is stronger and thus threatens tissue damage. These two processes are valuable in maintaining the organism in its everyday existence. Under normal conditions, the opposing process of habituation and sensitization function to maintain a balance between overreaction and underreaction to normal stimuli. When the inflammation process occurs, whether it is a minimal or maximal inflammation, the balances of habituation and sensitization are disrupted. The normal damping effects of habituation are shifted toward the sensitization process. This is caused by the larger and more extreme responses of the peripheral receptors to what would usually be a nonthreatening stimulus. The result is a larger than normal motor output to both the visceral and somatic structures innervated by the affected reflex pathways and thus to an overresponse to stimuli. The process disrupts the normal integration of physiological function.

Once the process of sensitization has begun, often over a few seconds of strong input, a secondary process begins to occur. Sensitization dissipates over a few seconds or minutes after the stimulus is gone. A longer lasting process, termed "long-term sensitization," begins to develop in the reflex pathways once sensitization has been in place for several minutes. This process precludes the excitability of the neural pathways from returning to normal for some time, often for hours.

The effects of this process can often be seen in laboratory experiments when the effects of bursts of stimulation are given, followed by an occasional stimulus pulse to test the responsivity of the reflex system. After the initial sensitization and the rapid fall of reflex excitability after stimulus termination, the response being tracked does not return to its prestimulation baseline but remains a small but significant amount above the base level. This hyperexcitability does not decay for varying amounts of time, depending on the time and strength of the stimulus. Unlike sensitization, long-term sensitization is thought to be a postsynaptic event, possibly involving the elaboration of proteins in the postsynaptic neuron, that remains active for some time after the initiating event.

Recently, Mantyh and his colleagues have shown dramatic changes in the substance P receptors and even structural reorganization of the dendrites of spinal interneurons after nociceptive inputs. These changes could be the basis for long-term sensitization.[52] Long-term sensitization involves a different mechanism than does the short-term process and can have effects that far outlast the originating stimulus.

Once a stimulus has acted on a reflex network for a longer time, the results can be even more dramatic. For many years, a process that became known as "spinal fixation" has been known but not fully recognized. First shown in anesthetized animals, spinal fixation was manifest as a remaining active leg flexion following 3–4 hours of limb flexion secondary to a cerebellar lesion. The lesion produced disrupted outflows from the postural centers in the cerebellum, resulting in sustained flexion of a limb. When the spinal cord was sectioned immediately following the lesion, the limb dropped to the usual flaccid paralysis of the spinal animal. However, if the animal was allowed to remain with the spinal cord intact after the lesion for 3–4 hours, then received a spinal transection, the limb remained flexed to some extent. The explanation was that the strong outflow from the injured cerebellum caused a hyperexcitability to develop in the target interneurons of the cord that remained active after the spinal transection, resulting in continued motor activity.

In the mid-1960s, research showed that the minimal time necessary for the "fixation" of this excitability was about 45 minutes. Animals receiving the spinal transection within 35 minutes showed no remaining flexion, while all those having 45 minutes between lesion and transection showed remaining flexion. This effect has now been shown to occur not only as a result of a cerebellar lesion but also with stimulation of the skin of the hind limb, and to occur in either intact or spinalized animals.[53-55] The change in the spinal reflexes produced by the cerebellar lesion was caused not by pain or nociceptive inputs but by changes in outflows from the postural centers.

This, along with more recent research, shows that changes in the reflex functions can occur with both nociceptive and nonnociceptive inputs, although nociceptive inputs are able to produce the changes more quickly than nonnociceptive inputs. The reflex excitability changes can be influenced by many factors, including:

Stress prior to the stimulation
Length and severity of stimulation
Whether the spinal cord is intact or sectioned

The changes have been traced for 3–7 days after only 45 minutes of fairly intense nociceptive stimulation and probably last even longer. With intense stimulus inputs, the effect is seen with as little as 20 minutes of stimulation. Obviously, strong inputs, especially nociceptive ones, can have rapid and long-lasting effects on the excitability of reflex circuits. While the locus of the changes seen in fixation is not yet known, it seems likely that the alterations being observed are a process akin to long-term sensitization—but one that lasts for a much longer time. It appears that the fixation process is also reliant on the elaboration of proteins in the postsynaptic cells and that it would affect the responsivity of those cells not only to the original inputs but to all inputs to the cell.

Another line of evidence of long-lasting increases in reflex excitability comes from studies of peripheral inflammation. They show that there are peripheral effects of inflammation on afferent inputs and receptive fields. Continued afferent inputs from peripheral inflammation produce dramatic changes in the responsivity of spinal interneurons. Interneurons upon which afferents from affected nociceptors synapse begin to respond much more easily to inputs from a variety of sources, such as touch, pressure, and even the movement of distant muscles. These dramatic changes in excitability also last for long periods, days and weeks, and develop during the initial inflammatory episode.

Knowing something about the mechanisms of the changes may allow us to restore the changes to more normal function. Dubner and Ruda[56] have summarized a series of intracellular changes that are linked to the excitability alterations seen with the inflammation process. The cells activated by the nociceptive inputs from inflamed peripheral structures begin to show enhanced activation of specific parts of the postsynaptic cell membrane called NMDA receptors. When these receptors become more active, the excitability of the cell is increased. If cellular activation continues even longer, changes in the activity of genes within the neuron are seen. A class of genes called intermediate-early genes, c-fos and c-jun, become more active, causing increased dynorphin release within the cell. Dynorphin is a substance that causes increased cell excitation. With more of it being produced, the cell is then held in a hyperexcitable state. Once the excitatory process is increased for a period of several days, some of the inhibitory interneurons in the network die away, further shifting the balance of activity toward hyperexcitation. There may be an increase in excitatory synapses due to cell sprouting, similar to that seen with some types of learning. The effects of injuries or dysfunctions that produce nociceptive or even nonnociceptive inputs to the spinal cord are to induce long-lasting or permanent excitability changes in the reflex networks. When the immediate challenge of responding to the cause of the injury is gone, the altered reflex networks remain in an altered state and no longer respond in concert with other networks, thus diminishing functional integration.

NON–IMPULSE-BASED INTEGRATION

Neurons convey not only impulses throughout the body to integrate function, but also a steady stream of material flowing from the neural cell body out the axon and dendrites. This flow is known as axoplasmic flow. It transports materials from where they are manufactured in the cell body down a complex microtubular structure within the axon. Materials to supply rebuilding of the axonic walls, resupply the transmitter substances, and so forth are carried on this system. Among the most common clinical effects of this transport can be seen when neural contact is withdrawn from an end organ, such as when a muscle is denervated by cutting its motor nerve, a relatively common occurrence. Not only does the muscle cease to contract, but unless the nerve regrows again to contact the muscle, the muscle fibers eventually lose their ability to contract. They change their structure to that of noncontractile connective tissue. Likewise, if an end organ is damaged, its nerve supply often retracts and the synapses are lost. The end organ supplies something to the nerve that allows the synapses to remain viable.

A great deal of study has been done on the uptake by nerve terminals of substances supplied by the end organ. A family of substances known as nerve growth factor (NGF) is essential to continued nerve contact with an end organ and for continued viability of contacts between nerves higher up the chain. If the end organ does not supply NGF, the synaptic contact is lost.

This factor is also essential in development, allowing appropriate nerves to reach and establish contact with the appropriate end organs. Loss of appropriate NGF causes deterioration of the nerve and its contacts. NGF is elaborated in the end organ and taken up by the presynaptic membranes, where it is transported up the axon to the cell body, a process called retrograde transport. There it regulates the function of the nerve and the nerve's ability to maintain synaptic contacts. Many other substances can be taken up and transported to the cell body, not all of them helpful to nerve function. The tetanus toxin, tetanospasmin, is made in peripheral structures after infection by the *Clostridium tetani* bacterium. The toxin is taken up by nerve terminals and transported to the central nervous system, where it affects neural function, causing the clinical signs of tetanus.

Many common nerve tracing techniques rely on the ability of the neuron to take up substances and transport them from the periphery of the nerve to the cell body. For example, horseradish peroxidase is used as a nerve tracer by injecting it into the area of nerve terminals, where it is taken into the cell and transported up the axon, eventually filling the cell body and even dendrites. A fixative can then be used to turn the horseradish peroxidase a dark brown-black, providing an easily visualized portrait of the cell. Many other dyes and materials are commonly used in this way to visualize nerve cells.

While much is known about the NGF family and some other substances, and about the actual transport mechanisms within the axon, less is known about the delivery of substances to end organs through transport from cell body to axon (anterograde flow), such as what is delivered to keep a muscle functional. In 1967, Korr et al.[57] published the results of a study that showed that amino acids placed on the cell bodies of the hypoglossal nucleus on the floor of the fourth ventricle were incorporated into the cell body and transported down the axon to the tongue muscle, where they were delivered into the muscle fibers. Later work showed that not only was the material transported but it was transported at several different rates of flow. That study and others since have shown that flow rates within an axon vary from as slow as 0.5 mm/day to as fast as 400 mm/day. The observed rates are[58]:

Slow (0.5–2 mm/day)
Medium (25 mm/day)
Fast (up to 400 mm/day)
Very fast (up to 2000 mm/day)

While much of the anterogradely transported materials are related to support of the neuron and synaptic functions, such as supply of neurotransmitter components, materials delivered by the nerve to its end organ are necessary for either its function or continued existence.[59]

The nervous system is not only the network for rapid communications within the body, but it serves as a vast network for a far slower two-way communication between the central

nervous structures and every part of the body. Disruption of this slow transport of materials has consequences for continued function that may not be evident immediately, but that range from subtle to disastrous. Complete withdrawal of NGF or of the materials delivered by the nerve to its end organ may result in loss of function. Disturbance of the flow of materials in either direction results in less than optimal function of the organs involved.

Many questions remain about the two-way communication of axoplasmic flow. What substances are being delivered? How necessary are they? What do the materials transported from the periphery to the nerve cell bodies do to the function of the cell or of the entire CNS? Are there crucial times for delivery of nerve factors to end organs for proper development? However these questions are answered, it is important to recognize the vast integrating nature of the non–impulse-based transport systems of the nervous system and the importance of proper function of this system.

Many things have been shown to affect the material flow within the nerve cells. Even small pressure on axons can impede proper axoplasmic flow. A sustained increased number of impulses carried by the neuron (as in those originating in facilitated areas of the cord) may decrease flow rates. Improper supplies of nutrients and oxygen to the cell body or axon alter the flow. The occurrence of the tissue tensions and fluid flow disturbances often associated with somatic dysfunctions can be factors in altering axoplasmic flows. The somatic dysfunctions treated by the use of manipulative treatment would be expected to have a positive effect on the flow of materials in axons of the area and hence to improve body function and integration.

CONCLUSION

In the normal integrative function of the nervous system, there are obviously a great number of influences acting on any neural pathway. Afferent inputs activate reflex outflows. Descending activities from higher nervous centers modulate excitability of interneurons. Ascending influences from lower spinal areas increase or decrease activity. Psychological effects are played out on all levels of the neuraxis. The nerves deliver to their end organs the materials necessary for normal function, while the end organs send to the nerves the substances necessary for continued synaptic viability.

These influences come together to determine the moment-to-moment excitability of any area of the central nervous system and to determine overall outflows to both somatic and visceral structures. If all of these influences are working in harmony, optimally integrated function can be expected from the various organs. If, however, one area is in a hyperexcitable state, the output from that area of the system will not be in harmony with the outputs of the other areas. In that case, the optimal function is disrupted, and the individual becomes increasingly prone to loss of function and to disease.

The long-term alterations in spinal reflex excitability now well-demonstrated by various studies seem almost certain to underlie the alterations demonstrated by Denslow and his colleagues. These breaks in the normal integration of the nervous system were shown to affect both visceral and somatic structures. The interactions between visceral and somatic inputs in the spinal cord provide the basis for that common effect. The changes shown in response to nociceptive inputs can easily account for the long-lasting nature of the "facilitation" identified in those studies. The facilitation was hypothesized by Korr to be the basis for the somatic dysfunctions long recognized by the osteopathic profession.

Since the neurons involved in the altered excitability are interneurons, the neurons upon which a variety of different pathways synapse, the data also support the effects of excitability changes on both somatic and autonomic outflows. The inputs from both visceral and somatic structures end on common interneurons. When the excitability of those interneurons is altered, the outflows are affected to all structures innervated by motoneurons to which those interneurons connect.

The reflex networks of the nervous system are not at all static, genetically determined entities. They are a vast network of highly interconnected pathways that are continually changing to meet local needs and to maintain integration of function. These processes allow the delicate moment-to-moment integration that characterizes optimal functional capacity. The integration, however, can be turned against the very system it serves. When abnormal or very strong inputs occur, the result can be a long-term disruption of the normal excitatory–inhibitory balances and a shift to excessive excitability (or in some cases, to excessive inhibition). The result, in either case, is the loss of functional integration and a decrease in functional capacity of the individual.

There are many factors that influence the total function of the individual, including their:

Accumulated effects of life
Habits
Living environment
Food
Psychological and spiritual makeup and state

The role of the state of the nervous system is but one of the factors influencing the total health of the person. An area of central excitation or facilitation, since it affects all organs and structures with which it communicates, delivers to the end organs the effects of all other stressors on the individual. In essence, it is the final common factor in communicating with the end organ. Most of the other stressors in a person's life are difficult to change, and the osteopathic physician has little impact on or control over them. However, the physician can directly affect the course of the facilitation and its effects by recognizing that it occurs and by using modalities, especially manipulative treatment, that alter it.

Rational therapy dictates the normalization of afferent inputs as quickly as possible. In chronic situations, use methods to reduce the abnormal inputs, thus allowing the body to restore normal balances of excitation and inhibition as fully as possible. In this way, the goal of total osteopathic treatment, to optimize each individual's function and to restore the individual's dynamic functional balance of optimal health, can be brought closer to reality.

REFERENCES

1. Still AT. *The Autobiography of A.T. Still.* Published by the author. Kirksville, Mo, 1897.
2. Sherrington CS. *The Integrative Action of the Nervous System.* New Haven, Conn: Yale University Press; 1906.
3. Eble JN. Patterns of response of the paravertebral musculature to visceral stimuli. *Am J Physiol.* 1960;198:429–433.
4. Sato A. Reflex modulation of visceral functions by somatic afferent activity. In: Patterson MM, Howell JN, eds. *The Central Connection: Somatovisceral/Viscerosomatic Interaction.* Indianapolis, Ind: American Academy of Osteopathy; 1992:53–73.
5. Rexed B. The cytoarchitectonic organization of the spinal cord in the cat. *J Comp Neurol.* 1952;96:415–495.
6. DeGroat WC. Spinal cord processing of visceral and somatic nociceptive input. In: Willard FH, Patterson MM, eds. *Nociception and the Neuroendocrine–Immune Connection.* Indianapolis, Ind: American Academy of Osteopathy; 1994:47–72.
7. Cervero R, Foreman RD. Sensory innervation of the viscera. In: Loewy AD, Spyer KM, eds. *Central Regulation of Autonomic Functions.* New York, NY: Oxford University Press; 1990:104–125.
8. Cervero F. Visceral and spinal components of viscero-somatic interactions. In: Patterson MM, Howell JN, eds. *The Central Connection: Somatovisceral/Viscerosomatic Interaction.* Indianapolis, Ind: American Academy of Osteopathy; 1992:77–86.
9. Sato A. The somatosympathetic reflexes: their physiological and clinical significance. In: Goldstein M, ed. *The Research Status of Spinal Manipulative Therapy.* Washington, DC: National Institutes of Health; 1975:163–172. DHEW publication NIH 76-998.
10. Hopkins DA, Armour JA. Localization of sympathetic postganglionic and parasympathetic preganglionic neurons which innervate different regions of the dog heart. *J Comp Neurol.* 1984;229:186–198.
11. Norris JE, Foreman RD, Wurster RD. Responses of the canine heart to stimulation of the first five ventral thoracic roots. *Am J Physiol.* 1974;227:9–12.
12. Wurster RD, Randall WC. Cardiovascular responses to bladder distension in patients with spinal transection. *Am J Physiol.* 1975; 228:1288–1292.
13. Wurster RD. Spinal sympathetic control of the heart. In: Randall WC, ed. *Neural Regulation of the Heart.* New York, NY: Oxford University Press; 1976:157–186.
14. Chung K, Chung JM, LaVelle FW, Wurster RD. The anatomical localization of descending pressor pathways in the cat spinal cord. *Neurosci Lett.* 1979;15:71–75.
15. Barman SM, Wurster RD. Visceromotor organization within descending spinal sympathetic pathways. *Circ Res.* 1975;37:209–214.
16. Geis GS, Wurster RD. Horseradish peroxidase localization of cardiac vagal preganglionic somata. *Brain Res.* 1980;182:19–30.
17. Geis GS, Wurster RD. Cardiac responses during stimulation of dorsal motor nucleus and nucleus ambiguus in the cat. *Circ Res.* 1980; 46:606–611.
18. Kalia M, Mesulam MM. Brain stem projections of sensory and motor components of the vagus complex in the cat, II: Laryngeal, tracheobronchial, pulmonary, cardiac, and gastrointestinal branches. *J Comp Neurol.* 1980;193:467–508.
19. Geis GS, Kozelka JW, Wurster RD. Organization and reflex control of vagal cardiomotor neurons. *J Auton Nerv Syst.* 1981;5:63–70.
20. Hopkins DA, Armour JA. Medullary cells of origin of physiologically identified cardiac nerves in the dog. *Brain Res Bull.* 1982;8:359–365.
21. Beacham WS, Perl ER. Background and reflex discharge of sympa-

thetic preganglionic neurons in the spinal cat. *J Physiol (Lond)*. 1964; 172:400–416.

22. Beacham WS, Perl ER. Characteristics of a spinal sympathetic reflex. *J Physiol (Lond)*. 1964;173:431–448.

23. Foreman RD, Wurster RD. Nerve conduction in descending pathways of the spinal cord initiated by activation of somato-sympathetic reflexes. *Am J Physiol* 1975;228:905–908.

24. Schoen RE, Finn WE. A model for studying a viscerosomatic reflex induced by myocardial infarction in the cat. *JAOA*. 1978;78:122–123.

25. Armour JA. Activity of in situ middle cervical ganglion neurons in dogs, using extracellular recording techniques. *Can J Physiol Pharmacol*. 1985;63:704–716.

26. Armour JA. Activity of in situ stellate ganglion neurons of dogs recorded extracellularly. *Can J Physiol Pharmacol*. 1986;64:101–111.

27. Boznjak ZJ, Kampine JP. Intracellular recordings from the stellate ganglion of the cat. *J Physiol (Lond.)*. 1982;324:273–283.

28. Gagliardi M, Randall WC, Bieger D, Wurster RD, Hopkins DA, Armour JA. Activity of in vivo canine cardiac plexus neurons. *Am J Physiol*. 1988;255:789–800.

29. Terui N, Koizumi K. Responses of cardiac vagus and sympathetic nerve to excitation of somatic and visceral nerves. *J Auton Nerv Syst*. 1984;10:73–91.

30. O'Toole MF, Wurster RD, Phillips JG, Randall WC. Parallel baroreceptor control of sinoatrial rate and atrioventricular conduction. *Am J Physiol*. 1984;246:H149–H153.

31. Koizumi K, Brooks CM. The integration of autonomic system reactions: discussion of autonomic reflexes, their control and their association with somatic reactions. *Ergeb Physiol Biol Chem Exp Pharmakol*. 1972;67:1–68.

32. Sato A, Schmidt RF. Somatosympathetic reflexes: afferent fibers, central pathways, discharge characteristics. *Physiol Rev*. 1973; 53:916–947.

33. Barman SM, Wurster RD. Interaction of descending sympathetic pathways and afferent nerves. *Am J Physiol*. 1978;234:H223–H229.

34. Quest JA, Gebber GL. Modulation of baroreflexes by somatic afferent nerve stimulation. *Am J Physiol*. 1972;222:1251–1259.

35. Geis GS, Wurster RD. Localization of ascending inotropic and chronotropic pathways in the cat. *Circ Res*. 1981;49:711–717.

36. Kozelka JW, Chung JM, Wurster RD. Ascending spinal pathways mediating somato-cardiovascular reflexes. *J Auton Nerv Syst*. 1981; 3:171–175.

37. Kozelka JW, Christy GW, Wurster RD. Somato-autonomic reflexes in anesthetized and unanesthetized dogs. *J Auton Nerv Syst*. 1982; 5:63–70.

38. Chung JM, Webber CL, Wurster RD. Ascending spinal pathways for the somatosympathetic A and C reflex. *Am J Physiol*. 1979; 237:H342–H347.

39. Chung JM, Wurster RD. Neurophysiological evidence for spatial summation in the CNS from unmyelinated afferent fibers. *Brain Res*. 1978;153:596–601.

40. Te Poorten BA. Spinal palpatory diagnosis of visceral disease. *Osteo Ann*. 1979;August:52–53.

41. Denslow JS, Hassett CC. The central excitatory state associated with postural abnormalities. *J Neurophysiol*. 1942;5(5):393–402.

42. Denslow JS. An analysis of the variability of spinal reflex thresholds. *J Neurophysiol*. 1944;7:207–215.

43. Denslow JS, Korr IM, Krems AD. Quantitative studies of chronic facilitation in human motoneuron pools. *Am J Physiol*. 1947; 105:229–238.

44. Korr IM. The neural basis of the osteopathic lesion. *JAOA*. 1947; 47:191–198.

45. Korr IM, Thomas PE, Wright HM. Patterns of electrical skin resistance. *J Neural Trans*. 1958;17:77–96.

46. Wright HM, Korr IM, Thomas PE. Local and regional variations in cutaneous vasomotor tone of the human trunk. *J Neural Trans*. 1960;22:34–52.

47. Schmidt RF. Neurophysiological mechanisms of arthritic pain. In: Patterson MM, Howell JN, eds. *The Central Connection: Somatovisceral/Viscerosomatic Interaction*. Indianapolis, Ind: American Academy of Osteopathy; 1992:130–151.

48. Schmidt RF. Nociception and pain. In: Schmidt RF, Thews G, eds. *Human Physiology*. 2nd ed. Heidelberg: Springer; 1987:223–235.

49. Payan DG. Peripheral neuropeptides, inflammation, and nociception. In: Willard FH, Patterson MM, eds. *Nociception and the Neuroendocrine–Immune Connection*. Indianapolis, Ind: American Academy of Osteopathy; 1994:34–43.

50. Groves PM, Thompson RF. Habituation: a dual process theory. *Psych Rev*. 1970;77(5):419–450.

51. Kandel ER, Brunelli M, Byrne J, Castellucci V. A common presynaptic locus for the synaptic changes underlying short-term habituation and sensitization of the gill-withdrawal reflex in *Aplysia*. *Cold Spring Harb Symp Quant Biol*. 1977;40:465–482.

52. Mantyh PW, DeMaster E, Malhotra A, Ghilardi JR, Rogers SD, Mantyh CR, et al. Receptor endocytosis and dendrite reshaping in spinal neurons after somatosensory stimulation. *Science*. 1995; 268:1629–1632.

53. Steinmetz JE, Cervenka J, Robinson C, Romano AG, Patterson MM. Fixation of spinal reflexes in rats using central and peripheral sensory input. *J Comp Physiol Psychol*. 1981;95(4):548–555.

54. Steinmetz JE, Patterson MM. Fixation of spinal reflex alterations in spinal rats by sensory nerve stimulation. *Behav Neurosci*. 1985; 99(1):97–108.

55. Patterson MM, Steinmetz JE. Long-lasting alterations of spinal reflexes: a basis for somatic dysfunction. *Manual Med*. 1986;2:38–42.

56. Dubner R, Ruda MA. Activity-dependent neuronal plasticity following tissue injury and inflammation. *Trends Neurosci*. 1992;15(3):96–103.

57. Korr IM, Wilkerson PN, Chornock FW. Axonal delivery of neuroplasmic components to muscle cells. *Science*. 1967;155:342–345.

58. Korr IM, ed. *The Neurobiologic Mechanisms in Manipulative Therapy*. New York, NY: Plenum Press; 1978.

59. Korr IM. The spinal cord as organizer of disease processes, IV: Axonal transport and neurotrophic function in relation to somatic dysfunction. *JAOA*. 1981;80(7):451–459.

Osteopathic Considerations in the Behavioral Sciences

INTRODUCTION

John A. Jerome

The chapters in this section discuss osteopathic considerations in the clinical and scientific application of biopsychosocial knowledge.

At the beginning of this century, the leading causes of death were diseases such as influenza, tuberculosis, pneumonia, diphtheria, and gastrointestinal infections. *"Since then, the yearly death rate from these diseases per 100,000 people has been reduced from 580 to 30!"*[1] Today, the major causes of death and morbidity result from behavioral factors such as accidents and violence or long-standing habits such as smoking, high-fat diets, lack of routine exercise, stress, and alcohol abuse.[2] The CDC of the U.S. Public Health Service has estimated that 50% of mortalities from the 10 leading causes of death in the United States can be traced to lifestyle factors.[3] Future improvements in health will come from managing the effects of unhealthy behaviors.[4,5]

From an osteopathic perspective, the behavioral sciences are the clinical and scientific application of biopsychosocial knowledge to the understanding and treatment of health and illness. Signs and symptoms of various types represent behavioral and physiologic imbalances and breakdowns in a patient's effort to adapt to and cope with change. Osteopathic philosophy is deeply rooted in the belief that a balance of physical, mental, and social systems are necessary for health. When one system is stressed or altered, the structure and function of other systems are stressed and altered as well. The primary care physician sees the repercussions from this imbalance as signs and symptoms of physical and behavioral illness. Somatic dysfunction and neuromusculoskeletal changes are common examples.

Most people wait until they feel something is wrong with them physically before they seek treatment. Over half of all patients in the United States with psychological problems are treated solely by a primary care provider.[6,7] These patients also have a higher incidence of organic illness.[8] During treatment, they use approximately twice as much routine medical care as those without psychological problems.[9]

Finally, all patients with physical illness of any kind have an emotional reaction to the illness. The consequences of these reactions and perceptions influence all aspects of their lives, at home, at work, and in society at large.

The goal of this section on behavioral sciences is to add clinical and scientific knowledge to the understanding and treatment of the patient as a unit of body, mind, and spirit. It includes a chapter on the management of pain, a common symptom in primary care. Other chapters explore:

Lifestyles
Life phases
Stress management
Health maintenance
Exercise
Psychoneuroimmunology

These chapters present some behaviorally based strategies for helping patients manage their physical health, thinking patterns and processes, emotional condition, and levels of functioning in relationships in the context of the patient's environment.

Osteopathically oriented patient care bases part of its philosophy on the understanding that biopsychosocial factors are interrelated and interdependently linked with disease and illness; a patient's health should be an optimal balance of physical, mental, emotional, and spiritual well-being.

REFERENCES

1. Centers for Disease Control and Prevention. *Ten Leading Causes of Death in the United States, 1977.* Washington, DC: Government Publishing Office; 1994.

2. National Center for Health Statistics. *Health of the United States, 1989.* Hyattsville, Md: Public Health Service; 1990.

3. Surgeon General. *Healthy People.* Washington, DC: Government Printing Office; 1979.

4. Surgeon General. *Report on Nutrition and Health.* Washington, DC: Government Printing Office; 1988.

5. Lalonde M. *A New Perspective on the Health of Canadians: A working document.* Ottawa: Government of Canada; 1974.

6. Regier D, Goldberg ID, Taube CH. The de facto U.S. mental health service system. *Arch Gen Psychiatry.* 1978;35:685.

7. Shapiro S, Skinner EA, Kessler LG, Von Korff M, German PS, Tischler G, Leaf PJ, Benham L, Cottler L, Regier DA. Utilization of health and mental health services: three epidemiologic catchment area sites. *Arch Gen Psychiatry.* 1984; 41:971.

8. Eastwood MR. Screening for psychiatric disorder. *Psychol Med.* 1971;1:197.

9. Hankin J, Oktay JS. *Mental Disorder and Primary Medical Care: An Analytic Review of the Literature.* Rockville, Md: Government Printing Office; 1979. National Institute of Mental Health, Series D No. (ADM) 78-661.

11. Lifestyles and Health Habits

GERALD G. OSBORN

Key Concepts

- **Impact of lifestyle and behavior on health and illness**

- **The importance of nutrition and health, including food pyramid**

- **Physical activity, and effects on disease and weight**

- **Obesity and disease, weight control and fitness**

- **Substance use, abuse, and treatment, including tobacco, alcohol, and illegal drugs**

- **Personal safety, especially in automobiles and homes**

- **Safe sexuality practices**

- **Healthy families and work satisfaction**

- **Stress anticipation and self-regulation**

- **Importance of personal support systems**

- **Doctor–patient relationship, and strategies for communication and change**

Historians of medicine describe in detail the dramatic changes that have taken place in medical education, practice, research, and technology in the 20th century. All agree that these changes in our system of health care have traded short-term mortality for long-term morbidity. It is ironic, however, that our modern high-technology advances in acute medical care have done little to improve overall human survival.

At the beginning of this century the average life expectancy was 47 years. Today it is 71.4 years for men and 78.4 years for women.[1] This increase results largely from a drastic reduction in infant mortality. Overall mortality has decreased because of effective public health measures aimed at disease prevention for large populations, not because of high technological medical procedures aimed at individuals. These fundamental preventive measures include those that provide us with clean air and water, high-quality affordable food, and safer work environments. Adding to this increased survival expectancy is a pharmaceutical industry providing us with immunizations to prevent the most common acute infectious diseases and with antibiotics to treat those infections we fail to prevent. Further strides in improving the long-term health of our patients depend on understanding the major impact of lifestyle and behavior on health and illness. This involves educating our patients, encouraging their active participation in and cooperation with health maintenance, and motivating them to make choices that promote healthy, vigorous, and enjoyable lives. Aging is inevitable, but for most people, ill health is not.

Assisting patients to live long and live well does not mean emphasizing prevention while neglecting high technological research and practice. Research and the development of new technologies are permanent and vital components in the continuum of health care. It does mean, however, that new preventive health care must be given at least equal status in the medical education and practice of the future if we as osteopathic physicians are to make a significant difference in the overall health of the population.

A systematic review of the ten most common causes of death in the United States reveals the importance of lifestyle and behavior, especially self-imposed risk, on health and illness (Table 11.1).[2]

NUTRITION

Science verifies Oscar Wilde's aphorism: *"You are what you eat."* Issues regarding nutrition need not generate the controversy and confusion so frequently portrayed in the popular media. Although controversies do exist, scientific nutritionists agree far more often than they disagree about what constitutes a healthy diet. Research consistently demonstrates that what

Table 11.1
The Leading Causes and Percentages of All Death in the United States

1. Heart disease	32.1%
2. Cancer	23.5%
3. Stroke	6.8%
4. Bronchitis and emphysema	4.5%
5. Accidents	3.9%
6. Pneumonia and influenza	3.6%
7. Diabetes mellitus	2.4%
8. HIV infection	1.6%
9. Suicide	1.4%
10. Chronic liver diseases	1.1%

Reprinted with permission from *The United States Surgeon General's Report on Nutrition and Health,* 1994.

157

people choose to eat is key to their general well-being as well as to specific illnesses, especially[3]:

Cardiovascular disease
Neoplastic disease
Diabetes
Osteoporosis

A diet consisting of the most currently determined proportions of protein, carbohydrate, and fat can radically improve one's overall level of health.

More useful than the former "Four Food Groups," which most patients learned in elementary school, is the more recently developed "Food Pyramid" (Fig. 11.1). The food pyramid helps clarify the newer and healthier proportions of proteins, carbohydrates, and fats in a more understandable visual construct. The typical American diet after World War II has been about right in the amount of protein, overly generous in simple carbohydrates and fats, and too meager in complex carbohydrates. The food pyramid helps guide patients toward these newer and healthier proportions (Table 11.2).

A simple readjustment of these proportions to current recommended levels offers significant protection from the development of cardiovascular disease and neoplastic illness. Further readjustment, encouraging foods lower in sodium and richer in calcium and potassium, offers protection against osteoporosis and hypertension.

Even patients who develop hypertension despite following these dietary recommendations experience better control with multimodal treatment, which includes becoming more aerobically fit and moderating alcohol use, along with the most current pharmacologic care.[4]

PHYSICAL ACTIVITY

Modern science consistently shows that a healthy life is an active life. Although the popular media provide many stories about people who compulsively exercise, these stories teach us nothing beyond the obvious consequences of fanaticism in any health endeavor. Health researchers in this area agree that higher levels of physical activity delay all-cause mortality primarily because of lower rates of cardiovascular disease and cancer. Their research shows also that physical activity is inversely associated with morbidity as well as mortality. The most recent comprehensive prospective study of physical activity and its relationship to health and specific illnesses demonstrated that the risk of all-cause and cause-specific mortality declines across physical fitness quintiles from the least fit to the most fit in both sexes.[5] These trends remained even after statistical adjustment for factors such as:

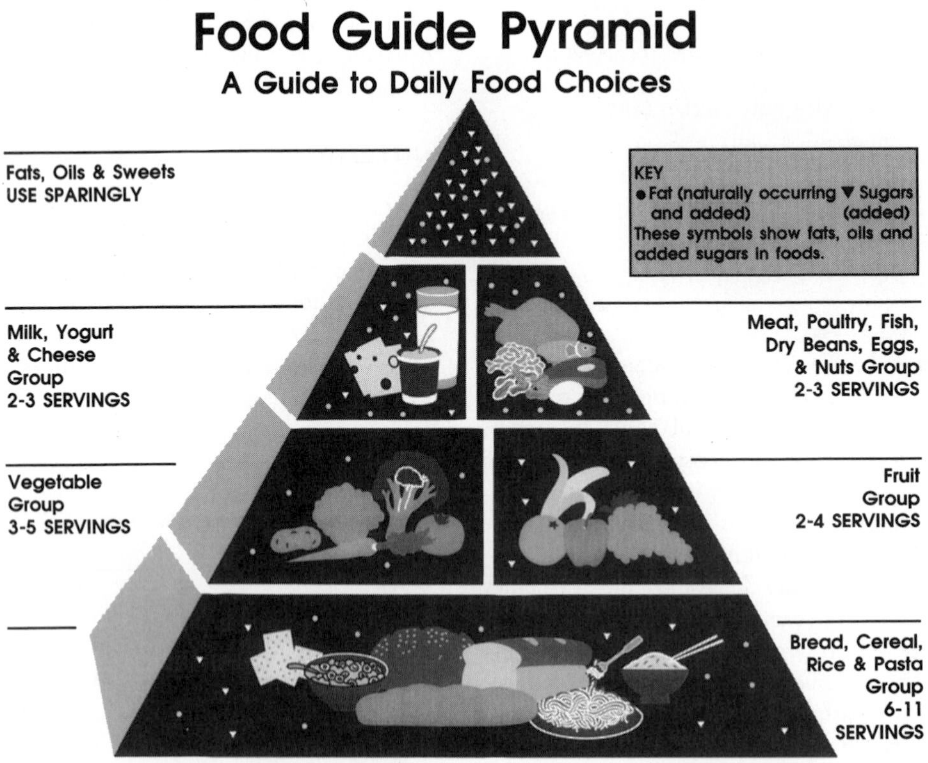

Figure 11.1. Use the Food Guide Pyramid to help you eat better every day...the Dietary Guidelines way. Start with plenty of Breads, Cereals, Rice, and Pasta; Vegetables; and Fruits. Add two to three servings from the Milk group and two to three servings from the Meat group. Each of these food groups provides some, but not all, of the nutrients you need. No one food group is more important than another—for good health you need them all. Go easy on fats, oils, and sweets, the foods in the small tip of the pyramid. (Reprinted with permission from U.S. Department of Agriculture. Human Nutrition Information Service; August 1992. Leaflet No. 572.)

Table 11.2
Percentage of Daily Calories Consumed

	Typical American Diet (%)	Recommended Diet (%)
Protein	15	15
Complex carbohydrates	20	40
Simple carbohydrates	25	15
Unsaturated fats	25	10
Saturated fats	15	20

Adapted from Pfeiffer GJ. *Taking Care of Today and Tomorrow. A Resource Guide for Aging and Long-Term Care.* Reston, Va; 1989. The Center for Corporate Health Promotion.

Age
Smoking
Cholesterol levels
Parental history of heart disease
Follow-up intervals

Like nutrition, the basic principles of exercise are straightforward and easy to understand for most people. Becoming more fit through exercise provides many benefits, which include reducing the risk of cardiovascular disease, osteoporosis, and noninsulin-dependent diabetes. General benefits of regular moderate exercise also include a reduction in feelings of anxiety and depression and even improvement in immune responses.

The most important principle to emphasize is fun and enjoyment. If all physicians would encourage their patients to pursue enjoyable physical activities, these activities would more likely become a component of a more healthy lifestyle. Most people find exercise more enjoyable when paired with a social activity. Therefore, physical activities that can be shared with family, friends, and colleagues are more likely to be continued as a part of ordinary social lives. The other important general principles include common sense, balance, and variety. The most systemically healthful types of physical activity are those that are aerobic. Aerobic exercise generally involves sustained, comfortable, submaximal effort as opposed to anaerobic short burst, quickly exhausting, "sprint-style" activities.

The first task is to begin almost regardless of initial level of fitness and then increase gradually. Most patients do not need cardiac stress tests or expensive, highly technical sports medicine evaluations. Patients should begin at a comfortable point consistent with their age and overall fitness level. They should then gradually increase to their self-determined level of maximal fun and enjoyment. Gentle stretching before warming up and after cooling down increases the likelihood of patients continuing their fitness programs. It does this by preventing injury, speeding up postexercise recovery, and decreasing the probability of delayed muscle soreness.

Americans spend approximately $8 billion per year on health spas and exercise clubs.[6] This might add to their social enjoyment, but becoming more fit need not be expensive. The most important expenses for any exercise program involve having proper shoes and safety equipment (such as a helmet for

bicycling, and wrist braces and elbow and knee pads for in-line skating) for the patient's selected activity. Careful attention must be paid to clothing when exercising in hot or cold weather. This is especially true for aged patients because of the increased risk of heat stroke, heat exhaustion, and hypothermia. Functional and protective clothing are essential. Style is optional. Other protective equipment important for safety involves protection from the sun. Good quality sunglasses and sun block should be part of most outdoor exercise equipment kits. Likewise, adequate hydration is extremely important. For aerobic exercise lasting less than one hour, cool water is generally sufficient. For longer periods of exercise or in hot, humid conditions, any of the popular "sports drinks" provide important additional glucose and electrolyte replacement, preventing dehydration and speeding postexercise recovery.

OBESITY

It is ironic that, along with the current emphasis on health and fitness, an increasing number of Americans are obese.[7] Health researchers and physicians engage in vigorous debate over the relative risks of being mildly to moderately overweight. They agree, however, that as patients become increasingly overweight, their health risks also increase. Both cross-sectional and cohort studies show associations between obesity and hyperlipidemia, hypertension, and hyperinsulinemia. These lead to the increased prevalence of coronary artery disease and noninsulin-dependent diabetes mellitus.[8–11] The following diseases are also more prevalent with increasing obesity[12,13]:

Some types of cancer
Degenerative joint disease
Sleep apnea
Gout
Gallbladder disease

An additional irony is that the caloric-restriction dietary treatments for obesity so often recommended are ineffective over time. Surveys of current literature indicate that dietary treatments alone do not work; some are detrimental and even dangerous. Recent surveys illustrate the complexity of the dilemma.[6,14] The definitive criteria for a risk/benefit analysis of the risk of obesity and the risks of weight loss diets are yet to be determined. The current approach to the problem is to suspend the singular concern for weight alone and focus on the overall level of fitness regardless of weight.

When patients ask about weight loss, include a complete discussion about physical fitness. Also emphasize the detrimental and ultimately ineffective results of caloric restriction diets. Remind patients frequently that nutritious food in the proportions shown in the Food Pyramid is the necessary fuel for healthy physical activity and basic body functions. Healthy eating, not calorie restriction, and daily aerobic activity are the cornerstones of living long and living well. A weight loss industry estimated at nearly $30 billion is supported more by the nearly universal American social stigma toward obesity than by a concern for health. Confronting our own aesthetic prejudices and those of our patients is an excellent place to start. The aesthetic ideal most promoted by the advertisement and fashion industries is simply unrealistic for most people.[6]

Following scientifically corroborated principles related to fitness is the best advice for the foreseeable future. Exciting research into the genetic controls involved in hunger, satiety, and lipid metabolism continues but new clinically applicable treatments are still far in the future.[15] Patients in the meantime are best served by deemphasizing weight and emphasizing fitness. Literature written by exercise physiologists for lay people emphasizes these points and is available to augment physicians' advice and counsel.[16]

SUBSTANCE USE AND ABUSE

Popular media attention and rancorous political debate tend to focus on illegal substance abuse. Yet the two legal substances, tobacco and alcohol, contribute more to the misery and ill health of our patients than do all the illegal substances combined. Focusing on those legal substances that constitute the most significant health hazards to our patients is central to primary care practice. Public health research on the matter is clear, despite political debate clouding the issues about the dangers of substance abuse.

Tobacco

The 1989 *U.S. Health & Prevention Profile* published by the CDC does not equivocate: *"Cigarette smoking is the single most preventable cause of death in our society."* The first Surgeon General's Report on Smoking was published in January of 1964. It created instantaneous, justifiable worldwide shock. The second report was issued in January of 1979. Joseph Califano, then Secretary of Health, Education, and Welfare, writing in the report's preface is even more forceful: *"this document reveals with dramatic clarity, that cigarette smoking is even more dangerous—indeed, far more dangerous—than was supposed in 1964."* The message to our patients must be clear, consistent, and firm: "If you don't smoke, please don't ever start; if you do, PLEASE STOP!"

This is clearly more easily said than done, but acting as an agent of change to promote our patients to stop smoking might be the best thing we ever do for them and their families. The vast majority of those who have stopped smoking have done so on their own, without formal or professional help of any kind (most by the "cold turkey" technique). The rest have required some level of professional guidance or a specific program. These people need the support of everyone to never quit quitting. Following are some useful methods to help people stop.[17]

1. Declare a date to stop and make it public. Many recommend a written statement including a request for the support and encouragement of family, friends, and coworkers. Some even publish this statement in a local paper.
2. Prepare to quit by making efforts to minimize stress, eat more

healthily than before, and begin a gradual and systematic program of physical fitness.
3. Attend to nicotine withdrawal by:
   - smoking fewer cigarettes per day, or only a portion of any cigarettes smoked;
   - switching to a different low tar and nicotine brand of cigarettes after each pack;
   - never buying more than one pack at a time;
   - continuing the gradual weaning process.
4. Break up learned smoking behavior patterns by:
   - waiting at least 10 minutes before lighting up when the craving begins;
   - distracting your attention from the craving to light up, i.e., go for a walk, drink water, relax, brush your teeth, etc.;
   - never offering or "bumming" a cigarette;
   - making smoking awkward and inconvenient, i.e., smoke only using the nondominant hand, and only while standing. Set the cigarette down between puffs, and lock up the cigarette pack between smokes.
   - thinking in terms of one-day-at-a-time. Rather than allowing yourself to think that you won't EVER be able to smoke again, tell yourself that TODAY you won't have a cigarette. One day is easier to manage than a lifetime.
   - staying positive and thinking of the endeavor as life enhancing rather than as a sacrifice.

On the quitting date and thereafter:

1. Make sure all cigarettes are gone.
2. Build in rewards: place the money you would have spent each week on smoking into a special savings account. To be fair, also figure spin-off savings, such as clothes, furniture, or car interiors damaged or ruined by cigarette burns, and place that amount into the account. Also place at least the cost of one visit to the doctor per year in the account.
3. Take your spouse or family out to dinner.
4. Prepare for times of craving by keeping substitutes handy, such as sugarless gum, sliced fruit, carrot or celery sticks.
5. Increase your fluid intake.
6. Keep a calendar or diary of your day-to-day progress.

Even with advice, some patients may require medications to assist their smoking cessation program. Medications useful for attenuating nicotine craving and the effects of withdrawal include nicotine polacrilex chewing gum and nicotine transdermal patches. Other medications include doxepin, a tricyclic antidepressant, and clonidine, a centrally-acting antihypertensive agent.[18,19] Other agents under investigation include corticotropin and citric acid aerosols.[20,21]

The most current comprehensive meta-analysis of smoking cessation interventions reveals that the most effective programs employ more than one modality for motivating behavioral change and involve both physicians and nonphysicians in an individualized face-to-face effort. These programs also provide a motivational message on multiple occasions, over the longest possible time period.[22]

As well as having a death rate 30 to 80% higher than nonsmokers, smokers consume a disproportionate share of health care resources. In 1985, the direct health care costs of smoking-related illnesses exceeded $16 billion. Calculations for the indirect costs such as lost productivity and earnings from excess mortality, disability, and premature death totaled more than $37 billion. Promoting smoking cessation for our patients is one of the most important primary prevention efforts.

Alcohol

The excessive use of alcohol accounts for a wide spectrum of health and social problems. Alcohol plays a causal or contributing role in deaths resulting from accidents, homicides, and suicides, as well as diseases such as cirrhosis and cancer. Beyond the negative effects on alcoholic individuals, alcoholism also has been estimated to negatively affect the lives and health of other people. Alcohol abuse is implicated in 50% of all divorces, in 45–68% of spouse abuse cases, and in up to 38% of child abuse cases. Alcohol abuse is especially harmful during pregnancy. Fetuses can be seriously harmed by alcohol. Fetal alcohol syndrome is now considered one of the three leading causes of prenatal mental retardation in the United States.

The alcohol abuser rarely changes this maladaptive behavior without strong, consistent, systematic, and long-term treatment. The first step involves accurate diagnosis so that the appropriate treatment can follow. A number of useful examiner and self-administered questionnaires are available, but the most useful diagnostic screen consists of four simple questions. The screen's acronym, CAGE, comes from the critical word in each question[23]:

1. Have you ever tried to *Cut* down on your drinking?
2. Are you *Angry or Annoyed* when people ask you about your drinking?
3. Do you ever feel *Guilty* about your drinking?
4. Do you ever take a morning *Eye* opener?

One positive response suggests the possibility of alcoholism and merits further exploration. Two positive answers make the likelihood extremely high. Three positive responses to questions 1 through 3, or a single positive response to question 4, is most likely diagnostic. The helpful features of these questions are their simplicity, sensitivity, and efficiency. These questions take under two minutes to ask and they should be included in every initial ambulatory and hospital admission workup. One of the most recent surveys of treatment options for alcoholism indicates that compulsory inpatient treatment followed by close monitoring for incipient relapse yields the best results.[24]

Alcohol abuse often is a symptom of psychiatric illness, most commonly anxiety and mood disorders. The ubiquity, social acceptance, and relative low cost of alcoholic beverages make drinking an effective short-term and maladaptive long-term manner of self-medication. If the alcohol problem is a primary disorder (alcohol-related disorder, DSM-IV),[25] substance abuse treatment alone suffices. If the alcohol problem is secondary to a psychiatric disorder (dual-diagnosis), specific attention to the underlying illness must be addressed simultaneously with the substance abuse disorder. The most useful recent method to diagnose psychiatric disorders efficiently and accurately in an ambulatory care setting is the Prime-MD (Primary Care Evaluation of Mental Disorders).[26] Prime-MD is a well-validated and highly reliable questionnaire that screens for psychiatric disorders. Patients fill out a questionnaire and the physician then follows up any positively endorsed target symptoms. It is specific for the most common psychiatric disorders presenting to primary care practice:

Mood
Anxiety
Somatoform disorders
Alcohol

If a psychiatric disorder is coexistent with alcoholism, referral for psychiatric consultation and comanagement is strongly recommended.

Illegal Substance Abuse

The effects of illegal substance abuse range from harmful to deadly; prevention is paramount. Efforts must be made on a spectrum of fronts, from governmental to personal, to discourage illegal substance use. Early diagnosis is imperative; in most cases treatment involves a lifelong recovery process. Self-help groups are useful; the most successful therapy usually involves multimodal treatment efforts by a multidisciplinary team. The primary care physician generally is the coordinator of the team-oriented treatment program.

PERSONAL SAFETY

Attending to personal and family safety is a major component of a preventive health program. Education, especially in the form of providing the best and most current information, is important for our patients. These issues can be incorporated into new patient screenings and provided for current patients in the form of pamphlets. Some safety videos are available.

Automobiles

Approximately 50,000 people in the United States die every year in automobile accidents. The automotive industry has made significant strides in making cars safer. Beyond seat belts, the two most important recent safety features are air bags and antilock brakes. Encourage patients to strongly consider these features when purchasing a car. The use of seat belts for everyone and extra protective seating for infants and small children in the rear seats are crucial. Other important points to emphasize include:

Keeping automobiles safer through proper maintenance, especially of brakes and tires
Obeying speed limits and all traffic regulations
Following all regulations when operating recreational vehicles
Wearing an approved helmet and protective clothing when operating a bicycle, moped, or motorcycle
Avoiding driving while taking sedative medications
Absolutely abstaining from drinking alcohol before driving

Home

Patients need to be provided with information about maintaining a safe environment in their homes. The following list is not inclusive of all issues; it represents significant areas where simple attention can make a major difference in household safety. The general nature of these recommendations do not minimize their importance for the health of our patients:

Keep medicines, harmful chemicals, and cleaning products secure and especially out of reach of children.

Prevent fires by judicious use of auxiliary home heating and by proper use of electrical appliances and outlets.

If fire should occur, minimize danger and damage by the use of smoke detectors and fire extinguishers. Also discuss and practice an escape plan with family members. Most local fire departments inspect and make recommendations at minimal cost.

Patients who choose to own guns should keep them in a secure place, unloaded, with appropriate locking mechanisms on the triggers. Ammunition likewise should be kept in a secure place separate from the weapons.

Keep power tools and lawn care equipment in good repair, especially their safety guards, and wear safety glasses and ear plugs during their operation.

Falls are a major cause of injury to older adults. Keep bathrooms and stairways free of obstacles and install appropriate lighting, handles, and banisters.

In winter, keep sidewalks and outdoor stairs clear of snow and ice. This can be a component of a family's fitness plan.

The home health checklist in Table 11.3 was specifically developed for elderly patients.[27]

SEXUALITY

Sexual behavior is a central component of healthy human functioning and a source of pleasure, comfort, and intimacy. Unfortunately, lack of knowledge about human sexuality can result in more than an unwanted pregnancy; it can result in illness and death. As well as providing the best possible counsel and information about contraception and family planning, physicians must also inform sexually active patients about safe sex practices. Risky practices should immediately be curtailed. These include:

Sex with an i.v. substance abuser

Sex with a prostitute, stranger, or person whose sexual history is unknown

Sex without the use of a condom

Sex with any person who engages in any of the above behaviors

Further advise patients that abstinence or sex with a noninfected person in a mutually monogamous relationship are the best methods for preventing all types of sexually transmitted diseases. For many people, however, this advice is not acceptable. In such cases, instruct them on minimizing risky behav-

Table 11.3
Home Hazard Checklist

Stairs
    Adequate illumination
    Top and bottom steps painted
    Nonskid treads
    Handrail: detached, graspable, end of rail shaped to signify bottom of stairway
    Risers painted in easily visible color
Living Areas—Carpets
    Edges tacked down completely
    Wall-to-wall with thick, shock-absorbent pads
    No throw rugs
Living Areas—Floors
    No highly polished floor surfaces
    Nonskid wax
    Thresholds removed
    No extension cords
    Access pathways free of low-lying furniture or other objects
    Baseboard lighting in halls
Other
    Emphasis on control of pets and small children to avoid causing trips
    No low couches, sharp-cornered furniture, or chairs on casters
    Light switches easily accessible to door or room
    Lighted switches
Bathroom
    Nonskid rubber mats in shower or bath
    Handrails in bath and by toilet
    Adequate lighting in bath and night light on access path
    Water temperature regulated at 43°C (110°F) or lower
    Clearly marked hot and cold faucets, preferably with separate controls
    Seat in tub
Kitchen
    Adequate illumination
    Stove controls large and clearly marked
    Large, easily grasped, protected handles on pots and pans
    Stored items easily accessible
Miscellaneous
    Smoke detectors with regularly checked, working batteries
    Adequate access and escape doors and windows
    Consider personal alarm system keyed to emergency system to be worn by high risk patient

Reprinted with permission from Snipes GE. Accidents in the elderly. *Am Fam Physician.* 1982;26:117–122.

ior. Although not 100% effective, consistent and correct use of condoms and other barrier contraceptives decrease risk and should be encouraged. Studies reveal that using contraceptives containing the spermicide nonoxynol-9 with condoms offers further protection if the barrier should fail.

FAMILY AND WORK

A healthy family life has long been seen as a source of comfort, joy, and inspiration. The family is the basic unit of society and needs the support of all. Fragmented, blended, or single-parent families need even more support. Families experiencing problems or who are in turmoil should be encouraged to seek help, whether it be support from caring relatives and friends, support groups, or professional family therapy. The primary care osteopathic physician should engage patients in constructive discussions about family health. A recent guide for health and long-term care[3] lists five qualities shared by healthy families:

A clear understanding of each member's role and responsibilities

An equitable distribution of power

Support and encouragement

Effective communication

A shared system of values or beliefs

It should become routine in osteopathic, family-oriented health care to inquire about these characteristics in medical history taking and to promote them at every therapeutic opportunity.

Doing work that one finds meaningful is a source of pride and personal fulfillment. The most tragic of work situations is to feel trapped in a work circumstance one despises. Many people, however, fail to take the steps necessary to make work more meaningful or to prepare themselves to change jobs or careers. If patients find that, despite their best efforts, they are unhappy in their work, they should be encouraged to survey their situation and develop a plan of change. Opportunities for alternative education and training are more abundant now than any time in the past. Even in the most difficult economic circumstances, education is the best investment a person can make.

Many people unhappy with their work never take full advantage of what the situation offers. Most larger employers have tuition-reimbursement plans for educational courses that go unused by the employees. Patients should also be encouraged to cultivate work friendships. If the work situations do not provide activities, patients can become agents of change who organize and develops work-related social or sports activities. Work need not be daily tedium and loathing; even planning for a change can be the activity that lifts patients' spirits and gives them hope and comfort.

STRESS

No life is without stress. There are, however, adaptive and maladaptive manners of coping even under the most stressful circumstances. Although there are many things that can happen in our patients' lives that are completely unexpected, many of life's difficulties can be anticipated and managed effectively. Many people accept high levels of stress in their lives but do not appreciate the high price they pay. Medical research has shown that a life lived in chronic stress can trigger and activate psychophysiologic disorders such as hypertension, peptic ulcer disease, and coronary artery disease.[28] More recent research in psychoneuroimmunology shows a relationship between stress and attenuation of immune responses.[29] Mental health researchers have long known that stress plays a strong role in various forms of anxiety and depression, as well as in many forms of substance use and abuse.

Most recently stress has been conceptualized as an organism's nonspecific response in an attempt to adapt to demands. Those demands can cover the spectrum of psychological, social, and physiologic functioning. Even ordinary day-to-day events, whether seen as positive or negative, involve adaptation to change. The concept of adaptation to change now dominates current thinking about stress. In 1967, Holmes and Rahe verified the stress of adaptation.[30] They developed a scale and assigned points to 43 life events to develop a stable and objective point of reference. They were not concerned with how people interpreted these events but merely with whether they happened. They demonstrated that the greater number of points a person scored over a 1-year period, the greater the probability of illness occurring within the next 2 years. The preventive implications are clear. Although a number of stress scales are now available, the Holmes & Rahe Social Readjustment Scale remains one of the most highly validated and widely used (Table 11.4).[30] This scale can be easily incorporated into medical practice and used liberally to help patients judge their own vulnerabilities and develop increasingly effective anticipatory coping strategies.

Stress can also be self-generated. The "Type A Personality" first described by Friedman and Rosenman has now become a household word.[31] Although it has been over-argued as a feature of coronary artery disease, the adaptive style of a person with these characteristics can hardly be envied. Research beyond Friedman and Rosenman's seminal work indicates that competitiveness, impatience, and difficulty dealing with anger and hostility are the core characteristics of coronary artery disease-prone personality styles. It might be difficult to completely alter these maladaptive styles, but counseling and education can modify them to the point where risks are significantly lowered.[32]

SUPPORT SYSTEMS

One of the major factors attenuating stress is an effective system of psychosocial support. Conceptualize a person's support system as a network of expanding concentric circles with one's closest confidant at the center. The importance of having a confidant cannot be overemphasized in buffering the effects of life stress. Most times this central confidant is a spouse or best friend, or it could be anyone who demonstrates care, concern, and respect for feelings and opinions. This confidant serves the preventive role of ensuring that all burdens and troubles can be shared. A system of support ranges from the confidence of having trusted advice available when planning a predicted transition to the comfort and nurturing of friends, neighbors, and community during unforeseen tragedy. The concept of the confidant includes helping professionals, such as the clergy or physicians, to provide assistance. Last, but certainly not least, religious faith provides the opportunity for a spiritual confidant. Patients for whom a spiritual dimension to life is important derive great comfort and benefit from their belief in power and meaning beyond what can be known in life in the world. Do not underestimate the positive healing power of spiritual belief systems.

Table 11.4
Social Readjustment Scale

Life Events	Holmes Points
1. Death of spouse	100
2. Divorce	73
3. Marital separation	65
4. Jail term	63
5. Death of close family member	63
6. Personal injury or illness	53
7. Marriage	50
8. Fired from job	47
9. Marital reconciliation	45
10. Retirement	45
11. Change in health of family member	44
12. Pregnancy	40
13. Sex difficulties	39
14. Having a baby	39
15. Business readjustment	39
16. Change in financial state	38
17. Death of close friend	37
18. Change to different line of work	36
19. Change in number of arguments with spouse	35
20. Mortgage large in relation to income	31
21. Foreclosure of mortgage or loan	30
22. Change in responsibilities in work	29
23. Son or daughter leaving home	29
24. Trouble with in-laws	29
25. Outstanding personal achievement	28
26. Spouse begins or stops work	26
27. Begin or end school	26
28. Change in living conditions	25
29. Change in personal habits	24
30. Trouble with boss	23
31. Change in work hours or conditions	20
32. Change in residence	20
33. Change in schools	20
34. Change in church activities	19
35. Change in recreation	19
36. Change in social activities	18
37. Small mortgage in relation to income	17
38. Change in sleeping habits	16
39. Change in number of family get-togethers	15
40. Change in eating habits	13
41. Vacation	13
42. Christmas	12
43. Minor violations of the law	11

Reprinted with permission from Holmes TH, Rahe RH. The social readjustment rating scale. *Jrnl Psychosomatic Research.* 1967;7:17–20.

DOCTOR–PATIENT RELATIONSHIP

The doctor–patient relationship remains the single most powerful healing tool of the physician. Technology is obviously important, but the power of the doctor–patient relationship allows "high tech" medicine to be used most wisely and to the greatest benefit. Primary and secondary prevention are two of the most important goals of the osteopathic physician, especially those in primary care practice. Physicians can do the most to encourage patients to become partners in their health care by using the power inherent in the doctor–patient relationship.

Most physicians agree that counseling is one of their most important tasks; paradoxically, most feel ineffective in this role. Many physicians feel generally pessimistic about their ability to motivate patients toward positive change. A recent review of doctor–patient relationship literature proposes four sequential strategies for motivating patient cooperation and encouraging patients to take more personal responsibility for their health.[33] The strategies are grounded in the patient compliance literature; they have also been expanded and integrated to include relevant social influences and psychotherapy research. A major contribution of this research has been the identification of the patient's health beliefs as a powerful predictor of cooperation with treatment. The review focuses on the critical importance of physician–patient relationship and interaction and then expands to the patient's relationship with the entire integrated primary care health team.

Patients who are not clear about what they are expected to do are unlikely to follow recommendations. A number of studies show major patient dissatisfaction with not receiving information from physicians; dissatisfied patients are less likely to cooperate (Table 11.5).[33]

Strategy 1: Informing the Patient

Never make assumptions about a patient's knowledge and understanding, regardless of socioeconomic class or level of education. First establish a confident level of baseline knowledge. Allowing patients time to explain their understanding of their problems allows for identification of incorrect or idiosyncratic perceptions as well as cultural beliefs. Keep verbal instructions clear; supplement them with pictures and printed materials if necessary. Avoid jargon whenever possible. Check patients' un-

Table 11.5
Communication Strategies for Behavior Change Encounters

Informing a patient
  Establish a baseline
  Explain and instruct
  Be clear, avoid jargon
  Check understanding
Obtaining a commitment to behavior change
  Make clear statement about desired behavior
  Explore readiness for change
  Obtain a commitment
Negotiating and tailoring regimen
  Identify congruence between physician's and patient's expectations
  Work toward plan that patient can agree to
  Tailor plan to patient's circumstances; disrupt routines minimally
  Consider a written contract
Attending to emotional responses
  Ask about and label feelings
  Legitimize feelings
  Support and encourage patient
  Be nonjudgmental
  Generate respectful statements

Reprinted with permission from Stoffelmayr B, Hoppe RB, Weber N. Facilitating patient participation: the doctor–patient encounter. *Primary Care.* 1989;16:265–278.

derstanding by asking them to repeat instructions or demonstrate how they might share the instructions with a third party.

Strategy 2: Obtaining Commitment from Patient

This involves the use of referent power, social power bestowed on a significant figure whose acceptance and approval are highly regarded and desired. The use of this referent power involves making direct and clear statements about a desired behavior change and eliciting the patient's commitment to cooperate. In the example of smoking, this would involve stating in a nonjudgmental but direct and authoritative manner the detrimental effects of smoking, and then asking the patient directly for a commitment to stop. Physicians' success in eliciting this commitment has been shown to be related to higher patient smoking cessation rates.

Strategy 3: Negotiating and Tailoring a Regimen

All treatment recommendations require a change from the patient's ordinary lifestyle. The more complex the changes recommended, the more difficult for the patient to cooperate. The goal of negotiation is to arrive at an agreement. Through negotiation and exploration of lifestyle and belief system issues, a regimen can be tailored to the individual life circumstance of each patient. When the negotiated agreement is written up as a mutually binding contract, it is more likely to be kept. A verbal agreement may also suffice.

Strategy 4: Attending to Patient's Emotional Responses

Here the quality of the doctor–patient relationship is crucial. Patients often complain, even bitterly so, about not being listened to or not having the opportunity to tell their story. Sto-

ries abound about technically competent but cold and aloof physicians. Research into doctor–patient relationships has shown patients' judgments about physicians are made on the basis of the physician's ability to recognize and respond to emotional concerns. Positive behavior change occurs more often in the presence of a high quality doctor–patient relationship. Patients in their distress and anxiety are not in the best condition to attend to the cognitive components of their instructions. Attending to emotions and setting patients at ease facilitates and promotes their understanding and cooperation.

Physicians also need to communicate their interest and concern for their patients nonverbally. Several tactics communicate care and interest:

Smiling
Sitting down
Using eye contact
Not appearing rushed

The osteopathic physician has a distinct advantage through the medium of touch and "the laying on of hands." Through the integrated verbal and nonverbal communication of care, trust is promoted, cooperation is maximized, and the doctor–patient relationship is strengthened.

The use of the integrated primary care team in this process is summarized in Table 11.6.[33]

CONCLUSION

Most of the task of providing the highest quality, cost-effective care involves teaching and motivating patients. The place to begin in creating the desired behavior we wish to see in our patients is to make them clearly reflected in our own. Many physicians have been successful in altering their personal health behavior habits for the better, but there is always room for

Table 11.6
Primary Care-Based Health Promotion

Activity	Outcome	Agent	Adjunct
Screening	Identification of risky behavior	Physician Nurses Other staff	Questionnaires Interactive Computer
Informing (Table 11.5)	Knowledge	Physician Nurse Health educator	Written materials Video station
Counseling (Table 11.5)	Commitment to behavior change	Physician	Written contract
Training/education	Skills to make short-term behavior change	Physician Nurses Other staff Health educator Nutritionists	Written materials
Emotional Support	Motivation	Entire PHCO team	Telephone calls/letters
Plan Adjustment/motivation	Long-term	Entire PHCO team	Telephone calls/letters Biologic measurement

Reprinted with permission from Stoffelmayr B, Hoppe RB, Weber N. Facilitating patient participation: the doctor–patient encounter. *Primary Care.* 1989;16:265–278.

improvement. Doctor means teacher, and the old maxim remains sound: "Example isn't the best way to teach, it is the only way to teach."

REFERENCES

1. National Center for Health Statistics. *United States Health and Prevention Profile.* Hyattsville, Md: U.S. Department of Health & Human Services; 1994. Public Health Service. (All statistics are taken from this source unless otherwise stated.)

2. *The United States Surgeon General's Report on Nutrition and Health, 1988.*

3. Adapted from: Pfeiffer GJ. *Taking Care of Today and Tomorrow: A Resource Guide for Aging and Long-Term Care.* Reston, Va: The Center for Corporate Health Promotion; 1989.

4. Gifford RW Jr, et al. The fifth report of the Joint National Committee on detection, evaluation, and treatment of high blood pressure (JNC-V). *Arch Intern Med.* January 25, 1993;153:154–183.

5. Blair SN, Kohl WH III, Paffenbarger RC Jr. Physical fitness and all-cause mortality. *JAMA.* 1989;262:2395–2401.

6. Garner DM, Wooley SC. Confronting the failure of behavioral and dietary treatments for obesity. *Clin Psychol Rev.* 1991;11:729–780.

7. Kuczmarski RJ. Prevalence of overweight and weight gain in the United States. *Am J Clin Nutr.* 1992;55:4955–5025.

8. Atkinson RL, et al. Weight cycling. National Task Force on the prevention and treatment of obesity. *JAMA.* 1994;272(15):1196–1202.

9. National Institutes of Health. Health implications of obesity: consensus development conference statement. *Ann Intern Med.* 1985;103:1073–1077.

10. Hubert HB, Feinlaub M, et al. Obesity as an independent risk factor for cardiovascular disease: a 26-year follow-up of participants in the Framingham heart study. *Circulation.* 1983;67:968–977.

11. Andres R, et al. Long-term effects of change in body weight on all-cause mortality. *Ann Intern Med.* October 1993;19(7):737–743.

12. Hubbard VS. *Overview of obesity and its health implications.* Nashville, Tenn: Health Implications of Obesity Series; 1992;5:1–13. Meharry.

13. Van Itallie TB, Lew EA. *Assessment of morbidity and mortality risk in the overweight patient. Treatment of the Seriously Obese Patient.* New York, NY: Guilford; 1992:3–32.

14. Brownell KD, Rodin J. The dieting maelstrom. Is it possible and advisable to lose weight? *Am Psychol.* 1994;49(9):781–791.

15. Zhang Y, et al. *Nature.* December 1994;372:425–432.

16. Bailey C. *Smart Exercise, Burning Fat, Getting Fit.* Boston, Mass: Houghton Mifflin Co; 1994.

17. Sees KL. Cigarette smoking, nicotine dependence, and treatment. *West J Med.* 1990;152:578–584.

18. Edwards NB, Murphy JK, et al. Doxepin as an adjunct to smoking cessation: a double-blind pilot study. *Am J Psychiatry.* 1989;146(3):373–376.

19. Franks P, Harp J, Bell B. Randomized controlled trial of clonidine for smoking cessation in a primary care setting. *JAMA.* 1989;262(21):3011–3013.

20. McElhancy JL. Repository corticotropin injection as an adjunct to smoking cessation during the initial nicotine withdrawal period: results from a family practice clinic. *Clin Ther.* 1989;11(6):854–861.

21. Rose JE, Hickman CS. Citric acid aerosol as a potential smoking cessation aid. *Chest.* 1987;92(6):1005–1008.

22. Kottke TE, Battista RN, et al. Attributes of successful smoking cessation interventions in medical practice. A meta-analysis of 39 controlled trials. *JAMA.* 1988;259(19):2883–2889.

23. Ewing JA. Detecting alcoholism, the CAGE Questionnaire. *JAMA.* 1984;252:1905–1907.

24. Walsh DC, Hingson RW, et al. A randomized trial of treatment options for alcohol abusing workers. *N Engl J Med.* 1991;325:775–782.

25. American Psychiatric Association. *Diagnostic and Statistical Manual of Mental Disorders.* 4th ed. Alcohol-Related Disorders. Washington, DC; 1994:194–205.

26. Spitzer RL, Williams JBW, et al. Utility of a new procedure for diagnosing mental disorders in primary care: the PRIME-MD 1000 Study. *JAMA.* December 1994;272(22):1749–1756. (PRIME-MD materials are available from Dr. Robert Spitzer, Biometrics Research Department, New York State Psychiatric Institute, Unit 74, 722 W. 168th Street, New York, NY 10032.)

27. Snipes GE. Accidents in the elderly. *Am Fam Physician.* 1982;26:117–122.

28. Kiecolt-Glaser JK, Glaser R. Psychosocial factors, stress, disease, and immunity. In: Glaser R, ed. *Psychoneuroimmunology.* New York, NY: Academic Press; 1991:849–867.

29. Cohen S, Tyrell DAJ, Smith AP. Psychological stress and susceptibility to the common cold. *N Engl J Med.* 1991;325:606–612.

30. Holmes TH, Rahe RH. The social readjustment rating scale. *J Psychosom Res.* 1967;7:17–20.

31. Friedman M, Rosenman RH. *Type-A Behavior and Your Heart.* New York, NY: Knopf; 1973.

32. Friedman M, Ulmer D. *Treating Type-A Behavior and Your Health.* New York, NY: Knopf; 1984.

33. Stoffelmayr B, Hoppe RB, Weber N. Facilitating patient participation: the doctor-patient encounter. *Prim Care.* 1989;16:265–278.

12. Introduction to Psychoneuroimmunology

DAVID A. BARON

Key Concepts

- **Effects of stress on health and disease, and field of psychoneuroimmunology**

- **Conceptualization of brain and immune functioning as an interactive system**

- **Integrated and similar functioning of central nervous, immune, and neuroendocrine systems**

- **Research on immunosuppression and taste aversion**

- **Alternative treatments**

- **Altered immune function with mood disorders**

- **Relationship between emotional stress and altered immune response**

- **Assessment and management of patient stress**

The concept of a connection between the mind and physiologic functioning is an old one. Hippocrates, the father of Western medicine, wrote in the 4th century BC that disease was the result of disharmony among the mind, the body, and the environment.

EFFECTS OF STRESS ON HEALTH AND DISEASE

Throughout history, medical researchers and clinicians have observed and reported the effects of stress on health and disease. Despite the general acceptance of this idea, it is difficult to define stress. Early concepts focused on stress as a universal force acting on a passive body, with all people reacting in the same way to a disruption. The modern concept emphasizes that stress is not what happens but rather how a person reacts to an event. Distress arises when a person perceives that imposed demands (stress) exceed his or her ability to cope. There is a physiologic response to stress. The stress response involves activation of the hypothalamic-pituitary-adrenal (HPA) axis; it is modulated by the autonomic nervous system (ANS). The ANS maintains balance through its two primary components, the sympathetic branch regulating arousal and the parasympathetic branch inducing relaxation. How stress and other noninfectious stimuli affect the body's defenses against disease is not yet completely understood.

PSYCHONEUROIMMUNOLOGY

This chapter introduces the field of psychoneuroimmunology (PNI). PNI conceptualizes the brain and immune functioning as an interactive system. As Rubinow[1] points out, the immune, neuroendocrine, and central nervous systems are stimulus response systems that are similar in the functions they subserve and tightly integrated in their actions. The reciprocal regulatory effects of these systems provide a basis (but not proof) for the belief that brain-immune interactions are clinically relevant and not reducible to characteristics of component systems.

Research

Research from the past decade confirms the tightly integrated and surprisingly similar functioning of the central nervous, immune, and neuroendocrine systems. Pert[2] suggested that the intimate integration of these three systems warrants their consideration as a single system. All three systems can function as sensory and effector organs, recognizing foreign antigen (immune) or incoming physiologic signals (endocrine or nervous). All three transmit signals and information as part of their basic function. Specifically, the immune response can be modulated by input from the nervous and neuroendocrine systems. Rubinow writes: *"The high degree of similarity and integration of the immune, central nervous, and neuroendocrine systems is teleologically sensible because their common task is to persevere homeostasis and assure the constancy and integrity of body cells and tissues, a task for which integration and regulatory redundancy are obligatory."*[1]

In many ways, this hypothesis is similar to osteopathic philosophy. In addition to musculoskeletal integrity, emphasis on total body homeostasis is a fundamental tenet of osteopathic teaching. The basic principles of PNI, like Engle's[3] biopsychosocial model, stress the interconnectedness or hard-wiring of emotions to the body's physiologic functioning.

Despite centuries of interest, research on the complex interactions between the central nervous system (CNS) and the immune system has only taken place in modern medicine. This is in part because of the lack of understanding of the complexities of immune functioning and the limited availability of biologic probes to measure the impact of one system on another. The term "psychoimmunology" was coined as recently as 1964 by George F. Solomon, in his classic paper, "Emotions, immunity, and disease: A speculative theoretical integration."[4]

In this paper, Solomon offers a theoretical explanation of how emotional states can diminish immunocompetence, ultimately resulting in physical disease. These speculations were of significant interest to the mental health community, particularly psychologists and psychiatrists. However, they did not enjoy a similar level of acceptance by the medical community at large, and especially not by immunologists. Without data derived from well-controlled research studies, the consensus was that something as imprecise and variable as emotion could not have an impact on a seemingly hard-wired physiologic response like immune functioning. No reasonable explanation existed regarding how these systems could talk to each other. There was no reason why they should. Despite repeated reports of illness following a significant emotional stressor, nothing more substantial than observational or anecdotal reports existed to convince the nonbelievers. It was Ader's[5] accidental finding that immunosuppression could be classically conditioned in mice, by pairing taste aversion (saccharin) with an immunosuppressive medication (cyclophosphamide), that ignited research interest in PNI.

Alternative Treatments

For the first time, direct evidence demonstrated the potential for external manipulation of the immune system. Intriguing questions followed. If immunologic response could be behaviorally conditioned to turn off, could it be conditioned to turn on or increase? Could this help explain the patient who dies shortly after giving up the will to live, or conversely, those who refuse to succumb and ultimately defy the odds to survive life-threatening conditions? These and related questions have driven PNI research and a plethora of mind–body and alternative treatments. Although controversial, PNI research might explain in part the therapeutic effects of many alternative medicine interventions. The establishment of the Office of Alternative Medicine by the National Institutes of Health underscored the clinical significance of PNI research. The goal of this new office is to promote and support research in mind–body medicine and unconventional treatment strategies.

Mood Disorders

In addition to conditioned immune suppression, altered immune function has been reported in patients with mood disorders. The relationship between clinical depression and physical illness was reported in the 2nd century by the Greek physician, Galen. He observed that melancholic (depressed) women were especially susceptible to breast cancer. In an effort to replicate and further explain this observation, Levy and colleagues[6] measured natural killer (NK) cell activity (a measure of immune competence) and psychological stress in women with breast cancer. They found NK activity to be a reliable and valid predictor of the patients' prognosis relative to their lymph node status. In a separate study, they reported that 51% of baseline NK activity changes could be accounted for by assessing a patient's adjustment to the diagnosis, depressive symptoms, and perceived lack of social supports.[6] They con-

cluded, based on multiple clinical trials, that differences in NK activity and overall prognosis could be predictably determined by assessing baseline stress as measured by emotional adjustment, depression or fatigue, and lack of social supports.

Emotional Stress

A number of studies over the past decade have explored the relationship between emotional stress and altered immune response. Stein[7] reported behavioral pathology and neuropsychiatric impairment of patients with autoimmune and viral conditions associated with systemic lupus erythematosus (SLE) and multiple sclerosis (MS). Early studies in the 1970s reported an increased prevalence of herpes simplex virus in patients with a psychotic depression when compared with age-matched nondepressed controls. Unfortunately, these studies did not monitor any specific immune parameters. Schleifer and colleagues[8] demonstrated that depressed patients had a decreased number of peripheral T cells compared with those of nondepressed control subjects. Their data suggested that the functional activity of lymphocytes, as well as the number of circulating immunocompetent cells, is reduced in patients with clinical depression. They also speculated that the altered immune functioning in patients with depression might be related to the severity of their depressive symptoms.

In addition to exploring the effect of stress on patients, studies have been reported on immunologic alterations in healthy people under stress. Kiecolt-Glaser et al.,[9] studying medical students at Ohio State University, found that examinations (a stressor for virtually all students) brought about a decline in NK activity. They observed a decrease by as much as 90% in interferon-γ production, a potent stimulator of NK cell growth and activity. L. Tamarkin (personal communication, 1992), using a similar study design, demonstrated a drop in cytokine functioning (another component of the immune system) in high school students at examination time. Although a decline of overall immunologic functioning is necessary to develop disease, this in and of itself is not sufficient. Few of these students became ill, yet their vulnerability to disease increased. To date, a temporary decline in immunocompetency has not been demonstrated to directly affect the onset of an illness. Although of paramount clinical importance, the answer to the question of how much of a drop results in a person getting sick remains elusive.

CONCLUSION

The primary goal of medical educators in the United States is to train medical students to diagnose and treat organic pathologic conditions. Much of what takes place in the practice of clinical medicine and surgery is based on conventional wisdom and long-standing patterns of practice. Mental health issues are often ignored and viewed as unimportant for treating physically ill patients. Too often psychiatrists are considered experts only in mental illness, rather than medical specialists. In the biopsychosocial model, psychosocial issues are seen as separate and distinct from biologic concerns. Yet consider the following facts:

Emotionally distressed patients visit the doctor and are hospitalized more frequently than nondistressed patients. People with emotional distress commonly visit their doctors with physical symptoms and complaints (dizziness, headaches, fatigue, pain, etc.) and never report mood symptoms.

Nearly two thirds of all physician visits fail to confirm a biologic diagnosis.

Medical illness can precipitate emotional distress, which complicates medical treatment and increases medical costs.

Emotional distress often goes unrecognized and untreated in medical encounters.

Appropriate mental health treatment reduces emotional distress, medical utilization, and costs. Savings from reduced medical costs can offset the cost of providing mental health treatment and result in lower overall health care costs.

Unfortunately, these facts are often ignored, leading to a striking mismatch between the true needs of patients and the health care services offered. The result is often ineffective care, frustration for both patient and physician, and the waste of ever-shrinking health care resources.

If nothing else, PNI research underscores the need to assess patients' emotional distress. Elicit information on stress levels and recommend appropriate stress reduction strategies; this might have a positive impact on a patient's overall health. For patients suffering from ongoing illness, attending to these issues can improve response to treatment. Emphasize the importance of lifestyle alterations such as cutting down on caffeine, maintaining a healthy diet, stopping smoking, and exercising regularly. Tailor other stress reduction strategies to the patient's lifestyle; they can be a key component in disease prevention. It is the responsibility of physicians to educate their patients about the importance of maintaining a healthy lifestyle. Make patients aware of target organs and areas particularly vulnerable to stress, such as the heart, kidney, gastrointestinal tract, and musculoskeletal system. This education should include protecting patients from claims of miracle cures or unsound, potentially dangerous interventions.

Be cautious not to overinterpret or overgeneralize clinical observations. A laboratory finding demonstrating a decrease in an immune parameter does not necessarily predict a change in health status. Our understanding of the intricate complexity of immunology and neuroscience is growing rapidly. The need to be open to new hypotheses is important, but one must still maintain a critical view. As with osteopathic concepts, the key to acceptance in the medical community, and ultimately to

enhancing the welfare of all people, is adherence to the principles of methodologically sound scientific research. Observation and case reports are an important preliminary step that must be followed by double-blind controlled trials. The challenge to the next generation of researchers and physicians is to continue and expand the work in progress in this exciting field.

REFERENCES

1. Rubinow DR. Brain, behavior, and immunity: an interactive system. *J Natl Cancer Inst.* 1990;(Monograph No. 10):79–82.
2. Pert CB, Ruff MR, Weber RJ, et al. Neuropeptides and their receptors: a psychosomatic network. *J Immunol.* 1985;135:820–826.
3. Engel GL. The need for a new medical model: a challenge for biomedicine. *Science.* April 8 1977;196:129–136.
4. Solomon GF, Moos RH. Emotions, immunity, and disease. *Arch Gen Psychiatry.* 1964;11:657–674.
5. Ader R, Cohen N. Behaviorally conditioned immuno suppression. *Psychsom Med.* 1975;37:333–340.
6. Levy SR, Lippman M, d'Angelo T. Correlation of stress factors with sustained depression of natural killer cell activity and predicted prognosis in patients with breast cancer. *J Clin Oncol.* 1987;5:348–353.
7. Stein M. Future directions for brain, behavior, and the immune system. *Bull N Y Acad Med.* July 1992;68(3):390–410.
8. Schleifer SJ, Keller SE, Siris SG, et al. Depression and immunity. *Arch Gen Psychiatry.* 1985;42:129–133.
9. Kiecolt-Glaser JK, Garner W, Speicher C, et al. Psychosocial modifiers of immunocompetence in medical students. *Psychosom Med.* 1984;46:7–14.

SUGGESTED READINGS

Benson H, Klipper MZ. *Mind Body Medicine.* Yonkers, New York: Consumer Reports Books; 1993.

Caudill MA. *Managing Pain Before It Manages You.* New York, New York: Guilford; 1995.

Fancher, Raymond E: *Pioneers of Psychology.* New York, New York: WW Norton & Company; 1979.

Laudenslager M, Ryan S, Drugan R, et al. Coping and immunosuppression: inescapable but not escapable shock suppresses lymphocyte proliferation. *Science.* 1983;221:568–570.

Monjan AA, Collector MI. Stress induced modulation of the immune response. *Science.* 1977;196:307–308.

Schleifer SJ, Keller SE, Bond RN, Cohen J, Stein M. Major depressive disorder and immunity: role of age, sex, severity, and hospitalization. *Arch Gen Psychiatry.* 1989;46:81–87.

Schleifer SJ, Keller SE, Meyerson AT, et al. Lymphocyte function in major depressive disorder. *Arch Gen Psychiatry.* 1984;41:484–486.

Solomon GF. Stress and antibody response in rats. *Int Arch Allergy Immunol.* 1969;35:97.

Weiner H. *Perturbing the Organism: The Biology of Stressful Experience.* Chicago, Ill: University of Chicago Press; 1992.

13. Pain Management

JOHN A. JEROME

Key Concepts

- **History and theories of pain management**

- **Different types of pain, including acute and chronic**

- **Areas of information flow with chronic pain: perceptual field, pattern recognition, pattern appraisal**

- **Use of medications and anesthetics in pain management**

- **Osteopathic approach to pain management**

Pain is the most common complaint for which individuals seek medical attention. The costs associated with this medical attention are estimated to be 60 to 90 billion dollars annually.[1-2] When successful, pain treatment that relies on the traditional medical model can be gratifying for both physicians and patients. Relief of discomfort can be accomplished safely and easily with nonprescription medications and/or spinal manipulation. However, effective treatment using this model depends on two factors:

1. Clearly identifiable and correctable biologic mechanisms underlying the pain
2. A straightforward treatment strategy that interrupts the pain signal

Unfortunately, only a small subset of pain cases meets these criteria. For the vast majority of patients with chronic pain, either the underlying cause cannot be clearly identified or medically corrected, or numerous attempts surgically or biochemically to decrease the pain signal fail to provide significant long-term relief.

The founding principles of osteopathic medicine are based on the observations that people possess a natural healing power and that there are inherent recuperative, restorative, and rehabilitative powers. As Irvin Korr writes in Section I, *"We recover from illnesses, fevers drop, blood clots and wounds heal, broken bones reunite, infections are overcome, skin eruptions clear up, and even cancers are known to undergo spontaneous remission."* Chronic pain is unique in that the organized, integrated unity and collaboration of body components are not functioning in a restorative manner. The person in pain has a wonderfully evolved endogenous opioid system built to relieve pain, and yet this natural ability to adjust and adapt has failed. Such pain problems are so remarkably resistant to conventional medical therapies that chronic pain is one of the most frequent causes of disability in the United States today.[2]

For the osteopathically trained physician, the musculoskeletal system is the primary means of pain expression. In the musculoskeletal system, unique sensory, affective, and evaluative expressions of pain and its related behavior are made possible by the coordinated contractions and relaxations of striated muscles. It is inevitable that continuous pain causes both structural and functional disturbances in the musculoskeletal system. In turn, pain causes repercussions elsewhere in the body and has an impact on the total functioning of the person in pain.

The osteopath recognizes that the person in pain is more than a biologic event. He or she is a thinking, feeling problem solver. That person, when confronted with pain, actively seeks information, makes decisions, and attempts to put forth his or her best effort possible in adapting to the painful condition. Osteopathic treatment is aimed at the person in pain, not the pain in the muscle or the pain in the head. The dualistic separation of mind and body, which currently is universally rejected in osteopathic philosophy, is still unfortunately the basis of much clinical medical practice and biomedical research.[3]

HISTORY OF PAIN THEORY

The modern history of pain theory began with Descartes (1596–1650), who first formally considered the brain, rather than the heart or some other organ, as the site where pain sensation was recognized. He described the sequence of a pain event in three stages:

1. Onset of tissue damage
2. Movement of a signal up a transmission line
3. Conscious experience of, and behavioral response to, the pain

Descartes wrote (Fig. 13.1), *"If for example fire (A) comes near the foot (B), the minute particles of this fire, which as you know move with great velocity, have the power to set in motion the spot of the skin of the foot which they touch, and by this means pulling upon the delicate thread (c, c) which is attached to the spot of the skin, they open up at the same instant the pore (d, e) against which the delicate thread ends, just as by pulling at one end of a rope makes to strike at the same instant a bell which hangs at the other end."* Continuous pain that could not be linked to a tissue-damaging event was considered a mystery, a punishment, or a mental problem.

The first systematic studies of pain did not take place until

Clinical practice guidelines* for the assessment and treatment of adults with acute low back pain problems.

The following are principal conclusions of this guideline:

- The initial assessment of patients with acute low back problems focuses on the detection of "red flags," which are indicators of potentially serious spinal or nonspinal pathologies.

- In the absence of red flags, imaging studies and further testing of patients are not usually helpful during the first 4 weeks of low back pain.

- Relief of discomfort can be accomplished most safely with nonprescription medication and/or spinal manipulation.

- While some activity modification might be necessary during the acute phase, bed rest over 2 days is not helpful and should be avoided.

- Low-stress aerobic activities can be safely started in the first 2 weeks of symptoms to help avoid debilitation; exercises to condition trunk muscles are commonly delayed at least 2 weeks.

- Patients recovering from acute low back problems are encouraged to return to work or to their normal daily activities as soon as possible.

- If low back symptoms persist, further evaluation might be indicated.

- Patients with sciatica might recover more slowly, but further evaluation can also be safely delayed in most cases. Loss of motor function in bladder and bowel is a major exception.

- Within the first 3 months of low back pain, only patients with evidence of serious spinal pathologic conditions, or severe, debilitating symptoms of sciatica, and physiologic evidence of specific nerve root compromise corroborated on imaging studies can be expected to benefit from surgery on a carefully selected basis.

- With or without surgery, 80% of patients with sciatica recover eventually.

- Nonphysical factors (such as psychological or socioeconomic problems) can be addressed in the context of discussing reasonable expectations for recovery.

*Acute Low Back Problems in Adults. Clinical Practice Guideline No. 14. Rockville, Md: Agency for Health Care Policy and Research, Public Health Service; December 1994. US Dept of Health and Human Services publication 95-0643.

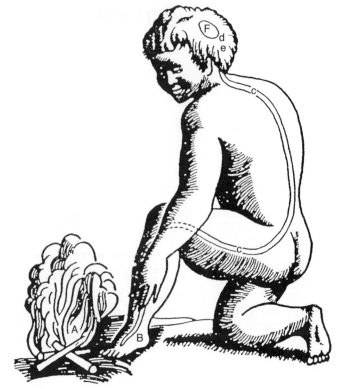

Figure 13.1. Descartes' (1664) concept of pain pathway. Fire (A), foot (B), thread (c, c), pore (d, e). (Reprinted with permission from Melzack R, Wall PD. Pain mechanisms: a new theory. *Science.* 1965;150:971.)

the early 19th century, when physiology emerged as a true experimental science. These early studies provided evidence that Descartes' theory of pain transmission lines and other mechanisms responsible for adverse pain signals were overly simplistic. Since that time, rather than focusing on the unity of mind and body, pain research has focused instead on mapping and describing the pain transmission (nociceptive) pathways. Consequently, the evolution of pain theory has closely paralleled the increasing knowledge of sensory physiology. Since current concepts of pain management are based on historical transmission theories, a brief outline of those theories follows.

Specificity Theory

Specificity theory asserts that pain is an independent sensation. Pain has its own sensory transmission apparatus that is associated with touch. The elements of touch are:

Itch
Pain
Heat
Cold

These sensations are a function of a direct system that conveys information from the sensory organ to the brain center responsible for that sensation.

Summation Theory

Summation theory argues that pain results from excessive stimulation of touch sensors. It asserts that any sensory stimulus is capable of producing pain if it reaches sufficient intensity.

Pattern Theory

Pattern theory suggests that all nerve endings at the periphery are alike, so that a pattern of impulses produces pain through the overstimulation of these sensory nerves.

Central Summation Theory

Central summation theory asserts that reverberatory activity in the spinal cord, which projects signals to brain mechanisms, is the process underlying the perception of pain in response to intense stimulation or tissue damage.

Fourth Theory of Pain

The "Fourth Theory of Pain" proposes that pain can be separated into two components: perception of pain and psychological reaction to pain. It assumes a one-to-one relationship between the intensity of the incoming noxious signal and the resultant experience of pain. The psychological reaction to the pain is assigned a minor role. This theory is another version and refinement of the earlier specificity and summation theories of pain. It differs from earlier theories in that the psychological perception of pain is recognized as a component of the pain experience. There has been no further research or conceptual development of this theory. Investigations into the psy-

chological components of the pain experience continue to lag behind the study of physical transmission mechanisms.

Sensory Interaction Theory

The sensory interaction theory identifies the existence of two systems involved in the transmission of pain and other sensory information:

1. A slow system that involves the thinly myelinated fibers
2. A fast system that involves the large myelinated fibers

According to this theory, both systems transmit signals into the spinal cord. The cord sums the inputs and produces a neural pattern that is transmitted to the brain, where it is perceived as pain.

Gate-Control Theory

The gate-control theory of pain[4-5] blends the scientifically agreed on elements of the earlier signal transmission theories and emphasizes signal modulation at the spinal cord. This theory predominates today. The model is heuristic and incorporates evidence of subcortical information processing mechanisms that can influence the experience of pain. This includes specialization, central summation, patterning, and modulation of inputs (Fig. 13.2). These mechanisms were all cornerstones of earlier theories. The gate-control theory also includes the influence of psychological events on the perception of pain.

A limitation of the gate-control theory of pain is that psychological events are not defined or differentiated from each other but are all placed under the umbrella term "Central Con-

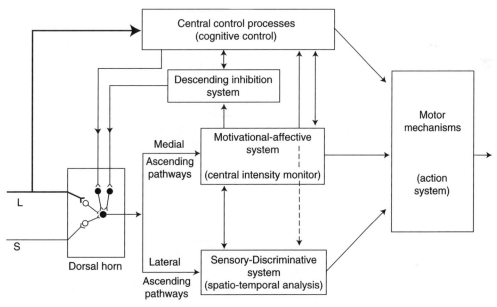

Figure 13.2. Conceptual model of sensory, motivational, and central control determinants of pain according to Melzack and Casey. Output of T cell in dorsal horn projects to sensory-discriminative system via lateral ascending system, and to motivational-affective system via medial ascending system. Central control "trigger" is represented by *heavy line* running from large fiber system to central control processes. Interaction between motivational-affective and sensory discriminative systems is indicated by *arrows*. (Slightly modified from Bonica JJ, sec. ed. *The Management of Pain, I.* Philadelphia, Pa: Lea and Febiger; 1990:90.)

trol Process." Since the advent of gate theory, research on the spinal thalamic tract and gating mechanisms has added to the development of this theory. The gate-control theory has been refined to incorporate developing knowledge of pain physiology.

Signal transmission is the main focus of all these pain theories. The consequence of this preference for transmission models of pain is that the central control processes become an inconsequential repository for the mysterious psychological "stuff" that is associated with the experience of pain. The psychological area includes:

Attention
Cognition
Perceptions
Affect
Personality traits
Early pain experiences
Social context
Cultural background
Information processing style
Mind
Self
Meaning of pain

The organization, let alone function, of the central control processes must be at least as complex as that of the physiologic pain systems studied thus far.[4]

Bonica took a significant step toward incorporating psychological components into chronic pain models. He included the brain stem pain inhibitory systems into the evolving blueprints of pain signal transmission within the brain. According to Bonica,[5] one structure of the descending inhibitory system, the periaqueductal gray, *"receives important input from such rostral structures as the frontal and insular cortex and other parts of the cerebrum that are involved in cognition"*[(p108)]. As understanding of the brain's involvement in pain transmission grows, a complete blueprint of the transmission system must include a description of how the conscious human mind processes pain information.

For the osteopathic physician, the mind and body are inseparable. The experience of pain as displayed in the musculoskeletal system is influenced by factors such as these:

Genetics
Lifelong learning and conditioning
Use and abuse of the body
Social and cultural factors that shape the individual's perception of pain

DEFINING PAIN

In 1979, the Subcommittee on Taxonomy of the International Association for the Study of Pain redefined pain by integrating both physiologic and psychological components. This modification was published in *Pain* (International Association for the Study of Pain[6]) as well as in the proceedings of the *Third World Congress on Pain*[7] and in *JAMA*[8]:

Pain: An unpleasant sensory and emotional experience associated with actual or potential tissue damage, or described in terms of such damage.

Note: Pain is always subjective. Each individual learns the application of the word through experiences related to injury in early life. Pain is the experience that we associate with actual or potential tissue damage. It is always unpleasant and therefore an emotional experience. Many people report pain in the absence of tissue damage or any pathophysiological cause; usually this happens for psychological reasons. This definition avoids tying pain to the stimulus. Activity induced in the nociceptor and nociceptive pathways by noxious stimulus is not pain, which is always a psychological state. . . .

Acute Pain

Acute pain is usually associated with a well-defined biologic cause and a rapid onset. It vanishes after healing has occurred. Acute pain follows an injury to the body and implies a natural healing process of short duration. It is only expected to persist as long as the tissue pathologic condition itself. Acute pain is also often, but not always, associated with objective physical signs of:

Increased cardiac rate
Increased stroke volume
Increased systolic and diastolic pressure
Increased pupillary diameter
Striated muscle tension
Decreased gut motility
Decreased salivary flow
Decreased superficial capillary flow
Changes in bronchiole diameter
Releases of glycogen, adrenaline, and noradrenaline

These changes in dynamic activity are assumed to be roughly proportional to the intensity of a noxious stimulus. The enormous biologic value of acute pain is a rapid orienting to the noxious stimulus and reacting to minimize or escape the damage being done by the tissue-damaging stimulus. Some acute pain during the healing process fosters rest, protection, and care of the injured area and thereby promotes healing and recuperative processes.

The overall behavioral signs of acute pain are agitation and the emerging flight-or-fight reaction. Patients with acute pain are anxious about the pain's intensity, meaning, and impact on themselves and their lifestyles. Drug therapy and allowing the natural healing processes to occur are the mainstay of treatments for the management of acute pain.

Chronic Pain and Suffering

Unfortunately, and rather often, pain persists after healing. It also persists after all conventional medical treatments and drugs have been tried. A constant barrage of erratic nociceptive impulses provide no new or useful information, but the adverse signal continues to reach consciousness. As an example, a failed back surgery patient 2 years postoperatively does not need to experience pain every time he moves his spine to remind him that he has scar tissue, adhesions, and functional changes in the structure of his back. Since he is no longer in the acute healing phase, the information provided by this type of redundancy is not useful and does not foster an adaptive response.

A pattern of objective signs also emerges as the chronic pain patient reports:

Sleep disturbance
Appetite changes
Decreased libido
Irritability
Depression
Decreased activity level
Deterioration in interpersonal relationships
Change in work status
Increased preoccupation with health and physical function

Over time, chronic pain patients become hypervigilant to all incoming stimuli, their behavior regresses, and they demand pain control from the medical community at any cost. The environment around the pain patient also often reinforces these ongoing pain behaviors. The pain behaviors are expressed through the musculoskeletal system and are integrated into the chronic pain patient's lifestyle. The result is that pain becomes the focal point of the individual's life. This leads to demoralization and suffering. The outcome of these structural and functional disturbances is the refractory, enduring pain experience commonly referred to as chronic pain syndrome.

These structural changes, functional disturbances, thoughts, feelings, and pain behaviors are all expressed by the person in pain through action of the musculoskeletal system. Much visceral, metabolic, and endocrine activity is also responding to the moment-by-moment changes of the musculoskeletal system in response to prolonged pain. With this rich afferent input of the musculoskeletal system into the central nervous system, it is inevitable that continuous redundant pain has profound consequences both physically and psychologically.

Nociception

Convincing arguments exist for the stance that chronic pain in some cases is caused, or at least set in motion, by a chronic physiologic, pathologic condition and prolonged permanent dysfunction of the peripheral and/or central nervous systems. Pain-generating mechanisms that can be self-sustaining produce complex, erratic nociceptive data that continually activate the biologic and psychological systems involved in the perception and expression of pain.[5] Examples include:

1. An abnormal neural hypersensitivity that results from prolonged nociception, such as when wide range dynamic neurons of the dorsal horn are activated in response to repeated intense stimulation
2. Tonic sensory inputs that originate in scar tissue, damaged nociceptive fibers, collateral sprouting, and peripheral neuropathies
3. Phasic sensory inputs that are brief, fast-rising (i.e., quickly reaching maximal intensity), intense, novel, or complex

4. Visceral and sympathetically maintained somatosensory and nociceptive inputs
5. All other sensory end organ inputs, particularly thermal-sensory and mechanical-sensory inputs that have become conditioned stimuli through repeated pairing with nociception
6. A lack of descending inhibitory tonic and phasic down-flow from supraspinal regions

Tissue-damaging stimuli activate specialized sensory receptors called nociceptors. These nociceptors are found in the:

Skin
Blood vessels
Subcutaneous tissue
Muscle
Fascia
Periosteum
Viscera
Joints
Other structures

When activated, end organs, like other receptors, generate impulses that are transmitted along peripheral fibers to the central nervous system (CNS). Some characteristics differentiate nociceptors from other somatosensory receptors:

1. Small receptive fields
2. High-response thresholds
3. Relatively persistent discharges without rapid adaptation
4. Location restricted to the endings of small afferent fibers

Two classes of peripheral nociceptors exist that cause subjectively different pains. The A-δ fibers produce sharp, well-localized, distinct pain associated with the injury itself. In contrast, C-fibers produce a dull, poorly localized, surprisingly persistent signal that evolves after injury. At the time of injury, pain is first created by A-δ fibers, and later by C-fibers. The pain information contributing to consciousness is transmitted along spinothalamic tracts and then to various parts of the brain from the thalamus. The final subjective pain experience is only weakly correlated with the degree of injury, the extent of damage, the number of receptors affected, or the energy of the noxious stimulus that provoked them. It is not the stimulus energy but the information contained in the stimulus that determines an individual's unique pain perception and response.

The spinothalamic system consists of two parts: the neospinothalamic tract and the paleospinothalamic tract. In addition to nociception, other sensory information is transmitted along these pathways, contributing to the information and raw data entering the brain in response to pain. The neospinothalamic tract rapidly delivers noxious impulses that give rise to the perception of sharp, well-localized pain, and an immediate warning of possible progressive injury.

The slower paleospinothalamic tract is composed of both long and short fibers projecting to the:

Reticular formation
Medulla
Midbrain

Periaqueductal gray
Hypothalamus
Medial thalamus

The pain perception is one of dull, aching, poorly localized pain sensations. Impulses arriving from the paleospinothalamic pathways synapse with neurons that reach the limbic forebrain structures. They then profusely project to many other parts of the brain. This pathway transports large amounts of general information that produces the long-term motivational and emotional dimensions of pain.

Although the spinothalamic transmission systems appear to correlate well with A-δ and C-fiber pain, one cannot assume that these structures simply represent subjective dimensions on a one-to-one basis. There are many interactions and feedback loops between them. Nor should it be assumed that the A-δ and C-fibers contribute solely to neospinothalamic and paleospinothalamic pathways, respectively. The nervous system can be closely approximated by such a model, but it is a comparatively simple transmission schematic.

Although nociceptive receptors can faithfully detect, transduce, and signal tissue injury, the afferent barrage is modulated at all levels of the nervous system by a multitude of cellular substances, tissue autocoids, spinal cord excitability, and structural reorganization. Long-term changes in sensory neurons create self-perpetuating neuronal activity before the signal reaches higher brain centers. Much of this modulation is activated by sympathetic and somatic efferent neurons, causing vasoconstriction and skeletal muscle spasm. In the higher brain centers, the synthesis of a complex pain perception from the incoming sensory information is further modified by anxiety and fear.

Most researchers and clinicians agree that chronic pain is a product of multiple interactions involving biologic, psychological, and social mechanisms. This synthesis of biopsychosocial factors into a network of interconnected causal agents helps to explain why chronic pain often persists. It also explains why the osteopathic emphasis on the musculoskeletal system and treating the entire person is relevant to the effective management of chronic human pain.

Central Control Processes

Central control processes such as the mind transform a noxious stimulus into cognitions, emotions, and behaviors that are appraised and acted on. The patient's responses to pain also are either reinforced or punished by the environment. That information is then fed back through the central control processes. This synthesis of nociceptive information across a series of mental events allows the individual to survive, adapt, and learn. The suffering associated with chronic human pain reflects an ongoing challenge to the information processing system. This is often a consequence of prolonged and erratic noxious stimulation. The end product is the patient's inability to integrate additional incoming noxious data into adaptive information processing routines or to elicit effective strategies for coping with pain. For the osteopathic physician, already well-versed

in the philosophy and practice of manual medicine, the realization comes quickly that the person in pain has a mind inseparable from the body and that the person actively thinks and has feelings about his or her pain. Becoming versed in how the pain information is organized psychologically allows the osteopath to bring his or her medical practice to fruition.

INFORMATION FLOW AND CHRONIC PAIN

Information flow implies that humans have the capacity to identify and incorporate potentially useful stimuli, to translate and transform the information received from the stimuli into meaningful patterns, and to use these patterns in forming an optimal response.[9–10] The information contained in A-fiber input immediately accesses and activates precise central control processes, which then rapidly and efficiently respond to a potential tissue-damaging stimulus. In contrast, C-fiber input supplies an ongoing status report after the injury and brings into focus all conditions that surround the injury.

As the individual thinks about the particulars of the tissue-damaging event, learning takes place. The individual anticipates damaging events and makes adjustments to optimize his or her chances for adaptation, learning, and long-term survival. Historically, the basic need to anticipate and avoid potential tissue-damaging events has set the stage for considerable complex higher-ordered thinking and innovative problem solving. Through evolution, humans have become good at anticipating, avoiding, or minimizing pain. When these skills are augmented with the ability to create symbols for communication, and to use language, reasoning, and abstract thinking, the result is the capacity for maximal adaptation.

When the person is unable to find an adaptive response, and redundant processing and reprocessing of the noxious stimuli is present, the integrity of the basic thinking, feeling, and problem-solving systems is threatened. As a result, the patient begins to "suffer," and the suffering continues until the threat of this disintegration has passed or the integrity of the information processing system is restored in some other manner. The patient continually seeks medical attention in search of treatment that will either interrupt the pain signal or help manage the impact of the pain on lifestyle.

The osteopathic profession has an historic opportunity to help suffering patients because of its philosophy of whole person, health-oriented care. Osteopathic physicians already recognize the relationship between the musculoskeletal system and pain expression. Osteopathic physicians understand and expect the interaction of mind and body systems. Osteopathic physicians know that systems both influence and are influenced by mental information processing systems, the manifestation of which—a patient's pain and suffering—is shaped by a history of learning experiences, culture, and environment. Osteopathic physicians are also learning how the musculoskeletal system processes pain information.

Information processing models of pain assert that a specific series of mental events occurs at the central control level, following prolonged noxious stimulation.[9–11] Figure 13.3 illus-

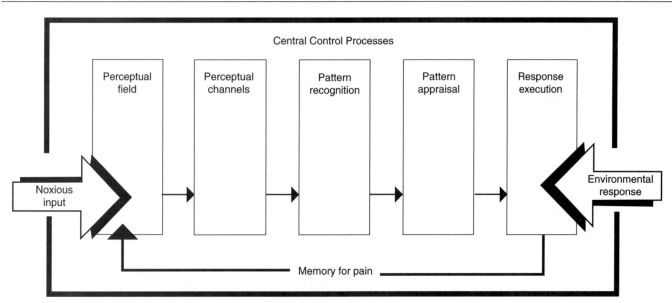

Figure 13.3. Flow chart for series of mental events that occur within central control processes following noxious input. (Reprinted with permission from Jerome JA. Transmission or Transformation? Information processing theory of chronic human pain. *American Pain Society Journal.* 1993;2(3):160–171.)

trates the flow of somatosensory data through these mental subsystems, as a noxious stimulus is transformed into information that facilitates pain perception, emotional appraisal, and musculoskeletal/behavioral responses. The consequences of these responses, reinforced within the individual's environment, are also appraised and fed back through the central control processes. This results in a dynamic-plastic system; dynamic in that the information processing systems continually respond to nociception, and plastic in that they also continually change as a result of nociception. The synthesis of pain information, coupled with the emotional appraisal, allows individuals to survive, learn, and adapt.

Perceptual Field

The perceptual field is a hypothetical construct used to describe the entire collection of all incoming stimulus events capable of being brought into conscious awareness for processing. The field consists of stimuli arising from:

1. Immediate, external, physical, and social environments
2. Immediate, internal, somatosensory environment
3. Central control processing itself
4. The noxious stimulus

The noxious stimulus is perceived among the many other sensory inputs that surround the painful event. Conscious attention is directed quickly toward noxious, novel, complex, or threatening sensory events. The central control processes scan this information for recognizable patterns in an effort to attach meaning, affect, and (eventually) a label to the nociceptive event. Included in the process is a search of stored memories of earlier pain experiences that are then integrated into a new pain experience for future reference. A reduced data stream of

salient sensory stimuli is then channeled to the pattern recognition subsystem of the central control processes for further analysis.

Only some of the data in the perceptual field is analyzed. The ability to focus selectively on some stimuli in the perceptual field, while ignoring others, is extremely important. If the flow of information were not restricted through many levels of preprocessing, we would be overwhelmed by the many extraneous events present in the perceptual field at the point of the tissue-damaging event.

Pattern Recognition

Pattern recognition is the psychological process that labels the nociceptive input and stores it in memory. This process, involving four steps, allows the individual to assign meaning to the pain experience and prepare for problem solving.

STEP 1: STIMULUS–RESPONSE (S–R) LEARNING

Over time, the experience of pain becomes associated with other stimuli in the environment that were not originally connected with the pain signal. The individual's response to the new associations, called conditioned stimuli, can elicit responses from the environment that are rewarding and that will expand and reinforce the pain responses. These expansive pain reactions are manifested as thoughts about pain, pain behaviors, and functional disturbances in the musculoskeletal system. They can then be elicited and maintained through other processes, including prior learning, conditioning, and cognitive mislabeling of somatosensory cues. An individual's beliefs and emotional reactions, over time, can also become conditioned stimuli that reinforce pain responses.

STEP 2: INFERENCE

The perception of pain reflects both a direct perceptual process and an inferential process. If a person reports symptoms A, B, and C surrounding pain, this does not necessarily mean that all three symptoms are directly perceived. Instead, it can mean that the first was perceived, and the other two were inferred from the first. For example, if a patient reports muscular stiffness, soreness, and pain, he or she actually might have felt stiffness, and then inferred soreness and pain from that sensation.

STEP 3: LABELING S–R RELATIONSHIPS

The stimulus–response relationships and inferences associated with pain experiences are then organized into memories. The pain memories are composed of all the mental factors that were active at the onset of pain. These factors include:

Thoughts
Images
Feelings
Musculoskeletal changes

When the pain memory is later activated, all of the mental factors and functional disturbances in the musculoskeletal system attached to it are also stimulated. This results in the re-experience of pain that is identical to the original experience at onset.

STEP 4: FORMING COGNITIVE STRUCTURES

Continuous pain and activation of pain memories encourage the assignment of global labels to pain experiences, lumping a large variety of pain experiences into a single pain construct. Memories that are associated with nociception are combined to form a pain schema, an expansive network, or neuromatrix, of pain-related information.[12–15] A pain schema can be thought of as a cognitive structure that forms the basis for personal beliefs about pain and for problem-solving strategies that develop in response to pain.

As pain becomes chronic, the pain schema expands and becomes more rigid. This is frequently a self-perpetuating process. As the pain schema expands, individuals begin focusing on schema-related and schema-consistent information and ignoring information or explanations that do not fit the schema. As a consequence, pain memories and perceptions are often revised to fit the pain schema, further expanding and solidifying it. Pain behaviors, such as reading about pain, seeing others in pain, and communicating with others about pain, can also influence the manner by which new pain experiences become structured and integrated into the general pain schema. In addition, the entire pain schema can be internally activated and/or driven by stimuli from central control processes, such as internal imagery and self-talk, and can therefore be expanded in the absence of direct external stimuli.[11]

Pattern Appraisal

Pattern appraisal is the psychological process that incorporates the individual's evaluation of the pain's personal meaning into the subsequent emotional response. Pattern appraisals become "hot" or emotionally charged when the current pain event is perceived as having a significant personal impact. There are four appraisal steps involved in this process. The outcome of each appraisal can assist in forming the foundation for the next appraisal. The entire appraisal process triggers significant emotional responses.

STEP 1: NOVELTY APPRAISAL

Novelty appraisal determines whether a novel nociceptor has occurred, or is expected, on the basis of information that has emerged from the scan of stimulus events in the perceptual field. Orienting and startle reflexes, and subsequent feelings of surprise or interest, prepare the individual to engage in further person–environment appraisals. For example, further appraisals might determine that the novel cause of the nociception is potentially dangerous, generating fear and hypervigilance.

STEP 2: HARM/HURT APPRAISAL

Harm/hurt appraisal determines whether the encounter with nociception is potentially damaging to the tissue or merely an unpleasant but benign somatosensory event.[16] From this harm/hurt appraisal, the individual decides either to avoid or approach the stimulus. If the event is appraised as potentially damaging, the individual might feel anxious, fearful, or disgusted and likely decide to avoid the stimulus. If the event is appraised as benign, the individual might experience interest, curiosity, anticipation, alertness, surprise, or amazement and decide to approach the stimulus.

STEP 3: COPING APPRAISAL

Coping appraisal evaluates the degree of control over nociception and its consequences, as well as immediate impact on the person and/or the person–environment relationship. Coping appraisal activates generalized autonomic arousal and motor responses, such as those that would be called on to fight or flee. If the individual tries unsuccessfully to control and cope, he or she might experience anger when the efforts are blocked or sadness from a sense of loss of control. Over time, the perceived loss of control over the pain experience leads to depression. The patient begins to feel trapped, helpless, or frustrated with the inability to overcome pain.

STEP 4: GLOBAL APPRAISAL

Global appraisal evaluates the overall state of the individual, including an appraisal of:

1. Long-term antecedents and consequences of nociception
2. Current level of adaptation to nociception

3. Possible interference nociception might have with future goals and needs

Global appraisal is an effort to understand the event, especially why it happened and its impact. Emotions attached to the outcome of global appraisal include shame, fostered by a sense that one has failed to reach an ideal standard for mastering and living with chronic pain. They also include guilt, fostered by a sense that one has transgressed personal, family, and/or cultural expectations for adequately coping with pain.

As a result of these dynamic appraisal processes, behaviors are selected, emotions are labeled and linked to painful musculoskeletal sensations, and the experience of pain reaches full perception and expression.

Response Execution

Response execution refers to preparing a correct mental response before taking action. Chronic pain patients have difficulty choosing the most productive response to prolonged erratic nociception because their resources for effective coping have been exhausted and/or because their customary pain coping strategies have become ineffective. To restore and/or develop effective pain coping responses, purposeful change in the following areas is required:

Personal meaning of pain
Emotional, behavioral, and musculoskeletal responses to pain
Relationships between individuals and their surroundings as they relate to pain

Information Processing Summary

Processing the information contained in a noxious stimulus requires that a person:

1. Selectively review information from the perceptual fields
2. Retain various aspects of the information to be analyzed and organized into meaningful patterns
3. Compare these new patterns to those already cataloged in memory
4. Transmit recognized pain patterns to specific information appraisal systems, including those responsible for attaching affect to the experience and those responsible for translating the information into behaviors, musculoskeletal reactions, and problem-solving routines
5. Optimally allow for successful adaptive responses, learning, and mastery

The pain patient continually selects and executes various problem-solving strategies in an effort to adapt and cope with pain. These strategies both influence and are influenced by the pain patient's musculoskeletal environment. A major player in the patient's musculoskeletal environment is the osteopathic physician, who often only sees the end product pain behaviors and the pain patient's demand for pain management.

PAIN MANAGEMENT

Successful treatment of chronic pain is often complicated by a patient's beliefs about medical science and the expectations that he or she consequently places on physicians. For example, many patients believe that complete pain relief is not only obtainable but is their right, and they expect physicians to provide that relief. Unfortunately, the underlying biopsychosocial mechanisms of chronic pain are not fully addressed. As a result, conventional treatments fail, leading to frustration for the patient, whose expectations are unfulfilled, and for the physician, whose goals are blocked. When this happens, the doctor–patient relationship often becomes strained, sometimes leading the physician to faulty assumptions about the patient, such as:

1. No physiologic cause for the pain can be identified, so the patient must either be imagining it or exaggerating its severity
2. The pain does not respond to medical treatment, so it must be psychogenic (i.e., the pain is a manifestation of emotional dysfunction)
3. The pain does not respond to treatment, so the patient will have to learn to live with pain for the rest of his or her life

These assumptions result in physician frustration, patient dissatisfaction, and, sometimes, litigation.

A large part of a physician's practice involves treating patients who have chronic pain. Conventional approaches to pain treatment rely primarily on:

1. Medications
2. Anesthetic blockade
3. Counter irritation
4. The osteopathic mission to restore function

Medications

Medications are an important management strategy, particularly for acute pain. The three main categories of medications are:

1. Nonopioid analgesics: aspirin, salicylate salts, acetaminophen, and nonsteroidal antiinflammatory drugs (NSAIDs)
2. Opioid analgesics
3. Analgesic adjuvants

These drugs are prescribed according to the World Health Organization's analgesic ladder. It involves choosing among these three groups based primarily on pain intensity. Many mild-to-moderate acute pains readily respond to nonopioid drugs alone; they are the obvious first choice. Some moderate-to-severe pains may require combining the nonopioid analgesics with a low dose opioid preparation, the second step in the analgesic ladder. The third step is the addition of a high-dose opioid preparation to the nonopioid analgesics. At any of these three steps, analgesic adjuvants might also be useful.

The American Pain Society (APS) and the International Association for the Study of Pain (IASP) outline a number of important concepts to remember when choosing drugs to manage pain:

1. Individualize route, dosage, and schedule
2. Administer analgesics on a regularly predetermined time schedule
3. Recognize and treat side effects
4. Do not use placebos to assess nature of pain
5. Watch for development of tolerance
6. Use analgesic adjuvants
7. Block pain transmission

These organizations are a constant source of updated information on the rapidly changing pharmacologic knowledge base regarding pain control with drugs.

INDIVIDUALIZATION

The oral route is optimal because of its convenience, safety, flexibility, and the relatively steady blood levels produced. It is especially optimal when compared with the intermuscular route, which has the disadvantages of painful administration, fluctuations in the absorption from muscle, an up to 60-minute lag to peak effect, and a rapid fall-off. Intravenous bolus administration provides the most rapid onset, with shorter time-to-peak-effect. Repeated boluses can be used to load to concentrations providing pain relief, followed by maintenance infusion for severe pain. Continuous infusions provide steady blood levels with fewer side effects.

Patients can also be given active responsibility and a sense of control over their medication by self-administering an analgesic bolus with a microprocessor controlled by infusion pump. The opioids can also be administered intraspinally (epidural or intrathecal). Described as patient-controlled analgesia (PCA), the patient can activate a demand switch that delivers a preset dose of opioid into the patient's i.v. line, if a predetermined time (the often called "lock out" interval) has elapsed since the previous dose. In some of the most severe and long-term chronic pain cases, the entire system can also be implanted in the individual and programed to deliver medication across a preset monthly schedule. The PCA is for severe, long-term chronic pain cases, such as cancer patients and the terminally ill, or when all other treatments have failed.

Another advance in the route of administration is transdermal patches that allow the medication to be absorbed through the skin. These patches provide continuous opioid infusion without pumps, needles, or internally-implanted devices. Children, in particular, would rather endure pain than have a shot or painful procedure. Fortunately, opioids in lollipops, nasal sprays, and rectal suppositories are now available. New, longer-acting topographical preparations are now available that can be applied to the skin an hour before a painful injection.

It is crucial not to create pain during the attempt to relieve pain. The old adage that "something has to hurt or taste bad to work" is out. Painful injections and procedures run the risk of provoking inflammation and muscle spasm in the vicinity of the injury, thereby generating central sensitization and even

more pain. Similarly, sympathetic reflexes can occur that decrease microcirculation in the injured tissue and adjacent muscle, producing some degree of ischemia and smooth muscle spasm. Because pain is a complex perception, many painful procedures performed to relieve pain can, over time, alter how pain information is processed mentally. This can lead to complex pain escape and pain avoidance behaviors that are then reinforced by the environment.

ANALGESICS

When pain medications are given on a PRN basis, it can take several hours and higher doses of opioids to relieve pain, leading to a cycle of undermedication alternating with periods of overmedication and drug toxicity. Administering opioids on a scheduled, around-the-clock basis also leads to fewer side effects. Although morphine is a strong opioid and often is a drug of choice, it is important to be familiar with the dose and time course of a variety of opioids. Patients must be followed closely, particularly when beginning or changing an analgesic regimen. Monitoring pain relief and side effects frequently, and adjusting the regimen accordingly, is crucial.

SIDE EFFECTS

The most common side effects of opioids include:

Sedation
Constipation
Nausea, vomiting
Itching
Respiratory depression

These side effects can escape recognition unless the patient is asked directly about them. Several ways to treat side effects are to:

1. Change the dose, regimen, or route on the same drug
2. Try a different opioid
3. Add another drug that counteracts the adverse effect
4. Use a route of administration that minimizes drug concentrations at the site producing the side effect

When choosing drugs, one should also be aware of the potential hazards of mixed agonist-antagonists.

PLACEBOS

The analgesic effect from intramuscular saline (or another placebo) does not provide any useful information about the genesis or the severity of the pain. In fact, many patients who have a documented organic basis for their pain obtain temporary relief from saline injection. There are many sufficient biologic and psychological reasons to explain a person's favorable response to placebos. It basically speaks to the strength of their central control processing mechanisms and their ability to recruit their descending inhibitory system. The brain produces a variety of morphine-like peptide substances, the most prevalent of which are enkephalins and endorphins. Derivatives of these compounds, metencephalon and β endorphin, are derived from pituitary β-lipotropin and have opioid agonist properties. Binding of enkephalins to specific receptors appears to inhibit the transmission of noxious impulses via peripheral unmyelinated fibers to the higher centers of the brain. These substances have also been found in higher centers of the CNS such as the hypothalamus, periaqueductal gray, and nucleus raphe magnus. Substances are easily produced in response to the manner in which pain information is processed. Conceptually, these naturally occurring peptides act like morphine, with the exception of being produced endogenously.

PSYCHOLOGICAL STATE

Remember that pain is a complex perception and not simply an alarm signal sent to the brain by injury-sensitive nerve endings. Pain perception is incomplete unless the emotional state and the cognitive and information processing routines are involved. Pain behaviors, including medication demands or excessive intakes, are often determined and shaped by the reinforcement, or consequences, of the patient's request for pain-relieving drugs. The patient exhibiting drug-seeking behaviors and becoming overwhelmingly involved with using and procuring pain-relieving drugs is demonstrating learned behaviors, some of which are learned in the doctor–patient relationship. In the usual medical setting, these learned behaviors take the form of:

Missed office appointments with subsequent off-hour calls for prescription renewals
Forgery of prescriptions, or solicitation of prescriptions from multiple physicians
Getting drugs from other patients or family members
Selling and buying drugs on the street
Use of prescribed drugs by bizarre means, such as i.v. administration of pills, tablets, or capsules

It is important to be alert to these cues.

TOLERANCE

Tolerance means that a larger dose of medication is required to maintain the original effect. This is an especially common occurrence in patients in all age groups who regularly take opioid analgesics. To delay the development of tolerance, and to provide effective analgesia on the tolerant patient, combine opioids with nonopioids or switch to an alternate opioid. Be aware of the development of physical dependence. Physical dependence means that an abrupt discontinuation of the opioid leads to withdrawal symptoms. It is difficult to compete with morphine for its analgesic efficacy, but this is a challenge that can be met.

ANALGESIC ADJUVANTS

A number of other classes of drugs can either enhance the effect of opioids or aspirin-like drugs, have independent analgesic activity in certain situations, or counteract the side effects of analgesics. The most common are the tricyclic antidepressants. In controlled trials, they have relieved pain related to neuropathy, postherpetic neuralgia, and chronic pain syndromes, regardless of whether the patient was depressed. The analgesic effect of tricyclics begins at lower doses. In animal studies, tricyclics potentiate opiate analgesia, possibly by blocking the reuptake of serotonin and norepinephrine at CNS synapses. However, there is no evidence to support the use of tricyclics in acute pain treatment. Interestingly, tricyclic antidepressants, which block the reuptake of norepinephrine and serotonin, are largely used for the treatment of neuropathic pain. Noradrenergic α_2 agonists are popular but they can produce side effects, especially hypotension and sedation. They are primarily limited to chronic long-term pain patients. The following have all been prescribed as analgesic adjuvants with varying and limited degrees of success:

Antihistamines
Benzodiazepines
Caffeine
Dextroamphetamine
Steroids
Phenothiazine
Anticonvulsants

As with all medications prescribed as analgesic adjuvants, these should provide an opportunity for:

Increasing activities of daily living
Participating in physical therapy
Decreasing pain behaviors
Developing long-term behavioral changes and pain coping strategies that are incompatible with prolonged pain

The patient should be actively moving into coping and adjusting to the pain condition, or actively participating in rehabilitation aimed at restoring functioning. Goals should be outlined for the patient that include a pharmacologic interruption of the pain process to allow behavioral changes and new cognitive strategies for pain control. Discuss treatment goals with the patient prior to and continuously during the administration of any drugs for pain control.

PAIN TRANSMISSION BLOCKING

To control acute pain, anesthetic blockade of neural transmission to virtually any part of the body can temporarily be achieved by direct application of local anesthetics (nerve blocks) such as procaine, lidocaine, tetracaine, or bupivacaine. In some severe cases, substances that destroy neural tissue can be injected (neurolytic block) in an effort to permanently obliterate the neural transmission mechanisms.

Diagnostically, nerve blocks determine specific pathways to aid in the differential diagnosis of the site or transmission mechanisms of a given pain. Prognostically, they partially predict the probable effectiveness of neurolytic or neurosurgical procedures. Interestingly, the pain-relieving effects of local anesthetics can often exceed the duration of the chemical blockade of neural transmission. The reason for this is not completely understood. It might be a result of decreasing sympathetic reflexes and skeletal muscle tension. Perhaps it results from the creation of a block of pain-free time during which the patient can restructure the pain informational processing routines or learn behavior patterns that help in coping with the pain. There are several anesthetic blockades that attempt to intercept the noxious input and thereby prevent its entry into the perceptual field.

Facet Injection

Facet injection temporarily decreases small fiber afferent activity by injection of a local anesthetic into the articular branches of Luschka, which innervate the zygoapophyseal joint capsules.

Facet Rhizotomy

Facet rhizotomy eliminates small fiber afferent activity through thermocauterization of the articular branches of Luschka.

Dry Needling of Trigger Points

Dry needling of trigger points produces a volley of small fiber afferent activity that causes brain stem inhibition of the ascending spinoreticular, spinothalamic, and spinocortical pathways.

Local Infiltration of Trigger Points

Local infiltration of trigger points with anesthetics causes a biphasic effect that initially decreases pain by the same mechanism as dry needling. Infiltration of the anesthetic decreases small fiber input from the trigger sites and central facilitory states. This decreases afferent activity associated with pain.

Counter Irritants

Counter irritants flood the perceptual field with many complex somatosensory stimuli, preventing the noxious input from being fully recognized and channeled into the higher levels of the central control processes. These treatments, prescribed by the physician, are often carried out by a physical therapist sensitive to the osteopathic model of treating simultaneously the biopsychosocial aspects of pain.

HOT PACKS

Hot packs promote local and reflexive decreases in sympathetic tone. Locally, this increases blood flow and washes out nociceptive metabolites. In general, it decreases segmental reflexes and sympathetic tone, decreasing afferent activity and promoting muscle relaxation.

TRANSCUTANEOUS NERVE STIMULATION

Transcutaneous nerve stimulation (TNS) involves peripheral nerve stimulation with small amounts of electric current. The mechanisms underlying the therapeutic effect are not clearly understood, but three theories have been proposed:

1. Electrical stimulation preferentially activates large myelinated fibers in the spinal cord, interfering with pain perception and increasing pain tolerance;
2. Electrical stimulation results in local axonal fatigue of A-δ fibers, reducing small fiber afferent (nociceptive input) activity;
3. Electrical stimulation activates the descending inhibitory system, which is involved in endogenous opioid production.

ICE

Ice causes a sudden increase in small fiber activity that floods the afferent pathways, causing the brain stem to inhibit further nociceptive input from the affected area.

VIBRATION

Vibration differentially stimulates large proprioceptive afferent fibers. This action is thought to interfere with pain perception.

ETHYL CHLORIDE

Ethyl chloride floods the ascending nerve pathways with small fiber input. When intense, it can result in supraspinal descending inhibition of small fiber afferents.

Osteopathic Approach

Current osteopathic thinking is far more than structural diagnosis and pharmacologic management. The mission of osteopathic medicine is to restore both physiologic and psychological function through multiple avenues of intervention.[17] The magnitude and vision of treatment must go beyond the conventional medical models of obstructing and/or flooding nociceptive pathways. The art and science of osteopathic medicine is best expressed in the treatment of the musculoskeletal system. Osteopathic manipulative diagnosis and treatment are extensively reviewed in Section VIII. The focus here is on other medical and psychological restorative treatments that complement the structural and functional management of the musculoskeletal system.

STRETCHING

Stretching produces relaxation of hypertonic muscles by increasing Golgi tendon organ discharge and reflex inhibition. Stretch of hypertonic muscles causes an increase in gamma afferent discharge that elicits brain stem descending inhibition, thereby facilitating muscular relaxation.

STRENGTHENING

Strengthening exercises hypotonic muscles. Muscle activity increases blood flow and produces a trophic response; i.e., healthy functioning is restored to the extent possible.

PROPRIOCEPTIVE NEUROMUSCULAR FACILITATION

Proprioceptive neuromuscular facilitation (PNF) involves the use of dynamic and static muscular contractions in the reacquisition of joint mobility and general flexibility. PNF stimulates proprioceptive and efferent impulses that promote more efficient muscle use, relaxation, and nutrition through improved neurocirculatory effects. PNF range-of-motion exercises use reciprocal inhibition concepts to relax muscles. The goal is to rehabilitate muscle groups and reinforce appropriate motor unit patterning.

GAIT TRAINING

Gait training is used to improve patterned motion behaviors (gait) through synergistic muscular activities that improve complex motor behavior.

BEHAVIORAL MODIFICATION

Behavioral modification includes classical and operant conditioning, desensitization, and direct suggestion for modifying "pain behavior" to alter the patient's perception and report of pain.

COUNSELING

Counseling uses interpretation to identify unrecognized factors underlying maladaptive pain processing routines. Some patients might unearth early traumas that are played out in their chronic pain experiences. For example, an individual might begin to understand that pain perceptions are triggered or amplified by feelings that originated in childhood but that later came to be labeled as "pain." Counseling also actively reinterprets the associations between pain and other feelings or affective states—especially depression, shame, and guilt—that sometimes arise out of the experience of pain itself. The primary purpose of counseling is to dismantle maladaptive information processing routines by bringing the underlying emotions into awareness and fostering insight into the links between pain perception, thoughts, and feeling states.

BIOFEEDBACK

Biofeedback therapy trains the patient to modify physiologic processes that are monitored by some instrument or device. Tension headaches appear to originate with sustained contraction of the musculature of the neck and possibly the scalp. Using an electromyograph to evaluate tension in frontalis and other muscles, investigators have developed biofeedback techniques for tension headache therapy. The patient is also taught general relaxation techniques, such as diaphragmatic breathing, progressive relaxation, and autogenic work formulas. In addition, other muscle tension pain syndromes throughout the body are amenable to electromyograph biofeedback.

SUPPORT GROUPS

Support groups rely on developing a strong therapeutic alliance among the group members and the physician or psychologist leading the group. These groups are an extremely powerful and low-cost strategy for managing large numbers of chronic pain patients.[18] The goal is to help patients cope with and adjust to their pain and condition. In the groups, the patients reconceptualize the meaning of the pain and their affective and evaluative responses to it. They review how the pain impacts themselves and their lifestyles and identify the events in the environment that would reinforce their pain behaviors and musculoskeletal reactions. If not used in a group therapy model, the following concepts form at least an outline for teaching coping strategies within the doctor–patient relationship. These concepts are also the foundational ideas for the advice given to the pain patient.

1. My pain is real. I will reject any notion that what I am feeling is all in my head.
2. I accept that I might need outside help to control my pain, and I refuse to quit or give in to the pain and the deterioration it causes.
3. At times my pain has had an overwhelming influence on my life, but I believe that I can and must choose how I react to it.
4. My best efforts and those of the medical community have not stopped my pain. This is not necessarily a fault of mine or a shortcoming of medicine. I will no longer fight with myself about this or blame medicine. No fight, no blame.
5. I will start coping with my pain by taking an inventory of the price I pay for pain, and the rewards I get from pain. This inventory must be done honestly and without fear of the findings. I will recognize some aspects of my coping with pain that I am doing well, and will also admit to myself mistakes that I have made in trying to cope with the pain.
6. I will forgive myself unconditionally for the past mistakes I have made while trying to adjust to the pain, and forgive others whom I perceive are responsible for my pain and troubles.
7. I will discuss my pain-driven behaviors, feelings, and thoughts openly with those I trust and when appropriate, be willing to make amends for any harm that I might have done.
8. I will hold two ideas in my head: (a) something might come along to relieve my pain and (b) at this time, I have to cope with the pain I have. In doing this, I will accept myself as I am; that is, as a worthwhile and fallible person who is living with pain at this point in my life. I will then move forward, with hope and courage, toward my primary goals of intimacy, bonding with others, and healthy interpersonal relationships.
9. I can choose to seek additional help at each step by developing a spiritually based program directed toward acceptance of my pain. I can then live by whatever spiritual principles promote wellness.
10. After gaining a reasonable level of functioning and pain control, I will recognize that there is still more to life than a

constant struggle to live with pain. Then, I will gradually separate myself from my pain management program or doctor, with the complete understanding that I may return at any time. I will realize that the pain problems I have are not my fault, and are, in part at least, a matter of probability and chance. I understand that I have more important primary goals in life, and that coping with pain is now a secondary issue—something I do to get to these primary goals.

CONCLUSION

Pain management options run along a continuum from noninvasive and low-risk to invasive and high-risk alternatives. Low-risk choices center on the osteopathic philosophy of compassionate care regarding the whole person in pain, with the primary emphasis on factors originating in the musculoskeletal system. In addition to osteopathic manipulative treatments, further low-risk choices include:

> Physical therapy
> Exercise
> Drugs
> Relaxation training
> Biofeedback
> Manual treatments of many kinds
> Counseling
> Behavior modification
> Support groups

Mild-risk options incorporate nerve blocks, and nonopioid and opioid analgesics. Moderate-risk alternatives include implantable therapies, particularly spinal cord stimulation and intraspinal drug infusion systems. The high-risk treatments consist of surgeries and nerve-destroying procedures. The most prudent overall treatment starts out and stays low-risk and noninvasive. Fortunately, osteopathic manipulative treatments and the other low-risk pain management options are also the most cost-effective and the most user-friendly to the patient. Patients in pain can be sedentary, deconditioned, overweight, tense, underexercised, and depressed. With encouragement from the physician, they can become physically fit, receive osteopathic manipulative treatment, be trained in relaxation training, and be enrolled as members of a chronic pain support group that will likely lead to adjustment to the pain condition.

Most chronic pain patients can be managed effectively when the treating physician uses a combination of these low-cost, conservative treatments. For the most difficult cases, nerve blocks and/or opioid analgesics might be necessary. With a pain that is severe and disabling, implantable therapies and neurodestructive procedures are always the last resort. They should only be carried out in consultation with other physicians and psychologists, as an orchestrated team effort. The choice of invasive therapeutic intervention for pain is determined largely by the severity of the patient's pain problem, resources available, comparative risk of the procedures under consideration, and emotional and physical state of the patient.[18–19]

Finally, it is of great importance for osteopathic physicians

---

Traps to avoid and guiding principles to manage high-risk chronic pain patients.

- *Failing to address patient fears.* **Rule out malignancy and communicate that clearly to the patient. Explain why the pain continues after damage and healing.**

- *Allowing the distressed patient to push you into procedures.* **These are often procedures that have a low chance of success, but the patient is desperate. In the end, your heroic efforts will be regretted by both you and the patient. Do not harm. Do not make a thick chart out of a thin chart.**

- *Assuming all problems are medical problems.* **Suffering for some patients might not be separated from social and psychological factors.**

- *Prescribing drugs that are not safe for long-term use.* **These patients have** *chronic* **problems and drugs started will be continued** *for years.*

- *Assuming the problem is psychological if there is no biologic diagnosis.* **Psychological problems are arrived at by examining psychosocial factors and by using psychodiagnostic procedures.**

- *Assuming that if you cannot stop the pain, it will be there for the rest of the patient's life.* **Some people get better on their own, and some pains go away with time.**

- *Failing to engage the patient to take responsibility for his or her pain.* **Patients' pain problems are** *their* **problems. You are doing what you can to help.**

- *Telling patients that their problem is "in their head."* **They will reject you, reject your treatment and continue to seek a physical diagnosis with which they can later confront you.**

- *Prescribing a mock regimen to "cure" the pain.* **Placebos are invaluable in clinical trials but have no diagnostic value in primary care. A placebo response does not discriminate psychogenic from somatic conditions.**

- *Setting "pain relief" as the solution.* **Complete cures and relief of all pain in this population are highly unlikely. Reducing the pain by perhaps 50%, restoring some function muscularly, socially, vocationally, and mentally, and adjusting to some pain and symptoms is more realistic.**

---

to distinguish between acute and chronic pain in their daily practice. Chronic pain can continue in an unrelenting fashion without ongoing evidence of tissue damage. Its persistence does not necessarily mean that the original organic damage has failed to heal or that the patient has significant psychiatric problems.

Chronic pain behavior might simply reflect the patient's experiences in other areas of life, such as:

Loss of intimacy
Difficult life situation
Vocational maladjustment
Economic hardship
Overwhelming social responsibility
Marital tension
Emotional or personality disorders
Organic brain syndrome
Deep emotional regrets, such as shame or guilt
History of childhood abuse or neglect
Dysfunctional family environment

Such high-risk chronic pain patients require psychological and social management in addition to medical care. There are a variety of traps[20–21] into which the well-intentioned but unwary primary care physician can fall when managing high-risk chronic pain patients. Refer such patients to a multidisciplinary pain service when a complex problem is encountered. These complex problems are more often the exception than the rule, and the vast majority of chronic pain patients can be treated easily by using the least invasive, conservative treatments.[22–23]

In summary, the physician's goal is to restore both physical functioning and adaptive musculoskeletal responses through the simultaneous use of physiologic and psychological interventions.[24] When managing chronic pain, it is routine to use:

Osteopathic manipulative techniques
Medications
Nerve blocks
Counter irritation
Physical therapies
Psychological counseling

Combining these elements into a comprehensive treatment approach increases the chances of a successful outcome. Intervention strategies that simultaneously address the biologic, psychological, and social factors of chronic pain are more likely to succeed and modify chronic pain perception and behavior.

Pain is the most common element in the symptoms presented to physicians. Successful management of chronic pain depends on much more than knowledge. Knowledge must be teamed with keen observation, patience, and compassion. Many physicians have come to believe that treating chronic pain, with all its biopsychosocial elements, reflects both the true art and the true science of osteopathic medicine.

REFERENCES

1. *Nuprin Pain Report.* New York, NY: Louis Harris and Associates; 1985.
2. Sternback RA. Survey of pain in the United States. *Clin J Pain.* 1986; 2:49–53.
3. Jerome JA. Theory leads: statistics follow. *American Pain Society Journal.* Fall 1995;4(3).
4. Melzack R, Casey KL. Sensory, motivational, and central control determinants of pain. In: Kenshalo DR, ed. *The Skin Senses.* Springfield, Ill: Charles C Thomas; 1968:423.
5. Bonica JJ. *The Management of Pain.* 2nd ed. Philadelphia, Pa: Lea & Febiger; 1990.
6. International Association for the Study of Pain. Pain terms: a list with definitions and notes on usage. *Pain.* 1982;14:205.
7. Mersky H. Development of a universal language of pain syndromes. In: Bonica JJ, Lindblom U, Iggo A, eds. *Advances in Pain Research and Therapy, V.* New York, NY: Raven Press; 1983:37–52.
8. de Jong RH. Defining pain terms. *JAMA.* 1980;244:143.
9. Jerome JA. Information processing theory of chronic pain. *America Pain Society Journal.* 1992;1:7–10. Bulletin.
10. Jerome JA. Life after pain. *Clin J Pain.* 1991;7:167–168.
11. Pennebaker JW. *The Psychology of Physical Symptoms.* New York, NY: Springer-Verlag; 1982.
12. Leventhal H, Everhart D. Emotion, pain and physical illness. In: Izard CE, ed. *Emotions and Psychopathology.* New York, NY: Plenum; 1979.
13. Melzack R. Phantom limbs, the self, and the brain. *Canadian Journal of Psychology.* 1989;30:1–14.
14. Melzack R. The gate control theory 25 years later: New prospectives on phantom limb pain. In: Bond MR, ed. *Proceedings of the 6th World Congress on Pain.* New York, NY: Elsevier; 1991.
15. Melzack R. Central pain syndromes and theories of pain. In: Casey KL, ed. *Pain and Central Nervous System Disorders.* New York, NY: Raven Press; 1991.
16. Fordyce WE. Behavioral Methods for Chronic Pain and Illness. St. Louis, Mo: CV Mosby; 1976.
17. Elkiss M, Jerome J. Chronic pain syndrome: an analysis of current therapies. *Michigan Osteopathic Journal.* 1978;43:8.
18. Turk DC, Meichenbaum D, Genest M. *Pain and Behavioral Medicine: A Cognitive Behavioral Perspective.* New York, NY: Guilford; 1983.
19. Turk DC, Melzack R. *Handbook of Pain Assessment.* New York, NY: Guilford; 1992.
20. Blazer DG. Psychopathology of Aging. *Am Fam Physician.* June 1977:15–16.
21. Hartwick CT. Tutorial 17: how to manage a difficult pain patient. *Pain Digest.* 1995;5:93–95.
22. Wall PD, Melzack R. *Textbook of Pain.* 3rd ed. New York, NY: Churchill Livingstone; 1994.
23. Acute Pain Management Guideline Panel. *Acute Pain Management: Operative or Medical Procedures and Trauma. Clinical Practice Guideline.* Rockville, Md: Agency for Health Care Policy and Research, Public Health Service; February 1992. US Dept of Health and Human Services publication 92-0032.
24. Jerome JA. Transmission or transformation? Information processing theory of chronic human pain. *American Pain Society Journal.* 1993; 2(3):160–171.

RESOURCES

IASP Press
International Association for the Study of Pain
909 NE 43rd St., Suite 306
Seattle, WA 98105
FAX: 206-547-1703

American Pain Society
Corporate Office
5700 Old Orchard Road, First Floor
Skokie, IL 60077-1057
Phone: 708-966-5595

14. Health Maintenance

JOYCE M. JOHNSON

Key Concepts

- **Patient's role in health maintenance and disease prevention**

- **Physician's role in patient education and coordination of health maintenance plan**

- **Innovative health maintenance strategies**

- **Physician as patient**

Health maintenance concepts can be defined as the aspects of physiology and behavior that maintain optimal functioning in the context of family, job, and social structure. As such, these concepts are essential elements in the practice of osteopathic medicine in general and primary care in particular. Health maintenance concepts focus on four factors:

Physical health
Emotional health
Lifestyle
Behavioral circumstances in relationship to self, job, and family

These factors, along with four osteopathic principles, are closely tied to health promotion[1]:

Concepts of body unity
Interdependence of structure and function
Concepts of self-regulation
General health maintenance

Osteopathic medicine has traditionally focused on holistic approaches to health care. It recognizes the intricate relationships among emotions, mind–body relationships, and physical health. Osteopathic principles outlined in Figure 14.1 embody these ideas.

Individual, patient-controlled behaviors have particular impact on homeostatic, health-maintaining mechanisms. For example, smoking damages regulatory mechanisms that control protective ciliary activities in the lungs, thereby reducing the ability to fight off respiratory infections. As A.T. Still noted, *"Diseases are effects. . .(not causes)."*[2] Recovery and self-healing capacities are often dramatic when allowed to work as they are intended.

Disease is a consequence of homeostatic breakdown. For example, potentially malignant cells occur under many circumstances. Most of the time, protective immune processes prevent

further development, and cancer is prevented. When the processes break down, cancer occurs (see Chapter 35, Oncology).

Patient education regarding the interdependent roles of individual behaviors, homeostasis, and health maintenance must be supplied by the practicing osteopathic physician.

PATIENT'S ROLE

The patient has enormous control over health maintenance and disease prevention. Sometimes this is recognized; often it is not. In today's complex society, one's personal health commonly depends on lifestyle decisions. Essential health maintenance strategies include:

Knowledgeable nutrition
Exercise
Stress management
Appropriate health screening

On the other hand, substance abuse, unsafe driving, unsafe sexual practices, and domestic abuse are among the most common reasons for entering the health care delivery system. All are within our individual control.

Ultimately, the patient is behaviorally accountable for health-maintaining decisions. If this is true, what is the role of the doctor–patient relationship? Cooperation is the key for developing a health maintenance plan. It emphasizes education and exploration of healthy and unhealthy alternatives.

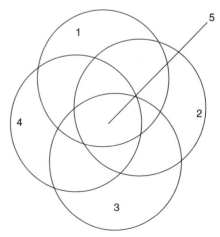

Figure 14.1. Some osteopathic concepts. 1: Body unity. 2: Capacity for self-regulation and health maintenance. 3: Capacity for recovery and self-healing. 4: Reaction of the musculoskeletal system to stress. 5: Disease as an effect or consequence of a breakdown in homeostatic mechanisms.

PHYSICIAN'S ROLE

Patient education is important to help optimize healthy behaviors. Physicians should look for the often dissimilar conscious and unconscious choices made in reaction to similar situations. Under these circumstances, changing risky behaviors is not without risk if behaviors and consequences are not understood and acted on in their immediate contexts and circumstances. For example, chronic pain and depression commonly mask complex family problems.

To carry out the physician's role in a knowledgeable way, one must be adequately educated and clinically alert to individual patient responses. For example, some patients prefer passive, more dependent roles, preferring to let the health care provider make decisions; others seek out more active and collaborative relationships. Still others wish to make all the decisions themselves. All these views are legitimate. Under stressful circumstances, however, perceptions and role expectations often change, so the physician must be clinically and behaviorally alert.

Cost–benefit research has demonstrated that the annual health maintenance physical may be unnecessary. As a result, many managed care plans no longer pay for such examinations. One outcome is that patients are more apt to have specific complaints that require a thorough history and physical. Under these conditions, the history and physical examination can be used for patient education. After specifics are identified and treated, and rather than focusing exclusively on a chief complaint, there is ample opportunity to elaborate on specifically tailored health maintenance strategies.

Older patients are apt to ignore or deny signs of serious, even life-threatening, illness, such as weight loss, chronic cough, or vaginal and rectal bleeding. Under these conditions, specific, age-appropriate examinations are required. Recommendations can be found in several places.[3–4]

Ultimately, the physician's role is to develop and coordinate a health maintenance plan that helps guide patient decisions and resource management.

INNOVATIVE HEALTH MAINTENANCE TOOLS FOR PHYSICIANS

Incorporating health maintenance strategies requires continuing education regarding health promotion and preventive services. Role modeling these activities with one's colleagues and employees is an important public relations tool. Table 14.1 outlines a number of strategies.

There are many physician roles. One role is to cure diseases through specific interventions. The physician is an integral part of the doctor–patient relationship. In the primary care setting, this role extends to both preventive services and health maintenance educational activities.

Transmission of facts by lecture and conversation are time-honored health education strategies. Individual responses are not built into the plan; the strategy is: "Let the facts speak for themselves." Scare tactics are common, and, not surprisingly,

Table 14.1
Innovative Health Maintenance Program

"Feeling focused" health education
Health maintenance plan with flow sheet
Patient-held minirecord
General interest seminars for patients
Focused seminars for selected patients
Ongoing patient study groups
"Disease of the month" campaigns
Office videotapes
Health maintenance clinic
Postcard reminders
Patient newsletters
Community seminars

outcomes are ineffective with generally low compliance using these methods.

Today, expert health educators focus on patient feelings and perceptions as parts of the educational process. For example, if a patient is hypertensive, explain the importance of continuing medication while listening carefully to the patient's reaction to the presentation. One common scenario is this: the patient feels that taking the medication is a sign of weakness if he or she takes it in front of colleagues at work. Such feelings often lead to noncompliance. Addressing these concerns can change the feeling and then the behavior, resulting in better compliance.

A formal health maintenance prescription and record can be readily developed for each patient. Separate parts of the medical record with flow sheets and calendars contain important call-back dates and times for such activities as blood pressure checks, blood sugars, Pap stains, and mammograms. Patient call-back schedules can be routinely used with these records. The health maintenance plan can also be held by the patient as a part of a personal medical record that summarizes the health history.[5] A postcard reminder system can help keep this program active.

Health maintenance examinations are ideal times for more formal consultations as problems arise. Together the patient and physician can review a range of lifestyle and environmental (family/work) issues that might be affecting overall health.

A number of sensitive and specific computerized health assessment questionnaires, such as the Cornell Medical Index, or other symptom checklists, such as the SF36, are available. Results can be used to tailor specific suggestions. An informal but systematic structured interview process can touch on such areas as:

Family circumstances and history
Nicotine use
Alcohol use
Illicit drug use
Exercise routines
Diet history
Job-related risks
Previous medical, trauma, sexual, and travel histories

Routine practices, such as seat belt use and the use of ear and skin protection, are also important as modifiable health maintenance strategies.

Patient seminars on topics of both general and situation-specific interest are often helpful. For example, a general discussion about postmenopausal hormone replacement advantages and disadvantages can help many individuals. On the other hand, specific topics, such as diabetes and fibromyalgia, will appeal to an interested subset of your population.

Support and discussion groups that meet periodically are often helpful, as are Disease of the Month programs highlighted by posters, brochures, and office videos. Videotapes in the waiting room are additional readily available patient resources. Topical areas include:

Adult and pediatric vaccinations
Stop smoking campaigns
Lipid awareness activities
Safe exercising

Medical students can be enlisted in planning and presenting the programs.

Special health maintenance clinics can be developed for screening activities on a scheduled periodic basis. The goal is to focus on patient education and routine preventive services. For busy acute practices, this is a good time to schedule an interdisciplinary team that can address multiple parts of complex problems in an organized way.

The physician's role commonly extends into the community. For example, periodic newsletters are good patient education aids. Articles can be written by the physicians involved or purchased commercially. Writing a regular newspaper column and appearing on television and radio are strong community education and public health services.

PHYSICIAN AS PATIENT

Of necessity, physicians tend to be independent individuals accustomed to controlling most situations. An extension of this role is that healthy physicians rarely willingly assume the role of patient. Regular checkups and health maintenance strategies are commonly overlooked; overwork and stress are common. Compared with most other professions, physicians have relatively high divorce and suicide rates, as well as alcohol and substance abuse problems.[6] Life and death responsibilities, coupled with long hours, contribute to unhealthy lifestyles adopted in response to the demands of medical education and residency training.

The trade-off for the joyous experience of helping patients and their complex, often life-threatening problems can be damage to a satisfying and rewarding family and social life. Primary care patients often sense this and respond to admonitions and education/compliance efforts with their physician's lifestyle in mind. They see their physician not as a role model but as an example of advice given and perhaps ignored. It is the physician's responsibility to change his or her own behavior and thus change this perception.

CONCLUSION

Practicing osteopathic medicine is challenging and rewarding. Balancing the stresses and rewards are forms of health maintenance.[7–9]

REFERENCES

1. Educational Council on Osteopathic Principles. *Osteopathic Principles Core Curriculum.* Washington, DC: American Association of Colleges of Osteopathic Medicine; 1989.
2. Truhalar R. *Sage sayings of AT Still.* Indianapolis, Ind: American Academy of Osteopathy; 1950:64.
3. US Preventive Services Task Force. *Guide to Clinical Preventive Services.* Baltimore, Md: Williams & Wilkins; 1989.
4. US Preventive Services Task Force. Guide to Clinical Preventive Services. *JAOA.* 1991;91(5)491–499. Special Pullout Section.
5. Dickey LL, Petitti D. Assessment of a patient-held minirecord for adult health maintenance. *J Fam Pract.* 1990;32(4):431–438.
6. Lowinson JH, Ruiz P, Millman RB, Langrod JG, eds. *Substance Abuse: A Comprehensive Textbook.* 2nd ed. Baltimore, Md: Williams & Wilkins; 1992.
7. US Department of Health and Human Services. *Healthy People 2000: National Health Promotion and Disease Prevention Objectives.* Washington, DC: U.S. Government Printing Office; 1991. DHHS publication (PHS) 91-50212. Full report with commentary.
8. US Department of Health and Human Services. *Healthy People 2000: National Health Promotion and Disease Prevention Objectives.* Washington, DC: U.S. Government Printing Office; 1991. DHHS publication (PHS) 91-50213. Summarizes the most important elements of 91-50212.
9. Battista RN, Lawrence RS, eds. *Implementing Preventive Services.* New York, NY: Oxford University Press; 1988. Supplement to American Journal of Preventive Medicine. 1988;4(4).

15. Life Phases and Health

JED G. MAGEN

Key Concepts

- **Definition of development**
- **Considerations of biologic influences, environmental effects, and discontinuous development**
- **Prenatal growth, and parental attachment to fetus**
- **Infancy, bonding, thriving, and adaptability**
- **Changes in years 1 to 5, including mobility, language, independence, toilet training, and sibling issues**
- **Cognitive development and socialization in school-age children**
- **Adolescent reorganization of cognitive, emotional, and biologic functioning**
- **Adulthood: creativity, procreativity, productivity**
- **Competing drives of integrity versus despair in the elderly**

A useful definition of development is *"a sequential increase in the structural or functional complexity of a system."*[1] Historically, the understanding of human development has also led from the less to the more complex. For example, infants were once thought of as being almost "blank slates." Early environmental experiences, especially with the primary caretaker, were assumed to result in the formation of the personality. Biologic influences were discounted. Individual development was thought of as a smooth upward reaching line that had a somewhat inevitable progression. The logical extension of this model was that early experiences and behavior should predict later behavior. In fact, early experiences do not seem to predict later behavior in any simple way.[2] Instead, it appears that human development is characterized by periods of time when behaviors change radically, and then there is relative stability until the next period of change. This discontinuous view of human development along with rapid advances in the neurosciences has helped alter our clinical approaches to behavior disorders in both children and adults.

CONTINUITIES AND DISCONTINUITIES IN DEVELOPMENT

Considerations of the process of development must take into account biologic influences, environmental effects, and the paradigm of discontinuous development. Rather than shifting smoothly from one phase to another, transitions are characterized by "biobehavioral shifts."[3] These times of transition involve fairly sudden reorganizations of the biologic, cognitive, affective, and social characteristics of the organism that result in new, more complex behaviors.[4] The timing and genesis of these shifts probably relates to repression and de-repression of genes, both as a result of internal timing factors and environmental influences. Furthermore, the organism is busily attempting to manipulate the environment in ways beneficial to itself. The move from childhood to adolescence is a particularly cogent example of a biobehavioral shift. Puberty is associated with an upsurge in sexuality with different behaviors toward the opposite sex, an increase in aggression, and striking physical changes.[5] Teenagers develop relationships with parents and peers that differ greatly from those same relationships during childhood. The epidemiology of various disorders also changes. For example, depression, which earlier is equally common in males and females, is now strongly predominant in females. These kinds of shifts in behavior are characteristic of growth and development.

PRENATAL PERIOD

Infants in utero respond to environmental influences in terms of both physical and behavioral development. A long list of factors can influence intrauterine growth and development.[6] Cigarette smoking and malnutrition are associated with decreased fetal growth. Alcohol use can result in fetal alcohol syndrome.

Just as the fetus grows and develops, the mother and other family members are likely to go through developmental steps in preparation for childbirth and caring for a new child. Mothers specifically are said to become more preoccupied with the self and with the neonate, especially after perceiving fetal movement. Fathers might also experience a beginning attachment once movement is palpable through the abdomen.

When this developmental process is not allowed to proceed to completion, parents might not be ready to interact with their infant in helpful ways. For example, parents of premature infants might not be ready to feed, nurture, and otherwise care for their infant. They might have difficulty in feeling that the baby is responding to them in any way. The perceived lack of

191

response can lead to fewer and fewer positive responses from the parents, putting the development of the relationship between infant and parents at risk. Interactional difficulties having their genesis in this early period have been implicated in the etiology of failure to thrive, and in various behavioral difficulties of infants and toddlers.

INFANCY

Infants come into the world with certain preprogramed capabilities that have evolved to help maximize their chances for survival. Rooting, sucking, grasping, and the Moro reflex are all adaptive in that they help the infant feed or maintain contact with the primary caretaker. Less obvious capabilities are also present. Newborns engage in complex visual activities. They scan patterns by means of eye movements going back and forth across edges.[7] By 1–4 months, they can discriminate many speech sounds.[8]

These innate preprogramed behaviors and capabilities are critical to the ability of the infant to develop and participate in the dyadic interaction between it and the primary caretaker, a phenomenon often termed "attachment." Attachment can also be defined as *an enduring emotional bond uniting one person with another.*[9] Klaus and Kennell used the term "bonding" for the first manifestation of this phenomenon as it occurs immediately after birth. They theorized that infants who were separated from their mothers and cared for in the newborn nursery did not bond as well as infants who were allowed to stay with their mothers.[10] Although this particular notion has not been substantiated, a process of bonding does take place, promoted by a variety of behaviors in which infants and parents engage. Holding infants at a distance that maximizes face-to-face contact, exaggerated greeting behaviors, and parental imitation of a newborn's facial and vocal expressions are all a part of this process.[11] For the newborn's part, eye contact with the primary caretaker, vocalizations, and the appearance of a social smile at approximately 8 weeks are all behaviors that will engage the caretaker and help promote reciprocal interaction.

Failure to thrive is a diagnosis made in infants who do not grow and do not achieve developmental milestones, such as the development of a social smile. Often this is the direct result of the failure to achieve a relationship with a caretaker who rarely handles or interacts with the infant. These infants also exhibit decreased growth hormone levels. On hospitalization, when given consistent care by hospital staff, growth hormone levels begin to elevate within hours. Experimental evidence suggests that touch in part operates as a soothing mechanism in animals by activating brain opiates. This mechanism might be operative in the therapeutic effect of osteopathic manipulative treatment. In summary, human infants are born with predispositions and tendencies to grow and learn in particular directions. This selective seeking of specific types of activities promotes brain growth and development.

Adaptability is a further important issue. The ability to modulate and change behaviors to match what might be going on in the environment is an important attribute. For instance, a parent who is unable to become calm and soothe an irritable, cranky infant is likely to have an infant who is, in fact, irritable and crying much of the time. The situation, sometimes labeled as colic, can be the result of a mismatch between what a parent is able to provide and what a particular child needs. Given at least average parenting ("the ordinary devoted mother"), most infants are able to obtain the stimulation and nurturance needed from the environment to progress developmentally.[12]

1- TO 5-YEAR-OLDS

Many changes occur from age 1 to 5. Brain growth and development continue. In fact, the number of synapses in the brain of a 1–2-year-old is 50% greater than the number present in an adult.[13] At approximately 1 year, children begin to walk. A sense of one's own body also begins to emerge in a coherent way. Gender identity seems to be set by approximately 2½ years.[14] Expressive language becomes evident. Babbling is present from approximately 6 to 18 months. Words first appear between 8 and 18 months, after which there is rapid acquisition of words.[15] Receptive language usually exceeds expressive language until age 4 or 5. With increasing independence and a developing ability to understand and evaluate social situations comes the appearance of behavior different from that desired by parents. Some parents begin having oppositional battles with their suddenly not-so-compliant 2- or 3-year-old. Talking with parents about consistent and calm limit-setting will often help parents through these difficult times.

Other common problems in this age group include toilet training and the birth of siblings. Most children will become interested in toilet training between 2½ and 4 years of age. There are many good texts and videos available on this subject. It is important to not develop battles of will around this issue.

The birth of siblings is a time when children feel displaced by a new intruder. They will often oscillate between excitement and anger at the new arrival. Opportunities to be with parents without the sibling and to engage in pleasurable activities are helpful, as are opportunities to vent anger in protected settings. A child who begins to throw dolls around the room after a new sibling arrives home is expressing anger in a way that will not hurt the sibling. As well, some regressive behavior can be expected. Bed-wetting, thumb sucking, or more oppositional behavior might be seen.

SCHOOL-AGE CHILDREN

Generally, children from kindergarten to puberty are considered to be school-age, or latency-age, children. The major tasks of this period are cognitive development and socialization. Cognitively, young school-age children are said to be dominated by "centration." They tend to view events as happening to them or in some way being affected by them. For example, children in this age group who experience parental divorce usually think that they in some way caused the divorce. It is not unusual to see depression, oppositional and angry behavior, and a decline in school performance as a result. As well, objects tend to be measured and defined by only a few of several possible dimensions and can be classified in idiosyncratic ways. For example, children might measure the volume of a column of water exclusively by its height or width without taking into account changes in the other parameter.[16] Cognitive psychologist Jean Piaget termed this preoperational thinking. When the school-age child achieves the ability to conserve, i.e., to recognize constant qualities or quantities of material even when the material undergoes changes in shape or color, he or she is said to have achieved the concrete operational level.[16]

School is a central experience for children. For the first time for many children, they spend the majority of the day with other children. This is often the first experience with adults other than parents in authority roles. A premium is placed on the ability to interact in socially appropriate ways with other children, as well as with adults. Rapid advances in interactional abilities take place. Children begin to learn strategies for continuing interactions and for reengaging after rejection and failure in groups. The development of self-concept as well as further internalization of a self-identity heavily depend on these early experiences in school.

Pediatricians and family practitioners are likely to see children with common problems, such as aggressive behavior, separation anxiety when going to school, academic problems, and the appearance of attention deficit hyperactivity disorder. Because school is a central experience and the family is still a center of activity, physicians need information from the parents, the child, and the school to evaluate these difficulties.

ADOLESCENCE

Adolescence marks a time of a profound biobehavioral shift, with a reorganization of cognitive, emotional, and biologic functioning. Adolescence generally coincides with the onset of puberty. In females, breast budding precedes menarche by approximately 1 year.[16] In males, the onset of puberty is marked by pubic hair and penile growth. Hormonal increases usually begin before these secondary sexual characteristics appear.[17] One of the triggers for the pubertal process might be related to a particular fat-to-lean body mass ratio.[18]

Cognitive and social-emotional changes are extremely important during this time. Cognitively, in Piagetian terms, the adolescent moves from the stage of concrete operations to formal operational processes. The individual begins to grasp highly abstract concepts and to manipulate them. The ability to formulate hypotheses and the use of deductive reasoning are formal operational processes that have obvious applications in school.

Perhaps the hallmark of adolescence is the process of separation-individuation.[19] During this time, it is said that the "final" crystallization of the adult personality is taking place along with a gradual separation from the family of origin. Many factors contribute to and interact in this developmental process. Cognitively, the adolescent can now conceive of a larger world

and others outside the family as having importance and relevance. The peer group begins to overtake parents in importance regarding matters of dress, opinion, and in numerous other areas. Relationships with the same and the opposite sex become of overwhelming concern. In short, the adolescent uses these relationships, and the ability to think independently, to separate from the family, build an increasingly independent lifestyle, and develop a character structure capable of self-regulation and independent action. Some conflict with parents is an inevitable result and can enhance this process to some extent. However, the traditional view of adolescence as a developmental period of turmoil does not seem to be true for a substantial number of adolescents. Offer documented a large group of male adolescents who seemed to go through this period of time in a "continuous growth" mode. There was little evidence of conflict or turmoil with family members. They were able to integrate various experiences of adolescence and to accept cultural and societal norms without conflict.[20]

Adolescents can also choose to separate in maladaptive ways. Individuals who engage in delinquent acts might be choosing an alternate path of separation from the family. In a chronic disease situation, such as diabetes, adolescents might need more care and be unable to become as independent as their peers. In reaction, they can become neglectful of diets or insulin injections. The adolescent diabetic with repeated ketoacidotic episodes might be engaging in a maneuver to express independence in the only effective way he or she knows for the moment.

The opposite—adolescents who never really separate and remain childish and enmeshed with parents—also occurs. In Western and especially American culture, adolescence is prolonged. College and professional education can extend into the late 20s or early 30s with continuing financial dependence on parents. This pattern can be particularly pertinent to medical students who undergo long periods of training, at first without any and then with minimal remuneration.

Other patterns of progression through adolescence do occur. That which we consider normative is, in part, culturebound. In some cultures, preadolescent and early adolescent male homosexuality is normative and does not seem to result in large numbers of homosexual adults. In many cultures, a sharp demarcation takes place between adolescence and adulthood with rites of passage.

For practitioners caring for adolescents, it is important to be supportive of the normal developmental process of the age group. Seeing the adolescent without the parents present for at least part of the medical visit is helpful. As well, teenagers often have concerns about confidentiality that will need to be discussed and respected.

ADULTHOOD

Although some personality development and change continues to occur in adulthood, for the most part, research in this area demonstrates that personality is fairly stable.[21–22] Based on this viewpoint, drastic personality changes in adulthood or old age should be viewed with a high index of suspicion. Similarly, cognitive changes should not be attributed to "aging" but should be investigated as a sign of a possible pathologic condition.[23]

Erik Erikson, as he did for childhood and adolescence, outlined a series of stages, including young adulthood, adulthood, and old age. He assigned a number of developmental tasks to each stage. In young adulthood, he contrasts competing drives of intimacy and isolation. Intimacy involves the development of a sharing mutual relationship, while isolation is a sense of being separate and unrecognized. The most important relationships are those that develop with potential partners. Developing a sharing, intimate relationship is of paramount importance.

In adulthood the core task is generativity, meaning creativity, procreativity, and productivity. There is a drive to have children, to succeed at one's career, and to be productive. One of the driving forces of adulthood is that of caring for and raising children. Passing on values and resources is a prime motivation.

However, as a consequence of increasing life spans, a competing dynamic seen in increasing frequency is that of the need to care for aging parents. Middle-aged adults may find themselves responsible for financial and perhaps physical care of elderly parents as well as their own children.[24] The stress and burden of this kind of situation can be significant.

Clinically, younger and middle-aged adults might present with depressions and anxiety disorders. Somatic symptoms as an expression of various stressors are even more commonly seen.

ELDERLY

Improved medical care is resulting in lengthening life spans. Formerly lethal disorders can now result in longer term chronic illnesses with morbidity and disability. It is appropriate that Erikson included a state of old age in his schema. In old age, the competing drives are said to be integrity versus despair. Despair and depression can be related to the knowledge that the life span is increasingly limited and to the loss of a spouse, friends, and career. Erikson does propose the competing drive of integrity, a sort of wisdom and perspective that comes with experience.

Many elders demonstrate the ability to adapt to changing circumstances over a long life span.[23] This set of coping mechanisms is extremely helpful in old age, when changes occur in many areas of social and individual functioning.

As individuals age, they might begin to expect to slow down and to develop some infirmities and disabilities. If expected, these problems can be taken in stride without too much upset or turmoil. Unexpected or catastrophic life events are especially stressful and less likely to be handled well.[25]

In many cultures, the elderly are viewed as carriers of culture and memory and as repositories of wisdom and judgment. This viewpoint comes close to the Eriksonian concept of an ideal old age. However, old age can degenerate into despair over continual losses of function, spouse, and friends. Thus, one of the primary concerns of elderly individuals is that of the quality of the physical and psychological care they receive. They can be increasingly demanding of health care professionals for care that promotes the best possible functioning. Older individuals have a justified concern with the quality of their final days. The avoidance of discomfort and long, drawn-out deaths while attached to various life support devices creates concern and should be discussed. Some physicians, however, are often uncomfortable talking about death and will actively try to avoid such discussions. Complete and compassionate care of elderly individuals requires that death and dying become topics of discussion.

CONCLUSION

The course of human development is characterized by an ever-increasing level of complexity with a series of biobehavioral shifts to new levels of organization. Although individual early experiences are important, it is not likely that any single incident will produce a radical alteration in personality. What seems to be important is consistent parenting and an adequate environment in which the individual can grow and develop. What is carried forward, what is continuous, is the pattern of consistent relationships that develops. Human development is a complex process that has no singular determinant of behavior or disorder. Development is truly a biopsychosocial process.

REFERENCES

1. Yates TT. Theories of cognitive development. In: Lewis M, ed. *Child and Adolescent Psychiatry: A Comprehensive Textbook.* Baltimore, Md: Williams & Wilkins; 1991:109–129.

2. Kagan J. Continuity and change in the opening years of life. In: Emde RN, Harmon RJ, eds. *Continuities and Discontinuities in Development.* New York, NY: Plenum; 1984:15–39.

3. Zeanah CH, Anders TF, Seifer R, et al. Implications of research on infant development for psychodynamic theory and practice. *J Am Acad Child Adolesc Psychiatry.* 1989;28(5):657–668.

4. Emde RN, Easterbrooks MA. Assessing emotional availability in early development. In: Frakenberg WK, Emde RN, Sullivan JW, eds. *Early Identification of Children at Risk.* New York, NY: Plenum; 1985.

5. Rutter M. Continuities and discontinuities in socio-emotional development: Empirical and conceptual perspectives. In: Emde RN, Harmon RJ, eds. *Continuities and Discontinuities in Development.* New York, NY: Plenum; 1984:41–68.

6. Smotherman WP, Robinson SR. Prenatal influences on development: behavior is not a trivial aspect of fetal life. *J Dev Behav Pediatr.* 1987;8(3):171–176.

7. Haith MM. *Rules That Babies Look By.* Hillsdale, NJ: Erlbaum; 1980.

8. Eimas PD, Siquelend ER, Josczyk P, et al. Speech perception in infants. *Science.* 1971;171:303–306.

9. Thompson RA. Attachment theory and research. In: Lewis M, ed. *Child and Adolescent Psychiatry: A Comprehensive Textbook.* Baltimore, Md: Williams & Wilkins; 1991:100–108.

10. Klaus MH, Kennell JH. Mothers separated from their newborn infants. *Pediatr Clin North Am.* 1970;17:1015–1037.

11. Emde RN. Development terminable and interminable: innate and motivational factors from infancy. *Int J Psychoanal.* 1988;69:23–42.

12. Winnecott DW. *Primitive Emotional Development.* New York, NY: Basic Books; 1945.

13. Huttenlocher PR. Synoptic density in human frontal cortex—developmental changes and effects of aging. *Brain Res.* 1979;163:195–205.

14. Money J, Hampson JG, Hampson JL. An examination of some basic sexual concepts: the evidence of human hermaphroditism. *John Hopkins Hospital Bulletin.* 1995;97:301–319.

15. Baker L, Cantwell DP. The development of speech and language. In: Lewis M, ed. *Child and Adolescent Psychiatry: A Comprehensive Textbook.* Baltimore, Md: Williams & Wilkins; 1991:169–174.

16. Combrinck-Graham L. Development of school-age children. In Lewis M, ed. *Child and Adolescent Psychiatry: A Comprehensive Textbook.* Baltimore, Md: Williams & Wilkins; 1991:257–266.

17. Brook CG. Endocrinological control of growth at puberty. *British Medical Bulletin.* 1981;37:281–285.

18. Friach RE, McArthur JW. Menstrual cycles: fatness as a determinant of minimum weight for height necessary for their maintenance or onset. *Science.* 1974;185:949–951.

19. Erikson EH. Elements of a psychoanalytic theory of psychosocial development. In: Greenspan SI, Pollock GH, eds. *The Course of Life: Psychoanalytic Contributions toward Understanding Personality Development, I. Infancy and Early Childhood.* Washington, DC: NIMH; 1980:11–61.

20. Offer D. Adolescent development: A normative perspective. In: Greenspan SI, Pollock GH, eds. *The Course of Life: Psychoanalytic Contributions toward Understanding Personality Development, II. Latency, Adolescence, and Youth.* Washington, DC: NIMH; 357–372.

21. Douglass K, Arenberg D. Age changes, cohort differences and cultural change in the Guilford-Zimmerman Temperament Survey. *J Gerontol.* 1978;33:737.

22. Costa PT Jr, McCrae RR. Personality in adulthood: a six-year longitudinal study of self-reports and spouse ratings on the NEO Personality Inventory. *J Pers Soc Psychol.* 1988;54:853.

23. Costa PT Jr, McCrae RR. Personality and aging. In: Hazzard WR, Andres R, Bierman EL, et al, eds. *Principles of Geriatric Medicine and Gerontology.* New York, NY: McGraw-Hill; 1990:101–107.

24. Brody EM. Parent care as a normative family stress. *Gerontologist.* 1985;25:19–29.

25. Neugarten BL. Social and psychological characteristics of older persons. In: Cassel CK, Riesenberg DE, Sorensen LB, et al, eds. *Geriatric Medicine.* New York, NY: Springer-Verlag; 1984:28–37.

16. Exercise, Fitness, and Health

RICHARD M. BUTLER AND FELIX J. ROGERS

Key Concepts

- **How the body adapts physiologically to dynamic exercise**

- **Intensity of exercise determined by measuring oxygen consumption**

- **Physiologic changes that constitute improvement in physical fitness**

- **Effects of exercise on specific illnesses and diseases such as coronary heart disease, hypertension, diabetes mellitus, serum lipoproteins, obesity, osteoporosis**

- **Effects of exercise on psychological health, especially anxiety and depression**

Exercise plays an important role in the osteopathic approach to health and disease. Much research data confirm that regular voluntary activation of the musculoskeletal system in the form of dynamic exercise provides numerous health benefits. The positive effects of exercise clearly supports the central role of the musculoskeletal system in the maintenance of health and the osteopathic concept that the body is capable of self-healing.

PHYSIOLOGIC ADAPTATIONS TO CHRONIC DYNAMIC EXERCISE

Dynamic exercise refers to the voluntary rhythmic contraction of flexor and extensor muscle groups against a constant load. Examples of dynamic exercise include walking, running, and swimming. Dynamic exercise when performed at lower intensities is primarily fueled by aerobic metabolism (oxidative phosphorylation) and can be maintained for prolonged periods. At higher intensities, both aerobic and anaerobic pathways are used, and duration of exercise becomes limited by the buildup of lactic acid in the exercising muscle groups.

Intensity of exercise is often measured by the increases in oxygen consumption resulting from aerobic metabolism. At rest, oxygen is consumed at a rate equal to approximately 3.5 mL/kg of lean body mass per minute. This resting level of oxygen consumption is defined as 1 MET. For simplicity, increases resulting from dynamic exercise are expressed in multiples of the 1 MET value. For example, an individual who has increased his or her oxygen consumption to a rate of 35 mL $O_2 \cdot kg^{-1} \cdot min^{-1}$ would be exercising at 10 METs. The de-

scription of oxygen consumption in terms of METs facilitates writing exercise prescriptions.

Physicians frequently ask, "How physically fit is a given individual?" The best index of fitness is maximal oxygen uptake measured at peak exercise. Maximal oxygen uptake is the result of the product of cardiac output (oxygen delivery to the tissues) and arterial-venous oxygen difference (oxygen use by the tissues). An individual who can increase oxygen consumption to 15 METs is more physically fit and has a greater exercise capacity than a person who can only achieve an increase of 10 METs. Maximal oxygen consumption depends on several factors, including:

Inherited physical endowment
Activity status
Age
Sex
Physical health of the cardiovascular system

For example, some individuals are born with a genetic potential to be more physically fit than others. No matter how intensely some individuals attempt to train, they are never able to achieve the maximum oxygen consumption needed to compete at an Olympic level. Also, as one ages, the body loses its capacity to consume oxygen. However, the performance of regular dynamic exercise increases maximal oxygen consumption, thereby improving physical fitness. This is true for individuals of all ages.

Improvement in physical fitness is achieved through regular dynamic exercise and occurs through both central (heart) and peripheral adaptations.[1] Well-trained individuals have several central adaptations in their hearts. Over time, there is an increase in left and right ventricular end-diastolic dimension with a "compensatory" hypertrophy.[2-5] This "eccentric" hypertrophy produces an increase in left ventricular mass without subsequent increases in myocardial wall stress and is believed to be a response to the volume load placed on the heart during dynamic exercise.[6]

An additional change at the central level involves the bradycardia seen in physically fit individuals. Not only are resting heart rates lower, but at any given work load they are also decreased as a result of training. These attenuated heart rates permit longer diastolic filling periods and consequent increases in stroke volume, preserving cardiac output (stroke volume × heart rate).

Another important consequence of this relative bradycardia is that the double product (heart rate × systolic blood pressure) remains lower throughout exertion. The double product is an indirect measure of myocardial oxygen consumption. The resultant lower levels of myocardial oxygen consumption for any given work load are particularly important for individuals with fixed coronary artery obstruction. Physical training allows these patients to perform greater work loads before experiencing angina.

Peripheral adaptations of the skeletal muscles include increases in capillary and mitochondrial density, oxidative enzyme activity, and more efficient regulation of blood flow. The net effect of these changes is an increase in the ability of skeletal muscles to extract and use oxygen, thereby increasing the arterial-venous oxygen difference. In addition, blood pressures are lower both at rest and at any given level of dynamic exercise,[7-8] which also contributes to lower myocardial oxygen consumption during exertion.

In summary, the net result of these central and peripheral adaptations is the delivery of greater amounts of oxygen-rich blood to tissues, with improved oxygen extraction capabilities at lower levels of myocardial oxygen consumption.

EXERCISE AND CARDIOVASCULAR DISORDERS

Primary Prevention of Coronary Heart Disease

As early as 1953, researchers observed that more physically active individuals had lower rates of cardiovascular morbidity and mortality than did their less active counterparts.[9] A subsequent large-scale study performed by Paffenbarger and colleagues[10] evaluated the relationship of reported levels of habitual physical activity levels with the future development of coronary heart disease mortality in 16,936 Harvard alumni. They found that individuals who reported expending over 2000 kcal/wk in physical activities had a reduced risk of coronary heart disease mortality over a follow-up period of 12 to 16 years.

Numerous other investigators, using both cross-sectional and longitudinal designs, confirm the association of increased levels of physical activity and measures of physical fitness with lower rates of coronary heart disease events.[11-19] Although not all studies confirm the beneficial association of physical activity,[20-21] the persuasiveness of the majority of observations has led the Centers for Disease Control and Prevention (CDC) and the American College of Sports Medicine to recommend promotion of an active lifestyle to improve the cardiovascular health for most individuals.[22-23]

Many researchers want to determine how much physical activity produces a physiologic benefit. Although beneficial effects can be obtained with low-level activities such as gardening[15] and walking,[24] a more consistent relationship appears when individuals participate in more vigorous activities such as running, swimming, and cross-country skiing. The total number of kcal expended is the most important factor in determining a protective effect.[25] A person can accumulate the total daily dose of exercise by doing 20–30 minutes of continuous dynamic activity daily. Alternatively, intermittent bouts of exercise, such as climbing stairs several times a day, also seem

to have a beneficial effect on cardiovascular health and might be easier to implement as a public health recommendation.

Secondary Prevention of Heart Disease

Physicians frequently recommend exercise training for persons with heart disease as part of a multidisciplinary program of cardiac rehabilitation. Such a program includes counseling, education, and a variety of risk factor modifications. The Agency for Health Care Policy and Research in 1995 developed guidelines for cardiac rehabilitation.[26] This group reviewed 114 scientific reports, 44 of which were randomized, controlled trials, that addressed the effects of cardiac rehabilitation exercise training on various outcome measures. A clear majority of trials demonstrated conclusive improvements in physical capacity and exercise tolerance without the occurrence of significant cardiovascular complications. These benefits occurred whether the exercise training was part of multidisciplinary cardiac rehabilitation, or an exercise-only program.

Other outcomes of cardiac rehabilitation exercise training seem to accrue only for participants in a multidisciplinary program. In this context, beneficial outcomes have been demonstrated for [26]:

Lipid lowering
Exercise habits
Symptoms of angina
Psychological status
Social adjustment

When combined with intensive dietary intervention, with and without lipid-lowering drugs, exercise training can regress or limit progression of angiographically documented coronary atherosclerosis.[27-29]

Beneficial outcomes have not been shown for the risk factors of cigarette smoking, body weight, or blood pressure when exercise training has been the primary intervention.[26] Exercise training as a sole intervention exerts less of an influence on rates of return to work than do nonexercise variables such as employer attitudes, prior employment status, and economic incentives.[30-31]

Two meta-analyses of randomized controlled trials[32-33] demonstrated significant mortality reduction for patients participating in cardiac rehabilitation exercise training. However, reduction in nonfatal reinfarction rates was not demonstrated as a consistent outcome. The results of these meta-analyses established an approximately 25% relative reduction in mortality at 10 years follow-up in rehabilitation versus control patients. The magnitude of this mortality reduction is similar to that seen with other interventions, such as the use of β blockade following myocardial infarction, or angiotensin-converting enzyme inhibitor treatment for myocardial infarction patients with left ventricular systolic dysfunction. The beneficial mortality outcome was greater in the controlled trials that involved multidisciplinary cardiac rehabilitation programs versus those that involved exercise only.

Elderly coronary patients represent a high percentage of patients sustaining myocardial infarctions or undergoing coronary artery bypass graft surgery and percutaneous transluminal coronary angioplasty. This subgroup of patients is also at high risk of disability following a coronary event. Elderly patients can safely participate in cardiac rehabilitation and show improvements comparable to their younger counterparts.[26]

Controversy has existed regarding the potential risks and benefits of exercise training for patients with left ventricular dysfunction and heart failure. Patients with congestive heart failure are often told to rest as much as possible and to avoid strenuous activities. However, evidence is accumulating that suggests that rehabilitative exercise training for patients with moderate-to-severe left ventricular dysfunction can improve functional capacity. A recent randomized crossover design study showed that participation in 8 weeks of exercise training resulted in significant decreases in submaximal exercise heart rate, rate pressure product, and symptoms of congestive heart failure compared with changes seen after 8 weeks of rest.[34] Peak oxygen consumption and exercise duration also increased significantly following exercise training.

Another randomized controlled study evaluated the effects of a 3-month training program in men with severe, compensated left ventricular dysfunction.[35] Compared with control patients, those involved in exercise training showed a 16% increase in exercise capacity. The improvements in functional capacity seen with exercise training appear mostly related to peripheral (skeletal muscle) adaptations[36]; changes in left ventricular function have not been demonstrated. Most importantly, studies to date have not demonstrated a deterioration in left ventricular function.

Hypertension

As many as 50 million Americans might have hypertension.[37] Increasing degrees of hypertension are associated with higher risks of[37]:

All-cause mortality
Coronary heart disease events
Stroke
Renal disease

Exercise is important both in the prevention[38] and treatment of hypertension.[37] Although pharmacologic agents are clearly effective antihypertensive agents, they can be associated with several side effects, including adversely affecting serum lipids.[39] Exercise as nonpharmacologic therapy has the potential advantage of lowering blood pressure while simultaneously improving other aspects of one's cardiovascular risk profile (as discussed below).

Cross-sectional[40] and longitudinal[41–42] observational studies have shown that more physically fit and active individuals have lower levels of blood pressure and lower risks of developing subsequent hypertension. Prospective experimental studies[43] have shown that exercise therapy is an effective intervention for lowering blood pressure. In addition to the use of aerobic exercise, low-intensity resistance exercises also appear to have

a beneficial effect on blood pressure.[44–46] Although early reports[47] suggested that blood pressure might increase to extreme levels during resistance training, subsequent studies have confirmed their safety for both normal[48] and cardiac patients.[49–51] These observations endorse prescribing exercise for most patients with hypertension, provided specific contraindications do not exist.

EXERCISE AND METABOLIC DISORDERS

Diabetes Mellitus

Exercise therapy has a positive impact on many aspects of diabetes mellitus, particularly those patients with type II diabetes mellitus. Obesity and insulin resistance are two important factors in the pathogenesis of type II diabetes mellitus. Exercise training can improve insulin sensitivity, decrease circulating insulin levels, and enhance glucose disposal for nonobese[52–53] and obese[54] individuals with diabetes. Beneficial improvement in lipid profiles has also been seen in physically active diabetic patients.[52,55] The increases in energy expenditure occurring during exercise also promotes weight loss and decreases obesity. These data confirm that prescribing exercise is an important component of the overall care of the diabetic patient.

Lipoprotein Alterations

The relationship between physical activity and serum lipoprotein levels has been controversial. Although numerous cross-sectional studies have found more favorable lipid profiles in active and physically fit persons compared with sedentary controls,[56–60] other studies have not confirmed this association.[61–65] In addition, many studies that have documented a positive association have not controlled for confounding variables, such as obesity and dietary fat consumption, known to influence total cholesterol levels. Prospective studies evaluating the influence of exercise on total cholesterol[66–79] have also shown conflicting results. In an attempt to clarify the role of exercise in alternations of lipid and lipoprotein levels, Tran and Weltman[80] performed a meta-analysis pooling the results of 95 studies evaluating 2926 subjects. They concluded that individuals who engaged in regular exercise could expect to lower their cholesterol an average of 10 mg/dL. However, changes in body weight and composition during exercise training can influence this relationship. Taken in total, it is clear that exercise therapy has an important role in patients with dyslipoproteinemias, but exercise programs should be individualized since not everyone receives a beneficial effect from it alone.

Obesity

Obesity has several adverse effects on health. It is known to be an independent risk factor for the development of[81–83]:

Coronary heart disease
Hypertension
Hyperlipidemia
Diabetes

Degenerative arthritis
Certain cancers

When only diet therapy is prescribed for weight loss, decreases in both body fat and lean body mass occur. However, a combination of diet and a dynamic exercise program can promote weight loss while preserving muscle mass.[84–87] Combined programs of exercise and dietary restriction appear to result in greater weight loss than either program alone.[88–90] Although lean persons often increase their caloric intake in response to vigorous exercise, this effect does not necessarily occur in obese men or women.[72,91–92] In addition, the ability to continue a program of regular physical activity assists patients in sustaining weight loss.[93] A program of moderate dietary restriction providing at least 1200 kcal/day, combined with regular physical activity resulting in a caloric deficit between 500 and 1000 kcal/day, should result in a weight loss of approximately 1 kg/wk while promoting a more desirable cardiovascular risk profile and improved functional working capacity.[94]

Osteoporosis and Skeletal Health

Osteoporosis is a cause of significant morbidity and mortality, particularly in elderly white women. The annual cost of osteoporosis and its complications to our health care system is estimated at $10 billion annually, with costs projected to double in the next 30 years.[95] Of the 1.5 million fractures occurring annually in the United States, the majority appear related to preexisting osteoporosis.[96] Interventions aimed at improving skeletal health could have a major impact on public health.

Regulation of bone metabolism and structure is a complex event involving the integration of several factors, including:

Parathyroid hormone
Activated vitamin D
Glucocorticoids
Local substances such as growth factors and cytokines

External mechanical forces also appear to influence bone metabolism. For example, it is known that immobilization results in significant bone reabsorption,[97–98] and the resumption of activity results in reaccumulation of bone mass.[99] Experimental models have shown that creating a mechanical strain across a segment of bone results in localized bone hypertrophy.[100–101] It follows from these observations that weightbearing exercise positively influences bone metabolism and slows or reverses the development of osteoporosis. However, the role of exercise in its prevention and treatment is not entirely clear.

Cross-sectional studies have found that increased levels of measured physical fitness,[102–104] reported physical activity,[105–109] and muscle strength[110] are correlated with higher measures of bone density. However, cross-sectional studies are unable to control for many factors that can bias these results. Prospective longitudinal studies have also given mixed results. Several investigators evaluating postmenopausal women performing aerobic exercise over time have found either a reduction in the rate of bone mineral loss[111] or a stabilization of bone density compared with more sedentary individuals.[112–116] Some investigators have even identified increases in bone mineral density in exercising postmenopausal women,[117–119] but these gains might reverse with cessation of an exercise program.[118] In contrast, not all investigators have been able to document the beneficial effects of moderate exercise programs.[120–122]

There are also potential negative consequences of exercise for individuals with osteoporosis, including stress fractures resulting from high-impact activities or excess strain across a given bone. Exercise programs should be individually tailored to each person. Recent data, however, continue to confirm that even frail elderly patients can safely perform high-intensity resistance exercises with marked improvement in functional capacity.[123] Therefore, the presence of osteoporosis is not a contraindication to exercise prescription; several exercises are considered safe and effective for patients with osteoporosis.[124–125]

EXERCISE AND PSYCHOLOGICAL HEALTH

Individuals who exercise on a regular basis often report that aerobic activities leave them with a sense of well-being, a feeling often termed a "runner's high." These subjective observations have led investigators to evaluate the potential influence of aerobic activities on mental health.

Anxiety and Anxiety Disorders

The experience of anxiety is common in normal individuals. It is characterized by the physical sensation of sympathetic activity and a cognitive process of worry or fear. For most individuals, the sensation of anxiety is associated with specific events, such as worrying about an upcoming test or a physical illness. With true anxiety disorders, however, the level of worry becomes more pervasive and begins to interfere with daily functioning.

Several controlled trials have shown that the performance of aerobic activity results in a decreased sensation of anxiety for normal individuals.[126–129] The mechanism by which these benefits occur is unknown; however, several hypotheses have been put forth. One hypothesis posits that exercise improves one's sense of self-efficacy and personal mastery.[130–131] Others have suggested that exercise acts as a cognitive diversion resulting in a decreased awareness of anxiety.[132–133] Another important factor might be that improvements in physical fitness result in a lower level of sympathetic hyperactivity in given situations.[134–135] Dishman[136] has suggested that the beneficial effect might be mediated through a sense of social reinforcement and support.

There is less information regarding the benefits of exercise therapy in individuals with true anxiety disorders.[137] One retrospective study of patients with anxiety disorders found increased reports of anxiety following exercise.[138] However, a prospective trial found that patients with panic disorder were able to undergo symptom-limited exercise testing; many of the subjects were reassured by the test.[139] These data are easily interpreted if one uses the cognitive behavioral model to conceptualize abnormalities in panic patients.[140] This model suggests that it is the cognitive misinterpretation of normal sympathetic activity that is key to the sense of impending doom characterized by panic disorder. The recreation of the sympathetic symptoms of a panic attack during exercise testing in a controlled environment with cardiac monitoring could be very reassuring to patients and can represent a powerful cognitive intervention. However, it remains to be determined if prescribing exercise has short- and long-term benefits for anxiety patients.

Depression

Feelings of sadness are a common experience for most individuals. Such feelings are usually related to specific life events and do not interfere with daily functioning to any great degree. If they become more intense and disruptive, they might meet criteria for a true depressive disorder.[141] Clinical depression is a common condition; one epidemiologic study reports a lifetime prevalence of 7.8%.[142]

There has been interest in the possible role of prescribed aerobic exercise in the treatment of both normal feelings of sadness and true depression. Some uncontrolled studies have found that normal individuals performing exercise report a reduction in feelings of depression.[143–146] However, there are few randomized studies and results have been mixed.[129,147–148] At this time, it is impossible to assert with any degree of certainty that the prescription of exercise improves depressed moods of normal individuals. However, a recent review[149] suggests that exercise might improve a broader concept of overall well-being. A sense of well-being can be influenced by many factors, including a comfort with one's physical appearance and sense of physical fitness. It is clear that exercise would have a positive impact on these factors.

Several randomized studies have evaluated the effect of exercise therapy in clinically depressed patients.[150–153] In general, it appears that exercise might be as effective as other forms of therapy, including meditation, progressive muscle relaxation, and interpersonal therapy for mild-to-moderately depressed outpatients. It might be that exercise alone or in conjunction with other forms of therapy should be part of the treatment of depressed patients who are candidates for outpatient therapy.

CONCLUSION

Despite the numerous benefits of exercise on emotional well-being, there is some concern that an excessive commitment to exercise can be associated with negative psychological consequences. Excessive competitiveness and overexertion have been reported to be associated with increased feelings of tension and anxiety.[154–155] There is also concern that some individuals could become "negatively addicted" to exercise.[156] However, it is unlikely that these observations apply to the majority of individuals who could benefit by adopting a more active lifestyle. These reports should not deter physicians from intervening with their patients and prescribing exercise to increase and maintain good health.

REFERENCES

1. Hammond HK, Froelicher VF. The physiologic sequelae of chronic dynamic exercise. *Med Clin North Am.* 1985;69:21–39.
2. Cox ML, Bennett JB, Dudley GA. Exercise training-induced alterations of cardiac morphology. *J Appl Physiol.* 1986;61:926–993.
3. Graettinger WF. The cardiovascular response to chronic physical exertion and exercise training: an echocardiographic review. *Am Heart J.* 1984;108:1014–1018.
4. Hauser Am, Dressendorfer RH, Vox M, et al. Symmetric cardiac enlargement in highly trained endurance athletes: a two-dimensional echocardiographic study. *Am Heart J.* 1985;109:1038–1044.
5. Maron BJ. Structural features of the athlete heart as defined by echocardiography. *J Am Coll Cardiol.* 1986;7:190–203.
6. Grossman W. Cardiac hypertrophy: useful adaptation or pathologic process? *Am J Med.* 1980;69:576–584.
7. Blomquist CG, Saltin B. Cardiovascular adaptations to physical training. *Annu Rev Physiol.* 1983;45:169–189.
8. Hammond HK, Froelicher VF. The physiologic sequelae of chronic dynamic exercise. *Med Clin North Am.* 1985;69:21–39.
9. Morris JN, Healy JA, Raffle PA, et al. Coronary heart disease and physical activity at work. *Lancet.* 1953;2:1053–1057, 1111–1120.
10. Paffenbarger RS Jr, Hyde RT, Wing AL, et al. Physical activity, all-cause mortality and longevity of college alumni. *N Engl J Med.* 1986;314:605–613.
11. Brunner D, Manelis G, Modan M, et al. Physical activity at work and the incidence of myocardial infarction, angina pectoris and death due to ischemic heart disease: an epidemiological study in Israeli collective settlements (kibbutzim). *J Chronic Dis.* 1974; 27:217–233.
12. Kannel WB, Sorlie P. Some health benefits of physical activity: the Framingham study. *Arch Intern Med.* 1979;139:857–886.
13. Garcia-Palmieri MR, Costas P Jr, Cruz-Vidal M, et al. Increased physical activity: a protective factor against heart attacks in Puerto Rico. *Am J Cardiol.* 1982;50:749–755.
14. Morris JN, Everitt MG, Pollard R, et al. Vigorous exercise in leisure time: protection against coronary heart disease. *Lancet.* 1980; 6:1207–1210.
15. Magnus K, Matroos A, Strackee J. Walking, cycling, or gardening, with or without seasonal interruption, in relation to acute coronary events. *Am J Epidemiol.* 1979;110:724–733.
16. Peters RK, Cady LD, Bischoff DP, et al. Physical fitness and subsequent myocardial infarction in healthy workers. *JAMA.* 1983; 249:3052–3056.
17. Leon AS, Connett J, Jacobs DR, et al. Leisure-time physical activity levels and risk of coronary heart disease and death. *JAMA.* 1987; 258:2388–2395.
18. Blair SN, et al. Physical fitness and all-cause mortality: a prospective study of healthy men and women. *JAMA.* 1989;262:2395–2401.
19. Eklund LG, et al. Physical fitness as a predictor of cardiovascular mortality in asymptomatic North American men: the Lipid Research Clinics mortality follow-up study. *N Engl J Med.* 1988; 319:1379–1384.
20. Keys A. *Seven Countries: A Multi Variant Analysis of Death and Coronary Disease.* Cambridge, Mass: Harvard University Press; 1980.
21. Punsar S, Karvonen MJL. Physical activity and coronary heart disease in populations from East and West Finland. *Adv Cardiol.* 1976;18:196–207.
22. Progress in chronic disease prevention: protective effect of physical activity on coronary heart disease. *MMWR.* 1987;36:426.
23. Pate RR, Pratt M, Blair SN, et al. Physical activity and public

health: a recommendation from the Center for Disease Control and Prevention and the American College of Sports Medicine. *JAMA*. 1995;273:402–407.

24. Rippe JM, Ward A, Porcari JP, et al. Walking for health and fitness. *JAMA*. 1988;259:2720–2724.

25. Rodriguez BL, Curb JD, Burchfiel CM, Abbot RD, Petrovitch H, Masaki K, Chiu D. Physical activity and 23-year incidence of coronary heart disease morbidity and mortality among middle-aged men. The Honolulu Heart Program. *Circulation*. 1994;89:2540–2544.

26. Wenger NK, Froelicher ES, Smith LK, et al. Cardiac Rehabilitation Clinical Practice Guideline, #17. Rockville, Md: US Dept of Health and Human Services, Public Health Service, Agency for Health Care Policy and Research, and the National Heart, Lung, and Blood Institute. AHCPR publication 95-0672, October 1995.

27. Ornish D, Brown SE, Scherwitz LW, et al. Can lifestyle changes reverse coronary heart disease? The Lifestyle Changes Heart Trial. *Lancet*. 1990;336:129–133.

28. Hambrecht R, Niebauer J, Marburger C, et al. Various intensities of leisure time physical activity in patients with coronary artery disease: effects on cardiorespiratory fitness and progression of coronary atherosclerotic lesions. *J Am Coll Cardiol*. 1993;22(2):468–477.

29. Haskell WL, Alderman EL, Vair JM, et al. Eeffects of intense multiple risk factor reduction on coronary atherosclerosis and clinical cardiac events in men and women with coronary artery disease: The Stanford Coronary Risk Intervention Project (SCRIP). *Circulation*. 1994;89:975–990.

30. DeBusk RF, Houston N, Haskell W, et al. Exercise training soon after myocardial infarction. *Am J Cardiol*. 1979;44:1223–1229.

31. Oldridge NB. Compliance with cardiac rehabilitation services. *J Cardiac Rehab*. 1991;11:115–127.

32. Oldridge NB, Guyatt GH, Fischer ME, et al. Cardiac rehabilitation after myocardial infarction. Combined experience of randomized clinical trials. *JAMA*. 1988;260:945–950.

33. O'Connor GT, Buring JE, Yusuf S, et al. An overview of randomized trials of rehabilitation with exercise after myocardial infarction. *Circulation*. 1989;80:234–244.

34. Coats AJ, Adamopoulos S, Meyer TE, et al. Effects of physical training in chronic heart failure. *Lancet*. 1990;335:63–66.

35. Keteyian SJ, Levine AB, Brawner CA, et al. Exercise training in patients with heart failure. A randomized controlled trial. *Ann Intern Med*. 1996;124:1051–1057.

36. Sullivan MJ, Higginbotham NB, Cobb FR, et al. Exercise training in patients with severe left ventricular dysfunction: hemodynamic and metabolic effects. *Circulation*. 1988;78:506–515.

37. The Fifth Report of the Joint National Committee on detection, evaluation, and treatment of high blood pressure (JNC V). *Arch Intern Med*. 1993;153:154–183.

38. National high blood pressure education program working group report on primary prevention of hypertension. *Arch Intern Med*. 1993;153:186–208.

39. Kasiske BL, Ma JZ, Kalil RSN, Louis TA. Effects of antihypertensive therapy on serum lipids. *Ann Intern Med*. 1995;122:133–141.

40. Fraser GE, Phillips RL, Harris R: Physical fitness and blood pressure in school children. *Circulation*. 1983;67:405–412.

41. Paffenbarger RS Jr, Wing AL, Hyde RT, et al. Physical activity and incidence of hypertension in college alumni. *Am J Epidemiol*. 1983;117:245–257.

42. Blair SN, Goodyear NN, Gibbons LW, et al. Physical fitness and incidence of hypertension in healthy normotensive men and women. *JAMA*. 1984;252:487–490.

43. Hagberg JM, Seals DR. Exercise training and hypertension. *Acta Med Scand*. 1986;711(Suppl):13.

44. Harris KA, Holley RG. Physiological response to circuit weight training in borderline hypertensive subjects. *Med Sci Sports Exerc*. 1987;19:246–252.

45. Wilmore JH, Pan RB, Ward P, et al. Strength, endurance, BMR and body composition changes during circuit weight training. *Med Sci Sports Exerc*. 1976;8:59–60.

46. Kelemen MH, Effron MB, Valenti SA, et al. Exercise training combined with antihypertensive drug therapy: effects on lipids, blood pressure, and left ventricular mass. *JAMA*. 1990;263:2766–2771.

47. MacDougall JD, Tuxen D, Sale DG, et al. Arterial blood pressure response to heavy resistance exercise. *J Appl Physiol*. 1985;58:785–790.

48. Gettman LR, Pollock ML. Circuit weight training: a critical review of its physiological benefits. *Physician Sports Med*. 1981;9:44–60.

49. Butler RM, Beierwaltes WH, Rogers FJ. The cardiovascular response to circuit weight training in patients with cardiac disease. *J Cardiopulmonary Rehabil*. 1987;7:401–409.

50. Keleman MH, Stewart KJ, Gillilan RE, et al. Circuit weight training in cardiac patients. *J Am Coll Cardiol*. 1986;7:38–42.

51. Butler RM, Palmer G, Rogers FJ. Circuit weight training in early cardiac rehabilitation. *J Am Osteo Assoc*. 1992;92:77–89.

52. Ruderman NB, Granda OP, Hohansen K. The effect of physical training on glucose tolerance and plasma lipids in maturity-onset diabetes. *Diabetes*. 1979;28(suppl 1):89–92.

53. Saltrin B, Lindgrarde F, Houston M, et al. Physical training and glucose tolerance in middle-aged men with chemical diabetes. *Diabetes*. 1979;28(suppl 1):30–32.

54. Bjorntorp P, DeJounge K, Krotklewski M, et al. Physical training in human obesity: III. Effects of long-term physical training on body composition. *Metabolism*. 1973;22:1467–1475.

55. Lampman RM, Santinga JT, Savage PJ, et al. Effect of exercise training on glucose tolerance, in vivo insulin sensitivity, lipid and lipoprotein concentrations in middle-aged men with mild hypertriglyceridemia. *Metabolism*. 1985;34:205–211.

56. Cooper KH, Pollock ML, Martin RP, et al. Physical fitness levels versus selected coronary risk factors: a cross sectional study. *JAMA*. 1976;236:166–169.

57. Hartung GH, Foreyt JP, Mitchell RE, et al. Relation of diet to high-density lipoprotein cholesterol in middle-aged marathon runners, joggers and inactive men. *N Engl J Med*. 1980;302:357–361.

58. Martin RP, Haskell WL, Wood PD. Blood chemistry and lipid profiles of elite distance runners. *Ann NY Acad Sci*. 1977;301:246–360.

59. Wood PD, Haskell W, Klein H, et al. The distribution of plasma lipoproteins in middle-aged male runners. *Metabolism*. 1976;25:1249–1257.

60. Wood PD, Haskell WL, Stern S, et al. Plasma lipoprotein distributions in male and female runners. *Ann NY Acad Sci*. 1977;301:748–763.

61. Adner MM, Castelli WP. Elevated high-density lipoprotein levels in marathon runners. *JAMA*. 1980;243:534–536.

62. Enger SC, Stromme SB, Refsum HE. High density lipoprotein cholesterol, total cholesterol and triglycerides in serum after a single exposure to prolonged heavy exercise. *Scand J Clin Lab Invest*. 1980;40:341–345.

63. Hunter R, Swale J, Peyman MA, et al. Some immediate and long term effects of exercise on the plasma lipids. *Lancet*. 1972;2:671–675.

64. Montoye HJ, Block WD, Goyle R. Maximal oxygen intake and blood lipids. *J Chronic Dis*. 1978;31:111–118.

65. Schane JA, Cundiff DE. Relationships among cardiorespiratory fitness, regular physical activity and plasma lipids in young adults. *Metabolism.* 1979;28:771–776.

66. Altekruse EB, Wilmore JH. Changes in blood chemistries following a controlled exercise program. *J Occup Med.* 1973;15:110–113.

67. Findlay IN, Taylor RS, Dangie HJ, et al. Cardiovascular effects of training for a marathon run in unfit middle aged men. *Br Med J.* 1987;295:521–524.

68. Lopez SA, Vial R, Balant L, et al. Effect of exercise and physical fitness on serum lipids and lipoproteins. *Atherosclerosis.* 1974;20:1–9.

69. Ruderman NB, Ganda OP, Johansen K. The effect of physical training on glucose tolerance and plasma lipids in maturity-onset diabetes. *Diabetes.* 1979;28(suppl 1):89–92.

70. Allison TG, Iammarino RM, Metz KF, et al. Failure of exercise to increase high density lipoprotein cholesterol. *J Cardiac Rehab.* 1981;1:257–262.

71. Freyman JF, McNeil DJ, Alanpovic P, et al. Effects of 12 weeks of exercise training on plasma lipids and apolipoproteins in middle-aged men. *Med Sci Sports Exerc.* 1982;14:103. Abstract.

72. Holloszy JO, Skinner JS, Toro G, et al. Effects of a six-month program of endurance exercise on serum lipids of middle-aged men. *Am J Cardiol.* 1964;14:753–760.

73. Leon AS, Conrad JC, Hunninglake DB, et al. Effects of a vigorous walking program on body composition, carbohydrate and lipid metabolism of obese young men. *Am J Clin Nutr.* 1979;32:1776–1787.

74. Lewis S, Haskell WL, Wood PD, et al. Effects of physical activity on weight reduction in obese middle-aged women. *Am J Clin Nutr.* 1979;29:151–156.

75. Wood PD, Haskell WL, Blair SN, et al. Increased exercise level and plasma protein concentrations: a one year randomized, controlled study in sedentary middle-aged men. *Metabolism.* 1983; 32:30–31.

76. Lipson LC, Nonow RO, Schaefer EJ, et al. Effects of exercise conditioning on plasma high density lipoproteins and other lipoproteins. *Atherosclerosis.* 1980;37:529–538.

77. Savage MP, Petraris MN, Thompson WH, et al. Exercise training effects on serum lipids of prepubescent boys and adult men. *Med Sci Sports Exerc.* 1986;18:197–204.

78. Streja D, Mymin D. Moderate exercise and high density lipoprotein-cholesterol: observations during a cardiac rehabilitation program. *JAMA.* 1979;242:2190–2192.

79. Wood PD, Stefanich ML, Preon OM, et al. Changes in plasma lipids and lipoproteins in overweight men during weight loss through dieting as compared with exercise. *N Engl J Med.* 1988; 319:1173–1179.

80. Tran ZV, Weltman A. Differential effects of exercise on serum lipid and lipoprotein levels seen with changes in body weight. *JAMA.* 1985;254:919–924.

81. Hubert HB, Feinleib M, McNamara P, et al. A 26-year follow-up of participants in the Framingham heart study. *Circulation.* 1983; 67:968–977.

82. Simopoulous AP, VanItalie T. Body weight, health, and longevity. *Ann Intern Med.* 1984;100:285–295.

83. Van Itallie TB. Health implications of overweight and obesity in the United States. *Ann Intern Med.* 1985;103(suppl 6, pt 2):983–988.

84. Hagen RD, Upton SJ, Wong L, et al. The effects of aerobic conditioning and/or caloric restriction in overweight men and women. *Med Sci Sports Exerc.* 1986;18:87–94.

85. Pavlou KN, Steffe WP, Leeman RN, et al. Effects of dieting and

86. Spoko RW, Leon AS, Jacobs DR Jr, et al. The effects of exercise and weight loss on plasma lipids in young obese men. *Metabolism.* 1985;34:227–236.

87. Weltman A, Matter S, Stanford BA. Caloric restriction and/or mild exercise: effects on serum lipids and body composition. *Am J Clin Nutr.* 1980;33:1002–1009.

88. Dudleston AK, Bennion M. Effect of diet and/or exercise on college women. *J Am Diet Assoc.* 1970;56:126–129.

89. Council on Scientific Affairs: treatment of obesity in adults. *JAMA.* 1988;260:2547–2551.

90. Weinsier RL, Wadden TA, Ritenbaugh C, et al. Recommended therapeutic guidelines for professional weight control programs. *Am J Clin Nutr.* 1984;40:865–872.

91. Woo R, Garrow JS, Pi-Sunyer FX. Effects of exercise on spontaneous intake in obesity. *Am J Clin Nutr.* 1982;36:470–477.

92. Woo R, Pi-Sunyer FX. Effect of increased physical activity on voluntary intake in lean women. *Metabolism.* 1985;34:836–841.

93. Miller PM, Sims KL. Evaluation and component analysis of a comprehensive weight control program. *Int J Obes.* 1981;5:57–65.

94. Hagen RD. Benefits of aerobic conditioning and diet for overweight adults. *Sports Med.* 1988;5:144–155.

95. Cummings SR, Rubin SM, Blank D. The future of hip fractures in the United States: numbers, cost, and potential effects of postmenopausal estrogen. *Clin Orthop.* 1990;252:163.

96. Riggs BL, Melton LJ III. The prevention and treatment of osteoporosis. *N Engl J Med.* 1992;327:620.

97. Uhthoff H, Jaworski Z. Bone loss in response to long-term immobilization. *J Bone Joint Surg.* 1978;60B:420–429.

98. Marcus R, Carte DR. The role of physical activity in bone mass regulation. *Adv Sports Med Fitness.* 1988;1:63–82.

99. LeBlanc A, Schneider VS, Evans HJ, et al. Bone mineral loss and recovery after 17 weeks of bed rest. *J Bone Min Res.* 1990;5:843–855.

100. Rubin CT, Lanyon LE. Bone remodeling in response to applied dynamic loads. *Trans Orthop Res Soc.* 1981;6:64.

101. Rubin CT, Lanyon LE. Regulation of bone mass by peak strain magnitude. *Trans Orthop Res Soc.* 1983;8:70.

102. Bevier WC, Wiswell RA, Pyka G. Relationship of body composition, muscle strength, and aerobic capacity to bone mineral density in older men and women. *J Bone Min Res.* 1989;4:421–432.

103. Pocock NA, Eisman JA, Yeates MG, et al. Physical fitness is a major determinant of femoral neck and lumbar spine bone mineral density. *J Clin Invest.* 1986;78:618–621.

104. Pocock NA, Pocock N, Eisman J, et al. Muscle strength, physical fitness, and weight but not age predict femoral neck bone mass. *J Bone Min Res.* 1989;4:441–448.

105. Chow RK, Harrison JE, Brown CF, et al. Physical fitness effect on bone mass in postmenopausal women. *Arch Phys Med Rehabil.* 1986;67:231–234.

106. Oyster N, Morton M, Linnell S. Physical activity and osteoporosis in postmenopausal women. *Med Sci Sports Exerc.* 1984;16:44–50.

107. Talmage RV, Stinnett SS, Landwehr JT. Age-related loss of bone density in nonathletic women. *Bone Min.* 1986;1:115–125.

108. Kanders B, Dempster DW, Lindsay R. Interaction of calcium nutrition and physical activity on bone mass in young women. *J Bone Min Res.* 1988;3:145–149.

109. Aloia JF, Vaswani AN, Yeh JK. Premenopausal bone mass is related to physical activity. *Arch Intern Med.* 1988;148:121–123.

110. Snow-Harter C, Bouxsein M, Lewis B. Muscle strength as a pre-

dictor of bone mineral density in young women. *J Bone Min Res.* 1990;5:589–595.

111. Block JE, Smith R, Friedlander A, et al. Preventing osteoporosis with exercise: a review with emphasis on methodology. *Med Hypotheses.* 1989;30:9–19.

112. Aloia JF, Cohn SH, Ostuni JA, et al. Prevention of involutional bone loss by exercise. *Ann Intern Med.* 1978;89:356–358.

113. Simkin A, Ayalon J, Leichter I. Increased trabecular bone density due to bone-loading exercises in postmenopausal osteoporotic women. *Calcif Tissue Int.* 1987;40:59–63.

114. White MK, Martin RB, Yeates RA, et al. The effects of exercise on the bones of postmenopausal women. *Int Orthop.* 1984;7:209–214.

115. Sandler RB, Cauley JA, Hom OL, et al. The effects of walking on the cross-sectional dimensions of the radius in postmenopausal women. *Calcif Tissue Int.* 1987;41:65–69.

116. Krolner B, Toft B, Pors Nielsen S, et al. Physical exercise as prophylaxis against involutional bone loss: a controlled trial. *Clin Sci.* 1983;64:541–546.

117. Smith EL, Reddan W, Smith PE. Physical activity and calcium modalities for bone mineral increase in aged women. *Med Sci Sports Exerc.* 1981;13:60–64.

118. Dalsky G, Stocke KS, Ehsani AA. Exercise training and lumbar bone mineral content in postmenopausal women. *Ann Intern Med.* 1988;108:824–828.

119. Chow R, Harrison JE, Notarius C. Effect of two randomized exercise programs on bone mass of healthy postmenopausal women. *BMJ.* 1987;295:1441–1444.

120. Cavanaugh DJ, Cann CE. Brisk walking does not stop bone loss in postmenopausal women. *Bone.* 1988;9:201–204.

121. Sanaki M, Wahner HW, Offord KP, et al. Efficacy of nonloading exercises in prevention of vertebral bone loss in postmenopausal women: a controlled trial. *Mayo Clin Proc.* 1989;64:762–769.

122. Rockwell JC, Sorsen AM, Baker S, et al. Weight training decreases vertebral bone density in premenopausal women: a prospective study. *J Clin Endocrinol Metab.* 1990;71:988–993.

123. Fiatarone MA, O'Neill EF, Ryan ND, et al. Exercise training and nutritional supplementation for physical frailty in very elderly people. *N Engl J Med.* 1994;330:1769–1775.

124. Sinaki M. Postmenopausal spinal osteoporosis: physical therapy and rehabilitation principles. *Mayo Clin Proc.* 1982;57:699–703.

125. Sinaki M. Beneficial musculoskeletal effects of physical activity in the older woman. *Geriatr Med Today.* 1989;8:53–72.

126. Lichtman S, Poser E. The effects of exercise on mood and cognitive functioning. *J Psychosom Res.* 1983;27:43–52.

127. Blumenthal JA, Williams RS, Needels TL, et al. Psychological changes accompany aerobic exercise in healthy middle-aged adults. *Psychosom Med.* 1982;44:520–536.

128. Fasting K, Gronningsaeter H. Unemployment, trait anxiety, and physical exercise. *Scand J Sport Sci.* 1986;8:99–103.

129. King H, Taylor CB, Haskell WL, et al. The influence of regular aerobic exercise on psychological health: a randomized, controlled trial of healthy middle-aged adults. *Health Psychol.* 1989;8:305–324.

130. Morgan W. Anxiety reduction following acute physical activity. *Psychiatr Ann.* 1979;9:141–147.

131. Long B. Aerobic conditioning and stress inoculation. A comparison of stress-management interventions. *Cognitive Ther Res.* 1984;8:517–542.

132. Hughes J. Psychological effects of habitual aerobic exercise: a critical review. *Prev Med.* 1984;13:66–78.

133. Morgan W. Effective beneficence of vigorous physical activity. *Med Sci Sports Exerc.* 1985;17:94–100.

134. Sinyor D, Golden M, Steinert Y, et al. Experimental manipulation of aerobic fitness and response to psychosocial stress: heart rate and self-report measures. *Psychosom Med.* 1986;48:324–337.

135. Cantor J, Zillman D, Day K. Relationships between cardiorespiratory fitness and physiological responses to films. *Percept Mot Skills.* 1978;46:1123–1130.

136. Dishman R. Medical psychology in exercise and sport. *Med Clin North Am.* 1985;69:123–143.

137. Taylor CB, Sallis JF, Needle R. The relation of physical activity and exercise to mental health. *Public Health Rep.* 1985;100:195–202.

138. Cameron O, Hudson C. Influence of exercise on anxiety level in patients with anxiety disorders. *Psychosom Med.* 1986;27:720–723.

139. Taylor DB, King R, Ehlers A, et al. Treadmill exercise testing and ambulatory heart rate measures in patients with panic attacks. *Am J Cardiol.* 1987;60:48J–52J.

140. Clark DM. Anxiety states: Panic and generalized anxiety. In: Hawton K, Salkovskis PM, Kirk J, Clark DM, eds. *Cognitive Behaviour Therapy for Psychiatric Problems. A Practical Guide.* Oxford, England: Oxford University Press; 1989.

141. American Psychiatric Association. *Diagnostic and Statistical Manual of Mental Disorders.* 3rd ed. Rev. Washington, DC: American Psychiatric Press; 1987.

142. Weissman MM, Bruce ML, Leaf PJ, et al. Affective disorders. In: Robins LN, Regier DA, eds. *Psychiatric Disorders in America: The Epidemiologic Catchment Area Study.* New York, NY: The Free Press; 1991.

143. Hayden R, Allen G. Relationship between aerobic exercise, anxiety, and depression: convergent validation by knowledgeable informants. *J Sports Med.* 1984;24:69–74.

144. Kowal D, Patton J, Vogel J. Psychological states and aerobic fitness of male and female recruits before and after basic training. *Aviat Space Environ Med.* 1978;49:603–606.

145. Berger B, Owen D. Mood alteration with swimming: swimmers really do "feel better." *Psychosom Med.* 1983;45:425–433.

146. Brown R, Ramirez D, Taub J. The prescription of exercise for depression. *Physician Sports Med.* 1978;6(Dec):34–49.

147. Moses J, Steptoe A, Mathews A, et al. The effects of exercise training on mental well-being in the normal population: a controlled trial. *J Psychosom Res.* 1989;33:47–6.

148. Folkings C. Effects of physical training on mood. *J Clin Psychol.* 1976;32:385–388.

149. Plante T, Rodin J. Physical fitness and enhanced psychological health. *Curr Psychol.* 1990;9:3–24.

150. Griest J, Klein MH, Eischens RR, et al. Running as treatment for depression. *Compr Psychiatry.* 1979;20:41–54.

151. Klein H, Eischens RR, Morgan WP, et al. A comparative outcome study of group psychotherapy versus exercise treatments for depression. *Int J Mental Health* 1985;13:148–177.

152. McCann I, Holmes D. The influence of aerobic exercise on depression. *J Pers Soc Psychol.* 1984;46:1142–1147.

153. McNeil JK, LeBlanc EM, Joyner M. The effect of exercise on depressive symptoms in moderately depressed elderly. *Psychol Aging.* 1991;6:487–488.

154. Morgan WP, Costill DL, Flynn MG, et al. Mood disturbance following increased training in swimmers. *Med Sci Sports Exerc.* 1988;20:408–414.

155. Steptoe A, Bolton J. The short term influence of high and low intensity physical exercise on mood. *Psychol Health.* 1988;2:91–96.

156. Morgan WP. Negative addiction in runners. *Physician Sports Med.* 1979;7:57–70.

17. Stress Management in Primary Care

JOHN A. JEROME

Key Concepts

- **Empathy for stress-related problems and their many manifestations**

- **Stress and related somatic complaints, including those related to somatic dysfunction**

- **Signs and symptoms of depression**

- **Signs and symptoms of anxiety**

- **Signs and symptoms of alcohol abuse**

- **Signs and symptoms of insomnia**

- **Adaptive methods for coping with stress**

- **Overview of treatment techniques**

- **Impact of the doctor–patient relationship**

In primary care, stress-induced somatic complaints are the mechanisms underlying the symptoms for 20–35% of all patients seeking treatment from physicians.[1–2] In the United States, more than 33% of the population is susceptible to acute or chronic stress and the physical and psychological disorders caused by stress.[3] The effects of stress include the following changes:

Biochemical
Physiologic
Behavioral
Psychological

Many of these changes are directly related to health. This chapter reviews the major theories of stress and presents a framework for understanding and treating the causes of stress. It includes guidelines for the cognitive–behavioral management of the effects of stress related to:

Anxiety
Depression
Alcohol abuse
Insomnia

CONCEPTUALIZING STRESS

Physicians often speak of stress as if it explains many unusual patient behaviors, signs, and symptoms. The term stress is also used as a catchall term for emotional reactions (such as anger, fear, and depression) or as an explanation for drug and alcohol abuse. Lay definitions are primarily concerned with the notion of environmental pressures and the belief that such pressures are aversive.

In the physical sciences, stress is a normalized force acting on an object. Osteopathic physicians learn to use palpation and manipulative treatment to physically manage stress-related effects. A narrow psychosocial focus occurs when patients and physicians talk about stress as an exclusive problem. Discussion often centers on stress-inducing environmental variables or on their biologic–psychological consequences. Stress is both.

Treating symptoms such as depression, anxiety, drug abuse, and insomnia does not alter environmental stressors or their underlying mechanisms. The treating physician is not able to directly control or change these psychosocially complex processes.

STRESS AS PROCESS

Stress is an interactive process in which the patient responds in predictable biopsychosocial ways to certain environmentally or internally mediated stressors. The process unfolds as a sequence of feelings, thoughts, and actions involving many interacting biopsychosocial factors. Stress is not a single precipitating event or the resulting biologic consequences. Stress involves:

Environmental stimuli
Psychological appraisals
Feelings
Behavioral and physiologic consequences

Physiologic responses to stressors are often linked to biochemical measurements of stress and tension in the musculoskeletal system. An osteopathically oriented examination for stress-related somatic dysfunction is one such measurement. Several objective measurements allow the physician to form impressions about the patient's emotional status and biologic condition and identify markers for the bodily systems most affected by stress. For example, catecholamines and corticosteroids, secreted by the adrenal medulla and cortex respectively, can be measured from urine and plasma levels. The secretion of catecholamines reflects sympathetic arousal because the adrenal medulla is innervated by the sympathetic nervous system.

Secretions of epinephrine and norepinephrine are also part of the sympathetic arousal process. The secretion of catecholamines leads to systemic reactions in the body such as increased

205

cardiovascular reactivity, and changes in cognitive, emotional, and behavioral functioning. These changes are often expressed as chronic muscle tension. Little doubt exists in the mind of the osteopathically trained physician that stress is reflected in the musculoskeletal system.[4–5]

By considering function along with structure, osteopathic concepts emphasize the role of the body's communication systems (nervous, circulatory, and endocrine) in both initiating and facilitating somatic dysfunction on a reflex basis. The term facilitation means the enhancement or reinforcement of otherwise subthreshold neuronal activities that stimulate effector units to carry out inappropriately whatever action they normally do.[6] Examples of effector sites are:

Muscle bundles
Muscle groups
Viscera
Other neural units and networks

Osteopathic treatment is designed to raise stimulus thresholds so that stressors are less likely to induce or maintain somatic dysfunction-related problems.

THEORIES OF STRESS

In 1932, Walter Cannon[7] was the first to write that the release of catecholamines and musculoskeletal arousal initially ease adaptation. Being aroused by stress provides a biologic advantage enabling the individual to respond rapidly to danger. Historically, these stress-related increases of catecholamines eased survival and adaptive responses. We ignored a pain, fought back, ran to safety on broken bones, and scrambled to the top of the food chain. We have survived as a species, but now survival depends on how we relate to our cortically driven society. That which was first described in Cannon's early work as our "fight-or-flight" strategy no longer serves us adequately in our ambiguous and increasingly complex world. Now we internalize the stressors and become distressed. We then present ourselves to the primary care physician requesting treatment for symptoms and problems.

Damaging stress levels are reached when perceived threats or dangers upset the biopsychosocial balance. When prolonged stress reaches critical levels, chronically increased concentrations of antiinflammatory corticosteroids and proinflammatory prostaglandins can alter immune responses, with increased vulnerability to immune-related problems. Damaging stress levels are reflected in the neuromusculoskeletal system as disruption of the body's homeostasis exhausts the patient. Diseases, impairments, and disabilities are apt to follow under certain circumstances.

Osteopathic philosophy teaches that structure and function are interdependent, that form follows function. Thoughts, emotions, and behaviors in response to stressors are in a blended and complex relationship that can affect both anatomy (structure) and physiology (function).

Hans Selye[8] first described the interdependent processes of

responding to stress as the general adaptation syndrome (GAS). Selye believed that our response to stress was a specific syndrome following certain patterns and affecting specific organs. Stress itself could be induced by a variety of internal or external stimuli.

When patients are continually stressed, they move through three response stages. First, there is a startle response and orienting reflex as the patient becomes aware of the stress and is biologically alarmed. Adrenal, cardiovascular, respiratory, and musculoskeletal functions increase.

Next is an attempt to cope and problem solve biologically, psychologically, and socially. The patient mobilizes all resources to meet and resist the stressor. If the patient is successful, mastery and learning occur. If the patient fails, he or she becomes exhausted physiologically, mentally, and emotionally.

The third stage, exhaustion, is what the osteopathic physician sees clinically as a variety of dysfunctional signs and symptoms affecting any and all organ systems, including the neuromusculoskeletal network. As coping responses fail, the exhaustion depletes adaptive reserves and resistance disappears. Common consequences of this failure to adapt include:

Fatigue
Depression
Anxiety
Insomnia
Musculoskeletal complaints
Drug seeking

When emotional and biologic reserves become depleted, patients often seek medical attention. Careful questioning is needed to uncover such problems as:

Family disruptions
Job dissatisfaction
Chronic overstimulation
Feeling overwhelmed
Being overweight
Lack of exercise
Poor relaxation habits

Because osteopathic theory emphasizes the interdependence of body structure and its overall function, osteopathic physicians commonly use palpatory diagnosis and osteopathic manipulative treatment in the primary care setting to help diagnose and manage somatic components of this syndrome.

Inquiries to the primary care physician are not about coping with stress, but more often:

"Why does my neck hurt?"
"I need something for my stomach."
"Can I have some time off work?"
"I need something for depression."
"Give me something to sleep."
"What should I do about my teenager?"

Clinically, two approaches are possible:

1. Change the stressor
2. Help the patient respond in healthy ways to the stress

Change Stressor

Before seeking medical treatment, the patient probably has made an independent effort to change the stressor without much success. Many studies illustrate that compliance with physicians' advice is low,[7] particularly in the current climate of health care delivery where the pace is hectic and often impersonal. As patients shift between physicians and insurance plans in a managed care environment, the personal relationships once forged between physician and patient disappear. Trusting relationships are difficult to establish under these circumstances, increasing the likelihood that professional advice will go unheeded.

Many patients who come to a primary care setting are looking for help with stress-related symptoms. A primary care osteopathically oriented approach assesses the disturbing psychosocial and organic problems, including the neuromusculoskeletal elements, so that a long-term treatment strategy can be developed. In such cases, after a detailed physical examination, the strategy incorporates all elements of the osteopathic philosophy. It includes:

Palpatory diagnosis
Manipulative treatment
Exercise
Appropriate medication
Coping strategy education

When hands-on procedures are used to identify stress-induced somatic dysfunction, the experienced osteopathic practitioner can determine whether the observed pattern of somatic dysfunction is associated with primary neuromusculoskeletal or a more complex behavioral dysfunction.

Directing all aspects of treatment toward modifying the biopsychosocial causes and maladaptive responses to stress is important. The primary care physician must be constantly aware that clinically evident stress reflects two realities:

1. A patient's response to stress-inducing environmental events produces biopsychosocial consequences.
2. A patient's stress management style is an important process in which the physician must intervene for long-term adaptive change.

Change Response to Stress

As previously mentioned, stress-related conditions are associated with at least 20% of primary care outpatients.[9–11] By changing the response to stress, one immediately treats some of the autonomic components of stress-related somatic dysfunction and their antecedents. Success is more likely when physicians educate patients, guide and mentor their adaptation, and teach them coping and stress-mastery skills. In a primary care practice, diagnosis begins by accurately diagnosing four of the most common behavioral consequences of stress[12–13]:

Depression
Anxiety
Substance abuse
Insomnia

When the diagnosis is made, carefully inform the patient and then guide him or her through a process of problem identification and problem-solving designed to either relieve or cope with the stress. The remainder of this chapter reviews the four stress-induced displays of stress from a cognitive–behavioral standpoint. Emphasis is on rapid techniques for diagnosis and on specific strategies to be employed within the doctor–patient relationship.

DEPRESSION

Feeling "down" is a universal experience. Being sad or "blue" accompanies disappointments, setbacks, or losses in life. The depressed mood usually lasts a short time and passes. For some people, however, the sadness becomes intense and long lasting, coloring every aspect of their existence. The future seems hopeless. They feel:

Powerless
Consumed by their helplessness
Overwhelmed
Unable to concentrate, sleep, or solve the routine problems of life

In the United States, clinical depression results in the hospitalization of 6% of all women and 3% of all men,[14–15] with 15% of all who are severely clinically depressed eventually committing suicide.[16]

The DSM-IV[17] and the *Guidelines for Detection and Diagnosis in Primary Care* [18–19] categorize mental health diagnoses. The word depression refers to a syndrome in which a variety of signs and symptoms occur. Typically, there is a change from previous adequate emotional functioning to a depressed mood and a loss of pleasure in life's usual activities. The depressed person feels sad or empty most of the time and often experiences impairment in interpersonal, social, or occupational functioning.

Associated symptoms include:

Fatigue
Feelings of worthlessness
Excessive guilt
Agitation
Diminished abilities to problem solve or concentrate
Indecisiveness
Insomnia or hypersomnia
Possible suicidal thoughts

If five or more of these symptoms are present for more than 2 weeks, a diagnosis of major depressive disorder is considered.

If over the last 2 years the patient reports having felt these symptoms and says that for more than half of that time it was hard to work, take care of simple things at home, or get along with people, the diagnosis is dysthymic disorder.

Measurement of Depression

There are many self-administered inventories, such as the Zung Depression Scale,[20–21] the Beck Depression Inventories,[22–23] and the MMPI Depression Scale.[24–25] These inventories provide reliable and valid measures of the severity of depression. The patient can initially be tested for a baseline measure and then repeatedly tested with the same instrument to measure progress. More recently developed structured interviews such as the PRIME-MD[26–27] allow one to quickly (i.e., in 8.4 minutes) determine the presence of pivotal signs and symptoms (Table 17.1). Medical disorders with intrusive symptoms of depression must be ruled out (Table 17.2). Depression has also been reported as a serious adverse effect of more than 100 commonly prescribed drugs (Table 17.3).

The tricyclic antidepressants and serotonin reuptake inhibitors are the gold standards for initiating management of many serious, possibly organic, depressions.[28–29] Recoveries are often dramatic as the patient reverts to predepression levels of functioning. Primary care physicians are exposed to a tremendous amount of publicity and marketing from drug companies to manage the symptoms of depression with various pharmacologic products. The belief is that as the symptoms are relieved,

the patient's physical complaints and general adaptation will improve. More commonly, however, problems do not subside entirely. When this is the case, other interventions can be used. General osteopathic care uses multiple strategies, such as:

Counseling
Drug therapy
Exercise
Osteopathic manipulative treatment designed to decrease the effects of stress-related disorders and somatic dysfunction

Cognitive Behavioral Factors in Depression

Depression can be understood in many ways within the framework of learning theory.[30–31] Deficits in social skills can set the stage for unrewarding social, vocational, and personal relationships causing subsequent feelings of depression. Studies with animals and humans[32] exposed over time to inescapable stress have shown that the subjects failed to demonstrate simple behaviors to escape or avoid the stress and subsequent punishment. In a laboratory setting when exposed to inescapable electric shock, dogs and humans felt helpless and both suffered from naturally occurring depression. Human and animal groups showed similar response patterns of:

Passivity
Slowed learning
Impaired problem solving
Loss of appetite

Their inability to stop the stressor or to escape from the stressor initiates cognitive processes that lead to a sense of powerlessness. Victims of inescapable stress lower their future expecta-

Table 17.1
Structured Interview Questions for Depression[a]

For the last 2 weeks, have you had any of the following problems *nearly every day?*

1. Trouble falling or staying asleep, or sleeping too much?	YES	NO
2. Feeling tired or having little energy?	YES	NO
3. Poor appetite or overeating?	YES	NO
4. Little interest or pleasure in doing things?	YES	NO
5. Feeling down, depressed, or hopeless?	YES	NO
6. Feeling bad about yourself, or that you are a failure or have let yourself or your family down?	YES	NO
7. Trouble concentrating on things, such as reading the newspaper or watching television?	YES	NO
8. Being so fidgety or restless that you were moving around a lot more than usual? If No: What about the opposite—moving or speaking so slowly that other people could have noticed?	YES	NO
9. In the last 2 weeks, have you had thoughts that you would be better off dead or of hurting yourself in some way? (Tell me about it.)	YES	NO

SCORING: If five or more of #1 to #9 are yes, one of which is #4 or #5, then consider *major depressive disorder.* If the condition has persisted over the last 2 *years* and the patient reports that it was hard to do their work, take care of things at home, or get along with other people, then consider *dysthymia.*

[a]Primary care evaluation for mental disorders (Prime-MD)

Modified from Spitzer RL, Williams JB. *PRIME-MD Clinical Evaluation Guide.* New York, NY: Biometrics Research, New York State Psychiatric Institute; 1994.

Table 17.2
Medical Illnesses and Conditions with Intrinsic Symptoms of Depression

Parkinson's disease
Normal pressure hydrocephalus
Multiple sclerosis/stroke
Brain tumors (temporal lobe)
Adrenal insufficiency syndrome
Hyperparathyroidism
Vitamin B_{12} or iron deficiency
Serum sodium or potassium reductions
Hypercalcemia
Cancer
Metal (thallium, mercury) intoxication
Chronic pain and disease (i.e., fibromyalgia, diabetes mellitus)
A common symptom in geriatric populations
20–24% of medical inpatients
Neurologic disorders (i.e., related to abnormal catecholamines or indoleamine metabolism)
Cardiac disease
Serious medical injury (i.e., spinal cord, end-stage renal disease)
Dementia, head trauma, seizure disorders

Modified from Derogatis LR, Wise TN. *Anxiety and Depressive Disorders in the Medical Patient. Clinical Practice No. 4.* Washington, DC: American Psychiatric Press; 1989:121.

Table 17.3
Drugs with Known Propensity to Induce Clinical Depression

Antihypertensives
    Reserpine
    α-methyldopa
    Guanethidine
    Clonidine
    Propranolol
    Hydralazine
Hormones
    Corticosteroids
    Progesterone
    Estrogen
Central Nervous System Depressants
    Benzodiazepines
    Barbiturates
    Alcohol
Neuroleptics
    Haloperidol
    Fluphenazine
Cardiovascular Agents
    Digitalis
    Procainamide
Anti–Parkinsonian Drugs
    L-Dopa
    Amantadine
Antimicrobials
    Cycloserine
    Gram-negative agents
    Sulfonamides

Reprinted with permission from Derogatis LR, Wise TN. *Anxiety and Depressive Disorders in the Medical Patient. Clinical Practice, No. 4.* Washington, DC: American Psychiatric Press; 1989:125.

Table 17.4
Faulty Reasoning Patterns Noted in Depression-Prone Patients

Arbitrary inference—drawing a specific conclusion in the absence of evidence to support the conclusion.
Selective abstraction—drawing a conclusion based on a detail taken out of context.
Overgeneralization—drawing a broad, global conclusion on the basis of one or more isolated pieces of information.
Magnification and minimization—exaggerating the significance of negative events and minimizing the significance of positive events.
Personalization—relating external events to oneself when there is no realistic basis for making such a connection.
Absolutistic, dichotomous thinking—placing all experiences in one of two opposite categories.

Reprinted with permission from Beck, AT, Rush AJ, Shaw BF, Emery G. *Cognitive Therapy of Depression: A Treatment Manual.* New York, NY: Guilford; 1979.

tions for control over stress and have measurably lower self-esteem and lower motivation.[33–35]

Aaron Beck [23,30] describes negative schemas as a learned maladaptive thinking process that often leads to depression. When faced with stressful events, some patients routinely employ negative views of themselves and their abilities (i.e, negative schemas) and are dominated by themes of failure and personal inadequacies. They have learned to expect their performance to be worse than that of others.[36–37] They view the world as an overwhelming place, laden with burdens and filled with excessive demands and daily defeats.[38]

Over time, negative depression schemas become stable, long-standing thought patterns. People with these patterns both organize experiences as depressing and selectively direct attention to the negative aspects of current and future stressors. These depression-prone personalities perceive the present as depressing, remember the past the same way, and respond to the future in a fixed, negative manner, independent of what occurs in their environments.

There are six basic cognitive errors in logic that a patient learns over time (Table 17.4). Insight into these faulty reasoning patterns is helpful for some depressed patients. Osteopathically trained physicians routinely work with their patients' cognitive coping styles in addition to pharmacologically managing their depressive symptomatology. Obviously, drug ther-

apy and cognitive behavioral treatments augment and complement each other. With major clinical depression, administering these strategies simultaneously often yields a superior result.[39–40]

ANXIETY

Anxiety is a generalized state of fear or apprehension in response to a perceived threat. The chronically threatened individual will eventually begin to experience anxiety and distress in everyday situations that would not normally have elicited such reactions in the past. An anxious reaction is a basic, genetically programed human response to a real or imagined threatening stressor. The biologic changes elicited by an anxious reaction have specific adaptive survival value. They represent alertness and arousal responses for better behavioral and biologic focusing and coping with the threat.

An anxious reaction represents one of several built-in stress programs that patients can use to adapt to and cope with new threats in their environment. Physically, anxiety is a generalized state of fear with especially strong manifestations in the hypothalamic, sympathetic, autonomic, adrenal, and reticular neuroendocrine networks. Physiologically, the symptoms reflect heightened autonomic arousal, including:

Elevated heart rate
Occasional heartbeat irregularities
Blood pressure changes
Sweating
Intestinal distress
Blood sugar changes
Generalized muscle tension
Altered pain perceptions

The last two are readily observed during an osteopathically oriented examination of the musculoskeletal system. Anxious individuals also report general symptoms such as:

Insomnia
Excessive worrying
Forgetfulness

Irritability
Difficulty concentrating

Experienced osteopathic physicians soon learn that chronic exposure to anxiety-inducing scenarios without adequate coping strategies often involve irrational cognitive appraisals of threats that, in turn, can lead to further and commonly excessive anticipatory anxiety.

Anxiety disorders occur in 15.4% of the patient population and account for 11% of all physician visits.[13] A study of 350 primary care physicians rated anxiety disorders as the most common psychiatric problem seen in their clinical practice.[41] Anxiolytic benzodiazepines are among the most commonly prescribed medications in the United States. Primary care physicians write 85% of these prescriptions. The diagnosis of anxiety is complicated by the fact that anxiety is often not the patient's chief complaint. Rather, patients experiencing anxiety generally complain of physical problems. Primary care physicians often focus exclusively on physical symptoms, failing to note that the patient's complaints are really created by unreported or unrecognized anxiety and chronic autonomic arousal including disturbed sleep–wake cycles. Hypervigilance is apparent with expressions of apprehensive expectations and generalized unfocused fears. Table 17.5 lists medical disorders and conditions associated with high amounts of anxiety.

Anxiety is also identified by diffuse and often severe panic attacks and general agitation that might not be related to any one particular situation or immediate stressor. The panic usually lasts anywhere from a few seconds to more than one hour. These dreaded feelings of being overwhelmed and out of control appear suddenly and climb to high intensities. The attacks are accompanied by intense feelings of apprehension over some presumed or pending distress or catastrophe. During panic attacks, one will experience:

Sweating
Trembling
Choking
Shortness of breath

Table 17.5
Medical Disorders and Conditions Associated with Disproportionately High Amounts of Anxiety

Hyperthyroidism
Cardiac disease (e.g., arrhythmias, paroxysmal tachycardias)
Mitral valve prolapse
Pernicious anemia
Respiratory disease
Endocrine disorders (e.g., hypoglycemia)
Porphyria
Depressive illness
Pre-senile or senile dementias
Effects of drug or alcohol use/withdrawal
Caffeine/tobacco use
Hypoglycemia
Pheochromocytoma
Epilepsy

Chest pain
Heart palpitations
Dizziness
Paresthesia

Measurement of Anxiety

Anxiety inventories such as the State-Trait Anxiety Inventory (STAI)[42] and anxiety subscales of the MMPI-2[24–25] measure individual differences in anxiety susceptibility and the patient's tendency to perceive a wide range of situations as threatening. The inventories also measure the patient's reported response to these situations with associated activation and arousal of the autonomic nervous system. Physiologic measurements of anxiety focus on:

Skin conductance
Heart rate
Blood pressure
Respiratory rate
Gastric motility symptoms
Pupillary diameter
Muscle tension

These measurements can also be routinely collected in the primary care setting. Structured interview questions to elicit information from the anxious patient seen in family practice settings are another tool (Table 17.6).

Anxiety Treatments

An osteopathically oriented approach for managing anxiety involves treating both the physical symptoms of chronic arousal and the mechanisms of learned and reinforced maladaptive arousal in response to prolonged stress. Benzodiazepines can be prescribed to reduce the paralyzing anxiety associated with a clear external stressor. These are most effective if prescribed on a temporary emergency basis with the goal of preventing dependence and iatrogenic withdrawal anxiety when medications are stopped. Avoid chronic use. Physical symptoms can also be controlled by relaxation, controlled diaphragmatic breathing, and biofeedback.[43–44] Anxiety-generating thoughts can be identified and techniques to counter them explored. These treatments attempt to reduce anxiety by enhancing coping abilities, providing interpersonal support, and training the patient to reduce learned anxiety associated with environmental stimuli.

All of these treatment modalities can be effectively used together or separately according to patient needs. Also, general measures to improve coping ability such as a healthy diet, moderate exercise, weight control, and mobilizing a support system of family and friends can set the stage for effective long-term anxiety management.[45] Positive outcomes of the proposed treatment will result when the primary care physician enters collaborative management relationships with anxious patients. The goal of these relationships is to alleviate overly aroused patients' fears as they learn new coping styles.

Table 17.6
Structured Interview Questions for Generalized Anxiety Disorder[a]

1. Have you felt nervous, anxious, or on edge on more than half the days in the last month?		YES NO

In the last month, have you *often* been bothered by any of these problems?

2. Feeling restless so that it is hard to sit still?	4. Muscle tension, aches, or soreness?	6. Trouble concentrating on things, such as reading a book or watching TV?
3. Getting tired very easily?	5. Trouble falling asleep or staying asleep?	7. Becoming easily annoyed or irritated?

8. Are three or more of #2 to #7 checked?	YES NO
9. In the last month, have these problems made it hard for you to do your work, take care of things at home, or get along with other people?	YES NO
10. In the last 6 months, have you been worrying *a great deal* about *different things, and has this* been on more than half the days in the last 6 months? (Count as yes only if yes to both.)	YES NO
11. When you are worrying this way, do you find that you can't stop?	YES NO
12. These current anxiety symptoms *are not* due to the biologic effects of a physical disorder, medication, or other drug?	YES NO

SCORING: Yes to 1, 8, 9, 10, 11, and 12 constitutes a probable diagnosis of *generalized anxiety disorder.*

[a]Primary Care Evaluation for Mental Disorders (PRIME-MD)

Modified from Spitzer RL, Williams JB. *PRIME-MD Clinical Evaluation Guide.* New York, NY: Biometrics Research, New York State Psychiatric Institute, 1994.

ALCOHOL USE AND DEPENDENCE

Medical care for alcohol abuse has become routine work in primary care practice. The use of alcohol as a coping strategy is uniquely human. As our society becomes more complex and ambiguous, more patients use and abuse alcohol. The reported use and abuse of intoxicating chemicals that alter the physiology of the body and the central nervous system dates back to the ancient Egyptian papyri and the Greek amphitheater at Delphi. Alcohol abuse and dependency have become a self-medication strategy for stress that is socially tolerated and modeled for our children.

Alcohol abuse adversely affects the lives of 10 million Americans and their families. Alcohol is involved in 10% of all deaths in the United States. Alcohol abuse and dependence are often prevalent in both partners where spousal and child abuse occur.[46–47] Physicians in primary care settings recognize only about half the problem drinkers they encounter and are even less likely to identify problems in women and the elderly.[48–51]

At one end of the drinking spectrum, alcohol is used in moderation without adverse consequences. At the other end of the spectrum are those drinkers who suffer medically, vocationally, and psychosocially from repeated abuse of alcohol. In the middle lie most of the drinkers with varying consumption patterns and risks of alcohol-related problems. Only 5% of the three-fourths of all Americans who drink acquire the disorder

of alcoholism.[48] Many people drink while under stress to anesthetize themselves and to experience the numbing effects of alcohol as a strategy for managing their own symptoms. Excessive problem drinking, in and outside the work place, costs U.S. industry approximately $15 billion a year.[49] Besides the significant economic consequences, alcohol also presents a significant health hazard and challenge to the osteopathic physician attempting to help his or her patients manage stress. Alcohol overuse is both a response to stress and a cause of further stress.

Alcohol As Response to Stress

It is important to distinguish between the effects of alcohol and the disease of alcoholism. Alcoholism is the consequence of the overuse of alcohol in people who are predisposed to addiction by genetic, physiologic, psychological, sociological, and other factors. The disease of alcoholism, regardless of the cause or whether the onset is acute or insidious, will eventually take over the life of the patient and his or her family.

Alcohol depresses the brain's neuronal and synaptic transmission systems, including inhibitory centers, in low concentrations.[52] These depressant effects create three basic psychological and behavioral patterns[53]:

Euphoriant effects
Disinhibiting effects
Anxiety-relieving effects

Initial euphoriant effects reflect central nervous system sedation, temporarily increasing self-esteem, courage, and confidence. To the alcoholic, these disinhibiting and anxiety-relieving effects seem almost magical. For example, alcohol's effects often allow a person to:

Talk to the opposite sex
Speak up at school or parties
Interact with the boss
Have fun playing with the children
Dance well
Be less sexually inhibited

As with any mood-altering drug, the individual returns to previous functional levels after he or she stops drinking.

A clear understanding of the drinking pattern is necessary to detect whether the problem is harmful or abusive or represents alcohol dependency. The DSM-IV[17] is the most widely used diagnostic framework for alcohol related disorders. Questions used in the PRIME-MD structured interview for alcohol use are useful as well (Table 17.7). The CAGE Questionnaire[54] is another simple diagnostic screen that consists of four questions:

1. Have you ever tried to **C**ut down on your drinking?
2. Are you **A**nnoyed when people ask you about your drinking?
3. Do you ever feel **G**uilty about your drinking?
4. Do you ever take a drink as a morning **E**ye opener?

Positive answers on three or four questions are significant diagnostically.

Table 17.7
Structured Interview to Elicit Information on Probable Alcohol Abuse/Dependence[a]

Opening Inquiries:

Have . . . . you thought you should cut down on your drinking? Why?

Has . . . . someone complained about your drinking? Who? Why?

Do . . . . you feel guilty or upset about your drinking? Why?

Have . . . . you had five or more drinks in a single day in the past month? How often have you had that much to drink in the past 6 months? Has that caused any problems?

1. Has a doctor ever suggested that you stop drinking because of a problem with your health? (Count as yes if patient has continued to drink in the last 6 months after doctor suggested stopping.)	YES	NO

Have any of the following happened to you *more than one time* in the last 6 months?

2. Were you drinking, high from alcohol, or hung over while you were working, going to school, or taking care of other responsibilities?	YES	NO
3. What about missing or being late for work, school, or other responsibilities because you were drinking or hung over?	YES	NO
4. What about having a problem getting along with other people while you were drinking?	YES	NO
5. What about driving a car after having several drinks or after drinking too much?	YES	NO

SCORING: Yes to most questions. (Consider responses to Opening Inquiries and other information known about the patient, such as information obtained from a family member.)

[a]Primary Care Evaluation for Mental Disorders (PRIME-MD)

Modified from Spitzer RL, Williams JB. *PRIME-MD Clinical Evaluation Guide.* New York, NY: Biometrics Research, New York State Psychiatric Institute; 1994.

Alcohol As Cause of Further Stress

Once alcohol use becomes a primary stress management strategy, further stress follows (Table 17.8). Alcohol might have been used initially to manage stress; disruption in work, personal, and social relationships, and isolation are the final consequences. The urgent need to drink concentrates the patient's remaining energies on securing and ingesting alcohol. Denial, minimization, and self-deception are used to explain the alcoholic's deterioration, especially when discussing alcohol use with the primary care physician. When the patient's self-esteem or prominence in the community are at risk, lying, evasion, and other manipulative behaviors emerge as strategies to avoid admitting the problem to the primary care physician and others. At the point of threatened or actual loss of job, family, home, or health, the physician may intervene and encourage the patient to enter an alcohol treatment program.

Primary care physicians refer patients with alcoholism to specialized treatment programs. Alcohol abuse is a chronic, relapsing disease, and these patients often require more consistent and involved treatment than primary care physicians can provide.[55] The recovering alcoholic will need a physician's guidance and family support to learn to face life's stressors without the use of intoxicants. With support from the physi-

Table 17.8
Alcohol-Related Stress-Induced Factors Affecting Somatic Dysfunction

Increased central nervous system excitability

Associated vitamin and nutritional deficiencies

Cirrhosis

Wernicke-Korsakoff syndrome

Alcoholic dementias

Functional gastrointestinal changes with and without gastrointestinal bleeding

Pancreatitis

Esophageal varices

Blackouts; brief amnesic periods

Ataxia and poor coordination

cian, the family, and a peer support group, the patient can change his or her maladaptive stress management style and abstain from alcohol. The tasks of the physician are to:

Develop a strong relationship built on trust

Make the diagnosis of alcoholism compassionately

Elicit the support of family and friends

Refer the alcoholic to a recognized recovery program

Reinforce the stress management techniques

STRESS MANAGEMENT TECHNIQUES

Social Support

The most powerful tool in the management of the patient's stress is his or her support network. This social network gives a person the feeling that he or she is valued and cared about. The idea that people need to be surrounded by groups of people who provide love and a sense of belonging is not new. The patient needs help to identify mentors and significant others in his or her environment whom he or she can trust and with whom he or she can share feelings. The osteopathic physician assumes an important role by providing this help and counseling the stressed patient. Referrals to self-help groups in the community such as Alanon and Recovery Inc. can help to reduce the patient's self-absorption. Participation in these groups also leads to the development of outside interests that are compatible with a lifestyle free of addictions.

Spiritual Support

For patients undergoing elective open heart surgery for coronary artery disease, those experiencing strength or comfort from their spiritual feelings are three times more likely to survive than are those without spiritual support. Those who participate in social and community groups (such as local government, senior centers, historical societies, etc.) also have three times the survival rate of those who do not take part in social activity. A 1995 study[56] involving 232 patients over age 55 found that seniors who had both "protective factors," i.e., spiritual and social support, enjoyed a tenfold increase in survival.

The amount or type of spiritual or social activity did not matter as much as the *"participation, comfort and support derived from the activity."*[56] Why and how spiritual feelings and social support extend life following open heart surgery is not understood. There are over 200 studies corroborating this health-enhancing, life-prolonging effect in a variety of circumstances and population groups. It is well-documented, for example, that Mormons (both clergy and devout members) have extremely long life expectancies. The physiologic mechanisms behind longevity and health are not well understood, however.

Sense of Control

Control is a powerful mitigator of stress. Patients can be given a sense that they can cope by learning to anticipate a potential stressor. The perception that a stressor can be accurately anticipated or stopped increases one's range of problem-solving possibilities and consequent feelings of control. By giving a patient information about stressors before the patient's exposure to them, researchers have reduced the threatening appraisals made when the stressor is experienced. Studies have determined that the stress of surgery or of common medical procedures can be reduced by giving patients accurate expectations of what they will experience.

Perceptions of Risk

Assessment of risk is influenced by certain biases and perceptions brought into the stressful situation by the patient and the health care provider. Many patients need to construct simplified models of the complex interaction of stressful factors in their environment to cope with stress effectively. Provide the patient with simplified models of how the world works and which risks must be taken to put the patient at ease. Many patients like to use general inferential rules to increase their understanding of health problems and the subtle and complex factors surrounding the risks posed by a stressor. Setting the stage for decreased anxiety and adaptive coping is as easy as taking a moment to listen to the patient's conceptual model of the stressors in his or her life. From there the physician can offer concrete explanations of the stressors and the risks imposed on the patient. One example is telling a patient with back pain that he or she has degenerative disk disease and osteoarthritis. This can sound intimidating and hopeless. To help the patient understand the diagnosis, the physician can describe the condition from the patient's own perspective. In this example, the patient's diagnosis could be described as "an aging back with stiffness that can be treated in many ways."

Observational Learning

Observational learning is learning that occurs without any apparent direct reinforcement. Many coping behaviors for stress can be learned if the patient observes another person modeling the behavior. Learning occurs without the individual patient making a response or receiving tangible external reinforcement for the behavior. This suggests the importance of our internalizations and cognitive abilities, which allow us to transform what has been observed into many new patterns of behavior.

Encourage your patient to become involved in settings and groups of people who are coping with stress. This can lead to new patterns of coping behaviors. For example, patients with intractable pain fear physical movement. Having them attend a group aquatic exercise program lets them observe others, perhaps older or in poorer health than themselves, moving without damage or injury. This vicarious learning lessens the patient's apprehension when the painful area is moved.

Progressive Relaxation

Progressive relaxation is based on the premise that muscle tension is closely related to anxiety. Individuals feel a significant reduction in experienced anxiety as their tense muscles are made to relax. The teaching of progressive muscular relaxation skills follows a standard procedure. The individual practices muscle relaxation after he or she decides which muscle groups are tense. For example, tell an individual to tighten his or her jaw and notice a pattern of feeling strain in these muscles. After maintaining the tension for approximately 10 seconds, tell the subject to let the muscle group completely relax, and then to notice a difference in sensation as the places that were previously tense and strained relax. After a few minutes of relaxation, repeat the sequence. The main goal of the training program is to teach individuals what it feels like to relax each muscle group and to provide practice in achieving greater relaxation. Once the individual can discriminate the pattern of tension in a particular muscle group, omit the instruction to tense before relaxing. Instead, the individual must relax the muscle from the present level of tension. The original relaxation procedure required months of training with hundreds of trained muscle sites. Clinical practice employs a much more abbreviated form of training and is easy to teach to the patient in a primary care setting.

Systematic Desensitization

Successful deep muscle relaxation inhibits stress-inducing anxiety as both nonthreatening and threatening scenarios are imagined. This treatment procedure employs a graded hierarchy of stressful scenes and images. It incorporates the patient's perception of the least stress-provoking situations to the most stress-provoking situations. Using imagery, the individual is first taught to relax individual muscles. When the imagery and muscle relaxations are mastered, work begins on an increasingly complex hierarchy of imagery and learning that moves gradually from low- to high-stress situations. As skills improve, instruction helps the learner tolerate increasingly difficult scenes during the relaxation process. As tolerance increases for anxiety-related imagery, the patient learns tolerance for anxiety-induced life situations. The therapeutic effectiveness of systematic desensitization has been shown with many anxiety-related disorders, such as phobias (including medical procedures), insomnia, and stress-related psychophysiologic disorders such as ulcers, asthma, and hypertension.[57]

Behavioral Rehearsal

Allowing individuals to act out or role play their interpersonal problems and usual manner of behavior is a method used in many different forms in primary care settings. The physician observes, listens to, and then often models or encourages the appropriate behaviors the patient might be lacking.

The physician often teaches assertiveness and problem-solving techniques. These techniques are most effective with individuals who experience stress as a result of difficulties in self-expression. A lack of appropriate interpersonal skills exacerbates stress-related physical symptoms. For example, an overwhelmingly demanding boss or spouse is a common cause of stress-related symptoms and health care seeking in a primary care setting. By teaching verbal strategies to more effectively deal with excessive and unfair demands, patients learn new and more effective coping behaviors.

Cognitive Restructuring

In cognitive restructuring, the physician determines and challenges specific thoughts or self-verbalizations that contribute to the stress-related disorder. Treatment is designed to help the patient modify negative, self-doubting statements by replacing them with self-enhancing declarations.[58] One cognitive restructuring method is called "thought stopping." Thought stopping is used when patients experience distress because of obsessive thoughts about stressors they have difficulty controlling. This also occurs with insomniacs, who cannot stop thinking long enough to fall asleep. The patient is asked to concentrate on the anxiety-induced thought and, after a short period, the physician suddenly and emphatically says, "stop." After this procedure has been repeated several times, the patient will report that the thoughts were interrupted by the word "stop." The physician then shifts control back to the patient. Specifically, the client is taught to utter a subvocal "stop" whenever he or she begins to engage in a self-defeating rumination.

Biofeedback

Using physiologic monitoring equipment, teach the patient to influence physiologic processes such as:

Blood pressure
Heart rate
Sweat gland activity
Skin temperature
Neuromuscular activity
Sphincter control
Penile tumescence

By receiving auditory or visual feedback, one learns about the close relationship between mind and body. The availability of sensitive recording devices for home use has made it possible

to work on these skills in a more organized and regular manner. There is a lack of systematic and well-controlled outcome studies that conclusively show the clinical effectiveness of some new monitoring devices. However, supportive literature for biofeedback-related muscle relaxation is slowly and cautiously appearing. Temperature biofeedback, which is also receiving positive support in the literature, controls Raynaud's phenomena and migraine headaches. From an osteopathic perspective, biofeedback makes it possible to extend voluntary control over some elements of somatic dysfunction by decreasing arousal responses affecting somatic and viscerosomatic reflex activities. Learning to master these responses helps develop a sense of control and improves confidence in one's self-healing abilities.

Psychophysiologic Insomnia Management

In the United States, approximately 10 million people annually consult their health care provider for sleep disorders, with half receiving prescriptions for sleeping medications.[59] Epidemiological studies suggest that 20–35% of respondents describe sleep problems as severe or constant for as long as 14 years. Other health problems are commonly identified as the primary complaints, however.[60] Persistent insomnia is not life threatening. When compared with good sleepers, however, insomniacs experience more[61–62]:

Hospitalizations
Anxiety
Depression
Fibromyalgia
Propensity for alcohol and other substance abuse

An inability to remain asleep is most common, followed by difficulty falling asleep and abnormal early morning awakening. Contributing factors appear divided among the following[60]:

Psychiatric (35%)
Psychophysiologic (15%)
Drug and alcohol dependency (12%)
Periodic limb movements (12%)
Medical, toxic, environmental (4%)
Various other (15%)

Typically, insomniacs are chronically aroused autonomically (anxious), or cognitively depressed and unable to stop thinking and worrying at bed time. They worry about not getting to sleep and then are too aroused at bed time to sleep. This worrying leads to fears that they will have poor daytime performance if they cannot make themselves sleep. Insomnia begets more insomnia and leads to poor learned sleep habits and routines. Insomnia lasting more than 3 weeks requires specific behavioral strategies to counteract the learned aspects of the insomnia. It also requires relaxation techniques and, if needed, intermittent use of sedatives or hypnosis.

Insomnia can be managed effectively by teaching sleep habit techniques that employ a variety of strategies (Table 17.9).

Table 17.9
Good Sleep Habits

Get up about the same time every day, regardless of when you go to bed.
Go to bed only when sleepy. Establish relaxing pre-sleep rituals.
Exercise regularly and keep active.
Organize your day around regular times for eating and outdoor activities with regular exposure to bright light, which synchronizes circadian cycles.
Avoid caffeine, nicotine, alcohol, excessive warmth, and hunger at bed time.
If you nap, try to nap at the same time every day.
When laying down to sleep, relax all your muscles, particularly your face and jaw, and breath slowly and evenly.
If you don't fall asleep in 20 minutes, get back up and return to bed when sleepy.

These techniques form the foundation for the guidance that the osteopathically trained physician gives to the patient. When sleep is restored, the patient feels more alert, and there are fewer vegetative and clinical signs of depression and anxiety during waking hours. Patients practicing good sleep habits report improved concentration, better problem solving, and more effective management of their stress.

Augmenting sleep habit strategies with medication for sleep during short intervals is another method used to manage insomnia. A prescription for exercise and a muscular relaxation training tape to be used in the evening hours will also promote better sleep. All this, coupled with encouragement by the physician, who functions both as educator and guide, will alleviate insomnia.

CONCLUSION

The osteopathically trained physician has many available tools to employ a broad approach to stress-related problems, including varieties of somatic dysfunction. Anxiety, depression, insomnia, and drug and alcohol abuse are common symptoms seen in primary care offices. Osteopathic management can be practiced in three ways:

1. By treating symptoms as they are reported and observed
2. By giving advice on managing stressors
3. By guiding and mentoring stress-related responses toward positive coping behaviors and strategies (the most rewarding)

Successful diagnosis depends on understanding the interactions of the biopsychosocial factors that lead to stress-induced problems. Successful treatment depends on giving clear explanations so that the patient understands the mechanisms that perpetuate his or her distress. The long-term goal is to assist the patient toward self-mastery and self-healing.

REFERENCES

1. Centers for Disease Control. *Ten leading causes of death in the United States.* Washington, DC: Government Publishing Office; 1980.

2. Surgeon General's Office. *Healthy people.* Washington, DC: Government Printing Office; 1979.

3. Surgeon General's Office. *Report on nutrition and health.* Washington, DC: Government Printing Office; 1988.

4. Korr IM. The sympathetic nervous system as mediator between somatic and supportive processes. In: *American Academy of Osteopathy Yearbook.* Indianapolis, Ind: 1970;170–175.

5. Korr IM. Sustained sympathicotonia as a factor in disease. In: *American Academy of Osteopathy Yearbook.* Indianapolis, Ind: 1978;207–221.

6. Ward R. Manual healing methods. In: Report to the National Institutes of Health on Alternative Medical Systems and Practices in the United States. Pub. 12–94: 113–119. 1995.

7. Cannon WB. *The Wisdom of the Body.* New York, NY: Norton; 1932.

8. Selye H. *The Stress of Life.* rev. ed. New York, NY: McGraw-Hill; 1976.

9. Anderson SM, Harthorn BH. The recognition, diagnosis and treatment of mental disorders by primary care physicians. *Med Care.* 1989;27;869–886.

10. Schulberg HC, Burns BJ. Mental disorders in primary care: epidemiologic, diagnostic, and treatment research directions. *Gen Hosp Psychiatry.* 1988:10.

11. Barrett JE, Barrett JA, Oxman RE, Gerber PD. The prevalence of psychiatric disorders in a primary care practice. *Arch Gen Psychiatry.* 1988;45:1100–1106.

12. Robins LN, Regier DA, eds. *Psychiatric Disorders in America.* New York, NY: Free Press; 1991.

13. Schurman RA, Kramer PD, Mitchell JB. The hidden mental health network: treatment of mental illness by nonpsychiatrist physicians. *Arch Gen Psychiatry.* 1985;42:89–94.

14. Secunda R, Friedman RlJ, Schuyler D. *The Depressive Disorders.* Washington, DC: Government Printing Office; 1973.

15. Beck AT. *Depression: Clinical, Experimental, and Theoretical Aspects.* New York, NY: Harper & Row; 1967.

16. Copas JB, Robin A. Suicide in psychiatric patients. The British. *J Psychiatry.* 1982;141:503–511.

17. American Psychiatric Association. *Diagnostic and Statistical Manual of Mental Disorders.* Rev. 4th ed. Washington, DC: American Psychiatric Association; 1987.

18. Depression Guideline Panel. *Depression in Primary Care, I. Detection and Diagnosis. Clinical Practice Guideline, No 5.* Rockville, Md: April 1993. US Dept of Health and Human Services, Public Health Service, Agency for Health Care Policy and Research publication 93-0550.

19. American Psychiatric Association. *Diagnostic and Statistical Manual of Mental Disorders.* Primary Care Version. Washington, DC: American Psychiatric Association; 1996.

20. Zung WWK. A self-rating depression scale. *Arch Gen Psychiatry.* 1965;12:63–70.

21. Zung WWK. A rating instrument for anxiety disorders. *Psychosomatics.* 1971;12:164–167.

22. Beck AT. *Depression: Clinical, Experimental and Theoretical Aspects.* New York, NY: Harper and Row; 1967.

23. Beck AT. *Cognitive Theory and the Emotional Disorders.* New York, NY: International Universities Press; 1976.

24. Hathaway SR, McKinley JC. *MMPI Manual.* Minneapolis, Minn: Psychological Corp; 1943.

25. Dahlstrom WG, Welsh GS. *An MMPI Handbook.* Minneapolis, Minn: University of Minnesota Press; 1972.

26. Spitzer RL, Williams JB, et al. *PRIME-MD Clinical Evaluation Guide.* New York State Psychiatric Institute, Biometrics Research Dept. 722 West 168th Street, Unit 74. New York, NY; 1994.

27. Spitzer RL, Williams JB. Utility of a new procedure for diagnosing mental disorders in primary care. *JAMA.* December 1994; 272(22):1749–1756.

28. Cameron OG. *Presentations of Depression.* New York, NY: John Wiley and Sons; 1987.

29. Nezu AM, Nezu CM. *Problem-Solving Therapy for Depression.* New York, NY: John Wiley and Sons; 1989.

30. Beck AT, Rush AJ, Shaw BF, Emery G. *Cognitive Therapy of Depression: A Treatment Manual.* New York, NY: Guilford; 1979.

31. Overmier JB, Seligman MEP. Effects of inescapable shock upon subsequent escape and avoidance learning. *J Comp Physiol Psychol.* 1967; 64:23–33.

32. Seligman MEP, Maier SF. Failure to escape traumatic shock. *J Exp Psychol.* 1967;74:1–9.

33. Abramson LY, Sackheim HA. A paradox in depression: uncontrollability and self-blame. *Psychol Bull.* 1977;84:835–851.

34. Abramson LY, Seligman MEP, Teasdale J. Learned helplessness in humans: critique and reformulation. *J Abnorm Psychol.* 1978;87:49–74.

35. Seligman MEP. Helplessness: *On Depression, Development, and Death.* San Francisco, Calif: Freeman; 1975.

36. Hollon SD, Beck AT. Cognitive therapy of depression. In: Kendall PC, Hollon, SD, eds. *Cognitive-Behavioral Interventions: Theory, Research and Procedures.* New York, NY: Academic Press; 1979:153–204.

37. Hollon SD, Kendall PC. Cognitive self-statements in depression: development of an automatic thoughts questionnaire. *Cognit Ther Res.* 1980;4:383–395.

38. Funabiki D, Calhoun J. Use of a behavioral-analytic procedure in evaluating two models of depression. *J Consult Clin Psychol.* 1979; 47:183–185.

39. D'Zurilla TJ. *Problem-solving Therapy: A Social Competence Approach to Clinical Intervention.* New York, NY: Springer-Verlag; 1986.

40. D'Zurilla TJ, Nezu AM. Development and preliminary evaluation of the social problem-solving inventory (SPSI). Paper presented at the meeting of the Association for the Advancement of Behavior Therapy. New York, November 1988.

41. Noyes R, Roth M, Burrows GD. *The Treatment of Anxiety, IV.* New York, NY: Elsevier; 1990.

42. Spielberger CD, Gorsuch RC, Lushene RE. *Manual for the state-trait anxiety inventory.* Palo Alto ,Calif: Consulting Psychologists; 1970.

43. Keabie D. *The Management of Anxiety.* New York, NY: Churchill Livingstone; 1989.

44. Kennerley H. *Managing Anxiety.* Oxford, England: Oxford Press; 1990.

45. Morris CG. *Psychology: An Introduction.* Englewood Cliffs, NJ: Prentice Hall; 1993.

46. West LJ, Cohen S. Provisions for dependency disorders. In: Hollant WW, Detels R, Knox G, eds. *Oxford Textbook of Public Health.* New York, NY: Oxford University Press; 1985;9:2.

47. Rankin JG, Ashley MJ. Alcohol-related health problems. In: Last JM, Wallace RB, eds. *Public Health and Preventative Medicine.* 13th ed. East Norwalk, Conn: Appleton & Lange; 1992;43.

48. Cleary PD, Miller M, Bush BLT, Warburg MM, Delbanco TL, Aronson M.D. Prevalence and recognition of alcohol abuse in a primary care population. *Am J Med.* 1988;85:4664–4671.

49. Buchsbaum DG, Buchanan RG, Poses RM, Schnoll SH, Lawton MJ. Physician detection of drinking problems in patients attending a general medicine practice. *J Gen Intern Med.* 1992;7:517–521.

50. Curtis JR, Geller G, Stokes EJ, Levine DM, Moore RD. Characteristics, diagnosis and treatment of alcoholism in elderly patients. *J Am Geriatr Soc.* 1989;37:310–316.

51. Dawson NV, Dadheech G, Speroff T, Smith RL, Schubert DSP. The effect of patient gender on the prevalence and recognition of alcoholism on a general medical service. *J. Am Intern Med.* 1992; 7:38–15.

52. Kissin B. The pharmacodynamics and natural history of alcoholism. In: Kissin B, Begleiter H, eds. *The Biology of Alcoholism, III: Clinical pathology.* New York, NY: Plenum; 1974.

53. Grenell RG. Effects of alcohol on the neuron. In: Kissin B, Begleiter H, eds. *The Biology of Alcoholism, II: Physiology and behavior.* New York, NY: Plenum; 1978.

54. Ewing JA. Detecting alcoholism. The CAGE questionnaire. *JAMA.* 1984;252:1905–1907.

55. Saunders JB, Aasland OG, Amundsen A, Grant M. Alcohol consumption and related problems among primary health care patients: WHO collaborative project on early detection of persons with harmful alcohol consumption. I. *Addiction.* 1993;88:349–362.

56. Oxman TE. Lack of social participation or religious strength and comfort as risk factors for death after cardiac surgery in the elderly. *Psychosom Med.* 1995;57:681–689.

57. Gatchel RJ, Baum A. *An Introduction into Health Psychology.* New York, NY: Random House; 1983.

58. Meichenbaum D, Turk D. The cognitive-behavior management of anxiety, anger and pain. In: Davidson PO, ed. *The Behavior Management of Pain.* New York, NY: Brunner/Mazel; 1976.

59. Lacks P, Morin CM. Recent advances in the assessment and treatment of insomnia. *J Consult Clin Psychol.* 1992;60:586–594.

60. Rosekind MR. The epidemiology and occurrence of insomnia. *J Clin Psychiatry.* 1992;53(suppl 6):4–6.

61. Lesch DR, Spire J-P. Clinical electroencephalography. In: Thorpy MJ, ed. *Handbook of Sleep Disorders.* New York, NY: Marcel Dekker; 1990:13–31.

62. Buysse DJ, Reynolds CF III. Insomnia. In: Thorpy MJ, ed. *Handbook of Sleep Disorders.* New York, NY: Marcel Dekker; 1990:375–433.

Osteopathic Considerations in Clinical Problem Solving

18. Clinical Problem Solving

SARAH A. SPRAFKA

Key Concepts

- **Four approaches to data gathering and synthesis, including pattern recognition, hypothetico-deductive method, problem-oriented perspective, and clinical decision analysis**

- **Problem-solving practices, including therapeutic touch, musculoskeletal pain, osteopathic manipulative treatment and medication, patient as a whole, and integrative thinking**

- **Osteopathic approach to clinical problem solving**

. . . in the long term, the osteopathic concept will survive because true principles never die. They may be averted, submerged, even denied, but they will emerge again, stronger than ever. They have only to be applied every day in patient care to show how fundamental and timeless they are.[1]

This chapter discusses clinical problem solving from an osteopathic primary care perspective. It begins by looking at four different approaches to clinical problem solving and discussing how each can be incorporated in the osteopathic family doctor's identification and explanation of a patient's problem. The second section discusses case vignettes to report and analyze an inquiry into osteopathic practitioners' self-reported problem solving processes. That inquiry is the source for the illustrative quotations used throughout this chapter. The third section summarizes a case illustrating application of the osteopathic approach to clinical problem solving. Throughout the chapter, the reader should keep in mind the following questions:

Is osteopathic clinical problem solving a prescriptive process, defined in part by established principles?

Alternatively, is osteopathic problem solving the same as what osteopathic physicians do when they tackle clinical problems?

Can osteopathic problem solving be a compromise occurring somewhere along that spectrum from principle to simple description of behaviors, describing a pattern that is different for each individual problem solver?

EXAMPLE CASE

Consider the following case. It is a Wednesday in mid-November. The setting is the office of A.B. Martin, DO, an osteopathic family practitioner. Mr. Johnson has made an appointment to see the physician. At the time of the patient's visit, Dr. Martin looks at the chart and notes that this is the patient's first visit to the office. One half hour has been allocated for the appointment. Based on preliminary examination, the following data have been entered in the chart:

Personal Data

Name: Richard Johnson
Age: 55
Ethnicity: White
Reason for visit: "I was raking leaves on Sunday and I got an aching sensation in my left shoulder. It still bothers me today."

Vital Signs

Ht: 6' 1"
Wt: 203 lbs.
BP: 160/110 mm Hg
P: 75 reg.
R: 16

Discussion

If you were Dr. Martin, what might you be thinking? At this point you have just the slightest bit of information about Mr. Johnson. He complains of shoulder pain. His weight is high relative to his height. You picture a large man. His blood pressure is elevated.

At this stage of your interaction with this patient (you have not met him yet), your first priority is clearly to conduct a thorough history and physical examination including a diagnostic palpatory examination, and to become acquainted with the patient as a person. As you plan for what you would like to learn from Mr. Johnson, you begin to consider some possible mechanisms for his presenting problem. These may be wide-ranging and include trauma to the shoulder or somatic dysfunction in the shoulder. He may have viscerosomatic reflex activity associated with cardiovascular and/or pulmonary disease.

At this point we leave the actual visit with Mr. Johnson, and consider some approaches you might take with this patient:

How you organize your data gathering and data synthesis

How you view this patient as an individual and as a member of a group

How you plan a short-term as well as longer-term strategy for your interaction with Mr. Johnson

DATA GATHERING AND SYNTHESIS

Data gathering and synthesis are at the heart of the problem-solving process for the clinician. The following sections elaborate on four major forms of data gathering and synthesis, and apply them to the example of Mr. Johnson.

Pattern Recognition

For the clinician, pattern recognition (also called pattern matching) is often invoked on those occasions when there is a clear, almost textbook picture, often of a diagnostic or causal nature, seen in the patient's presentation. For example, a clinician who is of a mind to consider a pattern for Mr. Johnson might think:

"Aha! White male, in his 50's, overweight, high blood pressure, presents with a variant on chest pain. Coronary artery disease, I'll bet you. And to complete the picture, I'll bet he smokes, has high cholesterol, and has a high stress sedentary job. I'll even bet you he has a positive treadmill test result."

Most of what we know about pattern matching comes from the work of Patel and colleagues[2-3] and Norman and colleagues.[4-7] The former have compared the diagnostic thought processes used by expert physicians with those of nonexperts, and those used with more and less complex problems. For example, expert physicians are described as employing a type of "forward reasoning" in solving straightforward problems; it involves going from highly selective data gathering directly to diagnostic conclusions. This process appears to be analogous to a sophisticated form of pattern recognition or pattern matching. It contrasts with what they call "backward" reasoning. Backward reasoning is employed when the diagnostician does more detective work by considering possible diagnoses and then checking back in the data to see whether there are supportive cues present, as well as using the diagnostic hypotheses to guide further data gathering. Novice problem solvers use backward reasoning (what others often refer to as the hypothetico-deductive method) much more than do expert problem solvers.

Norman and others have concentrated their research on recall and utilization of visual patterns such as those found in dermatologic problems and x-ray study interpretation. Problem solving by osteopathic primary care physicians corroborates and expands on this research. The following examples illustrate this type of reasoning.

VISUAL PATTERNS

Three types of visual patterns are common. One is the visual distinction of the presence of illness. Clinicians have described situations in which they walk into the examining room and the first thing they note is that the patient "looks sick." They use cues such as the patient's:

Coloring
Dullness of the eyes
Lethargy
Change in appearance since the last visit

Clinicians express the importance of visually assessing the apparent severity of the patient illness or "how sick" the patient looks. They note that this initial assessment often sets the tone for the subsequent workup. The assessment guides whether the workup is directed at identifying potentially serious physical illness or something that may be less serious or possibly lifestyle related, and whether it is more or less urgent for the physician to reach a preliminary conclusion and initiate treatment.

A second visual pattern particularly meaningful for osteopathic primary care physicians is that of the musculoskeletal system. On the first observation of the patient, the DO notes the patient's posture and movements. He or she is able to note where there are structural asymmetries (such as in levels of key bilateral landmarks), as well as observe symmetry, asymmetry, and any apparent restriction of the patient's natural spontaneous movements.

A third visual pattern noted by primary care physicians is identification of skin lesions. The experienced physician can tell by looking at a patient whether he or she has a disease such as chicken pox, whether there is a skin injury such as a burn, and whether there is one of the more common dermatologic problems such as psoriasis, squamous keratosis, or tinea crura.

SEASONAL/ENVIRONMENTAL PATTERNS

Common diagnostic patterns occur seasonally, and may be associated with the patient's living environment. Such problems are usually respiratory, for example:

Sore throats
Upper respiratory infections
Bronchitis
Sinusitis

In addition to visual and auditory cues such as runny nose, red eyes, and a distinctive cough, part of the diagnostic pattern is the season in which the presentation occurs. These problems are frequent in children in the fall and winter months when they are at school in an enclosed room with poor air circulation. Another common pattern is the child who, known to live in a home where members of the household smoke, presents with signs and symptoms of bronchitis.

ABDOMINAL PAIN

Abdominal pain is a frequent reason for visits to the family physician. It can occur in many forms, and some family physicians feel they have seen enough of certain distinctive presentations that they have become a diagnostic pattern. Two common presentations are:

1. The patient complains of colicky lower abdominal pain with radiation to the flank or groin, and feels more comfortable moving around than sitting or lying still. This pattern suggests a kidney stone.
2. The patient is a woman between the ages of 30 and 50, often with several children, who presents with right upper quadrant pain that radiates to the right side and often to the right shoulder, and with nausea, vomiting, and bloating. This pattern suggests gallbladder disease.

ESTABLISHED PATIENT

Patients often tell the physician what their problem is and what treatment is needed. This is particularly true for patients with chronic illnesses or for elderly patients with numerous health problems that are being managed by the physician. Here the pattern is not so much a visual or diagnostic one as it is the pattern of the individual patient, as he or she has interacted with the physician over time. When such a patient presents with a complaint, with or without his or her own explanation of the problem, the physician asks, "Does this problem fit the pattern for this patient? Would I expect this patient to have this problem given what I have learned about him or her over the years?" The answers to those questions help guide the interaction with the patient.

MUSCULOSKELETAL PATTERNS

Osteopathic physicians recognize patterns for musculoskeletal problems. Examples are:

1. The patient experiences sharp, highly localized pain in the thorax with inhalation, which worsens with a deep breath. This pattern suggests a rib restricted in inhalation.
2. The patient experiences low back pain with walking. This pattern suggests sacral torsion, or other pelvic somatic dysfunction.
3. The patient experiences headaches that start in the shoulder girdle or neck and progress upward to envelop the head. There is a feeling of the head being in a vise, or being squeezed by a stocking that is too tight. This pattern suggests a tension (or musculoskeletal) headache.

UNUSUAL BUT DISTINCTIVE PROBLEMS

At the opposite end of the spectrum for pattern recognition is the pattern formed for the uncommon problem. When patterns are formed for these problems it is often because they are serious, even life-threatening, and should not be missed under any circumstance. A salient example of such a problem is Reye's syndrome, a potentially life-threatening condition that occurs in some children as a consequence of aspirin ingestion, usually for a viral illness. As the pattern of signs and symptoms became clearer, i.e., as it took on the characteristics of a syndrome, health care providers as well as parents were encouraged to "think Reye's." Reference lists outlining the signs and symptoms of the syndrome were posted in emergency departments, physicians' offices, and other patient care areas. In a reasonably short time the pattern of this rather rare illness was internalized well enough by physicians and other providers that today it rarely goes unrecognized. And in recent years, thanks to improved parent and provider awareness of the causes of and treatments for Reye's syndrome, its occurrence has diminished to the point that it is now considered rare. Nonetheless, our awareness that it is potentially life-threatening does not allow us to forget about it.

CAVEATS

Although quick to admit that evoking a diagnostic pattern for common problems is hard to avoid and tends to increase with experience, clinicians often offer warnings against being trapped. Two examples are pertinent:

1. The patient is an elderly man, somewhat overweight, who presents with pain on the right side of his face, dizziness, and left ear pain. Physician examination reveals elevated blood pressure and inflammation of the left ear. The diagnostic pattern considered was otitis media for which ear drops and antibiotics would be prescribed. The patient subsequently suffers a cerebrovascular accident (CVA). The physician realizes there has been a mistake as a result of incomplete data gathering and interpretation. The significance of the elevated blood pressure had not been considered, nor had the fact that the patient felt more light-headed when he lay down. The physician included in his data interpretation only the cues that obviously fit the common pattern and did not give adequate attention to those cues that might have been indicative of another problem. The physician jumped to a convenient conclusion, and fell into a rather serious trap of erroneous or at least incomplete diagnosis.
2. The patient's chart lists several complaints as the reason for the visit. Examples are:

Headache
Dizziness
Dry mouth
Double vision
Emotional lability
Shortness of breath
Occasional muscle spasms

This patient expresses not only varied complaints but also complaints representative of several systems. The number and multisystemic nature of the complaints is a typical pattern for the patient who may be perceived as a hypochondriac, "crock," or "kook." The physician can easily fall into the trap of treating this patient superficially without gaining an understanding of his or her underlying problems.

Although practical instances of problem solving by pattern recognition reflect research findings, practitioners' experiences suggest a much more complex scenario than that created in the laboratory. The practitioner sees the pattern of the total patient in life's environment. The experience of the primary care practitioner with many patient encounters, as well as with several encounters with the same patient, allows him or her to develop pattern recognition habits not readily discovered in the controlled psychological study.

First is the pattern of perceived illness. Over numerous patient encounters, the seasoned practitioner learns to distinguish the visual and behavioral pattern of a patient who is ill. Primary care practitioners have a pattern for a patient who "looks sick." Key factors facilitating development and application of this pattern recognition skill that are particularly useful to the primary care physician (and awkward to effectively represent in psychological studies of clinical problem solving) are repeat visits and time. Especially in the instance of the established patient, any change from the patient's expected appearance raises a flag for the physician: "This patient looks sick."

Time and repeat visits also contribute to expecting and recognizing seasonal illness patterns. The primary care practitioner develops caveats around pattern recognition. A sixth sense, based on years of experience, warns against jumping to conclusions from recognition of a pattern. Although pattern matching is an efficient problem-solving method in primary care and is used frequently with success by family practitioners, there is always the feeling of "Yes, but what if . . . ," or "This solution seems deceptively simple. I sense something more complex." The potential dangers of pattern matching or instant diagnosis were summarized as follows by an osteopathic family practitioner: "Where you get into trouble is when you walk in (to the examining room) with the diagnosis already made. You can really get nailed."

Hypothetico-Deductive Method

We think about complex and not-so-complex problems in everyday life using a hypothetico-deductive method. Clinical problem solving is a specialized application of this method. Imagine one evening you come home after dark, let yourself into the house, flip on the kitchen light switch, and nothing happens. What do you think? Probably your first thought is that the bulb is burned out.

The problem situation has presented itself with your identification of an abnormal finding (no light at the flip of the switch). You then immediately generate a hypothesis about the cause of the abnormal finding (burned out bulb). One possible next step would be to replace the bulb and see if that solves the problem (test the hypothesis, in this case with an intervention). Another more conservative step would be to try other lights in the house to see whether they work (gather more data to further define the problem). You might even pause to consider whether there is a history of this or a similar malfunction occurring in the past. When did you last replace that bulb? Just recently? That would make "burned out bulb" a less likely hypothesis. Is this on the same circuit as the dehumidifier? Perhaps the surge from the dehumidifier coming on overloaded the circuit and tripped the breaker. That would suggest hypotheses in a whole different area, having to do with the fundamentals of how the house is wired, and/or where certain appliances are located. However, the probability is high that it

is the bulb and not something more extensive like an overload or a short circuit or a power outage affecting the whole house.

You can combine the high probability that it is the bulb with the knowledge that changing the bulb can do no harm. It can only solve the problem or fail to solve the problem. The thought processes we invoke are multiple and highly varied even for something as simple as a darkened kitchen.

Now let us go back to Mr. Johnson's case, identify the significant abnormal and normal findings, generate the hypotheses, and logically apply this hypothetico-deductive reasoning. Even before your interaction with Mr. Johnson, you have enough information to set you thinking. Based on the cues of the presenting complaint (gender, age, height, weight, and blood pressure), you probably generate some preliminary diagnostic hypotheses regarding the mechanism of the patient's illness. You are able to do this before you meet the patient.

Two major components of the hypothetico-deductive method are cue acquisition and hypothesis generation. Problem solving for a complex problem like this involves the early generation of several diagnostic hypotheses. Often the physician begins to consider diagnostic possibilities based on just a few cues, as you have done with Mr. Johnson. Frequently, several diagnostic hypotheses come to mind, or are retrieved from the physician's long-term memory, based on between one and five cues.

How many hypotheses? Since during the diagnostic workup hypotheses are carried in short-term memory while they are being evaluated, the number is limited. Usually the physician can expect to keep track of between three and seven diagnostic hypotheses during a complex clinical encounter.

What kind of hypotheses? Hypotheses can be general, such as the "cardiovascular problem" or "gastrointestinal problem" that you might be considering for Mr. Johnson. Or they can be specific, such as "pleurisy" or "myocardial infarction." The level of definition depends on several factors, such as the specificity of the data, how life-threatening the problem is, and the sophistication of the problem solver. With more detailed information the physician can entertain more focused hypotheses. For a patient presenting with diarrhea and abdominal cramping, a physician might differentiate between ulcerative colitis and Crohn's disease rather than simply hypothesizing a problem in the bowel.

That is not to say that clinical problem solving is predictably logical, going from general to specific. Specific hypotheses can be generated based on an extremely small data set, or the physician might have a substantial set of cues and still entertain global hypotheses. The sophistication of the physician is based on his or her knowledge base. The clinician who has been in practice longer has a larger knowledge base of problems, including more complex relationships, than the clinician with less experience. Although it would not appear that clinical problem solving in general is a learned skill, the ability to solve clinical problems increases with experience and the building of the clinical knowledge base.

Whether the problem is life-threatening is a variable that

often comes into play in clinical problem solving. It especially affects hypothesis generation when the physician realizes that the patient's symptom complex suggests a serious acute illness such as myocardial infarction. The physician's first duty is to ascertain the presence of a life-threatening condition and treat it, or at least stabilize the patient. Those situations can involve the immediate recognition of a sign-symptom pattern or the generation of a specific diagnostic hypothesis for which there might be a standard treatment protocol or algorithm.

Having generated one or more diagnostic hypotheses, the physician proceeds with more cue acquisition, which itself can be guided by the hypotheses. As with the example of the kitchen light, one expects certain findings to be present or absent if one or another hypothesis is true. For example, if the burned out bulb hypothesis is accurate, then the cue of non-functional bathroom light is unlikely (unless, of course, the bulbs had burned out in both rooms). However, if the hypothesis of tripped circuit breaker is true, and the bathroom and kitchen lights are on the same circuit, then one might test that hypothesis by trying the bathroom light.

Back to Mr. Johnson. As you elicit more data from the patient, you can relate the new cues to your working hypotheses, a process known as cue interpretation. Cues are usually interpreted as:

Positive (tending to support an hypothesis)

Negative (tending to refute an hypothesis)

Noncontributory (not helpful for the evaluation of an hypothesis)

Mr. Johnson was raking leaves when he experienced pain in the shoulder. If you later learn that Mr. Johnson's pain is not reproduced with movement of his arm, that cue may be interpreted as negative for trauma. If you learn he does not experience pain when climbing stairs, that cue could be interpreted as negative for exertional angina resulting from coronary artery disease. If you learn that he does not experience pain with deep breathing, that cue could be considered negative for a pulmonary hypothesis. It must be noted that a negative cue or even several negative cues do not rule out a hypothesis. Negative cues might cause the physician to move the hypothesis lower on his or her probability list. However, it takes substantial negative evidence or confirmation of a competing hypothesis for a diagnosis to be ruled out.

In conjunction with cue interpretation, an orderly data-gathering process allows you to generate new diagnostic hypotheses. With the iterative process of data gathering, hypothesis generation, and cue interpretation you begin prioritizing hypotheses. If all possible causes of the patient's problem are equally serious, give top priority to the most likely diagnosis, lower priority to the next most likely, and so on. Prioritizing diagnostic hypotheses is usually a much more complex process. When the physician is making the transition from the preliminary phases to hypothesis evaluation and prioritization, considerations such as treatability, severity of the illness (whether

it is life-threatening), and methods to be used for further hypothesis testing enter into the decision-making process.

In Mr. Johnson's case, a high priority might be given to the hypothesis of coronary artery insufficiency. Even though you discover cues in Mr. Johnson's data set negative for that hypothesis, experience suggests that given this patient's risk factors and the seriousness of the illness, this is a top-priority hypothesis. The primary care osteopathic physician can make creative use of the hypothetico-deductive model, beyond what has been elaborated on in ongoing studies of clinical problem solving. Most of the studies involve only one extensive (simulated) patient encounter. The primary care physician can plan multiple encounters with the patient (cue acquisition and interpretation opportunities) that might include implementation and assessment of the various phases of a management plan (hypothesis testing and hypothesis evaluation opportunities).

The hypothetico-deductive model for clinical problem solving typically involves four major steps:

Cue acquisition

Hypothesis generation

Cue interpretation

Hypothesis evaluation

There are some caveats for the osteopathic primary care practitioner in applying the hypothetico-deductive model in its purest form. Chief among those is that the model is oriented toward cause and effect. The cues the physician elicits from the patient are in a sense the effects of some disease or dysfunction, which may be viewed as the cause. Using the hypothetico-deductive model puts the clinician in the role of detective or analyst who draws from long-term memory hypotheses (such as normal anatomy, physiology, pathophysiologic states, specific disease entities, syndromes, etc.) that account for most if not all of the cues being offered by the patient. The ultimate objective, of course, is to use identification and solution of the diagnostic problem as the basis for development of a management plan that helps restore the patient to a healthy state. The goal is to resolve the patient's clinical problem.

There are other disadvantages or limitations to using this approach exclusively in considering diagnostic problems. In addition to being disease-oriented, the hypothetico-deductive model is extremely focused. In applying the model, the clinician is not encouraged to consider the whole patient. The model is highly cognitive, almost impersonal at times. Invoking the model does not necessarily prompt the clinician toward exercise of effective interpersonal skills or skills in patient education. The hypothetico-deductive model, if not supported by other effective clinical practices such as always keeping an open mind and listening carefully to the patient's whole story, can put blinders on the clinician, resulting in potentially serious errors. As Hunter[8] notes in her book, Doctors' Stories, the clinician who brings to the patient encounter his or her own perspective different from that of the patient runs the risk of transforming the patient's story into the doctor's story.

Through selective questioning, listening, and examination, the doctor risks gathering data that fit his or her preliminary impression of the patient's problem. Under those circumstances data can be missed, or worse, the doctor can make up cues that were not part of the patient's presentation. Even with thorough, orderly data gathering, cues can be over- or under-interpreted (interpreted as too strongly or not strongly enough related to a hypothesis), or they can be totally misinterpreted. The hurried physician who relies too heavily on the hypothetico-deductive model can be led down a primrose path. Properly applied, the hypothetico-deductive model of clinical problem solving can help the physician solve complex, difficult diagnostic problems. It is a method often seen in the hospital or consultation setting as well as used by the primary care practitioner faced with a complex diagnostic dilemma. For a thorough, academic discussion of the hypothetico-deductive problem solving model, see the book *Medical Problem Solving: An Analysis of Clinical Reasoning.*[9]

Problem-Oriented Perspective

In the 1950s, development of the problem-oriented medical system was begun by Lawrence Weed, MD. The system had several components, a key one of which was the Problem-Oriented Medical Record (POMR). A major goal of the problem-oriented medical system was to focus on the patient's problems and the interrelationships among them. The system was intended for use by primary care practitioners as well as specialists. The system places heavy emphasis on:

Establishment of a patient database
Problem identification
Patient education
Record keeping

Patient records, especially hospital charts, are usually source-oriented. The sections of the chart are organized by the source of the data. There is a section for physician's notes, for nursing notes, for laboratory notes, and others. In developing the POMR system, Weed sought to reorder the record keeping system so that it was organized around problems. If Mr. Johnson's chart contained a report of a chest x-ray study, it might be included under a Shortness of Breath on Exertion problem, if one had been identified for him, rather than under Radiology.

The POMR has four named components:

Defined database
Complete problem list
Initial plans
Progress notes

Narrative progress notes contain the following information:

Subjective data
Objective data
Assessment
Plan

The acronym SOAP makes the four sections easy to remember. Subjective data are those provided by the patient or another source of information (e.g., a parent) about the progress of the problem being addressed. These are usually history data. Objective data are those elicited by the physician, usually physical examination data. They can also be results of laboratory or imaging tests. In the assessment, the physician records his or her interpretation of the subjective and objective data. In the plan, the physician records any one or all of the following:

Diagnostic plan: what further diagnostic data are needed to understand the patient's problem
Therapeutic plan: what the physician intends to do to manage the problem
Patient education: what information needs to be discussed with the patient regarding the problem

The progress note or SOAP note has proved to be one of the most functional aspects of the problem-oriented system, as well as one of the least cumbersome to implement in a busy primary care practice.

In the 1960s and early 1970s, when the POMR system had its greatest visibility, physician accountability (in patient care as well as education) was a high priority. The problem-oriented system with its strong emphasis on comprehensiveness, avoidance of speculation about diagnoses, and patient education provided a method for audit and accountability that seemed ideal.

How does clinical problem solving relate to the problem-oriented system? That question has been a source of controversy since Weed introduced the system. Our natural tendency when confronted with a problem is often to formulate the problem and then immediately start generating hypotheses about its cause. That kind of cognitive speculation does not fit in well with the careful building-block process prescribed by the problem-oriented approach. Part of the reason for developing the problem-oriented system in the first place was Weed's and others' concerns that, in approaching clinical problems, physicians were making diagnostic and therapeutic errors because they were jumping to conclusions too quickly based on incomplete data. Through the problem-oriented system, Weed hoped to influence the development of orderly clinical problem-solving skills in student physicians. Part of his goal was to educate medical students and residents in the use of a highly structured thought process for clinical problem solving.

The process begins with the establishment of, if not a complete database, at least a partial database for the patient, from which the problem list and initial plans emerge. This approach provides a standard method for addressing each patient's problem complex. Shortcuts are not encouraged, or any steps skipped in problem identification and problem solving. A record is developed for the patient that is a direct reflection of the student's reasoning, and is used in evaluation of the student's clinical learning progress.

As researchers began to gain greater insight into the cognitive processes involved in clinical problem solving, it became clear that what Weed and the problem-oriented system were advocating involved a major transformation of age-old habits of diagnostic thinking. Physicians do not usually gather a complete database for a patient before forming impressions. Rather, they use preliminary impressions or hypotheses to guide data gathering. Physicians tend to see patterns, problem complexes, and interrelationships among problems that are centered on priorities (e.g., is this life-threatening, is it treatable) and pathophysiologic processes (what is the cause of this set of signs and symptoms). They might have trouble seeing problems as separate entities, only possibly to be combined later. As clinical trainers, they may have trouble teaching learners to think in ways that they find alien and inefficient. Resistance to the wholesale adoption of the problem-oriented system has been heavily influenced by the pragmatic stance that "if it ain't broke, don't fix it." For decades a traditional combination of approaches to clinical problem solving, record keeping, and accountability has been used that is effective and efficient. This new system would not only revolutionize thinking about clinical problems but also would turn the entire organization of record keeping systems and hospital audit systems on its ear. Even third party payers and medical education would be affected.

The problem-oriented medical system, although seemingly logical, proved difficult to implement. Several components are still frequently used, however, especially in family physicians' office records. For example, one might expect to see a numbered problem list at the front of the patient charts in some offices. The problem-oriented influence most likely to be seen in contemporary physicians' charts is the progress note or so-called SOAP note. Some medical education programs are problem-based rather than academic discipline or system-based. Although a wholesale transformation of clinical reasoning did not take place, the impact of the problem-oriented system is still felt. For a detailed explanation of the problem-oriented system, see *Your Health Care and How to Manage It*[10] and *Applying the Problem Oriented System*.[11]

Clinical Decision Analysis

The clinical decision analytic approach to diagnostic problem solving involves appreciating and using probabilities and their relationships in the diagnostic process. Looking back at our preliminary presentation for Mr. Johnson, even with the scant data we had before we met him, we could formulate a hypothesis of pain as a result of coronary artery insufficiency.

One test of the accuracy of that diagnostic hypothesis is a treadmill test or stress ECG. Our pattern matcher was already speculating about the anticipated outcome of that test before even meeting Mr. Johnson. Before performing the test, let us consider what we would learn from the results, and how much it would help us diagnostically. At the most basic level we can interpret the results of the test as either positive or negative, normal or abnormal. As with all tests, there are degrees of abnormal for this one, but for now we stick with just the two categories. A positive outcome tends to confirm the diagnosis and a normal outcome helps refute it.

Cost is also associated with the test. Although minimally invasive, the stress ECG involves not only patient and health care provider effort and time but also monetary cost. How much do we learn from the test, and does what we learn justify the cost? How much further history and physical examination data do we need before we feel comfortable deciding whether to order this test?

First the diagnostic perspective. Laboratory tests commonly used for diagnosis have predictive statistics associated with them based on the probability that a person with a certain disease will have a positive outcome on the test, as well as the probability that a healthy person will have a negative outcome on the test. The stress ECG is commonly used to test the diagnostic hypothesis of angina pectoris as a result of coronary artery insufficiency. Based on studies of large numbers of patients, we know the following about the test associated with coronary artery disease (CAD):

The probability that a patient with CAD will have a positive test result

The probability that a patient who does not have CAD will have a normal test result

For a given patient sample we can ascertain the probability that a patient with a positive test result has CAD, as well as the probability that a patient with a normal test result does not have CAD. Using these probabilities helps us decide whether our patient should undergo the test. Section 1 of the Appendix provides statistical properties of the stress ECG as it relates to CAD, details on definitions of terms, and an example.

In addition to applying our knowledge of test characteristics in judging the value of a test as it relates to a certain problem, we also use this probabilistic method to help us revise our thinking about a diagnostic hypothesis. We can assign a probability to the hypothesis of pain as a result of coronary artery insufficiency for Mr. Johnson. For example, on the basis of findings from the history and physical examination, we may be 70% sure that the hypothesis is true for this patient. Under these circumstances, we ask Mr. Johnson to undergo a treadmill test.

What do we learn if the test result is positive?

If the result is negative?

How do the test results help us evaluate our primary working hypothesis?

To relate the general information we have about the stress test to Mr. Johnson's special case, we use a method called Bayes' theorem, a formula for combining and revising probabilities based on new information, devised by Reverend Thomas Bayes in the 1700s. Section 2 of the Appendix gives an illustration of how Bayes' theorem is applied in thinking about Mr. Johnson's problem.

There are several schools of thought regarding the use of clinical decision analysis even at this simple level in diagnostic problem solving. Some clinicians, especially in fields such as cardiology where there is an extensive database on statistical properties of tests, frequently use clinical decision analysis to help decide whether to have patients undergo tests. Clinicians also use it, with the inclusion of utility estimates, to help in choosing management plans. An added benefit of decision analysis in the high technology fields is that it can help control costs if used conscientiously.

Another perspective, held more widely by primary care physicians, is more utilitarian. It states that regardless of the increment by which I might be able to improve my diagnosis with the result of a test whose statistical properties I know, I am (or am not) going to do the test anyway, because there is more to a test result than just diagnosis. For example, an argument in favor of doing a stress ECG for a patient with a high likelihood of CAD (meaning that I would learn little diagnostically from a positive test result) is that I can use the outcome to establish a target exercise heart rate for this patient, and thus a basis for developing a management plan. Similarly, an argument for doing such a test to assess a hypothesis with a low subjective probability ("I am quite sure this is not the patient's problem, but I don't want to miss it") is if the test proves positive, and the patient does indeed have the disease (not a necessary relationship, but it could happen), then it was worth doing the test. As one family physician put it: "If there are 95 negative tests out of 100, and of the 5 positive ones, one results in saving a patient's life, the other 99 were worth it."

A third perspective is what one might call the common sense approach. Here the clinician is aware of probabilistic relationships between test results and diagnoses. However, he or she uses them in an informal way. The clinician's reasoning might be: "I know this test helps me with the diagnosis. However, if it's negative, it won't tell me anything. A negative test result won't rule out this diagnosis. I'm quite sure this is not the patient's problem, so rather than risk wasting time and money on something that might have low yield, I'll do some other cheaper, less invasive tests to try to confirm another hypothesis, and use this test only if all else fails."

In this argument, the physician is considering several factors (cost and invasiveness as well as the potential value of alternatives), in addition to diagnosis, to reason against using a particular test.

We have considered the decision analytic approach to clinical problem solving from the perspective of how it can help the primary care physician use diagnostic tests efficiently and effectively in the problem-solving process. To use this method, the diagnostician must know a minimum of the statistical properties of the test he or she wishes to order, as well as, ideally, the prevalence in his or her patient population for the disease or problem being tested. Knowing that information and applying Bayes' theorem also allows the physician to estimate the change in probability of a diagnostic hypothesis under consideration, and thus have an idea of how the results of a test contribute to further understanding the patient's problem. Two references on clinical decision analysis are *Medical Decision Making*[12] and *Clinical Epidemiology*.[13]

We have presented several models for clinical reasoning. None of these models is used exclusively by clinicians in pondering diagnostic problems. However, all are used to some ex-

tent. The next part of this chapter presents some examples of osteopathic primary care physicians' reasoning about patient problems, accompanied by a discussion of their possible application to the problem-solving models we have discussed.

OSTEOPATHIC PHYSICIANS' CLINICAL PROBLEM SOLVING

Having considered several models of clinical problem solving, the reader may wonder if osteopathic physicians think that way. We conducted an inquiry into osteopathic physicians' impressions of their own problem solving processes. The subjects were for the most part family practitioners, as well as specialists and generalists who were not family doctors. Data from 13 family doctors were used in the study. Nonfamily practitioners were one each from the following practice areas:

Surgery
Pediatrics
General internal medicine
Cardiology
Sports medicine

Three academically-based family practitioners were included. The experimental method was a face-to-face interview with each subject, in which the following three major questions were posed and elaborated:

1. "Please tell me about a case or cases you have seen recently (or a type of case) where as soon as the patient presented you believed you knew what the nature of the patient's problem was." This question was intended to elicit a discussion of pattern matching problem-solving processes.
2. "Please describe for me a case or cases you have seen recently, or might still be working on, that for you have been a real diagnostic dilemma." This question was intended to elicit discussion of more complex problem-solving processes such as the hypothetico-deductive and decision analytic methods.
3. "Please discuss for me a case or cases you have seen recently where you were able to say: I handled that case the way I did because I am an osteopathic physician. There was something particularly osteopathic about the way I approached that patient." This question was intended to elicit subjects' perspective on what is distinctive about osteopathic physicians and how what they perceive as osteopathic is expressed in their clinical approach to their patients.

We analyzed the subjects' responses in an attempt to answer the question of whether practicing physicians actually use problem solving methods such as:

Pattern matching
Hypothetico-deductive thinking
Decision analysis
Problem-oriented process

Subjects' use of pattern matching is summarized in the earlier discussion of that model. This section focuses on diagnostic challenges or dilemmas, and what physicians saw as distinctively osteopathic about their thinking. Quotations are taken directly from physician interviews.

Complex Diagnostic Problem Solving

What are diagnostic dilemmas for osteopathic primary care practitioners? What problem-solving processes do they use in resolving the dilemmas?

Clinician problem solvers used the cyclical processes of data gathering, hypothesis generation, and cue interpretation (the hypothetico-deductive method) to clarify diagnostic problems and try to reach conclusions.

They used probabilistic thinking in two major ways. First, they used it to prioritize hypotheses to investigate based on their understanding of problem/disease prevalence combined with perceived cost of investigation. Second, they used probabilities to prioritize hypotheses for ruling out, or hoping to rule out, based for the most part on the perceived gravity or life-threatening potential of the disease or illness.

On occasion, clinicians called on knowledge of basic biologic principles (usually structure and function, occasionally biochemistry and microbiology) to trigger generation of diagnostic hypotheses as well as interpret cues in light of the hypotheses. The following sections discuss a series of cases that illustrate physicians' application of these three major forms of reasoning:

Hypothetico-deductive thinking
Probabilistic reasoning for purposes of prioritizing hypotheses based on prevalence, and gravity of illness
Application of basic biologic principles to the analysis of complex clinical problems

There are some contributors to the problem-solving process that are especially applicable in ambulatory care and that are not addressed in major psychological studies of clinical problem solving. The one key operating factor that separates the primary care practitioner's experience from that of an experimental subject is the return visit. The practitioner has an opportunity to interact with the patient on several occasions over a protracted period, thus introducing into the problem-solving process the variable of time and with it the natural course of an illness. The ambulatory care physician can use response to treatment as a key diagnostic variable. He or she can consider and assess more environmental, social, and psychological hypotheses as the underlying causes of a patient's illness than can the physician/researcher who sees the patient only once or for a short time period. Examples of our interviewees using these variables were frequent.

The most common diagnostic dilemma for the primary care physicians was abdominal pain, more specifically, abdominal pain in women patients. Abdominal pain as dilemma (what might be considered the opposite end of the diagnosis spectrum from pattern matching) attests to the frequency of abdominal pain as the reason for a visit to the physician. Statistics show that stomach pain, cramps, and spasms are the tenth most common reason for visits to U.S. physicians.[14] Of the problems

mentioned by our study group, abdominal pain was mentioned ten times; eight of the complaints came from women patients. Other diagnostic dilemmas mentioned were:

Fatigue (4)
Headaches (3)
Multisystem complaints (2)
Chest pain (1)
Tremor (1)
Back pain (1)
Leg swelling (1)

CASE ONE

The patient is a 33-year-old woman complaining of abdominal pain, bloating, and diarrhea. This is an established patient, and the physician noted she had undergone a dramatic change in appearance since her last visit. She was clearly sick. Following physical evaluation, which did not help reveal a particular cause, the physician entertained a hypothesis of viral gastritis, using the reasoning that the hypothesis explained the findings reasonably well, and it was a common underlying cause for this sign/symptom complex. The patient was treated conservatively with fluids and dietary management.

In the first round of clinical problem solving with this patient, the physician was able to recognize a change in the patient's expected pattern of appearance. He began using the hypothetico-deductive approach, probabilistic reasoning (a common cause for the sign/symptom complex), and time in developing and testing a diagnostic formulation.

The patient returned in one week. On return visit there was upper abdominal pain, bloating, and diarrhea as well as ankle edema. The physician now entertained a hypothesis of cardiovascular dysfunction as the cause for the edema, which might also explain the gastrointestinal problems, or which might be an additional underlying problem.

This is the second round of problem solving for the physician. There is a continuation of the problems seen on the first visit, plus a new symptom: ankle edema. The physician is still using hypothetico-deductive thinking to understand the patient's problems. He is generating hypotheses that together or separately might explain the findings. However, there is no indication that the physician was feeling able to resolve the problem. Rather than coming together, the problem was becoming more complex and diffuse. And the patient's condition was worsening.

As time passed, the patient became more seriously ill to the point where she was showing clinical and biochemical signs of severe malnourishment. An upper GI evaluation revealed a badly damaged small bowel, caused, as it turned out, by a gluten enteropathy that had progressed to the point of being life-threatening before it was discovered.

It took three rounds of clinical problem solving, plus time, to assess response to treatment and observe the development of the illness before the physician was able to generate the requisite hypotheses. The hypotheses combined with the gravity of the patient's illness indicated ordering the upper GI test that eventually revealed her underlying disorder. Technology did not diagnose the problem, however, as is often implied, particularly in specialty-oriented practice. Had the physician not reasoned the problem through to the point where he knew the test was indicated, he would never have had the opportunity to learn what the technology eventually revealed.

CASE TWO

The patient is a 34-year-old woman presenting with multiple complaints, centered in the abdominal area and lower back. The principal complaint on the first visit is episodic midepigastric pain. The patient also complains of occasional lower abdominal pain, low back pain, and constipation. The patient is obese. On examination there are decreased bowel sounds, but no rebound tenderness or guarding. There are no other abnormalities. There is a family history of gallbladder disease that, together with the patient's complaints and her appearance, triggered a general diagnostic hypothesis of gastrointestinal dysfunction. Included were the specific hypotheses of gallstones, along with possible reflux esophagitis and irritable bowel syndrome. The physician did not assign a high probability to the hypothesis of gallstones, thinking that the other two were much more likely, as well as less costly to treat. She chose to treat the symptoms conservatively (and, in part, use response to treatment to test hypotheses) with medication and diet. The patient did not respond to treatment.

This is another case where more than one round of problem solving is required. Here the physician starts by using hypothetico-deductive reasoning to generate diagnostic hypotheses based on a complex of signs and symptoms. She also uses probabilistic thinking to assign likelihood to her hypotheses; this helps with decision making about treatment. Although not discussed as one of our fundamental problem-solving approaches, the physician also calls on concepts of cost-effectiveness when she considers cost of testing and treatment in developing a management plan.

Before her next scheduled visit, the patient called the physician complaining of bloating, incapacitating pain, and no bowel movement for five days. Ultrasound of the gallbladder revealed no abnormality. The urgency of the patient's complaints suggested a more serious hypothesis, such as large bowel obstruction; the patient did not appear physically ill enough to support that hypothesis, nor was it supported by x-ray or laboratory findings.

The physician continues to think hypothetico-deductively. She feels she needs to dig deeper, be more invasive in her investigations, and incur more expense to understand the patient's problem. The physician generated at least one new hypothesis. She did not feel it was supported by enough data to be a strong contender. The physician appears to be balancing seriousness (if this is bowel obstruction it is extremely serious, and I had better not miss it) with likelihood (the hypothesis was not supported with sufficient cues, and although the patient expressed urgency about the problem, she did not appear ill enough to suggest that the problem was life-threatening).

On a subsequent visit the patient revealed she was at the top of the list for job cuts in her department. This was a turning point for the physician. She refrained from ordering additional expensive tests and chose rather to discuss the relationship of the patient's signs and symptoms with her anxiety over her job. The patient agreed there might be a relationship. The physician saw the patient's realization of the relationship between stress and physiologic symptoms as therapeutic. The patient improved once she understood how the threat of job loss could be the basis for physical illness.

In this case the physician used time, failure to respond to treatment, and her knowledge from previous acquaintance with this established patient as triggers for new diagnostic hypotheses and further data gathering. These eventually revealed what the physician thought to be the underlying problem. The case also exemplifies the primary care physician's ability to use repeat visits, time, and failure to respond to treatment as a basis for generating diagnostic hypotheses involving the patient's psychological and social environment as the underlying cause of physiologic complaints.

Physicians who discussed cases with us related several instances where the apparent underlying problem was social or environmental. These types of problems and the primary care osteopathic physician's role in assessing and developing management plans with patients are discussed elsewhere. Here we offer two composite scenarios discussed by several physicians.

In the first scenario, the patient is a woman in her 30s or 40s who is married or in a significant relationship. She comes to see the physician with a complaint, or brings her child with an illness. The complaint presented on any individual visit does not usually require the complex problem-solving process but rather calls on the physician's pattern recognition skills for common problems. The cue this prototypic patient presents that calls up complex problem-solving skills is that of multiple visits, with resolution of short-term problems and lingering evidence of an underlying long-term problem. For this complex patient presentation, the most common underlying causes are clinical depression and physical or psychological abuse. If the primary care physician can see the big picture and generate one of these hypotheses, he or she is well on the way to appropriate assessment and management of the patient's major problem. One study subject (a woman physician) related an extensive discussion of her discovery of this symptom complex and her subsequent realization of just how prevalent abuse and depression are among women patients.

In the second scenario, the patient presents with multisystem complaints. The patient is usually a woman. She has seen several physicians without a satisfactory outcome. She might or might not be married or in a relationship. She is usually in her 30s or 40s. The history may be rather complex, and usually involves pain. For example, the patient might have a history of migraine headaches for which she is taking medication, hypertension for which she is also taking medication, abdominal pain, and chronic diarrhea. She might also have episodes of back pain for which she takes medication. The abdominal pain might be intense and highly localized, e.g., in the right upper quadrant. On hearing this history, the physician in question focused her complex problem-solving process on the abdominal pain, entertaining hypotheses such as gallbladder disease or common bile duct stone, as well as abdominal distress of functional origin based on a history of abuse as a child, a failed marriage, and current involvement in a lesbian relationship. In the case related, the patient was vague about her extensive past medical and surgical history, prompting the physician to request her medical records from previous providers. The records revealed that the patient had been and is currently in a drug rehabilitation program. At this stage, the physician's perspective on the case changes dramatically because it is now apparent that the problem underlying the patient's physiologic complaints is the complex sociobehavioral problem of long-term unresolved substance abuse.

CASE THREE

The patient is a 19-year-old woman presenting with acute pelvic pain. She is sexually active. Physical examination reveals diffuse nonlocalized lower abdominal pain on palpation. Pelvic and rectal examinations revealed no abnormalities. The physician further analyzed the problem by considering basic anatomic structure, asking himself what is in the right and left lower quadrants of the abdomen. In women, the major structures in the lower quadrants of the abdomen are part of the uterus (which can be palpable if enlarged), the Fallopian tubes, and the ovaries. The cecum and appendix, and a portion of the ascending colon, are on the right. On the left are portions of the descending colon. The physician generates a diagnostic hypothesis set that includes primarily infectious and inflammatory processes because the onset of pain was acute:

Pelvic infection
Urinary tract infection
Inflammatory bowel disease

Appendicitis is also considered, but with low probability because the clinical cues did not support that hypothesis and did support the others. The patient is treated with a preliminary trial of antibiotics on the justification that not only might the treatment be appropriate for her problem, but also that the response to treatment would provide diagnostic information. Once the treatment regimen was completed, the patient's pain recurred and she came back to the physician.

This initially apparently straightforward infectious problem becomes complex when the patient fails to respond to treatment. The physician initially uses hypothetico-deductive reasoning apparently successfully, only to learn his standard medical approach to the problem has not brought resolution.

When the patient returned, having completed the initial treatment regimen, the physician chose to seek a second opinion and referred the patient to a specialist in gastroenterology who could not find signs of significant treatable pathophysiologic processes. The patient returned to the primary care physician.

In this third round of problem solving for this patient's problem, the primary care physician was able to use his unique perspective to further assess the patient. Unlike the specialist, the primary care physician had seen the patient on several occasions over many years. Thanks to the factor of time and return visits, he believed he knew the patient and believed her complaints were sincere.

On a subsequent visit, having exhausted all other logical possibilities, the physician sought a third opinion from a gynecologist who performed a laparoscopic investigation that revealed a chronically inflamed appendix. Surgical removal of the appendix resolved the problem.

The physician was clearly perplexed going into the last round of problem solving for this case. What had seemed to be an almost simple diagnostic and management problem had not resolved. Referral had not yielded satisfactory results. The problem's manifestation did not suggest any reasonable causes beyond those he had already considered. The physician's acquaintance with the patient as well as his need for resolution led him to pursue another avenue, that of structure and function, that finally proved fruitful, and he will probably never forget this extremely atypical example of an inflamed appendix.

CASE FOUR

The patient is a woman in her 30s who presents to the emergency department with multiple acute complaints. The primary problems are severe headache and abdominal pain, as well as chest pain and palpitations. The headache and abdominal pains were so intense that narcotics were administered in the emergency room to relieve them. The patient was admitted, and an attempt was made to ascertain whether the multiple symptoms were the result of multiple problems or one problem. For the headache the physician first entertained the hypotheses of subdural hematoma or tumor. Although on physical examination there were no neurologic signs to suggest either of those diagnoses, a CAT scan was done to be sure. It did not show any abnormalities. The patient had complained of palpitations, and physical examination in the emergency room showed sinus tachycardia. A treadmill ECG showed no abnormalities. The physician hypothesized that the cardiac symptoms and headaches were the result of stress or anxiety. The patient was treated with a short-term regimen of benzodiazepine (alprazolam), which relieved the headache and palpitations but had no effect on the abdominal pain.

At that point the physician believed he was dealing with two separate problems. One was the basis for the headaches and cardiac symptoms, which responded to treatment with an anxiolytic agent, and the other was an as yet undiagnosed abdominal problem. The patient's pain was localized in the upper abdomen, which triggered hypotheses of gallbladder disease or common bile duct obstruction, among others. The former was quickly ruled out as the patient's gallbladder had been surgically removed. Abdominal ultrasound showed a suspicious dilatation of the hepatic duct, which was confirmed by contrast dye radiographic evaluation (ERCP) to be a common duct stone. Removal of the stone resolved the abdominal pain.

The complex presentation in this case is what some might see as an internist's delight, even though part of the solution was surgical. The complex presentation triggered a variety of hypotheses, some of which were potentially life-threatening, and that the physician hoped to be able to rule out early on. The hypothesis set for this case included solutions that explained the combined data set (headaches, cardiac problems, and abdominal pain) and others that separated the problems. Response to the short-term treatment confirmed the hypotheses for more than one problem. The case is an excellent example of successful complex hypothetico-deductive reasoning in which hypothesis generation and evaluation from a single-problem as well as multiple-problem perspective yield resolution on essentially the first round. It is becoming more and more likely that primary care osteopathic physicians will see cases like this one. When they do, the cases should be cognitively satisfying.

CASE FIVE

The patient is a man in his 50s employed as a fire fighter who states he experienced an acute episode of chest pain approximately 1 week ago while fighting a house fire. The first and most likely hypothesis the physician generates is angina pectoris as a result of coronary artery disease. The patient has risk factors for CAD such as:

Age
Being overweight
Smoking
Having a stressful job

The patient does not appear in acute distress at the time of presentation. The physician prescribes sublingual nitroglycerine as needed to relieve the pain and has the patient undergo a stress ECG. After not one but two treadmill ECGs (one on being referred to a cardiologist), no abnormality is found. Neither treadmill test triggers the pain. An echocardiogram performed at a tertiary care center is interpreted as showing a valvular abnormality. The primary care physician is not satisfied that it is the cause of the patient's chest pain. During the testing period the patient experiences the pain occasionally, without relief from the nitroglycerine (failure to respond to treatment). Until now the physician has avoided asking the patient to undergo cardiac catheterization in favor of less costly, less invasive tests. Eventually cardiac catheterization reveals severe coronary artery disease requiring four-vessel bypass surgery.

In this case the physician expected a straightforward hypothetico-deductive reasoning sequence to yield the anticipated solution. This was almost a case for pattern recognition. The physician was tripped up in the hypothesis testing phase. The patient's failure to respond to treatment and successful execution of two treadmill tests constituted for the physician evidence against the hypothesis of angina pectoris as a result of CAD. Nonetheless, the physician would not rule out that

hypothesis and insisted on performing a more definitive (and much more costly) evaluation, results of which confirmed the hypothesis he had held all along.

The physician considered the negative treadmill test result as evidence against the hypothesis of coronary artery disease as the basis for the patient's chest pain. Nonetheless, the physician stuck by his original hypothesis using what appears to be intuition that he was on the right track. This is a perfect example of where probabilistic reasoning could have helped the physician resolve his ambivalence about the test results. Take a moment to consider the results using Bayes' theorem. Section 3 of the Appendix outlines how information about this case might be analyzed. We can readily see from that illustrative analysis that our physician's intuition was correct. Going through the formalities of probabilistic reasoning tells us that for a patient whom we are so sure has a diagnosis of coronary artery disease that we can assign a probability of 90%, even a negative stress ECG result only reduces our probability to just under 80%. In fact, for this patient, we probably didn't need the stress test to establish the diagnosis. If the result had been positive, it would not have helped that much.

This is a highly atypical case. In most cases such as this, the patient's presentation and course of illness are typical for the most likely diagnostic hypotheses, and diagnosis and management can proceed in an orderly fashion. The good primary care physician is alert to the atypical case and is able to use a combination of intuition and trust in the patient's sincerity to tell him or her when a case cannot be resolved "by the numbers."

SUMMARY

The primary care practitioner's thought processes reflect and expand those found in the controlled studies of clinical problem solving. Primary care osteopathic physicians regularly make informal use of hypothetico-deductive reasoning as well as probabilistic thinking. They also analyze problems using principles of structure and function. The primary care physician experiences a unique form of the complex problem-solving process as a result of his or her patient encounter pattern. In contrast to a specialist who might see the patient on a consultation or in the hospital setting during an intense period of a brief hospital stay, the primary care physician sees the patient for multiple comparatively short episodic visits. This encounter pattern allows the primary care physician to assess the patient's short-term response to treatment as well as his or her long-term health/illness pattern. The primary care encounter pattern provides the physician the unique opportunity to reasonably consider diagnostic hypotheses that are time dependent (e.g., depression, physical and psychological abuse, and hidden substance abuse) as part of a complex problem-solving methodology. The physician's problem-solving process is expanded to include the variables of repeat visits, time, and response to treatment, enabling him or her to place the problem-solving process for each patient in the context of the patient's life experience as well as that of the physician's practice experience.

Osteopathic Approach

The definition of what is osteopathic is different for every osteopathic physician. For some, primary care is a key factor in being osteopathic. Others may focus on the musculoskeletal system, palpatory diagnosis, and manual medicine as uniquely characterizing the osteopathic approach. In this text, the authors have agreed on four basic biologic principles particularly applicable in the practice of osteopathic medicine. The principles were formalized and related to osteopathic practice in a document produced by the Kirksville College of Osteopathic Medicine[15] and subsequently discussed in a report of a survey of osteopathic physicians.[16] The principles are as follows:

1. The body is a unit.
2. The body possesses self-regulatory mechanisms.
3. Structure and function are reciprocally interrelated.
4. Rational therapy is based upon an understanding of body unity, self-regulatory mechanisms, and the interrelationship of structure and function.

The principles are further articulated in Chapter 1, Osteopathic Philosophy.

Primary care practitioners in this study showed their awareness of osteopathic principles in a few instances by quoting verbatim precepts they used as a foundation for some aspect of their practice. More frequently, appreciation of osteopathic tenets was expressed through discussion of the role of the musculoskeletal system in diagnosis and treatment. By far the most prevalent theme was the more global ability of the osteopathic physician to consider the whole patient from functional, structural, sociobehavioral, and other perspectives.

OSTEOPATHIC PRECEPTS

Physicians quoted two precepts that affected their thinking: "The rule of the artery is supreme" and "The body heals itself" (a reference to the precept of self-regulation). A third precept, applied but not clearly articulated, was the interrelationship between structure and function as exemplified by the DO's use of viscerosomatic and somatovisceral reflexes in diagnosis and treatment.

Examples were given of applications of the self-regulation precept. First, the osteopathic physician's awareness that the body is a unit and is capable of self-regulation and self-healing helps him or her to gain a deeper understanding of the illness or dysfunction that might be the underlying reason for the patient's overt signs and symptoms of disease. The osteopathic physician is aware that there might be a more fundamental deviation from health that has compromised the patient's inherent functional dynamic equilibrium and allowed an illness or disease to develop.

Second, with regard to the restoration of health, the osteopathic physician's awareness of the body's capacity to heal itself helps him or her give more serious consideration to the treatment option of "do nothing," or "try managing this problem by supporting the body's function and avoiding medication for a while." The physician's understanding of the body's capacity for self-regulation and self-healing allows him or her to be comfortable with avoiding overmedication. The osteopathic physician is aware of the role of structural treatment in enhancing the body's self-regulatory capabilities.

Third, the physician respects the patient's (perhaps intuitive) understanding of the body's capacity for self-regulation and healing. One physician related a brief story about patients with a common cold. He noted, "Most people are competent." When dealing with an upper respiratory infection, most use over-the-counter medications, rest, and fluids to enable the body to heal itself.

The physician understands that treating the somatic component lets the patient's body heal itself, with or without medication. Expanding on the role of viscerosomatic reflexes in diagnosis and treatment, salient examples follow.

CASE SIX

The patient is a woman in her 30s or 40s who is employed as a secretary, a type of work that involves sitting in the same position for long hours, doing repetitive tasks such as keyboarding. The patient presents with hand numbness. There are no other symptoms. Palpation of the neck reveals changes in the musculoskeletal system from T1 to T4 bilaterally. Treatment of the cervical and thoracic areas resolves the hand numbness.

There are several possible interpretations of the structure–function relationships in this case. One interpretation has to do with the anatomic relationship of the first rib, the clavicle, and the brachial plexus. Another has to do with the fact that the arm receives primary sympathetic innervation from T2 to T8. The relationship might have to do with possible fascial tension at the thoracic inlet preventing good lymphatic drainage for the affected arm and hand.

Another physician described her evaluation of patients' backs. When she first performed the physical examination she looked for asymmetries (such as whether one side of the rib cage was more pronounced than the other) and for convexities or scoliosis. She noted how findings in patients' backs affect how they walk and how they do their jobs, and the impact findings have on their health. She was then able to use these initial cues in evaluating subsequent complaints the patient brings to her.

In these instances osteopathic physicians apply their understanding of the interrelationship of structure and function to diagnose and treat patients osteopathically.

MUSCULOSKELETAL SYSTEM IN DIAGNOSIS AND TREATMENT

Osteopathic physicians have an important diagnostic and therapeutic tool in the musculoskeletal system. Clinicians call on it in several ways.

From the patient evaluation perspective, palpatory diagnosis of musculoskeletal problems is a skill unique to the osteopathic physician. There are numerous examples of patients with musculoskeletal problems referred to osteopathic physicians by non-DOs who could not arrive at a satisfactory diagnosis with x-ray studies or EMGs and could not resolve the patient's pain with medication such as analgesics or muscle relaxants. The osteopathic physician is able to diagnose the patient's problems using palpatory skills and treat the problems with osteopathic manipulative treatment (OMT). The patient's pain is resolved with a simple noninvasive diagnostic and treatment approach. The next cases illustrate the osteopathic physician's special skills in musculoskeletal diagnosis.

CASE SEVEN

The patient is a domestic worker in her 40s. She presents with low back pain, which she attributes to an injury she sustained on the job. She states she fell backward into a bathtub and hurt her back. The physician is able to diagnose the problem as a sacral torsion. She treats the patient and relieves her pain. The patient seeks compensation, and the physician is called on for a deposition. Her ability to describe the palpatory findings and their relationship to the patient's story helps make the patient's case.

The next case is a counterexample.

CASE EIGHT

The patient is a woman in her 30s who presents with low back pain. The physician generates several hypotheses suggested by the acuteness and severity of the pain, chief among them being that the patient is passing a kidney stone. That hypothesis is supported not only by the patient's history (acute onset, localization of pain, family history of kidney disease), but also by physical examination (patient moving around on examination table, low back tender to palpation) and preliminary laboratory results (trace of blood in urine). The physician takes abdominal x-ray views with and without contrast medium, none of which shows any abnormality. She starts the patient on a regimen of antibiotics. The pain, still present, is localized on the right side, suggesting possible gallbladder disease. Ultrasound of the gallbladder reveals no abnormality. To quote the physician: "Finally it occurred to me that maybe the pain in her back is because she's got pain in her back." Palpatory diagnosis revealed somatic dysfunction at L1–L2, which the physician treated, relieving the patient's pain. "She skipped out of the office." The lesson here for the physician was that as a DO she should not forget her unique perspective. She needed to always remember to include the musculoskeletal system in her diagnostic formulation and treatment plan.

Musculoskeletal (osteopathic manipulative) treatment is seen by many osteopathic physicians as the sine qua non of osteopathic distinctiveness. For most primary care DOs it is a unique part of their treatment methodology, and, though characterized as adjunctive by some, plays a key role in patient management. The following cases are examples.

CASE NINE

This case illustrates osteopathic manipulative treatment and relief of stress. The patient is a woman in her 30s who is being treated by a non-DO for hyperthyroidism. She suffers intractable headaches for which the physician cannot provide relief. The patient is referred to the osteopathic physician, who describes her as a typical patient with hyperthyroidism: extremely thin, intense, slightly bulging eyes, quick birdlike movements, and rapid heartbeat. Musculoskeletal evaluation reveals the patient to be "stiff as a board." The DO treats the somatic dysfunction in the patient's neck and shoulders using osteopathic manipulation, with little effect. After several visits, however, the patient's headaches ease, and she begins to have more movement in her neck and shoulders. The patient lives in a stressful family environment that includes her terminally ill husband. The burden of family stress as well as the hyperthyroidism is reflected in her musculoskeletal system. Regular manipulative treatment in combination with ongoing medical therapy for the hyperthyroidism addressed the patient's disease process, increased the patient's comfort, and facilitated her ability to manage her life.

CASE TEN

The patient is an adult with sinusitis. The physician describing this case sees many of these patients, especially in the fall and winter, when people spend more time in an enclosed environment. In her office the physician has established a routine for managing a patient with this problem. She starts by doing a complete evaluation, including a structural assessment, checking especially the thoracic and cervical spine, and thoracic inlet. She treats with manipulative medicine those areas of the cervical and thoracic spine that need it, and performs a lymphatic pump technique. She notes the osteopathic manipulative treatment usually produces rather dramatic relief of symptoms and seems to improve the effectiveness of the medication she prescribes. She includes in her education to the patient instructions for administering saline solution nose drops, drinking lots of fluids, keeping the eustachian tubes clear if the ears are involved in the infection, and refraining from or minimizing smoking. She says, "I feel nice and osteopathic with cases like that." She notes that since these cases are not usually diagnostic challenges, she can focus during her time with the patient on structural diagnosis, manipulative treatment, and patient education.

CASE ELEVEN

The patient is a healthy man in his 30s. He works as a salesperson. Although his job requires that he be on his feet, he is not particularly active in his work. He might be characterized as a "weekend sportsman" who, though exercising little during the week, exercises vigorously on weekends. As a result he experiences back discomfort, which is then exacerbated by his work. The physician takes a focused history revealing no arthritis, injury, or underlying disease process that would express itself as back pain. The chief diagnosis is "musculoskeletal problem due to overuse." The patient's somatic dysfunction in the pelvis, lumbar, and thoracolumbar regions is treated with osteopathic manipulative treatment with good results.

THERAPEUTIC TOUCH

Osteopathic manipulative medicine, while useful in its own right as a treatment modality, is further effective as a form of therapeutic touch. This is particularly important to the primary care physician who seeks to know and treat the whole patient. Whether the patient is an elderly woman who comes in regularly for treatment of her stiff neck, or a postaccident patient with neck pain, the act of touching the patient to evaluate and treat the musculoskeletal system is therapeutic. One physician noted that her patients thought she listened to them better than another physician, and that might be because she touches them where it hurts rather than, for example, looking at x-ray films.

MUSCULOSKELETAL PAIN

Palpatory diagnosis and osteopathic manipulative treatment are particularly effective in evaluating and treating musculoskeletal pain, e.g., in postaccident patients. The vignettes outlined in Cases Seven and Eight are just two instances of the value of palpatory diagnosis in cases of musculoskeletal pain. The osteopathic physician's ability to put his or her hands on the patient and tell them where it hurts is not only a form of therapeutic touch but is also meaningful to patients, as well as being cost effective. The patient is comforted by diagnostic touch applied to a painful musculoskeletal area, and perceives it as a form of listening to their body. Furthermore, the ability to accurately interpret palpatory findings from the musculoskeletal system is perceived as a uniquely osteopathic skill. In one comparison between himself and a non-DO, a physician discussed referrals. He noted that the referral letters from non-DOs tended to focus on the immediate problem, such as a car accident or work injury. The osteopathic physician considers the injury in the context of the patient's total body mechanics:

Is the patient right or left handed?
Is this a woman with a young child?
What hip does she carry the baby on?
What is the patient's posture like?
What is the overall body condition?

Following treatment, further consideration of body mechanics can be used to assess its effectiveness.

OSTEOPATHIC MANIPULATIVE TREATMENT AND MEDICATION

One last category where palpatory diagnosis and especially osteopathic manipulative medicine are particularly helpful is in relation to medication. In Case Ten we offered a brief vignette where OMT was thought to relieve symptoms of upper res-

piratory infection (sinusitis), and enhance the effectiveness of medication. OMT may also help a patient avoid medication. Several physicians cited instances when they used this reasoning, particularly with elderly patients suffering from arthritis pain. One physician noted regular visits by elderly patients who sought manipulative treatment for neck and shoulder stiffness, enabling them to avoid medication. Another told of elderly women patients with osteoporosis who are hospitalized with a cardiac problem but also suffer musculoskeletal pain. Gentle osteopathic manipulative treatment to the spine makes them more comfortable. A third physician specifically instructs his elderly patients in exercise and stretching techniques to maintain mobility and avoid arthritic pain and stiffness. The physician treats these patients regularly with osteopathic manipulation. In his words: "It helps them avoid antiinflammatory medications that cause gastrointestinal problems. It's better for them to spend their money on a visit to the doctor for a manipulative treatment than on drugs."

PATIENT AS A WHOLE

The role of the musculoskeletal system in health and illness or injury and the osteopathic physician's skills in evaluating and treating the musculoskeletal system are important. By far the most distinctively osteopathic traits for the primary care physician, however, are the perception of the patient as a whole in an environment, and the capacity for integrative thinking. Examples are the best illustrations.

One woman physician had many women patients in her practice. Not infrequently they asked her about the pros and cons of hysterectomy. Her advice in nonmalignant cases was often to discourage them after considering the short- and long-term consequences of having the uterus surgically removed. In the short-term the patient must recover from the traumatic invasion of her body and likely experiences posthysterectomy depression. In the long-term the woman experiences permanent loss of reproductive function as well as loss of an important organ. The body is not simply a container for parts. The uterus is an integral part of a woman's bodily identity; its removal constitutes a partial loss of that personal identity.

A physician who practiced in an economically depressed area had many children in his practice who suffered frequent respiratory infections and sore throats. He saw the children as part of an unhealthy environment. They were usually poor, with a poor diet. They often did not have clean clothes, had not bathed recently, or did not have proper shoes (e.g., children who wore canvas sneakers without socks in the winter). The physician saw these characteristics of their life environment as contributing to his understanding of their illness and his ability to effectively treat them and restore them to health, or at least to more optimum functioning.

A woman physician managed many pregnant patients, including their deliveries. Her whole patient approach to the management of pregnancy and delivery involved awareness of the patient in her environment. On the initial encounter the physician considered with the patient the social context of her pregnancy and asked these questions:

Is the patient married to the father of the baby?

Is this her first pregnancy?

What is the family's reaction to the pregnancy?

What is the father's reaction?

If the patient is not married to the father, did he end their relationship when he found out she was pregnant?

What are the patient's expectations?

The physician emphasizes patient education on the first encounter. During prenatal care the physician treats musculoskeletal complaints with manipulative treatment. She finds that back pain, leg pain, stress at the pubic symphysis, and sacral somatic dysfunction seem to be the most common problems. During labor and delivery the physician is present. She finds that being there is therapeutic, especially if the patient is struggling. The physician provides coaching and companionship during this intense experience, sharing what she calls "a real space" with the patient. She is able to perform osteopathic manipulative techniques that are helpful, including a cranial technique (CV4) and sacral traction. Post partum the physician feels better able to manage the patient and her infant knowing she is thoroughly acquainted with the circumstances of the pregnancy. She has the patient's confidence, in addition to having been there and actively facilitated the delivery herself.

INTEGRATIVE THINKING

Exemplifying the osteopathic physician's distinctive capacity for integrative thinking, one physician expressed her approach literally: "You diagnose with all of your senses," she said. The physician looks, feels, and smells while listening to the patient. You look at the patient's body language, evidence of skin lesions, personal hygiene, and relate that to what the patient is telling you. She said, "The body doesn't lie. The patient may, but the body doesn't." If you question a patient's credibility, the use of all of your senses in patient evaluation helps elicit the patient's true history.

CASE TWELVE

A physician described a particularly troublesome case wherein the impact of the patient's environmental context was a significant factor in diagnosis and treatment.

The patient is a 27-year-old man presenting with abdominal pain on exertion. He is a basketball player, tall (6'8"), thin, usually healthy, and in good physical condition, who practices basketball three or four times a week. The abdominal pain occurred while playing basketball. The onset of pain was gradual, characterized as a cramping type of pain. It did not occur in association with eating or other activities. There was no history or evidence of sports injury. On learning of the reason for the visit, the physician considered the patient in his life context. This was a healthy individual who was seeing a physician for the first time with a complaint, on the advice of his father. Even before examining the patient, the physician,

knowing the family, believed the patient was legitimately, potentially seriously ill, or he would not have sought help. The physician attributed his ability to make those preliminary assessments to the fact that he was an osteopathic family practitioner in a relatively small community.

Physical examination revealed a large mass on palpation of the abdomen with no other abnormalities. The physician sought to further characterize and localize the mass with a flat plate of the abdomen, and a computed tomography (CT) scan. The flat plate showed accumulated stool in the left side of the large bowel, but no mass. Furthermore, the patient stated the pain was on the right, and he reported having a bowel movement every day. The data did not fit. At this point the physician's thinking ran along two lines. First, he believed there was a serious problem but did not want to alarm the family. He was aware that the patient's father-in-law, who was in his 50s, had passed away only three weeks before and the family was grieving his loss.

The physician considered several hypotheses to explain the anomalous data set, including the possibility of a hematoma on the muscle wall that had developed from an inadvertent or forgotten injury during basketball practice. The physician ordered an ultrasound of the abdomen that revealed a solid mass. It was now incumbent on him to inform the patient's family of his thinking. He was aware of the potential fear of cancer, especially since a family acquaintance (not a relative) had had a son (perhaps near the patient's age) die from cancer. The physician made a point of using probabilities to assure the family that the likelihood of a benign process was much higher than the likelihood of a malignancy. Surgical laparotomy was done, revealing a benign tumor approximately 5" in diameter that was removed, followed by uneventful recovery.

The physician described his problem-solving process for this case as occurring on two planes. One was the diagnosis and management of the medical problem; the other was the management of the interaction with the patient's family. He saw his ability to effectively integrate those two lines of thinking into effective overall patient management as particularly osteopathic.

SUMMARY

Osteopathic thinking is many things to many people. Osteopathic primary care practitioners seem to agree that there are a few key things about how they view patient care that makes them particularly osteopathic. First there is their ability to effectively use the musculoskeletal system in patient evaluation and management. They are able to bring those skills to bear in a range of areas, all the way from the most fundamental diagnosis and treatment of musculoskeletal complaints, to relating musculoskeletal intervention to the use of medications, to the realization of the power of therapeutic touch. They also show a keen awareness of the body's inherent capacity for self-regulation and self-healing through their understanding of the interaction of different therapeutic interventions, and their ability to use support of the musculoskeletal system to help restore the patient to health. Even more meaningful to those osteopathic primary care physicians, however, is their special understanding of the patient as a whole who exists in an environment, and their unique ability to think integratively about the patient in his or her life circumstance. This global sense of the whole person is for them far and away the greatest physician attribute that makes them distinctively osteopathic.

ILLUSTRATIVE CASE

We return to Mr. Johnson. We conclude this chapter by first recalling the information we presented about the patient earlier in the chapter, and then analyzing the case using an osteopathic approach to clinical problem solving.

Description

The patient is a white male, age 55, presenting with a complaint of aching in the left shoulder that he experienced while raking leaves. Other pertinent data are that the patient is overweight and hypertensive. You may wish to turn back to the initial patient presentation to recall the specific statement of the reason for the visit, as well as the vital signs.

STOP: If you were Dr. Martin, as you were planning to conduct a thorough history and physical examination including a diagnostic palpatory examination, what might you be thinking? What possible mechanisms might you be considering for his presenting problem?

The picture presented by the preliminary data suggests a life pattern that might have led to enough deterioration in the patient's ability to maintain homeostasis that it has culminated in this acute problem of pain. The pain could be of musculoskeletal origin, perhaps a strained ligament, muscle spasm, or swollen tendon, a myofascial trigger point, or even referred pain from the cervical or thoracic spine. Segmental facilitation (in this case in the thoracic spine) lowers the response threshold for many potential shoulder complaints. These are your most likely considerations at this point. However, other more potentially serious causes must be considered, such as a problem of cardiovascular origin involving ischemia, venous and lymphatic congestion, or referred pain from the arteries of the heart. The pain might also be referred from dysfunction of the gastrointestinal system, or perhaps be a problem of pulmonary origin, such as pleurisy. Less likely possibilities include immunologic disorders such as arthritis, connective tissue disease, or cancer. You also consider that there could be more than one mechanism that would explain most or all of the findings. For example, the elevated blood pressure may be a consequence of the pain experience or the patient's anxiety regarding his illness or his first visit to a new doctor, or it could be part of the same underlying problem that is causing the pain.

As you enter the examining room and greet Mr. Johnson, you note he is, as you expected, a large, heavy man who appears in no acute distress. You note an odor of cigarette smoke on the patient's clothing and hair. He is draped for examination, so you are unable to note whether he has a pack of cigarettes in his shirt pocket. As he shakes your hand you note he has a firm grip. His shoulders are level and he holds his head upright in the midline position. His coloring appears normal for a man his age. There is no evidence of hypoxia (bluish skin) or florid coloring. As he speaks you note he does not have any difficulty breathing at rest.

He describes his problem as follows. The shoulder discomfort occurred while he was raking leaves last Sunday afternoon. It was of gradual onset. He characterizes the discomfort as a heavy aching feeling. He indicates the frontal aspect of the upper chest on the left, and the left shoulder when you ask him to show you where the pain is. The pain does not seem to go anywhere outside of the left shoulder and upper chest. Specifically, it does not move to the sternal area or into the back.

He has had pain like this before on two occasions. The first one occurred last summer when he was using a post hole digger to help his son put in a new fence. The other occurrence happened approximately 2 months ago when he was helping a neighbor push her car out of the mud. On both occasions the pain subsided with rest and was completely gone by the following day. When the current episode happened, he rested, with relief after approximately 10 minutes. The pain recurred when he resumed the exertion of leaf raking. The discomfort seems to be more associated with exertion than with simple motion of the left arm and shoulder. The patient cannot reproduce the pain by moving the arm and shoulder while at rest. He has not noticed pain with any other form of exertion that does not involve the arms and shoulders, such as climbing stairs.

During the history of presenting complaint you ask him to take a deep breath and exhale fully. That does not reproduce the pain. The patient rates the pain when it was at its strongest as approximately a 7 on a scale of 1 to 10. It has not completely gone away, and he would currently rate the discomfort as a 2 or 3 on the same scale. Before continuing with a more detailed health history, you ask Mr. Johnson what it was that prompted him to seek help at this time. He responds that he has had aches and pains before that always went away. He sought help for this episode because it has not resolved as have previous episodes. Furthermore, he recalls a couple of years ago a coworker telling him her husband had pain in his left shoulder and arm while raking leaves, and it turned out he was having a heart attack. He admits he is concerned.

STOP: Review what you know about Mr. Johnson. First and foremost consider the impact the patient's life pattern has had on his health. His lifestyle, which has brought him to his current health status, has involved a steady challenge to and deterioration of his body's capabilities for self-regulation. The pain he has experienced on this most recent occasion as well as several previous ones is probably the manifestation of an acute medical problem. The problem results from a steadily decreasing ability on his part to maintain structural and functional balance and sustain a healthy dynamic equilibrium. The pain itself involves the musculoskeletal system but might not originate within these elements. Since moving the arm and shoulder at rest does not reproduce the pain, the joints of the shoulder are probably not the cause. Absence of pain with no-nexertional active motion of this region suggests that the pain probably does not originate with the muscles of the shoulder girdle. The fact that other forms of exertion such as stair climbing do not bring on the pain makes a cardiac problem such as coronary artery disease less likely as well. Deep inhalation and exhalation while at rest did not reproduce the pain, which would tend to weaken a pulmonary hypothesis. Further investigation is needed to evaluate the more remote possibility of a gastrointestinal problem. You continue the health history, guiding Mr. Johnson through a past medical history and review of systems.

PAST MEDICAL HISTORY

Mr. Johnson has not seen a physician in almost 10 years. His only significant past health problems have been gastrointestinal. Approximately 11 years ago he experienced periodic abdominal discomfort and intolerance to certain foods. After attempts at conservative management were unsuccessful, his gallbladder was removed with uneventful recovery. He has experienced no significant health problems since then. He has not had any further abdominal discomfort, nor problems with diarrhea, constipation, or bloody stools. His diet and weight are essentially unchanged since his surgery 10 years ago.

FAMILY HISTORY

Mr. Johnson is the third of four children. His father died 20 years ago at age 68 following a myocardial infarction. His mother is still living, age 85, and in relatively good health. His oldest brother died 3 years ago at age 60 following a myocardial infarction. He has one other brother, age 58, whom he has not seen in several years, and about whose health status he knows little. His sister, age 52, lives nearby, and is in good health.

CARDIOVASCULAR

He has had no difficulty breathing, nor experienced diaphoresis or shortness of breath with the chest discomfort. He sleeps on his back or side, and does not recall ever awakening feeling short of breath. He continues to smoke approximately two packs of cigarettes a day.

MUSCULOSKELETAL

He experiences occasional joint stiffness and low back pain; he attributes these to old age and being overweight. The back pain comes and goes, and has not changed in the last several years. The joint stiffness has worsened somewhat in the last year.

ENDOCRINOLOGIC

He has not experienced increased hunger or thirst in the last year. He has not experienced any night sweats, tremor, or intolerance of temperature changes.

GENITOURINARY

He has not had any urinary urgency, hesitancy, difficulty starting the stream, or change in force of the stream. He and his wife have intercourse approximately once a month. He has no difficulty achieving and maintaining an erection and orgasm. The chest discomfort does not occur during intercourse.

PULMONARY

He has not experienced hemoptysis, cough, phlegm, or pain with respiration.

EARS, NOSE, AND THROAT

He has occasional headaches that are relieved by ibuprofen. He has no difficulty hearing, or ringing in the ears. He has had no loss or blurring of vision. He wears glasses for reading only, which he purchases at a local department store. He has not had his eyes examined since the complete physical examination associated with his gastrointestinal problems several years ago.

SOCIAL HISTORY

Mr. Johnson tells you he is employed in a rather stressful, sedentary job. He has been married 25 years, and has two grown children who no longer live at home. His wife also works outside the home. Between them, they have a reasonable standard of living, and health insurance through his employer. Mr. Johnson smokes approximately two packs of cigarettes a day. He drinks between two and three 12-ounce beers a day during the week and approximately twice that many a day on weekends. Mr. Johnson does not exercise regularly, and his diet is high in fat.

STOP: Before continuing to the physical examination, establish some priorities for possible ways to explain the patient's deviation from health, as well as possible diagnostic hypotheses to explain his acute presenting problem. You see your most likely considerations and related cues as follows. There is long-term compromise of the body's ability to maintain health to the point that the patient's problem is now acute, and the health behaviors are significant risk factors for further damage. Supporting evidence includes:

> History of a high-fat diet
> Lack of exercise
> Stressful sedentary work
> Smoking
> Alcohol consumption

The presentation is an acute problem of pain suggesting a serious medical problem.

MUSCULOSKELETAL PAIN

He has musculoskeletal pain, possibly costochondritis from thoracic, cervical and/or shoulder somatic dysfunction, with possible radiculopathy or arthritis. The supporting evidence includes:

Pain location in upper chest and shoulder
Associated with exertion during use of associated muscles and joints
Patient is 55, overweight, has stressful job, sedentary lifestyle
Patient has experienced pain and stiffness in other joints

Controverting evidence includes:

Character of pain is heavy and aching
Rest does not completely relieve pain
Deep breath with complete exhalation does not reproduce pain
Movement of arm and shoulder does not reproduce pain
Patient describes pain as different than previous episodes

CARDIOVASCULAR REFERRED CHEST PAIN

The supporting evidence is:

Character of pain is heavy and aching
Association of this and previous episodes with upper body exertion
Failure to reproduce pain with simple movement
Acute phase of pain relieved by rest
Male, age 55, BP 160/110
Stressful job
Sedentary lifestyle
High-fat diet
Smokes
Family history of cardiovascular disease

Controverting evidence includes:

Location of pain
Pain not associated with coitus, climbing stairs, or other exertion
Pain not accompanied by shortness of breath or diaphoresis

GASTROINTESTINAL REFERRED PAIN

The supporting evidence includes:

Location in upper chest and shoulder
Patient is 55
Overweight
High-fat diet

Controverting evidence includes:

Partially relieved by rest
No apparent association with eating or foods
Gallbladder has been surgically removed

PULMONARY REFERRED PAIN

Supporting evidence includes:

Location in upper chest and shoulder
Brought on by upper body exertion
Patient smokes

The controverting evidence is:

Deep breath does not reproduce pain
Acute phase relieved by rest

You decide to order your preliminary differential diagnoses as follows (from most likely to least likely):

Chest pain, as a result of coronary artery insufficiency
Primary musculoskeletal pain
Gastrointestinal pain
Pulmonary referred pain

Your reasoning is that, although the pain is highly atypical for angina, Mr. Johnson has several risk factors for heart disease, and it would be a serious error to miss a cardiovascular problem in this patient.

PHYSICAL EXAMINATION

Repeat vital signs: Unchanged

Heart: Regular rate and rhythm without S3 or S4 murmurs.
Chest and lungs: Normal to percussion. Auscultation of lungs reveals scattered rhonchi.
Bruits heard over both femoral arteries. No carotid bruits.

Musculoskeletal findings that would aid in the diagnosis:

Tenderness to local palpation of paraspinal tissue at T2–T5 on the left
Tissue texture ropiness in that area
No pain on direct palpation of shoulder
Active and passive motion of shoulders and arms is symmetrical without restriction
Passive motion of shoulders and arms does not elicit pain on either side
Direct pressure applied over left glenoid fossa does not elicit pain
Range of motion of the cervical spine is full
Muscle strength testing in the upper extremities is symmetric and 5+/5+, and does not reproduce the pain
No trigger points are identified in the pectoral muscles
Costochondral joint pressure does not elicit pain or discomfort
No cyanosis or edema

STOP: Having completed the physical examination, take time to explain your thinking to the patient. What will you tell him? Take a few minutes to think through a possible explanation that he would understand.

Your explanation may include the following information:

1. Expression of empathy for the patient's concerns about his problem, and reinforcement for seeking care
2. Outlining of short-term and long-term plan based on your assessment of his immediate problem and your concerns about his overall health

Based on history and physical examination, possible sources of his acute medical problem are:

1. Coronary artery disease, supported by a history of pain with

exertion, as well as his lifestyle, smoking, and other risk factors. Although this seems like a problem of possible musculoskeletal origin, the fact that he could not reproduce the pain with motion, and you did not reproduce it with passive motion or direct pressure on the area, suggests that the musculoskeletal component of the pain is secondary to some other underlying process.

2. Gastrointestinal and pulmonary causes for the pain have not been completely ruled out, but they are much less likely at this time.

Your discussion of long-term considerations could include the following. Based on information about his lifestyle, as well as data such as his weight and blood pressure, you are concerned that he is at risk for more serious health problems. It appears his life pattern over the years has continuously challenged his body's ability to stay healthy. You wish to work with him once his immediate problem is managed, to develop some life habits that will improve his body's ability to return to and sustain optimum function, and thus reduce further health risks.

You decide to do the following additional tests:

Chest x-ray
CBC
Urinalysis
SMAC-20
ECG
Stress test

Your reasoning is that this is a new patient with significant health risks. These are low-cost high-yield sources of baseline data. Having these tests done for this patient is in keeping with the standard of care for your community. If you need to refer this patient to a cardiologist, for example, these data would be needed at a minimum.

You ask your office assistant to prepare Mr. Johnson for an ECG to be done in your office directly following the completion of the physical examination. You ask Mr. Johnson to schedule the other tests with your office staff person, and set up another appointment for 2 weeks from today, indicating that you will call him if results of the tests suggest he should see you sooner. In the meantime, you ask him to consider long-term management of his health, specifically how you and he can work together most effectively to begin to return him to a status of greater health and reduce his risks of subsequent illness and dysfunction.

The test results are as follows:

Chest x-ray film, ECG, and stress test show no abnormalities
Blood count, urinalysis, and SMAC are all within normal limits

STOP: In our presentation of Mr. Johnson's case, we have intentionally placed the clinician in a listening rather than questioning role. In a scenario portraying the physician as an active hypothesis tester, he or she asks numerous questions to elicit information specifically relevant to the hypotheses under consideration. Furthermore, the physical examination could

have focused on only the region of the complaint and on those regions that would yield data positive or negative for favored hypotheses. That pattern of data gathering is not usually functional for the osteopathic primary care physician, so we have not emphasized it here.

Now we have a reasonably complete preliminary data set for Mr. Johnson. A thorough evaluation of his illness is in order. The two major possible mechanisms for his presenting problem are chest pain atypical for angina with secondary musculoskeletal pain, probably as a result of coronary artery disease; and primary musculoskeletal pain.

The first explanation has the strongest support. The patient's pain could likely be of cardiac origin. It is a heavy, aching pain that is brought on by exertion and relieved by rest. It is not reproduced by direct pressure on or movement of the affected area. It does not seem to be related to eating (i.e., exacerbated by certain foods, or associated with gas or bloating), or breathing (e.g., brought on by taking a deep breath). The patient has many health risk factors for coronary artery disease. He is male, age 55, has a sedentary stressful job, does not exercise, is overweight, and smokes. Although the patient has few pertinent physical findings, those you did elicit are telling: elevated systolic and diastolic blood pressure, femoral artery bruits, and tenderness and tissue texture abnormalities at T2–T5, which have been shown to be associated with viscerosomatic reflexes from coronary artery disease.[17–18]

There are four characteristics used to establish a diagnosis of typical angina pectoris:

1. Chest discomfort brought on by exertion and/or stress
2. Location substernal or anterior chest wall
3. Pain feels heavy, like pressure or squeezing
4. Pain is soon (10 minutes or less) relieved by rest, or immediately with nitroglycerine

This patient has three of the four characteristics. Last, a normal chest x-ray film and ECG do not rule out coronary artery disease.

At this point you can assign approximately a 70% likelihood to a diagnosis of coronary artery insufficiency, with the diagnosis of primary musculoskeletal problem having a 20% likelihood, and other diagnostic possibilities combined in the remaining 10% probability range. You are now able to develop a management plan for the patient.

CONCLUSION

As we leave Mr. Johnson, consider what we have learned from his case and the many other brief cases presented here that could comprise an osteopathic approach to clinical problem solving. At the beginning of the chapter we posed several questions about the nature of osteopathic clinical problem solving. Is it a principle-based definable skill? Is it what osteopathic physicians do? How idiosyncratic is it? Predictably the answer lies somewhere in between.

Osteopathic problem solving is loosely couched in the four basic precepts of:

Body unity
Structure–function interrelationship
Self-regulation
Rational therapy

The application of those precepts by any given clinician problem solver to any given patient problem is not only idiosyncratic to the patient but also to the problem solver. The following considerations seem to be fundamental to osteopathic problem solving.

In considering a patient's problem, the osteopathic physician must be able to perceive the problem as having evolved from a compromise in the body's ability to maintain a healthy dynamic equilibrium or homeostatic state. The body's normal state, under circumstances of adequate nutrition, exercise, and physiologic and anatomic balance, is one of health. Health problems, whether or not they are amenable to labeling as disease processes, constitute deviations from that normal state of health. The goal of osteopathic problem solving is to ascertain the nature and source of the deviation from health.

The major problem solving models articulated here, which in various forms comprise most of what we know about clinical problem solving, can be considered to represent a subset of osteopathic problem solving. The problem-solving models and the osteopathic approach are far from being mutually exclusive. Rather, the osteopathic problem solver is seen as calling on the more restricted, reductionistic models to incorporate into his or her more global, holistic, conceptualization of health and illness, to achieve a more complete understanding of a patient's problem.

Not all osteopathic primary care physicians use osteopathic problem solving or are even cognizant of it. Therefore, it would be inaccurate to say that osteopathic problem solving is just what osteopathic physicians do. It is more than that. With further understanding and investigation we can characterize osteopathic problem solving to the point of articulating a model that is as applicable and teachable as the more allopathic models we have now.

REFERENCES

1. Astell Louise. Reflections and a forecast. *The DO.* 1981;21(5):155–159.
2. Groen GJ, Patel VL. The relationship between comprehension and reasoning in medical expertise. In: Chi MTH, et al., eds. *The Nature of Expertise.* Hillsdale, NJ: Erlbaum; 1988:287–310.
3. Patel VL, Groen GJ, Norman GR. Reasoning and instruction in medical curricula. *Cognition and Instruction.* 1993;10:335–378.
4. Schmidt HG, Norman GR, Boshuizen HPA. A cognitive perspective on medical expertise: theory and implications. *Acad Med.* 1990; 65:611–621.
5. Norman GR, Brooks LR, Allen SW, Rosenthal DR. The development of expertise in dermatology. *Arch Dermatol.* 1989;125:1062–1065.
6. Brooks LR, Allen SW, Norman GR. Rule and instance-based inference in medical diagnosis. *J Exp Psychol Gen.* 1991;120:278–287.
7. Schmidt HG, Boshuizen HPA. Encapsulation of biomedical knowledge. In: Evans D, Patel VL, eds. *Advanced Models of Cognition for Medical Training and Practice.* New York, NY: Springer-Verlag; 1993.
8. Hunter KM. *Doctors' Stories: The Narrative Structure of Medical Knowledge.* Princeton, NJ: Princeton University Press; 1991.
9. Elstein AS, Shulman LS, Sprafka SA. *Medical Problem Solving: An Analysis of Clinical Reasoning.* Cambridge, Mass: Harvard University Press; 1978.
10. Weed LL. *Your Health Care and How To Manage It.* Essex Junction, Vt: Essex Publishing Co; 1975.
11. Walker HK, Hurst JW, Woody MF. *Applying the Problem-Oriented System.* New York, NY: Medcom Press; 1973.
12. Sox HC Jr, Blatt MA, Higgins MC, Marton KI. *Medical Decision Making.* Boston/London: Butterworth's; 1988.
13. Sackett DL, Haynes RB, Tugwell P. *Clinical Epidemiology: A Basic Science for Clinical Medicine.* Boston/Toronto: Little, Brown and Co; 1985.
14. Schappert S. *National Ambulatory Medical Care Survey: 1990 Summary.* Hyattsville, Md: US Department of Health and Human Services, Public Health Service, Centers for Disease Control, National Center for Health Statistics; 1992.
15. Special committee on osteopathic principles and osteopathic technic of the Kirksville College of Osteopathy and Surgery. An interpretation of the osteopathic concept: tentative formulation of a teaching guide for faculty, staff, and student body. *Journal of Osteopathy.* October 1953:8–10.
16. Sprafka SA, Ward RC, Neff D. What characterizes an osteopathic principle? Selected responses to an open question. *JAOA.* 1981; 81(9).
17. Beal MC. Viscerosomatic reflexes: a review. *JAOA.* 1985; 85(12):786–801.
18. Kuchera M, Kuchera WA. *Osteopathic Considerations in Systemic Dysfunction.* Kirksville, Mo: KCOM Press; 1990.

APPENDIX TO CHAPTER 18

Section 1. Statistical properties of stress ECG as it relates to coronary artery disease

Diagnostic statistics for the stress ECG: a common method for displaying statistics is shown in Table 18.1 below, known as a 2-by-2 table.

We can analyze the table step by step as follows. Let's imagine we conducted an experiment on a sample of 500 patients. Furthermore, let's imagine that half, or 250, of our patients had CAD, as determined by the gold standard, an objective verification of the presence or absence of the disease in our patient

Table 18.1
Diagnosis of CAD

	Present	Absent	
Stress ECG +	150	22	172
Stress ECG −	100	228	328
	250	250	500

sample. That is our defined disease prevalence for this purpose. It is clearly unrealistically high; a change in prevalence to a more realistic level can change what we learn from test results. We have now established the values at the bottom of our "CAD present" and "CAD absent" columns. Now, let's say all 500 of our patients underwent a stress ECG. We would find that approximately 172 of them had positive test results, and test results for 328 of our patients would be normal. That would establish the values for the "Stress ECG +" and "Stress ECG −" rows of our table. We would also learn that, of the patients who had CAD, approximately 150 had a positive stress test result. Those are our true positives. Furthermore, approximately 228 of our healthy patients would have normal test results (true negatives). Clearly the test is not perfect, but it does identify a fair number of true positives and a large proportion of true negatives. To allow us to generalize from this study of 500 patients to other populations, we convert the number of true positives and true negatives to a proportion. In the first instance we divide true positives by total number of patients with CAD (150/250 = .60). That gives a statistic expressing the probability that a patient with CAD will have a positive stress ECG result, which is called the true positive rate or sensitivity of the test. Similarly, we divide the true negatives by the total of non-CAD patients (228/250 = .91). That statistic tells us the probability that a patient with no CAD will have a normal stress ECG result, which is the true negative rate or specificity of the test. Sensitivity and specificity remain constant for a test over time, and with changes in disease prevalence. They would only change if, for example, the quality of the test changed to increase or decrease its association with the presence or absence of this disease process.

Two other values of even greater interest to physicians than sensitivity and specificity are positive predictive value and negative predictive value. Those are the values that tell us for a known disease prevalence what the probability is of the disease being present given a positive test result (positive predictive value), and, conversely, what the probability is of a patient being disease free given a normal test result (negative predictive value). In our example above, these can be found as follows:

Positive predictive value = True positives/All positives or 150/172 = .87.

Negative predictive value = True negatives/ All negatives or 228/328 = .70

Thus, in a patient population where approximately half of the patients actually have coronary artery disease, any given patient with a positive stress ECG result will have an 87% probability of having the disease, and a patient with a normal stress ECG result will have a 70% probability of being disease free. However, unlike sensitivity and specificity, positive and negative predictive value are strongly affected by changes in disease prevalence. Consider the following example in Table 18.2.

As in the first example, we have a total patient sample of 500. However, we have revised the disease prevalence to 10%, or 50 out of 500 patients who have CAD, a level much more

Table 18.2
Diagnosis of CAD

	Present	Absent	
Stress ECG +	30	40	70
Stress ECG −	20	410	430
	50	450	500

likely to be seen by the primary care physician. We know that the true positive rate or sensitivity of the stress ECG is .60, so we can establish that for this patient population, 30 of our patients who have CAD by the gold standard will have a positive stress ECG result. We also know that the true negative rate or specificity of our test is .91, so we can establish that for this group, approximately 430 of our healthy patients will have a normal stress ECG result. Now, what if a patient in this group whose health status we didn't know had a positive stress test result? How sure could we be that he or she had CAD? We can ascertain that as follows:

Positive predictive value = True positives/Total positives or 30/70 = .43

Note how strongly the positive predictive value is affected by prevalence of the problem. In our previous examples where we arbitrarily decided that half of the patients had the target disease, our stress ECG had a positive predictive value of .87. However, if we decrease the disease prevalence to a more realistic level of 10%, we find that the positive predictive value of the test decreases also, to just over half of what it was in the previous example. Let us look at what happens to negative predictive value:

Negative predictive value = True negatives/All negatives or 410/430 = .95

Thus the negative predictive value of the stress test is also strongly affected by change in disease prevalence, only in the opposite direction. Its predictive power improves.

Section 2. Revising probabilities—Bayes' theorem

The formula version of Bayes' theorem we use in the example reads as follows:

$$p(D|+) = \frac{p(D) \times p(+|D)}{\{p(D) \times p(+|D)\} + \{p(\sim D) \times p(+|\sim D)\}}$$

What does it all mean? First, a brief introduction to the symbols we have used

Symbol	Meaning	Example
p	Probability	p(A) = probability of A
~	Not	p(~A) = probability of not A
|	Given	p(A|B) = probability of A given B

Looking first at the equation's numerator:

p(D|+) This is what we are trying to find. For this example it reads "the probability of the diagnosis given a positive test result." Or what is the probability that Mr. Johnson has CAD given that he has a positive test result. Conceptually it is the same as the positive predictive value, and could be calculated using a 2-by-2 table. In this instance it is being applied to a specific case rather than a patient population, and we are calculating it using Bayes' theorem.

p(D) The probability of the diagnosis. In this case let us consider a 70% probability of CAD for Mr. Johnson.

p(+|D) The probability of a positive test result given the diagnosis. We know that as well. It is the sensitivity of the test, equal to .60 for the stress ECG.

In the denominator of the equation we repeat the numerator—probability of disease times the true positive rate—and add the following:

p(~D) Probability of no disease, or our subjective probability that Mr. Johnson's chest pain is not the result of coronary artery disease.

p(+|~D) Which reads "the probability of a positive test result given no disease" that we determined earlier was the false–positive rate.

How do we determine the appropriate numbers to fill into Bayes' theorem for Mr. Johnson?

a. We have settled on a tentative diagnostic probability of coronary artery insufficiency of .70 for Mr. Johnson. So, for us, p(D) = .70

b. We know the sensitivity or true positive rate of the test to be .60. p(+|D) = .60

c. By subtracting we can establish the probability that Mr. Johnson's pain does not result from CAD: p(~D) = 1 − p(D) or, in our case, 1 − .70 or .30.

d. Last, we can look back at Table 18.1 and find the false–positive rate of our test to be 22/250 or .09. p(+|~D) = .09.

Substituting the numbers in the formula we obtain the expression:

$$p(D|+) = \frac{.7 \times .6}{(.7 \times .6) + (.3 \times .09)}$$
$$= \frac{.42}{.42 + .027}$$
$$= .94$$

Using Bayes' theorem, then, we have been able to learn that, starting with a diagnosis to which a probability of .70 was assigned (called the prior probability), and knowing the sensitivity and specificity of the stress ECG, we can improve our prediction of CAD for this patient from 70% to 94% if the result of the stress test is positive. Another way of saying this is the posterior probability of CAD for this patient is 94%. That is a reasonable improvement, and many diagnosticians would probably justify asking the patient to undergo the test.

Section 3. A firefighter in his 50s with chest pain

In sections 1 and 2, we obtain the necessary values for our formula. First we try to determine the probability that the patient has the disease, given a negative test result, or the negative predictive value of the test. To do that we use a combination of the following elements:

The probability that he does have the disease [P(D)], which, given the strength of his risk factors, we could set rather high, like at .90 (or 90% probability).

The probability of a negative test result given the disease, or the false–negative rate, which in this case is 1 − the sensitivity or .40

The probability that we think the patient does not have the disease, which is 1 − the probability that he does, or .10.

The specificity of the test, which we know to be .91.

Putting those numbers in our formula we get the following expression:

$$p(D|-) = \frac{p(D) \times p(-|D)}{\{p(D) \times p(-|D)\} + \{p(\sim D) \times p(-|\sim D)\}}$$
$$= \frac{.9 \times .4}{(.9 \times .4) + (.1 \times .91)}$$
$$= .798$$

We see from that illustrative analysis that our physician's intuition was correct. Going through the formalities of probabilistic reasoning tells us that, for a patient whom we are so sure has a diagnosis of coronary artery disease that we can assign a probability of 90%, a negative stress ECG result only reduces our probability for that diagnosis to just under 80%. In fact, for this patient we probably did not need the stress test to establish the diagnosis.

Osteopathic Considerations in Family Practice and Primary Care

INTRODUCTION

Richard L. Van Buskirk

Recently the public has become much more outspoken about its expectations for medical care. People demand that physicians treat them as individuals rather than as examples of diseases. Increasingly, people want physicians and other health care providers to pay attention to economic, social, and cultural factors when developing treatment plans. Patients prefer doctors who comfortably deal with personal and emotional concerns. Most prefer a physician with a healing touch; that is, one who is willing to use diagnostic and therapeutic touch as a part of diagnosis and treatment. Many transfer to other doctors in the hope of finding such a personal approach. Many insurers are including patient satisfaction as a significant quality-of-care criterion.[1] The osteopathic primary care physician is in an optimal position in these conditions. What are some of the defining characteristics of osteopathic primary care physicians that suit them so well for these complex roles?

DEFINING OSTEOPATHIC MEDICINE AND PRIMARY CARE

Osteopathic medicine is socially defined in three significant ways:

1. In the 19th century context in which the profession was founded
2. In a late 20th century biopsychosocial perspective that reinterprets the osteopathic philosophy in light of current knowledge
3. In terms of the integration of palpatory diagnosis and manipulative treatment into many aspects of diagnosis and case management

Osteopathic principles have been outlined in several ways. One of the more concise definitions is the 1953 Kirksville statement.[2] It consists of four statements:

"1. The body functions as a whole. It is regulated, coordinated, and integrated through multiple interactive biological and social systems.

2. The body is inherently self-regulating and self-healing. Responses to internal and external events are always modulated through feedback mechanisms. Equilibrium is a major function.

3. Structure and function are interrelated. They are inseparably linked at all levels.

4. Rational treatment is based on an understanding of body unity, self-regulatory mechanisms, and the interrelationships of structure and function. This principle unites the first three and is the basis for use of structural diagnosis and osteopathic manipulative treatment." (See also Chapter 1, Osteopathic Philosophy.)

From this perspective, osteopathic primary care has developed with the following defining characteristics. First, it is an approach that views the patient as a unique, integrated individual, united in mind, body, and spirit. Second, there is an orientation toward preventive medicine and health maintenance, as well as the diagnosis and treatment of disease. Third, osteopathy applies a view that the source of healing comes from within the patient, rather than from the physician and other external factors. Fourth, the osteopathic physician uses all rational diagnostic and treatment methods, including palpatory diagnosis and manipulative treatment. Each of these characteristics has a number of ramifications.

The integrated nature of body, mind, and spirit was emphasized by A.T. Still.[3-4] Sometimes called holism, the concept is one of the organizing themes of osteopathic philosophy. The idea implies that no organ or organ system exists in isolation. Disease, an unnatural state, always involves the whole body, rather than an isolated part; a normally well-integrated and balanced body-mind-spirit system has become dysfunctional. Generally, when a fundamentally healthy organism is confronted with disease, it heals itself, if given the opportunity.

OSTEOPATHIC PRIMARY CARE, HEALTH, AND DISEASE

For the osteopathic primary care physician, understanding the nature of health and disease requires a thorough knowledge of each patient's context, including factors such as:

Anatomic
Physiologic
Biochemical
Genetic
Psychological
Social
Cultural
Economic

Additional factors affecting health and disease include the stages of growth, development, maturation, and aging.

For example, a heart rate seen as normal in a child can signal a pathologic condition in an adult (see Chapter 15, Life Phases and Health). Prescribing medications calls on this general knowledge. For example, quinolone antibiotics cannot be used by children but are safe for adults. Others are safe for middle-aged adults but can be unsafe for the elderly.

Physiologic, biochemical, immunologic, and behavioral cyclic changes commonly influence both diagnosis and treatment recommendations. For example, blood sugar, digestive, and menstrual variations often affect drug dosing and spacing.

Psychosocial Factors and Compliance

The primary care physician often deals with deeply psychological problems, whether in the form of personality disorders, substance abuse, anxiety and depression, or the disruptive and stressful effects of personal, family, and job-related factors. The effects of such psychological variables on health and disease is significant for understanding a patient's willingness to comply with recommendations (see Chapter 14, Health Maintenance).

Even a patient's decision to seek help for a specific problem is always an open question. Common examples that often require careful psychosocial as well as physical assessment are headache, menstrual discomfort, and back pain, each of which is strongly influenced by one's basic personality and perceptions of disability and suffering. Some estimates suggest that as many as 60% of a symptomatic population for any of many diagnosable diseases, such as migraine and back pain, never see a physician for the complaint.[5]

Economic variables also play a large role in diagnostic and treatment processes. Income level and education, for example, are positively correlated with health. Just as importantly, disease manifestations are affected by the same issues. For example, clinical manifestations of migraine, diabetes, and hypertension can look different in a migrant worker and in a college professor.

Cultural, social, and insurance coverage factors significantly influence health care seeking. Those patients with low income, minimal insurance coverage, and lower socioeconomic status are discouraged from seeking health and medical care. In other situations, such as when workers' compensation and auto insurance accident coverages are available, more medical care is sought, some necessary, some not so necessary. Higher rates of utilization have regularly been associated with full-range insurance benefits. The ability to pay for prescription drugs and other treatments is affected by the same concerns.

Finally, the personality of the physician significantly affects the doctor–patient relationship. The importance of this element cannot be overemphasized. Patients often seek physicians for unconscious reasons, and vice versa; sometimes the interactions work, sometimes not. A well-versed osteopathic physician is continuously alert to the importance of this issue.

Health

Health is a dynamic equilibrium in which the body, mind, and spirit routinely restore balance in the face of various challenges. A corollary suggests that healing and health in their broadest senses are natural states. As individuals we are fundamentally healthy, rather than intrinsically unstable and subject to the depredations of disease. Intrinsic to the osteopathic philosophy and to osteopathic primary care is the concept that healing originates within the patient. Health is not a fixed state but a dynamically positive interaction with all aspects of one's life and circumstances. Criteria for a healthy life include:

1. Adequate food, shelter, education, and income
2. Adequate rest and exercise
3. Adequate physical strength and endurance
4. A mechanically balanced and flexible neuromusculoskeletal system
5. An ability to successfully maintain functional social and interpersonal relationships
6. Freedom from or healthy control of mental impairments and illnesses
7. Emotional and spiritual stability
8. Healthy coping strategies that withstand psychosocial, interpersonal, and biologic stresses
9. Healthy immune responses to biologic and psychosocial challenges
10. Healthy compensations for long-term genetic, mental, physical, emotional, and disease-related handicaps

An osteopathic focus on health starts with an understanding of its nature. Healthy individuals are hardy; they should be able to successfully resist the physical, biologic, psychological, and social challenges of daily living. They should be physically and mentally flexible, as well as adequately nourished and not overburdened by diseases and physical or mental handicaps.

Disease and Body-Mind-Spirit Triad

Most patients, some with diseases and many without, complain of problems relating to the body, mind, and spirit. Because of these issues, primary care physicians are commonly confronted with physical complaints associated with stressful life circumstances. Anxiety, depression, and somatoform complaints are particularly common (see Chapters 11, 12, 13, and 17). In many cases, symptom reports are associated with real physical changes, such as palpable muscle tension, blood pressure and blood sugar changes, or susceptibility to infections.

When treating diseases aggravated by preexisting stress-related factors, in which these factors are overlooked, symptom control and cure can lead to new symptom formation and reports, including physiologic changes in other organ systems. Multisystem somatoform disorders, fatigue, and pain reports are frequent examples. In most cases, the primary care physician can help the patient understand these naturally occurring body-mind-spirit checks and balances. A knowledgeable osteopathically oriented treatment program uses whatever means are appropriate to help the patient regain health, even when initial coping strategies are inadequate.

Under these circumstances, it is important that the osteopathic primary care physician maintain an insightful perspective when diagnosing and treating both functional disturbances and disease states. For example, most patients with chronic diseases, such as diabetes mellitus, hypertension, heart disease, and cancer, continue to function well most of the time, even when normal homeostatic balances are temporarily disturbed. Conversely, a disease or affliction, such as chronic pain and fatigue, can cause multiple complaints of anxiety and depression.

For the healthy patient, cure, control, or psychological acceptance of underlying medical and health problems often relieves anxiety and depression, and improves coping abilities. The net result of decreasing symptoms then leads to fewer physician contacts.

Examples of successful coping by intrinsic health-restoring homeostatic mechanisms are seen in many situations, such as adaptive immune system responses to microbial challenges, the maintenance of mental and psychological health under stress, and the tendency of the neuromuscu-loskeletal system to revert to normal when stress is relieved.

Treatment Strategies

In a general sense, osteopathic treatment involves using whatever means are appropriate to help the patient regain physical, mental, psychological, and spiritual health. Many methods are available, but palpatory diagnosis and manipulative treatment are readily available to every osteopathic primary care clinician. Other interventions can include:

Individualized or supervised exercise programs
Nutrition education
Individual and family counseling
Prescription or over-the-counter drugs
Surgery

Generally, the treatment goals are to restore and maximize function while minimizing disability and side effects of treatment.

Managed Care

The rapidly changing American health care delivery system has singled out primary care physicians as gatekeepers for most medical problems.[1] Under this concept, the primary care physician is explicitly expected to render the majority of diagnoses and treatments, including diagnostic and treatment procedures in many instances. Specialist referrals are made when available diagnostic and treatment options are outside the primary care physician's knowledge and skills.

As a rule, the primary care doctor signs a contract for services that requires her or him to maintain administrative control of all aspects of diagnosis and treatment, including referral specialty care. Because of her or his osteopathic whole-person orientation, managed care concepts present special opportunities for osteopathic primary care physicians.

CONCLUSION

The osteopathic primary care physician is well-suited to attend to patients as individuals and as members of social networks. He or she uses a personal, healing touch and pays attention to the economic, social, and cultural factors affecting patients' health, which meets the expectations of the public and leads to patient satisfaction.

REFERENCES

1. Alper PR. Primary care in transition. *JAMA*. 1995;272:1523–1527.

2. The osteopathic concept: an interpretation. *JAOA*. 1953;60:7–10.

3. Still AT. *The Philosophy and Mechanical Principles of Osteopathy*. Kansas City, Mo: Hudson-Kimberly Publishing Co; 1902.

4. Still AT. *Autobiography of Andrew Taylor Still*. Kirksville, Mo: AT Still; 1908.

5. Bergh KD, Asp DS, Calhaue-Pera KA. Sociocultural influences on medicine and health. In: Rakel RE, ed. *Textbook of Family Practice*. 4th ed. Philadelphia, Penn: WB Saunders; 1990:285–296.

19. Family Practice

RICHARD L. VAN BUSKIRK AND DAVID A. PLUNDO

Key Concepts

- **Foundations of osteopathic family practice**
- **Interdependent elements of illness, presentation of problems, and acceptability of diagnosis and treatment plan**
- **Integration of generalists' and specialists' skills**
- **Importance of psychoneuroimmunologic factors in disease**
- **Palpatory diagnosis and treatment in family practice**
- **Psychosocial considerations**

This chapter examines osteopathic family practice in a context that applies osteopathic philosophy and its principles. Osteopathic family physicians practice in many settings:

As solo practitioners
With one or two partners
In large health care systems such as the Kaiser-Permanente Health System
In all branches of the American military
In industrial, school, and sports medicine settings

American osteopathic family physician education and training programs are accredited by the American Osteopathic Association (AOA) and the American College of Osteopathic Family Physicians. The latter is the largest affiliated organization of the AOA and represents the majority of American osteopathic physicians.

FOUNDATIONS OF OSTEOPATHIC FAMILY PRACTICE

General practice, more recently called family practice, has been a fundamental part of American osteopathic medicine for more than 100 years. Rendering medical and health care for all segments of the population is its hallmark. Many central family practice concepts arise from osteopathic philosophy, contained in the 1953 Kirksville statement laying out its four basic principles[1] (see Chapter 1, Osteopathic Philosophy, and Section VI Introduction).

The philosophy states that all of us exist in a complex psy-

chosocial, biologic, and environmental matrix.[2-3] Within this matrix we function, maintain health, become ill, and cope with diseases. The osteopathic physician considers an array of factors affecting patient reports of illness and disease. Examples include:

Genetics
Biochemistry
Physiology
Anatomy
Environment
Sociocultural factors
Economic factors
Family
Job-related factors

All osteopathic physicians are taught to recognize and emphasize the importance of body unity in health and disease. Multiple family practice-related corollaries spring from this concept.

First, all diseases affect multiple organs and body systems. For example, a common sore throat creates both local and generalized body pain and malaise through nociceptive activation and generally altered neural activities. Inflammation arises from proinflammatory biochemistry with altered macrophage-lymphocyte/monocyte responses. Fever develops from altered temperature control mechanisms. Fatigue and loss of appetite are mediated through altered glucose-insulin, glucocorticoid, and tumor necrosis factor activities.

Second, there is general neuromusculoskeletal involvement in virtually all disease processes. This is the basis for osteopathically oriented palpatory diagnosis and manipulative treatment.

Third, the diffuse nature of illness and disease manifestations requires identifying and understanding ultimate causes rather than treating symptoms only.

Basic osteopathic preclinical and clinical education teaches all osteopathic physicians to consider psychological, social, familial, economic, environmental, and cultural contexts.[2-3] These complex but always interdependent elements affect:

The nature of an illness and its consequences
How and when problems are presented for health care in general
Whether a diagnosis is acceptable to the patient
Whether the proposed treatment plan is acceptable
Whether the treatment plan will be followed, i.e., a failure to assess and prescribe from such a complex viewpoint can slow down or even prevent recovery and restoration of health.[2-6]

Case Study

M.H. is a 17-year-old female who comes to the clinic with her mother, who is also a patient. Her last visit was six weeks ago. According to her mother, M.H.'s asthma is getting worse. Albuterol nebulizer use has increased to 10 times a day without relief. With the increase, symptoms of anxiety appeared, along with tachycardia and muscle tremors. After her last visit, she lost her prescription for a steroid inhaler and steroid nasal spray. Allergic rhinitis was an aggravating factor, as were obesity and gastroesophageal reflux. She had not followed instructions for controlling the reflux, nor had she tried to lose weight.

During the visit, M.H. rarely spoke, and then gave only short answers. Her mother carried most of the discussion, insisting that RAS (radioallergosorbent) testing be done to identify food sensitivities that she believed were the cause of her daughter's asthma. Neither mother nor daughter had kept a food log, as requested.

Because of continuing family contact, the family physician is aware that the mother, who is also asthmatic, has recently gone through a bitterly contested divorce, and M.H.'s two brothers had had some recent behavioral problems. There are financial problems, but the family is managing; the failure to obtain the prescribed medications is not financial because the family has insurance coverage.

PHYSICAL EXAMINATION

M.H.'s physical examination reveals the following:

Temperature: 99.2° F
Pulse: 92 and regular
Respirations: 20/min
Height: 66″
Weight: 192 lbs.
Blood pressure: 124/76

The nasal mucosa is pale and boggy with a bluish cast. Clear mucus is noted both in the nose and oropharynx. The lungs demonstrate mild bibasilar rhonchi with a prolonged expiratory phase. Palpatory examination of the neuromusculoskeletal system demonstrates general skeletal and myofascial involvement of the cervical and thoracic spine, diaphragm, and costal cage.

DISCUSSION

This case demonstrates a number of complex but interdependent physical and psychosocial elements. They are:

Failure to follow treatment recommendations
"Losing" prescriptions
High levels of family stress and dysfunction
Personality problems relating to self-worth and self-esteem

All of the elements influence not only the patient's health but also the physician's ability to recommend and assure compliance with an appropriate treatment plan. In this case, knowing and working with the family and its dysfunctional, stress-related problems can potentially help M.H. improve treatment compliance.

BASICS OF PRACTICE

The osteopathic profession has always had a strong preference for general practice. Some of the preference is personal, i.e., general practice-oriented students self-select into the profession. Some of this generalist orientation is also historical and cultural. These latter factors are discussed in Chapter 2, Major Events in Osteopathic History.

Nonetheless, American osteopathic medicine has always included strong roles for the medical specialties. This evolution has both personal preference and historical and cultural elements. From the outset, A.T. Still and his colleagues acknowledged the importance of safe surgical and obstetric practices carried out in a context that applies osteopathic philosophy and principles.

Osteopathic medicine has always used the interdependent knowledge and skills of generalists and specialists working together: the generalist with broadly developed skills in many different disciplines and the specialist with substantial in-depth knowledge and skills in more narrowly defined areas. The specialist can be likened to a master instrumentalist—perhaps even a soloist with great virtuosity—in the orchestra of health care. Conversely, the general practitioner/family physician-primary care provider is like a composer and conductor. His or her role is to artistically coordinate and direct the orchestra's performance, melding individual instrumental offerings into a single complex but unified production. In this analogy, the composer and conductor are not necessarily masters of every instrument in the orchestra. Instead, they know enough about each to weave richly complex sound forms and themes. The specialists (the instrumentalists) help the generalists (the composer and conductor) create the music.

Many other factors contrast primary care with specialty care. For the most part, the former implies the presence of personal accessibility, availability for a variety of medical and biopsychosocial problems, and willingness to coordinate most aspects of continuing personal and family-related medical and health care.[1,7]

In general, the primary care physician is more available, both in ease of access and in doctor–patient communication. For example, the family physician's communication style is more apt to be on a level that the patient can understand; i.e., the doctor is an interpreter of complex information in common terms.

A second area of emphasis in osteopathic family practice is continuity of care. Ongoing, long-term acquaintance with patients and family members, often across several generations, is the rule rather than the exception. In a literal sense, the physician becomes part of the extended family. This often includes an intimate knowledge of biopsychosocial and medical problems triggered by problems inside the family and its immediate environment. The physician deals not only with specific disease episodes but also with chronic illnesses often lasting years and decades.

Once established with a trusted family physician, patients tend to turn to that physician for most medical and health maintenance problems. Specialty care is sought when problems are beyond the generalist's knowledge and skill, or when patient satisfaction is an issue requiring consultation and clarification.

A fundamental commitment for the osteopathic family physician is to help patients and families maintain and restore health. This concept builds on the notion that the body is intrinsically capable of self-healing.[2,4-6,8-9] From this frame of reference, the physician provides a context for healing and health restoration, while the patient gets well according to his or her ability to adapt.

OTHER OSTEOPATHIC PERSPECTIVES

Other osteopathic perspectives are at the core of osteopathic family practice. Among the most important is the concept that diseases occur when individuals are vulnerable; i.e., disease is not a natural physical state.[4-6,8-9] A current interpretation of this aphorism comes from the emerging field of psychoneuroimmunology: diseases occur when there is an intersection of multiple stresses.[10] The body might be able to handle any single stressor in isolation, but when they accumulate, trouble often follows. Examples of factors influencing and producing stress are:

Age
Intelligence and educational background
Genetic vulnerability
Psychosocial and economic stresses
Coping style and hardiness
Previous experience with individual stresses
Unhealthy habits, including lack of seat belt and helmet use, smoking, drugs, and alcohol
Environmental toxins
Chronic organ-related dysfunctions, such as the neuromusculoskeletal and joint-related problems of special interest to osteopathically trained physicians
Specific diseases such as diabetes, hypertension, and cancer

In the osteopathic model, the normal, balanced, and integrated human organism can generally avoid infection, even though the body is colonized with pathogenic organisms. It can also both avoid and rapidly recuperate from most diseases, provided a healthy environment is maintained and stressors are controlled in a context of structural integrity and balance.[5-6]

Still another osteopathic concept suggests that any illness or disease inevitably affects the whole organism; i.e., unified functions of the mind, body, and spirit are modified and called on to adapt.[4-6] In medical school, physicians are often taught in such a way that individual organs and body systems seem to function as discrete entities. This teaching strategy makes it easier to communicate fact-based concepts and ideas. Its weakness, however, is in the lack of explicitly stated systems integration, which is left to the individual to figure out on her or his own. Ideally, general osteopathic education is at its best when it emphasizes integrative thinking and problem solving by highlighting the importance of interdependent structure and function concepts.

Case Study

An example of the complexity is represented by M.S., a 52-year-old hypertensive diabetic female with mild peripheral neuropathy. She also has mild hyperlipidemia, a hiatal hernia with gastroesophageal reflux, and multiple myeloma that has been in remission for the past 6 months. Because of her medical problems, she is on medical disability. She lives with her husband, a retired coal miner, and their 12-year-old daughter.

As the physician began an interim history and general physical assessment, the patient casually reported some intermittent left chest pain in the past 2 weeks. The pain involved her left shoulder and neck, and occurred with exertion and also at rest. There was no report of diaphoresis or shortness of breath. Fourteen months ago, prior to her cancer chemotherapy, she had a complete cardiac evaluation, including a thallium stress test. No heart disease was diagnosed, but it was noted that she had many risk factors.

On this day, her laboratory reports were generally within normal limits. Blood pressure was 142/87, pulse was 80/min and regular, respirations were 18/min, and temperature was 98.4° F.

Medications included an angiotensin-converting enzyme (ACE) inhibitor, a low dose sulfonylurea, intermediate-acting subcutaneous insulin once daily, omeprazole, gemfibrozil, and one pediatric aspirin daily.

Heart rate and rhythm were regular, and a previously known 2/6 systolic ejection murmur was noted over the apex. Her lungs were clear on auscultation. A mildly tender, obese abdomen showed no evidence of masses or hernia, and bowel sounds were normal. There was no guarding or rebound pain. A myelocytoma-related sternotomy scar was noted along with tenderness over multiple costochondral junctions anteriorly on the left. Palpation along the scar partially reproduced her previous pain.

Further palpatory examination identified segmental somatic dysfunction involving her cervical and thoracic spine, and also involving the left first, third, and fifth ribs. There was also palpable evidence of bilateral tissue texture changes in a barlike pattern at T4 and T8. Beal et al. have demonstrated that such changes often correlate with cardiac and esophageal/gastric abnormalities.[11-12] They observed that the findings can be used diagnostically when trying to separate cardiac and upper gastrointestinal dysfunctions on a viscerosomatic reflex basis.

An electrocardiogram demonstrated Q wave changes in leads 2, 3, and aVF. These were not present on her most recent ECG and suggested an interim inferior wall myocardial infarction. No ischemic changes were noted.

DISCUSSION

Clearly, M.S. has multiple potential sources for her complaints of chest pain. Unstable angina is an immediate concern, so immediate hospitalization is indicated. Because there is no chest pain at the moment, osteopathic manipulative treatment

(OMT) can be safely performed before admission. This will help in two ways. First, it can remove a potential neuromusculoskeletal source of chest pain. Second, it can remove a source of hyperactive somatovisceral reflexes (see chapters 5, 8, 9, 42, 66, 67). Other potential sources of her chest pain include esophagitis and reactivation of multiple myeloma.

As in any case management, a thorough knowledge of the patient's history is imperative. From an osteopathic perspective, a detailed knowledge of both the normal and abnormal is the key to clinical understanding and effective treatment.

OSTEOPATHIC DIAGNOSIS AND TREATMENT OF DISEASES

Although thorough knowledge is always ideal, it is rare that all details become known. Therefore, both diagnosis and treatment plans are sometimes imperfect. Knowing this, one must constantly be alert for any elements interfering with recovery. Because of such imperfections, experienced family physicians often use multiple strategies. Osteopathic family physicians have a special advantage when using palpatory diagnosis and manipulative treatment.[2,5]

Role of Palpatory Diagnosis and Manipulative Care

A basic osteopathic principle states that the neuromusculoskeletal system is functionally and inextricably linked with all body systems. A corollary of this idea implies that both health and disease inevitably involve musculoskeletal functioning.

More specifically, diseases are often the result of structural disorders relating to both the viscera and the somatic system.[4-6] In late 20th-century terms, there is close interweaving of visceral, autonomic, neural, immunologic, and musculoskeletal systems (see chapters 9 and 12). Perturbations in the immune system, for example, create effects at some level in all other body systems, and vice versa.[10-13] From this perspective comes the notion that manipulative treatment assists recovery from disease.[1,4-6,8-9] Some outcome studies have demonstrated differences in recovery rates from disease, but much work remains to scientifically confirm this osteopathic clinical experience with OMT. At a minimum, OMT is empirically useful in decreasing sources of neuromuscular and autonomic stress in an effort to improve the body's immune responses.

Having noted this clinical reality, it is also well-established that musculoskeletal dysfunction at some level is the rule, rather than the exception, even in the healthy population. Korr and his colleagues first demonstrated this in their published work with the sympathetic nervous system shortly after World War II.[13] Even though neuromusculoskeletal complaints might not be mentioned in the history, knowledgeable palpatory examination commonly identifies tender and painful sites associated with classically defined somatic dysfunction. Because such findings are so common, their origins and significance often require careful thought. It is common to have patients present with viscerally related clinical findings and associated asymptomatic sites of somatic dysfunction. It is reasonable to suppose that similar asymptomatic somatic dysfunction sites exist in the general population without clinical signs or symptoms. For such a group, one assumes that the somatic dysfunction represents either a potential disease trigger or a signal that latent or subclinical disease or impairment is present.

Osteopathic Manipulative Treatment in the Family Practice Setting

In some cases, manipulative treatment is sufficient for recovery and contraindications are few. Formal outcome studies supporting its use in other than neuromusculoskeletal disorders are sparse.[4-6,9,14-17]

Palpatory diagnosis and manipulative treatments of all types are fundamentally safe, and there are few reasons to avoid their use (see Chapter 73, Efficacy and Complications). Patient refusal tops the list of circumstances under which manipulation should be avoided. If the clinician's manipulative skills are inadequate for the complexity of the particular case, it might be appropriate to refer the patient to an osteopathic manipulative specialist, if one is available, just as one would do in other clinical situations where one's skills or knowledge are limited. Relative contraindications for thrusting (manipulation with impulse) maneuvers are:

Acute fractures or risk for fracture
Osteoporosis
Vertebral and carotid artery stenosis
Unstable spinal mechanisms
Acute torsional cervical trauma
Metastatic cancers

On the other hand, use of nonthrusting techniques are generally safe, when properly used, for many of the above problems (see Chapter 41, Part A; chapters 53, 54, 56–64, and 68). Many osteopathic techniques are soft and subtle in both their applications and whole body effects.

Culture is another consideration. The universal American exposure to modern medical and surgical diagnosis and treatment implicitly minimizes the roles for other forms of treatment, including osteopathic manipulative care for problems other than back pain. Limiting the role of osteopathic manipulative approaches in this fashion often unwittingly ignores a potentially powerful intervention. For example, many studies highlight probable efficacy in a number of rheumatologic, pulmonary, and cardiovascular problems (see Chapter 73, Efficacy and Complications).

Pharmacotherapeutics in Osteopathic Practice

Early in its history, osteopathic practices minimized the use of drugs. The reasons were obvious in that many were poisonous and often caused harm. At that time, most available treatments consisted of toxic, ineffective, or addictive chemical compounds, such as calomel, morphine, and laudanum. To his credit, A.T. Still found these repugnant.[5]

During the first 20 years of the 20th century, this parsimonious attitude among osteopathic practitioners toward pharmacotherapeutics shifted (see Chapter 2, Major Events in Osteopathic History). Osteopathic hospitals were springing up, and medical care in general was rapidly changing. By the middle 1920s, pharmacology courses were included in virtually all osteopathic curricula. In fact, the students at the Chicago College of Osteopathy staged a strike when the faculty vetoed its teaching in the middle 1920s.[18] Ultimately, the students prevailed, and the die was firmly cast for current, broadly practiced osteopathic pharmacology. Concurrently, important research and treatment breakthroughs radically changed management strategies for all types of diseases. World War II, the control of infections with antibiotics, and major advances in surgery and wound care were slightly more than a decade ahead.

Through all this, A.T. Still's students advocated health enhancement and restoration concepts that focused on correction of physical and structural abnormalities, as well as on environmental and psychosocial factors. If surgery was needed, it should be done.[4–6,8–9] Nevertheless, Still never changed his mind about the negative effects of medications. One major reason for the continuation of this point of view on the part of osteopathic physicians was the generally successful use of manipulative care during the worldwide flu pandemic of 1918[19] (see Chapter 2, Major Events in Osteopathic History).

During the last 60 years of the 20th century, osteopathic physicians have enthusiastically embraced the breadth and depth of all phases of the medical sciences. Today, medications and therapeutic protocols of all types are integral and valued elements of American osteopathic care.

Office Diagnosis and Treatment Procedures

Late 20th century practices have moved many surgical and diagnostic procedures away from the inpatient and toward the outpatient setting. Osteopathic family physicians generally include a variety of surgical and other office-based procedures in their practices. Common office gynecologic, obstetric, and gastrointestinal diagnostic procedures, including colonoscopy, biopsies, and even colposcopy, are performed by qualified physicians. Some might restrict themselves to procedures such as:

Simple excisional and incisional procedures
Arthrocentesis
Joint injections
Local nerve blocks
Uncomplicated casting

Others, particularly those in remote rural practices, are required to be proficient in more advanced procedures such as advanced cardiac life support and, on occasion, cesarean section.

DISEASE MANAGEMENT AND HEALTH RESTORATION

Five elements are the hallmarks of any treatment plan:

1. Symptom relief
2. Removal of offending organisms to the extent possible
3. Surgical removal of diseased parts when necessary
4. Replacement of substances no longer produced or absorbed

5. Restoration of emotional and psychosocial stability to the extent possible

The osteopathic physician's role is not only to recommend and perform appropriate interventions but also to proactively minimize negative side effects and complications by carefully weighing risks and benefits.

In many cases, there are relatively noninvasive interventions, such as:

Osteopathic manipulative care
Short-term use of medications
Lifestyle modifications
Avoidance of toxic environmental factors, such as smoking, alcohol, and abusive family and work relationships

PSYCHOSOCIAL CONSIDERATIONS

Traditional basic and clinical science education emphasizes the physiologic, biochemical, and genetic bases for health and disease. Modern osteopathic family practice also incorporates explicit psychosocial and cultural influences.[2] Some aspects are obvious, such as the interactive effects of personalities and interpersonal skills among physicians and patients. For example, the ability of patients to understand physician explanations and discussions depends on a variety of often subtle communication and individual personal styles (see Chapter 18, Clinical Problem Solving, and Section IV).

However, the seemingly simple decision to seek primary health care is often complicated by marginally understood individual, family, and work-related elements. These highly personal decisions can lead to such issues as overutilization and reluctance to accept treatment recommendations, resulting in lost wages and an increase in insurance, prescription, and physician costs.[3]

Family practitioners have long known that patient complaints often have origins in undiagnosed personality disorders, stress, dysfunctional family and work environments, and economic problems. For example, chronic head and neck pains often signal combinations of:

Family and interpersonal stress
Hormonal imbalances
Depression
Job-related ergonomic problems
Economic or interpersonal secondary gain
True migraine
Mechanical neck problems with somatic dysfunction
Intracranial vascular anomalies
Meningeal problems
Brain tumors
Impending strokes
Undiagnosed closed head injuries

Determining which of these many factors might be causing the presenting problem is a universal challenge for all physicians who deal with headaches. Emphasis on purely physical causes while ignoring those stemming from poor coping strategies commonly slows recovery.

FAMILY PRACTITIONER AS GATEKEEPER

As American health care delivery shifts toward increasing third-party insurance payment and managed care controls, primary care physicians are being asked to accept so-called "gatekeeper" roles.[7] The gatekeeper role revolves around the concept that the family practitioner or other primary care provider is in charge of diagnosing, managing, and directing the health care of patient panels. Responsibilities involve routine care for most medical and health problems in all age groups. When necessary, referral to appropriate specialists under contract with the same insurance carrier are approved on a case-by-case basis. A general gatekeeper goal is to provide quality medical and health care in the most cost-effective manner possible.[7]

Family practitioners are uniquely suited for these tasks because they routinely deal with all age groups and are most likely to treat whole families. The family practitioner is able to diagnose diseases and implement treatment strategies for a wide range of family-related problems and individual disease-related circumstances, generally without specialty referrals.[2–3]

Some argue that the family practitioner's knowledge and skills are less focused and of lower quality than those of comparable specialists. Recent outcome data from two hospital-based studies compared generalist versus specialist case outcome data. Each concluded that outcomes are virtually the same, and generalist care is often more cost-effective.[17,19–20] Some of this cost efficiency occurs because more care takes place in outpatient settings, with less use of high technology.

Another family practice advantage occurs when the generalist coordinates overall care: there is less transferring from one specialist to another when diagnosis and treatment are unclear. Of course, complex medical care, such as complicated cancer and AIDS management, might well require the services of several specialists. In general, however, specialist utilization and costs are lower where the gatekeeper model is employed.[7] As the population ages, whether this cost-saving differential continues remains to be seen. At the time of this writing, business and insurance considerations were extremely high profile.

Finally, even though economic factors are legitimate concerns for any physician, the ultimate focus must be on patients and their families. From an osteopathic viewpoint, the most effective version of the gatekeeper role occurs when the primary care physician can act as an:

Ombudsman
Advocate
Healer
Counselor
Patient educator

PREVENTIVE MEDICINE AND HEALTH MAINTENANCE

Osteopathic family practitioners emphasize preventive medicine and health maintenance.[2–3,21] This is in accordance with several points in the osteopathic philosophy, one of which states that diseases are mere effects; i.e., they reflect the body's failure to maintain normal compensatory mechanisms, both internally and in the environment.[5] Therefore, diseases are generally preventable, and it is an osteopathic physician's fundamental role to help patients understand and implement healthy lifestyles.

For instance, bacterial pneumonia rarely occurs because of simple exposure to an offending organism. The real cause is the immune system's failure to successfully respond. Preexisting problems can contribute to the immune failure, such as:

Smoking
Alcohol abuse
Drug abuse
Stress
Occupational exposure to air pollutants
Genetic susceptibility
Concurrent disease processes such as diabetes and cancer
Long-term neuromusculoskeletal stresses, often represented by somatic dysfunctions

Similarly, some cancers are best understood as the immunologic escape of genetically aberrant immortal cells.[22] Genetic alterations can result from a wide variety of environmental insults or inborn replication errors, or they can be spontaneous. Regardless, it is the failure of the immune system to destroy the aberrant cells that results in the cancer.

It is helpful to remember that, initially, all diseases and dysfunctions fall into four classes: immunologic, anatomic, genetic, and lifestyle. Immunologic dysfunctions are discussed in Section III. Anatomic dysfunctions and/or trauma, including sprains, strains, fractures, amputations, and organ death from traumatic ischemia, account for many family practice visits. Genetic problems are becoming increasingly high profile, as are lifestyle and self-defeating culturally based and biopsychosocially influenced behaviors. In all classes, there are multiple possibilities for long-range ameliorative and preventive/health maintenance interventions. It is in these contexts that osteopathic family practitioners can be particularly effective.[2,20]

CONCLUSION

This chapter examines the nature of late 20th century osteopathic family practice. Osteopathic family practitioners are uniquely able to deal with a wide spectrum of health and disease-related problems, including biologic, social, economic, and cultural influences. The emphasis is on resource mobilization, including medical and surgical care, osteopathic manipulative care, psychosocial and general family care. The role of the family physician in helping individuals and families maintain health while treating diseases is particularly important. Through appreciation for the osteopathic philosophy and its principles, the osteopathic physician is able to handle family physician tasks, particularly those that highlight the importance of self-healing and the importance of understanding as many disease and biopsychosocial variables as possible.

REFERENCES

1. The osteopathic concept: an interpretation. *JAOA.* 1953;60:7–10.
2. Model Program for Basic Standards for Residency Training in Fam-

ily Practice. *1994–1995 Membership Directory.* Arlington Heights, Ill: American College of Osteopathic Family Physicians, ACOFP; 1994.

3. Rakel RE. *Textbook of Family Practice.* 4th ed. Philadelphia, Pa: WB Saunders Co; 1994.

4. Still AT. *Osteopathy, Research and Practice.* Seattle, Wash: Eastland Press; 1992. (Reprint from The Journal Printing Co, Kirksville, Mo; 1910).

5. Still AT. *Autobiography of AT Still.* Reprint by American Academy of Osteopathy. Indianapolis, Ind; 1981.

6. Still AT. *The Philosophy and Mechanical Principles of Osteopathy.* Reprinted by Osteopathic Enterprise. Kirksville, Mo; 1986.

7. Alper PR. Primary care in transition. *JAMA.* 1995;272:1523–1527.

8. Hazzard C. *The Practice and Applied Therapeutics of Osteopathy.* Kirksville, Mo: Journal Printing Co; 1905.

9. Hulett GD. *A Textbook of the Principles of Osteopathy.* Kirksville, Mo: Journal Printing Co.; 1906.

10. Willard FH, Patterson MM, eds. *Nociception and the Neuroendocrine-Immune Connection. 1992 International Symposium.* Athens, Ohio: University Classics, Ltd; 1994.

11. Beal MC. Viscerosomatic reflexes: a review. *JAOA.* 1985;84:53–68.

12. Beal MC, Kleiber GE. Somatic dysfunction as a predictor of coronary artery disease. *JAOA.* 1985;85:70–75.

13. Denslow JS, Korr IM, Krems AD. Quantitative studies of chronic facilitation in human motoneuron pools. *Am J Physiol.* 1947; 150:229–238.

14. Chapman F. *An Endocrine Interpretation of Chapman's Reflexes.* Indianapolis, Ind: American Academy of Osteopathy; 1956.

15. Schmidt IC. Osteopathic manipulative treatment as a primary factor in the management of upper, middle, and pararespiratory infections. *JAOA.* 1982;81:382–388.

16. Riley GW. Osteopathic success in treatment of influenza and pneumonia. *JAOA.* 1919;18:565.

17. McGann KD, Bowman MA, Davis SW. Morbidity, mortality and charges for hospital care of the elderly: a comparison of internists' and family physicians' admissions. *J Fam Pract.* 1995;40:443–448.

18. Berchtold TA. *To Teach, To Heal, To Serve: A History of the Chicago College of Osteopathic Medicine.* Chicago, Ill: University of Chicago Printing Department; 1975; 84–85.

19. Safran DG, Tarlov AR, Rogers WH. Primary care performance in fee-for-service and prepaid health care systems. *JAMA.* 1994; 271:1579–1586.

20. Greenfield S, Nelson EC, Zubkoff M, Manning W, Rodgers W, Kravitz RL, Keller A, Tarlov AR, Ware JE Jr. Variations in resource utilization among medical specialties and systems of care. *JAMA.* 1992;267:1624–1630.

21. Inwald SA, Winters FD. Emphasizing a preventative medicine orientation during primary care/family practice residency training. *JAOA.* 1995;95:267–275.

22. Skolnick A. Essential components now in place for clinical testing of cancer vaccine strategies. *JAMA.* 1995;273:528–530.

20. General Internal Medicine

REGINA C. MOROZ

Key Concepts

- **Characteristics of osteopathic internal medicine physicians**

- **Methods for diagnosis and treatment, including holistic approach**

- **Change from hospital-based consultant to provider of ambulatory care**

This chapter explores how general internal medicine is practiced with an osteopathic perspective. Osteopathically oriented general internal medicine applies broadly conceived diagnostic and treatment approaches that include the in-depth diagnosis and management of all disease processes using holistic viewpoints. Care involves applying an extensive knowledge base and skills that deal with the diagnosis and treatment of all illnesses. Integrity, personal support, sensitivity, and compassion are essential skills. For osteopathic physicians, the knowledgeable and appropriate use of palpatory diagnosis and manipulative treatment are integral parts of these processes.

The general internist is a personal physician who provides long-term comprehensive care in the office and hospital. Primary care internal medicine incorporates an understanding and treatment of substance abuse and general mental health issues, as well as diagnosis and treatment of the following common problems:

Eye
Ear, nose, and throat
Neurologic
Reproductive
Dermatologic

Disease prevention, health maintenance, and wellness education are essential elements.

All internists train in the medical subspecialties, including emergency internal medicine and critical care, and often act as consultants to other specialists.[1]

HISTORY

The American Society of Osteopathic Internists was formed in 1923–1924 and met annually with the American Osteopathic Association. The first certifying board was formed in 1942. In 1943, the name was changed to the American College of Os-

teopathic Internists. A 2-year residency program was formed in 1943 and expanded to 3 years in 1945.[1–9]

In the first constitution, the founders' purpose was clear:

Article II, Section 2: Contributors purposes of this Society shall be to stimulate and carry on accurate and scientific research work pertaining to the diagnosis and treatment of disease; to write and to compile full and complete case records for study and statistical purposes; to develop the osteopathic concept with thoroughness and to apply it to the scientific study of health and disease; and to do such other things as may harmonize with and further the primary purpose of this Society.[10]

OSTEOPATHICALLY ORIENTED INTERNAL MEDICINE

An osteopathic internist's practice emphasizes an in-depth general history, physical examination, and detailed clinical diagnosis. It includes causes of diseases of internal organs and pathologies influenced both directly and indirectly by disordered neuromusculoskeletal mechanics. These pathologies can be, and often are, a mixture of somatic, visceral, and psychological elements. An internist's practice incorporates diagnostic and therapeutic measures applicable to specific diseases but generally does not include surgery, although an internist sometimes carries out minor surgery. Palpatory diagnosis and osteopathic manipulative treatment are integral parts of these processes. Surgical cases are included because they commonly require multispecialty services.

Hospital-Based Consultants

Historically, osteopathic internists have acted as hospital-based consultants for other specialists and general practitioners. They frequently deal with difficult diagnoses and case management issues. With increasing subspecialization, there has been a corresponding decline in the population of general internists. There is intellectual stimulation in both fields, however. Many of those who stay with primary care become personal physicians for the adult population, and a new emphasis on ambulatory education has recently emerged. Managed care and corporate practice have accelerated this phenomenon.

Mentors and Community Hospitals

Osteopathically based general internist education is mentor-oriented, and it generally occurs in community hospitals. This unique educational combination fosters a holistic approach to patient care that, in many cases, includes the use of osteopathic palpatory skills and manipulative treatment in a variety of case management situations. This education and training contrasts with allopathic internal medicine residencies, which are often university-based and subspecialty-oriented.

DIAGNOSIS AND TREATMENT

The osteopathic general internist uses multiple diagnostic and treatment methods and modalities, including palpatory diagnosis and manipulative treatment when indicated. The following cases illustrate the internist's methods.

Case One

HISTORY AND PHYSICAL EXAMINATION

A 43-year-old male construction worker presents to the general internist with complaints of epigastric pain. He admits a 2-week history of black, tarry stools, and drinks two or three six-packs of beer every night. He is recently divorced.

Physical examination reveals pale conjunctivae. The blood pressure is stable at 120/70, and heart rate is 123 beats per minute. There is exquisite epigastric tenderness. Stool examination is hemoccult positive; hemoglobin is 10.7; hematocrit is 30.3.

Palpatory musculoskeletal examination demonstrates classic somatic dysfunction across the midline from T5-T11.

COURSE

When first seen, the patient had been without food by mouth (NPO) for more than 12 hours and was a good candidate for esophagogastroduodenoscopy (EGD), which revealed a 1.5-cm antral ulcer that was not actively bleeding. Duodenal erosions were also noted.

The patient was informed of the findings and agreed to a course of H_2 blocker and dietary changes, with instruction to stop drinking alcoholic beverages. Because of the viscerosomatic reflexes represented by the middle and lower thoracic somatic dysfunction, a course of osteopathic manipulative treatment was incorporated as part of the management plan. Psychosocially, arrangements were made to help him deal with his alcohol dependency and accompanying depression.

Case Two

A 55-year-old male office worker appears in the emergency room with a 1-hour history of increasing chest pressure and diaphoresis. For the past several days he has been unusually fatigued and experienced two mild incidents of similar discomfort. There is no family history of heart disease.

He was a heavy smoker until 1 year ago, and has a long history of hypertension controlled by medication. There are no significant previous illnesses, except for a duodenal ulcer 4 years ago. He has a high stress lifestyle.

Physical examination reveals an anxious, ashen, middle-aged man with a blood pressure of 150/60 and a heart rate of 92. There is no jugular venous distension, and carotid pulses are normal. Pulmonary crackles and an S4 cardiac gallop are present. Palpatory findings reveal somatic dysfunction along the left cervical spine and left upper thoracic segments. An electrocardiogram demonstrates acute ST segment elevation in V1-V4 leads. CPK-MB is elevated at 20.

The most likely diagnosis is acute anterior wall myocardial infarction. Patients with ST segment elevation within the first 4 hours of a myocardial infarction have complete occlusion of the infarct-related artery in nearly 90% of all cases.

Early treatment that acutely reperfuses the infarct site limits infarct size. Techniques include:

Intravenous thrombolytic therapy
Percutaneous transluminal angioplasty (PTCA)
Emergency coronary artery bypass grafting (CABG)

The internist performs the first two techniques. After the acute intervention, the patient is often placed on nitrates, beta blockers, and slow-acting calcium channel blockers. Some evidence suggests that osteopathic manipulative treatment can decrease arrythmia complications, shock, and mortality if promptly and appropriately performed in the intensive care unit.[10]

Some osteopathic authors[11] suggest that

all . . . myocardial infarction . . . patients would benefit from cervical and thoracic manipulative treatment designed to reduce sympathetically-associated cardiocardiac reflex . . . activities as one strategy for preventing ventricular arrhythmias. Concern also exists for those with excessive parasympathetic activity which can lead to hypertension and subsequent diminished coronary blood flow to ischemic areas of myocardium. For patients in the intensive care unit following myocardial infarction, patients with angina, or patients with other serious cardiac insults, . . . osteopathic manipulative . . . treatment is, therefore, directed at calming sympathetic hyperactivity, especially in the upper thoracic spine . . . in order . . . to reduce inappropriate cardiocardiac reflexes, lower the incidence of ectopic foci and ventricular fibrillation, and to remove at least one factor which discourages development of . . . cardiac . . . collateral circulation.

In the long term, the patient needs lifestyle changes that deal with stress factors in his life, along with continuing management of his hypertension and diet.

PREVENTIVE MEDICINE AND HEALTH MAINTENANCE

The osteopathic general internist should be attuned to the need for counseling and for practicing preventive medicine and health maintenance strategies that explore health-related behaviors that include both behavioral and disease-related elements. Areas to explore include:

Family and work relationships, including harassment and abuse
Nutritional status and dietary habits
Exercise types and frequency
Tobacco type, past and present use
Alcohol type, past and present, including abuse

Illicit drug use

Substance abuse

Seat belt use

Sexual behaviors and sexually transmitted diseases

Dental health

Periodic physical examinations and treatment follow-ups include assessments of and for:

Lifestyle factors: diet, depression, anxiety, exercise, work status and satisfaction, smoking, alcohol, effects of trauma, sexual functioning

Rheumatologic disorders

Neurologic functioning

Orthopaedic functioning

Diabetes

Hypertension

Thyroid functions

General cardiovascular status

Pulmonary functions

Genitourinary functions

Lipid disorders

Gastrointestinal functions

Pain and sleep disorders

Breast, cervical, colorectal, and prostatic cancers

Other periodic cancer screens evaluate for these diseases:

Skin

Oral

Endometrial

Testicular

Ovarian

Thyroid

Postmenopausal, neurologic, and geriatric examinations of all kinds are common to the field. Neuromusculoskeletal health is an essential element in many situations. Because of her or his familiarity with palpatory diagnosis and manipulative treat-ment, the general osteopathic internist can assess these particular factors in relation to a variety of medical presentations.

CONCLUSION

The osteopathic general internist is personal physician to adolescent, adult, and elderly patients. He or she uses extensive disease-related and general medical knowledge, coupled with holistic and behavioral approaches that, in many instances, include the use of osteopathically oriented palpatory diagnosis and manipulative treatment. The rapidly changing health care delivery system in the United States has caused the osteopathic general internist to evolve from the primary role of hospital consultant to an important provider of ambulatory care. The internist integrates diagnosis and treatment with preventive medicine and health maintenance education.

REFERENCES

1. Marquis Who's Who. *The Official American Board of Medical Specialties Directory of Certified Medical Specialists.* New Providence, NJ: A Reed Reference Publishing Co; 1995;1:38–39.

2. Robuck SV. American Society of Osteopathic Internists. *JAOA.* 1932;31:463.

3. Robuck SV. Problems of the profession. *JAOA.* January 1923; 22:280–282.

4. Robuck SV. Impressions of the New York convention. *JAOA.* August 1923;22:728–729.

5. Tasker DL. Maturity of thought. *JAOA.* July 1924;23:849.

6. Kerr CV. The American Society of Osteopathic Internists. *JAOA.* December 1925;24:295.

7. Robuck SV. Convention of the American Osteopathic Internist Association. *JAOA.* July 1928;27:879.

8. American Osteopathic Association Roster, 1942–1943. *JAOA.* September 1942;41:88–90.

9. American Society of Osteopathic Internists. *JAOA.* September 1928; 27:69.

10. The osteopathic internist. *JAOA.* February 1928;27:461. Editorial.

11. Kuchera ML, Kuchera WA. *Osteopathic Considerations in Systemic Dysfunction.* 2nd ed. Kirksville, Mo: KCOM Press, 1990:60, 83.

21. Primary Care Pediatrics

JOSEPH A. ALDRICH

Key Concepts

- **Focus and scope of pediatric practice**
- **Special needs of children**
- **Palpatory diagnosis of children**
- **Effects of labor and delivery**
- **Research on osteopathic treatment of children's developmental and medical problems**

The osteopathic primary care pediatrician's responsibility is to assist his or her patients to maintain healthy growth and development. The pediatrician also recognizes and treats deviations from health (i.e., illness and disease) while using all available and appropriate methods in the patient's best interests. The osteopathic approach to these responsibilities highlights the somatic aspects of healthy structure and function that are integral parts of osteopathic philosophy and its guiding principles (see Chapter 1, Osteopathic Philosophy).

Conventional wisdom suggests that A.T. Still and his early colleagues used osteopathic manipulative treatment to treat many children for a variety of musculoskeletal and pulmonary problems, such as asthma. They also used it to treat more severe acute and chronic diseases that had proven resistant to standard treatments of that time, such as meningitis, cholera, and pneumonia.[1] Later in his life, Still wrote that his work helped convince him of the body's self-healing abilities and the importance of further developing and refining osteopathic concepts and their applications.[2]

An osteopathic pediatrician is trained to use all available diagnostic and treatment methods, including the psychomotor skills associated with palpatory diagnosis and manipulative treatment. These skills are particularly useful when diagnosing and treating infants and children because of their limited communication skills.

Pediatrics has always been an important discipline in the osteopathic profession. At first it had a natural alliance with obstetrics and general practice. With advancements in medical care of all kinds, many early medical and osteopathic clinicians and teachers acknowledged that neonates, infants, children, and adolescents had special needs. Thus the discipline of pediatrics was born.

The role of the osteopathic primary care pediatrician is to approach the patient as a whole, including her or his family and environmental elements, rather than dealing with single complaints. Clinically, the goal is to facilitate and maintain health; that is, preventive medicine is essential. Because infants and children grow rapidly, focus includes not only general health concerns and potential lifelong pathologies but also stresses the importance of psychosocial supports and their links with neuromusculoskeletal, circulatory, and immune functioning.

SCOPE OF PEDIATRIC PRACTICE

Osteopathic primary care includes all aspects of child care, from the neonatal period to age 18, i.e., throughout early growth and development. Often there are overlapping interests with other disciplines, such as internal medicine, orthopaedics, obstetrics and gynecology, and psychiatry. Age, maturity, and psychosocial variables generally determine the appropriate courses for diagnosis and treatment.

American College of Osteopathic Pediatricians

In recognition of the special educational and practice-related needs of pediatrics, the American College of Osteopathic Pediatricians was formed in 1940.[3] Its primary goal is to meet the special needs of osteopathic physicians who provide pediatric care, assuring the maintenance of a high degree of knowledge and skill for the discipline. Within the field, there are generalists and specialists. Most osteopathically based primary care pediatrics is carried out by generalists.

Neonates, Infants, Children, and Adolescents

Neonates, infants, children, and adolescents have special health-related requirements that vary with age, life stage, and levels of physical and psychosocial development. As an individual grows from infancy through adolescence, physical and emotional needs evolve from total dependency to the often turbulent independence of adolescence and young adulthood. Primary care pediatric practitioners are called on to understand and treat an array of problems associated with these rapid changes.

Infant and early childhood growth is truly astounding, as birth weight doubles by 6 months and triples by 1 year. Birth length doubles in 4 years. Throughout, the maturing musculoskeletal and nervous systems are active participants. Developmental variations and effects of birth trauma are more common than many realize.[4]

OSTEOPATHIC APPROACH

Palpatory diagnosis is particularly useful for infants and children because it is able to identify subtle changes of tissue tone and texture as well as cranial motion activities. These special skills augment the usual observations when dealing with developmental and behavioral benchmarks.

Effects of Labor and Delivery

It has been stated that osteopathy is both a science and an art dealing with the natural forces, and *"that order and health are inseparable, and when order in all parts is found, disease cannot prevail...."*[5(p21)] Early osteopathic physicians noted common adverse prenatal, perinatal, and early infancy effects associated with the strains and stresses of pregnancy, labor, and delivery. For example, Dr. Still was adamant in his belief that forceps delivery was harmful to the infant. On one occasion, he threatened to expel a student for using them. His position was to advocate the use of manipulative treatment during pregnancy and labor and delivery to *"treat the channels commonly known as the uterine arteries."*[6(p235)] In fact, a policy of watchful expectancy during the third stage of labor was a common osteopathic practice into the 1970s (Robert C Ward, DO, FAAO, personal communication).

During infancy, the adverse effects of prenatal positional strains along with the forces of labor can alter the infant's body mechanics and state of health. Perinatal suckling and sleep problems are relatively common, along with persistent asymmetrical positioning of the unfused cranial bones after the birthing process. From an osteopathic perspective, the goal is to treat the problems and restore healthy functions, using osteopathic manipulative treatment as an integral part of the process.

Osteopathically Oriented Research

Beginning in the 1960s, osteopathic physicians started publishing observational research suggesting that cranial osteopathic manipulation helps children with a variety of developmental and medical problems. Today and in the past, a few researchers have assessed the effects of osteopathic manipulative procedures on a range of infant and childhood problems associated with the following:

Birth trauma
Colic
Recurrent otitis media
Asthma
Learning disorders

In addition, recent basic science studies have identified clear evidence of cranial rhythms that were initially reported by Sutherland and his colleagues in the 1920s.[4,7-16]

General psychosocial, nutritional, and environmental factors play important roles in the management of pediatric and adolescent growth and development. Pediatricians, particularly those in primary care, are sensitive to these issues. In more technical areas, specialties such as pediatric intensive care, surgery, anesthesia, and radiology require highly trained physi-

cians because of the dramatic variations in patient maturity, physiology, and size. Imaging procedures, for example, can be procedurally difficult because of body size and need for sedation.

CONCLUSION

Pediatrics, as much as any area of medicine, places the physician-family-patient relationship in the spotlight. Well-developed communication and education skills are always high priorities. For example, securing pertinent information and background from those who cannot or will not talk is a continuing challenge. Knowing local colloquialisms and ethnic communication norms is an essential skill. Parent education and training can run the gamut from basic skills of infant care to dealing with issues of family abuse, as well as the normal, commonly misperceived developmental and behavioral changes of adolescence. Knowing the difference between normal development and abnormal deviation is of major importance, because earlier interventions generally have better outcomes. The osteopathic philosophy and its many applications have major roles to play in those outcomes.

REFERENCES

1. Trowbridge C. *Andrew Taylor Still: 1828–1917*. Kirksville, Mo: Northeast Missouri University Press; 1991:160–161.
2. Still AT. *Osteopathy, Research and Practice*. Kirksville, Mo: AT Still; 1910:28.
3. Bomboy RP. *The Golden Anniversary History of the American College of Osteopathic Pediatricians: 1940–1990*. Haddon Craftsmen, Inc; 1990.
4. Frymann VM. Relation of disturbances of craniosacral mechanisms to symptomatology of the newborn: study of 1250 infants. *JAOA*. 1966;65:1059–1075.
5. Still AT. *Philosophy of Osteopathy*. Indianapolis, Ind: American Academy of Osteopathy; 1899:21.
6. ibid, Still AT. p. 235.
7. Frymann VM, et al. Effect of osteopathic medical management on neurologic development in children. *JAOA*. June 1992;6:729–744.
8. Degenhardt B, Kuchera ML. The prevalence of cranial dysfunction in children with a history of otitis media from kindergarten to third grade. *JAOA*. 1994;94(9):754. Abstract.
9. Degenhardt B, Kuchera ML. Efficacy of osteopathic evaluation and manipulative treatment in reducing the morbidity of otitis media in children. *JAOA*. 1994;94(9):673.
10. DiGiovanni A (consultant). Fisons learning systems: asthma and its management, including an osteopathic perspective. Special paper developed for the osteopathic profession, 1993.
11. Frymann VM. The trauma of birth. *Osteopath Ann*. 1976;4:22–31.
12. Frymann VM. Learning difficulties of children viewed in the light of the osteopathic concept. *JAOA*. 1976;76:46–61.
13. Sutherland AS, Wales AL. *Contributions of Thought: Collected Writings of William Garner Sutherland, DO*. Indianapolis, Ind: Sutherland Cranial Teaching Foundation; 1967.
14. Frymann VM. A study of the rhythmic motions of the living cranium. *JAOA*. 1971;70:1–18.
15. Retzlaff EW, Mitchell FL Jr. *The Cranium and Its Sutures*. Berlin: Springer-Verlag; 1987.
16. Tetambel M. Recording of the cranial rhythmic impulse. *JAOA*. 1978:149. Abstract.

Osteopathic Considerations in the Clinical Specialties

INTRODUCTION

Felix J. Rogers

Osteopathic medicine is a comprehensive, integrated approach to patient care. Although the traditional strength of osteopathic medicine has been in primary care medicine, osteopathic physicians now provide health care within all specialties and most subspecialties of medicine and surgery.

The chapters that follow focus on dimensions of clinical practice that characterize or elucidate aspects of osteopathic philosophy or practice. Each chapter also reviews current and past research within the osteopathic profession. In some cases, additional scientific literature is incorporated because it directly pertains to issues central to osteopathic medicine. Each chapter provides a brief overview of the field of medicine described or discusses pertinent topics within the field; none are intended to represent a comprehensive description of the discipline.

DEFINING DISTINCTIVENESS

This section has 17 chapters representative of the clinical disciplines. Many subjects are not included, especially in the subspecialty areas of medicine and surgery. The topics included were chosen as examples of the manner in which osteopathic principles have been applied to these clinical areas. Other fields of study may not be included because of a paucity of osteopathic research in that area, because the implementation of osteopathic tenets is more complex or difficult to express, or because the osteopathic approach is so similar to another field that its inclusion would be redundant.

Medicine functions as a mix of clinical experience, expert opinion, and scientific evidence. Yesterday's expert opinion is regularly overturned by today's scientific evidence. More precise scientific evidence supersedes more general scientific evidence. Sometimes scientific evidence catches up with accepted clinical practice. It would be pleasant to think that we could define as scientific what we do every day in patient care, but this is not the case.

Osteopathic medicine, as a minority profession with certain philosophic emphases, especially feels pressured to prove itself in the scientific arena. There are inherent difficulties in this endeavor, however, because of the global nature of osteopathy's philosophic emphases. It is hard to define even small, measurable hypotheses to test such tenets as structure–function interrelationships, or the full nature of viscerosomatic or somatovisceral reflexes.

At the same time, osteopathic medicine is obligated to define its distinctiveness. One aspect of our profession is that we have defining characteristics; we endeavor as a group to establish guiding principles to represent a philosophic and scientific basis for health care. The following chapters describe the extent to which these principles can be applied to the practice of medicine in the clinical specialties. Other distinctive features of the osteopathic profession include:

Characteristics of students selected for admission to medical schools
The osteopathic educational process
An emphasis on primary care, especially in underserved areas
An orientation to clinical service as opposed to research and academic growth
A reliance on the patient–physician relationship as a key element in health care

These distinctive features are addressed in other sections of this textbook.

OSTEOPATHIC MANIPULATIVE TREATMENT AND CLINICAL PRACTICE

Osteopathic specialists must consider how osteopathic manipulative treatment, a modality distinct in this profession, might fit in with current clinical practice. Several clinical outcomes and related basic science research projects have suggested how and under what conditions manipulative interventions might work, but more extensive study is needed.

Because all medical practice is based on a significant proportion of clinical experience and expert opinion, osteopathic thought and, when appropriate, manipulative treatment are included in this introductory survey of clinical specialty correlations.

The chapters in this section represent a variety of approaches to osteopathic specialty practice and are different from one another. Each represents one or more tenets of traditional osteopathic philosophy: structure–function interrelationship, self-healing, and integration of systems. Some disciplines involve more obviously musculoskeletal problems than others; in other chapters other tenets are emphasized.

In practice, osteopathic medicine is a method of health care delivery implemented by an individual physician's approach to patient–physician relationships. In some cases, the relationship concentrates on the musculoskeletal system, either as the primary expression of disease or because of its integral relationship to health and/or a disease process. In this case, musculoskeletal palpatory diagnosis and osteopathic manipulative therapy (OMT) represent issues of such central importance that they are both necessary and sufficient for patient care. Other circumstances within the field of medicine are such that, while the musculoskeletal system might play a role in the patient's well-being, the application of palpatory diagnosis and OMT might be considered adjunctive rather than primary. For example, in obstetrics, sports medicine, physiatry, and pain management, there are clear indications for osteopathic manipulative therapy that allow for the most complete expression of comprehensive patient care management. Conversely, although OMT can be significantly beneficial in the treatment of the patient during pregnancy, labor, and delivery, the indications for OMT might be less frequently found in a general gynecology practice or in some of the medical specialties.

Recognizing the central role of the neuromusculoskeletal system in disease and health maintenance, osteopathic physicians have used OMT as a means to implement their philosophic principles. Remember that OMT is a tool for applying a philosophy, not the philosophy itself. Various approaches are now used to intervene with the neuromusculoskeletal system, including exercise, yoga, biofeedback, transcutaneous electrical nerve stimulation, acupuncture, and Tai Chi. Because each of these modalities, including manipulation, is used by health care practitioners outside the osteopathic profession, one might conclude that a defining characteristic of osteopathic medicine is not found in practice patterns that are in exclusive use. The key feature is the philosophic orientation behind the application of these methods of health care, with an emphasis on the role of the neuromusculoskeletal system.

The evolution of medicine in this century has also changed the way in which OMT is used. With the development of new technologies, including imaging techniques, new pharmacologic agents, and the growth of molecular medicine, palpatory diagnosis and OMT might play a proportionately smaller role in some fields than they did in the recent past. These facts do not deny their historical or present importance. If OMT did in fact save tens of thousands of lives during the influenza epidemic after World War I,[1] we would concede that it represented the best therapy available at that time. If genetic engineering were to provide a breakthrough to create specific antiviral agents to treat a similar influenza epidemic, we would all rejoice that more effective therapy is now available.

The development of effective antihypertensive agents has moved OMT to an adjunctive role in the treatment of hypertension, in contrast to a legitimate interest in studying the effectiveness of this modality a few decades ago. Ironically, the technological advance of cardiac transplantation might be seen as causing the opposite reaction: when patients on the waiting list for a heart transplant are enrolled in a program of cardiac rehabilitation exercise, a significant number show such improvement in their functional status that they are removed from the transplant list because of enhanced musculoskeletal function, not because of a change in their cardiac status.

In those clinical sciences in which highly technical developments have come to the forefront, the osteopathic physician might have the greatest relevance because he or she can provide the comprehensive perspective and integrated philosophies that characterize the best of medical care.

For example, diagnostic methods and therapies for patients with heart disease have proliferated dramatically in recent years. Unfortunately, so has the general tendency to apply all methods to all patients, even without scientific rationale. A clinical management strategy based on concepts of the unity of body, structure–function relationships, and the intrinsic ability of the body to heal still constitutes the most rational means of diagnosis and therapy as described in the following chapters.

The degree to which palpatory diagnosis and OMT are applied in each specialty varies considerably depending on the nature of that specialty, the applicability of manual medicine, and the scientific research to support use of these methods. Nonetheless, each chapter is based on the basic tenets of osteopathic medicine as defined 100 years ago.

CONCLUSION

Both the generalist and the specialist are obliged to use the best information available for the care of the patient. In some instances, this remains clinical experience, the tradition that has worked for osteopathic physicians throughout the profession's history. To make the best use of this experience, we rely on expert opinion. When scientific evidence is directly or indirectly available, it should be used. All three types of authority are reflected in these chapters. Each author has attempted to make clear the strength of the scientific evidence that underlies recommendations for treatment. The goal is always that of whole patient care, in itself one of the traditional values of the osteopathic profession.

REFERENCES

1. Smith RK. One hundred thousand cases of influenza with a death rate of one-fortieth of that officially reported under conventional medical treatment. *JAOA*. 1920;21:172–175.

22. Pediatrics

STEPHEN H. SHELDON

Key Concepts

- **History of pediatric care**
- **Osteopathic philosophy in pediatrics, including application of the four guiding principles**
- **Role of musculoskeletal system**
- **Relationship of child with environment**
- **Diagnosis of pediatric patients, including testing, history, and examination**
- **Osteopathic pediatrics as primary care**
- **Future of osteopathic pediatrics**

Pediatrics is the art and science of health care for children. It might be thought of as internal medicine for children, but this is not as simple as it appears. The scope of pediatric practice is vast because a child is not merely a small adult. Medicine for children focuses on a dynamically changing organism whose structure and function differ as dramatically between age groups as children do from adults. The discipline of pediatrics, however, does not focus only on the child patient. For many years the child fully depends on parents or caretakers to provide sustenance and nurturing to live and develop appropriately, and to gradually learn independence. The focus of pediatrics must be extended beyond the child to include care of the parent/child relationship and the family.

HISTORICAL PERSPECTIVE

The focus of pediatrics has changed remarkably over the years. There have been dramatic shifts in emphasis from diagnosis and expectant management of common infectious diseases to prevention and control of major illness during childhood. Immunizations, antibiotics, and modern fluid and electrolyte therapies have virtually eliminated diseases and conditions that had been responsible for major morbidity and mortality in infants and young children.

During the 17th century, mothers were the primary care providers for children. Few physicians had the ability and/or the inclination to care for sick children. Mothers were often assisted in this task by midwives, wet nurses, grandmothers, and wise elderly women.[1] Infant death was common; many

children died of common illnesses before reaching 1 year of age. Epidemics of diphtheria, scarlet fever, meningitis, diarrhea, and dehydration ran rampant through communities. Traditional medical practice was unable to cope with these common diseases of childhood; medical practitioners tended to shun sick children.

Medical care of the sick infant and young child was relegated to midwives. During the 17th and 18th centuries, midwives learned their trade by example. Most were women, but by the middle of the 18th century, male midwives began attending to birthing women as well. Schools for midwives began during the 19th century, initially as private enterprises established by obstetricians and later in medical schools. Because of the obstetric focus and immediate care provided to the mother, little attention was paid to the newborn infant.

Care of sick infants by midwives and of sick adults by internists left older pediatric patients with limited medical care. Internists reluctantly provided care to older children. It was not until the end of the 19th century and beginning of the 20th century that care of the newborn and young child became the responsibility of the few pediatricians of the time. Doctors Abraham Jacobi and Job Smith were among the first pediatricians in the United States.[1] These pioneers provided a framework for development of the specialty of pediatrics as a unique medical discipline.

Pediatrics in the osteopathic profession generally paralleled this development. A few osteopathic physicians began limiting their practices to children. Osteopathic diagnosis and techniques provided a much needed tool for the general practitioner in the management of sick children before the development of immunizations and antibiotics. The founding of the American College of Osteopathic Pediatricians in 1940 provided necessary standards for osteopathic pediatric education, procedures for review and credentialing, and continuing education of osteopathic pediatricians.[2]

OSTEOPATHIC APPROACH

The osteopathic approach to the practice of pediatrics adheres to the basic tenets of osteopathic philosophy. Osteopathic principles are applicable to children as well as to adults. However, because structure and function of the body during childhood are dynamically different from that of adults, diagnostic and therapeutic principles cannot be applied in the same manner. The pediatric patient must be approached differently. The following discussion addresses the application of guiding principles[3] to the pediatric patient.

267

I. The body functions as a whole. It is regulated, coordinated, and integrated through multiple interactive biologic and social systems.

This founding osteopathic principle remains true for children: their organ systems are interactive and function through highly integrated, regulated, and coordinated biologic and psychosocial processes. A child's body functions as a single unit, however, only when observing the infant and child at a given moment in time. What is true at one age might not be true at another.

Humans have the longest childhood of all mammals. Organ systems grow and develop at significantly different rates; these systems are at different levels of maturation at the time of birth. Although systems continue to interact, relationships change, regulation mechanisms vary, and coordination alters. The child as a unitary biopsychosocial system must be approached and observed longitudinally, in keeping with the ever-changing developmental precepts.

Because infants and small children are totally dependent on their parents or caretakers for sustenance and nurturing, the unitary concept must be extended. The healthy child must be considered biologically and psychologically as part of a dyad. During early years of development, this parent/child dyad functions as a single unit, although the child and the parent remain individuals.

II. The body is inherently self-regulating and self-healing. Responses to internal and external events are always modulated through feedback mechanisms. Equilibrium is a major function.

This principle applies even before birth; the fetus possesses an inherent ability to heal itself. Self-regulation and self-healing occur even during early stages of development. Inherent biologic rhythms appear at variable times throughout gestation. Some rhythms appear to be circadian while other are clearly ultradian. Rhythmic diurnal and nocturnal oscillations of biologic functions require development and maturation of specific feedback mechanisms. Variability in heart rate, respiratory movements, urine production, and sleep–wake cycling reveal circadian and ultradian cycling that is affected by both endogenous (e.g., regional CNS maturation) and exogenous (e.g., sunlight) factors.

Changes in physiologic parameters can be documented when the fetus is exposed to a variety of "environmental" influences. Even before birth, the immune system is functional and responds (although feebly) to infection in a highly reproducible, ontogenetic pattern. The integument heals. The heart rate increases in response to stress. Self-healing, self-regulation, and integration of organ systems transform as the fetus develops and approaches birth. Some systems are close to being fully mature at or soon after birth (e.g., the cardiovascular and lymphatic systems). Other systems reach relative maturity slightly later, during the first 12 months of life (e.g., the renal and hematopoietic systems). Still others only reach maturity many years after birth (e.g., the central nervous, genitourinary, and endocrine systems). A constantly changing internal milieu re-

quires the practitioner to pay attention to the various stages of maturation and to use continuity of longitudinal observations to differentiate health from disease.

Assess the parent/child dyad when addressing this osteopathic principle. Parent/infant bonding occurs early. This bonding is a complex phenomenon that functions to assure survival of the dyad. The strength of the parent/child dyad depends on the degree (and success) of bonding. Bonding creates a situation whereby the dyad functions as a single unit that becomes self-regulating. For example, a mother most often responds appropriately to her infant's needs based on the quality of the infant's cry, whether from hunger, pain, or simply to have a diaper changed. Self-regulation refers to communication and interaction between component parts of the dyad that might be unintelligible to others. When bonding is incomplete or dysfunctional, however, self-regulating of the dyad is difficult and might not occur without significant intervention.

III. Structure and function are interrelated; they are inseparably linked at all levels.

The principle of the interrelationship of structure and function is unique in pediatrics. During the earliest postconceptional stages of life, errors in genetic and/or structural organ development can occur that significantly affect function of one or many organ systems. Early developmental abnormalities, if severe, can compromise vital functions and might not be compatible with life in utero. Spontaneous termination of pregnancy can occur. Developmental errors in the structural formation of an organ or system that are less severe, or those that occur later in gestation, might be compatible with life but can significantly affect proper functioning of the organ system (e.g., congenital malformations of the heart). Because all systems are interrelated, abnormalities in the structure and function of one system affect the function of others. For example, a congenital cardiac defect can increase pulmonary blood flow, result in pulmonary hypertension, alter arterial oxygen saturation, and cause compensatory changes in the renal and hematopoietic systems.

IV. Rational treatment is based on an understanding of body unity, self-regulatory mechanisms, and the interrelationships of structure and function. This principle unites the first three principles and is the basis for use of structural diagnosis and osteopathic manipulative treatment.

Guiding principles of the structure and function of organ systems and self-regulation are based on maintaining a homeostatic state. Autoregulation moves physiologic processes to a homeostatic or neutral condition. The body functions best in this "normal" environment. During childhood, these principles are of major importance but must be approached in a developmentally appropriate manner. The fact that a child is a dynamically changing organism with differential rates of growth and maturation of component parts demands continuous reevaluation of interrelationships. Fundamental diagnostic and therapeutic principles applied to adults do not hold true for pediatric patients. Normative data and the neutral state are profoundly different in children and vary according to developmental levels. Therefore, the normal state is not distinct during childhood and varies from time to time depending on the postconceptional age of the child.

Musculoskeletal System

The position of the musculoskeletal system is of prime importance in the osteopathic approach to the pediatric patient. The musculoskeletal system has three basic functions:

1. Supporting all other organ systems
2. Transporting all other organ systems throughout the environment
3. Enabling the organism to manipulate the environment

This conventional definition of function of the musculoskeletal system is, however, incomplete. Other significant roles exist. For example, the musculoskeletal system is primarily responsible for heat production through interaction with the central nervous system; it participates in storage of metabolic substrates and takes part in proprioception. The physiology of the musculoskeletal system requires it to function as other organ systems in its ability to affect and effect changes in other organ systems. In this regard, dysfunction is not limited only to an inability to support, transport, or manipulate. The musculoskeletal system joins in regulation, coordination, modulation, and maintenance of a homeostatic state directly and/or indirectly and is mediated through the vascular and nervous systems.

During infancy and childhood, structure and function of the musculoskeletal system and nervous system are strikingly different from that of adults. At birth, the central and peripheral nervous system are incompletely myelinated. Myelinization progresses at a steady rate but is not complete until the middle to end of the second decade of life. Lack of complete myelinization results in profound variations in nerve conduction velocity and reflex patterns.

The musculoskeletal system is similarly maturationally incomplete at birth. Cartilaginous growth centers in membranous and long bones are present; bony and articular relationships change throughout development. Easily identifiable and palpable differences can be found in the infant's skull. Open fontanels, and flexibility and overriding of cranial bones make the infant's relatively large head malleable, permitting delivery through the mother's pelvic outlet. Encasement of the brain within a relatively inflexible, enclosed bony vault is not complete until the latter half of the first year of life. Radiographic demonstration of long bone growth centers provides a highly accurate assessment of bone age. Endocrine abnormalities can profoundly affect bone age and result in premature or delayed closure of epiphyseal growth plates. Identification of these changes can greatly assist in diagnosis. Bony and articular relationships do not attain adult relationships until after puberty.

Because of dynamically changing neural and skeletal relationships, structural diagnosis and osteopathic manipulative treatment are appreciably different in pediatric patients. Indeed, newborns, infants, toddlers, children, and adolescents differ remarkably. Structural diagnosis and management require considerable modification depending on the postconceptional age of the youngster. For example, as early as 1940, Barnes was teaching the importance of a thorough osteopathic structural examination as part of the postnatal assessment of every newborn. Barnes cautions, however, that it is easy to overtreat muscular lesions in babies and small children.[4] Heilig emphasizes that gentleness and specificity of location are essential in treating children.[5] Greenman advises annual complete structural examinations (or more frequently as indicated) because structural findings in growing children are not static and growth "spurts" can cause change in the postural structural pattern.[6] Shaping of bone and the functioning of joint surfaces depend on the whole body in motion. Changes in the vertebral areas result from abnormal stresses being brought to bear on cartilage, with subsequent ossification along the resultant synchondral planes.[5] These factors have significant implications on osteopathic diagnosis and treatment in infants and children.

Frymann has pioneered studies using somatic and cranial manipulative therapeutics in childhood.[7] Results in improving neurologic performance have been exciting. Future studies replicating Frymann's data are imperative because of the influence specific osteopathic pediatric care might have on developmental outcome and performance later in life. It has been demonstrated, however, in a cross-sectional blinded study that specific segmental motion cannot be appreciated by experienced examiners until the age of 6 months.[8] The development of segmental motion appears to parallel progressive myelinization of the innervation to postural muscles and develops at approximately the same time the infant develops the ability to sit without support. Before the appearance of this developmental landmark, horizontal posture predominates. Musculoskeletal relationships vary from the mature pattern because spinal articular surfaces do not become weightbearing until upright posture is achieved. Similar modification in spinal segmental relationships can also be identified when the ability to walk develops, although these changes are more subtle.

PEDIATRIC ECOLOGY

Organ systems do not function in isolation but contribute to a harmonious whole. This unitary philosophy of osteopathic medicine not only concerns the individual child but also can be expanded to include the external milieu in which the child exists. The human organism constantly responds to external influences that affect biopsychosocial function. A child is an ecologic unit within this context and functions in an ecologic matrix.

Ecology is the branch of science concerned with the complex relations between a specific organism and its environment.[9] The child, as an organism, is affected by an internal

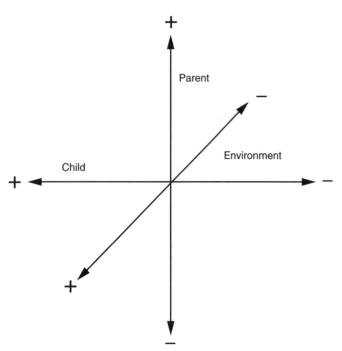

Figure 22.1. Ecologic matrix. +, vulnerabilities present. −, vulnerabilities absent. (Modified with permission from Levy HB, Sheldon SH, Conte JR. Special intervention programs for the child victims of violence. In: Lystad M, ed. *Violence in the Home.* New York, NY: Brunner/Mazel Inc; 1986:169–192.)

and external milieu. Relationships resulting in health and disease might be explained by movement within a four-dimensional matrix (Fig. 22.1).[10] The basic construct of this matrix includes:

Genetic, biologic, structural, physiologic, and psychological characteristics of the child (x axis)

Composition and characteristics of the caretaker(s) and family (y axis)

Social, cultural, and economic milieu in which the other two exist (z axis)

The fourth dimension of the matrix is time. Because developmental relationships are dynamically changing, continuity of care is required for optimal health assessment, management, and prevention. Vulnerabilities exist for each variable; the interaction of these vulnerabilities determines the presence (or absence) of abnormalities. For example, a child with an immunologic deficiency is more susceptible to infection when in an environment that can result in easy transmission of microorganisms (e.g., school classroom); family violence is more likely to occur when a parent is under significant stress, when the parent was abused as a child, when the social milieu permits corporal punishment of children, and when the child is hyperactive.

The concept of child ecology, therefore, requires the practitioner to identify vulnerabilities and modify, treat, or minimize vulnerabilities to place the ecologic unit in its most ho-

meostatic state. Continued monitoring and continuity of care are required to address the fourth dimension.

DIAGNOSIS

All experienced clinicians approach evaluation of the ill child in a virtually identical manner. The clinician begins by evaluating the patient situation (e.g., time of day, location of the patient encounter), perceiving cues (e.g., male or female patient, patient's age), and generating hypotheses. These initial steps in clinical problem solving occur instantaneously and unconsciously.[11] The clinician then tests hypotheses using an inquiry design driven by the initial hypothesis set. At the outset of the evaluation, hypotheses can be general guesses or hunches regarding a variety of possibilities or they can be nonspecific (e.g., the patient could have diabetes mellitus). The clinician then asks the patient's parent or caretaker to describe the problem and its natural history. One of the major differences in obtaining the pediatric history from that of adults is that it is most often second hand, because the child is unable to provide needed information. Consideration of the parent/child dyad as a single unit simplifies this task and renders information as reliable as possible. Parents provide the best historical information. Pay close attention to the details of the story; within the details lies the diagnosis.

The clinician next orders the hypothesis set in descending order of likelihood and tests each hypothesis in parallel. Hypothesis testing is done by first asking the parent questions that seek specific information. Ask questions to scan the history. Searching questions are designed to look for specific patterns of symptoms that support or refute each hypothesis. Scanning questions review the patient's history, are not specifically related to a hypothesis, and provide general information used for completeness and assurance that obscure details are not missed during the evaluation. At any time during the problem-solving process, new hypotheses may be added or deleted, or elevated or lowered on the list of diagnostic possibilities.

Searching and scanning a pediatric patient's history requires the inclusion of many specific areas of inquiry not present in a history obtained from an adult patient. First, information regarding the mother's pregnancy and the child's gestation can reveal clues to problems that might have affected the child during intrauterine life, such as:

Prematurity
Maternal drug or alcohol consumption
Preeclampsia

Other information provides important details regarding the health of the infant at the time of birth:

Birth weight
Birth length
Head circumference
Apgar scores
Gestational age by examination

Characteristics of the neonatal period and information about nutrition during the first few months can reveal meaningful data on parent/child bonding and on the child's general health. Obtain information regarding school performance and immunizations. A child's growth following an expected velocity and the attainment of normal developmental landmarks at expected chronological ages provide the most important information regarding the general health and well-being of the child. Children who suffer from significant chronic illnesses generally fall more than two standard deviations below the mean for age and sex on the growth curve (weight, height, head circumference) at a single point in time. They might exhibit longitudinal growth velocity that is slower than anticipated. Finally, clinical skills are used to perform comprehensive physical and structural examinations, further testing each hypothesis and searching for findings that support or refute viable hypotheses. The clinician identifies the problem; diagnostic closure results in a final working diagnosis and differential diagnosis; therapeutic closure results in a treatment plan.

PEDIATRICS AND PRIMARY CARE

Since its inception, osteopathic medicine has focused on primary care. Major areas of concentration in pediatric practice are health maintenance, health promotion, and disease prevention. Recommended schedules of health maintenance for the pediatric patient can be found in most pediatric textbooks.[12–13]

Examinations of well children are more difficult to perform than those of sick children because the initial hypothesis set is not guided by a specific complaint. Problem prevention and health maintenance are of prime importance in well child care. The history, physical examination, and clinical problem solving are instead guided by an extremely wide range of hypotheses related to disease states or disorders that are subclinical and not manifesting obvious signs or symptoms at that time.

The pediatrician focuses on primary, secondary, and tertiary prevention. Primary prevention refers to prevention of a disease process so that it will not affect the child; for example, immunizations to prevent:

Diphtheria
Tetanus
Pertussis
Polio
Measles
Rubella
Mumps
H. influenzae

Secondary prevention aims at identification of subclinical disease before the development of overt symptoms; e.g., at the time of the interim history, physical, and structural examination. In this way intervention can be provided to arrest clinical progression or eliminate the disease. Tertiary preventive practices consist of identification of clinical disease or disorder and alleviation of the disease or disorder through therapeutics and/or rehabilitation. Well child care and regularly scheduled visits

provide sufficient time for primary and secondary prevention of pertinent lifestyle disease. Take time to discuss issues of:

Normal child development
Accident prevention
Nutrition
Discipline
Parenting

CONCLUSION

The future of pediatrics will focus heavily on primary care and preventive medicine. As a primary care discipline, the pediatrician is in an ideal position to affect health and well-being. Lifestyle diseases that affect the majority of the population can be prevented or minimized by providing anticipatory guidance in epidemiologically important areas such as[11]:

Nutrition counseling for control of obesity and hypercholesterolemia
Behavior modification
Accident prevention
Smoking prevention

Osteopathic pediatricians are responsible for systematically investigating and documenting osteopathic concepts and principles during the early stages of child development. Early introduction of osteopathic care can affect and improve neurodevelopmental outcome significantly. Osteopathic diagnostic and therapeutic techniques used for children can be significant modalities for primary, secondary, and tertiary prevention. Unfortunately, little research on these modalities has been replicated. Osteopathic pediatrics provides a complete discipline of health care for children; the future requires the expertise of osteopathic pediatric specialists conducting scientifically based, randomized, and blinded clinical trials. Because much of osteopathic diagnosis is subjective, innovative techniques and methods of testing and analysis must be developed to provide replicable results.

A new morbidity has emerged. The challenge of the next decades includes:

Developmental disabilities
Learning disorders
Behavioral abnormalities
Environmental and lifestyle diseases

Major adult diseases, such as atherosclerosis, coronary artery disease, and hypertension, likely have roots in childhood. The challenge of improving the health and well-being of the general population requires attention during the earliest years of life.

The future of osteopathic pediatrics is clear: provision of the highest quality, complete pediatric care seated in a scientifically sound, replicable medical philosophy.

REFERENCES

1. Cone TE. *History of American Pediatrics.* Boston, Mass: Little, Brown & Co; 1979.

2. Bomboy RP. *The Golden Anniversary History of the American College of Osteopathic Pediatricians, 1940–1990.* Trenton, NJ: American College of Osteopathic Pediatricians; 1990.

3. The special committee on osteopathic principles and osteopathic technic, Kirksville College of Osteopathy and Surgery: an interpretation of the osteopathic concept. *J Osteopathy.* 1953;60:7–10.

4. Barnes M. Osteopathic treatment of infants. *JAOA.* 1941;40:242.

5. Heilig D. Osteopathic care of structural abnormalities. *JAOA.* 1949; 48:481.

6. Greenman PE. Structural abnormalities of children. *JAOA.* 1971; 71:157.

7. Frymann VM, Carney RE, Springall P. Effect of osteopathic medical management on neurological development in children. *JAOA.* 1992; 92:729.

8. Sheldon SH, Tettamble M, Kappler R. Child development and osteopathic diagnosis. *JAOA.* 1989;89:1357. Abstract.

9. Webster's Ninth New Collegiate Dictionary. Springfield, Mass: Merriam-Webster Inc; 1984.

10. Levy HB, Sheldon SH, Conte JR. Special intervention programs for child victims of violence. In: Lystad M, ed. *Violence in the Home.* New York, NY: Brunner/Mazel Inc; 1986:169–192.

11. Schulman JL, Hanley KK. *Anticipatory Guidance: An Idea Whose Time Has Come.* Baltimore, Md: Williams & Wilkins; 1987.

12. Behrman RE, Kliegman RM, Nelson WE, Vaughn VC III, eds. *Nelson Textbook of Pediatrics.* 14th ed. Philadelphia, Pa: WB Saunders; 1992.

13. Taeusch HW, Ballard RA, Avery ME. *Schafer and Avery's Diseases of the Newborn.* 6th ed. Philadelphia, Pa: WB Saunders; 1991.

23. Geriatrics

THOMAS A. CAVALIERI

Key Concepts

- **Historical perspective on geriatric medicine**
- **Theories and physiology of aging**
- **Comprehensive geriatric assessment, including medical, functional, psychological, and social components**
- **Special clinical concerns with the elderly: confusion, urinary incontinence, falling, and iatrogenesis**
- **Special contribution of osteopathic medicine to the elderly**

The elderly require a special approach; they are not just older adults. They also have needs stemming from aging physiology, the psychosocial impact of aging, and age-related diseases. The approach to the care of the elderly must be multidisciplinary and holistic; it must be driven by the goals of health maintenance and optimizing function. Osteopathic medicine is ideally suited to provide an approach to clinical care of the elderly aimed at achieving these goals.

HISTORICAL PERSPECTIVE

The "geriatric imperative" was promulgated in the 1970s and 1980s by the National Institute of Aging. It called for health care professions to respond to unmet clinical needs of the elderly.[1] It offered academic, attitudinal, demographic, and economic reasons to justify this concept. Academic reasons for the geriatric imperative centered on the absence of clinically relevant information on geriatrics and gerontology in the curricula of health professional schools and training programs. Attitudinal reasons for the geriatric imperative focused on negative stereotypes on aging believed to result in prejudice against the elderly and thought to be commonplace in our health care system.

Demographic and economic aspects of the geriatric imperative centered on the rapidly rising number of people aged 65 and over in this country and the impact of this population on health care costs. Representing approximately 12% of the total U.S. population today, this group is projected to increase to more than 18% of the population by the year 2030. The mean life span by the year 2040 will continue increasing and is projected to be well into the eighth decade of life for both sexes.

The "old old," those over age 85, are the most rapidly growing segment of the U.S. population. By the year 2040 it is projected that there will be one million centenarians in this country. With the elderly as the highest users of health care resources, these demographic changes will have an impact on the cost of health care.[2]

The past two decades have witnessed the impact of the geriatric imperative on the development of geriatric medicine in this country. While it is generally believed that we are still far from meeting the health care needs of the elderly, the geriatric imperative has succeeded in spawning much needed research in geriatrics and gerontology, influenced changes in medical education, and significantly altered our approach to the clinical care of the elderly. Osteopathic medicine has contributed greatly to the development of geriatrics in this country.

AGING PROCESS

The aging process itself is far from being completely understood. Recognizing the interrelationship among structure, function, and homeostasis with regard to the aging process is critical to the clinical care of the elderly. While aging and disease are distinctly different, the effects of the aging process on various organ systems are believed to reduce the organ's capacity to respond to increased demand. This has been called impaired homeostasis; it has significant clinical impact.

Theories of Aging

Various theories of aging have been proposed, but there is no consensus regarding the most likely explanation of biologic aging. The immunologic theory for aging attributes the decline in organ reserve seen with aging to the diminishing effects of the immune system. Thus, the thymus gland might be the master gland of the aging process, beginning with its involution at a young age. Numerous cellular theories of aging are still actively being investigated. The transcription theory attributes aging to the cell's limited ability to repair errors in transcription that occur in all cells.

The free radical theory for aging views highly charged molecules—free radicals—as the cause of the aging process. While present in the cell endogenously, effects of the atmosphere, such as ultraviolet light, might activate these chemicals to cause cellular damage leading to aging. Some research clinicians have proposed that antioxidants, such as vitamin C, block the effect of free radicals, thus slowing the aging process, but there are few data to support this. Other cellular theories of aging include the error theory, redundancy failure, and the cross-linkage theory.[3–4]

Physiology of Aging

The aging process itself is characterized by significant interindividual variation, manifested by the concept of chronologic age versus physiologic age. Thus, an individual can have a chronologic age of 75 but a physiologic age of 55. Another basic concept of physiologic aging is that the changes with age are linear, i.e., occurring at the same rate over time. Also, these changes are cumulative and actually begin at a young age, usually in the third decade. As such, an 80-year-old is not aging faster than a 40-year-old but has the cumulative effects of the aging process over three or four decades (Table 23.1).

Later sections in this chapter review age changes that have profound clinical impact. Understanding the relationship between structure and function, and taking into account age-associated altered homeostasis are vital to geriatric clinical care. With advanced age the body composition changes, causing a decrease in height, lean body mass, and body water, along with an increase in body fat. These changes, which alter the volume of distribution of certain drugs, have significant effects on pharmacokinetics with age and must be considered in prescribing drugs for the elderly. Dermatologic changes such as a decrease in subcutaneous fat, loss of sweat glands, and capillary fragility predispose the elderly to easy bruising, pressure sores, skin tears, and difficulty in body temperature regulation.[5]

Ophthalmic changes consist of a loss of elasticity of the lens, causing presbyopia, an increase in the near-point of vision. Thus, with age, ability to read fine print diminishes. Loss of auditory neurons and cochlear hair cells results in presbycusis, a diminished ability to hear high-pitched sounds. Changes in the central nervous system include:

Loss of brain weight
Diminution of many neurotransmitters
Decline in memory
Increased postural instability

These changes have been linked to the increased prevalence of delirium and falls in the elderly. Although these changes do occur, cognition shows little change with age, and dementia is not a normal concomitant result of these neural changes.

Aging changes in the musculoskeletal system include a loss of muscle mass and a decrease in bone mineral density. These effects on bone predispose the elderly to osteoporosis and fractures. This factor must be considered in the selection of certain osteopathic manipulative techniques in this age group.

Various changes take place in the cardiovascular system with age. Systolic blood pressure and, to a lesser extent, diastolic blood pressure increase with age, contributing to increased hypertension in the elderly. Calcification and sclerosis of the heart valves predispose the elderly to valvular stenosis and endocarditis. The cardiac output at rest is unaltered, but with increased exertion there is a decreased hemodynamic response. Pulmonary changes consist of a decline in alveolar surface area, a decrease in vital capacity, and a decrease in the partial pressure of arterial oxygen. These changes are believed to predispose the elderly to postoperative pulmonary complications.

With age there is a considerable decline in the number of nephrons of both kidneys, causing a significant decline in creatine clearance. This has an important clinical impact on drug prescribing for the elderly because many drugs are eliminated through renal excretion. Use caution in prescribing such medication to the elderly in view of diminished renal function. Immunologic changes consist of a decrease in T-cell function, a decrease in antibody production, and an increase in autoantibodies. These changes might account for the higher incidence of infections, malignancies, and autoimmune disorders in the elderly, as reflected in the immunologic theory of aging.[5]

COMPREHENSIVE GERIATRIC ASSESSMENT

Most medical care provided for the elderly is administered in primary care settings, an arena in which osteopathic physicians have been at the forefront. Primary care physicians skilled in the care of the elderly should recognize the importance of continuity of care and manage their patients, if possible, in all clinical sites where the elderly receive care, including the office, hospital, home, and nursing home. The physician skilled in geriatric medicine should be comfortable providing care in all these sites. Care is multidisciplinary. No one health care professional can meet all the multidimensional needs of the elderly. The physician must be willing to collaborate with multiple health care providers such as:

Nurses
Social workers
Physical therapists
Psychologists
Pharmacologists
Other medical specialists
Clergy

At the heart of geriatric care is the goal of optimizing function for the elderly, avoiding institutionalization, and maintaining the patient, as much as possible, in the community. This can be achieved through careful multidimensional evaluation coupled with a plan that stresses health maintenance and disease prevention.

The multidimensional evaluation of the elderly consists of a medical, social, functional, and psychological assessment. This has been called the comprehensive geriatric assessment and in geriatric assessment programs is performed by a geriatric multidisciplinary team consisting of a geriatrician, geriatric nurse practitioner, and gerontological social worker. The beneficial effects of this team approach have been well-documented, and include accuracy in diagnosis, decrease in unnecessary medications, avoidance of institutionalization, and increased longevity.[6] Comprehensive geriatric assessment usually incorporates the use of assessment tools to measure various aspects of the evaluation such as function, cognition, and affect.[7]

Table 23.1
Physiology of Aging and Clinical Impact

Age-Related Change	Clinical Predisposition
Body Composition and Conformation	
Decreased height	
Decreased lean body mass	Changes in pharmacokinetics
Decreased body water	
Increased body fat	
Aging Skin	
Thinning and sparseness of hair	Baldness
Hair follicles produce less melanin	Graying hair
Thin, fragile, wrinkled skin	Propensity to injury
Capillary fragility	Senile purpura
Decreased subcutaneous fat	Pressure sore
Atrophy of sweat glands	Difficulty in body temperature regulation
Decreased response to pain sensation and temperature	Accidents
Aging Eyes	
Loss of elasticity of lens	Presbyopia
Increased density of lens	Cataracts
Change in aqueous kinetics	Glaucoma
Decreased pupillary size	Falls and accidents
Sluggish light reflex	
Decreased color vision	
Increased glare sensitivity	
Aging Mouth and Teeth	
Loss of lingual papillae	Loss of interest in food
Poor taste sensation	Malnutrition and weight loss
Atrophy of olfactory bulbs and decline in sensation of smell	Decreased appetite
	Increased risk of gas poisoning
Resorption of gum and bony tissue surrounding teeth and bone of mandible	Loss of teeth and periodontal disease
Aging Ears	
Decrease in cerumen glands	Drier cerumen
Atrophy of cochlear hair cells	Presbycusis
Loss of auditory neurons	Presbycusis
Aging Cardiovascular System	
Increase in blood pressure	Hypertension
Aorta and large arteries lose elasticity and systemic vascular resistance increases	Left ventricular hypertrophy
Decreased baroreceptor reflex activity	Orthostatic hypotension
Calcification and sclerosis of heart valves	Valvular stenosis, endocarditis
Calcification and sclerosis of conduction system	Conduction abnormalities
Altered cardiac output	Decreased hemodynamic response to stress
Decreased heart rate	Decreased response to stress
Aging Respiratory System	
Calcification of costal cartilages	Decreased secretion clearance
Decline in alveolar surface area	Effects of hypoxemia
Alteration in pulmonary function tests	
Decreased vital capacity	Increased risk of pulmonary complications
Decreased maximum breathing capacity	
Increased residual volume	
Decreased PaO_2	
Aging Renal System	
Progressive loss of renal mass	Alteration in drug pharmacokinetics
Decrease in renal blood flow	
Decreased tubular function	Greater tendency toward dehydration
Decrease in creatinine clearance	Increased risk of adverse drug reactions

Table 23.1—*continued*

Age-Related Change	Clinical Predisposition
Aging Nervous System	
Decrease in brain weight	Drug toxicities, delirium
Alteration in CNS neurotransmitters	
Decrease in memory	"Benign senile forgetfulness"
Decreased reaction time	Decreased IQ scores
Altered sleep with decreased deep sleep and increased wakefulness	Increased sleep disturbances
Decreased vibratory sense	Altered gait
Decreased righting reflex	Falls, accidents
Increased postural instability	Falls, accidents
Altered gait	Falls, accidents
Aging Musculoskeletal System	
Loss of muscle mass	Decreased strength
Loss of bone mineral density	Osteoporosis
	Fractures
Osteoarthritis	Symptomatic arthritis
Aging Hematologic System	
Decreased lymphocyte production	
Decreased bone marrow cellularity	
Decreased hematopoietic functional reserve	Predisposition for anemia
Aging Endocrine System	
Impaired glucose tolerance	Diabetes mellitus
Increased insulin resistance	
Decreased estrogen	Menopause, predisposition to osteoporosis and coronary artery disease
Aging Immune System	
Decreased T-cell function	Predisposition to infections and malignancies
Decreased antibody production to new or old antigen	Predisposition to infection
Increased autoantibodies	Predisposition to autoimmune disorders
Aging Gastrointestinal System	
Decreased gastric HCl production	Altered drug absorption
Colonic motility diminished	Constipation
Decreased calcium absorption	Osteoporosis
Decreased hepatic biotransformation	Altered pharmacokinetics
Decreased hepatic albumin synthesis	Altered pharmacokinetics
Aging Genitourinary System	
Decreased bladder capacity	Urinary incontinence
Alterations in pelvic support	
Enlarged prostate gland	Prostate obstruction
Diminished vaginal and cervical secretion	Pruritus, dyspareunia
Decrease in sexual response	Fear of impotence

While not all elderly patients can or need to be evaluated in a comprehensive geriatric assessment program, this multi-dimensional approach to evaluation of the elderly can be incorporated into the primary care physician's practice.

Medical Assessment

The medical component of the comprehensive geriatric assessment includes the history, physical examination, and review of the baseline laboratory screening tests. There are significant differences between assessment of the elderly and assessment of younger adults. Keep in mind common obstacles when assessing the elderly. Atypical presentations of diseases are common. If this dimension is not considered, important clinical problems can easily be overlooked in the elderly. For example, delirium might be a manifestation of pneumonia, or a patient might appear to have dementia when the problem is actually depression.

Visual and hearing losses commonly contribute to communication problems. Use a quiet, well-lit room and speak slowly in a deep voice while facing the patient, when necessary.

It is a common myth that old people overreport problems. Actually, the elderly tend to underreport symptoms, possibly because of fear, embarrassment, misconceptions about normal aging, or cognitive impairment. Older persons might fail to report impotence because they believe it to be normal for their age or fail to report urinary incontinence because of fear of institutionalization. While the patient is the prime source for the history, other sources for history taking can be invaluable. This might be particularly necessary when the patient has cognitive disturbances. Sources can include family, other physicians, old medical records, visiting nurses, and other sources.

Because the elderly often have multiple concurrent problems, the history might be associated with multiple complaints. Use patience and clinical skill to prioritize and sort out each complaint. A careful medication history is vital in the assessment of the elderly and should include both prescribed and over-the-counter preparations. The elderly are the highest users of medication, using over 40% of all medications while representing 12% of the population. The elderly have the highest incidence of adverse drug reactions; view new complaints as possible drug reactions. Ask the elderly to bring in all prescribed and over-the-counter medications periodically to be evaluated by the primary care physician. This has been referred to as the "paper bag" test because it frequently results in a bag full of medications for the physician to review. Also, it is important when asking about allergies to differentiate true allergy from medication side effects, because older people frequently report a history of a drug side effect as an allergy.

The review of systems for the elderly is different because it must focus on questions that reflect common problems for which the elderly are not likely to report. Examples include:

Falling
Impotence
Depression
Change in bowel habits
Urinary incontinence

Because nutritional problems are so common in this age group, particularly for elderly men living alone, a dietary assessment is important. The history should also address ethical issues such as patients' views on advanced life support, their relationships with their families, and the presence of advance directives.

The physical examination can take longer with the elderly because of decreased mobility. Patience is required. Parts of the physical examination may be performed in an order different from the usual to accommodate special situations, such as wheelchair-bound or bed-bound patients. Because the elderly are frequently embarrassed about their situation or reluctant to undress for a physical, the physician should exert care to avoid unnecessary exposure.

Be aware of age-associated changes in physical findings that differentiate age and disease. Blood pressure evaluation should include both supine and standing measurements because of the frequency of orthostasis in the elderly. Because visual disturbances and hearing disorders are common in the elderly, it is important to assess vision and hearing. Weight should be monitored carefully because nutritional problems are common. Gait should be observed; gait disturbances are common and frequently lead to falls. Careful assessment of the carotid arteries for bruits is important because of the increased frequency of carotid artery disease.

The cardiac examination often reveals a grade I or II systolic ejection murmur as a result of age-related changes of the aortic valve. Bibasilar rales on examination of the lungs might not reflect pulmonary disease or heart failure but could indicate atelectasis, particularly in immobile, bed-confined patients. The abdominal examination should include deep palpation for the presence of an abdominal aortic aneurysm. Leg edema is commonly found and is usually the result of chronic venous stasis rather than heart failure.

The neurologic examination should include a careful assessment of cognitive status, using a standardized assessment discussed in a later section. Keep in mind that ankle jerks are frequently absent bilaterally in the elderly without clinical significance, and there is a diminution of vibratory sense of the lower extremities with age. Because musculoskeletal disorders increase significantly with age, predisposing the elderly to functional disability and immobility, the importance of the structural examination cannot be overemphasized. It is important to assess for somatic dysfunction, ranges of motion, postural disturbances, and abnormalities of gait. Developmental structural changes of the spine such as kyphosis and scoliosis are common in the elderly and should not be overlooked.

Because of physiologic changes with age, interpreting standard laboratory data is different for the elderly. Knowledge of age-associated alteration of various laboratory parameters is important to prevent overdiagnosis or underdiagnosis.[8] The erythrocyte sedimentation rate and blood glucose increase with age, for example, whereas creatinine clearance and serum albumin decline. Serum electrolytes and hemoglobin are unchanged with age (Tables 23.2 and 23.3).[9]

Functional Assessment

At the heart of comprehensive geriatric assessment is a determination of the patient's physical functioning. This consists of an evaluation of the patient's ability to perform the activities of daily living (ADLs) and the instrumental activities of daily living (IADLs). The ADLs include:

Bathing
Toileting
Feeding
Dressing
Grooming
Ambulation

The IADLs involve a higher level of functioning and include such tasks as:

Housekeeping
Meal preparation
Telephone use
Financial management
Shopping
Transportation
Medication administration

Table 23.2
Laboratory Values That Do Not Change with Age

Hepatic Function Tests
  Serum bilirubin
  AST
  ALT
  GGTP
Coagulation Tests
Biochemical Tests
  Serum electrolytes
  Total protein
  Calcium
  Phosphorus
  Serum folate
Arterial Blood Tests
  pH
  $PaCO_2$
Renal Function Tests
  Serum creatinine
Thyroid Function Tests
  T_4
Complete Blood Count
  Hematocrit
  Hemoglobulin
  RBC Indices
  Platelet Count

Reprinted with permission from Cavalieri TA, Chopra A, Bryman PN. When outside the norm is normal: interpreting lab data in the aged. *Geriatrics.* May 1992;47(5):66–70.

Table 23.3
Laboratory Values That Do Change with Age

Value	Degree of Change
Alkaline phosphatase	Increases 20% between 3rd and 8th decades
Biochemical tests	
Serum albumin	Slight decline
Uric acid	Slight decline
Total cholesterol	Increases 30–40 mg/dL by age 55 in women and age 60 in men
HDL cholesterol	Increases 30% in men; decreases 30% in women
Triglycerides	Increases 30% in men and 50% in women
Serum B_{12}	Slight decrease
Serum magnesium	Decreases 15% between 3rd and 8th decades
PaO_2	Decreases 25% between 3rd and 8th decades
Creatinine clearance	Decreases 10 mL/min/1.73 m² per decade
Thyroid function tests	
T_3	Possible slight decrease
TSH	Possible slight increase
Glucose tolerance tests	
Fasting blood sugar	Minimal increase (within normal range)
1-hr postprandial blood sugar	Increases 10 mg/dL per decade after age 30
2-hr postprandial blood sugar	Increases up to 100 mg/dL plus age after age 40
White blood cell count	Decreases

Reprinted with permission from Cavalieri TA, Chopra A, Bryman PN. When outside the norm is normal: interpreting lab data in the aged. *Geriatrics.* May 1992;47(5):66–70.

This information is essential to aid the physician in determining recommendations for patient placement such as the need for home care, a nursing home, or a residential care facility. The functional assessment can be obtained by questioning the patient or family or by direct observation. Direct observation is probably superior but is time consuming. Widely used standardized assessment tools enable the clinician to perform a functional evaluation.[10–11]

Psychological Assessment

The psychological assessment of the elderly evaluates both cognition and affect. Standardized, validated assessment tools are widely used both to screen for and measure dementia and depression. A careful assessment of cognition is an essential aspect of geriatrics. Orientation, registration, attention, recall, and language should all be tested. The most widely used cognitive assessment tool, the Mini-Mental State Exam, is easily administered and reproducible, and enables the clinician to measure and follow the mental status (Table 23.4).[12] Early dementia can easily be missed in the elderly if the clinician does not perform a cognitive assessment. Depression, which has its highest incidence in the elderly, can present atypically and be easily misdiagnosed. Assessing affect by questioning the patient about signs and symptoms of depression is important. The use of a

Table 23.4
Mini-Mental State Examination

Maximum Score	
	Orientation
5	What is the (year) (season) (date) (day) (month)?
5	Where are we (state) (county) (hospital) (floor)?
	Registration
3	Name three objects: one second to say each. Then ask the patient to repeat all three after you have said them. Give one point for each correct answer. Repeat them until he or she learns all three. Count trials and record number.
	Attention and Calculation
5	Begin with 100 and count backwards by 7 (stop after five answers). Alternatively, spell "world" backwards.
	Recall
3	Ask for the three objects repeated above in #3. Give one point for each correct answer.
	Language
2	Show a pencil and a watch and ask patient to name them.
1	Repeat the following: "no 'ifs', 'ands,' or 'buts'"
3	A three-stage command: "Take a paper in your right hand; fold it in half and put it on the floor."
1	Read and obey the following: (show subject the written item). CLOSE YOUR EYES
1	Write a sentence.
1	Copy a design (complex polygon as in Bender-Gestalt).
30	Total score possible

Reprinted with permission from Folstein MF, Folstein S, McHugh PR. Mini-Mental State: a practical method for grading the cognitive state of patients for the clinician. *Psychiatr Res* 1975;12:189–198. Elsevier Science Ltd, Oxford, England.

standardized assessment tool, the Geriatric Depression Scale, aids in recognizing and quantifying depression (Table 23.5).[13]

Social Assessment

Assessment of the patient's socioeconomic situation is essential to comprehensive geriatric care. Knowing the family structure and the patient's relationship with his or her family is important; most of the caregiving in the community is provided by families. Understanding the patient's values and attitudes toward various therapies is important. Identifying the patient's support system, whether it be informal, such as the family, or formal, such as community agencies, is likewise essential. The physician should be aware of the patient's financial resources to determine the feasibility of access to certain services. The physician must be aware of and actively interface with various community agencies or programs that provide vital support services for the elderly. These include the local area Agency on Aging, visiting nurses associations, Meals on Wheels, and Adult Protective Services.

SPECIAL CLINICAL CONCERNS

Geriatrics spans a broad spectrum of clinical concerns addressing issues ranging from preventive care for a healthy active elderly individual to the management of a frail 90-year-old person with multiple problems. Certain clinical problems for the elderly are of extreme importance because of both their profound clinical impact and increased prevalence. These problems include:

Confusion
Incontinence
Falling
Iatrogenesis

Until recently, these problems received little attention either from a clinical or a research perspective, yet they account for high morbidity and mortality in the elderly.

Confusion

Disturbances of cognition consist of dementia and delirium and are common in the geriatric population. While cognition remains relatively intact with normal aging, dementia affects more than 25% of those over the age of 80. For dementia to be diagnosed, it should have a gradual onset, cause dysfunction of multiple spheres of intellect such as memory, abstract thinking and judgment, not alter the state of consciousness, and occur to such a degree that the patient is unable to perform the activities of daily living (Table 23.6).[14]

Unlike dementia, delirium is a potentially life-threatening illness that is sudden in onset and is associated with a clouded state of consciousness and a disturbance of the sleep–wake cycle (Table 23.7). It is frequently a result of a toxic or metabolic disturbance.[15] Because delirium is a potentially life-threatening disorder, it is important that the clinician differentiate dementia from delirium (Table 23.8).

In addition to an increased prevalence in the elderly, dementia has a tremendous impact because it is a common reason for institutionalization and is one of the leading causes of mortality affecting the elderly. Alzheimer's disease accounts for approximately 50% of the causes of dementia; multi-infarct dementia accounts for another 25%. Fifteen percent are caused by irreversible disorders of the central nervous system, such as Pick's disease, Huntington's chorea, inoperable brain tumors, and Parkinson's disease. The remaining 10% result from treat-

Table 23.5
Geriatric Depression Scale (Short Form)

Choose the Best Answer for How You Felt Over the Past Week

1. Are you basically satisfied with your life?	yes/no
2. Have you dropped many of your activities and interests?	yes/no
3. Do you feel that your life is empty?	yes/no
4. Do you often get bored?	yes/no
5. Are you in good spirits most of the time?	yes/no
6. Are you afraid that something bad is going to happen to you?	yes/no
7. Do you feel happy most of the time?	yes/no
8. Do you often feel helpless?	yes/no
9. Do you prefer to stay at home, rather than going out and doing new things?	yes/no
10. Do you feel you have more problems with memory than most people?	yes/no
11. Do you think it is wonderful to be alive?	yes/no
12. Do you feel pretty worthless the way you are now?	yes/no
13. Do you feel full of energy?	yes/no
14. Do you feel that your situation is hopeless?	yes/no
15. Do you think that most people are better off than you are?	yes/no

Negative responses for questions 1, 5, 7, 11, and 13 indicate depression. The remainder of positive responses indicate depression.

Reprinted with permission from Yeasavage JA, Brink TL. Development and validation of a geriatric depression screening scale: a preliminary report. *J Psychiatr Res* 1983;17:1, 37–49. Elsevier Science Ltd., Oxford, England.

Table 23.6
Diagnostic Criteria for Dementia

A. The development of multiple cognitive deficits manifested by both:
    (1) memory impairment (impaired ability to learn new information or to recall previously learned information);
    (2) one (or more) of the following cognitive disturbances:
        (a) aphasia (language disturbance)
        (b) apraxia (impaired ability to carry out motor activities despite intact motor function)
        (c) agnosia (failure to recognize or identify objects despite intact sensory function)
        (d) disturbance in executive functioning (i.e., planning, organization, sequencing, abstracting).
B. The cognitive deficits in Criteria A1 and A2 each cause significant impairment in social or occupational functioning and represent a significant decline from a previous level of functioning.
C. The course is characterized by gradual onset and continuing cognitive decline.

Adapted from Diagnostic and Statistical Manual of Mental Disorders. DSM-IV. 4th ed. Washington, DC: American Psychiatric Association; 1994.

Table 23.7
Diagnostic Criteria for Delirium

A. Disturbance of consciousness (i.e., reduced clarity of awareness of the environment) with reduced ability to focus, sustain, or shift attention.
B. A change in cognition (such as memory deficit, disorientation, language disturbance) or the development of a perceptual disturbance that is not better accounted for by a preexisting, established, or evolving dementia.
C. The disturbance develops over a short time (usually hours to days) and tends to fluctuate during the course of the day.
D. There is evidence from the history, physical examination, or laboratory findings that the disturbance is caused by the direct physiologic consequences of a general medical condition.

Adapted from Diagnostic and Statistical Manual of Mental Disorders. DSM-IV. 4th ed. Washington, DC: American Psychiatric Association; 1994:132–133.

Table 23.8
Differentiating Delirium from Dementia

	Delirium	Dementia
Onset	Sudden	Insidious
Consciousness	Reduced	Clear
Attention	Globally disordered	Normal
Cognition	Globally disordered	Globally impaired
Hallucinations	Usually visual	Often absent
Delusions	Fleeting, poorly systemized	Often absent
Psychomotor activity	Increase or decrease	Usually normal
Speech	Often incoherent	Word-finding difficulty
Involuntary movements	Asterixis or coarse tremor	Often absent
Physical illness/drug toxicity	Present	Often absent

able causes of dementia such as various drugs, brain tumors, vitamin B_{12} or folate deficiency, depression, thyroid disturbances, and central nervous system infections.[16] Once dementia is diagnosed, a careful workup is needed to maximize treatment options and aid in prognosis. It is important to rule out the presence of a treatable dementia.

A comprehensive geriatric assessment is necessary to evaluate the multidimensional needs of the patient with dementia. The diagnostic workup involves a series of blood tests including:

Complete blood count
Blood urea nitrogen
Serum creatinine
Thyroid function tests
B_{12} and folate levels
Serologic test for syphilis

If indicated, a serologic test for HIV should be considered. A CT or MRI of the head should also be ordered. At times, an electroencephalogram, neuropsychological testing, and a lumbar puncture are useful in the workup. Because the problems of the patient with dementia span the dimensions of medical, behavioral, nursing, ethical, and social needs, management should be multidisciplinary. The physician must be an effective team leader to access and implement the plan of care. Osteopathic physicians, with their emphasis on holistic primary care, are well-suited for this role. Skillful management can contribute significantly to the well-being of the patient and his or her family.[17]

While the precise cause of Alzheimer's disease is still unknown, recent clinical and basic science research have expanded our understanding of this devastating disorder. Data suggest a genetic link to Alzheimer's disease probably related to the 14th, 19th, or 21st chromosomes. The diagnosis of Alzheimer's disease is still one of exclusion, but recent studies suggest the presence of a marker, ALZ-50, in the central nervous system that might prove to be a reliable diagnostic tool for confirming Alzheimer's disease. While pharmacologic treatment to reverse the dementia is still unavailable, multiple clinical trials aimed primarily at enhancing central nervous system acetylcholine are underway. One such agent, tacrine, was recently FDA-approved for treatment of Alzheimer's disease, but its role in the medical management of this disorder is yet to be determined.[18] Research in this area continues as a national priority.[19]

Urinary Incontinence

Urinary incontinence is a common disorder that is referred to as a hidden illness in the elderly because it is often overlooked by clinicians and because the elderly frequently do not report it out of fear of institutionalization. In fact, urinary incontinence is often the last event to occur before nursing home placement. This problem afflicts approximately 10% of the community-dwelling elderly, 30% of the elderly in acute care settings, and approximately 50% of nursing home residents. Its impact is seen in the psychological effects of isolation and depression, the potential for skin breakdown and infection, and the economic impact of institutionalization and costs of care. Although incontinence can occur acutely as a result of drugs or infection, we will focus here on persistent incontinence. An understanding of normal micturition is essential to understanding the mechanisms and management of this problem. There are four types of persistent urinary incontinence:

Urge
Stress
Overflow
Functional

Urge incontinence, the most common type in the elderly and representing approximately 65% of cases, is the result of an unstable bladder with uninhibited bladder contractions. Patients with this type of incontinence have the sudden urge to void but simply cannot make it to the bathroom in time. It is commonly the result of central nervous system conditions such as stroke, dementia, and multiple sclerosis. It can be successfully treated with anticholinergic drugs to relax bladder contractions and biofeedback to aid in bladder relaxation.

Stress incontinence occurs primarily in women and accounts for 15% of cases. It is manifested by incontinence with coughing or laughing and is related to weakness of the pelvic musculature and urethral incompetence. Treatment can be accomplished by estrogen cream to enhance the integrity of the urethra, exercise, biofeedback to improve strength and tone of the pelvic musculature, and α-adrenergic agonists to improve urethral tone. At times, surgical intervention is needed.

Overflow incontinence represents approximately 10% of cases and is often described as being associated with a diminished stream and leakage of small amounts of urine. It might be the result of urethral obstruction because of prostatic enlargement or a urethral stricture. It might also be the result of a distended acontractile bladder such as occurs in diabetes mellitus or as a complication of anticholinergic drugs. A urologic evaluation is essential to rule out obstruction. Cessation of anticholinergic medications is important, and if obstruction is ruled out, a trial of cholinergic agonists may be initiated.

Functional incontinence accounts for the remaining 10% of cases. This type is the result of the patient's physical inability to reach the toilet in time. It is usually a result of a problem with mobility, such as advanced arthritis, muscle weakness, or strokes. Treatment centers on making toilet facilities more readily available or obtaining a bedside commode.

The role of the primary care physician in the recognition and management of this disorder is essential, and particularly involves coordinating the involvement of the multiple disciplines of nursing, social work, and urology.[20] An indwelling Foley catheter should be avoided except in rare circumstances, such as with the presence of severe pressure sores. Significant advances have been made in clinical research in the treatment of the disorder. Once believed to be a disorder surgically treated by the urologist with little success, new data suggest that modalities initiated by the primary physician coupling medical treatment with exercise and behavioral management can result in improvement of most community-dwelling, cognitively intact elderly with incontinence.[21] While many osteopathic clinicians report increased efficacy when manipulative management is added to this regimen, this has not yet been proven in clinical trials. More research is needed in this area.

Falling

Gait disorders and instability often result in falls in the elderly, and have a profound impact on the clinical care of the aged. Accidents are the fifth leading cause of death in the elderly; approximately 70% of accidents result from falls. Considering the decrease in bone mineral density with age, fractures of the hip, femur, wrist, and humerus are not uncommon. Hip fractures lead to hospitalization, complications of surgery, and complications of immobility. There is a significant risk of institutionalization after hip fracture; some clinicians report mortality rates as high as 20%. Little attention has been focused on why the elderly fall and what measures can be taken to prevent falls and their consequences. Changes in postural control such as a decrease in proprioception and muscle tone, a slower righting reflex, and an increase in postural sway are all thought to contribute to falls. The increased incidence of various disorders with age, such as degenerative joint disease, strokes, peripheral neuropathy, muscle weakness, and impaired vision, are all believed to contribute to the increased frequency of falls. The causes for falls in the elderly are classified as either extrinsic or intrinsic. Extrinsic causes account for approximately 50% of falls and are largely a result of environmental factors such as poor lighting, throw rugs and frayed carpets, unstable furniture, and inappropriate bed or toilet heights. Intrinsic causes for falls include such problems as (Table 23.9)[22]:

Syncope
Drop attacks
Cardiac dysrhythmias
Strokes
Transient ischemic attacks
Seizures
Parkinson's disease
Orthostatic hypotension

Drugs such as antihypertensives, sedatives, antipsychotics, and hypoglycemics are also common causes of falls in the elderly.

Evaluation of the falling patient should include a careful

Table 23.9
Intrinsic Conditions Leading to Falls Among the Elderly

Condition	Symptoms Along with Fall
Orthostatic hypotension	Lightheadedness with postural change
	Palpitation or postural sway along with postural change
Diabetes mellitus	Reduced sensation of lower extremities
Vitamin B_{12} deficiency	Reduced proprioception
Cardiac arrhythmia	Palpitation, shortness of breath, dizziness, or syncope
Transient ischemic attack or cerebrovascular accident	Unilateral weakness, visual disturbance, or speech changes
Seizure	Aura, urinary or bowel incontinence, or syncope
Osteoarthritis of hips or knees	Weakness in quadriceps or knees (or both)
Hyperthyroidism/ hypothyroidism	Proximal muscle weakness of lower extremities
Polymyalgia rheumatica	Pelvic girdle weakness or quadricep muscle weakness (or both)
Normal pressure hydrocephalus	Ataxic gait, urinary incontinence, and dementia
Central nervous system lesion	Mental status change Focal neurologic deficit
Ménière's syndrome, labyrinthitis, or benign positional vertigo	Poor balance, ataxia, vertigo, dizziness
Hypoglycemia	Acute onset of mental status change, tremors, dizziness, weakness, or diaphoresis
Alcohol intoxication	Ataxic gait, mental status change, slurred speech

Reprinted with permission from Cavalieri TA, Gray-Miceli D. Evaluating and preventing falls among the elderly population. *JAOA.* 1994;94(7):610–614.

history of prior falls, a review of the patient's medical status, and a list of all current medications. The review of systems should include questioning the patient regarding symptoms suggesting transient ischemic attack, dysrhythmia, seizure, and so on. A careful physical examination should include supine and standing blood pressures for orthostasis, an assessment of visual acuity, evidence of joint or limb deformity, disorders of the feet, and evidence of muscle weakness or sensory deficits found in the neurologic examination. Gait should also be observed. A careful structural examination can reveal musculoskeletal abnormalities that might be contributory. Depending on the results of the history and physical, various laboratory studies such as a complete blood count, electrolytes, and blood urea nitrogen might be in order. Other studies that might be appropriate include an electroencephalogram, CT of the head, electrocardiogram, 24-hour Holter monitor, or carotid Doppler. An evaluation by a physical therapist and a home environmental assessment for hazards by a visiting nurse are often necessary.

Management consists of treating the primary underlying disorder if discovered. Physical therapy for gait training and use of an assistive device such as a walker or cane might be in order. Environmental manipulation such as improving lighting, increasing toilet height, and installing safety bars might also be necessary. The team approach to care of the falling patient, incorporating the nurse, physical therapist, occupational therapist, and others, can contribute significantly to the outcome. Recent research has revealed that this approach can reduce the frequency of falling for high-risk elderly fallers by 30%.[23]

Research is underway to demonstrate the impact of osteopathic manipulative treatment on falls prevention in the elderly. Specialized falls assessment programs have contributed to the much needed clinical research relevant to this important clinical syndrome in the elderly.[24]

Iatrogenesis

The elderly are particularly prone to iatrogenic disorders. Altered homeostasis coupled with the failure of physicians to recognize the special needs of the elderly contribute to the increased frequency of iatrogenesis in this age group. Common iatrogenic problems in the elderly include polypharmacy, immobility, and unnecessary hospitalization. The elderly have a high frequency of adverse drug reactions; studies show that the incidence of adverse drug reactions increases significantly with age. It has been reported that approximately 40% of hospitalized elderly patients develop an adverse drug reaction. Studies have also demonstrated that approximately 3% of all hospital admissions are the result of drug-induced disease, and the majority of these patients are elderly. Studies show that adverse drug reactions increase with the increase in the number of medications taken. These observations are believed to occur because of a decrease in the therapeutic window with age. Both pharmacokinetic and pharmacodynamic changes occur that predispose the elderly to adverse drug reactions. Changes in body

composition, such as a decline in serum albumin, altered hepatic metabolism, a decline in renal function, and changes in absorption, all contribute to the pharmacokinetic alterations. Changes in receptors with age result in altered sensitivity to certain drugs. All of these changes are compounded by the problem of polypharmacy, common with the elderly. Elderly people take approximately four to five medications; nursing home patients average eight medications. It is estimated that approximately 25% of medications prescribed for the elderly are unnecessary. Reflex drug prescribing has led to unnecessary medications. Appropriate and rational drug prescribing for the elderly is essential. Effective nonpharmacologic treatment modalities, such as osteopathic manipulative treatment, are particularly preferred for the care of the elderly when indicated.

Unnecessary bed rest and immobility are common iatrogenic problems for the elderly patient, particularly in hospitals and nursing homes. Physicians frequently fail to recognize the complications of immobility for their patients and neglect orders such as appropriate ambulation, rotating the patient, or physical therapy consultations. Consequences of prolonged immobility and bed rest include:

Pressure sores
Pneumonia
Venous thromboembolism
Constipation
Contractures
Urinary incontinence

Manipulative treatment might prevent many of the complications that immobile geriatric patients experience. The rib raising technique is easily performed and has a beneficial effect on the circulatory, respiratory, and nervous systems. The integral relationship of structure and function is the osteopathic concept most applicable to the consequences of immobility. Musculoskeletal activity is essential to maintain homeostatic mechanisms.

Hospitals can be dangerous places for any patient but are particularly dangerous for the elderly. Avoid unnecessary hospitalization. Aside from the potential complications of medication and bed rest, hospitalized patients experience increased hazards as a result of diagnostic and therapeutic procedures and nosocomial infections. Diagnostic procedures that incorporate contrast media, such as arteriography, cardiac catheterization, or intravenous pyelography, are potentially risky procedures for the elderly because of a higher incidence of contrast-induced renal disease in the aged kidney. Elderly patients with diabetes mellitus and dehydration have an even greater risk of developing contrast-induced renal disease. Hospitalized elderly patients are also at high risk of developing virulent nosocomial infections as a result of potential immunosuppression related to their underlying illness as well as age-related changes in immune function. Microorganisms such as *Staphylococcus* or Gram-negative rods rapidly colonize the oropharynx, skin, or urinary tract and predispose the elderly to hospital-acquired pneumonias, urinary tract infections, and wound infections. Consider every attempt to avoid hospitalization for the elderly patient in your management approach. Specialized geriatric assessment hospital units have been shown to be more effective for the management of elderly patients requiring admission to an acute care facility. Management is provided by a multidisciplinary team of health care professionals specially trained in the care of the elderly patient. Beneficial outcomes have included:

Decrease in medication use
Avoidance of nursing home placement
Improvement in functional status
Improved survival rate

More research is needed to determine the effectiveness of geriatric assessment units in acute care hospitals.[9]

GERIATRICS AND OSTEOPATHIC MEDICINE

The past few decades have seen enormous growth and development of the discipline of geriatric medicine in the United States. This has been an outgrowth of recognized unmet needs of the elderly within our health care system. Osteopathic principles and practice mesh nicely with basic concepts of geriatric medicine and offer osteopathic medicine a unique role in the growth and development of geriatrics in this country.

Incorporation of manipulative treatment into the clinical care of the elderly is an important modality of treatment that osteopathic physicians have as part of their therapeutic approach. Physicians often approach these patients with the use of pharmacologic treatment and fail to incorporate other modalities of treatment such as physical therapy or manipulative treatment. Medications such as nonsteroidal antiinflammatory agents frequently have adverse effects on the elderly, heightening the importance of including nonpharmacologic means of treatment. Manipulative techniques are beneficial to the elderly; as with any therapeutic modality, there might be a need to adjust certain approaches to fit the special needs of the elderly patient. The increased frequency of osteoporosis and decline in bone mineral density with age should dampen one's use of certain high-thrust, high-velocity techniques in the elderly. Soft tissue manipulation using muscle- and fascia-stretching techniques is particularly effective for many of the musculoskeletal complaints of the elderly.

Range of motion, respiratory, muscle energy, and craniosacral techniques are all beneficial approaches for geriatric patients. The craniosacral technique, CV4 compression, is an invaluable manipulative treatment for the elderly that has a multisystem effect and also helps patients relax. Although osteopathic manipulative treatment is a valuable tool in the management of geriatric patients, controlled, randomized studies are needed to document its efficacy and expand its acceptance.[25]

CONCLUSION

Many principles that have guided osteopathic medicine for decades are the same principles that are at the heart of geriatric medicine. The whole-person approach of osteopathic medicine is essential to geriatric care and involves a multidisciplinary, multidimensional approach to the evaluation and management of the elderly that considers the medical, socioeconomic, psychological, and functional aspects of the patient. The primary care setting is the best forum in which to implement this comprehensive care program. Primary care, stressing health maintenance, has been a true strength of osteopathic medicine and is vital to holistic geriatric care. The integral relationship of structure to function has been at the core of osteopathic medicine and is epitomized in the philosophy of geriatric medicine that has as its goal the maintenance of function. Osteopathic physicians are uniquely qualified to meet the health care needs of the elderly.

REFERENCES

1. Butler RN. Geriatrics and internal medicine. *Ann Intern Med.* 1979; 91:903–908.
2. Schneider EL, Guralnik JM. The aging of America. *JAMA.* 1990; 263(17):2335–2340.
3. Warner HR, Butler RN, Schneider EL. *Modern Biological Theories of Aging.* New York, NY: Raven Press; 1987.
4. Hayflick L. *How and Why We Age.* New York, NY: Ballantine Books; 1994.
5. Kenney A. *Physiology of Aging.* Chicago, Ill: Year Book Medical Publishers Inc; 1989.
6. National Institutes of Health. *Geriatric Assessment Methods for Clinical Decision-Making.* National Institutes of Health Consensus Development Conference Statement. Bethesda, Md: US Department and Health and Human Services. Public Health Service; October 1987;6(23).
7. Cavalieri TA, Chopra A, Gray-Miceli D, Shreve S, Waxman H, Forman L. Geriatric assessment teams in nursing homes: do they work? *JAOA.* December 1993;93(12).
8. Cavalieri TA, Chopra A, Bryman P. When outside the norm is normal: interpreting lab data in the aged. *Geriatrics.* May 1992; 47(5):66–70.
9. Kane R, Ouslander J, Abrass I. *Essentials of Clinical Geriatrics.* New York, NY: McGraw-Hill Co; 1989.
10. Kane RA, Kane RL. Assessing the Elderly: *A Practical Guide to Measurement.* Lexington, Mass: Lexington Books; 1981:46–49.
11. Schor EL, Lerner DJ, Malspeis S. Physician's assessment of functional health status and well-being. The patients' perspective. *Arch Intern Med.* 1995;155(3):309–314.
12. Folstein MJ, Folstein S, McHugh PR. Mini-Mental State: a practical method for grading the cognitive state of patients for the clinician. *J Psychiatr Res.* 1975;12:189–198.
13. Yeasavage JA, Brink TL. Development and validation of a geriatric depression screening scale: a preliminary report. *J Psychiatr Res.* 1983; 17(1):37–49.
14. Diagnostic and Statistical Manual of Mental Disorders. DSMV-IV. 4th ed. Washington, DC: The American Psychiatric Association; 1994.
15. Cavalieri TA. Acute confusional states in the geriatric population. *JAOA.* 1984;83(11):801–805.
16. Barry PP, Moskowitz MA. The diagnosis of reversible dementia in the elderly. *Arch Intern Med.* 1988;148:1914–1917.

17. Cain T, Jurivich DA. Primary care guidelines for the evaluation of confusion in the elderly. *JAOA.* 1994;94(7):601–605.

18. Davis KL, Thal LJ. A double blind placebo-controlled multicenter study of tacrine for Alzheimer's disease. *New Engl J Med.* 1992;337:1253–1259.

19. Katzman R. Alzheimer's disease. *New Engl J Med.* 1986;314(15):964–973.

20. Baumann MM, Jurivich DA. Office management of urinary incontinence: an algorithmic approach. *JAOA.* 1994;94(7):606–609.

21. Ouslander J. Urinary incontinence. *Clin Geriatr Med.* 1986;2(4):639–885.

22. Cavalieri TA, Gray-Miceli D. Evaluating and preventing falls among the elderly population. *JAOA.* 1994;94(7):610–614.

23. Tinetti ME, Baker DL, McAvary G, Claus EG, Garrett P, Gottschalk M, Koch ML, Trainor K, Horwitz R. A multifactorial interaction to reduce the risk of falling among elderly people living in the community. *New Engl J Med.* 1994;331(13):821–827.

24. Hazzard WR, Andres R, Bierman EL, Blass JP. *Principles of Geriatric Medicine and Gerontology.* Baskerville, NY: McGraw-Hill Information Services Company; 1990;7(3):115–119.

25. Dodson D. Manipulative therapy for the geriatric patient. *Osteopath Ann.* 1979;7(3):115–119.

24. Sports Medicine

THOMAS WESLEY ALLEN

Regular vigorous physical exercise is the cornerstone of health and the key to longevity.

Key Concepts

- **Special needs and unique attitudes of athletes**
- **Sports medicine physician's goal and skills**
- **Osteopathic approach to sports medicine**
- **Diagnosis and treatment of sports injuries**

During the 1970s and 1980s, the number of Americans engaging in regular vigorous physical activity increased. Adults reporting regular physical activity increased from 35% in 1978 to 41% in 1990.[1] However, the earlier "fitness boom" has not continued, and in 1991, fewer than 40% of adult Americans reported being physically active.[2] Van Camp was recently quoted as saying that only 22% of Americans were exercising enough to aid their health.[3]

At the same time, evidence of the beneficial effects of exercise in the maintenance of health and in the prevention of disease, especially coronary artery disease, continues to accumulate.[4–7] Furthermore, a reversal of coronary artery narrowing with a program of exercise, low-fat diet, and stress management has been observed[8] (see also Chapter 26, Cardiology). We also now recognize the benefits of exercise in the treatment of the following (see Chapter 16, Exercise, Fitness, and Health):

Hypertension
Obesity
Diabetes
Chronic pulmonary disease
Psychological disorders

The evidence of the positive contribution of exercise in the prevention and treatment of such a variety of common disorders provides the physician—especially the primary physician—with a powerful tool in the approach to the care of patients.

While most Americans remain sedentary, despite the clear evidence of the beneficial health effects of physical activity, millions exercise either regularly or sporadically. Patients with sports injuries are frequently ill-informed despite the wealth of information available to them. Regardless of the primary physician's interest in sports, he or she must be knowledgeable in the field of sports medicine to aid the athlete-patient in recovery and prevention of injuries.

The interest in exercise coupled with exercise-related stresses and demands on the physically active has led to a new area of interest and clinical practice: *sports medicine.* Sports medicine has evolved into a distinct medical specialty with an extensive and well-developed body of knowledge.

The American Osteopathic Academy of Sports Medicine describes sports medicine as *"that branch of the healing arts profession that utilizes a holistic, comprehensive team approach to the prevention, diagnosis, and adequate management of sport and exercise-related injuries, disorders, dysfunctions and disease processes."*

Ryan has noted that no other field of medicine involves so many related disciplines or has experienced such phenomenal growth in the past 30 years as sports medicine.[9]

HISTORY

Although the term "sports medicine" cannot be found in the literature until well into the 20th century,[9] physicians have been caring for athletes since ancient times. Greek physicians supervised the training and care of Olympic competitors: Herodicus (circa 400 BC), the teacher of Hippocrates, is the most well-known.

Galen (2nd century AD), who served as physician to the gladiators of Rome, has been called the first team physician. His contributions to the understanding of exercise physiology and his writings influenced the practice of medicine for more than a millennium.

When A.T. Still, the founder of the osteopathic medical profession, developed his revolutionary philosophy of medical care in the mid-19th century, he borrowed from some of the neglected philosophies of the past and made new applications to the practice of medicine of his day. The Hippocratic approach, with its central focus on body unity, was the key to Still's philosophy. He identified the musculoskeletal system as an essential element in the maintenance of health.

Coincident with Still's growing reputation as one highly skilled in providing relief for sprains, strains, and dislocations, professional and collegiate sports were becoming more popular. Many injured athletes came to Kirksville to be treated by Still; thus he became known as a pioneer in sports medicine.[10] Still was convinced of the importance of regular exercise in the maintenance of health and in the prevention of disease. Realizing that his students needed exercise, he recommended that they be encouraged to participate in athletic competition. For several years, football, baseball, and basketball teams represented the Kirksville College of Osteopathic Medicine in competition against major universities throughout the United States. Many of the graduates gained experience in treating athletic injuries while students at Kirksville and later became team doctors for colleges, high schools, and local teams, as osteopathic physicians do today.

SPECIAL NEEDS AND UNIQUE ATTITUDES OF ATHLETES

Who is an athlete? Athletes are "people in motion"—they are "dynamic"—they engage in "motion-oriented activity." Whether one participates in a team sport, an individual sport, or other physical activity, the key factor is motion. A physically active person is an athlete. As the late cardiologist and marathoner George Sheehan wrote, *"everyone is an athlete—only some of us are in training and some are not."*[11]

Athletes are usually highly motivated, healthy people. Their commitment to exercise stems from any number of motivating factors, including:

Maintenance of health
Prevention of disease
Body image
Weight control
Stress release or modulation
The "high" of competition

Their commitment can also be an overriding consideration in the treatment and rehabilitation of illness and injury. Illness or injury that might be minor or insignificant in a sedentary non-athlete can be a significant disability in the athlete. Remember that the athlete's interpretation of the problem is a critical factor for maximizing the recovery.

In addition, an injured athlete is probably at risk for reinjury. The same factors that contributed to the original injury will likely be present when the athlete resumes activity. Rehabilitation must focus not only on treatment of the current injury but also on progressive reconditioning and neuromuscular reeducation to prevent future injury. Also, cardiovascular and cardiopulmonary reconditioning must be addressed to prevent disuse if the athlete must be inactive a significant time during repair.

SPORTS MEDICINE PHYSICIAN

The sports medicine physician's goal is to help return the athlete to his or her pre-injury or pre-illness performance capacity. The sports medicine physician must understand the special importance that the athlete places on physical activity. He or she must understand what occurs during the activity and be able to plan or adjust the athlete's activity level to aid recovery with the goal of returning the athlete to the pre-injury or pre-illness performance. He or she must understand the psychological aspect of injury and illness for the athlete. An effective sports medicine physician will demonstrate an understanding of the special concerns and needs of the athlete and a willingness to be flexible in the therapeutic approach.

The special skills of the effective sports medicine physician are the general knowledge of medicine, the ability to make the diagnosis, familiarity with various therapeutic and rehabilitative approaches, and a knowledge of the sport itself including participation, field conditions, and equipment. The osteopathic physician, equipped with the skills of palpatory diagnosis and manipulative treatment techniques, holds a distinct advantage over physicians who have not developed these skills.

Which medical specialty or concentration is best suited for the practice of sports medicine? I believe that no other physicians are better trained and prepared than osteopathic primary care physicians to deal with the variety of medical and musculoskeletal problems common among athletes.

OSTEOPATHIC APPROACH

Principles

The problems of the athlete are particularly well-suited for osteopathic principles and concepts and their application. The basic tenets of osteopathic philosophy are clear in the approach to the athlete disabled by either illness or injury. One of the principles in osteopathic medicine is that health is based on the natural capacity of the human organism to resist and combat noxious influences in the environment and to compensate for their effects. The body is able to meet with adequate reserve the usual stresses of daily life and the occasional severe stresses imposed by injury or extremes of environment and activity. Osteopathic medicine recognizes that many factors impair this capacity and the natural tendency toward recovery. Among the most important factors are local disturbances of the musculoskeletal system. Athletes, who frequently exercise in temperature extremes and who experience profound physical stress, often sustain musculoskeletal system injuries. Musculoskeletal injuries account for the majority of sports-related problems.

However, since fewer than 5% of the musculoskeletal problems found in athletes require surgical intervention, the osteopathic physician with skills in musculoskeletal diagnosis and manipulative treatment is well-equipped to liberate the body's resources. Manipulative medicine alone or in combination with physical therapy modalities such as electrical stimulation, ultrasound, cryotherapy, etc., is most often the approach of choice.

Case History

The osteopathic physician's approach to the care of the athlete can be illustrated in the following example of shoulder dysfunction. The complaint of shoulder dysfunction, usually pain or a limitation of motion producing altered performance, can follow:

Minor or major physical trauma
Prolonged strain
Dysfunction of related neuromusculoskeletal structures
Viscerosomatic disorders

The diagnosis of the primary cause of shoulder complaints can be complicated because of complex anatomic relationships and the frequent occurrence of diseases and disorders distal to the shoulder that cause shoulder pain and dysfunction.

DIAGNOSIS

A systematic approach begins with determining the nature of the disability and the mechanism of injury:

When did symptoms appear?
Was there associated trauma?
Is there pain, stiffness, or limitation in the range of motion?
Are there contiguous areas (arm, neck, or thorax) of altered function or disability?

The next step is to search for complaints in the cardiac, pulmonary, or gastrointestinal systems because referred pain to the shoulder is often a characteristic symptom of disorders of these systems.

The many thoracoscapular muscles might be primary factors in the patient with shoulder complaints or might be secondarily disturbed by more distant primary pathologic conditions. Evaluate these muscles during the examination. Physicians often have found areas of significant dysfunction when examining areas distant to the painful shoulder. The cervical spine, thoracic spine, upper ribs, and clavicles with their associated muscular and neural structures can be implicated in the painful or dysfunctional shoulder. Perform a complete examination of the musculoskeletal structures not only adjacent to the area of discomfort but also in distant sites as well. Occasionally, the athlete is not aware of the primary area of dysfunction of the initial injury and has focused on a secondary area of dysfunction. A complete examination is essential to sort out the complaint.

The diagnostic approach to the patient with complaints referable to the shoulder must include a thorough and detailed physical examination and an inclusive history based on the interrelation of all body systems. The therapeutic and rehabilitative methods hinge on an accurate diagnosis.

TREATMENT

The first objective is to relieve the athlete's discomfort through appropriate analgesics, temporary immobilization and support, surgical repair, and/or manipulation to safely mobilize restricted areas. The "guarding" that the athlete performs to prevent exacerbating discomfort frequently results in somatic dysfunction of neighboring structures that must be addressed as part of the total care of the patient. The two major goals of manipulation of the shoulder girdle are to restore function and

to prevent motion loss.[12] Several techniques are available to the osteopathic physician, including passive assistive and active resistive applications. The well-known Spencer techniques are often of value.[12–13]

Follow this initial treatment by a detailed plan of rehabilitation, remembering the patient's particular needs and attitude toward the disability. Finally, working with the patient, determine a strategy to avoid or minimize the possibility of recurrence of the disability while maximizing the postdysfunction performance level. This strategy should consider the basic mechanism of the original dysfunction and might involve replacing the original physical activity with another, correcting a contributory structural imbalance, or continuing treatment of viscerosomatic abnormalities.

CONCLUSION

The care of athletes and of the problems associated with physical activity is in the province of the primary care physician who follows osteopathic principles and concepts. The ability to bring all accepted and scientifically validated methods to the care of the athlete is the key to success for both the athlete and the physician.

REFERENCES

1. McGinnis JM, Richmond JB, Brandt EN Jr, et al. Health progress in the United States: results of the 1990 objectives for the nation. *JAMA.* 1992:268(18):2545–2552.
2. Prevalence of sedentary lifestyle: behavioral risk factor surveillance system, United States, 1991. *MMWR.* 1993;42(29):576–579.
3. Roos R. Is Clinton's plan soft on exercise? *Physician Sportsmed.* 1994; 22(2):31–32.
4. Blair SN, Kohl HW III, Paffenbarger RS Jr, et al. Physical fitness and all-cause mortality. A prospective study of healthy men and women. *JAMA.* November 3 1989;262(17):2395–2401.
5. Paffenbarger RS Jr, Hyde RT, Wing AL, et al. A natural history of athleticism and cardiovascular health. *JAMA.* July 27 1984; 252(4):491–495.
6. Paffenbarger RS Jr, Hyde RT, Wing AL, et al. Physical activity, all-cause mortality, and longevity of college alumni. *N Engl J Med.* 1986; 314:605–613.
7. Thompson WG. Exercise and health: fact or hype? *South Med J.* 1994;87(5):567–574.
8. Ornish D, Brown SE, Scherwitz LW, et al. Can lifestyle changes reverse coronary heart disease? The lifestyle heart trial. *Lancet.* 1990; 336:129–133.
9. Ryan AJ, Allman FL, eds. *Sports Medicine.* San Diego, Calif: Academic Press; 1989.
10. Still CE Jr. *Frontier Doctor-Medical Pioneer: The Life and Times of A. T. Still and His Family.* Kirksville, Mo: Thomas Jefferson University Press; 1991.
11. Sheehan G. Sports medicine renaissance. *Physician Sportsmed.* 1990; 18(11):26.
12. DiGiovanna EL, Shiowiotz S. *An Osteopathic Approach to Diagnosis and Treatment.* Philadelphia, Pa: JB Lippincott; 1991.
13. Greenman PE. *Principles of Manual Medicine.* Baltimore, Md: Williams & Wilkins; 1989.

25. Ear, Nose, and Throat

HARRIET H. SHAW AND MICHAEL B. SHAW

Key Concepts

- **Structures and functions of the ear, nose, and throat (ENT) region**

- **Pathophysiology, diagnosis, and treatment options for common ENT problems seen in primary care settings, including sinusitis, allergic rhinitis, otitis media, and acute tonsillitis and pharyngitis**

- **The osteopathic approach to the diagnosis and treatment of ENT problems**

The ears, nose, and throat are not an autonomous system but rather are parts of at least three different systems. They are grouped together because they share several factors. These factors include:

Having respiratory mucosal lining
Containing organs of special senses
Having internal connections to each other
Being located in the head and neck

The nose, paranasal sinuses, mouth, and throat all function as part of the respiratory system. They are passageways for inspired and expired air. In addition, the nose and paranasal sinuses play an important role in conditioning and filtering inspired air. Olfaction is the special sense of the nose. The special senses of hearing and balance are housed in the ears. The mouth and throat function as part of the digestive system in chewing, swallowing, and in the special sense of taste. The throat and mouth also aid in speech.

Because of the diverse nature of this area, numerous and different clinical problems are associated with treating the ears, nose, and throat. Problems range from infectious processes, to vertigo, to difficulty swallowing or talking. Preventing and treating many of these problems requires an appreciation of these physiologic functions and anatomic relationships.

Several problems of the ENT are commonly encountered in the primary care setting. These include:

Allergic rhinitis
Sinusitis
Otitis
Tonsillitis

Treating this area from an osteopathic perspective uses the basic concepts of the structure–function relationship and the body's inherent healing capacity. In this chapter, the common problems noted above will serve as examples of how to approach the ENT patient osteopathically.

The respiratory system demonstrates the remarkable health maintenance systems within the body. With an understanding and appreciation of normal anatomy and function, the physician can effectively treat ENT patients to enhance the ability for recovery and the natural resistance to disease. It is the osteopathic physician's responsibility to consider the specific needs of the patient and to design a management plan de-emphasizing intervention in favor of promoting the body's ability to regulate itself toward health.

Patient education plays an important role in treatment and prevention of ENT problems. Increasing patients' awareness of medication abuse, pollutants, humidification, and allergies is a critical aspect of management.

Osteopathic manipulative treatment (OMT) is used empirically to treat ENT problems commonly encountered in primary care.[1–3] This treatment is based on the musculoskeletal system's impact on circulatory flow to and from all the tissues of the body, and its effects on physiologic function by way of the autonomic nervous system. Studies show that the physiologic function of various organs is affected by noxious somatic afferent stimulation.[4–5] Clinical experience shows that incorporating musculoskeletal treatment in the management of ENT patients improves recovery time and reduces the incidence of recurrence and complications.[6–7]

Medical intervention is most beneficial when the natural forces at work to maintain homeostasis are considered. Medications, surgery, and allergy desensitization can be most effective when based on specific diagnoses and combined with patient education and appropriate musculoskeletal treatment.

A general approach to the patient with a problem involving the ears, nose, or throat would include consideration of the following:

1. Anatomy of the area
2. Nervous supply
3. Venous and lymphatic drainage
4. Arterial supply
5. Built-in mechanisms for health maintenance
6. Predisposing factors for infection or disease

NOSE AND PARANASAL SINUSES

Anatomy and Physiology

The nose, an organ of respiration and olfaction, functions to filter, humidify, and regulate the temperature of inspired air.

The paranasal sinuses in the maxillary, frontal, sphenoid, and ethmoid bones are air-filled extensions of the nasal cavities and serve similar functions to that of the nose. Regardless of the temperature of outside air, the temperature of inspired air is changed to approximate body temperature during its passage through the nose. Similar changes are made in moisture content of inspired air so that it reaches the trachea at almost ambient humidity.

The superior, middle, and inferior turbinates, or conchae, are elevations on the lateral nasal walls. Heavily endowed with blood vessels, they help in the temperature control of inspired air. The nose provides a filter for particulate matter in the air. Much of the smoke, dust, pollens, and bacteria that one inhales is trapped and removed before the air enters the lungs. The nasal septum and the turbinates help create an airflow pattern in the nose that maximizes the air conditioning function of the nose and paranasal sinuses.

The nasal cavity and paranasal sinuses are covered by a pseudostratified, columnar, ciliated epithelium. Goblet cells and submucosal glands contribute to the mucus blanket that covers and protects the epithelium. This mucus film has two layers. The cilia beat within the inner, serous (sol phase) layer. The outer, more viscous (gel phase) layer is moved by the synchronized ciliary action. Secretions from the sinuses pass into the nasal cavity through the various ostia or openings in the sinuses. The outer layer of mucus traps dust and other particles, moving them through the ostia into the nasal cavity, where mucus is transported into the nasopharynx and swallowed. The process is referred to as mucociliary clearance. Pathogens are incorporated into the cells of the mucosa or destroyed by lysozymes and secretory immunoglobulin A (IgA) within the mucus.

The normal function of the paranasal sinuses depends on the effectiveness of mucociliary clearance. There are two basic drainage patterns of the sinuses. The anterior ethmoid, frontal, and maxillary sinuses are part of the anterior pattern draining to the ostiomeatal unit under the middle turbinate. The posterior ethmoid and sphenoid sinuses are in the posterior pattern draining to the sphenoethmoid recess (Fig. 25.1). The ostiomeatal unit is located superior to much of the maxillary sinus, making it necessary to actively move the mucus blanket "uphill" for effective drainage. This nondependent drainage situation exists with the sphenoid and, in some instances, with the ethmoid sinus as well. Conditions that create an obstruction to the normal flow of air and mucus predispose the sinuses to disease. They are described in standard references.

A proper balance of the autonomic nervous system is necessary for healthy mucosal function. The sympathetic nervous system regulates blood supply to the nasal mucosa. The sympathetic supply arises as the internal carotid plexus, which derives postganglionic fibers from the superior cervical ganglia. Fibers reach the pterygopalatine ganglion via the deep petrosal nerve, which joins the greater petrosal nerve to form the nerve of the pterygoid canal. Unopposed sympathetic stimulation leads to vasoconstriction accompanied by drying of the mucosa. Nasal mucus production is regulated predominantly by

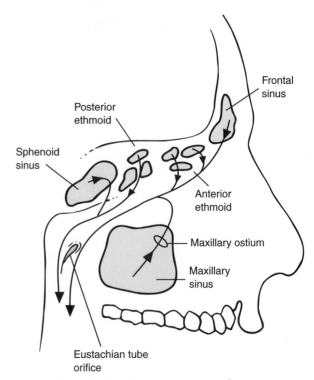

Figure 25.1. Drainage patterns of sinuses.

parasympathetic nerve fibers, but sympathetic fibers also reach the glands. Stimulation of parasympathetic fibers generally increases goblet cell secretions (Fig. 25.2).

The parasympathetic, secretomotor innervation comes from the facial nerve (cranial nerve VII), synapsing in the pterygopalatine ganglion. Tobacco smoke and other pollutants adversely affect mucus flow by inactivating cilia.[8] The quantity and composition of the mucus is influenced by such various factors as:

Temperature
Humidity
Oxygen concentration
Pollution
Irritants

Neuromediators, such as substance P, also appear to influence the function of the mucosal glands.[9]

Pathophysiology

Inflammation is a common cause of disease in the nose and paranasal sinuses (Table 25.1). Any of the following can initiate the inflammatory process:

Infections (viral or bacterial)
Allergy (food or inhalants)
Irritants (chemical or mechanical)

Inflammation is accompanied by swelling of the mucosa, excessive mucus production, and decreased ciliary motility. Symptoms include:

Obstructed breathing
Pain
Rhinorrhea
Epistaxis

Prolonged inflammation predisposes to recurrent infections and changes, such as thickening of the mucous membranes. These conditions impede the normal airflow and functioning of the mucosa.

Nasal obstruction and abnormal airflow can be the result of venous and lymphatic congestion causing engorgement of the mucosa, such as occurs with allergic rhinitis or upper respiratory infections. Structural defects such as polyps or a deviated

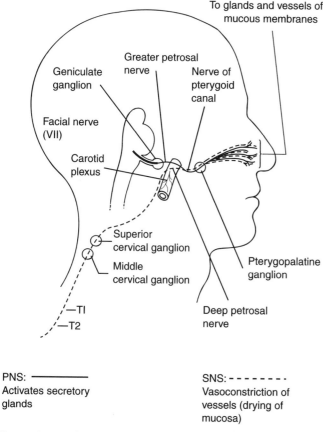

PNS: ————
Activates secretory glands

SNS: - - - - - - -
Vasoconstriction of vessels (drying of mucosa)

Figure 25.2. Autonomic nerve supply to glands and vessels of nasal and paranasal mucous membranes. PNS, parasympathetic nervous system; SNS, sympathetic nervous system.

Table 25.1
Common Disorders of the Nose and Paranasal Sinuses

Epistaxis	Deviated nasal septum
Nasal fractures	Unilateral nasal discharge
Acute rhinitis	foreign body
Allergic rhinitis	choanal atresia
Nonallergic vasomotor rhinitis	malignancy
Atrophic rhinitis	head trauma
Polyposis	Sinusitis

septum can also cause obstruction or abnormal airflow. When airflow patterns are disturbed, there is loss of normal function and the patient experiences discomfort. Changes in the mucosa and in airflow patterns have an adverse effect on the cleaning, humidifying, and temperature control of the air, as well as on the oxygen concentration in the sinuses. Sinusitis can result from prolonged derangement of airflow.

Obstructions resulting from mucosal changes are responsive to activities that alter sympathetic nerve discharge. Vigorous physical exercise improves nasal function for up to 60 minutes by reducing nasal airflow resistance and nasal blood flow.[10] One study showed that osteopathic manipulation resulted in significant improvement of nasal function as measured by nasal pressure curves in a group of 12 subjects serving as their own controls.[11] Addressing somatic dysfunction with osteopathic manipulation adds to patient comfort and aids the normal healing process.[6-7] Chronic conditions and progression of disease can be prevented by decreasing congestion and promoting good airflow.

Sinusitis

DIAGNOSIS

Sinusitis is one of the common manifestations of inflammation and obstruction in the upper respiratory tract. Patients often present with the following signs and symptoms:

Nasal congestion
Pain in the face or head
A feeling of fullness around the eyes
Occasional fever
A foul taste or smell
Postnasal drainage
Fatigue

Physical examination reveals tenderness to percussion over the sinuses. Nasal mucosa is often red and congested with drainage, either clear or purulent. Structural abnormalities such as septal deviation or hypertrophied turbinates are sometimes noted. Transillumination of the sinuses can reveal decreased light transmission, but this is not a definitive test. Edema and tenderness are frequently evident in the periorbital area. Numerous authors describe cervical soft tissue hypertonia with varying degrees of motion dysfunction.[1,12-13] Localized, small areas of tenderness and tissue tension have been noted. These correspond to Chapman's reflex points in the suboccipital area and inferior to the clavicle over the first rib.[14] Various other somatic dysfunctions occur that are unique to the individual patient.

Computerized tomography (CT) of the sinuses is replacing standard x-ray films for diagnosing sinusitis. CT is useful in identifying fluid levels and thickening of the mucosal lining. In cases of recurrent sinusitis, CT can delineate an anatomic blockage at the ostiomeatal complex that suggests the need for functional endoscopic surgery.

Chronic sinusitis can develop if the cause of inflammation is not removed. Steps must be taken to restore conditions that favor good physiologic function. It is important for the physician to determine whether infectious agents, allergens, or irritants are the primary cause. Local structural deformities causing poor aeration of the sinuses can predispose the patient to persistent infection. Decreased venous and lymphatic return can contribute to continued congestion and poor healing.

TREATMENT

Treatment falls under several categories:

Patient instruction and participation
Musculoskeletal
Medical
Surgical

First, determine the underlying pathophysiologic process, then tailor management in these four areas to the patient's particular needs.

In all cases, promoting mucociliary clearance is essential to the overall treatment and prevention of complications. Instruct patients to drink warm, clear fluids to hydrate the mucous membranes and increase mucociliary clearance.[10] Milk is believed to thicken secretions and is not recommended. No controlled clinical trials of antihistamines in sinusitis exist, nor is histamine known to play a role in this disease.[10] Consider antihistamine side effects of overdrying the mucosa and slowing of ciliary motion before using these medications. For patients with concomitant allergic disease, the availability of non-anticholinergic antihistamines, such as astemizole and terfenadine, has made it possible to avoid some of these complications. Mucoactive agents, such as guaifensin, hypertonic saline, and saturated solution of potassium iodide (SSKI), that alter the character, production, or movement of mucus can be helpful.[10]

When medications are used, select them for specific reasons. Treat inflammation resulting from infection with appropriate antibiotics. The most common pathogens involved in sinusitis are *Streptococcus pneumoniae, Haemophilus influenzae,* and *Moraxella catarrhalis.* In chronic sinusitis, *Staphylococcus aureus* is also encountered. Oral decongestants can be helpful when congestion and swelling are significant. Topical decongestants are often overused and lead to rebound swelling of the mucosa, known as rhinitis medicamentosa; therefore, limit their use.

The rationale for the use of OMT in sinus disease is to affect myofascial constraint on venous and lymphatic flow and to alter somatovisceral reflexes to the sinuses. Muscle activity is a recognized mechanism of increasing lymphatic flow. OMT to the neck, specifically those techniques involving muscle action (such as muscle energy and myofascial techniques), should contribute to increased lymphatic flow from the head. The expected result would be reduced swelling of the sinus mucosa. Use direct and indirect pressure techniques over the sinuses and sphenopalatine ganglion for assisting drainage of the sinuses.[15] If observed somatovisceral reflexes[4–5] also occur in the paranasal sinuses, accentuated somatic stimuli associated with somatic dysfunction of cervical and upper thoracic areas could impact the sympathetic vasomotor tone to the sinus area. One

of the goals of OMT in this area is to improve blood flow by altering the somatic component of this somatovisceral reflex.

Chemical irritants also cause inflammation of the respiratory mucosa. Tobacco smoke is the most prevalent irritant. Smokers suffer from frequent inflammatory conditions of the nose and paranasal sinuses. Children living in a home in which tobacco smoke is present are at higher risk of developing respiratory disorders.[16] Patient education is essential and often needs to be on-going. Judicious use of nicotine supplements and smoking cessation programs help some patients. Take a history to identify patients with hypersensitivity or overexposure to common chemicals such as formaldehyde and petroleum products. Increasing awareness of potential exposure is often sufficient treatment. Some cases, however, require substantial lifestyle and occupation changes.

An obstruction might exist as a result of local structural abnormalities. Evaluate the obstruction with a physical examination and, possibly, with further diagnostic tests (CT and endoscopy). In the presence of structural abnormalities such as deviated septum, nasal polyps, or enlarged turbinates, the patient might need surgery if conservative therapy fails to control recurrent infections.

Allergic Rhinitis

DIAGNOSIS

Symptoms of rhinorrhea, sneezing, itchy eyes, and watery eyes are associated with allergic rhinitis. This condition usually shows seasonal variation and recurrence. It is characterized in the physical examination by engorgement of the turbinates, which appear pale or violaceous rather than erythematous as in viral rhinitis. Nasal polyps are sometimes present and appear as yellowish boggy masses of mucosa. Signs of chronic rhinorrhea and postnasal drainage are also commonly seen.

TREATMENT

Inflammation as a result of allergy, associated with allergic rhinitis, can be treated with:

Antihistamines
Steroids (inhaled or systemic)
Cromolyn sodium
Hydration
Manipulative techniques that aid circulation

Antihistamines can counter the inflammation and vasomotor symptoms associated with allergic disease. Their anticholinergic side effects, particularly mucosal drying, can complicate the treatment. Many patients cannot tolerate the drowsiness associated with antihistamine use. Selective H_1 antihistamines (non-anticholinergic) minimize these side effects and offer a safer option for treating the allergic component of ENT problems.[10]

Inhaled steroids reduce local inflammation and associated symptoms. They are indicated for preventing recurrence of nasal polyps as well. They require 3 days to 2 weeks of regular use for symptomatic improvement to be apparent. Reserve systemic steroids for severe and/or resistant cases, and use them cautiously. Sodium cromoglycate (cromolyn sodium) serves as a mast cell stabilizer and has a suppressive effect on other inflammatory cells. It is best used prophylactically for allergic rhinitis. It also requires regular use for 1–2 weeks before benefits appear.[17]

To be effective and lasting, treatment must address the specific allergic cause. Responsible allergens can be foods or inhalants of the following types:

Dusts
Pollens
Molds
Animal danders

Take a history to determine the offending allergens. Year-round symptoms that are worse indoors suggest animal dander, dust, or dust mite allergy. Pollens are most common in the spring, grasses in the summer, and ragweed in late summer and fall. Often, allergy testing and elimination diets are necessary for specific diagnosis and treatment. Environmental control, particularly for dust, molds, and animal danders, is important in treating ENT disease with an allergic cause and requires educating and encouraging the patient, who could become discouraged by the need for lifestyle changes.

EARS

Anatomy and Physiology

The ear is a complex organ of hearing and balance. The temporal bone houses or provides attachment for all parts of the ear. The external ear consists of the pinna and external meatus. The pinna serves to collect and localize sound. The meatus is an air-filled tube through which sound waves travel to reach the middle ear.

The middle ear contains the tympanic membrane, separating the external from the internal ear, and the three bones, or ossicles—malleus, incus, and stapes. The middle ear is air-filled and transmits sound from an air media to the liquid media of the inner ear. It is lined by ciliated, respiratory mucosa. The inner ear consists of the liquid-filled cochlea for auditory sense and the vestibular system for the sense of equilibrium.

Connecting the middle ear to the nasopharynx is the auditory or eustachian tube, also lined by respiratory mucosa. The lateral one-third of the eustachian tube lies in the temporal bone, while the medial two-thirds is cartilaginous, opening only with swallowing or yawning. Air enters or leaves the middle ear cavity through this tube, providing balanced pressure between the atmosphere and middle ear. Swelling of the mucosa or hyperplasia of the adenoids causes obstruction that blocks the connection, resulting in poor functioning of the auditory system. Fluid then accumulates in the middle ear, and infection sets in. Children are often more susceptible than are adults to middle ear infections. Their eustachian tubes are

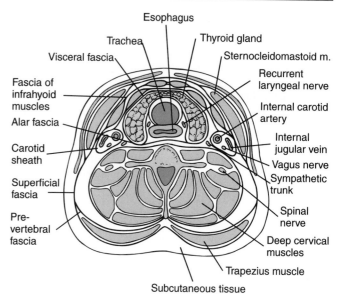

Figure 25.3. Cross-section of neck showing fascial layers.

Table 25.2
Common Disorders of the Ear

Hearing loss
  sensorineural
  conductive
External canal obstruction
  impacted cerumen
  exostoses/chondromas
  foreign bodies
External otitis
  bacterial
  fungal
	Otitis media
	  acute
	  with effusion
	Mastoiditis
	Tinnitus
	Vertigo and dizziness

shorter and more horizontal, and the supporting tensor veli palatini muscle is less efficient than in adults.

The cervical fascia contain the blood vessels and lymphatics supplying all the structures in the head (Fig. 25.3). The deep cervical lymph nodes lie in the reflection of the cervical fascia. The prevertebral fascia that invests many of the muscles of the neck lies over the sympathetic chain. The superficial lymphatics as well as the external jugular vein pierce the superficial fascia as they pass to join deeper structures. Myofascial structures have intimate relationships to the blood vessels, lymphatics, and ganglia serving the ear.[18] The influence of musculoskeletal manipulation in the treatment of ear problems is believed to exert some of its effect through these relationships.[1,15,19]

Pathophysiology

The ear is subject to numerous types of disorders involving the external, middle, or inner ear (Table 25.2). It can be affected by:

Infections
Inflammation
Neurologic disorders
Vascular problems

Pain, hearing loss, vertigo, and tinnitus are associated with these processes. Because the sensory innervation to the ear is derived from the trigeminal, facial, glossopharyngeal, vagal, and upper cervical nerves, otalgia is frequently a referred pain from other areas of the head and neck. Temporomandibular joint dysfunction and cervical dysfunction are common causes of ear pain.

The external ear is subject to infections, especially if persistently exposed to a moist environment. Infection or neurologic or vascular impairment can disturb the vestibular function of the inner ear. Hearing loss can result from various disturbances in the middle ear or from neurologic deficits. Chronic exposure to loud noise contributes to hearing loss (sensorineural) by traumatic damage to the receptors in the cochlea. Infectious and inflammatory processes in the eustachian tube and middle ear commonly cause hearing loss and ear pain.

Upper respiratory infections and allergy, with mucosal inflammation and lymphoid hyperplasia, can lead to eustachian tube dysfunction. Persistent obstruction of the eustachian tube pressure-equalizing system results in increasing negative pressure and decreased ventilation in the middle ear. Under these conditions, nasopharyngeal secretions can be aspirated into the middle ear, and drainage is impaired. The lowered PaO_2 impedes granulocyte formation, and bacterial colonization frequently results. Factors such as enlarged adenoids can aggravate the pooling of secretions in the middle ear. Reflux of nasopharyngeal contents into the middle ear is more likely to happen when swallowing occurs in the supine position. Bottle feeding has been associated with increased incidence of otitis media (infection of the middle ear), but evidence does not seem to warrant avoidance of bottle feeding.[20] There is evidence that attendance at day-care programs and exposure to tobacco smoke increase the risk of middle ear infections.[21]

Middle ear effusion can accompany acute infections and persist over several weeks or months. It is usually associated with hearing loss and, when present for extended periods, can lead to delays in receptive and expressive language development.[22]

Otitis Media

DIAGNOSIS

Otitis media is among the most common childhood diseases encountered in primary care. The incidence might be increasing as a result of larger numbers of children attending day-care centers. Acute otitis media often follows an upper respiratory infection. The patient complains of earache, fever, and hearing loss. Small children, unable to communicate these symptoms clearly, might display irritability, insomnia, or tugging at the ear. With the presence of pus in the middle ear, the tympanic membrane appears bulging and erythematous. It has decreased mobility with pneumatic otoscopy.

After the acute infection is resolved, effusion can persist in the middle ear. Patients complain of a painless hearing loss. The tympanic membrane can appear dull, and it is often retracted in chronic cases. Evidence of fluid can be observed in the middle ear as bubbles or as an air-fluid level. These signs are not always present, however, even though there is an effusion.

Eustachian tube dysfunction, often accompanying middle ear disease, is felt as tenderness just below the pinna, near the angle of the jaw. There might also be evidence of inflammation of the mucosa of the nasopharynx along with postnasal drainage in patients with otitis media. Lymphadenopathy and tenderness in the cervical soft tissues are also commonly seen. Cranial dysfunction is often present, particularly involving the temporal bones.[2,23]

TREATMENT

Informing patients and families regarding practices that lead to ear problems is part of total patient care. In the well baby examination, discuss infant feeding and avoidance of bottle feeding in the supine position. Encourage parents to protect their children from passive tobacco smoke.

Views are conflicting regarding treatment of acute otitis media.[24] It is generally held that prolonged hearing loss, especially in certain developmental stages, is detrimental to development of language and, possibly, reading skills. Pay attention to otitis media that becomes chronic or recurrent. Guidelines have been published by the U.S. Department of Health and Human Services for the management of uncomplicated otitis media with effusion in children ages 1 to 3.[20] The recommendations for the first 6 weeks of the condition are observation or oral antibiotics, and environment risk control. At 3 months, if significant hearing loss is present, tympanostomy with tube placement is an option. If the condition has been present for 4–6 six months with hearing loss, tube placement is indicated. According to the report, treatment in this age group should not include decongestants, antihistamines, or oral steroids.

Osteopathic manipulation, such as Galbreath's mandibular drainage, is easily performed. It can provide considerable benefit in reducing the congestion that leads to a chronic condition.[15,19] Swallowing and chewing open the eustachian tube and can be suggested as exercises for patients to help clear middle ear effusion.[25]

Recognizing causes of eustachian tube dysfunction can be critical to the treatment and prevention of otitis media. Allergic manifestations such as red, itchy eyes and persistent clear nasal discharge suggest a need for further allergic workup. Dietary questions regarding food intolerances or infant colic can suggest the influence of food sensitivities. Consider control of the allergic aspect of inflammation; discuss it with the patient or the patient's family.

Enlarged tonsils or adenoids are a cause of poor eustachian

tube drainage. Allergy as well as infection can play a role in the enlargement of these lymphoid organs. If acute bacterial infection is the cause, consider the common pathogens *Streptococcus pneumoniae, Haemophilus influenzae,* and *Streptococcus pyogenes.* Treat appropriately with antibiotics.

Decreasing the edema in and around the eustachian tube creates an environment for healthy function. Several manipulative techniques have been described to specifically address improved lymphatic and venous drainage from the head and neck.[12,15,19] The improved blood flow necessary for healing and for delivery of medications benefits infectious processes. Osteopathic manipulation in the treatment of respiratory infections should include techniques to:

Increase lymphatic flow
Address viscerosomatic and somatovisceral reflexes
Improve thoracic cage motion[26]

THROAT/PHARYNX

Anatomy and Physiology

The pharynx is divided into the:

Nasopharynx, which includes the portion above the soft palate
Oropharynx, from the soft palate to the hyoid bone
Laryngopharynx, from the hyoid bone to the lower border of the cricoid cartilage

The oral cavity lies immediately anterior to the oropharynx. The oral cavity and oropharynx are lined by squamous epithelium, whereas the nasopharynx and the laryngopharynx are lined by pseudostratified, ciliated columnar (respiratory) epithelium. A collection of lymphoid tissue referred to as Waldeyer's throat ring is located in the pharynx and plays an important role in immunity, especially in the first few years of life. The tongue and other structures in the oral cavity have important functions in digestion and speech (Fig. 25.4).

The palatine (faucial) tonsils are masses of lymphoid tissue located on either side of the oropharynx posteriorly. The adenoids (pharyngeal tonsils) are found on the upper and posterior walls of the nasopharynx. The tonsils and adenoids comprise the major portion of the lymphoid tissue of Waldeyer's ring encircling the pharynx. These structures, together with the lingual tonsil—an aggregate of lymph nodules on the posterior aspect of the tongue—and scattered lymphoid nodules beneath the mucous membranes of the pharyngeal wall, are the sites for B- and T-lymphocyte activity. All major classes of immunoglobulins are produced here by the B-lymphocytes, while the T-lymphocytes participate in cell-mediated immunity. With high demands for immune function placed on these lymphoid organs, hyperplasia can occur. Secondary obstruction of airflow through the nasopharynx and eustachian tubes results from significant lymphoid hyperplasia.

Blood supply to the tonsils derives from the external carotid system. Several arterial branches (typically three) go to the tonsils from the facial and lingual arteries. Venous drainage is ac-

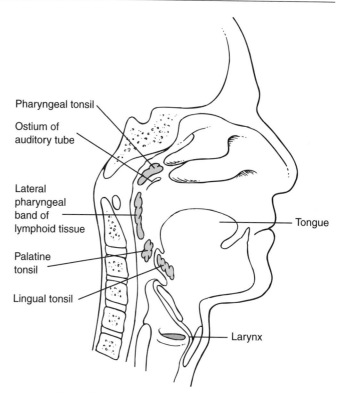

Figure 25.4. Lymphoid tissue in the pharynx.

Table 25.3
Common Disorders of the Throat

Pharyngitis	Thrush
Tonsillitis	Peritonsillar abscess
Epiglottiditis	Larynigitis
Infectious mononucleosis	

complished by a plexus around the tonsillar capsule, draining into the tonsillar branch of the lingual vein and connecting with the pharyngeal plexus.[27] Lymphatic drainage of the tonsils goes to the submandibular nodes to the superficial and upper deep cervical nodes. A node behind the angle of the mandible is especially associated with increased lymphatic activity from the tonsils.[28]

Pathophysiology

A variety of pathologic processes can occur in the pharynx (Table 25.3), but infection is the most common. Group A β-hemolytic streptococci and viruses are the common infectious agents. *Neisseria gonorrhoeae, Mycoplasma,* and *Chlamydia trachomatis* are also possible. Viral infections can cause ulcerative lesions of the tongue, lips, or buccal mucosa. Herpes simplex virus is responsible for herpes labialis or cold sores. Oral candidiasis (thrush) is common in denture wearers, in patients on corticosteroids or broad-spectrum antibiotics, and in diabetics.

It also occurs in those individuals with compromised immune systems, as caused by AIDS, chemotherapy, or local radiation.

Acute Tonsillitis/Pharyngitis

DIAGNOSIS

Sore throat is a common complaint, particularly in children. It is often accompanied by fever, odynophagia, and tender adenopathy. It is difficult to differentiate viral from bacterial infection on inspection. Typically, bacterial infection is exudative. Hoarseness, cough, rhinorrhea, and coryza are more often associated with viral infection. The appropriateness of using certain tests to identify group A β-hemolytic streptococci infections is under study.[29] Latex agglutination antigen tests and solid-phase enzyme immunoassays (ELISA) provide quick, but only moderately sensitive, screens for streptococcal infection. Throat cultures, although more sensitive, take longer for results to become available. All group A β-hemolytic streptococcal pharyngitis patients should be treated to prevent more serious consequences. Individual decisions for diagnosis and treatment should therefore take into account:

The patient's history
The local prevalence of and resistance to streptococcal infections
Potential for compliance
Availability and reliability of the laboratory

The differential diagnosis includes:

Infectious mononucleosis
Diphtheria
Fungal infections
Pharyngeal manifestations of systemic disease

TREATMENT

Group A β-hemolytic streptococcal pharyngitis requires a 10-day course of antibiotics. Penicillin V potassium and cephalosporins are effective. Erythromycin is a reasonable alternative for penicillin-allergic individuals. Ancillary treatment to control symptoms and make the patient more comfortable include:

Analgesics
Antiinflammatory agents
Salt water gargling
Osteopathic manipulation

Viral infections require only symptomatic treatment. Osteopathic manipulation to reduce swelling and improve lymphatic flow, probably stimulating the immune response, can particularly help provide symptomatic relief.[7,26]

OSTEOPATHIC APPROACH

The major principles to consider in treating ENT patients in terms of the musculoskeletal component of health and disease are as follows:

1. Assisting venous and lymphatic circulation
2. Promoting arterial flow
3. Normalizing spinal reflexes affecting function of the ear, nose, and throat
4. Relieving pain

The use of musculoskeletal diagnosis and treatment in these patients can aid healing, help the patient feel better, and improve overall resistance to disease.

As a guide, evaluate and treat somatic dysfunctions from central body areas to the periphery. The rationale for treating somatic dysfunction in the upper thoracic and cervical spine is to decrease somatic stimulation in the area of the sympathetic outflow and ganglia supplying the head and neck. Improving venous and lymphatic flow is the rationale for OMT to the cervical and thoracic inlet areas. Attempt to decrease myofascial tension in the areas through which lymphatic and venous vessels pass from the head to where they enter the central circulation at about the level of the first rib. Apply superficial drainage techniques (effleurage) to the face from medial to lateral to decrease tissue congestion in the sinus regions.

The mandibular drainage technique described by William Galbreath[19] is an effective lymphatic drainage procedure for the ear, eustachian tubes, and throat. Chapman's reflexes are small, nodular, tender areas that have been observed in relationship to inflammatory diseases of visceral structures. Used for diagnosis as well as treatment, they are believed to represent viscerosomatic reflexes and have been shown to be responsive to a rotary pressure technique.[14] Lymphatic pump techniques stimulate general lymphatic flow by affecting intrathoracic pressures. The osteopathic literature regarding treatment of infectious disease describes their use.[15,26]

CONCLUSION

In summary, the osteopathic physician can effectively treat ear, nose, and throat problems. Patient education and osteopathic manipulation are important for treatment and prevention of these problems. Medical intervention is most beneficial when the osteopathic physician combines it with education and musculoskeletal treatment.

REFERENCES

1. Blood HA. Infections of the ear, nose and throat. *Osteopath Ann.* 1978;6(11):1–18.
2. Woods DE. Management of ENT problems. *Osteopath Ann.* 1980; 8(5):31–41.
3. Moser RJ. Sinusitis, the effective osteopathic manipulative procedures in the management thereof. *Yearbook of Selected Papers.* Carmel, Calif: Academy of Applied Osteopathy; 1953:15–16.
4. Sato A. Reflex modulation of visceral functions by somatic afferent activity. In: *The Central Connection: Somatovisceral/Viscerosomatic Interaction.* Proceedings of 1989 American Academy of Osteopathy International Symposium. Athens, Ohio: University Classics; 1992:53–72.

5. Sato A, Schmidt RF. The modulation of visceral functions by somatic afferent activity. *Jpn J Physiol.* 1987;37:1–17.

6. Pintal WJ, Kurtz ME. An integrated osteopathic treatment approach in acute otitis media. *JAOA.* 1989;89(9):1139–1141.

7. Schmidt IC. Osteopathic manipulative therapy as a primary factor in the management of upper, middle, and pararespiratory infections. *JAOA.* 1982;81(6):382–388.

8. Wasserman SJ. Ciliary function and disease. *J Allergy Clin Immunol.* 1984;73:17–19.

9. Wagenmann M, Naclerio RM. Anatomic and physiologic considerations in sinusitis. *J Allergy Clin Immunol.* 1992;90:419–423.

10. Zeiger RS. Prospects for ancillary treatment of sinusitis. *J Allergy Clin Immunol.* 1992;90:478–495.

11. Kaluza CL, Sherbin M. The physiologic response of the nose to osteopathic manipulative treatment: preliminary report. *JAOA.* 1983;82(9):654–660.

12. Harakal JH. Manipulative treatment for acute upper-respiratory diseases. *Osteopath Ann.* 1981;9(7):30–37.

13. Hoyt WH. Current concepts in management of sinus disease. *JAOA.* 1990;90(10):913–919.

14. Owens C. An endocrine interpretation of Chapman's reflexes. *Acad Appl Osteopathy.* 1963.

15. Cathie AG. The sino-bronchial syndrome. *Yearbook of Selected Papers.* Fort Worth, Tex: Academy of Applied Osteopathy; 1968:9–11.

16. Charlton A. Children and passive smoking: a review. *J Fam Pract.* 1994;38(3):267–277.

17. Naclerio RM. Allergic rhinitis. *N Engl J Med.* 1991;325(12):860.

18. Greenman PE. Fascial considerations in treatment of the head and neck. *Osteopath Ann.* 1975;3(2):34–42.

19. Galbreath W. Manipulative structural adjustive treatment in middle ear deafness. *JAOA.* 1925;24:741.

20. U.S. Department of Health and Human Services. Managing otitis media with effusion in young children. *Arch Otolaryngol Head & Neck Surg.* 1994;120:793–796.

21. Froom J, Culpepper L. Otitis media in daycare children. A report from the International Primary Care Network. *J Fam Pract.* 1991; 32:289–294.

22. Updike C, Thornburg JD. Reading skills and auditory processing ability in children with chronic otitis media in early childhood. *Ann Otol Rhinol & Laryngol.* 1992;101:530–537.

23. Magoun H. *Osteopathy in the Cranial Field.* Kirksville, Mo: Journal Printing Company; 1976:213–215.

24. Browning G, Bain B. Childhood otalgia: acute otitis media. *Br Med J.* 1990;300:1005–1007.

25. Honjo I, Okazake N. Opening mechanism of the eustachian tube. *Ann Otol Rhinol & Laryngol.* 1980;89(3)(suppl 68, pt 2):25–27.

26. Rumney IC. Osteopathic manipulative treatment of infectious diseases. *Osteopath Ann.* 1974;2:29–33.

27. Krmpotic-Nemanic J, Draf W. *Surgical Anatomy of Head and Neck.* New York, NY: Springer Verlag; 1988.

28. Hollinshead WH. *Anatomy for Surgeons: The Head and Neck.* Philadelphia, Penn: Harper & Row; 1968.

29. Wegner DL, Witte DL. Insensitivity of rapid antigen detection methods and single blood agar plate culture for diagnosing streptococcal pharyngitis. *JAMA.* 1992;267(5):695–697.

26. Cardiology

FELIX J. ROGERS

Key Concepts

- **Components of screening evaluation for heart disease, including history, physical examination, electrocardiogram, and chest x-ray studies**

- **Pathophysiology, natural history, diagnosis, and treatment of ischemic heart disease**

- **Osteopathic approach to coronary heart disease**

- **Pathophysiology, natural history, diagnosis, and treatment of heart failure**

- **Osteopathic approach to heart failure**

Cardiology represents the largest component of internal medicine, and heart disease is the single most important cause of mortality in the United States. Screening for heart disease is an essential component of every evaluation performed by a general practitioner, surgeon, anesthesiologist, or internist. The components of a screening evaluation are the history, physical examination, electrocardiogram (ECG), and chest x-ray film. In this chapter, these components are starting points for the evaluation of patients with ischemic heart disease and congestive heart failure. These two categories represent more than 75% of the cardiac patients that practicing osteopathic physicians see. The pathophysiology of these disease processes is discussed along with the natural history, diagnosis, and therapy. The goal of this chapter is to review the field of cardiology to clarify the application of osteopathic concepts; important subjects such as arrhythmias, valvular heart disease, and congenital heart disease are not discussed.

It is appropriate to consider the cardiovascular system in terms of a modern interpretation of the basic tenets of osteopathic medicine.[1] The heart is well-innervated and participates in a broad range of reflexes,[2–12] including the viscerosomatic reflexes that are a major feature of classical osteopathic theory.

Research in the last two decades demonstrates the complex nature of neural regulation of cardiovascular function and the components of the systemic effects mediated by cardiac receptors. Integration of cardiovascular function and interactive mechanisms with other body systems is modulated by local and systemic neuroeffector, humoral, and immunologic responses.[13–17] Research has shown that these features have clinical significance in congestive heart failure.[18–23] Recent research

in therapy focuses on neuroendocrine modulation through exercise[24–27] and pharmacologic therapy[28–38] as an intermediate outcome, in addition to assessing health-related outcomes such as functional status and mortality.

Coronary artery disease (CAD) provides a clear example of inherent self-regulating and self-healing properties.[39–40] A century ago, the rule of the artery was supreme. The dramatic role of thrombolytic therapy for acute myocardial infarction makes this rule no less true today. The mechanism of atherosclerosis and the regulation of vascular smooth muscle tone are best understood in terms of the natural ability of the human organism to resist and combat harmful influences in the environment. Knowledge of self-regulation and self-healing forces at the arterial and arteriolar level forms the rational basis for the treatment of myocardial infarction, angina pectoris, and congestive heart failure, as discussed in the following sections.

The interrelation of structure and function is often used to establish the rationale for manipulative treatment. When applied to the cardiovascular system, this interrelationship is obvious yet so complex that it defies full explanation. Because this chapter is not intended to be encyclopedic, the reader is encouraged to refer to mechanisms of ventricular hypertrophy,[41–44] ventricular remodeling after myocardial infarction,[45–47] myocyte function in ventricular failure,[48–50] and myocardial and systemic responses to valvular heart disease[51–53] as four areas of modern investigation of this broad concept.

The specific challenges to osteopathic medicine in the field of cardiology are many. The musculoskeletal system manifests subtle changes in response to chronic CAD[54–55] or acute myocardial infarction,[56] which may be detected by a focused palpatory examination. These basic observations give rise to additional questions:

Can palpatory examination be used in a longitudinal manner to learn more about the natural history of patients with CAD?

Will an emphasis on the role of the musculoskeletal system in health and disease contribute to the effective treatment of patients with coronary heart disease or heart failure?

Will the osteopathic physician's traditional role as primary caregiver lead to improved therapy or more effective approaches to the prevention of ischemic heart disease?

CORONARY ARTERY DISEASE

Pathophysiology and Natural History

The pathophysiology of CAD has been investigated extensively on both sides of the Atlantic since the turn of the century. The

Figure 26.1. Natural history of coronary heart disease.

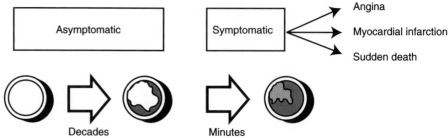

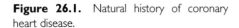

literature now clearly defines the pathophysiologic processes that underlie the development of the atherosclerotic lesion, from its beginnings as a fatty streak to the complex obstructive lesion that characterizes ischemic heart disease.[57–60] Similarly, cross-sectional and longitudinal epidemiologic surveys have clearly identified the role of risk factors in the development of coronary atherosclerosis, which have been summarized in recent reports.[61–62]

One of the most important clinical characteristics of ischemic heart disease is shown in Figure 26.1. Atherosclerosis typically begins as an insidious process, creating the atherosclerotic plaque over a period of decades. In response to some internal or external triggering factor, stable atherosclerotic disease becomes unstable. Of the three symptomatic presentations of the acute coronary syndromes, only angina pectoris does not carry the immediate threat of permanent morbidity or mortality. Atherosclerotic lesions can progress slowly for decades before they become symptomatic. Then, in a matter of moments, the lesions become symptomatic, with three manifestations:

Angina pectoris
Myocardial infarction
Sudden cardiac death

Angina is the only symptomatic presentation of ischemic heart disease in which there is neither permanent morbidity nor mortality, giving the physician the greatest opportunity to do the most good for the patient.

For decades, epidemiologic studies of ischemic heart disease have concentrated on risk factors for coronary atherosclerosis, the early detection of asymptomatic disease, and the role of primary and secondary risk factor modification for the prevention or amelioration of heart disease. Physicians are now calling for an investigation into the triggers that transform the atherosclerotic plaque from an asymptomatic lesion into a symptomatic lesion. The histopathologic events associated with the transformation of stable atheroma into one of the acute coronary syndromes are now well-defined from autopsy, angioscopic, and cardiac catheterization studies. The interrelationship of three vascular mechanisms causing acute myocardial ischemia is shown in Figure 26.2.

Herrick's classic description of coronary thrombosis was based on studies at the beginning of this century.[63] Since then, autopsy studies have defined the intracoronary events associated with acute myocardial infarction and unstable angina. The

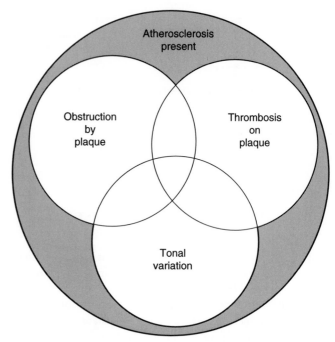

Figure 26.2. Interrelationship of three vascular mechanisms causing acute myocardial ischemia. (Reprinted with permission from Davies MJ. The pathophysiology of coronary atherosclerosis. In: Schlant RC, Alexander RW, eds. *The Heart, Arteries, and Veins.* New York, NY: McGraw-Hill, Inc; 1994.)

current era of studies was launched by the publication of the results of a meticulous autopsy study conducted in England on victims of sudden cardiac death.[40] This study documented the presence of plaque fissure associated with platelet aggregates or thrombus, and validated a prior landmark study on coronary atherothrombosis.[64] These data were later confirmed in studies on a large number of patients in Lithuania.[65] North American interest in this topic was aroused by the studies of patients subjected to cardiac catheterization immediately following acute myocardial infarction.[66] Later, the striking color video photography of intracoronary lesions viewed during angioscopy at the time of coronary bypass graft surgery provided the first view of the coronary arteries of living people,[67] and represented the opportunity to develop a simple yet comprehensive view of the continuum of acute coronary syndromes[39] (Figs. 26.3 and 26.4). The development of a fissure in an ath-

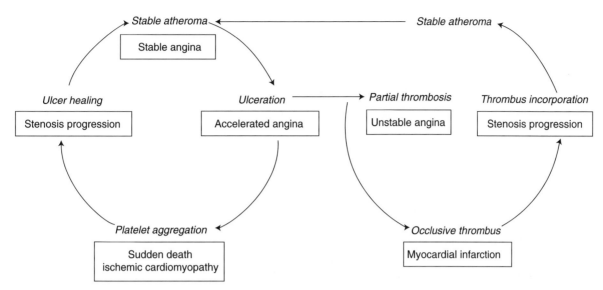

Figure 26.3. Ulceration-thrombosis cycle of coronary artery disease. (Reprinted with permission from Forrester JS, et al. A perspective of coronary disease seen through the arteries of living man. *Circulation.* 1987; 75:505–513.)

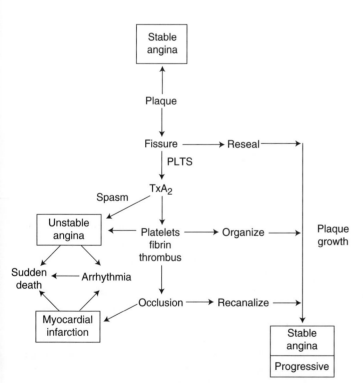

Figure 26.4. Angina (stable and unstable) and infarction clinical pattern and its relationship to vascular pathophysiologic changes. TxA$_2$, thromboxane A$_2$; PLTS, platelets. (Reprinted with permission from Davies MJ, Thomas A. Plaque fissuring—the cause of acute myocardial infarction, sudden ischaemic death and crescendo angina. *Br Heart J.* 1985; 53:363.)

erosclerotic plaque is now seen as common to crescendo angina, myocardial infarction, and sudden ischemic death.[68] The dynamic evolution of coronary atherosclerosis is well-described in clinical terms[59] and in terms of molecular biology.[69]

Despite this rather clear picture of the basic components that characterize the transformation of the coronary atherosclerotic lesion into unstable coronary syndromes, the nature of the triggering factors is incompletely defined. This area of clinical investigation focuses on the events that occur just before the onset of arterial thrombosis. Preinfarction ill health is a phenomenon of poorly defined malaise that precedes myocardial infarction by days, weeks, or months.[70–71] The subsequent demonstration of inflammatory reactions within atherosclerotic lesions with acute myocardial infarction[72] and the demonstration of more specific markers of infectious agents[73–75] raises the question of triggering events in patients with systemic infections.

A definite circadian pattern of onset of myocardial infarction was demonstrated in the Myocardial Infarction Limitation Study.[76] The increase in morning incidence of acute ischemic coronary events has been attributed to an increase in catecholamines and sensitivity of vascular receptors, increasing coronary vasomotor tone, and an increasing myocardial oxygen demand, all of which lower the threshold for ischemia.[77] Other triggering events include mental stress[78] and anger.[79] Although a period of strenuous physical activity is associated with a temporary increase in risk of myocardial infarction,[80] increasing levels of habitual physical activity were associated with progressively lower risk.[81] These data suggest that we have much to learn about the pathophysiology of acute coronary syndromes and would do well to observe carefully the events that occur on a systemic level at the same time that we study the molecular bases of the atherosclerotic lesion.

One view of the natural history of CAD is shown in Figure 26.3. The atherosclerotic lesion undergoes abrupt transformation with the development of plaque fissure and platelet aggregation. In one pathway, this process leads to the development of thrombus formation, which causes rest angina pectoris unless the thrombus is large enough to occlude the vessel and cause myocardial infarction. Coexisting coronary vasospasm may be a factor in initiating or exacerbating these events. If the thrombus occludes blood flow only transiently, a non–Q wave myocardial infarction occurs. If the patient survives this episode, the atherosclerotic lesion heals, progresses to stenosis, and then returns to the prior status of stable atheroma.

In a second pathway, plaque fissure and platelet aggregation leads to unstable angina with exertional chest pain and no rest component. The platelet aggregates may embolize distally, creating either ischemic cardiomyopathy because of repetitive insults or sudden arrhythmic cardiac death because of sudden plugging of an arteriolar vessel. If the patient survives this episode, the body's reparative processes will go from healing the acute coronary lesion, to stenosis progression, and then to stable atheroma.

There are two basic stages of ischemic heart disease. One stage involves stable coronary atherosclerosis, which may be symptomatic or asymptomatic. The second stage involves the unstable acute coronary syndromes. These syndromes include:

Unstable angina (including accelerated or resting angina)
Non–Q wave myocardial infarction
Q wave myocardial infarction
Ischemic sudden cardiac death

These four clinical syndromes are all part of a continuum in which the differentiating feature from a histopathologic standpoint is the size of platelet aggregate/thrombus that is formed at the site of plaque fissure.

The correlation of acute coronary syndromes with histopathologic events in the coronary lumen has led to a study of the endothelium as a key factor in the atherosclerotic process and natural history of patients with coronary disease. Atherosclerosis is far more than the mere accumulation of lipids within blood vessels; it is a disease of living arterial wall. Studies now show that events in the endothelial layer of coronary and other arteries set the stage for atheroma growth well before lesions or stenoses develop.[82] Likewise, angina, myocardial infarction, and sudden cardiac death are more than just downstream events in patients in whom the passive conduits (the epicardial coronary arteries) are plugged by atherosclerotic narrowing.

At the time Andrew Taylor Still formulated the axiom "The rule of the artery is supreme," arterial vessels were believed to be passive conduits for blood flow. Subsequently, vascular tone was thought to be controlled solely by vascular smooth muscle. A more dynamic view of the behavior of healthy and diseased coronary arteries focuses on endothelial function. The endothelium is a regulatory organ that mediates hemostasis, contractility, cellular proliferation, and inflammatory mechanisms in the vessel wall; it has a major role in atherosclerosis.[83]

The endothelium synthesizes several vasodilators and vasoconstricting substances. Endothelial-derived relaxing factor (EDRF) was discovered by Furchgott and Zawadski, based on the observation that intact endothelium was mandatory for acetylcholine-induced vasodilatation.[84] Atherosclerosis has been shown to impair endothelial cell vasodilator function and is associated with a paradoxical vasoconstrictor response to acetylcholine.[85] EDRF protects the artery against vasoconstriction and thrombus formation. Although there may be several relaxing factors, one is known to be nitric oxide. Endothelium-derived nitric oxide causes vasodilatation by binding to guanylate cyclase, an action identical to that of exogenously administered nitroglycerin. Endothelial function and EDRF are impaired by[81]:

Smoking
Hypertension
Hyperlipidemia
Diabetes mellitus
Atherosclerosis

Because EDRF can be considered as the blood vessel's own locally produced nitroglycerin, causing vascular smooth muscle to relax when a need exists for more blood flow,[86] ischemic heart disease might be viewed as an event that occurs when risk factors for atherosclerosis overwhelm the body's natural ability to resist disease.

Clinically, endothelial dysfunction can manifest as:

Vasospasm
Thrombus formation
Atherosclerosis
Restenosis following coronary balloon angioplasty[87]

Disorders of endothelial regulatory function may also explain previously enigmatic conditions such as syndrome X (chest pain with normal coronary arteries),[88] progression from coronary vasospasm to atherosclerotic narrowing,[89] and abnormal circulatory dynamics in patients with hypertension[90] or congestive heart failure.[91]

Other dynamic aspects of arteries include angiogenesis and remodeling in response to the development of atherosclerosis. Although the development of collateral blood vessels[92] and the recannulation of occluded arterial segments has a beneficial effect in terms of improving blood flow, angiogenesis itself has been broadly linked to cancer,[93] and the neovascularization of proliferating vasa vasorum has been postulated as a possible cause of plaque rupture.[94]

Vascular remodeling is the phenomenon of compensatory enlargement in the presence of atherosclerosis to preserve near normal lumen diameter (Fig. 26.5). Initially described in monkeys fed an atherogenic diet, this biologic response has now been demonstrated in human coronary,[95] carotid,[96] and femoral[97] arteries. Functionally important lumen stenosis may be delayed until the lesion occupies 40% of the internal elastic lamina area. The preservation of a nearly normal lumen cross-sectional area should be taken into account in evaluating atherosclerotic disease with angiography.[95] Lack of remodeling

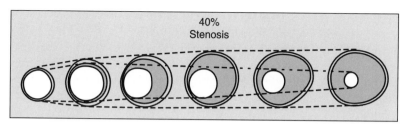

Figure 26.5. Possible sequence of changes in atherosclerotic arteries leading eventually to lumen narrowing. Artery enlarges initially (left to right in diagram) in association with plaque accumulation to maintain adequate, if not normal, lumen area. (Reprinted with permission from Glagov S, et al. Compensatory enlargement of human atherosclerotic coronary arteries. *N Engl J Med.* 1987;316:1371–1375.)

Table 26.1
Likelihood of Defining Coronary Artery Disease after Standard Treadmill Exercise Testing According to Age, Sex, and Symptoms in a Group of Patients with 1–1.5 Mm ST Segment Depression

Age	Asymptomatic		Nonanginal Chest Pain		Atypical Angina		Typical Angina	
Yr	Men	Women	Men	Women	Men	Women	Men	Women
30–39	3.9	0.6	10.4	1.7	37.7	8.5	83.0	42.4
40–49	11.0	2.1	25.8	5.8	64.4	24.5	93.6	72.3
50–59	18.5	6.5	36.7	16.3	75.2	50.4	96.1	89.1
60–69	22.9	14.7	45.3	32.6	81.2	71.6	97.2	95.3

Reprinted with permission from Diamond GA. Analysis of probability as an aid in the clinical diagnosis of coronary artery disease. *N Engl J Med.* 1979;300:1350–1358.

may be a major determinant in whether a person with coronary atherosclerosis develops its complications.[98]

Early stages of lesion development may be associated with overcompensation. At more than 40% stenosis, however, the plaque area continues increasing and involves the entire circumference of the vessel, and the artery no longer enlarges at a rate sufficient to prevent narrowing of the lumen.

DIAGNOSIS

The process of screening patients for heart disease involves the use of the:

History
Physical examination
ECG
Chest x-ray

The diagnosis of ischemic heart disease is most easily accomplished with patients who are symptomatic. When more fanfare was given to annual health screening evaluations, treadmill stress tests were often employed as part of executive physical examinations. Testing for asymptomatic CAD is not generally considered to be a fruitful endeavor, however, except in highly selected circumstances such as before noncardiac vascular surgery or in certain patients with multiple cardiovascular risk factors.

Diagnostic studies for patients with suspected or proven CAD fall into two general categories. The first consideration involves establishing the diagnosis of CAD. The history is the central element in this diagnosis. Numerous studies over the past two decades have validated Bayes' theorem, clarifying that virtually every cardiovascular study performed has little meaning by itself but is properly understood in the context of the patient's clinical presentation[99] (Table 26.1).

Table 26.1 shows that CAD has a wide range of probability in patients of the same age, dependent on whether they are asymptomatic or have chest pain believed to be of noncardiac origin, atypical for angina, or typical for angina. For patients with established heart disease, the second diagnostic consideration is to stage the patient and to define the patient's position on the continuum of stable or unstable coronary atherosclerotic syndromes described above. A high correlation exists between the clinical impression of stable angina, accelerated angina, resting angina, and acute myocardial infarction with the findings demonstrated on angiography[100] and angioscopy.[67] The initial classification should distinguish between those patients at low risk for myocardial infarction who can be further evaluated on an outpatient basis and those patients for whom immediate hospitalization is required.[101]

With the wide availability of highly sophisticated and expensive diagnostic studies for cardiovascular disease, the proper place for the ECG is often missed. An ECG performed during chest pain is of considerable value in the risk stratification of these patients in terms of the subsequent development of acute coronary events, regardless of whether myocardial infarction is proven at the time of that presentation. A completely normal ECG during prolonged chest pain can also provide useful diagnostic information. The bad name that resting electrocardiography obtained came from its inappropriate use as a single method to screen for heart disease in asymptomatic or mildly symptomatic patients and in symptomatic patients in whom the study was performed without correlation to symptoms of angina pectoris.

The general category of diagnostic studies for cardiovascular disease includes imaging techniques, tests of myocardial function, and physiologic assessments of cardiac performance. The new imaging techniques (magnetic resonance imaging, conventional or rapid sequence computed tomography, and echocardiographic studies) are expensive compared with plain chest x-ray films and cardiac fluoroscopy. Many tests (such as treadmill exercise stress testing) provide functional data; they may be supplemented by imaging techniques such as postexercise thallium imaging or postexercise echocardiography. Increasingly, pharmacologic stress testing with dobutamine or dipyridamole is substituted for exercise stress testing. Some studies, such as radionuclide ejection fraction, provide physiologic information alone.

The development of such a wide array of tests forces decision-making. Using all noninvasive studies is cost-prohibitive. If only a small number are to be used, they have to be carefully tailored to the patient's clinical state. These simple questions should be answered:

Is this study being performed to establish the diagnosis of heart disease or to stage known heart disease?

Will the study provide useful information concerning the patient's prognosis?

Is the study necessary to determine the best form of therapy for a patient, to assess the benefits of previously performed procedures, or to risk-stratify for noncardiac surgery?

Which test is the safest and the most feasible to perform and yields the most information, with the least possibility of confounding information?

Each of these issues is widely discussed in the medical literature.[102–105] Clinical experience and thoughtful judgment are the most important features of decision-making in this area.

TREATMENT

The ideal approach to patients with potential ischemic heart disease is primary prevention, so that they never develop symptomatic or significant coronary atherosclerosis. A holistic approach to the patient with CAD recognizes that a multifactorial disease process requires a comprehensive therapeutic plan. To prescribe an optimum therapy, patients should be risk stratified to determine the extent of myocardium at ischemic jeopardy and the state of left ventricular function. Likewise, each patient deserves the benefit of a multifactorial risk factor modification program. This includes:

Regular, progressive aerobic exercise
Weight loss when appropriate
Control of hypertension and diabetes
Cessation of cigarette smoking
Education about cardiovascular disease
Reduction of serum cholesterol
Modification of dietary cholesterol and fats
Control of stress and hostility

Emotional and psychological support are key features in successful risk factor modification programs.

Exercise is a particularly important component of a risk factor modification program. Exercise is recommended for healthy patients, patients identified at risk for CAD, patients with defined ischemic heart disease, and patients following myocardial infarction or revascularization.[106] The type of program a patient enters depends on his or her physiologic state and cardiovascular status at the time of enrollment. Many patients enter rehabilitation while hospitalized and continue in a phase II posthospital program that is monitored and supervised. Others begin with a phase III maintenance program that is supervised but not monitored. Recent information indicates that strength development through circuit weight training is both safe and feasible in selected patients with CAD.[107]

The primary goals of cardiac rehabilitation include a return to full functional status, resumption of previous occupation, and improved quality of life. Exercise itself has important additional benefits in terms of promoting the reduction of other cardiovascular risk factors such as obesity, hypertension, diabetes, and dyslipidemias.[106] The mechanism whereby cardiac rehabilitation works is not through improvement of coronary collaterals or myocardial blood flow but rather through enhancement of musculoskeletal efficiency. Because striated muscle represents the largest potential demand for cardiac output, improved functioning of this primary machinery of life has a significant effect on cardiovascular status.

All patients with ischemic heart disease should also have their spouse and family involved in this risk factor modification program. Family can be a significant source of support for the patient. Often, other family members have the same needs in terms of education, exercise, smoking behavior, and other risk behaviors. Lastly, ischemic heart disease is a frightening proposition. Even with an exercise program, many patients remain unable to break through the barrier of fear and return to fully functional lives. They represent clear examples of individuals who need psychological, social, and spiritual support as they cope with their illness.

Angina Pectoris

Patients with chronic stable angina pectoris are fortunate in that many effective pharmacologic agents are now available. Follow certain guiding principles. First, select a therapeutic agent based on the pathophysiology of the disease state—especially as it relates to coexisting disease processes—and on other cardiovascular characteristics. Although β-blocking agents, nitrates, and calcium entry blockers all represent effective first line agents for treating angina, some drugs may be superior to others in certain situations. For example, patients with coexisting hypertension would do well with a β-blocking drug; patients with coexisting heart failure would do best with nitrates; β-blocking agents should be used with caution in patients with diabetes or obstructive airway disease. Because the pathophysiology of ischemic heart disease involves healing of the intimal disruption in unstable angina, patients started on antianginal therapy during the acute phase of their illness may not require that medication indefinitely. Select a time to withdraw these drugs unless their continued use can be shown to be associated with a decreased risk of cardiovascular mortality.

The pathophysiology of acute coronary syndromes indicates that aspirin is appropriate for all patients with defined ischemic heart disease. Many physicians also advocate aspirin use for currently healthy individuals at risk, even without any evidence of CAD.

Unstable Angina

Unstable angina has three possible presentations[101]:

1. Symptoms of angina at rest (usually prolonged for more than 20 minutes)
2. New onset (less than 2 months) exertional angina of at least Canadian Cardiovascular Society Classification (CCSC) III in severity
3. Recent (less than 2 months) acceleration of angina reflected by an increase in severity of at least one CCSC class to at least CCSC Class III (Table 26.2).

The major treatment goals for patients with unstable angina are to control chest discomfort, relieve ischemia, and prevent the development of acute myocardial infarction. Guidelines for the diagnosis and treatment of angina have recently been developed by an expert panel, based on scientific and clinical evidence.[101]

Myocardial Infarction

The treatment of myocardial infarction today represents a combination of public health efforts, medical technology, and the application of molecular and cellular biology to patient care issues. Standard therapeutic interventions including β-blockers, thrombolytic agents, angiotensin-converting enzyme (ACE) inhibitors, balloon angioplasty, and the coronary care unit itself have all been developed only in the last few decades. Although controversy continues over specific issues related to optimal treatment, international multicenter trials and meta-analytic studies have established strong scientific evidence to support recommendations for therapy for myocardial infarction.[108–114] In the last decade, the strategy to treat myocardial infarction has shifted from an approach to prevent or manage malignant arrhythmias to efforts to reduce the extent of infarction, prevent reinfarction, and protect against deleterious effects of ventricular remodeling. Figure 26.6 summarizes the efficacy of various forms of treatment on mortality in acute myocardial infarction.

The role of early ambulation and cardiac rehabilitation is important to avoid complications of myocardial infarction and to maintain cardiovascular fitness before it is lost because of bed rest. Cardiac rehabilitation takes advantage of the patient being receptive to this intervention at this time, and it can be a part of a risk factor modification program that is begun in the hospital.

All patients should be offered a comprehensive treatment program for ischemic heart disease that includes multifactorial risk factor modification and cardiac rehabilitation, whether they present with unstable angina, acute myocardial infarction, or coronary bypass graft surgery.[106] Osteopathic manipulative treatment (OMT) should be provided for those patients who have open heart surgery because of the major disturbance of musculoskeletal function that they experience.[115]

OSTEOPATHIC APPROACH TO CORONARY HEART DISEASE

The application of the osteopathic concept[1] is most successful when it draws on traditional osteopathic practice, on scientific evidence from basic research and clinical trials, and on the relevant experience of other health care providers. In the field of cardiology, osteopathic physicians are able to incorporate a rich tradition of medical practice that can be used as they approach individual patients. This section touches on some of those features that seem particularly illustrative of the implementation of osteopathic concepts.

The history is a critical feature of the evaluation of patients suspected of having CAD. From the start, as J. Willis Hurst points out, the physician interview with the patient has a dual purpose: to obtain important medical information and to establish a bond between the patient and the physician.[116] Because the management of CAD involves lifestyle changes recommended by the physician, the initial history may also be considered as the first step in establishing the foundation for later risk factor modification programs.

The history of chest pain typical for angina pectoris may occur in a minority of patients with ischemic heart disease. Unusual somatic representation of chest pain to a site of previously experienced somatic pain may occur because of facilitation, convergence, or other mechanisms at the spinal level.[117–118] Until recently, episodes of angina were thought to be synonymous with myocardial ischemia, and chest pain was considered to be a reliable indicator of ischemia. Several reports have since demonstrated that episodes of asymptomatic myocardial ischemia are common in patients with known

Table 26.2
Grading of Angina Pectoris by the Canadian Cardiovascular Society Classification System

Class	Description of Stage
Class I	Ordinary physical activity does not cause angina, such as walking, climbing stairs. Angina [occurs] with strenuous, rapid, or prolonged exertion at work or recreation.
Class II	Slight limitation of ordinary activity. Angina occurs on walking or climbing stairs rapidly, walking uphill, walking or stair climbing after meals, or in cold, or in wind, or under emotional stress, or only during the few hours after awakening. Walking more than two blocks on the level and climbing more than one flight of ordinary stairs at a normal pace and in normal condition.
Class III	Marked limitations of ordinary physical activity. Angina occurs on walking one to two blocks on the level and climbing one flight of stairs in normal conditions and at a normal pace.
Class IV	Inability to carry on any physical activity without discomfort—anginal symptoms may be present at rest.

Reprinted with permission from Campeau L. Grading of angina pectoris by the Canadian cardiovascular society classification system. *Circulation.* 1976; 54:522–523.

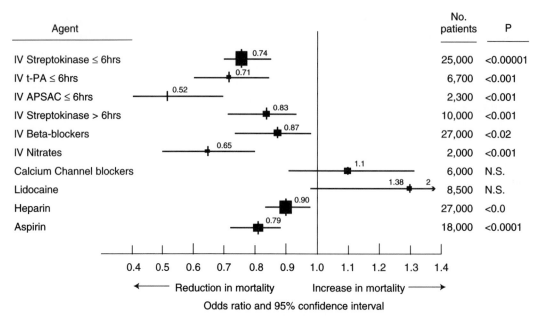

Figure 26.6. Effects of various treatments on mortality in acute myocardial infarction. Plot shows odds ratios and their 95% confidence. Size of the square is related to variance of data. Larger squares reflect more data; narrower confidence interval indicates more precise estimate of treatment effect. I.V., intravenous; t-PA, tissue plasminogen activator; AP-SAC, anisoylated plasminogen-streptokinase activator complex; N.S., not significant. (Reprinted with permission from Yusuf S, et al. Routine medical management of acute myocardial infarction. *Circulation.* 1990;82(suppl II):II-117–II-134.)

CAD.[119–121] Similarly, the Framingham Study has shown that unrecognized myocardial infarctions are common, numbering at least 1 out of every 4 infarctions. Half of the unrecognized infarctions are silent; the remainder are so atypical that neither the patient nor the physician entertains their possibility.[122]

Clinical studies on the manifestations of pain have been performed in a variety of cardiac conditions. At the opposite end of the spectrum from silent ischemia are patients with a "sensitive heart"[123] or syndrome X,[124] in whom an abnormal cardiac pain perception is a fundamental component of the clinical presentation.

The relationship between the myocardial locus of ischemia or infarction and the distribution of angina has been studied in several clinical circumstances. The distribution of cardiac pain during different locations of intracoronary stimulation by local injection of adenosine was experienced in the same body area by the majority of patients.[125] For all patients with Q wave myocardial infarction, pain location, radiation, duration, and severity were similar, although gastrointestinal symptoms were more common with inferior wall myocardial infarction.[126] For the same group of patients, a second myocardial infarction with a different location of pain was highly predictive of ischemia in a different cardiac region. In a study of palpatory findings of musculoskeletal changes with myocardial infarction, abnormalities of paraspinal soft tissue texture were more frequently associated with anterior than with inferior myocardial infarction.[127]

Clinical observations since the time of Sir William Harvey are consistent with the idea that myocardial nociceptors are sufficiently sparse that a certain mass of myocardium must be affected for pain to be perceived.[128–131] Studies that attempt to correlate pain perception with the extent of cardiac autonomic denervation by using meta-iodobenzylguanidine nuclear scanning have had inconsistent outcomes.[132–134] A prospective radiographic study that showed a higher incidence of cervical osteochondrosis in patients with painful ischemia compared with painless ischemia proposed summation of pain input from a musculoskeletal reflexogenic zone as a possible mechanism to explain pain perception in these patients.[135] (Osteophytic lipping of the lower thoracic spine has been shown to be more common in patients with coronary disease than in control patients,[136] but this study did not distinguish patients with painful and silent ischemia.)

Because cardiac pain is transmitted to the spinal cord by sympathetic afferent nerves, osteopathic physicians have examined the paraspinal musculature and soft tissue for a segmental somatic expression of this visceral disturbance. Beal[137] reviewed the osteopathic literature, noting a preponderance of changes in the areas of T1-T5. He found that an examination of the entire axial skeleton was only performed in two studies in which the status of the coronary arteries was defined by angiography.[54–55] In the study of patients with acute myocardial infarction,[56] the palpatory examination was restricted to the twelve thoracic segments.

Clinical protocols for the assessment of patients with chest pain have not yet included palpatory findings as a prospective aid for the diagnosis of coronary disease. The reproduction of chest discomfort by palpation is part of an algorithm for the evaluation of chest pain in the emergency room.[138] Because somatic factors can coexist with cardiac disease, and spinal segmental facilitation may augment the severity of chest wall pain,[139] the osteopathic profession could make a contribution to clinical medicine by a study of palpatory musculoskeletal findings in patients with chest pain.

OMT has been advocated on the basis that it reduces somatic dysfunction, interrupts the viscerosomatic reflex arcs, influences the viscus through stimulation of somatovisceral efferents, and reduces the potential preconditioning effect of somatic dysfunction to body stressors.[137] OMT has been recommended for the treatment of coronary heart disease based on a presumed mechanism to favorably alter autonomic nervous system function.[140] Two other modalities used to treat angina pectoris are related to somatovisceral reflexes: transcutaneous electrical nerve stimulation (TENS) and epidural stimulation.

TENS has been used with some success to treat chronic pain based on the mechanism whereby stimulation of large afferent A fibers reduces input to the brain from peripheral pain receptors via the small myelinated and unmyelinated C fibers. To treat angina, electrodes are placed over the area of pain and on the other side of the spine in the same dermatome to produce segmental stimulation. Neurostimulation is then employed to produce a tingling sensation or paresthesia; typically, patients employ TENS for 1 hour three times a day. Interventional trials on patients with angina refractory to maximal care demonstrated a reduction in angina episodes and an increase in exercise time until ischemia occurred.[141] With TENS, myocardial lactate production is improved and less pronounced ST segment depression is observed with atrial pacing, suggesting that TENS may decrease sympathetic activity directly or indirectly as a consequence of pain inhibition.[142] Intracardiac blood flow increased significantly in patients with CAD or syndrome X but not in cardiac transplant recipients.[143] Because transplant recipients have a denervated heart, these data might favor a mechanism that involves direct myocardial effects.

Epidural stimulation has also been employed as an adjuvant therapy for intractable angina pectoris. Subcutaneous electrodes are placed in the epidural space, in a location determined by sensation of paresthesias in an area that corresponds to anginal pain. This therapy has been shown to increase exercise duration, time to angina, and daily activity score, while decreasing angina episodes and nitroglycerin use.[144] De Jongste et al. postulate an electroanalgesic and anti-ischemic effect.

The implementation of osteopathic concepts to the treatment of patients with angina draws on clinical experience and a legacy of the application of physiology principles to the practice of medicine. Using viscerosomatic and somatovisceral reflexes effectively requires an expansion of osteopathic palpatory diagnosis and manipulative treatment. The information cited above should make clear the heterogeneity of patients with chest pain and the clinical spectrum that ranges from the hypersensitive heart to silent ischemia. Likewise, modification of the somatic component to angina has direct and indirect cardiac effects as well as systemic manifestations.

The osteopathic profession could make a strong contribution to these important areas of medicine with an expansion of past observations on paraspinal palpatory changes to include an examination of the area of pain perception in each patient. Likewise, a trial of the effects of OMT should not be restricted to spinal manipulation but should include treatment appropriate to the musculoskeletal changes identified in the soft tissue of the area of perceived pain.

Skilled practitioners of osteopathic palpatory diagnosis and manipulative treatment are greatly needed in hospitals. Specialists in osteopathic manipulative medicine are frequently helpful in the diagnosis of patients with chest pain atypical for angina. For patients without myocardial infarction, OMT is especially helpful for those with chest wall pain. For patients with proven myocardial infarction, OMT has been safely employed in the coronary care unit and the step down unit, with favorable clinical responses. Those patients receiving routine OMT after open heart surgery often respond dramatically to treatment. Unfortunately, these clinical observations have not been studied in controlled trials. Even a systematic recording of observations on a longitudinal or case control basis would be of significant interest.

Primary and secondary prevention of CAD are issues of critical importance. Because coronary atherosclerosis is a multifactorial disease, decades passed before the risk factors were placed in perspective.[145–146] Additional time elapsed before it was shown that risk factor modifications successfully reduced cardiovascular events, including mortality.[147–154] The last decade has seen research that demonstrates that lifestyle modifications with or without medications to lower serum cholesterol can halt or reverse the progression of atherosclerosis.[155–157] The level of exercise intensity,[158] diet,[159] and antioxidants[160] appear to be variables independent of serum cholesterol that can have favorable effects on coronary events or regression of atherosclerosis. Patients with normal serum cholesterol and CAD gain significant benefit from further lowering of serum cholesterol.[161] The rapid reduction in coronary events clearly precedes regression of atherosclerosis and is thought to represent a reestablishment of normal endothelial function.[162–164]

Although many physicians might contend that the most osteopathic approach is one that eschews drugs in favor of diet and exercise, others would argue that the most osteopathic approach is one that is individualized for the patient, according to the patient's values, resources, emotional needs, and social support.

HEART FAILURE

Heart failure is a clinical syndrome or condition characterized by[165]:

1. Signs and symptoms of intravascular and interstitial volume overload, including shortness of breath, rales, and edema
2. Manifestations of inadequate tissue perfusion, such as fatigue or poor exercise tolerance

Patients may have one or both of these features. The term "heart failure" has recently been recommended instead of the term "congestive heart failure" because many patients with heart failure do not manifest pulmonary or systemic congestion.[165]

More than 2 million U.S. citizens are estimated to have heart failure; approximately 400,000 cases are diagnosed annually. With the aging of the general population, heart failure has become an epidemic of the largest magnitude in North America, even with a reduction in mortality resulting from coronary heart disease and systemic arterial hypertension,[166] the two most common causes of heart failure.

Pathophysiology

In the United States, the most common cause of heart failure as a result of muscle damage is coronary heart disease; the most common cause of heart failure as a result of pressure overload of the heart is systemic arterial hypertension.[167] In South America, Chagas' disease is the most common cause of heart failure because of left ventricular damage; in Third World countries, volume overload because of rheumatic heart disease remains an important cause of heart failure. Often the disease entity is multifactorial, including features of hypertension, ischemic heart disease, and volume overload (Figs. 26.7 and 26.8).

Typically, heart failure involves systolic dysfunction with depression of contractile performance leading to depressed ejection fraction and cardiac output, and, frequently, ventricular chamber dilatation. Diastolic dysfunction is increasingly recognized as a significant feature in a minority of patients with heart failure.[168] This term implies impaired left ventricular filling and normal left atrial pressures, resulting in pulmonary and

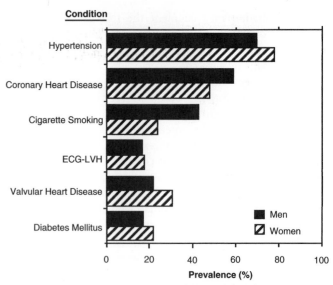

Figure 26.8. Prevalence of certain conditions among Framingham Heart Study subjects with congestive heart failure, by gender. ECG-LVH, electrocardiographic left ventricular hypertrophy. (Reprinted with permission from Ho KLL, et al. The epidemiology of heart failure: the Framingham Study. *J Am Coll Cardiol.* 1993;22(suppl A):6A–13A.)

systemic venous congestion with little or no systolic dysfunction. Diastolic dysfunction is especially common in patients with systemic arterial hypertension, ventricular hypertrophy, or infiltrative disease (Fig. 26.9). In systolic dysfunction, contractility is depressed and the end systolic pressure-volume line is displaced downward and to the right; there is diminished capacity to eject blood into a high pressure aorta. In diastolic dysfunction, chamber stiffness is increased and the diastolic pressure flow relation is displaced up and to the left; there is diminished capacity to fill at low diastolic pressures. The left ventricular ejection fraction is low in systolic dysfunction and normal in diastolic dysfunction.

Clinically significant left ventricular dysfunction activates neurohormonal mechanisms that promote fluid retention and that may perpetuate or worsen heart failure. Typically, these represent examples of compensatory mechanisms that are an exaggerated long-term response of a mechanism designed for short-term control. For example, the immediate hemodynamic response to hypotension caused by blood loss is intense vasoconstriction, elevation of systemic vascular resistance, and salt and water retention by the kidneys. A few decades ago, physicians believed that the endogenous mechanisms activated during heart failure played an advantageous, supportive role, and they were advised not to interfere with these compensatory mechanisms.[169] It is now thought that systemic vasoconstriction decreases left ventricular systolic performance and accelerates the progression of heart failure. The neurohumoral activation in heart failure includes alterations in the autonomic nervous system, including:

Baroreceptors and peripheral adaptation[13,19,170–171]
Adrenergic receptors[172–173]

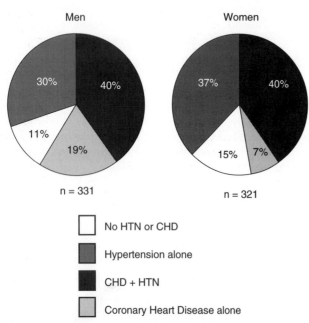

Figure 26.7. Prevalence of coronary heart disease (CHD) and hypertension (HTN) alone and in combination among Framingham Heart Study subjects with congestive heart failure, by gender. (Reprinted with permission from Ho KLL, et al. The epidemiology of heart failure: the Framingham Study. *J Am Coll Cardiol.* 1993;22(suppl A):6A–13A.)

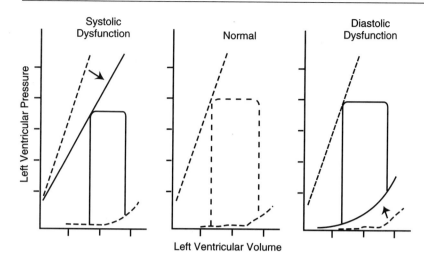

Figure 26.9. Left ventricular pressure-volume loops in systolic dysfunction and diastolic dysfunction. Normal left ventricular pressure and volume relationship is shown with a dashed line. (Reprinted with permission from Gaasch WH. Diastolic dysfunction. *JAMA.* 1994;271:1276–1280.)

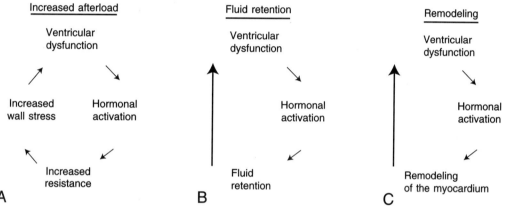

Figure 26.10. Three possible sequences that may cause progression of left ventricular dysfunction because of increased afterload, fluid retention, or ventricular remodeling. (Reprinted with permission from Poole-Wilson P. Pathophysiology of heart failure. *J Am Coll Cardiol.* 1993; 22(suppl A):22A–29A.)

Renin angiotensin-aldosterone system[174]
Atrial natriuretic factor[175–176]
Endothelial function[177–178]

The degree of activation of neurohormonal mechanisms appears to depend on the severity and acuteness of cardiac impairment as well as the status of extracellular fluid volume.[22,179] Local autocrine and paracrine systems in blood vessels and myocardium may also contribute to the long-term regulation of vascular tone and play a role in the pathogenesis of ventricular remodeling, dilatation, and progressive heart failure.[22] Besides these neurohormonal effects, heart failure also affects the kidneys, gastrointestinal system, and skeletal muscle. Figure 26.10 demonstrates three possible sequences that may cause progression of left ventricular dysfunction because of increased afterload, fluid retention, and ventricular remodeling.

Natural History

The natural history of heart failure is affected primarily by the underlying disease process that causes left ventricular dysfunc-tion. In some cases, this is idiopathic and irreversible. Some causes of primary muscle dysfunction may be spontaneously reversible, such as peripartum cardiomyopathy, alcoholic cardiomyopathy, or viral myocarditis. In other cases, the relentless deterioration of function may be interrupted by therapy for the underlying condition. For example, the treatment of systemic arterial hypertension, especially with ACE inhibitors, may not only control hypertension but also enhance cardiac performance and lead to regression of left ventricular hypertrophy. In the case of ischemic heart disease, although left ventricular dysfunction may be irreversible, therapy may halt or retard the progression of coronary atherosclerosis and the subsequent development of additional myocardial damage. Furthermore, ACE inhibitors may prevent or retard deleterious left ventricular remodeling[180] and thereby reduce mortality and morbidity.[181–182]

Patients with heart failure have a poor prognosis, with average mortality rates of at least 10% at 1 year and 50% at 5 years. Figure 26.11 shows the life expectancy in comparison with age-matched unaffected patients. The important predictors of survival are[183]:

Figure 26.11. Comparative life expectancy for men and women with clinical diagnosis of congestive heart failure and age-matched control patients; data from Framingham Study. (Reprinted with permission from McKee PA, et al. The natural history of congestive heart failure: the Framingham Study. *N Engl J Med.* 1971;285:1441–1446.)

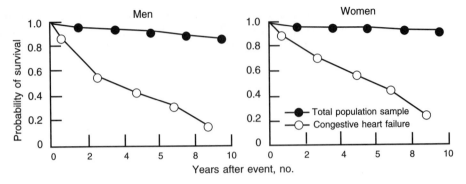

Cause of heart failure
Patient's symptomatic and functional status
Hemodynamic and pathologic findings
Neurohumoral activity
Presence of cardiac arrhythmias

DIAGNOSIS

The standard screen of history, physical examination, ECG, and chest x-ray are helpful to establish the diagnosis of congestive heart failure (Table 26.3). These modalities are best used to develop a composite assessment of the patient's status because pulmonary rales, jugular venous distension, and peripheral edema may be present in a minority of patients.[184] Likewise, the ECG is usually nonspecific.[185] In addition, complete blood count, serum electrolytes, creatinine, albumin, liver function tests, and urinalysis should be performed for all patients with suspected or clinically evident heart failure.[165] T_4 and TSH levels should be checked in all patients older than 65 years of age with heart failure and no obvious cause and in patients who have atrial fibrillation or other signs and symptoms of thyroid disease.[165]

To assess the patient's status, more specific data are needed concerning left ventricular systolic and diastolic function. Two-dimensional echocardiographic studies with Doppler is the diagnostic method of choice to assess patients with suspected heart failure. These studies provide the most information about the heart, including ventricular size, wall motion, and function, in addition to providing information about the cardiac valves, atrial chambers, right ventricle, and pericardium.[186] An estimation of ejection fraction is also possible from an echocardiographic study. The diagnosis of left ventricular diastolic dysfunction has been well-established using Doppler echocardiographic criteria.[187] Exercise testing is an emerging modality used to define the functional status of patients with heart failure.[188]

Because heart failure is the endpoint in a diverse group of clinical disorders, effort should always be made to establish a specific diagnosis. The cause is often reversible or treatable. It is unacceptable simply to use heart failure as the final diagnosis without reference to possible causes.

Table 26.3
Signs and Symptoms of Heart Failure

Symptoms Suggestive of Heart Failure
    Dyspnea on exertion
    Paroxysmal nocturnal dyspnea
    Orthopnea
    Acute edema
    Decreased exercise tolerance, easy fatigability
    Abdominal symptoms of swelling, bloating, or nausea, suggesting ascites or hepatic congestion
Physical Findings Suggestive of Heart Failure
    Distended neck veins
    Ventricular gallop
    Parasternal heave on palpation or laterally displaced apical impulse
    Pulmonary rales
    Ankle edema not due to venous insufficiency

TREATMENT

The goals of therapy for heart failure are to enhance survival, to improve the quality of life, and to improve symptoms, including exercise tolerance. Treatment components include patient and family education and counseling, restriction of dietary sodium and alcohol consumption, and pharmacologic management. Specific guidelines for the treatment of heart failure have been developed by an expert panel.[165] Cardiac rehabilitation programs are also recommended for patients with left ventricular systolic dysfunction.[106]

The Expert Panel on heart failure[165] has recommended the following guidelines with regard to pharmacologic therapy:

1. Patients with heart failure and signs of significant volume overload should be started immediately on a diuretic. Patients with mild volume overload can be managed adequately on thiazide diuretics, whereas those with more severe volume overload should be started on a loop diuretic.

2. Patients with heart failure resulting from left ventricular systolic dysfunction should be given a trial of ACE inhibitors unless the following specific contraindications exist: (a) history of intolerance or adverse reactions to these agents, (b) serum potassium level greater than 5.5 mEq/L that cannot be reduced, or (c) symptomatic hypotension. ACE inhibitors may be considered as the sole therapy in the subset of heart failure

patients who present with fatigue or mild dyspnea on exertion and who do not have any other signs or symptoms of volume overload. Diuretics should be added if these symptoms persist.

3. Digoxin can prevent clinical deterioration in patients with heart failure resulting from left ventricular systolic dysfunction and can improve patients' symptoms. However, its effects on mortality are unclear. Digoxin should be used routinely in patients with severe heart failure and should be added to the medical regimen of patients with mild or moderate heart failure who remain symptomatic after optimal treatment with ACE inhibitors and diuretics.

Other drug therapy for patients with heart failure often involves treatment for side effects created by the primary therapy. Potassium supplements are generally required for patients on high-dose diuretic therapy. Likewise, magnesium supplementation may be required for these patients. Long-term diuretic administration causes depletion of water-soluble vitamins, of which thiamin is the most important.

A special concern involves diastolic dysfunction as a characteristic of congestive heart failure, which was recognized for years in patients with obstructive cardiomyopathy. Only recently was the phenomenon of nonobstructive hypertrophic heart disease defined in elderly patients with hypertension.[189] It is now known that standard therapy with digitalis, diuretics, and arteriolar dilating agents may worsen or not improve the situation. Unfortunately, the natural history of this entity remains uncertain. Treatment goals for left ventricular diastolic dysfunction are described in Figure 26.12.

One of the ironies of medicine is that congestive heart failure is the epidemic of largest magnitude in internal medicine, yet little has been done to establish comprehensive treatment programs that might parallel the treatment plans available for patients with ischemic heart disease. In general, these patients do not receive the same psychological support given to patients with acute ischemic syndromes. The physiology of exercise is sufficiently different that these individuals are generally denied entrance to cardiac rehabilitation programs. Nutritional needs are greatly different from other forms of heart disease, not only because of salt restriction but also because of the malnutrition that is common with congestive heart failure. Osteopathic physicians could play a leadership role in developing a more comprehensive outpatient-based treatment program for patients with heart failure.

OSTEOPATHIC APPROACH TO HEART FAILURE

OMT has been studied only in a few groups of patients with heart failure. In those studies that looked at the hemodynamic markers of cardiac performance in patients with a variety of heart conditions, no change was demonstrated in hemodynamic parameters with manipulative treatment except for a change toward normalization of the total systemic vascular resistance in those patients who had elevated preintervention values.[190] One small study looked at markers of autonomic nervous system function in response to OMT. That pilot study showed an improvement in blood pressure responses to postural change, without beneficial effects on other indicators of autonomic function.[191] The effects of long-term OMT have not been investigated for patients with heart failure.

Given that few clinical studies have been performed that evaluate the efficacy of OMT, and that palpatory musculoskeletal findings have not been systematically evaluated for patients with heart failure, the osteopathic physician can focus on several other important issues in the approach to the patient with heart failure. These involve issues of prevention of heart failure, an emphasis on the musculoskeletal component of the syndrome of heart failure, and an orientation that considers diagnosis and therapy in the context of the integration of cardiac function with neurohumoral modulators of heart failure and the musculoskeletal system itself.

Prevention of heart failure in asymptomatic patients is the first area addressed by the AHCPR Expert Panel.[165] This guideline is restricted to asymptomatic patients who have moderately

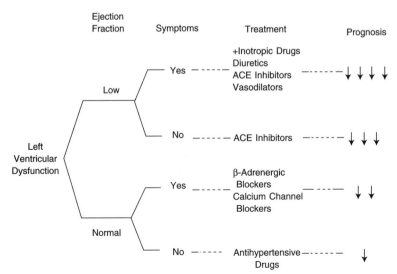

Figure 26.12. Classification of left ventricular dysfunction based on determination of the left ventricular ejection fraction. Within each category, treatment and prognosis related to presence or absence of symptoms. Significant differences exist in treatment recommendations for systolic as opposed to diastolic left ventricular dysfunction. (Reprinted with permission from Gaasch WH. Diastolic dysfunction. *JAMA.* 1994;271:1276–1280.)

or severely reduced left ventricular systolic function (ejection fraction less than 35–40%) for whom treatment with an ACE inhibitor is recommended to reduce the chance of developing clinical heart failure. Because systemic arterial hypertension and ischemic heart disease are clearly the most common causes of heart failure in the U.S., primary care physicians should consider the primary prevention of coronary atherosclerosis and the proper detection and treatment for hypertension to be manifestations of the primary prevention of heart failure as well. Although great strides have been made in terms of the percentage of hypertensive patients who are diagnosed, who are on medication, and who have proper control of hypertension, significant segments of the population are not beneficiaries of adequate control.[192] Furthermore, data from 6273 patients with heart failure or left ventricular dysfunction in the SOLVD Study Registry demonstrated the surprising finding that only 30% of patients were taking an ACE inhibitor, the most effective agent to use in managing heart failure. Substantial numbers were treated with agents controversial in the management of left ventricular dysfunction, such as calcium channel blocking agents, antiarrhythmic drugs, or β-blocking agents.[193]

As with the general population,[194] physical fitness confers a survival benefit to patients with heart failure.[195] In the general population, the reduction in mortality with improved levels of fitness is greatest for those persons who are unfit but who show a modest improvement in fitness (Fig. 26.13). In other words, unfit persons have the most to gain from an exercise program. Randomized controlled trials have not been conducted to show reduction in mortality in patients with heart failure who are enrolled in a program of exercise-centered cardiac rehabilita-

tion. Several studies have shown considerable improvement in terms of intermediate outcomes such as enhanced exercise capacity,[196–198] delayed anaerobic metabolism with exercise,[197] and improvements in dyspnea with exertion.[196]

Traditionally, heart failure was considered a contraindication to cardiac rehabilitation, or patients were not enrolled because of the perception that the primary limitation of their exercise tolerance was diminished skeletal muscle blood flow as a result of poor cardiac output. Although the latter does account for much of the fatigue with exercise, for many patients, their exercise limitation is the result of abnormal skeletal muscle fatigue, possibly related to muscle atrophy, abnormal metabolism,[25] or a cycle of deterioration related to a catabolic state provoked by tumor necrosis factor, insulin resistance, malnutrition, or inactivity.[26]

In the same way that cardiac output does not necessarily determine functional status, neither does the ejection fraction always determine exercise capacity or mortality. For example, Fig. 26.14 shows the lack of any relationship between ejection fraction and exercise tolerance in a group of patients with heart failure. Another concern involves the effect of vasodilators on ejection fraction and mortality. The combination of two direct-acting vasodilators, hydralazine and isosorbide dinitrate, is associated with significant increases in ejection fraction and exercise capacity as measured by peak oxygen consumption, compared with the ACE inhibitor enalapril. If the ejection fraction was to be the primary determinant of prognosis, this drug combination should also confer a superior survival advantage to enalapril. On the contrary, the results of a randomized trial comparing these two regimens demonstrated the clear mortality advantage of enalapril.[199]

Even though ejection fraction and cardiac output are key components to the syndrome of heart failure, by themselves

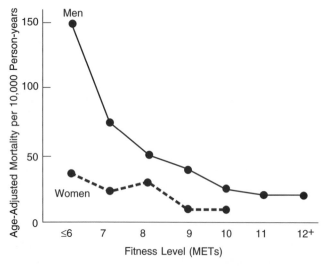

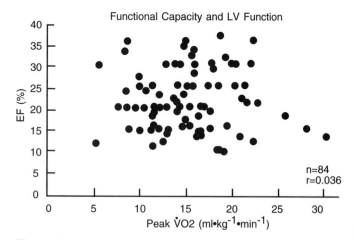

Figure 26.13.   Age-adjusted, all-cause mortality per 10,000 person-years of follow-up by physical fitness level (METs) achieved during maximal treadmill exercise testing. Survival advantage of higher fitness level is greatest at lowest level of physical fitness: unfit persons have the most to gain from exercise programs. (Reprinted with permission from Blair SN, et al. Changes in physical fitness and all-cause mortality. *JAMA.* 1989; 262:2395–2401.)

Figure 26.14.   Lack of correlation between functional capacity and left ventricular (LV) ejection fraction. Exercise capacity measured by metabolic gas analysis during exercise stress and expressed as peak oxygen consumption (Vo₂) in mL of O₂·kg⁻¹·min⁻¹. Note large range of exercise capacity in group of patients with severe LV dysfunction; ejection fraction (EF) is clearly not a major determinant of functional capacity in patients with heart failure. (Courtesy of T. Barry Levine, MD)

Table 26.4
History of Treatment of Heart Failure

Decade	Intervention	Target
Pre-1960	Digitalis	Heart
	Salt restriction	Volume overload
1970s	Loop diuretics	Volume overload
1980s	ACE inhibitors	Neurohormonal systems
1990s	Exercise	The whole person

they are an incomplete part of the picture. The full picture involves the whole patient with circulatory, neurohormonal, and musculoskeletal systems as an integrated unit. Table 26.4 provides a historical overview of treatments for heart failure. Using as many of these modalities as are suitable for the individual patient appears to be the optimal treatment.

REFERENCES

1. The special committee on osteopathic principles and osteopathic technic, Kirksville College of Osteopathy and Surgery: an interpretation of the osteopathic concept. *J Osteopathy.* 1953;60:1–10.
2. Linden RJ. Reflexes from the heart. *Prog Cardiovasc Dis.* 1975; 18:201–221.
3. Paintal AS. Vagal sensory receptors and their reflex effects. *Physiol Rev.* 1973;53:159–227.
4. Malliani A, Peterson DF, Bishop VS, Brown AM. Spinal sympathetic cardiovascular reflexes. *Circ Res.* 1972;30:158–166.
5. Malliani A, Lombardi F, Pagani M. Functions of afferents in cardiovascular sympathetic nerves. *J Auton Nerv Syst.* 1981;3:231–236.
6. Mark AL. The Bezold-Jarisch reflex revisited: clinical implications of inhibitory reflexes originating in the heart. *J Am Coll Cardiol.* 1983;1:90–102.
7. Wurster RD. Cardiac autonomic control—interaction of somatic and visceral afferents. In: Patterson MM, Howell JN, eds. *The Central Connection: Somatovisceral/Viscerosomatic Interaction. 1989 International Symposium.* Athens, Ohio: American Academy of Osteopathy, University Classics; 1989:266–276.
8. Lown B, Malliani A, Prosdocimi M, eds. *Neural Mechanisms and Cardiovascular Disease.* Fidia Research Series. Vol 5. Padova Italy: Liviana Press, Springer Verlag; 1986.
9. Hainsworth R, Kidd C, Linden RJ. *Cardiac Receptors.* Oxford, England: Cambridge University Press; 1979.
10. Abboud FM, Fozzard HA, Gilmore JP, Reis DJ. *Disturbances in Neurogenic Control of the Circulation.* Baltimore, Md: Williams & Wilkins; 1981.
11. Schwartz PJ, Brown AM, Malliani A, Zanchetti A, eds. *Neural Mechanisms in Cardiac Arrhythmias. Perspectives in Cardiovascular Research.* Volume 2. New York, NY: Raven Press; 1978.
12. Kobilka B. Adrenergic and muscarinic receptors of the heart. In: Roberts R, ed. *Molecular Basis of Cardiology.* Boston, Mass: Blackwell Scientific Publications; 1993:193–209.
13. Malliani A, Pagani M, Lombardi F, Cerulti S. Cardiovascular neural regulation explored in the frequency domain. *Circulation.* 1991;84:482–492.
14. Dzau VJ, Krieger JE. Molecular biology of hypertension. In: Rob-

erts R, ed. *Molecular Basis of Cardiology.* Boston, Mass: Blackwell Scientific Publications; 1993:325–353.
15. Korr IM. The spinal cord as organizer of disease processes: the peripheral autonomic nervous system. *JAOA.* 1979;79:82–90.
16. Zucker IH, Gilmore JP, eds. In: *Reflex Control of the Circulation.* Boca Raton, Fla: CRC Press; 1991.
17. O'Rourke ST, Vanhoutte PM. Vascular pharmacology. In: Loscalzo J, Creager MA, Dzau VJ, eds. *Vascular Medicine: A Textbook of Vascular Biology and Diseases.* Boston, Mass: Little, Brown & Co; 1992:133–155.
18. Zelis R, Flaim SF. Alterations in vasomotor tone in congestive heart failure. *Prog Cardiovasc Dis.* 1982;24:437–459.
19. Eckberg DL, Drabinski M, Braunwald E. Defective cardiac parasympathetic control in patients with heart disease. *N Engl J Med.* 1971;285:877–883.
20. Levin TB, Francis GS, Goldsmith SR, et al. Activity of the sympathetic nervous system and renin angiotensin system assessed by plasma hormone levels and their relation to hemodynamic abnormalities in congestive heart failure. *Am J Cardiol.* 1982;49:1659–1666.
21. Cody RJ. Neurohormonal influences in the pathogenesis of congestive heart failure. *Cardiol Clin.* 1989;7:73–86.
22. Dzau VJ. Contributions of neuroendocrine and local autocrine-paracrine mechanisms to the pathophysiology and pharmacology of congestive heart failure. *Am J Cardiol.* 1982;62:76E–81E.
23. Cohn JN, Levine TB, Olivari MT, et al. Plasma norepinephrine as a guide to prognosis in patients with chronic congestive heart failure. *N Engl J Med.* 1984;311:819–823.
24. Drexler H. Reduced exercise tolerance in chronic heart failure and its relationship to neurohumoral factors. *Eur Heart J.* 1991; 12(suppl C):21–28.
25. Uren NG, Lipken DP. Exercise training as therapy for chronic heart failure. *Br Heart J.* 1992;67:430–433.
26. Coats AJS, Clark AL, Piepoli M, et al: Symptoms and quality of life in heart failure: the muscle hypothesis. *Br Heart J.* 1994; 72(suppl):S36–S39.
27. Francis GS, Goldsmith SR, Cohn JN. Relationship of exercise capacity to resting left ventricular performance and basal plasma norepinephrine levels in patients with congestive heart failure. *Am Heart J.* 1982;104:725–731.
28. Cleland JGF, Oakley CM. Vascular tone in heart failure: the neuroendocrine therapeutic interface. *Br Heart J.* 1991;66:264–267.
29. Tuininga YS, van Veldhuisen DJ, Brouwer J, et al. Heart rate variability in left ventricular dysfunction and heart failure: effects and implications of drug treatment. *Br Heart J.* 1994;72:509–513.
30. Gheorghiade M, Ferguson D. Digoxin. A neurohormonal modulator for heart failure? *Circulation.* 1991;84:2182–2186.
31. Mark AL. Sympathetic dysregulation in heart failure: mechanisms and therapy. *Clin Cardiol.* 1995;18(suppl I):I3–I8.
32. Cody RJ. The effect of captopril on postural hemodynamics and autonomic responses in chronic heart failure. *Am Heart J.* 1982; 104:1190–1196.
33. Rouleau J-L, Packer M, Moyé L, et al. Prognostic value of humoral activation in patients with acute myocardial infarction: the effect of captopril. *J Am Coll Cardiol.* 1994;24:583–591.
34. Cody RJ, Franklin KW, Kluger J, Laragh JH. Sympathetic responsiveness and plasma norepinephrine during therapy of chronic congestive heart failure with captopril. *Am J Med.* 1982;72:791–797.
35. Kluger J, Cody RJ, Laragh JH. The contributions of sympathetic tone and the renin-angiotensin system to severe chronic congestive

heart failure: response to specific inhibitors (prazosin and captopril). *Am J Cardiol.* 1982;49:1667–1674.

36. Flapan AD, Nolan J, Neilson JMM, et al. Effect of captopril on cardiac parasympathetic activity in chronic heart failure secondary to coronary heart disease. *Am J Cardiol.* 1992;69:532–535.

37. Waagstein F, Caidahl K, Wallentin I, et al. Long-term β-blockade in dilated cardiomyopathy: effects of short- and long-term metoprolol treatment followed by withdrawal and readministration of metoprolol. *Circulation.* 1989;80:551–563.

38. Heilbrunn SM, Shah F, Bristow MR, et al. Increased β-receptor density and improved hemodynamic response to catecholamine stimulation during long term metoprolol therapy in heart failure from dilated cardiomyopathy. *Circulation.* 1989;79:483–490.

39. Forrester JS, Litvack F, Grunfest W, Hickey A. A perspective of coronary disease seen through the arteries of living man. *Circulation.* 1987;75:505–513.

40. Davies MJ, Thomas A. Thrombosis and acute coronary lesions in sudden cardiac ischemic death. *N Engl J Med.* 1984;310:1137–1140.

41. Komuro I, Yazaki Y. Control of cardiac gene expression by mechanical stress. *Annu Rev Physiol.* 1993;55:55–75.

42. Schneider MD, Parker TG. Molecular mechanisms of cardiac growth and hypertrophy: myocardial growth factors and proto-oncogenes in development and disease. In: Roberts R, ed. *Molecular Basis of Cardiology.* Boston, Mass: Blackwell Scientific Publications; 1993:113–134.

43. Schunkert H, Hense HW, Holmer SR, et al. Association between deletion polymorphism of the angiotensin-converting enzyme gene and left ventricular hypertrophy. *N Engl J Med.* 1994;330:1634–1638.

44. Morgan HE, Baker KM. Cardiac hypertrophy; mechanical, neural, and endocrine dependence. *Circulation.* 1991;83:13–25.

45. Pfeffer MA. Left ventricular remodeling after acute myocardial infarction. *Annu Rev Med.* 1995;46:455–466.

46. Pfeffer JM, Fischer TA, Pfeffer MA. Angiotensin-converting enzyme inhibition and ventricular remodeling after myocardial infarction. *Annu Rev Physiol.* 1995;57:806–826.

47. Vannan MA, Taylor DJE. Ventricular remodeling after myocardial infarction. *Br Heart J.* 1992;68:257–259.

48. Morgan HE. Cellular aspects of cardiac failure. *Circulation.* 1993; 87(suppl IV):IV-4–IV-6.

49. Maisch B. Local cardiac responses—alternative methods and control. *Am J Cardiol.* 1991;67:6C–10C.

50. Perreault CL, Williams CP, Morgan JP. Cytoplasmic calcium modulation and systolic versus diastolic dysfunction in myocardial hypertrophy and failure. *Circulation.* 1993;87(suppl VII):VII-31–VII-37.

51. Yun KL, Fann JI, Rayhill SC, et al. Importance of the mitral subvalvular apparatus for left ventricular segmental systolic mechanics. *Circulation.* 1990;82(suppl IV):IV-89–IV-104.

52. Yun KL, Miller DC. Mitral valve repair versus replacement. In: Carabello BA, ed. *Cardiology Clinics—Valvular Heart Disease.* Philadelphia, Penn: WB Saunders Co; 1991;9:315–327.

53. Carabello BA, Nakano K, Corin W, et al. Left ventricular function in experimental volume overload hypertrophy. *Am J Physiol.* 1989; 256:H974–H981.

54. Cox JM, Gorbis S, Dick L, et al. Palpable musculoskeletal findings in coronary artery disease. Results of a double blind study. *JAOA.* 1983;82:831–836.

55. Beal MC. Palpatory testing for somatic dysfunction in patients with cardiovascular disease. *JAOA.* 1983;82:822–831.

56. Nicholas AS, DeBias DA, Ehrenfeuchter W, et al. A somatic component to myocardial infarction. *Br Med J.* 1985;291:13–17.

57. Schwartz SM, Campbell GR, Campbell JH. Replication of smooth muscle cells in vascular disease. *Circulation Res.* 1986;58:427–444.

58. Geer JC. Fine structure of human aortic intimal thickening fatty streaks. *Lab Invest.* 1965;14:1764–1783.

59. Fuster V, Badimon L, Badimon JJ, Chesebro JH. The pathogenesis of coronary artery disease and the acute coronary syndromes. *N Engl J Med.* 1992;326:242–250, 310–318.

60. Ross R. Cell biology of atherosclerosis. *Annu Rev Physiol.* 1995; 57:791–804.

61. Summary of the second report of the National Cholesterol Education Program (NCEP) Expert Panel on the detection, evaluation, and treatment of high cholesterol in adults (adult treatment panel II). *JAMA.* 1991;269:3015–3023.

62. Grundy SM. National Cholesterol Education Program: second report of the Expert Panel on detection, evaluation, and treatment of high blood cholesterol in adults. *Circulation.* 1994;89:1329–1445.

63. Herrick JB. Clinical features of sudden obstruction of the coronary arteries. *JAMA.* 1912;59:2015.

64. Constantinides P. Plaque fissures in human coronary thrombosis. *J Atherosclerosis Res.* 1966;6:1–17.

65. Stalioraityte E, Pangonyte D. Sudden ischemic death. In: Bluzas J, ed. *Ischemic Heart Disease.* Vilnius, Lithuania: Mokslas Publishers; 1987:24–38.

66. DeWood MA, Sporer J, Notske R, et al. Prevalence of total coronary occlusion during the early hours of transmural myocardial infarction. *N Engl J Med.* 1980;303:897–902.

67. Sherman CT, Litvak F, Grundfest W, et al. Coronary angioscopy in patients with unstable angina pectoris. *N Engl J Med.* 1986; 315:913–919.

68. Davies MJ, Thomas AC. Plaque fissuring: the cause of acute myocardial infarction, sudden ischemic death, and crescendo angina. *Br Heart J.* 1985;53:363–373.

69. Libby P. Molecular basis of acute coronary syndromes. *Circulation.* 1995;91:2844–2850.

70. Report of the Inter-Society Commission for Heart Disease Resources: atherosclerosis study group and epidemiology study group. Primary prevention of the atherosclerotic disease. *Circulation.* 1970; 42:A55.

71. Soloman HA, Edwards AL, Killip T. Prodromata in acute myocardial infarction. *Circulation.* 1969;40:463.

72. van der Wal AC, Becker AE, van der Loos, Das PK. Site of intimal rupture or erosion of the thrombosed coronary atherosclerotic plaques is characterized by an inflammatory process irrespective of dominant plaque morphology. *Circulation.* 1994;89:36–44.

73. Kuo C-C, Shor A, Campbell LE, et al. Demonstration of *Chlamydia pneumoniae* in atherosclerotic lesions of coronary arteries. *J Infect Dis.* 1993;167:841–849.

74. Benditt EP, Barrett T, MacDougall JK. Virus in the etiology of atherosclerosis. *Proc Natl Acad Sci USA.* 1983;80:6386–6389.

75. Melnick JL, Adam E, DeBakey ME. Possible role of cytomegalovirus in atherogenesis. *JAMA.* 1990;263:2204–2207.

76. Muller JE, Stone PH, Turi ZG, et al. and the MILIS Study Group. Circadian variation in the frequency of the onset of acute myocardial infarction. *N Engl J Med.* 1985;313:1315–1322.

77. Rocco MB. Timing and triggers of transient myocardial ischemia. *Am J Cardiol.* 1990;66:18G–21G.

78. Bairey CN, Krantz DS, Rozanski A. Mental stress as an acute trigger of ischemic left ventricular dysfunction and blood pressure elevation in coronary artery disease. *Am J Cardiol.* 1990;66:28G–31G.

79. Taylor CB. Anger, angina and ischemia. *J Myocardial Ischemia.* 1994;6:11–17.

80. Willich SN, Lewis M, Löwel H, et al. The triggers and mechanisms in myocardial infarction study group. Physical exertion as a trigger of acute myocardial infarction. *N Engl J Med.* 1993;329:1684–1690.

81. Mittleman MA, Maclure M, Toffler GH, et al. Triggering of acute myocardial infarction by heavy physical exertion. Protection against triggering by regular exertion. *N Engl J Med.* 1993;329:1677–1683.

82. Vita JA, Treasure CB, Nabel EG, et al: Coronary vasomotor response to acetylcholine relates to risk factors for coronary artery disease. *Circulation.* 1990;80:491–497.

83. Nabel EG. Biology of the impaired endothelium. *Am J Cardiol.* 1991;68:6C–8C.

84. Furchgott RF, Zawadski JV. The obligatory role of endothelial cells in the relaxation of arterial smooth muscle by acetylcholine. *Nature.* 1980;288: 373–376.

85. Nabel EG, Sewyn AP, Ganz P. Large coronary arteries in humans are responsive to changing blood flow: an endothelium-dependent mechanism that fails in patients with atherosclerosis. *J Am Coll Cardiol.* 1990;16:349–356.

86. Healy B. Endothelial cell dysfunction: an emerging endocrinopathy linked to coronary disease. *J Am Coll Cardiol.* 1990;16:357–358.

87. McBride W, Lang RA, Hillis LD. Restenosis after successful coronary angioplasty—pathophysiology and prevention. *N Engl J Med.* 1988;318:1734–1737.

88. Egashira K, Inou T, Hirooka Y, et al. Evidence of impaired endothelium-dependent coronary vasodilatation in patients with angina pectoris and normal coronary angiograms. *N Engl J Med.* 1993;328:1659–1664.

89. Nobuyoshi M, Tanaka M, Nosaka H, et al. Progression of coronary atherosclerosis: is coronary spasm related to progression? *J Am Coll Cardiol.* 1991;18:904–910.

90. Panza JA, Quyyumi AA, Callahan TS, et al. Role of endothelium-derived nitric oxide in the abnormal endothelium-dependent vascular relaxation in patients with essential hypertension. *Circulation.* 1993;87:1468–1474.

91. Katz SD, Schwarz M, Yuen J, et al. Impaired acetylcholine-mediated vasodilatation in patients with congestive heart failure. Role of endothelium-derived vasodilating and vasoconstricting factors. *Circulation.* 1993;88:55–61.

92. Factor SM, Bache RJ. Pathophysiology of myocardial ischemia. In: Schlant RC, Alexander RR, eds. *The Heart, Arteries, and Veins.* New York, NY: McGraw-Hill, Inc; 1994:1036–1037.

93. Braunwald E. On future directions for cardiology. The Paul D. White Lecture. *Circulation.* 1988;77:13–32.

94. Barger A, Beeuwkes IR, Lainey L, Silverman K. Hypothesis: vasa vasorum and neovascularization of human coronary arteries. *N Engl J Med.* 1984;310:175–177.

95. Glagov S, Weisenberg E, Zarins CK, et al. Compensatory enlargement of human atherosclerotic coronary arteries. *N Engl J Med.* 1987;316:1371–1375.

96. Steinke W, Els T, Hennerici M. Compensatory carotid artery dilatation in early atherosclerosis. *Circulation.* 1994;89:2578–2581.

97. Lasordo DW, Rosenfeld K, Kaufman J, et al. Focal compensatory enlargement of human arteries in response to progressive atherosclerosis. In vivo documentation using intravascular ultrasound. *Circulation.* 1994;89:2570–2577.

98. Clarkson TB, Prichard RW, Morgan TM, et al. Remodeling of coronary arteries in human and non-human primates. *JAMA.* 1994; 271:289–294.

99. Diamond GA, Forrester JS. Analysis of probability as an aid in the clinical diagnosis of coronary artery disease. *N Engl J Med.* 1979; 300:1350–1358.

100. Ahmed WH, Bittl JA, Braunwald E. Relation between clinical presentation and angiographic findings in unstable angina pectoris and comparison with that in stable angina. *Am J Cardiol.* 1993;72:544–550.

101. Braunwald E, Mark DB, Jones RH, et al. *Unstable Angina: Diagnosis and Management. Clinical Practice Guidelines Number 10.* Rockwell, Md: Agency for Health Care Policy and Research and the National Heart, Lung and Blood Institute; March 1994. Public Health Service. US Department of Health and Human Services AHCPR publication 94-0602.

102. Shub C. Stable angina pectoris, 2. Cardiac evaluation and diagnostic testing. *Mayo Clin Proc.* 1990;65:243–255.

103. Fletcher GF, Schlant RC. The exercise test. In: Schlant RC, Alexander RW, eds. *The Heart, Arteries, and Veins.* New York, NY: McGraw-Hill, Inc; 1994:423–440.

104. Marcus MI, Schelbert HR, Skorton D, et al. *Cardiac Imaging. A Companion to Braunwald's Heart Disease.* Philadelphia, Penn: WB Saunders Co; 1991.

105. Moss AJ, Goldstein RE, Hall WJ, et al. Detection and significance of myocardial ischemia in stable patients after recovery from acute coronary event. Multicenter Myocardial Ischemia Research Group. *JAMA.* 1993;269:2379–2385.

106. Wenger NK, Froelicher ES, Smith LK, et al. *Cardiac Rehabilitation. Clinical Practice Guidelines Number 17.* Rockville, Md: Agency for Health Care Policy and Research and the National Heart, Lung, and Blood Institute; October 1995. Public Health Service. US Department of Health and Human Services AHCPR publication 96-0672.

107. Butler RM, Rogers FJ, Palmer G. Circuit weight training in early cardiac rehabilitation. *JAOA.* 1992;92:77–89.

108. LaFeuvre C, Yusuf S, Flather M, Farkouh M. Maximizing benefits of therapies in acute myocardial infarction. *Am J Cardiol.* 1993; 72:145G–155G.

109. Yusuf S, Sleight P, Held P, McMahon S. Routine medical management of acute myocardial infarction. Lessons from overviews of recent randomized control trials. *Circulation.* 1990;82(suppl II):II-117–II-134.

110. The GUSTO Investigators. An international randomized trial comparing four thrombolytic strategies for acute myocardial infarction. *N Engl J Med.* 1993;329:673–682.

111. ISIS-3 (Third International Study of Infarct Survival). Collaborative Group. ISIS-3: a randomized comparison of streptokinase versus tissue plasminogen activator versus anistreplase and of aspirin plus heparin versus aspirin alone among 41,299 cases of suspected acute myocardial infarction. *Lancet.* 1993;339:753–750.

112. Gruppo Italiano per lo Studio della Sopravivenza nell'Infarto Miocardico. GISSI-3: Effects of lisinopril and transdermal glycerol trinitrate singly and together on 6 week mortality and ventricular function after acute myocardial infarction. *Lancet.* 1994;343:1115–1122.

113. Ball SG, Hall AS, Murray GD. Angiotensin-converting enzyme inhibitors after myocardial infarction: indications and timing. *J Am Coll Cardiol.* 1995;25(suppl):42S–46S.

114. Rogers WJ, Dean LS, Moore PB, et al. Comparison of primary angioplasty versus thrombolytic therapy in acute myocardial infarction. *Am J Cardiol.* 1994;74:111–118.

115. Rogers FJ, Starzinski ME. The challenges of OMT in postsurgical management of cardiac patients. *JAOA.* 1989;89:1274–1275.

116. Hurst JW, Morris DC. The history: symptoms and past events related to cardiovascular disease. In: Schlant RC, Alexander RW, eds. *The Heart, Arteries, and Veins.* 8th ed. New York, NY: McGraw-Hill, Inc; 1994:205.

117. Ruch TC. Pathophysiology of pain. In: Ruch TC, Patton HD, eds. *Physiology and Biophysics. The Brain and Neural Function.* 20th ed. Philadelphia, Penn: WB Saunders Co; 1979:305–316.

118. Henry JA, Montuschi E. Cardiac pain referred to the site of previously experienced somatic pain. *Br Med J.* 1978;2:1605–1606.

119. Deanfield JE, Ribiero P, Oakley K, et al. Analysis of ST-segment changes in normal subjects: implications for ambulatory monitoring in angina pectoris. *Am J Cardiol.* 1984;54:1321–1325.

120. Deanfield JE, Maseri A, Selwyn AP, et al. Myocardial ischemia during daily life in patients with stable angina: its relation to symptoms and heart rate changes. *Lancet.* 1983;1:753–758.

121. Deanfield JE, Shea M, Kensett M, et al. Silent myocardial ischemia due to mental stress. *Lancet.* 1984;2:1001–1005.

122. Kannell WB, Cupples LA, Gagnon DR. Incidence, precursors, and prognosis of unrecognized myocardial infarction. *Adv. Cardiol.* 1990;37:202–214.

123. Cannon RO III. The sensitive heart. A syndrome of abnormal cardiac pain perception. *JAMA.* 1995;273:883–887.

124. Chauhan A, Mullins PA, Thuraisingham S, et al. Abnormal cardiac pain perception in syndrome X. *J Am Coll Cardiol.* 1994;24:329–335.

125. Crea F, Gaspardone A, Kaski JC, et al. Relation between stimulation site of cardiac afferent nerves by adenosine and distribution of cardiac pain: results of a study in patients with stable angina. *J Am Coll Cardiol.* 1992;20:1498–1502.

126. Pasceri V, Cianflone D, Finocchiaro ML, et al. Relation between myocardial infarction site and pain location in Q-wave acute myocardial infarction. *Am J Cardiol.* 1995;75:224–227.

127. Rosero HO, Greene CH, DeBias DA. A correlation of palpatory observations with the anatomical locus of acute myocardial infarction. *JAOA.* 1987;87:119.

128. White JC. Cardiac pain: anatomic pathways and physiologic mechanisms. *Circulation.* 1957;16:644–655.

129. Gettes LS. Painless myocardial ischemia. *Chest.* 1974;66:612–613.

130. Chierchia S, Lazzari M, Freedman B, et al. Impairment of myocardial perfusion and function during painless myocardial ischemia. *J Am Coll Cardiol.* 1983;1:924–930.

131. Shakespeare CF, Karitis D, Crowsher A, et al. Differences in autonomic nerve function in patients with silent and symptomatic myocardial ischemia. *Br Heart J.* 1994;71:22–29.

132. Hartikainen J, Mäntysaari M, Kuikka J, et al. Extent of cardiac autonomic denervation in relation to angina or exercise test in patients with recent acute myocardial infarction. *Am J Cardiol.* 1994;74:760–763.

133. Langer A, Freeman MR, Josse RG, Armstrong PW. Meta-iodobenzylguanidine imaging in diabetes mellitus: assessment of cardiac sympathetic denervation and its relation to autonomic dysfunction and silent myocardial ischemia. *J Am Coll Cardiol.* 1995;25:610–618.

134. Takano H, Nakamura T, Satou T, et al. Regional myocardial sympathetic dysinnervation in patients with coronary vasospasm. *Am J Cardiol.* 1995;75:324–329.

135. Sakalnikas RG, Gradauskas L. Cervical osteochondrosis and angina pectoris. In: Bluzas J, ed. *Ischemic Heart Disease. Diagnosis, Clinical Manifestations, and Presentation.* Kaunas, Lithuania: Institute of Cardiology Publishers; 1993:139–142.

136. Cox JM, Gideon D, Rogers FJ. Incidence of osteophytic lipping of the thoracic spine in coronary heart disease: results of a pilot study. *JAOA.* 1983;82:832–836.

137. Beal MC. Viscerosomatic reflexes: a review. *JAOA.* 1985;85:781–801.

138. Goldman L, Cook EF, Brand DA, et al. A computer protocol to predict myocardial infarction in emergency department patients with chest pain. *N Engl J Med.* 1988;318:797–803.

139. Kuchera ML, Kuchera WA. *Osteopathic Considerations in Systemic Dysfunction.* 2nd ed. Columbus, Ohio: Greyden Press; 1994:57.

140. Rogers JT, Rogers JC. The role of osteopathic manipulative therapy in the treatment of coronary heart disease. *JAOA.* 1976;76:71–81.

141. Mannheimer C, Carlsson CA, Emmanuelsson H, et al. The effects of transcutaneous electrical nerve stimulation in patients with severe angina pectoris. *Circulation.* 1985;71:308–316.

142. Emmanuelsson H, Mannheimer C, Waagstein F, et al. Catecholamine metabolism during pacing—induced angina pectoris and the effect of transcutaneous electrical nerve stimulation. *Am Heart J.* 1987;114:1360–1366.

143. Chahan A, Mullins PA, Thuraisingham SI, et al. Effect of transcutaneous electrical nerve stimulation on coronary blood flow. *Circulation.* 1994;89:694–702.

144. de Jongste MJL, Hautvast RWM, Hillege HL, et al. for the working group on neurocardiology. Efficacy of spinal cord stimulation as adjuvant therapy for intractable angina pectoris: a prospective randomized clinical study. *J Am Coll Cardiol.* 1994;23:1592–1597.

145. Keyes A, ed. Coronary heart disease in seven countries. *Circulation.* 1970;41(suppl 1):1–211.

146. Anderson KM, Castelli WP, Heartland MC, et al. Cholesterol and mortality: 30 years of follow-up from the Framingham Study. *JAMA.* 1987;257:2176–2180.

147. Lipid Research Clinics Program. The Lipid Research Clinics coronary primary prevention trial results, I. Reduction in incidence of coronary heart disease. *JAMA.* 1984;251:351–364.

148. Lipid Research Clinics Program. The Lipid Research Clinics coronary primary prevention trial results, II. The relationship of reduction and incidence of coronary heart disease to cholesterol lowering. *JAMA.* 1984;251:365–374.

149. Frick MH, Elo O, Haapa K, et al. Helsinki Heart Study: Primary-prevention trial with gemfibrozil in middle-aged men with dyslipidemia. Safety of treatment, changes in risk factors, and incidence of coronary heart disease. *N Engl J Med.* 1987;317:1237–1245.

150. Canner PL, Berge KG, Wenger NK, et al. Fifteen year mortality in Coronary Drug Project patients: long-term benefits with niacin. *J Am Coll Cardiol.* 1986;8:1245–1255.

151. Scandinavian Simvastatin Survival Study group: randomized trial of cholesterol lowering in 4,444 patients with coronary heart disease: the Scandinavian Simvastatin Survival Study (4S). *Lancet.* 1994;344:1383–1389.

152. Multiple Risk Factor Intervention Trial Research Group: Multiple Risk Factor Intervention Trial. Risk factor changes and mortality results. *JAMA.* 1982;248:1465–1477.

153. Aberg A, Bergstrand R, Johannson S, et al. Cessation of smoking after myocardial infarction. Effects on mortality after 10 years. *Br Heart J.* 1983;49:416–422.

154. Oldridge NB, Guryatt GH, Fischer ME, Rimm AA. Cardiac rehabilitation after myocardial infarction. Combined experience of randomized clinical trial. *JAMA.* 1988;260:945–950.

155. Ornish DM, Brown SE, Scherwitz LW, et al. Can lifestyle changes reverse coronary atherosclerosis? The Lifestyle Heart Trial. *Lancet.* 1990;336:129–133.

156. Haskell WL, Alderman EL, Fair JM, et al. Effects of intense mul-

tiple risk factor reduction on coronary atherosclerosis and clinical cardiac events in men and women with coronary artery disease: the Stanford Coronary Risk Intervention Project (SCRIP). *Circulation.* 1994;89:975–990.

157. Pitt B, Mancini GBJ, Ellis SG, et al. Pravastatin limitation of atherosclerosis in the coronary arteries (PLAC I). Reduction in atherosclerosis progression and clinical events. *J Am Coll Cardiol.* 1995;26:1133–1139.

158. Hambrecht R, Niebauer J, Marburger C, et al. Various intensities of leisure time physical activity in patients with coronary artery disease: effects on cardiorespiratory fitness and progression of coronary atherosclerotic lesions. *J Am Coll Cardiol.* 1993;22:468–477.

159. Verschuren WMM, Jacobs DR, Bloemberg BPM, et al. Serum total cholesterol and long-term coronary heart disease mortality in different cultures. Twenty-five year follow-up of the Seven Countries Study. *JAMA.* 1995;274:131–135.

160. Hodis HN, Mack WJ, LaBrec L, et al. Serial coronary angiographic evidence that antioxidant vitamin intake reduces progression of coronary artery atherosclerosis. *JAMA.* 1995;273:1849–1854.

161. Jukema JW, Bruschke AVG, van Boven AJ, et al. on behalf of the REGRESS Study Group. Effects of lipid lowering by pravastatin on progression and regression of coronary artery disease in symptomatic men with normal to moderately elevated serum cholesterol levels. The Regression Growth Evaluation Statin Study (REGRESS). *Circulation.* 1995;91:2528–2540.

162. Pearson TA, Marx HJ. The rapid reduction in cardiac events with lipid lowering therapy: mechanisms and implications. *Am J Cardiol.* 1993;72:1072–1073.

163. Treasure CB, Klein JL, Weintraub WS, et al. Beneficial effects of cholesterol-lowering therapy on the coronary endothelium in patients with coronary artery disease. *N Engl J Med.* 1995;332:481–487.

164. Anderson TJ, Meredith IT, Yeung AC. The effect of cholesterol-lowering and anti-oxidant therapy on endothelium-dependent coronary vasomotion. *N Engl J Med.* 1995;332:488–493.

165. Konstam M, Dracup K, Baker D, et al. *Heart Failure: Evaluation and Care of Patients with Left Ventricular Systolic Dysfunction. Clinical Practice Guidelines Number 11.* Rockville, Md: Agency for Health Care Policy and Research; June 1994. Public Health Service. US Department of Health and Human Services AHCPR publication 94-0612.

166. National Heart, Lung, and Blood Institute: *Morbidity and Mortality Chartbook on Cardiovascular, Lung, and Blood Diseases/1992.* US Department of Health and Human Services; 1992.

167. Ho KKL, Pinsky J, Kanne LWB, Levy D. The epidemiology of heart failure: the Framingham Study. *J Am Coll Cardiol.* 1993; 22(suppl A):6A–13A.

168. Stauffer JC, Gaasch WH. Recognition and treatment of left ventricular diastolic dysfunction. *Prog Cardiovasc Dis.* 1990;32:319–332.

169. Gaffney TE, Braunwald E. Importance of adrenergic nervous system in support of circulatory function in patients with congestive heart failure. *Am J Med.* 1963;34:320–324.

170. Creager MA. Baroreceptor reflex function in congestive heart failure. *Am J Cardiol.* 1992;69(suppl):10G–15G.

171. Ferguson DW, Abboud FM, Mark AL. Selective impairment of baroreflex-mediated vasoconstrictor responses in patients with left ventricular dysfunction. *Circulation.* 1984;67:451–460.

172. Bristow MR, Ginsburg R, Minobe W, et al. Decreased catecholamine sensitivity and beta-adrenergic receptor density in failing human hearts. *N Engl J Med.* 1982;307:205–211.

173. Anderson FL, Port JD, Reid BB, et al. Myocardial catecholamine and neuropeptide Y depletion in failing ventricles of patients with idiopathic dilated cardiomyopathy: correlation with β-adrenergic receptor down regulation. *Circulation.* 1992;85:46–53.

174. Lee WH, Packer M. Prognostic importance of serum sodium concentration and its modification by converting enzyme inhibition in patients with severe chronic heart failure. *Circulation.* 1986; 73:257–267.

175. Cody RJ. Atrial natriuretic factor in edematous disorders. *Annu Rev Med.* 1990;41:377–382.

176. Wei CM, Heublein DM, Perrella MA, et al. Natriuretic peptide system in human heart failure. *Circulation.* 1993;88:1004–1009.

177. Treasure CB, Alexander RW. The dysfunctional endothelium in heart failure. *J Am Coll Cardiol.* 1993;22(suppl):129A–134A.

178. Stewart DJ, Cernacek P, Costello KB et al. Elevated endothelin-1 in heart failure and loss of normal response to postural change. *Circulation.* 1992;85:510–517.

179. Benedict CR, Johnstone DE, Weiner DH, et al. for the SOLVD Investigators. Relation of neurohormonal activation to clinical variables and degree of ventricular dysfunction: a report from the registry of studies of left ventricular dysfunction. *J Am Coll Cardiol.* 1994;23:1410–1420.

180. Pouleur H, Rousseau MF, van Eyll C, et al. for the SOLVD Investigators. Cardiac mechanics during development of heart failure. *Circulation.* 1993;87(suppl IV):IV-14–IV-20.

181. Pfeffer MA, Braunwald E, Moye LA, et al. on behalf of the SAVE Investigators. Effect of captopril on mortality and morbidity in patients with left ventricular dysfunction after myocardial infarction: results of the survival and ventricular enlargement trial. *N Engl J Med.* 1992;327:669–677.

182. The SOLVD Investigators. Effect of enalapril on mortality and the development of heart failure in asymptomatic patients with reduced left ventricular ejection fractions. *N Engl J Med.* 1992;327:685–691.

183. Edwards BS, Rodeheffer RJ. Prognostic features in patients with congestive heart failure and selection criteria for cardiac transplantation. *Mayo Clin Proc.* 1992;67:485–492.

184. Harlan WR, Oberman A, Grimm R, et al. Chronic congestive heart failure in coronary artery disease: clinical criteria. *Ann Intern Med.* 1977;86:133–138.

185. Stapleton JF, Segal JP, Harvey WP. The electrocardiogram of myocardiopathy. *Prog Cardiovasc Dis.* 1970;13:217–239.

186. Echeveria HH, Bilisker MS, Myerburg RJ, et al. Congestive heart failure: echocardiographic insights. *Am J Med.* 1983;75:750–755.

187. Nishimura RA, Abel MD, Hatle LK, et al. Assessment of diastolic function of the heart: background and current applications of Doppler echocardiography, II. Clinical studies. *Mayo Clin Proc.* 1989;64:181–204.

188. Lipkin DP, Scriven AJ, Crake T, et al. Six-minute walking test for assessing exercise capacity in chronic heart failure. *Br Med J.* 1986; 292:653–655.

189. Topol EJ, Traill TA, Fortuin NJ. Hypertensive hypertrophic cardiomyopathy of the elderly. *N Engl J Med.* 1985;312:277–283.

190. Burchett GD, Dickey J, Kuchera M. Somatovisceral effects of osteopathic manipulative treatment on cardiovascular function in patients. *JAOA.* 1984;84:74. Abstract.

191. Rogers FJ, Glassman J, Kavieff R. Effects of osteopathic manipulative treatment on autonomic nervous system function in patients with congestive heart failure. *JAOA.* 1986;86:605. Abstract.

192. Drizd T, Dannenberg AL, Engel A. *National Center for Health*

Statistics: Blood Pressure Levels in Persons 18–74 Years of Age in 1976–1980 and Trends in Blood Pressure from 1960 to 1980 in the United States. US Government Printing Office; 1986. Vital and Health Statistics DHHS publication (PHS) 86–1684.

193. Bourassa MG, Gurné O, Bangdiwala SI, et al. for the Studies of Left Ventricular Dysfunction (SOLVD) Investigators. Natural history and patterns of current practices in heart failure. *J Am Coll Cardiol.* 1993;22(suppl):14A–19A.

194. Blair SN, Kohl HW III, Barlow CE, et al. Changes in physical fitness and all-cause mortality. A prospective study of healthy and unhealthy men. *JAMA.* 1995;273:1093–1098.

195. Bittner V, Weiner DH, Yusuf S, et al. for the SOLVD Investigators. Prediction of mortality and morbidity with a 6-minute walk test in patients with left ventricular dysfunction. *JAMA.* 1993;270:1702–1707.

196. Mancini DM, Henson D, LaManca J, et al. Benefit of selective respiratory muscle training on exercise capacity in patients with chronic congestive heart failure. *Circulation.* 1995;91:320–329.

197. Wilson JR, Mancini DM, Simson M. Detection of skeletal muscle fatigue in patients with heart failure using electromyography. *Am J Cardiol.* 1992;70:488–493.

198. Coats AJ, Adamopaulos S, Meyer TE, et al. Effects of physical training in chronic heart failure. *Lancet.* 1990;335:63–66.

199. Cohn JN, Johnson G, Ziesche S, et al. A comparison of enalapril with hydralazine-isosorbide dinitrate in the treatment of chronic congestive heart failure. *N Engl J Med.* 1991;325:303–310.

27. Hypertension

GARY L. SLICK

Key Concepts

- **Definition and classification of hypertension**
- **Epidemiology and benefits of treatment**
- **Diagnosis and treatment of hypertension, including pharmacologic and nonpharmacologic treatments**
- **Osteopathic approach to hypertension**

Elevation of systemic blood pressure can result from many disease processes. The majority of patients have no underlying cause for their hypertension, thus the term "essential hypertension." Hypertension, whether essential or secondary, will lead to cardiovascular complications and end organ damage if blood pressure elevation continues. End organ disease is the most devastating and potentially avoidable medical problem in the United States and in other developed countries.

Approximately 58 million Americans are hypertensive. Hypertension is the major factor underlying the 400,000 strokes and the 150,000 stroke deaths suffered annually, as well as the 1.25 million heart attacks and 490,000 heart attack deaths occurring each year. In addition to increasing the risk of stroke and heart attack, hypertension is also a significant risk factor for[1]:

Congestive heart failure
Chronic peripheral vascular disease
Aortic aneurysm
Renal failure

DEFINITION AND CLASSIFICATION OF HYPERTENSION

Diastolic Hypertension

Reliance on blood pressure levels to categorize individuals as hypertensive or normotensive has questionable validity. However, measuring blood pressure levels helps in determining severity and the need for therapy. Based on long-term studies, the severity of blood pressure elevation correlates well with the development of vascular complications. Diastolic blood pressure is usually referred to when defining the severity of hypertension and the risk of developing complications. Systolic levels, however, also correlate well with risk at any level of diastolic pressure. The Fifth Joint National Committee on Detection,

Evaluation and Treatment of High Blood Pressure (JNC-V) has defined hypertension as a diastolic blood pressure of 90 mm Hg or greater.[2] This is the most widely accepted definition of diastolic hypertension. Table 27.1 classifies hypertension according to severity as defined by the JNC-V.

Labile Hypertension

Labile hypertension is a blood pressure level that fluctuates across the dividing line from normotension to hypertension. Many patients with labile hypertension will later develop sustained hypertension.

Accelerated Hypertension

Accelerated hypertension is a progressive rise in blood pressure, usually greater than 110–120 mm Hg diastolic, with concomitant active end organ damage resulting from the elevated blood pressure. The end organ damage is usually manifested by:

Flame hemorrhages and exudates of the optic fundus
New onset or worsening azotemia
Hypertensive encephalopathy
Acute left ventricular failure

Malignant hypertension includes the same criteria as accelerated hypertension but includes the presence of papilledema.

Isolated Systolic Hypertension

Isolated systolic hypertension is a systolic blood pressure of 160 mm Hg or greater and a diastolic blood pressure less than 90 mm Hg (Table 27.1).

Essential or Secondary Hypertension

Hypertension can be classified as essential or secondary depending on the presence or absence of a recognizable underlying cause. Essential hypertension comprises by far most of the cases of hypertension, but the actual percentage of patients with secondary hypertension varies depending on the literature source. Most studies from large referral centers have grossly overestimated the true incidence of secondary hypertension. The true incidence of secondary hypertension most likely correlates with the results of the study at the Mayo Clinic.[3] It quoted the incidence of renovascular hypertension, pheochromocytoma, and primary aldosteronism as comprising 0.18%, 0.04%, and 0.01% of all hypertensives, respectively, after applying age- and sex-specific incidence figures from the U.S.

319

Table 27.1
Classification of Blood Pressure for Adults
Aged 18 Years and Older

Category	Systolic mm Hg	Diastolic mm Hg
Normal	<130	<85
High normal	130–139	85–89
Hypertension		
Stage 1 (mild)	140–159	90–99
Stage 2 (moderate)	160–179	100–109
Stage 3 (severe)	180–209	110–119
Stage 4 (very severe)	≥210	≥120
Borderline	140–159	<90
Isolated systolic hypertension	>160	<90

Reprinted from The Fifth Report of the Joint National Committee on detection, evaluation and treatment of high blood pressure. *Arch Intern Med.* 1993;153:154–183.

National Health Survey. The most common secondary causes of hypertension are drug-induced (oral contraceptives) and renal parenchymal hypertension. These cases probably comprise 2–5% of all cases of hypertension. The total percentage of essential hypertension, therefore, approaches 95–98% of all hypertensives.

HISTORY: EPIDEMIOLOGY AND BENEFITS OF TREATMENT

As mentioned above, hypertension is associated with increased cardiovascular morbidity and mortality. Pharmacologic reduction of blood pressure reduces these risks in mild, moderate, and severe hypertension. Several large clinical trials have reported beneficial results.

Veterans Administration Cooperative Study Group Trial

The first trial was the Veterans Administration Cooperative Study Group Trial,[4] which established the benefits of antihypertensive drug therapy in moderate and severe hypertension. This small trial established that treating a diastolic pressure of 115 mm Hg or greater in men (many with target organ damage) dramatically reduced morbidity and mortality. Benefits also appeared after 5 years of intervention in those individuals with diastolic pressures of 105–114 mm Hg.[5] There were fewer "morbid events" in those treated with diastolic pressures of 90–104 mm Hg. There was no significant effect in any group on coronary heart morbidity or mortality.

The Hypertension Detection and Follow-Up Program (HDFP)

The HDFP[6] studied over 10,000 subjects. It is the largest U.S. trial supporting the benefit of antihypertensive therapy in treating mild diastolic hypertension, with mild being defined as 90–104 mm Hg. The benefits might be more dramatic than the results reported because there was no untreated control

group. Patients receiving aggressive stepped-care therapy were compared with those receiving standard care. The results of the study showed a 20% decrease in coronary heart disease mortality in those patients with mild hypertension, a 45% reduction in stroke, and 46% fewer deaths as a result of myocardial infarction (MI). The reduction in mortality was greatest in those individuals with the mildest degree of hypertension (90–94 mm Hg). This study stands out because it demonstrated a significant reduction in the incidence of fatal and nonfatal MI. It emphasized the greater benefit of treatment if treatment is carried out before the emergence of target organ damage, such as left ventricular hypertrophy.

Australian Therapeutic Trial

The Australian Therapeutic Trial,[7] a placebo-controlled study, was moderate in size (3427 subjects) and included only those patients without target organ involvement. Patients with diastolic pressures less than 95 mm Hg were not included. There was a 30% reduction in mortality from all causes and in hypertension complications for those with entrance diastolic pressures of 95–99 mm Hg. Treatment did not significantly affect the incidence of MI.

Oslo Study

The Oslo Study[8] included subjects with diastolic pressures of less than 110 mm Hg and demonstrated a significant reduction in cerebrovascular events such as stroke and transient ischemic attacks. This study was the first to suggest an adverse treatment effect on coronary disease. Major coronary events, such as MI, were more frequent in the treatment group, which also eliminated the overall benefit on mortality.

Multiple Risk Factor Intervention Trial (MRFIT)

The MRFIT[9] enrolled more than 13,000 men and found no difference in mortality over 7 years between aggressively and conventionally treated groups. However, the study reported a 65% increase in mortality, primarily from coronary heart disease, in hypertensive men with abnormal resting ECGs who were treated aggressively with therapy that included diuretics. Despite this adverse effect, there was a 70% reduction in total mortality in the aggressively treated group when followed for a prolonged time.

Medical Research Council Trial (MRC)

The MRC[10] compared placebo to diuretic or propranolol therapy in 6000 patients with mild hypertension. Active treatment reduced the incidence of stroke and cardiovascular events but not coronary events. The study looked prospectively at the response of smokers versus nonsmokers and found that diuretics reduced strokes in all patients. Propranolol was effective in stroke reduction only in nonsmokers, and reduced coronary events in the same group.

Metoprolol Atherosclerosis Prevention in Hypertensives (MAPHY) Trial

The MAPHY[11] trial compared diuretics to metoprolol in 3234 middle-aged men with initial diastolic blood pressures of 100–130 mm Hg and no prior cardiovascular disease. The trial revealed a 48% reduction in total mortality at year four, and a significant reduction in coronary artery disease in the beta blocker-treated group. This was the first trial to demonstrate primary protection against complications of coronary artery disease. This protection was equally effective in smokers and nonsmokers, a result that differs from the MRC trial results. The MAPHY trial studied only men and did not have a placebo group. The coronary event protection therefore occurred when comparing diuretic treatment to metoprolol. The beta selectivity of metoprolol could account for the difference. Nonselective beta blockers might increase the catecholamine response with a resultant intermittent increase in blood pressure, negating the protective coronary effect of the beta blocker.

Possible explanations for the general lack of benefit of antihypertensive therapy on coronary events and coronary-related deaths might be related to several factors, such as:

Insufficient understanding of the multifactorial bases of coronary artery disease (CAD), in which hypertension might play a lesser role than in other cardiovascular events

Potentially adverse effects of lowering the blood pressure below a critical point (J point)[12] in which coronary events might actually be increased

Initiation of hypertensive therapy after coronary disease is too far advanced to result in any benefit

Differences and problems in study design

Other adverse effects of therapy on coronary morbidity, such as induced glucose intolerance, hyperlipidemia, hypomagnesemia, or hypokalemia-induced fatal arrhythmias

Currently, there are no large double-blind placebo-controlled trials on the long-term benefit of the newer classifications of antihypertensives. Such trials would determine if the angiotensin-converting enzyme (ACE) inhibitors and calcium channel blockers offer any greater advantage over the more frequently used agents in the previous trials (diuretics, beta blockers, reserpine, or hydralazine).

DIAGNOSIS

There are three major objectives for the clinical evaluation of the patient with confirmed hypertension:

1. Determine whether the patient has essential or secondary hypertension
2. Determine the presence and extent of the end organ involvement
3. Determine the presence of cardiovascular risk factors other than hypertension

A thorough medical history and physical examination are the core of the hypertensive evaluation.

Medical History

Only a few screening laboratory tests are necessary unless specific clues appear in the history and physical examination to warrant additional testing.

Obtain from the medical history information regarding:

Past history of cardiovascular disease
Cerebrovascular disease
Renal disease and diabetes mellitus
History of duration and severity of hypertension
Smoking
Hyperlipidemia
Level of exercise
Dietary habits (especially salt intake)
Fat and alcohol intake and weight gain
Family history of hypertension and cardiovascular complications
History of previous antihypertensive medication and other current prescription or nonprescription preparations that can alter the blood pressure or the effect of antihypertensive drugs

Table 27.2 includes a list of some of the medications that can alter blood pressure or the effect of antihypertensive drugs. Table 27.3 lists aspects of the medical history that may provide clues about secondary hypertension or target organ damage. Psychosocial and environmental factors such as stress, socioeconomic status, etc., can play a role in hypertension.[13–14] The osteopathic physician must consider the impact of these frequently ignored factors.

Physical Examination

Begin the physical examination by taking a proper blood pressure, with the patient in the supine, sitting, and standing positions. Blood pressure measurements sometimes vary considerably in an individual patient. This variation usually occurs as

Table 27.2

Medications that Might Alter Blood Pressure or the Effect of Antihypertensive Drugs

Drug	Effect
Sympathomimetics	Increase blood pressure
Antidepressants	Decrease effect of central acting agents and ganglionic blockers
Adrenal steroids	Increase blood pressure
Nonsteroidal anti-inflammatory agents	Interfere with effect of diuretics and ACE inhibitors
Nasal decongestants	Increase blood pressure
Oral contraceptives	Increase blood pressure
Cimetidine	Decrease bioavailability of hepatic-metabolized beta blockers
Ergot alkaloids	Increase blood pressure
Monoamine oxidase with inhibitors	Increase blood pressure in combination sympathomimetic amines
Appetite suppressants	Increase blood pressure

Table 27.3
Aspects of the Medical History and Physical Examination that Might Give Indications of Underlying Secondary Hypertension

Symptom/Sign	Cause of Hypertension/ End Organ Disease
History of spells with headache, pallor, perspiration, tachycardia, palpations, or feelings of doom	Pheochromocytoma
History of dyspnea, orthopnea, or paroxysmal nocturnal dyspnea	Hypertensive heart disease
History of hematuria/proteinuria	Renal hypertension
History of oral contraceptives	Oral contraceptive hypertension
Muscle weakness, nocturia, fatigue, and muscle cramps	Primary aldosteronism
Renal bruit (biphasic)	Renal artery stenosis
Difference between radial and femoral pulses or presence of femoral pulse delay	Coarctation of aorta
Palpable kidneys	Renal hypertension (polycystic kidneys)
Optic fundus changes: hemorrhages, exudates, papilledema	Accelerated/malignant hypertension

a result of the observer's techniques and the random biologic variation in the patient's own blood pressure level. Take the pressure at least twice, 5 minutes apart, and then average the values. Compare the blood pressure in the left and right arms. During the initial visit, measure it in the lower extremities to rule out coarctation of the aorta.

To obtain the correct systolic pressure, always inflate the blood pressure cuff while palpating the radial pulse until the pulse disappears. The incorrect method of inflating the cuff while auscultating over the antecubital area can reveal a falsely low systolic blood pressure. The Korotkoff sounds can disappear during the auscultatory gap. This phenomenon occurs particularly in individuals with wide pulse pressures. If the radial artery is easily palpable after amply inflating the cuff beyond the systolic blood pressure (Osler's maneuver), pseudohypertension might be present. Pseudohypertension can occur in elderly patients with hypertension who have rigid, noncompressible atherosclerotic vessels. It produces falsely high blood pressure results with cuff measurements.

Other portions of the physical examination that warrant special attention include the following:

Height and weight
Funduscopic examination
Carotid and femoral vessel examination for bruits
Cardiac examination
Abdominal examination for bruits, enlarged kidneys, masses or aneurysms
Extremity palpation for pulses and edema
Neurologic examination

An osteopathic structural examination is important for detecting musculoskeletal tension in the upper thoracic region

(C6-T6). Such tension has been a consistent somatic finding in a significant percentage of patients with hypertension.[15] Although not yet confirmed in clinical studies, musculoskeletal tension might indicate concurrent uncontrolled hypertension. Table 27.3 lists physical examination findings that can specifically indicate certain secondary causes of hypertension or target organ damage.

Only a minimum battery of diagnostic tests are necessary for the evaluation of most patients with hypertension (Table 27.4). Positive findings in the history or physical examination can necessitate additional tests to uncover a secondary cause of hypertension, target organ damage, or other cardiovascular risk factors. If an abnormal result occurs with the minimum battery of laboratory tests, additional evaluation is necessary depending on the abnormality. Table 27.4 lists abnormal results of the screening tests and what they might indicate. The general recommendation is to obtain the following:

Hemoglobin
Hematocrit
Serum potassium
Serum calcium
Serum creatinine
Serum cholesterol
Blood glucose
Serum uric acid

It is more cost-effective, however, to obtain an automated battery of tests (e.g., SMA-12 or SMA-24) that includes all the recommended parameters. Additional diagnostic procedures might be necessary for those patients whose blood pressures respond atypically or poorly to antihypertensive therapy, and for those whose blood pressures suddenly worsen or develop an accelerated or malignant phase.

TREATMENT

The goal of antihypertensive treatment is the prevention of morbidity and mortality associated with elevated blood pres-

Table 27.4
Minimum Laboratory Tests for the Initial Evaluation of Hypertension

Test	Detects
Serum creatinine	Renal parenchymal hypertension or hypertensive nephrosclerosis
Urinalysis	Renal parenchymal hypertension or hypertensive nephrosclerosis
CBC	Polycythemia or anemia from renal failure
Serum potassium[a]	Primary aldosteronism, Cushings' disease, renal artery stenosis, and accelerated hypertension
ECG	Hypertensive heart disease (LVH)
Chest x-ray	LVH
Serum cholesterol[a]/HDL	Coexistent risk factor for arteriosclerotic disease
FBS[a]	Coexistent cardiovascular risk factor for diabetes
Serum calcium[a]	Hyperparathyroidism

[a]Included on a blood chemistry profile test.

sure. The goal blood pressure should be 140/90 mm Hg or lower, if possible. Some recent controversy has arisen regarding how far the blood pressure should be lowered. Insurance company data have revealed that in the general population, cardiovascular mortality is inversely proportional to the blood pressure to values as low as 110/70 mm Hg.[16] Applying this inverse relationship to reducing blood pressure in the hypertensive population, however, may not hold true.

Several studies have shown a J-curve relationship between diastolic blood pressure and cardiovascular morbidity and mortality. This relationship demonstrates that morbidity and mortality fall with lowering of the diastolic blood pressure to a nadir (J point), and then begin to rise as blood pressure is lowered further (Fig. 27.1). This phenomenon may occur predominantly in hypertensive patients with a critical degree of coronary artery stenosis. For those patients, lowering the diastolic blood pressure below a critical point decreases coronary blood flow and results in myocardial ischemia and resultant coronary events. The J point appears to range between 85 and 90 mm Hg. Further studies are needed regarding this concept. A goal diastolic blood pressure of 90 mm Hg seems appropriate for most patients.

Nonpharmacologic Therapy

Nonpharmacologic therapy is generally appropriate for most patients. Because such therapy frequently involves more complex changes in lifestyle, physicians often are not aggressive in trying to achieve the appropriate goals of nondrug treatments. Some clinicians might unnecessarily refer the patient to other health providers for specific counseling related to lifestyle changes. Applying one of the basic concepts of osteopathic medical care—treatment of the whole patient—the osteopathic physician offers a unique contribution to patients with hypertension. Emphasize nonpharmacologic therapy. Table 27.5 lists those nonpharmacologic therapies that can be used as either definitive interventions or as adjuncts to pharmacologic therapy. For some patients with mild hypertension, nonpharmacologic therapy might be the only therapy needed to achieve adequate blood pressure control. Consider each mea-

sure in every patient; evaluate each patient for the nonpharmacologic measure that is appropriate and most effective. If nonpharmacologic therapy has been ineffective in attaining a goal blood pressure, institute pharmacologic therapy.

Pharmacologic Therapy

Once the decision has been made to employ pharmacologic intervention, one of several drugs can be used. In the general population, all antihypertensive agents are equally efficacious in lowering blood pressure. Approximately 50% of a cross-section of patients with mild hypertension respond to any one of more than 50 agents available. Factors such as side effects, lifestyle, and cost determine which agent is selected for a particular patient. Two general approaches to drug therapy have emerged over the last 20 years: the "stepped-care" approach and the "individualized-care" approach.

The stepped-care approach was originally described in 1977 in the first report of the Joint National Committee on the detection, evaluation, and treatment of high blood pressure.[17] Because so many antihypertensive agents are now available and suitable for initial drug therapy of hypertension, and because the stepped-care approach promotes a more regimented method of therapy, many physicians have abandoned this approach in favor of the individualized-care approach.

The individualized-care approach to hypertensive therapy is rooted in selecting an agent for a particular patient based on factors that predict which agent will be most suitable for the patient, such as:

Demographics
Associated diseases
Concomitant drug use
Economic factors
Quality of life issues

In essence, a physician develops a particular profile for each patient that indicates which drug is the best selection. Many times, however, the profile does not predict the best agent. It is then necessary to use a trial-and-error method to find the drug that controls the blood pressure, promotes adequate compliance, and allows an acceptable quality of life for the patient.

DIURETICS

Diuretics are one of two agents recommended in the JNC-V report as the primary therapy for hypertension. Thiazide diuretics are effective agents for many patients and are frequently recommended for elderly and black patients. Both of these populations tend to have lower renin values than do other patients with hypertension. Diuretics are particularly effective for patients who retain salt and water, such as those with congestive heart failure and other edema-forming states. For patients with chronic renal insufficiency, sodium retention frequently occurs; diuretics are usually needed unless the glomerular filtrate rate falls below 25–30 mL/min (serum creatinine greater than 2.0 mg/dL), at which time furosemide is indicated.

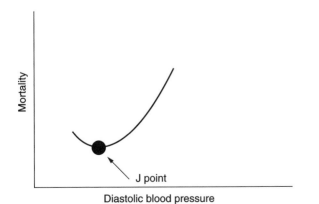

Figure 27.1. Diagrammatic representation of the J-curve relationship between diastolic blood pressure and mortality.

Table 27.5
Nonpharmacologic Therapy Modalities for
Treatment of Hypertension

Moderate dietary salt restriction—70–100 mEq sodium/day
Weight loss to within 15% of ideal body weight
Moderation of alcohol intake to 1 ounce/day or less
Cessation of smoking
Isotonic/aerobic exercise
Moderation of dietary fat intake—low intake of saturated fat
Osteopathic manipulative treatment (?)

Thiazide diuretics have become less preferable as initial therapy because of certain side effects and adverse reactions that can negatively impact morbidity and mortality. Thiazide diuretics are known to increase total cholesterol, LDL cholesterol, and triglycerides, which can adversely affect cardiovascular morbidity and mortality in the long term. Mild hypokalemia occurs in a significant portion of patients, although this usually is of no significance in otherwise healthy patients. However, for patients with ischemic heart disease, two large trials (MRFIT[9] and Oslo[8]) suggest that an increase in sudden death as a result of hypokalemia inducing ventricular arrhythmias can occur with patients taking diuretics. For this reason, diuretics are not generally recommended for patients with coronary artery disease as long as another agent can control blood pressure, and as long as a diuretic is not needed for sodium retention. This phenomenon is only an hypothesis, however, because a direct link among diuretics, hypokalemia, ventricular arrhythmias, and sudden death has not been substantiated.

β-ADRENERGIC BLOCKING AGENTS

β-Adrenergic blocking agents are effective in patients with hyperkinetic circulation, a condition most common in young white males. They are also effective in patients with high renin levels. Such levels play a pathophysiologic role in hypertension. Patients with specific concomitant diseases, such as coronary artery disease with angina and supraventricular arrhythmias, can be ideal candidates for beta blockers as initial therapy.

More recent studies indicate that beta blockers are effective as secondary preventive agents for patients who have had a previous MI. The MAPHY trial showed that beta blockers significantly reduce the incidence of coronary events, cardiovascular mortality, and overall mortality, compared with a cohort of patients on diuretics. When compared with diuretics, beta blockers offer primary prevention of coronary artery disease. Beta-blocking agents should be avoided in patients with:

Congestive heart failure
Conduction system disease
Hyperactive airway disease
Chronic obstructive pulmonary disease

They should be used with caution in patients with insulin-dependent diabetes mellitus and peripheral vascular disease.

Beta blockers (except for those with intrinsic sympathomimetic activity) decrease HDL cholesterol and increase triglycerides. Beta blockers have generally not been recommended for black patients. Numerous studies, however, indicate that when a diuretic is used in conjunction with a beta blocker, this combination is equally effective in both blacks and whites.

ACE INHIBITORS

Although not recommended as a primary therapy of hypertension by JNC-V, ACE inhibitors are frequently used as a first line treatment. They effectively lower blood pressure in more than 50% of people with mild hypertension when given as single agents and do not cause any significant degree of sodium retention. They are reportedly more effective in patients who do not have low-renin hypertension, especially young patients and whites, although many studies have demonstrated predictable and adequate responses in elderly and black patients. Much information has been published in the last 10 years on the specific benefit of ACE inhibitors. They offer renal protection against the progressive decline in renal function as a result of long-standing hypertension. The mechanism of this potential effect is still unresolved. Hypotheses have included reduction in intraglomerular pressure via efferent arteriolar dilatation, or a direct effect on glomerular capillaries by increasing permeability or reducing capillary wall stress. Similar mechanisms have been proposed for the potential renal protection offered by calcium channel blockers. To date, no long-term studies have reported any significant benefit for renal protection. Type I diabetic patients with diabetic nephropathy possess higher filtration rates and lower renal vascular resistance ("renal hyperfiltration"). Patients with high intraglomerular pressures may benefit most by ACE inhibitor therapy for their hypertension.

ACE inhibitor therapy seems to be one of the more desirable agents in treating patients with hypertension and congestive heart failure. A recent report emphasized the minimal negative effects on the quality of life when treating with ACE inhibitors. It compared them to other commonly used antihypertensives.[18] Side effects are few with these agents but can include:

Cough
Hyperkalemia
Acute decrement in renal function
Angioedema

The incidence of cough can be as high as 13–24%; coughing occurs more commonly at night. Hyperkalemia is more likely to occur in patients who have low renin states (the elderly) with chronic renal insufficiency and in those patients who are taking other drugs that can cause potassium retention, such as nonsteroidal antiinflammatory agents, potassium-sparing diuretics, and beta blockers. Diabetics could be more specifically prone to this complication, especially elderly patients with type II diabetes. The lack of side effects and efficacy make the ACE inhibitors attractive agents in the first and second line therapy of hypertension.

CALCIUM CHANNEL BLOCKING DRUGS

The newest class of agents are the calcium channel blockers. The proliferation of newer agents in this class continues. Although not recommended by JNC-V as primary therapy, they are effective as first line therapy and produce minimal side effects. The more recent sustained release preparations seem especially useful because they promote patient compliance. Calcium channel blockers seem to have a distinct advantage in the treatment of hypertension for patients with coexistent ischemic coronary artery disease and chronic arrhythmias. A secondary preventive role for diltiazem in patients who have experienced a non–Q wave MI and normal ejection fraction has been demonstrated over the short term (1–2 months). Because verapamil and diltiazem inhibit proximal conduction and increase the A-V node refractory period, they should not be used for patients with conduction system disease. The negative inotropic effect is manifested chiefly by verapamil and less so by diltiazem. The combination of verapamil or diltiazem with beta blocker, for patients with conduction system disease and heart failure, should be avoided because additive cardioinhibitory effects can occur.

Specific End Organ Preservation of Function

LEFT VENTRICULAR HYPERTROPHY

There are adverse morbidity and mortality statistics with the coexistence of hypertension and left ventricular hypertrophy (LVH). LVH represents an important independent risk factor for cardiac arrhythmias and sudden death.[19] In addition, LVH doubles the risk of death in patients with hypertension. Considerable attention has been focused on the possibility of reversing this abnormality by means of drug therapy. Regression of LVH as determined by echocardiography during short-term studies has been demonstrated with calcium channel blockers, ACE inhibitors, beta blockers, and methyldopa. Diuretics have essentially no effect on LVH regression. The direct vasodilators such as hydralazine and minoxidil may actually worsen it. It is unknown whether reversal of LVH with drug therapy of hypertension will also reduce the risk of morbidity and mortality associated with its presence.

DIABETES MELLITUS

The coexistence of hypertension and diabetes significantly worsens the morbidity and mortality of hypertension alone. Hypertension in a patient with type I or type II diabetes must be managed aggressively with control of the diastolic blood pressure at a level of less than 90 mm Hg. Diabetic patients with diabetic nephropathy are known to have hyperfiltration with a vasodilated renal circulation. This subjects the renal glomerular capillaries to a higher hydrostatic pressure and resultant damage to the renal glomerulus over time.

Recent evidence suggests that two groups of antihypertensives may offer specific renal protection in patients with diabetic nephropathy. The ACE inhibitors may offer specific protection by reducing efferent arteriolar tone by a reduction in angiotensin-II production, or through a direct antiproliferative effect on the glomerular capillary. The protective effect of calcium channel blockers in diabetic nephropathy remains controversial but could be related to reducing renal hypertrophy and glomerular capillary wall tension. Some of the calcium channel blockers have failed to produce any positive effect while others have resulted in renal protection, at least in experimental animals. To date, there are no long-term controlled studies to demonstrate any specific renal protection in humans other than that observed from blood pressure reduction alone.

Resistant Hypertension

A patient's failure to respond appropriately or at all to antihypertensive therapy presents a diagnostic dilemma. True "resistant" hypertension is unusual. In the majority of patients, it reflects a failure to follow the therapeutic regimen or the failure of the physician to place the patient on agents that are effective in lowering blood pressure. Table 27.6 lists the common factors that cause a poor response to antihypertensive therapy.

Of these factors, patient drug compliance and failure to restrict sodium are two of the most important factors that can be traced back to the patient. If the patient complies with drug therapy, collect a 24-hour urine sodium to determine whether excessive salt intake is a contributing factor. The recommended diet for hypertensives should contain 2 grams of sodium. If the patient has been ingesting excessive dietary sodium, restrict salt and/or institute a diuretic.

If the correct combination of antihypertensives is used and salt-dependent hypertension is not a factor, consider a secondary form of hypertension. For those patients in whom all of the factors in Table 27.6 have been eliminated and in whom a regimen of three or four drugs has failed, a course of a diuretic, beta-blocker, and minoxidil is probably necessary. In rare situations, some patients have responded to hospitalization and subsequently come under control with oral antihypertensives that previously were ineffective. This "resetting of the pressor receptors" has been proposed as a possible reason for this line of therapy being effective. It could also be a result of

Table 27.6
Common Factors Responsible for Resistant Hypertension

Pseudoresistance
   office hypertension
   pseudohypertension
   pseudotolerance (intravascular volume reexpansion)
Poor compliance with medication
Excessive salt intake
Alcohol ingestion
Drug interactions
Altered drug metabolism from cigarette smoking (beta blocker)
Obesity
Development of renal insufficiency
Secondary hypertension
Inadequate treatment

unrecognized previous patient noncompliance with oral therapy.

OSTEOPATHIC APPROACH

Few data are available regarding the supplemental benefit of osteopathic manipulative treatment in the treatment of hypertension. Data are also scarce on musculoskeletal palpatory findings in patients with hypertension. Various anecdotal reports have appeared in the past,[20–24] but none included a controlled trial until that of Morgan et al.[25] In that study, 29 patients with mild hypertension were randomly assigned to an 18-week cross-over controlled trial of manipulation versus sham manipulation. This study failed to demonstrate that either of the manipulative treatments could reduce or control hypertension.

Regardless of previously reported data, it is well-known that many individuals with essential hypertension demonstrate generalized increased sympathetic tone to the peripheral vasculature. One must consider that there may be a potential rationale for using osteopathic manipulative treatment in patients with hypertension in whom the treatment is aimed at facilitated segments to the kidney and so on. The recent study by Kelso and Johnson[26–27] demonstrating the musculoskeletal palpatory findings in patients with hypertension adds credence to the potential role of osteopathic manipulative treatment as adjunctive therapy. Further studies are needed to more thoroughly evaluate the overall benefit of manipulation on individuals with hypertension.

CONCLUSION

The greatest value of the osteopathic approach in the treatment of hypertension is related to the treatment of the whole patient and not just the hypertension. A detailed history that documents factors contributing to the elevated blood pressure is an advantage that the osteopathic physician may be able to offer. These factors include:

> Carefully reviewing with the patient not only past and present medical problems but also any significant psychological problems
>
> Identifying patterns of family relationships that might have contributed to the present situation
>
> Identifying living, working, and financial situations that may contribute to stress
>
> Identifying whether larger social issues partly cause problems and whether education or counseling can help alleviate their effects

Recognition and treatment of these factors by the primary care physician are an integral part of total patient management. The osteopathic physician's approach to the patient will aid significantly in gaining the confidence of the patient and will have a positive effect on his or her acceptance and response to the therapeutic plan. The patient's acceptance of the treatment plan and adherence to the physician's recommendations, in turn, reflect the nature of the patient–physician relationship.

This is the first step in effective management of the patient with hypertension, and it could be the osteopathic physician's greatest advantage.

REFERENCES

1. Kannel WB, Doyle JT, Ostfeld AM, Jenkins CD, Kuller L, Podell R, Stamler J. Optimal resources for primary prevention of atherosclerotic diseases. *Circulation.* 1984;70:153A–205A.
2. The Fifth Report of the Joint National Committee on detection, evaluation and treatment of high blood pressure. *Arch Intern Med.* 1993;153:154–183.
3. Tucker RM, Labarthe DR. Frequency of surgical treatment for hypertension in adults at the Mayo Clinic from 1973 through 1975. *Mayo Clin Proc.* 1977;52:549–555.
4. Veterans Administration cooperative study group on antihypertensive agents. Effects of treatment on morbidity in hypertension, I. Results in patients with diastolic blood pressures averaging 115 through 129 mm Hg. *JAMA.* 1967;202:1028–1034.
5. Veterans Administration cooperative study group on antihypertensive agents. Effects of treatment on morbidity in hypertension, II. Results in patients with diastolic blood pressure averaging 90 through 114 mm Hg. *JAMA.* 1970;213:1143–1152.
6. Hypertension detection and follow-up program cooperative group: five-year findings of the hypertension detection and follow-up program, I. Reduction in mortality of persons with high blood pressure. *JAMA.* 1979;242:2562–2571.
7. Management Committee, National Heart Foundation of Australia: the Australian therapeutic trial in mild hypertension. *Lancet.* 1980; 1:126–167.
8. Helgeland A. Treatment of mild hypertension: a five-year controlled drug trial: the Oslo study. *Am J Med.* 1980;69:725–732.
9. Multiple Risk Factor Intervention Trial Research Group: baseline rest electrocardiographic abnormalities, antihypertensive treatment, and mortality in the Multiple Risk Factor Intervention Trial. *Am J Cardiol.* 1985;55:1–15.
10. Medical Research Council Working Party: MRC trial of treatment of mild hypertension: principal results. *Br Med J.* 1985;291:97–104.
11. Wikstrand J, Warnold I, Olsson G, et al. Primary prevention with metoprolol in patients with hypertension: mortality results from the MAPHY study. *JAMA.* 1988;256:1976–1982.
12. Cruickshank JM, Thorp JM, Zacharis FJ. Benefits and potential harm of lowering high blood pressure. *Lancet.* 1987;1:581–584.
13. Dyer AR, Stamler J, Shebeller RR, Schoenberger J. The relationship of education to blood pressure: findings on 40,000 compiled Chicagoans. *Circulation.* 1970;54:987–992.
14. Keil JL, Tyrrer HA, Sandizer SH, Boyle E Jr. Hypertension effects of social, class and racial admixture: results of a cohort study in the black population of Charleston, South Carolina. *Am J Public Health.* 1977;67:634–639.
15. Johnston WL. Identification of stable somatic findings in hypertensive subjects by trained examiners using palpatory examination. *JAOA.* 1982;81:830–836.
16. Lew EA. High blood pressure, other risk factors and longevity: the insurance viewpoint. *Am J Med.* 1973;55:281–294.
17. A cooperative study: report of the Joint National Committee on detection, evaluation and treatment of high blood pressure. *JAMA.* 1977;237:255–261.
18. Croog SH, Levine S, Testa MA, et al. The effects of antihypertensive therapy on the quality of life. *N Engl J Med.* 1986;314:1657–1664.

19. Siegel D, Cheitlin M, Black D, Seeley D, et al. Risk of ventricular arrhythmias in hypertensive men with left ventricular hypertrophy. *Am J Cardiol.* 1990;65:742–747, 1990.

20. Downing JT. Observations on effect of osteopathic treatment on blood pressure. *JAOA.* 1914;13:257–259.

21. Anderson RA. An osteopathic method for normalizing blood pressure. *JAOA.* 1935;35:128–134.

22. Northup TL. Manipulation management of hypertension. *JAOA.* 1961;60:973–978.

23. Blood HA. Manipulation management of hypertension. In: *Yearbook of the Academy of Applied Osteopathy.* Newark, Ohio: American Academy of Applied Osteopathy; 1964:189–195.

24. Bayer JD. An osteopathic approach to management of hypertension. *The DO.* June 1971;11:143–151.

25. Morgan JP, Dickey JL, Hunt HH, Hudgens PM. A controlled trial of spinal manipulation on the management of hypertension. *JAOA.* 1985;85:308–312.

26. Johnston WL, Kelso AF, Babcock HB. Changes in presence of a segmental dysfunction pattern associated with hypertension. Part 1. A short-term longitudinal study. *JAOA.* 1995;95:243–255.

27. Johnston WL, Kelso AF. Changes in presence of a segmental dysfunction pattern associated with hypertension. Part 2. A long-term longitudinal study. *JAOA.* 1995;95:315–318.

28. Orthopaedics

RICHARD A. SCOTT

Key Concepts

- **Value of orthopaedic training to osteopathic physician**

- **Elements of an osteopathic orthopaedic examination**

- **Osteopathic orthopaedic approach to developmental dysplasia of the hip, hip fracture in the geriatric population, osteoarthritis of the knee, and low back pain**

- **Specifics of history and physical examination, pathophysiology, differential diagnosis, and management**

The study of orthopaedics is an integral part of osteopathic education. After residency, osteopathic orthopaedic surgeons make up one of the specialty colleges in the osteopathic profession. Orthopaedics is the specialty of medicine concerned with the preservation of the health and restoration of function of the skeletal system and its associated structures, i.e., spinal and other bones, joints, and muscles.[1] Orthopaedic training is essential to the osteopathic physician; orthopaedic knowledge extends the ramifications of somatic dysfunction into the structural and anatomicopathologic arena. Orthopaedic knowledge is vital in the differential diagnosis of patients presenting with musculoskeletal complaints; it offers unique insights into the diagnosis and treatment of traumatic and nontraumatic diseases of the musculoskeletal system. Many osteopathic orthopaedic physicians specialize in sports medicine or devote a portion of their practice to this field. They have skills and a special perspective in treating the structural and functional problems arising from sports injuries. Through prevention and rehabilitation, they want to encourage maximum function within the athlete's structure.

The emblem of the orthopaedic society is based on an 18th century drawing by Nicholas Andry (Fig. 28.1) that depicts a tree curved and twisted by the winds and weather, held upright by a series of ropes and splints.[2] This image continues to influence the orthopaedic community. By molding the growing skeleton, orthopaedic physicians help a child grow into a straighter and more functional adult. The etymology of the term "orthopaedics" reflects this perspective as well: "ortho" means to straighten, and "paedic" refers to the pediatric population. The osteopathic orthopaedic physician, with his or her emphasis on structure–function interrelationships, understands and respects this perspective.

The field of orthopaedics has subsequently been divided into orthopaedic medicine and orthopaedic surgery. Beginning in the 1930s, James Cyriax, MD, a British orthopaedist, applied the concept of interrelated structure and function and developed a diagnostic and treatment system that is now known as orthopaedic medicine, in contradistinction to orthopaedic surgery. He authored a series of original papers and the definitive text, *Textbook of Orthopaedic Medicine*, which describes the importance of making a precise anatomic diagnosis based on:

Joint range of motion patterns and their end-feel
Referred pain patterns
Differentiation of contractile and inert structures
Understanding of selective tension

He also created his own system of manual techniques to be incorporated into treatment.

Until his death in 1989, Cyriax believed that the intervertebral disk was the source of almost all spinal pain. While alive, his influence and his dogmatic teaching did not allow alternative ideas to compete.[3] Since his death, however, orthopaedic medicine in the United States has expanded its paradigm to embrace an understanding of myofascial and ligamentous pain. The American Association of Orthopaedic Medicine (AAOM) consists of MDs and DOs who find value in Cyriax's commitment to make a specific anatomic diagnosis using standardized physical examination of the somatic system and who wish to emphasize conservative management of orthopaedic cases. This organization embraces the diagnosis of somatic dysfunction and uses manipulative techniques in their treatment regimens; it is also the North American representative of the international organization of fully licensed physicians interested in manual medicine. AAOM has officially adopted the *Glossary of Osteopathic Terminology* to maintain consistency in their discussions of diagnoses amenable to manipulation. Treatment tools in orthopaedic medicine include:

Manipulation
Prolotherapy
Trigger point therapy
Orthotics
Exercise prescription
Commitment to an orthopaedic perspective

Orthopaedic surgery in the osteopathic profession is almost as old as the profession itself. At the American School of Osteopathy (ASO) in Kirksville at the turn of the century, surgeon

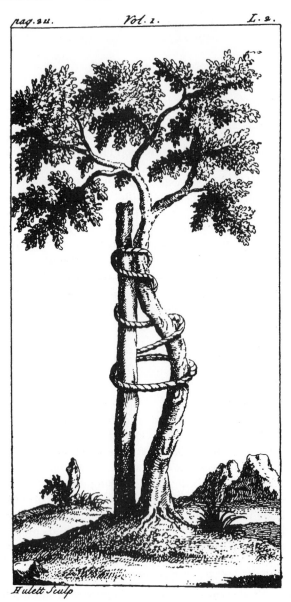

Figure 28.1. "An important basic orthopedic principle is embodied in the figure of the tree. The bone is not an inert, calcified, fibrous material. It is a growing, plastic, dynamic structure with an active metabolism that responds to a wide variety of stimuli, and is as truly "alive" as any other structure in our bodies." "Just as the twig is bent, the tree's inclined," wrote Alexander Pope.[40] (Reprinted with permission from Peltier LF. *Orthopedics: A History and Iconography.* San Francisco, Calif: Norman Publishing; 1993. Art from Andry N. *L'Orthopedie.* Paris: La veuve Alix, 1741.)

George Laughlin, DO, was gaining acclaim as an orthopaedic surgeon by applying European techniques to perform "bloodless surgery" on congenital hip dislocations and in other orthopaedic cases. The surgical team at the ASO at this time also included Andrew Taylor Still, MD, DO, who is credited with "revolutionizing the practice of surgery by osteopathy" by employing osteopathic manipulative treatment (OMT) in preoperative and postoperative care.[4] Research on the efficacy of the osteopathic approach for reducing postoperative surgical

complications with OMT was carried out many years later by another Kirksville orthopaedic surgeon, Edward Herrmann, DO.[5]

The osteopathic orthopaedic specialist has been influenced by adherence to the principles of osteopathic medicine. Even if most of the time in orthopaedics is spent in busy mechanical pursuits, equally important moments are spent practicing as an osteopathic physician. In this sense, the orthopaedist approaches patient care with a keen awareness that the orthopaedic problem is but one part of an entire medical and social paradigm. It is in these moments of interaction with internists, family practitioners, and patients' family members that the orthopaedist brings into play much of his or her osteopathic orientation. One of the goals in osteopathic orthopaedics is to inculcate this attitude of wholeness in treatment, lest the specialist in training take the easy route and forget that his or her area of expertise is only part of the whole.

An osteopathic physician treating an orthopaedic problem adjusts or modifies his or her approach in a manner different from that of a nonosteopathic physician. Osteopathic orthopaedic surgeons are in the subsection of orthopaedic surgeons who have been trained osteopathically, but they are essentially surgeons. The thought processes of surgeons, different from that of nonsurgeons and internists, involve an approach to problem solving that has an immediacy based on the need for urgent decision making. Farmer has studied the educational process and methodology used in training physicians to become surgeons and has noted differences in affect and approaches from that of general internal medicine, where the educational process has been studied more thoroughly (J.A. Farmer, unpublished work, 1992).

One of the things that may make orthopaedics alluring today is the tremendous advance in the ability of physicians to diagnose and surgically treat and thus modify diseases and problems that, in the past, could only be watched as they progressed. What differentiates the orthopaedist from other physicians and surgeons includes often lengthy technical procedures using saws, drills, and metallic implants, as well as the activities associated with fracture reduction and casting, juxtaposed to delicate repairs of tendons and nerves under magnification. Before a surgical procedure, the orthopaedic surgeon performs appropriate diagnostic examinations and tests and formulates a treatment protocol. After surgery, prevention of complications, education about postoperative nutrition, and rehabilitation necessitate a wide range of physician knowledge and skill.

One aspect of orthopaedics, both surgical and nonsurgical, deals with the diagnosis and treatment of traumatic and nontraumatic diseases of the musculoskeletal system. Many health professionals address these issues today. Who should examine and who should treat the injured or aching skeleton? Among the many who offer health care are:

Physician's assistants
Nurse practitioners
Specialty-trained registered nurses

Chiropractic physicians
Physical therapists
Massage therapists

In the hospital, the surgeon faces a bewildering, ever-changing number of possible procedures and implants with differing materials and engineering designs. The surgeon must also work closely with the medical managers and hospital administrators who control the expenditures for this technology. Ultimately, these procedures and tests are done for and on people who are not growing properly, have suffered traumatic injury, have developed arthritis, or have intractable pain.

INTEGRATED OSTEOPATHIC ORTHOPAEDIC EXAMINATION

The integrated osteopathic examination is detailed in other chapters, but certain principles bear summary here. Recognition of referred pain patterns from nerve roots, peripheral nerves, myofascial trigger points, and ligamentous structures is a prerequisite for the integrated osteopathic orthopaedic examination. A neurologic screening examination is also important for differential diagnosis and prognosis in patients referred for orthopaedic evaluation.

Use of selective tension in the examination relies on the observation that normal structures are painless and/or strong when stressed; inflamed or strained structures are painful or weak. Orthopaedic examination employs selective tension to evaluate muscle, meniscal, tendinous, and ligamentous structures and functions, looking for evidence of inflammation or strain. The physician isolates somatic structures and gently but specifically stresses them, looking for pain, weakness, and crepitus. McMurray's meniscal test and Yergason's test are examples of this form of examination.

The orthopaedic physical examination of the somatic system evaluates specific joint characteristics, including range-of-motion and the end-feel associated with major and minor joint motions. Often the same test of joint motion allows for structural and dysfunctional interpretations: excessive motion and/or a sloppy endpoint to the motion may suggest a ligamentous laxity, while a restrictive barrier at the end of motion testing may suggest a somatic dysfunction. It is important to recall that, in somatic dysfunction, the restrictive barrier appears in one combination of directions and is absent in the opposite combination of directions; the barrier is also reversible with manipulation. Restriction in all directions is characteristic of a capsular pattern seen in pathologic conditions such as arthritis or the fibrotic reaction to trauma or overwhelming stress. In such structural diagnoses, somatic dysfunction is also often secondarily present and can be appropriately treated to the patient's benefit. After the secondary somatic dysfunction is treated, the primary structural barrier characteristics remain.

This chapter is intended for generalists and primary care physicians and reviews a few types of orthopaedic disease while discussing how the orthopaedist sees these problems biologically, mechanically, and socially. The chapter discusses what may be distinctive aspects of an osteopathic practitioner's approach to four commonly seen orthopaedic problems:

Developmental dysplasia of the hip
Geriatric hip fractures
Osteoarthritis of the knee
Acute low back pain

Developmental Dysplasia of the Hip

The osteopathic physician, in examining the child at the time of birth and afterwards, first evaluates the whole child. In so doing, he or she looks for dysmorphic features that may be associated with multiple anomalies: the child who has cardiac or gastrointestinal abnormalities, failure to thrive, supernumerary digits, or the inability to bend limbs after delivery.[6] A child with multiple congenital anomalies may have abnormalities of the musculoskeletal system that occurred at the same moment in embryogenesis.

Instability of the hip is one of the more common problems in newborn children.[7] To evaluate hip stability, the physician observes any abnormalities in skin creases or gluteal folds, leg lengths, and inequalities, and watches for spontaneous motion and activities. The physician evaluates the hip while passing it through a range of motion, checks to see if there is easy and full abduction, and feels the placement and fluidity of motion of the femoral head in the acetabulum (the ball in the socket). An abnormality discovered in any of these observations or tests points to a problem.

Most physicians know the Ortolani sign, which is a palpable sensation of a rapid motion of the femoral head—or clunk—felt as the dislocated head is reduced into the hip socket from its dislocated position. Here, as Figure 28.2 shows, the femoral head is gently lifted over the labrum and into the socket. In the case of a reduced hip that is unstable, Barlow's test dislocates the hip as the femur is gently adducted with the hip flexed. The physician gently applies pressure over the medial proximal femur and, while doing so, can feel the femoral head slip out of the socket. As the hip is dislocated, gentle pressure on the thigh or knees gives the feeling that the head is not articulating with the socket but that there is a soft endpoint as the pressure is applied. Moreover, the thigh appears shorter. A positive result in any of these tests, performed routinely in the neonatal examination, suggests further studies or treatment. These tests are performed easily and simply by the osteopathic physician and are examples of the preeminence of a physical examination and the significance of palpatory findings in the evaluation. In the early period of neonatal development, these physical examination tests are more significant than are most imaging modalities, although the recent use of diagnostic ultrasonography has increased the accuracy and sensitivity of the diagnosis of the dysplastic hip. Ultrasonography is especially useful with abnormalities in the development of the soft tissues of the acetabular region, which are not visualized on x-ray films.[8] During treatment, various images such as x-ray studies and CT scans can be used to assess the accuracy and adequacy of the treatment as the child grows or to confirm the physical diagnosis.

Treatment of developmentally dysplastic and dislocated hips involves the application of a fundamental osteopathic precept: that growth and maturation of the skeleton follows function. A properly positioned joint with good, easy motion and adequate blood supply and muscle balance grows and develops normally. The orthopaedist's goal in the treatment of the dysplastic hip is to place that hip in a position whereby normal stimulation for growth of the acetabulum and proximal femur occurs. One can use external position devices such as casts or braces, internal fixation devices, or structural changes operationally to change the alignment of the bones so that they are allowed to grow and mature in an improved position.

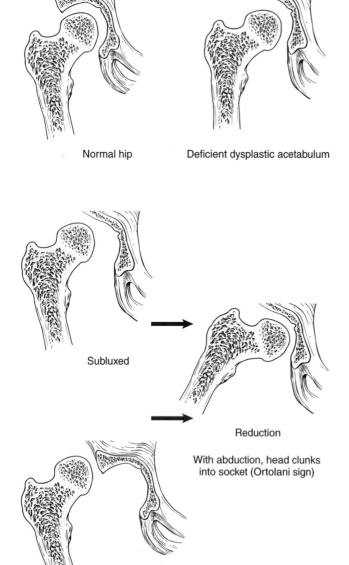

Normal hip

Deficient dysplastic acetabulum

Subluxed

Reduction

With abduction, head clunks
into socket (Ortolani sign)

Dislocated hip

Figure 28.2.   Ortolani sign.

In most cases, a dislocated or dislocatable hip can be either reduced shortly after birth or, if not reducible, held in a position in which the proximal femur is heading or pointing towards and centered over the triradiate cartilage, the middle portion of the acetabulum. Many orthopaedists today use the Pavlik harness to hold such a hip in a position of flexion and abduction while allowing the child to flex the hip and kick at will (Fig. 28.3). The position utilizes a safe zone whereby the femoral head is securely placed and at low risk of dislocation while the patient is harnessed and in which the pressures on the shaft are such that there is less risk for avascular necrosis of the femoral head than in those patients fixed in a rigid cast, which was the older method of treatment. The position in which the hips are placed is termed the human position, in contradistinction to older forms of immobilization in which the neonate's hip might be held in a position more akin to an amphibian or a frog. The principle is of essential importance: placing the hip within the socket in a stable position allows the body to continue to nourish the hip socket and allows its normal growth over a period of time. This has proven successful in most cases. The risk of complications such as femoral palsy from tight straps over the femoral nerve above the knee or of avascular necrosis from constriction of the epiphyseal blood supply are rare.

The second form of treatment of the growing child involves the realignment of the proximal femur and acetabulum to center the growing femoral head within the acetabulum. A typical case of a late unrecognized dislocation presents in a child of early walking age, at approximately 1 year. Such a toddler presents with a shortened leg or a waddling gait. As the child has grown with the hip in a dislocated position, the femur has progressed into a more valgus position at the femoral neck shaft angle (Fig. 28.4). The acetabulum is deformed and shallow, and the cartilaginous lip, or labrum, is defective. The axis of the femur has anteverted, or rotated anteriorly, and developed into a straighter than normal, or valgus, axis. The femur is now

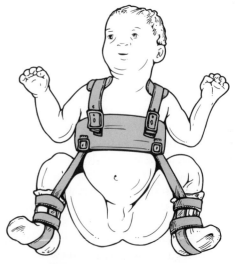

Figure 28.3.   Pavlik harness.

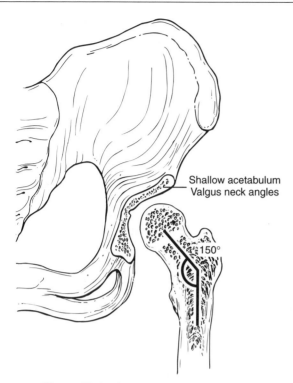

Figure 28.4. Long-standing hip dislocation.

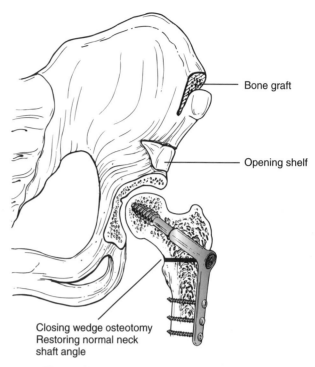

Figure 28.5. Open correction of late deformity.

too long relative to the muscle and capsular tissues surrounding the hip, thus forced manual reduction of the head into the acetabulum places too much tension on the growing bones and results in avascular necrosis of the femoral head. A serious insult to the blood supply of the articular surface of a joint results in collapse of the underlying subchondral bone with fractures that cannot heal because of the lack of nutrition. In lay terms, this is a "dead head," lifeless and unable to carry on its normal biologic function. Moreover, the acetabulum, which has not been stimulated by the femoral head acting within its cartilaginous tissues, has grown dysplastic with a deficient outer anterior and lateral rim. The cells for growth of the acetabulum have migrated proximal to the area of the true socket. The operative treatment for this condition is shown in Figure 28.5.

This operation requires that the superior and inferior sides of the hip joint, the femur and the acetabulum, be addressed simultaneously. In the femur, a shortening, varus osteotomy allows the femoral head to be reduced without undue pressure and changes the neck-shaft angle to a more normal degree from its valgus position. In the acetabulum, a more horizontal socket is formed by either placing a bone graft at the rim or performing an osteotomy above the rim and bending the growing cartilage. If the femoral head is kept reduced into the acetabulum and held there while the tissues heal, it stimulates joint growth and encourages continued normal development over time.

Bones and joints are plastic and develop as a result of the forces that are applied to them. One of the joys of treating young people is to watch the growing child mature over time. The physician can guide this development in many ways. The old saying, "As the twig is bent, so grows the tree," implies a

molding of the whole person. This image continues to influence the orthopaedic community: by molding the growing skeleton, orthopaedists help children grow into straighter, more functional adults.

The term dysplastic hip is used for the abnormality in appearance and congruity of the child's hip. The proper terminology is developmental dysplasia of the hip, which implies that dysplasia may occur not only at birth but also after birth. Congenital dysplasia implies that all dysplastic hips are present at birth. If that were the case, then all should be recognizable at birth. Some hips, however, are normal at birth but become dysplastic in the extrauterine environment. It is important that the physician routinely examine the well baby's hips at regular office visits. The physician should check the child's hips for symmetry, leg length, and equality of abduction at the first postpartum office visit, at 6 weeks of age, and at 6 months of age. The final examination is at 2 years of age, when standing ability and balance are included.[7]

The physician who treats the child with a dysplastic hip is treating not only a mechanical problem in a child but also a child in a family, a small member of a complicated social structure. For the young child, nutritional, educational, and emotional support are paramount. The physician needs to encourage the parents to provide the child with sufficient protein, minerals, and vitamins for growth. The physician also needs to encourage the parents to continue to supply intellectual stimuli or the school system to provide home-bound classes. Ensure that parents, siblings, and other nurturing family members provide emotional support to the child in a cast or in bed. A family with a child with hip dysplasia worries that the child will not walk and be active in life. They need encouragement that the child will probably be able to enjoy a lifestyle not unlike that of his or her friends'.

Hip Fracture in the Geriatric Population

One of the drawbacks of aging is the progressive loss of bone mineral universally noted in men and women after they enter their mid-70s. Weightbearing bones develop osteopenia and have a resultant structural weakness, particularly in the hip, that must withstand heavy forces. When the structural inadequacy of the hip bone is joined with diminished visual acuity, balance, and coordination, falls and fractures are common. In treating an aging population, each physician is involved with geriatric fracture problems.

The patient with a hip fracture presents with not only a mechanical problem to solve but also a personal and social problem. The personal upheaval in lifestyle and abilities as well as the severe economic hardships to the injured person and his or her family profoundly influences all caregivers, illustrating a major problem for public health providers. The number of aging persons with hip fractures is huge, and the costs of treatment for the fracture and its associated morbidity are staggering. It is estimated that 280,000 Americans suffered hip fractures in 1994. The cost in 1994 was nearly $10 billion. If a disease becomes a public health problem when it affects a significant portion of the population, it is incumbent on the public and on physicians to attempt to prevent or control the disease rather than simply treat the disease as it occurs.

In the aging population, fractures of the hip are of multiple types and are somewhat dependent on the forces that act through the hip. These fractures are described according to their location. There are subtrochanteric and intertrochanteric fractures and subcapital fractures. Each particular type of fracture has its own treatment approach. Those fractures that are within the cancellous bone of the intertrochanteric region, if not comminuted or broken into many fragments, generally heal rapidly with stable internal fixation.

Fractures in the subcapital region have multiple treatment protocols, and the approach is more difficult. The younger the patient, the more the physician's goal should be directed toward attempting to bring the bones to a physiologic healing. The blood supply to the femoral head is precarious. Simply aligning the bones and holding them together does not necessarily ensure healing. Just as in the growth of the immature skeleton, so does healing of fractures require adequate oxygenation, nutrition, and blood supply. For any patient with a subcapital fracture, the risk of avascular necrosis is high; nevertheless, with adequate protection and limited weightbearing, union can occur. The surgeon may try to reestablish circulation to the femoral head through a revascularization procedure in which a pedicle of bone attached to a blood supply is rotated into the proximal femur. One method I have used with success is the transfer of a pedicle of bone from the trochanteric region attached to the quadratus muscle along with its large artery. This pedicle is implanted into the femoral head and neck. For

younger patients, the surgeon tries to avoid prosthetic hip joint replacement, which is the alternative to internal fixation of the fracture. The younger the patient, the more likely it is that a prosthesis will fail before the patient has completed his or her active weightbearing life. To recapitulate, fractures in the subcapital region should be treated with internal fixation in the hope that healing will occur. However, if the fracture is severely displaced or if there appears to be a high risk of diminished blood supply to the femoral head, a prosthetic replacement is indicated.

As the population ages and the bone becomes more porotic, the subcapital fractures become more impacted or displaced, and the treatment protocol separates those that are stable or minimally displaced from those that are displaced. For the first group, internal fixation with cannulated screws is recommended; in the latter group, prostheses are recommended. As the population ages even more and the ability to ambulate or even get out of bed disappears, the protocol again becomes more complex because the physician needs to weigh the costs of hospital and surgical treatment and the high mortality rates against the possible alleviation of the acute fracture pain. Sometimes in very aged or cognitively impaired patients, a period of immobilization with traction may be sufficient for a fibrous healing because it allows turning and protection from bed sores; for others, a replacement with an endoprosthesis may allow an earlier discharge from the acute care hospital to the extended care facility with a lessened incidence of contractures, decubitus ulcers, heart failure, and pneumonia. In the treatment of the elderly patient with hip fracture, the osteopathic physician needs to address the respiratory, cardiac, and alimentary systems, as well as take steps to decrease the incidence of thrombophlebitis. He or she must realize that after a trauma such as a fracture and fracture surgery, derangements occur in all of the body systems. The physician must be vigilant and treat these derangements as they occur rather than simply pay attention to the hip alone. Mobilization of the thoracic spine frequently increases cardiorespiratory function and stimulates activity.

Osteopathic physicians need to use their skills and knowledge to help society as a whole in its efforts to increase the quality and quantity of life. Hip fractures occur partly because of biochemical changes associated with aging. The physician should understand how he or she can help the population of elderly people maintain their bony structure and integrity. The basic substrates needed for bone production include protein and calcium. Physicians understand that the absorption of calcium through the gastrointestinal tract partly depends on the interaction of vitamin D and its various active hydroxylated forms with circulating hormones such as calcitonin and estrogen. In nonsmokers, five years of estrogen use may reduce hip fracture rate by more than 50%.

Bone mineral production also is influenced by the basic principle that if an organ or structure is not used, it wastes away. If bone is not used or stressed, calcium is not deposited. A limb at rest or not stressed by gravity, as in a space station astronaut or in a person on bed rest, quickly becomes osteopenic. A physician can help patients maintain bone production by ensuring dietary and supplemental control of essential vitamins, minerals, and hormones. Patients should be encouraged to exercise, particularly in a weightbearing or an antigravity mode. Regular loading of the appendicular and axial skeleton is the best way to enhance sustained mineral production. To decrease the incidence of hip fractures in the elderly, the orthopaedic osteopathic physician should begin by encouraging middle-aged female patients to monitor their estrogen levels, replacing the estrogen particularly in those who are prematurely estrogen-depleted or who have proven accelerated bone loss. All bone will not be maintained strong enough not to fracture, despite these measures. The home and workplace must be made safer. Obstacles that may cause one to trip and fall should be removed. Finally, the balance and agility of the elderly should be evaluated regularly and appropriate steps taken to control seizures or to prevent vision loss.

The incidence of hip fractures is increasing as the population is aging. This is a population that is nutritionally and hormonally depleted. Moreover, it is a population that has forgotten to walk. Regulation of these factors as well as decreasing the extrinsic risk factors in the environment helps decrease the numbers of hip fractures. One of the ways in which the physician can decrease the risk of fractures is to decrease the amount of sedatives and drugs that can impair balance. A novel method for increasing stamina and balance has been proposed by Wolf. Based on a study performed by the National Institute of Aging, Wolf recommends that the elderly practice the ancient Chinese exercise, Tai Chi.[9]

The osteopathic physician has a major role in helping the individual patient as well as the population at risk for these fractures. In his or her treatment of a patient with a hip fracture, the goal is to control pain and return the patient to a nonhospital environment. How he or she treats or recommends treatment depends on the anatomic type of fracture as well as on the physiologic status of the patient.

Figure 28.6 represents the types of fracture and the treatment options. Fractures of the proximal femur are generally classified as intracapsular (occurring within the joint) or extracapsular (which are usually intertrochanteric), in which the fracture line goes between or through the greater and lesser trochanters. When possible, intracapsular fractures are treated with reduction and pin fixation. When this is not possible, prosthetic replacement is necessary. Intertrochanteric fractures are usually held in a reduced position with the use of a sliding compression screw.

Osteoarthritis of the Knee

To examine and treat the arthritic knee requires that one understand how arthritis affects the whole body. The term "arthritis" is used with little specificity and can refer to different types and causes of joint pain. Arthritis is joint inflammation. An arthritic problem can be the result of a systemic disorder that may be immunologically based, the effect of infection, or a metabolic disorder such as rickets. It can be a late effect of

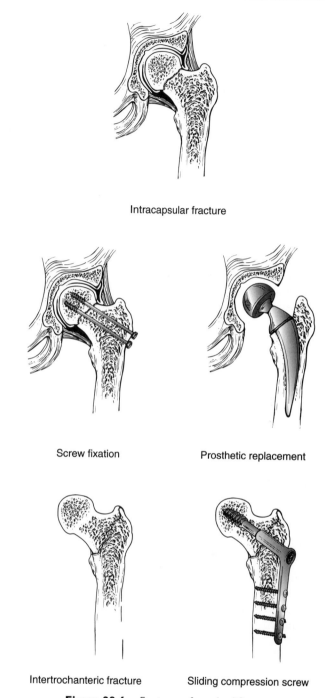

Intracapsular fracture

Screw fixation   Prosthetic replacement

Intertrochanteric fracture   Sliding compression screw

Figure 28.6. Fractures of proximal femur.

trauma such as a fall, a vehicular accident, or a sports ligamentous injury. Before evaluating the joint for which a patient presents to the office because of pain or swelling, the physician must first ascertain if there is a systemic cause for arthritis. Often the types and presentations of the common arthritides are recognizable with a thorough history and physical examination. A careful history allows the physician to recognize that a young female who presents with morning stiffness and symmetrical polyarticular disease might have rheumatoid arthritis or that a middle-aged man with a history of recurrent great toe pain associated with dietary indiscretions who presents with a hot, inflamed knee joint probably has gout. Examination of the gowned patient forces even the most casual examiner to recognize advanced psoriatic skin changes in an arthritic patient. To paraphrase one of the tenets of osteopathic medicine, a patient's disease affects his or her entire body system. It is appropriate and necessary that the osteopathic physician understand the relationship of an arthritic joint to the whole patient.

The most common kind of knee arthritis that presents to the orthopaedist is that of a wearing out or erosion of the articular surface of the medial compartment of the knee, called osteoarthritis. This is usually the result of repeated major and minor trauma or wear. Frequently this is coupled with a normal varus or mild bowlegged body habitus. As shown in Figure 28.7A, in this presentation, a line of weightbearing from the center of the axis of the femur passing to the center of the ankle joint passes inside of or medial to the center of the knee. In this case, the vast amount of forces and stresses that pass through the knee pass entirely through the medial compartment or through the medial femoral condyle and tibial plateau. If there has been an injury to the ligaments or cartilage of the

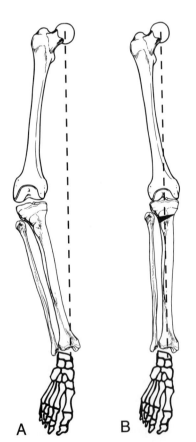

Figure 28.7.   Genu varum. **A**, A lower extremity with extreme genu varum in which the weightbearing line from the hip to the foot passes medial to the knee joint. **B**, A limb after a high tibial osteotomy in which the weightbearing line passes through a point lateral to the center of the knee joint.

knee, with time and the increase of stresses there is increasing wear and debris in the joint. To optimize treatment requires some understanding of how articular cartilage is nourished, what steps can be taken to decrease the wear debris or particulate gravel in the knee, and how to diminish stresses in the medial joint.

The articular surface, or the cartilaginous weightbearing element of a joint, is made up of a matrix of water-heavy proteins with a few living chondrocytes present. This anatomic area has no direct blood flow. The metabolites necessary for the nutrition and repair of the cartilage pass into the structure through the spongelike cartilage. With pressure from weightbearing or muscle contracture, the cartilage surfaces collapse, pushing the fluid into the joint. As the pressure is relieved, the joint fluid seeps back into the cartilaginous matrix, bringing the necessary metabolites and oxygen necessary for cell life. Therefore, it is important to maintain the motion and normal stresses to the knee. As part of the treatment of the arthritic patient, the osteopathic physician needs to encourage motion and activity. Some of the kinds of activities that are helpful in the maintenance of joint structure include low-impact aerobics, water exercises, and repetitive low-stress activities such as treadmills, cross-country skiing, and bicycling. Eccentrically loaded high-stress activities such as jumping are not recommended because the stresses across the joint are too great. Twisting or torquing motions, especially in a joint with weak ligaments, increase the forces and shear that occur across the cartilaginous area. If, as a result of previous trauma or the ravages of aging, the cartilage of the joint is damaged, then the irregularly shaped edges of this normally smooth articular cartilage may be easily ripped or torn with compression and shear. Judicious exercise is important to maintain the metabolic nutrition of the cartilaginous matrix, but overuse may cause serious problems. Assisting the patient to obtain and maintain a body weight within normal limits also helps to diminish the stresses in the joint.

Disabling unilateral medial knee arthritis has other effects as well. The patient with a painful joint has an antalgic gait: he or she limps. Limping causes a twisting motion to the joints above and below the painful joint. A common problem with limping is an imbalance in the sacroiliac articulation with a resultant somatic dysfunction in this joint. Often, as the knee bows medially, an effective leg length difference occurs that may need to be addressed with a lift. Patients with pronated feet increase the stresses over the medial knee joint. The use of a custom orthosis in the shoe frequently changes the dynamics, relieves pain, and allows the patella to track more normally in the patella-femoral trochlear groove.

With pain, the patient fails to exercise and becomes deconditioned; his or her entire cardiopulmonary status may deteriorate if left unattended. Many patients with pain cannot work as hard at their jobs and their hobbies as they would like and become depressed. Counseling and the use of antidepressant medications may be helpful.

At the present time in the development of orthopaedic implants, laboratory designed and manufactured biomaterials do not have the same degree of biologic function as do normal tissues. They are not self-reparative. They have different moduli of elasticity than the human tissues; they do not bend the same amount with forces as do human bones. The result of this is increased stress at the interface between the implant and the biologic tissue. Recently, researchers and clinicians have discovered that particles of wear debris that occur normally with time, particularly those of the high-density polyethylene that serves as the bearing surface in most prostheses, are read by the host cells as foreign. This causes an intense foreign body reaction in some patients. A side effect of this foreign body reaction is a release of biologically active mediators from the tissue macrophages and other immunologically competent cells of osteoclast-stimulating factors. These in turn cause the body, sometimes quickly, to resorb the bone surrounding the implant, weakening the junction between the prosthesis and the bone and allowing loosening, pain, and fracture to occur.

The choice of options for the physician treating osteoarthritis are difficult because no surgical implant can guarantee a relief of pain. As in the case of the younger patient with a hip fracture, replacement arthroplasty should be avoided for as long as possible. The following section and the accompanying diagrams describe the various braces used and surgical procedures done to alleviate discomfort. A physician recommends one modality for a particular patient with knee arthritis based on the understanding of that patient's physiology, age, life requirements, and goals as well as on his or her knowledge of the types of treatment available.

One of the simplest treatments is the application of a knee brace that applies pressure to the tibia below and the femur above, thereby increasing the forces applied over the lateral joint line. This brace is similar to those worn by athletes with torn ligaments; in fact, it was developed for use in arthritic patients through an offshoot of the sports medicine designs. For many the brace is successful for pain relief, although it may be cumbersome to apply and bulky under clothes.

For those who have an angular deformity that is severe and painful, osteotomy may realign the mechanical problems associated with genu varum. As depicted in Figure 28.7B, a simple form of osteotomy removes a wedge of bone from the lateral proximal tibia. If this wedge is properly calculated, when the osteotomy heals, the center of gravity or the forces acting through the knee pass through the lateral joint, thus diminishing the forces through the arthritic medial joint.

For many, as an adjunct to or substitute for osteotomy or bracing, arthroscopy may afford relief. If there is a degree of effusion and torn tissues with multiple loose particles floating inside the knee joint, a debridement or vacuuming of the knee can wash out the offending particles. While this is not curative, for many it affords a long period of pain relief.

For those whose knee joint is not a candidate for osteotomy and whose lifestyle and physiologic age are appropriate, joint replacement arthroplasty is indicated. Joint replacement arthroplasty requires adherence to a host of mechanical constraints. The joint must be in a normal and mechanically sound position, and the components need to be securely fixated to the bones of the knee joint. There are many options, ranging

from the unicompartmental hemi-arthroplasties that simply replace the damaged medial compartment to constrained systems in which the design attempts to substitute for damaged ligaments.

The osteopathic physician needs to understand some of the features of the implants and the physiologic changes that occur with implant arthroplasty. The risks of thrombophlebitis are high. Precautions are necessary, ranging from early activity and external compression devices to therapeutic anticoagulation with warfarin, heparin, or dextran derivatives. The risk of infection, both early and late, although not great is disastrous when it occurs. The risks are diminished through good surgical technique, by decreasing the number of bacteria that can come into contact with the wound, and with the use of appropriate antibiotics. Finally, the physician must recognize that a joint implant is a foreign body. With any systemic infection, circulating bacteria may adhere to the implant and cause a late infection. The judicious use of antibiotics in the face of systemic infections or bacteremias may decrease the incidence of infection. Many physicians recommend the prophylactic use of antibiotics with oral surgical procedures or at other times of predictable risk for bacteremia.

The osteopathic physician who evaluates the patient for a total joint arthroplasty must address the variety of problems that are involved in knee arthritis. Weight control, physical conditioning, exercise, and proper nutrition are helpful to encourage healing and to maximize the gains from the procedure. Ongoing research into the efficacy of osteopathic manipulative procedures in the preoperative period should encourage the physician to maintain a normalized spine. A recently performed study of the adjunctive use of OMT in the early postoperative period following joint arthroplasty showed that those who underwent OMT reported less pain, used fewer analgesic medications, and walked farther than those patients who were not manipulated.[10]

Low Back Pain

The most frequently seen problem for general orthopaedists today is low back pain. Back pain is ubiquitous in the population. The costs of treatment, the expenses of failed work, and the frequently associated problems with blame and the legal system make these problems of urgency. The patient and family need to have a return to work and normalcy; society needs some surcease from the huge costs necessitated by the disability structure. Every physician sees the patient with acute disabling back pain, unable to walk and unrelieved of discomfort. From the orthopaedist's point of view, today this urgency to relieve pain and disability quickly makes a dispassionate evaluation and treatment plan impossible. The new technological advances in imaging and in surgical technique have led many patients to believe that a rapid, easy, risk-free anodyne is available by surgery. Everyone has known someone who, following a back surgery, didn't get better but may have gotten worse. The litigants would have us believe it is because of faulty technique or poor technology or inadequate screws. Spine surgeons are still evolving techniques, materials, and methods to find out which patients with low back pain can benefit from which procedure. Other surgeons frequently do not want to examine, evaluate, or treat the patient with acute or chronic back pain because such patients are often difficult and demanding.

The osteopathic orthopaedic surgeon approaches the patient with low back pain with a systematic protocol. The primary objective for all physicians and surgeons is to define a distinct diagnosis: a diagnosis that has an accurate anatomic and pathologic basis. The great problem for surgeons in general and for orthopaedists in particular is to identify appropriate surgical pathologic conditions. Most back pain does not need to be treated surgically. In a great percentage of patients with low back pain, the final diagnosis is idiopathic. This means essentially that nobody knows what is the cause of the disease. Some estimates indicate that more than 50% of all patients with low back pain do not have a firm, accurate, anatomically defined reason for their pain. To operate is problematic if the diagnosis is uncertain.

Just because a surgeon may be predisposed to seek a surgical solution to a problem does not mean that the spine surgeon looks to operate first. Spine surgeons realize that for people with the same pathologic diagnosis, the long-term result of surgical and nonsurgical treatment may be the same. The outcome in equivalent groups of patients with low back pain and myelographically proven herniated disks is the same as for those who have undergone surgery and those treated nonsurgically. This does not mean that the patient with a frank neurologic deficit, weakness, numbness, and intractable pain over the ipsilateral dermatome should not be operated on. The immediate results of pain relief usually outweigh the fact that later, after the settling down of the disk space and the degenerative changes that occur in the surrounding structures, the postsurgical patient may subsequently have episodes of severe back and buttock pain. The spine surgeon approaches each patient who has been referred as having problematic back pain, pain that the referring physician thinks is severe enough to warrant consideration for operative treatment.

The orthopaedic spinal surgeon who evaluates the patient referred by the family practitioner, emergency room physician, internist, or family members first has to understand the reasons for referral. Back pain that is severe enough to make the bearer nauseous, that has defied the palliative or curative modalities that often prove successful, and that is unrelieved by narcotic medications, rest, and antiinflammatory shots, pills, and emollients must be a surgical disease. If pain is the anathema of life or, as Herkowitz has stated, *Life is the avoidance of pain"* (Annual Spine Session, 1993), then those who suffer and complain have an urgent imperative to seek the services of the surgeon. Patients and physicians are eager believers in the curative possibilities of the newer technologies. If magnetic resonance imaging (MRI) shows a bulging disk and a person has back pain, it follows that the excision of the disk will relieve the pain. That this does not always prove true and that the patient may not improve following a surgical experience does not necessarily mean that the surgeon was inept, but that the imaging

diagnostics may not have been as precise or as helpful as we would want, or that the acute episode is but one point in time of an ongoing process.

Asymptomatic herniations in the lumbar spine are common.[11] It is impossible for the person undergoing severe intractable back pain to think rationally about the nature of his or her pain. As compassionate as the physician-surgeon may be, it is his or her job to review the possible causes of back pain (Table 28.1) to be able to outline the appropriate steps to best understand and treat the acute episode.

Low back pain is so ubiquitous that its definition is elusive. In the context of this chapter, low back pain is that symptom complex in which the person experiencing pain describes it as encompassing the area of the lumbar spine and the associated musculature of the lumbar spine, as well as the sacrum and buttocks. Pain in the lumbar spine may be of local origin or may be referred. Disorders causing low back pain may, in turn, cause radiculopathy, which is a pain radiating through the peripheral nervous system usually into a defined dermatome or somatome. There are large lists of entities that can be associated with back pain. Lists in medicine are useful if only to refresh our memories of possibilities in diagnosis not readily at hand. Too often, however, they serve as diagnostic maps in which the observer-physician finds an easy way to choose tests for diagnostic possibilities. For instance, most people with back pain do not have myeloma. To run a gamut of blood and urine tests on an otherwise healthy 30-year-old to rule out myeloma is not reasonable until the more common and statistically significant clinical entities have been differentiated.

Tests should be chosen with a degree of scientific aplomb, using the test to help firm up a diagnosis only after a careful

Table 28.1
Causes of Back Pain

Mechanical	Tumor
Spinal arthritis	Primary
Degenerative disk disease	myeloma
Facet arthritis	sarcoma
Fracture	neural tumor
Spondylolysis	Secondary (metastatic)
Spondylolisthesis	prostate
Congenital	lung
genetic malformations	breast
achondroplasia	kidney
Nonmechanical	Rheumatologic
Viscerogenic	Seronegative spondyloarthropathy
renal colic	ankylosing spondylitis
inflammatory bowel disease	psoriatic arthritis
endometriosis	Reiter's syndrome
Vasculogenic	Behçet's syndrome
aortic aneurysm	fibromyalgia
ischemic spinal claudication	polymyalgia rheumatica
epidural venous anomalies	Rheumatoid arthritis
Infection	Metabolic
Diskitis	Osteoporosis
Herpes zoster	Paget's disease
Osteomyelitis	

history has been elicited and a physical examination has explored abdominal, pelvic, and spinal structures. In the recently published Clinical Practice Guideline *Acute Low Back Problems in Adults,*[12] the authors have included a series of red flags that help alert the examiner to responses or findings that merit detailed evaluation. Their algorithm (Fig. 28.8) outlines an approach to assessing low back pain symptoms. Throughout the patient evaluation, as the physician is considering the diagnostic tests and therapeutic regimens, he or she should be continually asking if there is some reason for this pain outside of or beyond the spinal area. The red flags that can suggest to the examiner that a serious underlying condition, such as cancer, is present include:

Age of 50 years or older
Previous history of cancer
Unexplained weight loss
Failure to improve with 1 month of therapy
No relief with bed rest

For a patient suffering from a known trauma or with a history of corticosteroid use, fracture is suspected. Intravenous drug abuse, urinary tract infection (UTI), or skin infection in a patient with back pain suggests osteomyelitis or diskitis. Sciatica suggests disk herniation and pseudoclaudication; the symptom of increasing leg pain or weakness that is eased with forward flexion or rest suggests spinal stenosis.[12]

HISTORY AND PHYSICAL EXAMINATION

As in most areas of medical care, the history is of primary importance. A quiet listening attitude on the part of the physician may encourage the patient to be more open and frank. Aspects of the history lead the interviewer to direct his or her questions and suggest further tests or examinations. Examples of questions that can help guide the examiner include:

When did the pain begin?
When is it worse?
What aggravates the pain?
What relieves the pain?
Have other family members had similar problems?
Was the onset associated with a traumatic episode?
Is litigation pending?

Although many of the tests are essential to confirm a diagnosis, the physical examination is crucial. Physical examination includes:

Observation
Palpation and manual motion testing
Neuromuscular examination
Vascular assessment

Although additional tests may later be employed, these four aspects of examination are essential. Many can be performed quickly and concurrently while distracting the patient. All require that the patient be properly attired so that his or her back

and legs can be observed and palpated. Examination of a fully clothed patient is inadequate.

Observation requires a keen eye. Watch the patient while he or she moves from chair to examining table and his or her ability to get off and on the examining table with or without assistance. Note the gait to ascertain if limp, foot drag or drop, or lurch exists. Note the use of an assistive device, cane or walker, as well as any alteration of muscle mass, tone, or atrophy, and the presence of any scars.

Palpation of the back and limbs can be performed in multiple positions. Note the tone of the muscles and the turgor of the skin in the extremities. Examine the spine in standing and supine positions, noting areas of discomfort, pain provocation, asymmetries, or muscle spasm. As the spine is placed through ranges of motion, note individual segments with abnormal findings and make measurements of the ranges of rotation, side-bending, and flexion. Perform percussion of the spinous process and palpation of contiguous areas such as ischial tuberosity, greater trochanter, and groin.

The neuromuscular examination tests motor power, particularly the strength of the ankle and toe flexors and extensors, hip flexors, gluteal muscles, and rectal tone. The ability to stand on toes or heels unassisted is a sensitive evaluator of leg strength and the presence of intact S1 or L5 nerve roots. Test for absent, present, or hyperesthetic sensation in legs, thighs, back, and perineum. Check deep tendon reflexes as well as the presence of clonus or a Babinski reflex. Assess the presence or absence of pressure on the nerve roots in the lumbar spine through the use of the straight leg-raising maneuver, which can be performed with the patient sitting and supine. This maneuver is performed by flexing the hip while keeping the knee extended. Record symptom provocation in the form of back or ipsilateral or contralateral thigh and leg pain. Vascular assessment includes palpation of peripheral pulses and auscultation of abdominal, iliac, and femoral vessels.

There are multiple tests and signs that can elicit symptoms and help the diagnostician. Examination of contiguous joints such as the hip may elicit a cause of referred pain. Frequently, the examiner finds patients with exaggerated complaints. Sometimes the patient may appear hysterical, to magnify the symptoms or to be a malingerer. Careful recording of these findings will help the examiner arrive at a meaningful conclusion. Waddell has listed tests and suggested evaluation for those with atypical findings.[13]

PATHOPHYSIOLOGY

The study of low back pain begins with an anatomic and pathologic consideration of the basis for pain. The basic structural element of the spine is the functional spinal unit (FSU). The FSU is the motion segment and is the "smallest segment of the spine that exhibits biomechanical characteristics similar to those of the entire spine. It consists of two adjacent vertebrae and the connecting ligamentous tissues."[14] How an FSU behaves depends on the structure of each of the elements and its characteristics, strength, flexibility, and responses to stress.

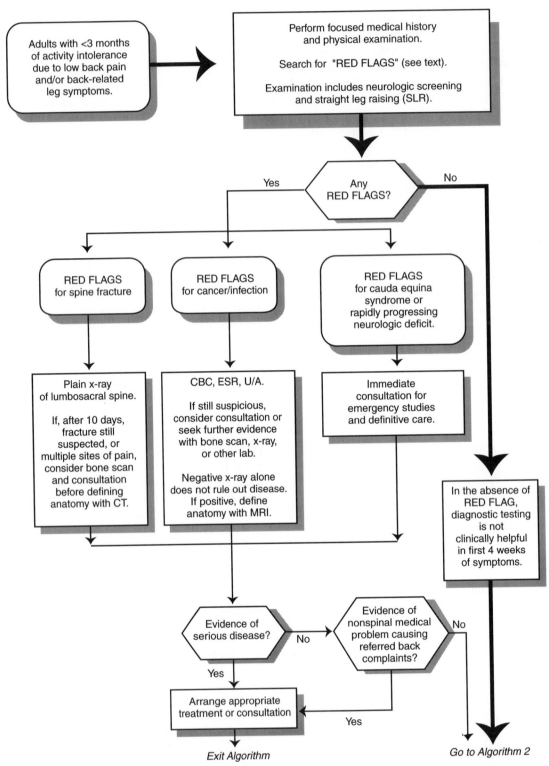

Figure 28.8.   Initial assessment of acute low back symptoms. CT, computerized tomography; CBC, complete blood count; ESR, erythrocyte sedimentation rate; U/A, urine analysis. (Reprinted from Bigos S, Bowyer O, Braen G, et al. *Acute Low Back Pain in Adults.* Clinical Practice Guideline, Number 14. Rockville, Md: US Department of Health and Human Services; December 1994. Public Health Service, Agency for Health Care Policy and Research AHCPR publication 95-0642.)

Each FSU is part of the entire axial skeleton from the inion to the coccyx, and each has a mechanical role to support the mass of the body as it moves in space and time.

The anatomic basis for disease encourages our understanding of the FSU. Disease can emanate from the bony structure, the synovial joints, and the ligaments constraining the adjacent vertebra. Moreover, disease can be caused by problems of the intervertebral disk. Figure 28.9 shows the anatomic basis of the FSU. The FSU contains the elements to contiguous spinal vertebra, their connecting disks, and the associated ligaments and muscles. The posterior elements consist of the spinous processes, ligaments, muscles, and facet joints. The middle segment contains the bony spinal canal and its contents, the neural elements, fat, and vasculature. The anterior elements include the vertebral bodies and the disk. In thinking about the spine as a source of pain, remember this anatomic image.

Figure 28.10 describes the type of motions the FSU undergoes in response to applied forces. This is a three-dimensional image. Over the last century, most physicians have relied on two-dimensional imaging such as x-ray and other modalities. Newer technology such as real time three-dimensional computerized technology scans allows us to better define what are the normal ranges for each of the motions. At present, definitions of measured abnormalities or segmental instability are unclear. The American Academy of Orthopaedic Surgeons offers this definition: *"Segmental instability is an abnormal response to applied loads, characterized by movement in motion segments beyond normal constraints."*[15] Concrete numbers based on an x-ray study or on goniometric measurement to define a pathologic instability and prove that it is associated with a painful problem are lacking, except in cases of gross luxation or angular change as seen in fractures. Palpatory diagnosis in which the endpoint of vertebral motion is ill-defined and either restricted from normalcy or lacking uniformity offers meaningful data to the examining physician.

The stability of the osseous spine depends on three zones, consisting of the anterior, middle, and posterior elements. This model, devised after a retrospective analysis of spinal fractures in the thoracic and thoracolumbar spine, has been widely adapted for use by spinal surgeons to arrange the thought processes in a more logical manner.[16] This discussion centers on the problems of the bony and soft tissue structures. The three columns as described by Denis include the posterior column formed by the posterior bony complex alternating with the posterior ligamentous complex (supraspinous ligament, interspinous ligament, capsule and ligamentum flavum). The middle column is formed by the posterior longitudinal ligament, the posterior annulus fibrosus, and the posterior wall of the vertebral body. The anterior column is formed by the anterior longitudinal ligament, the anterior annulus fibrosus, and the anterior part of the vertebral body.[16]

Denis designed his classification in an attempt to better understand the biomechanical changes found in the common and often devastating thoracic and thoracolumbar fractures. In his retrospective study, he described fractures at risk for neurologic compromise based on injury of the middle column. Although fractures of the "low back" or lumbar and lumbosacral spine are uncommon, the risk of damage to neural elements from middle column disruption in the lumbar spine is less because the cord usually stops above this area, the bony spinal canal is larger, and the cauda equina can be remarkably resistant to compressive damage from fracture fragments. For the anatomic basis of low back pain, the arbitrary separation of the spine into three segments is helpful. It allows the physician to focus on the anatomic element that is the pain generator.

Gunnar Andersson has divided the spine into anterior and posterior segments for ease in isolating causes of disease.[17] This author has labeled the central spinal canal as the middle column to isolate those entities that can cause back pain and may be present in the spinal canal alone (Fig. 28.9*B*).

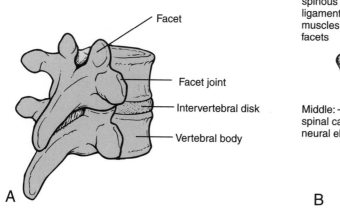

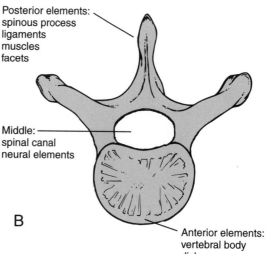

Figure 28.9. Functional spinal unit (FSU) seen from oblique projection (**A**) and end-on projection (**B**).

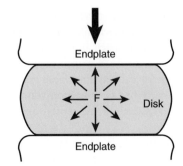

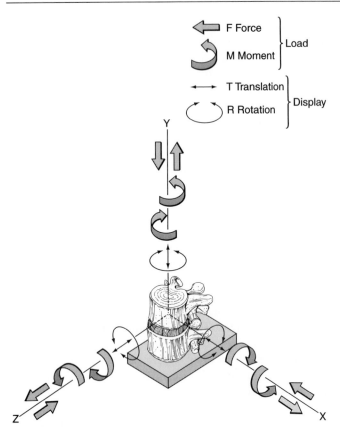

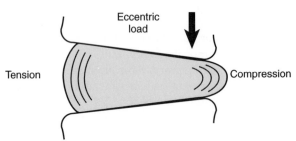

Figure 28.10. Three dimensional coordinate system fixed in space. Twelve-load components (forces or torques) depicted. Application of any one of load components produces displacement of upper vertebra with respect to lower vertebra, consisting of translation and rotation, further divisible with respect to coordinate axes.

Disk under compressive force-normal. Disk pushes, "bulges" annulus outward and compresses end plates.

With bending, eccentric loads cause tensile forces or unloading on one side and higher compressive loads on the flexion side.

Figure 28.11. Disk stresses. F, force.

Entities that may cause acute back pain in the anterior spine include fractures and invasive diseases of the vertebral body and disk, which include tumor, infection, and traumatic disk disruption. Traumatic disk disruption is often characterized by the Schmorl's node or herniation of the disk through the vertebral endplate. The disk has often been implicated as the major source of spinal pain. Certainly, as the disk ages, undue stresses may be placed on the facet joints and arthritic spurs may compress into the spinal canal. However, in the normal spine, the disk under load bulges as a viscoelastic shock absorber (Fig. 28.11). The normal disk behaves in a viscoelastic manner under pressure. During bending (flexion, extension, lateral bending), one side of the annulus is subjected to compression while the other side is put under tensile load. Although it is normal for the disk to bulge in a degenerated state or with a deficient annulus, the disk can herniate or protrude through the ligament and irritate, compress, or damage the neural structures.

Diseases of the middle column include those that compress the contents of the spinal canal; these can be either intrinsic or extrinsic to the canal. Examples of the latter are fragments of bone or disk that are herniated into or compress the thecal sac and neurofibromas or metastatic tumor masses that have entered the canal through the neural foramina and caused compression of the canal. Intradural tumors, meningeal infections, or the sequestered disk when free within the spinal canal can cause intrinsic compression of the spinal cord, as can extradural benign tumors or fibromas. Any narrowing of the spinal canal causes stenosis, a constricting and narrowing of the space available for the spinal nerves and the cauda equina.[18] Most often, spinal stenosis is a problem caused by bony changes, which are usually developmental and associated with aging and degenerative changes. These changes of stenosis rarely occur because of genetic problems, as in the achondroplastic dwarf whose ossification has prevented the development of a large enough spinal canal. The cauda equina syndrome is a syndrome of low back pain, characterized by involvement of the sacral nerves causing numbness around the perineum and loss of bladder and bowel function.[17]

Changes in the posterior column are common and frequently age-related or activity-related. The posterior elements contain the major motion segments of the spinal column including the apophyseal joints and the spinous processes. Fractures of the posterior elements may be associated with severe trauma; most often, severe sprains of the posterior elements are associated with rotatory and translational forces. Fractures, sprain, and somatic dysfunction are part of a spectrum of derangements of the FSU. Mechanical means such as manipulation or traction provide proper realignment of the FSU in these conditions.

The patient with acute low back pain often has a combination of preexisting problems associated with aging.[19] Such changes involve desiccation of the disk with loss of disk height and elasticity, the development of spurs at areas of excessive traction, and inflammation of the apophyseal joint with the production of synovial hypertrophy. For many patients, combinations of factors work together to summate the pain load at each of the areas that generate low back pain. Often, the bearable low back pain that is constant and caused by the inevitable aging process may be increased by a mechanically minor twisting in the posterior elements. When the threshold is reached, the resulting pain drives the patient to see the physician. More often than not, attention to the posterior elements with the use of manipulative techniques spares the expense of multiple diagnostic procedures and surgeries.

Spondylolysis is the most common structural problem found in the pediatric population; it often is not diagnosed until radiologic examination is performed on the adult patient. Spondylolysis is a defect in the pars intraarticularis, the bony bridge between the two facet joints; it is most often developmental or caused by a structural weakness. It may also be caused by an acute fracture, as in the gymnast who repetitively stresses the area in hyperextension activities or in the contact athlete who acutely loads the spine in lordosis. Although the radiologic findings in the oblique lumbar spinal x-ray view might suggest a more serious problem, most patients with acute low back pain and spondylolysis get better. With progressive motion, a vertebra can move or slip on the inferior vertebra; this is called spondylolisthesis. In the vertebra above the lumbosacral segment and most often in the aging spine, this is called pseudospondylolisthesis because it is not associated with a traumatic, developmental, or congenital weakness of the pars intraarticularis.

DIFFERENTIAL DIAGNOSIS

The thought processes involved in diagnosis require separating into definable groups the different known entities with which acute and chronic back pain are associated. One of the ways to separate the different types of back pain is to ask a few elementary questions:

Is the pain intrinsic or extrinsic to the spine?
Does the pain emanate from some deranged structure in the spine or is it directed to the spine from a distant or contiguous area?
Is the nature of the pain related to an injury, an inflammatory condition, an infection, a congenital anomaly, or compression of a neurologic structure?

The extrinsic causes of back pain are associated with viscerogenic and vasculogenic causes. Any visceral disease can manifest as back pain. The pain associated with pancreatitis is classic for unresolvable, unrelenting paroxysms of back discomfort. Prostatitis, renal colic from infection or an obstructed ureter, colitis, or perforated viscus and metastasis of cancer from colon, ovary, or other contiguous organs may all present as back pain. Most often a quick but deliberate palpatory examination of the abdomen and rectum differentiate these entities.

Vasculogenic causes of back pain are associated with claudication. Usually claudication presents with leg pain after or during exertion. It is uncommon but not rare for the ischemic spine to present with pain. The vasculogenic cause of low back pain that is the most urgent is that of the abdominal aortic aneurysm. Remembering that this is not an uncommon entity in the elderly population prone to atherosclerosis leads the physician to palpate and auscultate the abdomen.

Of the myriad other causes of back pain, those that are systemic in origin tend to act directly on the spine rather than from a distant focus. There are systemic diseases of inflammation, infection, and metastasis that cause back pain. Of the inflammatory diseases, the arthritides are most important; that which presents most insidiously is ankylosing spondylitis, one of the spondyloarthropathies. The diagnosis is difficult in the patient who has not developed the classic late radiologic changes but who presents with severe episodic nontraumatic low back pain and stiffness in bending. For this patient, the appropriate blood studies may help confirm the diagnosis. The other seronegative spondyloarthropathies and the inflammatory bowel diseases present with back pain for whom the treatment is nonsurgical.

Infections of the spine have been rare, but they may become more prevalent in the near future as viral diseases increase in a population with primary and secondary immunosuppression. In the proper host, any organism, if unchecked, is able to invade the paravertebral tissues, disk, or vertebral body. The paravertebral plexus of veins of Batson, for example, drains the organs of the pelvis and has been implicated as the conduit down which clusters of tumor cells or aggregates of bacterial organisms pass. These cells may then grow as a metastatic site in a vertebral body or in the epidural space. An awareness of the problem leads to appropriate differential diagnosis followed by controlled biopsy, aspiration, and culture.

Multiple myeloma is an example of a tumor that spreads to bone, particularly the marrow-rich vertebral body. Myeloma and all the myeloproliferative diseases are systemic diseases that tend to grow in the vertebral body, rendering it structurally weak and ready to fracture even with minimally applied force. The more common tumors to spread to bone are:

Breast
Prostate
Kidney
Thyroid
Lung

If faced with a middle-aged patient with low back pain and radiographic suggestions of a metastatic bone tumor, first ascertain whether the more common tumors have become metastatic. There are multiple tumors, benign and malignant, primary and metastatic, that can cause back pain. Figure 28.12 is an algorithm for diagnosis of spine tumors as proposed by James Weinstein, DO, a tertiary spine specialist.[20]

The physician and orthopaedist evaluating the patient with

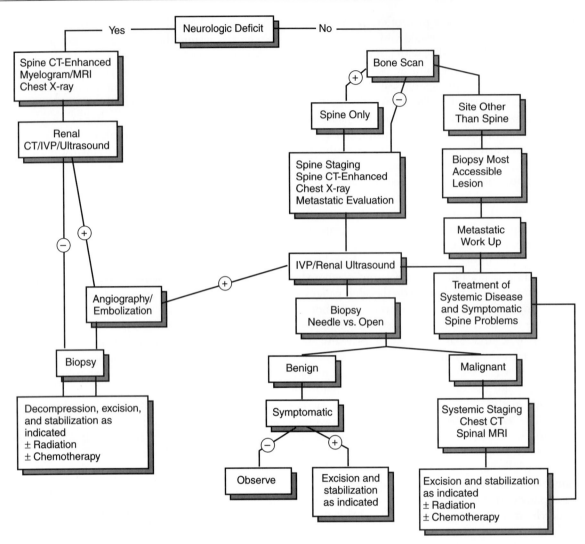

Figure 28.12. Algorithm of approach to spine tumors. (Reprinted with permission from Weinstein J. Differential diagnosis and surgical treatment of primary benign and malignant neoplasms. In: Frymoyer JW, ed. *The Adult Spine.* New York, NY: Raven Press, Ltd; 1991;41:851.)

low back pain must include tumor as a possible cause of the pain, realizing that it is an uncommon cause. All of the following should alert the physician that there may be a remote source of the low back pain:

Malaise
Fevers
Weight loss
Increased incidence of infections
Change in stool character
Blood in urine, sputum, or feces

A history of night or rest pain greater than pain with activity also is suggestive of tumor spread to bone. Of the various tests performed in physical examination, the most important is that of percussion. In tumor and infection of the spine, percussion of the spinous process of the affected vertebra causes severe pain out of proportion to that which might be expected.

The physician who meets a patient whose low back pain is a sign of metastatic disease may not find the diagnosis unexpected, although such a diagnosis usually startles the patient and the family. The patient with a somatoform disorder or psychogenic pain is not rare. Sometimes there are clues indicating a hysterical or hypochondriac pain pattern, such as frequent trips to the hospital or multiple operations, that may suggest some nonorganic cause of back pain. Hysterical paralysis, reputed to be common in Freud's time, is rarely encountered today. Nevertheless, we all see patients with executive back symptoms or back pain caused or amplified by the stresses of life. The terminology used by people to describe their symptoms is often suggestive of nonorganic pain. "My fellow worker gives me a headache," "My job is a pain in the buttocks," or "I feel like I'm carrying the weight of the world on my shoulders" are all examples of the kind of metaphors used by patients in describing their somatic complaints that may suggest that there are additional factors in back pain not associated with structural lesions. In my patient history form, I use a pain drawing in which the patient draws in the anatomic site of his or her pain (Fig. 28.13). For those who are hysterical, characteristic patterns of nonanatomic pain radiation are present.[21] If it is important for the examining orthopaedist to remember that metastatic disease is an omnipresent possibility and that a careful history and physical examination directs him or her to that possibility, it is equally important to remember that the sick patient can have disease. Patients with psychoses and neuroses also have infections, tumors, fractures, and diskogenic disease.[22]

Mark the area on your body where you feel the described sensations. Use the appropriate symbol. Mark areas of radiation. Include all affected areas.

| Numbness | — | Increased Sensitivity | 0000 |
| Constant, throbbing Ache | xxx | Sharp Twinge | /////// |

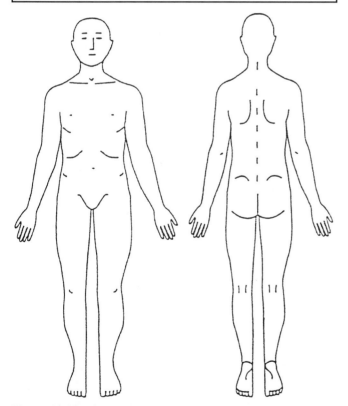

Figure 28.13. Pain drawing used by patient to depict severity, type, and location of pain. (Reprinted from Bigos SJ. *Acute Low Back Problems in Adults*. Clinical Practice Guideline, Number 14. Rockville, Md: US Department of Health and Human Services; December 1994. Public Health Service, Agency for Health Care Policy and Research AHCPR publication 95-0642.)

MANAGEMENT

Most often, the orthopaedist is encouraged to believe that the referring generalist has evaluated the possibility of nonlocalized origin of back pain. Although the orthopaedist runs through a checklist of nonlocalized possibilities during the interview and examination of the patient, the thoughts center on the kinds of problems that are mechanical or structural and might require some form of operative intervention. Most acute low back pain improves over a period of rest or over time. Many patients can be assisted by manipulative treatment. Certainly many of the acute episodes of low back myositis and fibromyalgia are amenable to fascial massage and mobilization, counseling, and tricyclic antidepressants.

Over the last 15 years, there have been major efforts to understand the nature of back pain—what are the sites or pain generators that transmit nociceptive impulses.[23] Operating orthopaedists are attempting to develop surgical[24] designs to stabilize the unstable spine, as well as to define what stability is. They have also been refining approaches and tools to decompress the stenotic spine or entrapped nerve root.

Strides are being taken to establish objective data regarding the efficacy of manipulative medicine. The osteopathic profession is challenged to perform objective studies carried out in a blinded prospective scientific manner. Accurate and reproducible data are difficult to obtain. For more information, review references[25–38] that exemplify current research in manipulative medicine, the majority of which support a beneficial effect of manipulative treatment in the management of low back pain.

Spinal surgeons who deal with complex curves in major adolescent and adult scoliosis must approach the skeleton as a whole as they plan their surgery to balance the weight of the body over the sacrum with an instrumented spinal fusion. The geometric designs require four-dimensional analyses using the x, y, and z axes as well as vector and torsional forces over time.[39] The approach to an 11-year-old with a paralytic curve and hydrocephalus is different from that of a 40-year-old with a 60° thoracic scoliosis resulting from Scheuermann's disease, a developmental disorder with progressive localized kyphosis. Most osteopathic physicians have been well-trained in the palpatory diagnoses of the small curves, rotations, and compensatory changes found remote from the primary lesion of somatic dysfunction. Osteopathic physicians should find the three-dimensional aspects of scoliosis easy to conceptualize.

CONCLUSION

This chapter on osteopathic orthopaedics is not meant to discuss in any detail the surgical aspects of orthopaedic treatment, even though these are the more exciting avenues for the surgeon. Despite the exciting approaches and materials now available, surgery is only useful to try to stabilize or decompress the spine. Most of the time, surgery is unnecessary. Just as treatment for disorders of the growing skeleton is directed toward helping the patient's body mature under guidance, in most cases of acute low back pain, restoration of nutrition, strength, and normal intersegmental motion alleviates pain. The use of algorithms or flow charts, although not foolproof, offer the clinician and the patient the greatest opportunity not to miss causes of back pain that are dangerous and life-threatening— such as fractures or tumors—or are unusual—such as aneurysm or spondylitis. Most often, based on the history and presentation, these life-threatening diseases that can be associated with back pain are ruled out. The nonoperative treatment consists of encouragement that the body will heal, medications to accelerate the healing, and manipulation and exercise to restore segmental normalcy and strength.

And so the reader is led back to the first illustration in this chapter, in which Andry likened the orthopaedic surgeon to the gardener who nurtured his fruit trees so that, by gentle, steady guidance, they grew strong and straight. Andry espoused principles of orthopaedic medicine that will always stay in favor.[40]

ACKNOWLEDGMENT

The author would like to express his gratitude for the help and guidance given by Michael L. Kuchera, DO, FAAO. His discussion of the field of orthopaedic medicine has been gratefully adopted and adapted.

REFERENCES

1. *"Micropedia."* The New Encyclopaedia Britannica. *Micropedia.* Vol VIII. Chicago, Ill: Encyclopedia Britannica Inc; 1987:1017.

2. Andry N. *L'Orthopedie.* Paris: La veuve Alix, 1741, as referenced in Peltier L. *Orthopedics: A History and Iconography.* San Francisco, Calif: Norman Publishing; 1993:22.

3. Gracer R. *Educational Committee Report.* American Association of Orthopedic Medicine (AAOM). Board of Directors, June 5–6, 1993.

4. Walter GW. *The First School of Osteopathic Medicine.* Kirksville, Mo: Thomas Jefferson University Press; 1992:63.

5. Herrmann E. Precepts and Practice. *The DO.* October 1965:163–164.

6. Goldberg MJ. *The Dysmorphic Child: An Orthopedic Perspective.* New York, NY: Raven Press; 1987.

7. Staheli LT. *Fundamentals of Pediatric Orthopedics.* New York, NY: Raven Press; 1992.

8. Hensinger R. The changing role of ultrasound in the management of developmental dysplasia of the hip (DDH). *J Pediatr Orthop.* November 1995;15(6):723–724 . Editorial. (This issue is a symposium discussing the complexities of DDH.)

9. Wolf S. In: Apple DF Jr, Hayes WC, eds. *Prevention of Falls and Hip Fractures in the Elderly.* Rosemont, Ill: American Academy of Orthopedic Surgeons; 1994:120.

10. Loniewski EG, Williams JL, Jarski R, et al. The effectiveness of osteopathic manipulative treatment after hip or knee arthroplasty: a prospective, controlled, randomized, single-blinded outcome study. *JAOA.* 1995;95:492. Abstract.

11. Herzog RJ. Magnetic resonance imaging of the spine. In: Frymoyer J, ed. *The Adult Spine.* New York, NY: Raven Press Ltd; 1991:475.

12. Bigos S, Bowyer O, Braen G, et al. *Acute Low Back Pain in Adults.* Clinical Practice Guideline, Number 14. Rockville, Md: US Department of Health and Human Services; December 1994. Public Health Service, Agency for Health Care Policy and Research. AHCPR publication 95-0642.

13. Waddell G, McCulloch JA, Kummel E, et al. Non-organic physical signs of low back pain. *Spine.* 1980;5:117–125.

14. White AA, Panjabi MM. *Clinical Biomechanics of the Spine.* 2nd ed. Philadelphia, Penn: J.B. Lippincott Co; 1990:45.

15. American Academy of Orthopedic Surgeons. A Glossary on Spinal Terminology. Quoted in: Frymoyer J, Pope MH. Segmental Instability. *Semin Spine Surg.* June 1991;3(2):109.

16. Denis F. The three-column spine and its significance in the classification of acute thoracolumbar spine injuries. *Spine.* 1983;8:817–831.

17. Andersson GB, McNeil T. *Lumbar Spine Syndromes, Evaluation and Treatment.* Wien, NY: Springer Verlag; 1989.

18. Mirkovic S, Garfin SR. Spinal stenosis: History and physical examination. In: Schafer M, ed. *Instructional Course Lectures.* Volume 43. Taunton, Mass: American Academy of Orthopedic Surgeons; 1994:435–439.

19. Frymoyer JW, Gordon SL. *New Perspectives on Low Back Pain.* Park Ridge, Ill: American Academy of Orthopedic Surgeons; 1989:217–241.

20. Weinstein J. Differential diagnosis and surgical treatment of primary benign and malignant neoplasms. In: Frymoyer JW, ed. *The Adult Spine.* New York, NY: Raven Press, Ltd; 1991;41:851.

21. Ransford AO, Cairns D, Mooney V. The pain drawing as an aid to the psychological evaluation of patients with low-back pain. *Spine.* June 1976;1(2):127–134.

22. Stein D, Floman Y. Psychologic approaches to the management and treatment of chronic low back pain. In: Weinstein JN, Wiesel SW, eds. *The Lumbar Spine.* Philadelphia, Penn: WB Saunders; 1990:811–827.

23. Fairbank J, Hall CT, van Akkerveeken H, et al. Diagnosis and neuromechanisms. In: Weinstein JN, Wiesel SW, eds. *The Lumbar Spine.* Philadelphia, Penn: WB Saunders; 1990:88–159.

24. Weinstein J, LaMotte R, Rudevile B. Nerve. In: Frymoyer JW, Gordon SL, eds. *Perspectives on Low Back Pain.* Park Ridge, Ill: American Academy of Orthopedic Surgeons; 1989;4:35–110.

25. Chrisman OD, Mittnacht A, Snook GA. A study of the results following rotatory manipulation in the lumbar intervertebral disc syndrome. *J Bone Joint Surg.* 1964;46:517–524.

26. Brodin H. Inhibition—facilitation technique for lumbar pain treatment. *Manual Medicine.* 1987;3:24–25.

27. Brunarski DJ. Clinical trials of spinal manipulation: a critical appraisal and review of the literature. *J Manipulative Physiol Ther.* 1984;7:243–249.

28. Dixon G. The current status of the scientific basis for manipulation. *Curr Concepts Rehabil Med.* 1985;2:3–5.

29. Di Fabio RP. Clinical assessment of manipulation and mobilization of the lumbar spine: a critical review of the literature. *Practice.* 1986; 66:51–53.

30. Anderson R, Meeker WC, Wrick BE, et al. A meta-analysis of clinical trials of spinal manipulation. *J Manipulative Physiol Ther.* 1992; 15:181–194.

31. Mac Donald R, Bell CMJ. An open controlled assessment of osteopathic manipulation in nonspecific low back pain. *Spine.* 1990; 15:364–370.

32. Greenland S, Reisbord LS, Haldeman S, et al. Controlled clinical trials of manipulation: a review and proposal. *J Occup Med.* 1980; 22:670–676.

33. Hadler NM, Curtis P, Gillings DB, et al. A benefit of spinal manipulation as adjunctive therapy for acute low back pain: a stratified controlled trial. *Spine.* 1987;12:703–706.

34. Jayson MIV, Sims-Williams H, Young S, et al. Mobilization and manipulation of low back pain. *Spine.* 1981;6:409–416.

35. Carey TS, Garrett J, Jackman A, et al. and the North Carolina Back Pain Project. The outcomes and costs of care for acute low back pain among patients seen by primary care practitioners, chiropractors, and orthopedic surgeons. *N Engl J Med.* 1995;333:913–917.

36. Deyo RA. Nonoperative treatment of low back disorders: differentiating useful from useless therapy. In: Frymoyer JW, ed. *The Adult Spine: Principles and Practice.* New York, NY: Raven Press; 1991:1567–1579.

37. Haldeman S, Phillips RB. Spinal manipulative therapy in the management of low back pain. In: Frymoyer JW, ed. *Adult Spine: Principles and Practice.* New York, NY: Raven Press; 1991:1581–1605.

38. Shekelle P, Adams A, Chassin M, et al. Spinal manipulation for low back pain. *Ann Intern Med.* 1992;117:590–598.

39. Asher MA, Strippgen, Walter, et al. Isola instrumentation. In: Weinstein SL, ed. *The Pediatric Spine.* New York, NY: Raven Press; 1994; 77:1619–1657.

40. Peltier LF. *Orthopedics: A History and Iconography.* San Francisco, Calif: Norman Publishing; 1993:21.

29. Obstetrics

MELICIEN A. TETTAMBEL

An up-to-date osteopath must have a masterful knowledge of anatomy and physiology. He [sic] must have brains in osteopathic surgery, osteopathic obstetrics, and osteopathic practice.

—ANDREW TAYLOR STILL[1]

Key Concepts

- **Somatic dysfunction in normal pregnancy, including low back pain, other musculoskeletal problems, fluid circulation, and hormonal changes**

- **Indications and contraindications for osteopathic manipulative treatment during pregnancy**

- **Examination, viscerosomatic reflexes, and exercise in first trimester**

- **Skeletal changes and carpal tunnel syndrome in second trimester**

- **Biomechanical changes in third trimester**

- **Evaluation of lumbosacral spine and pelvis for labor and birth; possible rupture of pubic ligaments**

- **Low back pain and wrist problems during postpartum period**

Osteopathic management of an obstetric patient requires knowledge of the influence of the maternal structural framework on her pregnancy, and the effect of the pregnancy on her structure. Somatic dysfunction, as defined in the American Osteopathic Association's glossary, is *"impaired or altered function of related components of the somatic (body framework) system; skeletal, arthrodial, and myofascial structures, and related vascular, lymphatic, and neural elements."*[2] Evaluation and treatment of somatic dysfunction enhances homeostasis, facilitates maternal adaptation to structural and hormonal changes, and may alleviate maternal discomfort caused by an enlarging uterus.

During the process of evaluating and treating somatic dysfunction, the osteopathic obstetrician monitors fetal well-being and addresses potential stresses in the mother's body that can occur as a result of pregnancy, labor, and birth. Physical changes and stresses in maternal structures, even apart from psychological aspects, are common. More than half of all pregnant women report some kind of musculoskeletal pain during pregnancy.[3–4] There are several aspects of the changing maternal-fetal structural relationships that may cause somatic dysfunction at any time from conception to postpartum. These relationships can be organized like pregnancy into trimesters. Obstetric conditions that may respond particularly well to os-

teopathic manipulative treatment (OMT) or that may be relative contraindications to such treatment are of special interest.

SOMATIC DYSFUNCTION IN NORMAL PREGNANCY

Three broad areas of somatic dysfunction effect changes in both mother and fetus. These include:

Changes in maternal structure and biomechanics as a result of the developing fetus
Changes in body fluid circulation
Hormonal changes

These changes are listed in descending order of our ability to treat osteopathically. Although most of these changes are reversible, wide variability exists among patients in the time interval after birth before complete reversion to the pregravid condition. The most obvious changes that occur during pregnancy are in the musculoskeletal system. The nongravid pelvis assumes a new angle when filled with a growing fetus and must be able to support the weight and volume of the enlarging uterus and fetal structures (often up to 6 kg). During fetal growth, the mother's center of gravity shifts forward. In compensation, the lumbar spine assumes an increased lordotic posture with a resultant increased pelvic tilt. This tilt is defined by the angle between the horizontal and the posterior superior and posterior inferior iliac crests (angle *theta* in Fig. 29.1).[5] The thoracic spine also increases its kyphotic posture. The changes in body fluid circulation and hormones during pregnancy are generally less obvious, less well-studied, and more controversial regarding their origins than are the changes in the musculoskeletal system.

Low Back Pain

One of the most common complaints and complications of pregnancy is low back pain, which has been traditionally accepted as inevitable by women and their physicians.[6] The majority of published reports regarding its cause are either anecdotal or reflect data taken from patient questionnaires. Only two studies have employed a traditional detailed physical examination of patients to properly diagnose the source of back pain.[7–8] Several studies have found that heavy manual labor and smoking are risk factors for the development of low back pain symptoms during pregnancy.[7–12] Parity, age, and previous history of low back pain have also been associated with such symptoms in most studies, but other reports have not supported these conclusions, perhaps because of limitations in study design, methods, and/or statistical power. The following have not been found to correlate with the development of low back pain symptoms during pregnancy[4]:

Race
Occupation
Fetal weight
Prepregnancy maternal weight
Weight gain
Exercise habits
Sleeping posture
Mattress type
Shoe heel heights[13]
Previous epidural anesthesia

The gravid uterus and the compensatory lordosis that it causes create a tremendous mechanical burden on the lower back.[14–15] This altered posture increases stress across the vertebral facets of the lumbar spine and increases shear forces across the intervertebral disk spaces. The paraspinal muscles shorten posteriorly and are unbalanced by overstretching abdominal muscles anteriorly. Fast et al. clinically illustrated the abdominal weakness in pregnancy by comparing the abilities of two groups (a 36-week pregnant cohort and an age- and weight-matched group of nonpregnant women) to perform a sit-up. Eighty-six percent of the pregnant women could not perform a single sit-up, compared with 11% of the nonpregnant controls.[16] This major difference in ability to perform a simple exercise with the abdominal muscles is indicative of the major change in normal structure and function during pregnancy.

Hyperlordosis is frequently implicated in the cause of low back pain. Although radiographic studies have not verified this to date, Bullock et al. used an inclinometer to measure the progression of kyphosis, lordosis, and pelvic tilt in 34 pregnancies.[17] In their study they found that thoracic kyphosis increased by an average of 6.6%, lumbar lordosis by 7.2%, and pelvic tilt by only 1.9% throughout the course of pregnancy. These small degrees of increase and tilt did not correlate with development of low back symptoms in their study group. Snijders et al. studied 16 pregnant women, using a combination of reflectometers and mathematical modeling to measure curvature of the spine in the weeks just before and just after birth.[18] Their patients were an average of 10 mm taller before birth; kyphosis and lordosis were less marked before birth than after. They postulate that these findings are a result of a relaxation of the psoas muscle, which allows the lordosis normally present to flatten. Östgaard et al. have concluded that pregnant women compensate for intrapelvic changes by subtle lumbar lordosis. These investigators postulate that lumbar lordosis results from hip joint, upper trunk, and neck extension rather than from lumbar spine extension.[19]

Pain in the sacroiliac region has been suggested to result from excessive connective tissue stretch and microtrauma. This pain is a consequence of the trunk extensor muscle forces that balance the anterior tilt of the pelvic brim caused by the growing uterus.[20] Pelvic distension further increases mobility of the sacroiliac joints (Fig. 29.1). The transition between physiologic and pathologic pelvic relaxation, resulting in pain, is indistinct. At first, the main symptoms of pelvic relaxation are spontaneous pain and tenderness of the sacroiliac joints elicited by

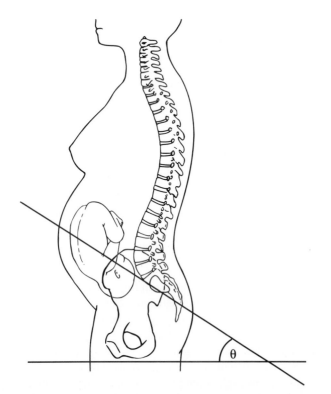

Figure 29.1. Spinal and pelvic changes in pregnancy. (Adapted from DiGiovanna EL, Schiowitz S. *An Osteopathic Approach to Diagnosis and Treatment.* Philadelphia, Penn: JB Lippincott Co; 1992.)

direct or indirect pressure.[21–22] Later, sacroiliac relaxation results in lumbar backache that radiates down the back of the thighs. Occasionally, pain may radiate over the anterior aspects of the lower part of the abdomen and thighs.[23–24]

Another type of back pain that commonly affects a large group of pregnant women is located in the posterior part of the pelvis, distal and lateral to the lumbosacral junction. Pain radiates to the posterior part of the thigh and may extend below the knee, and thus may be interpreted as sciatica or posterior joint syndrome. A study by Östgaard et al. of 436 pregnant women revealed that this condition, given the name "posterior pelvic pain," is different from sciatica. It is less specific than the nerve root syndrome in distribution and does not extend down into the ankle and foot.[25] This pain is different from posterior joint syndrome because it does not emerge from the lumbar area. Additionally, posterior pelvic pain does not include muscle weakness or sensory impairment, and reflexes are unchanged. Therefore, posterior pelvic pain associated with pregnancy should not be treated as low back pain or sciatica.

Radicular symptoms frequently accompany low back discomfort associated with pregnancy.[6] Despite increased shear placed across the disk space (which varies among individuals), herniated nucleus pulposis during pregnancy is uncommon, having an incidence of only 1:10,000.[26] It has been postulated that direct pressure on nerve roots or plexi by the gravid uterus is responsible for many of the radicular symptoms.[27] "Parietal neuralgia of pregnancy" was first described by Bushnell in 1949.[28] He proposed that mechanical pressure of ligamentous structures of the spine on nerve roots (resulting from increased lordosis of pregnancy) was responsible for radicular pain of pregnancy. The symptoms are primarily paresthesias in the distribution of the ilioinguinal and iliofemoral nerves.

Lightening, an event that generally occurs during the final four weeks of pregnancy, is also occasionally associated with radicular symptoms. The presenting part of the fetus settles into the pelvis, thus "lightening" the pressure against the diaphragm and upper abdominal cavity.[29] Although breathing becomes much easier for the mother, she may also experience radicular symptoms, which have been attributed to direct pressure of the gravid uterus on components of the lumbosacral plexus that coalesce into the sciatic nerve. A recent study using magnetic resonance imaging demonstrated that bulges or herniations of lumbosacral disks are common in women of childbearing age and that pregnant women do not have an increased prevalence of disk abnormalities.[30]

There is concern that pregnancy may cause preexisting scoliosis to progress. Berman et al. identified an increased progression of the curve in three of eight patients who had idiopathic scoliosis.[31] They proposed a link between the effects of the hormone relaxin and the mechanical stress of pregnancy that causes scoliotic curves of more than 25° to progress. In contrast, in a large retrospective review of 355 women who had idiopathic scoliosis (175 of whom had been pregnant and 180 of whom had not), Betz et al. concluded that pregnant scoliotic patients are not at risk for an increase in the progression of spinal curvature.[32] Scoliotic curves tend to progress in adulthood, but pregnancy does not seem to aggravate the rate of increase. In addition, mild-to-moderate idiopathic scoliosis does not appear to create problems with pregnancy. The rate of successful pregnancy outcomes in women who had scoliosis did not differ from those without scoliosis.[32] However, one recent review suggested that patients with scoliosis had more premature births than were expected.[33] Women with previous posterior spinal fusion for idiopathic scoliosis have also been shown to have no increased risk of development of low back pain during pregnancy.[32]

Other Musculoskeletal Problems

Although certain musculoskeletal changes occur during pregnancy, pregnancy itself may affect some preexisting musculoskeletal conditions such as rheumatoid arthritis and ankylosing spondylitis. Pregnancy may have ameliorating effects on most women who have rheumatoid arthritis, usually beginning as soon as they become pregnant and continuing until approximately 6 weeks after birth.[34] The signs and symptoms of the disease may recur with a flare in the postpartum period. Some investigators have speculated that rheumatoid arthritis tends to improve in pregnancy because of increased cortisol secretion.[35] Others have proposed that increased α-glycoprotein in the maternal serum decreases inflammation.[36–37] Some researchers also assert that substances derived from the fetal tissues alter the severity of this autoimmune disease, perhaps through secretion of cortisol or other substances.[38]

Whereas rheumatoid arthritis generally improves with pregnancy, ankylosing spondylitis is often aggravated by pregnancy, perhaps because of the increased stresses on the sacroiliac joints during enlargement of the nearby uterus.[39] Overall, the course of the disease (over decades) is not affected positively or negatively by one or more pregnancies.[39] Even though ankylosing spondylitis often limits motion of the pelvic joints, it is usually not a hindrance to vaginal birth.[40–42]

Changes in Body Fluids and Circulation

Increased circulation to the pelvic organs is necessary to meet the metabolic needs of fetal development. Unfortunately, this increase is sometimes accompanied by insufficient return of fluid into maternal systemic circulation. Either of these can result in congestion or edema of maternal organs and tissues. Fluids increase an average 6.5 liters over the course of pregnancy.[43] Hemorrhoids or varicosities of the vulva or lower extremities may occur as a result of sluggish venous return influenced by pressure of the uterus on the venous plexi in the pelvis. Back pain may also be related to development of varicosities.[43–45] Some women complain of night back pain 1–2 hours after lying down, which may awaken the patient from sleep. Fast et al. noted that dependent edema accumulates when a pregnant woman is in the upright position during the day.[43] When she lies down at night, the changes in osmotic forces allow some of this fluid to return to the intravascular space, resulting in increased venous return. This increased venous return, coupled with venous blockage that occurs by pressure of the fetus on the vena cava, results in decreased blood flow through the pelvis. A delayed, stagnant hypoxia of the neural tissue and the vertebral bodies ensues, producing the delayed low back pain (and sometimes radicular symptoms) that awaken the patient.[45]

Physical factors of pulse and respiration changing pressure gradients between the abdomen and thorax alter venous flow dynamics, causing congestion (Fig. 29.2).[46] Because of this flow alteration, a change in volume of abdominal organs (e.g., liver, pancreas) also occurs, which tends to increase abdominal cavity pressure. This reversal of venous flow into vertebral and spinal membranes causes central nervous system congestion, resulting in complaints of headache, nausea, and lightheadedness. Because the venous system of the spine is valveless,[47] blood from the spinal cord, membranes, and spine passes through communicating veins to the azygous and hemizygous systems (which do not have individual veins for all thoracic and lumbar spinal levels). Venous blood from these areas usually drains into the heart via the superior vena cava. Decreased efficiency of this closed system may decrease oxygen and cardiac output as arterial blood volume is influenced by cardiac contractions "pushing" venous blood, and as respiration "pulls" venous blood with breathing effort. Nausea, headache, and congestion of the liver and pancreas may result from venous stasis also caused by the gravid uterus on the vena cava, as well as the venous plexi emanating from the spine.[48]

Hormonal Changes

During pregnancy, alterations in hormonal levels cause physical changes in many parameters. One of the most dramatic of these changes is the widening and increased mobility of the sacroiliac joints and the symphysis pubis, which begins at the 10th to 12th week of pregnancy. The increased width of the symphysis pubis can be detected radiographically as early as the first trimester and becomes maximum near term. The hormone relaxin has been identified as a major contributor to these changes in joint laxity during pregnancy.[15] Relaxin is secreted by the corpus luteum of pregnancy.[49–50] Concentrations of relaxin are elevated during the first trimester and then decline early in the second trimester to a level that remains stable throughout the rest of the pregnancy until labor.[49] Interestingly, the level of relaxin is not increased with twin gestations. Lower concentrations have been found, however, after 43 weeks gestation and in women in premature labor.[50] Primary target tissues are the cervix, uterus, and ligamentous structures of the pelvis. Relaxin promotes relaxation of the articulations of the pelvis in preparation for passage of the fetus during the birthing process.[51] MacLennan et al. reported that women who have been incapacitated by low back pain during pregnancy have extremely high levels of relaxin,[52] suggesting that excessive relaxin is not innocuous.

Another important change during pregnancy that is related to hormonal alterations occurs in the respiratory system. Dur-

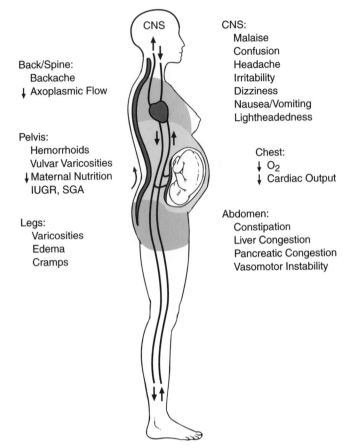

Figure 29.2. Pathophysiologic effects of congestion during pregnancy. CNS, central nervous system; IUGR, intra-uterine growth retardation; SGA, small for gestational age. (Adapted from Kuchera M, Kuchera W. *Osteopathic Considerations in Systemic Dysfunction.* 2nd ed. Kirksville, Mo: KCOM Press; 1992.)

ing pregnancy, there are relatively large changes in the mechanical configuration of the thoracic cage, most of which occur before the uterus enlarges sufficiently to account for such increases. The chest circumference increases 5–7 cm, the subcostal angle increases from 68 to 103°, and the diaphragm is pushed superiorly by approximately 4 cm but increases in excursion by 1–2 cm.[53] These changes lead to a 30–40% increase in tidal volume and a similar increase in minute ventilation because the respiratory rate is essentially constant. These changes are usually attributed to the effects of higher levels of circulating progesterone in pregnancy (based on physiologic studies of progesterone-treated, nonpregnant animals), but relaxin possibly also plays an important role.

Elevations in steroid hormonal levels (especially progesterone) may promote fluid retention, which enhances congestion in both local tissues (e.g., periuterine) and distant sites (e.g., pedal edema, exacerbated by gravity). This congestion may decrease oxygenation and metabolism at the cellular level, leading to accumulation of metabolic waste products in soft tissues as well as in the gastrointestinal tract.[54]

FIRST TRIMESTER

At the initial prenatal visit (usually after the first or second missed menstrual period), the obstetrician obtains a full health inventory and performs a complete physical examination.[54] In addition to performing a traditional pelvic examination, the osteopathically trained obstetrician may also perform further palpatory structural examination to identify somatic dysfunction that could affect the outcome of pregnancy. Asymmetry of bony landmarks, joint motion tests, tissue texture changes, and local tenderness are used to confirm areas of somatic dysfunction. Palpatory examination of the paraspinal tissues is performed to identify areas of tissue texture changes that represent viscerosomatic reflex sites.[55] Special attention is given to evaluation of any tissue texture change at the costotransverse area because of the belief that autonomic nerve effects on segmental muscles are specific. Spinal segmental sites for somatic dysfunction associated with visceral disease are related to the autonomic nervous system supply for various organs.[47,56–62] Hansen and Schliak have identified spinal reflex sites at thoracolumbar levels of T10-L2 (Fig. 29.3)[63] affecting these organs:

Large bowel
Appendix
Kidney
Ureter

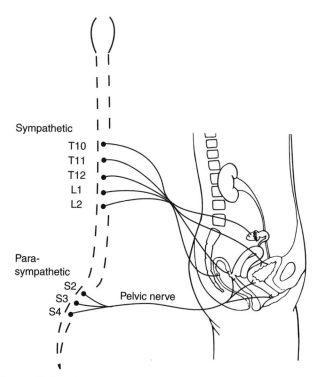

Figure 29.3. Sympathetic and parasympathetic innervation of female pelvis. (Adapted from DiGiovanna EL, Schiowitz S. *An Osteopathic Approach to Diagnosis and Treatment.* Philadelphia, Penn: JB Lippincott Co; 1992.)

Adrenal medulla
Testes
Ovaries
Urinary bladder
Uterus

Woods reported that presurgical palpatory findings of a viscerosomatic reflex correlated with the diagnosis in 10 of 13 patients who had acute abdominal disorders.[64] Palpatory diagnosis of viscerosomatic reflexes should assist the physician in the differential diagnosis of somatic pain. When combined with other historic or physical evidence, a positive reflex may enhance the predictive value of the diagnosis of visceral disease.

OMT of viscerosomatic reflexes has been advocated on the basis that it is designed to reduce residual effects in the somatic structures following a visceral disorder or to influence the viscus through stimulation of somatovisceral effects.[65] Osteopathic physicians have advocated manipulative treatment as a part of the treatment regime for organic problems, as well as for preoperative and postoperative management of patients with organic disease.[66–69]

In the first trimester of pregnancy, "morning sickness," or hyperemesis, is a common complaint. The precise cause of the nausea and vomiting remains unclear.[54] Viscerosomatic reflexes may be identified on structural examination and often respond to OMT.[61] Chapman's reflexes[70] are anterior and posterior myofascial tender points related to organ function that have been "geographically" charted on the body (Fig. 29.4). Evaluation of C2 and T5-T9 may identify digestive disturbances.[71] Use tenderness of a Chapman's anterior point for diagnosis as well as an indicator to evaluate the degree of success in relieving organ dysfunction. Posterior points are less sensitive to palpation and are usually used for treatment. Use anterior points for treatment when attempts at a posterior approach are unsuccessful. The indications and contraindications for OMT during pregnancy are summarized in Table 29.1.

Pregnant women often inquire about exercise at the first prenatal visit. Selection of exercises should reflect a consideration of the changes in the patient's weight, body habitus, and balance to minimize the risk of injury to the patient and her fetus.[3,23,72] Maintenance of good abdominal tone should be encouraged.[73] Current recommendations from the American College of Obstetricians and Gynecologists are that pregnant women exercise for no longer than 15 minutes at a time and that they maintain a pulse rate of less than 140 beats per minute and a core body temperature of less than 38° C.[74] It has been shown that the second stage of labor lasts only half as long in athletes as in nonathletes.[75] Of course, regimens should be individualized. High-risk patients, such as those who have diabetes, hypertension, defects of the cervix, or a history of miscarriage, may not be able to exercise.[76] In addition to exercise, weight gain has been advised to be limited to a total of 9.1–13.6 kg (approximately 1.4 kg/month) during the course of pregnancy.

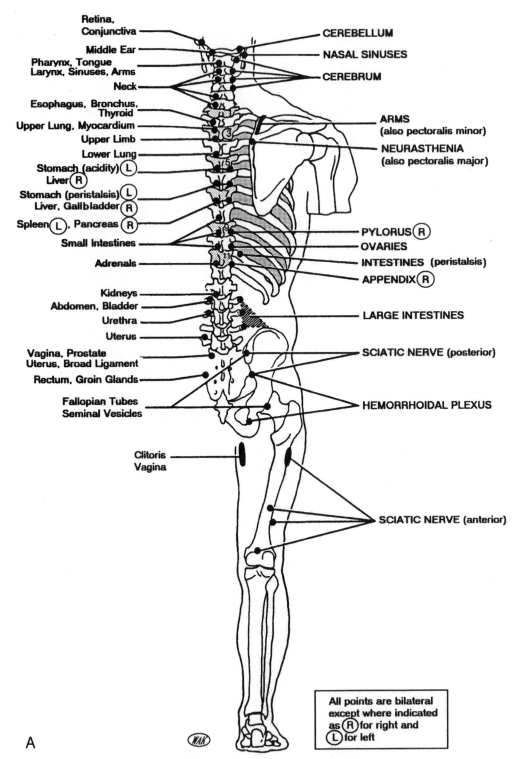

Figure 29.4. Chapman's reflexes. **A,** Posterior points. **B,** Anterior points. (Adapted from Kuchera M, Kuchera W. *Osteopathic Considerations in Systemic Dysfunction.* 2nd ed. Kirksville, Mo: KCOM Press; 1992.)

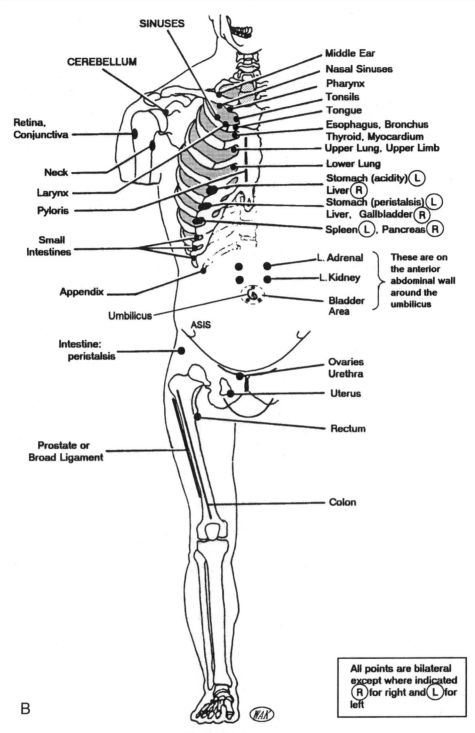

SINUSES

CEREBELLUM

Middle Ear
Nasal Sinuses
Pharynx
Tonsils
Tongue
Esophagus, Bronchus
Thyroid, Myocardium
Upper Lung, Upper Limb
Lower Lung
Stomach (acidity) (L)
Liver (R)
Stomach (peristalsis) (L)
Liver, Gallbladder (R)
Spleen (L), **Pancreas** (R)

Retina,
Conjunctiva

Neck

Larynx

Pyloris

Small
Intestines

Appendix

Umbilicus

Intestine:
peristalsis

Prostate or
Broad Ligament

L. Adrenal
L. Kidney
Bladder Area

These are on
the anterior
abdominal wall
around the
umbilicus

ASIS

Ovaries
Urethra
Uterus

Rectum

Colon

All points are bilateral
except where indicated
(R) for right and (L) for
left

B

WAK

Figure 29.4—*continued*

SECOND TRIMESTER

In the second trimester of pregnancy, the uterus is emerging from the pelvis into the abdomen. The woman may become aware of fetal motion, as well as note stretching pains above the pubic symphysis. If the woman has had abdominal or pelvic surgery, pain may be augmented by stretching of previously formed adhesions. Fascial release (direct or indirect) treatment may provide some relief in this situation.

Structural examination of the pelvis at this time may address restrictions of motion of the sacrum and related ligamentous and muscular structures that could result in backache, sciatica, cramps, or posterior pelvic pain.[25] The patient may be treated in the sitting, standing, prone, or supine position—whichever position she can best tolerate. Almost any type of treatment modality (both direct action or indirect method) can be used, depending on operator skill and patient acceptance.

Table 29.1
Indications and Contraindications for Osteopathic Manipulative Treatment During Pregnancy

Indications
    Somatic dysfunction during pregnancy
    Scoliosis or other structural condition associated with pregnancy
    Edema, congestion, or other pregnancy-associated condition amenable to
        osteopathic manipulative treatment
Contraindications
    Undiagnosed vaginal bleeding
    Threatened or incomplete abortion
    Ectopic pregnancy
    Placenta previa
    Placental abruption
    Premature rupture of membranes (preterm)
    Preterm labor (relative contraindication)
    Prolapsed umbilical cord
    Eclampsia and severe preeclampsia
    Surgical or medical emergencies (other than those listed above)

Although complaints related to skeletal changes continue in the second trimester, the second most frequent area of musculoskeletal symptoms during pregnancy is pain in the hands and wrists.[3] Carpal tunnel syndrome (CTS) occurs most frequently in the second trimester and is the cause of these symptoms for many women. Symptoms of CTS often include the classic triad of numbness, tingling, and pain at night, usually bilaterally.[28,77] CTS probably results from localized edema and swelling in the carpal tunnel. It occurs twice as commonly in pregnant patients who have swelling of the fingers as in those who do not. It also occurs more commonly in those women with preeclampsia and hypertension.[78] In one study, CTS occurred in 2% of 2358 pregnant women.[79] In another study, 25% of 1000 women had median nerve compression at some time during pregnancy.[78] These symptoms are somewhat more common in older primiparous women who have generalized edema.[79]

CTS in pregnancy virtually always resolves completely soon after birth.[80] Palliative management is indicated for patients who are sufficiently symptomatic to warrant any treatment. Nighttime splinting of the wrist to support it in neutral or slight dorsiflexion has been reported to be successful.[79] Sucher has demonstrated improvement of nerve conduction studies and magnetic resonance changes resulting from osteopathic treatment with myofascial technique.[81–82]

THIRD TRIMESTER

In the last 3 months of pregnancy, gravitational effects on the uterus and its contents accentuate abdominal fascial drag on inguinal tissues, causing pressure on the venous and lymphatic return flow from the lower extremities and also on the inferior vena cava. Leg edema and hemorrhoids are common complaints. The pregnant woman may find it difficult to lie in a supine position without experiencing nausea or dizziness from hypotension that results from vena caval compression.

During the third trimester, the mechanical and structural changes in the woman become maximal. As a result of these changes in biomechanics, complaints attributable to loss of balance, changes in gait, and especially low back pain are common. Constipation and reflux esophagitis are also frequent, again as a result of near-maximal changes in structure, fluid, and/or hormones. Use myofascial or soft tissue osteopathic treatment to mobilize fluids from extremities to the systemic circulation. A specific palpatory structural examination to identify gastrointestinal viscerosomatic reflexes for treatment may also be helpful.

Osteopathic treatment to relieve somatic dysfunction should focus on spinal segmental levels of T10-L2, the sympathetic nerve supply that influences adrenal and ovarian function as well as uterine contractility. Gitlin and Wolf[83] provoked uterine contractions in a small group of women with term pregnancies following use of osteopathic cranial manipulation. Additional case histories pertaining to osteopathic management of pregnancy, with discussion of treatment techniques, may be found in *Osteopathy in the Cranial Field.*[84]

LABOR AND BIRTH

After the 36th or 37th week of gestation, before active labor, perform a pelvic examination to evaluate fetal size, presentation, and pelvic outlet accommodation for the fetus. An assessment of the woman's chances for delivering vaginally can be made by interpreting the examination of the "true pelvis" (inlet, midpelvis, and outlet). The pelvic inlet is bounded anteriorly by mentally constructing a line from the iliopectineal lines along the pectineal eminence and pubic crest to the symphysis. Posteriorly, the inlet is bounded by the sacrum at the level of termination of the iliopectineal lines. The sacral base is not included because it is superior to this territory. The plane of the pelvic inlet is a flat surface bounded similarly, but usually inclined horizontally (with the patient in a standing position) at a 40–60° angle. The pelvic outlet is bounded by the pubes, ischial tuberosities, and coccyx. The midpelvis contains all structures between the pelvic inlet and outlet.

Caldwell-Moloy's classification of pelvic types provides the standard for the identifying features of four basic pelvic types[85]:

    Gynecoid
    Android
    Anthropoid
    Platypelloid

This classification is based on normal variation in the following pelvic features (Figs. 29.5–29.7):

    Shape of inlet
    Splay of pelvic sidewalls
    Prominence of ischial spines
    Height of pubic symphysis
    Transverse diameter of pelvic outlet
    Width of pubic arch
    Curvature and inclination of the sacrum

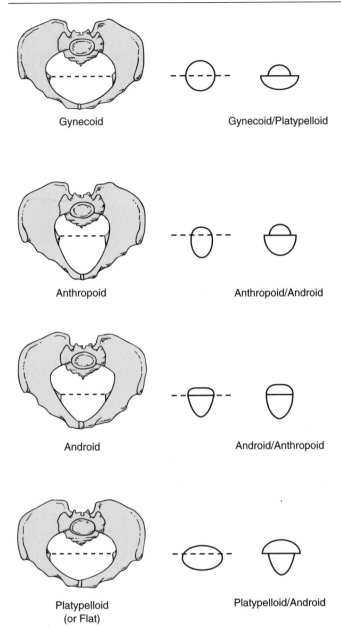

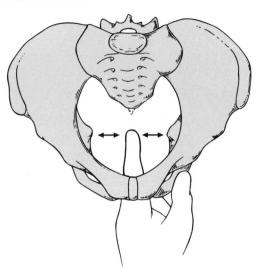

Figure 29.6. Evaluation of transverse diameter. Lateral motion (*arrows*) of gloved finger limited by transversely narrowed pelvis. (Reprinted with permission from Steer CM. Moloy's evaluation of the pelvis. In: Steer CM, ed. *Obstetrics.* Philadelphia, Penn: JB Saunders; 1959.)

Figure 29.5. Pelvic types. **Left column,** Four "classical types," as defined by Caldwell-Moloy's classification of pelvic types. **Center column,** Shapes of pelvic space for each type. **Right column,** "Mixed" pelvic types named by posterior shape/anterior shape.

Early pelvic typing may become necessary if there is a past history of trauma or fracture or if the fetus' size seems greater than that indicated by menstrual date. Definitive pelvic typing is not clinically helpful before 32 weeks' gestation. If birth occurs before this time, the baby may be so small that bony architecture may not be a major factor in the labor and birth process. The closer to term the pelvis is evaluated, the less patient discomfort there is likely to be, as pelvic tissues become more softened and relaxed as a result of hormonal and physiologic effects of pregnancy on the musculoskeletal system.

In individuals, "pure" pelvic types are unusual. Despite a

great variation in individual features of the bony pelvis, the birth canal is curved anteriorly in nearly all women (Fig. 29.8). To be born, the fetal presenting part must negotiate both the pelvic curve and any narrow areas that may be present in the pelvis. Other maternal and fetal variables to contend with during labor are the quality of uterine contractions, head molding ability, and head flexion capability. Most normal labors require minimal intervention.

Osteopathic structural evaluation of the labor patient should focus on the lumbosacral spine and pelvis, especially on mobility of the sacrum. Manipulative management considerations might include gentle techniques (such as soft tissue or myofascial stretching) that cooperate with natural forces of labor; women do not tolerate active or aggressive manual procedures at this time. A posterior sacral base provides ample space throughout the course of fetal descent; however, the fetal occiput may maintain the posterior position at birth. If the sacral base is restricted anteriorly in its lower portion, the occiput tends to rotate into the anterior pelvis, usually maintaining the occiput anterior position for birth. If the entire sacrum persists in an anterior position throughout its long axis (i.e., a flat pelvis), the head descends through the midpelvis in the transverse position. Sometimes a cesarean section becomes necessary for birth because the head cannot descend any further or cannot rotate for a vaginal birth. OMT of the maternal pelvis with the objective of addressing sacral motion restrictions may assist the labor and birth process.

Despite the variety of pelvic types and distortions, the fetal head may traverse the pelvis uneventfully if the pelvis is large enough to accommodate the size of the infant.[86] The most deleterious conditions are those encountered when an average-sized head attempts to squeeze through an average-sized android, or "funnel" pelvis in which the spines are prominent,

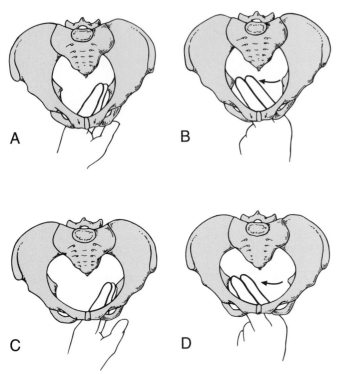

Figure 29.7. Estimation of width of subpubic arch. **A** and **B**, Method of examination to determine narrowed diameters in mid and lower pelvis. **C** and **D**, Estimation of wide diameters of mid and lower pelvis. (Reprinted with permission from Steer CM. Moloy's evaluation of the pelvis. In: Steer CM, ed. *Obstetrics*. Philadelphia, Penn: JB Saunders; 1959.)

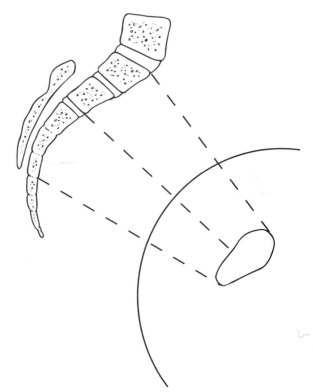

Figure 29.8. Axis of pelvis in sagittal section. Note that curve is relatively straight throughout inlet but curves anteriorly in the midpelvis. *Dashed lines*, top to bottom: Planes of pelvic inlet, midpelvis, and outlet. (Reprinted with permission from Scott JR, DiSaia P. *Danforth's Obstetrics and Gynecology*. 7th ed. Philadelphia, Penn: JB Lippincott; 1994:105–128.)

sidewalls convergent, lower sacrum anterior, and subpubic arch narrow. When the subpubic arch is wide, the occiput may position itself with ease. If the arch is narrowed, the occiput remains posterior, in the area of the sacrum. With prolonged maternal pushing, in addition to possibly unsatisfactory placement of the maternal legs in stirrups, iliac dysfunction, sacral base restriction, back and leg pain with resultant neuropathy, and even pubic symphysis separation may occur.[87–88]

True rupture of the ligaments supporting the symphysis pubis during labor does occur. Lindsey et al. believed that rupture is caused by the wedge effect of the forceful descent of the fetal head against the pelvic ring, usually during birth, creating a separation of more than 1 cm.[89] Normal physiologic separation has been reported to not exceed 10 mm; this amount of separation causes no or only slight symptoms.[90] Characteristically, when the pubis ruptures, there is often an audible "crack," with acute pain in the region that may radiate to the back or thighs. The pain is aggravated by walking and bending, and the patient develops a waddling gait. On examination, a distinctive gap may be palpable at the symphysis. There may also be soft tissue swelling and tenderness over the area. Treatment usually consists of conservative measures: bed rest in the lateral decubitus position and a restrictive pelvic binder to reduce the separation and to maintain the reduction.[3] Additional osteopathic structural evaluation of the spine and pelvis, and ma-

nipulative treatment of additional areas of somatic dysfunction, may help to stabilize the pelvis and to reduce soft tissue swelling. Although subsequent pregnancies are generally unaffected,[91–92] some patients may experience pain in the suprapubic region during subsequent pregnancies, especially in the third trimester.

POSTPARTUM

The osteopathic physician can maximize the successful birth experience for the mother. She may also need treatment for residual somatic dysfunction in the postpartum period. The most obvious challenge is to assist the woman in returning her pelvis, axial skeleton, and the supporting soft tissues to their pregravid state; this often calls for OMT. Although carpal tunnel syndrome usually occurs in the second or third trimesters, Wand reported its development in 18 patients, not during pregnancy but while they were nursing.[80] These symptoms resolved when breastfeeding ceased. Snell et al. reported similar findings in the puerperium in five patients and attributed the problem to fluid retention caused by the hormone prolactin.[93]

Another frequently encountered cause of pain in the hand and wrist is de Quervain's tenosynovitis, which results from compression and irritation of the extensor pollicis brevis and abductor pollicis longus tendons as they pass through the first dorsal compartment of the wrist near the styloid process of the radius.[3] Fluid retention has been suspected as an initiator of this problem, which is intensified by the use of the hand and fingers and by movement of the wrist.[94–95] Patients who have persistent symptoms have reported that infant care activities,[94] as well as breastfeeding,[95–96] aggravate the condition.

Although back pain is the most common complaint of expectant mothers, persistent back pain can also become a problem during the postpartum period. Russell et al. investigated factors associated with long-term backache after childbirth in 299 patients, especially those factors that may have been associated with epidural anesthesia during labor.[97] They concluded that, although new long-term backache was reported by the women given epidural analgesia in labor, the pain tended to be postural and not severe. Also, no differences existed in the nature of the backache between those who did or did not receive epidurals during labor. Although back pain during or after pregnancy may be common, it should not be dismissed on the basis that it is a normal accompaniment of pregnancy.

CONCLUSION

A systematic approach by the osteopathic obstetrician who has been trained to identify and treat somatic dysfunction may discover underlying sources of discomfort for pregnant, birthing, and postpartum women. In this situation, osteopathic manipulative treatment may be used to effect a more comfortable and enjoyable childbearing experience.

REFERENCES

1. Still AT. *The Philosophy and Mechanical Principles of Osteopathy.* Kansas City, Mo: Hudson-Kimberly Publishing Co; 1902.
2. Allen TW. *1995 Yearbook and Directory of Osteopathic Physicians.* 86th ed. Chicago, Ill: American Osteopathic Association; 1995.
3. Heckman JD, Sassard R. Musculoskeletal considerations in pregnancy. *J Bone Joint Surg Am.* 1994;76:1720–1730.
4. Rungee JL. Low back pain during pregnancy. *Orthopedics.* 1993; 16:1339–1344.
5. DiGiovanna EL, Schiowitz S. *An Osteopathic Approach to Diagnosis and Treatment.* Philadelphia, Penn: JB Lippincott Co; 1992:459.
6. Mantle MJ, Greenwood RM, Currey HLF. Backache in pregnancy. *Rheumatol and Rehabil.* 1977;16:95–101.
7. Berg G, Hammar M, Moller-Nielson J, Linden U, Thorblad J. Low back pain during pregnancy. *Obstet Gynecol.* 1988;71:71–78.
8. Daly JM, Frame PS, Rapoza PA. Sacroiliac subluxation: a common, treatable cause of low back pain during pregnancy. *Fam Pract Res J.* 1991;11:149–159.
9. Nwuga VC. Pregnancy and back pain among upper class Nigerian women. *Aust J Physiother.* 1982;28:8–11.
10. Östgaard HC, Andersson GBJ, Karlsson K. Prevalence of low back pain during pregnancy. *Spine.* 1991;16:549–552.
11. Östgaard HC, Andersson GBJ. Previous back pain and risk of developing back pain in a future pregnancy. *Spine.* 1991;16:432–436.
12. Svensson H-O, Andersson GB, Hagstad A, Jansson P-O. The relationship of low back pain to pregnancy and gynecologic factors. *Spine.* 1990;15:371–375.

13. Bendix T, Sorensen SS, Klausen K. Lumbar curve, trunk muscles, and line of gravity with different heel heights. *Spine.* 1984;9:223–227.
14. Freeman WS. Common complaints during pregnancy. *Res and Staff Physician.* 1979;25:69–73.
15. RK Laros Jr. Physiology of normal pregnancy. In: Willson JR, Carrington ER, eds. *Obstetrics and Gynecology.* St. Louis, Mo: Mosby Year Book; 1991:242.
16. Fast A, Weiss L, Duccommun E, Medina E, Butler JG. Low back pain in pregnancy—abdominal muscles, sit up performance, and back pain. *Spine.* 1990;15:28–30.
17. Bullock J, Juli GA, Bullock M. The relationship of low back pain to postural changes during pregnancy. *Aust J Physiother.* 1987;33:10–17.
18. Snijders CJ, Seroo JM, Snijder JG, Hoedt HT. Change in form of the spine as a consequence of pregnancy. *Digest of the 11th International Conference on Medical and Biological Engineering.* 1976:670–671.
19. Östgaard HC, Andersson GB, Schultz AB, Miller JA. Influence of some biomechanical factors on low-back pain in pregnancy. *Spine.* 1993;18:61–65.
20. McGill S. A biomechanical perspective of sacro-iliac pain. *Clin Biomech.* 1987;2:145–151.
21. Epstein JA, Benton J, Browder J, Lavine LS, Rosenthal AH, Warren R. Treatment of low back pain and sciatic syndromes during pregnancy. *NY State J Med.* 1959;59:1757–1768.
22. Hagen R. Pelvic girdle relaxation from an orthopaedic point of view. *Acta Orthop Scand.* 1974;45:550–563.
23. Lotgering FK, Gilbert RD, Longo LD. The interactions of exercise and pregnancy: a review. *Am J Obstet Gynecol.* 1984;149:560–568.
24. Sands RX. Backache of pregnancy: a method of treatment. *Obstet Gynecol.* 1958;12:670–677.
25. Östgaard HC, Zetherstrom G, Roos HE, Svanberg B. Reduction of back and posterior pelvic pain in pregnancy. *Spine.* 1994;19:894–900.
26. LaBan MM, Perrin JCS, Latimer FR. Pregnancy and the herniated lumbar disc. *Arch Phys Med Rehab.* 1983;64:319–321.
27. Wells J. Osteitis condensans ilii. *AJR.* 1956;76:1141.
28. Bushnell LF. The postural pains of pregnancy, part I: parietal neuralgia of pregnancy. *West J Surg Obstet Gynecol.* 1949;57:123–127.
29. American College of Obstetricians and Gynecologists. Pregnancy and the postnatal period. In: *ACOG Home Exercise Program.* Washington, DC: ACOG Press; 1985a:1–5.
30. Weinreb JC, Wolbarsht LB, Cohen JM, Brown CE, Maravilla KR. Prevalence of lumbosacral intervertebral disk abnormalities on MR images in pregnant and asymptomatic nonpregnant women. *Radiology.* 1989;170:125–128.
31. Berman AT, Cohen DL, Schwentker EP. The effects of pregnancy on idiopathic scoliosis: a preliminary report on eight cases and a review of the literature. *Spine.* 1982;7:76–77.
32. Betz RR, Bunnell WP, Lambrecht-Mulier E, MacEwen GD. Scoliosis and pregnancy. *J Bone Joint Surg.* 1987;69A:90–96.
33. Visscher W, Lonstein JE, Hoffman DA, Mandel JS, Harris BS, I. Reproductive outcomes in scoliosis patients. *Spine.* 1988;13:1096–1098.
34. Heckman JD. Managing musculoskeletal problems in pregnant patients. *J Musculoskel Med.* 1984;1:35–40.
35. Rhodes P. Orthopaedic conditions associated with childbearing. *Practitioner.* 1958;181:304–312.
36. Kangilaski J. Why does arthritis pain diminish with pregnancy? *JAMA.* 1981;246:317.

37. Kay NR, Park WM, Bark M. The relationship between pregnancy and femoral head necrosis. *Br J Radiol.* 1972;45:828–831.

38. Froelich CJ, Goodwin JS, Bankhurst AD, Williams RC Jr. Pregnancy, a temporary fetal graft of suppressor cells in autoimmune disease? *Am J Med.* 1980;69:329–331.

39. Østensen M, Husby G. Seronegative spondylarthritis and ankylosing spondylitis: Biological effects and management. In: Scott JS, Bird HA, eds. *Pregnancy, Autoimmunity, and Connective Tissue Disorders.* New York, NY: Oxford University Press, 1990;163–184.

40. Østensen HC, Romberg Ø, Husby G. Ankylosing spondylitis and motherhood. *Arthritis Rheum.* 1982;25:140–143.

41. Pregnancy worsens course of ankylosing spondylitis. *Orthop Rev.* 1980;9:81.

42. Steinberg CL. Ankylosing spondylitis and pregnancy. *Ann Rheum Dis.* 1948;7:209–215.

43. Fast A, Weiss L, Parich S, Hertz G. Night backache in pregnancy—hypothetical pathophysiological mechanisms. *Am J Phys Med & Rehab.* 1989;68:227–229.

44. Fast A, Shapiro D, Ducommon EJ, Friedman LW, Bouklas T, Floman Y. Low back pain in pregnancy. *Spine.* 1987;12:368–371.

45. LaBan MM, Wesolowski DP. Night pain associated with diminished cardiopulmonary compliance. A concomitant of lumbar spinal stenosis and degenerative spondylolisthesis. *Am J Phys Med & Rehab.* 1988;67:155–160.

46. Kuchera M, Kuchera W. *Osteopathic Considerations in Systemic Dysfunction.* 2nd ed. Kirksville, Mo: KCOM Press; 1992:149.

47. Gray H. *Gray's Anatomy.* 35th ed. Philadelphia, Penn: WB Saunders Co; 1973.

48. Zink JG, Lawson WG. Pressure gradients in the osteopathic manipulative management of the obstetrical patient. *Osteopath Ann.* 1979;7:208–214.

49. Sherwood OD. Relaxin. In: Knobil E, Neill J, eds. *The Physiology of Reproduction.* New York, NY: Raven Press; 1988:585–658.

50. Szlachter BN, Quagliarello J, Jewelewicz R, Osathanondh R, Spellacy W, Weiss G. Relaxin in normal and pathogenic pregnancies. *Obstet Gynecol.* 1982;59:167–170.

51. Cunningham FG, MacDonald PC, Gant NF. *Williams' Obstetrics.* 18th ed. San Mateo, Calif: Appleton & Lange; 1989:134–135.

52. MacLennan AH, Nicolson R, Green RC, Bath M. Serum relaxin and pelvic pain of pregnancy. *Lancet.* 1986;2:243–245.

53. Cugell DW, Frank NR, Gaensler ER, Badger TL. Pulmonary function in pregnancy, I. Serial observations in normal women. *Am Rev Tuberc Pulm Dis.* 1953;67:568–584.

54. Scott JR, DiSaia P. *Danforth's Obstetrics and Gynecology.* 7th ed. Philadelphia, Penn: JB Lippincott; 1994:105–128.

55. Beal MC. Viscerosomatic reflexes: a review. *JAOA.* 1985;85:786–801.

56. Bonica JJ. Autonomic innervation of the viscera in relation to nerve block. *Anesthesiology.* 1968;29:793–813.

57. Head H. On disturbances of sensation with special reference to the pain of visceral disease. *Brain.* 1893;16:1–133.

58. House EL, Pansky B. *A Functional Approach to Neuroanatomy.* 2nd ed. New York, NY: McGraw-Hill; 1967.

59. Crosby EC, Humphry T, Lauer EW. *Correlative Anatomy of the Nervous System.* New York, NY: MacMillan Co; 1962.

60. Bhagat BD, Young PA, Biggerstaff DE. *Fundamentals of Visceral Innervation.* Springfield, Ill: Charles C Thomas; 1977.

61. Pottenger FM. *Symptoms of Visceral Disease.* 5th ed. St. Louis, Mo: CV Mosby Co; 1938.

62. White JC, Smithwick RH, Simeone FA. *The Autonomic Nervous System.* 3rd ed. New York, NY: MacMillan Co; 1952.

63. Hansen K, Schliack H. *Segmental Innervation.* Stuttgart, Germany: G Thieme; 1962.

64. Woods ER. The viscerosomatic reflex in acute abdominal disorders. *JAOA.* 1962;63:239–242.

65. Hix EL. Reflex viscerosomatic reference phenomena. *Osteopath Ann.* 1976;4:496–503.

66. Conley GJ. The role of the spinal joint lesion in gallbladder disease. *JAOA.* 1944;44:121–123.

67. Larson NJ. Manipulative care before and after surgery. *Osteopath Med.* 1977;2:41–49.

68. Young GS. Gently applied manipulation eases post-op convalescence. *Clin Trends Osteopath Med.* 1978:4–7.

69. Drew EG. The role of the secondary lesion from the surgical standpoint. *JAOA.* 1939;38:377–378.

70. Owens C. *An Endocrine Interpretation of Chapman's Reflexes.* 2nd ed. Chattanooga, Tenn: Chatanooga Printing & Engraving Co; 1937.

71. Taylor G. The osteopathic management of nausea and vomiting of pregnancy. *JAOA.* 1949;48:581–582.

72. Huch R, Erkkola R. Pregnancy and exercise—exercise and pregnancy: a short review. *Br J Obstet Gynecol.* 1990;97:208–214.

73. Wiskstrom J, Haslam ET, Hutchinson RH. Backache during pregnancy—its etiology and management. *J La State Med Soc.* 1955;107:490–494.

74. Mersy DJ. Health benefits of aerobic exercise. *Postgrad Med.* 1991;90:103–107, 110–112.

75. Women say running helped pregnancy, labor. *Phys and Sportsmed.* 1981;9:24–25.

76. Pregnant women advised to consider exercise risks. *Phys and Sportsmed.* 1982;10:27.

77. Nygaard IE, Saltzman CL, Whitehouse MB, Hankin FM. Hand problems in pregnancy. *Am Fam Physician.* 1989;39:123–126.

78. Voitk AJ, Mueller JC, Farlinger DE, Jonston RU. Carpal tunnel syndrome in pregnancy. *Can Med Assoc J.* 1983;28:277–281.

79. Eckman-Ordeberg G, Sälgeback S, Ordeberg G. Carpal tunnel syndrome in pregnancy: a prospective study. *Acta Obstet Gynecol Scand.* 1987;66:233–235.

80. Wand JS. Carpal tunnel syndrome in pregnancy and lactation. *J Hand Surg.* 1990;15B:93–95.

81. Sucher BM. Myofascial manipulative release of carpal tunnel syndrome: documentation with magnetic resonance imaging. *JAOA.* 1993;93:127–128.

82. Sucher BM. Palpatory diagnosis and manipulative management of carpal tunnel syndrome. *JAOA.* 1994;94:647–663.

83. Gitlin RS, Wolf DL. Uterine contractions following osteopathic cranial manipulation—A pilot study. *JAOA.* 1992;92:1183.

84. Magoun H. *Osteopathy in the Cranial Field.* Kirksville, Mo: Journal Printing Company; 1966.

85. Steer CM. Maloy's evaluation of the pelvis. In: Steer CM, ed. *Obstetrics.* Philadelphia, Penn: JB Saunders; 1959.

86. Frymann V. Relation of disturbances of cranio-sacral mechanisms to symptomatology of the newborn: study of 1250 infants. *JAOA.* 1966;65:1059–1075.

87. Whiting L. Osteopathic prevention of certain complications of labor and the puerperium. *JAOA.* 1945;44:495–498.

88. McCormick J. Some variations can be made in the "obstetrical workshop". *JAOA.* 1944;44:195–197.

89. Lindsey RW, Leggon RE. Separation of the symphysis pubis in as-

sociation with childbearing: a case report. *J Bone Joint Surg.* 1988; 70A:289–292.

90. Young J. Relaxation of the pelvic joints in pregnancy: pelvic arthropathy of pregnancy. *J Obstet Gynaecol Br Emp.* 1940;47:493.

91. Cibils LA. Rupture of the symphysis pubis: a case report. *Obstet Gynecol.* 1971;38:407–410.

92. Dhar S, Anderton JM. Rupture of the symphysis pubis during labor. *Clin Orthop.* 1992;283:252–257.

93. Snell NJ, Coysh HL, Snell BJ. Carpal tunnel syndrome presenting in the puerperium. *Practitioner.* 1980;224:191–193.

94. Schned ES. De Quervain tenosynovitis in pregnant and post-partum women. *Obstet Gynecol.* 1986;68:411–414.

95. Schumacher HR Jr, Dorwart BB. Occurrence of De Quervain's tendonitis during pregnancy. *Arch Intern Med.* 1985;145: 2083–2084.

96. Johnson CA. Occurrence of De Quervain's disease in post-partum women. *J Fam Pract.* 1991;32:325–327.

97. Russell R, Groves P, Taub N, O'Dowd J, Reynolds F. Assessing long term backache after childbirth. *BMJ.* 1993;306:1299–1303.

30. Gynecology

MELICIEN A. TETTAMBEL

What diseases does woman have that man does not have? Such diseases as belong to the womb and its appendages ... It matters not whether the cause is far remote or in close proximity to the uterus; we must find it, or we will be found in the antediluvian tribe of speculum cranks of all the blind female doctors' ages.

—A.T. STILL[1]

Key Concepts

- **Anatomy of the pelvis**
- **Patient evaluation for pelvic pain, including history and physical examination**
- **Causes of pelvic pain**
- **Pelvic floor disorders**

The osteopathic obstetrician-gynecologist has the opportunity to integrate the influences of the musculoskeletal system in the management of a variety of health care concerns experienced by female patients. Because of the large scope of gynecology, this chapter does not address all diagnostic and treatment topics involving the female reproductive system. It focuses instead on two common women's health care issues frequently encountered by primary care providers—pelvis pain and pelvic disorders—that may have a component of somatic dysfunction or musculoskeletal influence. In gynecology, palpatory expertise in evaluation of the female pelvis and its contents is a prerequisite for ancillary testing and patient management.

PELVIC PAIN

Anatomy

Evaluation of pelvic pain requires extensive knowledge of the anatomy and physiology of the female pelvis. Although standard references[2-4] completely discuss the anatomy of the female pelvis, salient points helpful to osteopathic physicians are summarized here to illustrate the possible causes of somatic dysfunction.

The striated muscles of the vaginal introitus and skin of the perineum receive somatic motor and sensory fibers from the lumbosacral plexus. The pelvic viscera are supplied by the autonomic plexuses, conveying sympathetic and parasympathetic nerves to these organs. Ventral roots of the lumbar and sacral

nerves originate from the lumbosacral plexuses. The obturator nerve, the lumbosacral trunk (of the plexus), and the entire sacral plexus lie in proximity to the pelvic organs. Only particular branches of the plexuses are directly involved in pelvic innervation (Fig. 30.1).

Muscular contraction and vasoconstriction are mediated by sympathetic innervation, while muscle relaxation and vasodilation are caused by parasympathetic innervation. Most autonomic fibers enter the pelvis via the superior hypogastric plexus, which runs from the 4th lumbar vertebra to the hollow of the sacrum. It descends into the base of the broad ligament to join the parasympathetic fibers from the pelvic plexuses. The motor fibers and accompanying sensory nerves arrive at the pelvic plexus from S2-S4 by way of the nervi erigentes. The sensory nerves from the uterus, which escort the sympathetic nerves to enter the cord at T11 and T12, cause referred pain to the abdomen. Cervical afferent nerves, S2-S4, refer pain to the lower back and lumbosacral regions.

Autonomic innervation to the pelvic organs includes these sensory fibers:

Sympathetic
Parasympathetic
Motor
Visceral

The uterus, vagina, ureter, bladder, and rectum are supplied by the inferior hypogastric plexus. Visceral afferent pain path-

Figure 30.1. Nerves of uterus and perineum. (Reprinted with permission from Ponsky B. *Review of Gross Anatomy*, 5th ed. New York, NY: Macmillan Publishing Company; 1984:459.)

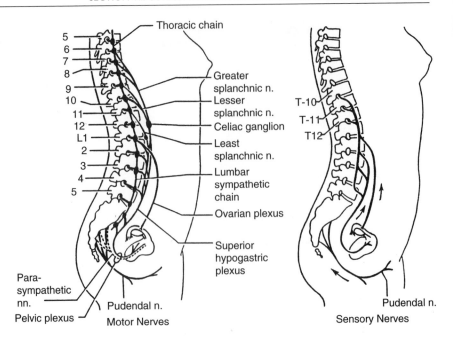

ways of the ovary, uterine tube, fundus, body of the uterus, and cervix connect with the spinal cord at the level of T11-T12. Pain is referred to corresponding skin dermatomes, usually from the lower abdomen. Sacral plexus injury can cause disabling changes of a motor or sensory nature, as Beal discusses in his review of viscerosomatic reflexes.[5]

The genitofemoral nerve (L1-L2) traverses across the belly of the psoas major muscle to the anterior thigh to supply the labia majora. Injury results in sensory changes. The obturator nerve (L2-L4) supplies motor branches to the adductor muscles of the leg, hip, knee joint, and medial thigh. Injury results in loss of thigh adduction, loss of internal and external rotation capability, and sensory losses to these areas. Table 30.1 summarizes nerves that cause painful impulses from the pelvic organs.

Patient Evaluation: History and Physical Examination

The history should include the patient's description of pain with reference to:

Localization
Quality
Intensity
Radiation
Duration
Aggravation
Alleviation

The relationship of the pain to the menstrual cycle, bowel movements, urination, sexual activity, and physical activity should also be discussed. Similar painful episodes in the recent or distant past should be explored, along with other possible related somatic complaints such as anorexia, weight gain, or other gastrointestinal or urologic symptoms.[6] Also note mus-

culoskeletal complaints that may or may not accompany pelvic pain, such as low back pain.

Ascertain the influence of pain and its ability to disrupt everyday activities, as well as other concurrent events that may have occurred with the acute onset of pain. Examples include cramps with IUD placement, sexual trauma, or strain from lifting heavy objects.[7]

Whereas acute pelvic pain may be of sudden onset and localize within 24 hours, chronic pelvic pain differs in both duration and location. As described by Glintner,[8] chronic pain is pain that has been present for 6 months, is diffuse and intermittent in nature, and involves no organic pathologic findings. Fifteen to thirty percent of women presenting with this complaint undergo laparoscopy; 10–15% undergo hysterectomies.[9–10] Some women may have associated stressors such as depression over pregnancy loss, employment issues, or personal relationships. The perceptions that both the patient and her partner have about the illness are also important.[11] Elicit information about medications or other attempts to relieve the pain. Psychological evaluation may become necessary but should not preclude other diagnostic studies, especially when the pain itself becomes the disease rather than a symptom of the disease.[12–13]

Additional gynecologic history should include inquiries about:

Infertility
Infection
Contraceptive methods used
Endometriosis
Last pelvic examination

The surgical history should include not only pelvic procedures but also any other procedures, such as orthopaedic, urologic, or neurologic operations. The medical history should include

Table 30.1
Nerves Carrying Painful Impulses from Pelvic Organs

Spinal Segments	Nerves	Organ
T9–T10	Sympathetic via renal and aortic plexus and celiac and mesenteric ganglia	Ovaries
T9–T10	Sympathetic via aortic and superior mesenteric plexus	Outer two-thirds of fallopian tubes, upper ureter
T11–T12, L1	Sympathetic via hypogastric plexus	Uterine fundus, proximal fallopian tubes, broad ligament, upper bladder, cecum, appendix, terminal large bowel
S2–S4	Pelvic parasympathetic	Upper vagina, cervix, lower uterine segment, posterior urethra, bladder trigone, uterosacral and cardinal ligaments, rectosigmoid, lower ureters
S2–S4	Pudendal, inguinal, genitofemoral, posterofemoral cutaneous	Perineum, vulva, lower vagina

conditions that could manifest as pelvic pain, such as colitis or cystitis.

The physical examination should focus on careful and gentle palpatory evaluation of the abdomen to avoid guarding. Attempt to reproduce and localize the pain during the pelvic examination to discover findings that may correspond to specific pelvic pathology.[14] Consider endometriosis if the uterus is fixed and if there is uterosacral nodularity that is also tender to palpation. Adnexal enlargement may suggest a cyst, ectopic pregnancy, or infection. A backache may be the result of a uterine prolapse.[15]

Consider psychological evaluation if an obviously traumatic event is directly associated with the onset of pain or if there is concomitant neurosis, psychosis, or aberrant behavior.[16] Table 30.2 summarizes some of the more common causes of pelvic pain.

DIFFERENTIAL DIAGNOSIS OF PELVIC PAIN

Dysmenorrhea

Painful menstruation, or dysmenorrhea, can be primary or secondary to organic pelvic disease. Approximately 50% of menstruating women are affected by dysmenorrhea; 10% may require bed rest. The peak age of incidence is 20–24 years of age.

Primary dysmenorrhea usually appears within 6–12 months of the menarche and may be a feature of ovulatory cycles. Dysmenorrhea may be caused by uterine contractions or ischemia, psychological factors, and cervical factors.[17–18] Psychological factors may alter pain perception. Cervical stenosis has been cited as a painful stimulus but has little support in the literature as an important factor.[19]

Women with dysmenorrhea may have increased frequency or duration of uterine contractility. Cramping usually begins a few hours before menses and can persist for hours or longer. The pain is localized to the lower abdomen and may radiate to the thighs and lower back. The pain may also be associated with nausea, fatigue, dizziness, headache, or altered bowel habits.

Table 30.2
Causes of Pelvic Pain

Gynecologic
  Endometriosis
  Pelvic inflammatory disease
  Abdominopelvic adhesions
  Severe pelvic relaxation
  Uterine myomata
  Benign ovarian neoplasms (solid and cystic)
  Ovarian remnant
  Cyclic pelvic pain (primary or secondary dysmenorrhea)
Urologic
  Urinary tract infection
  Cystitis (interstitial and acute)
  Renal calculi
Gastrointestinal
  Irritable bowel syndrome
  Crohn's disease
  Diverticulitis
  Constipation
  Bowel obstruction
Musculoskeletal
  Somatic dysfunction
  Hernias
  Muscular strains/sprains
  Herniated disk
  Fibromyositis (with or without trigger points)
  Pelvic bone tumors
Psychogenic
  Psychosexual trauma/abuse
  Depression
  Somatization

Treatment options include:

Nonsteroidal antiinflammatory drugs (NSAIDs)[20–21]
Oral contraceptive pills
Calcium blockers (e.g., nifedipine)
Progestogens
Osteopathic manipulative treatment[22–24]

If a patient fails to respond to medical therapy, consideration should be given to a secondary cause of dysmenorrhea. Laparoscopy and/or hysteroscopy with endometrial curettage may be performed to exclude pelvic disease.

Secondary dysmenorrhea is not limited to menstrual pain, is less related to the first day of bleeding, develops in women 30–40 years of age, and may be associated with other symptoms. Some of these symptoms may include dyspareunia, infertility, and abnormal bleeding.[25] Table 30.3 summarizes possible causes of primary and secondary dysmenorrhea. Management focuses on treatment of the specific underlying disease. Some of these diseases are discussed in the following sections.

Premenstrual Syndrome

Premenstrual problems have been formally described since Frank in 1931.[26] They include but are not limited to:

Bloating of the abdomen and pelvis
Weight gain
Irritability
Mood swings
Depression
Fatigue
Difficulty concentrating

The term premenstrual syndrome (PMS) was first used by Greene and Dalton in 1953.[27] However, the current term "ovarian cycle syndrome" better describes the syndrome because many symptoms also occur around the time of ovulation. Approximately 5–10% of women experience severe PMS symptoms that interfere with normal daily life.

The cause of PMS has not been entirely determined.[28] Table 30.4 lists proposed hypotheses that attempt to explain the syndrome. Most healthy women report occasional symptoms before menses. The syndrome is associated with ovulation and therefore does not occur before puberty, during pregnancy, or after menopause. Nor does it occur in anovulatory women. Menstruation is incidental, as cyclic symptoms continue to be bothersome if the ovaries are still present in a woman who has had a hysterectomy. Extensive metabolic and psychological studies have yet to identify a specific abnormality. Treatment options have included:

Medication to suppress cyclic ovarian activity[29]
Psychotherapy to help patients develop coping skills[30]
Diet or food supplements such as pyridoxine or oil of primrose (which may interfere with prostaglandin synthesis and lessen cramps)[31]
Diuretics to reduce bloating[32]
Diets with reduced fat, caffeine, or salt to avoid irritability or water retention[33–34]

Uterine Pain

Pelvic pain is not usually the result of variations in uterine position in the pelvis. Deep dyspareunia may occasionally be associated with retroversion, whereby the pelvic nerves are irritated by stretching of the uterosacral ligaments and pelvic veins become congested from uterine heaviness and position.[25]

Table 30.3
Clinical Features of Primary and Secondary Dysmenorrhea

Primary Dysmenorrhea
Initial onset—within 2 years of menarche.
Pain—cramplike, lasting 48–72 hr after onset of menses; strongest in intensity over lower abdomen. May radiate to back or inner thigh.
Associated symptoms—nausea and vomiting, fatigue, diarrhea, lower backache, headache.
Pelvic examination findings—normal.

Secondary Dysmenorrhea
Endometriosis—pain occurs in premenstrual or postmenstrual phase or may be continuous. Patient may experience dyspareunia, premenstrual spotting, or have cul-de-sac nodularity on examination. Age of onset in the 20s or 30s.
Pelvic inflammation—initially pain may be menstrual, but may extend into premenstrual phase with subsequent cycles. Patient may have intermenstrual bleeding, dyspareunia, and pelvic tenderness.
Fibroids, adenomyosis—pain is a dull, heavy ache in pelvis. Uterus enlarged on examination and may be tender.
Ovarian cysts—unilateral tenderness, radiating into thigh. Adnexal enlargement on examination.
Pelvic congestion—dull, ill-defined ache that worsens premenstrually but improves with menses. Patient may have history of sexual dysfunction.

Table 30.4
Proposed Hypotheses for Causes of Premenstrual Syndrome

Abnormal estrogen secretion
Excess deficiency of progesterone
Excess deficiency of cortisone, androgens, or prolactin
Excess deficiency of prostaglandin
Excess of antidiuretic hormone
Abnormality of endogenous opiates or melatonin secretion
Deficiencies of vitamins A, B_1, B_6, or minerals such as magnesium
Hypoglycemia
Hormone allergy
Menstrual toxin
Psychological, social, evolutionary, and genetic factors

A tender uterus that is noted on pelvic examination to be fixed in retroversion should arouse suspicions of other intraperitoneal pathologic conditions, such as endometriosis or pelvic inflammatory disease. Laparoscopy is indicated to evaluate pelvic structures. Pelvic heaviness and low back pain may be present with advanced degrees of uterine prolapse. Before deciding on hysterectomy as a course of treatment, some of these symptoms may be remedied by using a pessary.

The concept of pelvic congestion syndrome has a variety of proponents.[3] This syndrome has been described in multiparous women who have pelvic vein varicosities and congested pelvic organs.[35] Pain is worse premenstrually and is aggravated by fatigue, standing, and sexual intercourse. In the clinical examination, the uterus is mobile, usually retroverted, soft and boggy, and slightly enlarged. There may be associated menorrhagia and urinary frequency.[36] Dilated veins may be seen on venographic studies.[37] Additional and independent factors other than venous congestion may be involved, as some women with pelvic varicosities have no pain. Surgery is not usually beneficial for this condition.[38] There have been some uncontrolled observations of similar symptoms of pain and metrorrhagia occurring after tubal ligation; no prospective studies have been performed.[25]

Uterine leiomyomas (fibroids) are smooth muscle tumors of the uterus that are the most common indication for major surgery in women. Twenty percent of women develop uterine fibroids by age 40.[3] Fibroids have the potential to grow to an enormous size but have low malignant potential. The majority cause no symptoms and may require no treatment other than careful observation. Occasionally, the patient may become aware of a lower abdominal fullness or mass above the pubic symphysis. Symptoms develop insidiously as the fibroid competes with neighboring organs for space in the pelvis. Symptoms include:

Pressure
Congestion
Bloating
Urinary frequency or retention
Dysmenorrhea

Other causes of pain are the result of fibroid infarction with degeneration, torsion on the fibroid's pedicle, or compression of pelvic nerves. Occasionally, a submucous leiomyoma may attempt to protrude through the cervix, causing pain akin to that of vaginal childbirth.

Management of this condition includes addressing the patient's desire for preserving future fertility, along with careful observation.

Myomectomy may be performed to maintain the uterus for future pregnancy.[39–40] Uterine curettage may control menometrorrhagia. Gonadotropin-releasing hormone (GnRH) agonists have been used to shrink myomas to enhance fertility, as well as to reduce blood loss during surgery.[41–43] Oral contraceptives also reduce menstrual flow, preserve fertility, and control dysmenorrhea. Hysterectomy is reserved for the symptomatic patient for whom reproductive capability is not an issue.

Adenomyosis may cause dysmenorrhea and menorrhagia, but rarely does it cause chronic intermenstrual pain. Adenomyosis is defined as the extension of endometrial glands and stroma into the uterine musculature. Approximately 15% of women develop varying degrees of adenomyosis in their late 30s and early 40s, and they may have associated endometriosis.[25] Patients express that their dysmenorrhea is of a colicky nature. In 30–40% of patients with adenomyosis, the disease is an unexpected pathologic finding in a hysterectomy patient who did not experience menorrhagia or uterine enlargement.[44] In the case of a large adenomyoma, pressure on the bladder or rectum may be reported by the patient. On pelvic examination, the uterus is symmetrically enlarged; occasionally the uterus may enlarge asymmetrically, suggesting the presence of a fibroid. However, the adenomyomatous uterus is softer than a uterine myoma. Treatment depends on the specific symptoms and on the exclusion of other uterine pathologic conditions.

Menorrhagia and dysmenorrhea, if not too severe, may be treated palliatively with NSAIDs, oral contraceptive pills, or GnRH agonists.[20] Otherwise, hysterectomy may be indicated. The ovaries should be preserved if they are normal and if the patient is not menopausal.

Endometriosis

Endometriosis is a benign condition in which endometrial glands and stroma are present outside the endometrial cavity. Other locations include the ovary, bowel, bladder, peritoneum, and sites outside the pelvic boundaries. Endometriosis is a challenge to gynecologists because it is a diagnostic and surgical enigma. More than 15% of women have some degree of the disease. It is noted in approximately 20% of gynecologic surgical procedures, with a 50% rate of unexpected findings.[44]

The characteristic triad of symptoms associated with endometriosis is dysmenorrhea, dyspareunia, and dyschezia. Secondary dysmenorrhea first appears or escalates in the late 20s or early 30s. If the endometriosis is associated with obstructive genital anomalies, severe dysmenorrhea may occur at menarche.[25]

Dyspareunia is generally associated with deep coitus, irritating the endometrial implants located in the cul-de-sac, on the uterosacral ligaments, or in portions of the posterior vaginal fornix. On pelvic examination, the cul-de-sac may feel gritty and be exquisitely tender to the touch.[45]

Dyschezia is experienced with uterosacral, cul-de-sac, and rectosigmoid colon involvement. As stool passes between the uterosacral ligaments, the patient experiences pain. This symptom is highly characteristic and is more common with endometriosis than with chronic salpingo-oophoritis, a condition mistaken for endometriosis.[46]

If the ovarian capsule is involved with endometriosis, ovulatory pain and midcycle vaginal bleeding are reported by the patient. However, the nature of pelvic pain caused by endometriosis is variable. Some investigators have found that the degree of pain is inversely proportional to the extent of the disease.[44] Minimal endometriosis in the cul-de-sac may be more painful than a large ovarian endometrioma that can expand freely into the abdominal cavity. Frequently, pelvic examination yields no signs of endometriosis.

The diagnosis of endometriosis should be suspected in an afebrile patient with the previously mentioned characteristic endometriosis symptom triad: a firm, fixed tender adnexal mass and tender nodularity in the cul-de-sac and uterosacral ligaments. Pelvic ultrasound may indicate an adnexal mass of complex echogenicity. The definitive diagnosis is made by the characteristic gross findings of "blueberry" spots, chocolate cysts, or "powder burns," or by histologic findings of endometrial tissue at laparoscopy or laparotomy.[47–49]

Management of endometriosis depends on the following considerations[46]:

Certainty of the diagnosis
Severity of symptoms
Extent of the disease

Preservation of fertility
Compromised function of the gastrointestinal and/or urinary tracts

If reproductive capacity is not a concern, total abdominal hysterectomy with bilateral salpingo-oophorectomy should be considered.[50] Menopause can be managed with hormone replacement therapy. If future fertility is a consideration, pursue conservative surgery, including resection of the disease, lysis of adhesions, ovarian resection, or electrocautery or laser treatment of small lesions.[47–48]

Medical therapy may be considered if the endometriosis is minimal in extent and the symptoms are tolerable. NSAIDs are recommended to address dysmenorrhea. Oral contraceptive pills or hormonal manipulation may decrease the intensity and duration of dysmenorrhea and menses. Temporary suppression of menstruation and endometrial implant formation can be achieved through short-term use of danazol or GnRH agonists.[51–52] Fertility is preserved by involution of implants.[53] However, when a palpable endometrioma is present, the likelihood of a complete response to medical therapy is small.[54]

Pelvic Inflammatory Disease

Pelvic inflammatory disease (PID) comprises a constellation of inflammatory disorders of the upper genital tract, including:

Endometritis
Salpingitis
Tubo-ovarian abscess
Pelvic peritonitis

The two most common conditions of PID in the nonpregnant patient are salpingo-oophoritis and tubo-ovarian abscess.

The diagnosis of acute salpingo-oophoritis is often made inappropriately.[55] The patient usually presents with lower quadrant abdominal pain that is frequently bilateral. She may have started her menstrual period recently. Additional symptoms may include nausea, dysuria, and purulent vaginal discharge. Abdominal examination reveals generalized tenderness without palpable masses. Bimanual examination reveals cervical motion tenderness and bilateral adnexal tenderness. Usually there are no adnexal masses. Differential diagnoses must include:

Acute appendicitis
Urinary tract infection
Adnexal torsion
Endometriosis
Hemorrhagic corpus luteum ovarian cyst
Ectopic pregnancy

The definitive diagnosis is confirmed by laparoscopy or laparotomy, especially when the patient is unresponsive to antibiotic therapy. If surgery is not indicated, empirical treatment with broad spectrum antibiotics may be initiated on an outpatient or inpatient basis until the infectious agent is identified.[56] Medication alterations are then based on laboratory results.

Patients with acute tubo-ovarian abscess experience:

Severe pelvic and lower abdominal pain
High fever
Nausea and vomiting
Impending septic shock

Abdominal examination reveals marked tenderness with muscular rigidity, a pelvic mass, and rebound tenderness. Bimanual pelvic examination is extremely difficult because of the abdominal pain. An adnexal mass may be discovered. It may be easier during a rectal examination to recognize a pelvic mass that may be directed into the cul-de-sac.

The differential diagnosis may include the following:

Septic incomplete abortion
Uterine rupture
Acute appendicitis with possible rupture
Peritonitis from abscess formation
Diverticular abscess (especially if left-sided pain is present)
Adnexal torsion
Perforated peptic ulcer
Pancreatitis
Mesenteric artery thrombosis

Laboratory results of any vaginal cultures confirm the infectious cause. Ultrasonography may demonstrate adnexal pathology or cul-de-sac flocculation.

The treatment plan includes hospitalization with intravenous hydration, analgesics, and systemic antibiotics. Abscesses may resolve without need for acute surgical intervention. Timing of surgical intervention requires clinical judgment. Should the patient not respond to 72 hours of multi-agent broad spectrum antibiotics and have persistent spiking fevers, urgent laparotomy may be necessary to remove affected pelvic organs that have become infected by the ruptured abscess. Drainage and lavage of the peritoneal cavity may conserve pelvic organs.

Chronic PID may cause pain because of recurrent exacerbations that require antibiotic therapy or because of hydrosalpinges and adhesion formation around the tubes, ovaries, and intestines. Endometriosis is the most frequently encountered differential diagnosis, particularly if there is no well-documented history of acute infection. Before ascribing pain symptoms to adhesions, one should note adhesions specifically in the area of pain localization. Some patients with extensive pelvic adhesions may be asymptomatic. Laparoscopy or laparotomy may be required to identify the adhesions.

Ovarian Pain

Ovarian cysts are usually asymptomatic, but pain may occur as a result of rapid distension of the ovarian capsule. Some women may develop recurrent hemorrhagic ovarian cysts that apparently cause pain and dyspareunia. Impaired blood supply to the ovaries has been implicated, especially after previous pelvic surgery such as partial oophorectomy or hysterectomy.[57] Bimanual examination reveals an adnexal enlargement with tenderness. Ultrasound may determine whether the cystic structure is complex or contains clear fluid. Resultant cyst formation may become painful. An ovary or ovarian remnant may become retroperitoneal secondary to inflammation or previous surgery.[58]

Other Organic Causes

Besides the reproductive organs, the pelvis also contains elements of the urinary and gastrointestinal systems. Many genitourinary problems result in pelvic pain. Urinary retention, urethral syndrome, and trigonitis are rather common causes.[59] These causes are often associated with uterine prolapse, vaginitis, and endometriosis. Gastrointestinal sources of pelvic pain may include:

Penetrating neoplasms of the GI tract
Irritable bowel syndrome
Partial bowel obstruction
Inflammatory bowel disease
Diverticulitis
Hernia formation

Because the innervation of the lower intestinal tract is shared by the uterus and fallopian tubes, pelvic pain can also be nongynecologic in origin.[60]

Neuromuscular Pain

Low back pain of neuromuscular origin usually increases with activity and stress. Chronic low back pain without lower abdominal pain is seldom of gynecologic origin. Occasionally, a pelvic mass accompanied by neuromuscular symptoms may be revealed during surgical exploration to be a neuroma or bony tumor.[61]

PELVIC FLOOR DYSFUNCTION

Pelvic floor muscle dysfunction can contribute to many conditions, including:

Urinary stress incontinence
Fecal incontinence
Sexual dysfunction
Pelvic relaxation
Levator ani syndromes

These problems are underreported, embarrassing, and undertreated.[62] Symptoms of these problems may limit a woman's ability to function in daily living activities. Pelvic floor dysfunctions are often preventable; emphasis should be placed on prevention through education and exercise before problems arise.[63]

A review of pelvic floor anatomy with specific muscle functions follows, along with a discussion of the diagnosis and treatment of pelvic floor dysfunction.

Anatomy

The most common terms used to refer to the pelvic floor are levator ani and the pelvic diaphragm complex.[64] The pelvic floor complex consists of the visceral pelvic fascia and pelvic diaphragm, and the urogenital anal triangles with superficial and deep genital muscles. The sphincters of the urethra are also included.

The levator ani group forms the deepest layer of striated muscles, which are laterally bordered by the arcus tendineus, the pyriformis muscle, and the obturator internus muscle. The fascia of this group is continuous with these pelvic diaphragm muscles. The anterior pubic portion of the levator ani muscles includes the pubococcygeus, with the puborectalis and pubovaginalis portions. The iliococcygeus forms the posterior iliac portion. The ischiococcygeus muscle lies adjacent but more superior to the levator ani group, assisting the levator ani in its supportive function.

The perineum can be divided into the urogenital triangle regions and the anal triangle regions[65] (Tables 30.5 and 30.6).

Table 30.5
Pelvic Diaphragm (the Pelvic Floor and Walls)

Muscle	Action
Levator ani	
Anterior pubic portion	
Pubococcygeus (pubovisceral)	Supports the pelvic viscera
Pubovaginalis	Sphincter of vagina and urethrae
Puborectalis	Loops around rectum, elevates and helps constrict anal canal
Posterior illiac portion	
Fibococcygeus	Assists in support of pelvic viscera
Coccygeus ischiococcygeus	Flexes coccyx, assists in support of pelvic viscera, and stabilizes the sacroiliac joint
Obturator internus	Lateral or external rotator of hip
Pyriformis	External rotator of hip, stabilizes hip joint

Table 30.6
Urogenital and Anal Triangles

Muscle	Action
Urogenital Triangle Region (superficial layer)	
Ischiocavernosus ischial tuberosity	Erection of clitoris
Bulbocavernosus (bulbospongiosis)	Vaginal sphincter and assists in erection of clitoris
Superficial transverse perineals	Fixes perineal body
Deep layer/perineal membrane Striated urogenital sphincter muscles	
Upper portion	
Sphincter urethrae (rhabdosphincter)	Constrict urethral lumen
Lower portion (deep transverse perineal)	
Urethrovaginal sphincter	Compresses ventral wall, assists incontinence mechanism
Compressor urethrae	
Anal Triangle Region	
External and sphincter	
Subcutaneous part	Voluntary sphincter of the anal canal and assists the puborectalis
Superficial part	
Deep part	

Superficial external genital muscles form a figure-eight around the vagina and urethra and around the anus (Fig. 30.2). Deeper in the urogenital triangle is the urogenital diaphragm. It is anterior to and more superficial than the pelvic diaphragm. It is also incorporated transversely with muscle and fascia that span across the ischiopubic rami bilaterally. The urogenital diaphragm consists of the striated urogenital sphincters.

The female urethral sphincters include the striated sphincter urethrae and the distal intrinsic and external sphincters. The levator ani and the compressor urethrae muscles assist the sphincters in urethral closing.[66]

The pelvic floor performs three important functions: supportive, sphincteric, and sexual. The pelvic floor, in conjunction with the pelvis bones, muscles, and connective tissues, provides support of the pelvic organs against gravity and any increases in abdominal pressure. Support and tone for vaginal walls are also provided. Sphincteric function aids in control of perineal openings. Pelvic floor muscles prevent incontinence by increasing intraurethral pressure and stabilizing endopelvic fascia during sphincter contraction. The muscles also relax for defecation and contract to control flatus. They contribute to fecal continence by keeping the anorectal angle closed.[67] A functional pelvic floor stabilizes the proximal urethra, improves severe lower tract symptomatology, and assists in the ability to delay urination via bladder reflex inhibition.[66] The sexual function consists of contraction of perivaginal muscles during coitus to enhance sexual activity. The muscles also respond reflexively during orgasm. Decreased pubococcygeal strength and awareness impede sexual response.[68]

Pelvic Floor and Incontinence

Incontinence affects 10–11 million people of all ages. Women are twice as likely as men to be incontinent.[69] Denial is common because many patients believe that it is an inevitable result of childbirth and aging. Involuntary loss of urine during physical activity is called stress urinary incontinence. Nygaard et al. studied the relationship between exercise and incontinence and found that 47% of regularly exercising women experienced some degree of incontinence.[70] Of 326 women, 22% of the subjects were nulliparous. High-impact exercises (running and jumping) resulted in more episodes of incontinence than did low-impact activities.

In another study, Nygaard et al. discussed the possibility of a urine continence threshold.[71] Incontinence was common in young highly fit, nulliparous women. Women who frequently exercised addressed their incontinence by wearing protective pads, staying close to a toilet, and limiting fluid intake.

Urogynecologic dysfunctions have multifactorial causes that require medical evaluation and urodynamic testing. When an evaluation indicates muscle dysfunction, an osteopathic physician may gain additional insight from his or her understanding of the interrelationship between structure and function of the pelvis. Although treatment includes surgical, pharmacologic, and structural options, all treatment plans should incorporate exercises aimed at improving the neuromuscular function of the pelvic floor muscle complex.[72] The success of manipulative treatment and exercise depends on the condition of the sensory and motor system of the patient.

Numerous resources are available that discuss incontinence.[69] However, a routine pelvic examination may identify opportunities for education and prevention of poor performance of pelvic floor muscles. Further examination should include visual inspection of the perineum during a pelvic floor contraction to note whether the proper muscles are contracting and relaxing, and digital palpation to detect muscle strength or pain. Note any cystocele, rectocele, or poorly repaired episiotomies. Uterine or vaginal prolapse should also be documented.[67]

Pelvic relaxation with decrease in normal pelvic floor sup-

Figure 30.2. Pelvic floor muscles as seen from below in supine female. (Reprinted with permission from Travell J, Simons D. *Myofascial Pain and Dysfunction: The Trigger Point Manual, Vol 2,* Baltimore, Md: Williams & Wilkins, 1992.)

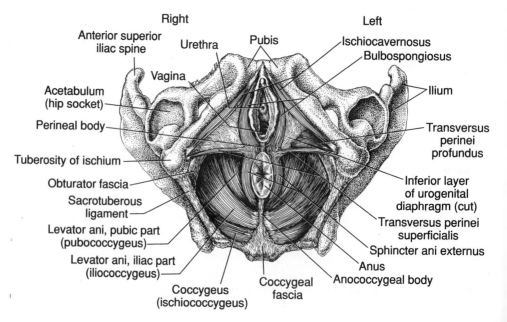

port can occur with congenital or developmental weakness of the supportive structures, or when pelvic structures (especially the pudendal nerve) are damaged in childbirth.[73–74] Even if the pelvic floor muscles are not damaged in vaginal delivery, the muscles must accommodate the passage of the fetus through the pelvis. Scar tissue may limit muscle contractility.[75] Postpartum patients are often afraid to recondition the perineum because of pain, and they usually fail to perform the Kegel exercises taught in childbirth classes.[76–77]

The fascia and support structures are also influenced by menopause and aging.[64,78] Changes in the pelvic floor from chronic constipation and straining during defecation can lead to anorectal incontinence with outstretched perineum and sphincter denervation.[79] Chronic cough also strains the muscles of the pelvic floor.[80] Kegel exercises, developed in the 1950s, were meant to address early stages of pelvic relaxation, not to prevent the need for surgery.[76] Although the mechanism by which these exercises alleviate dysfunctions is not fully understood, the patient benefits from regular contraction and relaxation of isolated muscle groups to increase motor recruitment abilities.

Pelvic Floor Pain

Hypertonus dysfunctions of musculoskeletal and urogynecologic systems are known as the levator ani syndrome.[81] Poorly localized pain is the primary symptom. The pain may be located in perivaginal or perirectal areas, in lower abdominal quadrants, and in the pelvis. Vulvar or clitoral burning may sometimes be present. Pain can also be located in suprapubic or coccyx regions, even down the posterior thigh. More specific symptoms reported by women with hypertonus dysfunction include[82]:

Dysmenorrhea
Dyspareunia
Sexual dysfunction
Voiding difficulty
Frequency and urgency of urination

Tension myalgia of the pelvic floor is a spectrum of diagnoses of various syndromes of pelvic musculature, including pyriformis syndrome, levator ani syndrome, coccygodynia, and vaginismus.[83] Other diagnoses with a component of hypertonus dysfunction include[63,73]:

Chronic low back pain
Endometriosis
Chronic pelvic pain with negative laparoscopy findings
Interstitial cystitis
Urethral syndrome
Sphincter dyssynergia

Chronic pelvic pain is the second most common complaint in gynecologic practice. Musculoskeletal postural dysfunction has been implicated and can lead to levator ani syndrome by maintaining inefficient holding patterns of muscles that contribute to persistence of pain.[73,84] Somatic dysfunction of the pelvis, if untreated, may cause hypertonus as a result of restriction of motion of pelvic joints and their related structures. Myofascial pain syndromes create pain, tenderness, and autonomic phenomena from myofascial trigger points. Simons and Travell have identified trigger points in the[85]:

Coccygeus
Levator ani
Obturator internus
Adductor magnus
Pyriformis or oblique abdominals

Chapman's reflexes may also be used to identify and treat somatic dysfunction of the female pelvis.[86] Osteopathic manipulative treatment in conjunction with posture education and a directed pelvic floor exercise program should remedy hypertonus dysfunction that is not caused by other, more serious pelvic pathologic conditions.

CONCLUSION

Assessment and treatment of some pelvic floor dysfunctions requires working knowledge of pelvic anatomy, physiology, and biomechanics. Although gynecologists are trained to perform surgery on female patients, osteopathically trained gynecologists are trained in the architecture and engineering of the female pelvis. They have the opportunity to both diagnose and prevent dysfunctions that have been influenced by the musculoskeletal system, through use of skilled palpatory evaluation of the female patient's entire body structure.

REFERENCES

1. Still AT. *The Philosophy and Mechanical Principles of Osteopathy.* Kansas City, Mo: Hudson-Kimberly Publishing Co; 1902:156.
2. Clemente CD. *Gray's Anatomy.* 30th ed. Philadelphia, Penn: Lea & Febiger; 1985.
3. Scott JR, DiSaia P. *Danforth's Obstetrics and Gynecology.* 7th ed. Philadelphia, Penn: JB Lippincott; 1994.
4. Mattingly RF, Thompson JD. *Te Linde's Operative Gynecology.* Philadelphia, Penn: JB Lippincott; 1985.
5. Beal MC. Viscerosomatic reflexes: A review. *JAOA.* 1985;85:786–800.
6. Walker E, Katon W, Harrop-Griffiths J, Holm L, Russo J, Hickok LR. Relationship of chronic pelvic pain to psychiatric diagnoses and childhood sexual abuse. *Am J Psychiatry.* 1988;145:75–80.
7. Smith RP. Identifying the causes of pelvic pain. *The Female Patient.* 1993;18:41–51.
8. Glintner KP. Chronic pelvic pain. *JAOA.* 1974;74:335–340.
9. Gambone JC, Lench JB, Slesinski MJ, Reiter RC, Moore JG. Validation of hysterectomy indications and the quality assurance process. *Obstet Gynecol.* 1989;73:1045–1049.
10. Reiter RC, Milburn A. Exploring effective treatment for chronic pelvic pain. *Contemp OB/GYN.* March 1994:84–89.
11. Perez-Stable EJ, Miranda J, Munoz RF, et al. Depression in medical outpatients: under-recognition and misdiagnosis. *Arch Intern Med.* 1990;150:1083–1089.
12. Walker EA, Katon WJ, Hansom J, et al. Psychiatric diagnoses and sexual victimization in women with chronic pelvic pain. *Psychosomatics.* 1995;36:531–540.

13. Harrop-Griffith J, Katon W, Walker E, et al. The association between chronic pelvic pain, psychiatric diagnosis, and childhood sex abuse. *Obstet Gynecol.* 1988;71:589–594.

14. Reiter RC. A profile of women with chronic pelvic pain. *Clin Obstet Gynecol.* 1990;33:130–136.

15. Rapkin AJ, Reading AE. Chronic pelvic pain. *Curr Probl Obstet Gynecol.* 1991;49:99–106.

16. Wood DP, Wiesner MG, Reiter RC. Psychogenic chronic pelvic pain, diagnosis, and management. *Clin Obstet Gynecol.* 1990;33:179–195.

17. Pickles VR. A plain muscle stimulant in the menstruum. *Nature.* 1957;180:1198–1199.

18. Rosenwaks Z, Seegar-Jones G. Menstrual pain: its origin and pathogenesis. *J Reprod Med.* 1980;25(suppl):207–212.

19. Kumazawa T. Sensory innervation of reproductive organs: visceral sensations. *Prog Brain Res.* 1986;67:115–131.

20. Chan WY, Dawood MY, Fuchs F. Prostaglandins in primary dysmenorrhea: comparison of prophylactic treatment and ibuprofen and use of oral contraceptives. *Am J Med.* 1981;70:535–541.

21. Dawood MY. Dysmenorrhea and prostaglandins. In: Gold JJ, Josimovich JB, eds. *Gynecologic Endocrinology.* New York, NY: Plenum; 1987:405–422.

22. Boesler D, Warner M, Alpers A, Finnerty EP, Kilmore MA. Efficacy of high velocity, low amplitude manipulative technique in subjects with low back pain during menstrual cramping. *JAOA.* 1993;93:203–214.

23. Hitchcock ME. The manipulative approach to the management of primary dysmenorrhea. *JAOA.* 1976;75:109–118.

24. Chapman JD. Progress in scientifically proving the benefits of OMT in treating symptoms of dysmenorrhea. *JAOA.* 1993;93:196. Editorial.

25. Hacker N, Moore JG. *Essentials of Obstetrics and Gynecology.* Philadelphia, Penn: WB Saunders Co; 1992.

26. Frank RT. The hormonal causes of pre-menstrual tension. *Arch Neurol Psychiatry.* 1931;26:1053–1064.

27. Greene R, Dalton K. The premenstrual syndrome. *Br Med J.* 1953;1:1007–1009.

28. Magos A, Studd JWW. The premenstrual syndrome: A review. In: Studd JWW, Whitehead MI, eds. *The Menopause.* Oxford, England: Blackwell Scientific Publications; 1988:271–288.

29. West CP. Inhibition of ovulation with oral progestins—effectiveness in premenstrual syndrome. *Eur J Obstet & Gynecol Reprod Biol.* 1990;34:119–128.

30. Smith S, Schiff I. The premenstrual syndrome diagnosis and management. *Fertil Steril.* 1989;52:527–543.

31. Khoo SK, Munro C, Battistutta D. Evening primrose oil and treatment of premenstrual syndrome. *Med J Aust.* 1990;153:189–192.

32. O'Brien PM, Craven D, Selby C, Symonds EM. Treatment of the premenstrual syndrome by spironolactone. *Br J Obstet Gynaecol.* 1979;85:142–147.

33. Starzinski M. Premenstrual syndrome: update and osteopathic approach to treatment. *Osteopath Ann.* 1987;14:39–42.

34. Abraham GE. Nutritional factors in the etiology of the premenstrual tension syndrome. *J Reprod Med.* 1983;28:7–12.

35. Taylor HC. Vascular congestion and hyperemia: their effect on structure and function of the female reproductive system: parts I and II. *Am J Obstet Gynecol.* 1949;57:211–221.

36. Taylor HC. Pelvic pain based on a vascular and autonomic nervous system disorder. *Am J Obstet Gynecol.* 1954;67:1177–1182.

37. Mathis BV, Miller JS, Lukens ML, Paluzzi MW. Pelvic congestion syndrome: a new approach to an unusual problem. *Am Surg.* 1995;61:1016–1018.

38. Duncan CH, Taylor HC. A psychosomatic study of pelvic congestion. *Am J Obstet Gynecol.* 1952;64:1–8.

39. Babakania A, Rock JA, Jones HW Jr. Pregnancy success following abdominal myomectomy for infertility. *Fertil Steril.* 1978;30:644–647.

40. Baggish MS, Sze EHM, Morgan G. Hysteroscopic treatment of submucosal myomata uteri. *J Gynecol Surg.* 1989;5:27–30.

41. Conn PM, Crowley WF Jr. Gonadotropin-releasing hormone and its analogues. *N Engl J Med.* 1991;324:95–103.

42. Friedman AJ, Rein MS, Harrison-Atlas D, Garfield JM, Doubilet PM. A randomized, placebo-controlled, double-blind study evaluating leuprolide acetate depot treatment before myomectomy. *Fertil Steril.* 1989;52:728–733.

43. Lumsden MA, West CP, Hawkins RA, Bramley TA, Rumgay L, Baird DT. The binding of steroids to myometrium and leiomyomata (fibroids) in women treated with the gonadotropin releasing hormone agonist, Zoladex (ICI 118630). *J Endocrinol.* 1989;12:389–396.

44. Adamson G. Diagnosis and clinical presentation of endometriosis. *Am J Obstet Gynecol.* 1990;162:568–569.

45. Ranney B. The prevention, palliation, and treatment of endometriosis. *Am J Obstet Gynecol.* 1975;123:778–785.

46. Moore JG, Binstock MA, Growdon WA. The clinical implications of retroperitoneal endometriosis. *Am J Obstet Gynecol.* 1988;158:1291–1298.

47. Ranney B. Endometriosis I: conservative operations. *Am J Obstet Gynecol.* 1970;107:743–753.

48. Surrey ES, Halme J. Effect of peritoneal fluid from endometriosis patients on endometrial proliferation in vitro. *Obstet Gynecol.* 1990;76:792–797.

49. Revised American Fertility Society classification of endometriosis: 1985. *Fertil Steril.* 1985;43:351–352.

50. Ranney B. Endometriosis III: complete operations. Reasons, sequelae, treatment. *Am J Obstet Gynecol.* 1971;198:1137–1144.

51. Ansbacher P. Treatment of endometriosis with danazol. *Am J Obstet Gynecol.* 1975;121:283–284.

52. Henzl MR. Gonadotropin-releasing hormone (GnRH) agonists in the management of endometriosis: a review. *Clin Obstet Gynecol.* 1988;31:840–856.

53. Cedars MI, Lu JK, Meldrum DR, Judd HL. Treatment of endometriosis with a long-acting gonadotropin-releasing hormone agonist plus medroxyprogesterone acetate. *Obstet Gynecol.* 1990;75:641–645.

54. Meldrum DR, Pardridge WM, Karow WG, et al. Hormonal effects of danazol and medical oophorectomy in endometriosis: enigmas in diagnosis and management. *Obstet Gynecol.* 1983;62:480–485.

55. Toth A. Alternative causes of pelvic inflammatory disease. *J Reprod Med.* 1983;28:699–702.

56. American College of Obstetrics and Gynecologists (ACOG). Technical Bulletin 153: Antimicrobial therapy for gynecological infections. Washington, DC: ACOG; 1991.

57. Dicker RC, Greenspan JR, Strauss LT, et al. Complications of vaginal and abdominal hysterectomy among females of reproductive age in the United States. The collaborative review of sterilization. *Am J Obstet Gynecol.* 1982;144:841–848.

58. Pettit PD, Lee RA. Ovarian remnant syndrome: diagnostic dilemma and surgical challenges. *Obstet Gynecol.* 1988;71:580–583.

59. Vereekin RL. Chronic pelvic pain of urologic origin. In: Ranaer MR,

ed. *Chronic Pelvic Pain in Women.* New York, NY: Springer-Verlag; 1981:155–161.

60. Rapkin AJ, Kames LD. The pain management approach to chronic pelvic pain. *J Reprod Med.* 1987;32:323–327.

61. Malinak LR. Operative management of pelvic pain. *Clin Obstet Gynecol.* 1980;23:191–200.

62. Physicians hear about incontinence. *JAMA.* 1990;264:2381–2382. Editorial.

63. Benson JT. *Female Pelvic Floor Disorders: Investigation and Management.* New York, NY: WW Norton; 1992.

64. DeLancey J, Richardson AC. Anatomy of genital support. In: Benson JT, ed. *Female Pelvic Floor Disorders: Investigation and Management.* New York, NY: WW Norton; 1992.

65. Moore K. *Clinically Oriented Anatomy.* 2nd ed. Baltimore, Md: Williams & Wilkins; 1985.

66. Mostwin J. Current concepts of female pelvic anatomy and physiology. *Urol Clin North Am.* 1991;18:175–195.

67. Spence-Jones C, Kamm MA, Henry MM, Hudson CV. Bowel dysfunction: a pathogenic factor in uterovaginal prolapse and urinary stress incontinence. *Br J Obstet Gynaecol.* 1994;101:147–152.

68. Graber B. Kline-Graber G. Female orgasm: role of pubococcygeus muscle. *J Canadian Psychiatry.* 1979;40:348–351.

69. Urinary Incontinence in Adults: Clinical Practice Guideline. Rockville, MD: Agency for Health Care Policy and Research; 1992. Public Health Service. US Department of Health and Human Services. AHCPR publication 92-0038.

70. Nygaard I, DeLancey JO, Arnsdorf L, Murphy E. Exercise and incontinence. *Obstet Gynecol.* 1990;75:848–851.

71. Nygaard I, Thompson FL. Prevalence of urinary incontinence in college varsity athletes. Proceedings from the American Uro-Gynecologic Society. San Antonio, Tex: 1993.

72. Wallace K. Female pelvic floor functions, dysfunctions, and behavioral approaches to treatment. *Clin Sports Med.* 1994;13:459–481.

73. King PM. Musculoskeletal factors in chronic pelvic pain. *J Psychosomat Obstet Gynaecol.* 1991;12:87–98.

74. Sampselle C, Brink CA, Wells TJ. Digital measurement of pelvic muscle strength in childbearing women. *Nurs Res.* 1989;38:134–138.

75. Snooks S, Swash M, Henry MM, Setchell M. Risk factors in childbirth causing damage to the pelvic floor innervation. *Br J Surg.* 1985;72:S15–S17.

76. Kegel A. Early genital relaxation: new technique of diagnosis and nonsurgical treatment. *Obstet Gynecol.* 1956;8:545–550.

77. Bump RC, Hurt WG, Fantl JA, Wyman JF. Assessment of Kegel pelvic muscle exercise performance after brief verbal instruction. *Am J Obstet Gynecol.* 1991;165:322–329.

78. McGuire E, Delancey J. Age-specific urinary tract problems: The postmenopausal woman. In: Buchsbaum HJ, Schmidt J, eds. *Gynecologic and Obstetric Urology.* Philadelphia, Penn: WB Saunders; 1993.

79. Halligan S, Bartram CI. Evacuation proctography combined with positive contrast peritoneography to demonstrate pelvic floor hernias. *Abdom Imaging.* 1995;20:442–445.

80. Staskin DR, Zimmern PE, Hadley HR, Raz S. The pathophysiology of stress incontinence. *Urol Clin North Am.* 1985;12:271–278.

81. Salvati E. The levator syndrome and its variant. *Gastroenterol Clin North Am.* 1987;16:71–78.

82. Klock SC. Female sexuality and sexual counseling. *Curr Probl Obstet Gynecol Fertil.* 1993;16:107–139.

83. Sinaki M, Merrit J, Stillwell GK. Tension myalgia of the pelvic floor. *Mayo Clin Proc.* 1977;52:717–722.

84. McCandless S, Mason G. Physical therapy as an effective change agent in the treatment of patients with urinary incontinence. *J Miss State Med Assoc.* 1995;36:2714.

85. Travell J, Simons D. *Myofascial Pain and Dysfunction: The Trigger Point Manual, Volume 2: The Lower Extremities.* Baltimore, Md: Williams & Wilkins; 1992.

86. Owens C. *An Endocrine Interpretation of Chapman's Reflexes.* 2nd ed. Chattanooga, Tenn: Chattanooga Printing & Engraving Co; 1937.

MARK E. EFRUSY AND RICHARD M. ROTNICKI

Key Concepts

- **Alimentary tract as integration of mind and body**

- **Diagnosis and treatment of esophageal disorders, including gastroesophageal reflux disease, diffuse esophageal disease, achalasia, and esophageal cancer**

- **Diagnosis and treatment of motility disorders of the stomach**

- **Diagnosis and treatment of gastric inflammatory diseases, including peptic ulcer and gastric cancer**

- **Physiology, diagnosis, and treatment of disorders of the small intestine and colon**

- **Diagnosis and treatment of diarrheal illnesses, including inflammatory bowel disease, irritable bowel syndrome, diverticular disease, and colorectal cancer**

For the osteopathic physician, the alimentary tract represents the essence of the integration of the mind and body. No other system so aptly demonstrates the close intricate relationship among the central nervous system, neuromuscular system, and visceral organs of the body. More than 50% of patients presenting to family physicians with gastrointestinal problems have no demonstrable structural abnormality of the digestive system. Their problems are a reflection of disorders of the central nervous system or the neuromuscular structure of the body. The symptoms are often attributed to stress, emotional lability, depression, or any number of vaguely defined environmental causes.

The elucidation of the function of the enteric nervous system and more than 20 gut peptides and amines has greatly increased our understanding of the relationship of the central nervous system and the gut to the remainder of the body.[1–3] These recently established hormones and neurotransmitters play an important role in gut function. The hormones gastrin, secretin, cholecystokinin, 5-hydroxytryptamine, and others act as central hormones or as local paracrines.[1–2] Most of these substances, now isolated in the gut, are found in great quantities in the central nervous system, i.e., in the brain and spinal cord.[3] Interestingly, the enkephalins, also isolated originally in the brain and central nervous system, are being found in large quantities in the digestive system.[2] Understanding the control of the alimentary tract function has become complex and can no longer be considered solely in terms of primary autonomic function, i.e., sympathetic and parasympathetic or functions isolated in any way from the remainder of the body.[4]

Somatic dysfunction in the mid and upper thoracic areas is generally recognized in disturbances of the upper gastrointestinal system.[4–5] These findings are usually explained as the effect of disturbed function. The osteopathic physician knows that normalization of these changes in tissue, mobility, and tenderness is associated with clinical improvement, suggesting that these findings are also a cause and not just an effect. In this chapter, we keep these principles in mind when discussing specific disorders of the digestive system and integrate their effect on the entire body, particularly on the musculoskeletal system.

This discussion of the gastrointestinal system includes only the hollow viscera; additional reading on disorders of the pancreas and liver is strongly suggested.

ESOPHAGEAL DISORDERS

The majority of disorders of the esophagus manifest as disorders of the normal sequence of motility. The three major problems that can result from disorders of motility include:

1. Lower esophageal sphincter disorder (LES)
2. Diffuse esophageal spasm and its variants
3. Achalasia

There are numerous subtypes that fall either in or among these three categories; all are related to disturbances of motility.

Gastroesophageal Reflux Disease

Gastroesophageal reflux disease is probably the most common disorder, not only of the esophagus but also of the entire alimentary system.[6] Its clinical presentation, heartburn or pyrosis, is experienced by virtually everyone at one time or another. Many individuals require occasional symptomatic treatment; a significant few require intensive medical attention. Gastroesophageal reflux is simply the excessive regurgitation of gastric and occasionally duodenal contents into the distal esophagus. This reflux is generally a consequence of a lowering of the physiologic high pressure zone between the stomach and the esophagus known as the lower esophageal sphincter. When pressures in the sphincter are less than 10 mm Hg, significant gastroesophageal reflux occurs from the stomach into the negative pressure of the thoracic cavity.[7]

The structural relationship of the lower esophageal sphincter, above or below the diaphragm, can be a contributing factor in promoting gastroesophageal reflux (i.e., the presence or absence of a hiatal hernia). The displacement of the lower esophageal sphincter or the proximal stomach above the diaphragm decreases the ability of the physiologic sphincter to prevent reflux. However, the mere presence of a hiatal hernia is not synonymous with reflux. The degree of tissue damage of the distal esophagus that occurs with reflux depends not only on local tissue resistance but also on the ability of the peristaltic wave in the distal esophagus to clear the reflux contents. Hence, the syndrome of gastroesophageal reflux is generally a combination of disorders of motility and mucosal resistance, including acid clearance, lower esophageal sphincter incompetence, and anatomic position.[6–7]

The consequence of persistent gastroesophageal reflux is an inflammatory process of the squamous epithelium of the distal esophagus that causes a leukocytic infiltration of the mucosa and submucosa, leading to mucosal ulceration and disruption.[8] Persistence and recurrence of this event can result in scar formation and collagen deposition, causing stricture and dysphagia.

The clinical spectrum of gastroesophageal reflux ranges from a mild syndrome to serious inflammatory disease leading to nutritional deficiency and possibly neoplasia. The symptoms of reflux are rather straightforward: heartburn or pyrosis, a burning sensation generally localized to the substernal area, commonly with radiation to the suprasternal notch and exacerbated by the recumbent or stooping position.[7,9–10] Typically, it occurs anywhere from 20 minutes to 1-1/2 hours after meals; often, if not always, it is at least transiently relieved with ingestion of an alkali.

The symptoms are rather specific while the physical findings are remarkably few. Substernal tenderness, although nonspecific, is often noted. For the osteopathic physician, somatic dysfunction of the mid and upper thoracic areas is typically found on palpatory evaluation.[4]

The management of gastroesophageal reflux of mild to moderate degree is supportive and symptomatic using the combination of antireflux maneuvers relying primarily on gravity, diet adjustment, and the addition of antacids or acid suppressors or inhibitors to the regimen. Concomitantly, osteopathic manipulative treatment can be supportive and symptom-relieving. Most therapy continues for 4–8 weeks, at which time one expects a substantial clinical improvement. Lasting improvement often necessitates a change in lifestyle, including:

Weight reduction
Dietary modification
Cessation of smoking
Elimination of heavy ethanol consumption

If symptoms persist or do not respond effectively, further investigation is required. This includes an endoscopic assessment of the upper gastrointestinal tract and appropriate photography, biopsy, and cytology as indicated. If the latter does not yield a specific diagnosis and gastroesophageal reflux is still suspected, 24-hour pH monitoring above the distal esophageal sphincter and esophageal manometry are available diagnostic modalities. The 24-hour pH monitoring presently is the gold standard in establishing the diagnosis of gastroesophageal reflux.[11]

Moderate to severe disease requires specific therapies for this disorder once the diagnosis is established. These therapies include rigid adherence to a caloric-restricted diet with a low percentage of fat and avoidance of chocolate, peppermint, alcohol, caffeine, and cigarettes. The majority of the caloric intake should occur in the earlier part of the active day with the avoidance of a large evening meal or a bed time snack. Avoiding the recumbent position after meals and elevating the bed with various devices or wedges is helpful. Histamine type 2 receptor (H_2) blockers such as cimetidine or ranitidine are indicated.[12] In refractory cases, omeprazole (Prilosec), a proton pump inhibitor, is extremely effective, particularly in cases of severe reflux associated with stricturing.[13] When this medical regimen fails in reasonable-risk patients, consider surgically correcting the lower esophageal sphincter incompetence with a fundoplication procedure.[14] Advancement in laparoscopic surgical technique has resulted in resurgent interest and use of this procedure.

The long-term sequelae of untreated gastroesophageal reflux include:

Chronic gastrointestinal hemorrhage
Gastroesophageal ulceration
Stricturing of the distal esophagus
Development of gastric or intestinal metaplasia of the distal esophagus (known as Barrett's esophagus)[15]

This latter condition has been implicated as a potential precursor for the development of adenocarcinoma of the esophagus.[16] However, early recognition of the symptoms of gastroesophageal reflux and their effective management in the context of general health can prevent these complications from occurring.

Diffuse Esophageal Spasm

Noncardiac chest pain is a manifestation of the common disorders of esophageal motility. Diffuse esophageal spasm is the classic clinical syndrome in this group. It manifests as intermittent bouts of spontaneous high-amplitude nonprogressive contractions of the esophagus producing episodic chest pain and/or dysphagia to both liquids and solids. These contractions are generally segmental but are seldom defined on routine radiographic examination of the esophagus. This disorder, more common in young people, is intermittent and presently has no defined neuromuscular basis.[17]

Variants of this disorder, for example, the nutcracker esophagus and nonspecific esophageal motility disorders, produce a similar but wider range of motility disturbances and symptoms. The condition often manifests as a severe chest pain with radiation to either the back or occasionally the jaw, lasting for several minutes. The initiating event can be a cold liquid, ingestion of food, or stress. Evaluation for coronary artery disease generally finds little support for a cardiac origin. The diagnosis is difficult to establish unless the symptoms can be reproduced during a motility assessment of the esophagus with esophageal manometric testing.[17]

Achalasia

The third type of esophageal motility disorders is achalasia, an uncommon but serious disorder. It is characterized by aperistalsis of the body of the esophagus, generally associated with a slightly to moderately elevated lower esophageal sphincter tone that fails to completely relax with swallowing.[18] The barium x-ray study generally shows a dilated esophagus often approaching the dimensions of a colon ("sigmoid esophagus") that tapers into a rattail configuration as it enters the stomach. This disease is thought to be an idiopathic degeneration of the neuromuscular apparatus of the mid and distal esophagus with degeneration of the ganglion cells of the myenteric plexus as well as a retrograde deinnervation of the vagus nerve in this area.[19]

Diagnosis of achalasia is made by use of an upper GI barium study, upper endoscopy, and esophageal manometry. Medical treatment of achalasia involves using nitrates and calcium channel blockers. Patients refractory to medical treatment require either pneumatic dilatation or surgical myotomy.

The esophagus has an overlooked propensity to refer pain to the mid and upper thoracic areas. It is not rare for a patient with an esophageal disorder, either inflammatory or motility-related, to present with pain in the upper back, mainly at T4-T6, with soft tissue and skin changes that can be palpated on careful physical examination.[20] Manipulative techniques can be applied in the correction of these changes.

Esophageal Cancer

Esophageal cancer remains generally an incurable disorder with low 5-year survival rates. Its cause is primary esophageal disease, i.e., chronic gastroesophageal reflux with the development of Barrett's esophagus (gastric metaplasia of the distal 3 cm or greater of the tubular esophagus) or the excessive ingestion of environmental toxins, especially smoking and alcohol abuse, in genetically susceptible individuals.[21] Discussion of this disorder is beyond the scope of this chapter.

STOMACH DISORDERS

The primary functions of the stomach are to store ingested foods and solids temporarily and to secrete pepsinogens, acid, gastrin, and intrinsic factor. The stomach facilitates the initial digestive process by mixing foods with secretions, reducing solids to small particles, and delivering this material in a controlled fashion to the duodenum and jejunum for further digestion and absorption. The rate of this delivery depends on the osmolarity, pH, and lipid concentrations reaching duode-

nal receptors. The proximal stomach is where receptive relaxation occurs and little active motility is evident. The mid and distal portions of the stomach empty with progressive peristalsis controlled by duodenal feedback, as well as an intrinsic gastric pacemaker located on the greater curvature of the stomach at the junctions of the proximal and middle thirds of the stomach. The normal frequency of this electrical pacemaker is 3 peristaltic contractions per minute.

Motility Disorders

Aberrant motility of the stomach has been the source of a number of disorders, reflecting systemic disease, intrinsic abnormalities of the gastric pacemaker, or smooth muscle contraction. These disorders are well-recognized and are frequent clinical problems confronting the physician. The symptomatology caused by abnormal gastric motility is often vague, leading to a misdiagnosis of a functional illness or nervous stomach that often frustrates both patient and physician. The symptoms of dyspepsia, postprandial bloating, unexplained nausea and emesis, and fullness often are early indicators of abnormal gastric motility.

A number of drugs and systemic illnesses affect gastric emptying either through their action on smooth muscle or through vagal innervation of the stomach:

Diabetes mellitus
Progressive systemic sclerosis
Anticholinergic medications
Psychotropic medications

It is important to be aware of the broad spectrum of influences on gastric emptying during the history and physical examination. Diabetes mellitus, particularly in young people, can manifest a gastrointestinal motility disorder involving the stomach, referred to as gastroparesis diabeticorum.[22]

Surgical alteration of the innervation of the stomach, such as truncal vagotomy, pyloroplasty, or partial resection, affects gastric motility and should not be overlooked in a careful history and physical examination. Finally, there is a motility disorder of the stomach that is becoming more frequently recognized in which the gastric pacemaker ineffectually discharges or causes antegrade and retrograde propagation of waves leading to poor gastric emptying and unexplained nausea and vomiting. This latter entity is often referred to as tachygastria.[23]

Often the only clues to motility disorders of the stomach on physical examination are viscerosomatic reflexes that lead to somatic dysfunction in the mid and upper thoracic area, particularly on the left side.[24] Although not well-defined, somatic dysfunction is commonly found by osteopathic physicians who carefully assess musculoskeletal function in patients presenting with ill-defined internal disorders such as abnormal gastrointestinal motility.

Medical treatment is aimed at eliminating or treating the underlying disorder, specifically if it is a systemic illness such as diabetes or systemic sclerosis, or discontinuing the offending drug. Primary gastric motility disorders, however, are more difficult to manage, but there has been some benefit with pro-kinetic agents such as bethanechol (a cholinergic agonist), metoclopramide, doperidone, and, most recently, cisapride.[25]

GASTRIC INFLAMMATORY DISEASE

Gastritis (inflammation of the gastric mucosa) is one of the more common diagnoses assigned to patients complaining of nonspecific dyspepsia or indigestion. When better defined, however, the term gastritis has relatively specific clinical and pathophysiologic implications. Acute gastritis is an inflammatory response of short duration, usually initiated by exogenous agents (most commonly alcohol and drugs), particularly the nonsteroidal agents and aspirin.[26] It seldom progresses to chronic disease but can present clinically with vague abdominal discomfort or more commonly with blood loss, often in the form of hematemesis or melena. When assessed endoscopically, one generally finds superficial erosions of the stomach, most typically in the medial and antral portions. When this is associated with the use of nonsteroidal antiinflammatory drugs (NSAIDs), it is often referred to as NSAID-induced gastropathy.

There are two broad categories of chronic gastritis. The first, type A, which diffusely involves the fundus but usually spares the antrum, is commonly a disorder of aging and affects approximately 20% of the adult population older than 65 years. In its severest form, type A chronic gastritis is associated with pernicious anemia.

Type B gastritis involves mainly the antrum of the stomach initially but later involves more proximal portions as it spreads. It is much more common, accounting for approximately 80% of the chronic gastritis seen in the United States. This is a disorder related to aging. More recently it has been related to the finding of a gastric spirochete, *Helicobacter pylori.*[27–28] This agent is presently found in approximately half of the adult population older than 50 years of age and is frequently associated with type B chronic gastritis.[28] A possible association of this agent with the development of intestinal metaplasia and gastric carcinoma is the subject of numerous ongoing trials.[29]

The clinical presentation of chronic gastritis, either type A or type B, is vague. Often, nonspecific postprandial dyspepsia or pain is the only clinical clue, unless the chronic gastritis evolves into an actual peptic ulcer of the stomach or duodenum. The diagnosis generally requires endoscopic survey of the stomach and appropriate biopsy of tissues to confirm the inflammatory response histologically and to search for *H. pylori* organisms with the Giemsa stain. The *H. pylori* also produce urease, which can be detected by various tests for urease on the gastric mucosal tissue and, more recently, by breath test analysis.[30]

Management of chronic gastritis depends on the degree of symptoms, the presumed underlying cause, and the mindset of the physician. There is an art to evaluation and management of these patients. Clinical experience supports the observation that upper thoracic manipulation to relieve visceral somatic reflexes often suffices to relieve the patient's symptoms and is

reassuring.[31] When *H. pylori* is confirmed as a causal agent, the decision to treat becomes more complicated. There are many studies that have shown this agent to be susceptible to numerous antibiotic agents and bismuth compounds.[32] The current consensus is to treat those individuals who demonstrate *H. pylori* on biopsy or urease testing and who have a gastric or duodenal ulcer present.[33]

Several regimens are used to treat *H. pylori.*[32,34] More recently, omeprazole in combination with either amoxicillin or clarithromycin has been used, achieving 80–85% eradication rates.[35]

Peptic Ulcer

Peptic ulcer of the stomach or duodenum results when the aggressive factors of acid and pepsin overcome the defensive mechanisms of the gastroduodenal mucosa. These defensive mechanisms for the most part are related to gastric mucosal integrity. Endogenous prostaglandins are major factors in protection through the maintenance of:

Mucous secretion
Bicarbonate secretion
Epithelial cell turnover rate
Gastric mucosal blood flow

The aggressive factors are:

Acid
Pepsin
NSAIDs
Alcohol
H. pylori

When an imbalance occurs between the defensive factors and the aggressive factors, either a deficiency of the former or an excess of the latter, peptic ulcer disease is a consequence. The ulcer crater is a reflection of a multitude of disorders manifesting themselves in a final common pathway.

Potential causes of this disorder include these agents:

Genetic
Environmental
Hormonal
Medicinal
Infectious

The dictum of Schwartz, "no acid, no ulcer" is as applicable today as it was when originally stated in 1913. Acid is essential for the formation of peptic ulcer disease; its removal or inhibition generally allows healing. There is a significant tendency for patients with peptic ulcer disease, particularly duodenal ulcers, to have hypersecretion of acid. In many individuals this is related to an excessive parietal cell mass that is under genetic control. Similarly, there is an elevated serum pepsinogen I in many individuals with duodenal ulcer disease, particularly in the individual with a strong family history of duodenal ulcer. Interestingly, many gastric ulcer patients are normal secretors or hyposecretors of acid, suggesting that there might be a different physiology for ulcer development in the stomach than in the duodenum. However, both require the presence of acid and both respond to similar medical programs. "No *H. pylori*, no ulcer" supplements "no acid, no ulcer" as the dictum of the 1990s. Elimination of this spirochete usually prevents recurrence.[36]

The clinical presentation of peptic ulcer disease depends on its location, the age of the patient, and complicating events. Generally, pain is the presenting symptom: a burning sensation in the epigastrium or left upper quadrant. Pain precipitated by meals suggests a gastric location of the ulcer. Discomfort relieved by meals or associated with hunger pains and relieved by eating suggests a duodenal location. There is considerable overlap in these presentations; reliance on the clinical history alone can be misleading.

Peptic ulcer pain is relieved by the ingestion of alkali or agents that inhibit acid production. The pain occasionally radiates to the back and the mid and upper thoracic areas, if it has a posterior location in the stomach or the duodenum. The reported osteopathic findings in the musculoskeletal examination generally include increased tension in the mid and upper thoracic areas and lesions of the 5th through 7th thoracic vertebrae, with some restricted movement as well.[37–38] The pain of untreated peptic ulcer disease lasts from 2 to 8 weeks; there is generally a prompt response to treatment. The morbidity of peptic ulcer disease lies in the recurrent nature of this disorder and in the secondary complications that develop because of recurrence. The primary complications of peptic ulcer disease include gastrointestinal hemorrhage (7–11%), perforation (2–4%), and gastric outlet obstruction (1–3%).[39]

The medical management of peptic ulcer disease has been revolutionized since the advent of the H_2 receptor antagonist, cimetidine, in 1977. For the most part, it has replaced the standard acid-neutralizing technique of antacid administration. With the H_2 receptor antagonist, acid secretion is stopped at the parietal cell level by blocking the histamine receptor. These agents have led to better compliance by patients and accelerated ulcer healing. Recent studies have shown that maintenance therapy with H_2 receptor antagonists often prevents or diminishes the frequency of recurrence of the ulcer as well as bleeding complications.

Antimicrobial treatment is the standard for treating *H. pylori*-positive ulcers, both gastric and duodenal.[33] Multiple regimens are available, including the standard triple therapy consisting of bismuth, tetracycline, and metronidazole. Newer combinations include omeprazole in combination with either amoxicillin or clarithromycin. Most of these regimens offer an 80–85% success rate.[33–35] The proton pump inhibitors, which block the final common pathway of acid secretion in the parietal cell, create an environment of complete achlorhydria. These compounds have been effective in treating difficult and refractory peptic ulcer patients, particularly hypersecretors, and those with the rare syndrome of Zollinger-Ellison. This latter condition is generally related to adenomas of the pancreas, duodenum, or other areas of the gastrointestinal tract that autonomously secrete gastrin or a potent secretagogue, which in

physiologic amounts is part of the mechanism of acid production in the stomach.[40]

Diet therapy plays a much smaller role today than in the past. The avoidance of salicylates, nonsteroidal drugs, and cigarettes is advisable. Smoking has been shown to be not only a possible causal factor in ulcer production but also a contributor to excessive recurrence and delayed healing. Surgery remains an option in managing the complications of peptic ulcer.

Empiricism has become a more accepted technique in the overall management of peptic ulcer disease, particularly in an era when cost-effectiveness is of prime importance in our medical programs. The majority of patients presenting with uncomplicated dyspeptic symptoms, whether they are thought to be caused by peptic ulcer, non-ulcer dyspepsia, gastritis, or gastroesophageal reflux, can be managed holistically. Osteopathic physicians use an approach relying primarily on history, physical examination, and measures to exclude peptic ulcer complications, i.e., stool assessment for occult blood, blood counts, and chemistry profiles. If there is no evidence of an extraordinary or complicating event, the routine use of the aforementioned medical agents, along with osteopathic manipulative treatment (OMT) for symptomatic relief, generally suffices.[37] However, when one suspects a complication or is dealing with a patient older than 50 years of age in whom a suspicion of a gastric origin of an ulcer is high, endoscopic documentation is essential mainly to exclude gastric carcinoma. The history and physical examination, including osteopathic examination, in the initial assessment of the patient with esophageal or gastrointestinal inflammatory disease often obviate the need for more expensive technical intervention and allow a symptomatic therapeutic approach effective for most patients.

Gastric Cancer

Gastric cancer has become less of a clinical problem in recent years. There has been a dramatic decrease in the incidence of this disease over the last three decades. The incidence has dropped from 38 per 100,000 to a present level of approximately 8 per 100,000.[41] This decline has been attributed to a change in environmental factors, including better refrigeration, less use of nitrates, and better general sanitation and health measures. Nonetheless, this disease still accounts for substantial morbidity and a mortality in high-risk population groups. Risk factors for gastric carcinoma are listed in Table 31.1.[42]

Table 31.1
Risk Factors for Gastric Carcinoma

Chronic atrophic gastritis and intestinal metaplasia
Gastric polyps
Gastric dysplasia
Helicobacter pylori
Postgastrectomy states
Pernicious anemia
Hypertrophic gastropathy (Ménétrier's disease)

SMALL INTESTINE AND COLON DISORDERS

The function of the small intestine is to absorb fluids and nutrients. This process is extremely efficient, allowing for the absorption of 95% of fat and protein and almost 99% of carbohydrates, water, and electrolytes. For this absorption to occur, there must be digestion of the more complex forms of food presented to the small intestine. This process of absorption requires integration of gastric, duodenal, pancreatic, and liver function at the cellular level. Malabsorption or maldigestion can occur with dysfunction of any one of these major organs.

Digestion products presented to the cellular level of the small intestine are rapidly absorbed, with active transport of these materials through the epithelial cell. Most nutrients are efficiently absorbed along the entire length of the small intestine; disease of the small bowel must be extensive to produce defects sufficient to cause appreciable malabsorption. Conjugated bile salts and vitamin B_{12} are absorbed only in the terminal ileum or the distal small bowel. Destruction of this area, surgically or by a disease such as ileitis or radiation, causes malabsorption of these substances. Of the three major food substances—carbohydrates, protein, and fats—the last requires the most work for absorption. Inefficiency in any one of the major digestive organs almost invariably leads to fat malabsorption, i.e., steatorrhea; it is generally the first sign of a clinical malabsorption syndrome. Fat absorption requires not only the function of the stomach, pancreaticobiliary system, and small intestine but also the formation of micelles, which are water-soluble aggregates of bile salts, phospholipids, and the products of lipid digestion. These micelles are efficiently transported to the epithelial cell, where further transport occurs through the gut lymphatics. Further along in the process of fat absorption is a breakdown of the triglyceride and a resynthesization of the triglyceride in the cellular compartment of the small intestine. Almost all nutrient absorption occurs in the small intestine, as evidenced by the excellent nutrition of patients who have had colectomies. The colon itself plays a minor role in carbohydrate absorption through the colonic breakdown of unabsorbed carbohydrates to organic acids. These are rapidly absorbed in the colonic epithelium. The caloric salvage by this mechanism is minimal in normal physiology.[43]

Disorders of Digestion and Absorption

Chronic diarrhea with weight loss, edema, or evidence of vitamin deficiency states (hypoprothrombinemia, hypocalcemia, or anemia) should lead the clinician to consider a disorder of digestion or absorption. Often these clinical signs are subtle, and a thorough assessment for a nutritional defect is required to unmask these conditions.

Malabsorption in the form of lactase intolerance from lactose deficiency is common, particularly among non–Europeans. It occurs at a relatively early age and is a common pediatric illness in many areas of the world. The spectrum of lactase deficiency varies from mild gastric distension, bloating, and nonspecific diarrhea, to a full-blown nutritional deficiency

state. The other disaccharidase deficiencies and monosaccharide malabsorption syndromes are rare in adult medicine and are primarily pediatric diseases.[44]

The major manifestation of malabsorption or digestion in the adult patient is steatorrhea. Normally, there are less than 8 gm of fat excreted in the stool/24 hr; amounts in excess of this indicate fat malabsorption. The gold standard for quantitation of fat is a 72-hour stool measurement. The qualitative method, a simple fecal smear for fecal fat staining with Sudan black stain, often suffices as a screening test to detect steatorrhea.[45] Several disorders with steatorrhea as a major clinical feature lead to significant nutritional deficiency (Table 31.2).

The workup of disorders of absorption and digestion generally begins with a thorough history and physical examination. A careful osteopathic assessment is essential because it often unmasks malnutrition through evidence of muscle wasting and motion restriction in the thoracic areas, as well as through skin abnormalities such as scaling, edema, and nonspecific rashes. Oral pharyngeal changes of cheilosis and glossitis suggest the combination of nutritional and vitamin deficiencies. Once malabsorption is suspected, assess the stool for fat with either a Sudan stain or quantitative analysis. If steatorrhea is identified, the physician should next determine what organ system is at fault. A barium evaluation is performed to assess the integrity of the stomach and small intestine and, occasionally, the right colon. The D-xylose test, a pentose sugar rapidly absorbed at the mucosal level without the requirements of the pancreaticobiliary system, evaluates mucosal integrity of the small bowel. A normal D-xylose test result would suggest a disorder of the pancreas, liver, or stomach.[46]

A small intestine biopsy, performed via a multipurpose suction tube or, more commonly today, through endoscopic techniques, establishes with a reasonable degree of certainty the diagnosis of:

Adult celiac disease
Nontropical sprue
Whipple's disease
Immunodeficiency syndromes
Abetalipoproteinemia
Lymphoma
Lymphangiectasia
Eosinophilic infiltration
Amyloidosis
Inflammatory bowel disease
Parasitic infestations[47]

Table 31.2
Disorders of Malabsorption

Chronic pancreatic insufficiency
Chronic cholestatic liver and biliary disease
Terminal ileal disease (Crohn's disease, radiation enteritis)
Drugs that bind bile salts (cholestyramine)
Bacterial overgrowth (deconjugation of bile salts)
Short bowel syndrome
Small bowel mucosal disease (celiac disease, Whipple's disease)

If the small bowel biopsy findings are normal or if evidence points toward a disease of the other digestive organs (i.e., the pancreas, stomach, or liver), specific investigations in these areas are undertaken. For example, the pancreas is initially best assessed through imaging techniques such as plain film of abdomen for calcifications, ultrasonography, CT scanning, and endoscopic retrograde cholangiopancreatography (ERCP).

If the liver appears to be the source of the malabsorption, through a deficiency of bile salt production or obstruction of flow, imaging techniques such as CT scanning or ultrasonography are recommended in the initial evaluation. Assessment of stomach function is still best done through fluoroscopic and endoscopic techniques. Occasionally, abnormal motility of the small intestine allows bacterial overgrowth that can deconjugate bile salts, leading to malabsorption. Assessment of bacterial overgrowth through small intestinal intubation and culture is occasionally done. Often, empirical therapy with antibiotics is tried when this disorder is suspected.

DIARRHEAL ILLNESSES

In the normal individual, approximately 9 liters of fluid are presented to the duodenum each day, 8 of which are absorbed on the transit through the small bowel. Approximately 1 liter of fluid reaches the colon with approximately 90% being absorbed, leaving 100 mL in stool per day. When 100 mL is exceeded, a diarrheal state results. Diarrhea is generally described as the passage of more than 200 mL stool/day or more than a 250 gm stool/day. Two types of diarrhea are generally recognized: osmotic and secretory. Osmotic diarrhea generally results from the failure to absorb water and fluids normally. Secretory diarrhea results from excessive secretion by either the small or large intestine of fluids and electrolytes. These types of diarrhea can be differentiated by measurements of fecal sodium and potassium. Fasting diminishes the volume of osmotic diarrhea, while in secretory diarrhea it has little or no effect.[48]

The importance of the two major types of diarrhea is in categorizing the differential diagnosis and management of diarrheal illnesses. Lactose intolerance and ingestion of nonabsorbable solutes such as magnesium and sorbitol are probably the leading causes of osmotic diarrheas. This is commonly seen with the excessive ingestion of antacid preparations or over-the-counter laxatives. Secretory diarrheas, conversely, are more common and are caused by bacterial enterotoxins, bile salts, fatty acid, and many laxatives that contain rinoceoloic acid (castor oil). The first prototype of secretory diarrhea was the *Vibrio cholerae* toxin, whose mechanism is the release of adenocyclates and the secondary stimulation of water and electrolyte secretion by both the colon and small intestine. Since that time, it has become apparent that many microbiologic agents secrete toxins and enterotoxins that turn on intestinal secretion in a similar manner, overwhelming the colon's capacity to absorb the excess fluid. The colon's absorptive capacity is generally 4 L/day; when this threshold is overwhelmed, diarrhea usually occurs.[46]

Clinically, most secretory diarrheas are of high-volume output with large, watery stools not significantly exacerbated by eating. A subcategory of invasive diarrheas is a combination of mucosal disruption by invading organisms such as shigellosis or *Campylobacter jejuni*. These organisms invade epithelial cells, particularly in the colon, and impair the ability to absorb the excessive fluid. They also turn on colonic and small bowel secretion. The presentation of a patient with this invasive type of diarrhea is one of small, frequent volume stooling containing many fecal leukocytes. Recently, toxigenic *Escherichia coli* organisms, a common cause of traveler's diarrhea, have been identified in the southern hemisphere. In the United States, a subtype of *E. coli* has been identified with both secretory and invasive properties leading to a high frequency/small volume bloody diarrhea. The differentiation of toxigenic diarrheas from invasive organisms is important because the latter often require antibiotic therapy. Identification of fecal leukocytes in the early part of evaluation of a patient with diarrhea suggests an invasive diarrhea.[49]

Although stool cultures can occasionally identify an offending organism in mild toxigenic diarrheas, particularly those secondary to *E. coli* and several viruses, they are seldom helpful and often misleading. Ninety percent or more of diarrheal illnesses caused by infectious agents are self-limiting, requiring no specific therapy. The 5–10% that require specific therapy generally present with constitutional symptoms such as fever, rigors, chills, and, often, signs of toxicity. A diffuse viscerosomatic reflex can often be detected on palpation of the lower thoracic and upper lumbar areas. There are nonspecific soft tissue changes not reflecting a specific site or limitation of motion.[50] The identification of a possibly invasive diarrheal illness requiring therapy can be expedited by careful history and physical examination and analysis of the stool. For the most part, diarrheal illness can be managed by appropriate food and oral electrolyte repletion, if the dehydration is not too severe. Symptomatic treatment with bismuth subsalicylate, diphenoxylate, and loperamide often improves symptoms and does not significantly worsen the course of the diarrhea.

If a diarrheal illness persists for more than 1 week, a more intensive investigation is generally required. This usually starts with a flexible endoscopic examination of the colon for assessment of the mucosa and appropriate biopsy of tissue. Often this is followed by a barium evaluation of the small bowel. It should be stressed that barium has no place in the initial management or evaluation of diarrhea because it often interferes with stool cultures and assessment.[51]

Diarrhea in AIDS patients is a frequent and significant problem. Approximately 50% of AIDS patients present with some degree of bowel habit changes, generally watery diarrhea. This can become extremely debilitating. An organism is identified only 40% of the time. There is growing recognition that the protozoan *Cryptosporidium* and the mycobacterium *avium intracellulare* are pathogens for increasing numbers of AIDS patients. Unfortunately, there is no good therapy for these organisms; most of the treatment in the diarrhea of AIDS is supportive and symptomatic. The liberal use of loperamide, difenoxylate, and oral glucose electrolyte solutions is being emphasized. In severe refractory cases, a trial of octreotide (somatostatin) can be undertaken.[52-53]

Diarrhea associated with *Clostridium difficile* toxin is frequently related to antibiotic use. Almost any antibiotic is capable of allowing the overgrowth of *C. difficile* and the production of toxin. This type of diarrhea runs the spectrum from a mild, self-limiting disorder to a full-blown pseudomembrane type of colitis that can be life-threatening. It typically occurs 1 week to 2 months after exposure to an antibiotic. *C. difficile* diarrhea is frequently found in nursing home patients and is a common cause of hospital-acquired diarrhea. It is treated by removal of the antibiotic and by the use of either vancomycin or metronidazole for *C. difficile* overgrowth. Metronidazole is as equally efficacious as Vancomycin and is the first drug of choice because of its lower cost.[54] Treatment is usually started after *C. difficile* toxin A has been identified in the stool on specific assay. This assay has become widely available and should be part of the management and workup of diarrheal illnesses, particularly when an antibiotic history can be elicited.

Diarrhea associated with malnutrition and severe electrolyte depletion can lead to suspicion of an endocrine-producing tumor. These tumors often secrete vasoactive intestinal peptide (VIP), a potent secretagogue that causes a massive outpouring of fluid and electrolytes. Diagnosis is made by assay for the specific secretagogue. Recently, octreotide has been used for treatment with moderate success.[55]

Inflammatory Bowel Disease

Inflammatory bowel disease refers to ulcerative proctitis, ulcerative colitis, and Crohn's ileocolitis, a group of idiopathic, chronic inflammatory disorders of the intestine. They represent a continuum of diseases ranging from mild superficial involvement of the rectum to severe transmural disease involving the large and small intestine and occasionally the stomach and esophagus. Inflammatory bowel disease has emerged as a major chronic health problem, particularly in young people in the Western world. This group of disorders is a clinical manifestation of the interaction of environmental, genetic, and immunologic factors in the production of abnormal intestinal permeability and inflammatory responses leading to a chronic, recurrent illness primarily manifesting itself as a diarrheal disorder.[56]

The two major subtypes of inflammatory bowel disease are Crohn's disease and ulcerative colitis. The clinical manifestations vary with the site involved. Ulcerative colitis involves only the mucosa of the colon, beginning in the rectum and proceeding proximally. This proximal extension generally determines disease severity. Clinically, there is an urgent diarrhea with rectal tenesmus (the painful urgency to defecate), often with small volume, blood, and mucus diarrhea. Colectomy is curative in ulcerative colitis but not in Crohn's disease.

Crohn's disease can involve the entire GI tract from mouth to anus but generally targets the distal small bowel and right colon. Macroscopic involvement of the colon only, small bowel only, or other areas of the GI tract occurs less commonly. Crohn's disease is a transmural disease in which all the layers of the small and large intestine are involved, in contrast to ulcerative colitis. Recurrence of inflammation after surgical resection of Crohn's disease is extremely high (70–80% within 1–2 years), and generally this is an incurable, lifelong illness. The diarrhea of Crohn's disease is more insidious, generally of higher volume, and less often associated with blood and mucus in the stools. More commonly, there is evidence of chronic malabsorptive disorders, chronic blood loss, and weight loss.[57]

Inflammatory bowel disease is a systemic disorder with several extraintestinal manifestations (Table 31.3). Of particular interest for the osteopathic physician is the arthropathy of inflammatory bowel disease. Both ulcerative colitis and Crohn's disease have as part of their constitutional presentation a migratory inflammatory disorder of the large joints of the body. This could be a knee or ankle; sometimes the hands or shoulders are involved. Ankylosing spondylitis of the axial skeleton, particularly the low back, is involved. Sacroiliitis is not an uncommon manifestation of Crohn's disease, and this might be the first and most outstanding clinical symptom in inflammatory bowel disease.[58] Recognition of these facts by the osteopathic physician occasionally allows an early diagnosis of inflammatory bowel disease to be made based primarily on low back or peripheral joint pain. Inflammatory bowel disease should always be considered when a young person presents to the physician with a history of a recurrent, low back pain with no obvious cause and constitutional signs such as malnutrition, weight loss, or diarrhea.

Skin and ocular structures are also involved in inflammatory bowel disease, and can be a clue to the underlying condition. Erythema nodosum and pyoderma gangrenosum are two common cutaneous manifestations of inflammatory bowel disease. Iritis, episcleritis, and uveitis are ocular complications.[58]

The diagnosis of Crohn's disease or ulcerative colitis depends on a history and physical examination. Endoscopic assessment of the colon is combined with radiographic evaluation of the upper GI tract and small bowel. All possible treatable or self-limiting forms of diarrhea need to be excluded with careful stool analysis for ova and parasites along with culture and sensitivity tests before a specific diagnosis of inflammatory bowel disease is made. Several weeks or even months of observation might be necessary before a definitive diagnosis can be

Table 31.3
Extraintestinal Manifestations of Inflammatory Bowel Disease

Skin:	Erythema nodosum and pyoderma gangrenosum
Mouth:	Aphthous ulcers
Eyes:	Episcleritis, anterior uveitis, and conjunctivitis
Joints:	Acute arthropathy, sacroiliitis, and ankylosing spondylitis
Liver disease:	Primary sclerosing cholangitis

made. This delay does not alter the natural history of inflammatory bowel disease and can prevent unnecessary anguish and the socioeconomic consequences of labeling a patient with inflammatory bowel disease.[59]

The long-term consequence of inflammatory bowel disease, particularly ulcerative colitis, is colorectal cancer. Ulcerative colitis is recognized as a premalignant condition. Once the disease has been present more than 7 years, surveillance examinations are indicated, particularly if the disease involves more than just the distal rectum and colon.[60] There is an increased incidence of cancers in Crohn's disease but it does not approach the frequency seen in ulcerative colitis. Routine surveillance is not recommended at this time for patients with Crohn's disease.[61]

The treatment for inflammatory bowel disease is directed primarily at suppression of the end-stage of the inflammatory cascade process, generally involving the use of immunosuppressives. Corticosteroids still remain the cornerstone of treatment of acute inflammation in both disorders in which sulfasalazine is a first line maintenance therapy. More recently, the 5-aminosalicylate compounds, olsalazine, and mesalamine are used when the disorder is limited to the colon. Pentasa (a brand of mesalamine) is a sustained-release product currently used to treat inflammatory bowel disease involving the small bowel and colon.[62] More recently, a number of more potent immunosuppressive agents have shown promise in both ulcerative colitis and Crohn's disease, including 6-mercaptopurine and azathioprine.[63] Cyclosporine, a potent immunosuppressive, is currently undergoing trials for the treatment of inflammatory bowel disease.[64] Further discussion of these interesting approaches is beyond the scope of our text.

Irritable Bowel Syndrome

Irritable bowel syndrome is a functional condition of the digestive system, usually emanating from the small bowel or colon, that produces symptoms of abdominal discomfort and is often associated with altered bowel habits, usually diarrhea alternating with constipation. Commonly, passage of hard stools is followed by periods of days or weeks of high-frequency, low-volume diarrhea. The latter is a misnomer in that the total amount of stool passed per 24 hours is generally less than 200 mL. Hyperdefecation would be a more accurate term for the frequency of bowel movements. This is a condition generally starting early in life, waxing and waning through most of the adult years, often coinciding with life's stresses. The abnormalities associated with this syndrome have been attributed to a number of neuropsychiatric disorders, motility disturbances, and altered individual pain thresholds. To date, there has been no well-defined pathophysiology of this condition. Irritable bowel syndrome is for the most part a catch-all term to describe disorders of the digestive system for which no obvious organic lesion can be defined.[65]

The most common motor abnormalities associated with irritable bowel syndrome have included altered myoelectric ac-

tivity of the smooth muscle of the left colon, delayed, blunted, or prolonged postprandial motor activity of the colon, and increased response to cholecystokinin and cholinergic hormones. Recently, a number of paracrine disturbances as well as hormonal influences have been considered as contributing factors.[66] Much work remains to better elucidate the roles of these agents or factors in contributing to this functional group of disorders. When clinical studies are undertaken in association with personality profiles, many of the patients with irritable bowel syndrome appear to have a significant psychoneurosis—most commonly anxiety and depression. The importance of this syndrome, however, should not be deemphasized because of a lack of measurable organic disease because it accounts for 40% or more of the referrals to a gastroenterology practice.[65,67]

Exclude serious organic disease before making a diagnosis of irritable bowel syndrome. This is best done with a history and physical examination and a personality interview. Routine screening of stools for occult blood, occasionally a flexible sigmoidoscopy, and possibly even barium evaluation of the GI tract is necessary to exclude inflammatory bowel disease or colorectal tumor. Interestingly, from the osteopathic point of view, there are few associated viscerosomatic reflexes with irritable bowel syndrome. The symptomatology appears to be out of proportion to the physical findings and osteopathic lesions noted in these individuals.[67–68]

Treatment of this disorder remains difficult. It should be centered on reassurance from the physician, the judicious use of mild anticholinergics, antispasmodics, avoidance of foods clearly related to symptoms, normalizing bowel function with fiber supplements (particularly psyllium preparations), and increasing physical exercise. The role of the physician in reassurance and support cannot be overemphasized in managing this benign but often debilitating disorder.

Diverticular Disease

On the continuum of motility disorders of the bowel, diverticulosis coli is on the point just beyond irritable bowel syndrome. Many investigators feel that the motility disorder underlying many of the irritable bowel syndromes eventually culminates in a development of colonic diverticulosis, which are herniations of mucosa and submucosa through colonic muscle at sites where arteries penetrate the muscle. This is an extremely common disorder, affecting approximately one-third of Americans more than 60 years of age, and is often seen at earlier ages. Its high prevalence has been attributed to our lifestyle, particularly the lack of fiber in our diet and, as mentioned, an increased colonic pressure, possibly related to irritable bowel syndrome. There appears to be a hereditary predisposition in many of these individuals.[69]

There are four recognized clinical presentations of diverticular disease:

Asymptomatic disease (the most common)
Painful diverticular disease

Diverticulitis
Diverticular bleeding

The latter three are the most important clinically and require attention. Painful diverticular disease is generally the result of a contraction of hypertrophied sigmoid muscle and is probably a manifestation of the underlying motility disorder or irritable bowel syndrome.[69]

True diverticulitis is a microperforation occurring as a complication in fewer than 10% of patients with diverticulitis. The inflammation that arises from the microperforation is local, involving pericolonic tissue, although occasionally an abscess can develop and fistula to the bladder or bowel can occur. Perforation is rare. The clinical manifestations of diverticulitis are left lower quadrant abdominal pain, usually with rebound tenderness, fever, and leukocytosis; it is often associated with constipation. Treatment of diverticulitis usually consists of an intravenous antibiotic and bowel rest.[69]

Diverticular bleeding is more common in the elderly, presenting with an abrupt onset of lower gastrointestinal hemorrhage usually in the form of maroon-colored stools. The bleeding, at least 50% of the time, emanates from diverticula involving the right colon. Determination of the bleeding site is usually accomplished through colonoscopy, the tagged RBC nuclear medicine scan, or angiography.[70–71] Approximately 80% of these bleeding episodes stop spontaneously; the rest require either radiographic or surgical intervention.

There are several characteristics of diverticular disease as they relate to the practicing physician. Diverticulosis coli is extremely common and for the most part benign and inconsequential. Diverticulitis and diverticular bleeding require urgent medical treatment and often surgical intervention. The symptomatic diverticular patient without complications can be managed the same as the patient with irritable bowel syndrome, with diet, fiber, and reassurance.[72] Osteopathic lesions associated with diverticular disease are primarily those associated with the complicating factors, i.e., nonspecific lower left lumbar restrictive motion and soft tissue changes.[73] Investigations of symptomatic diverticular disease should be undertaken not necessarily to confirm the diagnosis but to exclude other diseases in this age group that mimic this onset, particularly colorectal cancer.

Colorectal Neoplasm

Colorectal cancer has now become the second most frequent cause of death from cancer in the United States. The Western diet, high in animal fats and generally low in fiber, appears to be a predisposing risk factor. Most of the identifiable risk factors include[74]:

Advancing age (older than 50 years)
Family history of colorectal cancers or polyps
Ulcerative colitis
History of familial polyposis or nonpolyposis family cancer

syndromes, such as Lynch syndromes 1 and 2 (the latter associated with breast, uterine, and ovarian cancer)
History of previous colon cancer

There appears to be a well-defined sequence of progression from adenomatous polyp to cancer. The greater the size and villous component of the polyp, the higher the likelihood of degeneration into a malignancy. Most polyps, however, do not become malignant. The progression from an adenoma to a carcinoma takes from 5 to 10 years, and it is during this progression that surveillance can allow successful intervention. Surveillance reduces mortality for colorectal cancer.[75]

Colon cancer and polyps in their early stages are generally symptom-free, with the only finding being occasional occult blood in the stool. Because of this, fecal occult blood testing has become a major screening technique for large populations. The currently impregnated guaiac slides remain the gold standard for testing, but newer techniques using radio-labeled antibody to hemoglobin and porphyrin derivatives are on the horizon. Presently, the tools used by the physician in detecting adenomatous and colorectal cancers in the early stages are yearly fecal occult blood testing, flexible sigmoidoscopy, and, when appropriately applied, colonoscopy. The last is used as a surveillance or screening technique in high-risk individuals as described above.[76]

The general schemes being recommended at this time are yearly fecal occult blood testing in individuals between the ages of 40 and 50, and a flexible sigmoidoscopy beginning at age 50 and repeated every 5 years thereafter. In higher-risk individuals, screening at an earlier age is recommended, particularly in familial polyposis syndromes and family cancer syndromes. Much controversy remains regarding the application of these surveillance techniques to various risk groups, particularly the use of colonoscopy. A colonoscopy is time-consuming and expensive, particularly when applied to a large population group. There is hesitancy in making recommendations for its widespread use at this time.[76–77]

The natural history of colorectal cancer as our population ages appears to be that of a more proximal lesion. The percentage of tumors being found in the right colon is increasing, suggesting that colonoscopy could indeed be the final answer to early detection of this lesion. With early detection, colorectal cancer found in its early stages within the confines of the bowel is curable in 80–90% of the cases. Beyond this, the cure rates in surgery are dramatically reduced to 30–40%.[78]

Radiation and chemotherapy have limited roles in management of surgically incurable disease. There is a developing role for adjuvant chemotherapy, particularly in tumors confined to the bowel. Preoperative and postoperative radiation of rectal tumors is used to reduce tumor bulk.

Colorectal cancer remains a major public health hazard; the impact physicians can have in this area is in early detection. Changes in our diet and lifestyle, such as increasing dietary fiber, lowering fat content, possibly the addition of calcium supplements, and attainment of ideal body weight can help to lower the incidence of colorectal cancer for future generations.[79]

CONCLUSION

This brief description of the hollow viscera of the GI tract is intended to increase the osteopathic physician's understanding of the integration of visceral and somatic pathways in relation to the application of osteopathic principles.

REFERENCES

1. Solcia E, Capella C, Buffa R, Usellini L, Fiocca R, Sessa F. Endocrine cells of the digestive system. In: Johnson LR, Christensen J, Jacobson MJ, Walsh JH, eds. *Physiology of the Gastrointestinal Tract.* New York, NY: Raven Press; 1987:111–130.

2. Costa M, Furness JB, Llewellyn-Smith IJ. Histochemistry of the enteric nervous system. In: Johnson LR, Christensen J, Jacobson MJ, Walsh JH, eds. *Physiology of the Gastrointestinal Tract.* New York, NY: Raven Press; 1987:1–40.

3. Nicoll RA, Malenka RC, Kaver JA. Functional comparison of neurotransmitter receptor subtypes in mammalian central nervous system. *Physiol Rev.* 1990;70:530.

4. Harakall J, Burns C. An osteopathic approach to disease of the upper gastrointestinal tract. *Osteopath Ann.* February 1978;6(2):51–54.

5. Alexander C. The role of the osteopathic lesion in functional and organic gastrointestinal pathology. *JAOA.* September 1950; 50(1):25–27.

6. Nebel OT, Fornes MF, Castell DO. Symptomatic gastroesophageal reflux: incidence and precipitating factors. *Am J Dig Dis.* 1976; 21(11):953–956.

7. Richter JE, Castell DO. Gastroesophageal reflux: pathogenesis, diagnosis, and therapy. *Ann Intern Med.* 1982;97:93.

8. Ismail-Beigi F, Horton PF, Pope CE II. Histological consequences of gastroesophageal reflux in man. *Gastroenterology.* 1970;58:163.

9. Johnson F, Joelsson B, Gudmundsson K, Greiff L. Symptoms and endoscopic findings in the diagnosis of gastroesophageal reflux disease. *Scand J Gastroenterol.* 1987;22:714.

10. Klauser AG, Schindlebeck NE, Muller-Cissner SA. Symptoms in gastro-oesophageal reflux disease. *Lancet.* 1990;335:205.

11. DeMeester TR, Wang CI, Wernly JA, et al. Technique, indications, and clinical use of 24-hour pH monitoring. *J Thorac Cardiovasc Surg.* 1980;79:656.

12. Sontag SJ. The medical management of reflux esophagitis; role of antacids and acid inhibition. *Gastroenterol Clin North Am.* 1990; 19(3):683.

13. Klinkenberg-Knol EC, Jansen JBMJ, Lamers CBHW, Nelis F, Snel P, Melinissen SGM. Use of omeprazole in the management of reflux esophagitis resistant to H₂-receptor antagonists. *Scand J Gastroenterol.* 1989;24(suppl 166):88.

14. Rosetti M, Hell K. Fundoplication for the treatment of gastro-esophageal reflux in hiatal hernia. *World J Surg.* 1977;1:439.

15. Thompson JJ, Zinsser KR, Enterline HT. Barrett's metaplasia and adenocarcinoma of the esophagus and gastroesophageal junction. *Hum Pathol.* 1983;14:42.

16. Cameron AJ, Ott BJ, Payne WS. The incidence of adenocarcinoma in columnar-lines (Barrett's) esophagus. *N Engl J Med.* 1985; 313:857.

17. Katz PO, Dalton CB, Richter JE, Wu WC, Castell DO. Esophageal testing of patients with non-cardiac chest pain or dysphagia. *Ann Intern Med.* 1987;106:593.

18. Cohen S, Lipshutz W. Lower esophageal sphincter dysfunction in achalasia. *Gastroenterology.* 1971;61:814.

19. Woolam GL, Maher FT, Ellis FH Jr. Vagal nerve function in achalasia of the esophagus. *Surg Forum.* 1967;18:362.

20. Walton WJ. The digestive system: esophagus. In: *Textbook of Osteopathic Diagnosis and Technique Procedures.* St. Louis, Mo: Matthews Publishing Co; 1972:71.

21. Katlic MR, Wilkins EW Jr, Grillo HC. Three decades of treatment of esophageal squamous carcinoma at the Massachusetts General Hospital. *J Thorac Cardiovasc Surg.* 1990;99:929.

22. Kassander P. Asymptomatic gastric retention in diabetics (gastroparesis diabeticorum). *Ann Intern Med.* 1958;48:797.

23. Camillieri M, Malegelada JR. Abnormal intestinal motility in diabetics with the gastroparesis syndrome. *Eur J Clin Invest.* 1984; 14:420.

24. Walton WJ. The digestive system: stomach. In: *Textbook of Osteopathic Diagnosis and Technique Procedures.* St. Louis, Mo: Matthews Publishing Co; 1972:72.

25. Richter JE. Efficacy of cisapride on symptoms and healing of gastro-oesophageal reflux disease: a review. *Scand J Gastroenterol.* 1989; 24(suppl 165):19.

26. Price AB. The Sydney system: histological division. *J Gastroenterol Hepatol.* 1991;6:209.

27. Marshall BJ, Warren JR. Unidentified curved bacilli in the stomach of patients with gastritis and peptic ulceration. *Lancet.* 1984;1:1311.

28. Dooley CP, Cohen H, Fitzgibbons PL, Bauer M, Appleman MD, Perez-Perez GI, Blaser MJ. Prevalence of *Helicobacter pylori* infection and histologic gastritis in asymptomatic persons. *N Engl J Med.* 1989;321:1562.

29. Cornea P. Is gastric carcinoma an infectious disease? *N Engl J Med.* 1991;325:1170.

30. Hazell SL, Borody TJ, Gal A, Lee A. *Campylobacter pyloridis* I: Detection of urease as a marker of bacterial colonization and gastritis. *Am J Gastroenterol.* 1987;82:292.

31. Bondies OI, Stillman CJ. Notes on the diagnosis and treatment of ulcerative gastritis. *JAOA.* 1936;35:568–571.

32. O'Connor HJ. Eradication of *Helicobacter pylori*: Therapies and clinical implications. *Postgrad Med J.* 1992;68:549–557.

33. NIH consensus development panel on *Helicobacter pylori* in peptic ulcer disease. *JAMA.* 1994;272:65–69.

34. Chibi N, Rao BV, Rademaker JW, et al. Meta-analysis of the efficacy of antibiotic therapy in eradicating *Helicobacter pylori. Am J Gastroenterol.* 1992;87:1716–1727.

35. Bayerdorffer E, Mannes GA, Sommer A, et al. High dose omeprazole treatment combined with amoxicillin eradicates *Helicobacter pylori. Eur J Gastroenterol Hepatol.* 1992;4:697–702.

36. Graham DY, Lew GM, Klein PD, et al. Effect of treatment of *Helicobacter pylori* infection on the long term recurrence of gastric or duodenal ulcer. A randomized, controlled study. *Ann Intern Med.* 1992;116:705–708.

37. Magoun H. Gastroduodenal ulcers from the osteopathic viewpoint. *Yearbook. Acad Appl Osteopathy.* 1962:117–120.

38. Bruer W. The osteopathic concept of peptic ulcer. *JAOA.* 1950; 49(7):343–345.

39. Sleisenger MH, Fordtran JS. Ulcer complications and their nonoperative treatment. In: Sleisenger MH, Fordtran JS, eds. *Gastrointestinal Disease. Pathophysiology, Diagnosis, and Treatment.* Philadelphia, PA: WB Saunders Co; 1993:698–708.

40. Zollinger RM, Moore FT. Zollinger-Ellison syndrome comes of age. *JAMA*. 1968;204:361.

41. Howson CP, Hiyama T, Wynder EL. The decline in gastric cancer: epidemiology of an unexplained triumph. *Epidemiol Rev*. 1986;8:1.

42. Cornea P. Is gastric carcinoma an infectious disease? *N Engl J Med*. 1991;325:1170.

43. Sleisenger MH, Fordtrand JS. Digestion and absorption of nutrients and vitamins. In: Sleisenger MH, Fordtrand JS, eds. *Gastrointestinal Disease, Pathophysiology, Diagnosis, and Treatment*. Philadelphia, PA: WB Saunders Co; 1993:977–1008.

44. Buller HA, Gravel RJ. Lactose intolerance. *Annu Rev Med*. 1990; 41:141.

45. Drummey GD, Benson JA, Jones CM. Microscopical examination of stool for steatorrhea. *N Engl J Med*. 1961;264:85.

46. Craig RM, Athinson AJ Jr. D-xylose testing: a review. *Gastroenterology*. 1988;95:223.

47. Mee AS, Burke M, Vallon AG, Newman J, Cotton PB. Small bowel biopsy for malabsorption: comparison of the diagnostic accuracy of endoscopic forceps and capsule biopsy specimens. *Br Med J*. 1985; 291:769.

48. Fordtran JS. Speculations on the pathogenesis of diarrhea. *Fed Proc*. 1967;26:1405.

49. Pickering LK, Dupont HL, Olarte J, Conklin R, Ericsson C. Fecal leukocytes in enteric infections. *Am J Clin Pathol*. 1977;68:562.

50. Northup TL. Diarrhea, Technique for Relief. *American Academy of Osteopathy Yearbook*. 1977;42:28. Monograph.

51. Guerrant RL, Shields DS, Thorson SM, Schorling JB, Groschel DH. Evaluation and diagnosis of acute infectious diarrhea. *Am J Med*. 1985;78(suppl 6B):91.

52. Malenbranche R, Gumein JM, Laroche AC. Acquired immunodeficiency manifestations in Haiti. *Lancet*. 1983;2:873.

53. Cello JP, Grendell J, Basuk P, Simon D, Weiss L. Controlled clinical trial of octreotide for refractory AIDS-associated diarrhea. *Gastroenterology*. 1990;98:163.

54. Teasley DG, Gerding DN, Olson MM, Peterson LR, Gebhard RL, Schwartz MJ, Lee JT Jr. Prospective randomized trial of metronidazole versus vancomycin for *clostridium difficile*—associated diarrhea and colitis. *Lancet*. 1983;2:1444.

55. Maton PN, Gardner JD, Jensen RT. Use of long-acting somatostatin analogue SMS 201-995 in patients with pancreatic islet cell tumors. *Dig Dis Sci*. 1989;34:285.

56. Mendeloff AI, Calkins BM. The epidemiology of idiopathic inflammatory bowel disease. In: Kirsner JB, Shorter RG, eds. *Kirsner Bowel Disease*. 3rd ed. Philadelphia, PA: Lea & Febiger; 1988:3.

57. Crohn B, Yarnis H. *Regional Ileitis*. 2nd ed. New York, NY: Grune and Stratton; 1958:42.

58. Snook J, Jewell DP. Management of the extra-intestinal manifestations of ulcerative colitis and Crohn's disease. *Semin Gastrointest Dis*. 1991;2:115.

59. Sleisenger MH, Fordtrand JS. Ulcerative colitis: diagnosis. In: Sleisenger MH, Fordtrand JS, eds. *Gastrointestinal Disease, Pathophysiology, Diagnosis, and Treatment*. Philadelphia, PA: WB Saunders Co; 1993:1313–1318.

60. Collins RH, Feldman M, Fordtran JS. Colon cancer, dysplasia and surveillance in patients with ulcerative colitis. *N Engl J Med*. 1987; 316:1655.

61. Shorter RG. Risk of intestinal cancer in Crohn's disease. *Dis Colon Rectum*. 1983;26:686.

62. Thompson ABR. Review article: new developments in the use of 5-aminosalicylic acid in patients with inflammatory bowel disease. *Aliment Pharmacol & Ther*. 1991;5:449.

63. Goldstein F. Immunosuppressant therapy of inflammatory bowel disease: pharmacologic and clinical aspects. *J Clin Gastroenterol*. 1987;9:645.

64. Sandborn WJ, Tremaine WJ. Subject review: cyclosporine treatment of inflammatory bowel disease. *Mayo Clin Proc*. 1992;67:981.

65. Manning AP, Thompson WG, Heaton KW, Morris AF. Towards positive diagnosis of the irritable bowel. *Br Med J*. 1978;2:633.

66. Harvey RF, Read AE. Effect of cholecystokinin on colonic motility and symptoms in patients with irritable bowel syndrome. *Lancet*. 1973;1:1.

67. Magliocco J. Irritable bowel syndrome. *Osteopath Ann*. 1987; 14(4):16–20.

68. Lindberg RF, Strachan WF, Koehleon WO. Relation of structural disturbances to irritable colon ("colitis"). *JAOA*. Feb. 1941;40:253–257.

69. Almy TP, Howell DA. Diverticular disease of the colon. *N Engl J Med*. 1980;302:324.

70. Casarella WJ, Kanter IE, Seaman WB, et al. Right-sided colonic diverticula as a cause of acute rectal hemorrhage. *N Engl J Med*. 1972; 286:450.

71. Harris R. Radionuclide evaluation of lower gastrointestinal hemorrhage: a review. *JAOA*. April 1986;86(4):226–234.

72. Hyland JM, Taylor I. Does a high fiber diet prevent the complications of diverticular disease? *Br J Surg*. 1980;67:77.

73. Walton WJ. Visceral efferent findings of colon, sigmoid, and rectum. In: *Textbook of Osteopathic Diagnosis and Technique Procedure*. St. Louis, Mo: Matthews Publishing Co; 1972:72, 137.

74. Moore JR, LaMont T, et al. Colorectal cancer: risk factors and screening strategies. *Arch Intern Med*. 1984;144:1819.

75. Winawer SJ, Prorok P, Macrae F, Bralow SP. Surveillance and early diagnosis of colorectal cancer. *Cancer Detect Prev*. 1985;8(3):373–392.

76. American College of Physicians. *Clinical Efficacy Assessment Project. Screening for Colorectal Cancer*. Philadelphia, PA: American College of Physicians; 1990. Monograph.

77. Eddy DM. Screening for colorectal cancer. *Ann Intern Med*. 1990; 113:373.

78. Beahrs OH. Colorectal cancer staging as a prognostic feature. *Cancer*. 1982;50:2615.

79. Uritchevsky D. Diet, nutrition and cancer. The role of fiber. *Cancer*. 1986;58:1830.

32. General Surgery

SYDNEY P. ROSS

Key Concepts

- **Foundations of osteopathic concept in surgery**

- **Osteopathic principles in abdominal and chest wall surgery**

- **Management of postoperative complications using osteopathic methods**

- **Somatic dysfunction and the alimentary tract; use of osteopathic manipulative treatment for ileus**

- **Use of counterstrain for postoperative ileus**

The practice of surgery is almost as old as humanity. With the use of tools, Neolithic men and women became craftspeople. They might have also used implements for surgical purposes because examples of trepanation (removal of a segment of bone from the skull) have been discovered in France dating to the Neolithic period. Signs that skull wounds healed indicate that a fair proportion survived the operation.[1] Surgical procedures were highly developed among some of the pre-Columbian peoples. Wounds were cleaned and closed with an astringent vegetable concoction or egg substances from diverse birds and then covered with feathers or bandages made of skin. Among the Incas and other pre-Columbian peoples, the surgeon was often a separate practitioner who looked after wounds and performed bloodletting and other lesser surgical procedures.[2] The ancient Egyptians employed cauterization and the fire drill as surgical tools. They made a type of adhesive tape by impregnating gums into linen strips used to pull gaping wounds together.[3]

In the early years of the 19th century, the principal therapies open to European and American physicians were general regimens of:

Diet
Exercise
Rest
Baths and massage
Bloodletting
Scarification
Cupping
Blistering
Sweating
Emetics
Purges
Enemas
Fumigations

Many plant and mineral drugs were available, but only a few rested on sound physiologic or even empirical foundations. For the most part, practitioners permitted illnesses to run their course without interference; careful observers noted little benefit from the therapies available. When anesthesia became commonplace and the limitations of pain disappeared, surgical procedures multiplied in number and complexity. The potential benefits of surgery were overshadowed, however, by the frequent, devastating infections that often resulted in death. Only when the bacterial origin of disease was discovered and the necessity for keeping germs away from the operative field was proved (notably by Lister) could surgery safely enter the interior regions of the body.[4]

Before 1926, the general use of the term "surgery" implied allopathic surgery. In June of 1926, 52 years after Andrew Taylor Still founded the first school of osteopathy, 10 osteopathic physicians met in Louisville, Kentucky, to form a new surgical educational association. On January 26, 1927, the American College of Osteopathic Surgeons (ACOS) was incorporated as a not-for-profit corporation. Until then, osteopathic physicians were almost exclusively primary care physicians whose practices concentrated on manipulative treatment. Although they might have had skills in suturing wounds or performing minor surgical procedures, formal programs in training did not begin until this time. The founding members of ACOS wanted to incorporate osteopathic concepts into the practice of surgery. They all believed that Dr. Still's teachings improved the care of surgical patients.

Surgery is usually defined as that branch of medicine that treats diseases, injuries, and deformities by manual or operative methods.[5] Using this definition, no branch of the healing arts owns surgery. No surgical incision or procedure can be called osteopathic or allopathic. Society at large does not ask for a political definition of surgery but rather accepts it as a medical practice based on the sciences of anatomy and physiology. There is no osteopathic surgery; however, there are osteopathic physicians who are trained in surgical disciplines and perform surgical procedures within the context of osteopathic medicine. Osteopathic surgeons today believe, as did the original founders of the American College of Osteopathic Surgeons, that the application of osteopathic principles improves the care of surgical patients. In 1983, the Board of Governors of the American College of Osteopathic Surgeons[6] approved the following definition of general surgery:

General Surgery is a specialty that encompasses a wide field of practice. It requires cognitive and procedural skills for treating a broad variety of diseases, injuries and deformities. General surgeons are thoroughly trained in the preoperative and postoperative care of surgical patients as well as in the technical performance of surgery. These principles of general surgery are the basis of all the surgical subspecialties. The core areas include surgery of the abdominal wall, alimentary tract, breast, endocrine organs, and trauma. In addition, the general surgeon has knowledge and experience in gynecological, oncologic, orthopedic, pediatric, peripheral vascular, plastic and urological surgery. The general surgeon is also trained and experienced in the management of the critically ill patient with multiple organ system failure including but not limited to cardiopulmonary resuscitation, nutritional support, endoscopic procedures, management of sepsis and coagulopathies. A comprehensive training (residency) is the basis for this definition.

Osteopathic general surgery residents continue to learn and apply osteopathic principles[7] during their residency programs. The educational foundation of these osteopathic principles is established during medical school and internship programs. Up until approximately 25 years ago, many of the individuals who entered general surgery residency programs had the opportunity to hone their skills in osteopathic principles and practice when they practiced primary care medicine before their residency. Presently, nearly all surgical residents enter a residency directly after their internship.

The basic tenets of osteopathic medicine are comprehensive philosophic principles that are incorporated into each aspect of surgical care, including:

Preoperative evaluation of a patient
Intraoperative management
Postoperative care

As in the other specialties of osteopathic medicine, these tenets are integrated into the regular practice of medicine and its training programs and are not an add-on to conventional surgical practice.

The core areas of general surgery are the basic blocks for training in all surgical disciplines. This chapter does not attempt to cover each of those but instead focuses on the common areas of abdominal, chest wall, and alimentary tract surgery. In this chapter we examine how osteopathic principles are implemented in the approach to the patient and in the management of common postoperative complications.

ABDOMINAL AND CHEST WALL SURGERY

Osteopathic physicians historically have accepted the precept that structure and function are integrally interrelated and that if one part of the body is affected, the entire organism is affected. Although practitioners of allopathic medicine might not disagree with these precepts, they represent active principles for osteopathic surgeons.

The patient is approached for surgery with the recognition that the patient's entire clinical context is as important as the surgery itself. Osteopathic physicians accept the idea that a patient's mental state is a critical feature in the outcome of the surgery. Conducive factors leading to a favorable outcome include a patient who is confident in his or her surgeon, is satisfied that the surgical procedure has been adequately explained, has a solid understanding of the expected morbidity of the procedure, and has realistic expectations for recovery and home care. The family plays a significant role in determining the success of major surgical operations.

Traditionally, osteopathic surgeons have been aware of the entire family and how that family relates to the patient. Many surgeons, including this author, feel that this can have a profound effect on the success or failure of a well-performed surgical procedure.

Management of Postoperative Complications

Major surgical procedures that involve the chest wall and the abdominal wall have a relatively high mortality. Table 32.1 lists the serious complications that can occur after a variety of major surgical procedures. Sabiston[8] stated that pulmonary complications can occur in 5–7% of all major surgeries performed with general anesthesia. The incidence of complications can double in abdominal surgery, triple for smokers, and quadruple for patients with chronic obstructive pulmonary disease. Atelectasis, a collapse of alveoli that renders them unable to be involved in gas exchange, is the most frequent pulmonary complication following surgery. This complication generally sets the framework for subsequent pulmonary infections.

The most popular mechanical method for prevention of postoperative atelectasis in the United States is an incentive spirometer. It is used extensively because it encourages deep breathing and requires minimal supervision and personnel to administer.[9–10] The beneficial effects of incentive spirometry in the prevention of postoperative complications have recently been challenged, however.[11–12] Just changing the angle of the patient's recumbency from 60° to 30° altered the effectiveness of postoperative incentive spirometry. This finding suggests features other than just lung mechanics involving the major

Table 32.1
Postoperative Complications of Major Surgical Procedures

Wound infections
Intraabdominal sepsis (peritonitis)
Subphrenic and subhepatic abscess
Empyema
Mediastinitis
Pneumonia
Acute respiratory insufficiency (including adult respiratory distress
    syndrome (ARDS))
Renal failure
Postoperative jaundice
Postoperative ileus
Bowel obstruction
Acute gastric hemorrhage
Multiple organ failure
Myocardial infarction

airways. One of the suggestions for the alteration in air flow with a change in recumbency is fluctuating diaphragmatic motion.[13] In the presence of diaphragmatic dysfunction, incentive spirometry can have little effect in improving gas exchange. The change in recumbency angle alone is believed to result in an improved diaphragmatic link tension relationship and a shift in compartment compliance as the patient reclines.[14-15]

The earliest osteopathic physicians incorporated their understanding of viscerosomatic and somatovisceral reflexes into their management of patients in the postoperative period. The visceral motor, visceral sensory, and visceral tropic reflexes that arise from stimuli originating in the lungs appear to manifest themselves in tissue supplied by nerves arising in most of the cervical segments; the reflexes are most marked in those tissues supplied by neurons arising in the 3rd to 5th cervical segments. Pottinger[16] stated that the visceral motor reflex caused by inflammation in the lungs shows itself in the contraction of the fibers of those muscles that receive their origin from the cervical portion of the cord and particularly from the 3rd to 5th cervical segments. This manifests clinically as an increased tone or spasm in the paraspinal tissues involved.

Osteopathic surgeons have presumed that this viscerosomatic reflex might be clinically significant and could have important implications for the possibility that modifying a somatovisceral reflex could be beneficial in the postoperative state.[17-22] In 1963, Henshaw[23] published the results of an interventional trial of surgical patients initiated in 1961. A total of 1031 surgical patients were studied. Of this total, 109 (10.6%) had preexisting somatic dysfunction at the level of the 3rd, 4th, and 5th cervical vertebra before surgery. This cohort formed the study group for investigation. Seventy-five of the 109 patients were given osteopathic manipulative treatment (OMT) for these lesions. In this group, three patients (4%) developed postoperative pulmonary complications. In the 34 patients who had cervical spine somatic dysfunction but did not receive OMT, 29 (85%) developed some form of pulmonary complication.

Unfortunately, the external validity of such a study is diminished in our era because the patients were not randomized. In addition, the definition of pulmonary complications was so broad that a high percentage of the defined entities (emphysema, pulmonary edema, cough) are of such sufficiently vague endpoints that they do not represent meaningful outcomes. There would be considerable interest in knowing the outcome of the 922 patients who had surgery in the absence of preexisting cervical spine somatic dysfunction.

The Henshaw study was conducted according to research methods and employed statistical methodology that was typical for that time period. Although the study does not withstand modern scientific scrutiny, the described results are so impressive that a current study to replicate these findings is warranted.

Another form of OMT that is described as effective in the prevention of atelectasis in the postoperative period is the thoracic lymphatic pump (TLP). The TLP is a ventilator assist technique that uses passive and active rib excursion. The TLP technique is reported to have reduced the mortality from the 1918 influenza outbreak from 5% in the general population to 0.25% in 100,000 treated patients.[24]

A recent study indicated that TLP can be equally as effective as incentive spirometry in reducing the postoperative occurrence of atelectasis.[25] This study also indicated that patients treated with the TLP had an earlier recovery and faster return to preoperative values for both the forced vital capacity and FEV$_1$ (forced expiratory volume at 1 second) compared with patients who did not receive TLP. OMT has been recommended in the postoperative median sternotomy patient to promote faster return to normal chest and diaphragmatic dynamics.[26] This is particularly important because there are more than 250,000 patients annually undergoing coronary bypass grafting through a median sternotomy incision.

ALIMENTARY TRACT

Many osteopathic physicians believe that treating the somatic component of a viscerosomatic reflex can improve a visceral pathologic condition. The diagnosis of a viscerosomatic reflex is based on a documentation of visceral disease and the objective findings of somatic dysfunction on palpatory examination. The finding of somatic dysfunction should lead to a review of the patient's clinical status to determine whether symptoms of a visceral disorder can be elicited.

Beal defines the somatic component of a viscerosomatic reflex to have the following findings[27]:

Two or more adjacent spinal segments that show evidence of somatic dysfunction located within the specific autonomic reflex area
A deep confluent muscle reaction
Resistance to segmental joint motion
Skin and subcutaneous tissue changes consistent with the acuity or chronicity of the reflex

However, the predictive value of palpatory findings in the differential diagnosis of visceral disease has not been established for clinical practice. The results can be variable, dependent on interobserver differences or issues related to the interpretation of musculoskeletal findings. At the same time that the clinical utility of musculoskeletal findings is incompletely defined, the effectiveness of manipulative treatment for somatic manifestations of chronic organ disease has not been established. Many osteopathic physicians have advocated manipulative treatment as part of the treatment regimen for organic problems of the heart and gallbladder. Although postoperative manipulative treatment has been recommended as promoting a shorter, smoother convalescence from the effects of visceral disease, prospective studies have not been conducted to test this hypothesis.

One of the major postoperative problems that can affect any type of surgery is postoperative ileus. Ileus is defined as the functional inhibition of propulsive bowel activity, regardless of the pathogenic mechanism. This is differentiated from motility disorders resulting from structural abnormalities, which is called a mechanical bowel obstruction. Ileus following surgery is further classified into postoperative and paralytic ileus. Postoperative ileus is the uncomplicated ileus that occurs following surgery and resolves spontaneously within 2–3 days. It most likely results from the temporary inhibition of extrinsic motility regulation and is more severe in the colon. In contrast, postoperative paralytic ileus lasts for more than 3 days following surgery. It affects all segments of the bowel and probably results from further inhibition of local, intrinsic contractile systems. Patients who have this disorder accumulate gas and secretions in the intestinal system leading to bloating, distension, emesis, and pain.

In spite of major advances in many areas of medicine, relatively few improvements have been made in the understanding of ileus. The most important advance was made over a century ago with the introduction of nasogastric suction in 1884.[28] The earliest studies of bowel motility focused on mechanisms for reduction and stimulation of intestinal contractions. Early in this century, the role of inhibitory sympathetic reflexes mediating ileus was recognized. With the inhibitory reflex efferent limb clearly established, investigators searched for the afferent system. Many possibilities exist, including peritoneal or cutaneous stimulation, release of inhibitory humoral agents, inhibition of smooth muscle by inflammation, or muscle or nerve inhibition by anesthetic agents.

Parasympathetic fiber stimulation increases motility and stimulation of sympathetic fibers inhibits it. Vagal nerve section in animals does not alter small intestinal motility, whereas splanchnic nerve division increases contractility. Sympathetic chronic inhibitor control predominates in the gut. Sympathetic activation occurs with stress and surgery and is thought to significantly alter bowel motility during the postoperative period.

The treatment for ileus has changed little in the past 100 years. Nasointestinal intubation and suction is the only proven effective therapy. Coupled with intravenous hydration or total parenteral nutrition, patients are maintained until ileus resolves spontaneously.

OMT has been used in the management of postoperative ileus for years. The following are a few of the OMT techniques that are used in treating postoperative ileus:

1. Gentle inhibition of hypertonic paravertebral muscles to the point of tissue relaxation (2–5 minutes total time)
2. Gentle inhibition of hypertonic paravertebral muscles in the thoracic region; this is most effectively directed toward spinal segments that are associated with the surgical site via supplying sympathetic innervation to the involved viscera
3. Indirect method fascial release manipulation of the diaphragm, thoracic inlet, and midcervical spine

In 1968, Herrmann[29] reported the results of a study in which he performed a chart review of 317 consecutive patients undergoing major surgery who received routine postoperative OMT, compared with a subsequent series of 92 patients who underwent major surgery but did not receive OMT postoperatively. In this study, the description of adynamic ileus used the following criteria:

1. Absence of bowel sounds
2. Abdominal distension
3. Tympany to percussion of the abdomen
4. Absence of flatus being passed per rectum

For those patients in whom adynamic ileus was diagnosed, OMT was then performed in the following manner. With the patient supine, intermittent pressure was applied to the paravertebral tissues of the lumbar and lower thoracic spine, producing extension of those areas, in addition to deep pressure. This was done for approximately 2 minutes. The treatment was repeated every 2 hours. Each patient was periodically reexamined to observe the effect, if any, that the treatment had on the criteria used for the diagnosis of postoperative adynamic ileus.

Only one case of ileus was noted in the series of 317 patients who received OMT postoperatively. This represents an incidence of 0.3%. Seven patients (7.6%) in the group of 92 patients who did not receive OMT postoperatively developed ileus. In these seven cases, the age range was from 9 to 73 years. After the administration of OMT, six of these patients showed improvement, as manifest by a resumption of bowel sounds or passage of flatus. This study was not a controlled, randomized trial, and the report provides scant details of the study design and methodology. It suggests that postoperative OMT aids in prevention of postoperative ileus. Because this viewpoint is widely held by practitioners of OMT, a randomized trial is warranted to investigate the efficacy of OMT in the treatment of this and other postoperative complications.

Jones[30] has described a form of OMT called counterstrain method. This method has been used in the severely traumatized postoperative patient. It uses tender points for the specific diagnosis of somatic dysfunction. Jones described the tender point as being a discrete, approximately pea-sized bundle or swelling of fascia, muscle tendrils, connective tissue, and nerve fibers, as well as some vascular elements. Counterstrain can be done without assistance from the patient and can be configured to be performed in patients who are severely injured.[31] Postoperative ileus and pulmonary dysfunction have been treated using the counterstrain method.

CONCLUSION

Osteopathic principles are widely implemented in the surgical treatment of patients today. The formal development of this process began with the establishment of regular surgical training programs in the osteopathic profession in 1926. The primary focus has centered on the osteopathic concepts of:

1. The interrelationship between structure and function
2. The need to treat the patient as a regulated, integrated, and coordinated unit

The first precept represents the rationale for the application of osteopathic manipulative treatment in the preoperative or postoperative period. The second precept is expressed in the surgeon's approach to the patient, his or her family and social support, and his or her own psychological state as critical features related to the overall outcome of any surgical procedure.

Osteopathic manipulative treatment is underused in the treatment of surgical patients. The challenge for the osteopathic surgeon is to translate years of clinical experience with osteopathic palpatory diagnosis and treatment into research protocols that determine the effectiveness of these methods for the surgical patient. Specific areas for investigation include the possibility that thoracic lymphatic pump or other techniques might reduce the overall incidence of pulmonary atelectasis, that OMT might reduce postoperative adynamic ileus, or that counterstrain techniques could assist in the recovery of patients following trauma or major surgical procedures. More remote areas of investigation involve how osteopathic manipulative treatment might affect the immune system in a manner that could aid the recovery of patients undergoing oncological surgical procedures.

REFERENCES

1. Lyons AS. Prehistoric medicine. In: Lyons AS, Petrucelli RJ, eds. *Medicine, An Illustrated History*. New York, NY: Harry N Abrams; 1978:27.

2. Bosch J, Petrucelli RJ. Medicine in the pre-Columbian Americas. In: Lyons AS, Petrucelli RJ, eds. *Medicine, An Illustrated History*. New York, NY: Harry N Abrams; 1978:50–55.

3. Lyons AS. Ancient Egypt. In: Lyons AS, Petrucelli RJ, eds. *Medicine, An Illustrated History*. New York, NY: Harry N Abrams; 1978:98.

4. Lyons AS. The beginning of modern medicine. In: Lyons AS, Petrucelli RJ, eds. *Medicine, An Illustrated History*. New York, NY: Harry N Abrams; 1978:523–533.

5. *Dorland's Medical Dictionary*. Philadelphia, Penn: WB Saunders; 1981.

6. Minutes of the meeting of the Board of Governors of the American College of Osteopathic Surgeons; October 1983.

7. The special committee on osteopathic principles and osteopathic technic. Kirksville College of Osteopathy and Surgery. The osteopathic concept: an interpretation. *J Osteopathy*. 1953;60:7–10.

8. Sabiston DD Jr. *Essentials of Surgery*. Philadelphia, Penn: WB Saunders; 1987.

9. Dohi S, Gold MI. Comparison of two methods of postoperative respiratory care. *Chest*. 1978;73:592–595.

10. Jung R, Wight J, Nusser R, Rossoff L. Comparison of three methods of respiratory care following upper abdominal surgery. *Chest*. 1980; 78:31–35.

11. Schweiger I, Gamulin Z, Forster A, et al. Absence of benefit of incentive spirometry in low risk patients undergoing elective cholecystectomy. *Chest*. 1986;89:652–656.

12. Stock MC, Downs JB, Gauer PK, et al. Prevention of post operative pulmonary complications with C-pap, incentive spirometry and conservative therapy. *Chest*. 1985;87:151–157.

13. Froese A, Bryan AC. Effect of anesthesia and paralysis on diaphragmatic mechanics in man. *Anesthesiology*. 1974;41:242–255.

14. Braun NMT, Aurora NS, Rochester DS. Force length relationship of the normal human diaphragm. *J Appl Physiol*. 1982;53:405–412.

15. Sharp JT, Goldberg NB, Druz WS, Danson J. Relative contribution of the rib cage and abdomen to breathing in normal subjects. *J Appl Physiol*. 1975;39:608–618.

16. Pottinger FF. *Essentials of Surgery*. 5th ed. St. Louis, Mo: CV Mosby; 1938.

17. Brock WW. Osteopathy and surgery. *J Osteopathy*. April 1905:111–113.

18. Downing WJ. Osteopathic manipulative treatment of nonsurgical gallbladder. *Academy of Applied Osteopathy Yearbook*. Carmel, Calif: American Academy of Osteopathy; 1965:196–199.

19. Koogler P. Osteopathic care of surgical cases. *J Osteopathy*. April 1949:21–24.

20. Larson NJ. Manipulative care before and after surgery. *Osteopath Med*. 1977:41–49.

21. Stiles ET. Osteopathic treatment of surgical patients. *Osteopath Med*. September 1976:21–23.

22. Young GS. Postoperative osteopathic manipulation. *Academy of Applied Osteopathy Yearbook*. Carmel, Calif: American Academy of Osteopathy; 1970:77–82.

23. Henshaw RE. Manipulation and post operative pulmonary complications. *DO*. September 1963:132–133.

24. Smith RK. 100,000 cases of influenza with a death rate 1/40th of that officially reported under conventional medical treatment. *JAOA*. January 1920:172–173.

25. Sleszynski SL, Kelso AF. Comparison of thoracic manipulation with incentive spirometry in preventing post operative atelectasis. *JAOA*. 1993;93:834–835.

26. Dickey JL. Post operative osteopathic manipulative management of median sternotomy patients. *JAOA*. 1989;89:1274–1277.

27. Beal MC. Viscerosomatic reflexes: a review. *JAOA*. 1985;85:787–801.

28. Livingston EH, Passaro EP. Post operative ileus. *Dig Dis Sci*. 1990; 35:121–132.

29. Herrmann E. Precepts and practice. *DO*. 1965:163–164.

30. Jones LH. Spontaneous release by positioning. *DO*. 1964;4:109–116.

31. Schwartz HR. The use of counterstrain in an acutely ill in-hospital population. *JAOA*. 1986;86:433–442.

33. Nephrology

CARMELLA D'ADDEZIO

"Just as a filthy sewer will produce disease in the whole city, so the failure of one organ will produce disease of the whole body, and the salvation of the city or body depends on your mechanical philosophy and work."

—A.T. STILL[1]

Key Concepts

- **Description, classification, and differentiation of acute renal failure, chronic renal failure, and end-stage renal disease**

- **Physiology, causes, and types of renal osteodystrophy**

- **Diagnosis and treatment of osteodystrophy**

- **Neurologic disorders resulting from CRF**

- **Pathogenesis, diagnosis, and treatment of renal anemia**

- **Diagnosis and treatment of cardiovascular disease secondary to renal failure**

- **The relationship between renal failure and musculoskeletal dysfunction**

This chapter applies the basic tenets of osteopathic medical philosophy and health care delivery to the treatment of patients with renal disease. It focuses on renal failure to develop an approach to management of nephrology problems in general.

Acute renal failure (ARF) is the rapid decline in glomerular filtration rate (GFR) that can occur over hours, days, or weeks, and the retention of nitrogenous waste products (Fig. 33.1). ARF occurs in approximately 5% of all hospital admissions. ARF is usually found on screening laboratory testing of hospitalized patients and is frequently asymptomatic. For the purposes of diagnosis and management, ARF is divided into three categories (Table 33.1):

1. Pre-renal failure: disorders of renal hypoperfusion, in which the kidney is intrinsically normal (approximately 55% of total cases)
2. Intrinsic renal failure: diseases of the renal parenchyma (approximately 40% of total cases)
3. Post-renal failure: acute obstruction of the urinary tract (approximately 5% of total cases)

ARF, although usually reversible, is a major cause of in-hospital morbidity and mortality because of the high incidence of associated complications.

Chronic renal failure (CRF) results from loss of renal structure and function from progressive injury. Uremia generally is associated with a cornucopia of signs and symptoms related to CRF, regardless of its cause. Because of a "compensatory" hypertrophy of nephrons, clinical manifestations of CRF rarely occur until the GFR drops below 20–25% of normal.

End-stage renal disease (ESRD) affects all segments of the United States population. According to the United States Renal Disease Study 1993 Annual Data Report, diabetes mellitus is the most common cause of ESRD (34.2%). The second most common cause is hypertension (29.4%), followed by glomerulonephritis (14.2%), cystic renal disease (3.4%), and interstitial nephritis (3.4%).[2]

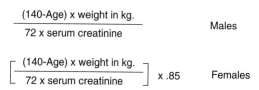

Figure 33.1. Estimation of glomerular filtration rate: Cockcroft and Gault equation.

Table 33.1
Causes of Acute Renal Failure (Potentially Reversible Renal Failure)

Pre-Renal	Renal	Post-Renal
Definition: an oliguric state resulting from inadequate perfusion of the kidneys.	*Definition:* a decrease in GFR resulting from intrinsic renal disease.	*Definition:* mechanical obstruction distal to the glomeruli.
Reduced vascular volume:	Primary glomerular injury:	Obstruction:
hemorrhage	acute poststreptococcal GN	nephrolithiasis
extracellular volume depletion	acute GN	tumors
sweating	serum sickness	retroperitoneal fibrosis
burns	hemolytic-uremic syndrome	prostate enlargement
intestinal losses:	thrombotic thrombocytopenic purpura	ureteral instrumentation
vomiting, diarrhea,	systemic lupus erythematous	surgical accident
gastrointestinal or biliary	vasculitis	
drainage	Goodpasture's syndrome	Rupture of the bladder
urinary losses:	non–Goodpasture's syndrome	
diuretics, osmotic diuresis, renal	bacterial endocarditis	
salt wasting	Primary tubulointerstitial injury:	
"third spaces":	ischemic	
pancreatitis, peritonitis,	papillary necrosis	
gastroenteritis	nephrotoxic	
cardiac pump failure	heavy metals	
congestive heart failure	anesthetic agents	
cardiogenic shock	antibiotics	
cardiac tamponade	methanol	
Hepatorenal syndrome	hypercalcemia	
Sepsis	hyperuricemia	
	myoglobin	
	light chain disease	

GN, glomerulonephritis.

The following sections consider the effect of renal failure (whether acute or chronic) on these systems:

Endocrine
Neurologic
Hematologic
Cardiovascular
Musculoskeletal

THE NEPHRON IN CHRONIC RENAL FAILURE

Patients with CRF demonstrate only minimal changes in body fluid composition until the GFR decreases to 10% of normal function. Bricker[3] examined diseased kidney function in the presence of a normal contralateral kidney. The remaining "normal" kidney was found to adapt its handling of solutes, which is directed toward conservation of normal body fluid composition. A feature of the failing kidney is that each solute is regulated independently. For example, phosphorous concentration rises when the GFR reaches 25% of normal, whereas sodium regulation is maintained until the GFR reaches 10% of normal.[4]

Our goal in osteopathic medicine is to enhance the body's inherent ability to heal itself. In the case of renal disease, the goal is to assist the patient to support the natural adaptive mechanisms of the kidney to preserve renal function and provide the patient with a better quality of life. Table 33.2 outlines the basic management of CRF.

ENDOCRINE MANIFESTATIONS: RENAL OSTEODYSTROPHY

This section looks only at the problem of renal osteodystrophy. Bone is not a stagnant body organ. Approximately 400 mg of calcium enters and leaves the bony skeleton daily. Phosphates and bicarbonate, as well as other minerals, follow the movements of calcium. Therefore, deficiencies of calcium, phosphate, and bicarbonate increase bone reabsorption and inhibit bone formation. Other principle factors that have direct effects on bone are parathyroid hormone and vitamin D. The effect of parathyroid hormone is primarily to stimulate osteoblast function. There are lesser effects from other hormones such as thyroid.

Aluminum toxicity can be a cause of significant bone disease. Figure 33.2 outlines the genesis of renal osteodystrophy.

There are four types of renal osteodystrophy:

1. High turnover disease
2. Ostitis fibrosa
3. Low turnover disease, such as osteomalacia
4. Mixed osteodystrophy, which is a combination of osteomalacia and ostitis fibrosa

High turnover bone disease is the predominant form of osteodystrophy found in CRF. The primary agent in this form of bone disease is a gradual increase in parathyroid hormone. This complex event involves increased parathyroid hormone

Table 33.2
Basic Management of Chronic Renal Failure

Search for any reversible component of the renal failure.
Correct intravascular volume deficit or excess.
Correct extracellular fluid volume deficit or excess.
Restrict dietary protein to 0.5–0.6 gm/kg body weight/24 hr.
Restrict sodium and potassium to 2 gm/24 hr if the patient is having difficulty with these.
Prescribe multivitamins; include folic acid, iron, and vitamin C.
Control hyperkalemia (alkali, kayexalate).
Control hypertension, particularly with ACE inhibitors and calcium channel blockers.
Evaluate the anemia; correct any nonrenal factors. If the patient is symptomatic and/or the hematocrit drops below 25%, begin erythropoietin therapy.
Prescribe phosphate binders with meals.
Adjust all drug doses to the degree of the patient's renal function.
Control metabolic acidosis (alkali treatment).
Monitor secondary hyperparathyroidism closely; calcium supplements and vitamin D supplements are frequently necessary.
Refer early to an ESRD program.
    options: hemodialysis
             continuous ambulatory peritoneal dialysis (CAPD)
             continuous cycled peritoneal dialysis (CCPD)
             transplant
             none of the above

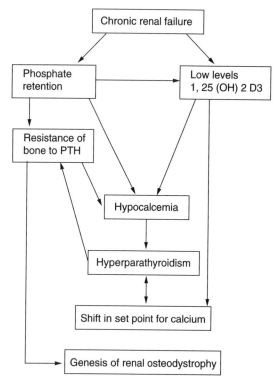

Figure 33.2.   Renal osteodystrophy in chronic renal failure.

secretion, delayed renal excretion of this hormone, direct effects of phosphate, and a decrease in 1,25-dihydroxy vitamin D receptors.[5]

Low turnover bone disease is characterized by damage to the bony matrix from aluminum and iron, except in diabetes when it can occur without evidence of aluminum or iron deposition.[6]

Diagnosis

The differential diagnosis of renal osteodystrophy can be difficult. The need for cost containment requires physicians to employ a diagnostic plan at low cost, with minimal inconvenience to patients.

Imaging techniques cannot precisely determine the cause of renal bone disease. In particular, plain films are a poor tool. Dual-beam photon densitometry, which measures bone density, appears to be the single most useful imaging study.

Serum calcium and phosphorus levels are nonspecific indicators of the disease cause. However, alkaline phosphatase is elevated in the presence of high turnover disease or mixed renal osteodystrophy, and is typically normal in low turnover bone disease. Serum parathyroid hormone levels vary according to methodology. Significant elevations of the N terminal or C terminal parathyroid hormone favor the presence of high turnover disease. The results of aluminum assays also vary according to methodology. In general, the diagnosis of aluminum toxicity and subsequent low turnover bone disease is supported by an elevated serum aluminum above 300 μg/L as measured by most laboratories.

There are other promising tests for the measurement of parathyroid hormone, and other assays such as β_2-microglobulin. At the present time, if the diagnosis remains obscure, a bone biopsy might be the best method to distinguish high turnover from low turnover disease in renal osteodystrophy.[6–7]

Treatment

The goal of therapy is to prevent renal osteodystrophy from occurring in the first place. One wishes to preserve bone and prevent the symptoms of bone pain, weakness, and bone fracture, which contribute to a decreased quality of life and a decreased potential for rehabilitation of the CRF patient.

Phosphate retention directly relates to hypocalcemia, secondary hyperparathyroidism, and decreased 1,25-dihydroxy vitamin D production. Therefore, a major thrust of therapy is to reduce serum phosphate levels. Aluminum hydroxide has been the mainstay of dietary phosphate binders in the past. However, aluminum toxicity itself can cause the low turnover bone disease. Physicians have turned to alternative dietary phosphate binders in the form of calcium carbonate and calcium acetate. These are not taken like antacids after meals but instead must be taken with all meals and snacks simultaneously if the patient is to have the dietary phosphate binding effect.[8]

Aluminum overload bone disease can be limited if the clinician remembers that certain treatments are the primary agents in initiating this disease. Therapeutic interventions for aluminum toxicity depend on the severity of the symptoms.

These interventions vary from the use of dietary phosphate binders to adjusting dialysate concentrations.

Prescribe a low protein diet to help decrease the phosphates pre-dialysis. The usual protein restriction is 0.5–0.6 gm/kg of body weight daily. For dialysed patients, the restriction is more liberal: 0.7–1.0 gm/kg of body weight daily.[9]

Based on extensive animal model work, R. W. Shrier et al.[10] have proposed increased nephron oxygen consumption as a potential factor in the progression of CRF. There appears to be a 2.2-fold increase in oxygen consumption per nephron that is consistent with the tubular adaptation that occurs with nephron loss. Over time, this increased workload across the nephron damages it. Protein restriction has been shown to decrease oxidant stress and can provide protection against CRF progression.

In conclusion, there are alterations in parathyroid hormone function and inactivation of 1,25-dihydroxy vitamin D in the failing kidney. Combined, they cause calcium-phosphorous alterations that affect the normal bony mechanics. By intervening with dietary interventions and dietary phosphate binders, one can slow the onset of renal osteodystrophy. The injudicious use of oral aluminum hydroxide phosphate binders, however, can enhance low turnover bone disease and aluminum toxicity inadvertently.[11]

NERVOUS SYSTEM MANIFESTATIONS

The patient with CRF can present with a variety of neurologic disorders. The patient on maintenance dialysis might have neurologic dysfunction, some of which is unique to dialysis and some of which can be attributed to CRF itself. The discussion here concentrates on disorders of renal failure, not those of maintenance dialysis. Our goal again is prevention and recognition of disease processes.

The central nervous system disorders associated with renal failure vary in intensity with the rapidity of the onset of renal failure. Patients with slowly progressive renal failure might first have mild cognitive dysfunction and mild clouding of the sensorium, which can proceed to severely impaired mentation, delirium, and ultimately coma.

Uremic Encephalopathy

Uremic encephalopathy is an organic brain syndrome that occurs in acute or chronic renal failure when the GFR falls below 10% of normal.

DIAGNOSIS

The symptom complex of the neurologic manifestations spans cognitive, neuromuscular, autonomic, and sensory functions. These symptoms can include but are not limited to:

Easy fatigue
Insomnia
Slurred speech
Anorexia

Central vomiting
Altered memory
"Restless leg syndrome"
Asterixis
Confusion
Bizarre behaviors
Vertigo
Nystagmus
Coma
Convulsions

Causes other than uremia can result in any of these symptoms, however. Electrolyte disturbances, drug intoxications, and vitamin deficiencies can present in a similar manner. The physician should rule out other possible causes, particularly drug intoxications (always look to see what you might have introduced that might cause the disease), and correct those before diagnosing uremic encephalopathy (Table 33.3).[12]

TREATMENT

If the physician has corrected vitamin deficiencies, drug intoxications, and electrolyte imbalances and the symptoms persist, dialysis is the appropriate therapeutic intervention.

Uremic Neuropathies

Uremic neuropathies are common by the time the patient is in end-stage renal failure. Approximately 65% of patients in end-stage renal failure have peripheral neuropathies. Uremic neuropathies are usually bilateral, distal polyneuropathies.

Motor and sensory tracts are affected. Motor nerve conduction and sensory nerve conduction velocities can be affected even without clinical manifestations. Patients might demonstrate autonomic dysfunctions such as impotence and postural

Table 33.3
Commonly Employed Therapies or Diagnostic Tests That Can Lead to Rapid Deterioration of Renal Function

Use of NSAIDs in the face of dehydration, hyperkalemia, or renal insufficiency
Use of ACE inhibitors in patients with bilateral renal artery stenosis
Use of iodinated radiocontrast agents in patients with one or a combination of the following:
  volume depletion
  hypokalemia
  diabetics with proteinuria
  patients with impaired renal function
  the elderly
  patients who had previous nephrotoxicity from radiocontrast
Indiscriminate treatment of edema without thought to cause. For example, congestive cardiomyopathies, cirrhosis, nephrotic syndrome, and malnutrition
  a hypo-osmotic state can manifest as edema; removing the edema further depletes intravascular volume, which can exacerbate renal failure
Antibiotics and antibiotic combinations, particularly aminoglycosides in combination with cephalosporins

hypotension. As with uremic encephalopathies, the peripheral neuropathies do not usually manifest until the GFR falls below 10% of normal. The lower extremities are more profoundly affected than are the upper extremities. The physical signs of peripheral neuropathy frequently commence with impaired vibratory sensation. Loss of the deep tendon reflexes will ensue, and the patient will commonly develop anesthesias in a "stocking" distribution in the lower extremities. The molecular basis for the disturbance is still unclear. It might be related to uremic toxins, chief of which is the parathyroid hormone. Current research is assessing the effects of parathyroid hormone on calcium transport across axonal membranes.[13–17]

DIAGNOSIS

Electrolyte disturbances, drug toxicities, and vitamin deficiencies can mimic the symptoms of uremic neuropathies. Therefore, rule them out first. Motor and sensory nerve conduction studies will demonstrate impaired and slowed conduction.

TREATMENT

Pre-dialysis treatments are aimed at reducing the uremic toxins, primarily through dietary restrictions of protein.[18–21] Vitamin supplementation, including folic acid and the B complex vitamins, is part of every dietary prescription for patients with peripheral neuropathies from uremia. If the symptoms are not controlled, dialysis is indicated.

HEMATOLOGIC MANIFESTATIONS IN RENAL FAILURE

Renal Anemia

Anemia is present in patients with both acute and chronic renal failure. In ARF, the severity of the anemia is associated with multiple factors, such as concurrent hemorrhage, degree of hydration, and type of renal failure (e.g., hemolytic-uremic syndrome). Erythropoiesis is impaired in both acute and chronic renal failure.

Anemia can be the first clinical finding in a patient with CRF. The anemia worsens as renal function deteriorates. It can become difficult to distinguish uremic symptoms from anemic symptoms because they can be similar, such as decreased exercise tolerance, increased angina pectoris, and fatigue. Remember that the uremic symptoms can be controlled by dialysis and diet, but not those attributed to the anemia.

The primary pathogenesis of the renal anemia is a result of depressed secretion of erythropoietin by the damaged kidney. Some data suggest that there is uremic impairment of hematopoiesis. Other contributors to the anemia of renal disease include[22]:

Hemolysis
Blood loss
Aluminum toxicity
Folate deficiencies
Hyperparathyroidism

DIAGNOSIS

Base the diagnosis on the complete blood count and peripheral smear showing a depressed hematocrit and normochromic normocytic anemia. Other laboratory tests to help distinguish the anemia include:

Serum iron
Transferrin
Ferritin
Folate
B_{12} levels
Reticulocyte count

Always rule out the possibility of intercurrent gastrointestinal hemorrhage. Platelet dysfunction is associated with CRF and can predispose the patient to subclinical gastrointestinal hemorrhage. Patients can be unaware of occult gastrointestinal bleeding if they are taking a multivitamin including iron.

TREATMENT

Treatment today relies not on frequent red blood cell transfusions but on exogenous administration of erythropoietin. Erythropoietin treatment helps prevent iatrogenic disease (like hemosiderin deposition) from frequent transfusion, or the development of hepatitis and HIV. The one caveat associated with erythropoietin treatment is the possibility of the development of hypertension.[23] The intervention of erythropoietin administration greatly enhances the quality of life of the patient with CRF.

CARDIOVASCULAR MANIFESTATIONS OF RENAL FAILURE

Hypertension

Hypertension can cause renal failure, or it can be caused by renal failure. This section focuses on the latter form of hypertension and on treatment rationales to control blood pressure. The primary goal is to preserve renal function in the impaired kidney by decreasing the hydrostatic pressure gradient across the filtration membranes in the glomerular capillary loops. There are many potential mechanisms for increased blood pressure in CRF. Blood pressure equals cardiac output times total peripheral resistance. There might be expanding intravascular volume in renal failure, which increases cardiac output and hence systemic blood pressure. Controversy exists regarding how the renin angiotensin system (RAS) interacts with the development of hypertension. For a more detailed discussion of the RAS and treatment of hypertension, see Chapter 27, Hypertension.

A new development with CRF is the extensive use of erythropoietin for anemia control, which can elevate blood pressure. Close monitoring of the blood pressure in patients treated with erythropoietin is highly recommended. Adjust the dose of the erythropoietin to the hematocrit and the blood pressure levels.

The vascular endothelium might play a more significant role in hypertension associated with renal disease than was previously considered. Vascular endothelial cells release endothelin 1, a potent vasopressor. Endothelin 1 also acts to release aldosterone and catecholamines.[24] It has been reported that renal failure patients with essential hypertension have high circulating levels of endothelin 1, compared with normotensive patients with renal failure.

The vascular endothelial cells also release relaxing factors. The currently identified vascular endothelial-relaxing factor is nitric oxide. Animal models of essential hypertension show that levels of vascular endothelial smooth muscle relaxant factors are depressed. It appears, then, that endothelial dysfunction could also contribute to the hypertension associated with CRF.[25–27]

TREATMENT

The treatment of hypertension in CRF has been shown to prolong the life of the functional remaining nephrons.[28–29] Because 80–90% of the patients with ESRD have hypertension, early intervention in the course of the disease process is necessary to prolong the life of nephrons.

Early interventions include dietary changes, such as salt and water restrictions, to maintain a dry weight state for the patient. When dietary interventions fail, many antihypertensive medications are available. Make the choice of an antihypertensive with reference to the patient as a whole, as discussed in Chapter 27, Hypertension. By controlling the blood pressure, one can prolong the life of the remaining nephrons substantially.[28–30]

Myocardial Function

CRF can adversely affect myocardial function. The renal anemia increases cardiac work while decreasing oxygen supply to the myocardium. With severe anemia, overt heart failure and left ventricular dilatation can ensue. In vivo and in vitro studies implicate chronic elevations of parathyroid hormone as having adverse effects on the myocardial function.[31–32] Metastatic calcium accumulations can occur in heart muscle and valves, causing deleterious affects on myocardial function and rhythm. Parathyroid hormone has also been shown to inhibit mitochondrial function in heart cells, causing a decrease in adenosine triphosphate synthesis.[31] This impaired cellular activity can worsen left ventricular contractility.[33]

Electrolyte and acid-base abnormalities can depress myocardial contractility and lead to arrhythmias. Hyperkalemia can lead to asystole.[34] Calcium is an essential element in the contractile mechanism of the heart, and heart failure has been associated with severe hypocalcemia.[35] Hypomagnesemia can precipitate digitalis toxicity.[36] Hypermagnesemia has been associated with arrhythmias, hypotension, and cardiac arrest.[37] Metabolic acidosis can adversely affect the heart, particularly when coupled with other electrolyte abnormalities.

Effusive-constrictive pericarditis can depress cardiac function by restriction of ventricular filling. One of the causes of pericarditis in CRF appears to be related to uremic toxins. In the patient with CRF who develops pericarditis, dialysis is the recommended therapy.[38]

Diagnosis might consist of assessment of the patient's pulse, blood pressure, and cardiac auscultation, or it might be more sophisticated, involving color Doppler echocardiography.

As with other clinical manifestations of renal impairment, correct the metabolic abnormalities first. If the symptoms persist, dialysis is indicated.

MUSCULOSKELETAL MANIFESTATIONS

Musculoskeletal manifestations of renal failure range from generalized muscle dysfunctions, such as cramping, to specific viscerosomatic dysfunctions. The viscerosomatic component of renal disease has been reported in osteopathic literature for some time. Nelson reported on the relationship of postural spinal mechanics and urinary tract infections. In pyelonephritis with ureteral spasms, he found the spinal lesion at the level of the 4th and 5th lumbar segments. The diagnosis was confirmed by cystoscopy.[39]

Conn noted a viscerosomatic lesion in the lower thoracic and lumbar regions with nephritis.[40] In patients with renal failure, Johnston and Hollandsworth et al. compared dialysis patients with hypertension to a similarly matched group who had no hypertension or renal failure. They demonstrated both structural abnormalities and tissue temperature changes at T9-T12.[41–42]

The place for osteopathic manipulation in renal failure is unclear. If we ascribe to Dr. Still's tenet, the rule of the artery must be absolute or disease will follow; thus, treating a facilitated or compensatory segment should improve function. To date, a double-blind controlled study has not been done to test the effect of osteopathic manipulative treatment on renal function.

CONCLUSION

Enhancement of quality of life involves the individual's perception. The clinician should be able to determine what each patient's perception of quality of life is and develop a plan to meet that patient's goals. For example, in several end-stage renal disease centers, exercise programs have been shown to enhance both activity levels and patients' perceptions of well-being. A scientific study has not been reported as yet on the effects of exercise in end-stage renal disease patients. However, the anecdotal reports are promising.[43]

Therapeutic interventions are directed at improving quality of life for the patient by controlling disease symptoms and delaying the start of dialysis. To maximize this effort, be involved in the education of the patient. Establish access to community resources to assist patients in better understanding the nature of their disease process and its multisystem effects.

REFERENCES

1. Still AT. *Osteopathy: Research and Practice.* Seattle, Wash: Eastland Press; 1992.
2. Ismail N, Becker BN. Treatment options and strategies in uremia:

current trends and future directions. *Semin Nephrol.* 1994;14(3); 282–299.

3. Bricker NS, Klahr S, Rieselbach RE. The functional adaptation of the diseased kidney. I. Glomerular filtration rate. *J Clin Invest.* 1964; 43:1915–1921.

4. Bricker NS, Klahr S, Libowitz H, Rieselbach RE. Renal function in chronic renal disease. *Medicine.* 1965;44:263–288.

5. Massry SG, Coburn JW, Popvtzer MM, et al. Secondary hyperparathyroidism and chronic renal failure: the clinical spectrum in uremia, during dialysis and after renal transplantation. *Arch Intern Med.* 1969;124:431–441.

6. Hodsman AB, Sherrard DJ, Alfrey AC, et al. Bone aluminum and histomorphometric features of renal osteodystrophy. *J Clin Endocrinol & Metab.* 1982;54(3):539–546.

7. Hurkska KA, Tietelbaum SL, Kopelman R, et al. The predictability of histologic features of uremic bone disease by noninvasive techniques. *Metab Bone Dis.* 1978;1:39.

8. Saltopolsky E, Delmez JA. Pathogenesis of secondary hypoparathyroidism. *Am J Kidney Dis.* 1994;23(2):229–236.

9. Mitch WE. Dietary protein restriction in patients with chronic renal failure. *Kidney Int.* 1991;40:326–341.

10. Shrier RW, Shapiro JI, Chan L, et al. Increased nephron oxygen consumption: potential role and progression of chronic renal disease. *Am J Kidney Dis.* 1994;23(2):176–182.

11. Massry SG, Smogorzewski M. Mechanisms through which parathyroid hormone mediates its deleterious affects on organ function in uremia. *Semin Nephrol.* 1994;14(3):219–231.

12. Mahoney CA, Arief AI. Central and peripheral nervous system effects on chronic renal failure. *Kidney Int.* 1983;24:170.

13. Akmal M, Massry SG. Role of parathyroid hormone in the decreased motor nerve conduction velocity of chronic renal failure. *Proc Soc Exp Biol & Med.* 1990;9195:202–207.

14. Dyck PJ, Johnson EJ, Lambert EH, et al. Segmental demyelination secondary to axonal degeneration in uremic neuropathy. *Mayo Clin Proc.* 1971;46:400–431.

15. Goldstein DA, Chui LA, Massry SG. Effect of parathormone in uremia on nerve calcium and motor nerve conduction velocity. *J Clin Invest.* 1978;62:88.

16. Ochs S. Calcium and the metabolism of axoplasmic transport. *Fed Proc.* 1982;40:2301.

17. Thomas PK, Hollinrake K, Lascelles R, et al. The polyneuropathy of chronic renal failure. *Brain.* 1971;94:761.

18. Green T, Bourgoinie JJ, Habwe V, et al. Baseline characteristics in the modification of diet in renal disease. *J Am Soc Nephrol.* 1993; 3:1819–1834.

19. Klahr S, Levery A, Beck GJ, et al. The modification of diet and renal disease study group: effects of dietary protein restriction and blood pressure control on the progression of chronic renal failure: the modification of diet in renal disease study. *New Engl J Med.* 1994; 330:877–884.

20. El Nahas AM, Masters-Thomas A, Brady SA, et al. Selective effective low protein diets on chronic renal diseases. *Br Med J.* 1984; 289:1337–1341.

21. Laidlaw SA, Berg RL, Kopple JD, et al. Patterns of fasting plasma amino acid levels in chronic renal insufficiency: results from the feasibility phase of the modification of diet in renal disease study. *Am J Kidney Dis.* 1994;23(4):504–513.

22. Basu TK, Stein RM. Erythrocytosis associated with chronic renal disease. *Arch Intern Med.* 1974;133:442.

23. Buckner FS, Eschbach JW, Haley NR, et al. Hypertension following erythropoietin therapy in anemic hemodialysis patients. *Am J Hypertens.* 1990;3:947.

24. Shichiri M, Hirata Y, Ando K, et al. Plasma endothelin levels in hypertension and chronic renal failure. *Hypertension.* 1990; 15(5):493–496.

25. Vanhoutte PM. Endothelium and control of vascular function. State of the art lecture. *Hypertension.* 1990;15:498.

26. Panza JA, Quyyumi AA, Brush JE Jr, et al. Abnormal endothelium dependent vascular relaxation in patients with essential hypertension. *New Engl J Med.* 1990;323:22–27.

27. Luscher TF, Raij L, Vanhoutte PM, et al. Endothelium dependent vascular responses in normotensive and hypertensive Dahl rats. *Hypertension.* 1987;9:157–163.

28. Hannedouche T, Albouze G, Chauvear P, et al. Affects of blood pressure and anti-hypertensive treatment on progression of advanced chronic renal failure. *Am J Kidney Dis.* 1993;21(suppl 2):131–137.

29. Morgensen CE. Long term anti-hypertensive treatment inhibiting progression of diabetic nephropathy. *Br J Med.* 1982;285:685–688.

30. Schulman NB, Ford CE, Hall WD, et al. Prognostic value of serum creatinine and effective treatment of hypertension on renal function. *Hypertension.* 1989;13(suppl 1):80–93.

31. Bogin E, Levi J, Harary I, Massry SG. Effects of parathyroid hormone on oxidative phosphorylation of heart mitochondria. *Miner Electrolyte Metab.* 1982;7:151–156.

32. Drueke D, Fauchet M, Fleury J, et al. Effect of parathyroidectomy on left ventricular function in hemodialysis patients. *Lancet.* 1980; 1:112.

33. McGonigle RJ, Fowler MB, Timmis AB, et al. Uremic cardiomyopathy: potential role of vitamin D and parathyroid hormone. *Nephrology.* 1984;36:94–100.

34. Kim KE, Swartz C. Pathophysiology, diagnosis, and management of hyperkalemia. In: *Emergency Medical Management.* New York, NY: Grune and Stratton; 1971:113.

35. Feldman AM, Fivush B, Zahka KG, et al. Congestive cardiomyopathy in patients on continuous ambulatory peritoneal dialysis. *Am J Kidney Dis.* 1988;11:76.

36. Neff MS, Mendelssohn S, Kim KE, et al. Magnesium sulfate and digitalis toxicity. *Am J Cardiol.* 1972;29:377–382.

37. Rardon D, Fish C. Electrolytes in the heart. In: Hurst WJ, Schlant RC, Rackley CE, et al, eds. *The Heart, Arteries and Veins.* 7th ed. New York, NY: McGraw-Hill; 1990:1557.

38. Ribot S, Frankel HJ, Gielchinsky I, Gilbert L. Treatment of uremic pericarditis. *Clin Nephrol.* 1974;2:127.

39. Nelson CR. Symposium: urologic manifestations of man's constitutional inadequacies; structural diagnosis and treatment. *JAOA.* 1954;53(5):255–257.

40. Conn RW. Osteopathic principles supporting manipulative treatment in nephritis. *JAOA.* 1941:494–496.

41. Johnston WJ, Kelso AF, Hollandsworth DL, Karrat JJ. Somatic manifestations in renal disease: a clinical research study. *JAOA.* 1987; 87(1):22–35.

42. Beal MC. Viscerosomatic reflexes: a review. *JAOA.* 1985; 85(12):786–801.

43. Painter P. Exercise for individuals with end-stage renal disease. In: Goldberg L, Elliott DL, eds. *Exercise for Prevention and Treatment of Illness.* Philadelphia, Penn: FA Davis Company; 1994;14:289–300.

34. Neurology

MITCHELL L. ELKISS AND LOUIS E. RENTZ

Key Concepts

- **Overview of neurologic structures**
- **Headaches, including migraine, cluster, and tension-type**
- **Treatment for headache**
- **Spinal disorders**
- **Peripheral nerve entrapments, including carpal tunnel syndrome and chronic pain syndrome**

The specialty of neurology deals with the structure, function, disease, and dysfunction of the neuromusculoskeletal system. The neuromusculoskeletal system includes the brain, spinal cord, and peripheral and autonomic nervous systems, as well as the muscular system. The early development of osteopathic medical concepts emphasized the role of the nervous system as an integrator of function between the various systems of the body.[1]

This chapter provides an overview of neurology as practiced by osteopathic physicians, focusing on some common neurologic disorders in which the application of osteopathic concepts is straightforward. The syndromes of headaches, spinal disorders, peripheral nerve entrapments, and chronic pain are described in more detail.

OVERVIEW

The central nervous system (CNS) is particularly unique in the human animal. It allows us the potential to pursue rational thought, experience the deepest emotional states, perform complex motor functions with little or no conscious attention, and have mechanisms for integrating a multitude of bodily functions. The system includes segmental mechanisms for regulating sensory and motor functions. It includes primitive brain centers responsible for posture and locomotion, more evolved systems of personality and feeling, and the most evolved system of the capacity for human mindfulness. All functions of the human organism are under some form of neural control; the maintenance of normal nervous system activity is essential for health. Relevant to the osteopathic physician is the intimate relation between the nervous system and manifestations of somatic dysfunction.[2] As we dissect the nervous system into its component parts, we must remember that the subtotal of nervous system activity is a complex of electrophysiologic and neurochemical phenomena, demonstrating features of instability superimposed on tonic activity at multiple levels of the nervous system, resulting in the complex neurobiology of humans.

The structure of the nervous system can be clinically divided into reasonably circumscribed areas that correspond to specific neurologic functions. For purposes of discussion, these divisions are the:

Brain, including the cerebral cortex, basal ganglia, cerebellum, and brainstem
Spinal cord
Peripheral nerves and muscles

These areas are discussed more comprehensively in other texts.[3]

The cerebral cortex contains the primary motor system for the initiation of conscious motor activity, the primary sensory system for the appreciation of conscious sensory input, and the centers for memory, speech, and visuospatial integration. Lesions in these areas produce contralateral defects in motor and sensory functions. Compromise of the dominant hemisphere disturbs speech and language functions while nondominant hemispheric disruption influences visuospatial processing and the potential for visual imagery.

The basal ganglia are intermediate nuclear structures that act as relay stations between the other sensorimotor control systems. The primary clinical functions of the basal ganglia include the inhibition of segmental reflexes, such that resting muscles can remain at rest. They control automatic and associated movements that occur without conscious processing (i.e., swinging the arms while walking, or smiling while talking). Disorders of the basal ganglia typically produce tremors at rest, rigidity, loss of associated movements, and posture disturbances.

The cerebellum functions to match proprioceptive inputs (state of the muscles and joints) with cortical output (motor intent) to control muscles during movement to ensure smooth motor transitions and to maintain posture and balance. Clinical disorders of the cerebellum manifest as tremor during movement, postural abnormalities, imbalance, and ataxia.

The brainstem acts as a connection between the cerebral cortex, the basal ganglia, the cerebellum, and the spinal cord, through which all impulses traveling into or out of the CNS are transmitted to the spinal segmental level. The brainstem also contains the nuclei of the cranial nerves and the autonomic centers.

The spinal cord extends in segments from the brainstem. The segments exist in relation to each nerve root and contain the anterior horn cells from which arise the peripheral motor nerves and the dorsal horns into which sensory neurons enter. In essence, the motor roots supply all the muscles related to that segment (myotome) and similarly receive the sensory input from that segment (dermatome). The peripheral nerves transmit impulses to the muscles for movement and contain the sensory fibers for pain, temperature, touch, and proprioception.

The autonomic nervous system, sympathetic and parasympathetic, controls the visceral functions of the body. With rapidity and intensity, the autonomic nervous system can influence visceral functions. Each autonomic pathway comprises a preganglionic and postganglionic neuron. Preganglionic sympathetic neurons originate in the intermediolateral column of the thoracolumbar spinal cord and exit through the ventral roots and spinal nerve to pass into one of the chain ganglia. There they either synapse or pass through to one of the outlying sympathetic ganglia. From the sympathetic chain ganglia or the outlying ganglia, postganglionic neurons originate and course to their organ of destination. The parasympathetic division originates in the brainstem and the sacral cord. Their preganglionic neurons pass uninterrupted to the organ that is to be controlled. The postganglionic neurons are located in the wall of the target organs.

These summary descriptions of the anatomy of the nervous system illustrate that each of these systems is interdependent and exerts its ultimate effect in either the facilitation or inhibition of the spinal cord segments.[4] The nervous system continually receives information about the organism's internal and external environment through the afferent sensory system arising from the musculoskeletal system and the viscera. This information is processed centrally, transmitted in the CNS in some form, and stored as learned or retained information. The nervous system output is transmitted through the efferent limb to the somatic and visceral compartments of the body. It is through the motor unit that the dominant effects of the motor system are manifest and through the peripheral autonomic system that efferent nervous functions are played out on the viscera. Through this process, the neuromuscular system helps to preserve and maintain total body functional integrity.

Practically speaking, the assumption of the upright stance involves an intricate interaction of the basic neurologic centers, with particular reference to the descending supraspinal pathways, the cooperation of the basal ganglia and cerebellum, the limbic system, and the lobes of the neocortex. This evolutionary accomplishment frees the human hands for manipulation of its environment and for further development. Biomechanical dysfunction can be a consequence of an imperfect adaptation to a continually changing center of gravity in the upright stance. The neuromusculoskeletal system provides the human with its behavioral repertoire; dysfunction of the neuromusculoskeletal system results in the clinical phenomenon of somatic dysfunction.

The next section elaborates on the concept of the osteopathic lesion and common neurologic disorders that illustrate osteopathic concepts in the genesis of symptoms and signs, as well as in therapeutic management.

CONCEPT OF OSTEOPATHIC LESION

The actual mechanism of the interrelationship between the spinal cord and the musculoskeletal abnormalities known as the "osteopathic lesion" is based on the concept of segmental facilitation. J. Stedman Denslow, DO, originally defined this concept in the early 1940s using a new investigational technique of the time: electromyography. The concept of segmental facilitation, as described by Denslow, was that *"motor neuron pools in spinal cord segments related to areas of somatic dysfunction were maintained in a state of facilitation."*[5] That is, they were chronically hyperirritable and therefore hyperresponsive to impulses reaching them from any source in the body. The sources of these inputs included proprioceptive and nociceptive stimuli from the periphery under the influence of the supraspinal centers described above. Denslow went on to conclude that *"muscles innervated from these segments are, therefore, kept in a state of hypertonus much of the day with inevitable impediment to spinal motion and with structural and functional consequences to the muscle and person over a period of time."*[6]

Stated another way, the facilitated segments are believed to be related specifically to the osteopathic lesion complex such that areas of localized pain, tenderness, increased muscle tension, or limitation of motion in a spinal segment influence that part of the nervous system to which they are connected. Conversely, the musculoskeletal phenomena can be influenced by the segmental nervous system behavior itself, which can be produced by facilitation originating from peripheral, central, and visceral pathways.[7]

The concept of segmental facilitation is an extension of general concepts of neuronal facilitation. In segmental facilitation, a spinal segment receives exaggerated input from either a somatic or visceral structure. The efferent motor and autonomic components of the spinal segment are maintained in a state of excitement, such that further stimulation results in additional activation with somatomotor and sympathetic manifestations that are clinically recognizable. The segment is hyperirritable and, like a lens, shows qualities of focusing the input. In this way, ascending or descending inputs tend to converge and locally increase the activity at the facilitated segment. A decreased threshold to stimuli is applied above or below the segment and can result in increased efferent somatic (muscle contraction) and autonomic (sweat, vasomotor) activity at this level. In this way, the spinal cord can be seen as an organizer and active participant in the disease process.[8–11] The involved muscles can be maintained in a hypertonic state and thereby affect spinal motion, contributing to the restrictive musculoskeletal pattern typical of somatic dysfunction. Likewise, excess sympathetic segmental efferent activity can affect related somatic and visceral structures. The pathophysiologic consequences of local sympathetic hyperactivity are documented[12] and could play a role in the signs and symptoms of somatic dysfunction.

Segmental dysfunction of the neuromusculoskeletal system becomes visible when it manifests signs of somatic and/or sympathetic hyperactivity. Afferent stimuli from internal and external sources are organized by spinal cord mechanisms and manifest clinical features unique to the individual. Individuals have uniquely different responses to a general increase in psychic or physical stress. The common presence of increased somatic and sympathetic activity results in tissue texture abnormalities (TTA), one of the cardinal features of osteopathic palpatory diagnosis.[13] It is the pattern of somatic dysfunction and its relationship to visceral disease that becomes particularly relevant as a diagnostic tool.[14–15] Manipulative treatment influences the neural mechanisms responsible for the aforementioned reactive tissue changes; therapeutic success can be assessed through changes in these same factors.

Impulse-based electrical activity is not the only mechanism whereby the nervous system can influence bodily functions. The presence of trophic substances produced by the nerve cell and transported along its axon and microtubular structures are critical in maintaining the vitality of the organism.[16] These substances transsynaptically affect a variety of target end organs. The antegrade and retrograde flow of axoplasm suggests that the communication is bidirectional. This normal axoplasmic flow is disturbed by primary disease of the neuron (motor neuron disease) or in those conditions that produce mechanical deformation of the nerve by entrapment, stretch, angulation, or pressure.[17]

Perceptions and feelings can influence the state of the body's muscular activity, autonomic activity, and the capacity of its homeostatic mechanisms to respond to exogenous influences— even the ability to respond to osteopathic manipulative treatment (OMT). Neuroendocrine mechanisms allow the affective tone of individuals, their feeling state, and their personality to have an impact on their neuromusculoskeletal system. These mechanisms can be localized to the limbic system, the hypothalamus, the pituitary gland, and the neuroendocrine circuits.

In the early stages, continued afferent barrage (nociceptive, proprioceptive, autonomic) and a widening zone of involvement maintains the state of chronic facilitation. With chronic lesions, a more lasting mechanism must be at work. Sustained patterns of excitability and synaptic transmission become learned behavior in the spinal cord and brain.[18] The facilitated segment is the focus of efferent neuronal hyperexcitability. Metaphorically speaking, the zone of somatic dysfunction continues to represent the squeaky wheel. Additional local or general afferent stimulation results in an increased somatic and sympathetic efferent outpouring to those tissues innervated through the facilitated segment, manifesting as increased signs and symptoms of somatic dysfunction.

The osteopathic point of view considers wellness or health a positive state. It appreciates the organizational unity, inherent healing capacity, and self-regulating ability of the human body. Crucial is the concern for the interrelationship between structure and function.

HEADACHES

Headaches are one of the most frequent presenting complaints to both the general practitioner and the neurologist. Table 34.1 represents the current International Headache Society classification of headaches.[19] This classification is useful for establishing a clinical diagnosis of headache type; good scientific models exist for only some of the headache types, and there could be overlap between categories of headache in a given patient. Most headaches are mixed tension-type and migraine. This presentation is complicated by the multifactorial nature of headache, including these features:

Physical
Psychological
Familial
Ethnic
Cultural

The osteopathic physician is uniquely situated to evaluate the headache patient and to manage diagnostic and therapeutic resources.

Pain can result from noxious stimulation of the eyes, ears, mouth, and nasal cavities. Pain-sensitive intracranial structures include the venous sinuses and their tributaries, the dura (particularly at the base of the brain), and the arteries of the pia-arachnoid and dura mater. Some extracranial structures are also pain-sensitive, including the:

Skin
Subcutaneous tissues
Fascia
Muscles
Arteries
Cranial periosteum
Regional articulations

Acute head pain is often the result of dysfunction, displacement, or encroachment on one of the above structures. Cranial nerves V, VII, IX, and X, and upper cervical nerve roots II and

Table 34.1
International Headache Society Classification of Headaches

1. Migraine
2. Tension-type headache
3. Cluster headache and chronic paroxysmal hemicrania
4. Miscellaneous headaches unassociated with structural lesion
5. Headache associated with head trauma
6. Headache associated with vascular disorders
7. Headache associated with nonvascular intracranial disorder
8. Headache associated with substances or their withdrawal
9. Headache associated with noncephalic infection
10. Headache associated with metabolic disorder
11. Headache or facial pain associated with disorder of other facial or cranial structures
12. Cranial neuralgias, nerve trunk pain, and deafferentation
13. Headache not classifiable

Reprinted with permission from International Headache Society. Classification of headaches. *Cephalgia.* 1988;8(suppl 7).

III convey impulses from the head and face. The afferent signal is carried along A-δ and C fibers of the peripheral nervous system, predominantly with the cells in the spinothalamic and trigeminal spinal tracts in laminae I, II, V, and X. The nociceptor fibers transmit synaptically using glutamate, substance P, and other neuropeptides.[20]

A description of the quality and location of the headache is useful in establishing a cause. Investigate these questions:

Does it pound like a vascular headache or squeeze like a tension headache?

Does it localize to the region of the extracranial arteries, sinuses, teeth, tendinomuscular attachments, temporomandibular joint, or cervical vertebrae?

What is the severity and the time course of the pain?

Is there an acute, severe onset as is typically seen in subarachnoid hemorrhage?

Is it chronic and nagging, more typical of tension-type headache?

Does it tend to reoccur like migraine?

Is it a "once in a lifetime" event like most CNS infections?

For example, migraines often occur in the morning and rarely last more than a day or two. Cluster headaches typically occur at night and rarely last for more than 30–120 minutes. Tension headaches can last for weeks or months.

The associated features of a headache include its relation to:

Menstruation
Activities
Head position
Time of day
Exercise
Sleep habits
Environmental toxicity
Food and drink intake

It is important to know the age of onset, relevant family history, and exacerbating and relieving factors. A psychosocial assessment and thorough history and physical examination can reveal the symptoms and signs of anxiety, depression, and anger that can increase and heighten pain awareness.

The physical examination of these patients includes a thorough general examination and a comprehensive neurologic examination including:

Mental state
Cranial nerves
Strength
Reflexes
Coordination
Sensation
Appropriately detailed musculoskeletal assessment

The musculoskeletal assessment is most rewarding for patients with chronic or acute recurring headache.

The neuromusculoskeletal assessment includes active and static body analysis. Observe and palpate the facial and mandibular attachments, the temporomandibular joints, and the temporalis, masseter, buccinator, and pterygoid muscles, evaluating levels of muscle contraction and local tenderness. Direct superficial and deep cervical palpation from the skin to the synovial joints. Assess rotational characteristics of the head, cervical, and upper thoracic regions, as well as the basioccipital attachments at the atlas for anterior, lateral, and posterior asymmetry. In addition, carry out a screening of the total musculoskeletal system; the screening can include evaluation of:

Leg length and lower extremity symmetry
Sacropelvic base analysis
Cranial rhythmic activity
Suture mobility analysis

In clinical practice, the relationship between symptoms and signs and the ability to reproduce the painful symptoms during the examination is helpful in clinical localization. This is particularly true for the biomechanical syndromes, such as[21–23]:

Temporomandibular joint syndrome
Malocclusive dental syndromes
Cervical spine syndromes (spondylosis, disk degeneration, facet dysfunction)
Cranial neuralgias
Cranial suture syndrome
Short leg syndrome
Nerve encroachment syndrome
Myofascial pain syndromes

This type of evaluation supplies information that can be essential to formulating comprehensive therapeutic objectives.

Therapeutic success can be optimized by multimodality evaluation and treatment. The psychosocial model can suggest whether cognitive, behavioral, or psychotherapeutic intervention is needed. The pharmacologic model attempts to describe the problem neurochemically and offers a logical interventional protocol based on differential pharmacotherapeutic profiles (such as serotonergic, dopaminergic, noradrenergic, gabaergic, cholinergic). The biomechanical model provides a rational basis for choosing among manipulative treatment methods (i.e., direct action, indirect action, or myofascial techniques).

Furthermore, therapies directed at enhancing the self-healing capacities of an individual are important in the overall therapeutic formulation. These therapies include nutritional evaluation and counseling, evaluation and education in sleep hygiene, instruction and prescription of appropriate relaxation and stress reduction therapies, the use of therapeutic exercise, and the promotion of a positive attitude through education about the nature of headaches, the realistic objectives of management, and the use of positive visual imagery.[24]

Migraine Headaches

In migraine headaches, disordered neurogenic control of the craniocerebral circulation accompanies the attack.[25] The trigeminal vascular system (the trigeminal neuron whose unmyelinated axon surrounds a cephalic blood vessel) functions in pain transmission and in promoting inflammation in the affected blood vessels via the neurochemical activity of substance P.[26] Cerebral, meningeal, basilar, and vertebral arteries can be affected through the trigeminal, vagal, and upper cervical axons, which all converge in the trigeminal nucleus caudalis of the brainstem.[27–28] The inflammatory response is associated with norepinephrine and serotonin release of brainstem origin, and histamine, adenosine, and bradykinin of local origin.

When the migraine is triggered, the intrinsic brainstem noradrenergic system (from the locus ceruleus) is activated and triggers enhanced neuronal firing in the susceptible cerebral cortex. This firing in the cerebral cortex originates a spreading wave of cortical depolarization that ultimately reaches pain-sensitive blood vessels, resulting in depolarization of the associated trigeminovascular axon. This depolarization triggers a sterile inflammatory reaction through the release of substance P and the activation of mast cells and prostaglandin synthesis.[25–26]

Migraine can be accompanied by an aura consisting of neurologic changes, typically in a vascular distribution, lasting from 10 to 90 minutes, that mimics and sometimes results in transient cerebral ischemia. In rare cases, the neurologic aura resolves and the migraine becomes complicated as the patient suffers cerebral infarction. The most common auras are ocular and can involve scintillating scotomata or flashing lights, often occurring in jagged lines—the so-called fortification spectrum.[29] The visual phenomena can be multicolored and typically changes size, shape, and distribution during the evolving aura. The aura usually precedes the actual headache but can occur during and even after. On occasion, the aura is separate from the headache component or the headache can be absent.[30]

Multifocal neurologic symptoms can occur in the basilar artery distribution (the Bickerstaff syndrome) and include[31]:

Cranial nerve changes
Dysarthria
Facial paresthesia
Ataxia
Vertigo

In the middle cerebral artery distribution, migraine can have manifestations of hemiparesis, hemisensory loss, or aphasia. In general, the aura presents with visual phenomena, atypical for cerebrovascular insufficiency. A clue to migraine symptoms is a gradual progression of symptoms, unlike the rapid march of a focal seizure or the sudden onset of cerebral vessel thrombosis or embolism.

Migraine can begin in childhood, adolescence, or adulthood. In women, it can be associated with hormonal fluctuation. Migraine is typically a throbbing pain, following a vascular distribution of the superficial or deep cerebral vessels, lasting for several hours. It is often associated with nausea or vomiting, and sensitivity to bright lights, loud noises, or strong smells. For some patients, tenderness, tightness, pain, and limitation of motion in the suboccipital and cervical musculature accompanies migraine. Characteristically, migraine is relieved by sleep.

On initial presentation of migraine, it is not always possible to be certain of the diagnosis, and a well-designed differential diagnostic process is appropriate (Table 34.2). Although the risk of aneurysm, brain tumor, arteriovenous malformation, or vasculitis is slight, enhanced brain computed tomography, magnetic resonance imaging (MRI), or cerebral angiography is useful to exclude these possibilities and should be used if the diagnosis is uncertain.[32]

Migraine can acutely respond to vasoactive drugs such as sumatriptan, dihydroergotamine, ergotamine, isometheptene, and even caffeine. The serotonin 1-d receptor agonists (sumatriptan, dihydroergotamine) are particularly effective in aborting a migraine. Simple agents like aspirin or acetaminophen are often combined with barbiturates and/or narcotics. Other nonsteroidal antiinflammatory drugs (NSAIDs) are also used with variable success. The parenteral use of phenothiazines is helpful; unfortunately, they are frequently associated with unacceptable side effects.[33]

When migraine headaches are frequent or severe, prophylactic use of medications is indicated. These are medications used regularly to help prevent the migraines and include β-blockers (e.g., propranolol), calcium channel blockers (e.g., verapamil), tricyclic antidepressants (e.g., amitriptyline), serotonin antagonists (e.g., cyproheptadine, fluoxetine), ergot derivatives (e.g., methysergide), and anticonvulsants (e.g., valproic acid).

Nonpharmacologic approaches, including OMT, are often valuable. Osteopathic management of migraine can include OMT. In the active phase of migraine, vigorous treatment can, theoretically, increase blood flow to an already inflamed vascular bed, thereby explaining the clinical exacerbation that can follow treatment. Gentle therapy with indirect techniques, and venous and lymphatic drainage techniques are likely more helpful during the attack. Because of the prominent autonomic involvement, evaluate and treat at the sympathetic sites of lower cervical and upper thoracic vertebrae, associated ribs, and myofascial attachments. Treatment can be directed at joints of the head and neck, muscles, and myofascial restrictions of the head, neck, and shoulders. Behavioral techniques like biofeedback, relaxation therapy, and programs that teach stress reduction and coping skills have also been successfully used to reduce the frequency and severity of migraine attacks.[34] For some patients, musculoskeletal triggers or prodromes exist for their migraines.[35–36]

The possible role of musculoskeletal triggers is further suggested in posttraumatic migraine. In such cases, trauma to the skull, cervical spine, or myofascial elements is followed by a unilateral, throbbing migraine.[21,37] These headaches can recur for days, weeks, and months. OMT can be used in an attempt to modify these triggers that arise from bony, ligamentous, and myofascial structures. In practice, OMT is especially useful between migraine events, when the patient is more tolerant of manipulation.

Applications of local heat, cold, massage, acupressure, trigger point therapy, acupuncture, traction, or local anesthetic blockade can be used in these regions that typically harbor

Table 34.2
Headaches Resulting from Systemic Disease or Primary Neurologic Disorder

Disorder	Pathophysiology	Clinical Features	Paraclinical Features (lab, x-ray, etc.)	Treatment
Glaucoma[61]	Increased intraocular pressure	Dilated pupil, disturbed vision, general headache	Abnormal tonometry	Medication, surgery
Cerebral aneurysm, ruptured or unruptured[62]	Berry aneurysm, hypertension	Explosive headache, nuchal rigidity, abnormal neurologic	Blood in the CSF, abnormal angiogram	Neurosurgery
Temporal arteritis[63]	Inflammation	Throbbing headache, >55 years old, tender temporal artery, blurred vision, jaw claudication	Elevated ESR, positive biopsy for arteritis	Glucocorticoids
Optic neuritis[64]	Inflammation, demyelination	Orbital pain, loss of vision, worse with eye motion, papillitis	Abnormal visual evoked response, abnormal MRI	Glucocorticoids
Dissection of carotid, vertebral arteries[65–67]	Drugs, trauma	Severe, local pain, tender artery, Horner's syndrome	Angiogram, ultrasound, MRI	Surgery, anticoagulants
Temporomandibular joint syndrome, internal derangement, myofascial[68]	Joint degeneration, muscular imbalance	Pain in jaw, click in joint, locking of joint, pain with lateral or vertical movement, tight muscles	Abnormal MRI	Dental, physical therapy, exercise
Trigeminal neuralgia[69]	Irritation of CN-5, vascular loop, mechanical	Sharp, stabbing pain in trigeminal zone, triggers: wind, eating, chewing	Rarely abnormal MRI	Medication (anticonvulsants), neurosurgery
Herpes zoster trigeminalis cervicalis	Infection	Burning pain hypersensitive rash/vesicles	Virus identification	Antiviral therapy
Meningitis encephalitis	Usually infection bacterial, viral, etc.	Nuchal rigidity acute headache, fever, signs of infection	(+)CSF pleiocytosis, low glucose, high protein	Antibiotics, corticosteroids, supportive
Sinusitis, facial osteomyelitis[70]	Infection	Nasal obstruction, tender bone, fever	Leukocytosis, abnormal CT/MRI	Antibiotics
Intracranial hypertension from a mass	Traction, displacement of painful structures, block of CSF, hydrocephalus	Recent onset, headache, worse at rest, papilledema	Abnormal CT/MRI	Glucocorticoids, furosemide, mannitol, neurosurgery
Benign intracranial hypertension[71]	Altered CSF dynamics	Young, female, obesity, hormone fluctuating sight papilledema	Increased CSF pressure, small ventricles, enlarged blind spot	Glucocorticoids, acetazolamide, CSF removal, neurosurgery
Exertional headache, strain, lift, cough, exercise, coitus[72]	Posterior fossa mass, Chiari malformation, migraine variant	Abrupt, severe, lasts 15–20 minutes, men > women	CT/MRI	If no mass, precede activity with NSAIDs
Normal pressure hydrocephalus	Communicating, block in CSF absorption	Ataxia, incontinence, dementia	Hydrocephalus, cisternography	Ventricular shunt, CSF removal
Myofascial pain syndrome[23]	Trauma	Bands, nodules, trigger points, poor sleep	—	OMT, spray/stretch, needling

CSF, cerebrospinal fluid; ESR, erythrocyte sedimentation rate.

tender points referring pain to the headache zone. These applications might help to decrease the afferent activity from the painful site and reduce the primary and secondary muscle spasms.

Cluster Headaches

Cluster headache is a distinctive vascular syndrome characterized by attacks that tend to occur daily for weeks at a time only to vanish again for months or years. Approximately 20% of patients develop a chronic form, called chronic paroxysmal hemicrania or hemicrania continua.[38] Clinicians believe that cluster headaches are the result of neurogenic inflammation affecting the vascular plexus of the cavernous sinus, its tributaries, and its autonomic nervous supply.[39–40] The headaches tend to occur at certain times of the day; most notably, they develop 2–3 hours after going to sleep. Like migraine, cluster headaches often occur when the individual is switching from rapid eye motion (REM) sleep to non—REM sleep. This is accompanied by a shift from parasympathetic, cholinergic activity to sympathetic, aminergic (catecholamine, serotonin, norepinephrine) activity.[41]

Cluster headaches tend to be periorbital in location and characteristically develop rapidly, reaching severe intensity within minutes. They are associated with autonomic vasomotor features including:

Ptosis
Miosis
Conjunctival injection
Unilateral lacrimation
Rhinorrhea
Nasal stuffiness

Distinct from migraine, cluster headaches are much more common in men. They can occur several times a day and can even awaken the sufferer from sleep. Cluster headaches can be seen following trauma and, at times, can refer pain to the cervical and upper thoracic paraspinal region, as well as to the suprascapular region.[42–43]

The carotid-cavernous vasculature is involved along with its autonomic innervation. This includes the pterygopalatine ganglion and the cervical sympathetic ganglia. Patients often have a tender carotid artery, called carotidynia. Attempts to anesthetize the pterygopalatine ganglion with cocaine or lidocaine have been somewhat successful. Cluster headaches might respond acutely to parenteral sumatriptan or dihydroergotamine, both of which are serotonin 1-d receptor agonists.[44] Many respond to inhaled oxygen via facial mask (5–7 L/min for 5–10 minutes.) Prophylactically, β-blockers, calcium channel blockers, and tricyclic antidepressants are used along with short courses of high-dose steroids or NSAIDs. For the more chronic cluster, lithium is a potent therapy. Not surprisingly, OMT is best directed to the upper ribs, the cervicothoracic spine, the associated soft tissues, and the relevant craniofacial structures.

Tension-Type Headaches

Tension-type headaches are classified by the International Headache Society as episodic or chronic. They are further divided by the presence or absence of involvement of the pericranial muscles. Involvement can be demonstrated by electromyography or palpation.[45–46]

Tension-type headache is the most frequent headache type. It is characterized by mild-to-moderate intensity pain, described as pressing or tightening, typically bilateral and usually occipital in location. In distinction from migraine, it is not aggravated by exercise or routine physical activity. Like migraine, it runs in families, is more common in women, and can be affected by hormonal cycles. It is episodic if it occurs less than half the days of the month and chronic if it occurs more than half the days of the month.[47]

The International Headache Society distinguishes between tension-type and migraine headaches. Many believe, however, that these headache types are related disorders. In fact, most patients with migraines have tension-type headaches, and many patients with tension-type headaches have migraines. Both migraine and tension-type headaches might be the result of abnormalities in central pain control mechanisms, as well as trigeminal neuronal hypersensitivity. Both might be associated with muscle tenderness, electromyographic abnormalities, and abnormal platelet serotonin levels. When severe, they both can be associated with depressed cerebrospinal fluid β-endorphins.[47]

Clinicians theorize that there might be a vascular, supraspinal, and myogenic integrated model for migraine and tension-type headache.[48] The trigeminal nucleus caudalis is a major relay nucleus for head and neck pain. Nociceptive inputs from the pericranial muscles and the cephalic arteries converge at this nucleus, which has excitatory and inhibitory outputs. When the afferent nociceptive signal is intense, sensitization of the entire pain pathway, peripheral and central, can occur. This facilitation creates a painful sensitivity to typically nonnoxious stimuli. In the migraine, the nociceptors are vascular and the nonnoxious stimuli are vascular pulsations. In the tension-type headache, the nociceptors are myofascial and the nonnoxious stimuli are muscle contractions. In either case, supraspinal facilitation is likely to be present and neuronal sensitization can occur.

Some neurologists would modify the classification of the International Headache Society to include chronic daily headache, which is further differentiated as a daily or near-daily type of headache with superimposed migraine. Patients with chronic headaches are prone to overusing multiple drugs and have a high rate of treatment failure. The headaches can be primary, as a transformed migraine, a chronic tension-type headache, a new daily headache, or a hemicrania continua. Secondary causes of chronic daily headache can exist, including posttraumatic headache, cervical spine dysfunction, vascular disorders, and nonvascular intracranial disorders.[35,49–51] Frequently, an episodic problem becomes chronic as a result of analgesic medication overuse.

Treatment begins with a close look to identify any medication overuse, drug dependency, or depression, which require specific intervention. Inquire for a past history of emotional, physical, or sexual abuse and incorporate that information into the treatment rationale. Every effort is made to identify and eliminate potential sources for triggers, such as the:

Teeth
Jaw
Sinuses
Cranial and cervical bones
Joints
Ligaments
Associated myofascial structures

These, too, demand specific interventions. Physical, psychological, and pharmacologic therapies can operate concurrently.[52]

Treatment

In headache management, the presence of somatic dysfunction is systematically identified and handled with OMT. Cervical vertebral segmental disorders, focal and regional myofascial disorders, and craniosacral disorders are common.[53–54] Exercise particular care with regard to manipulation of the cervical spine. Infrequently, cervical manipulation has been reported to aggravate a herniated intervertebral disk or a spinal cord injury[55]; most critically, cervical manipulation has been associated with vertebral artery laceration, intimal dissection, thrombosis, and thromboembolic infarction in the vertebrobasilar distribution of the posterior circulation.[56–58] Most of the complications have been seen with hyperextension and hyperrotation of the upper craniocervical segments, often in the course of a thrusting technique.[59]

Pharmacologic therapy is best served with a clearly limited (symptomatic) regimen to prevent drug-induced headaches. Preventive therapy is usually begun with a tricyclic antidepressant, especially useful when there is an associated sleep disturbance. More recently, sodium valproate has been found to have prophylactic value in chronic daily headache.

Nonpharmacologic therapies are also prescribed. Patients can be evaluated and educated regarding proper sleep hygiene. A therapeutic exercise program should be customized to the patient. Nutritional evaluation and recommendations can be given. Relaxation strategies and visual imagery techniques can be taught to each patient. It is important to involve the patient as an active participant in his or her own therapy.

Being able to assess the patient more completely permits a more comprehensive diagnosis. Multifactorial problems allow the formulation of a more thorough and multifaceted treatment program, increasing the potential for success. The osteopathic approach offers a successful model for an integrated multidimensional treatment with the patient as the focus and the physician as the facilitator.[60]

In addition to primary headache syndromes, a wide variety of neurologic and systemic disorders present with headache. These disorders must be considered when evaluating the patient en route to establishing a working and differential diagnosis, before proceeding with any therapeutic intervention. Table 34.2 is a collection of some of those conditions, highlighting clinical, diagnostic, and therapeutic features.

In general, the less specific the symptoms, the greater the suspicion that something more than benign headache is present. Consider further diagnostic studies, MRI, computerized tomography, electroencephalography, cerebral angiography, blood and cerebrospinal fluid analysis, and neurologic consultation when the patient does not respond promptly and appropriately to osteopathic medical management.

SPINAL DISORDERS

The practice of neurology frequently involves problems affecting the spine. This can involve the spinal column and its structural elements (spondylopathy), the nerve roots (radiculopathy), and even the spinal cord (myelopathy).

The spinal column includes the vertebral body, the intervertebral disk, the facet joints, the ligaments, and the myotendinous structures. The pathophysiology of spinal column disorders often involves a degenerative process such as spondylosis (osteoarthritis) of the vertebral body, which is frequently seen in association with degeneration of the intervertebral disk. The degeneration ultimately affects the adjacent related facet joints and results in strain in ligaments and myotendinous structures. Trauma commonly underlies this process.[73]

The spinal column can be also be affected by malignancy arising in the bone or more commonly from secondary metastasis of systemic cancer. Infection of the spinal column can result from systemic infection such as mycobacterial, fungal, or bacterial sepsis. Spinal pathologic conditions can also occur with osteoporosis and other metabolic abnormalities of bone or from less common arthritic diseases such as ankylosing spondylitis or rheumatoid arthritis. Disease processes adjacent to the spine can also result in spinal column destruction, including paraspinal tumors and abscesses.[74–77]

A common pathophysiologic process affecting the spinal column is the process of somatic dysfunction. Somatic dysfunction can affect single segments or multiple spinal segments and accompany any of the aforementioned spinal column pathologies.

The spinal nerve roots are affected by their location within the spinal canal. They are exposed to trauma from[78–80]:

Extruding disks
Fractured fragments
Spinal and paraspinal tumors
Degenerative changes in the vertebral elements
Intraspinal ligaments
Frank avulsions

In addition, the nerve roots lack the tight endothelial junction of the blood-brain barrier; the result is lowered protection from infection (e.g., herpes zoster, syphilis), neoplastic invasion, inflammatory demyelination (e.g., Guillain-Barré syndrome), or toxic exposure to chemotherapy agents, myelographic contrast agents, or anesthetic agents. The nerve roots are also susceptible to vascular insufficiency in the form of vasculitis, diabetes mellitus, and radiation exposure.[81]

Spinal cord syndromes can result from an intrinsic pathologic condition or from injury to the spinal cord from extrinsic compression. Intrinsic spinal cord pathologic conditions include myelitis—typically as a result of a virus, vasculitis, or multiple sclerosis—and neoplasms of the glial elements of the cord. Nutritional deficiencies can also result in degeneration of the spinal cord, typically subacute combined degeneration from cobalamin deficiency. CNS degenerative diseases affecting the spinal cord include motor neuron disease and multisystem degeneration. The spinal cord is vulnerable to ischemia if there is disruption in the anterior spinal artery circulation. Severe spinal trauma can result in hemorrhage or laceration of the spinal cord. Extrinsic compression of the spinal cord can result from the same conditions that cause nerve root compression, typically tumors that are primary or metastatic in the spinal canal, and from epidural infections or hematomas. Compression fractures of the vertebral bodies can result in subluxation and spinal cord compression. When the spinal cord is compressed from epidural tumor or infection, the spinal cord symptoms are preceded by vertebral pain.[82–85]

The symptom of vertebral bone or ligament disease is usually pain. Typically, patients complain of deep and aching pain in the affected region of the spine. Often, the pain is worse in certain positions or with certain activities. For example, patients with intervertebral disk disease commonly complain that their back pain is worse with prolonged sitting or standing, whereas acute problems are made worse with activity and improved with rest. The pain can refer locally to paraspinal segments. This referral pattern most likely has to do with nociceptors converging on a common dorsal horn projection neuron.[86] In the cervical region, the pain can involve the upper arm, shoulder, and scapulothoracic region. In the lumbar region, it involves the low back, hip, and upper leg. Numbness, weakness, and other neurologic symptoms are notably absent when only the bone and ligamentous vertebral elements are affected.

Patients with radiculopathy might complain of pain, numbness, tingling, or other sensations that typically are described as radiating from proximal to distal. In the cervical region (C-2–T-2), the radiation is in a dermatomal pattern in the arm and occiput. In the lumbosacral region (L-1–S-5), it is in a dermatomal pattern in the buttock and leg; in the thoracic region, the radiation is in a dermatomal pattern in the chest or abdomen. Because the pain is generated in the nerve root, patients describe a variety of pain sensations including electric, burning, stabbing, dull, sharp, or tearing pain. Patients also describe impulses of pain with coughing, sneezing, lifting, or moving the bowels. The pain is often worse with positions that either compress the nerve root (side-bending of the spine) or stretch the nerve root (forward bending of the spine). The pain can be relieved by maneuvers that take the pressure or stretch off of the nerve root. Spinal stenosis can produce radicular symptoms on the basis of intermittent ischemia to the nerve roots, typically related to walking.

When the motor fibers are affected, patients with radiculopathy can complain of weakness localized to the muscles innervated. In the lumbosacral region, the nerves supplying bladder, bowel, and sexual function can be affected; patients might complain of urinary hesitancy or retention, constipation, or impotence.

The pain of spinal tract origin is diffuse and referred several segments below the level of the lesion. The location of motor and sensory complaints depends on the area of the spinal cord involved. Unilateral lesions of the spinothalamic tract cause contralateral numbness to pain and temperature, whereas lesions of the posterior columns cause ipsilateral loss of position sense, light touch, and vibration. Bilateral lesions of the sensory fibers result in bilateral sensory disturbances below the level. Limb weakness results when there is an abnormality in the anterior horn cells or corticospinal tracts. The weakness can be accompanied by atrophy if it is in the lower motor neuron or spasticity if in the upper motor neurons. Bladder, bowel, and sexual functions are often compromised.

On physical examination, test sensation with pain, temperature, and touch. With radiculopathy, the sensory loss is dermatomal, and the margins of sensory loss might not be as demarcated as seen in peripheral nerve lesions. The motor deficits are in muscle groups with a common myotomal innervation. The weakness of individual muscles is usually partial rather than complete. Because the ventral roots contain the lower motor neurons, radicular weakness is often associated with fasciculations, decreased muscle tone and bulk, and decreased reflexes. In the upper extremities, the root innervation is checked by the deep tendon reflexes of the biceps (predominantly C-5), brachioradialis (predominantly C-6), triceps (C-7), and the finger flexors (C-8). In the lower extremities, the root innervation is checked by the deep tendon reflexes of the quadriceps (predominantly L-4), biceps femoris (L-5), and gastrocnemius (predominantly S-1). Unilateral sacral root lesions can cause numbness but usually do not affect muscle control. However, when bilateral sacral roots are involved, the rectal sphincter becomes weak. Test muscle strength for all of the major muscle groups of the upper and lower extremities.

Provocative maneuvers can be of great diagnostic value in patients with radiculopathy. In cervical or lumbar nerve root compression syndromes, side-bending of the involved spine can narrow the intervertebral foramina and increase radicular complaints (Spurling sign). Conversely, applying manual traction to the cervical or lumbar region usually offers relief. Stretching the nerve roots of the sciatic nerve with straight leg raising can provoke radicular symptoms (Lasègue's sign). Manual compression of the external jugular veins can cause an increase in intraspinal pressure. Compression aggravating radicular symptoms in either the upper or lower extremity (Naffziger's sign) can be a sign of nerve root compression.[87]

Many diagnostic tools are available for evaluating the functional and structural aspects of nerve roots. MRI offers the best noninvasive view of the nerve roots and surrounding structures. Computerized tomography has some value when bone details are needed. Invasive myelography, with the instillation of intrathecal contrast, continues to have a role diagnostically, especially when combined with postmyelogram computerized tomography. Sometimes it is important to evaluate the cerebrospinal fluid for signs of infection, inflammation, neoplasia, or hemorrhage by determining the cell count along with protein, glucose, and microbiologic studies.[88–90]

The functional status of nerve roots can be tested with nerve conduction studies that include antegrade and retrograde response to stimulus (F responses and the H reflexes). Nerve conduction studies and electromyography can reveal the presence of radiculopathy, but the abnormalities detected are a function of the chronicity of the lesion. Electrophysiologic testing of the nerve roots can also be done with somatosensory evoked potentials.[91-93]

The physical findings in myelopathy classically reveal a sensory level. Spinothalamic-mediated pain and temperature, and dorsal column-mediated touch, vibration, and position sense are disturbed below the level of spinal cord disturbance. Typically, this affects pain and temperature beginning several segments below the actual level of the lesion. Usually both sides are affected. Because primarily upper motor neurons are involved, the motor examination reveals a spastic increase in tone and an increase in the muscle stretch reflexes below the level of the lesion. Weakness is diffuse and can be mild or severe. The distribution of weakness reflects the pathologic condition in the anterior horn cells or corticospinal tracts. Depending on the level of the lesion, the patient can have positive Babinski signs and ankle clonus in the lower extremities and positive Hoffman's signs in the upper extremities. Sphincter tone can be increased. Gait can be disturbed by spasticity, weakness, or sensory ataxia. Patients with dorsal column sensory loss lose their balance and fall when asked to stand unaided with their eyes closed (Romberg's sign). If the patient's neck is flexed, he or she could experience an electric sensation traveling the spinal cord and the extremities (Lhermitte's sign), the result of stretching the long dorsal column fibers.[87]

When specific disease of the spinal column is identified, institute appropriate treatment. When there is structural weakness, supportive bracing can be used. Physical therapies are often valuable. Therapeutic exercise regimens are an essential component to all comprehensive treatment plans. Consider nutritional assessment and supplementation when necessary. Use medications with analgesic, antiinflammatory, and bone supportive properties. Anesthetic blocks of locally irritable structures (or facets) can be effective.[94]

OMT is useful in a wide range of vertebral column disorders, including those of somatic dysfunction.[95-100] MacDonald[101] demonstrated responses to osteopathic manipulation for low back pain of 14 to 28 days' duration on the basis of outcome studies. The Agency for Health Care Policy and Research (AHCPR) recently concluded "manipulation to be safe and effective for patients in the first month of acute low back pain symptoms without radiculopathy."[102] Osteopathic treatment is derived from the more comprehensive nature of the osteopathic neurologic evaluation. The examination can yield information local to the area of chief complaint as well as more general information on the effects of interrelated problems. For example, a person with mechanical low back pain could have an associated visceral disease (such as endometriosis) that can contribute viscerosomatically to the physical findings that the patient presents. Likewise, a similar low back pain could be related to a problem with the foot or leg. By identifying contributing elements, a more complete diagnostic understanding can be reached and a more comprehensive treatment undertaken.

Standard treatment of radiculopathy is appropriately directed to the specific pathologic condition involved. For example, antiviral agents are used for herpes zoster infection, or antineoplastic agents for carcinomatous radiculopathy. For degenerative spine conditions causing radiculopathy, physical measures to reduce compression and deformation with traction, physical therapy, and therapeutic exercise are beneficial. Attempt to decrease inflammation with oral corticosteroids or nonsteroidal antiinflammatory medication. Sometimes the corticosteroids, along with anesthetic agents, are introduced into the epidural space, usually lumbar but occasionally thoracic or cervical.[103-104] Patients are given extensive education about provocative aspects of their lifestyle, work, and habits with a goal of minimizing aggravating factors. If persistent radiculopathy causes progressing sensory or motor findings, or pain that cannot be controlled, surgical decompression is advisable. When the cauda equina is affected, a particular urgency exists to diagnose and decompress. In these cases, a delay in treatment can be associated with a marked increase in morbidity, with lingering bladder, bowel, sexual, and lower extremity dysfunction.

Specific intervention with OMT has to be undertaken cautiously, if at all, for patients with radiculopathy. Any manipulative procedures that increase nerve root compression or deformation can be potentially injurious. Nonetheless, in careful hands, the use of knowledgeably applied gentle manipulative forces might improve conditions for the nerve root and could potentially affect arterial, venous, and lymphatic circulation, as well as improve local biomechanical factors. At the least, OMT can be useful in alleviating some of the secondary musculoskeletal reaction that develops in the face of nerve root pathologic conditions.

PERSONAL APPROACH TO NEUROLOGIC DIAGNOSIS

When patients present with variable complaints of pain, sensory disturbance, or weakness, it is the neurologist's job to answer three questions. These are:

1. Is there a neurologic abnormality?
2. Can the neurologic abnormality be localized?
3. Can a differential diagnosis be generated for the abnormality in question?

For example, if a patient presents with neck or back pain, the physician attempts to localize the symptom by history. An effort is made to differentiate spinal cord disorders, nerve root syndromes, or vertebral disorders.

In the general history, it is necessary to know the patient's past personal history of illness, trauma, and surgery. Knowing the family history is valuable as a potential source of hereditary or constitutional susceptibility. The general history includes a search into the history for abuse (substance, physical, sexual, emotional). At the same time, explore the psychosocial background of the patient and his or her family. Inquire into the patient's nutrition, work, and exercise habits, sleep patterns, and potential risk exposures. A mental status examination to evaluate the higher cortical functions and arousal system should be followed by a complete neurologic examination.

This examination includes evaluation of the cranial nerves and the motor and sensory system. Test coordination and gait. Motor examination includes an assessment of muscle tone, muscle strength, muscle bulk, and the activity of the associated myotendinous reflexes. Sensory examination includes tests of light touch, pain, temperature, vibration, and proprioception. In addition to a routine neurologic examination, perform a musculoskeletal structural examination for patients with spinal complaints, including[105]:

1. Inspection of the patient walking and standing, from an anterior, posterior, and lateral view, looking for static and kinetic structural asymmetries
2. Performance of the standing flexion test
3. Performance of the standing lateral flexion test
4. Performance of the seated flexion test
5. Assessment of seated trunk rotation
6. Assessment of seated lateral flexion
7. Seated cervical assessment for flexion, extension, lateral flexion, and rotation
8. Supine rib testing
9. Supine upper extremity testing
10. Supine and prone lower extremity testing

The musculoskeletal structural examination provides structural signs of asymmetry (e.g., scoliosis, an increase in kyphosis or lordosis, or significant deviation from balance gravitational centering). In addition, the limbs and vertebral complex can be assessed for characteristics of motion by adding a palpatory examination of the soft tissue (muscles, ligaments, tendons, deep and superficial fascia, and the subcutaneous structures). The site of the primary musculoskeletal problem can often be determined. It is possible to know what biomechanical problems are helping to create, maintain, and aggravate the primary problem. In the areas of clinical interest, make the soft tissue examination, the motion testing, and the static structural examination precise to identify the local elements of dysfunction.

The musculoskeletal findings are often secondary to another disease of the musculoskeletal system, a reaction to internal disease, or a compensatory response to the presence of pain. Being able to assess the patient more thoroughly allows a more inclusive diagnosis with the possibility of a more extensive treatment program, increasing the potential for success. The ability to exclude the more unusual and potentially morbid conditions can only result from such an osteopathic evaluation. Additionally, this approach offers the ability to choose among multiple and costly diagnostic possibilities.

ENTRAPMENT NEUROPATHIES

Entrapment neuropathies represent a localized injury or irritation to one of the peripheral nerves. They are caused by the mechanical effects of the impinging adjacent tissues. The typical anatomic causes include entrapment within the osseofibrous tunnels where the nerve changes course against fibrous and muscular bands. Entrapment can be precipitated by trauma; once the trauma occurs, the local anatomic configu-

ration often causes a repetition of a mechanical injury. This local anatomic configuration can result in local compressive injury to the neural elements. The neural elements at risk include both the axon and the associated myelin. It can compromise local circulation, including arterial venous and lymphatic influences. Table 34.3 represents specific sites of nerve entrapment.[106–107]

Carpal Tunnel Syndrome

Carpal tunnel syndrome is the result of entrapment of the distal branches of the median nerve as it passes through the carpal tunnel. The tunnel is formed by the carpal bones and the carpal ligaments. The contents of the tunnel are flexor tendons and the median nerve. Either strong flexion or extension of the wrist can impact the median nerve. There can be acute compression with mechanical deformation and ischemic change. Chronic progressive compression can result in vascular compromise. The first effect of increased compression is an obstruction of venous return from the nerve, which leads to increased capillary distension and further increases in intratunnel pres-

Table 34.3
Sites of Nerve Entrapment and Treatments

Nerve	Site of Entrapment	Treatment
Median	Carpal tunnel, pronator teres, anterior interosseous syndrome	OMT, splint, exercise, surgery
Ulnar	Elbow, cubital tunnel, canal of Guyon, thoracic outlet	OMT, exercise, surgery
Radial	Supinator muscle	OMT, exercise, surgery
Brachial	Thoracic outlet scalenes, pectoralis minor, cervical rib	OMT, exercise, surgery
Sciatic	Pelvic outlet piriformis muscle	OMT, exercise, surgery
Posterior tibial	Tarsal tunnel	OMT, exercise, surgery
Common peroneal	Fibular head	OMT, exercise, surgery
Obturator	Obturator foramen	OMT, exercise, surgery
Femoral	Pelvic brim inguinal ligament	OMT, exercise, surgery
Ilioinguinal	Abdominal wall	OMT, exercise, surgery
Intercostal	Rib cage	OMT, exercise, surgery
Trigeminal	Foramen ovale, foramen rotundum, petrosphenoid ligament, Meckel's cave	OMT, surgery
Cranial nerves II, III, IV, V, VI	Orbital apex, exit foramina, reciprocal tension membrane, cavernous sinus	OMT, surgery
Cranial nerves VIII, IX, X, XI, XII	Basisphenoid, basiocciput, jugular foramina, hypoglossal canal	OMT, surgery
Cranial nerves VII, VIII	Temporal bone, internal auditory meatus	OMT, surgery
Cranial nerve I	Ethmoid, cribriform plate, sphenoid, lesser wing	OMT, surgery

sure. In a cyclic fashion this continues to self-amplify, impairing nutrition to the nerve. The large myelinated fibers are most vulnerable. At this stage, symptoms appear with pain and paresthesia is usually transient and reversed by restoring proper circulation. As things get worse, the capillary circulation is sufficiently slowed to create endoneurial edema, epineural edema, and intratunnel edema. This edema can still be reversed if adequate decompression is obtained. In the final stages, there is arterial insufficiency and increasing mechanical deformation, resulting in nerve fiber destruction and ultimate fibrous replacement.

Carpal tunnel can be caused by trauma to the wrist, hypertrophic arthritides, or thickening of the flexor retinaculum. Hypertrophic neuropathy, local edema, ganglion cysts, and tenosynovitis can all compromise the carpal tunnel. Some systemic diseases are predisposing, such as:

Hypothyroidism
Diabetes mellitus
Pregnancy
Leukemia
Paraproteinemia
Gout

The diagnosis depends on a careful history to differentiate local disease from systemic disease. With systemic disease the symptoms are frequently bilateral. The history is important in understanding predisposing biomechanical factors. These factors are often related to work, hobbies, or chronic behaviors. The patient complains of pain and paresthesias in the thumb, index, and long finger. Aching can spread proximally, to the arm and forearm. Early, the pain is transient; later, it becomes permanent. Commonly, it is worse at night or during provocative activities. In the earliest stages, a shake of the hand can restore circulation and relieve symptoms. Later, immobilization with a splint can be relieving. Vague weakness, often described as "dropping things," is common.

Physical examination reveals a sharply demarcated median nerve sensory deficit, confined to the palm, often splitting along the long or ring finger. Motor examination reveals a weakness of the thumb abductor, thumb opposer, and distal thumb flexor. In the more advanced stages, atrophy of the thenar eminence is evident. Tinel's sign is often positive, with percussion of the nerve at the wrist producing a tingling into the hand. Phalen's test, forced wrist flexion, can reproduce the pain and paresthesias. Even a reversed Phalen's test, forced wrist extension, can be provocative.

Electrodiagnostic tests are helpful in corroborating the diagnosis and quantifying the degree of abnormality. The findings of prolongation of the distal motor and/or sensory latencies is an early sign of demyelination. Axonal involvement and degeneration are demonstrated by the appearance of neurogenic atrophy on electromyography. The electromyogram can be useful to rule out more proximal lesions, such as a radiculopathy. The carpal tunnel itself may be demonstrated on plain radiogram, computed tomogram, and even better with MRI, which can reveal the structural consequences of an anatomic compression.

The standard treatment has consisted of immobilization with wrist splints and avoidance of the provocative activities related to the carpal tunnel syndrome. Paraneural infiltration with local anesthetics and corticosteroids is sometimes used. When conservative measures fail, surgical decompression is the appropriate treatment.[108]

The osteopathic neurologist begins with a more thorough evaluation. Not only is the biomechanical function of the wrist examined, but also the biomechanics of the fingers, hand, forearm, elbow, arm, shoulder, cervical and thoracic spine, and rib cage are assessed. This assessment is performed in the context of a complete osteopathic structural examination. Restrictive lesions along the upper extremity and shoulder girdle can influence circulation (venous, lymphatic, and arterial) and mechanical deformation of the median nerve that begins at the nerve root, runs through the brachial plexus, and terminates in the median nerve that runs through the arm and forearm before passing through the carpal tunnel. Whole body mechanical issues, like slumped posture, can influence the local conditions at the carpal tunnel. The veins and lymphatics drain proximally into the superior vena cava and thoracic duct. Mechanical dysfunction in the rib cage and cervicothoracic region are as relevant as the mechanics of the arm itself. Arterial insufficiency can be affected similarly at multiple levels. The sympathetic component, often understated, can be influenced from the root of the neck, where the sympathetic ganglia are found, through the upper extremity itself.

The treatment, then, is to treat general structural problems with OMT and exercise. Direct manipulation to the functional releasing of biomechanical barriers at the:

Neck
Upper back
Shoulder
Rib cage
Thoracic inlet and outlet
Upper arm
Forearm
Wrist
Hand
Fingers

The techniques can be direct or indirect; numerous examples of osteopathic treatment approaches have been proposed. These include myofascial release, muscle energy, thrusting, and functional techniques.[97,100,109] Sucher[109] has demonstrated a model for clinically, electrophysiologically, and graphically evaluating the carpal tunnel syndrome. He has shown the pathologic changes on neurologic examination, through distal nerve latency studies, and by obtaining MRI images of the carpal tunnel to measure its volume. He has then proceeded to treat these patients with OMT. He retests his patients and demonstrates objective changes in neurologic findings, distal nerve latencies, and carpal tunnel volume, as measured by

MRI. Sucher presents strong evidence for the therapeutic value of osteopathic management techniques.[110]

Another syndrome of nerve entrapment is thoracic outlet syndrome. This is a syndrome affecting the brachial plexus at the level of the cervicobrachial junction. It is associated with abnormal cervical ribs and most often with disturbed myofascial relations. Thoracic outlet syndrome most typically affects the lower trunk of the brachial plexus. Compression can occur over the slope of the first rib, in the triangle made by the scalenus anterior and medius, along fibrotendinous attachments of any of the scalenes, along fibrosseous cervical rib rudiments, or under the pectoralis minor.

Patients might also complain of pain and numbness of the upper extremity typically extending along the ulnar aspect of the hand. The pain is usually worse with the arm elevated or abducted. Thoracic outlet syndrome can be associated with pain, weakness, and a variety of sensory complaints. Physical findings include sensory loss, particularly in the ulnar distribution. Weakness of intrinsic, ulnar innervated muscles is an unusual late finding in thoracic outlet syndrome. Provocative tests are helpful to diagnose and localize the syndrome. Depending on the site of entrapment, there might be localized tenderness. For example, with symptoms elicited on isometric scalene contraction, the entrapment can be localized to the scalene triangle and is associated with localized tenderness of the brachial plexus at this site. When hyperabduction with extension is the culprit, the site of entrapment is often the tendon of the pectoralis minor and local pectoral hypertonicity; tenderness is typical. Sometimes a bruit of the subclavian artery can be auscultated at the site of its compression.[111]

Electrodiagnostic confirmation is frequently difficult. Prolonged nerve conduction velocity across the thoracic outlet can be demonstrated; in more advanced cases, axonal involvement might be encountered on electromyography. Somatosensory evoked potentials of the upper extremity can be localizing.[112] Imaging of the region in question is best attempted with MRI; however, MRI findings are frequently inconclusive. Simple cervical spine radiograms might reveal the presence of cervical ribs.

Standard management includes exercises to improve posture, reduce mechanical stress, lengthen shortened muscles, and avoid symptom-producing circumstances. Analgesics, antiinflammatory agents, muscle relaxants, and physical therapies are used. Progressive stretching exercises are included when indicated. When conservative measures fail, surgical intervention remains.

Osteopathic management of thoracic outlet syndrome includes appropriate structural evaluation with particular attention to the cervical, thoracic, costal, scapular, and brachial mechanical relationships. In comparison with carpal tunnel, the thoracic outlet syndrome involves a more widely affected area. It is therefore more difficult to define the inciting event and to establish targeted therapy. Evaluation of posture reveals a high incidence of posture with head forward and with rounded, upward, and anterior displaced shoulders. Evaluation of the work station and of the habits of the patient can reveal a subset of behaviors that are dysfunctional. OMT consisting of myofascial-releasing maneuvers to the restrictive musculoskeletal structures can be useful. When they are only temporarily useful—symptoms return when the patient resumes his or her unaltered lifestyle—efforts to modify the patient's life circumstances are employed. These efforts include modification and elimination of occupational and avocational mechanical stressors and the promotion of postural awareness with training in postural modification. The most important long-term aspects are the identification of the specific biomechanical restrictors and the prescription and training of the patient in the performance of self-administered stretching exercises.[113–116] As a general concept, the temporary beneficial response to manipulative therapies can be understood using this model. When the pathologic process involves chronically-acquired, well-learned maladaptive somatic behaviors, it is not surprising that a single manipulation does not eradicate such a process. Multiple strategies are necessary. Patient education, instruction, and performance in a protracted therapeutic exercise program is often most useful. In this way the neuromusculoskeletal system can be reeducated.

A particularly osteopathic approach to the cranial neuropathies can be based on the early writings of Sutherland and Magoun.[107] In these works, the anatomy of the nerves and their relationship to dural investments, nearby vasculature, bony foraminae, and osseoligamentous structures were elaborately described. The naturally mobile aspect of these cranial and intracranial structures was appreciated. Sutherland and Magoun recognized the potential for vulnerability to mechanical distortion and compression with the resultant production of symptoms, often directly localized to individual cranial nerves. Such symptoms can be related to trauma, developmental phenomena, inflammation, or ischemia.

Chronic Pain Syndrome

There is a difference between patients suffering acute pain and those suffering chronic pain (see Chapters 10, 13, and 36). Patients with acute and subacute pain syndromes typically have some degree of tissue injury with nociceptive activation. These can be recurring events as in rheumatoid arthritis, migraine headache, or trigeminal neuralgia. Ongoing acute pain is usually the result of continued nociceptive input from a destructive type of lesion, such as a malignant neoplasm.

Conversely, chronic benign nonmalignant pain syndromes last for more than 6 months without obvious signs of ongoing tissue damage. These chronic pain syndromes can be associated with adequate or inadequate coping by the patient. When coping is insufficient, the pain becomes the central focus for the patient. Patients with this problem are believed to have continuous low-level nociceptive barrage or alteration of central processing pathways. This nociceptive barrage can be the result of musculoskeletal or other peripheral pathologic processes with nociceptor activation. It can also reflect a pathologic condition of the nociceptors, their axons, and their central connections.[117]

Clinical experience demonstrates a high incidence of biomechanical dysfunction in the patient with the chronic pain syndrome. It is not uncommon that patients with this type of pain syndrome are underrecognized as having a significant structural pathologic condition. In fact, significant biomechanical dysfunction can be present, representing either a primary or secondary process. This information can go unrecognized by the majority of evaluators who use only standard neurologic and medical evaluation. Patients can begin with one pathologic problem and over time develop secondary somatic dysfunction. Conversely, patients can begin with a primary biomechanical insult that eludes recognition. In either event, the recognition of somatic dysfunction and its appropriate management are helpful in the global management of the patient with chronic pain.

One outcome of a good structural examination is the diagnosis of the common and often overlooked myofascial pain syndrome (see Chapters 65 and 66). This syndrome requires the palpatory identification of tender trigger points in muscles that, when palpated, cause pain to be referred to distant sites. These patterns of referral have been meticulously detailed by Travell and Simons.[23] The muscles can harbor painful nodules and bands that act as trigger points and are associated with pain, stiffness, limitation of motion, and weakness. Identified appropriately, the muscles are responsive to a variety of different treatments directed at the active trigger point. When these trigger points are deactivated by deep pressure, dry needling, local infiltration, stretching, or OMT they no longer serve as a source for pain generation.[118]

Nonpharmacologic therapies focused on enhancing the self-healing capacities of an individual are particularly important in the overall therapeutic formulation. These nonpharmacologic therapies include:

Nutritional evaluation and counseling
Evaluation and education in therapeutic sleep hygiene
Instruction and prescription of appropriate relaxation
Stress reduction techniques
Therapeutic exercise
Positive visual imagery
Promotion of a positive attitude through education about the nature of their pain problem
Formation of realistic objectives of management

All of these techniques involve the patient as an active participant in his or her own therapy.

CONCLUSION

It is clear that assessing the patient more completely generates a more comprehensive diagnosis. This fosters the prescription for a multifaceted treatment program that increases the potential for success. An additional advantage includes an ability to exclude more unusual yet potentially morbid causes of chronic pain. Furthermore, it offers the osteopathic neurologist the tools to rationally choose among the multiple and costly diagnostic and therapeutic possibilities. The osteopathic approach offers a successful model for integrated multidimensional treatment with the patient as the focus and the physician as the facilitator.[119]

REFERENCES

1. Still AT. *Autobiography of A.T. Still.* Kirksville, Mo: AT Still; 1897
2. Denslow JS. Neural basis of the somatic component in health and disease and its clinical management. *JAOA.* 1972;72:149–156.
3. Brodal A. *Neurological Anatomy In Relation to Clinical Medicine.* New York, NY: Oxford University Press; 1981.
4. Kandel E, Schwartz J, Jessell T. *Principles of Neural Science.* New York, NY: Elsevier Science Publishing Co, Inc; 1991:326–380.
5. Denslow JS. An analysis of the variability of spinal reflex thresholds. *J Neurophysiol.* 1944;7:207–216.
6. Denslow JS, Korr IM, Krems AD. Quantitative studies of chronic facilitation in human motoneuron pools. *Am J Physiol.* 1947; 150:229–238.
7. Korr IM. Somatic dysfunction, osteopathic manipulative treatment, and the nervous system: a few facts, some theories, many questions. *JAOA.* 1986;86:111–114.
8. Patterson MM. A model mechanism for spinal segmental facilitation. *JAOA.* 1976;76:62–72.
9. Korr IM. The spinal cord as organizer of disease processes, I. Some preliminary perspectives. *JAOA.* 1976;76:35–45.
10. Korr IM. Spinal cord as organizer of disease processes, II. The peripheral autonomic nervous system. *JAOA.* 1979;79:82–90.
11. Korr IM. Spinal cord as organizer of disease processes, III. Hyperactivity of sympathetic innervation as a common factor in disease. *JAOA.* 1979;79:232–237.
12. Johnson R, Lambie D, Spalding J. The autonomic nervous system. In: Baker AB, Baker LH, eds. *Clinical Neurology.* New York, NY: Harper and Row; 1985:57.
13. Adams T, Steinmetz M, Heisey S, Holmes K, Greenman P. Physiologic basis for skin properties in palpatory physical diagnosis. *JAOA.* 1982;81:366–377.
14. Beal MC. Viscerosomatic reflexes: a review. *JAOA.* 1985;85:786–800.
15. Johnston W, Hill J, Elkiss M, Marino R. Identification of stable somatic findings in hypertensive subjects by trained examiners using palpatory examination. *JAOA.* 1982;81:830–836.
16. Schwartz J. Synthesis and trafficking of neuronal proteins. In: Kandel E, Schwartz J, Jessell T, eds. *Principles of Neural Science.* New York, NY: Elsevier Science Publishing Co, Inc; 1991:57–65.
17. Korr IM. The spinal cord as organizer of disease processes, IV. Axonal transport and neurotrophic function in relation to somatic dysfunction. *JAOA.* 1981;80:451–467.
18. Denslow JS. Pathophysiologic evidence for the osteopathic lesion: the known, unknown, and controversial. *JAOA.* 1975;74:415–421.
19. International Headache Society. Classification of headaches. Cephalgia. 1988;8(suppl 7).
20. Jessell T, Kelly D. Pain and analgesia. In: Kandel E, Schwartz J, Jessell T, eds. *Principles of Neural Science.* New York, NY: Elsevier Science Publishing Co. Inc; 1991:389–392.
21. Magoun H. Trauma: a neglected cause of cephalgia. *JAOA.* 1975; 74:400–410.
22. Lay E. Osteopathic management of trigeminal neuralgia. *JAOA.* 1975;74:373–389.
23. Travell JG, Simons DG. *Myofascial Pain and Dysfunction: The Trigger Point Manual.* Baltimore, Md: Williams & Wilkins; 1983.
24. Rossman M. *Healing Yourself.* New York, NY: Bantam Books; 1987.

25. Welch KMA. Migraine: a biobehavioral disorder. *Arch Neurol.* 1987;44:323–327.

26. Moskowitz MA. The neurobiology of vascular head pain. *Ann Neurol.* 1984;16:157–168.

27. O'Connor T, Vanderkoop D. Pattern of intracranial and extracranial projections of trigeminal ganglion cells. *J Neurosci.* 1986; 6:2200–2207.

28. Brodal A. The cranial nerves. In: *Neurological Anatomy in Relation to Clinical Medicine.* New York, NY: Oxford University Press; 1981:508–513.

29. Bowles DB. Visual field effects of classical migraine. *Brain and Cognition.* 1993;21:181–183.

30. Pederson DM, et al. Migraine aura without headache. *J Fam Pract.* 1991;32:5–7.

31. Bickerstaff ER. Basilar artery migraine. *Lancet.* 1961;1:15–20.

32. Blend R, Bull J. The radiological investigation of migraine. In: Smith R, ed. *Background to Migraine: First Migraine Symposium.* London, England: Heinemann Medical Books Ltd; 1967:1–10.

33. Davidoff RA. Treatment of the acute attack. In: *Migraine: Pathogenesis, Manifestations, and Management.* Philadelphia, Penn: FA Davis; 1995:194–220.

34. Davidoff RA. Trigger factors and non-pharmacologic approaches. In: *Migraine, Manifestations, and Management.* Philadelphia, Penn: FA Davis; 1995:183–193.

35. Kidd RF, Nelson R. Musculoskeletal dysfunction of the neck in migraine and tension headache. *Headache.* 1993;33(10):566–569.

36. Blau J, Macgregor E. Migraine and the neck. *Headache.* 1993; 33(10):88–91.

37. Weiss H, Stern B, Goldberg J. Post-traumatic migraine: chronic migraine precipitated by minor head or neck trauma. *Headache.* 1991;31:451–456.

38. Kudrow L. Cluster headaches—new concepts. *Neurol Clin.* 1983; 2:369–384.

39. Hardebo J. How cluster headache is explained as an intracavernous inflammatory process—lesioning sympathetic fibers. *Headache.* 1994;34:125–126.

40. Gawel M, Krajewski A, Luo Y, Ichise M. The cluster diathesis. *Headache.* 1990;30:652–655.

41. Graham J. Cluster headache: the relation to arousal, relaxation, and autonomic tone. *Headache.* 1990;30:145–148.

42. Sanin L, Matthew N, Ali S. Extratrigeminal cluster headache. *Headache.* 1993;33:369–370.

43. Matthew N, Rueveni V. Cluster-like headache following head trauma. *Headache.* 1988;28:297–299.

44. Hardebo J. Subcutaneous sumatriptan in cluster headache. *Headache.* 1993;33:18–19.

45. Langemark M, Olesen J. Pericranial tenderness in tension headache—a blind, controlled study. *Cephalgia.* 1987;7:249–256.

46. Schoenen J, Jamart B, Gerard P, Lenarduzzi P, Delwaide PJ, et al. Exteroceptive suppression of temporalis muscle activity in chronic headache. *Neurology.* 1987;37:1834–1836.

47. Silberstein S. Tension-type headaches. *Headache.* 1994;34:S2–S7.

48. Olesen J. Clinical and pathophysiological observations in migraine and tension-type headache explained by integration of neural, vascular, and myofascial inputs. *Pain.* 1991;46:125–132.

49. Meloche J, Bergeron Y, Bellavance A, et al. Quebec Headache Study Group. Painful intervertebral dysfunction: Robert Maigne's original contribution to headache of cervical origin. *Headache.* 1993;33:328–332.

50. Michler R, Bovim G, Sjaastad O. Disorders in the lower cervical spine: a cause of unilateral headache. *Headache.* 1991;31:550–551.

51. Hack G, Koritzer R, Robinson W, Hallgren R, Greenman P. Anatomic relation between the rectus capitis posterior minor muscle and the dura mater. *Spine.* 1995;20:2484–2486.

52. Olesen J, Rasmussen B. Management of acute nonvascular headache—the Danish experience. *Headache.* 1990;30:541–543.

53. Miller H. Head pain. *JAOA.* 1972;72:135–143.

54. Upledger J, Vredevoogd J. *Craniosacral Therapy.* Chicago, Ill: Eastland Press; 1983:297–299.

55. Vick DA, McKay C, Zengerle CR. The safety of manipulative treatment: review of the literature from 1925 to 1993. *JAOA.* 1996; 96:113–115.

56. Raskind R, North CM. Vertebral artery injuries following chiropractic cervical spine manipulation: case reports. *Angiology.* 1990; 41:445–452.

57. Powell F, Hanigan W, Olivero W. A risk/benefit analysis of spinal manipulation therapy for relief of lumbar and cervical pain. *Neurosurgery.* 1993;33:73–79.

58. Hart R, Easton J. Dissections of cervical and cerebral arteries. *Neurol Clin.* 1983;1:155–182.

59. Okawara S, Nibbelink D. Vertebral artery occlusion following hyperextension and rotation of the head. *Stroke.* 1975;5:2–3.

60. Elkiss M. Chronic headache pain, an osteopathic perspective. Washington, DC: Testimony before the Agency for Health Care Policy and Research; October 31, 1995. Transcript of Open Forum, Duke University, Durham, North Carolina.

61. Lowe R. Aetiology of the anatomical basis for primary angle closure glaucoma. *Br J. Ophthalmol.* 1970;54:161–169.

62. Day J, Raskin N. Thunderclap headache: symptom of unruptured cerebral aneurysm. *Lancet.* 1986;11:1247–1248.

63. Buchbinder R, Detsky A. Management of suspected giant cell arteritis. *J Rheumatol.* 1992;19:1120–1122.

64. Herndon R, Rudick R. Multiple sclerosis and related conditions. In: Baker AB, Baker LH, eds. *Clinical Neurology.* New York, NY: Harper and Row; 1987;33:45–46.

65. Kokkinos J, Levine S. Neurologic complications of drugs and alcohol abuse. *Neurol Clin.* 1993;11:577–590.

66. Fisher CM. The headache and pain of spontaneous carotid dissection. *Headache.* 1982;22:60–65.

67. Mokri B, Sundt T, Houser D. Spontaneous internal carotid dissection, hemicrania, and Horner's syndrome. *Arch Neurol.* 1979; 36:677–680.

68. Weinberg S, Lapopinte H. Cervical extension:flexion injury (whiplash) and internal derangement of the temporomandibular joint. *J Oral Maxillofac Surg.* 1987;45:653–656.

69. Dubner R, Sharov Y, Gracely R, Price D. Idiopathic trigeminal neuralgia: sensory features and pain mechanisms. *Pain.* 1987; 31:23–24.

70. Moore J, Patcher M, Waldenmaier N, et. al. High field magnetic resonance imaging and perinasal sinus and inflammatory disease. *Laryngoscope.* 1986;96:267–271.

71. Wall M. Idiopathic intracranial hypertension. *Neurol Clin.* 1991; 9:73–95.

72. Martin E. Headache during sexual intercourse (coital cephalgia): a report of 6 cases. *Irish J Med Sci.* 1974;148:342–345.

73. Salter RB. Degenerative disorders of joints and related structures. In: *Textbook of Disorders and Injuries of the Musculoskeletal System.* Baltimore, MD: Williams & Wilkins; Baltimore, 1970:200–230.

74. Henson RA, Urich H. Involvement of the vertebral column and spinal cord. In: *Cancer and the Nervous System.* Oxford, England: Blackwell Scientific Publications; 1982:120–150.

75. Salter RB. Inflammatory disorders of bones and joints. In: *Textbook of Disorders and Injuries of the Musculoskeletal System.* Baltimore, Md: Williams & Wilkins; 1970:165–166.

76. Finneson B. The lower back in the diagnosis of rheumatic diseases. In: *Rheumatic Diseases—Diagnosis and Management.* Philadelphia, Penn: JB Lippincott Co; 1977:114–135.

77. Salter R. Generalized and disseminated disorders of bone. In: *Textbook of Disorders and Injuries of the Musculoskeletal System.* Baltimore, Md: Williams & Wilkins Co; 1970:129–149.

78. Davis C. Extradural spinal cord and nerve root compression from benign lesions of the lumbar area. In: *Youmans Neurological Surgery.* Philadelphia, Penn: WB Saunders; 1982:2535–2555.

79. Arbit E, Patterson R. Extradural spinal cord and nerve root compression from benign lesions of the dorsal area. In: *Youmans Neurological Surgery.* Philadelphia, Penn: WB Saunders; 1982:2562–2568.

80. Ehni G. Extradural spinal cord and nerve root compression from benign lesions of the lumbar area. In: *Youmans Neurological Surgery.* Philadelphia, Penn: WB Saunders; 1982:2574–2604.

81. Bradley W. Diseases of the spinal roots. In: Dyck P, Thomas P, Lambert E, Bunge R, eds. *Peripheral Neuropathy.* Philadelphia, Penn: WB Saunders; 1984:1368–1382.

82. Mulder D, Dale A. Spinal cord tumor and disks. In: Baker AB, Baker LH, eds. *Clinical Neurology.* New York, NY: Harper and Row; 1975;44:1–25.

83. Moossy J. Vascular disease of the spinal cord. In: Baker AB, Baker LH, eds. *Clinical Neurology.* New York, NY: Harper and Row; 1988;46:1–14.

84. Doyle W, Cooper P, Wilmot C, Faden A, Hall K. Trauma of the spine and spinal cord. In: Baker AB, Baker LH, eds. *Clinical Neurology.* New York, NY: Harper and Row; 1991;47:1–44.

85. Kincaid J. Myelitis and myelopathy. In: Baker AB, Baker LH, eds. *Clinical Neurology.* New York, NY: Harper and Row; 1989;48:1–28.

86. Jessell T, Kelly D. Pain and analgesia. In: Kandel E, Schwartz J, Jessell T, eds. *Principles of Neural Science.* New York, NY: Elsevier Science Publishing Co; 1991:388–389.

87. DeJong R. *The Neurologic Examination.* Hagerstown, Md: Harper and Row; 1979.

88. Wagle W. Neuroradiology. In: Baker AB, Baker LH, eds. *Clinical Neurology.* New York, NY: Harper and Row; 1990;2:178–233.

89. Latchaw R, Taylor S, Meyer J, et. al. The spine. In: *Computed Tomography of the Head, Neck, and Spine.* Chicago, Ill: Year Book Medical Publishers Inc; 1985:595–695.

90. Norman D. The spine. In: Brant-Zawadzki M, Norman D, eds. *Magnetic Resonance Imaging of the Central Nervous System.* New York, NY: Raven Press Books Ltd; 1987:289–328.

91. Aminoff M. Electromyography. In: Aminoff M, ed. *Electrodiagnosis in Clinical Neurology.* New York, NY: Churchill Livingstone; 1980:197–220.

92. Daube J. Nerve conduction studies. In: Aminoff M, ed. *Electrodiagnosis in Clinical Neurology.* New York, NY: Churchill Livingstone; 1980:229–260.

93. Chiappa K, Jayakar J. Evoked potentials in clinical medicine. In: Baker AB, Baker LH, eds. *Clinical Neurology.* New York, NY: Harper and Row; 1989;7:1–48.

94. Bonica J, Buckley P. Regional analgesia with local anesthetics. In: *The Management of Pain.* Philadelphia, Penn: Lea & Febiger; 1990:1883–1960.

95. Greenman P. Manipulation with the patient under anesthesia. *JAOA.* 1992;92:1159–1170.

96. Shepelle P, Adams A, Chassin M, et. al. Spinal manipulation for low back pain. *Ann Intern Med.* 1992;117:590.

97. Greenman PE. *Principles of Manual Medicine.* Baltimore, Md: Williams & Wilkins; 1989.

98. Stiles E. An osteopathic approach to low back pain. *Osteopath Ann.* 1976;4:44–48.

99. Stoddard A. *Manual of Osteopathic Technique.* London, England: Hutchison Medical Publications; 1961.

100. Ward R. *Myofascial Release Technique: Tutorials on Level I, II, and III.* Michigan State University, College of Osteopathic Medicine, East Lansing, MI; 1992.

101. MacDonald R, Bell C. An open controlled assessment of osteopathic manipulation. *Spine.* 1990;15:364–370.

102. Bigos S, Bowyer O, Braen G, et al. *Acute Low Back Problems in Adults. Clinical Practice Guideline.* Rockville, Md: US Department of Health and Human Services. Public Health Service. Agency for Health Care Policy and Research; 1994.

103. Anderson KH, Mosdal C. Epidural application of corticosteroids in low back pain and sciatica. *Acta Neurochir.* 1987;87:52–53.

104. Bush K, Hiller SA. Controlled study of caudal epidural injections of triamcinolone plus prosoine for the management of intractable sciatica. *Spine.* 1991;16:72–75.

105. Moran P, Pruzzo N. In: Mitchell FL Jr, ed. *An Evaluation and Treatment Manual of Osteopathic Manipulative Procedure.* Kansas City, Mo: Institute for Continuing Education in Osteopathic Principles; 1973:15–17.

106. Sunderland S. *Nerves and Nerve Injuries.* London, England: Churchill Livingstone; 1978:653–1021.

107. Magoun HI. *Osteopathy in the Cranial Field.* Kirksville, Mo: The Journal Printing Co; 1966:95, 184, 207, 251, 259, 294.

108. Sunderland S. The carpal tunnel syndrome. In: *Nerves an Nerve Injuries.* London, England: Churchill Livingstone; 1978:711–723.

109. Sucher BM. Palpatory diagnosis and manipulative management of carpal tunnel syndrome. *JAOA.* 1994;94:647–663.

110. Sucher BM. Myofascial manipulative release of carpal tunnel syndrome: documentation with MRI. *JAOA.* 1993;93:1273–1278.

111. Sunderland S. Disturbances of brachial plexus origin associated with unusual anatomical arrangements in the cervico-brachial region: The thoracic outlet syndrome. In: *Nerves and Nerve Injuries.* London, England: Churchill Livingstone; 1978:901–917.

112. Synek VM. Diagnostic importance of somatosensory evoked potentials in the diagnosis of thoracic outlet syndrome. *Clin Electroencephalogr.* 1986;17:112–116.

113. Sucher BM. Thoracic outlet syndrome: a myofascial variant, I: Pathology and diagnosis. *JAOA.* 1990;90:686–704.

114. Sucher BM. Thoracic outlet syndrome: a myofascial variant, II: treatment. *JAOA.* 1990;90:810–823.

115. Sucher BM, Heath DM. Thoracic outlet syndrome: a myofascial variant, III: structural and postural considerations. *JAOA.* 1993;93:334–345.

116. Dobrusin R. Osteopathic approach to conservative management of thoracic outlet syndromes. *JAOA.* 1989;89:1046–1057.

117. Bonica J. General considerations of chronic pain. In: *The Management of Pain.* Philadelphia, Penn: Lea & Febiger; 1990;8:180–195.

118. Sola A, Bonica J. Myofascial pain syndromes. In: *The Management of Pain.* Philadelphia, Penn: Lea & Febiger; 1990;21:352–366.

119. Elkiss M, Jerome J. Chronic back pain syndrome: an analysis of current therapies. *Mich Osteopathic J.* 1978:21–28.

35. Oncology

MICHAEL I. OPIPARI

He taught us that the treatment of the patient was the most important element in the treatment of disease, that the patient not the disease was the entity.[1]

—THAYER, ON SIR WILLIAM OSLER

Care more particularly for the individual patient than for the special features of the disease.[1]

—SIR WILLIAM OSLER

Key Concepts

- **Malignancies that appear as disease involving bone and soft tissue structures, the central nervous system, or the peripheral nervous system, including renal cell cancer, lung carcinoma, and plasma cell neoplasm**

- **Manifestations of malignancy in musculoskeletal system, including back pain, joints, muscle, and skin**

- **Manifestations of malignancy in central nervous system, including cerebral and indirect paraneoplastic malignancies**

- **Manifestations of malignancy in peripheral nervous system, including remote peripheral manifestations, spinal cord compression, and other causes of peripheral neuropathy**

- **Viscerosomatic-type oncologic responses**

- **Presenting diagnostic and treatment options to patients**

- **Supportive care of cancer patients, including symptom and pain relief, blood and blood products, and general supportive care**

- **Philosophic principles of care of cancer patient**

- **Stress and treatment**

- **Osteopathic approach, including indications and contraindications for osteopathic manipulative treatment**

The patient with a cancer diagnosis presents a complex series of events for the primary care physician. The clinical manifestations of the cancer family of diseases are many. They can occur secondary to altered structure or function at the primary site of tumor involvement. They can occur as a result of involvement of a secondary site with metastatic disease or remote tumor effects such as paraneoplastic syndromes. Often the malignant process is accompanied by signs or symptoms unrelated to the primary site, without any clinical evidence of metastasis. Metastasis occasionally can be present and subclinical yet produce symptoms, or it can be totally absent with the primary tumor manifesting itself through a paraneoplastic mechanism.

Through this mechanism, a malignancy can affect a hormonal, cytokine, or metabolic process to exert effects at distant sites or within other organ systems without metastasis being present.

This chapter discusses malignancy as a disease entity with an emphasis on its manifestations and effects on the neuromusculoskeletal system. The relationship of the neurostructural presentation of a patient with malignancy compared with a nonneoplastic structural lesion can be interesting and deceiving.

Three different malignancies are presented here as index tumors and serve as prototypes for the variety of neuromusculoskeletal presentations to be discussed. All three of these malignant diseases have the potential to appear as disease involving bone and soft tissue structures, the central nervous system (CNS), or the peripheral nervous system.

INDEX TUMORS

Renal Cell Cancer

Renal cell cancer (hypernephroma, Grawitz' tumor) is elusive and unpredictable, accounting occasionally for prolonged delays in diagnosis. Renal cell carcinoma makes up only 2–3% of all malignant disease.[2] The classic triad of presenting symptoms including hematuria, flank pain, and abdominal mass is infrequent, occurring in less than 10% of patients.[3–4] The presenting symptoms are more commonly associated with distant manifestations, either metastatic or paraneoplastic. As many as 34% of patients have metastasis at the time of diagnosis.[5] When present, metastases occur most commonly in lung, bone, liver, and lymph nodes.[6–7] This tumor is commonly referred to as the "internist's tumor" because of its presenting humoral or systemic signs and symptoms of a medical rather than urologic nature. The systemic manifestations can include:

    Anemia
    Erythrocytosis
    Fever of unknown origin
    Weight loss
    Hypercalcemia

These manifestations can occur in the absence of metastatic disease. The hypercalcemia is often related to elaboration of an ectopic parathormone-like substance from the tumor (parathyroid hormone-related peptide, PTHrP). In addition, a hepatic dysfunction syndrome occurs in up to 15% of patients without metastasis, manifesting as significantly altered hepatic enzymes.[8]

The natural history of renal cell carcinoma is unpredictable. Patients with metastatic disease can remain stable for months to years and then suddenly develop progressive metastasis leading to death. Patients with progressive disease can likewise suddenly stabilize for a prolonged time. Renal cell carcinoma is one of the most common tumors reported to undergo spontaneous regression after removal of the primary site.[9] The majority of these cases have not been histologically confirmed.

Neuromusculoskeletal metastasis can occur to the spine (producing back pain) or to soft tissue areas as a mass. It can occur as a compression of spinal cord or nerve root producing peripheral neuropathic symptoms, or it can produce CNS signs and symptoms as a result of direct metastasis or paraneoplastic effects (hypercalcemia).

The diagnosis of renal cell cancer is most commonly accomplished by radiologic techniques (intravenous pyelogram, ultrasonography, and/or renal arteriography). Treatment with surgery is most effective when the disease is localized. If metastatic disease is present, the extent and location dictate whether surgery is appropriate. Radiation and chemotherapy are palliative and of limited benefit. Immune modulating therapy with IL-2 and/or α-interferon hold some promise.

Lung Carcinoma

Lung cancer is the most common cancer and the most common cause of cancer death in males and females. The rapid rise in female lung cancer incidence and death is attributed to increased smoking among women. In males, the rate has stabilized and might be showing early evidence of reversal as a result of smoking cessation. At the time of diagnosis, the disease generally has spread to regional lymph nodes or distant sites.

Small cell lung cancer (oat cell cancer) is one of the four major cell types of lung cancer arising from the bronchial surface epithelium and originating as a submucosal growth. Epidermoid (squamous) cancer, adenocarcinoma, and large cell carcinoma make up the other major varieties. Small cell cancer is generally an aggressive, rapidly growing neoplasm making up approximately 20–25% of lung cancers. Once the most common variety of lung cancer, epidermoid comprises 25–30%, adenocarcinomas 40%, and large cell cancer 15% of lung tumors.[10] Analysis shows survival to be the best in epidermoid cancers. However, with the recent advent of intensive combination chemotherapy, small cell cancer is involved in a small fraction of long-term survivals. Because of its aggressive behavior, small cell cancer has regional lymph node involvement at the time of surgical resection in 70% of cases.[11] At autopsy, lung cancer metastasis is present in every body organ, with small cell cancer having absolute likelihood of extrathoracic metastasis. Common clinical problems related to distant metastasis include:

    CNS metastasis with neurologic deficits
    Bone metastasis presenting with bone or back pain and pathologic fracture
    Liver metastasis
    Adrenal metastasis
    Lymph node metastasis
    Skin metastasis

Paraneoplastic syndromes occur commonly with lung cancer. Some occur more specifically with individual histologic varieties of lung cancer. These can be the presenting symptoms in patients without metastasis, or prior to the diagnosis of the primary lung cancer. Paraneoplastic syndromes include:

    Cushing's syndrome
    Syndrome of inappropriate antidiuretic hormone (SIADH)
    Nonmetastatic hypercalcemia (PTHrP)
    Subacute cerebellar degeneration
    Dementia syndromes
    Peripheral neuropathies
    Polymyositis and dermatomyositis

Any of these syndromes can appear as altered CNS function and can create difficulty in discussing appropriate treatment options and decisions. A frequent musculoskeletal paraneoplastic manifestation is hypertrophic pulmonary osteoarthropathy. While the endocrine syndromes considered above, except for PTHrP production, are particularly common with small cell carcinoma, the osteoarthropathy is most commonly seen with adenocarcinoma. Lung cancer should be included as a part of the differential diagnosis for all patients with paraneoplastic syndromes.

A type of paraneoplastic syndrome occurring with lung cancer involves the ectopic production of bombesin, a multi-amino acid neuropeptide hormone. Since bombesin was first isolated from amphibian skin, the mammalian equivalent, gastrin-releasing peptide (GRP) or human bombesin, has been found in tumors of neuroendocrine and some nonneuroendocrine origin.[12] Bombesin-like immunoreactivity has been found in human brain, spinal cord, gastrointestinal mucosa, and pulmonary neuroendocrine cells. High levels of this immunoreactivity are noted in up to 50% of pulmonary carcinoid tumors and in many small cell lung cancers.[13] This substance is particularly interesting because of its apparent autocrine growth-enhancing ability imposed on the tumors.

The diagnosis of lung cancer requires tissue confirmation by biopsy, surgical resection, or cytology of sputum or selected bronchial washings. Therapy varies with the specific cell type and stage but commonly involves a combination of surgery, radiotherapy, and/or chemotherapy. Overall survival at 5 years after surgical resection for all resectable stage cell types varies between 30% and 80%, although the previously noted negligible survival rates for small cell cancer are improving as a result of intensive combination chemotherapy.[14]

Plasma Cell Neoplasm (Multiple Myeloma)

Plasma cell neoplasm is a neoplasm of B-lymphocytes of monoclonal origin that progresses to a large cellular population. The plasma cells produce immunoglobulins or immunoglobulin fractions that can be distinguished and detected in blood and urine as monoclonal or M protein on a protein electrophoresis pattern. The diagnosis of this neoplasm is made by the demonstration of[15]:

Bone marrow plasmacytosis
Monoclonal immunoglobulin detection
Anemia
Bone pain

This disease is the most common primary tumor to involve medullary bone and is often overlooked in a patient presenting with back pain. Often the symptoms are vague and nonspecific. Typical lytic "punched out" bone lesions can be absent; a diffuse osteoporosis pattern might be seen on x-ray films. The incidence of myeloma is reported at two to four per 100,000 population, with a higher rate in blacks than in whites. Plasma cell tumors can originate in extramedullary sites as well. They have been known to arise in almost any organ; the upper airway passages (nasal sinuses, nose, nasopharynx, tonsil) are the most frequent extramedullary sites. These tumors can also arise in skin and subcutaneous tissue, presenting as soft tissue masses. At least two-thirds of patients present with a skeletal symptom of bone pain, especially in the spine and ribs. Pathologic fractures are common. Spinal cord compression and nerve root compression are common complications of this disease and can

produce radicular pain. Peripheral neuropathies can occur as a result of amyloid deposition in nerves or perineural vasculature.

Other clinical problems common in the myeloma patient include hypercalcemia, reported in at least 35% of patients at presentation.[16] The progressive confusion and drowsiness in these patients can resemble CNS disease. Gastrointestinal symptoms of nausea, vomiting, and constipation together with polyuria can signal the onset of hypercalcemia. A hyperviscosity syndrome is also a complication of myeloma and is the result of a change in concentration, size, and shape of the monoclonal globulin. If the serum viscosity relative to water rises above four, symptoms occur. These symptoms include:

Cephalgia
Visual disturbance
Fatigue
Vertigo
Nystagmus
Paresis
Confusion
Coma

This combination of symptoms can closely resemble CNS metastasis. Hyperviscosity is treated by plasmapheresis and specific chemotherapy including steroids and alkylating agents.

Make attempts to diagnose myeloma before the patient experiences a pathologic fracture. Anemia, proteinuria, and rouleau formation on a peripheral smear report or a report of bone demineralization are early clues.

Myeloma usually enters a chronic phase easily responsive to steroids and alkylating drugs. Pathologic fractures can be surgically treated with pinning for long bone disease. Irradiate impending fractures and spinal cord or nerve root compression. Maintaining activity and ambulation is essential in treating this disease. Fluid hydration is beneficial for the renal complications and for preventing hyperviscosity. Eventually these patients enter an acute phase characterized by packing of the marrow with plasma cells producing pancytopenia leading to infection. Infection and renal failure are frequently terminal events.

We have evaluated two relatively common malignant diseases and one extremely common malignant tumor. All three were selected for inclusion here because of their frequent signs or involvement of the nervous, muscular, or skeletal system. These tumors can affect soft tissue and bone simultaneously, sequentially, or not at all. Any physician following or treating a patient with malignancy must be aware of the natural history potential of such presentations.

UNIQUE NEUROMUSCULOSKELETAL MANIFESTATIONS OF MALIGNANCY

The manifestations discussed in this section are divided into musculoskeletal, central nervous, and peripheral nervous systems. The presence of metastasis can frequently influence the presenting symptoms within these systems. The presence of metastasis is often overlooked because of the site of involvement. The major mechanisms of metastasis involve direct tumor extension and lymphatic and hematogenous dissemination. The specific vasculature invaded during metastasis can determine the site involved in the distribution of the blood-borne metastasis.[13–14] This is typified in prostatic carcinoma and in other pelvic tumors by metastatic spread to the vertebral spine, or in carcinoma of the breast by spinal metastasis in the absence of pulmonary spread.[17–18] This metastatic pattern to vertebral bone can occur as a result of the vertebral venous plexus, a system of valveless vessels extending along the spine and forming anastomoses with veins extending from the brain to the pelvis. Batson, who described the anatomy of this system now carrying his name, demonstrated extensive retrograde-antegrade vascular flow potential in the venous system as related to posture and abdominal pressure.[17–18]

Musculoskeletal System

BACK PAIN

The bony skeleton is the second most common metastatic site of malignancy.[19] Over 80% of the metastatic tumors originate within these organs[20]:

Breast
Prostate
Lung
Kidney
Thyroid gland

Microscopically, at autopsy, a much higher rate of metastasis to bone is present than is noted clinically, in more than 80% of cases of breast and prostate cancer, 50% of thyroid cancer, and 40% of lung and kidney cancers.[20] The spine is involved most often, with a reducing order of frequency extending from lumbar to dorsal to cervical areas of the spine.[21–23] Metastatic bone disease is much more common than are primary bone tumors. Metastatic bone disease in the spine can be lytic (clastic or destructive) or blastic (sclerotic) or a mixture of both, depending on the predominant process of formation or destruction of bone that occurs in metastases.

Back pain is often the first indication of metastatic disease. Back pain can be present for varying periods of time before the onset of neurologic signs or symptoms, which usually occur secondary to compression of a nerve root or the spinal cord. The origin of back pain can be difficult to localize in the skeletal system because of the vagaries of available diagnostic tests. Radionuclide scans visualize osseous changes earlier than do radiographs. Scans depend on osteoblastic activity for demonstration of abnormalities.[24] Actual bone density loss of at least 50% is required to demonstrate metastasis on x-ray films.

Without the osteoblastic process, and in purely lytic bone disease, a false–negative bone scan can occur. In elderly patients, a reactive or inflammatory process such as arthritis or degenerative vertebral disease can mimic the metastatic process and create a false–positive bone scan. Bone scan abnormalities require radiographic, computerized tomography (CT), or magnetic resonance imaging (MRI) confirmation of metastases.

Often, two procedures are indicated for comparison before the diagnosis is made and treatment is begun. CT and MRI, which have greater degrees of resolution, are often helpful in detection of otherwise silent lesions. With a high index of clinical suspicion and without imaging documentation, localization by specific sensory or dermatomal level can focus an area to permit treatment by radiation therapy.

When evaluating the patient with back pain, always consider malignancy, especially prostate cancer in a male age 60 years or older. Additional systemic manifestations include weight loss, pain unrelated to motion or position, and pain unresponsive to analgesic medications. Often there is an urgency in considering spinal metastasis so that appropriate therapy and maintenance of neurologic function can be maintained in patients with spinal cord compression.

Leptomeningeal carcinomatosis is seen most often in small cell lung cancer, breast cancer, and leukemia. In these patients, a variety of diagnoses can precede the diagnosis of leptomeningeal disease. They include:

Cerebral tumor
Meningitis
Psychoses
Hysteria
Polyneuritis[25]

This manifestation of systemic malignancy can occur as a presenting symptom. The symptoms often include[26]:

Low back pain
Nonspecific leg pain (radicular)
Headache
Mental status change
Extremity weakness
Neck pain
Nuchal rigidity

The diagnosis is confirmed by finding malignant cells in the cerebral spinal fluid (CSF) as well as elevated CSF protein and low CSF glucose levels.[26] The evaluation of these patients, without knowledge of the presence of a related malignancy, can easily lead to mistaken diagnosis for the back and leg pain resulting from a musculoskeletal somatic lesion rather than from malignancy.

JOINTS

The joints can be involved with malignancy by either a primary tumor or metastatic process to the bone or synovium. This joint involvement presents as asymmetric arthritis or diffuse articular changes caused by an indirect humoral-related process as in hypertrophic osteoarthropathy. Leukemia in children presents as localized or diffuse bone pain associated with joint swelling and pain.[27] Bronchogenic carcinoma likewise presents as symmetric painful swelling of the digits, resembling early rheumatoid arthritis, as a result of metastasis.[28] Undiagnosed renal carcinoma has been reported by Ritch in three cases to present and be treated as shoulder arthritis, prior to discovery of metastasis to the clavicle or upper humerus.[29]

Hypertrophic pulmonary osteoarthropathy (HPOA) is a paraneoplastic syndrome presumed to result from secretion of estrogen, growth hormone, or neurogenic factors in patients with intrathoracic tumors.[30] This syndrome produces a symmetric clubbing of fingers and toes, periostitis of long bones, and polyarthritis resembling rheumatoid arthritis.[31] The joints most frequently involved are the knees, ankles, and wrists. The presenting symptoms are pain, tenderness, and swelling of the affected joints. Involvement of the metacarpal-phalangeal and proximal interphalangeal joints has been reported. A classic finding is periosteal tenderness and radiographic evidence of periosteal elevation. Lung cancer is the most frequent malignancy associated with HPOA, which occurs in 12% of patients with adenocarcinoma and less frequently in patients with squamous cancers.[31] Osteoarthropathy is negligible in small cell cancer of the lung. Synovial fluid analysis generally produces a noninflammatory fluid finding.[32–33] The rheumatoid factor is absent in HPOA. Perhaps the most characteristic finding is the dramatic symptom relief that can occur within hours of primary tumor resection.[27]

MUSCLE AND SKIN

A wide spectrum of skin, muscle, and connective tissue manifestations are associated with previous, current, or undiagnosed malignancies. These can be secondary to direct or metastatic involvement or the result of a paraneoplastic effect. Adenocarcinoma of bronchial origin has been discovered as a mass of the calf.[34] Previously undiagnosed renal carcinoma has been reported as a large growing vascular mass of the biceps muscle.[7] Metastatic soft tissue or muscle masses can occur and have been reported in any anatomic area. These can produce pain and affect function as a result of compression of muscle or nerve invasion. Because these masses are occasionally small, deep seated, and not readily detectable, they are often overlooked and/or treated inappropriately.

Dermatomyositis and polymyositis have been associated with up to a 50% incidence of malignancy[31]; they can precede the malignancy by days or years. The skin manifestations, when present, include a purplish erythema. The predominant clinical complaint is a progressive proximal muscular weakness developing over weeks to months. The diagnosis is made by muscle biopsy, elevated erythrocyte sedimentation rate and muscle enzymes, and abnormal electromyography (EMG). This syndrome, more common in men, is often labeled carcinomatous myopathy or neuromyopathy because of the diminished to absent deep tendon reflexes. The predominant associated malignancies are lung and gastric cancer.

Acanthosis nigricans, a hyperpigmented, hyperkeratotic skin lesion in intertriginous or flexor areas of axillary, neck, or anogenital areas is frequently associated with gastric carcinoma or other abdominal malignancies.

Asymmetric shoulder girdle and arm pain can occasionally present as a structural problem simulating cervical nerve root irritation or brachial plexopathy as in thoracic outlet syndrome. This can be seen in lung cancer with apical involvement and brachial plexus compression by a superior sulcus (Pancoast) tumor.

Central Nervous System

Although the CNS is a composite of both brain and spinal cord, only those manifestations related to the brain are discussed here. This includes malignant disease involvement of the brain and those manifestations associated with primary malignancy that give rise to CNS symptoms without a direct metastatic relationship.

DIRECT CEREBRAL MALIGNANCY

Malignant disease can occur in the brain as either a primary tumor or a metastasis from an extracranial primary site. The symptoms noted are referable to the region of the brain involved. Of the extracranial tumors that frequently spread to the brain, lung and breast are the most common. Autopsy studies have shown that of all cerebral metastasis, approximately 65% are multiple in occurrence,[35] providing a rationale for whole brain irradiation as therapy rather than surgery. Surgical therapy is limited to selected situations (true solitary lesions) in metastatic brain disease. In most circumstances, adequate control of symptoms, as well as maintenance of CNS function, are attained with whole brain irradiation until the primary disease progresses.

INDIRECT PARANEOPLASTIC

Various syndromes have been described that affect the CNS indirectly. These syndromes affect the CNS less frequently than they affect the peripheral nervous system.[36] One of the most common syndromes is subacute cerebellar degeneration, which manifests as a progressive symmetric disabling cerebellar failure and clinically includes ataxia and dysarthria.[37]

Other cerebellar features can occur. Dementia is frequently associated with the cerebellar degeneration. There is generally progressive clinical deterioration with an occasional report of clinical improvement with removal of the primary tumor.[36] The most frequent malignancies associated with subacute cerebellar degeneration are lung, prostate, and colorectal cancer. Other dementia syndromes can also occur and are often associated with hematologic malignancies (progressive multifocal leukoencephalopathy).

A number of endocrinologic manifestations of malignancy occur in which there are indirect CNS signs. These are not a result of metastasis but instead are the result of polypeptide hormone-like substances or cytokines produced by the primary tumor. These hormones are autonomous in their production and are not regulated by normal hormonal feedback control. The three most frequent of these syndromes are:

Cushing's syndrome
Syndrome of inappropriate antidiuretic hormone (SIADH)
Nonmetastatic hypercalcemia

The ectopic adrenocorticotropic hormone (ACTH) syndrome (Cushing's) is most commonly associated with lung cancer, especially small cell (oat cell) lung cancer. In small cell cancer of the lung, 25% of patients have either the clinical syndrome or significant elevations of ectopically produced ACTH.[31] This is clinically manifested by the signs of corticoid excess such as:

Muscle weakness
Hypokalemia
Edema
Hyperglycemia
Hypertension
Neurologic syndromes of altered mental status

The same syndrome can occur in other tumors as well. Treatment of the primary tumor is the most effective therapy.

The syndrome of inappropriate antidiuretic hormone also occurs most commonly in lung cancer, especially the small cell variety, with 8–10% of these patients having the clinically evident syndrome.[31] The tumor produces high quantities of the hormone arginine vasopressin (AVP). The major laboratory features are hyponatremia, reduced serum osmolality, and increased urine osmolality relative to serum. The significant clinical symptoms include:

Altered mentation
Confusion
Lethargy
Psychosis
Seizures
Coma

These symptoms can mimic a primary CNS tumor.

Hypercalcemia is the most frequent metabolic complication associated with malignancy. It occurs commonly with:

Breast carcinomas
Lung carcinomas
Renal carcinomas
Head and neck cancers
Multiple myeloma

This entity occurs in approximately 10% of patients with cancer. Fifteen to 20% of this group of patients do not have evidence of bone metastasis.[31] Hypercalcemia is associated with breast carcinoma; in multiple myeloma it is usually secondary to bone metastasis with calcium release from bone into the serum. Lung cancer, especially epidermoid and large cell varieties, and kidney cancer are most frequently associated with the nonmetastatic hypercalcemia. Both of these tumors account for more than 50% of the cases of tumor-produced parathyroid hormone-related peptide (PTHrP). It is not unusual for either of these tumors to present symptoms as a result of hypercalcemia before a diagnosis of malignancy has been made or suspected.

The major clinical signs and symptoms of hypercalcemia occur with serum calcium levels in excess of 14 mg/dL. Serum calcium levels measured as ionized calcium or total calcium must be adjusted by a formula based on serum albumin levels. It is only the ionizable (free or unbound) portion that is clinically significant. The clinical effects of hypercalcemia are predominant on four systems. The gastrointestinal system effects include:

Nausea
Emesis
Anorexia
Constipation

The renal manifestations are polyuria, and polydipsia with a late effect of nephrocalcinosis. Cardiovascular effects include:

Significant ECG alterations
Arrhythmias
Hypertension
Marked increase in digitalis sensitivity

The neurologic effects, which can resemble metastatic CNS disease, include:

Depression
Lethargy
Hyporeflexia
Progressive stupor
Eventual coma
Possible death

Treatment should begin promptly and include intravenous hydration, avoidance of calcium administration, and selected use of osteoclast inhibitors such as mithramycin, calcitonin, and bisphosphates. In addition, definitive treatment of the primary tumor by surgical resection, radiation, or chemotherapy is essential.

Peripheral Nervous System

This section discusses the direct and remote effects of the malignant process from the standpoint of symptoms related to peripheral motor or sensory nerve involvement in the extremities. Although many of these problems have their origin within the CNS, often the end effects manifest themselves peripherally in the extremities. Therefore, these considerations occur from the point of signs and symptoms rather than from origin.

REMOTE PERIPHERAL MANIFESTATIONS

Peripheral neurologic problems are common in the typical cancer patient. The most frequent etiology of these problems is direct invasion by primary or metastatic tumor. Neuropathic symptoms (carcinomatous neuropathy) resulting from remote effects of the malignancy on the peripheral nervous system can occur but are uncommon. In addition to discussing myasthenic syndrome and sensory motor polyneuropathy, this section also describes spinal cord disease with nerve root and plexus involvement.

Myasthenic syndrome, also known as Eaton-Lambert syndrome, is especially associated with small cell lung carcinoma. This disorder is characterized by proximal pelvic girdle muscle weakness. Other muscle symptoms can occur, and other tumors can be associated with it. This syndrome is unlike myasthenia gravis in that the EMG muscle potential and clinical strength improve with repeated stimulation or with exercise.[38–39] The Tensilon test (diagnostic for myasthenia gravis by instant relief of muscle weakness after Tensilon administration) is not responsive as it is with myasthenia gravis. Treatment of this disorder rests essentially with treatment of the primary malignancy (small cell lung cancer with chemotherapy).

Mixed sensory-motor polyneuropathy is most commonly associated with malignancy. This entity is most frequently seen with lung, breast, and gastrointestinal malignancies.[40] The involvement produces distal extremity muscle weakness and wasting of muscles associated with distal sensory loss and areflexia. EMG studies have shown denervation of muscle and slowed nerve conduction time, while histologically, axonal degeneration and demyelination is noted.[36] Recovery is rare.

SPINAL CORD COMPRESSION

Epidural metastasis and spinal cord compression occur in 5–10% of cancer patients.[41] The vertebrae are the most common sites of bone metastasis; this can lead to vertebral collapse and compressive involvement of the spinal cord and nerves. It occurs with great frequency; effects are devastating if the signs and symptoms are not recognized in time to intervene. Patients with vertebral metastasis commonly present to emergency rooms or primary care physicians with low back pain and are seen as having a structural or somatic problem. Spinal cord compression, a true oncologic emergency, must be considered clinically and evaluated carefully. Certain signs should direct one's attention to this consideration, including[41]:

Age older than 50 years
Recent weight loss
Presence of lymphadenopathy
Pain unresponsive to previous treatment measures
Neurologic deficits in a patient with a history of malignancy

Constans et al. reported on a review of 600 cases of spinal metastases with neurologic manifestations and noted 53% had thoracic spine localization, 32% had lumbosacral spine localization, and 15% had localization in the cervical spine.[42] It appears appropriate to recommend x-ray evaluation for patients with thoracic back pain without a known cause. This recommendation does not apply to patients with lower back discomfort, the most common back pain complaint heard by primary care physicians. In the Constans review, the most common primary tumor in males was lung cancer, at 19.17%; the most common primary tumor in females was breast cancer, at 53.31%.[42]

Tumor metastasis to the vertebrae occurs most commonly because of a system of valveless, small veins known as Batson's plexus. These are richly connected to other venous systems with the pelvic, retroperitoneal, extraabdominal, and thoracic areas allowing freedom of movement of tumor cells to implant and metastasize within the spine. Blood flow alone does not account for the osteotropism of some tumors, notably prostate and breast cancers.

The primary presenting symptom of spinal cord compression is back pain; in most cases it is localized to the involved area of vertebral damage. In studies in which x-ray and surgical findings are noted, osteolytic lesions are usually present (71%), with osteoblastic lesions in 21% and mixed lytic-blastic lesions in 8%.[42] The back pain might have been present for days to weeks or longer; rarely is it a major reason why patients seek medical attention. The progression of symptoms to motor weakness, numbness (sensory loss), and finally bladder or rectal dysfunction (autonomic loss) concerns the patient. The entire process has a variable rate of progression. The significant pathophysiologic process is related to spinal cord and nerve infarction as a result of arterial or venous occlusion by the compression process.

As the progression of neural compression occurs, the symptom focus shifts from that of back pain to localization of neurologic symptoms in the extremities with pain, weakness, or numbness. Radiculopathy is identified by pain referred from the primary spinal site, dermatomal sensory changes, and altered deep tendon reflexes. It is common especially in the lower extremities. This process can be bilateral or unilateral. If bilateral, it is not unusual for one side to progress more rapidly than the other. Occasionally, an entire nerve plexus (cervical or lumbar plexopathy) is involved, producing pain or aching in a single extremity only, without a dermatomal pattern.

The anatomic site of the radiculopathy or plexopathy can be determined by the primary tumor. Most cervical spinal cord compression is noted with lung cancer (40%), followed by breast cancer. Brachial plexus involvement occurs most often in association with lung cancer. Apical or superior sulcus tumors of the lung commonly predispose the patient to brachial plexopathy with resulting arm and hand symptoms of pain, swelling, and loss of function.

Lumbar plexopathy most frequently is associated with pelvic tumors, especially colorectal cancer and sarcomas.[43] The symptom complex presented is generally the same as with spinal cord compression, with pain the first and predominant symptom. The pain is radicular in approximately 85% of cases.[44] Plexopathy in the lumbar area can also present as unilateral or bilateral lower extremity symptoms. Specific areas of paresis, paresthesia, or pain can help to localize tumor involvement to a specific portion of the plexus.

Diagnostic tests beyond x-ray films are needed to localize the tumor and to plan therapy. MRI is the modality of choice in spinal cord compression and can often provide the necessary information for treatment planning. When suspicion exists for spinal cord or plexus compression, diagnostic imaging studies should be done quickly.

Initiate treatment for suspected spinal cord compression with corticosteroids such as high dose dexamethasone. Administer it as soon as the diagnosis is suspected and before diagnostic studies are completed. The beneficial effect of steroids might only be short term and can result in pain relief by relieving inflammatory edema. Steroid administration is usually continued through the immediate therapy period and then tapered off. Definitive therapy requires surgical laminectomy and/or radiotherapy. Surgery is preferred in radioresistant tumors (such as renal carcinoma) or in cases of tumor recurrence after previous radiation. Thus far, most radiation results are comparable to surgical results. The responses are variable and must be judged by the degree of symptoms and neurologic deficit with which the patient presents at diagnosis. Most patients with significant paresis or paraplegia at diagnosis do not regain neurologic function. Patients who maintain neurologic function at diagnosis generally retain function after therapy. Consider spinal cord compression in any cancer patient with back pain and/or lower extremity symptoms.

OTHER CAUSES OF PERIPHERAL NEUROPATHY

Other phenomena can produce peripheral neuropathy with direct tumor or paraneoplastic involvement. Neurotoxic chemotherapy (with Vinca alkaloids, cisplatin, taxanes) can produce paresthesia, muscle weakness, and hyporeflexia. Other neuropathic effects have been reported, such as neuronal deposition of amyloid in multiple myeloma, or hemorrhage into nerves in leukemia.

In conclusion, it is not uncommon for malignant tumors to present at onset or through the course of disease progression as neurologic, muscular, or skeletal symptoms. Often the symptoms mimic osteopathic musculoskeletal lesions with or without accompanying neurologic components.

VISCEROSOMATIC-TYPE ONCOLOGIC RESPONSE

Tumor Necrosis Factor (Cachectin)

A variety of cytokines can act as immune system modulators and have been shown in vitro and in vivo to have antitumor effects. These include the interleukins, interferons, and tumor necrosis factor (TNF). TNF can serve as an example of a potential viscerosomatic antineoplastic response. TNF is a polypeptide hormone secreted principally by macrophages.[44] This substance is produced in the body in response to various stimuli, including neoplasms and infection. After attack of an organ or system, it is speculated that the body responds in a self-protective manner by signaling between cells involved in immunity and inflammation.[45] Multiple biologic responses can occur that can be either beneficial or harmful to the body. The responses depend on the level of TNF released, the duration of the exposure, and other factors.[46] Excessive production and exposure associated with infection is believed to lead to tissue destruction and endotoxic shock.[46] Cachexia, frequently associated with malignancy, infection, and other processes, is believed to be secondary to TNF, hence the name cachectin. Antineoplastic activity of TNF has been noted against a wide variety of tumors.[47] The cytolytic effect of TNF is directed toward tumor cells but not normal cells.[44] The mechanism of action might be related to a direct cellular attack as well as indirectly through tumor vascular damage.[47] In addition to these antitumor effects, TNF might also exert mitogenic properties as well as inflammatory properties such as fever induction. TNF appears to be a prime mediator of the immune system interacting with immune responses such as[44]:

Enhanced cytolysis when combined with interferon
Enhancement of macrophage and neutrophil function
Activation of T cells
Controlling some leukocyte precursor differentiation

In addition, evidence now exists that TNF has antibacterial and antiviral properties.

The area of cytokines creates potential treatment opportunities. Combinations with immune modulators or even chemotherapeutic agents are being attempted for possible enhanced synergistic response.[46] Burgers has reported an increased antitumor activity against renal cell carcinoma metastasis in an animal model by combining recombinant human TNF and VP-16 chemotherapy.[47]

TNF is an excellent example in oncology of a somatic response to stimulation of a viscera or organ system by invasion of tumor or infection. The response, in addition, provides evidence for the self-regulatory and self-protective healing capacity of the somatic structure.

PRESENTATION TO PATIENT OF DIAGNOSTIC AND TREATMENT OPTIONS

Use knowledge and understanding of the patient when presenting the diagnosis of cancer and discussing the disease and its prognosis, diagnosis, and treatment options. This aspect of patient care is extremely significant. As an osteopathic physician, one has a distinct advantage in these discussions because of the osteopathic philosophy of treating the whole patient rather than only the disease. Most patients continue to perceive a future with cancer as a short, lonely, painful, and helpless prospect. The initial discussion with the patient and family may be by the oncologist or the primary care physician, using a philosophy based on:

Hope
Realistic goal setting
Honesty
Integrity
Knowledge that the individual is more than his or her disease

It is important to inform the patient and family that the diagnosis is malignancy or cancer. Use of the term tumor should be avoided because it is often confusing and can be deceiving. Ask the patient whether to include the spouse or other family members in the initial discussion. In most instances, the patient already has a strong suspicion and might prefer support from spouse or family. It is important to sit with the patient and discuss the diagnosis in a supportive, unhurried fashion. The understanding and support offered at this time set the tone and pattern for the remainder of the treatment relationship with the patient. A fully informed, trusting, and cooperative patient will, in most cases, remain cooperative and trusting.

After informing the patient of the diagnosis, make a distinction for the patient about the cure and control of disease based on realistic expectations of what is possible. Patients and families need an opportunity to think, ask questions, discuss the diagnosis, and express their feelings. They might feel abandoned if they are hurried through a brief one-sided discussion, informed they will be referred to an oncologist, and hurried on their way before they can ask a question. Ask them what they have been told before beginning the discussion. Speak in lay language no matter what the educational level of the patient. Stress that something positive can be done for the patient. The greatest fear of the patient is that he or she will be sent out being told there is nothing that can be done. Even in the case of a medically untreatable cancer, the patient can be given hope of support, comfort, and caring. A supportive attitude is sometimes difficult for the patient to accept from a family member; this attitude must be conveyed from the physician. If surgery, radiation, or chemotherapy is to be offered, inform the patient, but always accompany this with the information that general supportive care is available at the same time if needed.

In the event of metastatic disease that cannot be cured, stress the potential long-term control from the chemotherapy or radiation to be used. Indicate that the purpose of the systemic therapy is at least to stabilize the disease at present levels and to prevent further growth or spread, if not shrink the disease. Throughout the entire interaction, create an atmosphere of concern for the whole patient rather than only an interest in the disease. The patient is to be cared for while the disease is attacked. Throughout the course of the conversation, do not hesitate to hold the patient's hand, arm, or shoulder, or to pat his or her hand or arm. Patients and families have indicated that touching conveys more sincerity in caring about the whole patient.

Often when discussing therapy, especially chemotherapy, a patient is resistant to discuss treatment options because of unfounded "horror stories" they have heard. It is appropriate to be assertive in encouraging chemotherapy when it has a known good outcome in a particular malignancy and when the likelihood is high of a beneficial effect. Otherwise, therapy, including investigational or cooperative group protocols, can be offered in an objective manner while informing the patient of all benefit and risk potentials. If the patient is strongly opposed to the uncertain benefit of a treatment program, reassure the patient and allay any guilt by informing the patient, and especially the family, that there is no definite right or wrong therapy in many malignancies. This is the reason investigational treatment protocols are available. The right choice is the choice that leaves the patient and family comfortable with their decision and does not create conflict between patient and family, especially in the later phases of the disease process.

The physician must support the patient's choices, unless the patient is depriving himself or herself of proven benefit. This might not apply at the time of initial discussion and presentation of therapy options, but can apply later when searching for a subsequent therapy or when choosing to discontinue an ineffective or toxic therapy. The physician's support of the patient's choices reaffirms the care and importance of the patient in the total treatment of the disease. The patient's needs must be met.

Discussion of prognosis is generally avoided at the initial consultation with the patient. Address this question by a statement indicating the need to wait to observe the response of the planned treatment. The presence or absence of a response and the type of response influence and can change the prognosis.

Often during the initial discussion, it is helpful to sit beside or across from the patient, without a desk separating you, or at the side of the hospital bed. Several strategies create an integral relationship between patient and physician:

Closeness to the patient
Body language
Verbal communication consistent with empathic discussion of support and concern
Agreement to work as a partner in treating the patient

The key element of the future relationship with a patient must be the treatment of the whole patient rather than a diseased organ. The patient must know that throughout the course of the disease and treatment, the less than can be done for the disease, the more that is done for the patient.

Often at the initial consultation or at subsequent visits after discussion of response or suggested changes in treatment protocol, the patient has a desire to take the physician's hand or embrace the physician in gratitude. One may participate in this gesture with the patient. Patients who have been treated with the holistic philosophy discussed here have been observed to have improved longevity and function over comparable patients who have been treated with only an objective, rigid, scientific philosophy of an investigational study without personalization (Michael I. Opipari, personal observation).

SUPPORTIVE CARE OF CANCER PATIENT

Equally as important as the specific antineoplastic therapy is the supportive care that the patient might require at some time. For patients who decline specific antitumor therapy or who terminate such therapy after a trial, supportive care is of paramount importance during the patients' remaining life with the disease.

Supportive care consists predominantly of three categories:

Symptom control and pain relief
Blood and blood products
General supportive medical care

The latter category includes:

Infection prevention and treatment
Nutrition support
Rehabilitative support

Psychosocial support
Legal support
Pastoral care support

The last three are all components of hospice care.

In the following sections, the discussion of medical management of pain control, use of blood and its products, nutrition, and infection therapy is limited. These subjects are well-reviewed and documented in the medical literature. These subjects are discussed here instead from the philosophic viewpoint of a medical oncologist with an osteopathic background and experience.

Symptom and Pain Relief

Symptoms other than pain and discomfort are important to the cancer patient. Anxiety and apprehension can be addressed by spending time in discussion with the physician, social worker, nurse, psychiatrist, or psychologist. Simple treatment program adjustments can be made to correct the symptom. Pain should always be treated. This is the least a physician can do for a patient, especially if the disease cannot be cured. The patient must not be forsaken in favor of the disease process. Many traditional modalities are available to treat pain, including analgesics and various delivery methods to improve effectiveness (intrathecal or intraventricular injections, continuous infusion pumps, self-delivery pumps, etc.). In addition, neurosurgical procedures such as cordotomy and rhizotomy are available, as are anesthetic blocks.

Although no scientific data are yet available, another modality is also useful for selected patients to alleviate anxiety and pain symptoms. Simple, gentle, soft tissue manipulation without any pressure or thrust can be effective, especially for late-stage, inactive, and bed-bound patients. The procedure permits the physician to touch the patient and commit time to care for the patient in addition to treating the disease.

Blood and Blood Products

Red blood cell transfusions to correct anemia, granulocyte transfusions during prolonged suppression in sepsis, and platelet transfusions to prevent bleeding during bone marrow suppression are all supportive measures occasionally needed. These transfusions might be needed during periods of disease complications or during toxicity from systemic therapy. This support is often lifesaving. Continued support with expensive or scarce blood products must be balanced, however, with the benefit to be attained for end-stage patients in the terminal phase of the disease.

General Supportive Care

Nutritional support of the patient with malignancy is essential, whether the patient is actively being treated or not. Malnutrition is part of a general failure to thrive syndrome commonly associated with cancer. The patient might need other supportive care such as antibiotics, blood products, and psychosocial support to assist with nutrition. In addition, nutritional counseling with a dietitian can be helpful, as well as nutritional supplements that are available as commercial products for high-protein enteral support. Total parenteral nutrition administered through percutaneous or surgically placed venous access can also be used for hospitalized patients for whom the enteral approach is not possible because of small intestine problems or other specific circumstances.

Antiinfective therapy can be lifesaving during periods of increased risk such as granulocytopenia after chemotherapy. It can also be provided as combination antibiotic therapy to treat documented infection, sepsis, or fever during granulocytopenia. Specific antimicrobial therapy is guided by culture and sensitivity results.

Movement and bowel or bladder functions are areas of general supportive care not only for the cancer patient but also for any critically ill or geriatric patient. Encourage all patients to be active out of bed as much as possible. A positive attitude on the patient's part can be maintained to a greater degree with increased mobility that, in turn, can lessen stress and anxiety and even support the immune system in its attack on the disease. In addition, staying active enhances venous blood return and reduces the risk of venous thrombosis, decubitus ulceration, edema, and constipation. Many cancer patients have prolonged periods of bed rest because of bone pain, pathologic fracture, or paraplegia as a result of spinal cord compressive disease. For these patients, activity is essential to maintain even minimal functional ability. If assisted ambulation is possible, encourage it. If ambulation is impossible because of pain, fracture, weakness, or neurologic deficit, chair sitting might be possible. For the totally bed-bound patient, offer side-to-side moving with mild soft tissue manipulation.

Bowel function can be maintained with appropriate hydration, nutrition, and activity. Stool softeners and other medications or maneuvers such as manual (suppository or digital) stimulation can be used. Constipation can be uncomfortable for an immobile patient, especially one with bone pain or fracture.

Bladder function and control are also essential for patients confined to bed. If incontinence is present, an indwelling catheter can be useful. Every attempt should be made to remove the catheter and resume normal function if possible. If it is not necessary, a catheter only keeps patients tied to a bed and inactive for prolonged periods and restricts the benefits of physical activity.

Rehabilitative care is frequently an essential element in symptomatic and supportive management of the cancer patient. Rehabilitation can include physical, occupational, and speech therapy and might be indicated after management of spinal cord compression syndrome, cerebral metastasis, and head and neck malignancies. Often rehabilitative care assists with functional palliation for patients who have 6 months or more of life expectancy.

Hospice care is becoming widely recognized and used as an effective modality in the care of terminal persons. Hospice focuses on meeting the needs of the patient and the family after there is no longer effective therapy for the disease. The hospice philosophy is centered on effective pain and symptom management while also meeting other physical, social, emotional, and spiritual needs with the aid of a multidisciplinary team of specialists in each area. The patient is maintained in an environment of warmth and caring with family, in the home, except when this is not possible or is unavailable. Dealing with pain and preparation for death is extremely difficult or impossible for some physicians; it represents a deficiency in medical training. Hospices meet this need so that death can be accepted as a natural phase of life.

PHILOSOPHIC PRINCIPLES OF CARE OF THE CANCER PATIENT

Traditional cancer therapy includes surgery, radiation therapy, and drug therapy. Continue to use each and all of these modalities, but never forget to care for the person rather than the tumor. Patient decisions and actions are often based on their thoughts, feelings, and perceptions.

To Treat Or Not To Treat

Many physicians assume that all cancer must be treated, regardless of whether there is any effective treatment to offer. Remember, we must treat every patient, but we have no need to treat every cancer. In many cases, more benefit can be provided to the patient with careful understanding, supportive therapy, and meeting his or her needs than with definitive antineoplastic therapy. Honesty with the patient is necessary—honesty regarding the availability of effective treatment modalities and regarding cure. Discuss a life-threatening disease such as metastatic renal cell cancer in a positive and optimistic fashion. Inform the patient of the unpredictable natural history of the disease, which can have long-term stable control in some patients. Discuss and offer immunotherapeutics such as interferon and IL-2 if the patient is an appropriate candidate. The patient, however, must be reassured that the physician is available throughout the treatment course. Reassure patients that they are not permitted to remain uncomfortable and that multiple modalities are available for relief of discomfort. Reassure them that the physician will discuss all decisions regarding therapy with them and will assist them in decision making. Inform and support the family if the patient wishes. Throughout the discussion, which can become more frequent and personal as the relationship develops, touching the patient is important. The patient must leave the physician after each visit confident that a partnership has developed.

Touching As Communication

Some patients complain that the only time a physician has touched them in the past was in the process of physical examination or in placing a stethoscope on their chest. Cancer patients feel comforted by an appropriate touch of a hand or even, on occasion, a tear shed with theirs. Touching is a nonverbal communication with the patient that says, "I recognize you as a whole person, not only a diseased body or organ or

an interesting case." Recognition of the whole person encompassing the cancer is to recognize the integration of all of the body systems. No system can alone become diseased or healthy without impact or benefit to the whole person or other systems. They must all get well and survive together. The basic osteopathic philosophy emphasizes the need to treat the person as a whole. This approach must consider the patient with the disease as well as the patient's environment. The full embodiment of supportive care facilitates patient care and provides patient benefit to a greater degree than does traditional anticancer therapy.

STRESS AND TREATMENT AS MODULATORS OF BIOLOGIC RESPONSE

Psychoneurobiology examines the interrelationships between emotions, the CNS, and somatic cellular biologic responses. There is little argument that the immune system plays a significant role in the initiation and course of malignant disease. The role of T-cell and B-cell lymphocytes, helper, suppressor, and natural killer (NK) cells together with interferons has been extensively reviewed in the literature. The connection between the CNS and the systemic response to illness is often mediated by the endocrine system with the assistance of cortisol, the endogenous opiates (endorphins and enkephalins), and other steroids and hormones that regulate some aspects of cellular biologic response.[48] Nerve endings have been demonstrated within lymphoid organs (nodes and spleen). In addition, receptors have been demonstrated on the surface of lymphocytes for hormones such as ACTH.[48] It is conceivable that certain stresses on the human body alter the biologic response in terms of enhanced or suppressed output or function of substances including interferon, NK cells, etc.[49–50]

One can then speculate on the effect of the cancer process, which can produce further suppression of an already suppressed immune system. Although interesting to speculate, the concept of immunologic surveillance has not been confirmed in clinical or human research definitively, particularly as applied to the effect of stressors. Stress and anxiety can lead to increased output of cortisol and catecholamines through pituitary ACTH. The cortisol then can initiate an immune suppressive response.[48,51] Glaser and Glaser have demonstrated depressed interferon production by leukocytes concomitant with a reduced interferon regulation of NK activity at times of increased stress.[52] The endogenous opiate polypeptides, β-endorphin, and the enkephalins have been demonstrated to enhance NK cell production and activity as well as inhibit metastasis in laboratory animals.[53–54]

Although no definitive scientific evidence yet exists, it appears possible that alterations in the emotional state and spirit of the cancer patient, assisted by the physician through optimism, support, and empathy, can result in an enhanced biologic response. This alteration in the patient's emotional status can be produced by recognition and treatment of the whole person. The oncologist frequently encounters a patient with advanced metastatic disease who, without specific antitumor therapy, is able to continue to live and function while waiting for a child to graduate or be married or to witness a grandchild's birth. The emotional state and the will to live apparently affect the biologic behavior of the disease and the well-being of the patient.

OSTEOPATHIC APPROACH

Many osteopathic physicians have mistakenly believed that manipulative treatment is contraindicated for patients with cancer. While this might be true for some techniques or for some patients, other techniques can be helpful for:

Relieving pain
Improving visceral function
Reducing tension and stress
Improving the doctor–patient relationship through touch

This section reviews the contraindications, indications, and specific techniques for osteopathic manipulative treatment (OMT) of the patient with cancer.

Contraindications for OMT

While OMT in general is not contraindicated, treatment of the area immediately surrounding a cancer is contraindicated because of the risk of hematogenous spread. This is particularly true for the vertebral column where Batson's venous plexus, a system of valveless vessels anastomosing with brain and pelvic veins, provides a two-way route of metastasis. OMT for the entire vertebral column is therefore contraindicated when there is known or suspected vertebral tumor. Suspect a primary or metastatic vertebral cancer when there is acute back pain associated with systemic symptoms such as:

Fever
Chills
Night sweats
Fatigue
Weight loss

Persistent back pain despite adequate treatment also raises a possibility of vertebral tumor. Back pain in a patient with another known cancer or a suspected cancer at a site that commonly metastasizes to the spinal column should raise the index of suspicion (Table 35.1).

Two types of manipulative techniques do pose some risk when used for the cancer patient. Manipulative techniques that are contraindicated in oncology patients include:

Thrust near bone or joint cancer
Lymphatic pumps
Any technique in immediate vicinity of cancer

High-velocity low-amplitude (HVLA) techniques have been reported to cause pathologic rib fractures in patients with osteoporosis. Presumably, these thrust techniques could result in fracture of a rib or other bone weakened by a primary or metastatic tumor. HVLA technique is therefore contraindicated for

Table 35.1
Primary Malignancies That Commonly Metastasize to Vertebral Column and Spinal Cord, Listed In Order of Frequency

Vertebrae	Spinal Cord
Breast	Lung
Prostate	Breast
Lung	Colon
Kidney	Sarcoma
Thyroid	

joints associated with bones that have known or possible cancer.[55] Thrust technique can be safely applied to the oncology patient as long as metastasis to the area being considered for treatment has been ruled out by MRI, CT scan, or bone scan. Other techniques such as muscle energy or indirect techniques can be safely applied for joint somatic dysfunction even when there is documented bony involvement, as long as there is no direct extension of tumor into the area being treated.

The other contraindicated technique for patients with known or suspected cancer are the lymphatic pumps, including the thoracic pump and the pedal or Dalrumple pump. Because one route of metastasis is lymphogenous spread, these active lymphatic pump techniques could theoretically contribute to spread of cancer, although this has never been documented by animal studies or case reports. Passive lymphatic treatment using indirect techniques for the thoracic outlet and inlet followed by pectoralis lift technique can be safely substituted for an active pump in cancer patients with pneumonia, congestive heart failure, or other problems for which a lymphatic pump is considered.[56]

Indications for OMT

OMT, if judiciously applied, can be a valuable tool for the care of oncology patients, who have the same potential for noncancer somatic dysfunction and pain as anyone else but have more psychosocial stress. In addition, a patient with cancer can be experiencing postsurgical pain as well as cancer pain. Furthermore, a terminal patient can have immobility-related visceral dysfunction amenable to OMT. Indications for OMT in cancer patients include:

Pain and somatic dysfunction
Constipation
Atelectasis
Pneumonia
Postsurgical lymphedema

For patients with known cancer, the primary indication for OMT is musculoskeletal pain associated with somatic dysfunction but not directly related to the tumor. The somatic dysfunction can be unrelated to or secondary to the cancer or its treatment. For instance, a patient who underwent median sternotomy and resection of a lung cancer might develop thoracic and intercostal pain from a preexisting somatic dysfunction made worse by the surgery, from a viscerosomatic reflex from the lung to the thoracic spine, or from surgical trauma to the costovertebral or costochondral joints. The choice of techniques for treating somatic dysfunction in cancer patients with musculoskeletal pain is highly individualized. It depends on:

Patient's age
Severity of illness
Previous injuries
Other diseases
Time since surgery

In general, indirect methods such as myofascial release and counterstrain techniques are more applicable when there is acute or severe illness and with advancing age. Direct methods such as thrust and muscle energy should be reserved for stable patients and when metastasis to the area being treated has been definitively ruled out.

OMT is also indicated for prevention or treatment of immobility-related complications in bedridden terminal cancer patients. Prolonged immobility can cause atelectasis predisposing to pneumonia or constipation, which might already be present as a side effect of narcotic analgesics. To prevent and treat atelectasis or constipation, thoracolumbar soft tissue and rib-raising treatment can be applied daily, in many cases by family members instructed to do these techniques at home. The initiation of rib raising should be preceded by treatment of significant vertebral and rib somatic dysfunction to prevent exacerbation of visceral facilitation.

Extremity lymphedema with swelling and pain, especially common after radical mastectomy for breast cancer, can be helped by OMT. Effleurage of the extremity following indirect or muscle energy treatment of the thoracic inlet and shoulder girdle for arm edema can be applied once or twice a week. Likewise, for leg lymphedema, the manipulative procedure can be directed to the diaphragmatic structures as well as to the thoracic inlet. The intent is to relieve lymph flow by normalizing fascial relationships. Thoracic or pedal pumps that could provide further lymphatic drainage are contraindicated unless complete surgical cure of the cancer has been achieved, except in end-stage patients for palliation and comfort.

Pain, immobility and its consequences, and postsurgical lymphedema are common problems in cancer patients that can be readily treated with OMT. An additional benefit of treatment is an improved sense of well-being that is reported by many patients. It is entirely possible that this period of well-being is the result of enhancement of the immune system with elevated output of cellular immune substances, NK cells, or endogenous opiates. It has been demonstrated that prognosis can be predicted for patients with breast cancer by the sustained level of natural killer activity.[57] A future study to measure serum and CSF levels of various immune substances in response to OMT would be an invaluable addition to the osteopathic literature.

CONCLUSION

The osteopathic physician has a special opportunity and obligation to treat the cancer patient as a whole person, not just a disease. Practitioners of the osteopathic approach, with its emphasis on touch and healing, can provide cancer patients and their families with the information and support they need.

ACKNOWLEDGMENT

David Reed Beatty, DO, is greatly appreciated for his assistance in reviewing this chapter and for providing material for the section "Osteopathic Manipulative Treatment for the Cancer Patient."

REFERENCES

1. Bean RB, Bean WB. *Sir William Osler—Aphorisms.* New York, NY: Henry Schuman Inc; 1950.
2. Parker SL, Tony T, Bolder S, Wingo PA. Cancer statistics. American Cancer Society. *CA-A Cancer Journal for Clinicians.* 1996;46:1.
3. Cherukuri SV, Johenning PW, Ram MD. Systemic effects of hypernephroma. *Urology.* 1977;10:93–97.
4. Bellinger MF, Koontz WW, Smith MJV. Renal cell carcinoma: twenty years of experience. *VA Med Mon.* 1979;106:819–824.
5. Paulson DF, Perez CA, Anderson T. Genito-urinary malignancies. In: DeVita VT, Hellman S, Rosenberg SA, eds. *Cancer: Principles and Practice of Oncology.* Philadelphia, Penn: JB Lippincott; 1982; 23:733.
6. Paulson DF, Perez CA, Anderson T. Genito-urinary malignancies. In: DeVita VT, Hellman S, Rosenberg SA, eds. *Cancer: Principles and Practice of Oncology.* Philadelphia, Penn: JB Lippincott; 1982; 23:733.
7. Chandler RW, Schulman I, Moore TM. Renal cell carcinoma presenting as a skeletal mass: a case report. *Clin Orthop Relat Res.* 1979; 145:227–229.
8. Chisolm GD. The systemic effects of malignant renal tumors. *Br J Urol.* 1971;43:687–700.
9. Richie JP, Garneck MB. Primary renal and ureteral cancer. In: Rieselbach RE, Garnick ME, eds. *Cancer and the Kidney.* Philadelphia, Penn: Lea & Febiger; 1982;17:665.
10. DeVita VT, Hellman S, Rosenberg SA. *Cancer: Principles and Practice of Oncology.* Philadelphia, Penn: JB Lippincott; 1993;23:673.
11. DeVita VT, Hellman S, Rosenberg SA. *Cancer: Principles and Practice of Oncology.* Philadelphia, Penn: JB Lippincott; 1993;24:731.
12. Alexander RW, Upp JR, Poston GJ, Gupta V, Townsend CM, Thompson JC. Effects of bombesin on growth of human small cell lung carcinoma in vivo. *Cancer Res.* 1988;48:1439–1441.
13. Sunday ME. Weekly clinicopathological exercises, case 5-1986. *N Engl J Med.* 1986;314(6):375.
14. Holland JF, Frei E, Bast R, Kufe D, et al. *Cancer Medicine.* Philadelphia, Penn: Lea & Febiger; 1993;28:1285.
15. Tula CJ, Berman L, Alexanian R. Connective tissue disease manifested as multiple myeloma. *South Med J.* 1984;77:1580–1581.
16. Hoffman R, Benz EJ, Shattil SJ, Furie B, Cohen HJ, Silberstein LE. *Hematology, Basic Principles and Practice.* New York, NY: Churchill Livingstone; 1991:1026–1031.

17. Batson OV. The function of the vertebral veins and their role in the spread of metastases. *Ann Surg.* 1940;112(1):138–148.

18. Batson OV. The role of the vertebral veins in metastatic processes. *Ann Intern Med.* 1942;16:38–45.

19. Hendrickson FR, Sheinkop MB. Management of osseous metastases. *Semin Oncol.* 1975;2:399–404.

20. Cadman E, Bertino JR. Chemotherapy of skeletal metastases. *Int J Radiat Oncol Biol Phys.* 1976;1:1211–1215.

21. Behallia KS. Metastatic disease of the spine. *Clin Orthop.* 1970; 73:52–60.

22. Drew M, Dickson RB. Osseous complications of malignancy. In: Lokich JJ, ed. *Clinical Cancer Medicine: Treatment Tactics.* Boston, Mass: GK Hall; 1980:97.

23. Berrettoni BA, Carter JR. Mechanisms of cancer metastasis to bone. *J Bone Joint Surg.* 1986;68-A(2):308–312.

24. Swanson DA, Bernardino ME. "Silent" osseous metastasis in renal cell carcinoma: value of computerized tomography. *Urology.* 1982; 20(2):208–212.

25. Willis RA. *The Spread of Tumours in the Human Body.* 3rd ed. London, England: Butterworths; 1973:259–268.

26. Smalley RV. The management of disseminated breast cancer. In: Carter SK, Glatstein E, Livingston RB, eds. *Principles of Cancer Treatment.* New York, NY: McGraw-Hill; 1982:327–341.

27. Schaller J. Arthritis as a presenting manifestation of malignancy in children. *J Pediatr.* 1972;81(4):793–797.

28. Karten I, Bartfeld H. Bronchogenic carcinoma simulating early rheumatoid arthritis. *JAMA.* 1962;162:170–172.

29. Ritch PJ, Hansen RM, Collier BD. Metastatic renal cell carcinoma presenting as shoulder arthritis. *Cancer.* 1983;51:968–972.

30. Jao JY, Barlow JJ, Krant MJ. Pulmonary hypertrophic osteoarthropathy, spider angiomata and estrogen hyperexcretion in neoplasia. *Ann Intern Med.* 1969;70:581.

31. Minna JD, Higgins GA, Glatstein EJ. Cancer of the lung. In: DeVita VT, Hellman S, Rosenberg SA, eds. *Cancer: Principles and Practice of Oncology.* Philadelphia, Penn: JB Lippincott; 1982;14:396–474.

32. Schumacher H Jr. Articular manifestations of hypertrophic pulmonary osteoarthropathy in bronchogenic carcinoma. *Arthritis Rheum.* 1976;18:629–636.

33. Rooney TW. Musculoskeletal manifestations associated with malignancy. *Osteopath Ann.* 1983;11(10):437–442.

34. Alburquerque TL, Ortin A, Cacho J. Metastases in deep calf muscles as first manifestation of bronchus adenocarcinoma. *Am J Med.* 1987; 83:606–607.

35. Sugarbaker PH, Dunnick NR, Sugarbaker E. Diagnosis and staging. In: DeVita VT, Hellman S, Rosenberg SA, eds. *Cancer: Principles and Practice of Oncology.* Philadelphia, Penn: JB Lippincott; 1982; 11:232.

36. Riddoch D. Neurological manifestations of cancer. *Practitioner.* 1981;225:819–826.

37. Brain WR, Wilkinson M. Subacute cerebellar degeneration associated with neoplasms. *Brain.* 1965;88:465.

38. Lambert EH, Eaton LM, Rooke ED. Defect of neuromuscular condition associated with malignant neoplasms. *Am J Physiol.* 1956; 187:612.

39. Lambert EH, Rooke ED. Myasthenic state and lung cancer. In: Brain WR, Norris FH Jr, eds. *The Remote Effects of Cancer on the Nervous System.* New York, NY: Grune and Stratton; 1965:67–80.

40. Croft PB, Urich H, Wilkinson M. Peripheral neuropathy of sensorimotor type associated with malignant disease. *Brain.* 1967;90:31–66.

41. Bates DW, Reuler JB. Back pain and epidural spinal cord compression. *J Gen Intern Med.* 1988;3:191–197.

42. Constans JP, DeDiviths E, Donzelli R, Spaziante R, Meder JF, Haye C. Spinal metastasis with neurological manifestations. *J Neurosurg.* 1983;59:111–118.

43. Jaeckle KA, Young DF, Foley KM. The natural history of lumbosacral plexopathy in cancer. *Neurology.* 1985;35:8–15.

44. Van Der Merwe PA. Tumor necrosis factor. *S Afr Med J.* 1988; 74:411–417.

45. Abraham E. Tumor necrosis factor. *Crit Care Med.* 1989;17:590–591.

46. Tracey KJ, Vlassara H, Cerami A. Cachectin/tumor necrosis factor. *Lancet.* 1989;1:1122–1126.

47. Burgers JK, Marshall FF, Isaacs JT. Enhanced anti-tumor effects of recombinant human tumor necrosis factor plus VP-16 on metastatic renal cell carcinoma in a xenograft model. *J Urol.* 1989;142:160–164.

48. Glaser R, Kiecolt-Glaser J. Stress-associated immune suppression and acquired immune deficiency syndrome (AIDS). *Adv Biochem Psychopharmacol.* 1988;44:203–215.

49. Glaser R, Kiecolt-Glaser JK, Stout K, Tarr KL, Speicher CE, Holliday JE. Stress-related impairments in cellular immunity. *Psychiatry Res.* November 1985;16(3):233–239.

50. Glaser R, Kiecolt-Glaser JK. Stress and immune function. *Clin Neuropharmacol.* 1986;9(suppl 4):485–487.

51. Southam CM. Emotions, immunology and cancer: how might the psyche influence neoplasia? *Ann NY Acad Sci.* 1969;164(2):473–475.

52. Glaser R, Rice J, Stout JC, Speicher CE, Kiecolt-Glaser JK. Stress depresses interferon production by leukocytes concomitant with a decrease in natural killer cell activity. *Behav Neurosci.* 1986; 100(5):675–678.

53. Faith RE. Inhibition of pulmonary metastasis and enhancement of natural killer cell activity by methionine-enkephalin. *Brain Behav Immun.* 1988;2:114–122.

54. Williamson SA, Knight RA, Lightman SL, Hobbs JR. Differential effects of B-endorphin fragments on human natural killing. *Brain Behav Immun.* 1987;1:329–335.

55. Kuchera WA, Kuchera ML. *Osteopathic Principles in Practice.* 2nd ed. Kirksville, Mo: KCOM Press; 1992:295.

56. Kuchera ML, Kuchera WA. *Osteopathic Considerations in Systemic Dysfunction.* 2nd ed. Kirksville, Mo: KCOM Press; 1992:28.

57. Levy S, Herberman R, Lippman M, d'Angelo T. Correlation of stress factors with sustained depression of natural killer cell activity and predicted prognosis in patients with breast cancer. *J Clin Oncol.* 1987;5(3):348–353.

36. Physical Medicine and Rehabilitation

NEIL SPIEGEL

Key Concepts

- **Therapeutic modalities, including heat, cold, electrical stimulation, osteopathic manipulative treatment, trigger point injections, and acupuncture**

- **Therapeutic exercise**

- **Uses of orthotics and prosthetics**

- **Electromyography and nerve conduction studies**

Physical medicine and rehabilitation, also known as physiatry, can be broadly defined as that branch of health care that delivers care to the disabled population. *"Rehabilitation is defined as the development of a person to the fullest physical, psychological, social, vocational, avocational, and educational potential consistent with his or her physiological anatomic impairment and environmental limitations."*[1] The common "disabilities" encountered by physiatrists are:

Orthopaedic
Neurologic
Neuromuscular
Cardiovascular
Pulmonary

The principal role of the physiatrist is to act as both physician and allied health team coordinator. This team also includes:

Physical and occupational therapists
Speech pathologists
Psychologists
Social workers
Rehabilitation nurses
Vocational counselors
Nutritionists

An essential activity of the physiatrist is to establish lines of communication among the team, patient, family members, other involved physicians, employer, and third-party payors if necessary. Assess any disability with a fundamental osteopathically oriented structure–function concept because treatment goals must actively involve patients in their own self-healing processes as they move toward independence and autonomy.

Impairment is defined as the loss of, the loss of use of, or the derangement of any body part, system, or function.[2] Disability is defined as loss of function(s) together with effects on one's quality of life. Disability includes loss of the individual's capacity to meet personal, social, or occupational demands, or to meet statutory or regulatory requirements.[2] Handicap is a disadvantage for a given individual resulting from an impairment or a disability that limits or prevents the fulfillment of a normal role (depending on the age, sex, and social and cultural factors) for that individual.[1] These concepts are important because rehabilitation focuses on the disability and handicap in addition to the impairment. The existence of impairment does not necessitate disability. One can have a severe limp, for example, without being functionally disabled.

THERAPEUTIC MODALITIES

The physiatrist often uses several modalities in the management of various disorders. Heat, cold, electrical stimulation, and osteopathic manipulative treatments (OMT) are commonly prescribed:

To manage acute and chronic pain
To augment strengthening following central and peripheral nerve injuries
To augment skin and bone healing, repair, and remodeling

These modalities are most effective when used with other therapeutic strategies in a total approach.

Therapeutic Heat

Apply therapeutic heat using principles of conduction, convection, or conversion, and to penetrating, superficial, or deep depths (Table 36.1). Superficial heating by conduction includes the use of hot (hydrocollator) packs and paraffin. Hydrotherapy uses principles of convection as water flows over body surfaces. Deep heating methods raise temperatures by:

Conversion
Microwaves
Short waves
Ultrasound
Laser energy

In general, heat increases collagen tissue extensibility by changing its viscoelastic properties.[3] It is most effective when used with concomitant and posttreatment stretching. Joint stiffness decreases, blood flow increases, and hypertonic muscles relax because of decreased muscle spindle sensitivity,[3] while inflammatory infiltrates, exudates, and edema are reduced. Counterirritant effects often decrease pain, possibly by increasing endorphins.[3]

**Table 36.1
Heating Modalities Subdivided According to
Primary Mode of Transfer**

Primary Mode of Heat Transfer	Modality	
Conduction	Hot packs	
	Paraffin bath	
Convection	Fluidotherapy	
	Hydrotherapy	Superficial heat
	Moist air	
Conversion	Radiant heat	
	Laser	
	Microwave	
	Shortwave	Deep heat
	Ultrasound	

Reprinted with permission from Lehmann JF, Basmajian JV. *Therapeutic Heat and Cold.* 4th ed. Baltimore, Md: Williams & Wilkins; 1990:444.

Contraindications to therapeutic heat include:

Heating of anesthetized sites because of poor patient monitoring and potential for tissue breakdowns
Inadequate blood supply
Bleeding tendencies
Malignancy at treatment site (not to be confused with hyperthermic treatments for certain cancers)
Fluid-filled sacs at risk for swelling or rupture
Male gonads (because of damage to spermatogenesis)
A developing fetus

Figure 36.1 outlines the change in temperature with time at various depths below the surface of the skin during application of a hydrocollator pack.

Therapeutic Cold

Therapeutic cold is commonly used for anesthetizing and relaxing acutely hypertonic muscles, minimizing the effects of mechanical trauma and bruising, burns, pain in general, and some types of arthritis. Theoretically, cold decreases muscle tone by lowering muscle spindle sensitivity. Figure 36.2 demonstrates the effect cooling has on the amplitude of ankle clonus.[3] Nerve conduction decreases, thereby slowing synaptic and myoneural junction activities, which, in turn, alter descending central neural effects. Cold also decreases swelling and bleeding because of vasoconstriction. It indirectly changes sympathetic tone, making it useful in pain control.

Figures 36.3 and 36.4 demonstrate the change in temperature of the skin, subcutaneous tissue, and muscle during the application of ice on a human thigh. The change in temperature at the muscle level decreases with increased thickness of the subcutaneous tissue.[3]

Electrical Stimulation

Physiologic responses to electrical stimulation include:

Relaxation of hypertonic muscles
Endorphin production[4]

Circulation enhancement by muscle contractions
Immune system responses[4]

Recently, the controversial use of electrical stimulation to augment strength training has been employed by some clinicians. However, several studies fail to support any advantage of electrical stimulation over conventional strength training as long as the individual can perform a maximum voluntary contraction (i.e., when the nerve supplies are intact).[4] Tables 36.2 and 36.3 provide various indications and uses for transcutaneous electrical nerve stimulation (TENS). Contraindications include fresh fractures, bleeding, phlebitis, and demand pacemakers.

Osteopathic Manipulative Treatment and Manual Medicine

Musculoskeletal pain syndromes are frequently the reason for a consultation with a specialist in physical medicine and rehabilitation. In these syndromes, the musculoskeletal system may be involved directly or indirectly through reflex mechanisms in which many other organ systems may be compromised. A detailed osteopathic structural examination assists in the diagnosis. Manual OMT management procedures are often effective in the treatment.[5] Whether used by physicians or allied health professionals, OMT has an important role in the rehabilitation of the disabled. Examples of clinical use are detailed in the case histories presented later in this chapter. Manual treatments and peripheral stimulation techniques are commonly used by physical or occupational therapists to treat neurologic conditions, such as encouraging active motion in a hemiparetic shoulder or attempting to desensitize the distal stump of an amputated limb. How these treatments work has been the subject of much speculation. Generally, it appears that both central and peripheral inhibitory reflexes are activated through stimulation of mechanoreceptors.

Trigger Point Injections and Acupuncture

Physiatrists commonly use both trigger point injections and acupuncture to treat pain syndromes. Acupoints relevant to a particular condition are generally tender to palpation. Melzack, Stillwell, and Fox demonstrated a high degree of correspondence between trigger points and acupuncture points (71%).[6] Trigger points are one of the hallmarks of some myofascial pain syndromes. They are defined as a hardened or fibrotic band within a muscle that is tender to palpation and that usually refers pain to a reference zone (Fig. 36.5). Figure 36.6 demonstrates the anatomy of a taut band/trigger point.[7]

Treatment strategies can include injection of the trigger points with local anesthetic[5] or the use of acupuncture[8] or acupressure (local pressure). There are not yet quality controlled studies about these strategies in the literature.

THERAPEUTIC EXERCISE

The exercise prescription is often the responsibility of the physiatrist, since exercise plays a role in almost every aspect of the

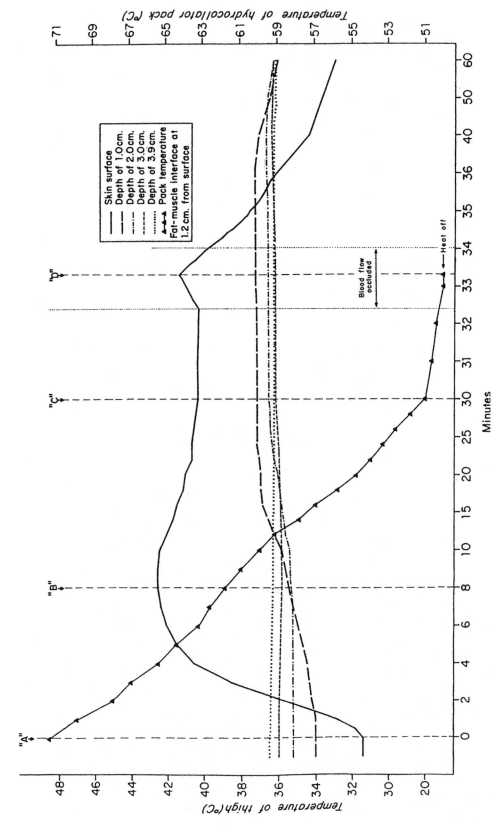

Figure 36.1. Temperatures recorded in the human thigh and heat source during application of a hydrocollator pack. A, Temperature distribution before heat is applied. B, Peak temperature at skin surface. C, Temperature equilibrium approached throughout specimen. D, Blood flow obstructed by tourniquet just before heat is discontinued. (Reprinted with permission from Lehmann JF, Silverman DR, Baum BA, Kirk NL, Johnston VC. Temperature distributions in the human thigh produced by infrared, hot pack, and microwave applications. *Arch Phys Med Rehabil.* 1966;47:291–299.)

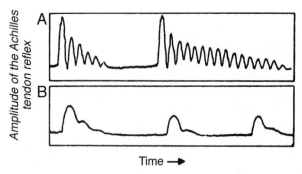

Figure 36.2. Effect of cooling on amplitude of ankle clonus before (A) and after (B) 20 minutes of cold application. (Reprinted with permission from Petajan RH, Watts N. Effect of cooling on the triceps surae reflex. *Am J Phys Med.* 1962;41:240–251.)

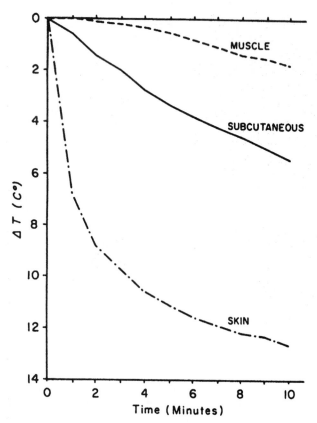

Figure 36.3. Change in temperature of skin, subcutaneous tissue, and muscle during application of ice on human thigh with less than 1 cm of subcutaneous fat. (Reprinted with permission from Lehmann J, de Lateur BJ. Therapeutic heat. In: Lehmann JF, ed. *Therapeutic Heat and Cold.* 3rd ed. Baltimore, Md: Williams & Wilkins; 1982.)

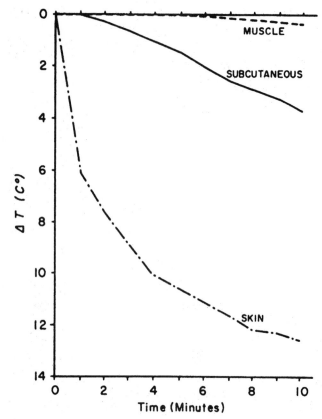

Figure 36.4. Change in temperature of skin, subcutaneous tissue, and muscle during application of ice on human thigh with greater than 2 cm of subcutaneous fat. (Reprinted with permission from Lehmann JF, de Lateur BJ. Therapeutic heat. In: Lehmann JF, ed. *Therapeutic Heat and Cold.* 3rd ed. Baltimore, Md: Williams & Wilkins; 1982.)

rehabilitation process.[7] *"Therapeutic exercise may be defined as the prescription of bodily movement to correct an impairment, improve musculoskeletal and cardiovascular function, or maintain a state of well-being."*[9]

Basic exercise to maintain or regain mobility and range of motion includes passive, active, and active-assisted exercise. Passive motion means that the therapist is providing the entire force and the patient is "passive." The intensity of the force varies depending on the diagnosis. For example, in a patient with acute rheumatoid arthritis, passive range of motion should be carried out slowly and gently. If range of motion is not maintained, irreversible contractures can develop.[10] Active range of motion is movement performed by the patient without the assistance of a therapist. An example is self-stretching exercise to improve flexibility after a period of immobilization. Stretching exercise is often beneficial in the treatment of various pain syndromes. Active-assisted exercise is a combination of passive and active. A classic example of this type of exercise is the muscle-energy osteopathic manipulative technique.

Exercise is often used to develop or increase strength and endurance. Strength is defined as the maximal force that can be exerted by a muscle. There are static and dynamic forms of strength. Static or isometric strength is the maximal force that can be exerted against an immovable object. Dynamic strength is either isotonic or isokinetic. By definition, isotonic exercise is a force exerted by a muscle that remains constant throughout the entire arc of movement.[11] In isokinetic exercise, the resistance and force may vary throughout the arc of movement but the speed of the movement is constant.[12] The indications for specific types of exercise are beyond the scope of this chapter.

Table 36.2
TENS Analgesia—Surgery and Trauma

Indication	Number of Subjects	Experimental Design	Summary of Results
General Surgery			
Abdominal surgery	102	Randomized	77% good or excellent results in TENS group; 50–67% reduction in medication usage in TENS group
Abdominal and thoracic surgery	288	Randomized	TENS groups had less pain, improved pulmonary function, less ileus, and shorter ICU stays
Mixed surgery and trauma	20	Uncontrolled	80% relieved of protracted ileus within 24 hours
Orthopedic Surgery			
Total hip replacement	40	Randomized	Reduced medication use in TENS group
Hand surgery	44	Double-blind controlled	23% reduction in anesthesia requirements in TENS group
Knee surgery	34	Consecutive patients, no controls	Increased range of motion and reduced use of narcotics
Low back surgery	52	Consecutive randomized	TENS group reduced narcotic consumption 57%
Podiatric surgery	125	Controlled	TENS group required fewer narcotics; 74% with TENS noted excellent pain relief compared with 17% of controls
Obstetrics			
Labor and delivery	249	Variable	78–88% reported some relief, best relief in first stage; 70% required pudendal or epidural blocks
Postcesarean pain	9	Controlled	50–60% reduction of pain with TENS; deep pain, such as uterine contractions, was not affected

Reprinted with permission from Basford JR. Electrical therapy. In: Kottke FJ, Lehmann JF, eds. *Krusen's Handbook of Physical Medicine and Rehabilitation.* 4th ed. Philadelphia, Penn.: WB Saunders; 1990:376.

Table 36.3
TENS Analgesia—Miscellaneous Indicators

Indication	Number of Subjects	Experimental Design	Summary of Results
Acute rib fractures	24	Randomized	Statistically significant increases in PaO_2 and peak expiratory flow rates in the TENS group
Brachial plexus avulsion	58	Uncontrolled	60% with dramatic responses
Chronic interstitial cystitis	23	Uncontrolled	78% good to excellent reduction of pain; 35% had urinary frequency return to normal
Rheumatoid arthritis	20	Blinded	90% of patients doubled lifting endurance while using 70 Hz TENS
Burns	24	Double-blind	TENS and morphine equally effective for analgesia during enzymatic burn debridement
Hemophiliac joint pain	36	Controlled	71% of TENS patients vs. 25% of controls reported at least 50% pain relief
Osteoarthritis (knee)	30	Randomized double-blind	TENS appeared more effective than paracetamol but results were obscured by placebo effects
Angina	44	Variable multiple studies	Increased work capacity; decreased ST depression
Phantom limb pain	3	Case reports	Contralateral electrode placement; all 3 patients felt TENS to be beneficial
Acute minor trauma	100	Double-blind controlled	TENS equivalent to acetomorphine-codeine
Dysmenorrhea	21	Controlled	66% received some benefit from TENS, but majority felt Naprosyn to be equally or more effective
Spinal cord injury pain syndrome	31	Uncontrolled	35% of treatments successful
Headache (musculoskeletal)	60	Uncontrolled	70% of subjects received 60% reduction in headache severity and frequency

Reprinted with permission from Basford JR. Electrical therapy. In: Kottke FJ, Lehmann JF, eds. *Krusen's Handbook of Physical Medicine and Rehabilitation.* 4th ed. Philadelphia, Penn.: WB Saunders; 1990:377.

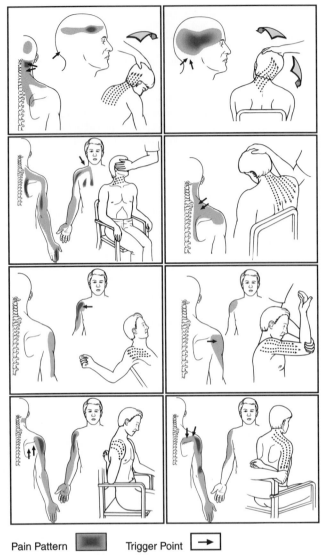

Pain Pattern ▨   Trigger Point →

Figure 36.5. Location of common trigger points and reference pain patterns. (Reprinted with permission from Simons DG. Myofascial pain syndromes. In: Basmajian JV, Kirby RL, eds. *Medical Rehabilitation.* Baltimore, Md: Williams & Wilkins; 1984.)

ORTHOTICS AND PROSTHETICS

Orthotics and prosthetics are frequently prescribed by the physiatrist. These devices are usually used to address functions in relation to mobility, i.e., joint and muscle group activities. An orthotic device is any device used to improve or maintain function. It may be necessary, however, to immobilize an area secondary to trauma of any type (e.g., fractures and inflammatory processes). These devices are commonly used for the rehabilitation process in strokes, neck and low back pain, entrapment neuropathies, in lower motor neuron problems such as peripheral neuropathies, and in postpolio syndromes. (A clinical example, carpal tunnel syndrome, is discussed later in the chapter.)

A prosthetic device replaces a missing anatomic structure such as following an amputation. Congenital and acquired skeletal deficiencies commonly require these devices. A working knowledge of biomechanics is essential for prescribing such devices.

ELECTROMYOGRAPHY AND NERVE CONDUCTION

Electromyography and nerve conduction studies make up a significant part of physiatric practice. These studies provide specific information about both musculoskeletal and neurologic functioning. They are used along with the history and physical examination when further clarification is needed.

Nerve conduction studies are performed on peripheral nerves and are particularly useful in diagnosing nerve entrapment syndromes. They help differentiate a neuropathic from a myopathic process and assist in subclassifying neuropathies into types, such as axonal and demyelinating. They also assist in diagnosing other neuromuscular diseases such as multiple sclerosis and myasthenia gravis. Somatosensory, auditory, and visual evoked potentials assess more proximal and central nerve conduction capacities, helping to identify such problems as brainstem lesions, acoustic neuromas, and a variety of upper motor neuron lesions. The evoked potentials are also useful for monitoring surgical procedures such as scoliosis surgery, when nerve root or spinal cord damage is a risk.

Electromyography is especially useful for precisely defining peripheral nerve dysfunction, including nerve root lesions such as radiculopathies, and for identifying the levels of involvement. It is also useful for determining whether regeneration has occurred after nerve injuries.

The following are some typical cases that physiatrists see that illustrate these fundamentals.

CASE HISTORY I

A 32-year-old right-handed woman who works as a computer programmer presents with complaints of right hand numbness, tingling, and pain over the past 2 to 3 weeks.

Given her occupation and symptoms, carpal tunnel syndrome and repetitive strain injuries are possible diagnoses. More questions should be asked to determine the extent of her disability.

Generally, however, isokinetic exercises are used in a more advanced setting during the rehabilitation process, such as when returning an athlete to a sport. Reserve isometrics for early use in treatment or when joint disease is present (arthritis). Dynamic strengthening exercise depends on the type of contraction: shortening or concentric contraction, and lengthening or eccentric contraction.

Endurance is generally considered as the ability to continue performing a specific task. Endurance exercise usually involves reciprocal and dynamic use of larger muscle groups[11] for a period of time instead of numbers of repetitions as with static and dynamic strengthening. Exercise can be used to treat a variety of ailments commonly seen by physiatrists. The publications referenced in this chapter provide a more detailed discussion of exercise.

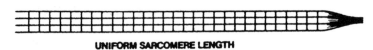

Figure 36.6. Schematic diagram comparing the anatomy of muscle fibers in a taut band/trigger point with normal muscle fibers. Shortened sarcomeres in trigger point area increase tension and restrict stretch range of motion. (Reprinted with permission from Goodgold J. *Rehabilitation Medicine.* St Louis, Mo: Mosby; 1988.)

In addition to hand pain, she also complains of bilateral neck and shoulder problems and frequent headaches. The right hand frequently cramps and "falls asleep" while she is working. (These same symptoms sometimes awaken the patient at night.) Shaking and massaging relieve symptoms temporarily. Additional complaints are clumsiness and sleep disturbances.

The extent of her disability is now more defined. Note that a similar patient with left-sided complaints who is also right-handed would have the same impairment but would be disabled to a different extent.

Physical Examination

There is decreased sensation to pin prick with altered two-point discrimination along the right median nerve distribution. Tinel's volar surface distal wrist percussion sign is positive for tingling in the flexor distribution of the long finger. Phalen's wrist flexion and median nerve stretch test also reproduce the hand symptoms. Manual muscle testing demonstrates normal distal hand strength, but there is considerable proximal rhomboid, middle and lower trapezius, and rotator cuff weakness. A structural/biomechanical examination of the right upper limb and shoulder girdle and neck demonstrates myofascial pain and tension in the upper trapezius and scalenes with tight wrist flexors, extensors, transverse carpal ligament, and forearm muscle groups. The right first rib is superior at the posterior attachments with a right convex T2-T6 group curve. C5-C6 is extended, rotated, and side-bent right, with limited passive range of motion to right side-bending and rotation. Neurovascular (Adson's maneuver) and foraminal compression signs (Spurling's maneuver) are negative.

This osteopathically oriented structural examination is consistent with a diagnosis of carpal tunnel syndrome with considerable additional evidence of proximal involvements of the neck, shoulders, upper thoracic spine, upper costal cage through the first rib, and rotator cuff.

Additionally, one might choose to perform electromyography (EMG) and nerve conduction studies (NCS/EMG) to confirm the diagnosis and determine the extent of nerve involvement, if any. Ruling out other disease processes such as pernicious anemia, multiple sclerosis, diabetes, and hypothyroidism are further considerations.

Treatment

Treatment is designed for these identified problems:

Carpal tunnel syndrome as a result of cumulative trauma disorder/repetitive strain injury
Associated cervical, shoulder, and upper limb somatic dysfunction
Mild right-sided proximal muscle weakness
Problems associated with the work environment and improper ergonomics

Treatment might include right wrist and distal forearm splints to decrease median nerve irritations, along with a course of nonsteroidal antiinflammatory drugs (NSAIDs). Prescribe regular breaks from the repetitive activity. Repetitive activity should not be done for more than 6 hours a day or should be avoided completely. OMT designed to release the myofascial and joint-related problems should be considered in the management strategy.[13]

Physical therapy is commonly used to help the patient deal with movement limitations and weak muscle groups. The occupational therapist helps evaluate the work site with recommendations for improving computer and seating ergonomics. Cumulative trauma disorder accounts for more than 50% of all occupational illnesses in the United States today.[14] A letter to the employer may be needed to document the need for work site changes. Detailed job descriptions are often helpful in making recommendations. If conservative treatment fails, surgery may be needed, particularly if functional losses and nerve degeneration continue.

CASE HISTORY II

A 40-year-old male who manages a fast food outlet presents with complaints of neck pain and headaches of increasing severity over several months. He is also bothered by numbness and tingling in all four extremities.

This is a rather ambiguous presentation that requires more detailed information about factors such as:

Job stress
Social life and habits

Alcohol and caffeine use
Family history

Diabetes mellitus and thyroid disorders are real possibilities. Further questioning reveals extremely high stress levels at work. Division and store profits are down and his job is in jeopardy. Sleep disruption has been a problem for several months. There is no diabetes or thyroid history in the family. Weekend binge drinking, mostly beer, has been part of his lifestyle for many years. He does not smoke or use caffeinated beverages.

Peripheral neuropathy, cervical myelopathy, and fibromyalgia or myofascial pain syndromes are considerations.

Physical Examination

The sensory and motor neurologic examination has normal results except for mildly diminished Achilles tendon reflexes. The structural examination demonstrates multiple bilateral myofascial tender spots and trigger points in the neck, shoulders, and upper back. These painful sites replicate his chief complaints.

Further workup includes a routine blood profile that includes:

Complete blood count
Fasting blood sugar
Liver function tests
Thyroid screen

If symptoms persist, an EMG/NCS would be considered to rule out peripheral neuropathy. Notably, all these test results are normal for this individual.

Diagnostically, this patient most likely has a myofascial pain/fibromyalgia syndrome, although his male gender would make the diagnosis unusual since more than 95% of such cases occur in women. Because of his alcohol habits, subclinical peripheral polyneuropathy may be an additional factor. The alcoholism, previously undiagnosed, and his high stress-dependency issues need special attention.

Treatment

Treatment strategies for this type of patient are often complex, drawn out, and potentially frustrating. Nonadherence to therapy is common with such patients. A coordinated team effort is necessary in this case, including consultation with a psychologist to assist with stress, pain management, and dependency issues, and a physical therapist to encourage a regular, well-rounded exercise program that substitutes for alcohol.

Cardiovascular and aerobic fitness with emphasis on stretching tight muscles is essential for the long term. Some medications, such as the tricyclic amitriptyline in low doses, often help both sleep disruption and painful muscles during the exercise and fitness program.[15] They are not particularly useful in the long term for this type of problem, however. Manual treatments of different types are sometimes useful for fibromyalgia but are more helpful for myofascial pain problems. Manual treatments are particularly helpful in designing specific

patient problem-based exercises. Because dependency needs are an issue, members of the team should not allow the patient to become dependent on either physical therapy or OMT. The real goal is to develop and nurture new coping skills coupled with appropriate treatment to encourage independence and autonomy, the self-healing that is a basic osteopathic principle.[15]

CASE HISTORY III

A 45-year-old left-handed woman arrives on the rehabilitation ward from the acute care hospital service. She was hospitalized 5 days ago when she presented to the emergency room following a sudden onset of right-sided weakness. Echocardiography demonstrated an atrial septal defect, and a brain MRI showed a left middle cerebral artery thrombosis thought to be embolic. She was placed on Coumadin, an anticoagulant, and moved to the rehabilitation unit where her medical condition stabilized.

Both diagnosis and impairment have been identified. The physiatrist's role and goal is to minimize the disability. A detailed psychosocial history will help in molding the treatment plan.

Social History

The patient works full-time as a sign maker for a grocery store chain. Her peers see her as a hard worker. She has a 50-pack/year history of cigarette smoking, and she drinks 10–12 cups of coffee daily. She has two children, a 13-year-old girl and a 10-year-old boy. Importantly, she is a single parent with no support from her ex-husband. Her mother, however, is extremely supportive.

Issues requiring attention are:

Child care
Work habits
Work modifications
Possible vocational retraining
Attempts at modifying her smoking and caffeine intake

The physical examination focuses on functional assessments since the medical components had been clarified previously. Specific attention is paid to:

Communication skills
Ambulation and transfer skills
Eating
Dressing
Self-care
Personal hygiene

Vocational skills and general social issues are integral parts of the process.

The patient walks with a cane in her left hand. She has exaggerated right knee flexion during the left leg push-off phase of her gait. Her endurance is poor, and she fatigues after approximately 50 feet, needing frequent verbal and visual cues for encouragement. Learning and carry-over are fair to poor. (Carry-over is the ability to repeat a part of a task after being taught.) She needs moderate assistance in standing because of right proximal leg weakness. Her eating is adequate after a tray is set up for her. She has considerable difficulty with personal hygiene and dressing skills because of poor hand and forearm coordination. Proximal right shoulder and arm mobility testing demonstrates some movement, but there is a lot of "spasticity" interfering with normal movement patterns. Her speech pattern is dysarthric (slurred), with fair to poor intelligibility. She does not demonstrate visual, language, or auditory aphasias, however. Both bowel and bladder function are intact.

Treatment

Treatment is designed around the following problem list:

Right hemiplegia with both mobility and communication difficulties

Atrial septal defect with concurrent need for anticoagulation; future heart surgery may be necessary to repair the atrial septal defect

Tobacco and caffeine abuse, the former being particularly problematic

Social and vocational disruptions with additional money problems facing her as a single parent

A well-coordinated team effort is necessary. Her prognosis for at least some functional recovery is quite good because of her age, left-handedness, degree of early recovery, and the maintenance of normal bowel and bladder functions.

Despite this prognosis, however, there is considerable risk for another embolic episode because of the open septal defect. A second event would disable her further. These realities need to be clearly communicated to her and her family as part of the treatment and rehabilitation effort. Long-term adherence to lifestyle and behavioral changes, with particular efforts aimed at smoking cessation to lessen the possibility for further embolization, is a major goal.

CONCLUSION

These three cases are representative of physiatric practice. Clearly, rehabilitation medicine and osteopathic philosophy and principles have much in common and complement one another. Concentrating on broad-based treatment approaches to address whole body concerns from a functional standpoint is important with both physiatric and osteopathic practitioners. Promotion of self-healing, another osteopathic concept, is always a goal of rehabilitation.

Providing care for the disabled population requires the physiatrist to have a broad array of skills. An in-depth knowledge of biomechanics, interdependence of organ functions, and

psychosocial concepts, in addition to those discussed above, is essential. The additional advantage of using structural diagnosis and manipulative treatment in this context is of special interest because of their beneficial diagnostic and therapeutic effects.

REFERENCES

1. Delisa J. *Rehabilitation Medicine, Principles and Practice.* Philadelphia, Penn: Lippincott; 1993;1:3.
2. Barry DT. Quantitative assessment of physical performance. In: Kottke FJ, Lehmann JF, eds. *Krusen's Handbook of Physical Medicine and Rehabilitation.* 4th ed. Philadelphia, Penn: WB Saunders; 1990:61–71.
3. Lehmann JF, De Lateur BJ. Diathermy and superficial heat, laser and cold therapy. In: Kottke FJ, Lehmann JF, eds. *Krusen's Handbook of Physical Medicine and Rehabilitation.* 4th ed. Philadelphia, Penn: WB Saunders; 1990:283–367.
4. Basford JR. Electrical therapy. In: Kottke FJ, Lehmann JF, eds. *Krusen's Handbook of Physical Medicine and Rehabilitation.* 4th ed. Philadelphia, Penn: WB Saunders; 1990:375–401.
5. Andary M, Tomski M. *Physical Medicine and Rehabilitation. Clinics of North America. Office Management in Pain Syndromes.* Philadelphia, Penn: WB Saunders; 1993:41–125.
6. Melzack R, Stillwell DM, Fox EJ. Trigger points and acupuncture points for pain: correlation and implications. *Pain.* 1977;3:3–23.
7. Ma DM. Needle electromyography and nerve conduction studies in clinical electrodiagnosis. In: Goodgold J, ed. *Rehabilitation Medicine.* St. Louis, Mo: Mosby; 1988:45–60.
8. Lee MHM, Liao SJ. Acupuncture in physiatry. In: Kottke FJ, Lehmann JF, eds. *Krusen's Handbook of Physical Medicine and Rehabilitation.* 4th ed. Philadelphia, Penn: WB Saunders; 1990:402–432.
9. Knapp ME. Massage. In: Kottke FJ, Lehmann JF, eds. *Krusen's Handbook of Physical Medicine and Rehabilitation.* 4th ed. Philadelphia, Penn: WB Saunders; 1990:433–435.
10. Kottke FJ. Therapeutic exercise to maintain mobility. In: Kottke FJ, Lehmann JF, eds. *Krusen's Handbook of Physical Medicine and Rehabilitation.* 4th ed. Philadelphia, Penn: WB Saunders; 1990:436–451.
11. De Lateur BJ, Lehmann JF. Therapeutic exercise to develop strength and endurance. In: Kottke FJ, Lehmann JF, eds. *Krusen's Handbook of Physical Medicine and Rehabilitation.* 4th ed. Philadelphia, Penn: WB Saunders; 1990:480–519.
12. Ciccone CD, Alexander J. Physiology and therapeutics of exercise. In: Goodgold J, ed. *Rehabilitation Medicine.* St. Louis, Mo: Mosby; 1988:759–772.
13. Sucher B. Myofascial manipulative release of the carpal tunnel syndrome—documentation with MRI. *JAOA.* 1993;93:12.
14. Rempel DM, Harrison RJ, Barnhart S. Work-related cumulative trauma disorders of the upper extremity. *JAMA.* 1992;268:787–788.
15. Carettes S, McCain GA, Bell DA, Fam AG. Evaluation of amitriptyline in primary fibrositis: a double-blind placebo control trial. *Arthritis Rheum.* 1986;29:655–659.

37. Respiratory System

GILBERT E. D'ALONZO, JR. AND SAMUEL L. KRACHMAN

Key Concepts

- **Respiratory functions, including ventilatory measurement, patterns and control, and pulmonary circulation and gas exchange**

- **Viscerosomatic reflex and lung disease**

- **Thoracic lymphatic drainage**

- **Osteopathic manipulatory effects on pulmonary function and thoracic lymphatic pump**

- **Prevention and treatment of lung disease, including pneumonia, chronic obstructive pulmonary disease, respiratory distress syndrome, and postoperative pulmonary complications**

The respiratory system includes the lungs, central nervous system, chest wall (with the diaphragm and intercostal muscles), and pulmonary circulation. The central nervous system performs as a system controller, regulating the activity of the respiratory muscles that function as a pump. The pumping action of this organ system is the body's mechanism to exchange oxygen for carbon dioxide. This system provides adequate oxygenation, which is vital to end-organ function, releases at least one end product of metabolism, and participates in the homeostasis of acid-base metabolic balance. Malfunction of an individual component of the respiratory system or alterations of the relationships among various components can lead to disturbances in end-organ function and, eventually, in total body performance.

The respiratory system, like other body components, is constructed to preserve function and maintain health. It depends on the proper function of other systems, and, of course, other systems depend on the process of respiration. Additionally, the lungs are organs that interface with the environment through the exchange of air that occurs with each breath. Each day, the lungs are exposed to more than 10,000 liters of ambient air that may contain microorganisms, dusts, and chemicals. The exposure to these noxious agents is likely responsible in part for a wide variety of diseases, including infections, inflammatory conditions, and malignancies. However, the lungs possess certain defenses that reduce the likelihood that injury and disease will develop. The lungs and the entire breathing process

participate moment to moment in the body's self-regulatory, self-healing, and health maintenance processes.

The process of respiration is complicated and consists of four major related events:

Ventilation
Gas exchange
Gas transport to and from body tissues
Regulation of breathing

Proper respiratory function depends on a delicate harmony with other systems, notably but not exclusively the cardiovascular, neuromuscular, and skeletal systems. Disease cannot occur in one system without affecting other body systems. The eventual extent generally depends on the severity of the initial disruption. In essence, the body attempts to function as a unit with a cadre of purposeful interrelationships and interdependencies between structure and function. Its goal is to enhance optimal function, ensure health, and prolong survival.

Four major aspects of disturbed respiratory function should be considered. They are disturbances in:

1. Ventilatory function
2. Pulmonary circulation
3. Gas exchange
4. Control of respiration

RESPIRATORY FUNCTION

Ventilation

Ventilation consists of the movement of air from outside the body through the upper air passages and the subdivisions of the conducting airways into the terminal respiratory units, and back out again. The amount of inspired air that reaches the sites of gas exchange is determined by many factors, including lung parenchymal distensibility and the way in which air moves or flows through the tracheobronchial tree. A pumping action, requiring a neuromuscular and skeletal effort, is necessary to expand the lungs and to cause air to flow through the respiratory system. Therefore, ventilation depends on the capabilities of the following:

Respiratory muscles
Mechanical properties of the airways
Lung parenchymal respiratory units

Respiration occurs at the level of the terminal respiratory unit and the alveoli. Respiration is defined as the process of gas

441

exchange between the body and its environment. The exchange of gases depends on:

Volume and distribution of blood flow through the pulmonary circulation

Volume and distribution of ventilation within the lungs

Diffusion characteristics of oxygen and carbon dioxide across the air-blood barrier

Regulation of breathing influenced by a variety of neurologic and metabolic factors

The lungs can be expanded and contracted in two ways:

1. By downward and upward movement of the diaphragm to lengthen or shorten the chest cavity
2. By elevation and depression of the ribs to increase and decrease the anteroposterior diameter of the chest cavity

Normal breathing at rest is accomplished almost entirely by the first of the two methods. During inspiration, contraction of the diaphragm pulls the lower surfaces of the lungs downward. During expiration, the diaphragm relaxes and the elastic recoil of the lungs, chest walls, and abdominal structures compresses the lungs. When ventilation has to increase, as with exercise, rapid expiration is necessary, and the elastic forces of the respiratory system are not sufficient enough to meet the demands of respiration. Abdominal muscle contraction occurs, forcing the abdominal contents upward against the bottom of the diaphragm. Additionally, when minute ventilation increases, recruitment of the accessory respiratory muscles raises the rib cage. Raising the rib cage, in turn, expands the lungs to a greater degree than that found at rest and augments inspiration. The major accessory muscles that raise the rib cage include the:

Sternocleidomastoid muscles

Anterior serrati

Scaleni

External intercostals

The muscles that pull the rib cage downward during expiration are the abdominal recti and the internal intercostals.

When the chest wall is opened during surgery, the lungs have a continual elastic tendency to collapse, pulling away from the chest wall, whereas the chest wall tends to recoil outward. These movements in opposite directions are responsible for the development of negative pleural pressure when the respiratory system functions in the intact state. The expansibility of the lungs and thoracic cage is called compliance. Compliance is expressed as the volume increase in the lungs for each unit increase in alveolar pressure, or for each unit decrease in pleural pressure. Because compliance is an expression of the distensibility of the elastic respiratory system, measured values of compliance depend on the elastic recoil properties of the lungs and chest wall.

If we think of the respiratory system as two completely collapsible elastic balloons, supported by a rigid Y-shaped tube (Fig. 37.1), we can better understand the relationship between compliance and elastic recoil. As volume is added through the tube to expand the collapsed balloons, pressure is generated within the system because of the tendency of the elastic walls to recoil inward. As more volume is added, the balloons continue to expand, and the volume-pressure curve begins to flatten as the elastic elements reach their limits of distensibility. Because compliance is defined as the change in volume resulting from a change in pressure, it is derived from the volume-pressure curve as the slope of the line at any point along the line. The position of the line depends on the elastic recoil of the lungs.

The lungs of patients with emphysema are more distensible, and the lungs of patients with diffuse lung fibrosis or other infiltrative inflammatory diseases are less distensible, or stiffer, than normal lungs. Volume-pressure curves from adults with normal lungs, with emphysema, and with lung fibrosis are shown in Figure 37.2. All three patients are assumed to be of similar age and body build, so they would have thoracic cages with similar vital capacities. Note that emphysematous lungs are larger than normal and fibrotic lungs are smaller than normal. The curve from the patient with emphysema is shifted to the left and above that of the normal curve, whereas the curve from the patient with fibrosis is flatter and shifted downward. When expressed at any given lung volume as a percent of the vital capacity (VC), compliance is lower with fibrosis.

Another factor that must be considered during breathing is resistance to airflow in the respiratory system. Resistance is computed from simultaneous measurements of the airflow and the pressure difference causing the airflow. Airflow is easy to measure, but measuring the pressure differences that cause the air to flow requires specialized equipment. The flow-resistance properties of individual components of the respiratory system can be analyzed separately, i.e., the airways and the tissues of the lungs and chest wall.

Figure 37.3 graphically illustrates three types of work that are associated with the inspiratory effort:

Compliance

Tissue resistance

Airway resistance

During normal quiet breathing, most of the work performed by the respiratory muscles is used simply to expand the lungs. Conversely, during heavy breathing when air movement must flow through the respiratory passages at very high velocity, the greater proportion of work is then used to overcome airway resistance. In pulmonary disease, all three of the different work components can be vastly increased. Compliance work and tissue resistance work are especially increased by diseases that diffusely involve the lung parenchyma and/or involve the chest wall. Airway resistance work is especially increased in diseases that obstruct the airways, such as asthma and other forms of chronic obstructive pulmonary disease. However, even diseases that involve the airways, often with increasing severity, affect tissue resistance work. In advanced obstructive airway diseases, malnutrition, deconditioning of the respiratory muscles, and somatic dysfunction can lead to enhanced tissue resistance work.

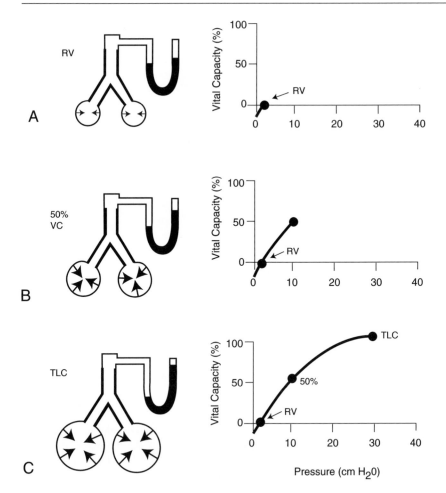

Figure 37.1. Schematic representation of volume-pressure relationships of isolated lungs. **A**, Because excised lungs collapse to less than residual volume (*RV*), at RV a small recoil pressure (*arrows*) is evident. This pressure is reflected in slight deflection of column in manometer and value on horizontal (*pressure*) axis. **B**, At 50% vital capacity (*VC*), recoil pressure is increased (*arrows*), thus more pressure is reflected in manometer and on horizontal axis. **C**, At total lung capacity (*TLC*), recoil pressure is maximal (normally about 30 cm H_2O).

During normal quiet breathing, no muscle work is performed during expiration because expiration results from passive elastic recoil of the lungs and chest. In heavy breathing or when airway resistance and tissue resistance are increased, expiratory work does occur and at times can be greater than inspiratory work.

Normally, the lungs sit within the chest wall. The pressures and forces acting on the structures are interrelated. At the end of normal exhalation during quiet breathing (measured as the functional residual capacity, or FRC), the lungs are partially inflated. The elastic recoil exerts a force that tends to empty the lungs. At the same time, chest wall volume is such that its elastic recoil promotes outward expansion. FRC occurs at the lung volume at which the tendency of the lungs to collapse is opposed by the equal and opposite tendency of the chest wall to expand.

For the lungs and the chest wall to achieve a volume other than the FRC, or resting volume, the respiratory muscles must actively oppose the tendency of the lungs and the chest wall to return to FRC. During inhalation to volumes above FRC, the inspiratory muscles must actively overcome the tendency of the respiratory system to decrease volume back to FRC. During active exhalation below FRC, expiratory muscle activity must overcome the tendency of the respiratory system to increase

volume back to FRC. At peak inspiration (total lung capacity, or TLC), the force applied by the inspiratory muscles to expand the lungs is balanced by the inward recoil of the lungs. The major determinants of TLC are the stiffness of the lungs and inspiratory muscle strength. If the lungs become stiffer or less compliant, the TLC decreases; if the lungs become more compliant, such as in patients with emphysema, the TLC increases. If the inspiratory muscles are significantly weakened, however, they are less able to overcome the inward elastic recoil of the lungs and the TLC is reduced.

At the end of a maximal expiration (residual volume, or RV), the force exerted by the expiratory muscles to decrease lung volume further is balanced by the outward recoil of the chest wall. The wall becomes extremely stiff at low lung volumes. The volume of gas found within the lungs at RV is influenced by two factors.

The first factor is the ability of the subject to exert a prolonged expiratory effort. This is often related to muscle strength and the ability of the patient to override certain sensory stimuli from the chest wall. These stimuli create a sensation that tends to stop the expiratory effort. The second factor is the ability of the lungs to empty to a smaller volume. In lungs with diseased airways, flow limitation or airway closure can limit the amount of gas that is expired. Additionally, weak

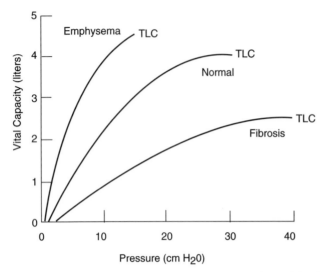

Figure 37.2. Representative volume-pressure curves from adult subjects of same age, sex, and body size, showing changes caused by emphysema and pulmonary fibrosis compared with normal lungs.

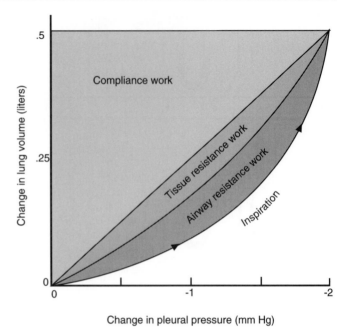

Figure 37.3. Graphical representation of three different types of work accomplished during inspiration: (1) compliance work, (2) tissue resistance work, and (3) airway resistance work.

chest wall muscles or airflow obstructive disease can result in an elevated RV.

MEASUREMENT OF LUNG FUNCTION

Lung function is most commonly measured under "static" conditions for determination of lung volumes and under dynamic conditions for determination of expiratory flow rates. The expiratory flow rates are generally determined during a forced expiratory maneuver. Figure 37.4 demonstrates the various lung volumes measured during spirometry under less than forceful conditions. VC, expiratory reserve volume (ERV), and inspiratory capacity (IC) are measured by having the patient breathe into and out of a spirometer. A spirometer is a device used to measure expired or inspired gas volume while plotting volume as a function of time. Other volumes, namely RV, FRC, and TLC, cannot be measured in this way because they include the volume of gas present in the lungs after a maximal expiration. Generally, one of two techniques is used to measure these volumes, either helium dilution or body plethysmography. These techniques measure FRC. When using slow spirometry measurements, one can mathematically determine the RV and, hence, the TLC (Fig. 37.4).

During a forced expiratory maneuver using a spirometer, one can determine the forced vital capacity (FVC) and the expiratory rates at 1-second intervals after the initiation of the forced expiratory maneuver. The forced expiratory volume in 1 second (FEV_1) is the most important parameter for determining the presence of airflow obstruction, especially when compared with the FVC as a ratio (FEV_1/FVC).

PATTERNS OF ABNORMAL FUNCTIONS

The two major patterns of abnormal ventilatory function, as measured by static lung volume measurement and forceful spirometry, are the restrictive and obstructive ventilatory patterns. A decrease in expiratory flow rates is the hallmark of the obstructive pattern (Fig. 37.5). The TLC is either normal or increased. The RV is often elevated as a result of the trapping of air during expiration. Finally, the VC is frequently decreased in obstructive disease, not because of low lung volumes but because of a marked elevation in RV.

The hallmark of a restrictive pattern is a decrease in lung volumes, principally in the TLC and FVC. When the restrictive ventilatory defect is the result of pulmonary parenchymal disease, the RV is generally decreased and forced expiratory flow rates are preserved. Extraparenchymal restrictive disease is the result of either inspiratory muscle weakness or a stiff chest wall. As a result, TLC is reduced, but the RV is often not significantly affected and expiratory flows are generally well-preserved. Certain patients with restrictive disease can have expiratory muscle weakness or a deformed chest wall that is abnormally rigid at volumes below the FRC. The ability to expire to a normal RV is then limited. Therefore, RV is often elevated, unlike the pattern observed in the other restrictive subcategories. One reason to establish a ventilatory diagnosis is to characterize the functional disorder, which can often provide diagnostic information (Table 37.1).

Pulmonary Circulation

The principal function of pulmonary circulation is to deliver blood in a thin film to terminal respiratory units so that the exchange of carbon dioxide for oxygen can occur. Other functions occur besides gas exchange. This circulation acts as a filter of the venous drainage from virtually the entire body. Pul-

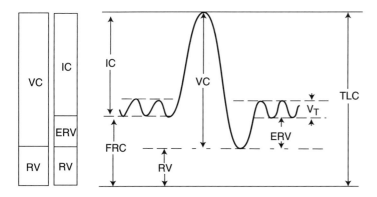

Figure 37.4. Lung volumes, shown by block diagrams (left) and by a slow spirographic tracing (right). *TLC*, total lung capacity; *VC*, vital capacity; *RV*, residual volume; *IC*, inspiratory capacity; *ERV*, expiratory reserve volume; *FRC*, functional residual capacity; *V*$_T$, tidal volume.

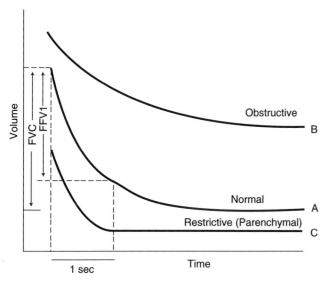

Figure 37.5. Spirographic tracings of forced expiration, comparing a normal tracing (*A*) and tracings in obstructive (*B*) and parenchymal restrictive (*C*) disease. Calculation of FVC and FEV$_1$ is shown only for normal tracing. Because there is no measure of absolute starting volume with spirometry, curves are artificially positioned to show relative starting lung volumes in different conditions.

Table 37.1
Alterations in Ventilatory Function

	TLC	RV	VC	FEV$_1$/FVC
Obstructive	N to ↑	↑	↓	↓ [a]
Restrictive				
Pulmonary parenchymal	↓	↓	↓	N to ↑
Extraparenchymal—inspiratory	↓	N to ↓	↓	N
Extraparenchymal—inspiratory + expiratory	↓	↑	↓	Variable

[a]Mild obstructive (small airways) disease may have ↓ MMFR with normal FEV$_1$/FVC. See text for abbreviations. N, normal; MMFR, maximum midexpiratory flow rate.

monary circulation provides nutritional substrates to the lung parenchyma that are important for the synthesis of surfactant. The blood present in the lungs serves as a reservoir or sump for the left ventricle. Finally, pulmonary circulation modifies a variety of circulating hormones by biochemical transformation.

The pulmonary vasculature must normally accommodate the entire output of the right ventricle. The thin-walled pulmonary vasculature has minimal resistance to blood flow and is capable of handling large volumes of blood at low perfusion pressures compared with that of the systemic circulation. The distribution of blood flow throughout the lungs principally depends on hydrostatic forces. Pulmonary arterial pressure is lowest at the apex of the lungs and highest at the lung bases in the upright position. With an increase in blood flow during exercise, the pulmonary vasculature is capable of recruiting and distending underperfused vessels. Therefore, the pulmonary vasculature is capable of handling large increments in blood

flow with a minimal change in vascular resistance and pressure.

Certain neurogenic, humoral, and chemical stimuli cause active pulmonary vasomotor reactions. Pulmonary arteries and veins are innervated with nerve fibers from the sympathetic trunks and the vagus nerves. The degree of influence that the autonomic nervous system exerts over the pulmonary circulation in the normal human adult is uncertain.

Several naturally occurring humoral agents can cause either vasoconstrictor or vasodilator responses of the pulmonary vascular bed. Vasoconstrictors have been shown to influence the human pulmonary vascular bed. These include catecholamines, angiotensin, and prostaglandins. Certain vasodilators, such as prostacyclin and acetylcholine, also influence the pulmonary vascular bed. The role of these substances in the control of the pulmonary circulation in health and disease remains speculative. Alveolar hypoxia, at a local level, induces pulmonary vasoconstriction. A synergistic relationship exists between the effects of alveolar hypoxia and acidosis on pulmonary vascular resistance (Fig. 37.6). In the presence of acidosis, as hypoxia becomes more significant, the increase in pulmonary vascular resistance accelerates.

Pulmonary vascular resistance also increases if thrombi or vascular proliferation diminishes the intraluminal cross-sectional area. Pulmonary vascular resistance can also increase in any disease state in which the small pulmonary vessels are oblit-

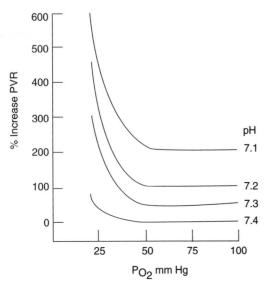

Figure 37.6. Effect of changes in inspired PO_2 on pulmonary vascular resistance (*PVR*) under conditions of different arterial blood pH. As inspired PO_2 is decreased, pulmonary vascular resistance increases; this effect becomes exaggerated and occurs at progressively higher PO_2 values as pH is decreased.

Table 37.2
Classification of Pulmonary Hypertension Based on Anatomic Site of Underlying Disease

Anatomic Site	Underlying Disease
Postcapillary	Left ventricular dysfunction
	Mitral valve stenosis
	Atrial myxoma
	Constrictive pericarditis
	Constrictive mediastinitis
	Pulmonary veno-occlusive disease
Mixed capillary and precapillary	Airway and parenchymal disease
	COPD
	Interstitial lung disease
	Pulmonary vascular disease
	Pulmonary embolism
	Congenital heart disease (left-to-right shunt)
	Vasculitis
	Primary pulmonary hypertension
	Chest wall disease
	Kyphoscoliosis
	Fibrothorax
Normal or near-normal lungs	High altitude sickness
	Chronic alveolar hypoventilation
	Sleep-disordered breathing
	Neuromuscular diseases

erated. Over time, the pulmonary arterial pressure rises, and cardiac output eventually decreases as the right ventricle fails.

Pulmonary hypertension may be the result of respiratory or cardiovascular disease and may complicate the course and management of the primary disorder responsible for its development. It may also result from certain hematologic, infectious, and inflammatory conditions not solely involving the cardio-respiratory system, or it may occur in the absence of an identifiable precipitating disorder. Regardless of whether pulmonary hypertension is primary or secondary, this pathophysiologic alteration usually remains clinically silent until the process is advanced. Patients then often present with signs of right heart failure.

Two major anatomic categories of pulmonary hypertension are postcapillary, and combined (or mixed) capillary and precapillary. Postcapillary pulmonary hypertension refers most commonly to diseases of the left heart that cause the pulmonary venous pressure to be elevated with a passive increase in pulmonary arterial pressure. Mixed capillary and precapillary pulmonary hypertension is a category that is generally associated with:

Normal left ventricular end-diastolic pressure
Normal left atrial pressure
Normal pulmonary venous pressure
Normal pulmonary capillary wedge pressure

The pulmonary hypertension in this category is secondary to an increase in pulmonary vascular tone, vascular remodeling, or a combination of these pathologic changes (Table 37.2).

Pulmonary hypertension may occur secondary to diseases of the airways, parenchyma, or vessels, in which the cross-sectional vascular bed surface area is decreased and blood flow through the lungs remains constant. Pulmonary hypertension may also occur with left-to-right intracardiac shunts, in which the pulmonary blood flow is increased and vascular anatomic remodeling may result. Extrapulmonary diseases, such as severe kyphoscoliosis and fibrothorax, produce distortion of the chest cavity, mechanical compression of lung parenchyma, and alveolar hypoventilation. These changes often lead to substantial degrees of pulmonary hypertension.

Some patients with normal or near-normal lungs may have pulmonary hypertension. Patients who have sleep-related breathing disorders with transient but severe hypoxemia during sleep are at risk for the development of pulmonary hypertension. These conditions are associated with alveolar hypoxia, pulmonary vasoconstriction, and vascular remodeling that eventually leads to pulmonary hypertension.

With diseases affecting the pulmonary vessels, a decrease in the cross-sectional area of the pulmonary vascular bed is responsible for the increased pulmonary vascular resistance. Patients who experience recurrent pulmonary emboli and patients with an idiopathic or primary form of pulmonary arteriopathy have an intraluminal obliterative process that increases pulmonary vascular resistance, and both develop substantial, often life-threatening, pulmonary hypertension.

Pulmonary Gas Exchange

The primary function of the respiratory system is to remove the appropriate amount of carbon dioxide from blood entering the pulmonary circulation and to provide adequate oxygen to the blood leaving the pulmonary vascular bed. Therefore, there must be an adequate supply of fresh air to the alveoli and an appropriate degree of ventilation to remove carbon dioxide from the lungs and, hence, from the circulation. For these functions to occur, there must be:

Adequate ventilation or delivery of oxygen to the alveoli and removal of CO_2 from the alveoli

Adequate circulation in terms of both perfusion and distribution of blood flow through the vascular bed

Adequate gas movement across the membranes that make up the alveoli and pulmonary capillaries

Appropriate matching of ventilation and perfusion

Hypoxemia is associated with a variety of diseases that affect the lungs or other components of the respiratory system. The four basic mechanisms of hypoxemia are:

1. Decrease in the inspired concentration of oxygen
2. Hypoventilation
3. Shunt
4. Ventilation-perfusion inequality

Diffusion impairment contributes to hypoxemia in only select clinical circumstances, which are generally extreme in character and rare in occurrence. The most common cause of hypoxemia is ventilation-perfusion inequality. Lung regions with low ventilation-perfusion ratios are most important for the development of arterial hypoxemia.

The essential mechanism underlying hypercapnia is inadequate alveolar ventilation for the amount of carbon dioxide that is being produced. The causes of arterial hypercapnia include:

Increased carbon dioxide production

Decreased ventilatory drive

Disease of the respiratory pump

Increased airway resistance making it difficult to sustain an adequate ventilation

Inefficiency of gas exchange resulting from an increase in dead space and/or excessive ventilation-perfusion inequality

For many patients with disease, more than one mechanism is responsible for the hypercapnia.

Different clinical situations are generally associated with a certain mechanism that is responsible for hypoxemia. Hypoventilation as a cause of hypoxemia is always associated with an elevated arterial P_{CO_2}. A loss of respiratory drive and a variety of neuromuscular diseases are associated with this mechanism of hypoxemia. Shunt as a cause of hypoxemia can result from the movement of blood from the right to the left side of the heart without entering the pulmonary circulation, as occurs with intracardiac shunts. Shunting of blood through the pulmonary parenchyma can also occur and is most frequently the result of disease in which there is an absence of ventilation in areas of lung that remain perfused. Atelectasis and alveolar filling diseases, such as pneumonia and pulmonary edema, often increase the shunt fraction of blood that goes through lung parenchyma.

As mentioned, ventilation-perfusion inequality is the most common cause of hypoxemia clinically. Lung airway and parenchymal diseases, including asthma, emphysema, chronic bronchitis, and interstitial lung diseases, and including all of the infiltrative diseases, demonstrate hypoxemia by this mechanism. Finally, a low mixed venous saturation can also influence the arterial blood in patients with an increased shunt fraction and/or ventilation-perfusion inequality made worse by hypoxemia.

Ventilatory Control

The many influences that affect breathing and gas exchange are mediated by a control system that incorporates peripheral and central receptors in a complex network of nerve pathways and integrating centers in the brain and spinal cord. The neurologic respiratory control system contains three principal interconnecting components:

A controller located within the central nervous system that initiates signals of its own, in addition to integrating information from sensing units

A group of effectors in the lungs, airways, and muscles of respiration that carry out commands from the controller

Different central and peripheral sensors that monitor the adequacy of breathing

Control of respiration by the central nervous system is functionally and anatomically partitioned. The brainstem regulates automatic respiration, whereas the cerebral cortex affects voluntary breathing. Integrating neurons in the spinal cord possess efferent information from both upper and lower respiratory centers in the brain as well as afferent information from peripheral proprioceptors. The neurons send the final signals to the muscles of respiration. Efferent autonomic impulses also travel in the vagus nerves from the central nervous system to the airways and lung parenchyma.

The medulla is the center for spontaneous respiration, whereas the respiratory activity found in the pons serves to smooth the transition from inspiration to expiration. The pons also contains two important regulatory centers: the apneustic center and the pneumotaxic center. These centers also play a role in modulating respiratory activity. The apneustic center appears to contain the normal inspiratory inhibitory mechanism. The pneumotaxic center is believed to act as a fine tuner of the pattern of breathing by influencing the response to afferent stimuli generated during hypoxia, hypercapnia, and lung inflation. Stimulation of respiratory components of the cortex inhibit respiratory movements and, in other areas, increases respiratory frequency. Behavior-related activities involving breathing, such as talking, swallowing, crying, and laughing, cause marked changes in ventilation that may completely override the autonomic control, which responds chiefly to chemical stimuli and to changes in lung inflation.

The descending neurologic tracts that originate in the cortical breathing centers and control voluntary breathing are separate from those that originate in the brainstem that involve involuntary breathing. The neurologic influence in these descending tracts is integrated with local reflex information at the level of the spinal cord from which the segmental motoneurons that innervate respiratory muscles emerge. These interrelated processes at the segmental level are complex and might differ in various respiratory muscles.

The main effectors of breathing are the muscles of respiration. Other central neuromechanisms regulate both the participation in breathing of skeletal muscle in the upper airways and the responses of smooth muscle and mucous glands within the tracheobronchial tree.

The respiratory system must be responsive to a wide variety of needs for ventilation. Therefore, it is desirable to have suitable sensors to initiate changes and to monitor whether any correction that occurs in ventilation is appropriate. Four sets of well-defined sensors have been described. The carotid bodies and aortic bodies function as chemoreceptors, monitoring the chemical composition of the arterial blood. Immediate hyperventilation is one of the principal compensatory responses to sudden hypoxemia. Chemoreceptor activity from the carotid bodies is increased by a decrease in arterial Po_2, an increase in arterial Pco_2, or a decrease in arterial pH. The aortic body chemoreceptors act in a similar fashion. Stimulation of the carotid body causes bradycardia and hypotension, whereas, stimulation of the aortic body induces tachycardia and hypertension.

Certain central receptors work to maintain acid-base balance in the central nervous system. The lungs and upper airways are equipped with a multitude of receptors that, when stimulated, have profound effects on breathing as well as on the circulation of other visceral and somatic systems. Receptors in the skeletal muscles of respiration help regulate muscle behavior at the spinal segmental level. Afferent impulses that originate from these sensors and go to the brain in the ascending spinal tract likely have some influence on the control of breathing. Muscle sensors have been linked to the sensation of dyspnea.

Located in the walls of the airways throughout the lungs are stretch receptors that transmit signals through the vagal system into the central nervous system when the lungs become overstretched. These signals affect inspiration in a similar way as signals from the pneumotaxic center; i.e., they limit the duration of inspiration. This breathing control process is called the Hering-Breuer inflation reflex. This reflex helps protect the lungs from overinflation and from the development of barotrauma.

THE OSTEOPATHIC APPROACH

We have reviewed various components of the respiratory system and discussed certain disturbances that are commonly encountered in patients with respiratory disease. As mentioned previously, breathing is a dynamic process involving moment-to-moment active gas exchange at the level of the lungs. The thoracic cage acts as a pump coordinated by a complex central controller mechanism and influenced by coordinated neural reflex activity. When the thorax acts as a pump, it involves complex muscular relaxation and contraction, motion of fascial planes, and the movement of nearly 150 joints of the body.

It is possible that the thoracic viscera affect the thoracic musculoskeletal pump. Likewise, the thoracic pump, when dysfunctional, must negatively affect the thoracic viscera. Maintaining normal respiratory motion during inspiration and expiration inherently tends to create a healthy environment for the thoracic viscera. Dysfunction of the thoracic cage, therefore, must have a negative influence. Unimpeded physiologic motion of the thoracic cage is important to maintain:

Sufficient arterial supply
Adequate venous drainage
Efficient lymphatic drainage
A sensitive and responsive autonomic regulatory influence on the respiratory system

Branches from the vagus nerves, containing both afferent and efferent components, make up the parasympathetic innervation of pulmonary structures, particularly the bronchi and bronchioles. The principal vagal effects are mainly secretory and bronchoconstrictive in character. The sympathetic supply to the lungs originates in the first to the fourth or fifth thoracic spinal cord segments (Fig. 37.7). The postganglionic fibers are derived from the stellate ganglion and the upper thoracic paravertebral ganglions. At times, the middle and superior cervical ganglia also contribute to the sympathetic innervation of the pulmonary system. The sympathetic innervation supplies vasomotor fibers to the trachea, bronchi, and pulmonary blood vessels.

Visceromotor reflexes from the lungs express themselves in the somatic area of the upper thoracic region. Viscerosensory reflexes can be found in the same region. The most common clinical response to enhanced reflex activity is muscle rigidity in the upper thoracic area, involving mainly the paravertebral musculature but also the sternocleidomastoid, scaleni, and diaphragm muscles.

The neuroregulation of the diaphragm is the function of the phrenic nerves. The autonomic nerves found in the diaphragm are probably vasomotor afferents. Again, the sympathetic nerves arise from the first four thoracic segments of the spinal cord, the parasympathetic supply is derived from the vagus nerves, and the neurons pass through both the thoracic and abdominal plexuses before innervating the muscle (Fig. 37.7).

The excursion of the diaphragm is important for proper pulmonary function. Additionally, its rhythmic pumping action with respiration is likely to favorably affect abdominal organ function. The rhythmic motion of the diaphragm may have a positive influence on gastrointestinal function and perhaps even enhances venous drainage of other visceral organs such as the liver and spleen. Certainly, proper diaphragmatic motion is necessary for optimized lung function. With inhibition of diaphragmatic motion, there is marked disruption in pulmonary gas exchange secondary to lung parenchymal atelectasis. Likewise, viscerosomatic reflexes will affect movement of the thoracic cage. This restrictive movement process could

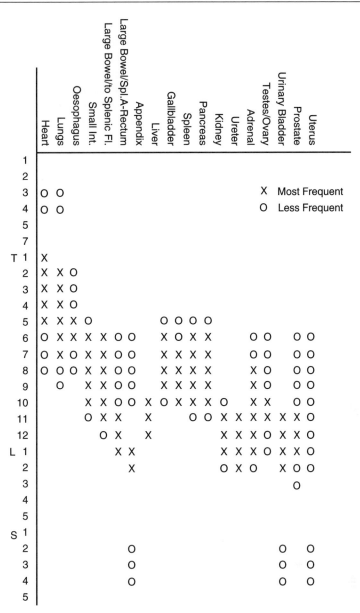

Figure 37.7. Site location of segmental sympathetic nerve supply.

induce a splinting effect, asymmetric movement of the chest, and intercostal hyperalgesia. It could also induce pain on palpation and, in severe cases, on voluntary motion. This reduced thoracic cage motion can also influence gas exchange by the induction of lung parenchymal atelectasis.

Reduction or impairment of thoracic cage mobility influences lymphatic drainage. A reduction in lymphatic drainage from the thoracic viscera may help contribute to the development of pulmonary congestion and a higher likelihood of lung inflammation and infection.

The Viscerosomatic Reflex and Lung Disease

Studies have confirmed the existence of somatovisceral and viscerosomatic reflexes.[1-2] The viscerosomatic reflex is the result of afferent stimuli arising from a visceral disorder affecting somatic tissue. Afferent impulses from visceral receptors are transmitted to the dorsal horn of the spinal cord, where they synapse with interconnecting neurons. These neurons convey the stimulus to sympathetic and peripheral motor efferents, resulting in sensory and motor changes in skeletal muscle and the overlying tissue, including skin. Skeletal muscle spasms resulting from nociceptive visceral stimuli have been observed clinically in patients. These spasms can be detected as a muscle contraction or as localized paravertebral muscle splinting. It is possible that presymptomatic signs of visceral disease may be evident in the somatic system. The intensity and the extent of the tissue response differs among individuals and disease states. Preliminary studies suggest that the intensity of the somatic dysfunction is greater in patients with cardiac disease who present with symptoms of severe pain than in patients with pulmonary disease who are more apt to present with symptoms of dyspnea.[2–3]

Spinal segmental sites for somatic dysfunction associated with visceral disease are related to the autonomic nervous system supply for various organs. Viscerosomatic reference sites for the lungs are generally C3 and C4, and T2-T9 (Fig. 37.8).[4–6] Areas of somatic dysfunction associated with visceral disease have been identified by palpatory examination by a number of investigators.[6] Osteopathic physicians have shown a particular interest in the identification of somatic dysfunction related to organic disease.[7] For the most part, these findings are similar to charted autonomic nerve supply data.

In a 5-year, double-blind study of 5000 hospitalized patients who were examined for evidence of somatic dysfunction and its relationship to diagnosis, most visceral diseases appeared to have more than one region with an increased frequency of segmental findings.[8] Unpaired viscera were also found to have an increased frequency of findings on one side, and the number of spinal segments involved appears to be related to the duration of the disease. In a subsequent report, Kelso et al.[9] observed an increased incidence of palpatory findings in the cervical spine in patients with upper airway diseases. Upper thoracic involvement was seen in patients with lower respiratory disease.

In a study by Beal and Morlock,[3] 40 patients with a diag-

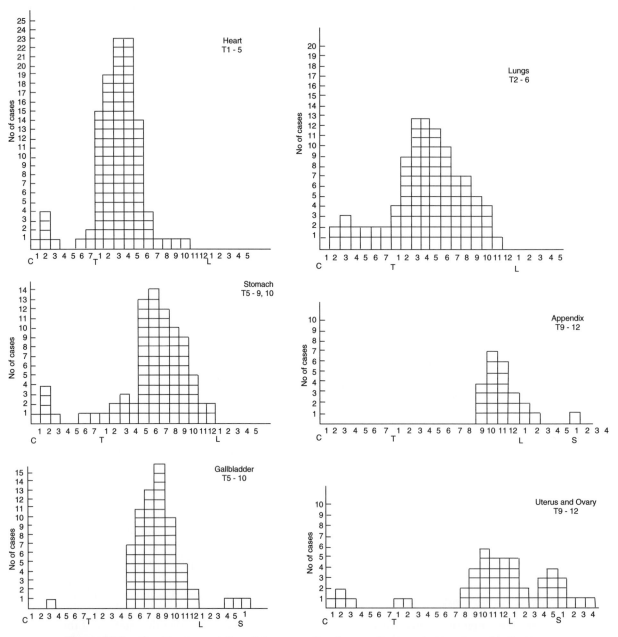

Figure 37.8. Graphic representation of viscerosomatic reference sites reported in osteopathic literature.

nosis of pulmonary disease—mainly chronic obstructive lung disease—were examined for evidence of somatic dysfunction. A prevalence of spinal findings was found in the T2-T7 paraspinal area. The somatic dysfunction that was found generally involved two or more adjacent spinal segments, deep-muscle splinting, and resistance to a compression motion test (Fig. 37.9). Other investigators have reported similar findings in patients with respiratory disease.[10–13] Nicholas evaluated 10 patients with respiratory disease and found an increased incidence of paravertebral muscle tension at C4-C7 and T2-T9 bilaterally.[12] In patients with chronic obstructive pulmonary disease, a palpatory examination tested skin drag, red reaction, sidebending, and hypermobility. The greatest number of findings were seen in the spinal segments T1-T9.[13]

With lung disease, especially if inflammation is present, visceral afferent nerve activity likely increases. This increase results in a change in the paravertebral muscular anatomy from the T1-T7 cord levels. When the lungs are irritated, the seven upper thoracic cord segments have been found to have low reflex thresholds that discharge easily. Viscerosomatic reflexes likely occur even with subthreshold stimuli. This low threshold phenomena is termed facilitation. Viscerosomatic reflexes from the lungs may be responsible for initiating the facilitated cord segments in this example. These reflexes will also interact with somatic nerves in the spinal cord to initiate reflexes, allowing the physician to palpate the paravertebral musculature and discern changes that indicate lung dysfunction. Even though there are two lungs in each thorax, the palpable musculoskeletal findings of lung disease in the upper thoracic area are more frequently found on the left side than on the right side.[3]

During states that produce an increase in sympathetic tone in the lung, certain hypersympathetic effects are speculated to occur. Increased sympathetic tone results in lung vasoconstriction with regional hyperperfusion and airway epithelial hyperplasia. With airway epithelial hyperplasia, an increase in goblet cells occurs and luminal secretions increase.

The musculoskeletal effects described often restrict chest cage excursion and further interfere with respiration. The cer-

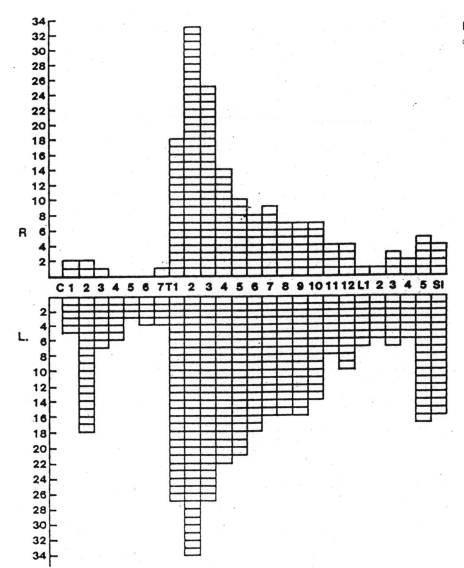

Figure 37.9. Somatic dysfunction in 40 cases of pulmonary disease.

vical paravertebral area is another high-incidence area of somatic dysfunction in respiratory disease. This area of spinal facilitation could interfere with appropriate diaphragmatic function. Diaphragmatic function is already stressed by the relative immobility of the ribs and spine as influenced by the viscerosomatic reflex in the thoracic area. The increased workload on the diaphragm could result in enhanced fatigability. In patients who have recruited use of the secondary muscles of respiration (often patients with advanced respiratory disease), fatigue of the scaleni and sternocleidomastoid muscle may result in dysfunction of the high thoracic rib cage, including the first rib. This mechanical disruption likely further impairs breathing efficiency.

Thoracic Lymphatic Drainage

Osteopathic physicians have long been concerned with optimal lymphatic drainage from tissues.[14-15] The maintenance of proper lymphatic drainage is thought to encourage proper tissue activity and metabolism and have a particular importance in providing for a proper immunologic environment.

Normally, contraction of the diaphragm and thoracic cage movement during respiration influences lymphatic drainage. Proper movement and lymphatic drainage throughout the lungs are considered important for the maintenance of normal function and a disease-free existence. Additionally, proper movement is essential for fighting infection and for reducing healing time. Tissue congestion is thought to decrease the effectiveness of medical therapy. Therefore, osteopathic medicine uses manipulative treatment to enhance movement and lymphatic drainage, with both preventive and curative influences on disease.

Osteopathic Manipulative Treatment

Many musculoskeletal patterns may arise as a reflex or mechanical consequence of pulmonary disease; they may serve to exacerbate or complicate the disease. Therefore, the treatment options of the osteopathic physician include not only pharmacologic and surgical therapies but also the use of osteopathic manipulative treatment (OMT). If OMT can reduce the pain and immobility that is associated with somatic dysfunction as it relates to pulmonary disease, then this treatment modality should enhance thoracic excursion. OMT should not only improve breathing and respiration but also enhance the healing process in patients with inflammatory and infectious diseases involving the lung. Additionally, if manipulative treatment can enhance thoracic lymphatic drainage, then this process could also be associated with accelerated healing. Prophylactic rib elevation and thoracic pump techniques are likely useful in the prevention of venous stasis. They should play a role in prophylaxis of deep venous thrombotic disease and pulmonary embolism in patients at bed rest.

OMT may do more than improve motion and enhance blood and lymphatic flow related to the thoracic cage. Improving thoracic motion may have a positive influence in maintaining proper lung function and enhancing healing. Manip-

ulation has possible direct effects on the lung parenchyma itself. OMT likely affects the neurohumoral system in a way that benefits the lungs. Osteopathic research can make a major contribution to the health care of patients suffering from respiratory disease. Through the use of manipulative treatment, patients with respiratory disease could have improved functional performance during the daytime. They could also enjoy enhanced sleep at night, with or without the concomitant use of standard medical therapy.

PULMONARY FUNCTION

Attempts have been made to determine how OMT alters physiologic function. Eggleston[16] and Detwiler[17] observed the immediate effects of OMT on vital signs, including respiratory rate. The design of these studies lacked proper controls, however, making it difficult to draw conclusions from their data.

A more carefully controlled study by Ortley et al.[18] designed experiments to determine, in healthy subjects, if measurable physiologic changes resulted from manipulation. Healthy male medical students were selected and participated in five interventional sessions, which included two control periods. There was an emphasis on observing the effects of OMT on respiration. High-velocity, short-amplitude manipulation was used as osteopathic intervention. A decrease in heart rate in a number of subjects and a decrease in skin resistance and respiratory rate in four of six subjects was found. In the four subjects who showed a drop in respiratory rate, three had a compensatory increase in tidal volume (V_T). The increase in V_T appeared to be the result of a greater abdominal movement component. Manipulation had no effect on expiratory or inspiratory reserve volumes, VC, forced expiratory volumes, and maximal midexpiratory flow rate as determined by pulmonary function testing. One obvious problem with the study was that the subjects were healthy and only a few were studied.

A series of experiments observing the effects of OMT on pulmonary function was conducted by Murphy.[19-21] Restricted breathing, including a loss in lung compliance, has been associated with altered lung gas exchange and the eventual development of hypoxemia. Improving restricted breathing improves gas exchange.

Murphy attempted to examine the influence of thoracic mobilization on selected pulmonary functions.[19] Pulmonary function tests were performed before and after each thoracic mobilization or restriction procedure. Her early findings indicated that thoracic mobilization techniques in healthy subjects tend to decrease the FRC and RV, while increasing the total thoracic compliance. Restriction techniques tend to decrease the FRC and total compliance. RV appears to be increased, and it may be that air-trapping or uneven lung ventilation distribution is responsible for this change. In further studies, Murphy found that there is an increase in V_T and respiratory rate after thoracic mobilization, which results in an increase in alveolar ventilation.[20]

In a technique that restricts breathing and thoracic mobilization, a decrease in V_T and an increase in respiratory rate are noted. At times there are minute ventilation increases, but overall alveolar ventilation remains decreased. Looking at the effect of nitrogen clearance from the lungs, thoracic mobilization clears nitrogen from the lungs faster. Any procedure that restricts breathing, creating a rapid shallow breathing pattern, reduces the clearance rate of this gas.

Murphy used a subsequent mathematical model to analyze the various factors that may have influenced the clearance of nitrogen from the lung. She concluded that, for nitrogen clearance to be enhanced, it is important to increase V_T and improve the distribution of gas in a homogeneous fashion throughout both lungs. This means that manipulation likely not only improves movement but also may improve ventilation homogeneity. In other words, OMT not only may improve movement factors of the thorax—increasing bulk airflow with each breath—but also may, with each breath taken, distribute air more evenly through the lungs, improving ventilation-perfusion relationships.

Finally, in her effort to further study this observation, Murphy used ^{131}I-labeled human albumin to study the effect of thoracic mobilization on pulmonary capillary circulation.[21] This method was used to look at the distribution of blood flow throughout the lungs. In healthy subjects, blood flow distribution may reflect the distribution of ventilation, since ventilation usually matches perfusion in healthy subjects. Murphy reported that thoracic mobilization increases the density of radioactivity throughout the lungs. This finding suggests that enhanced movement of the chest will likely improve not only perfusion but also ventilation in a more homogeneous pattern. This process should lead to improved lung gas exchange.

Doran and colleagues[22] studied the role of spinal curvature on respiratory mechanics. They hypothesized that an alteration in lumbar lordosis induces changes in respiration. Their experience had been that many patients in the initial physical examination have an increased lumbar lordosis that manipulation can decrease. Experiments were performed to establish the reproducibility and variability of a table that they constructed to quantify the degree of lumbar lordosis. Once the reliability of their measurement table was determined, they recruited young adult volunteers. They assessed how osteopathic manipulative treatment would affect respiratory function.

The test was administered using high-velocity, short-amplitude techniques with emphasis placed on the transitional areas of the spine. Respiratory function was measured for 15 minutes using both a pneumotachograph and a respiratory plethysmography, which assesses thoracoabdominal motion and timing. Following manipulative treatment, which often successfully decreased the lumbar lordotic curvature, there is a corresponding decrease in respiratory rate and an increase in V_T. A larger abdominal component to each breath, as compared with the thoracic component, is noted.

Doran et al. concluded that one of the significant factors that correlate with impairment of respiration is the lordotic curve, and that osteopathic manipulative treatment can alter this curve and affect the mechanics of respiration favorably.

These investigations, reported in abstract form, are hard to interpret. Most of the conclusions are based on minimal published data. A need exists for extensive controlled studies exploring the effect of OMT on pulmonary mechanics and gas exchange.

THORACIC LYMPHATIC PUMP

The thoracic lymphatic pump has been investigated for its effect on respiratory function and its immunomodulating effect by a variety of techniques. Since the early reports of Miller in the 1920s,[23–24] the thoracic lymphatic pump technique has been used as a research and treatment tool. More recently, Allen has been responsible for readdressing the potential value of the lymphatic pump technique. He proposed a study to investigate the effects of this intervention on respiratory function in healthy subjects.[25] The results of this study have yet to be published, but results have been obtained for some patients with respiratory disease who have received thoracic lymphatic pump intervention. These patients have shown an improvement in VC, improved mobilization of the thoracic cage and spine, and more rapid clearing of airway secretions.[26]

In a subsequent editorial, Allen and Kelso stated that patients who have been treated with the thoracic pump and mobilization of the thoracic cage and spine nearly uniformly experience a sense of well-being and relief from pulmonary congestion, dyspnea, and the milder forms of air hunger.[27] They claim that physicians have also observed improved sputum expectoration. In this same editorial, the authors provoke the osteopathic profession's interests in establishing a national clinical trial to explore not only the physiologic changes that occur with this form of manipulative intervention but also how these changes improve the quality of care of our patients.

Additional proposed mechanisms for the effectiveness of thoracic lymphatic pump therapy center on an enhancement of immune function. In a preliminary investigation, Measel studied the effect of the lymphatic pump on the immune response of normal male medical students by measuring how two serologic tests changed in response to pneumococcal polysaccharide antigen, administered subcutaneously.[28] The students, once treated by the thoracic lymphatic pump technique, had an increased immune response on the basis of testing for polysaccharide 1, 3, 4, 6, 8, 14, 23, 25, and 56 by passive hemagglutination. This study suggests that the lymphatic pump had a significant effect on the humoral or B-cell component of the immune system.

On follow-up, Measel and Kafity in a double-blind study evaluated the effect of the thoracic lymphatic pump technique on peripheral blood, bone marrow, and thymic-derived cells, again in medical students.[29] Preliminary results indicate that white cell counts rose and lymphocyte numbers decreased following lymphatic pump intervention. Additionally, the percentage of circulating T cells and B cells increased following therapy.

Therefore, thoracic lymphatic pump therapy seems to significantly change the peripheral leukocyte blood picture in healthy individuals. In a pilot study, Paul et al.[30] attempted to determine whether interferon, an antiviral and antibacterial chemical, could be released or induced by thoracic lymphatic pump manipulation. Twelve healthy adults were studied in a controlled fashion. Serum samples were drawn immediately before and at different times during the 24-hour period after manipulative intervention. Interferon levels were determined by a tissue culture technique that used a reduction of cytopathic effect as the endpoint variable. Mean pretreatment serum interferon levels were no different than the posttreatment levels in this acute study. This study does not discount the effectiveness of the lymphatic pump maneuver in the treatment of infectious lung disease. It is possible that the classic agents necessary for interferon production may be required to initiate stimulation of interferon production and that the thoracic lymphatic pump served to augment or enhance the response. Further research is necessary to clarify the usefulness of the thoracic lymphatic pump technique for the augmentation of body interferon production.

A more recent study used a guinea pig model to explore the effect of thoracic lymphatic pump technique on macrophage activity during lung infection with *Streptococcus pneumoniae*.[31] This study may or may not relate to humans, but the sequence of experiments performed indicate that the thoracic lymphatic pump technique has an effect on macrophage enzyme activity that could be important for the control of pneumonia with this organism in humans. Again, further controlled studies are necessary.

Prevention and Treatment of Lung Disease

Osteopathic physicians typically treat respiratory disease by conventional means, but their options expand to a new level and intensity with the appropriate use of OMT. As discussed earlier, a variety of manipulative techniques are useful in relieving thoracic cage discomfort, in facilitating inspiration and expiration, and in improving overall ventilation and perfusion of the lungs. In addition to techniques that concentrate on paravertebral muscle disease, other techniques concentrate on improving rib motion and enhancing the performance of the secondary muscles of respiration, such as the cervical strap muscles and the superficial muscles of the thorax.

Thoracic lymphatic pump techniques have been used to enhance the elimination of airway secretions and perhaps even increase the movement of fluids from lung parenchyma. The thoracic pump techniques are often employed with rib elevation techniques. This combination of techniques has been proposed to prevent venous stasis and to enhance fluid movement from the parenchyma of the lung.

Most osteopathic physicians do not treat specifically for the thoracic problem that is present but expand their therapy to treat the entire body. Although special attention might be directed at the cervical and higher thoracic area, for patients with respiratory disease it is not unusual to also treat the lower thoracic, lumbar, and sacral areas. The patient's condition and response to manipulation should govern the frequency and in-

tensity of each osteopathic manipulative intervention. Optimal timing has not been established.

Clinical studies of the effectiveness of the use of osteopathic manipulative treatment in visceral disease are limited. The use of manipulation has been explored in patients with a variety of infectious diseases of the airways and lungs and with chronic obstructive pulmonary disease, including asthma and emphysema. Limited information is available on using manipulative techniques in the management of respiratory distress syndrome and for the prevention of postoperative pulmonary complications.

PNEUMONIA

The early osteopathic literature is full of anecdotal case reports and information discussing the use of OMT in the treatment of acute and chronic pneumonia. From the turn of the 19th century to the middle of this century, pulmonary tuberculosis was frequently treated adjunctively with manipulative intervention.[32–38]

The older literature also has many articles focusing on using manipulative treatment for the treatment of bacterial pneumonia other than tuberculosis.[39–61] Most notably, several articles taught the effectiveness of osteopathic manipulative support for patients suffering from influenza pneumonia during the great flu epidemic of 1918.[48–53] These older studies are primarily anecdotal; no data are presented. Nonetheless, osteopathic physicians at that time and even today are convinced that manipulative treatment improves the course and outcome of patients with both acute and chronic infections of the chest. The literature cited in this chapter contains excellent descriptions of the techniques of manipulation used in treating pneumonia.

Initial manipulative treatment in pneumonia has three main goals:

1. Reduced parenchymal lung congestion
2. Reduced sympathetic hyperreactivity to the parenchyma of the lung
3. Increased mechanical thoracic cage motion

An explanation of the rationale[62–63] for and how OMT should be used in the treatment of pneumonia can be found elsewhere.[58–61, 64–66] Clinical studies on the effectiveness of osteopathic manipulative treatment in visceral disease are limited. Data concerning the use of this therapy in the treatment of lower respiratory tract disease are few.

An early study by Kurschner[67] compared chloramphenicol therapy with combined chloramphenicol and OMT in the treatment of children with whooping cough. This study was poorly controlled and the number of patients enrolled was small, but the use of OMT was associated with a lower daily cough average and a quicker recovery and return to school compared with those who had not received manipulation.

Purse performed a retrospective analysis of the use of manipulation in the treatment of upper respiratory tract infection in children.[68] Purse reviewed 4600 cases of upper respiratory tract infection, in which 780 incidences of complications were found. These complications ranged from simple conjunctivitis and acute otitis media to acute pneumonia and bronchitis. The nearly 17% complication rate was below the 33–50% rates commonly associated with standard medical treatment at that time. Schmidt[69] reported her anecdotal experience in treating 100 cases of upper respiratory tract disease using OMT. The majority of patients had pharyngitis, rhinitis, or sinusitis. The investigator concluded that manipulation reduced duration of symptoms and complications, but the data presented were uncontrolled and entirely anecdotal. Nevertheless, the study's greatest value is the detail in which patient management is described.

Kline studied 252 children who had been hospitalized for respiratory infection over an 18-month period.[70] All patients received supportive therapy. One group received OMT, another group received antibiotics without manipulation, and a third group received a combination of therapies. The investigator found that patients who received supportive therapy, manipulative treatment, and antibiotics recovered faster than the patients who received manipulation or antibiotics alone.

Recently, the efficacy of osteopathic manipulative treatment in elderly hospitalized patients with acute pneumonia has been reported.[71] In a small group of patients older than 60 years of age with acute pneumonia, osteopathic manipulative treatment was effective in reducing the duration of antibiotic use and the duration of worrisome leukocytosis.

CHRONIC OBSTRUCTIVE PULMONARY DISEASE

The use of OMT for the treatment of asthma and other forms of chronic obstructive pulmonary disease has been suggested in the osteopathic literature from as early as 1902, when the *Journal of the American Osteopathic Association* first appeared.[72–73] One of the 1902 articles[72] stresses the relevance of environmental control measures as part of the treatment plan for asthma, a unique concept for that time. The importance of manipulative intervention was also stressed. In 1912, Louisa Burns, DO, published her experiences in diagnosing and treating asthma in patients at the Pacific College of Osteopathy.[74] She reviewed 21 cases of asthma and also carefully described a multitude of structural findings associated with reactive airways disease, the importance of avoiding irritant gases and dusts, and how osteopathic manipulative treatment is effective in attenuating the chronic symptoms of this disease.

Perhaps the first clinical study of manipulation and pulmonary disease was that by Wilson.[75] Published in 1925, his study included 20 patients with asthma who had received a type of vaccine treatment and who were given manipulative intervention. This study, albeit poorly controlled, showed that 15 of these patients had some temporary relief; 10 patients had 50% fewer asthmatic attacks over an extended time period. Additionally, the study demonstrated the reproducibility of certain palpatory findings in patients with asthma. Wilson con-

cluded that *"this study tells a cold, hard, cash story to employers and insurance companies"* about the benefit of this form of therapeutic intervention. Dr. Wilson's specific manipulative techniques for asthma were eventually published the following year,[76] and an even more in-depth treatise of his techniques was published 21 years later.[77]

One of the most concise descriptions of the osteopathic management of asthma was published in 1959 by Kline.[78] His management plan was based on personal experience with patients having acute asthma and others with a variety of chronic lung diseases. During acute asthma, *"lesions will always be found in the 2nd to 4th thoracic vertebrae and the 4th rib of the right will always be elevated."* The only other constant finding is *"a lesion of the 3rd cervical vertebrae with rotation to the left."* Dr. Kline's manipulative interventions were active, involving treatments that focused on improving cervical and thoracic mobility and on using the thoracic lymphatic pump. Kline emphasized not only relaxation of the thoracic cage but also improvement of diaphragmatic function. He strongly urged physicians to continue manipulative treatment on a regular basis, even during periods of asthma stability.

Belcastro et al.[79] hypothesized that osteopathic manipulative treatment may be effective in the treatment of bronchiolitis. To investigate this theory, they enrolled 12 patients in this study, ages 2–11 months, with a clinical diagnosis of bronchiolitis. They randomly assigned each infant to a treatment scheme, comparing OMT with postural drainage and bronchodilator therapy with placebo. A sequence of osteopathic manipulative treatments was developed; outcomes were measured by the number of hospital days and the daily respiratory rate. Although data were inconclusive because of the small number of study patients, this study did establish a research protocol and discussed the treatment of bronchiolitis from an osteopathic standpoint.

Other forms of chronic obstructive pulmonary disease have been treated by OMT. Over a 9-month period, Howell et al.[80] evaluated 17 patients with chronic obstructive pulmonary disease who received OMT. The effect of this intervention was assessed by measuring pulmonary function tests, including arterial blood gases. Improvement was shown in the arterial carbon dioxide tension, in arterial oxygen saturation, in TLC, and in RV, especially in those patients who were hyperinflated and barrel-chested (typical features of emphysema). However, in another study[81] involving patients with chronic obstructive pulmonary disease (COPD), manipulation did not change VC or RV. Nonetheless, manipulation may have improved work capacity and dyspnea, both at rest and during exertion. The patients who received OMT also had fewer upper respiratory tract infections than did the patients who did not receive manipulation.

In a case report by Howell and Kappler,[82] OMT was directed toward mobilization of a COPD patient's "rigid thoracic spine and chest cage." During 16 months of therapy, thoracic cage mobility improved. Specifically, high thoracic paraspinal "tissue reactivity" diminished. Clinically, walking tolerance increased and episodes of difficult breathing became less frequent. Additionally, the oxygen saturation of arterial blood improved but hyperinflation as determined by pulmonary function testing increased. The increase in TLC in this patient likely represents progressive emphysema, a process that would be difficult to influence with any therapeutic intervention. More importantly, these authors discussed the importance of exploring new clinical endpoint variables for evaluating OMT. These include:

Parameters of functional performance
Compliance and distensibility of the thoracic cage
Lung ventilation and perfusion relationships
Spinal and thoracic cage mobility

Finally, at least two authors have outlined many of the factors that must be considered when a clinical study exploring the effects of manipulation on COPD patients is being considered.[83–84]

The role of osteopathic manipulative treatment in treatment algorithms for acute and chronic asthma and for the management of other chronic obstructive pulmonary disease needs to be better defined by well-controlled clinical investigations. Manipulative treatment should be beneficial for these groups of patients. An intervention that improves thoracic mobility and favorably affects the regulatory mechanisms of the autonomic nervous system should be beneficial in patients with asthma and COPD. The clinical experience of some osteopathic physicians appears encouraging,[85] but carefully designed clinical investigation is needed.

RESPIRATORY DISTRESS SYNDROME

Only one study exists in which OMT was used in the treatment of respiratory distress syndrome in the newborn.[86] A rib-raising technique was used and a variety of treatment endpoint variables were assessed. This study lacked proper control but it suggested that the use of OMT could favorably affect outcome, mainly by reducing deaths. The death rate in the study group was lower than that found using historical controls.

PREVENTION OF POSTOPERATIVE PULMONARY COMPLICATIONS

Generally speaking, pulmonary complications are the most frequent cause of morbidity postoperatively. Atelectasis, a collapsed or airless segmental lung condition, is the most common pulmonary complication. Surgeries that are commonly associated with the development of lung atelectasis include high abdominal surgery and thoracic surgery. Aggressive pulmonary toilet measures, including patient-generated incentive spirometry, have been important in reducing the incidence of this complication postoperatively. From an osteopathic standpoint, it is important to point out that these surgeries often have a musculoskeletal component, even when postoperative pulmonary complications do not exist. The existence of a pulmonary complication enhances the probability of a musculoskeletal component developing. Osteopathic physicians have been treating patients with manipulative treatment, both preopera-

tively and postoperatively, to prevent respiratory complications from occurring.[87]

Henshaw[88] not only defined the presence of postoperative somatic dysfunction but also clearly pointed out the high incidence of preoperative somatic dysfunction in patients undergoing either low or high abdominal surgery. Recently, Sleszynski and Kelso[89] have studied the effects of thoracic lymphatic pump administered on the first postoperative day in patients that had undergone cholecystectomy. They compared this manipulative modality with the use of incentive spirometry in the prevention of atelectasis. In preventing atelectasis, the thoracic lymphatic pump-treated patients had similar occurrences as those patients treated with incentive spirometry. However, the thoracic lymphatic pump-treated patients had an earlier recovery and a quicker return toward preoperative values for FVC and FEV_1 than did patients treated with incentive spirometry.

CONCLUSION

The respiratory system is a beautifully designed pump whose chief purpose is to exchange carbon dioxide for oxygen in the respiratory process. A disease that affects any component of this physiology generally disrupts the entire pump system. Whether the disease affects the lung parenchyma, vascular circulation, lymphatic circulation, or a neuromuscular component, alterations of the musculoskeletal system will be found in the physical examination. These alterations cannot be ignored. They must be used in a way in which they can help detect the presence of visceral disease. These alterations must eventually be treated to enhance the likelihood of cure and improve the time to complete disease resolution. Proper medical care and OMT should be combined to support the respiratory system. The osteopathic physician's knowledge and skills in providing effective manipulative treatment often optimize thoracic cage motion, improve diaphragmatic function, enhance lymphatic drainage, and stabilize autonomic influences.

Osteopathic physicians are convinced of the efficacy of manipulative treatment. Our experience has been that this form of therapy is helpful for our patients. There are limited data demonstrating the clinical efficacy of manipulative intervention in certain disease states. It is imperative that further clinical investigation be pursued to advance the science of osteopathic medicine.

ACKNOWLEDGMENTS

We would like to thank the *JAOA* staff for helping us in our search for the older osteopathic literature. Kim Williams was invaluable in her efforts in preparing this manuscript.

REFERENCES

1. Kolzumi K, Brooks McC C. The integration of autonomic system reactions. A discussion of autonomic reflexes, their control and their association with somatic reactions. In: *Ergebnisseder Physiologic*. Berlin: Springer-Verlag; 1972.

2. Beal MC. Palpatory testing for somatic dysfunction in patients with cardiovascular disease. *JAOA.* 1983;82:822–831.

3. Beal MC, Morlock JS. Somatic dysfunction associated with pulmonary disease. *JAOA.* 1984;84:179–183.

4. Pottenger FM. *Symptoms of Visceral Disease.* St. Louis, Mo: CV Mosby Co; 1938.

5. Bhagat BD, Young BA, Biggerstaff DE. *Fundamentals of Visceral Innervation.* Springfield, Ill: CC Thomas; 1977.

6. Hansen K, Schliack H. *Segmental Innervation.* Stuttgart, Germany: G Theime; 1962.

7. Beal MC. Viscerosomatic reflexes: a review. *JAOA.* 1985;85:786–801.

8. Kelso AF. A double-blind clinical study of osteopathic findings in hospital patients—Progress report. *JAOA.* 1971;70:570–592.

9. Kelso AF, Larson NJ, Kappler RE. A clinical investigation of the osteopathic examination. *JAOA.* 1980;79:460–467.

10. Long FA. Study of the segmental incidence of certain spinal changes in various disorders. *Osteopathic Digest.* 1940;6:11–13.

11. Deming GS, Kruener VC. Study of the segmental incidence of certain spinal palpatory findings in disorders of the respiratory tract. *JAOA.* 1943;43:264–267.

12. Nicholas NA. Correlation of somatic dysfunction with visceral disease. *JAOA.* December 1975;75:425–428.

13. Miller WD. *Treatment of Visceral Disorders by Manipulative Therapy. The Research Status of Spinal Manipulative Therapy.* Bethesda, Md: US Department of Health, Education, and Welfare; 1975.

14. Millard FP. Applied lymphatics of the chest. *JAOA.* 1912;21:22–23.

15. Millard FP. Drainage of the intercostal spaces. *JAOA.* 1923;22:262–265.

16. Eggleston AA. The effect of manipulative treatment on body function. A preliminary report. *JAOA.* 1940;39:279–284.

17. Detwiler ES. Some immediate effects of osteopathic manipulative treatment. Studies on four hundred cases. *JAOA.* 1950;49:391–395.

18. Ortley GR, Samwick RD, Dahle RE, et al. Recording of physiologic changes associated with manipulation in healthy subjects. *JAOA.* 1980;80:228–229.

19. Murphy AJ. Preliminary studies of the influence of pulmonary and thoracic mobilization procedures on pulmonary function. *JAOA.* 1965;64:951–952.

20. Murphy AJ. Comparison of nitrogen washout curves from human experiments and from a mathematical model of the lung. *JAOA.* 1967;66:1023–1024.

21. Murphy AJ. Continuation of the study of the effect of thoracic mobilization on the distribution of ^{131}I in the lungs. *JAOA.* 1971;70:1057–1058.

22. Doran J, Freiburger L, Zink G, Kilmore M. Relationship of osteopathic manipulative treatment, lordosis, and respiration. *JAOA.* 1982;82:139–140.

23. Miller CE. Osteopathic principles and thoracic pump therapeutics proved by scientific research. *JAOA.* 1927;26:910–914.

24. Miller CE. The mechanics of lymphatic circulation. *JAOA.* 1923; 22:397–398.

25. Allen T. A pilot study on the effect of the thoracic pump on respiratory function. *JAOA.* 1963;62:839.

26. Allen TW, Pence TK. The use of thoracic pump in treatment of lower respiratory tract disease. *JAOA.* 1967;67:408–411.

27. Allen TW, Kelso AF. Osteopathic research and respiratory disease. *JAOA.* 1980;79:360.

28. Measel JW. The effect of the lymphatic pump on the immune response: I. Preliminary studies on the antibody response to pneumococcal polysaccharide assayed by bacterial agglutination and passive hemagglutination. *JAOA.* 1982;82:28–31.

29. Measel JW. The effect of the lymphatic pump on the B and T cells in peripheral blood. *JAOA.* 1986;86:608.

30. Paul RT, Stomel RJ, Broniak FF, Williams BB. Interferon levels in human subjects throughout a 24-hour period following thoracic lymphatic pump manipulation. *JAOA.* 1986;86:92–95.

31. Boyer JM, Davis M, Cashon G, et al. Effects of thoracic pump technique on macrophage activity during infection of guinea pigs with *Streptococcus pneumoniae. JAOA.* 1987;87:698–699.

32. Keene WB. Some possibilities in the treatment and prevention of tuberculosis from an osteopathic standpoint. *JAOA.* 1904;4:147–154.

33. Meacham WB. On pulmonary tuberculosis. *JAOA.* 1905;4:315–322.

34. Bolles NA. The osteopathic and physical examination of a case of pulmonary tuberculosis. *JAOA.* 1906;5:283–288.

35. Hayden WJ. Tuberculosis. *JAOA.* 1906;5:288–293.

36. Meacham WB. Pulmonary tuberculosis. *JAOA.* 1908;7:201–205.

37. Terrell AP. Tuberculosis—A study. *JAOA.* 1910;9:332–335.

38. Johnson FE. Osteopathy and tuberculosis. *JAOA.* 1936;35:319–327, 341.

39. Hulett MT. Osteopathic lesions in acute respiratory diseases. *JAOA.* 1907;6:381–384.

40. Ivie WH. The treatment of pneumonia. *JAOA.* 1909;8:279–281.

41. Link EC. Osteopathic care of pneumonia. *JAOA.* 1910;9:521–527.

42. Overton JA. The treatment of pneumonia. *JAOA.* 1912;11:1033–1037.

43. Webster GV. The treatment of pneumonia. *JAOA.* 1914;14:128–131.

44. Laughlin GM. Osteopathic treatment of pneumonia. *JAOA.* 1916; 15:271–276.

45. Connor RF. Treating and aborting lobar pneumonia. *JAOA.* 1916; 15:336–343.

46. Fulham CV. Pneumonia. *JAOA.* 1917;16:917–921.

47. LaRue JB. Pneumonia. *JAOA.* 1919;18:206–208.

48. Tuttle LK. Influenza and pneumonia treatment. *JAOA.* 1919; 18:211–214.

49. Fulham CV. Treatment of pneumonia. *JAOA.* 1920;20:175–177.

50. Burns L, Perry AE. Osteopathic treatment and laboratory findings. *JAOA.* 1920;20:179–181.

51. Crane RM. Experiences with pneumonia. *JAOA.* 1922;21:347–350.

52. Miller CE. The specific cure of pneumonia. *JAOA.* 1924;24:99–101.

53. Death statistics reveal comparative values of osteopath and drug treatments. *Osteopathic Physician.* December 1918;34:1–2.

54. Peckham FF. Osteopathic care and management of lobar pneumonia. *JAOA.* 1927;27:180–181.

55. Fischer RL. Treatment of lobar pneumonia. *JAOA.* 1929;29:354–358.

56. Conley GJ. Treatment. *JAOA.* 1937;36:316–318.

57. Watson JO, Percival EN. Pneumonia research in children at Los Angeles County Osteopathic Hospital. A preliminary report. *JAOA.* 1939;39:153–159.

58. Horton ER. Osteopathic manipulative treatment in pneumonia. *JAOA.* 1940;39:511–513.

59. Litton HE. Manipulative treatment of pneumonia. *Yearbook Acad Applied Osteopathy.* 1965;1:136–138.

60. Medaris CE. The osteopathic treatment for lobar pneumonia. *Yearbook Acad Applied Osteopathy.* 1947:124–130.

61. Facto LL. The osteopathic treatment for lobar pneumonia. *JAOA.* 1947;46:385–392.

62. Burns L. Osteopathic pathology of the lungs. *JAOA*. 1933;32:474–478.
63. Grainger HG. Lobar pneumonia and the segmental plane. *JAOA*. 1951;50:255–263.
64. Fryman VM. The osteopathic approach to cardiac and pulmonary problems. *JAOA*. 1978;77:668–673.
65. D'Alonzo AF, Evans DJ. Disorders of the respiratory system. In: Hoag JM, ed. *Osteopathic Medicine*. New York, NY: McGraw-Hill; 1969:465.
66. Hèilig D. *Illustrative Points in Technique*. New York, NY: McGraw-Hill; 1969:197–203.
67. Kurschner OM. A comparative clinical investigation of chloramphenicol and osteopathic manipulative therapy of whooping cough. *JAOA*. 1958;57:559–561.
68. Purse FM. Manipulative therapy of upper respiratory infections in children. *JAOA*. 1966;65:964–972.
69. Schmidt IC. Osteopathic manipulative therapy as a primary factor in the management of upper, middle, and pararespiratory infections. *JAOA*. 1982;81:382–387.
70. Kline CA. Osteopathic manipulative therapy, antibiotics, and supportive therapy in respiratory infections in children: comparative study. *JAOA*. 1965;65:278–281.
71. Noll DR, Bryman PN, Gebhardt GP, Masterson EV. The efficacy of OMT in the elderly hospitalized with acute pneumonia. *JAOA*. 1992;92:1179.
72. Forbes HW. Bronchial asthma. *JAOA*. 1902;1:106–109.
73. Coffman KW. Asthma. *JAOA*. 1902;1:188–190.
74. Burns L. Clinic reports from the Pacific College of Osteopathy. *JAOA*. 1912;11:1054–1056.
75. Wilson PT. Experimental work in asthma at the Peter Bent Brigham Hospital. *JAOA*. 1925;25:212–214.
76. Wilson PT. Specific technic for asthma. *JAOA*. 1926;25:473.
77. Wilson PT. The osteopathic treatment of asthma. *JAOA*. 1959;45:491–492.
78. Kline JA. An examination of the osteopathic management of bronchial asthma. *Yearbook Acad Applied Osteopathy*. 1946:127–131.
79. Belcastro MR, Backes CR, Chila AG. Bronchiolitis: a pilot study of osteopathic and manipulative treatment, bronchodilators, and other therapy. *JAOA*. 1984;83:672–676.
80. Howell RK, Allen TW, Kappler RE. The influence of osteopathic manipulative therapy in the management of patients with chronic obstructive lung disease. *JAOA*. 1975;74:757–760.
81. Miller WD. *Treatment of Visceral Disorders by Manipulative Therapy. The Research Status of Spinal Manipulative Therapy*. Bethesda, Md: US Department of Health, Education, and Welfare; 1975:295–301.
82. Howell RK, Kappler RE. The influence of osteopathic manipulative therapy on a patient with advanced cardiopulmonary disease. *JAOA*. 1973;73:322–327.
83. Hoag JM. Project in the study of chronic obstructive lung disease. *JAOA*. 1970;69:1031–1033.
84. Mall R. An evaluation of routine pulmonary function tests as indicators of responsiveness of a patient with chronic obstructive lung disease to osteopathic health care. *JAOA*. 1973;73:327–333.
85. Hoag JM. Musculoskeletal involvement in chronic lung disease. *JAOA*. 1972;71:698–706.
86. Bailey WP. Evaluation of rib raising technique in respiratory distress syndrome. *JAOA*. 1963;62:924–928.
87. Still GA. Advantages and necessity of osteopathic post-operative treatment. *JAOA*. 1919;18:481–486.
88. Henshaw. *The DO*. September 1963:132–133.
89. Sleszynski SL, Kelso AF. Comparison of thoracic manipulation with incentive spirometry in the prevention of post-operative atelectasis. *JAOA*. 1993;93:834–845.

38. Rheumatology

BERNARD R. RUBIN

Key Concepts

- **Clinical evaluation of the patient, including history, physical examination, laboratory tests, x-rays, and other tests**

- **Diagnosis and description of clinical syndromes, including inflammatory and noninflammatory arthritis, and connective tissue diseases**

- **Treatment of rheumatic diseases with medications and manipulative therapy**

Rheumatology can be defined as the subspecialty of internal medicine that deals with the medical evaluation and treatment of the musculoskeletal system. Rheumatologists are subspecialists in internal medicine who devote themselves to additional training in the rheumatic diseases. Musculoskeletal complaints are ubiquitous in society and are frequently cited as one of the most common reasons why patients visit physicians. The Arthritis Foundation reports that there are more than 100 different forms of arthritic diseases.[1] The osteopathic physician must differentiate among these conditions. The importance of making a correct diagnosis ensures that the most cost-effective tests will be performed, appropriate therapy will be recommended to the patient, and focused guidance with counseling will be offered to the patient. Because the fastest growing portion of the United States' population is individuals older than 85 years of age, the cumulative incidence of rheumatic diseases in the population and their importance in an aging population will increase over the next several decades. This review of rheumatology is in no way exhaustive; it is intended as a general overview.

CLINICAL EVALUATION OF PATIENT

The history and physical examination of the person with a probable rheumatic disease requires careful questioning, observation, and hands-on examination.

History

The most important answer to be gained from the history is whether an inflammatory or noninflammatory rheumatic disease is causing the patient's problem.[2] Questions useful in distinguishing inflammatory from noninflammatory rheumatic diseases include the following examples:

1. Are the joints stiff in the morning?
2. What is the duration of morning stiffness?
3. Does the stiffness improve during the day?
4. Is there joint swelling rather than simply joint pain?
5. What types of activities make the pain better, and what types of activities make the pain worse?
6. Over what period of time has the joint pain been present? Is it a matter of hours, days, weeks, or months?
7. What is the pattern of the joint pain and/or swelling? Is it symmetric, asymmetric, or located in only one joint?
8. Is the pain actually *in* a joint or is it diffuse and located around the area of the joint?

A knowledge base of clinical rheumatic disease presentations helps the physician categorize answers to these questions and differentiate among different illnesses. A "functional" history is often helpful in determining the nature of a patient's disability as a result of rheumatic disease.[3] For example, asking if someone can dress unassisted, stand up from a commode without assistance, walk stairs unattended, comb his or her hair, etc., helps the physician gain a more accurate picture of the extent of disability present. In general, persons with rheumatic complaints and rheumatic diseases are more often concerned about potential disability than they are concerned about death.[2] Many patients with rheumatic diseases are previously healthy until they suffer a constellation of musculoskeletal complaints that render them unable to adequately perform their activities of daily living. These concerns and fears must be dealt with early on to achieve an effective doctor–patient relationship.

Physical Examination

The physical examination is divided into two parts:

1. General physical examination
2. Specific musculoskeletal examination

An adequate examination of the musculoskeletal system can usually be done fairly rapidly.[4] The patient should be completely undressed. As a general guideline, the physician performs observation, then palpation, and finally the movement of joints through their range of motion. A typical history and physical form is included as a guide (Figs. 38.1–38.4). Because most individuals present with a chief complaint of pain, the purpose of the physical examination is to try to locate the site of the pain and determine whether the pain is truly related to an underlying rheumatic disease. The history attempts to define whether an arthritic disease is inflammatory or noninflam-

Chief complaint _____

Present illness _____

_____

_____

Past medical history _____   Past surgical history _____

_____

Current medications _____   Allergies _____

_____

Family history _____   Social history _____

_____

Figure 38.1. Initial rheumatology history.

matory, and therefore the physical examination should help determine if the impression gained from the history is correct.

In general, examine each joint looking for warmth, redness, synovial thickening, deformity, and effusion. Perform active and passive range of motion on all joints.[5] Use the general physical examination to determine whether any systemic or extraarticular features are present that would lend weight to a diagnosis of a rheumatic disease. Apply basic osteopathic principles during the course of the history and physical examination, particularly for noninflammatory rheumatic diseases. Palpatory findings can lead to specific diagnoses and subsequent manipulative treatment.[6–7]

Laboratory Evaluation

The laboratory evaluation of rheumatic diseases includes the use of routine laboratory tests such as complete blood count, chemistry panel, and urinalysis. Examine synovial fluid in selected individuals; it can provide diagnostic information. Last, sophisticated autoantibodies and immune complex assays are performed when specific inflammatory rheumatic diseases are suspected. Remember that the purpose of laboratory tests in the evaluation of a possible rheumatic disease is to support the clinical diagnosis that has been derived from the history and physical examination.[8] Rarely will the laboratory tests surprise the accomplished physician. In general, a test should not be ordered unless one has a specific idea of what to do with the anticipated result. For example, patients with rheumatoid arthritis might have a positive antinuclear antibody; persons older than 60 years of age might have rheumatoid factor in their blood in the absence of rheumatoid arthritis; an elevated sedimentation rate can indicate the presence of any type of inflammation or infection, even unrelated to a rheumatic disease; an abnormal creatine phosphokinase (CPK) value is not necessarily diagnostic of someone with polymyositis. Laboratory tests can be helpful and useful in confirming the diagnosis of a rheumatic disease when it is suspected, but they can be confusing if ordered in a random fashion.

X-rays and Other Diagnostic Tests

The radiographic examination of joints is important to differentiate inflammatory from noninflammatory rheumatic diseases. In general, inflammatory rheumatic diseases appear "subtractive" on x-ray films. Inflammation of a joint, whether from infection or an autoimmune process, can lead to osteopenia, joint erosions, and typically, a loss of bone substance. Noninflammatory rheumatic diseases are "additive." There is an increase in bone as a result of subchondral sclerosis, osteophyte formation, and bridging of the joint space. The pattern of involvement in x-ray studies is typically a mirror of the involvement that one would suspect clinically. X-ray films are often used to stage patients and to follow their progress once therapy has been instituted. In the last several years, the use of magnetic resonance imaging (MRI) scans, computerized tomography (CT) scans, and other radiographic modalities have helped refine our understanding of the underlying process in some of the rheumatic diseases. X-ray studies are used to reinforce and substantiate the clinical impression already gained from a careful history and physical examination.

CLINICAL SYNDROMES

Clinical syndromes have three major types: inflammatory arthritis, noninflammatory arthritis, and connective tissue disease.

Inflammatory Arthritis

Four different inflammatory arthritic conditions are discussed briefly. These include:

Rheumatoid arthritis
Crystal-induced arthritis
Seronegative spondyloarthropathies
Infectious arthritis

General/Constitutional

_____ Fatigue
_____ Fever
_____ Intercurrent illness
_____ Shaking chills
_____ Weight loss
_____ Anorexia

Skin

_____ Alopecia
_____ Photosensitivity
_____ Psoriasis
_____ Purpura
_____ Rash (malar)
_____ Rash (other)
_____ Raynaud's phenomenon
_____ Skin tightening
_____ Skin ulcers (digital)
_____ Skin ulcers (nondigital)
_____ Nail pitting

HEENT

_____ Conjunctivitis
_____ Dry eyes
_____ Dry mouth
_____ Headache
_____ Mucosal ulcers
_____ Nasal complaints
_____ Ocular inflammation (other)
_____ Salivary gland enlargement
_____ Sore throat
_____ Tinnitus

Cardiopulmonary

_____ Chest pain
_____ Chest pain (pleuritic)
_____ Cough (persistent)
_____ Dyspnea or orthopnea
_____ Edema (dependent)
_____ Hemoptysis
_____ Palpitations
_____ Wheezing

Endocrine

_____ Calcium intake
_____ History of thyroid disease
_____ Heat/cold intolerance

Gastrointestinal

_____ Abdominal pain (other)
_____ Diarrhea
_____ Dysphagia
_____ Hematemesis or melena
_____ Peptic ulcer symptoms
_____ Nausea or vomiting

Genitourinary

_____ Genital ulceration
_____ Hematuria by history
_____ Proteinuria by history
_____ Renal stone
_____ Menstrual abnormality
_____ Urethral discharge
_____ Dysuria
_____ Prostatitis
_____ Urinary infections
_____ Infertility/Miscarriages

Hematologic

_____ Anemia by history
_____ Leukopenia by history
_____ Thrombocytopenia by history
_____ Bleeding disorder

Neuropsychiatric

_____ Muscle pain
_____ Muscle weakness
_____ Paresthesias
_____ Psychiatric (specify)
_____ Seizures
_____ Visual loss
_____ Difficulty sleeping

Articular

_____ Morning stiffness
_____ Arthralgias
_____ Joint swelling
_____ Heel pain
_____ Night pain
_____ Neck pain
_____ Low back pain

Figure 38.2. Review of systems for rheumatologic examination.

RHEUMATOID ARTHRITIS

Rheumatoid arthritis is one of the most common inflammatory rheumatic diseases. It occurs in approximately 1% of the population of the United States, primarily in women during their childbearing years. Rheumatoid arthritis should be differentiated from the seronegative spondyloarthropathies. The sero-negative spondyloarthropathies include diseases such as ankylosing spondylitis, Reiter's syndrome, psoriatic arthritis, and the arthritis of inflammatory bowel disease. The key distinguishing features between these two major groups of inflammatory rheumatic diseases are that rheumatoid arthritis patients have a symmetric polyarthritis and they frequently have rheumatoid factor in their blood. Persons with seronegative

Description of patient: _____

Ambulatory status: _____ Weight _____ Height _____

Blood pressure: _____ Temp _____ Pulse _____

Skin

_____ Abnormal pigmentation

_____ Alopecia

_____ Calcinosis

_____ Digital ulcers (scars)

_____ Gottron's papules

_____ Erythema nodosum

_____ Periungual erythema

_____ Heliotrope eyelids

_____ Keratoderma blennorrhagicum

_____ Nail pitting

_____ Psoriasis

_____ Purpura

_____ Discoid lupus

_____ Malar rash

_____ Rash, other (specify) _____
      _____

_____ Scleroderma, generalized

_____ Telangiectasias

_____ Ulcerations, other

_____ Urticaria

_____ Splinter hemorrhage

Eyes

_____ Cataract

_____ Conjunctivitis

_____ Episcleral or scleral disease

_____ Fundi (abnormal)

_____ Iritis, acute

_____ Uveitis, chronic

ENT

_____ Oral ulcers

_____ Salivary gland enlargement

_____ Temporal artery tenderness

_____ Thyroid (abnormal)

_____ Xerostomia

Chest

_____ Pleural effusion

_____ Pleural rub

_____ Rales

_____ Wheezing

_____ **Breast masses**

Heart

_____ Abnormal P2

_____ Cardiomegaly

_____ Murmur, diastolic

_____ Murmur, systolic

_____ Pericardial rub

_____ Gallop (specify)

_____ Arrythmia

Abdomen

_____ Hepatomegaly

_____ Jaundice

_____ Peritoneal signs

_____ Splenomegaly

_____ Tenderness

Genitalia

_____ Pregnancy

_____ Ulcerations, Rashes (balanitis)

_____ Urethral discharge

_____ **Extremities**

_____ Absent pulses

_____ Clubbing

_____ Edema

_____ Raynaud's phenomenon

_____ Sclerodactyly

Neuropsychiatric

_____ Muscle atrophy

_____ Muscle tenderness

_____ Muscle weakness, proximal

_____ Muscle weakness, distal

_____ Neuropathy, entrapment

_____ Neuropathy, motor

_____ Neuropathy, sensory

_____ Personality change

_____ Phalen's sign

_____ Psychosis

_____ Tinel's sign

DTRs

_____ Biceps   _____ Ankle

_____ Triceps   _____ Babinski

_____ Brachioradialis

_____ Knee

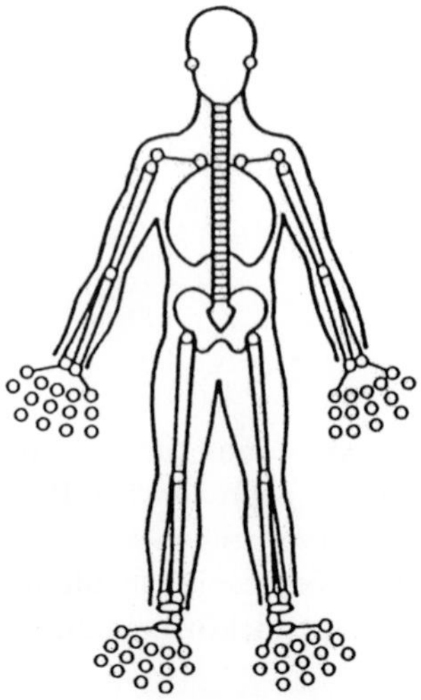

Figure 38.3. Physical examination form for rheumatologic examination.

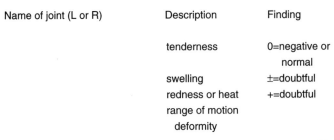

Name of joint (L or R)	Description	Finding
	tenderness	0=negative or normal
	swelling	±=doubtful
	redness or heat	+=doubtful
	range of motion	
	deformity	

Figure 38.4. Joint examination form for articular index. Assess 33 joints on each side, recording the results using the system shown here, representing an overview of rheumatologic findings.

spondyloarthropathies classically have an asymmetric polyarthritis; by definition, rheumatoid factor is absent from their blood. There is an association with the HLA-B27 gene and seronegative spondyloarthropathy.

Rheumatoid arthritis can begin abruptly or insidiously. Most patients with rheumatoid arthritis have periods of exacerbations or remissions that are of variable lengths of time. The remissions might or might not be influenced by treatment, whether pharmacologic therapy, manipulative treatment, or physical therapy. Almost half of all patients with rheumatoid arthritis are disabled within 10 years of their diagnosis.[9] Rheumatoid arthritis is not a morbid condition only; many persons with rheumatoid arthritis actually have increased mortality. Increased mortality might result not only from the disease itself but also from some of the therapies used.[10]

Extraarticular features are found in both rheumatoid arthritis and the seronegative spondyloarthropathies; a careful history and physical examination are necessary when a physician suspects inflammatory rheumatic disease. The presence of peripheral neuropathy, muscle atrophy, subcutaneous nodules, skin rashes in various locations, and eye inflammation, among other features, help not only to secure a diagnosis of inflammatory arthritis but also to differentiate between rheumatoid arthritis and a seronegative spondyloarthropathy.

Juvenile rheumatoid arthritis (JRA) is a type of arthritis that occurs in patients younger than 18 years of age. Approximately 70,000 children in the United States have juvenile rheumatoid arthritis.[11] JRA takes many forms, including systemic-onset JRA, also known as "Still's disease." Still's disease is associated with negative rheumatoid factor, negative antinuclear antibody, high fevers, and a rash. A small percentage of these patients will go on to have chronic destructive arthritis. Pauciarticular JRA occurs in half of all patients with juvenile rheumatoid arthritis. Pauci means few, and generally four or fewer joints in total are affected. Most of these children are negative for rheumatoid factor. Young girls with positive antinuclear antibody and pauciarticular JRA are at risk for iridocyclitis, which can cause potentially serious insidious eye inflammation. These young girls must be examined regularly by an ophthalmologist with slitlamp examinations until they reach adulthood. Older boys with pauciarticular JRA who are HLA-B27–positive might have a form of juvenile ankylosing spondylitis manifested by sacroiliitis and asymmetric lower extremity arthritis.

CRYSTAL-INDUCED ARTHRITIS

Other forms of inflammatory polyarthritis include crystal-induced arthritis. The two primary categories are gout and calcium pyrophosphate deposition disease (pseudogout). Both of these conditions occur in middle-aged or elderly individuals. Clinically they present as an acute monarthritis. The diagnosis is confirmed by performing polarized microscopy of synovial fluid and identifying the appropriate crystal. Gout is probably the second most common cause of inflammatory arthritis in the United States.[12]

INFECTIOUS ARTHRITIS

Infectious arthritis is a true rheumatologic emergency. The major subsets are gonococcal or nongonococcal infectious arthritis. Infectious arthritis causes pain, tenderness, and swelling of the affected joint. Gonococcal arthritis is the most common cause of acute bacterial arthritis. The classic presentation is a young, sexually active individual who presents with an acute monarthritis preceded by a migratory pattern of polyarthralgias associated with fevers and chills. Skin lesions, either vesicular or target lesions, can be present in this disseminated gonococcal infection (DGI).[13] The diagnosis of gonococcal arthritis is highly suspected by the history and physical examination because the ability to grow gonococcus in culture medium is difficult, whether from synovial fluid or blood. Nongonococcal bacterial arthritis is caused by Gram-positive organisms in up to 85% of patients, unless the patient is immunosuppressed or has other complicating medical factors. Clinically, patients present with an acute monarthritis in a joint previously affected by arthritis. Organisms are usually seen on Gram stain; appropriate therapy is begun depending on the clinical setting. Rare causes of infectious arthritis include viral organisms, fungi, and anaerobic bacteria. Mortality and morbidity of infectious arthritis have both markedly decreased in the last 20 years primarily as a result of physicians' enhanced awareness of the necessity for early joint fluid drainage coupled with aggressive antibiotic therapy.

Noninflammatory Arthritis

OSTEOARTHRITIS

Osteoarthritis is the most common arthritic disease, usually affecting both men and women older than 50 years of age. Weightbearing joints are usually involved. Osteoarthritis has several distinct forms, including nodal arthritis, which seems to be a disorder transmitted by autosomal dominant genes in women. The recent discovery of genetic defects in joint collagen in a family with osteoarthritis underscores the idea that osteoarthritis is not simply the result of wear and tear in the joint.[14] A variant called erosive osteoarthritis seems to be associated with self-limited inflammation of the distal interphalangeal joints, erosions at the margins of these joints, and a tendency towards fusion of the inflamed joints.[15] Primary generalized osteoarthritis affects the hands, knees, hips, and feet, and could just represent a more severe form of osteoarthritis. Isolated joints can be affected, usually in those individuals in occupations that impose stress on the joints, such as jackhammer operators and miners. Evidence suggests an increased incidence of osteoarthritis on the long leg side of a patient with leg length discrepancy.[16]

Exercise has a controversial association with osteoarthritis;[17] studies are underway to examine this issue in more detail. Osteoarthritis affects the spine; the topic of back pain is covered in detail in Chapter 28, Orthopaedics. From a rheumatologic standpoint, osteoarthritis is not simply wear and tear of the joint. Local inflammation occurs, and alterations in the lubricating properties of synovial fluid combined with changes in resiliency of cartilage can play more of a role in the pathophysiology of osteoarthritis than has been previously noted. Pain usually is the presenting manifestation of osteoarthritis. Laboratory test results should be normal. Synovial fluid has a low white cell count, a good mucin clot, and normal viscosity. X-ray studies show features of an additive disease consistent with noninflammatory arthritis.

SOFT TISSUE RHEUMATISM

Soft tissue rheumatism includes myofascial pain syndromes, fibromyalgia, and localized bursitis and tendinitis. Fibromyalgia syndrome has been reported to occur in up to 5% of the population. It might be associated with a specific sleep abnormality: alpha wave intrusion into stage IV delta wave non–REM sleep. Clinically, fibromyalgia is a chronic musculoskeletal syndrome characterized by diffuse pain and tender points, without evidence of synovitis or myositis. Laboratory tests and x-ray films are normal. The physical examination is highlighted by reproducible tenderness at specific tender points.[18] Fibromyalgia is one rheumatic disease that has particularly been embraced by osteopathic physicians.[19] The diffuse nature of the musculoskeletal pain coupled with anatomically distinct tender points has encouraged controlled studies[20–22] examining the use of osteopathic manipulation in the management of this condition. Myofascial pain syndromes and repetitive strain syndromes can overlap clinically with fibromyalgia syndrome. Myofascial pain syndromes are often locally painful and follow physical trauma. If local treatment is not helpful, the trigger points of myofascial pain can broaden, and the condition can take on more characteristics of fibromyalgia syndrome.[23]

Repetitive strain syndrome is a chronic pain syndrome that occurs after activities involving repetitious movement. The pain is located in the arm and tends to be constant. Often numbness and tingling are found in a nondermatomal distribution in the affected arm. Repetitive strain syndromes have been noted in epidemics[24] but can be differentiated from fibromyalgia syndrome because the symptoms are localized to the arms.

OSTEOPOROSIS

Osteoporosis is epidemic in America. Although not a traditional rheumatologic condition, the fact that pain is a presenting manifestation has caused many rheumatologists to become interested in this illness. Standard x-ray studies are not helpful in making the early diagnosis of osteoporosis, compared with assessing bone density by dual photon absorptiometry and dual energy x-ray absorptiometry (DEXA). The clinical history and physical examination coupled with bone density measurements determine which female patients have postmenopausal osteoporosis, reflecting a long-term imbalance between bone resorption and formation. Secondary causes such as corticosteroid use, malignancy, and nutritional disorders enter into the differential diagnosis and require specific therapy as indicated.

Connective Tissue Diseases

Rheumatology is also concerned with connective tissue diseases. These are uncommon illnesses, but appropriate diagnosis and subsequent therapy can be lifesaving.

POLYMYOSITIS

Polymyositis and dermatomyositis present with severe proximal muscle weakness, coupled with low-grade fevers, malaise, and fatigue. The diagnosis rests with laboratory evaluation of muscle enzymes, electromyography (EMG) to detect muscle abnormalities, and abnormal muscle on biopsy. Scleroderma is a rare rheumatologic condition that begins with an early edematous phase associated with puffy hands or puffy extremities and slowly evolves into thickened skin with tight hidebound appearance. Skin is either hyperpigmented or hypopigmented and taut and shiny. Prognosis in scleroderma is usually related to the presence of underlying hypertension and renal disease secondary to vascular inflammation.

VASCULITIS

The vasculitides include many syndromes such as periarteritis nodosa, Churg-Strauss vasculitis, and Wegener's granulomatosis. Once again, these rare conditions are characterized by autoimmune inflammation and destruction of multiple organs. Diagnosis is difficult, and treatment usually requires immunosuppressive medications.

SYSTEMIC LUPUS ERYTHEMATOSUS

Systemic lupus erythematosus (SLE) is a prototypic connective tissue disease. Approximately one-tenth as common as rheumatoid arthritis, it is more common in African-Americans. Diagnosis can be difficult because, although multiple laboratory tests are currently available, the diagnosis is made on clinical grounds. Most patients with SLE have dermatologic features such as a malar rash, discoid rash, or photosensitivity. Arthritis can look superficially like rheumatoid arthritis; erosions are usually absent in x-ray studies.[25] Visceral organ damage can occur in SLE, including pleurisy, pericarditis, renal disease, and neurologic conditions such as seizures, psychosis, or peripheral neuropathy. Laboratory features such as anemia, thrombocytopenia, or leukopenia are frequent. A positive antinuclear antibody (ANA) test result is almost uniformly present in patients with lupus. Other autoantibodies such as double-stranded DNA, anti-SM, anti-RO, and anti-LA antibodies can be present or absent in any given patient. Although autoantibody tests are important from a research standpoint and perhaps in some clinical settings, the diagnosis of SLE remains clinical.[26] Recently, osteopathic manipulative treatments (OMT) have been applied to the treatment of patients with SLE in combination with traditional medical therapy.[27]

Soft tissue rheumatism, fibromyalgia syndrome, and myofascial trigger points occur more commonly in individuals with an underlying rheumatic disease such as rheumatoid arthritis, osteoarthritis, or SLE.[28] Therefore, pains causing an individual to present to a primary care practitioner's or rheumatologist's office might not be the result of primary rheumatic disease but of coincidental fibromyalgia or myofascial pain syndrome. OMT is useful in managing the soft tissue rheumatic complaints.

TREATMENT OF RHEUMATIC DISEASES

Treatment of rheumatic diseases is based on the diagnosis and the severity of illness. Treatment follows from a careful history and physical examination, coupled with appropriate laboratory tests and x-ray studies. Treatments can be divided into pharmacologic and nonpharmacologic methods.

Medications

Pharmacologic therapies are nonspecific. Nonsteroidal antiinflammatory drugs (NSAIDs) are fundamental to the treatment of most rheumatic diseases. They are useful as both analgesic and antiinflammatory agents. Local injection of corticosteroids into affected joints and/or trigger points can produce dramatic improvement. Antibiotic therapy is necessary for treatment of infectious arthritis; the antibiotic of choice depends on the organism cultured or clinically implicated in the condition. Systemic corticosteroids and other immunosuppressant medications are reserved for patients who fail with more conservative measures. These drugs are used judiciously. Long-term side effects of steroids include:

Cushingoid appearance
Osteoporosis
Hypertension
Diabetes mellitus
Cataracts
Depression

In general, rheumatologists now treat inflammatory rheumatic diseases more aggressively earlier in the course of the illness, hoping to alter or prevent joint and internal organ destruction if possible. This treatment philosophy is controversial but is a trend that has been evolving over the past decade.[29] One can argue convincingly that the greatest advance in the management of end-stage osteoarthritis and rheumatoid arthritis over the past 25 years has been the ability to surgically replace destroyed joints. Orthopaedic surgical intervention as a component of a team approach to the management of rheumatic diseases adds a totality to the pharmacologic, nonpharmacologic, surgical therapy continuum.

Manipulative Therapy

Nonpharmacologic therapy for rheumatic diseases is rewarding. Physical therapy and occupational therapy are fundamental to the treatment of most rheumatic diseases; this subject is covered more extensively in Chapter 36, Physical Medicine and Rehabilitation. OMT has been effective in the treatment of fibromyalgia syndrome, specifically with regard to strain-counterstrain techniques.[19–20] Several controlled studies have been performed using manipulative treatment in conjunction with tricyclic antidepressants, NSAIDs, and minor tranquilizers for the therapy of fibromyalgia syndrome.[20–21]

Patients appear to experience improved quality of life when offered OMT, as opposed to more traditional pharmacologic therapy. Research studies involving large numbers of patients followed for months or years have not yet been done. The long-term benefits of OMT are unknown in these conditions. A study examining the use of OMT as an adjunct in the management of SLE has begun.[27] Results have not been finalized, but one would anticipate that patients with SLE and associated fibromyalgia-like complaints would benefit from OMT. One does see improvements in their overall sense of well-being and quality of life, but whether manipulative treatment alters immune function in this situation has yet to be determined.

Tucker published a paper examining the treatment of osteoarthritis using manual therapy.[30] He believed that the early use of manipulative treatment might be beneficial, but if symptoms persisted after 6 months, more aggressive traditional therapy should be considered. His paper, published almost 30 years ago, has conclusions that are valid today regarding the early use of physical measures for the treatment of osteoarthritis followed by more traditional pharmacologic therapy. In general, osteopathic physicians treat rheumatic diseases with pharmacologic therapy in addition to OMT. The specific manipulative techniques used depend on the patient's age, presence of osteoporosis and/or vertebral fracture, the extent of the arthritis, and the presence or absence of complicating systemic extraarticular features.

CONCLUSION

Osteopathic physicians have a modality—osteopathic manipulative treatment—that benefits individuals who suffer from rheumatic diseases. With the possible exception of infectious arthritis, no rheumatic disease can truly be cured. It is clear that the body is a unit, and that structure and function are intimately interrelated. The body might well have an inherent ability to heal itself. Combining appropriate diagnosis with pharmacologic therapy and manipulative treatment allows patients to experience an overall improved sense of well-being and hopefully achieve a better outcome. Clinical research is the key to answering questions regarding the potential benefit of osteopathic manipulative treatment in the management of the rheumatic diseases. Recent studies cited in fibromyalgia and systemic lupus erythematosus are the first efforts to examine osteopathic manipulative treatment in a defined population. More controlled studies of this nature must be done to logically and appropriately answer questions raised regarding the benefits of manipulative treatment. Further clinical investigation should continue so that the science of osteopathic medicine and its benefit on the outcome of these diseases can be proven.

ACKNOWLEDGMENTS

This chapter is dedicated to my daughter, Sarah E. Rubin. Her smiles brighten every day. The intellectual support and patience of my co-worker, Cynthia Ann Jimenez, RN, helped me find the time in an overworked schedule to complete this project. Not to be forgotten are the other members of the Rheumatology Division, Doctors Raymond Pertusi and Mitchell Forman, who offered important suggestions. Lastly, Kristi Ramos, a secretary who has been a delight to work with.

I thank each of you for your support in helping to bring forth this chapter.

REFERENCES

1. Decker JL and the Glossary Subcommittee of the ARA Committee on rheumatologic practice. American Rheumatism Association nomenclature and classification of arthritis and rheumatism. *Arthritis Rheum.* 1983;26:1029–1032.
2. Liang MH, Sturrock RD. Evaluation of musculoskeletal symptoms. In: Klippel JH, Dieppe PB, eds. *Rheumatology.* London, England: Mosby; 1994:2.1.1.–2.11.6.
3. American College of Rheumatology Glossary Committee. *Dictionary of the Rheumatic Diseases, III: Health Status Measurement.* New York, NY: Contact Associates International Ltd; 1988:1–65.
4. Ball GV, Koopman WJ. *Clinical Rheumatology.* Philadelphia, Penn: WB Saunders; 1986:60–62.
5. Gall EP. History and Physical Examination. In *Primer on the Rheumatic Diseases.* 10th ed. Atlanta, Ga: Arthritis Foundation; 1993:60–64.
6. Pringle M, Tyreman S. Study of 500 patients attending an osteopathic practice. *Br J Gen Pract.* January 1993:15–18.
7. Kuchera ML, Kuchera WA. *Osteopathic Considerations in Systemic Dysfunction.* 2nd ed. rev. Columbus, Ohio: Greyden Press; 1994:159–167.
8. Shmerling RH, Liang MH. Laboratory Evaluation of Rheumatic Diseases. In *Primer on the Rheumatic Diseases.* 10th ed. Atlanta, Ga: Arthritis Foundation; 1993:64–66.
9. Kushner I. Does aggressive therapy of rheumatoid arthritis affect outcome? *J Rheumatol.* 1989;16:1–3.
10. Pincus T, Callahan LF. Taking mortality in rheumatoid arthritis seriously: predictive markers, socioeconomic status and comorbidity. *J Rheumatol.* 1986;13:841–845.
11. Singsen BH. Epidemiology of the rheumatic diseases of childhood. *Rheum Dis Clin North Am.* 1990;16:581–599.
12. Lawrence RC, Hochberg MC, Kelsey JL, et al. Estimates of the prevalence of selected arthritic and musculoskeletal diseases in the United States. *J Rheumatol.* 1989;16:427–441.
13. Goldenberg DL, Reed JI. Bacterial arthritis. *N Engl J Med.* 1985; 312:764–771.
14. Knowlton RG, Katzenstein PL, Moskowitz RW, et al. Genetic linkage of a polymorphism in the type II pro-collagen gene (COL2A) to primary osteoarthritis associated with mild chondrodysplasia. *N Engl J Med.* 1990;322:526–530.
15. Ehrlich GE. Inflammatory osteoarthritis, I. The clinical syndromes. *J Chronic Dis.* 1972;25:317–328.
16. Panush RS, Schmidt C, Caldwell JR, et al. Is running associated with degenerative joint disease? *JAMA.* 1986;255:1152–1154.
17. Grofton JP, Trueman GE. Studies in osteoarthritis of the hips: Part II. Osteoarthritis of the hip and leg length disparity. *Can Med Assoc J.* 1971;104:791–799.
18. Goldenberg DL. Fibromyalgia syndrome: an emerging but controversial condition. *JAMA.* 1987;257:2782–2787.
19. Backstrom G, Rubin BR. *When Muscle Pain Won't Go Away.* 2nd ed. Dallas, Tex: Taylor; 1995:49–59.
20. Rubin BR, Cortez CA, Gamber R, Shores J. Treatment options in fibromyalgia syndrome. *JAOA.* 1990;90(9):844.
21. Rubin BR, Gamber R, Shores J, Davis G, Cortez C. The effect of treatment options on perceived pain in fibromyalgia syndrome. *Arthritis Rheum.* 1991;34(5):R33.
22. Lo KS, Kuchera ML, Preston SC, Jackson RW. Osteopathic manipulative treatment in fibromyalgia syndrome. *JAOA.* 1992;92(9):177.
23. Wolfe F, Simons DG, Fricton JR, et al. The fibromyalgia and myofascial pain syndromes: a preliminary study of tender points and trigger points in persons with fibromyalgia, myofascial pain syndrome and no disease. *J Rheumatol.* 1992;19:944–951.
24. Hocking B. Epidemiological aspects of "repetition strain injury" in Telecom Australia. *Med J Aust.* 1987;147:218–222.
25. Reilly PA, Evison G, McHugh NJ, Maddison PJ. Arthropathy of hands and feet in systemic lupus erythematosus. *J Rheumatol.* 1990:17;777–784.
26. Gladman DD, Urowitz MB. Systemic lupus erythematosus. B. Clinical features. In: Schumacher HR, ed. *Primer on the Rheumatic Diseases.* 10th ed. Atlanta, Ga: Arthritis Foundation; 1993:106–111.
27. Pertusi RM, Rubin BR, Davis GC. Instruments to assess quality of life in SLE. *JAOA.* 1993;93(9).
28. Smythe H, Lee D, Rush P, Buskila D. Tender shins and steroid therapy. *J Rheumatol.* 1991;18:1568–1572.
29. Wilske KR, Healey LA. Remodeling the pyramid—a concept whose time has come. *J Rheumatol.* 1989;16:565–567.
30. Tucker WE. Treatment of osteoarthritis by manual therapy. *Br J Clin Pract.* 1969;23(1):3–8.

Osteopathic Considerations in Palpatory Diagnosis and Manipulative Treatment

Part A. Overview: Evaluation and Management

Part B. Regional Examination and Treatment

Part C. Palpatory Diagnosis and Manipulative Treatment

Part D. Goals and Expectations

INTRODUCTION

John M. Jones III and Robert E. Kappler

The following chapters contain detailed descriptions of musculoskeletal examination and various treatment techniques commonly taught at osteopathic medical colleges in the United States. We would like to gratefully acknowledge the contributions made by the faculties of those colleges.

Andrew Taylor Still never taught what he called techniques and explicitly recommended against teaching osteopathy in that fashion. He felt that if the physician knew anatomy, it was unnecessary to teach techniques, because the method to be used for a particular patient's problems should be obvious. So why do we teach techniques at our colleges today?

In 1892, when Still founded the American School of Osteopathy, he established a curriculum dominated by anatomy. This was partly because he discarded much of the standard medical curriculum; it was of little use to the physician and largely harmful to the patient. There has been an explosion of knowledge in both the basic and clinical sciences since that time. To the medical student, it often seems that all the knowledge accumulated in the past century has been retained in the curriculum, without the deletion of a single element of medical minutiae. This may be true to an extent. Currently, only about 10% of the curriculum in the first 2 years of osteopathic education is reserved for teaching the philosophy, principles, and mechanics of osteopathic manipulative diagnosis and treatment.

FORMS OF TREATMENT

There are many forms of osteopathic manipulation. Only the basic types taught during the first 2 years at United States colleges of osteopathic medicine are presented in the following chapters. Other forms of osteopathic manipulation, such as visceral manipulation, are left for later work. Also, not every possible form of a particular technique is included. For example, there are at least six ways to do high-velocity low-amplitude thrust technique on a typical cervical vertebra. Only representative samples of the techniques are included.

These samples of treatment can be classified as soft tissue techniques, articulatory techniques, or direct and indirect methods of treatment. Techniques named according to the activating forces used are muscle energy, springing, or high-velocity low-amplitude (HVLA) thrust. Those referring to a concept of treatment are called strain/counterstrain, myofascial release, or osteopathy in the cranial field. Related topics of release by positioning are discussed, as well as Simon and Travell's system of trigger points. Though trigger point diagnosis and treatment is not classified as osteopathic, it fits well into the practice of musculoskeletal medicine and is used by many osteopathic physicians.

MODELS

In each of these classifications of treatment techniques, the diagnosis and treatment are based on a mental model, a cognitive system of reference that is workable when applied to patients with somatic dysfunctions. Models have limitations. They cannot explain everything; that is not their purpose. They are designed to correlate certain gathered information with a diagnosis and to relate this diagnosis to a successful treatment. The muscle energy model of sacral torsion does not delineate the exact biomechanics of the sacrum or which specific muscle(s) are involved in the treatment. However, if the physician collects data, arrives at a diagnosis, and treats the disorder as indicated, the somatic dysfunction should resolve. The muscle energy model relates to the body in terms of simplified biomechanics. Many physicians use the muscle energy model not because it is perfect but because it works and they are pragmatic.

Models that survive the test of time and propagate are those that have empirically proven themselves by benefiting the patients. The models in the following chapters are examples of ways to accomplish biomechanical changes and achieve treatment goals. They are not the only way. If you understand anatomy, you can use a variety of ways to achieve the same objective. If you do not understand anatomy, following a protocol may do the patient no good; the patient's physique may not conform to the 5'10", 170-pound model on which the protocol was based. Knowing anatomy, however, is not enough by itself.

You may, for instance, adapt a technique by using muscle energy activation on a position normally followed by HVLA. You base this on what you palpate and sense happening with the patient and on the patient's unique response to past or current treatment. You may use treatment in two planes rather than three, because of positional limitations imposed on the patient because of surgery, trauma, or the formation of osteophytes in osteoarthritis. You might more appropriately make a completely different choice of treatment technique because of the positional limitation. For example, the muscle energy model requires flexion to confront an extension lesion. If the surgeon wants the head to remain flat, you may elect to use indirect myofascial release at the cervical segment level, requiring only a few degrees of motion, which would not raise the head off the pillow.

PHYSICIAN KNOWLEDGE AND EXPERIENCE

The choice of technique depends on the knowledge and experience of the physician as well as the limitations of the patient. When a patient has a diagnosable somatic dysfunction in the cervical region, you have many treatment options. Some may be contraindicated, as illustrated by the case of a male septuagenarian who was in the hospital for cardiac electrophysiologic studies. He had lost consciousness several times before admission, when he turned his head. During provocative testing, his heart stopped beating for 6 seconds, until defibrillation was used to restart cardiac performance. Normally, one would think that use of strain/counterstrain techniques would be much easier on a patient than most other treatments. However, in this case, treatment by strain/counterstrain is contraindicated. Muscle energy, HVLA, or articulatory treatment would also be inadvisable. Osteopathic diagnosis and treatment provide the alternatives of indirect segmental treatment or osteopathy in the cranial field (with caution in this case). Carefully consider your patient's limitations, along with your own skill level, when choosing which technique to use. Clinical judgment about "when to use what" is often difficult until one acquires a certain body of clinical experience, largely by observing decisions made by other physicians.

TECHNIQUE VERSUS TREATMENT

Another problem is making the jump between performing a technique and doing an osteopathic treatment. Osteopathic manipulation can be reduced in scope to the point where it appears to be a series of specific treatments for specific problems. If it is carried out in this fashion, however, it loses its identity as osteopathic manipulation and becomes merely manual medicine. The term manual medicine implies a form of treatment applied by the hands. The term osteopathic manipulation indicates more than that; it indicates that the physician is applying the four basic principles of osteopathic philosophy. One of these principles is that the body is a unit. The true osteopathic approach cannot be broken down into isolated procedures specific for particular complaints; the osteopathic approach treats the patient as a unit.

It is often said that when you see an osteopathic physician for treatment of a low back problem, the doctor might check your feet, your knees, and your neck. The goal of osteopathic treatment includes consideration of the entire person, not a specific dysfunctional muscle. Though its success helps the patient overcome the dysfunction or disease, the osteopathic treatment is performed to support the patient, in whatever way is indicated.

That is the osteopathic ideal. Realistically, there are many times in medical practice where the dictates of time, resources, and energy direct you to apply this ideal in limited form. The effects of applying specific procedures to a specific dysfunction have far less profound effects than a total treatment. The degree to which you apply osteopathic philosophy is determined by the degree to which you are practicing osteopathy. To offer an analogy, an engine sometimes needs an overhaul but sometimes only a minor adjustment or a single part. In the same way, time constraints may indicate that a specific procedure should be provided today, with a more thorough treatment in the scheduled follow-up visit. A single procedure that treats the body's needs may be preferable to no treatment at all, or to merely writing a prescription to treat the disease. At no time should you lose sight of the impact of that procedure on the total body. The body is constantly trying to maintain optimal homeostasis, using its self-healing ability and self-regulatory mechanisms. By directing the osteopathic manipulation to a prime site, the body may be able to continue improvement. At the next visit, you can reevaluate body needs and administer further treatment as necessary.

Beginning physicians often hesitate to use manipulation on hospital patients. There is the fear of treating an already debilitated patient. Always bear in mind that a physician is expected not to use techniques that could hurt the hospital patient but to use common sense and clinical judgment as to what the patient needs and is able to tolerate. Particularly if you are working in a nonosteopathic institution, or with preceptors who learned only direct methods of treatment, there is the supposition on the part of the preceptor that you would use HVLA without proper consideration. There are many osteopathic techniques; always discuss which techniques are best for the particular patient with the best risk:benefit ratio for treatment.

The verbalization of osteopathic manipulative treatment is always limited in scope. We attempt to put into words an experience that includes:

> Palpatory assessment
> Other tactile and proprioceptive input
> Integration of that data on a nonverbal level
> Kinesthetic response through our hands and/or other parts of the anatomy.

We do all of this based on cognitive knowledge. We do it to change the motion characteristics, fluid flow patterns, and sensorimotor responses of our patients. It is not always possible to verbalize everything we do, partially because so many things happen simultaneously. This makes it difficult to describe each factor adequately. Proprioception is difficult to describe, because the feeling of where one is in space is unique to each individual. Because language is linear and sequential, the description of two synchronous events might be perceived in a sequenced linear fashion. Since most mental processing is on a nonverbal level, it is often difficult to describe portions of it at all. Korr has described the experience of diagnosis and treatment as a nonverbal dialogue between the osteopathic physician and the patient.[1]

ART OF OSTEOPATHIC MEDICINE

Osteopathic manipulative diagnosis and treatment are part of a complex process involving three domains:

> Affective
> Cognitive
> Psychomotor

The physician must have enough interaction with the patient to achieve relaxation and trust. The physician's brain must receive proper palpatory, visual, and auditory input. This is processed through previously gained cognitive knowledge. Reacting to this input, the physician's processing and kinesthetic output take place in a real-time, ongoing fashion. This all occurs simultaneously, and in many forms of treatment, without stop.

The art of medicine is not strictly fact-oriented. From initial observation and facts, a diagnosis may appear accurate, but further observation can show otherwise. A diagnosis may be accurate for a limited time, after which different characteristics prevail. Patience and persistence help you adapt, accepting art in medicine as well as science. Learning manual medicine skills is not like learning facts of biochemistry. Only a small portion of the data can be grasped by memorization of facts. As with any psychomotor skill, seeing or doing something once is only a beginning. Repeated practice of the technique is necessary to gain skill.

Different patients also respond in different ways to the same technique. An individual also has a unique response to different technique types. Each practitioner becomes part of this human equation and is also unique. The way you are taught a skill during training may be different than the way you finally employ that skill. As you practice, you master the skill. An old story is told about an education professor who was approached by a teacher. "I've taught second grade for 20 years," she told the professor, who replied, "Have you really taught second grade 20 years? Or have you taught 1 year 20 times?" Attention to variations in input from patients, as well as following the results of research, leads to constant refinement in skills. Merely learning treatment protocols and applying them in the same fashion never produces improvement. The human being who is your patient is both your school and one of your teachers.

In a simplistic way, each osteopathic technique system could probably be assigned to deal better with certain types of physical ailments. However, this analogy ignores the complex human factor. Physicians who use one type for all problems may have selected it because it is the one with which they are most comfortable or at which they are most adept. Their practices may be self-selecting for patients who benefit from what they do, with others leaving to find help elsewhere. A physician practicing the highest form of osteopathy is one who uses the approach, method, techniques, or plan that best matches the patient asking for help. If the indicated osteopathic manipulative treatment is HVLA, that becomes the highest form of treatment for that patient. If it is osteopathy in the cranial field, then that is the one that is most appropriate.

Some may feel that OMT is singularly effective for a wide range of clinical problems. Other are somewhat skeptical, often because they have not seen a patient who presented to a physician with a clinical problem.

Some patients, often those with problems associated with motion loss from a nonrecurring physical force or trauma, respond immediately and dramatically. Some resolutions take longer, as the body requires time to respond; healing takes time. Observe the effects of watering a brown lawn. Immediately after watering, the lawn is still brown, but it turns green with time.

Sometimes somatic dysfunction is secondary to postural, mechanical, or visceral disorders. In these cases, OMT provides temporary relief, but the somatic dysfunction tends to return because the cause is still present. A psychic or emotional component is sometimes the major cause. These patients do not get better until the emotional component is resolved.

In some cases, OMT is used to provide maintenance treatment. The term maintenance is prejudicial because insurance companies won't pay for maintenance, even though this treatment enables better function and quality of life. The treatment is indicated and is proper.

On occasion, patients just don't get better in spite of the best efforts of the physician. The physician must constantly reexamine such cases, analyzing the data to see if a different approach or type of treatment is more effective. The only way to know what OMT does is to try it and gain clinical experience by following the patients. Remember as you use this approach that you are promoting the efficiency of natural function in your patients, enabling the human organism to function at its individual optimal level.

ANATOMY

To diagnose and treat a patient efficiently and effectively, you must know anatomy. There are several ways to know anatomy. One way is by being able to locate and name every structure. Another is by being able to successfully palpate and mentally interpret the response of tissues from the proprioceptive input from your hands. All osteopathic techniques produce functional and physiological changes in tissue, in the following ways:

Lengthening
Shortening
Increase in tone in some muscles
Corresponding decrease in tone of their antagonists
Increase in motion in one or more directions
Decrease in other directions

The effects of osteopathic manipulation go beyond their obvious impact on the neuromusculo-skeletal system, such as a decrease in pain or an increase in motion. Profound changes are seen in:

Blood and lymphatic fluid flow
Neural system
Endocrine system
Respiration
Autonomic balance

Improvement of homeostatic mechanisms increases functional efficiency of the tissues, enhances quality of life, and increases resistance to illness and injury.

ASPECTS OF LEARNING

When learning and practicing, remove as many distractions from the situation as possible. See that neither your own needs nor the environment distract you. If you are training the sense of touch, remove the distraction of sight and sound by closing your eyes and focusing on palpation in a quiet environment. If you are focusing on the need to go to the lavatory, you are not able to concentrate on sensory input related to the patient, because your brain is directing attention to your own internal sensations. Hunger or thirst can be tremendously distracting. An emotional upset may make it temporarily impossible for you to effectively receive input unless you can put the distraction out of your mind. Thinking about how much time you are taking or how much you have to do may block immediate proprioceptive interpretations.

You may be learning a new field, in an area totally different from the cognitive skills at which you have excelled. Be patient with yourself and realize that your learning may not proceed at the same pace as the learning of others. Sometimes it may be rapid; other times, slow. Continuous progress should be your goal, but be patient with yourself as you learn this challenging integrative process.

Is any one method or type of activation the most profound form of manipulative treatment in osteopathy? Which one gets the best results from the body? Is direct treatment superior to indirect treatment? At times, listening to one physician or a special interest group of physicians makes it seem as if this were so. However, the original question makes as much sense as asking if the knife, fork, or spoon is the superior instrument for dining. Each has its place. Each has its function, to which the others are less well adapted. Can you use a knife to pick up peas? Certainly. However, most of us prefer one of the other instruments, because they are better adapted to that function.

CONCLUSION

An osteopathic physician looks upon the study of osteopathic diagnosis and treatment as a lifelong discovery process that combines art and science. Your understanding and application of these principles will, because of your commitment and receptivity to new input, continue to develop and refine over your professional life.

REFERENCES

1. Korr I. Somatic dysfunction, osteopathic manipulative treatment and the nervous system: a few facts, theories, many questions. JAOA. February 1986;86:109–114.

39. **Palpatory Skills**

AN INTRODUCTION

ROBERT E. KAPPLER

Key Concepts

- **Art of palpation, including practice using hands and fingers**

- **Identification of dominant eye and hand in palpatory technique**

- **Development of finely tuned sensory perception and mental filters in palpatory skill**

- **Motion perception**

- **Palpation of acute and chronic somatic dysfunction**

This chapter introduces the art of palpation. Being efficient and accurate with palpation is an asset for any physician regardless of specialization. Palpation is especially important to osteopathic manipulative diagnosis and treatment because it is fundamental to functional and structural evaluation. Two of the essentials of effective practice are palpatory skill in locating and defining somatic dysfunctions and manipulative skill to appropriately treat them. The "Glossary of Osteopathic Terminology" defines palpation as *"the application of variable manual pressure to the surface of the body for the purpose of determining the shape, size, consistency, position, inherent motility and health of the tissues beneath."*[1] Another definition (DiGiovanna E. New York College of Osteopathic Medicine. OPP course syllabus, 1992) puts it another way: *"Palpation consists of lightly placing the hands or fingers on the patient's body in order to discover changes in the normal condition of soft tissues, bones, or organs beneath the surface of the skin, as well as the skin itself."* Still another definition includes the descriptive words "gentle handling," an important point to remember when applying this skill. Skill in recognizing normal tissue movement(s) along with changes that signal dysfunction or disease can be acquired with continued practice.

ART OF PALPATION

The art of palpation requires discipline, time, patience, and practice. To be most effective and productive, palpatory find-

ings must be correlated with a knowledge of functional anatomy, physiology, and pathophysiology. It is much easier to identify frank pathologic states, a tumor for example, than to describe signs, symptoms, and palpatory findings that lead to or identify the pathologic mechanisms.[2] This is analogous to learning to read an electrocardiogram or a sonogram: it takes time to develop the "vocabulary of sight" that allows a person to distinguish and describe true pathologic patterns. Through repetitive palpatory experiences, physicians realize ranges of normal and correlate significant findings with:

Past and present history
Tissue texture changes
Restriction of motion
Asymmetry
Subjective tenderness
Related symptomatology

Considering all of these together strengthens the differential diagnostic decision (Frymann V. College of Osteopathic Medicine of the Pacific. Syllabus for workshop on palpation, 1990). Treatment then follows.

Palpation with Fingers and Hands

Palpation with the fingers and hands provides sensory information (Frymann V. Syllabus for workshop on palpation, 1990) that the brain interprets as:

Temperature
Texture
Surface humidity
Elasticity
Turgor
Tissue tension
Thickness
Shape
Irritability
Motion

To accomplish this task, it is necessary to teach the fingers to feel, think, see, and know. One feels through the palpating fingers on the patient, one sees the structures under the palpating fingers through a visual image based on a knowledge of anatomy, one thinks what is normal or abnormal, and one knows with a confidence acquired by practice that what is felt is real and accurate.

Through complex peripheral and central processing, the smallest sensory perception can be amplified to the point of conscious recognition and analysis. Mitchell[2(p.882)] calls palpation *"a two-way **communication** system in which the patient's tissues react to the presence of the palpator's hand."* This is more likely to occur when palpation has been practiced over a period of time.

Three steps define the process. The first is detection, the second is internal amplification or magnification, and the third is analysis and interpretation. This last step translates palpatory findings into meaningful anatomic, physiologic, or pathologic states"(Frymann V. Syllabus for workshop on palpation, 1990). Familiarity with osteopathic terminology permits description of palpatory findings in consistent terms.

Learning Palpatory Technique

Effective palpatory technique cannot be learned by observation. Watching another physician palpate a patient indicates where the hands are placed but gives little or no indication of the feel of tissues being palpated. Some believe that palpation and the interpretation of palpatory findings are more accurate if palpation is performed with the dominant hand. It is also believed that results are more consistent if the examiner has the dominant eye over the area that is being palpated.

Many individuals have a dominant hand with which they prefer to palpate or motion test. This may or may not be the hand with which they write. Recognition of a dominant hand will allow the individual to develop a compensatory mechanism to obtain accurate information when using both hands. For example, if one hand is stronger than the other, practice in applying equal pressure over equivalent structures can result in accurate interpretation of such manual information. Interpretation of dominant and nondominant proprioceptive feedback from each hand is also a response that the individual can adjust. Recognition of dominance, if it exists, and development of a compensatory mechanism is the main issue here; in time, apparent palpatory ambidexterity may result.

To find the dominant eye, look at a distant object with both eyes open (Fig. 39.1). Extend your dominant hand and make a circle with your thumb and index finger that encircles your view of the distant object. Now, close one eye; open it and close the other eye. The eye that saw the object encircled with the fingers of your dominant hand is generally your dominant eye.[2(p.882)]

There are more touch (kinesthetic) nerve endings in the pads of the fingers than elsewhere in the hand. It is generally agreed that the thumb and/or the first two finger pads, rather than the finger tips, are the most sensitive part of the hand to train and use for palpation (Frymann V. Syllabus for workshop on palpation, 1990).

Some physicians find that variations in skin temperature are best perceived by the dorsum of the hand, especially the dorsum of the middle phalanges of fingers 2, 3, and 4; others use

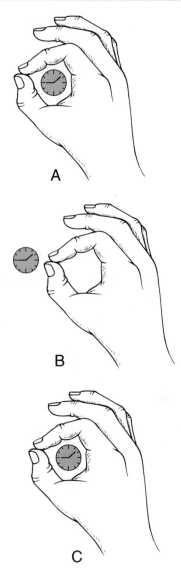

Figure 39.1.   Right eye dominance. **A.** Both eyes open. **B.** Right eye closed; left eye open. **C.** Left eye closed; right eye open. (Modified from W.A. Kuchera.)

the palmar surface. Try both and see which is more effective for you. The coordinated use of the palms and the fingers around an object is best suited for obtaining a stereognostic sense of contour.[3]

Since the hands are so important to a physician, they should be carefully protected and cared for. They are sensitive diagnostic instruments.

Flexibility of the joints of the elbows, wrists, hands, and fingers is important. Relaxation is also important to eliminate any muscle tension that would block perception. Strength of hands and fingers can be increased by using a finger exerciser, squeezing a ball, or playing a musical instrument that requires fingering.

When examining a patient, tell the patient in general terms about the procedure as it goes along. This is especially important if significant tenderness might be elicited during deep palpation. Take the necessary time, moving gently and deliberately. Initially it is common to apply too much pressure in an attempt to feel the tissue. Avoid poking, prodding, tickling, or "stirring" the tissue. These actions can cause reflex irritation.[3(p.113)]

Louisa Burns, DO, a noted early osteopathic researcher, made the following suggestions to those beginning to develop palpatory skills:

Palpate the objects with the lightest possible touch, scarcely touching the surface

Be aware of surface elevations and temperature differences

Using slightly more contact, palpate the surface

Try to ascertain the qualities or characteristics of the substance of the object

Describe perceptions as accurately as possible

Palpatory skill involves more than a mechanism for finely tuned sensory perception. These skills might be enhanced by trying to palpate a hair through several pages of a telephone directory. A more significant component is to be able to focus on the mass of information being perceived, paying close attention to those qualities associated with tissue texture abnormality, and bypassing many of the other palpatory clues not relevant at the time. This is a process of developing mental filters. Consider an analogy in music, where the orchestra conductor focuses on the violins. The conductor is aware of the entire orchestra playing, but is diverting attention to a specific portion of sound that he or she is perceiving.

The brain cannot process everything at once. By concentrating only on the portion you want, it becomes easy and fast to detect areas of significant tissue texture abnormality. In a comparison of student musculoskeletal examinations with experienced examiners, Kappler et al.[4] observed that the experienced examiners recorded fewer findings than student examiners, but the experienced examiner's findings were more significant. This shows that experienced physicians apply a filtering process to their palpatory data, rejecting insignificant findings without being consciously aware that they are doing this. The student is overwhelmed with the mass of palpatory data and has not yet developed this filtering process to reduce the data to a manageable component.

Motion Perception

If any motion is present, describe the sensations transmitted through the fingers. Also, estimate the weight of objects, the amount of pressure needed to move them, and the resistance or force exerted against your pressure.

Perception of motion is an essential component of palpation. A major difference in palpation of living tissue is this sensed motion. Motion of the body is described as passive, active, and inherent.[5]

Passive motion is brought about by the physician; it is movement done to the subject. Active motion is performed by the subject; it is deliberate, conscious muscular activity. Inherent motion is activity unconsciously generated within the body

(Goodridge J. Michigan State University College of Osteopathic Medicine. Biomechanics syllabus, 1986), such as respiratory motion or peristalsis.

Inherent motion is postulated to occur in any of several ways:

Biochemically, at the cellular or subcellular level

As part of multiple electrical patterns

As a combination of a number of circulatory and electrical patterns

As some periodic pattern not yet understood

Experts agree that individuals can perceive tissue movement as minute as 1 μm.[6] With practice and patience, inherent motion may be palpated.

By varying the palpation pressure, successive layers of tissue can be palpated. In palpating superficial tissue, use the lightest effective touch. To palpate successively deeper layers, apply only as much additional pressure as necessary. As a general rule, this means palpating to the depth of the tissue or structure to be examined, that is, down to but not through the structure being examined. The use of various depths of touch differs from physician to physician, usually depending on the model of diagnosis and treatment chosen.

Somatic Dysfunction Palpation

The osteopathic physician uses all palpatory skills to diagnose somatic dysfunction. The definition of somatic dysfunction is *"impaired or altered function of related components of the somatic (body framework) system: skeletal, arthrodial, and myofascial structures, and related vascular, lymphatic, and neural elements."*[1]

The osteopathic diagnostic criteria for somatic dysfunction is discerned through palpation and can be conveniently recalled through the mnemonic TART. These letters stand for:

T: Tissue texture abnormalities

A: Asymmetry (static, motion, tonicity, turgor, color, temperature)

R: Restriction of motion

T: Tenderness (in the area of the abnormality)

By grouping these palpatory findings according to the characteristics of acute and chronic inflammation, somatic dysfunction can be further classified, as shown in Table 39.1.

ACUTE SOMATIC DYSFUNCTION

Palpate with light to somewhat firmer touch. Several types of change may be present; biochemically mediated tissue texture changes often predominate. First, the skin over the somatic dysfunction may feel warmer. The skin and deeper tissues directly over the area of somatic dysfunction may be tender. The skin and subcutaneous tissues may also feel tense and less mobile. Superficial muscle tension may be detected through a slight increase in palpatory pressure. Finally, there may be fullness caused by edema.

Deep palpation, defined as pressure sufficient to contact the periaxial soft tissues of the spinal column, can also identify

Table 39.1
Classification of Somatic Dysfunction

Acute	Chronic
History: recent; often an injury	History: long-standing
Pain: acute pain, severe, cutting, sharp	Pain: dull, achy; paresthesias (crawling, itching, burning, gnawing)
Vascular: vessels injured, release of endogenous peptides = chemical vasodilation, inflammation	Vacular: vessels constricted because of sympathetic tone
Skin: warm, moist, red, inflamed (via vascular and chemical changes)	Skin: cool, pale (via chronic sympathetic vascular tone increase)
Sympathetics: systemically increased sympathetic activity but local effect overpowered by bradykinins so there is local vasodilation due to chemical effect	Sympathetics: has vasoconstriction due to hypersympathetic tone. Regional sympathetic hyperactivity. Systemic sympathetic tone may be reduced toward normal
Musculature: local increase in muscle tone, muscle contraction, spasm, increased tone of the muscle spindle	Musculature: decreased muscle tone, flaccid, mushy, limited range of motion because of contracture
Mobility: range often normal, quality is sluggish	Mobility: limited range, with normal quality in the motion that remains
Tissues: boggy edema, acute congestion, fluids from vessels and from chemical reactions in tissues	Tissues: chronic congestion, doughy, stringy, fibrotic, ropy, thickened, increased resistance, contracted, contractures
Adnexa: moist skin, no trophic changes	Adnexa: pimples, scaly, dry, folliculitis, pigmentation (trophic changes)
Visceral: minimal somatovisceral effects	Visceral: somatovisceral effects are common

From Kuchera WA, Kuchera ML. *Osteopathic Principles in Practice.* 2nd ed. Columbus, Ohio: Greyden Press; 1994:25.

several types of change. Pain or tenderness over acute areas of dysfunction is common. It is also common to find swelling in the deep periarticular tissues, giving the area a soggy, swollen texture. Muscles directly concerned with the affected vertebral segment demonstrate a doughy tightness or hypertonicity. Finally, there are perceptible changes in interosseous relations, best evaluated by motion testing a vertebral unit. This reveals restricted motion in one direction and a preference or freedom of movement in the other direction.

CHRONIC SOMATIC DYSFUNCTION

Palpation with light to slightly more firm touch may elicit evidence of several types of chronic tissue changes. The skin may be somewhat immobile and tense in the presence of chronic fibrotic changes beneath the skin. These changes reduce the skin's elasticity. Temperature changes in the skin may be present or absent. Usually the skin is cool to touch. The muscles have a hard, ropy, and nonresilient texture as a result of fibrotic changes. When the dysfunction is very chronic it may actually have lost its tone and not feel fibrotic. The amount of tenderness is less than that found in acute dysfunction, often described as a dull, uncomfortable, or burning pain. In the absence of irritation, inflammation may subside and there may be little or no tenderness.

Deeper palpation reveals additional changes. Most notably there is a decreased range of motion between the vertebral segments. As stated before, often there is little or no tenderness. It is helpful to evaluate mobility changes and interosseous changes together, using each to check the other. At this level, too, fibrotic changes replace edema. When a chronic somatic dysfunction has reached an advanced stage, fibrotic changes result in dysfunction of the surrounding fascias, musculature,

and ligaments, sometimes to a point of producing contractures and joint ankylosis.

CONCLUSION

Position your dominant eye over the structure being palpated. Place thumbs or finger pads over the area to be palpated. To ensure greater accuracy, mentally transfer your thoughts to the interface of your hand with the patient's body. Realize that resiliency or resistance to motion can be sensed in the initial movement during motion testing. You can miss these subtle findings and get hung up on gross motion restrictions, for example, how far a vertebral joint or tissue moves rather than the quality of the movement. Avoid these common errors in palpation:

Lack of concentration
Too much pressure
Excessive movement

These palpatory skills provide a method of obtaining practical experience in developing the art of palpation. There are many other exercises. Initially, palpation is practiced on a partner in the skills laboratory. During clinical clerkships, one gains additional experience by examining attending physicians' patients. Ultimately, palpatory experience is gained from palpatory examination of the physician's own patients. The physician continues to learn and never stops gaining experience. The preceding section shows how to get started in the process of obtaining palpatory data from the patient.

Remember that development of a high level of palpatory skill is an ongoing process, requiring patience and practice.

ACKNOWLEDGMENTS

Barbara Peterson collected the materials and Judith McPherson organized and assisted with the writing of this chapter.

REFERENCES

1. The Glossary Review Committee of the Educational Council on Osteopathic Principles. Glossary of osteopathic terminology. In: Allen TW, ed. *AOA Yearbook and Directory of Osteopathic Physicians.* Chicago, Ill: American Osteopathic Association; 1993.
2. Mitchell F Jr. The training and measurement of sensory literacy in relation to osteopathic structural and palpatory diagnosis. *JAOA.* June 1976;75:881.
3. Kuchera WA, Kuchera ML. Palpation of soft tissue. In: *Osteopathic Principles in Practice.* 2nd ed. rev. Columbus, Ohio: Greyden Press; 1994:111.
4. Kappler RE, Larson NJ, Kelso AF. A comparison of osteopathic findings on hospitalized patients obtained by trained student examiners and experienced osteopathic physicians. *JAOA.* June 1971; 70(10):1091–1092.
5. Van Allen P, Stinson J. The development of palpation. *JAOA.* January 1941;40(5):207, 208.
6. Greenman PE. *Principles of Manual Medicine.* 2nd ed. Baltimore, Md: Williams & Wilkins; 1996.

40. Progressive Exercises for Developing the Sense of Touch

ROBERT E. KAPPLER

Key Concepts

- **Perception of tactile differences in tissue texture and motion**

- **Perception on palpation of layers and structures of the body**

- **Palpation of thoracic and lumbar areas with passive flexion**

- **Palpation for somatic dysfunction in cervical, thoracic, lumbar and sacroiliac areas**

This chapter presents progressive exercises for developing palpatory skills. The exercises should help to refine and improve beginning practitioners' sense of touch.

EXERCISE 1: PALPATING INANIMATE OBJECTS

Goal

The goal is to perceive slight tactile differences of tissue texture and motion. Exercises on inanimate objects serve to sharpen tactile concentration and attention. Concentration is essential. Close the eyes to eliminate extraneous stimuli. Pay attention to kinesthetic sensations received through the fingers.

Procedure

1. Put a mixture of coins in a pocket or purse. By touch, distinguish between heads and tails, and between pennies, dimes, nickels, and quarters. Identify date lines on the coins.
2. Locate a hair that has been placed under a sheet of paper; attempt to estimate its length. Add sheets of paper until you can no longer palpate the hair.
3. Palpate several types of human bones. Identify the bones and their component parts, envisioning the tissue that normally surrounds them.
4. Palpate a human bone and a solid plastic imitation of the same bone. Identify the characteristics of the human bone that distinguish it from the replica.

EXERCISE 2: LAYER PALPATION

Goal

The goal is to concentrate and perceive various layers and structures of the body by varying the pressure of palpation.

Light touch is thought by many experienced palpators to be the most useful and easy to use.

Very light touch, or light touch, consists of laying the hands passively on the skin or moving the hands lightly over the skin. Such light touch can be used to determine skin temperature, texture, moistness, oiliness, resistance, tone, and elasticity.

Pass the hand just above the skin to determine skin temperature.

Firmer pressure communicates with the deeper cutaneous layers and fascial sheaths. It explores superficial muscles to determine their tone and mobility.

Firm pressure and compression explore deeper muscle, fascia, and bony relationships.

Palpate your own tissues. Close your eyes and relax. Concentrate your attention through the palpating fingers of one hand.

Procedure

1. Lightly palpate the dorsum of the other hand. Scarcely touching the surface, feel the contour of the hand. Test the dorsal and palmar aspects of the palpating fingers to determine which is most sensitive to temperature.
2. Using very light touch, palpate and describe skin texture, moisture, and thickness. Gently pinch the skin on the back of the hand. Elevate it and release it. How long did it take for the skin to resume its normal configuration? Evaluate skin drag on both the palm and dorsum of the hand. Skin drag is the estimation of the amount of resistance experienced when the pads of the fingers are lightly applied and moved (dragged) over the skin surface. On which aspect of the hand do the palpating fingers move most easily? Why? Describe any increase in skin drag that is due to excessive dryness, slight perspiration, or edema. Describe any decrease in drag resulting from excessive perspiration, oiliness, or atrophy.
3. Locate the veins and note their size and texture. Make a fist several times to engorge the veins and then describe the differences observed. Locate the radial artery and describe the differences between it and a vein.
4. Increase the contact between your palpating fingers and the skin of your hand so that you create a shearing stress in the subcutaneous tissues. Shearing in this context refers to movement of tissues between layers. Note that with this palpation one can shear only so far before the palpating fingers slide on the skin. Shear across the hand in various directions describing what you feel. Does the skin move equally and easily in all directions?

5. Palpate the extensor tendon of the ring finger. Place two fingers along the length of the tendon; flex the ring finger, and palpate the sense of the linear movement along the tendon.

6. Palpate the tendon of the biceps at the elbow. How does it feel? It should be ropelike, smooth, and firm.

7. Place the thumb and index finger of the palpating hand on either side of the midphalangeal articulation of a finger on the opposite hand. Note the quality and range of various elements during flexion and extension. Now lighten your touch while performing the same movements. Notice how little contact is needed to distinguish flexion and extension.

8. Place your palpating fingers on the anterior surface of the proximal third of your other forearm. Use slightly more pressure than that used for skin, palpating the muscles used to flex the fingers. Now maintain palpatory contact during flexion of the middle finger. Describe the feel of these flexor muscles and fascia during the maneuver.

EXERCISE 3: PALPATE PARTNER'S FOREARM

Procedure

This exercise requires a partner. Sit facing one another across a narrow table. Examine your partner's left forearm and then have your partner in turn examine your left forearm.

1. Lightly place the palm and fingers of the palpating hand over the dorsal forearm of your partner, just distal to the elbow. Close your eyes, relax, and concentrate your attention through the palmar surface of your fingers. Without moving your hand, think skin. Try to perceive and describe skin temperature, texture, thickness, and moistness.

2. Next, compare the dorsal and palmar aspects of the forearm, and describe the differences. Which aspect is smoother? Thicker? Warmer? Drier?

3. Now, with a slightly firmer touch, concentrate on the second layer, the subcutaneous fascia. Gently move the skin of the forearm longitudinally and horizontally. How thick is it? How loose? Many of the tissue texture changes associated with somatic dysfunction are within this layer.

4. Gently and slowly increase the depth of touch until you feel the deep fascial layer that forms a sheath around the underlying structures. Think deep fascia. Is it smooth? Continuous? Firm? Palpate the deep fascial layer; then slowly move the hand horizontally across the forearm to identify areas of thickening that form fascial compartments between bundles of muscles. Identifying enveloping layers of deep fascia is often helpful in separating one muscle from another; use it to work with even deeper structures.

5. Palpating through the deep fascia, concentrate on the underlying muscle. Is it soft and compliant? How is its elasticity? Pay attention to individual muscle fibers and the directions in which they run. Have your partner slowly open and close the hand as you note the quality and range of movement created by the contracting and relaxing muscle. Describe the difference. Palpate the forearm muscles as the hand is clenched. This sensation simulates the feel of the most common tissue texture

abnormality at the level of muscle or in areas of somatic dysfunction.

6. Still palpating at the level of muscle, move your hand slowly down your partner's forearm until you feel the musculotendinous junction, an area or region where the muscle is vulnerable to injury. Move past the musculotendinous junction toward the wrist. Note the transition from muscle to musculotendinous junction to the smooth, round, firm feel of tendons.

7. Follow the tendons distally until you feel a structure that binds them at the wrist. This is the transverse carpal ligament (flexor retinaculum) and palmar carpal ligament (a thickening of the deeper anterolateral fascia). Note fiber direction, thickness, and firmness. How does it feel in comparison with the tendon? Compare the palpatory sensation over this area with that over tendons that are more superficially located.

8. Now place your index finger over the proximal radiohumeral joint at the dimple of the elbow. Place your thumb opposite your index finger, on the ventral side over the lateral side of the humeroulnar attachments. You should now be palpating the head of the radius. Describe the characteristics. Compare the feel of this living bone with a plastic model or with your memory of bone from a cadaver.

9. Move your thumb and index finger proximally until you locate the joint space. Your finger and thumb fall into it. You should not be able to feel the joint capsule. The joint capsule is not palpable because palpable joint capsules signal pathologic changes.

EXERCISE 4: PALPATING SPINAL MOTION AND PARAVERTEBRAL TISSUE TEXTURE

Goal

The following provides a general idea of how to palpate living tissue and assumes a classroom situation with an instructor available to demonstrate and interpret as needed. This process uses palpation of the thoracic and lumbar spinal areas to test the relative resistance of the vertebrae and their spinous processes when passive flexion is introduced. The partner sits with the examiner standing behind.

Procedure

1. Using your finger pads, place the first three fingers of your palpating hand between the spinous processes of T1 and T2, T2 and T3, and T3 and T4. Remember to use the pads of your fingers. Locate the spinous processes and interspinous ligaments, noting how they feel. Compare differences between the feel of the bone and the feel of the ligament.

2. Place your other hand on the top of the partner's head. Passively flex the head and neck, while feeling increasing tension of the interspinous ligaments. Note: One spinous process may move more easily than another (Fig. 40.1).

3. Using the fingers of both hands, palpate for temperature differences along the paravertebral thoracic and lumbar spine. Use either the palmar or dorsal surface of your fingers, depending

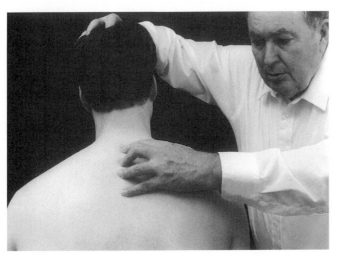

Figure 40.1. Palpating upper thoracic flexion-extension.

which you find to be more sensitive. Using both hands simultaneously, stroke the back from C7 to L5. Which areas are warmer? Try to find a segment within the thoracic area that is either warmer or cooler than another segment. Compare left with right sides, and superior with inferior. Stroking of this type is useful in identifying changes in contour as well as identifying areas of edema and increased tissue tension. Also palpate for moisture differences, noting stickiness, dryness, wetness, waxiness, and slipperiness.

4. Proceeding from T2 to L5, lightly compress the paravertebral soft tissues. Then use deeper pressure, but less than that required to palpate bone. You may notice that in some areas tissues compress more easily, while in others there is more resistance. Significant resistance indicates an area of tissue texture abnormality (TTA)[1] bearing further investigation. Lightly palpate the skin and subcutaneous tissue over the resistant site. This helps you to identify the outer limits of tissue texture involved.

EXERCISE 5: PALPATION FOR SOMATIC DYSFUNCTION

Goal

These exercises deal with palpation of each area of the spine and the tissue changes that may be perceived in areas of somatic dysfunction. Review the types of tissue changes that are encountered in patients with vertebral somatic dysfunction before undertaking the final exercises in this section. These exercises assume a classroom situation, in which partners take turns acting as the patient.

Cervical Area

PROCEDURE

1. Stand or sit at the head of the table behind your supine patient. Cradle the patient's occiput in your palms. This position frees

the fingers for checking cervical soft tissue and vertebral mechanics.
2. Lightly palpate the posterior cervical skin. If you identify an area of localized tissue tension, palpate for swelling, deep muscle tension, and interosseous mobility.
3. Straighten the cervical curve by passively flexing the neck. Place the pads of the fingers of one hand between the spinous processes and check for separation of the spinous processes.
4. Reverse the procedure with passive backward bending of the head and neck. What happens to the spinous processes?
5. Assess side-bending and translatory movements.[1] With the pads of the fingers on either side of the articular column and directly across from each other, assess side-bending by translating to the right, then left (Fig. 40.2).
6. Using deep pressure, over the posterolateral margin of the articular column, translate anteriorly (both right and left sides), checking for spontaneous vertebral rotation capability.

Thoracic Area

PROCEDURE

1. Stand behind your seated patient. The pads of the thumbs are most effective for palpation in this exercise.
2. Lightly stroke the skin over the thoracic area, noting any temperature difference. For this part of the exercise, you may find that the dorsal surfaces of the middle phalanges are more sensitive to temperature change (Fig. 40.3).
3. With a slightly deeper touch, palpate the subcutaneous and myofascial structures, noting soft tissue changes such as muscle tension and swelling.
4. Increase the depth of touch until you can feel the periarticular tissue changes; note the deeper tissue characteristics.
5. Examine the facets and transverse processes, one side at a time and together, along with the spaces between spinous processes.
6. Check motion response during passive flexion, extension, rotation, and side-bending of the thoracic area.

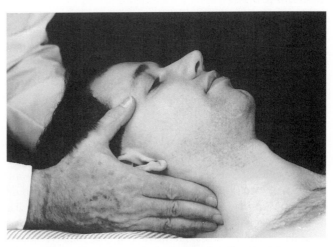

Figure 40.2. Assessing cervical spine side-bending translation.

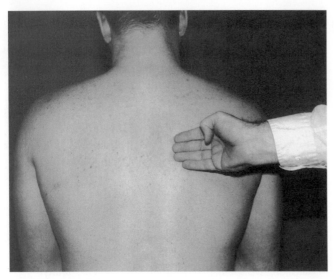

Figure 40.3.   Checking temperature using back of hand and fingers.

Lumbar Area

PROCEDURE

1. Stand to the side of your prone patient, at the level of the patient's hips.
2. Using light touch, palpate bilaterally for lumbar contour and any tissue texture abnormalities. Systematically compress the tissues over the transverse processes until you feel bony resistance.
3. Test passive and active motion capability of individual vertebrae. Induce rotation by direct anterior pressure over one transverse process while no pressure is on the contralateral side. Then test rotation to the opposite side (Fig. 40.4).
4. Induce side-bending to one side by applying lateral translatory force to one transverse process; then test the other direction.
5. Note differences in the mechanical response when the patient is seated and prone. Maximum spinal loads occur when seated and are the least when supine.

Sacroiliac Area

PROCEDURE

1. Stand to the side of your prone patient, at the level of the hips.
2. Palpate the entire gluteal area. The palm of the hand is useful for palpating gross muscle changes. Ask the patient to extend the opposite hip as you palpate the contraction of the gluteus maximus muscle. Compare the right and left sides.
3. Now assess the superficial tissues overlying and lateral to the superior and inferior poles of the sacroiliac joint, noting any tension in the gluteal muscles. Adjust your depth of touch as needed to assess various tissue layers. The pads of the thumbs are best used for this deep palpation, although other methods may be used. Bilaterally check the posterior superior iliac spines for asymmetry. Use the pads of each thumb, placed directly caudad to the posterior superior iliac spines (PSIS) and note their levels. The PSIS are called pure landmarks because they can be affected only by the position of the innominate.

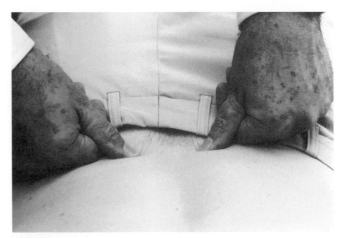

Figure 40.4.   Testing lumbar spine rotation.

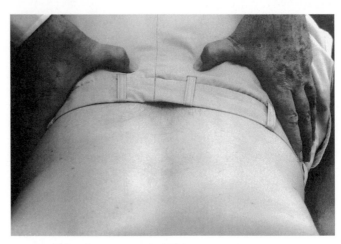

Figure 40.5.   Checking level of PSIS with patient prone.

The level of the PSIS is a clue to possible innominate rotation. Is one more cephalad or more caudad (Fig. 40.5)?
4. Check depth of the sulcus between the posterior surface of the PSIS of the ilium and the posterior surface of the sacrum. This sulcus depth is called a mixed landmark because its depth can be affected by the innominate or the sacrum.
5. To determine rotation of the sacrum, palpate deeply in the sulcus using the tips of the thumbs. Is the sacral base level or is one side more anterior or posterior than the other side? This is a pure landmark that indicates sacral base rotation. Check for rotation of the innominates by evaluating the anteroposterior levels of the posterior superior iliac spine on both right and left.

ACKNOWLEDGMENT

Judith McPherson organized and assisted with the writing of this chapter.

REFERENCE

1. The Glossary Review Committee of the Educational Council on Osteopathic Principles. Glossary of Osteopathic Terminology. In: *AOA Yearbook and Directory of Osteopathic Physicians.* Allen TW, ed. Chicago, Ill: American Osteopathic Association; 1995.

41. Diagnosis and Plan for Manual Treatment

A PRESCRIPTION

ROBERT E. KAPPLER, JOHN M. JONES III, AND WILLIAM A. KUCHERA

Key Concepts

- **Definition of somatic dysfunction, and possible causes**

- **Essential elements of diagnosing somatic dysfunction, including observation, screening tests, palpation, and motion testing**

- **Effects of somatic dysfunction on range of motion and "end feel"**

- **Decisions physician must make after diagnosis of somatic dysfunction**

- **Answers to "When is it important to use manipulative treatment?"**

- **Considerations when developing a treatment plan, including sequence in which somatic dysfunctions should be treated, dose and frequency of treatments, and choice of techniques**

Many treatment procedures follow the principles of osteopathic philosophy. The use of manual intervention to remove impairment of normal body function was emphasized by A.T. Still. This intervention, osteopathic manipulative treatment (OMT), requires a careful evaluation and diagnosis of the patient before, during, and after treatment. The evaluation of the patient leads to a precise and individual plan for his or her treatment.

The plan is the guide for the patient's treatment developed from observations and findings about him or her at that moment. The plan is written in the record for later reference. A note is recorded stating whether the procedure was effective or ineffective.

Osteopathic examination methods and procedures have been categorized. Dinnar[1,2] listed four:

General impressions
Regional motion testing
Superficial and deep tissue evaluation
Local characteristics of motion

DIAGNOSIS

Somatic dysfunction is an impaired or altered function of related components of the somatic (body framework) system, such as these elements:

Skeletal
Arthrodial
Myofascial
Vascular
Lymphatic
Neural

Four criteria are used for diagnosis of somatic dysfunction:

1. Tissue texture abnormalities (T)
2. Asymmetry of bony landmarks (A)
3. Restriction of motion (R)
4. Tenderness or soreness to examiner pressure (T)

These form the acronym TART.

The following is a plan for conducting an osteopathic evaluation for diagnosis of somatic dysfunction. The physician first looks at the whole person, noting characteristics of gait and evidence of asymmetries. Screening tests are performed. Abnormal findings on general impression tests such as asymmetrical bony landmarks or regional motion suggest regions that require further palpatory evaluation for tissue texture changes and asymmetry of segmental motion characteristics.

Palpation reveals localized areas that stand out from surrounding areas by exhibiting temperature differences, swelling, hyperesthesia, or firmness, which can be identified as tissue texture changes (TTC). Palpation of these areas is almost always tender (T).

The segmental areas of TTC and tenderness are then tested for motion characteristics. Motion testing may be active or passive. The characteristics of motion of a joint and its tissues can be described in various ways (Fig. 41.1). It may involve rotation around one of three axes (vertical, transverse, anteroposterior) or translation in one of the three planes of the body, or it may be a shearing of myofascial tissue layers.

For the spine, forward and backward bending indicates motion in the sagittal plane about a transverse axis. Pressure on the transverse process initiates rotation in a horizontal plane about a vertical axis; side-to-side translation of the vertebral body produces side-bending. Regardless of how the segments of a region are tested, the questions that must be answered are:

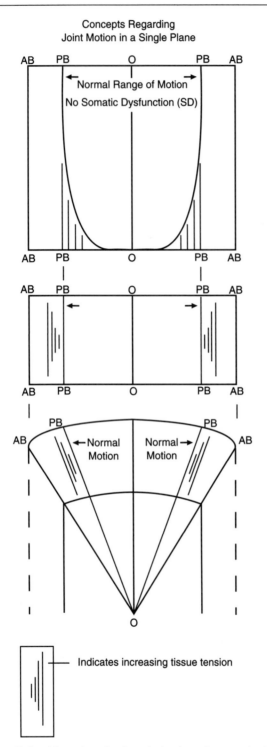

Figure 41.1. Normal motion in a single plane: three methods of illustration. *AB*, anatomic barrier; *PB*, physiologic barrier; *RB*, restrictive barrier.

Does it move?
Does it move appropriately? (Is it restricted in motion?)
What is the quality of motion?
What does the end range of motion feel like?

Motion has direction, range, and quality. Visual observation measures the range of motion; palpation reveals the quality of motion. The quality of motion is described as:

Smooth
Ratcheting
Restricted
Exhibiting resistance to the motion introduced

The presence of normal passive motion in one direction of one plane of motion and resistance in the other is presumptive evidence of somatic dysfunction.

The range of motion with somatic dysfunction is decreased. This decrease of motion occurs within the normal range of motion for the joint. The quality of motion can be shown in a graph (Fig. 41.2). The joint will move farther in the direction in which the somatic dysfunction occurred; its movement is restricted in the opposite direction. There is a restriction to motion in one direction, called a restrictive barrier. As the joint is moved in the direction of the restrictive barrier, the curved line of resistance rises at a much more rapid rate than the resistance encountered when moving toward the physiologic barrier in the opposite direction. The restrictive barrier of the joint occurs before motion reaches the physiologic barrier on that side.

Kappler[3] describes the resistance near the limits of motion as "end feel." The end feel of motion in a direction toward the somatic dysfunction (restrictive barrier) is different from the end feel away from the direction of the somatic dysfunction. The end feel in a normal joint should be the same in either direction. End feel characteristics may be used to differentiate which of the many manipulative procedures to use.

TREATMENT

Approach

Somatic dysfunction is identified with the following diagnostic findings:

Asymmetry of tissue texture
Range of motion
Perception of tenderness
Characteristics of the end feel

The physician makes further decisions based on the answers to these questions:

1. Are the findings significant and related to the patient's problem(s)?
2. Should the findings be altered by manipulation?
3. If so, which of the many techniques are indicated and likely to be effective for this patient?

Additional questions relate to the areas of restricted motion. Are they:

1. A primary somatic dysfunction related to the musculoskeletal system?
2. A somatosomatic reflex related to some other musculoskeletal problem?
3. A viscerosomatic reflex from a dysfunctional or diseased organ? Clinical investigations[4] have found the presence of somatic components related to visceral disturbances.
4. A mechanism protecting some damaged tissue or weakened

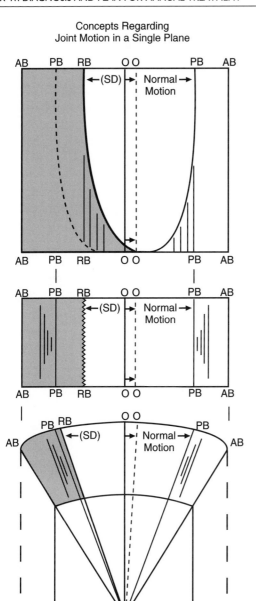

Concepts Regarding
Joint Motion in a Single Plane

— Indicates Motion Loss

Figure 41.2. Somatic dysfunction in a single plane: three methods of illustrating the "restrictive barrier" (the restrainer). *AB*, anatomic barrier; *PB*, physiologic barrier; *RB*, restrictive barrier; *SD*, somatic dysfunction.

structure? Treatment of the somatic dysfunction in this situation is not indicated at this time; strengthening of the weakened area is indicated.[5]

The positional and motion aspects of somatic dysfunction can be described using two parameters:

1. The position of a body part as determined by palpation and referenced to its adjacent defined structure (the upper segment is named in relation to the lower).
2. The directions in which motion is more free and the directions

in which motion is restricted.[6] The goal of treatment is to enhance movement to resolve somatic dysfunction.

Hoag[5] asked, *"When is it important to use manipulative treatment?"* He answered the question as follows:

"When the challenge is not overly severe but the body is not responding adequately to the appropriate treatment regimen," or *"when appropriate (manipulative) treatment may aid the body's response or may accelerate the healing process."*

"When the body is critically ill and life's continuance is in the balance, a more optimal musculoskeletal reaction to illness may be the factor that tips the balance of recovery in favor of the patient."

Zink and Lawson[7] answered, *"The findings are significant to treat until a physiologic state existed that included eupnea in the supine position."* The osteopathic physician focuses on the whole person. While the person's symptom may be localized, the major influence can be elsewhere.

Methods

1. The dose of treatment is limited by the patient's ability to respond to the treatment. The physician may want to do more and go faster; however, the patient's body must make the necessary changes toward health and recovery.
2. The physician's ability to execute a technique effectively is a major factor in determining which techniques to use. There are many different technique approaches. The physician must choose from the various techniques that are effective in his or her hands.
3. There must be an objective to be accomplished by the treatment. Treatment should be outcome-oriented, meaning that the intended objective is accomplished. Do not allow OMT to become oriented only to the process, meaning that once you have given the OMT, the process is viewed as completed. Examples of objectives are: mobilize the sacrum, decrease rib tenderness, improve motion at T5, relax cervical muscles.
4. The objective is the constant; the method is the variable.
5. The technique chosen must be safe and potentially effective. Risk/benefit relationships must always be considered.
6. The physician must be able to execute the technique effectively. The technique must be modified to meet the needs of the patient and the physician.

Sequence

There are different opinions regarding what should be treated first. Absolute rules for sequencing do not exist. Patients' problems vary and may require deviation from the physician's usual approach. One school of thought suggests that the initial approach is to balance the pelvis. Another opinion suggests that, since the sacrum is the base of support, the sacrum should be treated first. A sample sequence is as follows:

1. For low back pain, and especially with psoas involvement, treat the lumbar spine first.
2. Treat the upper thoracic spine and ribs before treating the cervical spine.

3. Treat the thoracic spine before treating specific rib dysfunctions.
4. For very acute somatic dysfunctions, treat secondary or peripheral areas to allow access to the acute area.
5. Cranial treatment can produce relaxation and allow OMT to work in other areas.
6. For extremity problems, treat the axial skeletal components first (spine, ribs, sacrum).

These guidelines on sequencing are not absolute rules. Each physician, after gaining experience, develops his or her own approach.

Dose and Frequency

A quotation frequently repeated in osteopathic circles is attributed to A.T. Still: *"Find it, fix it, and leave it alone."* The statement addresses dosage, with the admonition to resist continuing treatment but give the patient time to respond. The ability of patients to respond is variable. Pediatric patients respond quickly, while geriatric patients respond more slowly. Patients who are very ill and debilitated respond slowly; they cannot respond appropriately to a treatment dose appropriate for an ambulatory patient. Some forms of osteopathic manipulative treatment, such as thoracic pump, may be performed several times a day. Soft tissue stretching may be performed frequently. Specific joint mobilization is an example of a treatment approach that requires a longer interval between treatments.

The frequency of visits for ambulatory patients has several guidelines, as well as some confounding factors. The availability of time in the physician's appointment schedule is a practical factor in the scheduling of the next visit. The physician may work at more than one site and not be available at a particular location every day. Patient availability must be considered, as well as factors such as travel distance, work, and prior commitments. Apart from physician or patient availability, the acuteness of the patient's problem is a major consideration in the scheduling of the next visit. The ambulatory patient disabled with an acute low back problem would be reevaluated in 24–48 hours. A patient with chronic low back discomfort might be seen every 2 weeks. Consider response to treatment in a decision for timing the next visit. A favorable response suggests lengthening the interval. A poor response might suggest that the patient is not yet able to respond appropriately and should be seen again soon when the ability to respond improves.

At times, the patient may exhibit more dysfunctions than can be appropriately handled in one visit. A plan of treatment involves immediate objectives along with longer-term objectives. Provide palliative treatment with the understanding that the real task is yet to be addressed.

DOSE GUIDELINES

1. The sicker the patient, the less the dose.
2. Caring, compassionate novices often err on the side of overdose.
3. Allow time for the patient to respond to the treatment.
4. Do not waste the dose on insignificant areas. Concentrate on key areas needing treatment.
5. Chronic disease requires chronic treatment.
6. Pediatric patients can be treated more frequently; geriatric patients need a longer interval to respond to the treatment.
7. Acute cases should have a shorter interval between treatments; as they respond, the interval is increased.

Direct or Indirect Method

Two major factors determine choice of technique:

The ability of the patient to respond to the treatment
The ability of the physician to execute the technique

We lack precise answers for when to choose one technique instead of another. There are only general guidelines. Sometimes certain techniques are inappropriate to achieve the intended objective. There are times when the risk/benefit relationship is such that certain techniques should be avoided. The use of forceful high-velocity technique in a patient with advanced osteoporosis might lead to pathologic fracture. This text contains chapters on a number of technique types and their use.

The ability of the physician to execute the technique is probably the greatest factor in determining choice of technique. For many years, direct action thrust techniques were taught and were used very successfully by osteopathic physicians in the treatment of their patients. Those physicians did not face the challenge of trying to decide which type of technique to use. They knew thrust techniques and learned how to modify the techniques to make them work.

Some osteopathic physicians tended to use one type of technique approach, other than high-velocity low-amplitude force (HVLA) direct action thrust. Some physicians used only muscle energy. Others used only functional or indirect techniques. Many of these physicians were considered experts in their field. This illustrates the reality that there is more than one method to achieve the objective. Precise answers to choice of technique do not exist. Indirect technique is of no value to a physician who lacks skills in using indirect technique. HVLA is of no value to a physician who lacks skills to use that technique.

The model for today's osteopathic physician is eclectic, with knowledge and skill in a broad spectrum of techniques. The more methods available, the greater the chance of success in treating a wide range of patients and patient problems.

Techniques are classified as direct and indirect. Direct technique means that the initial positioning of the patient's somatic dysfunction is in the direction of the restrictive barrier, then a final activating force is applied. Indirect technique involves positioning away from the restrictive barrier.

Indirect technique is usually comfortable for the patient because the physician is moving the tissues in a direction that is freer, in a direction the tissues want to go. Most of these procedures involve holding in the proper position; release is by inherent forces rather than physician forces. Examples of the indirect method are Sutherland's ligamentous release technique,[8] functional technique, and counterstrain technique.

Direct technique usually involves a greater amount of force. Procedures of this type are soft tissue, articulation, myofascial, muscle energy, and thrust techniques. Descriptions of these techniques are found in other chapters in this text.

A muscle energy procedure for the treatment of a patient with an acute, stiff neck is clinically effective, but the initial positioning is not toward or away from the restrictive barrier. The neck is positioned in a neutral, pain-free position and held while the physician instructs the patient to turn the neck in a direction which it will not move. The muscles that are contracting are not the shortened, painful muscles, but the antagonist nonpainful group. After the patient completely relaxes this contraction, the physician rotates the neck a few degrees toward the new barrier, being careful to avoid a painful position. This procedure is repeated several times and usually results in significant improvement of the patient's condition.

An osteopathic manipulative treatment has been described as a transaction between two unique persons.[9] The amount of HVLA used for one patient may be inappropriate for another. The presence of osteoporosis suggests a lesser force. Thus, thrust or impulse must be titrated. How much force should be used in a HVLA thrust? Kimberly states, "... *enough to effect a physiologic response (increased joint mobility, produce a vasomotor flush, produce palpable circulatory changes in periarticular tissues, and/or provide pain relief) but not enough to overwhelm the patient.*"

Plan of Intervention

A plan of intervention requires a specific diagnosis. Decisions must be made based on the answers to these questions:

What doesn't move?
What direction will it move?
In which direction doesn't it move?

The plan includes the decision to use a direct or indirect method of treatment to improve the movement. It considers in what direction the treatment can most effectively be applied. It includes choosing the best technique for the patient from the variety of therapeutic procedures available.

The plan of treatment and the patient's response to the treatment should be recorded in the chart's progress note. A review of the record at a follow-up visit can change the plan for the next visit. The record also is used for purposes of research, reimbursement, or legal documentation. One example of the SOAP—subjective, objective, assessment, plan—note method of recording an osteopathic office call follows:

SOAP

S: Subjective

A 28-year-old woman complains of a cold with coughing, difficulty getting a deep breath, fatigue, and low back pain. The symptoms have been present for 5 days. She complains of nasal discharge and postnasal drip. She has had a mild fever. She has no known allergies,

has otherwise been very healthy, and has had OMT in the past with no complications. There has been no change in bowel or bladder activity.

O: Objective

The patient's heart rate is 88 and regular, blood pressure is regular at 130/72, temperature is 99° orally, and respirations are 16 and not labored but shallow. There is anterior and posterior tender lymphadenopathy, the pharynx is hyperemic, and the nasal passages are congested and contain thick creamy mucus. The umbo of the tympanic membranes are conjested and hyperemic, but no fluid is seen and there is a normal cone of light. The chest is clear to auscultation over all lobes, and auscultation of the heart revealed no murmurs or adventitious sounds. There is decreased diaphragmatic breathing with best motion on the left side; C2-4 is R_R S_R, the thoracic inlet is side-bent and rotated left; T12 is N R_L S_R. ASIS are inferior and PSIS are superior on the left.

A: Assessment

1. Acute upper respiratory infection
2. Somatic dysfunction of the cervical, cervicothoracic, thoracolumbar, and pelvic regions

P: Plan

1. Cervical soft tissue
2. Direct action side-bending thrust to C3
3. Indirect action myofascial unwinding to thoracic inlet
4. Effleurage of face and neck provided. Soft tissue to thoracolumbar region and direct action–muscle energy to T12 SD. Diaphragm redomed with indirect method. Classic lymphatic pump soft tissue given
5. Counterstrain treatment of anterior innominate
6. Prescribe amoxicillin 250 mg, 30 tabs, 2 tabs four times a day

Manipulation was successful and the patient left the clinic improved with this note: "Take all of Rx and expect to be improved in 24 hours and know you are better in 48 hours. If this is not the case or you have any problem with medications, call me or come to clinic for recheck."

(Personal Signature, DO)

CONCLUSION

There are several parts to a treatment plan, including the sequence in which somatic dysfunctions should be treated, the dose and frequency of treatments, and the choice of techniques. Such intervention requires a careful evaluation and diagnosis of the patient before, during, and after treatment. The evaluation of the patient leads to a precise and individual plan for his or her treatment.

REFERENCES

1. Dinnar U. Classification of diagnostic tests used with osteopathic manipulation. *JAOA*. March 1980;79:451–455.

2. Dinnar U. Description of fifty diagnostic tests used with osteopathic manipulation. *JAOA*. January 1982;81:314–321.

3. Kappler RE. Direct action techniques. *JAOA*. December 1981; 81(4):239–243.

4. Beal MC. Viscerosomatic reflexes: a review. *JAOA*. December 1985; 85:786–801.

5. Hoag JM. The musculoskeletal system: a major factor in maintaining homeostasis. *1977 Yearbook American Academy of Osteopathy*, Newark, Ohio: American Academy of Osteopathy; 1979:5–16.

6. The Glossary Review Committee of the Educational Council on Osteopathic Principles. Glossary of osteopathic terminology. In: Allen TW, ed. *AOA Yearbook and Directory of Osteopathic Physicians*. Chicago, Ill: American Osteopathic Association; 1990:675.

7. Zink JG, Lawson WB. An osteopathic structural examination and functional interpretation of the soma. *Osteopath Ann*. December 1979;7:12.

8. Lippincott H. The osteopathic techniques of Wm. G. Sutherland, D.O. In: Northup TL, ed. *AOA Yearbook*. Indianapolis, Ind: American Academy of Osteopathy; 1949:1–24.

9. Korr IM. Somatic dysfunction, osteopathic manipulative treatment and the nervous system: a few facts, some theories, many questions. *JAOA*. February 1986;86:109–114.

42. Musculoskeletal Examination for Somatic Dysfunction

WILLIAM A. KUCHERA, JOHN M. JONES III, ROBERT E. KAPPLER, AND JOHN P. GOODRIDGE

Key Concepts

- **Elements, procedure, and interpretation of initial osteopathic musculoskeletal screening examination**
- **Additional, more focused, screening examination**
- **Musculoskeletal examination of hospitalized and outpatient clients**
- **Examination of ambulatory patients**
- **Recording of examination findings**

The osteopathic musculoskeletal examination is preceded by recording the patient's history. The purpose of the osteopathic musculoskeletal evaluation is to gain:

Information about the musculoskeletal system
Musculoskeletal clues to dysfunction of other systems or of the general health status of the patient

An osteopathic examination is unique in that palpation integrated with motion testing is the major component of the structural examination. Discovery of musculoskeletal dysfunction often provides additional clues that direct, focus, and/or expand the examination. The musculoskeletal diagnosis also expands the logical conclusions that can be drawn from that examination. Several researchers have discussed aspects of the musculoskeletal examination.[1-8]

A physician's skilled hands are the primary tools; they are used to gather the information necessary to evaluate and assess tissue texture change, and quality as well as quantity of motion. Tenderness is a relatively objective response of the patient elicited by the physician's palpation.

Osteopathic diagnostic criteria for identifying somatic dysfunction can be recalled with the mnemonic "TART":

T: *Tissue texture abnormalities.* This is a palpatory assessment of quality of tissues, usually paraspinal. Tissue changes accompany somatic dysfunction. Tissue texture change is evaluated in layers, from superficial or skin to deep, such as deep muscle. Tissue texture changes are described as acute or chronic.

A: *Asymmetry of position of bony (or other) landmarks.* Findings are discovered by inspection. Though the key element in determining the presence or absence of asymmetry is observation, or visual inspection, palpatory asymmetry is also evident.

R: *Restriction of motion.* Active motion testing involves instructing the patient to move, with the physician observing and recording range of motion. Passive motion testing involves the physician slowly introducing motion (with the patient inactive or passive). The quantity of motion is assessed by taking the joint to the endpoint of motion in both directions, or in all directions if multiple planes of motion are being assessed. Quality of motion is assessed by palpation, that is, the physician introduces motion and assesses compliance or resistance to the motion being introduced.

T: *Tenderness.* Tenderness is said to be present when the physician applies a stimulus, usually palpatory pressure, and the patient reports discomfort, flinches, has a facial change, or otherwise indicates discomfort. The test is objective in that the physician applies a measured force to the patient. Patient response involves a degree of subjectivity, depending on the individual's sensitivity or threshold for pain. Tenderness differs from pain. Pain is a totally subjective cerebral (cortical) perception of nociceptive input reported by the patient in the absence of palpatory stimulus.

A musculoskeletal examination for somatic dysfunction is best performed in stages, progressing from an overview screening examination to a more detailed and finally segmental definition of TART at a specific joint, facet, or vertebral unit. The progressive approach, from screening examination to a more detailed examination, is applicable in most situations. The patient may be a hospitalized patient, an ambulatory outpatient, or a patient with a specific musculoskeletal problem who is referred to a physician with a special proficiency in osteopathic manipulative medicine.

A multistep musculoskeletal scanning examination is presented here first. For the purpose of simplicity, the components of this examination are identified as stage I (general) or stage II (more focused) tests. An example of a simple musculoskeletal examination form for recording results of this examination is included. Following this more complete presentation, examples of applying simple musculoskeletal screening examinations to ambulatory or to bedfast hospital patients are presented.

An osteopathic musculoskeletal examination is a prerequisite for manipulative treatment and determines where to treat and how to treat. Rarely, if ever, will a physician include all of these test procedures in a single examination. If a problem is suspected in a specific region, use as many of the tests as indicated to gather as much information as is needed while the patient is in a specific position. Develop an examination sequence, related to your experiences and preference for treatment procedures.

For efficiency, it is important to use an examination sequence that is organized and responsive to the chief complaint and that does not require frequent change of patient position. The examination must identify obvious significant musculoskeletal changes (false-negative results must be minimized). Have a sufficient database of findings to develop a treatment plan. With experience, one better understands how the various findings are interrelated.

Some musculoskeletal examinations may not lead to a musculoskeletal treatment plan at the time of examination. A screening examination may be used to identify potential problem areas to be further evaluated and treated later. Sometimes examinations may be conducted for the purpose of collecting osteopathic research data to be analyzed at a later date in accordance with the research protocol.

An organized total body musculoskeletal screening examination includes inspection, palpation, and motion testing to identify a problem or problems in one or more of the body's regions:

Cranial
Cervical
Thoracic
Costal
Lumbar
Abdominal
Pelvic
Appendages

Consider these questions and relationships as you examine the patient:

1. Is a problem (a dysfunction) present?
2. Is there a problem with the base of support or is it a weight-bearing problem?
3. Is the problem in one or more regions of the body, and if so, which ones?
4. Is there tissue texture abnormality (temperature, turgor, tension, or discomfort with compression)?
5. Is there asymmetry?
6. Is there a restriction of active, passive, or inherent motion?
7. Is there tenderness?
8. How do the findings correlate with known medical, personal, and social histories?
9. How do these areas correlate with the areas of sympathetic or parasympathetic innervation to the viscera, that is, can they be attributed to or result from a visceral dysfunction or disease?
10. Are there other objective findings associated with the same segmental level?
11. How do the findings correlate with a common or known pattern, such as the common compensatory pattern of the fascias of the body?[9]
12. What are the identified problems and can I list them clearly?

The initial examination is a brief scan of all areas of the body, while focusing attention on the area involved in the patient's history of the chief complaint and/or the viscerosomatic region or regions related to it. Record the end result on the patient's chart, documenting that all areas were examined and that somatic dysfunction was diagnosed or not diagnosed in a given region. Include a specific segmental diagnosis in the report to support somatic dysfunction in the region and to aid in planning for specific osteopathic manipulative treatment.

Musculoskeletal Screening (Scanning) Examination

What follows is an abbreviated outline form of an organized multistep musculoskeletal screening (scanning) examination (Table 42.1). Note: Finding any abnormalities during this screen warrants a more detailed evaluation of the region and your assessment of how those findings affect the total patient.

Stage I Examination

GENERAL APPEARANCE

GAIT

STANDING

Static Findings

Observe for Symmetry

This includes the levels of the trochanter, posterior superior iliac spine (PSIS), iliac crests, scapula, acromion, and mastoid planes.

1. Posterior observation
2. Lateral observation
3. Anterior observation

Observe for Curves

1. Anteroposterior (AP): cervical lordosis, thoracic kyphosis, lumbar lordosis
2. Lateral: rotoscoliosis

Motion Findings

Flexion Test

Lumbar Range of Motion

Forward bending, backward bending, side-bending.

Hip Drop Test

Pelvic Side Shift

SEATED

Static Findings

Observe for Symmetry

Observe for Curves

Did they change from the standing position?

Table 42.1
Primary Scanning Examination

The following charts are divided into a left side and a right side. The left side presents information that may be found on a primary scanning examination. The right side presents additional tests and observations that can be performed to gain further information regarding a preliminary finding. Additional information can be found in each of the regional sections.

Another form of the musculoskeletal examination: The physician performs the primary screening examination. Positive findings require a more complete examination of the area using the secondary screening examinations.

Primary Scanning Examination	Secondary Screening Examination
General Appearance	General appearance
	Body type, muscle development, weight, height, nutritional status
Gait	Is weight transferred in a continuous manner from heel to toe for push off.
	Is there a limp?
	Is there toeing in, toeing out, excessive pronation or supination?
	Is either leg internally or externally rotated?
	Is there symmetrical motion?
	through pelvis and lumbar area?
	through thoracic area, shoulders?
	arm swing present and equal bilaterally?
Standing: Static Findings	
Observe symmetry—trochanters, PSIS, crests, scapula, acromion, mastoid planes.	Standing: Posterior observation
A. Posterior observation	Observe: angulation of head carriage, level of shoulders, scapulae, symmetry of paraspinal muscles, carrying angle of elbows, Achilles tendon. Unilateral fullness indicative of hypertonicity (tight); hypotonicity (loose); left and right muscle groups (i.e., trapezius, erector spinae mass (ESM), gluteus maximus, hamstrings, gastrocnemius).
	Palpate: level of shoulders, inferior border of scapulae, iliac crests, trochanters; hypertonicity or hypotonicity of trapezias, ESM, iliolumbar ligament attachments, gluteus maximus, iliotibial bands, hamstrings, quadriceps, gastrocnemius muscles; tension and height of arches of feet.
B. Lateral observation	Laterally:
	Observe: A P cervical, thoracic, and lumbar curves for increased lordosis/kyphosis; evaluate the gravitational line (through external auditory meatus, acromioclavicular joint, greater trochanter, lateral malleolus); any sway or rotation of the pelvis? Are knees flexed or hyperextended?
C. Anterior observation	Anteriorly:
	Observe: head carriage (rotation of side-bending in relation to shoulders), shoulder levelness, rib cage configuration (pectus carinatum, pectus excavatum), sternal deformities, clavicular deformities or elevation, supraclavicular fossae depth or fullness, linea alba hair patterns, scars, iliac crest heights, ASIS, patellae, anterior tibial tuberosities, upper extremities for internal/external rotation, antecubital fossae for angles of fullness
Standing: Spinal Motion Findings	Standing Motion Tests
A. Forward bending (FB) Backward bending (BB), and Side-bending (S)	Truncal forward bending: observe range of motion, group restrictions, accessory motions, "rib hump."
	Standing flexion test: (Do at same time as truncal test.) Observe when the patient bends forward to approximate fingertips to toes, for a change in asymmetry of position of PSISs from that before the movement and that at the end of movement. The patient stands erect with knees extended and feet acetabular distance apart. If leg length inequality is suspected because the iliac crests or the PSISs are not level with the transverse plane, a shim may be placed under the shorter leg to level the iliac crests, or the PSISs, before performing the tests and changes in flexion test observed.
T = tissue texture changes	
A = asymmetry	
R = restriction motion	
T = tenderness	
	The medial surface of your thumbs are placed contacting the posterior superior iliac spines at their inferior notch and ride with the iliac spines as the patient flexes. Assessment is made of the position of the left and right PSISs relative to a transverse plane before and at the terminal position of forward bending from the waist. If motion of one thumb over the PSIS continues after termination of motion of the other thumb, a positive standing flexion test is recorded.

Table 42.1—*continued*

Primary Scanning Examination	Secondary Screening Examination
B. Lumbar range of motion tests: (FB, BB, Side-bending)	Lumbar motion testing:
	Lumbar forward bending: This can be measured in several ways. Forward bending may be assessed by visual observation. The position of the patient's fingertips in relation to the floor can be measured. An inclinometer can be used over the lumbar spine and the number of degrees of forward bending recorded. A horizontal line can be drawn on the patient's skin at the sacral base and at L1. The distance between these lines can then be measured with a tape measure between these two lines before and after bending over.
	Lumbar backward bending: This is usually measured by inspection. A goniometer or inclinometer may be used for more precise measurement.
	Lumbar side-bending: (Active) Observe for presence or absence of thoracic and lumbar lateral curves while the patient side-bends as far as possible to the left and the right by sliding hand down the lateral aspect of the thigh toward the knee [R]
	Lumbar horizontal levelness: palpate on both sides of the body.
C. Hip drop test Used to compare with side-bending test to identify a contralateral curve in the lower lumbar area, especially LS. Observe for side with greatest drop of hip bone toward floor	Hip Drop Test: (Active) Normal = 20–25° hip drop. Place your hands, palms parallel with the floor, superior to patient's iliac crests; observe their relationship to a transverse (horizontal) line. To do a *right hip drop test*: direct patient to stand on the right leg and let the left hip drop by bending the left knee without lifting the heel from the floor (do not let the patient rotate the pelvis in the transverse plane, nor translate the pelvis in a coronal plane). Record the *right hip drop* by observing the level of your hands (at iliac crests) relative to the transverse plane and compare with previous position. Now do a *left hip drop test* by having the patient stand on the left leg and dropping the right hip. Interpretation: The crest that drops the most is on the side of the increased convexity of a lumbar curve. If that is on the same side as the increased convexity of the trunk side-bending curve, a "C" curve is present in the thoracolumbosacral vertebral column. If the trunk side-bending increased convexity is on the opposite side, an "S" curve is present in the lumbar area. Where these contralateral curves meet at the midline of the vertebral column suggests the possibility of a localized, segmental, somatic dysfunction.
D. Pelvic side shift (passive) The purpose of this test is to evaluate the position of the sacrum (which is the base of support for the spine) in relation to the midline.	Pelvic Side Shift Motion Test: Is the sacrum in the midline, or is the sacrum deviated to one side? If the deviation to one side is obvious, inspection of this lateral deviation of the sacral position is all that is necessary. If not obvious, proceed with the side-shift motion test. This is done by standing behind the patient, placing one hand on the hip area and stabilizing the opposite shoulder with the other hand. The pelvis is translated laterally by pushing on the hip. The hand position is reversed and the pelvis is translated in the opposite direction. The test is positive on the side of freer translation. The sacrum (base of support) is positioned on the side of freer motion.
Seated: Static Findings	Static Findings: Observe Symmetry and Cervical, Thoracic and Lumbar Curves: patient seated
Seated Spinal Motion Tests A. Seated flexion test (Active)	Seated Motion Tests Your thumbs are placed at PSISs as described above. The patient is seated upright with the feet flat on the floor and then bends forward reaching for the floor. Assessment is again made before movement begins and at the end of movement.
B. Trunk side-bending (and rotation) tests (Active)	With the patient seated, ask the patient to flex (forward bend) the trunk, extend (backward bend) the trunk, rotate to each side, side-bend to the left and right. Observe and record any restriction of motion. (Passive) Flex the patient's neck into FB, BB, side-bending, and rotation.
C. Trunk rotation test	Place your hands on patient's shoulders lateral to the body of the scapula with your fingers on the anterior aspects of the shoulders. With your hand behind the patient's shoulder, initiate a rotary motion and feel the resistance and observe the range, first in one direction, then in the other. Compare for symmetry.

Table 42.1—*continued*

Primary Scanning Examination	Secondary Screening Examination
D. Acromion drop test (Fig. 42.10)	This is a passive test for lateral flexion of the upper thoracic spine. Place one hand superior to the acromioclavicular joint and press inferomedially. (With the same hand, further pressure toward the hip on the same side will determine the thoracolumbar side-bending.) Repeat for other side and note any asymmetry of resistance or range.

E. Cervical motion testing	Active flexion/extension
	Active side-bending
	Active rotation
	These motions may also be done passively with expected motion being symmetrical and FB 90°, BB 90°, rotate right 90°, rotate left 90°. There are a variety of physician hand contacts to passively explore the above movements with the patient seated. The hand contact should sense the beginning of restriction before the patient experiences discomfort. Note both the sense of resistance and the range of movement.
	Note the following:
	  Any sensation of resistance to motion
	  Unilateral restriction of motion
	  The range of motion

Seated Spinal Palpation Cervical, thoracic, and lumbar spine	Seated Palpation With the patient in the seated position, the cervical, thoracic, and lumbar spine regions can be palpated for tissue texture abnormality and tenderness. A screening palpation is done using several fingers covering a broad expanse of the patient's back. Palpation of local areas is ordinarily done with one or two fingers. See section of palpation with the patient in the prone position for a detailed description of palpatory findings.
Seated Upper Extremity Testing Extend arms above the head	Seated Upper Extremity: Observation seated and palpation Patient's arms are actively abducted in the coronal plane and extended over the head. The medial surface of the upper arms touch the ear on the respective side while the head is in a neutral position. Elbows should be straight. The dorasl surface of the hands should be equally approximated. If the above is accomplished, the test is negative. However, if the patient is unable to bring the arms to the ears, the shoulders, upper ribs, upper thoracic area, and the large muscle groups affecting the shoulder need to be specifically examined. If the dorsal surface of the hands cannot be equally approximated, the elbows and wrists need to be examined specifically for motion restriction. Hypertrophied shoulder or associated myofascial trigger points in the muscles also prevent this.
Supine Testing for Lower Extremity and Ribs A. Observation	Observe levelness of iliac crests, ASIS, pubic tubercles, and the medial malleoli. Instruct patient to "hip flop"—used to place patient on table without undue deformity due to tension. Have patient flex hips and knees with feet together and flat on the table. Then have the patient lift the hips high off the table and drop the hips back to the table.
B. Motion testing of lower extremity	With the patient's knees extended, grasp the calcanei and ankles and passively internally and externally rotate the lower extremity. Compare symmetry of motion. Flex one of the patient's legs at the knee and at the hip and then passively test for internal and external rotation of the hip joint. Compare symmetry of motion and end-feel.
C. Supine—costal cage motion Four quadrant screen	Evaluate durationof inhalation and exhalation motions of ribs 2-6 by placing hands lateral to sternum; fingers should follow in intercostal spaces. Thumbs should touch each other as they rest on the sternum. Place hands more laterally to evaluate the bucket-handle motions of ribs 7-10. Operator's hands are passive as patient breathes, first normally, and then with exaggeration if necessary. Palpate ribs 11 and 12 (floating ribs) at their anterior ends; note and compare the intercostal spaces above each of these ribs. Have the patient breathe in and out and check the symmetry of pincer motion of the floating ribs.

Motion Findings

Flexion Test

Other Motion Tests

1. Cervical, upper extremity: shoulder, elbow, wrist, hand
2. Torso: thoracic and lumbar side-bending, rotation, flexion, extension

Tissue Texture Abnormality and Tenderness

Palpation

Tissue texture abnormality, tenderness, motion.

SUPINE

Static Findings

Settle the pelvis before proceeding by performing the "hip flop" procedure. In the hip flop procedure, have the patient flex the knees and hips, pick the buttocks up, and then relax the muscles and let the pelvis drop to the table. You then passively bring both legs to the table in full extension. This will reduce asymmetry caused by poor initial alignment on the table or asymmetry caused by minor muscle spasm.

Observe for Symmetry

Includes levels of ASIS, iliac crests, superior pubic rami, malleoli.

Motion Findings

Cervical

See Chapter 45, "Cervical Spine," for supine segmental motion testing of the cervical spine.

Costal Motion

Four-quadrant screen: costal cage.

Lower Extremity

Includes observation, motion of the hip, knee, ankle, and foot.

Tissue Texture Abnormality and Tenderness

Palpation

Tissue texture abnormality and tenderness.

Stage II Examination

These examinations are performed on those failing the regional screen (scan) (Table 42.1).

GENERAL APPEARANCE

Body type, muscle development, weight, nutritional status.

GAIT

Is weight transferred in a continuous manner from heel to toe for push off? Is there a limp? Is there toeing in, toeing out, or excessive pronation or supination? Is either leg internally or externally rotated? Is there symmetrical motion through the pelvis and lumbar area, through the thoracic area, the shoulders? Is arm swing present and equal bilaterally?

STANDING

Static Findings

Observe Posteriorly for Horizontal Asymmetry (Fig. 42.1)

Observe angulation of head carriage; level of shoulders and scapulae; asymmetry of paraspinal muscles; carrying angle of elbows; relative thickness and tension of the Achilles tendons (unilateral fullness is indicative of congestion, tension is indicative of increased weight bearing on that side); and relative

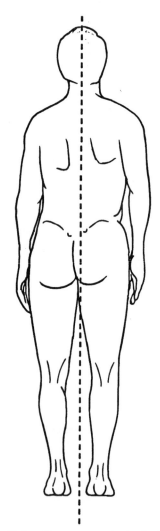

Figure 42.1. Observe posterior body alignment.

tension of the right and left muscle groups, such as the trapezius, erector spinae, gluteus maximus, hamstrings, and gastrocnemius. Palpate level of shoulders; level of inferior borders of scapulae; level of iliac crest; level of PSIS; level of greater trochanter.

Palpation

Palpate for hypertonicity (tight) or hypotonicity (loose) of left and right trapezius, erector spinae, iliolumbar ligament attachments, gluteus maximus, iliotibial bands, hamstring, and gastrocnemius. Palpate arches of feet for height and tension.

Observe Laterally for Anteroposterior Asymmetry (Fig. 42.2)

Observe AP spinal curves for increased lordosis or kyphosis in cervical, thoracic, and lumbar areas. Observe gravitational line (external auditory meatus, acromioclavicular joint, greater tro-

chanter, lateral malleolus) and position of pelvis for asymmetrical rotation. Observe knees partially flexed or hyperextended.

Observe Anteriorly and Palpate for Horizontal Asymmetry (Fig. 42.3)

Observe head carriage (rotation or side-bending in relation to shoulders), shoulder levels, rib cage configuration (pectus carinatum, pectus excavatum), sternal deformities, clavicular deformities or elevation, supraclavicular fossae for fullness and depth, linea alba hair patterns, or scars.

Palpation

Palpate for iliac crest levelness, anterior superior iliac spine (ASIS) levels, quadriceps muscles, patellar levelness, anterior tibial tuberosity levelness, upper extremities for internal and external rotation, and antecubital fossae for angles and fullness.

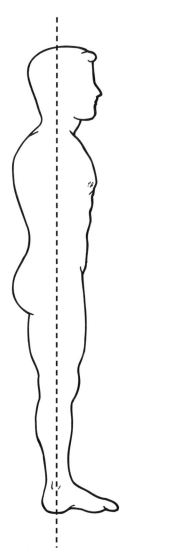

Figure 42.2. Observe lateral body alignment.

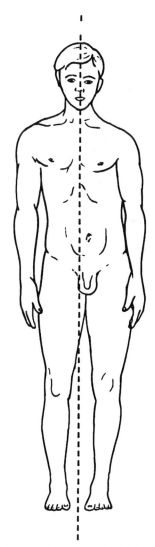

Figure 42.3. Observe anterior body alignment.

Motion Tests

Truncal Forward Bending (Fig. 42.4)

Observe range of motion, group restrictions, accessory motions, and "rib hump" and do a standing flexion test. The truncal and forward bending tests can be performed as one maneuver.

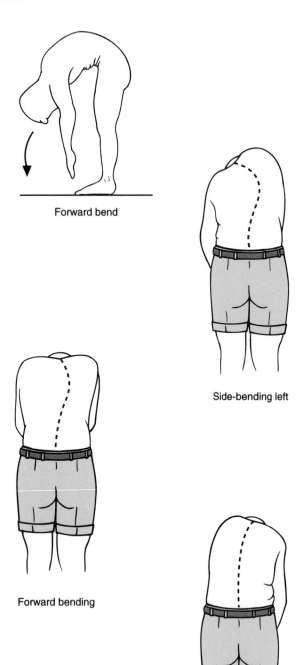

Forward bend

Side-bending left

Forward bending

Side-bending right

Figure 42.4. Standing forward bending test.

Flexion Test (Fig. 42.5)

This is an active flexion test at PSISs. As the patient bends forward to approximate fingertips to toes, observe for a change in asymmetry of position of PSISs from their position before the movement and their position at the end of forward bending.

PROCEDURE

1. The patient stands erect with knees extended and feet acetabular distance apart.
2. Place the medial surface of your thumbs to contact the posterior superior iliac spines at their inferior notch and ride with the iliac spines as the patient flexes.
3. Assess the position of the left and right PSISs relative to a transverse plane before and at the terminal position of forward bending from the waist.
4. The PSISs may be level or unlevel before the test begins. If motion of one thumb at the inferior notch of the PSIS continues to rise after termination of motion of the other thumb, a positive standing flexion test is recorded for that side.

INTERPRETATION

A positive standing flexion test indicates that there is somatic dysfunction somewhere in the leg or the pelvis (usually the innominate) on the side of the positive test.

Lumbar Range of Motion Tests

Forward Bending (Fig. 42.4)

This can be measured in several ways. Forward bending may be assessed by visual observation. The position of the patient's fingertips in relation to the floor can be measured and recorded

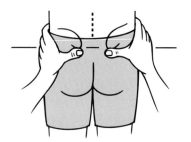

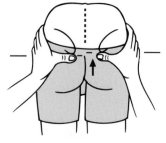

Figure 42.5. Standing flexion test: positive on right.

as an objective test and used to determine the effect of certain types of treatment. An inclinometer can be placed over the lumbar spine, and the number of degrees of forward bending are recorded. A horizontal line can be drawn on the patient's skin at the sacral base and at L1. The distance between these lines is measured with a tape measure with the patient in the upright position and in a forward-bent position.

Backward Bending

This is usually measured by inspection. A goniometer or inclinometer may be used for a more precise measurement.

Side-bending Test (Active) (Fig. 42.6)

Observe for the presence of a smooth curve, abrupt changes in the curve, or the absence of thoracic and lumbar lateral curves, while the patient side-bends as far as possible to the left and the right, by sliding hand down the lateral aspect of the thigh toward the knee.

Hip Drop Test (Active) (Fig. 42.7)

The hip drop test screens for the ability of the lumbar and lumbothoracic region (especially the lumbosacral region) to side-bend away from the side of the hip drop.

PROCEDURE

1. Place your hands, palms parallel with the floor, superior to the most lateral portion of the patient's iliac crests; observe their relationship to a transverse (horizontal) line.

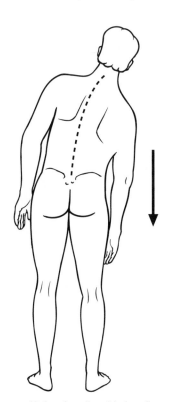

Figure 42.6. Standing side-bending test.

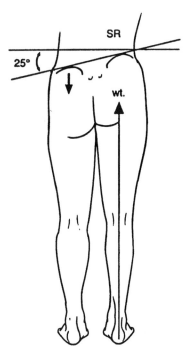

Figure 42.7. Negative left hip drop test. *SR*, S$_R$, where the lumbar spine is side-bent right; *wt.*, weight-bearing side.

2. Direct the patient to bend one knee without lifting that heel from the floor (in a manner that does not rotate the pelvis in the transverse plane, nor translate the pelvis in a coronal plane)
3. Observe the level of your hands (at iliac crests) relative to the transverse plane and compare with the previous position.
4. Repeat with the other knee.

INTERPRETATION

The hip or iliac crest that drops the most during a hip drop test is the side that can obtain the greatest convexity of lumbar/thoracolumbar curve. A *negative hip drop test* indicates normal side-bending ability of the lumbar and thoracolumbar regions of the spine to the contralateral side of the hip drop test; there is a hip drop of 20–25° and a smooth curve away from the side of the hip drop (its convexity is on the same side as the hip drop). A *positive hip drop test* indicates that there is some somatic dysfunction or pathology in the lumbars or thoracolumbar junction that prevents the region of the spine from side-bend normally to the side opposite the hip drop. An example of a positive left hip drop test: With weight being supported on the right leg, the left hip drops *less than* 20–25° and the lumbar and thoracolumbar spine does not side-bend smoothly, is flat, or is angled in its attempt to side-bend to the right side. It indicates that this region of the spine should have a segmental examination to determine the cause of the side-bending dysfunction.

The hip drop test can also be used to estimate the type of scoliosis present in a patient. If you observe a left scoliosis (thoracic region side-bent to the right) in a patient and the left hip drop test is negative, a "C" curve (side-bent right) is most likely present. If the left hip drop test is positive and the right hip drop is negative in that person, an "S" spinal curvature is most likely present. The area of flattened or angled spinal curvature seen in this patient with the positive left hip drop test is probably where the contralateral curves meet and is often called a crossover point. Somatic dysfunction at a crossover has expanded significance because it is more likely to be associated with visceral dysfunction in organs receiving sympathetic innervation from that level of the spinal cord.

Pelvic Side Shift Test (Passive) (Fig. 42.8)

In perfect posture as viewed from the back, the midline of the sacrum should be in the mid-heel line (vertical gravitational line) and should not deviate to the right or left.

PROCEDURE

1. Stand behind the patient and inspect for lateral deviation.
2. Place your left hand on the pelvis and right hand on the shoulder. Translate the patient's pelvis to the right side while stabilizing the shoulder.
3. Switch hands and translate the pelvis to the left side.
4. Compare the resiliency to movement of one side with the other.

INTERPRETATION

This test determines whether the sacrum, as the center of the pelvis, is in the midline. The test is positive on the side of freer translation; that is, the positive test indicates that the pelvis is shifted to that side. The sacrum (base of support) is positioned on the side of the freer motion. If the deviation to one side is obvious, inspection of this lateral deviation of the sacral position is all that is necessary.

SEATED

Observe for Symmetry, Curves

Observe for symmetry with the patient in the seated position.

Motion Tests

Flexion Test (Fig. 42.9)

Flexion test at PSISs (active). Your thumbs are placed at PSISs as described above for the standing flexion test.

PROCEDURE

1. The patient is seated upright with the feet flat on the floor.
2. Have patient bend forward, reaching for the floor.
3. Assess the levelness of the PSISs before movement begins and at the end of movement.

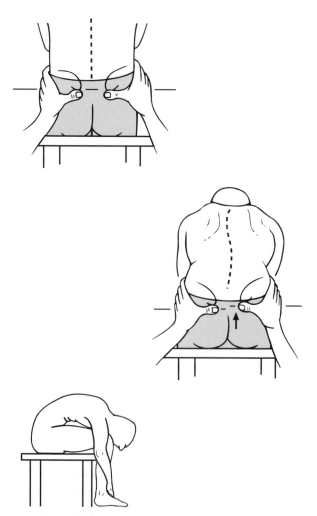

Figure 42.9.   Seated flexion test: positive on right.

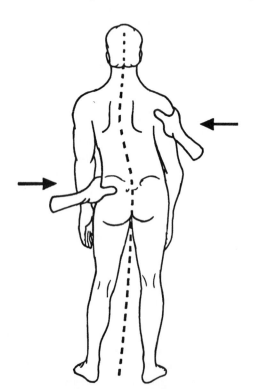

Figure 42.8.   Left pelvic side-shift test.

INTERPRETATION

Interpretation is the same as for the standing flexion test. Since the patient is seated, the positive test indicates somatic dysfunction somewhere in the pelvis on the side of the positive test, that is, in the sacrum or innominate (usually in the sacrum).

Cervical Motion Test (Active)

PROCEDURE

With the patient seated, ask the patient to flex the head and neck, extend the head and neck, rotate to each side, side-bend to the left and right. Note: Passive cervical testing is also a good test.

INTERPRETATION

Observe and record any restriction of motion.

Trunk Side-bending, Rotation, and Sagittal Plane Motion Tests (Active)

PROCEDURE

Ask the patient to flex (forward bend) the trunk, extend (backward bend) the trunk, rotate to each side, side-bend to the left and right.

INTERPRETATION

Observe and record any restriction of motion.

Trunk Side-bending and Rotation Tests (Passive) (Fig. 42.10)

Feel with the pushing hand for the direction of greater resistance.

PROCEDURE

For lateral flexion, place one hand superior to the acromioclavicular joint and press the patient's shoulder toward patient's hip on the same side to assess ease and ability of the upper thoracic region to side-bend. Repeat for the other side and note any asymmetry of resistance or range.

For rotation, place your hands on the patient's shoulders lateral to the body of the scapula with your fingers on the anterior aspects of the shoulders. With your hand behind the shoulder, initiate a rotary motion and feel the resistance and observe the range, first in one direction, then in the other. Compare for asymmetry.

An additional method of testing the upper thoracic spine is to place one hand on the patient's head and introduce motion. The other hand contacts the upper thoracic area and monitors the motion being introduced through the head and neck. For rotation and side-bending, contact the transverse process area on both sides. (For flexion and extension, monitor the spinous process-interspinous area.)

There is a variety of physician hand contacts to passively

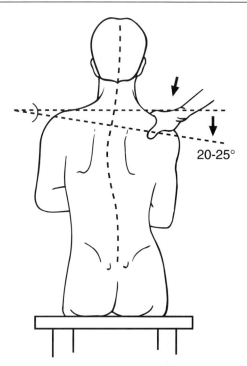

Figure 42.10.   Right trunk side-bending test: acromion drop test.

explore the above movements with the patient seated. The hand contact should sense the beginning of restriction before the patient experiences discomfort. Note both the sense of resistance and the range of movement.

INTERPRETATION

Note any sensation of resistance to motion or unilateral restriction of motion, and record the range of motion.

Palpation

With the patient in the seated position, the cervical, thoracic, and lumbar spine regions can be palpated for tissue texture abnormality and tenderness. A screening palpation is performed using several fingers covering a broad expanse of the patient's back. Palpation of local areas is ordinarily done with one or two fingers. Description of tissue texture abnormality may be found in Chapter 39, "Palpatory Skills."

Upper Extremity Observation

Palpation

Motion Tests

Extend Arms over Head, Active (or Passive) (Fig. 42.11)

PROCEDURE

The patient actively abducts both arms in the coronal plane and extends them over the head. The medial surface of the upper arms touches the ear on the respective side while the head is in a neutral position.

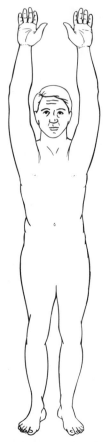

Figure 42.11.   Arm screening examination: arm extension test.

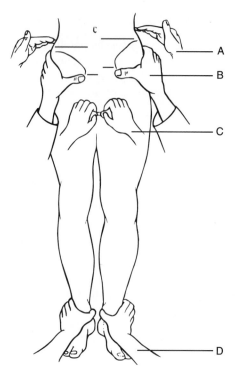

Figure 42.12.   Static assessment of anterior pelvis and legs.

INTERPRETATION

The elbows should be straight and the medial surface of the upper arms should touch the ears. The dorsal surface of the hands should be equally approximated. If the above is accomplished, the test is negative. However, if the patient is unable to bring the arms to the ears, the test is positive; and the shoulder joints including the clavicles and scapulae, the upper ribs, upper thoracic area, and the large muscle groups affecting the shoulder need to be specifically examined.

If the dorsal surface of the hands cannot be equally approximated, the elbows and wrists need to be examined specifically for motion restriction. Hypertrophied shoulder or associated myofascial trigger points in the muscles can also prevent this.

SUPINE

Observe for Asymmetry

Observation of Leg and/or Pelvic Asymmetry (Fig. 42.12)

PROCEDURE

1. Assess iliac crests with transverse plane (Fig. 42.12*A*).
2. Assess ASIS levels with transverse plane (Fig. 42.12*B*)
3. Assess pubic tubercles with transverse plane (Fig. 42.12*C*).
4. Assess malleoli levels with transverse plane of the body (Fig. 42.12*D*).

Motion

Passively internally rotate lower limbs (knees extended) by grasping calcanei and ankles; note asymmetry of motion.

Costal Cage Motion

Four Quadrant Screen for the Ribs

PROCEDURE

1. Evaluate duration of inhalation and exhalation motions of ribs 2-6 by placing hands lateral to sternum; fingers should follow in intercostal spaces. Thumbs should touch each other as they rest on the sternum.
2. Place hands more laterally to evaluate the bucket-handle motions of ribs 7-10.
3. Keep hands passive as patient breathes, first normally, and then with exaggeration if necessary.
4. Apply pressure posteriorly over ribs 11-12 (floating ribs), gently springing them. Have the patient breathe fully to evaluate pincer (caliper) motion of these two ribs with inhalation and exhalation.

Cervical Motion

See Chapter 45 for supine segmental motion testing of the cervical spine.

SCREENING MUSCULOSKELETAL EXAMINATIONS FOR OUTPATIENT AND HOSPITALIZED PATIENTS

A 3- to 5-minute osteopathic structural screening examination is part of the standard history and physical examination performed by osteopathic physicians on all patients admitted to a hospital. To develop an organized approach to an osteopathic structural examination, sample screening examinations are provided for outpatients, ambulatory inpatients (Table 42.2), and hospitalized patients unable to stand (Table 42.3). A recording form for a hospital musculoskeletal examination is shown in Table 42.4.

In the present health care environment, people are usually hospitalized for delivery, major surgery, a systemic disorder, or a disease. A musculoskeletal screening examination is used to determine spinal regions that are not functioning properly. These regions are then examined segmentally to identify specific somatic dysfunctions. Somatic dysfunctions are associated with related facilitated spinal cord segments when there is continuous somatic or visceral dysfunction. They can also identify dysfunction in homeostatic mechanisms (thoracic inlet, abdominal diaphragm, regions of sympathetic outflow). Osteopathic manipulative treatment designed to remove these somatic dysfunctions will therefore aid the patient in his or her natural ability to recover.

Osteopathic manipulative treatment of somatic dysfunctions benefit the patient's general well-being and the medical, preoperative, or surgical healing mechanisms. The American Osteopathic Association presently requires that three positions be used in the osteopathic musculoskeletal examination if possible. Record the positions for the examination at the beginning of the physical report. If the patient cannot achieve some position or some of the examinations can not be completed, record the reasons in the progress notes or the physical examination.

The following screens fulfill the current standards required by the American Osteopathic Association. While not the only acceptable approaches, they are comprehensive and easy to perform.

SCREENING MUSCULOSKELETAL EXAMINATIONS FOR AMBULATORY OUTPATIENTS OR HOSPITALIZED PATIENTS

The following examination for ambulatory patients (W.A.K. contribution) is provided as a screen of all key areas of the musculoskeletal system and includes a screen for musculoskeletal clues of possible viscerosomatic dysfunction (Table 42.2). Use the results to formulate a plan to provide osteopathic manipulative support for the patient with primary and/or secondary somatic dysfunction.

Hospitalized patients are often unable to move or change positions comfortably. Primary musculoskeletal problems do not lead to a large number of admissions to the hospital these days. Treatment of somatic dysfunctions in the hospital is directed toward support of the patient's own homeostatic mechanisms. If the patient does have a primary musculoskeletal problem, it is usually obvious and the examination can be altered accordingly (Tables 42.3 and 42.4).

Most patients are not in the hospital for primary musculoskeletal disorders; secondary involvement is, however, common. The osteopathic examination integrates musculoskeletal findings, viscerosomatic reflexes, and other tissue texture changes with a thorough history and physical, providing a comprehensive clinical approach and unique insights into the differential diagnosis. Detailed knowledge of functional anatomy, visceral innervation, the importance of the sympathetic and parasympathetic components of the nervous system, and awareness of the lymphatic drainage distribution helps the physician decide where to focus the physical examination.[10] Evaluate key areas affecting homeostatic balance to determine if musculoskeletal findings indicate health status change in the patient and whether OMT might make a difference in the healing process. Include the:

Thoracic inlet
Abdominal diaphragm
Paraspinal regions from T1 to L2
Occipitoatlantal and sacroiliac regions

In a screening structural examination, do a minimal examination unless there is indication for seeking additional data. The osteopathic musculoskeletal screening should not take more than 3–5 minutes; it is integrated with other aspects of the history and physical examination. As mentioned before, screening, as defined by the American Osteopathic Association, includes examination in three positions, with inspection, palpation, and regional and segmental motion testing of the spine and pelvis. Also include major findings in the extremities. Note:

Anteroposterior spinal curves
Any lateral curves
Limitations of motion
Muscle hypertonicity or spasm
Tenderness

The patient's history draws attention to areas of potential involvement, including viscerosomatic relationships. An adequate examination should reveal significant positives and negatives important in arriving at an accurate diagnosis. Although this is a screening examination, note specific segmental diagnoses if they are found and are significant. The end result is a chart recording all areas examined and the somatic dysfunction that has been diagnosed as and related to the patient's complaints and problems.

Have a routine approach to the patient, modifying it as the situation warrants, fitting the individual patient's needs, time allowed, and environmental constraints. The form offered here (Table 42.4) is for recording purposes and does not specify a particular sequence. Develop a routine sequence as indicated in Tables 42.2 or 42.3. Doing so makes it less likely that portions of the examination will be inadvertently omitted.

When doing the regional examinations for TART changes, remember that motion limitation is more important than static asymmetry. The combination of motion asymmetry with any one additional TART criterion is sufficient to diagnose somatic

Table 42.2
Screening Musculoskeletal Examination for the Ambulatory Patient

Tests	Neg.	Pos.	Explanation
Body Planes	Neg.	Pos.	Estimates levelness of horizontal planes under the mastoid bone, shoulder, inferior scapular angle, iliac crests, PSIS, greater trochanter Positive = unlevel horizontal planes. This indicates postural change that could be related to compensatory mechanisms, visceral dysfunction, and/or scoliosis. Follow-up for evidence of scoliosis, unlevel sacral base, chronic tissue congestion problems, complaints of postural stress.
Arms	Neg.	Pos.	The patient raises his/her arms above the head; upper arms touch ears, back of hands are together. Positive = unable to fully extend the extremity with upper arms along side of the ears. Indicates dysfunction in any one or a combination of the joints of the upper extremity and also includes the upper back and upper thoracic region. Individual joints listed above are specifically examined according to the patient's history and concerns.
Legs	Neg.	Pos.	The patient squats down and returns to upright position. Tests hips, knees, ankles, and strength of flexors and extensors of the hips, knees, and legs. Positive = inability to flex legs while weight bearing to a point where the thighs are at least level with the ground or to be able to return to upright position without assistance. Individual joints listed above are specifically examined *according to the patient's history and concerns.*

Table 42.2—*continued*

Tests	Neg.	Pos.	Explanation
Standing Flexion Test	Neg.	Pos.	The operator monitors the inferior notches of the PSIS as the patient bends forward with arms hanging toward the floor. Localizes pelvis and leg somatic dysfunction to one side. (Can also visualize "hump" if rotoscoliosis is present.) Positive = the PSIS rises asymmetrically with forward bending and/or there is a "rib hump." Because of weight bearing, this test indicates dysfunction *in the leg and/or the pelvis on the "positive" side.* ("A rib hump indicates rotoscoliosis often due to an unlevel sacral base.)
Seated Flexion Test	Neg.	Pos.	The operator monitors the inferior notches of both PSISs while the patient bends forward with arms hanging toward the floor. The test localizes somatic dysfunction to one side of the pelvis. (Can also visualize a "rib hump" if rotoscoliosis is present.) Positive = the PSISs rises asymmetrically with forward bending and/or there is a "rib hump." Because the patient is *not* weight bearing, the positive side indicates some problem with the innominate or the sacral joints on the positive side. ("Hump" indicates rotoscoliosis.)
Trunk Rotation	Neg.	Pos.	Passive rotation of the trunk to the right and to the left. Positive = unilateral reduced rotation, i.e., restriction in rotation R or L. (N = 90°) Indicates restriction to rotation somewhere in the thoracolumbar or lumbar spine. If there is a problem in rotation, there is also problem with side-bending. If fail screen, follow with segmental diagnosis of joint somatic dysfunction and correlate findings with neurological evaluation.
Acromion Drop Test	Neg.	Pos.	The physician depresses the shoulder on one side and then the other. This action tests side-bending of the upper thoracic spine. Positive = acromion does not drop as far on one side. (N = 25°) Indicates that the upper thoracic area of the spine is restricted in side-bending toward the side of the positive acromion drop test. In neutral somatic dysfunctions, this would mean there is also some problem in rotating to the opposite side in that region and rotation to same side in a nonneutral somatic dysfunction. The function of the fascial thoracic inlet may also be compromised.

Table 42.2—*continued*

Tests	Neg.	Pos.	Explanation
Cervical Rotation	Neg.	Pos.	Passive rotation of the head and neck to the right and to the left. Positive = Head and neck has less rotation to one side compared with that of the other side. (N = 90°C) Indicates restriction to rotation somewhere in the cervical spine. If rotational dysfunction is noted, typical cervical vertebral motion will be restricted in side-bending to the same side. Test segmentally.
Collateral Ganglion Palpation	Neg.	Pos.	Steady digital pressure over the collateral sympathetic ganglia of the abdomen: Tests for tenderness of the celiac, superior mesenteric, and inferior mesenteric ganglia. Tenderness indicates possible dysfunction of one or more of the organs innervated by the tender collateral ganglia. Positive = tissue texture change and/or pain to palpation; correlate celiac, superior mesenteric or inferior mesenteric ganglion with appropriate organ history, more specific physical findings, and/or laboratory work.
Fascial Patterning			The physician passively tests rotation preference or restriction of fascias at specific total body reference zones, i.e., occipitoatlantal, cervicothoracic, thoracolumbar, and lumbosacral regions. (Classification is either compensated or uncompensated according to the classification patterns of Zink) Positive = Uncompensated pattern (areas do not alternate) indicates greatest hindrance to fluid movement in the body; compensated patterns (areas alternate) are less of an obstruction. Equal ease of rotation in either direction at all four reference zones is considered ideal. Correlate variances in the pattern with sites of congestion; next step is osteopathic manipulative treatment.

Protocol of W.A. Kuchera.

dysfunction. Motion asymmetry may be noted passively (with physician-controlled motion) and/or actively (patient-controlled motion). Passive motion testing may be more reliable for actual possible range of motion of a joint, since a patient may not achieve full active range of motion if fearful or uncomfortable. However, active motion testing may be more indicative of the actual functional limitations of the patient because of its associated induced pain.

Adapt the approach to the examination according to whatever positional or motion limitations are imposed on the patient by his or her condition or treatment protocol. When the patient cannot stand or cannot sit, examination is obviously limited to that which is possible, such as in the prone, supine, or lateral recumbent positions. When the history and physical examination are completed, the osteopathic physician arrives at one of four conclusions:

Table 42.3
Screening Musculoskeletal Examination for the Hospitalized Patient

Screen		Neg.	Pos.	Explanation
Arms Extended	Active Passive	Neg. Neg.	Pos. Pos.	This screens shoulder, elbow, forearm, and wrist motion combinations. Positive = unable to bring arms above the head with upper arms touching ears and backs of hands together. More focused examination of restricted joints in that extremity and upper thoracic region.
Fascial Patterning		Neg.	Pos.	Screens rotational preference of the fascias at specific reference areas described in the fiscal patterning described by Zink. Regional Sites = occipitoatlantal, cervicothoracic, thoracolumbar, and lumbosacral junctions. Positive = uncompensated pattern (sites do not alternate preferences) indicates greatest hindrance to fluid movement in the body; compensated patterns (sites alternate preferences) pose less of an obstruction to fluid flow. Correlate with sites of congestion; next step is segmental diagnosis and manipulative treatment of the somatic dysfunctions present.
Collateral Ganglion Palpation Anterior view		Neg.	Pos.	Screens for collateral ganglion tenderness indicating dysfunction of organ groups segmentally innervated within the region by celiac, superior mesenteric, or inferior mesenteric ganglia. Positive = palpable tissue texture change and tenderness of a ganglion area. Correlate this with the organs that each collateral ganglion services (sympathetic innervations). Correlate collateral ganglion with appropriate organ history and more specific physical findings and/or laboratory tests.
Paraspinal Segmental Palpation		Neg.	Pos. T1–4 T1–6 T5–9 T10–T11 T12–L2	Screens for dysfunction of organ groups (this screen is more specific than collateral ganglion screen) Positive = palpable asymmetry of tissue texture and motion and tenderness. Head and neck Heart and lungs Upper GI (GB-R, liver-R, pancreas-R*, spleen- L, stomach-L, duodenum-L) Small intestines, proximal colon, adrenal, kidneys, upper ½ ureter, gonads. Distal colon, lower ½ ureters, bladder, pelvic organs. Correlate with visceral dysfunction; next step is rib raising.

This is an AP transparent diagram revealing anterior and spinal landmarks superimposed.

Table 42.3—*continued*

Screen		Neg.	Pos.	Explanation
	Active	Neg.	Pos.	Screens hip, knee, and ankle combinations
	Passive	Neg.	Pos.	Positive = restricted extension of ankle, flexion of knee or flexion of hip.
				More focused examination of restricted joints in that extremity and somatic innervation to the lower extremity.

Leg Flexion

Protocol of W.A. Kuchera.

*a*Some believe that the pancreatic reflex can be found bilaterally, i.e., right and left.

1. There is a significant somatic component related to the patient's condition.
2. There is no significant somatic component of the patient's condition.
3. There is a significant somatic component not related to the patient's presenting problem but that requires evaluation and consideration in the treatment plan.
4. There is significant somatic dysfunction that is not directly related to the patient's present problem but that should be addressed at a later time to result in an improved overall level of health.

If there is a significant somatic component, note a diagnosis of somatic dysfunction as one of the patient's problems and incorporate appropriate OMT in the treatment protocol. It is likely, for instance, that a patient entering the hospital for cholecystectomy will have a viscerosomatic reflex inducing somatic dysfunction in the thoracic region. An efficient screening should reveal that information. The diagnoses entered in the chart on this particular patient would include:

1. Chronic cholecystitis with cholelithiasis
2. Thoracic somatic dysfunction secondary to item 1

Guidelines may be useful for organizing knowledge into a practical and useful form. The following are guidelines to include elements important in the osteopathic hospital screening examination.

SAMPLE HISTORY AND OSTEOPATHIC MUSCULOSKELETAL EXAMINATION

A 38-year-old male, complaining of low back pain of insidious onset and of 3 months duration, is examined in the standing, seated, prone, and supine positions. Review of systems reveals no relevant information. The back pain is worse at the left lumbosacral area. Neurological examination reveals no deficits.

In the standing position, the left iliac crest, trochanter, and PSIS planes are low on the right. There is a positive right standing flexion test. A right lumbar paravertebral humping is observed, with the apex at L2. AP curves appear normal.

In the seated position, there is a positive right-seated flexion test. Lumbar rotation left and side-bending left are restricted. A tissue texture abnormality is present at T6-8 on the right; T6-8 is also backward bent. Thoracic rotation is equal bilaterally.

In the prone position, the right sacral sulcus is deep with tenderness and tissue texture abnormality present. The right inferolateral angle of the sacrum is posterior and inferior. The lumbar paravertebral muscle mass is prominent on the right, with tenderness and tissue texture abnormality at L2. L2 is rotated right (restricted in left rotation).

In the supine position, the right ASIS is superior, and the left ASIS is inferior. Abdominal tenderness is present in the subxiphoid area only. Screening examinations of the cranium and cervical spine are negative.

RECORDING FINDINGS

Musculoskeletal findings are physical findings and should be recorded as such (Table 42.5). Motion disturbances in somatic dysfunction can be recorded in three ways.[11]

Where is it? (position)
What will it do? (direction of more free motion)
What won't it do? (direction of restriction)

The goal of recording the musculoskeletal screening examination for all inpatients and outpatients is to be able to answer the following questions:

1. Are there significant somatic dysfunctions related to the patient's problems?
2. Can I locate the regions involved for further study and for administration of osteopathic manipulative treatment to support the patient?
3. Could there be a viscerosomatic or somatovisceral connection?

Table 42.4
Example of Charting: Musculoskeletal Examination of the Patient Described on page 506

(STANDING) (Circle as appropriate):			"X" ☐ IF UNABLE TO STAND	
DATE:			↑ = Increased	↓ = decreased
Cervical Lordosis	*Normal*		↑	↓
Thoracic kyphosis	*Normal*		↑	↓
Lumbar lordosis	*Normal*		↑	↓
Rotoscoliosis	(*Dextro lumbar*)		Levo (L)	(Apex = *L2*)

OTHER POSITIONS EXAMINED (Circle as appropriate):				
(Seated)	(Prone)		Fowler's	
Supine	Lateral recumbent		(Supine)	

EXAMINATION OF SPINE AND EXTREMITIES

No.	Regions	TTA	A	R	T
1.	Cranium				
2.	Cervical				
3.	Thoracic				
—	T1-5				
—	(T5-9)	(X)	(X)	(X)	(X)
—	T-10-L2				
4.	Costal				
5.	(Abdomen)	(X)	(X)	(X)	(X)
6.	(Lumbar)	(X)	(X)	(X)	(X)
7.	Sacrum	(X)	(X)	(X)	(X)
8.	Innominate (hip bone)				
9.	Upper extremity				
10.	Lower extremity				

TTA = Tissue texture abnormalities
A = Asymmetry
R = Restriction of motion (side-bending/rotation)
T = Tenderness

ᵃThe patient is a 38-year-old male, complaining of low back pain of insidious onset and of 3 months duration. Examiners choices are indicated in italics.

CONCLUSION

The osteopathic musculoskeletal evaluation provides information about the musculoskeletal system and musculoskeletal clues to dysfunction of other systems or of the general health status of the patient. It is unique in that palpation integrated with motion testing is the major component of that portion of the examination. Discovery of musculoskeletal dysfunction often provides additional clues that direct, focus, or expand the examination; the musculoskeletal diagnosis also expands the logical conclusions that can be drawn from that examination.

Table 42.5
Chart for Musculoskeletal Examination of the Hospitalized Patient

STANDING (Circle as appropriate):			"X" ☐ IF UNABLE TO STAND	
DATE:			(↑ = Increased)	(↓ = decreased)
Cervical Lordosis	Normal		↑	↓
Thoracic kyphosis	Normal		↑	↓
Lumbar Lordosis	Normal		↑	↓
Rotoscoliosis	Dextro (R)		Levo (L)	Apex =

OTHER POSITIONS EXAMINED (Circle as appropriate):		
Seated	Prone	Fowler's
Supine	Lateral recumbent	

EXAMINATION OF SPINE AND EXTREMITIES

No.	Regions	TTA	A	R	T
1.	Cranium				
2.	Cervical				
3.	Thoracic				
—	T1-5				
—	T5-9				
—	T-10-L2				
4.	Costal				
5.	Abdomen				
6.	Lumbar				
7.	Sacrum				
8.	Innominate (hip bone)				
9.	Upper extremity				
10.	Lower extremity				

	TTA = Tissue texture abnormalities
	A = Asymmetry
Relevant Segmental Diagnosis AND Elaborate on Findings:	R = Restriction of motion (side-bending/rotation)
	T = Tenderness

Form composed by John M. Jones III.

REFERENCES

1. Dinnar U. Classification of diagnostic tests used with osteopathic manipulation. *JAOA.* March 1980;79:451–455.

2. Dinnar U, et al. Description of fifty diagnostic tests used with osteopathic manipulation. *JAOA.* January 1982;81:314–321.

3. Johnston WE. Hip shift: testing a basic postural dysfunction. *JAOA.* 1964;63:923–930. Reprinted in Peterson B, ed. *Postural Balance and Imbalance.* Newark, Ohio: American Academy of Osteopathy; 1983:109–112.

4. Kappler RE. Postural balance and motion patterns. *JAOA.* May 1982;81:598–606. Reprinted in Peterson B, ed. *Postural Balance and Imbalance.* Newark, Ohio: American Academy of Osteopathy; 1983:6–12.

5. Mitchell FL Jr, Moran PT, Pruzzo NA. *An Evaluation and Treatment Manual of Osteopathic Muscle Energy Procedures.* 1st ed. Valley Park, Mo: published by authors; 1979.

6. Sutton SE. Postural imbalance: examination and treatment utilizing flexion tests. *JAOA.* February 1978;77:456–465. Reprinted in Peterson B, ed. *Postural Balance and Imbalance.* Newark, Ohio: American Academy of Osteopathy; 1983:102–108.

7. Sutton SE. An osteopathic method of history taking and physical examination, Part I. *JAOA.* June 1978;77:780–788.

8. Sutton SE. An osteopathic method of history taking and physical examination, Part II. *JAOA.* July 1978;77:845–858.

9. Zink JG, Lawson WA: An osteopathic structural examination and functional interpretation of the soma. *Osteopathic Ann.* 1979; 7(5):208–214.

10. Kuchera ML, Kuchera WA. *Osteopathic Considerations in Systemic Dysfunction.* 2nd ed. rev. Columbus, Ohio: Greyden Press; 1994.

11. Glossary Review Committee of the Educational Council on Osteopathic Principles. In: Allen TW, ed. Glossary of osteopathic terminology. *AOA Yearbook and Directory of Osteopathic Physicians.* Chicago, Ill: American Osteopathic Association; 1994.

43. **Examination and Diagnosis**

AN INTRODUCTION

MICHAEL L. KUCHERA

Key Concepts

- **An integrated osteopathic neuromusculo-skeletal regional examination links structure and function, in an expanded database for diagnosis and treatment.**

- **This examination provides information about primary musculoskeletal dysfunction, termed somatic dysfunction, and provides somatic clues to internal or systemic disease. Sometimes findings make a diagnosis of an impending problem before there is subjective evidence of the disease process.**

- **Information from an integrated osteopathic examination can be used in a management program to direct specific treatment of the neuromusculoskeletal dysfunction, which is directed toward support of homeostatic mechanisms that aid the patient's own body defenses in the fight against a systemic disease.**

The osteopathic perspective provides unique insights into physical examination and differential diagnosis. This orientation begins on the first day of anatomy class and continues throughout a lifetime of osteopathic practice. Osteopathy emphasizes the interrelationship between structure (anatomy) and function (physiology), which leads to physical examination skills many consider second to none. Without specific knowledge of pertinent anatomy and physiology, the osteopathic approach could be thought too "time-consuming." With this knowledge, however, it is not only time-efficient but also cost-effective. A true diagnosis is reached quickly, with fewer unnecessary expensive tests; disorders are identified at the earliest dysfunctional state, when prognosis is good and treatment costs are relatively minimal.

THE OSTEOPATHIC EXAMINATION

Emphasis on the neuromusculoskeletal system, supported by an in-depth knowledge of functional anatomy and physiology, provides osteopathic practitioners the opportunity to incorporate additional viscerosomatic and somatovisceral reflex clues largely unavailable in many other health care systems.

Integration of these physical findings is further enhanced by our emphasis on understanding body unity as completely as possible. A survey of patient stressors and the individualized response to those stressors is necessary, along with information on the following:

Symptoms
Pain patterns
Activities of daily living
Nutritional and environmental data

These can all be translated or interpreted with an understanding of their anatomic and/or physiologic impact on the patient's body unity. This provides insight into the unique individual who is placing his or her trust in the physician's skill and judgment. A hands-on approach and the willingness to listen to the patient (often cited by patients as a characteristic of an osteopathic physician) initiate therapeutic mechanisms of healing even as data is being gathered to make a diagnosis. Patients are highly satisfied with this type of attention, examination, and synthesis.

The osteopathic physician examines the homeostatic reserve of each patient. "*To find health is the object of the physician; anyone can find disease.*"[1] This portion of the examination is essential for determining prognosis and treatment design when host mechanisms are compromised. It is also helpful in the examination of noncompromised or compensated hosts, in designing preventive strategies, or in directing a patient toward optimum health levels. In an osteopathic approach to examination and diagnosis, it is not enough to study the disease and its byproducts; an intimate and thorough knowledge of the individual is essential.

An osteopathic examination cannot just be the traditional history and physical examination with a palpatory diagnosis of somatic dysfunction added to it. An osteopathic examination strives to provide all pertinent information needed for diagnosis. The osteopathic physician practicing osteopathic medicine must diagnose beyond the disease; osteopathic diagnosis strives to know all about the whole person. A whole person is one who encompasses structure–function interactions, self-healing mechanisms, and unique responses to stressors, all within the patient's internal and external environments.

CHAPTER SCOPE AND DESIGN

The following regional chapters emphasize the functional anatomy and diagnostic tests that form the building blocks of an osteopathic examination. Information in these chapters is included to provide selected representative structural and functional considerations that may produce symptoms or compromise homeostasis. This text does not attempt to replace standardized texts on physical examination or medical and surgical differential diagnosis, nor does it attempt to replace exhaustive anatomy and physiology texts. Instead, the chapters in this section are designed to augment and focus the osteopathic physician's synthesis of skills needed to perform an osteopathic medical examination. The physician must recognize functional disturbances that influence a patient's progress and therefore require additional attention.

The definition of somatic dysfunction requires an assessment of the function and physiological interrelationships between certain anatomic structures, including:

Skeletal tissues
Arthrodial tissues
Myofascial tissues
Arteries
Veins
Nerves
Lymphatics[2]

The physical examination of somatic dysfunction, which is not covered in other texts, is a central component (but not the only component) in the osteopathic examination. The chapters in this section therefore center on the anatomic and physiologic information that is provided by discovering somatic dysfunction in a body region. Reviewing Chapters 41 and 42 on palpation may be beneficial as preparation for these chapters. The following regional chapters in this section have a similar format, including the issues described in the following sections here.

Functional Anatomy

To understand each region appropriately, an overview of pertinent skeletal, arthrodial, and myofascial structures is provided. Functional anatomy is emphasized.

Functional relationships of somatic structures with related neural, lymphatic, and other vascular elements are also discussed for each region.

Anatomy and Somatic Dysfunction

STRUCTURES PREDISPOSING TO SOMATIC DYSFUNCTION

Many congenital abnormalities require functional compensation. An example is the presence of a wedge vertebra causing a group curve, postural disorder, and muscle imbalance; this same problem can create autonomic disturbance and compro-

mise respiratory and circulatory function. Congenital abnormalities may also cause altered functional activity because of altered structural design. They may place the patient at risk for injury by certain functional challenges, including certain forms of treatment.

Several degenerative or traumatically acquired disorders, such as arthritis or destruction of joint supportive structures, alter joint function.

SOMATIC DYSFUNCTION AND PHYSIOLOGY

Somatic dysfunction modifies physiology. Tissue texture changes are important in an osteopathic physical examination because they reflect a patient's autonomic and trophic functions. Important physical findings include:

Myofascial and reflex points
Sympathetic activity differences
Warmth or coolness of the skin
Cutaneous humidity
Lymphatic congestion
Systemic consequences

Findings discussed in each region include myofascial trigger and tender points. These can be palpated in each region and are often the cause of referred pain phenomena as well as lymphatic congestion, neural entrapment, and/or autonomic sequelae.[3]

Effects of sympathetic and parasympathetic hyperactivity can often be traced to systemic dysfunction.[4] The following chapters identify some important syndromes or systemic changes that illustrate this relationship. They identify significant viscerosomatic reflex findings. Spinal somatic dysfunction may also occur as a consequence of visceral dysfunction or disease at levels segmentally related to the visceral autonomic innervation. Spinal cord facilitation is one way of explaining how this crosstalk between the somatic and the visceral systems occurs.

Lymphatic congestion is commonly associated with somatic dysfunction. The chapters identify lymphatic drainage pathways and locations of sites where early dysfunction of this mechanism can be palpated. Anatomical structures pertinent to the movement of lymph, or which might especially impede lymph flow, are highlighted.

SOMATIC DYSFUNCTION AND STRUCTURE

Functional demand on dysfunctional structure often causes structural change to occur. Wolff's law[2] observes that calcium is laid down along lines of stress resulting in bony spurs, joint immobility, and calcified ligaments. Osteoarthritic changes following regional trauma should be suspected and an appropriate examination performed. Muscle hypertrophy occurs in overworked muscles; disuse atrophy occurs in those not worked adequately. Chronic skin changes (dryness, scaling, cracking, thickening, pimples, etc.) occur when trophic substances (carried via vascular channels or by axoplasmic flow) do not provide adequate nutrition.

Osteopathic Manipulative Treatment

Knowledge of functional anatomy is important to the successful performance of osteopathic manipulative treatment.

The accurate diagnosis of somatic dysfunction, using motion characteristics, is vital for designing appropriate osteopathic manipulative treatment (OMT). The arthrodial component of somatic dysfunction often affects the minor motions of the joint. The minor motions then affect the major motions. The major and minor motions for each region are discussed in these chapters.

OMT often requires that an activating force be applied in the plane of the joint. When necessary, joint facings and the alignment of the joint spaces are discussed. In addition, different types of joints have different palpatory characteristics and permit different motions. Where this is important, the regional chapters discuss what classification of joints is involved. For example, diagnostic and treatment approaches with OMT are very different for a synchondrosis compared with approaches for a synovial joint.

Common Clinical Conditions

Common clinical problems can provide insights into the value of the osteopathic approach to regional examination.

Each chapter in this section offers a discussion of common clinical conditions and presents a process applicable to arriving at a differential diagnosis for the conditions common to each region.

Each chapter includes a few characteristic conditions that are discussed in more depth to provide a greater understanding of osteopathic problem solving.

Table 43.1 lists clinical conditions that are more completely discussed in the following regional chapters.

PRINCIPLES OF SPINAL MOTION

Spinal and vertebral mechanics can be described according to a number of conventions. The following discussion touches on three: Fryette's concepts, neutral and nonneutral mechanics, and a right-handed orthogonal coordinate system. The latter is mentioned for the sake of completeness because its concepts permit mathematical modeling of spinal movement. It is important to remember that physical laws, such as Wolff's law, are always at work.[a]

GENERAL SPINAL MOTIONS

All spinal and vertebral movements are described in relation to motions of their anterior and superior surfaces.

---

[a]Wolff's law: Bones and soft tissues deform (are strained) according to the stresses (forces applied over an area) placed on them.

Table 43.1
Clinical Conditions by Region

Head and neck	Thoracic cage
Headache	Gastritis
Temperomandibular joint dysfunction	Pneumonia
Otitis media	Costochondritis
Acute torticollis	(Also see scoliosis)
Cervical radiculopathy	
Lumbar/abdomen	Pelvis/sacrum
Psoas syndrome	Sacral shear
Lumbar radiculopathy	Innominate shear
Quadratus lumborum triggers	Pubic shear
Ileus post lumbar fracture	Piriformis syndrome
(Also see spondylolisthesis)	Dysmenorrhea
Upper extremity	Lower extremity
Thoracic outlet syndrome	Acute sprain
Carpal tunnel syndrome	Pes planus
Radial head somatic dysfunction and	Osgood Schlatter disease
trauma	Genu valgus
Tennis elbow	

A single vertebra is called a *vertebral segment* (see Glossary: segment).

Two adjacent vertebrae and their associated arthrodial, ligamentous, muscular, vascular, neural, and lymphatic elements make up a *vertebral unit* (see Glossary).

Vertebral units demonstrate *coupled motions*, which are two segments moving in relation to each other. For example, side-bending and rotation always occur together rather than separately, i.e., they are coupled.[5] Coupled motions are conventionally characterized as neutral/type I or nonneutral type II responses.

Origin of Type I and Type II Concepts as Simple and Compound Coupled Motions

Harrison H. Fryette, DO, with credit to Dr. Robert Lovett,[6] was an early osteopathic physician who discussed two fundamental physiologic spinal motions, labeling them simple and compound movements.[6(p29)] In his system, simple movements referred to free and easy forward and backward bending activities with minimal facet and ligamentous/bony interferences.[6(p19)] Compound movements, on the other hand, involve increasingly complex combinations of coupled vertebral unit activities that link side-bending and rotation with both spinal and vertebral unit flexion and extension.[6(p28)] He labeled them as combinations of "extension–rotation–side-bending" (ERS) and "flexion–rotation–side-bending" (FRS).[6(19)]

Although somewhat controversial and difficult to follow, a variant of his convention is still widely referenced in osteopathic literature and elsewhere, the type I and type II labeling system. The method has considerable practical utility because, as Fryette noted, facet joints are *"in control in any area of the spine"* and they *"govern rotation. . .and side-bending."*[6(p21)]

More recently, nomenclature has evolved toward use of the terms neutral and nonneutral mechanics and their responses in relation to a right-handed x, y, z orthogonal coordinate system, where the z-axis is in the craniocaudad direction. The following integrates some of this thinking.

Neutral (Type I) Mechanics

Neutral, type I, mechanics typically occurs in the thoracic and lumbar spine in the presence of free and easy articular and soft tissue motion (see Figures 12 and 14 in Ref. 2, p 698).[2,5(p61)] Side-bending movements are accompanied by vertebral segment rotations away from formed concavities and toward the convexities. Clinically, the transverse processes rotate posteriorly on the side of the formed convexity. For example, neutral right lumbar side-bending creates left rotation of one or more vertebral segments. A typical neutral, type I, response involves three or more segments.

Nonneutral (Type II) Mechanics

Nonneutral, type II, coupling rotates one or more vertebral segments toward the formed concavity as varieties of bending and twisting are introduced. Under these conditions, forward and backward bending are generally symmetrical, while side-bending movements rotate vertebral segments and units toward the formed concavity. In this situation, facets and their surrounding soft tissues are asymmetrically engaged as the forward and backward bending process unfolds. The sooner facets and soft tissues asymmetrically engage, the earlier the nonneutral, type II, responses begin.

Nonneutral/type II, ERS/FRS segmental motions commonly occur throughout the thoracic and lumbar spine when vertebral facets, soft tissues, and costovertebral attachments are asymmetrically engaged during compound movements (Figure 13 from Glossary, p 698). Under these conditions, the involved segments and units unit rotate into the formed concavity. If functional compromise occurs in other components of the involved vertebral unit, such as the neutral, vascular, and lymphatic elements, somatic dysfunction is present.

For those wishing more background, complicated combinations of interacting neutral and nonneutral mechanics are described by Hoover in a 1950 paper.[7]

A third principle, described by Beckwith and Hoover and Nelson, came later.[8,9] It suggests that initiation of vertebral segment motion in any plane modifies and reduces movement in all other planes. The idea is well-discussed in Greenman's second edition of *Principles of Manual Medicine* (Table 43.2).[5(p62–63)]

CONCLUSION

Considering the close and clinical relationship of structure and function offers a refreshing and unique insight into patient examination and assessment. Dysfunction of the soma and its related elements plays a significant role in the production of a variety of patient complaints, signs, and/or symptoms and is frequently accompanied by visceral dysfunction. For these reasons, a conscious search for somatic dysfunction through the

Table 43.2
Vertebral Motion

Segment(s)	Type(s)
C0–C1 (occipitoatlantal)	(Neutral) I (always)
C1–C2 (atlantoaxial)	(Rotation)
C2–C7 (typical cervical)	(Nonneutral) II
C7–L5 (typical thoracic and lumbar)	(Neutral) I and (nonneutral) II

Reprinted with permission from Greenman PE. *Principles of Manual Medicine*. 2nd ed. Baltimore, Md: Williams & Wilkins, 1996:63.

use of palpation and motion testing is an important part of a patient examination. Information obtained through a regional neuromusculoskeletal examination is integrated with the history and all other findings related to the entire individual. This approach provides the data essential for making a differential diagnosis and a working diagnosis and for developing a rational and total treatment program to promote the patient's health or to support the patient with disease or dysfunction.

By studying anatomy and physiology from the philosophical vantage point needed to formulate 'rational osteopathic treatment,' the osteopath discovers a unique and valuable perspective of health and disease. Interpretation of somatic clues through understanding of the physiology underlying symptom development allows the physician to surmise the dysfunction or pathophysiology occurring in a given individual patient. It offers direction and information for the physical examination and the differential diagnosis. Rather than simply diagnosing and treating symptoms or symptom complexes, the osteopathic physician seeks to augment the health that is found within the individual.[4]

REFERENCES

1. Truhlar RE. *Sage Sayings of A.T. Still*. Indianapolis, Ind: American Academy of Osteopathy; 1994.

2. The Glossary Subcommittee of the Educational Council on Osteopathic Principles. Glossary of Osteopathic Terminology. In: Allen TW, ed. *AOA Yearbook and Directory of Osteopathic Physicians*. Chicago, Ill: American Osteopathic Association; 1994.

3. Travell JG, Simons DG. *Myofascial Pain and Dysfunction: The Trigger Point Manual, II*. Baltimore, Md: Williams & Wilkins; 1992.

4. Kuchera ML, Kuchera WA. *Osteopathic Considerations in Systemic Dysfunction*. 2nd ed. Columbus, Ohio: Greyden Press; 1994.

5. Greenman PE. *Principles of Manual Medicine*. 2nd ed. Baltimore, Md: Williams & Wilkins; 1996:61–63.

6. Fryette HH. *Principles of Osteopathic Technic*. Indianapolis, Ind: American Academy of Osteopathy; (1918) 1966:15, 19, 21, 28, 29.

7. Hoover HV. Complicated lesions. In: *American Academy of Osteopathy Yearbook*. Indianapolis, Ind: American Academy of Osteopathy; 1950:67–69.

8. Beckwith CG. Vertebral mechanics. *JAOA*. Jan 1944. Reproduced in *American Academy of Osteopathy Yearbook*. Indianapolis, Ind: American Academy of Osteopathy; pp 93–98.

9. Hoover HV, Nelson CP. Basic physiologic movements of the spine. In: *American Academy of Osteopathy Yearbook*. Indianapolis, Ind: American Academy of Osteopathy; 1950:63–66.

44. **Head**

DIAGNOSIS AND TREATMENT

ROBERT E. KAPPLER AND KENNETH A. RAMEY

Key Concepts

- Cranial motion in terms of flexion and extension of certain bones, and how to do a cranial motion assessment

- Origin and location of trigger points in musculature of head and neck

- Role of connective tissue in craniosacral motion and role of dural continuity in referred pain

- How somatic dysfunction can alter arterial supply, leading to symptoms, and venous flow, producing congestion

- Routes of lymphatic flow in head and neck and possible points of blockage

- Parasympathetic and sympathetic innervation of head and neck and consequences of parasympathetic hyperactivity or altering sympathetic input

- Function and location of cranial nerves (CN) I–XII, including possible dysfunctions

- Effects of compressing fourth ventricle

- Understanding and treatment of sinus, eye, and ear disorders

- Goals and methods of osteopathic treatment of common cold

- Four major classifications of headaches

- Physiology of migraines, cluster headaches, and tension headaches, and osteopathic treatment of whole person

- Physiology and causes of traction and inflammatory headaches

- Presentation of trigeminal neuralgia

- Anatomy, motion, diagnosis, and muscle energy treatment of temporomandibular joint (TMJ) dysfunction

Symptoms involving the head, ears, eyes, nose, and throat (HEENT) structures are frequently seen and may be sources of significant functional disability. Consideration of structural and functional relationships allows the clinician to more accurately diagnose various conditions and implement appropriate treatment.

SKELETAL STRUCTURES

The adult skull is composed of 29 bones (Figs. 44.1–44.7). There are eight in the cranial group:

Occiput
Sphenoid
Ethmoid
Frontal
Paired temporals
Paired parietals

There are 14 in the facial group:

Vomer
Mandible
Paired maxillae
Palatine
Zygomatic
Lacrimal
Nasal
Inferior conchae bones

Seven are in the miscellaneous group: six inner ear ossicles and the hyoid. From a craniosacral perspective, they can be divided into midline and paired bones. During craniosacral flexion, the midline bones (sphenoid, occiput, ethmoid, and vomer) move into flexion around their respective transverse axes. The paired bones externally rotate during craniosacral flexion. During craniosacral extension the reverse occurs.[1]

MUSCLES

The myofascial system is frequently involved in head symptoms. Travell and Simons have described various myofascial trigger points (TPs) that may refer pain to and/or cause dysfunction of structures of the head.[2(p.8)] Somatic dysfunction and TPs are closely related and potentiate one another. Emotional stress may be associated with clenching of the teeth and may produce TPs in the masseter and pterygoid muscles. Frowning or squinting may set up TPs in the orbicularis oculi

515

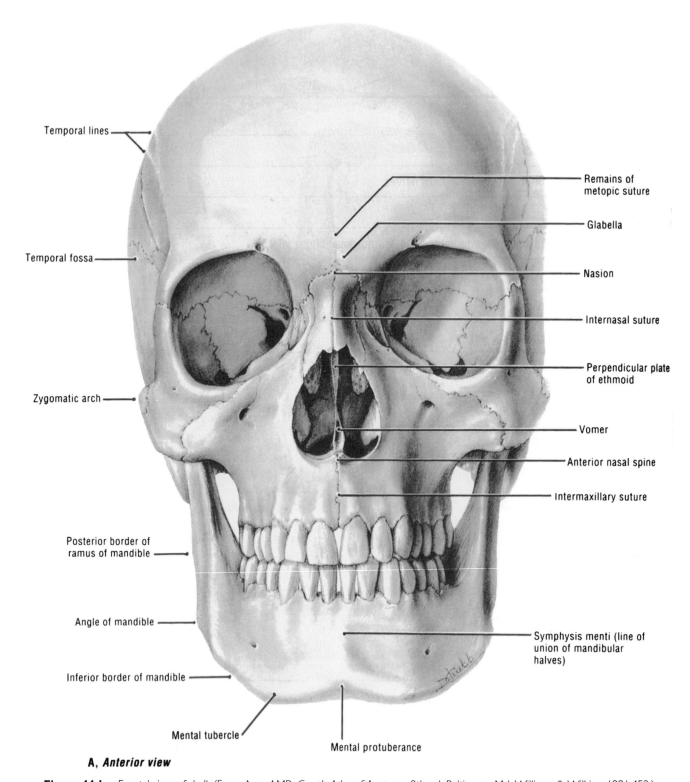

Temporal lines

Temporal fossa

Zygomatic arch

Posterior border of
ramus of mandible

Angle of mandible

Inferior border of mandible

Mental tubercle

Remains of
metopic suture

Glabella

Nasion

Internasal suture

Perpendicular plate
of ethmoid

Vomer

Anterior nasal spine

Intermaxillary suture

Symphysis menti (line of
union of mandibular
halves)

Mental protuberance

A, *Anterior view*

Figure 44.1.   Frontal view of skull. (From Agur AMR. *Grant's Atlas of Anatomy*. 9th ed. Baltimore, Md: Williams & Wilkins; 1991:452.)

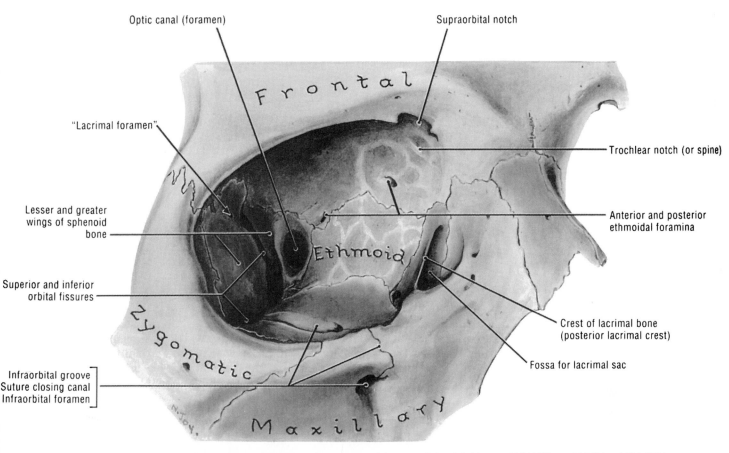

Figure 44.2.   Orbital view of skull. (From Agur AMR. *Grant's Atlas of Anatomy.* 9th ed. Baltimore, Md: Williams & Wilkins; 1991:482.)

and occipitalis muscles. TPs in the sternocleidomastoid muscle may refer pain to the eye. Motor vehicle accidents, especially from the rear, may produce TPs in the sternocleidomastoid, splenius cervicis, and trapezius muscles. TPs in the orbicularis oculi muscle may produce such ipsilateral visual disturbances as blurred vision, decreased light perception, tears, and conjunctival reddening. TPs in the occipitalis muscle may refer pain behind the eye and orbit. TPs in the trapezius muscle may refer pain to the orbit. A more complete list of trigger points is listed in Table 44.1 and Figure 44.8.[2(p.9)]

CONNECTIVE TISSUE

The dura mater lines the skull and produces folds, or intracranial membranes, that act as partitions between, and support for, the cerebral hemispheres and cerebellum (Figs. 44.9 and 44.10).[1(p.27)] These structures form the reciprocal tension membrane (RTM) and are integrally involved in craniosacral motion. The dura lining the skull extends through the cranial sutures and becomes continuous with the periosteal covering of the skull. The falx cerebelli extends inferiorly from the straight sinus and firmly attaches to the foramen magnum. It attaches to the bodies of the second and third cervical vertebrae and extends downward as a tube that ultimately attaches to the

second sacral segment (Fig. 44.11). The dura becomes continuous with the extracranial fascia at various foramina in the base of the skull and continues outward as sheaths (perineurium) surrounding various cranial and spinal nerves. Extracranial and intracranial dural continuity may help explain why dysfunction in the periphery is referred to the head.[1(p.15)]

ARTERIAL SUPPLY

The face and scalp are supplied by branches of the external carotid artery (primarily the facial artery).[3(p.665)] The internal structures of the head are primarily supplied by the internal carotid and vertebral arteries (Fig. 44.12). The internal carotid artery passes through the carotid canal in the petrous portion of the temporal bone. The internal carotid arteries supply the anterior portions of the cerebrum.[3(p.804)] Cranial dysfunction in the areas where the temporal bones articulate with the occiput and sphenoid may alter the normal function of these arteries.[3(p.150)] This may produce symptoms (weakness and altered sensation) on the opposite side of the body. The vertebral arteries arise from the subclavian artery and ascend through the transverse foramen of C6-C3. At C2 they make several right angle turns before piercing the dura to enter the skull through the foramen magnum.[3(p.804)] The vertebral arteries supply the

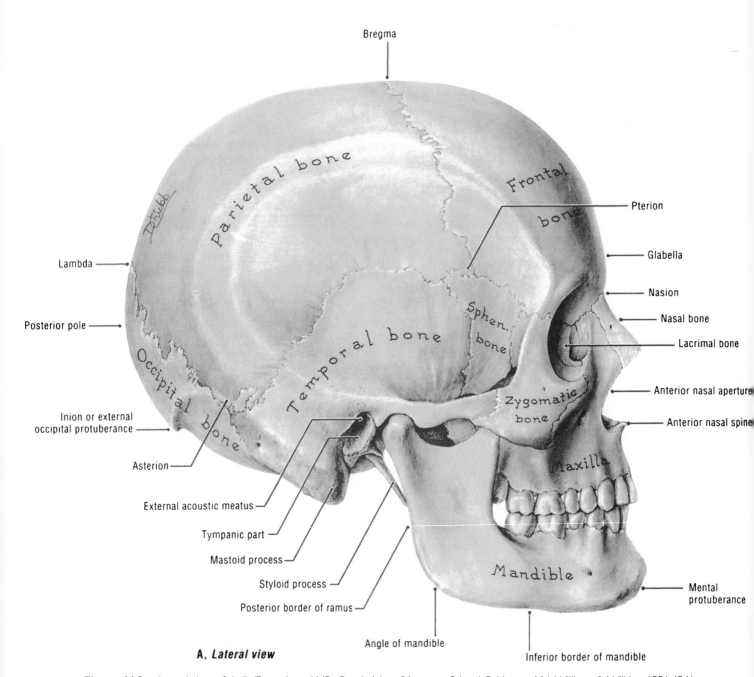

A, Lateral view

Figure 44.3.   Lateral view of skull. (From Agur AMR. *Grant's Atlas of Anatomy*. 9th ed. Baltimore, Md: Williams & Wilkins; 1991:454.)

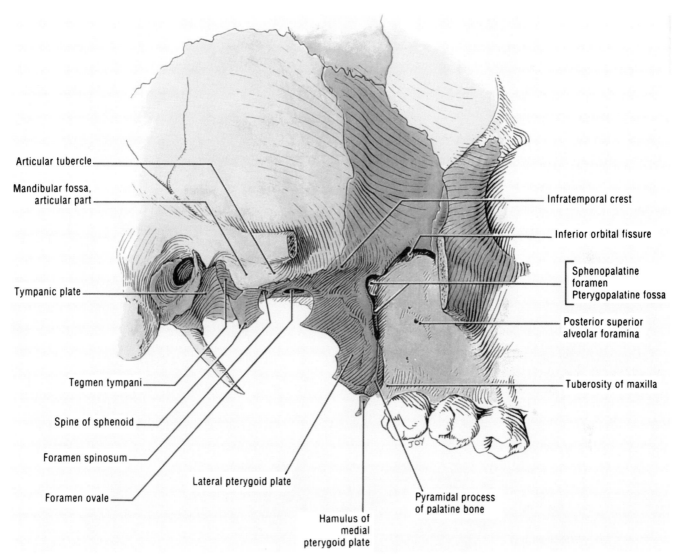

Articular tubercle

Mandibular fossa,
articular part

Tympanic plate

Tegmen tympani

Spine of sphenoid

Foramen spinosum

Foramen ovale

Lateral pterygoid plate

Hamulus of
medial
pterygoid plate

Pyramidal process
of palatine bone

Tuberosity of maxilla

Posterior superior
alveolar foramina

Sphenopalatine
foramen
Pterygopalatine fossa

Inferior orbital fissure

Infratemporal crest

Figure 44.4.   Lateral view of skull (close-up of sphenoid and temporal bones). (From Agur AMR. *Grant's Atlas of Anatomy*. 9th ed. Baltimore, Md: Williams & Wilkins; 1991:502.)

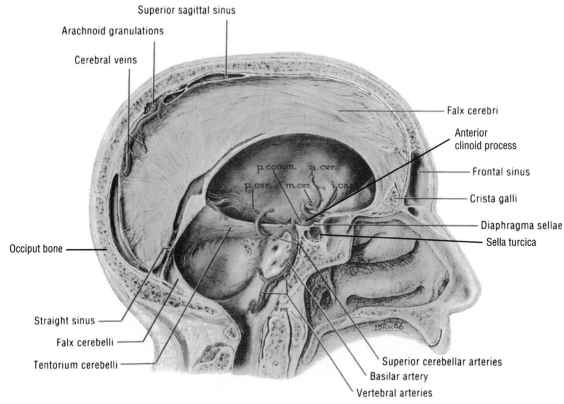

Figure 44.5.   Lateral view of interior of skull. (From Agur AMR. *Grant's Atlas of Anatomy.* 9th ed. Baltimore, Md: Williams & Wilkins; 1991:466.)

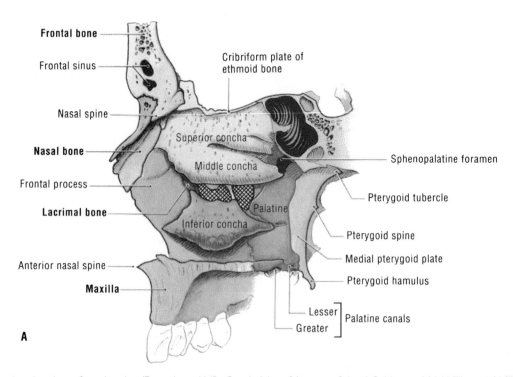

Figure 44.6.   Interior view of nasal cavity. (From Agur AMR. *Grant's Atlas of Anatomy.* 9th ed. Baltimore, Md: Williams & Wilkins; 1991:519.)

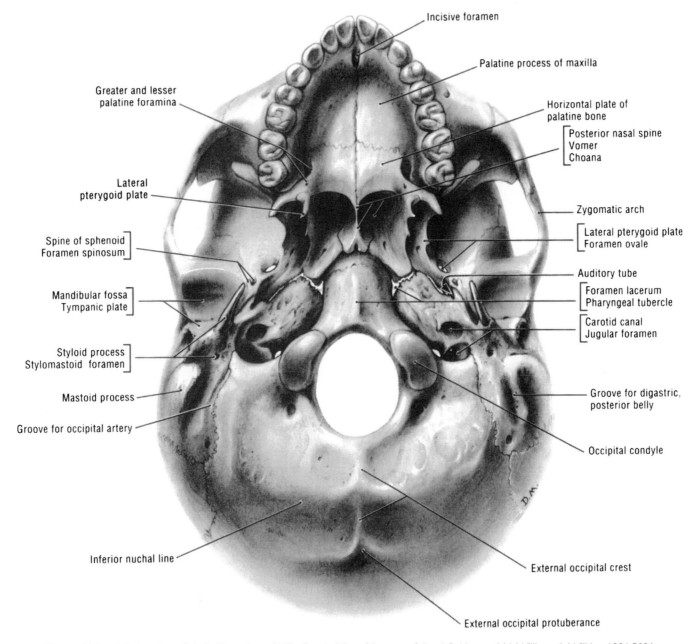

Figure 44.7.   Inferior view of skull. (From Agur AMR. *Grant's Atlas of Anatomy*. 9th ed. Baltimore, Md: Williams & Wilkins; 1991:582.)

visual area of the cerebrum (occipital lobe), brainstem, and cerebellum. Dysfunctions affecting this artery may lead to visual abnormalities and dizziness.[3(p.701)]

VENOUS DRAINAGE

Approximately 85% of the venous drainage from the head occurs via the internal jugular veins (Fig. 44.13). They pass through the jugular foramina, located along the occipitomastoid suture between the occipital and temporal bones. Dysfunction of these bony structures and/or the associated regional connective tissue may impair venous flow, leading to congestion.[2(p.6)]

LYMPHATIC DRAINAGE

A knowledge of lymphatic drainage patterns may assist in the localization of pathological conditions in the head (Fig. 44.14). Lymphatic vessels in the forehead and anterior part of the face drain into the submandibular lymph nodes. Lymph vessels from the lateral face and eyelids drain inferiorly toward the parotid lymph nodes and ultimately drain into the deep cervical lymph nodes.[3(p.668)] The superficial lymph nodes include the submandibular, occipital, retroauricular, and superficial parotid lymph nodes.

Lymph from the forehead drains into the submandibular lymph nodes. The occipital region of the scalp drains into the

Table 44.1
Myofascial Trigger Points

Eye symptoms and/or pain
    Sternal division of the sternocleidomastoid muscle
    Splenius cervicis muscle
    Occipitalis muscle
    Orbicularis oculi muscle
    Trapezius muscle
Ear pain, tinnitus, and/or diminished hearing
    Deep portion of the masseter muscle
    Clavicular portion of the sternocleidomastoid muscle
    Medial pterygoid muscle
    Occipitalis muscle
Eustachian tube dysfunction
    Medial pterygoid muscle
Nose pain
    Orbicularis oculi muscle
Maxillary sinus pain and/or sinus symptoms
    Lateral pterygoid muscle
    Masseter muscle
    Sternal division of the sternocleidomastoid muscle
Throat pain and/or difficulty swallowing
    Medial pterygoid muscle
    Digastric muscle
Cranial nerve entrapment
    V: (buccal nerve branch), lateral pterygoid muscle
    XI: sternocleidomastoid muscle

occipital lymph nodes. The temporoparietal region drains into the retroauricular lymph nodes. The frontoparietal region drains into the superficial parotid lymph nodes. Lymph from the superficial lymph nodes eventually drains into the cervical lymph nodes. The deep cervical lymph nodes are located along the internal jugular vein. Lymph from the deep cervical structures passes through the jugular trunk into the left (thoracic duct) and right lymphatic trunks (Fig. 44.15).[3(p.675)]

All drainage from the head must pass through the neck, cervical fascias, and thoracic inlet to return to the general circulation. Dysfunction in any of these structures may lead to lymphatic congestion. Increased sympathetic stimulation to the head and neck may also decrease lymphatic drainage.[2(p.3)]

PARASYMPATHETICS

Parasympathetic nerve fibers to the pupil are supplied by cranial nerve (CN) III (oculomotor nerve) (Fig. 44.16). They innervate the ciliary muscle and cause contraction of the pupil. Parasympathetic activity may affect the lens and lead to a shortening of focal length. Parasympathetic fibers to the lacrimal gland and nasopharyngeal mucosa travel via CN VII (facial nerve). They synapse in the sphenopalatine ganglion (Fig. 44.17). Parasympathetic hyperactivity may lead to excessive tear production and profuse, clear, thin secretions from the mucosa of the nasopharynx and sinuses. Parasympathetic nerves to the thyroid arise from the superior and inferior laryngeal nerves and a branch from the main vagus nerve (CN X).[2(pp.4–5)]

SYMPATHETICS

The structures of the head and neck obtain their sympathetic innervation from cell bodies located at spinal cord levels T1-T4 (Fig. 44.18). The preganglionic and postganglionic fibers synapse in the upper thoracic region and/or cervical sympathetic ganglia. The sympathetics to the head generally follow the course of the arterial supply.[2(p.2)] The superior, middle, and inferior cervical ganglia lie in the cervical tissues at C2, C6, and C7, respectively.

Visceral afferent nerves stimulated by organ dysfunction frequently follow the same pathways as sympathetic innervation. Excessive input from head and neck structures may produce facilitation in the upper thoracic cord segments. Facilitation may result in excessive sympathetic outflow from the affected segments to the associated viscera (T1-T4 to head and neck) and may produce physiologic changes in somatic tissues innervated by the involved cord segments.[2(p.170)] Relevant palpatory changes mediated by viscerosomatic reflexes from EENT structures can therefore be found in T1-4 paraspinal tissues and in predictable anterior Chapman's points on the anterior chest wall above rib 4.[2]

Palpatory changes in the upper thoracic and cervical paraspinal tissues may indicate structural or functional involvement of the sympathetic nervous system. Conditions such as Horner's syndrome (constricted pupil, ptosis, and facial anhidrosis on the affected side) may indicate significant structural involvement or blockage of the sympathetic nervous system. Increased sympathetic tone may also lead functionally to photophobia, unsteadiness, and tinnitus. Hyperesthesia of the pharyngeal tissues may cause patients to cough and expectorate in an attempt to rid themselves of an imaginary foreign body in the throat.[2]

Increased sympathetic activity to the structures of the head and upper thoracic musculature may alter the normal physiologic responses the tissues can provide. Vasoconstriction commonly results in decreased nutrient supply and reduced lymphatic and venous drainage from target tissues. The body's ability to mount an immune response and obtain effective concentrations of medications is reduced in areas of vasoconstriction and tissue congestion.[2]

Prolonged sympathetic stimulation may allow the nasal and pharyngeal secretions to become thick and sticky, thereby reducing effective clearing. This is due to a relative increase in the activity and number of goblet cells in the nasal epithelium, constriction of arterioles, and decreased vascular and lymphatic drainage of the tissues. Sympathetic stimulation also produces vasoconstriction and inhibits secretion, leading to dryness of the nasopharyngeal mucosa. Dryness and cracking of the mucosa may result in the breakdown of normal mucosal defenses, thereby permitting secondary bacterial infection.[2]

Dilation of the pupil (mydriasis) occurs with increased sympathetic activity to the eye. This may elevate intraocular pressures in patients with narrow angle glaucoma. Prolonged upper thoracic and cervical dysfunctions have been associated with the development of lens cloudiness.[2(p.4)] The Barr-Lieou syndrome (vertigo, ataxia, vasodilation, and eye pain) results from

Pain Guide

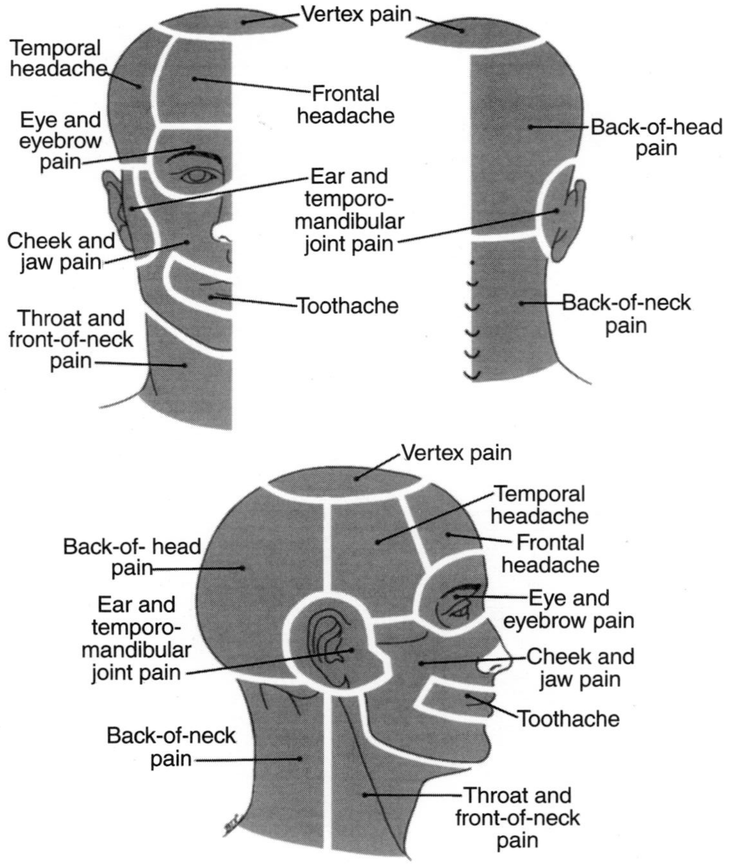

Figure 44.8. Muscle trigger points pain guide (*left*) and areas of referred pain (*right*) in the head and neck. (From Travell JG, Simons DG. *Myofascial Pain and Dysfunction: The Trigger Point Manual. The Upper Extremities.* Vol I. Baltimore, Md: Williams & Wilkins; 1983:166–167.)

Vertex Pain

Sternocleidomastoid (sternal)
Splenius capitis

Back-of-Head Pain

Trapezius (TP$_1$)
Sternocleidomastoid (sternal)
Sternocleidomastoid (clavicular)
Semispinalis capitis
Semispinalis cervicis
Spenius cervicis
Suboccipital group
Occipitalis
Digastric
Temporalis (TP$_4$)

Temporal Headache

Trapezius (TP$_1$)
Sternocleidomastoid (sternal)
Temporalis (TPs$_{1,2,3}$)
Splenius cervicis
Suboccipital group
Semispinalis capitis

Frontal Headache

Sternocleidomastoid (clavicular)
Sternocleidomastoid (sternal)
Semispinalis capitis
Frontalis

Zygomaticus major

Ear and Temporomandibular Joint Pain

Lateral pterygoid
Masseter (deep)
Sternocleidomastoid (clavicular)
Medial pterygoid

Eye and Eyebrow Pain

Sternocleidomastoid (sternal)
Temporalis (TP$_1$)
Splenius cervicis
Masseter (superficial)
Suboccipital group
Occipitalis
Orbicularis oculi
Trapezius (TP$_1$)

Trapezius (TP$_1$)
Trapezius (TP$_2$)

Trapezius (TP$_3$)
Multifidi
Levator scapulae
Splenius cervicis
Infraspinatus

Throat and Front-of-Neck Pain
Cheek and Jaw Pain

Sternocleidomastoid (sternal)
Masseter (superficial)
Lateral pterygoid
Trapezius (TP$_1$)
Masseter (deep)
Digastric
Medial pterygoid
Platysma
Orbicularis oculi
Zygomaticus major

Toothache

Temporalis (TPs$_{1,2,3}$)
Masseter (superficial)
Digastric (anterior)

Back-of-Neck Pain

Sternocleidomastoid (sternal)
Digastric
Medial pterygoid

hypersympathetic activity and proprioceptive dysfunction arising from cervical trauma as is often seen in whiplash injuries.

The sympathetics innervate blood vessels that supply the thyroid and innervate the cells that produce thyroid secretions. Increased sympathetic stimulation may increase thyroid gland secretion.[2]

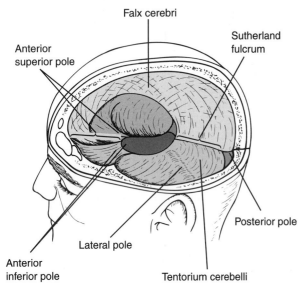

Figure 44.9. Dural reflections within skull.

CRANIAL NERVES

There are several important cranial nerves (Fig. 44.19).

Olfactory Nerve (I)

The nerve of smell has olfactory neurosensory cells located in the olfactory neuroepithelium covering the superior concha of the nasal cavity and superior portion of the nasal septum. The axons of these cells form nerve bundles that pass through the foramina of the cribriform plate of the ethmoid bone and eventually travel to the olfactory areas of the brain (anterior perforated substance and uncus).[3(p.853)] Dysfunction of CN I may lead to an altered sense of smell or an impression of an odor that does not exist.[2(p.70)] CN I may be affected at the point where it crosses the lesser wing of the sphenoid or by dysfunction of the frontoethmoid articulation.[1(pp.119,167)]

Optic Nerve (II)

Fibers arise from the ganglion cells of the retina and unite to form the optic nerve. The optic nerves pass through the optic canal (in the lesser wing of the sphenoid) and unite in the middle cranial fossa to form the optic chiasma. From there optic tracts continue dorsolaterally around the midbrain to the lateral geniculate bodies of the thalamus. Optic radiations from there relay information to the visual cortex in the occipital lobes of the brain.[3(pp.854–857)] This nerve may be affected by

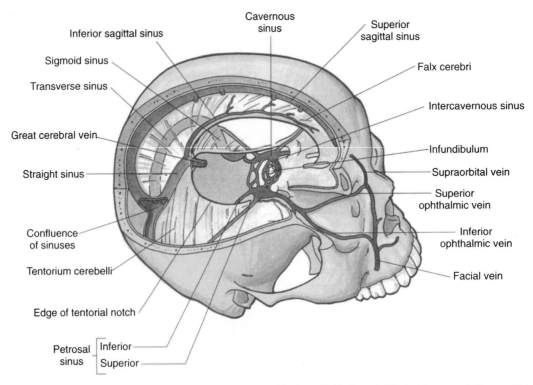

Figure 44.10. Median section of head and relationship of dural folds to intracranial structures. **A.** Lateral view. **B.** Superior view. (From Moore KL, Agur AMR. *Essential Clinical Anatomy.* Baltimore, Md: Williams & Wilkins; 1996:359.)

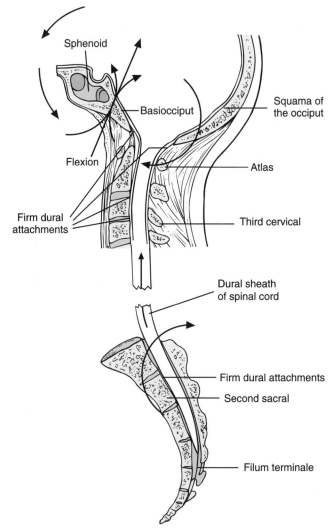

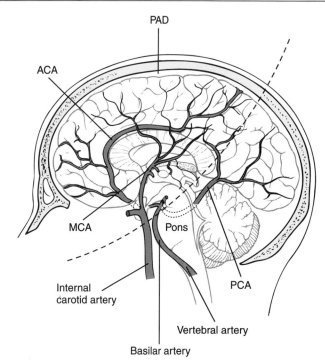

Figure 44.11. Dural continuity of skull, cervical vertebrae, and sacrum. (Adapted from Magoun H. In: *Osteopathy in the Cranial Field.* 3rd ed. Kirksville, Mo: The Journal Printing Co; 1976.)

Figure 44.12. Major arterial supply to brain. *Areas above dotted line* are supplied by internal carotid arteries; *areas below dotted line* are supplied by vertebral arteries. *ACA,* anterior cerebral artery; *MCA,* middle cerebral artery; *PCA,* posterior cerebral artery; *PAD,* pia, arachnoid, and dura.

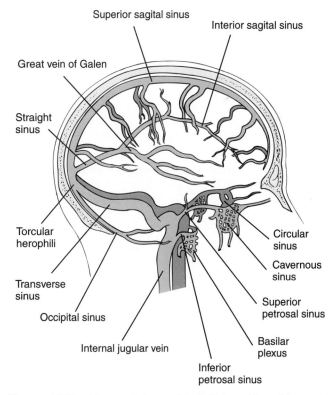

Figure 44.13. Venous drainage of skull. (Adapted from Magoun H. In: *Osteopathy in the Cranial Field.* 3rd ed. Kirksville, Mo: The Journal Printing Co; 1976.)

lesions of the sphenoid or membranous tension anywhere between the sphenoid and occiput.[1(pp.205–207)]

Oculomotor Nerve (III)

The oculomotor nerve arises from the midbrain, passes through the lateral wall of the cavernous sinus after passing over the top of the petrosphenoidal ligament and enters the orbit via the superior orbital fissure (opening between the greater and lesser wings of the sphenoid). It supplies the levator palpebrae and all of the extraocular muscles of the eye except the superior oblique and lateral rectus. By way of parasympathetic ganglion, it supplies the smooth muscle in the sphincter pupillae and ciliary muscles.[3(p.859)] Tension on the petrosphenoid ligament (anterior aspect of the tentorium cerebelli), especially from dysfunction affecting the temporal or sphenoid bones, may affect functioning of this nerve. This can cause

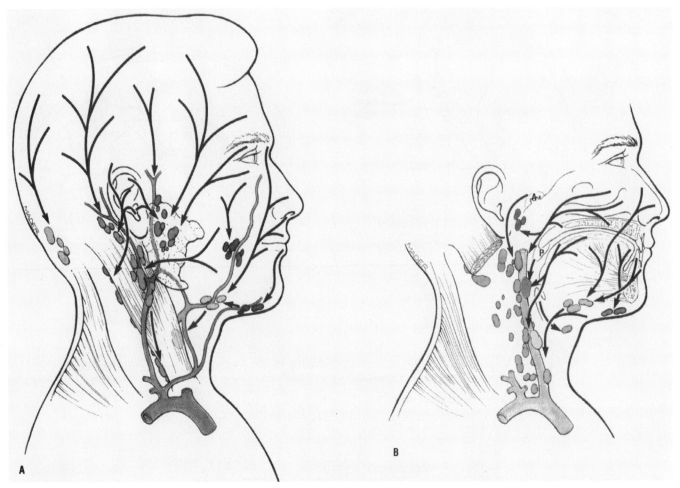

Figure 44.14.   Lymph nodes of head (**A**) and neck (**B**). *A,* pharyngeal tonsil; *P,* palatine tonsil. (From Agur AMR. *Grant's Atlas of Anatomy.*
9th ed. Baltimore, Md: Williams & Wilkins; 1991:548.)

symptoms of double vision, ptosis, or accommodation dysfunction. Back pressure from restriction at the jugular foramen
may cause overdistension of the cavernous sinus, causing dysfunction in CN III, IV, V, and VI.[1(pp.205–207,293)]

Trochlear Nerve (IV)

The trochlear nerve emerges dorsally from the midbrain, enters
the lateral wall of the cavernous sinus after passing through the
petrosphenoidal ligament, and enters the orbit via the superior
orbital fissure. This nerve has a long course and is more easily
torn during head injury.[3(p.861)] The dysfunctions listed under
the oculomotor nerve may also affect this nerve.[1(pp.205–207,293)]
The most common symptom, diplopia, occurs when the patient looks downward.

Trigeminal Nerve (V)

The trigeminal nerve, arising from the pons, consists of three
large sensory nerves from the face:

Ophthalmic (V¹)
Maxillary (V²)
Mandibular (V³)

The ophthalmic (V¹) nerve passes through the lateral wall of
the cavernous sinus and enters the orbit through the superior
orbital fissure. It supplies these areas:[3(pp.205–207,293)]

Upper eyelid
Scalp
Forehead
Eyeball
Ethmoid sinus
Nasal cavity
Lacrimal gland
Adjoining conjunctiva

The dysfunctions listed under the oculomotor nerve may also
affect the ophthalmic nerve.[3(p.863)]

    The maxillary nerve (V²) is a pure sensory nerve and runs
anteriorly in the inferior portion of the cavernous sinus. It

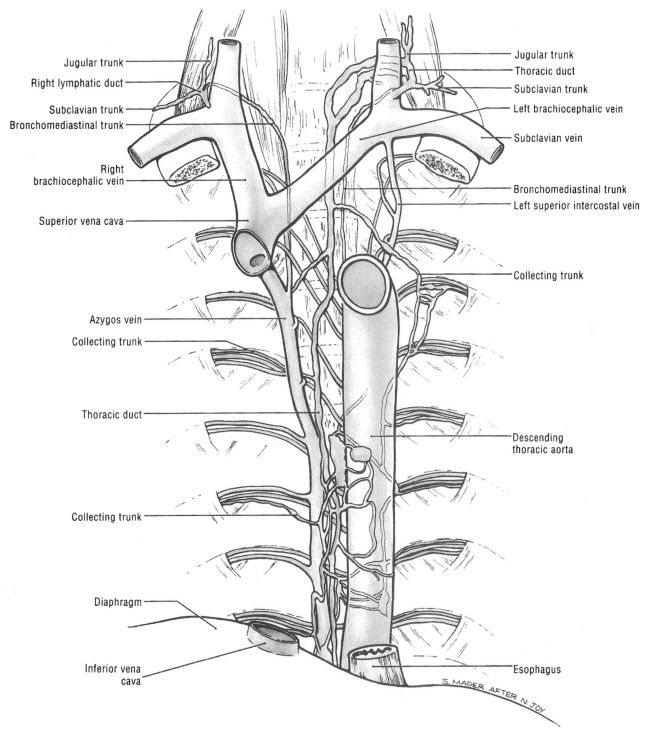

Jugular trunk
Right lymphatic duct
Subclavian trunk
Bronchomediastinal trunk
Right brachiocephalic vein
Superior vena cava
Azygos vein
Collecting trunk
Thoracic duct
Collecting trunk
Diaphragm
Inferior vena cava

Jugular trunk
Thoracic duct
Subclavian trunk
Left brachiocephalic vein
Subclavian vein
Bronchomediastinal trunk
Left superior intercostal vein
Collecting trunk
Descending thoracic aorta
Esophagus

S. MADER AFTER N. JOY

Figure 44.15.   Lymphatic drainage through thoracic inlet. (From Moore KL. *Clinically Oriented Anatomy*. 3rd ed. Baltimore, Md: Williams & Wilkins: 1985:78.)

leaves the middle cranial fossa via the foramen rotundum in the greater wing of the sphenoid. It courses through the pterygopalatine fossa and the infratemporal fossa and enters the orbit via the inferior orbital fissure. V² supplies portions of:[3(p.863)]

Dura
Maxillary sinus
Roots of the maxillary premolar and molar teeth
Nasal septum
Lower eyelid

Nose
Upper lip

The sphenopalatine ganglion is located in the pterygopalatine fossa. Tic douloureux may be associated with dysfunction of the V² division of the trigeminal nerve and may result from lesions of the temporals, sphenoid, maxillae, and mandible.[3(p.294)]

The mandibular nerve (V³) exits the middle cranial fossa via the foramen ovale of the sphenoid. It contains both motor and sensory roots. V³ supplies these areas:[3(p.865)]

Teeth
Gingiva of the mandible
Skin of the temporal region
Part of the auricle
Lower face

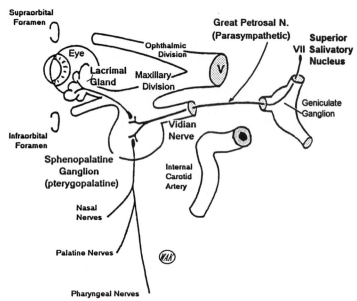

Figure 44.16. Parasympathetic nerves to orbital and nasal areas. (Modified from Kuchera ML, Kuchera WA. *Osteopathic Considerations in Systemic Dysfunction*. 2nd ed. rev. Columbus, Ohio: Greyden Press; 1994.)

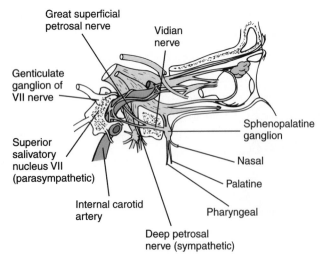

Figure 44.17. Sphenopalatine ganglion. (Modified from Kuchera ML, Kuchera WA. *Osteopathic Considerations in Systemic Dysfunction*. 2nd ed. rev. Columbus. Ohio: Greyden Press; 1994.)

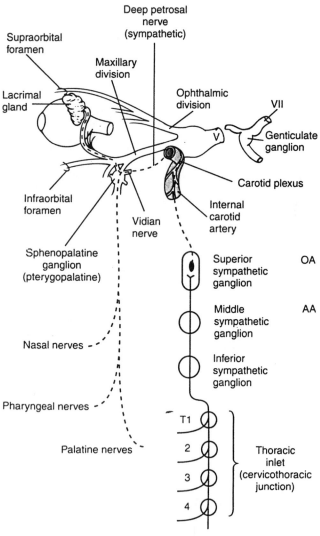

Figure 44.18. Sympathetic nerves to head. *OA*, occipitoatlantal; *AA*, atlantoaxial. (Modified from Kuchera ML, Kuchera WA. *Osteopathic Considerations in Systemic Dysfunction*. 2nd ed. rev. Columbus, Ohio: Greyden Press; 1994.)

Muscles of mastication
Floor of the oral cavity
Part of the tongue

It may be affected by sphenoid dysfunction.[1(p.330)]

Trigeminal neuralgia in this division may be precipitated by TMJ dysfunction, shaving, or even poor-fitting dentures.

The extensive interconnections of the trigeminal nerve with other cranial nerves play an important role in a variety of reflexes. Sensory afferent information from innervated structures (such as the sinuses) is often perceived as headache in the anterior or middle cranial fossae, behind the eyes, or at the vertex of the head.

Abducens Nerve (VI)

The abducens nerve supplies the lateral rectus muscle of the eye. It arises from the pons, ascends the clivus, runs underneath the petrosphenoid ligament, courses through the cavernous sinus, and enters the orbit via the superior orbital fissure.[3(p.865)]

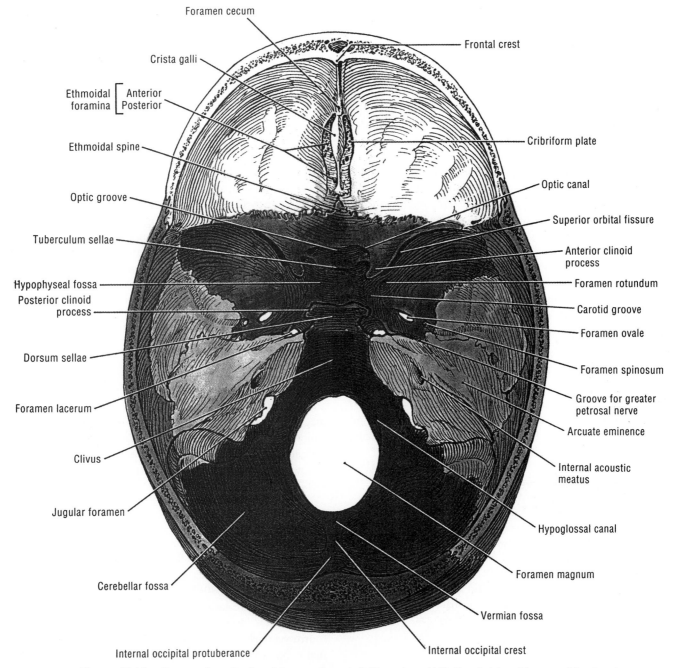

Figure 44.19. Foramen for exit of cranial nerves from skull. (From Agur AMR. *Grant's Atlas of Anatomy.* 9th ed. Baltimore, Md: Williams & Wilkins; 1991:477.)

Dysfunction of this nerve may be secondary to petrosphenoid ligament tension resulting from severe lesions of the sphenoid or temporals.[1(p.206)] Of three nerves passing in proximity to the petrosphenoidal ligament (III, IV, VI) and innervating the extraocular muscles, the abducens nerve is most often affected and may result in medial strabismus and diplopia.

Facial Nerve (VII)

The motor root supplies the muscles of facial expression and muscles of the:

Scalp
Auricle
Buccinator
Platysma
Stapedius
Stylohyoid
Posterior belly of the digastric muscle

The sensory root conveys fibers for taste buds in the anterior two-thirds of the tongue, soft palate, and a small area around the external acoustic meatus. It supplies secretory stimulus to the submandibular, sublingual, and intralingual salivary glands and lacrimal glands. The facial nerve arises from the pons, enters the internal acoustic meatus of the temporal bone, joins the facial canal, and exits the skull via the stylomastoid foramen.[3(p.866)] This nerve may be affected by dysfunction of the sphenoid, occiput (especially condylar parts), temporals, and cervical fascia.[1(p.150)] Both temporal and upper thoracic dysfunctions may play a significant role in the genesis of Bell's palsy (facial nerve paralysis).[1(p.269)]

Vestibulocochlear Nerve (VIII)

This has two parts: a vestibular nerve involved in the maintenance of equilibrium and a cochlear nerve involved with hearing. Both divisions arise in a groove between the pons and medulla and course through the internal acoustic meatus with the facial nerve.[3(p.869)] Lesions of the sphenoid, occiput, and temporals may affect the functioning of this nerve, producing vertigo or hearing dysfunctions.[1(p.150)]

Glossopharyngeal Nerve (IX)

The glossopharyngeal nerve supplies the stylopharyngeus muscle. It sends secretomotor fibers to the parotid gland and carries sensory fibers from the pharynx, tonsils, and posterior portion of the tongue. It arises from the medulla and leaves the skull through the jugular foramen.[3(p.869)] Dysfunctions affecting the jugular foramen (temporal, occiput, occipitomastoid suture or cervical fascia) may interfere with normal function of this nerve.[1(p.119)]

Vagus Nerve (X)

The vagus nerve supplies structures in the:

Head (dura of posterior cranial fossa)
Neck (pharynx, soft palate, carotid sinus, and larynx)
Thorax (heart and lungs)
Abdomen (stomach, liver, pancreas, duodenum, and smooth muscle of the gut up to the left colic flexure)

The vagus nerve arises from the medulla and exits the skull via the jugular foramen.[3(p.871)] Dysfunction anywhere along its course through the head (especially jugular foramen), neck (especially OA, AA, and C2), thorax, and abdomen may affect normal function. Extensive direct interconnections with C2 and several other cranial nerves result in a number of referred pain and parasympathetic reflexes. Common symptoms include:

Posterior headaches (often referred from throat, lung, heart, or bowel)
Bradyarrhythmias
Cough
Accentuated gag reflex
Vomiting
Shallow respiration patterns

Accessory Nerve (XI)

The accessory nerve supplies the sternocleidomastoid and trapezius muscles; it also supplies muscles in the pharynx and palate. It arises from both the cervical spinal cord and medulla, and exits the skull through the jugular foramen. Dysfunctions affecting the jugular foramen (temporal, occiput, occipitomastoid suture, or cervical fascia) may interfere with normal function of this nerve.[1(p.119)] Sternocleidomastoid dysfunction and/or trigger points often accompany somatic dysfunction affecting this cranial nerve. Torticollis is an associated clinical condition that benefits from osteopathic manipulative treatment (OMT).

Hypoglossal Nerve (XII)

The hypoglossal nerve is the motor nerve of the tongue. It arises from the medulla and exits the skull via the foramen magnum. It courses through the hypoglossal canal in the occipital bone.[3(p.873)] Dysfunction of the condylar parts of the occipital bone may affect functioning of this nerve,[1(p.234)] resulting in suckling disorders in infants and in dysphagia and swallowing difficulties in adults.

FOURTH VENTRICLE

The fourth ventricle is a diamond-shaped opening in the pons that acquires cerebrospinal fluid (CSF) from the third ventricle via the cerebral aqueduct and transmits it into the subarachnoid space (Fig. 44.20).[3(p.699)] Many of the nuclei of cranial nerves V–XII are located in the floor of the fourth ventricle (Fig. 44.21). Dysfunctions affecting CSF flow through the fourth ventricle may have a significant impact upon those cranial nerves whose nuclei are located there. Compression of the fourth ventricle is an osteopathic manipulative treatment technique that may be used to normalize fluctuation of the CSF, postulated to improve functioning of the associated nuclei.[1(p.110)] The technique is performed by holding the occiput

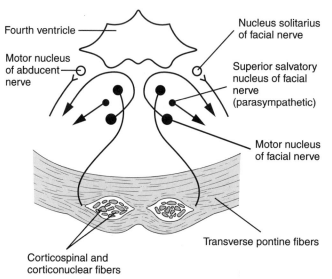

Figure 44.20. Floor of fourth ventricle. (Modified from Snell RS. *Clinical Neuroanatomy for Medical Students.* 2nd ed. Boston, Mass: Little, Brown and Co; 1987.)

(or temporals or sacrum) in craniosacral extension and resisting flexion until a still point and release are perceived.[1(p.155)]

ADJUNCTS FOR SINUS, EYE, AND EAR DISORDERS

Paranasal Sinuses

These are air-filled extensions of the nasal cavity into the following cranial bones:

Frontal
Ethmoid
Sphenoid
Maxillae

The sinuses are lined with mucous membranes continuous with those of the nasal cavities. All of the paranasal sinuses drain directly or indirectly into the nasal cavity. Frontal and sphenoidal sinuses are absent at birth, although a few ethmoid cells and small maxillary sinuses are present. The ethmoid and maxillary sinuses enlarge during childhood. The frontal and sphenoidal sinuses develop during childhood and adolescence. Sinus headache referral patterns are predictable because the sinuses are innervated by branches of the trigeminal nerve.

FRONTAL SINUSES

These drain into the middle meatus. They are innervated by branches of the supraorbital nerves (CN V[1]).

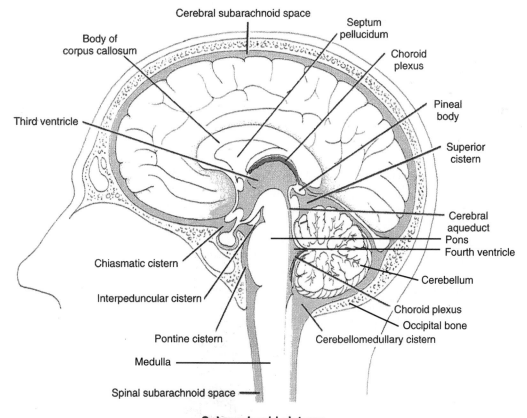

Subarachnoid cisterns

Figure 44.21. Lateral view of fourth ventricle. (Modified from Moore KL, Agur AMR. *Essential Clinical Anatomy.* Baltimore, Md: Williams & Wilkins; 1996:365.)

ETHMOID SINUSES

The anterior and middle ethmoid cells drain into the middle meatus. The posterior ethmoid cells drain into the superior meatus. They are innervated by branches of the ophthalmic nerves (CN V[1]).

SPHENOID SINUSES

These drain into the sphenoethmoidal recess in close approximation to the cavernous sinuses and are innervated by the posterior ethmoid nerve (CN V1). Infections of the sphenoid sinus are especially dangerous because of close association with the pituitary, brainstem, cavernous sinus, and cranial nerves.

MAXILLARY SINUSES

The largest of the paranasal sinuses drain into the middle meatus. They are innervated by branches of the maxillary nerve (CN V2).[3(pp.759–762)]

Sinus dysfunction (acute and chronic sinusitis and chronic postnasal drip) may result from dysfunction in the cranium. Focus on improving the general health of the mucous membranes by correcting ventilation and circulation, restoring autonomic balance, and eliminating stagnant secretions by removing mechanical hindrances.[1(p.290)] See *Osteopathy in the Cranial Field* by Magoun[1] and *Osteopathic Considerations in Systemic Dysfunction* by the Kucheras[2] for specific techniques.

Eye

Each orbit is composed of seven bones (Fig. 44.2):[1(p.205)]

Frontal
Sphenoid
Maxilla
Zygoma
Palatine
Ethmoid
Lacrimal

Four of the eye muscles (superior, inferior, medial, and lateral rectus) originate from a common tendinous ring surrounding the optic canal (lesser wing of the sphenoid). The superior oblique muscle arises from the body of the sphenoid bone superomedial to the common tendinous ring. The inferior oblique muscle originates on the maxilla in the floor of the orbit. All are involved in eye control (Fig. 44.22).[3(p.715)] Dysfunction of the frontal, sphenoid, and maxillae may produce muscle imbalance in the eye.[1(p.206)] Cranial dysfunction may affect the nerves innervating the eye. Restrictions of the orbital bones may contribute to venous stasis.[1(p.206)] Dysfunction of the occiput can obstruct the jugular foramen, leading to backpressure in the orbit. These factors may contribute to such conditions as:[1(pp.267–306)]

Amblyopia
Astigmatism
Diplopia
Hyperopia
Myopia
Strabismus

These conditions may benefit clinically from removing somatic dysfunction. Gentle eye mobilization using indirect techniques may also decrease ocular tension resulting from glaucoma.

Ear

The ear serves two major functions: maintenance of equilibrium and hearing.[3(p.866)] Most of the structures of the ear reside within the temporal bone. Hence, dysfunction of the temporal bone may contribute to impaired hearing and vertigo (Fig. 44.23). The eustachian tube connects the middle ear to the nasopharynx (Fig. 44.24).[3(p.772)] It equalizes middle ear pressure with atmospheric pressure. Fixed internal rotation of the temporal bone maintains partial or complete closure of the eustachian tube. This may have two effects: perception of high-pitched noises or impaired drainage from the middle ear, thereby producing a medium for recurrent ear infections. Fixed external rotation maintains patency of the eustachian tube and may result in the perception of a roar or low-pitched noises.[1(p.150)] Eustachian tube dysfunction is the most common cause of otitis media and benefits from OMT to the cranium, medial pterygoid muscle, and cervical fascias.

COMMON COLD

Viral illness decreases host resistance and produces uncomfortable symptoms. Inflammation may help predispose the patient to secondary bacterial infection. Visceral afferent impulses from the upper respiratory tract facilitate the upper thoracic spinal cord segments, resulting in excessive sympathetic output to the head, neck, and bronchial tubes. Osteopathic treatment:

1. Improves the blood supply
2. Increases venous and lymphatic drainage from the affected area
3. Relieves muscle spasm, thereby improving breathing
4. Relieves pain
5. Reduces reflex disturbances
6. Improves circulation to and from the reticuloendothelial system and thereby improves immune function

Correction of cranial dysfunctions assists in sinus drainage. Circular pressure applied to the supraorbital and infraorbital nerves may ease sinus pain. Treatment of the upper thoracic spine (rib raising) may reduce sympathetic outflow to the nose, sinuses, and bronchial tubes, producing thin, saliva-like secretions. This assists in cleansing the structures of the head and upper airways. Treatment of cervical myofascial and articular dysfunctions and fascial torsions at the thoracic inlet improves lymphatic and venous drainage.[2(p.27)] Facial effleurage and lymphatic pump procedures augment drainage.

HEADACHE

Headache is one of the most common conditions seen in a primary care practice. Every year, 40–50 million Americans

Figure 44.22. Extraocular muscles and nerves. **A.** Anterior view of muscles. **B.** Posterior view of muscles. **C.** Nerves of the orbit. *CN,* cranial nerve. (From Agur AMR. *Grant's Atlas of Anatomy.* 9th ed. Baltimore, Md: Williams & Wilkins; 1991:486.)

A

Superior rectus

Sclera

Cut edge of conjunctiva

Pupil

Iris

Seen through cornea

Lateral rectus

Medial rectus

Inferior rectus

B

Superior rectus

Superior oblique

Medial rectus

Lateral rectus

Dural sheath

Inferior oblique

Subarachnoid space

Optic nerve

Inferior rectus

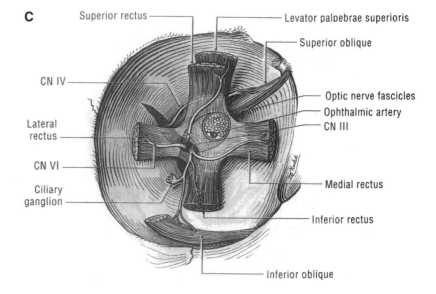

C

Superior rectus

Levator palpebrae superioris

Superior oblique

CN IV

Optic nerve fascicles

Ophthalmic artery

CN III

Lateral rectus

CN VI

Medial rectus

Ciliary ganglion

Inferior rectus

Inferior oblique

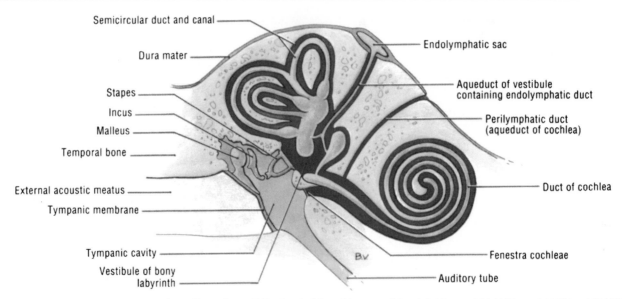

Figure 44.23.   Internal structures of ear. (From Agur AMR. *Grant's Atlas of Anatomy*. 9th ed. Baltimore, Md: Williams & Wilkins; 1991:534.)

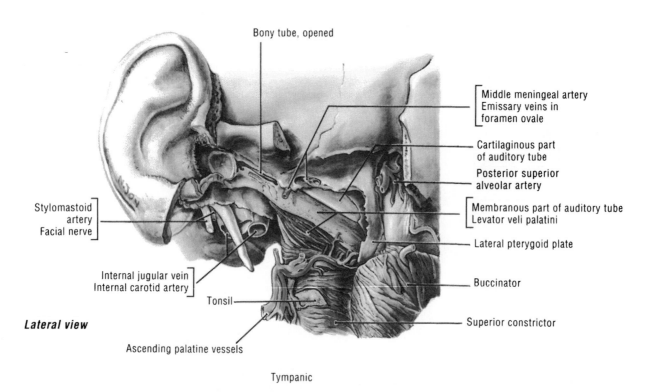

Figure 44.24.   Connection of middle ear to nasopharynx. Lateral view. (From Agur AMR. *Grant's Atlas of Anatomy*.
9th ed. Baltimore, Md: Williams & Wilkins; 1991:541.)

seek treatment for headaches.[4(p.2)] This condition may be caused by a number of intracranial and extracranial abnormalities. The underlying cause is frequently described as unknown. A thorough knowledge of anatomy and physiology allows the osteopathic physician to diagnose structural abnormalities contributing to headache and, in many cases, allows one to logically explain previously "unknown" causes of headache. The implementation of a rational treatment plan signif-

icantly reduces suffering and improves the overall functioning of the patient.

The head and scalp contain many pain-sensitive structures. These include:

Skin and its blood supply
Muscles of the head and neck
Great venous sinuses and their tributaries

Portions of the dura mater at the base of the brain
Dural arteries
Intracranial arteries
Cervical nerves
Trigeminal (V), abducens (VI), and facial (VII) nerves

The brain parenchyma is not sensitive to pain. For structures above the tentorium cerebelli, pain pathways travel via the trigeminal nerve. Pain referred from structures above the tentorium cerebelli are therefore perceived in the frontal, temporal, and parietal regions of the head. For structures below the tentorium cerebelli, pain pathways travel via the glossopharyngeal (IX) and vagus (X) nerves and the upper cervical spinal nerve roots. Pain referred from structures below the tentorium cerebelli are generally perceived in the occipital region.[4(p.4)]

Structural abnormalities may place tension on pain-sensitive structures and cause discomfort. For example, parietal bone dysfunction may place strain on the superior sagittal sinus, thereby causing discomfort in the parietal region. Upper cervical dysfunction may lead to discomfort in the occipital region. Gastrointestinal abnormalities may produce headache in the occipital region through the vagus nerve.

A detailed history is vital to the diagnosis and treatment of headache. Information regarding the patient's birth history (mother's pregnancy, labor, method of delivery, use of forceps) and childhood growth and development may shed light on the causes of headache. A history of trauma is frequently important. Family history should be obtained,[4(p.4)] including information about:

Headache: onset, frequency, location, duration, and severity
Associated symptoms
Trigger factors
Previous medical and surgical history
Prior headache therapy

Perform a complete physical examination, including a neurologic evaluation, in addition to the structural examination. It is always important to rule out serious organic causes of headache:

Brain tumor
Aneurysm
Arteriovenous malformation
Hemorrhage
Temporal arteritis

Neuroradiologic studies such as computerized tomography (CT) and magnetic resonance imaging (MRI) may be needed to rule out more serious and life-threatening pathologies.[4(p.4)]

There are four major classifications of headache:[4(p.2)]

1. Vascular (migraine and cluster)
2. Tension (muscle contraction)
3. Traction and inflammatory type (brain tumor, infection, cerebrovascular disease)
4. Cranial neuralgias (trigeminal neuralgia, temporomandibular joint)

Migraine

Migraine headaches are recurrent and vary widely in intensity, frequency, and duration. The pain is frequently described as a unilateral throbbing, pounding pain. It may later radiate to the opposite side. Migraine may be associated with:

Nausea
Vomiting
Diarrhea
Vertigo
Tremors
Photophobia
Phonophobia
Sweating
Chills

Migraine headaches may be preceded by:

Aura
Scotomas (blind spots)
Photopsia (flashing lights)
Paresthesias
Visual, olfactory, and auditory hallucinations
Vertigo
Syncope

The initial episode most frequently occurs during puberty but can occur at any age between 5 and 40 years. Migraine headaches may be triggered by:[4(pp.7–10)]

Head injury
Stress
Hormone fluctuations
Fasting
Oversleeping and undersleeping
Vasoactive substances in foods (wine and cheese, cold foods)
Changes in weather and temperature (bright light, poor ventilation)
Physical stimuli (smoking)

The production of migraine symptoms involves two major events: vasoconstriction and vasodilation. The cerebral blood vessels can be divided into two major systems. The large arteries at the base of the brain and the pial arteries make up the innervated vascular system, which has a rich adrenergic nerve supply. These arteries respond to catecholamines. The noninnervated vascular system consists of the parenchymal arteries and the terminal high-resistance arteries; they respond to local metabolic factors.

Trigger factors (listed above) produce unilateral cerebral vasoconstriction via the adrenergic nervous system. Platelets systemically aggregate and release serotonin, which augments vasoconstriction of the adrenergically innervated blood vessels. The overall result of this vasoconstriction is a reduction in cerebral blood flow. If blood flow is sufficiently reduced, an aura develops. The vasoconstriction phase causes local anoxia and acidosis and a systemic drop in serotonin. In response to local metabolic factors (anoxia and acidosis), the noninnervated arteries dilate, increasing cerebral blood flow and promoting local vasomotor changes that result in dilation of the innervated extracranial and intracranial arteries on the same side. Serotonin sensitizes the pain receptors in the blood vessels. This vasodilation, along with the sensitization of pain fibers, produces the pain of migraine.[4(p.10)]

The trigeminal vascular reflex may also explain some of the events seen in the production of migraines. The cortex, thalamus, hypothalamus, and cervical roots C1-C3 may send afferent pain stimulation to the spinal nucleus of the trigeminal nerve. These impulses may then travel via the facial nerve (CN VII) to produce parasympathetic dilation of the internal and external carotid arteries. This dilation feeds back into and causes further afferent pain stimulation in the spinal nucleus of the trigeminal nerve. Stimulation of the trigeminal ganglion, through vasodilation, may produce edema in the dura.[4(pp.13–14)]

How might somatic dysfunction play a role in the genesis of migraines? Somatic dysfunction in the upper thoracic spine increases the level of sympathetic tone to the innervated blood vessels of the head. Increased sympathetic tone produces vasoconstriction and a resultant decrease in cerebral blood flow. This results in a relative anoxia and may lower the threshold for vasodilation, thereby leading to the production of migraine symptoms. Cranial dysfunction affecting the cortex, thalamus, and hypothalamus, and upper cervical dysfunction affecting cervical roots C1–C3 may result in the transfer of afferent pain stimuli to the spinal nucleus of the trigeminal nerve. This may produce vasodilation and resultant symptoms via the facial nerve (CN VII).

The trigeminal nerve courses through various portions of the sphenoid bone. An elevated greater wing of the sphenoid (torsion) may irritate the trigeminal nerve, thereby feeding into the trigeminal vascular reflex. The facial nerve courses through the temporal bone. Dysfunction of the temporal bone (internal rotation) may result in reflex vasodilation of the internal and external carotid arteries via the facial nerve. Occipitomastoid compression may reduce venous drainage through the jugular foramen, thereby producing congestion and dysfunction in the cortex, thalamus, and hypothalamus.

These dysfunctions are listed as generalizations. Somatic dysfunction in areas not directly adjacent to the head (lumbar spine, sacrum, pelvis) may produce fascial strains that are transmitted to the head and may play a key role in the genesis of migraines. Treat the whole patient with an osteopathic approach.

Cluster Headache

Cluster headaches occur in series or groups lasting several weeks to several months with pain-free intervals of 14 or more days. The average age at onset is 20–30 years. They are more common in men than in women. The pain is typically unilateral and is described as an excruciating, boring sensation behind or around one eye that may radiate over the entire side of the head. The opposite side may be affected in a subsequent series. Associated symptoms include:

Conjunctival injection
Tearing
Nasal congestion
Rhinorrhea
Partial Horner syndrome
Sweating
Flushing on the same side of the head

Cluster headaches may be triggered by alcohol consumption and cigarette smoking.

Extracranial vasodilation and increased cerebral blood flow are associated with cluster headache attacks. This may result from similar mechanisms seen with migraine headaches. Somatic dysfunction listed in the preceding section on migraine headaches may also be involved in the genesis of cluster headaches (upper thoracics, upper cervicals, sphenoid, temporals, etc.). The associated Horner syndrome (unilateral miosis, ptosis, sweating, and flushing) may be due to an abnormality with the sympathetic nerve supply to the orbit. This may occur as a result of compression of the cervicothoracic (stellate) ganglion secondary to upper thoracic or upper rib (elevated first rib) dysfunction. Compression of the pterygopalatine ganglion (dysfunctions of the sphenoid, palatine, and maxilla) may also affect sympathetic supply to the orbit.[1(p.183)]

Tension Headache

Tension (muscle contraction) headaches are the result of the body's response to:

Stress
Anxiety
Depression
Fatigue
Emotional conflicts (work, school, family, marriage)

This response includes contraction of the skeletal muscles of the head, neck, and face and some reflex vasodilation of the extracranial vessels. Women experience these headaches most commonly; they generally begin between the ages of 20 and 40 years. Tension headaches usually occur bilaterally and may be described as a fullness, tightness, or pressure in the forehead, temples, or back of the head and neck. They may occasionally be described as a bandlike tightness around the head. Tension headaches are not usually associated with nausea and vomiting. They may be associated with sleep disturbances. Headaches associated with anxiety may cause difficulty falling asleep. Headaches associated with depression may cause early and frequent awakening. Decreased levels of serotonin in the brain may make the patient susceptible to depression. The reduced levels of endorphins seen in depression may make the patient susceptible to chronic pain.[4(p.19)]

Postural imbalance may significantly contribute to tension headaches. Somatic dysfunction in the upper thoracics, cervicothoracic junction, and cranium (internally rotated temporal bone) may result in increased levels of sympathetic tone. Increased levels of sympathetic tone may result in increased muscle tone and vasoconstriction, thereby reducing blood supply to the muscles of the upper back, neck, and head. This may produce a relative ischemic muscle tenderness.

Traction and Inflammatory Headache

Headaches can be produced when pain-sensitive structures are distended, displaced, or inflamed. Early diagnosis is vital for effective treatment of these conditions and to prevent complications associated with late diagnosis.

Cerebrovascular disease may produce headache. Hypertension headaches can develop when hypertension becomes moderate or severe. Headaches caused by hypertension are usually located in the occipital region and are described as moderately severe, nagging, and throbbing. They usually begin in the morning and decrease when the patient stands up. They may become severe and persistent when the diastolic blood pressure rises to 130 mm Hg. They may be associated with episodes of blurred vision, confusion, and drowsiness. Adequate blood pressure control may help prevent the development of strokes. Hypertensive encephalopathy may develop if this condition goes untreated.[4(pp.2–33)]

Headaches may be associated with transient ischemic attacks (TIAs). They are usually described as a pressure sensation and can develop both during and after the TIA. They generally persist for several minutes, rarely for hours. Similar headaches may occur between TIA episodes. Carotid TIAs usually cause unilateral frontal headaches associated with:

Transient hemiplegia
Hemiparesthesia
Unilateral blindness
Speech abnormalities

Vertebrobasilar TIAs may cause:[4(pp.24–33)]

Occipital headaches
Dizziness
Diplopia
Impaired vision
Numbness
Dysarthria

Aneurysms can cause headaches and extraocular muscle abnormalities. These headaches are noted in the eye or frontal area and may be associated with:

Miosis
Ptosis
Decreased vision
Carotid bruit

Extraocular muscle abnormalities occur through compression of the oculomotor nerve (CN III). The symptoms may be similar to those seen with cluster headache but are of a more prolonged duration.[4(pp.24–33)]

Large lobar hemorrhages more frequently cause headaches than smaller hemorrhages into the thalamus or basal ganglia. The headache most commonly occurs on the same side as the hemorrhage. Frontal hemorrhage commonly produces pain in the forehead and eyes. Occipital hemorrhage frequently produces headache in the occipital region and neck. Subarachnoid hemorrhages (SAH) typically have a sudden onset and incapacitating severity. They may be described as the "worst headache of my life" and may be associated with exertion. The pain may persist for hours to days. The patient may be completely asymptomatic immediately prior to bleeding or may experience a warning headache days to weeks before the rupture. The associated headache is usually generalized and may spread to involve the neck, back, and lower extremities. Nuchal rigidity may develop. Associated symptoms may include:

Photophobia
Pain with eye movement
Confusion
Autonomic disturbances (elevated temperature, pulse, blood pressure)
Focal neurologic symptoms
Visual abnormalities

Funduscopic examination may reveal papilledema.[4(pp.24–33)]

Arteriovenous malformations are abnormal blood vessels connecting the arterial and venous systems. Most are located in the cerebral hemispheres, primarily in the distribution of the middle cerebral artery. Prior to rupture, the symptoms may remain localized in the area of the malformation. The headaches may be accompanied by auras and may mimic a migraine. A skull bruit may be auscultated. Rupture may not be associated with exertion and may result in a sudden, lateralized, severe headache. Confusion and neurologic deficits may develop.[4(pp.24–33)]

Brain tumors can be a cause of headache. The pain is usually intermittent, deep, aching, nagging, and pressurelike. Throbbing is not usually noted. Coughing and straining may worsen the headache. Changing positions may induce a headache. The pain worsens as the tumor grows and the intracranial pressure increases.[4(pp.24–33)]

Acute hydrocephalus occurs secondary to ventricular obstruction or shunt malfunction. A severe headache and visual disturbances may occur. Emergency ventricular drainage must be performed.[4(pp.24–33)]

Temporal arteritis is a condition resulting from inflammation of a scalp artery (usually the superficial temporal artery). This condition is generally seen in patients over age 50. The affected artery is swollen and tender. The associated headache is severe, throbbing, or stabbing and is localized over one temple. The pain is worse when the patient stoops or lies flat. The pain decreases when pressure is applied over the common carotid artery. Other symptoms include:

Fever
Weight loss
Night sweats
Joint pain

Visual disturbances may develop secondary to ischemic optic neuropathy. The diagnosis is confirmed by biopsy.[4(pp.24–33)]

Trigeminal Neuralgia

Trigeminal neuralgia is associated with unilateral recurring pain over the distribution of the trigeminal nerve. It usually affects the maxillary division but may include the ophthalmic division late in the disease. The pain is described as intermittent, severe, short, sharp, momentary bursts that are similar to electric shocks. Patients may cry or twitch in response to severe

pain. Mild stimulation to trigger zones can stimulate attacks.[4(pp.24–33)] Dysfunction of the temporals, sphenoid, maxillae, and mandible can lead to trigeminal nerve irritability and subsequent symptoms. Trigeminal neuralgia may appear following dental extraction.[1(pp.295–300)]

Temporomandibular Joint

ANATOMY AND MOTION REVIEW

The temporomandibular joint (TMJ) is formed by the head of the mandible and mandibular fossa of the temporal bone. These two structures are separated by a fibrocartilaginous articular disc. The stylomandibular ligament connects the angle of the mandible to the styloid process of the temporal bone. The sphenomandibular ligament connects the lingula (medial aspect) of the mandible to the spine of the sphenoid (Fig. 44.25). When the mouth is opened, the head of the mandible and articular disc move anteriorly on the articular surface of the temporal bone while the head of the mandible rotates on the inferior surface of the articular disc about a transverse axis (Fig. 44.26). During protraction and retraction, the heads and articular discs slide anteriorly and posteriorly, respectively. The temporalis, masseter, and medial pterygoid muscles close the mouth. The mandible is protracted by the lateral pterygoid muscle and retracted by the posterior fibers of the temporalis muscle. Gravity normally opens the mouth but may be assisted by the lateral pterygoid, suprahyoid, and infrahyoid muscles.[3(pp.731–733)]

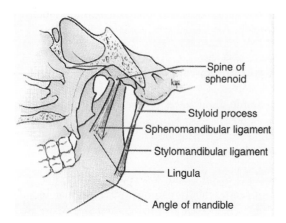

Figure 44.25. Ligamentous attachments of sphenoid and temporal bones to mandible. Medial view. (From Moore KL, Agur AMR. *Essential Clinical Anatomy.* Baltimore, Md: Williams & Wilkins; 1996:384.)

Figure 44.26. Opening motion of temporomandibular joint. (After Blaschke DD, reproduced with permission from Solberg WK, Clark GT. *Temporomandibular Joint Problems: Biologic Diagnosis and Treatment.* Chicago, Ill: Quintessence Publishing; 1980:73.)

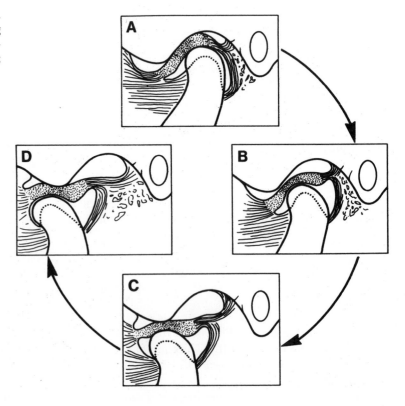

Frequently, the anterior gliding motion of the mandible and articular disc is restricted. Assume that the patient has a left TMJ restriction. As the mouth opens, the right side of the mandible and right articular disc glide anteriorly while the left side is restricted. This results in deviation of the chin to the left side (side of restriction). Cranial dysfunction may affect TMJ motion. As the temporal bone externally rotates, the mandibular fossa moves posteriorly and medially. Internal rotation allows the mandibular fossa to move anteriorly and laterally. The mandible may deviate toward the side of the externally rotated temporal bone or away from the side of the internally rotated temporal bone. Sphenoid dysfunction may affect the TMJ through its direct articulation with the temporal bone or by its articulation with the mandible through the sphenomandibular ligament. Short leg syndrome has also been associated with TMJ.[2(p.161)]

DYSFUNCTION: DIAGNOSIS

Place your hands on either side of the patient's head with your index fingers anterior to the external auditory meatus (area of the TMJ). Instruct the patient, "Open your mouth slowly." Observe the chin (or midincisural line) for deviation from the midline while palpating the TMJs. Remember that deviation occurs to the side of the restricted TMJ.

MUSCLE ENERGY TREATMENT

Assume that the patient has a left TMJ restriction. The chin deviates to the left as the mouth is opened.

1. Use your right hand to support the right side of the patient's head. Contact the left side of the mandible with your left hand.
2. Instruct the patient, "Open your mouth"; have him or her stop when mandibular deviation occurs to the left. Use your left hand to apply a force directed to the right against the mandible.
3. Instruct the patient, "Push your chin to the left against my hand." Maintain a counterforce to resist motion.
4. Maintain muscle contraction for 3–5 seconds. Then instruct the patient to relax. Wait 2 seconds and then engage the new barrier. Repeat the process a total of three times.
5. Reevaluate the motion.

CRANIAL MOTION ASSESSMENT

The vault hold is used both to assess and normalize motion of the bones of the cranium. The patient should be in the supine position, comfortable and relaxed. Glasses, nonfixed dental appliances, and bulky objects in pockets should be removed. The physician should be seated at the patient's head, forearms resting comfortably on the treatment table. The fingers of both hands must be relaxed.

Hand placement is specific. Incorrect placement may give improper information and may disrupt the patient's mechanism. Place the pads of your fingers in the following positions:

1. Little finger on the squamous portion of the occiput
2. Ring finger behind the ear on the mastoid region of the temporal bone
3. Middle finger in front of the ear on the zygomatic process of the temporal bone
4. Index finger on the greater wing of the sphenoid
5. Thumbs resting gently (crossed or uncrossed) over the top of the head (Fig. 44.27)

Assess amplitude, flexion, extension, and specific motion of the individual bones. Treat the entire cranium. Pay special attention to the temporal bones. Dysfunctions may be treated with indirect technique or direct techniques applied to specific articular restrictions. Remember, you can progress only as fast as the patient's body can respond.

The sacrum has an involuntary motion pattern that is closely related to the motion of the head. This motion occurs

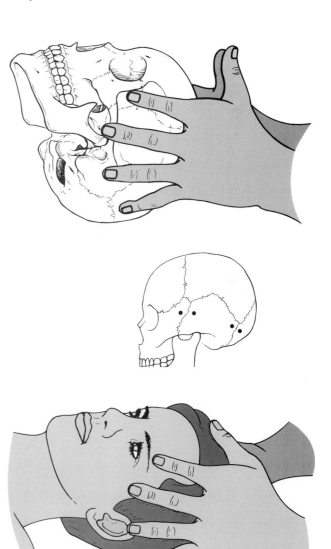

Figure 44.27. Finger position for vault hold.

about the respiratory axis located at the level of the second sacral segment. During craniosacral flexion, the base of the sacrum moves posterosuperiorly and the apex moves anteriorly (anatomic extension). During craniosacral extension, the base of the sacrum moves anteroinferiorly and the apex moves posteriorly (anatomic flexion).[1(pp.70–72)] Dysfunctions in sacral motion can affect the cranium and vice versa. Sacral motion can be assessed as follows:

1. Position the patient supine. Sit at the level of the patient's pelvis facing toward the head. Palpate with your dominant hand. If you are right-handed, sit on the patient's right side. If you are left-handed, sit on the patient's left side.
2. Place your dominant hand between the patient's legs and under the sacrum. The base of the sacrum should rest on your terminal phalanges.
3. Relax your hand and palpate the inherent motion. Follow the sacrum into flexion and extension. Is the motion smooth and symmetrical or is a dysfunction pattern present.

Sacral dysfunction can be treated using both direct (engage the barrier) or indirect (moving toward the direction of freer motion) technique. Continually listen with your fingers until a release occurs. Again, you can only progress as fast as the patient's body allows.

CONCLUSION

Symptoms in HEENT structures are frequently seen and may be sources of significant functional disability. Consider the structural and functional relationships between the structures of the head to diagnose more accurately various conditions and to implement appropriate treatment.

REFERENCES

1. Magoun HI. *Osteopathy in the Cranial Field.* 3rd ed. Kirksville, Mo: The Journal Printing Co; 1976.
2. Kuchera ML, Kuchera WA. *Osteopathic Considerations in Systemic Dysfunction.* 2nd ed. Columbus, Ohio: Greyden Press; 1994.
3. Moore KL. *Clinically Oriented Anatomy.* 3rd ed. Baltimore, Md: Williams & Wilkins; 1992.
4. Diamond S. *Clinical Symposia: Head Pain, Diagnosis and Management.* Summit, NJ: Ciba-Geigy Corp; 1994.

45. **Cervical Spine**

ROBERT E. KAPPLER

Key Concepts

- **Functional anatomy of the cervical spine, including skeletal, muscular, ligamentous, neural, vascular, and lymphatic aspects and motion biomechanics**

- **Diagnosis of cervical spine, using active and passive motion testing**

- **Occipital and C2-7 motion testing of the cervical spine**

- **Clinical information on cervical spine problems**

- **Treatment of symptomatic, unstable cervical spine complaints**

The cervical spine is of great significance to those who employ manipulative treatment. The cervical region is a pathway between the head and the thorax with neural, vascular, and musculoskeletal communication. Injury, pathology, or dysfunction may interfere with these vital communications.

FUNCTIONAL ANATOMY

Skeletal

The cervical spine consists of seven vertebral segments. The atlas (C1) and axis (C2) are atypical. The vertebral body of C2 is modified superiorly to form the dens (odontoid process). The atlas does not have a vertebral body; instead it rotates around the dens.[1] The superior surface of the atlas contains bilateral joint surfaces that articulate with the occipital condyles. The transverse processes of the atlas, called lateral masses, are modified and palpable. The spinous process of axis (C2) is palpable.

The articulation between C2 and C3 as well as the remainder of the cervical joints is considered typical. The facets are in a plane that points toward the eye. Rotation motion of the typical cervical segments follows the plane of the facets. Anterior or forward rotation is toward the eye rather than rotation in a horizontal plane.

A specialized set of synovial joints is present on the lateral surface of the vertebral bodies of the midcervical spine. They are known as uncovertebral joints (or uncinate) joints of Luschka. They provide stability to the cervical spine and de-

crease the likelihood of herniated nucleus pulposis in the cervical region.

There are no typical transverse processes. The anterior and posterior tubercles, which serve as muscle attachments, are the true transverse processes. The bone between the facets, which we palpate and consider as a transverse process, is known as the articular pillar. The lateral portions of the atlas are known as lateral masses.

The lateral portions of the cervical vertebra are modified to contain a foramen through which the vertebral artery passes. While this provides protection for the vertebral artery, it also creates the possibility of trauma to the artery from bony insult.

Muscular

The posterior spinal muscles are continuous from the cervical spine to the sacrum. Significant modification of these muscles occurs at C2, with a group of oblique muscles traversing from atlas and axis to the occiput. The anterior spinal muscles (prevertebral muscles) traverse from T3 to the occiput. The scalene muscles that go from the lateral portions of the cervical spine to the first and second rib act as lateral stabilizers as well as accessory muscles of respiration. The levator scapula muscle goes from the posterior tubercles to the upper medial border of the scapula. The general investing fascia splits to cover the sternocleidomastoid muscle anteriorly (mastoid process to sternum and clavicle) and the trapezius muscle posteriorly. Since the trapezius muscle attaches to the scapula, it is the primary connection between the head and neck and the shoulder girdle. The process of lifting with the upper extremity distributes force to the cervical spine. Anteriorly there are muscles that travel from the mandible to the hyoid to the sternum and clavicle.

Ligamentous

The cervical spine contains the usual spinal joint ligaments. The ribs do not attach to the cervical spine. The transverse ligament portion of the cruciate ligament supports the atlas in rotating about the dens. The anterior surface of the spinal cord lies immediately posterior to the transverse ligament. Rupture of this ligament (or laxity, which may occur with rheumatoid arthritis) creates the possibility of the dens contacting the spinal cord and causing catastrophic neurologic damage.

Neural

The spinal cord extends from the medulla in the brain through the cervical and thoracic spine to the L2 level of the lumbar

541

spine. Spinal cord injuries may occur from a number of different traumatic events, including:

Automobile and motorcycle accidents
Gunshots and stabbings
Diving into an empty swimming pool
Football and other violent contact sports

Damage to the cord may be ischemic as much as physical. Cervical spinal stenosis is a condition in which the spinal cord has insufficient room in the neural canal. Osteophyte formation contributes to stenosis, as does instability with excess fore-to-aft or side-to-side translation. A cervical disc may protrude posteriorly into the cord.

Disturbance of the vascular supply produces neurologic symptoms and damage. The vertebral artery may become occluded by thrombosis, which may be precipitated by injury to the artery as it passes through the intervertebral foramina and over the atlas, then enters the cranium through the foramen magnum. Arteriographic studies have shown that, in normal subjects, extension and rotation of the occiput produce a functional occlusion of the opposite vertebral artery.

The cervical cord gives rise to the cervical plexus and the brachial plexus. Since the brachial plexus innervates the upper extremity, nerve root impingement at the cervical intervertebral foramen produces not only neck pain but upper extremity neurological symptoms. Impingement of the nerve roots can occur from disc protrusion or osteophyte impingement.

Proprioceptive reflexes from the cervical spine create a muscle response in the lower extremity. Rotation of the cervical spine in unconscious subjects causes involuntary external rotation of the lower extremity in the direction of cervical rotation.[2] Another phenomenon is cervical vertigo[3–6] in which proprioceptive input from suboccipital muscles and ligaments or the sternocleidomastoid muscle can produce vertigo.

The sympathetic paraspinal trunk extends from the thoracic spine to the cranium and contains the superior, middle, and inferior cervical ganglia. In addition to efferent fibers, the small nociceptive afferents (C fibers) travel with the sympathetics and synapse in the upper thoracic cord; the cord contains intermediolateral cell columns. Nociceptive input from the cervical spine produces palpable musculoskeletal changes in the upper thoracic spine and ribs, as well as increased sympathetic activity from this area.[7–8] Upper thoracic and upper extremity problems may have their origin in the cervical spine.

Vascular

The arterial supply to the head and neck comes from the subclavian, carotid, and vertebral arteries. The carotid arteries lie anterior to the cervical vertebra. The carotid pulse may be palpated for diagnostic purposes. Avoid pressure over the carotid arteries while palpating the cervical spine.

Thoracic outlet syndromes involve neurovascular compression. Three anatomic sites are often considered:

1. Compression between anterior and middle scalene
2. Compression between clavicle and first rib
3. Compression between pectoralis minor and the upper ribs

Venous return from the upper extremity is not impaired by scalene tension, as the veins pass in front of the anterior scalene muscle.

Lymphatic

The brain is devoid of lymphatic channels; vascular return from the cranium is venous. However, cervical lymphatic drainage is important. Superficial nodes must penetrate the general investing fascia to connect with the deep channels that return lymph to the vascular compartment in the thorax. Infections and inflammation from the head, ear, nose, and throat require effective lymphatic drainage. Use fascial stretching/release to facilitate return as lymph channels pass through the general investing fascia. Use special lymphatic pump techniques in treating the neck. As always, the thoracic inlet must be free to allow lymph to return.

Motion Biomechanics

The major motions at the occiput (0-A joint) are flexion and extension. Side-bending and rotation are considered minor movements. The occiput rotates and side-bends in opposite directions. The occipital condyles converge anteriorly. The lateral portion of the atlas articulation is higher (more cephalad) than the medial portion. Posterior movement of the occiput causes a glide to the superior lateral portion, creating side-bending to the opposite side. Anterior rotation is associated with a medial, inferior glide. This gliding motion is considered a minor movement of the joint and is the motion involved in occipital joint restriction.

The major motion of the atlas–axis joint is rotation. Half of the rotation of the cervical spine occurs at the atlas. Cineradiographic studies show that there is a significant amount of flexion–extension of the atlas.[9–10] This motion does not seem to be involved in somatic dysfunction of the atlas. Side-bending is not a significant component of atlas movement. Cineradiographic studies have shown that during rotation, anteriorly or posteriorly, the atlas moves inferiorly on both sides, maintaining a horizontal orientation.[11] Side-bending restriction is usually not diagnosed or treated. The atlas rotates about the dens, and motion restriction of the atlas involves rotation. Motion testing involves rotation testing.

Motion of the typical cervical segments (C2 through C7) is similar to type II mechanics. Cineradiography shows that the cervical spine rotates and side-bends to the same side. Type I (neutral) mechanics have not been identified on cineradiography.[12–13] The vertebral bodies of typical cervical segments are saddle-shaped rather than flat on the superior and inferior surfaces. Side-bending of the cervical spine can produce lateral translation into the convexity. Some osteopathic physicians call this motion side-slip.

DIAGNOSIS

Inspection

Observe the skin for color changes. Look for asymmetry of position, including:

Flexion or extension
Side-bending to the right or left
Rotation to the right or left
Anterior posterior curves
Relationship of the head to the lateral weight-bearing line

Active Motion Testing

With the patient seated, ask him or her to:

Rotate to the right and to the left
Side-bend right and left (attempt to touch the ear to the shoulder)
Flex or touch the chin to the chest
Extend or backward bend

Occasionally, extension may produce lightheadedness. Record these motions in degrees. Measure the range with a goniometer. Osteopathic physicians may elect to bypass active motion testing and proceed directly to passive motion testing. If the patient has neck complaints or has sustained trauma, first determine the amount the patient can move.

PALPATION

The cervical spine may be palpated in the seated position as well as in the supine position. Tissues on the anterior and lateral portions of the neck can be comfortably assessed with the patient seated and the physician standing behind the patient. Palpate muscle tension, tenderness, and tissue texture abnormality (scalenes, sternocleidomastoid, trapezius). The examination of the neck with the patient seated and the examination of the upper thoracic spine are often integrated. Passive motion testing to evaluate the ability of muscles to lengthen is sometimes done (for example, side-bend cervical spine to evaluate scalene tension).

Palpation of the cervical spine with the patient supine allows for a detailed evaluation of tissue texture abnormality and tenderness surrounding the cervical spine. The suboccipital region contains muscles that are more lateral than the mid and lower cervical region, so paraspinal palpation must involve a more lateral placement of the fingers. Significant suboccipital tissue texture abnormality is usually associated with changes in the ipsilateral upper thoracic and rib angle area; look for them. Palpation over the posterior portion of the articular pillars reveals local muscle hypertonicity, tenderness, and tissue texture abnormality associated with segmental dysfunction. These changes are usually apparent with rotational restriction.

Palpation over the lateral margins of the articular pillars (locate fingers laterally; direct the palpatory force medially) reveals tenderness and tissue texture abnormality over the convex (anterior component) side of segmental dysfunction. For example, given C4 rotated and side-bent right with restriction of left rotation and side-bending, the posterior portion of the articular pillar is tender on the right side; the lateral margin of the articular pillar is tender on the left side.

The terms open facet and closed facet are sometimes applied as positional descriptors of cervical spine somatic dysfunction. Flexion motion (in a normal spine without motion restriction) causes the facets to open, while extension motion closes the facets. Side-bending motion with coupled rotation to the same side produces a concave side and a convex side. The facets on the concave side are closed, while the facets on the convex side are open. Given a condition of C5 extended, rotated, and side-bent right (restriction of flexion, rotation, and side-bending left), the right side is the concave side and the left side is the convex side. In motion testing, extension is free so both facets close. During flexion motion testing, the facet on the right side is closed and resists opening. This produces palpable asymmetry in which the right transverse process (technically, the articular pillar) is more posterior, and the paraspinal muscle over C5 right is tight and palpable. This concept can be applied to C2-7 segmental motion testing. If a segment is extended (flexion restriction), rotated, and side-bent right (restriction of rotation and side-bending left), flexing this segment, which is engaging the barrier, intensifies the palpable posterior transverse process on the right as well as the palpable muscle change. From this position of flexion, motion testing reveals a dominant restriction of left rotation and side-bending. If this segment is extended, the motion restriction is significantly less. Engaging the barrier in flexion or extension intensifies the rotation and side-bending restriction.

Passive Motion Testing

REGIONAL MOTION

Test the range of regional cervical rotation, side-bending, flexion, and extension with the patient in the supine position. Evaluate these motions by contacting the head bilaterally and introducing the motions through the head. The range of extension may be difficult to evaluate with the patient supine because the table gets in the way.

SEGMENTAL MOTION

A novice may test every segment. The experienced clinician tests those segments in which palpation and screening motion tests suggest that there is a problem.

The suboccipital area can be confusing. Neurologically, C1 and C2 are considered a common neurologic segment. Hyperactivity of the C1-2 segment potentially involves three joints: the occipitoatlantal (OA) joint, the atlantoaxial (AA) joint, and C2/C3. Therefore, positive palpatory findings in the suboccipital region demand testing of these three joints. Each joint is different in its motion, so they must be individually tested.

Occipital Motion Testing of C0-1

LATERAL TRANSLATION TEST

The physician stands or sits at the head of the supine patient. Grasp the head with both hands, with the finger tips of index and middle finger over the occipital articulation (Fig. 45.1). Translate the head to the right and to the left, evaluating freedom or resistance. A more precise method is to perform the lateral translation test in flexion and in extension. Flex the occiput (0-A), then translate to the right and to the left. Then extend the occiput and translate to the right and to the left. Restriction of right translation with freedom of left translation suggests an occiput rotated left and side-bent right (occiput posterior left). If translation is done in flexion and extension, restriction is encountered when the barrier is engaged. Restriction of right translation in the flexed position suggests an occiput that is extended, rotated left, and side-bent right with restriction of flexion, rotation right, side-bending left.

There are two OA joints, one on each side. Given a condition of occiput rotated right and side-bent left, the dominant restriction, tenderness, and tissue texture abnormality may be on the right side or it may be on the left side. In treating this dysfunction with high-velocity technique, it may be appropriate to localize force precisely to one side or the other side. The terminology that has been used by the osteopathic profession for years is positional terminology. *This in no way implies that positional diagnosis is preferred; identification of motion restriction is imperative.* In the above example of the occiput rotated right and side-bent left, the right side is called posterior occiput and the left side is called anterior occiput. A posterior occiput right exhibits motion restriction, tissue texture abnormality, and tenderness on the right side. An anterior occiput left exhibits motion restriction, tissue texture abnormality, and tenderness left. Do confirmatory motion tests. Focusing on one side at a time, assess freedom of flexion and extension. The posterior occiput

side exhibits restriction of extension. The anterior occiput side exhibits restriction of flexion.

ATLAS MOTION TEST

The atlas rotates in relation to the axis and becomes restricted in rotation. The motion test of atlas function is a rotation test. It is convenient to isolate cervical rotation to the atlas by flexing the cervical spine prior to rotation. This produces physiologic locking of C2-7. This is an example of the third principle of physiologic motion of the spine. Flexion of C2-7 effectively eliminates rotation in this area.

Stand or sit at the head of your supine patient. Grasp the head with the fingertips contacting the lateral mass of the atlas. Flex the cervical spine. Rotate to the right and to the left, assessing the range of motion, and freedom or resistance. (Fig. 45.2). A right-rotated atlas exhibits restriction of left rotation. Osteopathic positional terminology for this dysfunction is posterior atlas right. Flexion and extension and side-bending motions are not tested.

Some osteopathic physicians refer to an anterior atlas. The anterior side is opposite the posterior atlas. Given an example of atlas rotated right with restriction of left rotation, the right side would be the posterior atlas side. If the left side exhibited tenderness and tissue texture abnormality, it would be referred to as an anterior atlas left. These are not common, but when present are very symptomatic and tender. Retroorbital pain is often associated with an anterior atlas.

C2-7 Motion Testing

FLEXION AND EXTENSION TEST

At a segmental level, C2-7 motion is difficult to assess by directly flexing and extending, although this has been the method used by many osteopathic physicians in the past. The lateral

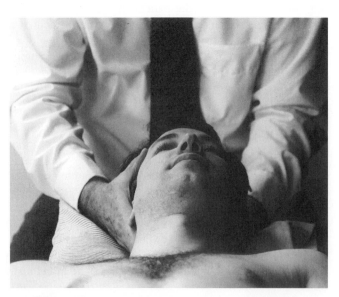

Figure 45.1. Lateral translation test for occipital motion.

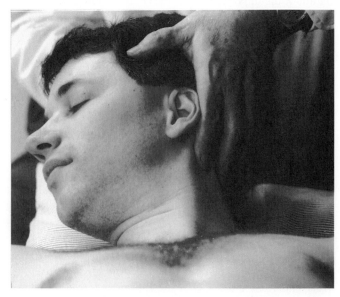

Figure 45.2. Rotation test for occipital motion.

translation test, which was used extensively by the Muscle Energy Tutorial Committee,[14] provides a more precise method of evaluating flexion and extension while evaluating side-bending.

LATERAL TRANSLATION TEST

The lateral translation test is similar to the occiput lateral translation test, except that the hand placement is on the cervical region with the fingertips over the lateral portion of the articular pillars. Stand or sit at the head of the supine patient. Support the patient's head with your hands, while palpating the lateral border of the articular pillars. Localizing the force to one segment, test lateral translation to the right and to the left with the segment flexed and with the segment extended. Restriction of right translation in the flexed position suggests extension. Right side-bending suggests right rotation with restriction of flexion, left side-bending, and left rotation (Fig. 45.3).

ROTATION TEST

A rotation test can be done, applying force to one segment at a time. Rotation movement should follow the planes of the facets, so the force is directed up toward the eye, rather than rotation in a horizontal plane. Stand or sit at the head of the supine patient. Support the patient's head, with your fingertips contacting the posterior surface of the articular pillars. Rotate (following the plane of the facets) to the right and to the left, assessing restriction or freedom. Remember, any normal segment should rotate both ways with equal range and freedom. Restriction of right rotation of C5 suggests a positional diagnosis of C5 left rotated, left side-bent with restriction of right rotation, right side-bending. The posterior transverse process is on the left (Fig. 45.4).

CLINICAL INFORMATION

Clinical information is available on cervical spine problems.

Suboccipital symptoms of tension and tissue change are al-

most always associated with upper thoracic and rib problems on the same side. It is important to treat the upper thoracic area first because of sympathetic influence and muscle connections. Testing the suboccipital area before and after treatment of the upper thoracics reveals a significant decrease in suboccipital findings.

The cervical prevertebral muscles (scalenes, longus group) are usually involved in acute neck problems. Gross cervical motion testing reveals restriction of rotation and side-bending to the same side. Sternocleidomastoid shortening causes rotation and side-bending to opposite sides. Treatment of scalene and prevertebral muscles must start with treatment of the upper thoracic spine. The functional base of the neck is the upper thoracic spine and ribs.

Acute extension trauma (whiplash) with actual injury to flexor muscles takes prolonged time to treat. Counterstrain, indirect fascial release, and cranial techniques are more appropriate for initial treatment. Look for an extended (flexion restriction) upper or mid thoracic somatic dysfunction as part of the injury. The sequence of treatment is as follows: first, the thoracic spine; second, the suboccipital area; and third, the rest of the cervical spine.

Acute torticollis with massive neck muscle spasm causes motion to be painful and limited. Use a muscle energy technique. Position the head at the midpoint of pain-free motion. Hold the head, and ask the patient to turn the head toward the restriction. Relax. Reposition the head a few degrees toward the restriction and repeat. Sometimes a significant improvement in range of motion is achieved. This technique is not classified as direct or indirect, in that the barrier is not engaged nor is the neck positioned in the other direction. Instead, the neck is positioned in the middle, with the ultimate objective of reaching the barrier.

Cervical root irritation or compression from osteophyte or disc produces nerve-related symptoms in the upper extremity, such as pain, numbness, or muscle weakness. Careful neurologic testing reveals the nerve root dysfunction. Remember that

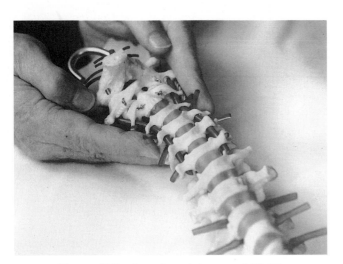

Figure 45.3. Lateral translation test of C2-C7.

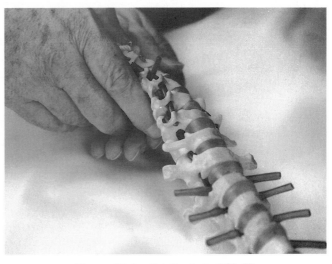

Figure 45.4. Rotation test of C2-C7.

the thumb is innervated by the upper portion of the brachial plexus, the little finger by the lowest portion. Look for sensory loss and motor weakness with decreased deep tendon reflexes. The biceps reflex tests C5, the triceps reflex tests C7. Palpable flaccidity of arm muscles may be present. Sometimes the nerve root irritation is intermittent and insufficient to produce any neurologic deficit.

Cervical root irritation usually produces a reflex change in the interscapular area, which then produces arm symptoms. A recalcitrant interscapular problem might be due to a reflex from the cervical spine. Many patients with cervical root problems experience shoulder pain when they lie supine on the table. Often, extension of the neck exacerbates the symptoms. Oblique cervical spine x-ray views reveal osteophytes (cervical spondylosis). Electromyography confirms any neurological findings. Magnetic resonance imaging is an outstanding method of imaging cervical discs. CT scans also reveal encroachment. Cervical myelograms are not being done as often as before, as this is an invasive test and noninvasive tests are now available.

TREATMENT

The following are treatment guidelines for symptomatic, unstable cervical spine problems:

1. Avoid high-velocity manipulation of the cervical spine.
2. Decrease muscle tension. Treatment of the upper thoracic spine and ribs is essential to accomplish this goal.
3. Counterstrain, cranial, and indirect techniques are the least traumatic to the neck. Muscle energy technique, if done without pain, is appropriate.
4. Traction, with proper direction of force, is appropriate.

CONCLUSION

Manipulative treatment of the cervical spine can greatly assist healing of injury, pathology, or dysfunction of the cervical region. This region serves as a pathway between the head and the thorax with neural, vascular, and musculoskeletal communication.

REFERENCES

1. Warwick R, Williams PL, eds. *Gray's Anatomy*. British 35th ed. Philadelphia, Pa: WB Saunders Co; 1973:235.
2. Aston-Jones G, Valentino R. Brain noradrenergic neurons, nociception and stress: basic mechanisms and clinical implications. In: Willard FH, Patterson MM, eds. *Nonciception and the Neuroendocrine–Immune Connection, 1992 International Symposium*. Indianapolis, Ind: American Academy of Osteopathy; 1992:107–132.
3. Wing L, Hadephobes WW. Cervical vertigo. *Aust N Z J Surg*. 1974; 44(3):275–277.
4. Jepson O. Dizziness origination in the columna cervicalis. *J Can Chiropractic Assoc*. 1967;11(1):7–8.
5. Hargrave WW. The cervical syndrome. *Aust J Physiotherapy*. 1972; Dec 18:144–147.
6. Greenman P. *Principles of Manual Medicine*. Baltimore, Md: Williams & Wilkins; 1989:125.
7. Payan D. Peripheral neuropeptides, inflammation and nociception. In: Willard FW, Patterson MM, eds. *Nociception and the Neuroendocrine–Immune Connection, 1992 International Symposium*. Indianapolis, Ind: American Academy of Osteopathy; 1992:34–46.
8. deGroat W. Spinal cord processing of visceral and somatic nociceptive input. In: Willard FW, Patterson MM, eds. *Nociception and the Neuroendocrine–Immune Connection, 1992 International Symposium*. Indianapolis, Ind: American Academy of Osteopathy; 1992:47–73.
9. Hosono N, Yonenobu K. Cineradiographic motion analysis of atlantoaxial instability in os odontoideum. *Spine*. 1991;16(suppl 10)Oct:S480–S482.
10. Van Mameren H, Sanches H. Cervical spine motion in the sagittal plane II. *Spine*. 1992;May17(5):467–474.
11. Kirksville College of Osteopathic Medicine. *Cineradiographic Studies of the Atlas* [film]. Kirksville, Mo: Kirksville College of Osteopathic Medicine; 1970. (This tape was later erased and lost.)
12. Felding J. Cineroentgenography of the normal cervical spine. *J Bone Joint Surg*. 1957;39A:1280–1288.
13. Ochs C, Romine J. Radiographic examination of the cervical spine in motion. *United States Naval Med Bull*. 1974;64:21–29.
14. Mitchell F Jr. *The Muscle Energy Manual, I*. East Lansing, Mich: MET Press; 1995:166–167.

46. **Upper Extremities**

ROBERT E. KAPPLER AND KENNETH A. RAMEY

By extensive study, I have formed in my head a perpetual image of every articulation in the framework of the human body.[1]

—A.T. STILL

Key Concepts

- **Functional anatomy of upper extremities, including assessment of range of motion**

- **Muscle groups and innervations of glenohumeral and scapulothoracic joints, and elbow and wrist**

- **Arterial and venous supply to the area**

- **Lymphatic drainage of upper extremities**

- **Sympathetic innervation and brachial plexus**

- **Diagnosis by history and physical examination, including observation, palpation, pulses, several reflexes, motor strength, and sensation**

- **Motion testing of shoulder, and costovertebral, costosternal, sternoclavicular, acromioclavicular, and scapulothoracic joints**

- **Configuration, physiologic motion, and somatic dysfunction of elbow and forearm**

- **Configuration, physiologic motion, and somatic dysfunction of wrist and hand, including intercarpal, carpometacarpal, metacarpophalangeal, and interphalangeal joints**

- **Special tests, including Adson's, Yergason, drop arm, apprehension, bicipital; tendinitis, Apley "scratch," Tinel's sign, Palen, Allen's, and tennis elbow tests**

- **Treatment of carpal tunnel syndrome, reflex sympathetic dystrophy, adhesive capsulitis, and thoracic outlet syndrome**

The upper extremities are vital to a person's ability to perform the activities of daily living. Even minor injuries may produce disabilities significantly affecting a patient's overall function. Effective diagnosis and treatment necessitates a thorough understanding of the structure and function of this important region.

FUNCTIONAL ANATOMY

Skeletal and Arthrodial Structures

The bones of each upper limb include the:

Clavicle
Scapula
Humerus
Radius
Ulna
Eight carpal bones
Five metacarpal bones
Fourteen phalanges

Functionally, the upper extremity can be divided into the:[2]

Scapulothoracic joint
Acromioclavicular joint
Sternoclavicular joint
Glenohumeral joint
Elbow
Wrist
Intercarpal, carpometacarpal, metacarpophalangeal, and interphalangeal joints

The scapulothoracic joint is formed by the articulation of the anterior surface of the scapula with the posterior thorax. Considerable motion is possible:

Elevation
Depression
Protraction

Retraction
Rotation about a transverse axis

The sternoclavicular joint is formed by the articulation of the medial end of the clavicle with the manubrium of the sternum. This joint may become sprained by clavicular displacement in relation to the sternum.

The acromioclavicular joint is formed by the articulation of the lateral end of the clavicle with the acromion of the scapula. Functionally, this joint acts as a ball and socket providing anteroposterior, superoinferior, and rotational motion.

The glenohumeral joint is formed by the articulation of the head of the humerus with the glenoid fossa of the scapula. The motions of this joint include flexion–extension, abduction–adduction, and internal–external rotation.

The elbow joint is formed by the articulation of the humerus, ulna, and radius. The true elbow joint is the ulnohumeral joint. The proximal ulnohumeral joint, which allows supination and pronation of the forearm, is also located on the lateral side of the elbow joint. Possible motions include flexion–extension and abduction–adduction of the ulna on the humerus; the pivotal motion for pronation and supination of the forearm is provided by the proximal radioulnar joint.

The wrist is formed by the junction of the ulna, radius, and the carpal bones. The true wrist joint is the radiocarpal joint, formed by the distal end of the radius and the three proximal carpal bones: the scaphoid, lunate, and the triquetral. Possible motions include flexion–extension and abduction–adduction, as well as supination and pronation of the hand and forearm.

Articulations in the hand include the

Intercarpal joints
Carpometacarpal joints
Metacarpophalangeal joints
Interphalangeal joints

Osteopathic diagnosis largely involves the assessment of both quality and quantity of motion. General ranges of motion permit effective screening of the skeletal and arthrodial components of this region.

There is a ratio of movement between abduction of the arm at the glenohumeral joint and rotation of the scapulothoracic articulation: for every 3° of abduction measured at the glenohumeral joint, 2° actually occurred at the glenohumeral joint and 1° occurred at the scapulothoracic articulation. When the arm is fully abducted to 180°, 120° was due to the glenohumeral joint motion alone and 60° was due to rotation of the scapula and clavicle to elevate those structures 60° (Tables 46.1–46.3).

Somatic dysfunction typically involves restriction and the end of a range of motion. It is most likely to be found in the minor motion(s) of each joint. Orthopaedic problems associated with disruption of joint stabilizers commonly involve laxity and instability at the end of a range of motion. The most time-effective yet thorough examination involves screening ranges of motion with careful attention to end-motion palpatory finding.

Muscles

Muscles generally act in groups to produce specific motions. Detailed assessment of the upper extremity necessitates an understanding of these groups and their innervations.[2] Tables 46.4–46.7 present the muscles of the following joints:[2]

Glenohumeral joint (Table 46.4)
Scapulothoracic joint (Table 46.5)
Elbow (Table 46.6)
Wrist (Table 46.7)

Arterial Supply

The left subclavian artery arises from the posterior part of the arch of the aorta. It passes posterior to the left sternoclavicular joint. The right subclavian artery arises from the brachiocephalic trunk.[3] The subclavian arteries pass over the top of the first rib between the anterior and middle scalene muscles. The subclavian artery becomes the axillary artery at the lateral border of the first rib. The axillary artery passes posterior to the pectoralis minor muscle and becomes the brachial artery at the inferior border of the teres major muscle. Branches from the axillary and brachial arteries supply structures of the shoulder, arm, forearm, and hand. Somatic dysfunction of the following structures may affect arterial supply:

Anterior and middle scalenes
Upper thoracic vertebrae

Table 46.1
Major Motions of the Shoulder, Elbow, Wrist, and Metacarpophalangeal Joints

Glenohumeral Joint	Elbow	Wrist	Metacarpophalangeal
Abduction 180°	Flexion 135°	Supination 90°	Flexion 90°
Adduction 45°	Extension 0–5°	Pronation 90°	Extension 30–45°
Flexion 90°		Flexion 80°	
Extension 45°		Extension 70°	
Internal rotation 55°		Ulnar deviation 30°	
External rotation 40–45°		Radial Deviation 20°	

Reprinted with permission from Hoppenfeld S. *Physical Examination of the Spine and Extremities.* New York, NY: Appleton-Century-Crofts 1976.

Table 46.2
Major Motions of the Proximal and Distal Interphalangeal (IP) Joints

Proximal Interphalangeal Joint	Distal Interphalangeal Joint
Flexion 100°	Flexion 90°
Extension 0°	Extension 20°

Reprinted with permission from Hoppenfeld S. *Physical Examination of the Spine and Extremities.* New York, NY: Appleton-Century-Crofts 1976.

Upper ribs
Clavicles
Fascia of the upper extremity

Venous Supply

The axillary vein lies on the medial side of the axillary artery. The axillary vein receives tributaries that correspond to the branches of the axillary artery and receives venae comitantes of the brachial artery. It ends at the lateral border of the first rib where it becomes the subclavian vein.[3] The subclavian vein passes over the first rib anterior to the anterior scalene muscle.[3] The subclavian vein unites with the internal jugular vein to become the brachiocephalic vein.[3] The left brachiocephalic vein passes posterior to the left sternoclavicular joint and crosses the midline. The right brachiocephalic vein passes posterior to the right sternoclavicular joint. The right brachioce-

phalic vein joins the left brachiocephalic vein to form the superior vena cava.[3] Dysfunction in the upper thoracic vertebrae (causing increased sympathetic tone to the upper extremities), upper ribs, clavicles, and fascia of the upper extremities may impair venous return. Since the vein passes anterior to the scalene muscles, scalene tension does not create venous distention of the upper extremity.

Lymphatic Drainage

The major lymph nodes of the upper extremities are found in the fibrofatty connective tissue of the axilla. They are arranged into five groups, four of which lie inferior to the pectoralis minor tendon and one superior to it. These are the:

Pectoral
Lateral
Subscapular
Central
Apical

The pectoral group of axillary lymph nodes lies along the medial wall to the axilla. This group receives lymph mainly from the anterior thoracic wall and breast. The efferent vessels from these nodes pass to the central and apical groups of axillary lymph nodes.[3]

The lateral group of lymph nodes lies along the

Table 46.3
Major Motions of the Joints of the Thumb

Thumb	Thumb Metacarpophalangeal Joint	Thumb Interphalangeal Joint
Palmar abduction 70°	Flexion 50°	Flexion 90°
Palmar adduction 0°	Extension 0°	Extension 90°

Table 46.4
Muscles of the Glenohumeral Joint and Shoulder

Primary flexors	Deltoid (anterior portion) muscle	Axillary nerve,	C5
	Coracobrachialis muscle	Musculocutaneous nerve	C5–6
Secondary flexors	*Pectoralis major muscle (clavicular head)*		
	Biceps		
Primary abductor	Deltoid (midportion) muscle	Axillary nerve,	C5–6
	Supraspinatus muscle	Suprascapular nerve	C5–6
Secondary abductors	*Deltoid muscle (anterior, posterior)*		
	Serratus anterior muscle via scapula		
Primary adductor	Pectoralis major muscle	Anterior thoracic nerve (medial, lateral)	C5–T1
	Latissimus dorsi muscle		
Secondary adductors	*Teres minor muscle*		
	Anterior deltoid muscle		
Primary extensors	Latissimus dorsi muscle	Thoracodorsal nerve	C6–8
	Teres major muscle	Lower subscapular nerve	C5–6
	Deltoid (posterior portion)	Axillary nerve	C5–6
Secondary extensors	*Teres minor muscle*		
	Triceps (long head) muscle		
Primary external rotators	Infraspinatus	Suprascapular nerve	C5–6
	Teres minor	Axillary branch	C5
Secondary external rotators	*Deltoid muscle (posterior portion)*		
Primary internal rotators	Subscapularis muscle	Subscapular nerves (upper and lower portion)	C5–6
	Pectoralis major muscle	Anterior thoracic nerves (medial and lateral)	C5–T1
	Latissimus dorsi muscle		
	Teres minor muscle		
Secondary internal rotators	*Deltoid muscle (anterior portion)*		

Table 46.5
Muscles of the Scapulothoracic Joint

Primary elevators	Trapezius muscle	Accessory nerve	CN XI
	Levator scapulae muscle	Dorsal scapular N. C5 (plus)	C3–4, C5
Secondary elevators	*Rhomboid major muscle*		
	Rhomboid minor muscle		
Primary protraction	Serratus anterior muscle	Long thoracic N.	C5–7
Primary retraction	Rhomboid major muscle	Dorsal scapular	C5
	Rhomboid minor muscle	Dorsal scapular N.,	C5
Secondary retractor	*Trapezius muscle*		

Table 46.6
Muscles of the Elbow Joint

Primary flexors	Brachialis muscle	Musculocutaneous nerve	C5–6
	Biceps muscle	Musculocutaneous nerve	C5–6
Secondary flexors	*Brachioradialis muscle*		C6
	Supinator muscle		
Primary extensor	Triceps muscle	Radial nerve	C7
Secondary extensor	*Anconeus muscle*		

Table 46.7
Muscles of the Wrist

Primary flexors	Flexor carpi Radialis muscle	Median nerve	
	Flexor carpi Ulnaris muscle	Ulnar nerve	
Primary extensors	Extensor carpi Radialis longus m.	Radial nerve	C6 (7)
	Extensor carpi Radialis brevis m.	Radial nerve	
	Extensor carpi Ulnaris muscle	Radial nerve	
Primary supinators	Biceps muscle		
	Supinator muscle	Radial nerve	
Secondary supinator	*Brachioradialis m.*		
Primary pronator	Pronator teres muscle	Median nerve	C6
	Pronator quadratus m.	Median n. (ant. interosseous branch)	
Secondary pronator	*Flexor carpi radialis m.*		

lateral wall of the axilla. This group receives lymph from most of the upper limb.

The subscapular group of axillary lymph nodes is located along the posterior aspect of the thoracic wall and scapular region. Efferent vessels pass from here to the central group of axillary lymph nodes.

The central group of axillary lymph nodes is situated deep to the pectoralis minor near the base of the axilla. This group receives lymph from the other axillary lymph nodes. Efferent vessels pass lymph to the apical lymph nodes.

The apical group of axillary lymph nodes is situated in the apex of the axilla. This group receives lymph from the central lymph nodes. The efferent vessels from this group unite to form the subclavian lymphatic trunk. The right subclavian lymphatic trunk drains into the right lymphatic duct. The left subclavian lymphatic trunk drains into the thoracic duct. Somatic dysfunctions affecting the venous system may also affect lymphatic drainage, thereby producing congestion in the upper extremity.

Sympathetics

The sympathetic innervation to the upper extremities arises from the upper thoracic spinal cord. The sympathetic ganglia lie anterior to the rib head, in the fascia common to both structures. Dysfunction in the upper thoracic spine and ribs may increase sympathetic tone to the upper extremity and produce altered motion, nerve dysfunction, and lymphatic and venous congestion. Increased sympathetic tone is accompanied by palpatory findings in the upper thoracic/rib area. It also increases the sensitivity to painful stimulus and reduces both arterial blood getting to the structures of the arm and lymphatic fluids returning from the arm via the lymphatic vessels. The cause of these musculoskeletal findings may be viscerosomatic; they may be primary somatic in the area, or they may be reflex from the cervical spine. Nociceptive afferents from the cervical spine travel in the sympathetic chain and synapse in the intermediolateral cell columns of the upper thoracic cord. This produces an irritable focus in the cord, with resulting somatic and sympathetic hyperactivity.

Brachial Plexus

Nerve roots C5–8, and T1 form the brachial plexus. These nerve roots pass through the intervertebral foramen of the cervical vertebrae and pass between the anterior and middle scalene muscles. The roots unite to form successive trunks, divisions, cords, and branches. The nerve trunks extend from the scalene triangle (formed by the anterior and middle scalenes and the clavicle) to the clavicle. Nerve divisions extend from a position posterior to the clavicle to the axilla. Nerve cords are found in the axilla. Nerve cords divide into branches that innervate various structures in the upper extremity. The neurovascular bundle of the arm contains the subclavian artery, subclavian vein, brachial plexus, and the sympathetic nerve plexus.

DIAGNOSIS

History

When is arm pain something more? Upper extremity discomfort cannot always be attributed to dysfunction in this area. A good clinician must determine whether the discomfort is primarily caused by dysfunction in the extremity or referred from another area.

If the cause lies in the upper extremity itself, there is generally restricted motion. Pain is usually localized to specific dermatomes and may be described as acute, sharp, and severe. Discomfort is usually improved by rest, is frequently reproduced by motion, and may lead to the perception of strength loss.

If the discomfort is referred from another area (lungs, diaphragm, stomach, intestines, heart, cervical spine), passive motion does not appear restricted. Pain is diffuse and poorly localized and may be described as nagging, achy, or dull. Discomfort is usually worse at night. Discomfort is frequently related to symptoms in other areas (difficulty breathing, chest pain, cough, gastrointestinal upset) and may not be reproduced by motion. Motion is generally good, but decreased strength or muscle atrophy is possible (e.g., disk herniation).

Observation

Observation begins the moment the patient walks into the room. Observe the patient's overall posture and motion. Is there any abnormality? Observe the patient in the standing position. Look at the height of the shoulders. A low shoulder may be the result of a short leg or a lateral curve. Look at the spine from the side. Is the thoracic kyphotic curve normal, increased, or decreased? An area of thoracic spine flattening may indicate the presence of an extended somatic dysfunction. Dysfunction in the upper thoracic spine may alter sympathetic tone and produce dysfunction in the upper extremity. Begin at the shoulder and examine the skin of the upper extremity. Is there any asymmetry? Areas that appear reddened or have pigment changes may have somatic dysfunction. Observe the various muscle groups bilaterally. Is there evidence of hypertrophy or atrophy? Look for the presence of fasciculations (small tremors) in the muscle.

Palpation

Begin by palpating the superficial tissues of the shoulders. Palpate into the deeper tissues. Look for signs of acute or chronic tissue texture change. Remember to compare the right side with the left side and areas located superiorly with areas located inferiorly. Compare muscle groups bilaterally for size and tone.

Pulses

Thorough examination of the upper extremities necessitates an examination of the brachial and radial pulses. The brachial pulse is found on the medial surface of the arm just medial to the biceps tendon. The radial pulse is best palpated over the lateral and ventral side of the wrist. Examine the arterial pulses with the distal pads of the second, third, and fourth fingers. Palpate firmly but not so hard that the artery is occluded. Arterial pulses can be examined for:

Heart rate and rhythm
Pulse contour (wave form)
Amplitude (strength)
Symmetry

Lack of symmetry between the left and right extremities suggests impaired circulation. The amplitude of the pulse can be described on the scale shown in Table 46.8.[4]

Reflexes

The three basic reflexes that evaluate the integrity of the nerve supply to the upper extremity are the biceps reflex, the brachioradialis reflex, and the triceps reflex. Each of these is a deep tendon reflex (lower motor neuron reflex) transmitted to the cord as far as the anterior horn cells and returning to the muscle via the peripheral nerves. Reflexes may be increased in the presence of an upper motor neuron lesion or may be decreased in the presence of a lower motor neuron lesion (bulging disk).

BICEPS REFLEX

This primarily tests the integrity of neurologic level C5. Place the patient's arm over your opposite arm so that it rests upon your forearm. With your elbow supporting the patient's arm under the elbow's medial side, place your thumb on the tendon of the biceps in the cubital fossa. Instruct the patient to rest the arm on your forearm and relax. Tap your thumbnail with a neurologic hammer. The biceps should jerk slightly. You should be able to see or feel its movement.

BRACHIORADIALIS REFLEX

This tests neurologic level C6. Support the patient's arm in the same manner used to test the biceps reflex. Tap the brachioradialis tendon at the distal end of the radius with the neurologic hammer.

TRICEPS REFLEX

This reflex tests neurologic level C7. Use the same position as above. Tap the triceps tendon where it crosses the olecranon fossa.[2] Remember to compare both sides. Reflexes may be graded as shown in Table 46.9.

Table 46.8
Standard Method for Recording Amplitude of the Pulse

4/4	Bounding
3/4	*Full, Increased*
2/4	Expected
1/4	*Diminished, barely palpable*
0	Absent, not palpable

Table 46.9
Standard Method for Recording Amplitude of a Reflex

0	Absent
1/4	Decreased but present
2/4	Normal
3/4	Brisk with unsustained clonus
4/4	Brisk with sustained clonus

Table 46.10
Standard Method for Recording Motor Strength

5/5	Normal	Complete range of motion against gravity with full resistance
4/5	Good	Complete range of motion against gravity with some resistance
3/5	Fair	Complete range of motion against gravity
2/5	Poor	Complete range of motion with gravity eliminated
1/5	Trace	Evidence of slight contractility. No joint motion
0	Zero	No evidence of contractility

Motor Strength

The strength of various muscle groups can be evaluated by applying force in a manner that loads the muscle as the patient resists. Remember to test the uninjured side first. Table 46.10 shows a standard method of recording motor strength.

Differences in muscle strength may be subtle. Compare the strength of various groups in different positions to get the full clinical picture. There are some simple screening procedures that are useful. Palpation for flaccidity, while not a test of strength, may reveal muscles that should be tested. For cervical root or brachial plexus problems, perform a grip strength test by asking the patient to squeeze two of your fingers. Another simple test is to ask the patient to squeeze the thumb and index finger together, and then you try to pull them apart. If normal strength is present, it is difficult to pull them apart.

Sensation

This can be tested by light touch, pinprick, or two-point discrimination. Compare both sides and areas located superiorly with areas located inferiorly. Look for areas of either decreased or increased sensation. Sensation around the upper extremity is controlled by five different nerve supplies:

1. C5 controls the lateral arm
2. C6 controls the lateral forearm
3. C7 controls the index finger
4. C8 controls the medial forearm
5. T1 controls the medial arm

Motion Testing

SHOULDER MOTION

Shoulder motions can be screened by using gross motion analysis or by the seven motions of Spencer. Gross motions can be screened by having the patient:

Abduct the arm to put the palms together overhead
Abduct the arm to put the back of the hands together overhead
Reach across the chest to touch the opposite shoulder
Reach behind the body to scratch the opposite shoulder (Apley's scratch test)

Internal and external rotation may be tested as follows:[5]

1. With the arm at the side, the forearm is flexed 90° at the elbow and the elbow is supported. The forearm is turned medially to test internal rotation and laterally to test external rotation.
2. With the arm abducted 90° at the shoulder, the forearm is flexed 90° at the elbow and the elbow is supported. An anterior arc of the forearm produces internal rotation, and a posterior arc produces external rotation.

Testing of the shoulder can be localized to the glenohumeral joint by stabilizing the scapula with one hand as the arm is moved with the other. A gross test of stability of the glenohumeral joint is to stabilize scapula and translate the head of the humerus anteriorly and posteriorly. Compare both sides. An unstable joint moves too freely; with adhesive capsulitis, there is no motion. Motion of the entire shoulder girdle is evaluated without stabilizing the scapula to isolate glenohumeral motion. In evaluating total shoulder girdle motion, observe the amount of scapulothoracic motion as the shoulder girdle moves. Most shoulder problems involve dysfunction of muscles. Malposition of the scapula alters the working length of a shoulder girdle muscle. Treatment of shoulder problems necessitates and often starts with evaluation and treatment of scapulothoracic position and motion.

The seven motions of Spencer systematically test all shoulder motions and can be expanded to include a treatment mode should any restrictions be identified. During testing and treatment, the scapula is fixed in position to permit movement only at the glenohumeral joint:

1. Extend the upper extremity 90°.
2. Flex the upper extremity 180°.
3. Circumduct the upper extremity while compressing the glenohumeral joint (tests joint surfaces).
4. Circumduct the upper extremity while applying traction (tests the capsule).
5. Abduct the upper extremity 90°.
6. Place the patient's hand behind the small of the back and gently test internal rotation by pulling the elbow forward.
7. Extend the upper extremity and apply traction and caudal glide to the humerus while holding the proximal end of the humerus.
8. Sometimes the physician finishes by holding the patient's hand with the upper extremity extended and shaking the upper extremity up and down while carrying the upper extremity through an arch in a parasagittal plane to the limits of comfort.

If the seven gross motions tested using Spencer's techniques are normal, then the shoulder is considered to have good function.[5]

COSTOVERTEBRAL JOINTS

These are the true costovertebral and costotransverse joints of the first rib. Both of these joints are synovial. The first rib is an atypical rib and articulates only with the body of T1. The common somatic dysfunction of the first rib is elevation: the rib moves freely in elevation and has a restriction of motion to depression. Motion is tested by placing your thumbs over the posterior aspect of the rib and instructing the patient to take a deep breath. Assess the quality of motion in both inhalation (elevation) and exhalation (depression). Frequently T1 is rotated and side-bent to the side opposite to the side of the elevated first rib.

COSTOSTERNAL JOINT OF THE FIRST RIB

This is a synchondrosis, not a synovial joint. It is therefore very stable. Its functional purpose is more for support than for motion. Because of this stability, somatic dysfunction is not often found in this area.

STERNOCLAVICULAR JOINT

This is a complex synovial joint that contains a cartilaginous meniscus. The subclavius muscle depresses and pulls the medial end of the first rib forward when the lateral end of the clavicle is elevated. There are three axes of motion in the sternoclavicular joint. These are tested by having the patient shrug the shoulders up and down, forward and backward, and internally and externally rotating the shoulder while bridging and palpating the joint with your fingers.

ACROMIOCLAVICULAR JOINT

This joint also has motion about three axes; motion about each axis is difficult to palpate. Separation of the joint is palpated by placing your fingers over the joint and adducting the arm across the thorax. The most common somatic dysfunction of this joint involves a functional glide of the clavicle upward and laterally along the acromion. Acromioclavicular (AC) separation goes beyond somatic dysfunction and is a true sprain. The extent of injury can be easily evaluated by palpating the AC joint and applying a downward traction to the humerus. The extent of gaping is a measure of the injury. This physical examination test is also very useful in evaluating healing. Treatment of AC separation is usually a matter of taking care of the accompanying thoracic cage problems, which are always present. The joint heals itself, and surgery is rarely needed.

SCAPULOTHORACIC JOINT

This pseudojoint allows the scapula to glide medially and laterally, superiorly, and inferiorly, and rotate over the posterolateral chest cage. The position of the scapula can be evaluated in a seated or standing examination. Asymmetry of position of the scapula usually indicates asymmetry of motion. Scapular motion can be tested with the patient lying on his or her side.

Grasp the scapula with both hands and take it through the various motions. The scapula can:[5]

1. Glide forward and separate each vertebral border 15 cm and glide backward to bring the vertebral borders closer
2. Glide 10–12 cm superiorly and inferiorly
3. Rotate to elevate or depress the glenoid fossa 30° each way

ELBOW AND FOREARM

Configuration and Physiologic Motion

The ulnohumeral joint is the true elbow joint.[6] The head of the radius at the proximal end of the radial bone near the elbow is not a part of the elbow joint. Primary motion of the normal elbow is 160° of flexion and 0° of extension about a transverse axis (10° of hyperextension is found in some individuals). The elbow joint is stable medially and laterally but weak anteriorly and posteriorly. Its anteroposterior stability and strength depends on the muscles that pass anteriorly and posteriorly to the elbow joint and on how firmly the trochlea of the humerus fits into the trochlear notch of the ulna. The medial side of the ulnar notch is anatomically elongated and there is a slight ridge in its joint surface. There is also a grooved spiral in the humeral joint surfaces. The groove–spiral anatomical characteristic causes the hand to normally move toward the mouth when the elbow is flexed and to the lateral side of the hip during extension of the elbow. This structural configuration also produces the normal carrying angle of the arm, greater in the female than in the male. This carrying angle is not very noticeable if the arm is hanging at the side of a person because in this position the forearm has a natural partial pronation.

The elbow also "wobbles" into ulnar adduction during its normal motion. An abduction somatic dysfunction of the ulna increases the carrying angle, and adduction somatic dysfunction decreases the carrying angle (Fig. 46.1). As the distal end of the ulna is abducted, the olecranon process glides more medially. This reciprocal movement of the two ends of the ulna also occurs with adduction. It is restriction in one of these glides and ease in the opposite glide that constitutes ulnar somatic dysfuncion. Somatic dysfunction of the elbow joint is named according to the motion that is present, that is, ulnar abduction or ulnar adduction (Fig. 46.2).

The true wrist is the ellipsoid synovial radiocarpal joint (Fig. 46.3) formed by a concavity in the distal end of the radius, three proximal carpal bones of the wrist (the navicular or scaphoid bone in the snuff box of the wrist, the lunate, and the triquetral bones), and an articular disk. The articular disk separates the true wrist joint from the distal radioulnar joint; the head of the ulna (the distal end of the ulna) is not a part of the true wrist joint.

The true elbow and wrist joints are functionally linked with the radius by proximal and distal synovial radiocarpal joints and a fibrous middle radiocarpal joint called the interosseous membrane (Fig. 46.4). The interosseous membrane maintains functional symmetry and stability of the forearm while the proximal and distal radioulnar joints allow pivot action, per-

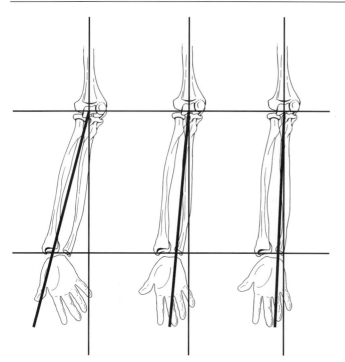

Figure 46.1. Carrying angle and parallelogram effect. (Illustration by W.A. Kuchera.)

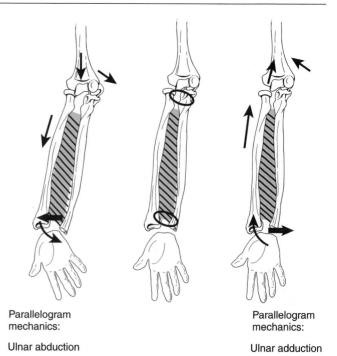

Parallelogram
mechanics:

Ulnar abduction

Parallelogram
mechanics:

Ulnar adduction

Figure 46.2. Ulnar abduction (*left*) and adduction (*right*). (Illustration by W.A. Kuchera.)

mitting supination and pronation of the hand. The fibers of the interosseous membrane extend cephalad from attachment on the ulna to a more proximal attachment on the radius. This arrangement allows the bones of the forearm to share the forces of compression whether they occur from the hand upward or the shoulder downward. Note the reciprocal glide of the radial head in response to the direction of movement at the distal end of the radius in Figure 46.7.

The radius and ulna are held in a parallelogram arrangement by the radiocarpal joints (Fig. 46.5). The ulna is part of the elbow joint, and the radius is part of the wrist joint. The radius is able to move more freely than the ulna. With the ulna relatively fixed at the ulnohumeral joint and the radius fairly fixed at the radiocarpal joint (especially with the scaphoid), abduction or adduction of the ulna results in a reciprocal positioning of the hand (Fig. 46.2). During abduction of the ulna, the radius glides distally and the wrist is literally pushed into increased adduction. During adduction of the ulna, the radius glides proximally and the wrist is pulled into a more abducted position, compared with the position of the opposite wrist. If this reciprocal positioning principle of the elbow and the wrist is incorporated in the direct and indirect treatment of ulnar abduction or adduction somatic dysfunctions, these techniques will become more effective and efficient. The parallelogram arrangement of the forearm bones with the action of the proximal and distal radioulnar joints permits forearm/wrist motions. The interosseous membrane (a radioulnar fibrous joint) provides stability to the forearm and prevents stress of the ligaments and/or bony compression in the forearm or the wrist as these motions occur.

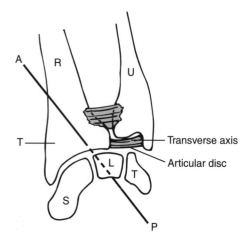

Figure 46.3. Right radiocarpal joint (true wrist joint) and distal radioulnar joint. *R*, radius (bone); *U*, ulna (bone); *S*, scaphoid (bone); *L*, lunate (bone); *T* triquetral (bone). (Illustration by W.A. Kuchera.)

There is reciprocal motion of the radius. When the hand is pronated, the distal end of the radius crosses over the ulna as it moves anteriorly and medially (Fig. 46.6). Near the end of full pronation, the head of the radius glides posteriorly, that is, there is reciprocal motion of the radial head relative to the distal radius.

Motion in an arc opposite from the position of the pronated hand is called supination (Fig. 46.7). When the forearm is supinated, the distal end of the radius moves posteriorly and the radial head glides anteriorly.

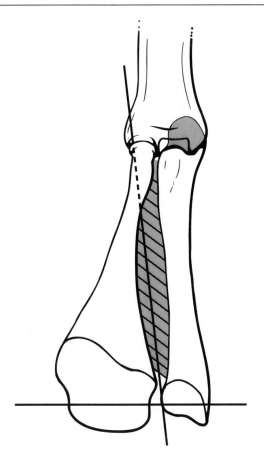

Figure 46.4. Forearm: interosseous membrane. (Illustration by W.A. Kuchera.)

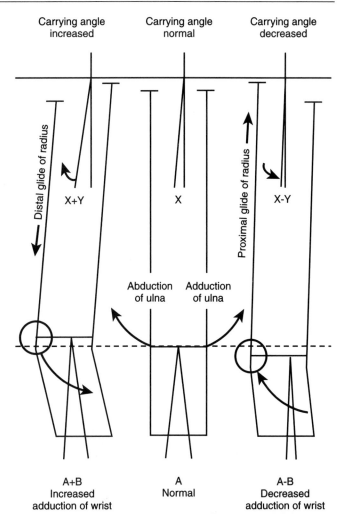

Figure 46.5. Right forearm: parallelogram effect. (Illustration by W.A. Kuchera.)

These motions are best palpated near the end of full supination or pronation of the hand. They are palpable if the operator's fingers are under the elbow and the thumb of that hand is palpating the radial head while the other hand supinates or pronates the patient's hand. Motion in the symptomatic forearm is compared with motion in the opposite or "normal" forearm.

The mechanism for strain of the forearm, wrist, or elbow can very easily also strain the interosseous membrane. Interosseous membrane dysfunction can perpetuate elbow or wrist disability long after proper orthopaedic care and apparently complete healing of strains, sprains, or fractures of the elbow or wrist should have taken place. In some unknown way, the collagen tissues often retain stress patterns of past injury. In such cases, palpation of the interosseous membrane reveals increased tension and elicits areas of subjective tenderness. Interosseous strains may be removed by direct or indirect fascial treatments.

Somatic Dysfunction of Elbow Joint Area

Several principles govern the elbow joint area:

1. Somatic dysfunction of the extremity is found in the minor gliding motions of the joint, not the major motions.

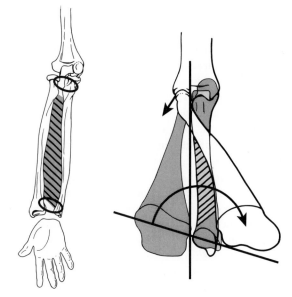

Figure 46.6. Forearm: pronation. (Illustration by W.A. Kuchera.)

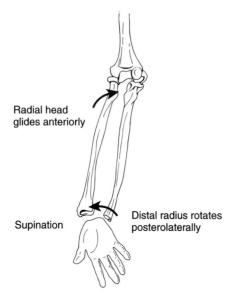

Figure 46.7.   Forearm: supination. (Illustration by W.A. Kuchera.)

2. Somatic dysfunction of the ulnohumeral joint is usually primary, and somatic dysfunction of the radioulnar joints is usually secondary.
3. Impaired function of any joint of the arm produces compensatory changes in all other joints. If total functional demand overtaxes any one of the other joints, secondary somatic dysfunction is produced in those joints as well.

Somatic Dysfunction of Forearm

Inspection by itself is usually not very helpful. It may be helpful when the carrying angle has been affected by somatic dysfunctions of the ulnohumeral joint. Increased abduction of the ulna would increase the carrying angle and encourage adduction of the hand at the wrist. Increased adduction of the ulna at the elbow encourages some abduction of the hand at the wrist. This is noticed as less adduction of the hand at the wrist.

Patient history may direct the physician to the site of the somatic dysfunction and often indicates the region in the upper extremity. Comparing minor passive gliding motions of the right and left upper extremities is the most helpful way of finding the exact somatic dysfunction.

If the wrist hurts, look at the elbow. The only sign of somatic dysfunction of the elbow may be a complaint of pain in the patient's wrist.

If all ulnohumeral joint somatic dysfunction has been treated, there is no inflammation in the elbow joint, and the elbow still cannot be flexed completely, the problem is most likely one of the radioulnar joints, usually the proximal one. The interosseous membrane may also be involved.

Reciprocal motions of the ends of the radius are preserved even when radial stress results in somatic dysfunction. A posterior radial head somatic dysfunction is usually produced by a fall forward onto the palm of an outstretched hand because

the anterior motion of the distal radius, started by the pronation, is accentuated. Though a fall forward is on the hand, the hand is in a pronated position and the forward vector of the hand and body pushes the distal radius into a more anterior rotation causing the radial head to move posteriorly (Fig. 46.8).

An anterior radial head somatic dysfunction is likely to result from a fall backward where the patient extends the arm posteriorly to break the impact of the fall, lands on the palm, and forces the distal end of the radius posteriorly. In this type of injury, the forearm is in the supinated and anatomical position (Fig. 46.9).

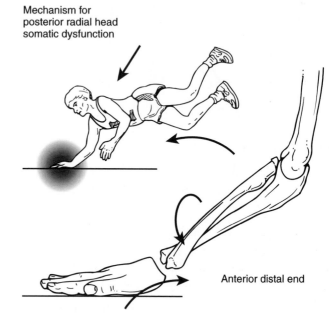

Figure 46.8.   Forward fall on outstretched hand. (Illustration by W.A. Kuchera.)

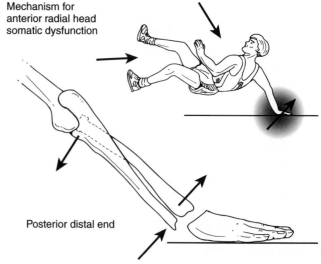

Figure 46.9.   Fall backward on extended arm. (Illustration by W.A. Kuchera.)

WRIST AND HAND

Configuration and Physiologic Motion

The hand joins the forearm by way of the true wrist joint. This is a stable joint composed of the radius, three carpal bones, and the attached cartilage. The basic configuration of the true wrist (the radiocarpal joint) is illustrated in Figure 46.3. This joint has two major axes of motion: the transverse axis, around which there is flexion and extension, and an anteroposterior axis, about which there is abduction and adduction. All motions are named according to the anatomical position of the joint and not according to the position in which the physician is holding the hand in relation to the body of the patient. Movement of the wrist toward the thumb side is abduction and toward the little finger is adduction.

Each motion of the wrist has a normal range of motion. The wrist can flex 90° and extend 70° about its transverse axis and can abduct 20° and adduct 50° about its anteroposterior axis. Combined motion about both of these axes permits a motion called circumduction. Figures 46.10 and 46.11 illustrate normal motion of flexion and extension.

Somatic Dysfunction of Wrist

Somatic dysfunction (SD) is not related to the gross motions of the wrist but to dysfunction of the slight gliding motions of the carpal bones on the radius as the wrist is moved. In Figures 46.10 and 46.11, notice the direction of glide of the carpal bone during each of these wrist motions.

Somatic dysfunction of the wrist is named according to the direction of motion preference. If a wrist extends and is restricted in its full flexion, it is an extension somatic dysfunction

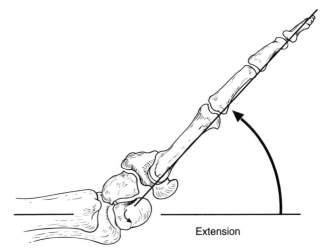

Extension

Figure 46.11. Wrist extension: anterior (ventral) glide of proximal carpal bones. (Illustration by W.A. Kuchera.)

(Fig. 46.12). You would say that the wrist was restricted in flexion. In this extension somatic dysfunction the three carpal bones glide ventrally and are restricted in gliding dorsally. The opposite is true for a flexion somatic dysfunction of the wrist; similar relationships occur for the other wrist motions.

Several principles describe somatic dysfunction of the wrist:

1. Observation is not very helpful when looking for somatic dysfunction; swelling of the wrist is an inconsistent sign.
2. Painful compression means dysfunction is present, but this test does not diagnose the specific problem that is present.
3. Radial glide and limited parallelogram motions are not obvious until the opposite motion is attempted. If there is an adduction somatic dysfunction at the wrist with a proximal shift of the radius, the problem may not be evident until abduction of the wrist is tested and the results are compared with the opposite side.
4. Flexion–extension somatic dysfunction of the wrist is usually caused by a trauma that overcomes the ligamentous restraints and opposing muscle pull. This can often result if a strain or sprain exceeds the extent of a somatic dysfunction. Restricted extension of the wrist is its most common major motion loss caused by dysfunction.

Somatic Dysfunction of Hand

INTERCARPAL JOINTS

Intercarpal somatic dysfunction often occurs from a fall on an outstretched hand. For this reason, somatic dysfunction in these areas is very likely to have a compression component. If the wrist joint is swollen, the physician must rule out fracture of the navicular bone (scaphoid). This is also true if there is pain on pressure over the snuff box or if there is persistent pain and dysfunction following proper conservative care, even if the initial posttrauma x-ray studies showed "no evidence of fracture." Sometimes the scaphoid does not reveal evidence of frac-

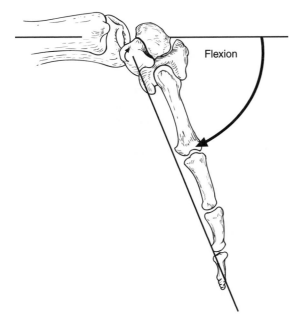

Flexion

Figure 46.10. Wrist flexion: dorsal glide of proximal carpal bones. (Illustration by W.A. Kuchera.)

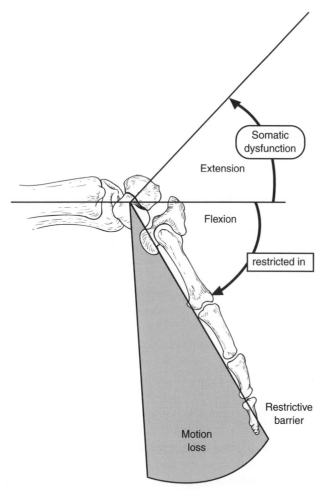

Figure 46.12. Wrist extension: somatic dysfunction. (Illustration by W.A. Kuchera.)

ture until the disruption in its blood supply slowly produces degeneration of the bone.

CARPOMETACARPAL JOINTS

All of these joints except the thumb are classified as plane synovial joints, which share a common joint cavity with the intercarpal joints. Their main type of somatic dysfunction is a dorsal glide with restriction in ventral glide.

The carpometacarpal joint of the thumb is different; it is a separate saddle-type joint, having both a concave and a convex articular surface. This configuration permits angular movements in almost any plane with the exception of limited axial rotation. Only a ball and socket joint has more motion than the carpometacarpal joint of the thumb. Because it has very good motion, it is more likely to have compression strain or sprain of the ligaments than to have somatic dysfunction.

METACARPOPHALANGEAL AND INTERPHALANGEAL JOINTS

The metacarpophalangeal (MP) joints and all the interphalangeal (IP) joints of the hand are gliding joints. The fifth MP

joint has the most motion; there is less motion in the fourth MP joint, and the third and second MP joints have the least motion. The MP and IP joints may develop somatic dysfunction in any one of a combination of six gliding motions:

    Anteroposterior glide
    Mediolateral glide
    Internal–external rotational glide

All of these motions are minor motions and cannot be initiated directly by muscle action.

Diagnosis

Compression is always part of MP and IP somatic dysfunctions, as when a ring on a finger gets caught as the person is jumping over a wire fence. Intermetacarpal cramps and pain may be a sign of MP or IP somatic dysfunction. Pain in the metacarpal joints may be referred from an ulnohumeral joint somatic dysfunction.

SPECIAL TESTS FOR THE UPPER EXTREMITY

Adson's Test

Adson's test is used to determine the state of the subclavian artery, which may be compressed by an extra cervical rib or by tightened anterior and middle scalene muscles. To perform Adson's test, take the patient's radial pulse at the wrist. Continue to feel the pulse while abducting, extending, and externally rotating the arm. Then instruct the patient to take a deep breath and turn the head toward the side being tested. Marked diminution or absence of the radial pulse indicates compression of the subclavian artery.[2]

Yergason Test

The Yergason test determines whether the biceps tendon is stable in the bicipital groove. Instruct the patient to fully flex the elbow. Grasp the flexed elbow in one hand while holding the wrist with your other hand. To test the stability of the biceps tendon, externally rotate the patient's arm as he or she resists, and at the same time pull downward on the elbow. If the biceps tendon is unstable in the bicipital groove, it pops out of the groove and the patient experiences pain. If the tendon is stable, it remains secure and the patient experiences no discomfort. This procedure may also be performed using one hand to palpate the tendon and the other hand to introduce motion.[2]

Drop Arm Test

The drop arm test detects whether or not there are any tears in the rotator cuff. First, instruct the patient to fully abduct the arm. Then instruct the patient to slowly lower the arm to the side. If there are any tears in the rotator cuff (especially in the supraspinatus muscle), the arm drops to the side from a position of about 90° abduction. The patient is not able to lower the arm smoothly and slowly no matter how many times they try. If the patient is able to hold the arm in abduction, a gentle tap of the forearm causes the arm to fall to the side.[2]

Apprehension Test

The apprehension test detects chronic shoulder dislocation. Abduct and externally rotate the patient's arm to a position where it might easily dislocate. If the shoulder is ready to dislocate, the patient has a noticeable look of apprehension or alarm on his or her face and resists further motion.[2]

Bicipital Tendinitis

The long head of the biceps muscle extends intraarticularly under the acromion through the rotator cuff to insert at the top of the glenoid. Impingement may result in inflammation of the tendon. This condition may also result from subluxation of the tendon out of the bicipital groove. Pain is usually localized to the proximal humerus and the shoulder. Resistive supination of the forearm aggravates pain. The distal portion of the biceps tendon is palpated in the cubital fossa medial to the tendon of the brachioradialis muscle. If the tendon is inflamed, the area may feel "puffy" and may be sensitive to touch. Also examine the coracoid process of the scapula as the tendon of the short head of the biceps attaches there.

Apley "Scratch" Test

The Apley scratch test is used to evaluate a patient's range of shoulder motion. First, to test abduction and external rotation, ask the patient to reach behind his or her head and touch the superior medial angle of the opposite scapula. To test the range of internal rotation and adduction, instruct the patient to reach in front of the head and touch the opposite acromion. To further test internal rotation and adduction, instruct the patient to reach behind the back and touch the inferior angle of the opposite scapula. Observe the patient's movement during all phases of testing for any limitation of motion or for any break of normal rhythm or symmetry.

Alternatively, instruct the patient to abduct the arms to 90°, keeping the elbows straight. Then instruct the patient to turn the palms up in supination and continue abduction until the hands touch overhead. This tests full bilateral abduction and provides instant bilateral comparison. Next, instruct the patient to place the hands behind the neck and push the elbows out posteriorly to test abduction and external rotation. Finally, test adduction and internal rotation by instructing the patient to place the hands behind the back as high as they go as if to scratch the inferior scapular angle.[2]

Tinel's Sign

Tinel's sign is used in the diagnosis of carpal tunnel syndrome. Attempt to elicit or reproduce pain or tingling in the distribution of the median nerve by tapping over the transverse carpal ligament.[2]

Phalen's Test

Phalen's test is also used in the diagnosis of carpal tunnel syndrome. Attempt to elicit or reproduce symptoms by flexing the patient's wrist to its maximum degree and holding it in that position for at least 1 minute.[2]

Allen's Test

Allen's test determines whether or not the radial and ulnar arteries are supplying the hand to their full capacity. Instruct the patient to open and close the fist several times and then squeeze the fist tightly so that the venous blood is forced out of the palm. Place your thumb over the radial artery and your index and middle fingers over the ulnar artery. Press both arteries against the underlying bones to occlude them. Instruct the patient to open the hand. The palm of the hand should be pale. Release one of the arteries at the wrist while maintaining pressure on the other one. Normally, the hand flushes immediately. If it does not react or flushes very slowly, the released artery is partially or completely occluded. Test both arteries.[2]

Tennis Elbow

This is also known as lateral epicondylitis. This condition is an inflammatory response to overuse of the extensor muscle group attached to the lateral epicondyle of the humerus. It is usually caused by repeated overload of the musculotendinous units attaching to the epicondyle. This condition produces pain that may be localized to the lateral epicondyle or may radiate down the forearm extensor group or up into the brachioradialis muscle. The pain is intensified by resistive extension of the wrist and fingers or by shaking hands. Pressure over the lateral epicondyle is painful.[7,8]

TREATMENT

Carpal Tunnel Syndrome

This condition is most commonly described as an entrapment neuropathy of the median nerve at the wrist producing paresthesias and weakness of the hands.[9] Carpal tunnel syndrome is frequently associated with repeated or sustained activity of the fingers and hands. Incidence rates are reported as high as 25.6 cases per 200,000 work hours[10] and involving 10% of workers. Medical cost estimates vary from $3,500 to $60,000 per case.[11]

Patients experience numbness or paresthesias on the palmar surface of the thumb, index, and middle fingers, and radial half of the ring finger. Numbness and paresthesias of the whole hand may occur. Pain may be referred to the forearm and less commonly to the neck and forearm regions. Pain or tingling of the fingers often occurs at night and is relieved by shaking or exercising the hand. Weakness and atrophy of the thenar muscles usually appear late and can occur without significant sensory symptoms. On examination, symptoms may be reproduced by percussion over the volar surface of the wrist (Tinel's sign) or by full flexion of the wrist for one minute (Phalen's maneuver). Decreased touch may be demonstrated over the fingers supplied by the median nerve. Nerve conduction studies are considered to be the gold standard for the diagnosis of this condition.[9]

The syndrome is traditionally described as resulting from pressure on the median nerve where it passes with the flexor tendons of the fingers through the tunnel formed by the carpal bones and the transverse carpal ligament.[9] Additional explanations exist. Single compressions of dog sciatic nerves have failed to produce significant conduction loss. Both proximal and distal compressions have produced conduction blocks in 50% of test animals.[12]

In 1973 Upton and McComas proposed the existence of the "double crush syndrome." This syndrome hypothesizes that neural function is impaired when single axons that are compressed on one region become especially susceptible to damage in another area. The authors report that "a slight compression may cause a reduction in axoplasmic flow too small to result in denervation changes, but when coupled with the onset of a slowed lesion might further reduce axoplasmic flow below the safety margin for prevention of denervation at a distal lesion and clinical symptoms ensue.[13] Abramson demonstrated that decreased blood supply to a nerve alters conduction.[14] Larson suggested that upper thoracic dysfunction alters upper extremity vasomotion.[15] Hurst demonstrated a relationship between cervical arthritis and bilateral carpal tunnel syndrome.[16] Sunderland has suggested that lymphatic and venous congestion contribute to this disorder.[17]

The treatment of carpal tunnel syndrome has traditionally involved the use of wrist splints, antiinflammatory drugs, and local injection of steroids. Surgical decompression of the carpal tunnel with release of the transverse carpal tunnel ligament is used if symptoms persist or motor abnormalities are present.[9,18] Evidence in the preceding paragraph suggests that the hand symptoms may be related to dysfunctions in the upper extremity, and cervical and thoracic spine. Osteopathic treatment incorporates the modalities described above and should also include:

1. Reducing sympathetic tone to the upper extremity by correcting upper thoracic and upper rib dysfunctions. This directly affects nerve function by improving blood flow and reducing congestion by improving lymphatic and venous drainage. An internally rotated temporal bone may be associated with increased sympathetic tone in the upper thoracic spine and, if it is diagnosed, should also be treated.
2. Removing cervical somatic dysfunction to improve brachial plexus function.
3. Removing myofascial restrictions in the upper extremity, thereby removing potential sites of additional compression.
4. Increasing space within the carpal tunnel using direct release techniques.

Reflex Sympathetic Dystrophy

Reflex sympathetic dystrophy (RSD) is characterized by pain and tenderness usually of the distal extremity accompanied by vasomotor instability, trophic skin changes, and rapid development of bone demineralization. A precipitating event can be identified in two thirds of the cases. These include:

Trauma
Myocardial infarction
Stroke
Peripheral nerve injuries

RSD is observed most often in individuals over the age of 50. An entire hand or foot is usually affected. The pathogenesis of RSD is poorly understood. The vasomotor manifestations are thought to be caused by abnormal stimulation of the sympathetic nervous system.[9] Larson implicates the upper thoracic spinal segments with facilitating a vasomotor response in the upper extremity.[15]

RSD evolves through three clinical phases. The clinical manifestations of the first phase are pain and swelling that develop weeks to months following the precipitating event. The pain has an intense, burning quality. The involved extremity is warm, edematous, and tender especially around the joints. Increased sweating and hair growth occur. In 3–6 months, the skin gradually becomes thin, shiny, and cool (second phase). Clinical features of the first two phases overlap. In another 3–6 months, the skin and subcutaneous tissues become atrophic, and irreversible flexion contractures of the hand or foot develop (third phase). Motion of the shoulder on the affected side is frequently painful and greatly restricted, a condition referred to as the shoulder–hand syndrome.[9]

Early recognition and treatment are important to prevent permanent disability. RSD may be reversible in its early phases. Appropriate mobilization of the patient following a myocardial infarction, stroke, or injury may help prevent this condition. Pain should be properly controlled. Exercises are helpful. Sympathetic nerve blocks may be initially effective, but the response may not be sustained. High-dose prednisone has benefited some patients.[9] Osteopathic treatment should focus on reducing sympathetic tone to the extremity. This includes correcting cervical, upper thoracic, and upper rib dysfunctions. Apply gentle articulation and mobilization techniques. Always treat the whole patient.

Adhesive Capsulitis

This is also known as "frozen shoulder." This condition is characterized by pain and restricted movement of the shoulder usually in the absence of intrinsic shoulder disease. Adhesive capsulitis may follow bursitis or tendinitis of the shoulder or be associated with systemic disorders such as chronic pulmonary disease, myocardial infarction, and diabetes mellitus. Prolonged arm immobility contributes to the development of this condition. Reflex sympathetic dystrophy is thought to be a pathogenic factor. The capsule of the shoulder is thickened, and a mild, chronic, inflammatory infiltrate and fibrosis may be present.

Pain and stiffness usually develop gradually over several

months to a year, but may progress rapidly in some patients. Pain may interfere with sleep. The shoulder is tender to palpation, and both active and passive motion are restricted.[9]

Early mobilization following an injury to the arm or shoulder may help prevent the development of this condition. Local injection of corticosteroids and administration of nonsteroidal antiinflammatory drugs and physical therapy may help.[9] Osteopathic manipulation should be directed to the upper thoracics, upper ribs, and entire shoulder complex. The objective is to improve motion. Avoid taking the patient into the crampy pain zone. This only slows progress. Only progress as fast as the patient's body can respond. Indirect techniques may be especially effective in the initial treatment phases.

Myofascial Triggers

See Chapter 66, "Travell and Simons' Myofascial Trigger Points."

Chapman's Points

See Chapter 67, "Chapman's Reflexes."

Thoracic Outlet Syndrome

This condition results from compression of the neurovascular bundle (subclavian artery, subclavian vein, and brachial plexus) as it courses through the neck and shoulder. Several dysfunctions may compress the neurovascular bundle as it passes from the thorax to the arm, including:

Cervical ribs
Excessive tension in the anterior and middle scalene muscles
Dysfunctions of the clavicle, upper ribs, or upper thoracics
Abnormal insertion of the pectoralis minor muscle

Patients may develop:

Shoulder and arm pain
Weakness
Paresthesias
Claudication
Raynaud's phenomenon
Ischemic tissue loss
Gangrene

Examination is often normal unless provocative maneuvers are performed. Occasionally distal pulses are decreased or absent and digital cyanosis and ischemia may be evident. Tenderness may be present in the supraclavicular fossa.[9] Some forms of thoracic outlet syndrome are associated with sympathetic autonomic dysfunction, which produce upper extremity symptoms. Sympathetic dysfunction has accompanying palpatory findings in the upper thoracic or rib area. Most patients can be managed conservatively. Patients should avoid positions that aggravate symptoms. Osteopathic treatment should be directed toward improving mechanics in the:

Cervical region
Upper thoracics
Upper ribs
Clavicles
Scalene muscles
Muscles of the shoulder and pectoral girdle

Surgical intervention is a last resort.

CONCLUSION

Understanding the structure and function of the upper extremities leads to effective diagnosis and treatment of disabilities in this area and therefore improves the overall function of the patient.

REFERENCES

1. Truhlar RE. *Doctor A.T. Still in the Living.* Published by the author, 1950.
2. Hoppenfeld S. *Physical Examination of the Spine and Extremities.* Norwalk, Conn: Appleton & Lange; 1976:25.
3. Moore KL. *Clinically Oriented Anatomy.* 3rd ed. Baltimore: Williams & Wilkins; 1992:528.
4. Seidel HM, Ball JW, Dains JE, Benedict GW. *Mosby's Guide to Physical Examination.* St. Louis, Mo: CV Mosby Co; 1987:309–311.
5. Kuchera WA, Kuchera ML. *Osteopathic Principles in Practice.* 2nd ed. rev. Columbus, Ohio: Greyden Press; 1994:539.
6. Kuchera WA, Kuchera ML. *Osteopathic Principles in Practice.* 2nd ed. rev. Columbus, Ohio: Greyden Press; 1994:615–629.
7. Roy S, Irvin R. Throwing and tennis injuries to the shoulder and elbow. In: *Sports Medicine: Prevention, Evaluation, Management, and Rehabilitation.* 1983:38, 221–222.
8. Gunter-Griffin, Letha Y. *Athletic Training and Sports Medicine.* 2nd ed. Rosemont, Ill: The American Academy of Orthopedic Surgeons; 1991:274.
9. Wilson JD, et al. *Harrison's Principles of Internal Medicine.* 12th ed. New York: McGraw-Hill; 1991:1487.
10. Armstrong TJ. *An Ergonomics Guide to Carpal Tunnel Syndrome.* Ergonomics Guide Series. Akron, Ohio: American Industrial Hygiene Association; 1983.
11. Hiltz R. Fighting work-related injuries. *National Underwriter.* 1985; 89:15.
12. Nemoto K. Experimental study on the vulnerability of the peripheral nerve. *Nippon Sea Gakkai Zasshi.* 1983:57, 1773–1786.
13. Upton A, McComas AJ. The double crush in nerve entrapment syndromes. *Lancet.* 1973;2:359.
14. Abramson DI, Rickert BL, Alexis JT, Hlavova A, Schwab C, Tandoc J. Effects of repeated periods of ischemia on motor nerve conduction. *J Appl Physiol.* 1971;30:636–642.
15. Larson NJ. Osteopathic manipulation for syndromes of the brachial plexus. *JAOA.* 1972;72:94–100.
16. Hurst LC, et al. The relationship of double crush syndrome to carpal tunnel syndrome (an analysis of 1000 cases of carpal tunnel syndrome). *J Hand Surg.* 1985;10:202.
17. Sunderland S. The nerve lesion in the carpal tunnel syndrome. *J Neurol Neurosurg Psychiatry.* 1976;39:615.
18. Anonymous. Carpal tunnel syndrome: getting a handle on hand trauma. *Occup Hazards.* February 1987;42:45–47.

47. Thoracic Region and Rib Cage

RAYMOND H. HRUBY, JOHN P. GOODRIDGE, AND JOHN M. JONES III

Key Concepts

- **Importance of thorax and rib cage for normal function**

- **Structure and function of thoracic area, including lymphatics, connective tissues, neural connections, and motion**

- **Clinical characteristics of thoracic movements**

- **History and physical examination including observation, palpation, and motion testing**

- **Assessment, diagnosis, and treatment of structural dysfunctions**

Because the heart and lungs are contained in the thorax, this region's unique significance in life has long been recognized. The inability to draw breath or the perception of pain in the thorax often constitute real or imagined immediate and life-threatening problems. Movement of the thorax is necessary for normal function in both obvious and not so obvious ways. Because much of the regulatory outflows of the sympathetic nervous system originate in the thoracic spinal cord, disturbances in the muscles and joints of the thoracic region often mimic life-threatening problems. Injury to thoracic vertebrae can cause long-term sequelae for health and survival. Efficient chest movement involves over 100 joints. The complexities of the thoracic cage and the vital importance of its organ systems underscore the necessity for the osteopathic physician to understand its many functions, diagnoses, and potential treatment approaches.

The thoracic region is bounded by the cervical region above and the lumbar region below. In diagnosis and treatment, it cannot be considered separately from the other body regions, since dysfunctions in it or other regions are always interdependent.

ANATOMY AND PHYSIOLOGY

Thoracic and Costal Skeleton

The thoracic cage includes 12 thoracic spinal vertebrae, 12 pairs of ribs, and the sternum. Although the scapula overlies the posterior portion of the rib cage and is connected to the sternum through the clavicle, these two structures are more properly considered a part of the upper extremity (see Chapter 46, "Upper Extremities") even though they are often involved in thoracic injuries and pain syndromes.

White and Panjabi[1] divide the thoracic spine into three anatomical regions:

Upper (T1-4)
Middle (T4-8)
Lower (T8-L1)

It is also helpful to divide the thoracic and upper lumbar spine into four functional divisions that roughly correspond to the thoracolumbar outflow of the sympathetic system:

T1-4: Sympathetics to head and neck; with T1-6 to the heart and lungs.
T5-9: All upper abdominal viscera: stomach, duodenum, liver, gall bladder, pancreas, and spleen.
T10-11: Remainder of small intestines, and kidney, ureters, gonads, and right colon.
T12-L2: Left colon and pelvic organs.

This functional division is often very useful to the osteopathic physician because visceral afferent (generally nociceptive; see Chapter 5, "Autonomic Nervous System") neurons usually follow the same pathway as the sympathetic outflows. Visceral disturbances often cause increased musculoskeletal tension in the somatic structures innervated from the corresponding spinal level through the viscerosomatic reflexes (see Chapter 10, "Neurophysiologic System"). Manipulative treatment at that spinal level is used to reduce somatic afferent input from the associated facilitated segments, which, in turn, reduces somatosympathetic activity to the affected viscus.[2]

Generally, the thoracic spine has a mildly kyphotic, forward-bending curve that varies from person to person. In the osteoporotic or elderly patient, the angle of this curve can become more acute, causing biomechanical problems and necessitating compensatory adaptation in other regions of the spine and in general posture. Individual thoracic vertebrae are parts of a continuum with the cervical and lumbar vertebrae, with size increasing from cervical to lumbar to account for increased weight bearing. The spinous processes of the thoracic vertebrae are particularly large and easily palpated, pointing increasingly caudad from T1 through T9 and back to an almost anteroposterior orientation from T10-T12.

Thoracic vertebral facet joints are plane-type synovial joints. The interarticular surfaces of these interarticular joints are smooth, shiny, compact bone, covered with hyaline cartilage, and are surrounded by a thin, loose articular capsule, lined with synovial membrane. The facet joints guide and limit gross, segmental, and coupled movements. The superior facets of each thoracic vertebra are slightly convex and face posteriorly (backward), somewhat superiorly (up), and laterally. Their angle of declination averages 60° relative to the transverse plane and 20° relative to the coronal plane. Remember the facet facing by the mnemonic, "BUL" (backward, upward, and lateral). This is in contrast to the cervical and lumbar regions, where the superior facets face backward, upward, and medially ("BUM"). Thus, the superior facets are BUM, BUL, BUM from cervical to thoracic to lumbar. In the lower portion of the thoracic spine, the superior facet surface begins to face more posteriorly than laterally, and at T12 it may even face medially, as part of a functional transition to the lumbar spine. The inferior facet of each thoracic vertebra faces in the opposite direction from the superior and has a slightly concave surface.

The thoracic vertebrae are separated by disks, as are the cervical and lumbar vertebrae. The disks act as shock absorbers and permit flexibility between the vertebrae. Each disk is composed of an outer annulus fibrosus and an inner nucleus pulposus, a gel at the center of the disk that acts like a semifluid hydrophilic ball bearing that becomes less hydrated and broader under sustained compression. The annulus fibrosus is composed of concentric lamellae of fibrocartilage, running at right angles to the fibers of adjacent layers. Its structural arrangement is more vulnerable to tears posteriorly, where the lamellae are thinner and less numerous. However, the restricted motion of the thoracic spine due to the attachments of the rib cage and the fairly broad posterior longitudinal ligament make ruptured thoracic disks relatively uncommon. On the other hand, discopathy from trauma, aging, and degenerative disease is relatively common in the thoracic area.

The 12 sets of ribs correspond with the 12 thoracic vertebrae. All ribs are composed of a bony segment and a costal cartilage. Each rib has a cup-shaped depression in its bony segment where the costal cartilage fits into the costochondral joint and where the periosteum of the rib joins the perichondrium of the rib cartilage. The rib heads join with the thoracic vertebrae at the costovertebral articulations. The heads of ribs 2-9 articulate with a demifacet on the vertebra above and below. For example, rib 2 articulates by demifacets with T1 and T2. The heads of ribs 1 and 10-12 articulate with unifacets on their corresponding vertebrae. The transverse processes of vertebrae TI-T10 also have synovial costotransverse joints with the tubercle of the corresponding rib.

Ribs 1, 2, 11, and 12 are called "atypical ribs." Rib 1 is the flattest, shortest, broadest, strongest, and most curved. The subclavian artery and the cervical plexus are vulnerable to muscular compression where they pass over the first rib between the tubercles and attachments of the anterior and the middle scalene muscles, the so-called scalenus anticus syndrome. The latter is one of a number of conditions clinically labeled as thoracic outlet syndrome; see Chapter 34, "Neurology"). The subclavian vein may also be compressed between the first rib and the clavicle. Rib 2 is considered anatomically atypical because of its tuberosity that attaches to the proximal portion of the serratus anterior muscle. Ribs 11 and 12 are anatomically

atypical because they do not have tubercles, do not attach to the sternum or other costal cartilages, and have tapered ends. These two ribs are also called floating or vertebral ribs. Rib 10 is sometimes considered atypical because of its single articulation between the rib head and T10.

Anatomically typical ribs (3-9 and in most respects 10) have heads, necks, tubercles, angles, and shafts that connect directly or via chondral masses to the sternum. Rib 1 and ribs 2-7 connect directly with the sternum by their own individual cartilaginous synovial joints (rib 1 with a stable synchondrosis) and so are often called the true ribs. Ribs 8-10 merge into a single cartilaginous mass that attaches to the sternum and so are called vertebral chondral ribs. Ribs 11 and 12 do not connect with the sternum and hence are called floating ribs. Because ribs 8-12 do not connect directly to the sternum, they are often called the false ribs.

The costovertebral joints between the heads of the ribs and the vertebral bodies allow gliding or sliding costal motions. The costotransverse joints at the tubercle of the typical ribs, with the facets at the tip of the transverse processes of their own vertebra, a synovial membrane, and a thin articular capsule, allow gliding and slight rotational motions. When these motions are restricted, respiratory movements are commonly impeded.

The sternum has three parts:

Head or manubrium
Body or gladiolus
Tail or xiphoid process

The superior portion of the manubrium cradles the clavicles at the sternoclavicular joints, forming the manubriosternal notch or jugular notch, which is a landmark for several anterior thoracic strain/counterstrain tender points. The sternal notch lies almost directly anterior to the T2 vertebral body. The manubrium joins the sternal body via a fibrocartilaginous symphysis, or secondary cartilaginous joint called the sternal angle or angle of Louis. This joint lies anterior to the fourth thoracic vertebra. Because the second rib attaches to the manubrium and sternal body with a synovial joint, the sternal angle is an anterior landmark for counting the ribs. The xiphisternal joint is located anterior to the ninth thoracic vertebra. It is also a hyaline cartilage symphysis that fuses into a synostosis in the fifth decade.

Muscles of Thoracic Area

The muscles of the thoracic area are involved in:

Actions of the ribs and vertebrae
Posture
Head and neck control
Breathing
Locomotion
Stabilization of the extremities
Visceral function

Table 47.1 lists the major muscles of the thoracic area, with the action, proximal and medial attachments, distal and lateral

Table 47.1
Regional Thoracic Muscles

Muscle	Action	Proximal/Medial Attachments	Distal/Lateral Attachments	Innervation
Pectoralis major	1. *Clavicular head:* flexion, adduction, horizontal flexion and medial rotation of the humerus at the shoulder 2. *Sternocostal head:* flexion, adduction, medial rotation and horizontal flexion of the humerus at the shoulder. Also extends flexed humerus. Through its action on the humerus it depresses, protracts and rotates downward	1. Clavicular division: anterior surface of the medial ½ of the clavicle 2. Sternocostal head: sternum to 7th rib, cartilages of true ribs and aponeurosis of external abdominal oblique muscle	1. Clavicular division: lateral lip of the intertubercular groove of the humerus. 2. Sternal division: lateral lip of the intertubercular groove of the humerus.	1. Clavicular head: lateral pectoral, C5, C6 2. Sternocostal head: lateral and medial pectoral, C7, C8, T1
Pectoralis minor	Depresses scapula and rotates scapula inferiorly. Important anterior shoulder stabilizer	Anterior surfaces of 3rd, 4th, and 5th ribs near the costal cartilages	Coracoid process of the scapula	Medial pectoral, C6, C7, C8
Teres major	Adducts and medially rotates humerus at the shoulder. Extends the shoulder joint	Dorsal surface of inferior angle of the scapula	Medial lip of intertubercular groove of humerus. Medial to latissimus dorsi tendon	Lower subscapular, C6, C7
Teres minor	Lateral rotation of humerus at the shoulder. Stabilization of head or humerus	Superior ⅔ of dorsal surface of lateral border of scapula	Inferior aspect of greater tubercle of the humerus, capsule of the shoulder joint	Axillary, C5, C6
Trapezius	1. *Lower fibers:* depresses the scapula. Retracts the scapula. Rotates the scapula upward so the glenoid cavity faces superiorly. Gives inferior stabilization of scapula. Aids to maintain spine in extension. 2. *Middle fibers:* retracts and aids in elevation of scapula 3. *Upper fibers:* elevates the scapula as in shrugging the shoulders. Rotates the scapula upward so the glenoid cavity faces superiorly, when acting with the other sections of the trapezius it retracts the scapula.	1. *Lower fibers:* spinous processes of 6th–12th thoracic vertebrae 2. *Middle fibers:* spinous processes of 1st–5th thoracic vertebrae 3. *Upper fiber:* external occipital protuberance, medial ⅓ of superior nuchal line, ligamentum nuchae and spinous process of the 7th cervical vertebra	1. *Lower fibers:* medial ⅓ of spine of the scapula 2. *Middle fibers:* superior border of spine of scapula 3. *Upper fibers:* lateral ⅓ of clavicle and acromion process	1. *Lower division:* spinal root of accessory and anterior primary rami C3, C4 2. *Middle division:* spinal root of accessory and anterior primary rami C3, C4 3. *Upper division:* spinal root accessory and anterior primary rami C3, C4
Latissimus dorsi	Extends, retracts, and medially rotates the humerus at the shoulder. Through its action on the humerus it depresses, retracts, and rotates the scapula downward. Assists in forced expiration.	Flat tendon that twists upon itself to insert into the intertubercular groove of the humerus, just anterior to and parallel with tendon of pectoralis major	Broad aponeurosis that originates on the spinous processes of lower 6 thoracic and all lumbar vertebrae; posterior crest of ilium, posterior surface of sacrum, lower 3 or 4 ribs, and an attachment to the inferior angle of the scapula	Thoracodorsal C6, C7, C8
Levator scapulae	Elevates the scapula and rotates the scapula downward so the glenoid cavity faces inferiorly. Working with the upper fibers of the trapezius, elevates and retracts the scapula. *Reversed action:* when scapula is fixed, laterally flexes and slightly rotates cervical spine to the side.	Transverse processes of first four cervical vertebrae	Vertebral border of scapula between superior angle and scapular spine	Dorsal scapular C5 and anterior primary rami C3, C4

Table 47.1—*continued*

Muscle	Action	Proximal/Medial Attachments	Distal/Lateral Attachments	Innervation
Rhomboid	1. *Minor:* retracts and elevates the scapula. Assists in rotating the scapula downward 2. *Major:* retracts and elevates the scapula. The inferior fibers aid in rotating the glenoid cavity inferiorly.	1. *Minor:* lower part of ligamentum nuchae, spinous processes of C7 and T1 2. *Major:* spinous processes of 2nd–5th thoracic vertebrae	1. *Minor:* medial border of scapula at the root of the spine of the scapula 2. *Major:* medial border of scapula from spine to inferior angle	1. *Minor:* dorsal scapular, C4, C5 2. *Major:* dorsal scapular, C4, C5
Quadratus lumborum	Lateral flexion of lumbar vertebral column; helps action of the diaphragm in inspiration	Iliolumbar ligament, posterior part of the iliac crest	Inferior border of the 12th rib and transverse processes of the upper 4 lumbar vertebrae	Anterior primary rami T12, L1, L2, L3
Serratus anterior	1. Accessory muscle of respiration 2. Protraction of the scapula	Superior lateral surfaces of upper 8 ribs at the side of the chest	Costal surface of the medial border of scapula	Long thoracic, C5, C6, C7
Serratus posterior (superior/inferior)	Accessory muscles of inspiration. Superior elevates superior ribs; inferior depresses inferior ribs	1. *Superior:* lower portion of ligamentum nuchae and spinous processes of the 7th cervical and 1st, 2nd, and 3rd thoracic vertebrae 2. *Inferior:* spinous processes of 11th and 12th thoracic and 1st, 2nd, and 3rd lumbar vertebrae, and the thoracolumbar fascia	1. *Superior:* superior borders of 2nd–5th ribs distal to the angles 2. *Inferior:* inferior borders of lower 4 ribs just beyond their angles	1. *Superior:* anterior primary rami T2–5 2. *Inferior:* anterior primary rami T9–12
Intercostals	1. Keep the intercostal spaces from bulging and retracting with respiration 2. Elevate the ribs anteriorly with inspiration			
External intercostals				
Internal intercostals				
Innermost intercostals				
Subcostal muscles	Depress the ribs			
Transversus thoracis	Depress the second to sixth ribs			
Levatores costarum	Elevate the ribs	Transverse processes of the 7th cervical and upper 11 thoracic vertebrae	The outer surface of the rib immediately below the vertebrae from which it takes origin, between the tubercle and the angle	Anterior primary rami of the corresponding intercostal nerves
Splenius	1. *Capitis:* acting bilaterally, extends the head and neck. Acting unilaterally, laterally flexes and rotates the head and neck to the same side. 2. *Cervicis:* laterally bends and rotates the neck	1. *Capitis:* spinous processes of C7–T3, inferior half of ligamentum nuchae 2. *Cervicis:* Spinous processes of 3rd–6th thoracic vertebrae	1. *Capitis:* mastoid process and lateral third of the superior nuchal line 2. *Cervicis:* transverse processes of 1st, 2nd, 3rd, and 4th cervical vertebrae on the posterior aspect	1. *Capitis:* posterior primary rami of the middle cervical spinal nerves 2. *Cervicis:* posterior primary rami of the lower cervical spinal nerves

Table 47.1—*continued*

Muscle	Action	Proximal/Medial Attachments	Distal/Lateral Attachments	Innervation
Spinalis	1. *Cervicis:* laterally bends and rotates the neck 2. *Thoracis:* acting unilaterally, lateral flexion of the spine. Acting bilaterally, extension of the spine.	1. *Cervics:* lower portion of ligamentum nuchae, spinous processes of the 7th cervical and 1st and 2nd thoracic vertebrae 2. *Thoracis:* spinous processes of the 1st and 2nd lumbar vertebrae, thoracic vertebrae 11 and 12	1. *Cervicis:* spinous process of the axis and the 3rd and 4th cervical spinous processes 2. *Thoracis:* spinous processes of upper thoracic, vertebrae T4–T8	1. *Cervicis:* posterior primary rami of the spinal nerves 2. *Thoracis:* posterior primary rami of the spinal nerves
Semispinalis	Extends the thoracic and cervical region and rotates it toward the opposite side.	1. *Capitis:* between superior and inferior nuchal lines of the occipital bone 2. *Cervicis:* spinous processes of 2nd–5th cervical vertebrae 3. *Thoracis:* spinous processes of the 1st–4th thoracic vertebrae and 6th and 7th cervical vertebrae	1. *Capitis:* 7th cervical and 1st–6th thoracic transverse processes and articular processes of 4th, 5th, and 6th cervical vertebrae 2. *Cervicis:* transverse processes of the 1st–6th thoracic vertebrae 3. *Thoracis:* transverse processes of 6th–10th thoracic vertebrae	1. *Capitis:* posterior primary rami of cervical spinal nerves 2. *Cervicis:* posterior primary rami of cervical spinal nerves 3. *Thoracis:* posterior primary rami of thoracic spinal nerves, T1–6
Longissimus	1. *Capitis:* acting bilaterally, extends the head; acting unilaterally, laterally flexes and rotates the head to the same side. 2. *Cervicis:* acting unilaterally, laterally flexes the neck. Acting bilaterally, laterally flexes the vertebral column. Acting bilaterally, extension of vertebral column; draws ribs down.	1. *Capitis:* transverse processes of the 1st–5th thoracic vertebrae and the articular processes of the 4th–7th cervical vertebrae 2. *Cervicis:* transverse processes of the 1st–5th thoracic vertebrae 3. *Thoracis:* the common broad thick tendon with the iliocostalis lumborum, fibers from the transverse and accessory processes of the lumbar vertebrae and thoracolumbar fascia	1. *Capitis:* the posterior margin of the mastoid process 2. *Cervicis:* transverse processes of the 2nd–6th cervical vertebrae and transverse process of the atlas 3. *Thoracis:* the tips of transverse process of all thoracic vertebrae and the lower 9 or 10 ribs between the tubercles and angles	1. *Capitis:* posterior primary rami of spinal nerves 2. *Cervicis:* posterior primary rami of spinal nerves 3. *Thoracis:* posterior primary rami of spinal nerves
Iliocostalis	1. *Cervicis:* acting bilaterally, extension of the spine; acting unilaterally, laterally flexes the vertebral column 2. *Thoracis:* acting bilaterally, extension of the spine; acting unilaterally, laterally flexes the spine 3. *Lumborum:* acting bilaterally, extension of the spine; acting unilaterally, laterally flexes the spine	1. *Cervicis:* the posterior tubercles of the transverse processes of the 4th, 5th, and 6th cervical vertebrae 2. *Thoracis:* into the angles of the upper 6 or 7 ribs and into the transverse process of the 7th cervical vertebra 3. *Lumborum:* inferior borders of the angles of the lower 6 or 7 ribs	1. *Cervicis:* superior borders of the angles of the 3rd–6th ribs 2. *Thoracis:* superior borders of the angles of lower 6 ribs medial to the tendons of insertion of the iliocostalis lumborum 3. *Lumborum:* anterior surface of a broad and thick tendon, which originates from the sacrum, spinous processes of the lumbar and 11th and 12th thoracic vertebrae, and from the medial lip of the iliac crest	1. *Cervicis:* posterior primary rami of spinal nerves, C6, C7, C8 2. *Thoracis:* posterior primary rami of spinal nerves 3. *Lumborum:* posterior primary rami of spinal nerves

Table 47.1—*continued*

Muscle	Action	Proximal/Medial Attachments	Distal/Lateral Attachments	Innervation
Rotatores	Rotate the vertebral column	1. *Brevis:* bases of the spinous processes (lamina) of the 1st vertebra above 2. *Longus:* bases of the spinous processes (lamina) of the 2nd vertebra above	1. *Brevis:* transverse processes of the vertebrae 2. *Longus:* transverse processes of the vertebrae	1. *Brevis:* posterior primary rami of spinal nerves 2. *Longus:* posterior primary rami of spinal nerves
Multifidus	1. Rotate the vertebral column toward the opposite side 2. Stabilize the vertebral column	Spinous processes of all the vertebrae except the atlas	Posterior surface of the sacrum, the dorsal end of the iliac crest, the mammary and transverse processes of lumbar and thoracic vertebrae and the articular processes of the 4th–7th cervical vertebrae	Posterior primary rami of spinal nerves
Interspinales	1. Unite the spinous processes 2. Produce slight extension of the vertebral column	Pairs of small muscles joining the spinous processes of adjacent vertebrae, one on each side of the interspinous ligament. Continuous in the cervical region extending from the axis to the 2nd thoracic vertebra and in the lumbar region from the 1st lumbar vertebra to the sacrum	*See proximal/medial attachment*	Posterior primary rami of spinal nerves
Intertransversarii	1. Unite the transverse processes 2. Produce lateral bending of the vertebral column	Unite transverse processes of consecutive vertebrae. Well developed in the cervical region	*See proximal/medial attachment*	Anterior and posterior primary rami of spinal nerves
Diaphragm	Contracts into the abdomen with inhalation and relaxes into the thorax with exhalation	The central tendon, which is an oblong sheet forming the summit of the dome	An approximately circular line passing entirely around the inner surface of the body wall: 1. *Sternal portion:* two slips from the back of the xiphoid process 2. *Costal portion:* the inner surfaces of the cartilages and adjacent portions of the lower 6 ribs on either side, interdigitating with the transversus abdominis 3. *Lumbar portion:* medial and lateral arcuate ligaments and right and left crura from the anterolateral surfaces fo the bodies and discs of the upper three lumbar vertebrae	Phrenic nerve, C3, C4, C5
Obliquus capitis inferior	Rotates the atlas, turning the face toward the same side	Apex of the spinous process of the axis	The inferior and dorsal part of the transverse process of the atlas	Posterior primary rami of C1
Subclavius	Depresses clavicle, draws it medially	1st rib at junction with costal cartilage	Groove on the inferior surface of the clavicle, between the costoclavicular and conoid ligaments	Subclavius C5, C6

attachments, and innervation of each. It is especially important to note the action of each muscle, since altered tone can affect the function of not only the bones to which the muscle is attached but other body areas as well. In addition, increased and decreased tone has the capacity to alter both general and microcirculation in myriad ways, such as altered homeostatic regulation and cellular immunity.

As with all muscles, the thoracic muscles are fed not only by circulatory elements but by physiologically active trophic substances delivered directly by nerves themselves.[3] In addition, there is evidence that the sympathetic nerve supply to striated and smooth muscles alters muscle tone and contractile forces. Attention to the palpatory cues associated with altered muscle tone therefore implies the presence of any of many differential diagnostic factors that are discussed throughout this text.

The larger muscles of the head, neck, shoulder girdle, and thorax control not only much of the activity of the thoracic cage but help stabilize the cervical and cranial areas, as well as the arms and shoulder girdle. For example, the splenius capitus and cervicis muscles originate on the lower cranial and upper cervical areas, while attaching distally along the middle thoracic spine, as low as T6-T8 in some cases. Vertebral dysfunctions in the upper thoracic areas can affect the action of these muscles, causing problems with motion outside the thoracic area in the head and neck. Lower down, the internal and external oblique muscles are generally viewed as trunk rotators but also attach to the lower ribs along with the diaphragm. Altered tone in these muscles can alter diaphragmatic and respiratory function and vice versa. Experienced palpation readily identifies these relationships.

Of special note in the thoracic muscles are the erector spinae groups that extend and side-bend the vertebral column and allow smooth flexion by gradually decreasing resistance to forward bending. These muscles are often involved in group or multiple movement dysfunctions, i.e., altered coupling or non-neutral vertebral unit dysfunctions, and are vulnerable to insult with unplanned movements or trauma. Also implicated in this type of problem are the deep back muscles, especially the rotatores and multifidus. These small muscles are richly innervated with muscle spindles that provide proprioception. In fact, one of their primary tasks is to signal position and speed of motion of the vertebral column. (This task makes them important in the maintenance of posture and in directing movement. They are also very vulnerable to sudden stretch and unplanned movement, which appears to alter the sensory inputs to the spinal cord and brain, with resultant development of altered motion and pain typical of vertebral somatic dysfunction.)[4-6]

The abdominal diaphragm is the primary muscle of respiration. It forms the floor of the thorax, attaching to the xiphoid process, the internal surface of the inferior six ribs, the upper two (left) or three (right) lumbar vertebrae, and their intervertebral disks. Its fibers converge into a common central tendon that has no bony attachment. When the diaphragm contracts with inhalation it descends into the abdomen; when it relaxes during exhalation it moves upward into the thorax. This up and down movement produces pressure gradients between the thoracic and abdominal cavities and is important for both efficient respiration and circulation. Because there are one-way valves in the larger lymphatic vessels, the pressure gradients also enhance the movement of lymph and venous blood toward the heart. When the dome of the diaphragm is flattened because of asymmetrical load and/or tonus, respiration and lymphatic drainage from anywhere in the body becomes less efficient.

There are three apertures in the diaphragm: one for the vena cava at about the level of T8, another for the esophageal hiatus at T10, and the third for the aorta at the level of T12. Diaphragmatic muscle fibers are arranged so that, when it contracts in inspiration, the vena caval opening dilates, permitting more venous blood to pass from the abdomen to the thorax; at the same time, the esophageal hiatus constricts to prevent gastric contents from rising in the esophagus. Its contraction has no influence on the aortic hiatus, which lies posterior to the diaphragm and so does not truly pierce the diaphragm.

The diaphragm is able to do most of the work of breathing under normal conditions and during moderately forced inspiration. With increased respiratory demands, accessory muscles of respiration become involved to move the ribs even more. The scalene muscles, attached to the upper two ribs, assist inhalation. Hypertonicity and/or hypotonicity of segmental intercostal muscles alters rib behavior, making breathing less efficient. Actual spasm in these muscles can result in pain at rest or especially with each deep breath or cough. Quiet exhalation creates passive recoil of the lung as the diaphragm relaxes. Forced exhalation also involves the inferior internal intercostal and abdominal muscles, including the trunk rotators and erector spinae.

Osteopathic manipulative treatments can often restore or partially rehabilitate altered diaphragmatic function. These treatments are designed to increase motion of the lower costal cage by freeing the diaphragm for better excursion. This, in turn, helps improve breathing mechanics and assists in venous blood return and lymphatic flow. This approach can be especially helpful for individuals with asthma, respiratory infections, loss of general lung compliance, and associated disorders.

Lymphatics

As blood moves through the capillaries, fluid filters into the interstitial tissues. The return of interstitial fluid through the lymphatic system is necessary for health and proper function and is even more important when the patient has disease. Lymphatic drainage from the lower half of the body is supplied by the thoracic duct (or left lymphatic duct (LLD)). Smaller lymphatic vessels drain into the cisterna chyli in the abdomen. Trunks from the left side of the head, the left arm, and the thoracic viscera also empty into the thoracic duct before it drains into the junction of the left internal jugular and the left subclavian veins. In approximately 20% of the population, three trunks—the right jugular, the right subclavian, and the right transverse cervical trunks—join to form the right lymphatic duct (RLD). The remainder of the population varies in the way the three trunks empty into the jugulosubclavian junction in the anterior neck. The RLD enters the junction of the right internal jugular and right subclavian veins.[7]

Pressure gradients between the thorax and the abdomen during the respiratory cycle play an important role in venous and lymphatic return to the heart. Inappropriate muscle tone (spasm or hypertonicity), as well as constrictive effects of connective tissue (fascia), can impede lymphatic return. Osteopathic manipulative treatment removes these mechanical impediments and increases the efficiency of lymph flow (see Chapter 68, "Lymphatic System").

Connective Tissues and Fascia

Connective tissue unites and surrounds all other tissues. It is found between the cells of organs, as tendons of muscles, and as ligaments joining skeletal parts. Of special importance to the osteopathic physician are the fascias of the body. These connective tissues surround virtually all organs, muscles, and vessels of the body.[8] Fascial elements called the pericardium and pleura even surround the heart and lungs, respectively. Fascia is a fibrous tissue that is effectively wound around the invested organs at various winding angles.

Trauma, chemical alterations of the bathing fluids (immune changes), and other pathologic agents alter the winding angles of the fascial bands and change cross-linkages between the bands, causing altered tensions of the fascias throughout the body. An increase in tension in the fascial sheets leads to altered interstitial fluid (lymph) flows, decreased blood flow, and decreased efficiency of organ function. Normalization of the fascial tensions assists the body to a more efficient function, thereby using less energy. Osteopathic manipulative techniques including direct and indirect myofascial release have been developed to address these problems in ways not generally found to be effective with most other manipulative techniques. The thoracic fascias are often involved in dysfunctions due to thoracic trauma and the detrimental effects noticeable because of heart and lung involvement.

Neural Connections of Thoracic Area

The neural connections of the thoracic area are of vital importance to all body functions. Not only do the usual connections to the musculoskeletal system exit the spinal cord in the thoracic region, but a large part of the sympathetic nervous system originates in the thoracic region. An understanding of the relationships of the thoracic nerves and their relationships to the bony landmarks is vital to understanding neurological problems associated with the thoracic region.

The spinal cord, which runs from the brainstem to about the level of L3, is a continuous structure with no segmentation. During embryologic development, the spinal nerve bundles are gathered into spinal nerve roots with formation of the vertebrae to pass out between the encircling bones through the intervertebral foramina. This imposes what appears to be a dermatomal segmentation effect. Inherently, however, the function of the spinal cord is not segmented.

The spinal nerves exit through the intervertebral foramina, which identify their vertebral level. Each spinal nerve is numbered at the level at which it exits, except in the cervical region, since there are eight cervical nerve roots, and seven cervical vertebra. Spinal nerve C1 exits above the atlas, and the eighth root exits below C7. All other roots exit below their corresponding vertebrae. Since the intervertebral foramen is a bounded space and the nerve roots share that space with other tissues, the roots are especially vulnerable to pressure from herniated nucleus pulposus and even edema. Somatic dysfunction in a thoracic area may cause local edema and tissue tightening that can exert pressure on the nerve root and, importantly, can alter blood and fluid flows to and from the nerve sheaths. Such pressure can alter neural conductivity in the affected roots, while the lack of proper blood and fluid flow to the sheaths can cause irritability in the nociceptors of the sheath, causing pain along the nerve distribution.[9] Local disturbances can often be relieved with proper manipulative treatment, designed to restore proper motion and fluid flow to the region. As stated previously, radiculopathy is somewhat rare in the thoracic region, although discopathy is less rare. These problems in the thoracic area are not easy to diagnose because of overlapping dermatomes and a lack of readily testable deep tendon reflexes (see Chapter 34).

The abdominal diaphragm receives its motor innervation through the phrenic nerves coming from C3-5. Perhaps more importantly, sensory nerves of the diaphragm innervate the mediastinal pleura, the fibrous pericardium, and the parietal layer of the serous pericardium.[10] This relationship helps explain the very common palpatory findings of cervical tensions and somatic dysfunctions associated with pericardial or diaphragmatic irritation that are mediated via the viscerosomatic reflexes (see Chapter 10). Manipulative treatment of the involved cervical segments is designed to ameliorate thoracic and diaphragmatic dysfunction through somatovisceral reflex pathways.

Parasympathetic innervation to the thoracic viscera as well as to many of the abdominal viscera comes through the vagus nerve (cranial nerve X). These relationships are shown in Table 47.2 (and discussed in Chapter 5). Treatment of problems encountered in the function of the thoracic viscera must include assessment and treatment of cranial and cervical areas to normalize vagal function.

The majority of the outflows of the sympathetic system originate in the thoracic region (Table 47.2 and see Chapter 5). The distribution of the sympathetic system to almost every tissue and area of the body makes this system a very important one for all body functions. It is even becoming evident that the sympathetic system is vitally important in regulating immune function[11] (see Chapter 9, "Neuroendocrine–Immune System and Homeostasis"). The importance of the sympathetic nervous system for all body functions suggests that disturbances within the thoracic vertebra and their associated musculature that affect the function of the sympathetic system

Table 47.2
Composite Autonomic Innervation

Parasympathetic Innervation: Craniosacral	Viscera	Thoracolumbar	Sympathetic Innervation			
			Regional Areas	Cord Level	Splanchnic Nerves	Collateral Ganglia
			Head and neck	T1–4		(Cervical ganglia)
Cranial III	Pupils					
Cranial VII	Lacrimal and salivary glands		Heart			(Cervical ganglia)
Cranial VII	Sinuses	T1–4		T1–6		
Cranial IX, X	Carotid body and carotid sinus		Lungs			—
	Thyroid					
	Trachea/bronchi	T1–6				
	Mammary glands	T1–6				
	Esophagus lower ⅔					
	Aorta	T1–6	Upper GI tract	T5–9	Greater splanchnic	Celiac ganglion
	Heart					
	Lungs and visceral pleura		Small intestines, right colon, adrenal, and ovary or testes	T10–11	Lesser splanchnic	Superior mesenteric ganglion
	Stomach	(L)				
Cranial X Vagus	Duodenum		Appendix, left colon, and pelvis	T12	Least and lumbar splanchnics	Inferior mesenteric ganglia
	Liver	T5–9				
	Gall bladder and ducts					
	Spleen		Entire GI tract	T5–L2		
	Pancreas					
	Right colon[a]		Entire colon	T10–L12		
S2–4	Ovary and testes					
	Small intestines	T10–11	Entire GU tract (kidney, ureters, and bladder)	T10–12		
	Kidney	T10–L12	Adrenal	T10–11		
	½ Transverse colon					
	Left colon	T12–L2	Upper ureter	T10–11		
(None)	Adrenal	T10–11	Lower ureter	T12–L1		
(Vagus)	Upper ureter	T10–11				
	Lower ureter	T12–L1	Bladder	T12–12		
	Bladder (body)					
S2–4	Bladder trigone and sphincter	T12–L2				
	Uterine body					
	Prostate					
	Genital cavernous tissues					
(None)	Arms	T2–8				
(None)	Legs	T11–L2				

Adapted from Kuchera WA, Kuchera ML. *Osteopathic Principles in Practice.* 2nd ed. rev. Columbus, Ohio: Greyden Press; 1994:68–69.

[a]Right colon and right half of transverse colon.

can have widespread consequences. Identification and treatment of somatic dysfunction in the thoracic region is especially important in treating problems ranging from infectious processes to functional abnormalities.

Visceral dysfunction that alters inputs to the spinal cord not only increases the sympathetic outflows back to the visceral areas through viscerovisceral reflex pathways but also alters somatic outflows in often unexpected patterns. Understanding this phenomenon provides insight on how to treat many painful and/or functional problems. Due to the overlap of visceral afferents onto spinal pathways that also receive somatic afferents, the sensory experience of visceral irritation is often one of referred pain to a somatic structure, with concomitant increased somatic muscle tone. One of the most common such patterns is that of the shoulder pain and muscle tension associated with acute myocardial infarction. The nociceptive inputs from the compromised myocardium is experienced as shoulder or chest pain. Often there is a vicious circle of increased somatic involvement, when increased somatic activity also increases sympathetic outflows to the heart, further exacerbating the pathologic process. Treating the somatic component of the process, while obviously not the only course of treatment, can be of benefit. Recognition of the visceral origin of referred pain patterns can save the osteopathic physician much time and missed diagnoses. Likewise, recognizing that osteopathic treatment of the involved somatic structures can help the course of the problem. Understanding the somatic areas likely to show effects of underlying visceral pathological conditions through viscerosomatic reflexes[2] provides the osteopathic physician with another important diagnostic and treatment tool.

VARIATIONS AND DYSFUNCTIONS

Vertebral and Costal Cage Motion

Thoracic spinal and costal cage movements are integral parts of total body movements that include intimately detailed interdependent functions with both the craniocervical and lumbopelvic systems. Both bony and general configurational anomalies are common; Wolff's law is always at work. Wolff's law states that bones and soft tissues deform (are strained) according to the stresses (forces applied over an area) that are placed on them. Examples of general configurational alterations affecting both shape and movement characteristics are seen with scoliosis, kyphosis, the arthritides, and leg length inequalities.

General body shapes and movement characteristics are also affected by growth, aging, and lifestyle factors. For example, experienced tennis players tend to develop costothoracic alterations in association with repetitive twisting and stressing from the dominant hand side. So also do automobile assembly line workers as they bend, twist, and turn in the same direction hundreds of times a day. On the other hand, age-induced osteoporosis and arthritic changes also affect these same characteristics. Interdependent spinal and costal cage movements are always changing as life processes unfold.

Thoracic Spinal Motion

Available thoracic spinal motion is generally less than in either the cervical or lumbar areas. This is because all planes of motion are affected by costal cage mechanics and their complicated relationships with head, neck, shoulder girdle, and lumbopelvic anatomy. Thoracic spinal motion is further complicated by a number of other factors that go beyond basic costovertebral configuration and mechanics. A few of the elements include configurational characteristics of the anteroposterior curves in the sagittal plane such as:

Kyphosis
Costal cage asymmetries such as pectus excavatum and carinatum

Osteoporosis/osteoarthritis effects
Increased chest wall diameter associated with a variety of cardiopulmonary problems
Cervical, shoulder girdle, rotator cuff influences; e.g., anterior muscles are generally tighter than are posterior groups. Under these circumstances, anteroposterior curves tend to become more kyphotic
Effects of lifestyle and affective states such as slumping with depression

Characteristics of primary and secondary lateral deviations include:

Scoliosis with and without kyphosis
Effects of upper and lower motor neuron lesions
Effects of repetitive motion activities
General thoracic spinal motion characteristics

Because of configurational changes in size and shape, thoracic spinal motion characteristics vary markedly from the cervicothoracic to thoracolumbar junctions. The upper and middle portions demonstrate greater rotation than elsewhere in the spine with the exception of the atlantoaxial (AA) joint. Generally, flexion capability is greater than for extension. Side-bending capability is even less because of rib cage constraints. In the lower portions, flexion and extension capacities are greatest, while side-bending abilities exceed those of rotation; that is, they are more like lumbar spine mechanics.

Upper thoracic coupling is typically neutral/type 2 and generally occurs as low as T4; movements are similar to normal cervical spine behavior. Some suggest that these motions are associated with the interdependent combination of asymmetrical vertebral and upper rib shapes and attachments and their interactions with cervical muscle extensors and side-benders that attach as low as T5 and T6 (splenius mechanics).

Middle thoracic coupling is commonly a mix of neutral/type I and nonneutral/type II movements that may rotate to either the formed convexity or to the formed concavity.

Lower thoracic coupling is more apt to accompany lumbar neutral/type I mechanics.

Clinical Characteristics of Thoracic Movement

Clinically, there is a constant tendency for spinal flexion because of the effects of gravity and the tendency for the back extensors to become inhibited while flexors tend toward contraction. Clinically, it seems that the rotatores, intertransversarii, and multifidi are often involved in postural stress, somatosomatic, and viscerosomatic reflexes (see Chapters 10 and 34). When these muscles are reflexly affected by facilitation, they are often responsible for maintaining nonneutral somatic dysfunction of the vertebral units innervated by the involved muscle, neural network, or viscera. Some refer to this phenomenon as the "somatic component" of impairment, illness, or disease (see Chapter 77, "Somatic Dysfunction").

Both neutral/type I and nonneutral/type II vertebral unit dysfunctions are common in the thoracic spine. Neutral/type I asymmetries typically involve three or more segments that are either flexed or extended; they are mildly scoliotic. Nonneutral/type II vertebral unit dysfunctions generally involve a single vertebral unit with both proximal and distal neutral/type I responses.

Neurologic pathological conditions, trauma, visceral disease, and intrinsic mechanical asymmetries are common sources of spinal dysfunctions. Trauma, for example, often flexes, extends, and/or twists the spine simultaneously in such a way that the accumulated forces localize around a vertebral unit, thereby disturbing the mechanics of both single vertebral segment and vertebral units. (See Glossary for clarification.) Deforming injuries of this type often alter physical shapes; that is, they cause plastic deformations with permanent stretching of ligaments and distortions in facet joints and osseous-ligamentous relationships. Not surprisingly, recurring nonneutral/type II vertebral unit dysfunctions are common under these circumstances. This type of vertebral unit change is sometimes associated with altered visceral functions; for example, somatic dysfunction is superimposed on vertebral segment and vertebral unit changes with resulting facilitated peripheral, autonomic, and centrally mediated reflex activities (see Chapters 10 and 34). Patients report many clinical symptoms when these processes occur.

Rib Mechanics

During inhalation, the thoracic cage widens its vertical, transverse, and anteroposterior dimensions as the diaphragm contracts. With deep inhalation, the anterior ends of the superior ribs move more anteriorly and superiorly along with the sternum (Fig. 47.1).

Typical ribs are attached to the sternum by the costal cartilage and move primarily in pump-handle movements that move the anterior component of the costosternal system up-

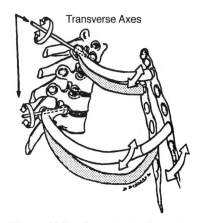

Figure 47.2. Pump-handle rib motion.

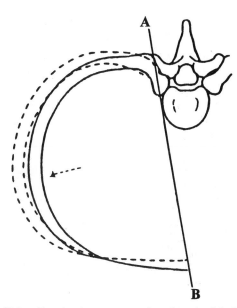

Figure 47.3. Functional anteroposterior rib axis. (Modified from *Gray's Anatomy*. 35th ed. Edinburgh: Churchill Livingstone; 1973:421.)

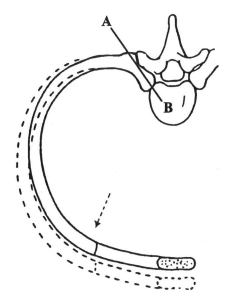

Figure 47.1. Functional transverse rib axis. (Modified from *Gray's Anatomy*. 35th ed. Edinburgh: Churchill Livingstone; 1973:421.)

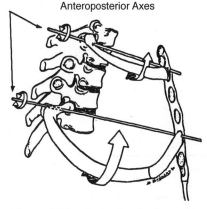

Figure 47.4. Bucket-handle rib motion.

ward and anteriorly. (See Glossary for more detailed definition.) The rib shaft is the handle of the bucket and the vertebral column is the pivot point (Figs. 47.1 and 47.2).

Atypical ribs, the vertebrocostal ribs 1 and 2 and 8-12, move in a bucket-handle manner (Figs. 47.3 and 47.4). In this case, the rib moves more laterally and superiorly with functional pivot points posteriorly and anteriorly. Functionally, the shafts move laterally and superiorly during inhalation as the transverse diameter of the costal cage increases.

HISTORY AND PHYSICAL EXAMINATION

The evaluation of the thoracic region and rib cage includes:

Elements of history taking
Observation
Auscultation
Percussion
Palpation
Motion testing

The following sections focus on aspects of the history and examination that are uniquely osteopathic in nature.

History

Ask standard questions of the patient as part of the total evaluation of the thoracic region. Do a history of the systems most closely associated with the thoracic cage. This includes such systems as the cardiac, pulmonary, and gastrointestinal systems. Ask if there has been any history of trauma. This information is particularly important to the osteopathic physician, as trauma to the thoracic region may have produced disturbances in structural relationships that have resulted in disturbances in visceral function. Historical information should also include when the complaint first appeared, whether a similar complaint has occurred in the past, and whether there are any underlying predisposing conditions. If there is pain, ask:

About its location
About its duration
Whether it is constant or intermittent
Whether anything has ameliorated or exacerbated it
The quality (stabbing, aching, burning, or like an electrical shock)
Whether it radiates to any other location
How much stress the patient has recently been experiencing

Information gathered during history taking helps one begin formulating hypotheses as to the nature of the patient's problem. Combined with the physical examination findings, the history allows development of a working diagnosis and an appropriate comprehensive treatment approach that includes osteopathic manipulative treatment.

Observation

Observe certain aspects of the thoracic region with the patient in standing, seated, supine, and prone positions. These observations help determine whether more detailed examination is warranted. Observations include:

1. The skin, noting such characteristics as color, skin rashes or eruptions, and hair distribution
2. The relationship of the neck to midline. This gives information about rotation and side-bending abilities of both the neck and upper thoracic regions.
3. The sternum, observing for pectus excavatum (hollow chest, depressed sternum) or pectus carinatum (pigeon chest, protruding sternum)
4. The clavicular heads for levelness
5. The shoulders for excessive rounding
6. The nipple heights

In the standing position, observe the patient from the front, noting shoulder heights and the general shape and contour of the thoracic cage. Also observe the patient from the back, taking note of shoulder heights, position of the scapulae, contour and shape of the thoracic cage, and any observable evidence of lateral spinal curvature such as scoliosis. Observing the patient from each side, note shape and contour of the thoracic cage including observable evidence of changes in the sagittal spinal curves such as lordosis and/or kyphosis. Make the same observations with the patient seated.

Evaluate the patient for trunk side-bending abilities. With the patient standing, observe right and left side-bending from the back without forward bending. Observe for symmetry of motion of the induced spinal curve. A normal curve should be a smooth C-shaped curve with paravertebral muscle fullness on the side of the convexity. Lack of a C-shape to the induced spinal curve suggests the presence of vertebral motion segment dysfunction in the region.

Again from the back, observe forward bending as the patient attempts to touch the floor. Follow the formed contour of the spine and thoracic cage. Asymmetrical changes anywhere along the spine and rib cage raise the suspicion of vertebral motion segment and possibly somatic dysfunction in the area. Observe lateral posture using an imaginary vertical line that lies along a path drawn from the external auditory meatus to the tip of the acromion, through the middle of the femoral trochanter, ending just anterior to the lateral malleolus (see "postural line" in Glossary). Thoracic kyphosis and lordosis suggest the need for more detailed evaluation.

Prone and supine observations assess general thoracocostal shape, symmetry, and contour. Respiration is best observed with the patient supine. Is respiratory effort mostly thoracic or abdominal, or a combination of each? Altered patterns often indicate any of many somatic, visceral, or neurosensory problems reflected partially as somatic dysfunction in the thoracic region.

Examination

When the history and screening examination indicate a thoracic regional dysfunction, look for more specific signs of vertebral motion segment or soft tissue myofascial dysfunction. The following points are helpful in learning to identify and describe pertinent thoracic anatomical landmarks.

Vertebral motion segments are identified by the letter T followed by a number from 1 to 12, for example, T1, T2, and so on. The ribs are identified by the letter R followed by a number from 1 to 12, for example, R1, R2, and so on.

It is important to be able to distinguish C7 from T1 when evaluating the thoracic region. This can easily be done using the following method. Ask the patient to bend the head forward. With the head in this position the seventh cervical vertebra (C7) usually has the most prominent spinous process in the cervicothoracic region. Place a finger on the tip of this spinous process and ask the patient to backward bend the head. In this position, the spinous process of C7 translates anteriorly. The spinous process of the vertebra just below this one is then identifiable at that of T1.

The sternal notch is located at the superior border of the manubrium between the two sternoclavicular (SC) joints. This structure is anterior to and at the same horizontal level as the second thoracic vertebra.

The sternal angle is the point at which the sternum and manubrium unite. It is located anterior to and in the same horizontal plane as the fourth thoracic vertebral segment. The costal cartilage of rib two (R2) inserts at the sternal angle. This is a clinical guide to the numbering of the ribs. The sternal angle lies anterior and in the same horizontal plane as the fourth thoracic vertebra. The xiphisternal angle is located at the inferior end of the sternum and is also anterior to and in the same horizontal plane as the ninth thoracic vertebra.

The spine of each scapula is usually at the level of the spinous process of T3. The inferior angle of each scapula is usually at the level of the spinous process of T7.

A useful way of identifying the thoracic vertebrae involves the rule of threes. This rule is a generalization that is only approximate but positions the palpating fingers in the approximate position for locating individual thoracic vertebrae:

1. The spinous processes of T1, T2, and T3 project directly posteriorly so that the tip of each spinous process is in the same plane as the transverse processes of its associated vertebra.
2. The spinous processes of T4, T5, and T6 project in a slightly caudal direction so that the tip of each spinous process is in a plane that is approximately half the way between the transverse processes of its associated vertebra and those of the vertebra immediately below.
3. The spinous processes of T7, T8, and T9 project caudally at a sharper angle so that the tip of each spinous process is in the same plane as the transverse processes of the vertebra immediately below it.
4. For the T10, T11, and T12 vertebrae the spinous processes are placed as follows. The spinous process of T10 is similar to those of T7-T9. The spinous process of T11 is similar to those of T4-T6. T12 is similar to those of T1-T3.

Palpation

Observation and the screening examination provide information about body regions that may have significant somatic dysfunction. Palpation is used to further investigate these areas and to further localize and identify the somatic dysfunctions that may be present. Somatic dysfunctions may be representative of musculoskeletal dysfunction, viscerosomatic reflex changes, or both.

Palpation of the thoracic spine and rib cage can find tissue texture abnormalities and restricted motion. When either is found, more palpation may be used to identify somatic dysfunction in specific vertebral segments and/or ribs.

Palpate for tissue texture changes by lightly stroking the paravertebral soft tissues in a cephalocaudal direction, either bilaterally or unilaterally. The search is for changes in tissue texture defined as:

Increased tone or tension (hypertonicity)
Spasm
Fasciculation
Ropiness
Bogginess (indicative of edema)
Increased or decreased temperature
Moisture

Warm, moist, and boggy tissue usually suggests acute somatic dysfunction, while cold, dry, ropy tissue suggests chronic somatic dysfunction. When an area is interpreted as having abnormal tissue texture, asymmetry, restricted motion, or tenderness, perform a more detailed assessment.

Perform the red reflex test by firmly but with slight pressure stroking two fingers on the skin over the paraspinal tissues in a cephalad to a caudad direction. The stroked areas briefly become erythematous and then almost immediately return to their usual color. If the skin remains erythematous longer than a few seconds, it may indicate an acute somatic dysfunction in the area. As the dysfunction acquires chronic tissue changes, the tissues blanch rapidly after stroking and are dry and cool to palpation.

In addition to palpating the paravertebral tissues, assess the tips of the spinous processes and the interspinous ligaments for evidence of gross asymmetry, edema, or tenderness. Palpation also extends laterally to the transverse processes, the costotransverse articulations, and the rib angles; look for tissue texture changes and tenderness.

MOTION TESTING

Thoracic region motion testing further identifies areas of altered movement of the vertebrae, ribs, and soft tissues. Use more detailed palpation of vertebral motion segments and surrounding ribs and soft tissues to assess areas where gross motion restriction are located.

Motion restriction evaluation involves both active and passive motion testing. Active motion testing assesses voluntary motions produced by the patient. Passive motion testing is induced while the patient remains as passive and relaxed as possible.

Active Motion Testing of Thoracic Spine

FLEXION/EXTENSION: SAGITTAL PLANE BENDING

The patient sits on the examination table or on a stool with the feet on the floor. Ask the patient to bend forward and backward as you palpate for asymmetries and vertebral motion segment restrictions.

SIDE-BENDING

The patient side-bends right and left as you palpate for restriction in spinal curves and vertebral motion segments for neutral and nonneutral dysfunctions. Identify the level of the apex of any curve where limitation is seen.

ROTATION

The patient rotates right and left as you note restriction in spinal and vertebral unit motion segments, both unilaterally and bilaterally, to identify the spinal segmental level where limitation occurs.

Active Motion Testing of Vertebral Motion Segment

Place the thumbs over the sites immediately posterior to the left and right thoracic transverse processes at the level to be evaluated. Then ask the patient to slightly flex, extend, side-bend right, side-bend left, rotate right, and rotate left as palpation determines the site(s) of greatest restriction in comparison with vertebral segments above and below.

Passive Motion Testing

REGIONAL EXAMINATION OF UPPER THORACIC SPINE

Flexion and Extension

Place one hand posteriorly on the patient's upper thorax and the other on top of the patient's head. Bend the head and neck forward until flexion creates movement in the upper thorax (T1-T4). Note flexion restrictions as the process proceeds. Then bend the head backward until extension creates movement in the upper thorax, again noting any movement restrictions.

Side-bending

With a hand on the patient's upper thorax, bend the head and neck to one side then the other side, noting any lateral flexion restrictions.

Rotation

With one hand on the patient's upper thorax, use the other hand to rotate the head and neck right and left while palpating for upper thoracic rotation restrictions.

REGIONAL EXAMINATION OF LOWER THORACIC SPINE

Flexion/Extension

Place the palmar surface of one hand on the patient's lower thorax. Place the other hand on the opposite shoulder. Bend the torso forward and backward, noting any flexion and extension restrictions with the hand palpating the lower thorax.

Rotation and Side-bending

Carry out rotation and side-bend right and left lower thoracic assessment with the same hand positions.

SEGMENTAL EXAMINATION OF UPPER THORACIC SPINE

Segmental motion tests are most commonly done with the patient seated.

Flexion/Extension

Place the fingertips of the long and ring fingers of one hand between the spinous processes of the first four thoracic vertebrae. Use the other hand passively to move the head and neck into flexion and extension. Assess each vertebral motion segment as the process unfolds. Typically, the spinous process of the superior vertebra moves anteriorly and superiorly before those that are more distal. If a vertebral motion segment does not move freely into flexion, it is defined as being caught in an extended position, such as an ERS vertebral unit dysfunction that is restricted during flexion movements.

Examine extension in a similar manner, but with passively induced backward bending. If a vertebral motion segment does not extend well, it is being caught in a flexed position. If it does not extend well, it is because that vertebra is in a flexed position, and is a FSR vertebral unit dysfunction with restriction in extension.

Side-bending

Passive right and left side-bending are similarly assessed with the palpating fingers in the same areas between the upper four thoracic transverse processes. If the transverse process of one segment does not approximate the transverse process of the segment below, it is restricted in side-bending right or left in accordance with the restriction.

Rotation

A T1 rotation example follows: Place the index and long fingers over the transverse processes of T1. Then rotate the head passively right or left until T1 begins to rotate in the same direction. Right rotation restriction suggests that T1 is positionally rotated left. The same procedure is effective for the upper four thoracic vertebral motion segments.

Diagnosis

Use active and passive motion testing to formulate a specific positional diagnosis for a given spinal segment. For example, if T2 does not extend, it is in a flexed position and moves into flexion most easily. If it does not easily rotate left, it is rotated right. If it does not easily side-bend left, it is side-bent right.

SEGMENTAL EXAMINATION OF LOWER THORACIC SPINE

Motion testing is performed with the same maneuvers used on the upper thoracic segments. However, instead of using the head and neck as a lever, use the nonpalpating arm wrapped anteriorly over the shoulders, palm on the opposite shoulder, axilla over the near shoulder, to use the upper trunk as a lever to move T5-T12

Examine all the lower thoracic segments for flexion/extension, right and left side-bending, and right and left rotation movements.

The principles of physiologic motion of the spine are used to identify any specific segmental motion restrictions noted. For example, if in flexion and left side-bending a transverse process becomes much more posterior on the left, this indicates that the vertebra is extended, rotated and side-bent to the left (ERLSL).

If the motion restriction is most noticeable with the patient in the neutral position (that is, motion improves in flexion and extension), then the motion restriction is described as a neutral vertebral motion segment dysfunction. For example, if the vertebrae are rotated to the left and side-bent to the right in the neutral position, the segmental dysfunction is recorded as NRLSR.

Prone Segmental Motion Testing

Also examine the patient in the prone position. First test individual segments by placing the thumb of each hand over the transverse process at a particular spinal level. Pressing anteriorly first on one side and then the other, vertebral displacement is readily assessed. If the transverse process goes forward more easily on the left and resists movement on the right, the vertebra is rotated right.

Evaluate side-bending by placing the thumbs over the region of the transverse processes of the vertebra to be examined and the one immediately below. This places the thumbs approximately at the disk space between the two. Translatory and rotational stressing to each side induces side-bending; that is, translation left encourages side-bending to the right and vice versa. For example, if right translation is induced more easily, the vertebra is side-bent to the left.

Sphinx or Television-Watching Maneuver

Ask the patient to prop up on the elbows with weight resting on the elbows so that backward bending arches the spine. If a motion segment is restricted with extension, the motion segment is considered to be flexed.

If the motion at the dysfunctional segments improves with both flexion and extension, then motion segment dysfunction is occurring in the neutral position.

Costal Region

Motion dysfunctions of the ribs are designated as either structural or respiratory. Specific structural dysfunctions include:

Anterior or posterior subluxations (the first rib may have a structural dysfunction known as superior subluxation)
External rib torsions
Anteroposterior compression
Lateral compressions
Laterally flexed ribs

Respiratory dysfunctions are classified as either inhalation or exhalation dysfunctions and may involve either single ribs or groups of ribs.

Evaluation for Structural Rib Dysfunctions

With the patient seated, first stand behind and then in front of the patient while palpating over the rib angles in the upper, middle, and lower rib cage regions. Make assessments over the rib angles to decide whether one rib angle in a group of ribs is more or less prominent than another. Also evaluate the contour of rib shafts. Normally the inferior border of each rib is palpated more easily than the superior border. Evaluate the width of each intercostal space anteriorly, laterally, and posteriorly. Each interspace should be symmetrical throughout. Finally, note any tenderness, hypertonicity, or other tissue texture abnormalities.

If a given rib angle is more or less prominent than the others, an anterior or posterior subluxation may be present (see Glossary). If the superior border of a rib is more easily palpated than the inferior border, an external rib torsion may be present.

If there is less prominence of a rib shaft anteriorly and posteriorly with accompanying increased prominence along the midaxillary line, an anteroposterior costal cage or individual rib compression is present.

Conversely, if there is more prominence of a rib shaft in the anterior and posterior dimensions along with less prominence along the midaxillary line, a lateral rib compression is present.

Prominence of the rib shaft in the midaxillary line along with asymmetry of the interspaces immediately above and below the rib indicates the presence of a laterally flexed rib.

EVALUATION OF FIRST RIB

The first rib should be assessed for superior subluxation. To do this, stand behind the seated patient and grasp the anterior and superior borders of the trapezius on each side to retract the tissue posteriorly. Direct fingertip pressures caudally on each side to contact the posterior and lateral shaft of the first ribs. If there is a superior subluxation of one of the ribs, tenderness and unleveling of the dysfunctional rib is present.

EVALUATION OF RIBS 1–10

With the patient supine, stand at the side of the patient so that your dominant eye is over the patient's midline. Then place your hands over the patient's upper anterior thoracic cage so that the tips of the middle fingers contact the inferior borders of the clavicles. Ask the patient to inhale deeply and then exhale fully; assess pump-handle motion of the upper ribs, looking for asymmetry of motion between the left and right sides of the upper rib cage (see Glossary).

Evaluate the upper rib cage in the same manner, but along the midaxillary line. This maneuver assesses bucket-handle motion (also called bucket bail motion) of the upper rib cage (see Glossary). The process is repeated for the middle and lower rib cage regions.

Asymmetry of motion in any of the rib cage areas indicates the presence of respiratory rib dysfunction in that region. Respiratory rib dysfunctions are described as having either inhalation or exhalation restriction. There is usually one rib within a group of ribs that is responsible for maintaining the inhalation or exhalation restriction. This rib is referred to as the key rib and is the rib that must be identified and treated in order to remove the group restriction.

To identify the key rib within a group of ribs, examine each rib in the group individually. This is done by placing a finger on each pair of ribs in the group, first at the parasternal area (for pump-handle restriction) and then in the midaxillary line (for bucket-handle restriction). For each placement, ask the patient to inhale and exhale. Palpate successive pairs of ribs within the group until symmetry of motion on respiration is noted. With inhalation restriction, the key rib is found at the top of the group, but it is located at the bottom of the rib group with exhalation restrictions.

In summary, inhalation restrictions involve a rib or group of ribs that first stops moving during inhalation. The key rib is the top rib in the group. Exhalation restrictions involve a rib or group of ribs that stops moving first during exhalation. The key rib is the bottom rib in the group.

EVALUATION OF RIBS 11–12

Ribs 11 and 12 have no anterior cartilaginous attachment and therefore do not exhibit pump-handle or bucket-handle movement. Instead, they move posteriorly and laterally with inhalation, and anteriorly and medially during exhalation. This motion is sometimes described as caliper motion.

Assess for respiratory dysfunction of these ribs with the patient in the prone position. Stand at the side of the patient, with the dominant eye over the patient's midline. Place your hands over the 11th and 12th ribs, contacting the rib shafts with the thumbs and thenar eminences. Ask the patient to inhale and exhale fully; note any asymmetry of motion in the ribs. If either of the ribs does not move posteriorly with inhalation, it is described as having an inhalation restriction. Conversely, if the ribs do not move anteriorly with exhalation, exhalation restriction is present.

Diaphragm Evaluation

One method of examining the diaphragm for motion restriction is as follows. Stand behind the seated patient and pass your hands around the thoracic cage under the arms of the patient. By gently but firmly introducing the finger pads upward and medially under the costal margins, assess diaphragmatic motions. Testing is easier when the patient leans slightly backward against your chest in a slightly slumped position. This position lessens tension of the muscular attachments on and around the costal margins, making palpation a good deal easier. Assess motion restriction and asymmetry by passively rotating the diaphragm gently right and left.

Sternum Evaluation

Compression and decompression of the sternum can be a valuable diagnostic test, for many reasons. Two common examples are sternocostal problems associated with seat belt injuries in car accidents and mechanical chest wall problems secondary to coronary artery bypass surgery.

STERNAL COMPRESSION

Testing the sternum involves gentle compression and release with particular attention to respiratory, mechanical, and pain-related responses arising both locally and from points distant. Functional and myofascial approaches are particularly useful (see Chapters 57–63).

To test the sternomanubrial joint, place the thenar eminence of one hand on the superoanterior edge of the manubrium, and that of the other hand on the body of the sternum. Compress slightly, noting any indication that the tissue moves more easily in one or more directions as the patient goes through the respiratory cycle.

Perform the same test at the xiphisternal joint using one thenar eminence on the sternum and a single finger (or the thumb and a finger) on the inferior border of the xiphoid. Maintain slight pressure on the sternum while depressing and then lifting the xiphoid with slight anterosuperior pressure, and note any tendency for the tissues to move toward a position of ease.

OTHER DIAGNOSTIC INDICATORS

Palpation that elicits tenderness, complaints of pain, wincing, grunting, or grimacing provides valuable assessment information. For example, point tenderness over a bone may be an indication of a fracture, sprain, infection, or even cancer. Pain in muscle and connective tissue in the absence of trauma is more indicative of musculoskeletal dysfunction or connective tissue disorder. Palpating for tender spots and trigger points is often helpful (Chapters 65–67).

ASSESSMENT AND TREATMENT

After the history and physical examination are completed, apply the osteopathic philosophy by assessing the type and amount of osteopathic manipulative treatment the patient needs. Whether it is administered immediately often depends on the setting and circumstances. For example, an acute hospital or emergency room typically calls for an approach different from a primary care setting. The choice of manipulative treatment depends on the expertise of the physician as well as the patient's condition and response to previous treatment. All manipulative treatment is performed in a context that interdependently includes the whole body and the person as a whole.

Having a primary treatment plan is essential. The treatment prescription depends on the diagnosis and expected outcomes; it may be medical, surgical, manipulative, reassurance-based, or any combination. Since the focus of this chapter is on neuromusculoskeletally based thoracic region problems, it is assumed that all other aspects of diagnosis and standard medical care have been integrated. Under these circumstances, osteopathic manipulation is then provided as either a primary intervention or as a method for supporting intrinsic homeostatic mechanisms, ameliorating pain, and/or assisting the patient to attain and maintain an optimal state of health.

Problems that have been particularly responsive to osteopathic manipulation of the thoracic region include:

Costovertebral joint dysfunctions
Neuromuscular imbalances
Myofascial disorders
Painful problems associated with somatic dysfunction related viscerosomatic and somatosomatic reflexes, neurovascular and lymphatic circulatory changes

The following two examples illustrate these problems.

Example 1: Primarily Neuromusculoskeletal

A 35-year-old female patient presents with chest pain. After a careful history eliminated other causes, the physician concludes that the problem is primarily musculoskeletal. Palpatory diagnosis indicates that there are multiple levels of thoracic somatic dysfunction at T4 (FSRRR) and T7 (ESLRL). There is decreased inhalation-related movement involving ribs 7-10 on the left along with decreased left-sided diaphragm motion.

Treatment might consist of soft tissue techniques followed by high-velocity, low-amplitude (HVLA) techniques for the thoracic segments and strain and counterstrain for the ribs, as well as indirect myofascial release of the diaphragm.

Example 2: Somatic Components of Visceral Disease

A 65-year-old patient is hospitalized for pneumonia. Both structural and respiratory rib dysfunctions are found throughout the rib cage along with multiple thoracic, cervical, lumbar, and diaphragmatic problems. Appropriate antibiotics, muco-

lytics, and other indicated procedures are used. In an osteopathically oriented setting, osteopathic manipulation is used with an eye toward improving sympathetic/parasympathetic factors, diaphragm excursion, spinal and rib mechanics, and also vascular and lymphatic flow to improve the work of breathing. The goal is to decrease sympathicotonia and energy wasted on inefficient breathing by decreasing abnormal mechanoreceptor and nociceptive inputs to the central nervous system (decreasing pain) and assisting the body in mobilizing the immune system.

Seriously ill and hospitalized patients are more commonly treated with indirect treatment. However, rib raising and direct articulatory technique is often indicated. For ICU/CCU patients, indirect myofascial techniques are appropriate as are strain and counterstrain or craniosacral approaches.

CONCLUSION

The thoracic cage is a complex region of the body, containing and protecting many vital organs. Osteopathic physicians must understand the proper function, diagnosis, and treatment of the thoracic area.

REFERENCES

1. White AA, Panjabi MM. *Clinical Biomechanics of the Spine.* Philadelphia, Pa: JB Lippincott; 1978:44–56.
2. Patterson MM, Howell JN, eds. *The Central Connection: Somatovisceral/Viscerosomatic Interaction.* Indianapolis, Ind: American Academy of Osteopathy; 1992.
3. Korr IM. The spinal cord as organizer of disease processes, IV: axonal transport and neurotrophic function in relation to somatic dysfunction. *JAOA.* 1981;80(7):451–459.
4. Korr IM. Proprioceptors and somatic dysfunction. *JAOA.* 1975; 74(7);638–650.
5. Patterson MM, Steinmetz JE. Long-lasting alterations of spinal reflexes: a basis for somatic dysfunction. *Man Med.* 1986;2:38–42.
6. Van Buskirk RL. Nociceptive reflexes and the somatic dysfunction: a model. *JAOA.* 1990;90(9):792–804.
7. Gallaudet BB. *A Description of the Planes of Fascia of the Human Body.* New York, NY: Columbia Press; 1931.
8. Budgell B, Sato A. Somatoautonomic reflex regulation of sciatic nerve blood flow. *J Neuromusculoskeletal System.* 1994;2:170–177.
9. Moore KL. *Clinically Oriented Anatomy.* 2nd ed. Baltimore, Md: Williams & Wilkins; 1985.
10. Warwick R, Williams P, eds. *Gray's Anatomy.* 35th ed. Edinburgh: Churchill Livingstone; 1973.
11. Willard FH, Patterson MM, eds. *Nociception and the Neuroendocrine–Immune Connection.* Indianapolis, Ind: American Academy of Osteopathy; 1994.

48. Lumbar and Abdominal Region

WILLIAM A. KUCHERA

Key Concepts

- **Functional anatomy of lumbar and abdominal areas, including skeleton, ligaments, muscles, fascia, vasculature, lymphatics, and nerves**

- **Motion and dysfunction in lumbar and abdominal areas**

- **Aids to diagnosis, including patient history, physical examination, observation, auscultation, palpation, and motion testing**

- **Reflexes and muscle strength**

- **Treatment of specific problems, including postural stress or decomposition, psoas syndrome, postfracture or postoperative ileus, radiculopathy, and quadratus lumborum myofascial triggers**

The lumbar region links the pelvis with the thoracic region. Its functional connections link it with the head and neck, the upper extremities, lower extremities, and even the viscera. Back and/or abdominal pain and dysfunction do not necessarily arise from a symptomatic area. Problems in the pelvis, abdomen, and lumbar regions need to be considered.

Facets of the thoracic region are oriented in a coronal plane. The region should provide more motion in all planes than should the sagittal plane orientation of the lumbar facets, but in fact its motion is limited. The rib cage hinders the ability of the thoracic region to rotate, side-bend, flex, or even to extend. Analysis reveals that it is the lumbar and thoracolumbar regions that provide most of these motions of the trunk.

The lumbar and pelvic regions are frequent sites of strain, pain, and disability. Low back dysfunction makes up a large part of worker's compensation claims and is often the reason for absences from work, insurance claims, and disability payments. Despite mechanical problems, including somatic dysfunction, being responsible for 90% of the complaints of backache,[1(p.148)] the physician must always consider the functional connections of the back. This is important so that the treatment offered is directed toward the primary cause and not to the symptom of a backache or a back problem.

The lumbar region is the posterior boundary for almost the entire abdomen. Primary sympathetic fibers for innervation of all organs below the diaphragm, except the descending colon and pelvic organs, pass from the intermediolateral cells in the thoracic spinal cord through the thoracoabdominal diaphragm (Fig. 48.1). In the abdomen these primary fibers enter the celiac, superior mesenteric, and the inferior mesenteric collateral ganglia where they synapse. Secondary or postganglionic fibers continue on to innervate specific groups of organs in the abdomen and pelvis. Parasympathetic innervation is supplied from the craniosacral outflow. All abdominal organs down to the midtransverse colon are supplied by cranial nerve X (CN X, or vagus nerve); the rest of the abdominal organs and all of the pelvic viscera receive their parasympathetic innervation from the pelvic splanchnic nerves (sacral roots 2, 3, 4).

The first three lumbar vertebrae serve as primary posterior attachments for the crura of the abdominal diaphragm. These vertebrae also supply attachments for the erector spinae mass of muscles that extend from the pelvis all the way to the neck and head. The latissimus dorsi muscle connects the pelvis and the lumbar region with the upper extremity. Through a lumbosacral aponeurosis and fascia, the lumbar region is functionally attached to the hamstrings, the gluteal muscles, and the iliotibial band into the lower extremity; through the oblique abdominal muscles, the posterior lumbar region is functionally related to the anterior abdominal wall.

Lumbar spinal nerve roots L1-4 are the main components of the lumbar plexus. The nerves of the lumbar plexus innervate and form in the psoas muscle, anterior to the transverse processes of the lumbar vertebrae. The psoas muscles extend from vertebral bodies and the anterior surface of the transverse

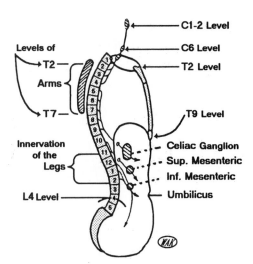

Figure 48.1. Anatomic levels and sympathetic innervation to organs below diaphragm, head/neck, and arms and legs.

581

processes in the lumbar vertebra. They then pass along the superior border of the true pelvis where they pick up the iliacus muscles. The iliopsoas muscle then attaches to the lesser trochanter of the femur via common tendons. The lumbar plexus also forms the femoral, obturator, ilioinguinal, and the iliohypogastric nerves. Lumbar dermatomes are located in the posterior lumbar paraspinal region, but then extend into the anterior part of the thigh, leg, and foot. Pain or paresthesias of these areas of skin provide clues to the location (level) of possible lumbar nerve dysfunction and/or irritation.

Visceral pain from the left colon, ureters, and pelvic structures (except the cervix), as well as musculoskeletal pain and somatic dysfunction from the pelvis, may be referred to the upper lumbar and thoracolumbar paraspinal regions. Pain from cervical dilation refers pain to the sacral region via visceral afferents that follow the pathways of the pelvic splanchnic nerves. Referred pain from the left colon and ureters can be clearly understood by the origin of the sympathetic innervation, but referred pain from the pelvic viscera and somatic dysfunction from the sacrum and other pelvic structures have only recently been explained. Spinal nerves with white rami are found only from T1 to L2. Visceral afferent and nociceptive reflexes from the pelvic area follow the pathway of the sympathetic chain (Fig. 48.2) up to the paraspinal ganglia of the L2 or L1 level. They then enter the cord, facilitate the cord, and then reflex out the somatic nerves at the thoracolumbar region. Spasms of the uterine muscles or contractions of the uterus during labor refer this discomfort to the thoracolumbar

paraspinal region (area of sympathetic innervation to the uterus). Because visceral afferent pain fibers from the cervix uteri travel the pathways of the pelvic splanchnic nerves (parasympathetic from roots S2, 3, 4), pain from cervical dilation refers to the posterior sacral region.

These examples of lumbar and abdominal myofascial and neural interconnections with other regions of the body illustrate that back and/or abdominal pain and dysfunction does not necessarily arise from a symptomatic area. Problems in the pelvis, abdomen, and lumbar regions need to be intelligently pursued. Some examples of these connections are presented here in greater detail.

FUNCTIONAL ANATOMY

Skeletal

The lumbar region forms the posterior skeletal and myofascial border of the true abdomen. The five vertebrae are distinguished by their larger size and the absence of costal facets and transverse foramina. The body of a lumbar vertebra is wider transversely and deeper from front to back than any other spinal vertebra.[2(p.322)] Its large cross-sectional area is designed to sustain longitudinal loads. It also acts as an accessory site for hematopoiesis and contains longitudinal and vertical bony trabeculae, arranged to increase its stability. The posterior element or arch of a lumbar vertebra, easily visualized on an AP lumbar x-ray view, is especially adapted to stand the forces that act upon it. The posterior element attaches to the body via the pedicle, a landmark that aids in the identification of other posterior elements in x-ray images. Using the pedicle as a base, one can identify the transverse process, the superior articular process, the inferior articular process, and the lamina. By following the lamina to where it joins the lamina on the other side, one identifies the spinous process (Fig. 48.3).

Lumbar spinous processes are distinguished by their palpable, thick, quadrangular, spadelike shape. This is in contrast to the fingertip-sized palpatory characteristic of thoracic spinous processes. The body of the vertebra, its two pedicles, and the laminae enclose the triangular lumbar vertebral canal that contains the spinal cord and its associated elements. When one lamina fails to fuse with the lamina from the opposite side, a spina bifida results (Fig. 48.4).

The most common deformity of this type is called a spina bifida occulta, meaning that it is "hidden." Spina bifida occulta is frequently found at the L5/S1 level of the spine. The only physical clue of this anomaly may be a patch of coarse hair over the site of the spina bifida occulta. This congenital anomaly does not have meningeal components and is not considered to be a condition that should keep a person from employment. It may modify muscle attachments, however, and be associated with the finding of a higher incidence of other posterior vertebral anomalies, such as spondylolisthesis. In the severe form of spina bifida, the spinal membranes protrude (with or without cord tissue) and are known as a meningocele or a meningomyelocele.

The spinal cord usually terminates between the levels of L1

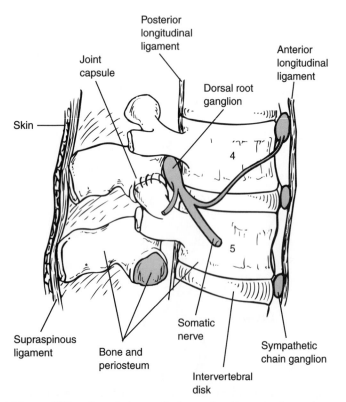

Figure 48.2. Paraspinal sympathetic ganglia of lower lumbar region.

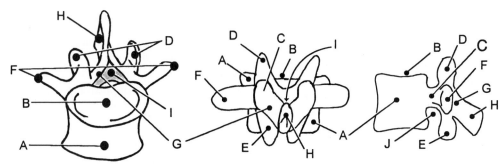

Figure 48.3. Vertebral components using a lumbar vertebra as an example. *A,* body; *B,* centrum; *C,* pedicle; *D,* anterior articular process; *E,* posterior articular process; *F,* transverse process; *G,* lamina; *H,* spinous-process; *I,* spinal canal; *J,* intervertebral foramen. (Courtesy of W.A. Kuchera.)

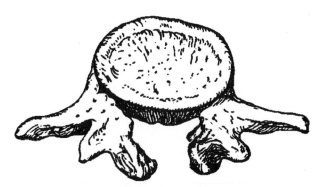

Figure 48.4. Spina bifida occulta.

and L2, with a range as high as T12 and as low as L3. The vertebral canal, with the posterior longitudinal ligament running along its anterior surface, contains the conus medullaris (terminal end of the spinal cord), the filum terminale, and the nerves of the cauda equina. It normally decreases in its anteroposterior dimension as one progresses from L1 to L5. As a person ages, the diameter of the lumbar canal may be compromised by factors such as:

Hypertrophy of the posterior longitudinal ligament
Thickening of the ligamentum flava on its posterior wall
Osteoarthritis
Exostoses
Osteophytes
Tumors
Ruptured lumbar intervertebral disk

Edema can also compromise the nerves in a canal that is deformed. If there is enough pressure on the cord or the nerves of the cauda equina, weakness and paralysis of the lower extremities and the sphincters of the bladder and rectum may occur. This symptom complex is a severe form of spinal stenosis called cauda equina syndrome. It is considered to be a surgical emergency if progressive paralysis of the lower extremities occurs. The paralysis begins in the feet and progresses upward. This paralysis may progress slowly or occur very rapidly with complete paralysis of the lower extremities within an

hour. If cauda equina syndrome is suspected, surgical consultation and decompression should be obtained immediately. A timely emergency surgical decompression should provide full use of the lower extremities. If surgery is delayed too long, motor function of the lower extremities and/or sphincters may never return, even though there is complete decompression of the nerves and cord.

Between the lumbar vertebrae is a large intervertebral disk, built to transmit or tolerate heavy loads. All of the intervertebral disks taken together account for about one fourth of the length of the spinal column. They are composed of:

Glycosaminoglycans
Mucopolysaccharides
Proteoglycans
Collagen

Each disc has an annulus at its center, surrounded by a nucleus pulposus. The annulus, composed of concentric lamellae of collagenous fibers oriented 65° from vertical and alternating in right to left successive layers, encircles and contains the nucleus pulposus. The nucleus pulposus is semifluid, composed 70–90% of water, and is deformable but not compressible. With weight bearing, the nucleus loses its water, resulting in 1.5 mm of creep in the first 2–10 minutes. Rest in the supine position with the lower extremities flexed and raised is the optimum position for returning the disc to its full or optimal height. The weakest region, and therefore the region most likely to rupture, is located on its posterior side, where it is poorly enforced by the narrowed posterior longitudinal ligament, which is narrower in the lumbar than in the cervical region.

An intervertebral foramina for passage of a lumbar nerve is defined by the:

Adjacent pedicles
Vertebral bodies
Common intervertebral disc
Articular processes
Synovial joint of the two adjacent vertebrae

Because the pedicles on a lumbar vertebra are located on the superior third and posterior side of a lumbar vertebra, a lumbar nerve that exits the cauda equina wraps around the pedicle and passes through the intervertebral foramen of its number before it crosses its disc space (Fig. 48.5). This is why L5 radiculopathy is usually produced by a ruptured L4 disc and a S1 radiculopathy from a lumbosacral (L5) disk herniation.

Forward bending, side-bending, and rotation away from the location of a ruptured and protruding intervertebral disc are uncomfortable for the patient. These positions displace the nucleus pulposus toward the site of rupture and a lumbar nerve root. In contrast, lumbar extension is more likely to be uncomfortable to a person who has radiculopathy caused by the narrowing of an intervertebral foramen, as this positioning narrows the foramen. These people are more comfortable with flexion, because flexion enlarges an intervertebral foramen.

In neutral, the lumbar spinal region normally forms a smooth backward bending curve with a L2-L5 lumbolumbar lordotic angle averaging 43° (ML Kuchera, personal research). Functionally, this curve permits more extension than flexion before the sagittal plane reaches a position where normal nonneutral multiple plane operation is expected to occur. A facet on a superior articular process of a typical lumbar vertebra faces posteromedially and is lateral to the facet of the inferior articular process of the vertebra above. The joint space between two lumbar vertebrae should generally lie in a coronal plane orientation, best seen on an anteroposterior (AP) x-ray view of the lumbar spine. The most common congenital abnormality, called zygapophyseal tropism, with an incidence of 30%, is asymmetry of the lumbar facets. This means that a facet on one side is "twisted" and does not match the orientation of the facet on the other side of that same vertebral unit. Asymmetry of lumbar facets should not be a cause for an employer's rejection of an applicant for a job. Clinically, however, asymmetric joints at the same level produce asymmetric muscle tensions and motions. This apparently stresses the back at that level and clinically is found to lengthen the recovery period of those patients.

Ligaments, Muscles, and Fascias

Two ligaments directly connect the lumbar vertebral bodies: the anterior and the posterior longitudinal ligaments. The posterior longitudinal ligament becomes narrower in the lumbar region and is not as supportive to the posterolateral margins of the intervertebral lumbar disk. The main ligaments of the posterior arch are the:

Ligamentum flava between the lamina
Interspinous ligaments between the lumbar spinous processes (weak and often absent)
Supraspinous ligaments (degenerated in the adult lumbar spine and possibly ruptured)

The iliolumbar ligament is a unique ligament of the lumbosacral region and deserves special attention. It attaches to the transverse processes of L4 and L5 and the iliac crest (Fig. 48.6), and the anterior and posterior regions of the sacroiliac joint (See Fig. 72.4). This ligament is represented by muscle fibers in neonates and children and is gradually replaced by ligamentous tissue by the third decade of life.

When stressed, the iliolumbar ligament becomes tender. *The iliolumbar ligament is typically the first ligament to become tender when there is lumbosacral postural decompensation.* This tenderness is sometimes not evident to the patient until it is lightly palpated. The most common tender area is located 1 inch up and lateral to the posterior superior iliac spine (PSIS) on the iliac crest.

All of the muscles and the bones are compartmentalized and protected by the deep fascias that then form the thoracolumbar aponeurosis (Fig. 48.7). This fascia gives attachment to the latissimus dorsi muscle, extending to the upper/proximal humerus. Next to the spine, this fascia compartmentalizes the interspinalis, multifidi, and rotatores muscles. More laterally and yet near the midline, it encloses the longissimus muscle,

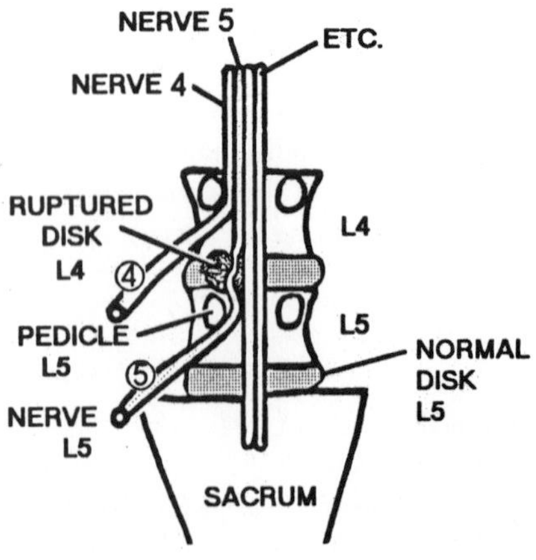

Figure 48.5. Relationship of lumbar radiculopathy to ruptured lumbar disk. (Courtesy of W.A. Kuchera.)

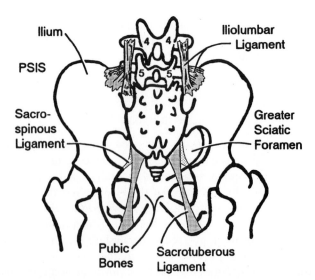

Figure 48.6. Iliolumbar ligament. (Courtesy of W.A. Kuchera.)

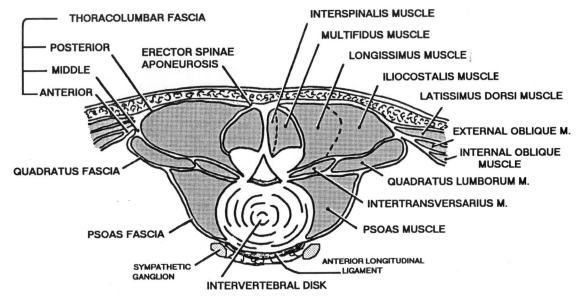

Figure 48.7. Thoracolumbar aponeurosis and deep lumbar fascia.

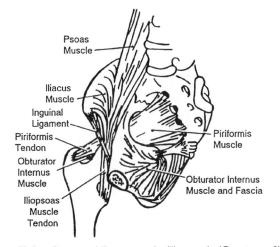

Figure 48.8. Psoas and iliacus muscle (iliopsoas). (Courtesy of W.A. Kuchera.)

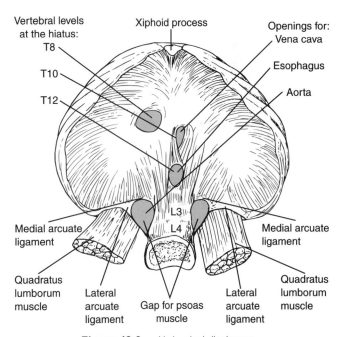

Figure 48.9. Abdominal diaphragm.

and more laterally, the iliocostalis muscle group that inserts on the angles of the ribs in the thoracic region. Its deeper layers form compartments for the intertransversarii and the quadratus lumborum muscle. The quadratus lumborum muscle can be clinically and functionally thought of as the posteroinferior extension of the abdominal diaphragm. The fascia continues anteriorly to attach to the transverse processes and then proceeds further anteriorly to enclose the psoas muscle.

Arising from the anterolateral surface of the T12-L4 vertebrae and their transverse processes, the psoas muscle joins the iliacus muscle from the inner surface of the ilium and inserts by a common tendon into the lesser trochanter of the femur (Fig. 48.8). The lumbar plexus (lumbar nerve roots L1-4) forms within the belly of the psoas muscle. The thoracolumbar aponeurosis is also continuous with the fascia of the abdominal

wall, the fascia over the gluteus muscle, and the fascia lata of the lower extremity.

The abdominal diaphragm forms the superior boundary of the abdominal area (Fig. 48.9). It attaches by right and left crural attachments to the first two lumbar vertebrae on the left and the first three lumbar vertebrae on the right. Slips of muscle attach to the lower six ribs and then to the xiphoid process. In some ways, the diaphragm is functionally continuous with the action of the quadratus lumborum muscle. This muscle is structurally a lumbopelvic extension of the abdominal diaphragm. A well-domed relaxed diaphragm produces much bet-

Figure 48.10. Abdominal diaphragm and pressure gradients.

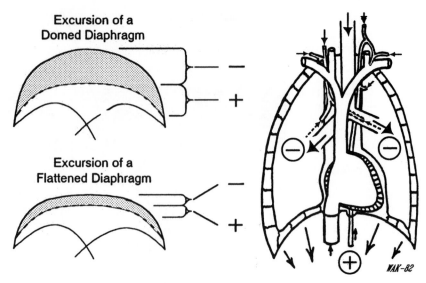

ter pressure gradients between the thoracic and abdominal areas than a flattened diaphragm and therefore improves the return of lymph and venous blood back to the thoracic area venous system and the heart (Fig. 48.10).

Parietal peritoneum, lining the abdominal cavity, angles from the posterior wall of the abdomen to form very defined mesenteric connections to the abdominal viscera (Fig. 48.11). These mesenteries carry the:

Sympathetic fibers
Parasympathetic fibers
Arteries
Veins
Visceral afferent fibers
Lymphatic vessels of the viscera

The root of the mesentery for approximately 30 feet of small intestines is only 6 inches long and is located on the posterior wall of the abdominal cavity, posterior to a point about one-inch to the left and one-inch above the umbilicus. The root of the mesentery runs inferolaterally to a second point just anterior to the right sacroiliac joint. Mental visualization of these mesenteries allows a physician to determine more accurately the origin of palpable masses and the origin of auscultated abnormal sounds. It is also important when performing visceral manipulation to free fascial pathways and improve visceral function.

Abdominal mesenteric lift is applied by manipulation to affect the mesenteries (refer to Figure 48.18) and is directed toward improving:

Intestinal function
Innervation
Circulation
Nutrition
Removal of waste products

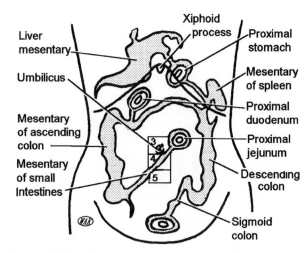

Figure 48.11. Posterior attachments of abdominal mesenteries.

This is performed by placing the flattened fingers along the side of a bowel segment in line with the mesentery of that segment of intestine. The intestine is then gently "lifted" at right angles to the attachment of its mesentery, to the point of balanced tension. This position is held, and the patient is asked to take half of a deep breath and hold the breath while the palpatory balance is maintained. When the patient has to breathe, you feel a slight relaxation of the mesentery. Take up the slack and repeat a few times until no more improvement is palpated.

Vasculature and Lymphatics

The thoracic aorta lies along the anterior and left anterolateral side of the thoracic vertebrae. It enters the abdominal cavity through the aortic hiatus in the abdominal diaphragm at the level anterior to the 12th thoracic vertebra. Here it becomes the abdominal aorta. Its main lumbar branches are the following:

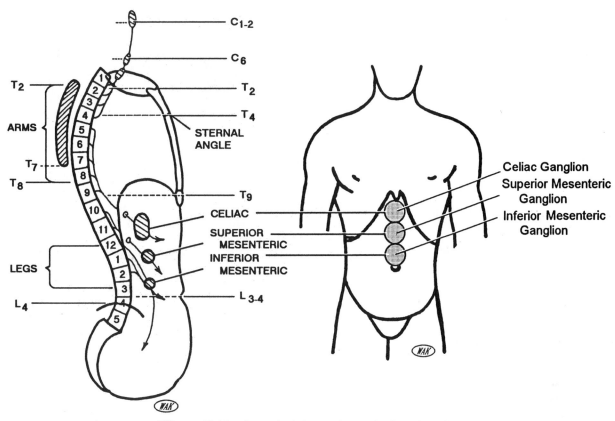

Figure 48.12. Sympathetic innervations and collateral ganglia.

Celiac
Superior mesenteric
Renal
Inferior mesenteric

Lying on its anterior surface and associated with the arterial branches with the same names are the celiac, superior mesenteric, and inferior mesenteric collateral sympathetic ganglia (Fig. 48.12). In these collateral (midline) ganglia, primary sympathetic fibers synapse with secondary sympathetic fibers, which then continue on to innervate the abdominal viscera.

The left lymphatic duct (the thoracic duct) drains interstitial fluids from the lower extremities, the pelvic and abdominal viscera, the left arm, and the left side of the head (Fig. 48.13). It begins as the cisterna chyli, a 2-inch, yellowish, cigarette-shaped structure in the abdomen. This structure lies just to the left of the thoracolumbar junction and the first lumbar vertebra. It receives lymphatic vessels that drain interstitial fluids from all the abdominal organs, the pelvic organs, the lower extremities, and all of the superficial lymphatic vessels located below a horizontal plane of the body running through the umbilicus (Fig. 48.14). The superficial lymphatic vessels drain lymph into superficial inguinal nodes. Lymph then travels into the deep nodes, the deep trunks along the common iliacs and aorta, and finally into the cisterna chyli. It should be noted that lymph from the ovary, testicles, and prostate does not drain into the inguinal nodes but drains into the deep pelvic

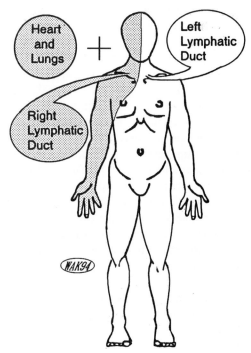

Figure 48.13. Main lymphatic ducts of body.

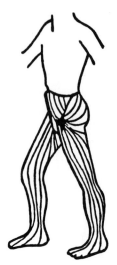

Figure 48.14.   Lymphatic drainage of lower half of body. (Courtesy of by W.A. Kuchera.)

nodes. That is why the only palpable, nonsubjective clue to early ovarian or testicular cancer is palpable mass on a pelvic, testicular, or prostatic examination.

The umbilicus is located approximately anterior to and in a horizontal plane running through the L3-4 disc space. Since the abdominal aorta divides into the common iliac arteries at about the level of the umbilicus, bruits from the aorta, an abdominal aortic aneurysm, or the renal arteries are identified by auscultation near the midline between the umbilicus and the xiphoid process. Renal artery bruits are usually auscultated best in the epigastric region.

Anatomical relationships and a good history help a physician determine the cause of a patient's complaints. For example, an older hypertensive patient, complaining of severe back pain, numbness of the lower extremities, and a palpable abdominal mass, with a bruit over the abdominal aorta, could have either an abdominal aneurysm or renal artery stenosis. Back pain produced by a dissecting abdominal aneurysm is a surgical emergency.

It is more likely, however, that back pain is due to lumbosacral strain and/or somatic dysfunction. In every case, the more serious medical problems must also be considered by evaluating the history and physical findings. In highly suspicious cases, ordering and reviewing special radiological and laboratory tests or magnetic resonance imaging (MRI) may be indicated. After surgical emergencies are ruled in or ruled out, osteopathic manipulation of the patient's somatic dysfunction may become the primary treatment. It gives the patient comfort, improves the effectiveness of other necessary treatment, and/or speeds recovery by improving structure–function relationships.

The abdominal cavity is separated from the thoracic cavity by the abdominal diaphragm. The diaphragm is necessary not only for breathing but also for the production of pressure gradients between the thoracic and abdominal cavities. It helps move venous and lymphatic fluids from the tissues back to the venous circulation and the heart. The diaphragm attaches posteriorly to L1-3 on the right and L1-2 on the left. To permit more efficient movement of the rib cage and diaphragm, the quadratus lumborum anchors the 12th rib and in this way extends the anchorage of the diaphragm to the iliac crest.[3] A well-domed diaphragm (relaxed, with a high and smoothly curved profile) produces very effective pressure gradients when it contracts and relaxes, improving lymphatic flow from all parts of the body (Fig. 48.10).

The external and internal veins of the vertebrae, the spinal canal, and the cranium do not have valves to direct fluid flow; they are devoid of valves. The valves of the intervertebral veins accompanying the spinal nerves through the intervertebral foramen may be ineffective.[4(p.703)] This would permit blood flow to be reversed, indicating that blood flow through these channels depends on the pressure within the various cavities of the body. A Valsalva maneuver can reverse the flow of blood within the vertebral column (Fig. 48.15). This functional anatomical fact is used to explain how pelvic and abdominal neoplasms may metastasize to vertebral bodies and to the brain.[4(pp.703–707),5] It also explains why poor lymphatic and venous drainage may be associated with chronic congestive headaches and contribute to back pain symptoms.

Nerves

The lumbar plexus is composed of nerves derived from lumbar roots 1-4 and a branch from T12. As previously mentioned, lumbar spinal nerve roots enter directly into the psoas muscle where the lumbar plexus is formed, and its nerve branches emerge from the muscle borders and surfaces.[2(p.635)] The nerves can generally be divided into these functional divisions:

- The femoral nerve (L2, 3, and 4), which exits the femoral canal to supply innervation to the quadriceps muscles of the thigh and sensory fibers to the skin of the anterior thigh
- The obturator nerve (L2, 3, and 4), which exits the obturator foramen to innervate the adductor muscles of the thigh and to carry sensory fibers to the medial portion of the thigh
- A group of muscular branches (lumbar), which innervate the psoas major and minor, the iliacus, and the quadratus lumborum muscles
- The iliohypogastric (L1), ilioinguinal (L1), and genitofemoral (L1 and 2) nerves, which supply sensation to the lateral skin of the gluteal area, the root of the penis or mons and the upper part of the scrotum and labia, the inguinal and femoral triangle areas, and the cremasteric muscle, respectively
- Lateral femoral cutaneous nerve (L2 and 3), which emerges from the psoas muscle just superior to the iliac crest, runs over the iliacus muscle, passes just medial to the anterior superior iliac spine (ASIS), and passes through or posterior to the inguinal ligament to enter the thigh. It supplies sensory fibers for a large oval dermatome over the anterior and lateral part of the thigh.

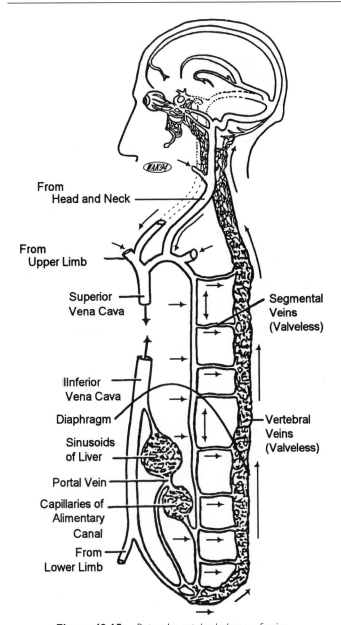

Figure 48.15. Batson's vertebral plexus of veins.

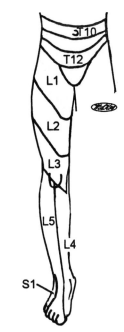

Figure 48.16. Lumbar dermatomes.

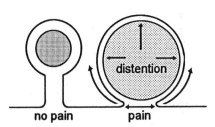

Figure 48.17. Visceral pain from distention of an abdominal organ. (Courtesy of by W.A. Kuchera.)

Dermatomal patterns for the lumbar nerves are located in the anterior portion of the lower extremity (Fig. 48.16). Hoppenfeld[6] provides the easiest pattern to remember. He advises to construct mentally three oblique lines on the anterior thigh that divide the thigh into three equal sections. These lines start from a superior position on the lateral thigh and extend to a more inferior position on the medial thigh. The inferior oblique line must go through the patella. These lines delineate L1, L2, and L3 dermatomes. Then construct a line from the patella to the big toe to delineate the L4 dermatome medially and the L5 dermatome laterally. Take a small section on the lateral side of the foot to indicate part of the S1 dermatome. Remember, however, that these lines are approximate and not rigidly followed by the actual nerve distribution.

Areas of sensitivity may recede from or exceed the boundaries as drawn.

Myotomal symptoms from lumbar nerve dysfunction, irritability, or radiculopathy are evidence by cramps and/or weakness of the muscles innervated by that root (see Chapter 50, "Lower Extremities").

Sclerotomal pain, described as deep toothachelike pain, arises from ligaments, bones, or joints. Knee pain, for example, can be caused by a lesion of the L3 vertebra, ligaments in the L3 area, the hip, or the knee. All of these sites have the same L3 sclerotomal distribution. (See the sclerotomal chart in Chapter 50.)

Mesenteries from the posterior wall of the abdomen (Fig. 48.11) carry the sympathetic fibers, parasympathetic fibers, and arteries to the viscera. They also carry visceral afferent fibers, veins, and lymphatic vessels away from the viscera. The visceral peritoneum is sensitive to stretch. It produces visceral pain only when the distention of the viscus exceeds the length of the visceral peritoneum on the outside of the mesentery (Fig. 48.17). The mesenteries are palpated for tension or tenderness by placing the extended fingers of the hands flat over the lateral margin of the ascending or descending colon and moving this viscera toward the midline of the body. The physician monitors continuously for changes in resistance to this movement. The mesentery of the sigmoid colon is moved toward the umbilicus. The 6-inch mesentery, along with 30 feet of small intestines, is palpated by placing the extended fingers carefully into the lower left abdominal quadrant to obtain as much of the small intestines as possible, and moving this toward the upper right quadrant of the abdomen. The mesenteries are treated in a similar manner. The fingers are extended and placed flat over the lateral margin of the mesentery you wish to treat. Medial pressure is then placed over the section of the bowel at right angle to its posterior, mesenteric, abdominal wall attachment (Fig. 48.18). The tension is held as the patient takes a half-breath and holds it. When air hunger occurs, palpate an increase lengthening and relaxation of the mesentery. The process is repeated two or three times.

Inflammation can produce three types of pain referral to the soma from abdominal and pelvic viscera. Fibers carrying afferent impulses from an inflamed visceral organ tend to synapse at the same cord segment levels that provide the sympathetic innervation for the organ that is dysfunctioning.

VISCERAL PAIN

Visceral afferent impulses travel back to the cord using the same course used by the sympathetic efferent nerves to that organ. This pain tends to be vague and gnawing, deep, poorly localized, and midabdominal (Fig. 48.19).

VISCEROSOMATIC PAIN

Somatic afferent fibers from the root of the mesentery report to the somatic cord segment of that organ's sympathetic innervation (Fig. 48.20). This type of sensory input produces the

paraspinal somatic clues that help you to locate the viscera that is most likely dysfunctional. The clues are tenderness, asymmetry, restriction, and tissue texture changes (TART). The pain and tissue texture changes are primarily localized at the paraspinal level consistent with the organ's sympathetic innervation.

SOMATIC PAIN CAUSED BY PERCUTANEOUS REFLEX OF MORLEY

This type of somatic pain, caused by the percutaneous reflex of Morley, is usually located directly over the inflamed organ and is produced by direct contiguous irritation of the parietal peritoneum and the somatic abdominal wall (Fig. 48.21). It is responsible for rebound tenderness and abdominal guarding associated with more severe abdominal pain.

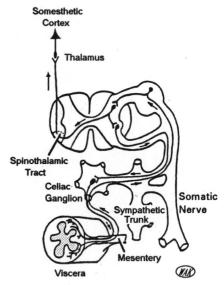

Figure 48.19.   Pathway of visceral pain: vague midline pain.

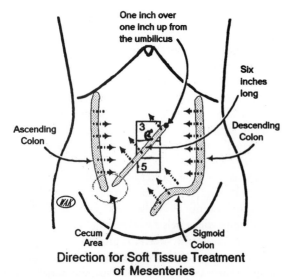

Direction for Soft Tissue Treatment of Mesenteries

Figure 48.18.   Treatment pattern for abdominal mesenteries.

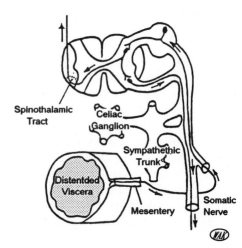

Figure 48.20.   Pathway of viscerosomatic pain: paraspinal pain in area of sympathetic innervation of dysfunctional organ or system.

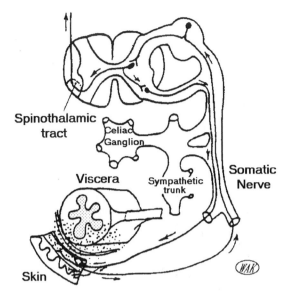

Figure 48.21. *Pain from reflex of Morley: direct extension; pain over organ.*

MOTION AND DYSFUNCTION

There seems to be very little motion of the lumbar spinal region when one attempts to move two lumbar vertebrae. Much more motion is possible when the lumbar vertebrae move as a group. In the lumbar spine, rotation and side-bending are closely coupled.

The expected motions of the lumbar spine are:

Flexion
Extension
Side-bending
Rotation

Side-bending and rotation are coupled motions; one cannot occur without the other. Translatory motion in three planes is also permitted. The pattern of multiple plane motion that occurs in the lumbar spine depends on the position of the sagittal plane when the vector of rotation or side-bending is introduced. In the neutral sagittal plane range, side-bending and then rotation occur to opposite sides and in a group of vertebrae. If the sagittal plane were in the nonneutral range defined as flexion or extension of a degree sufficient to engage the facets as prime movers of the spine, side-bending and rotation would occur to the same side. This type of motion usually takes place at a single vertebral unit and is called Fryette (type II) motion.

Because of lumbar vertebral construction and joint facings, neutral (type I) pattern of motion[7] results in a group of vertebrae when directed by the vertebral bodies and discs. In the lumbar region, this multiple plane motion is possible in a greater range of sagittal plane extension than flexion.

It takes very little flexion to stabilize the lumbar spine and disks, where motion is directed by the facets; this pattern of motion is called nonneutral or type II motion.[7] It occurs in one, or rarely two, vertebral units. Though nonneutral motion

(type II motion) is more likely to be produced when the lumbar spine is flexed, it is possible to produce nonneutral lumbar motion with forced hyperextension. Examples of forced hyperextension are a high-diver entering the water, a gymnast doing a back walkover, or a painter painting a high ceiling.

Myofascial trigger points in the gluteus medius,[8(pp.150–165)] the rotatores and multifidi,[9] the iliopsoas,[8(p.89–108)] quadratus lumborum, or the piriformis muscles produce pain patterns in the lumbar region and sometimes with sacral and lower extremity referral patterns (Fig. 48.22). Again, it is important clinically to consider that lumbar dysfunction and pathologic processes may produce symptoms in other areas of the body, such as:

Iliolumbar ligament syndrome
Meralgia paresthetica
Shoulder dysfunction from lumbosacral somatic dysfunction via the latissimus dorsi muscle
Dermatome, myotome, or sclerotome patterns of pain in the lower extremity

If somatic dysfunction of the lumbar spine influences the lumbosacral junction, it may be responsible for persistent sacroiliac (sacral torsion) somatic dysfunctions.

TART findings,[7] especially in the upper two lumbar segments, may be related to viscerosomatic reflexes from primary dysfunction of the descending colon or organs in the pelvis. It is also possible that they are secondarily related through the nociceptive reflexes now believed to be carried by nociceptive afferent fibers traveling up the sympathetic chain to the T12-L2 segments of the cord. Since L1 and L2 are the only nerves in the lumbar spine that have white rami, lumbosacral and sacral pain may be experienced in the L1 and 2 somatic dermatomes and the lumbothoracic region of the back.

Lumbar somatic dysfunction often results from normal motion that becomes arrested during routine activities of daily living. This is especially true when muscles are previously fatigued or stressed in some way by thermal, biochemical, or biomechanical stress such as overuse, postural strain, or excessive load.

An osteopathic physician, adept at finding and treating somatic dysfunction, must always remember that approximately 10% of back pain patients have some medical cause of their back pain, such as:

Kidney dysfunction
Ureteral obstructions
Prostate or bladder irritation
Primary cancers that metastasize to bone
One of the two surgical emergencies presenting as backache (dissecting abdominal aneurysm and cauda equina syndrome)[1]

These conditions require medical and/or surgical care. The same caution can be given to a medical internist or surgeon who must realize that not all conditions require only medicine or surgery. This also means that approximately 90% of patients

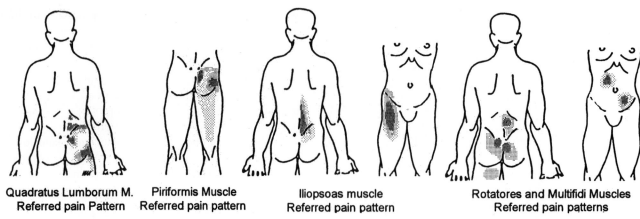

Quadratus Lumborum M.   Piriformis Muscle   Iliopsoas muscle   Rotatores and Multifidi Muscles
Referred pain Pattern   Referred pain pattern   Referred pain pattern   Referred pain patterns

Figure 48.22.   Pain referred from myofascial trigger points. (Modified from Travell JG, Simons DG. *Myofascial Pain Dysfunction: The Trigger Point Manual.* Vol. I., Baltimore, Md: Williams & Wilkins; 1992.)

have some musculoligamentous or "idiopathic" cause for their back discomfort, with palpable musculoskeletal clues and related somatic dysfunctions. Many of these people have somatic dysfunction and/or postural decompensation as their primary diagnosis.

Somatic clues provide further information to help confirm a diagnosis and direct a more efficient workup. They indicate osteopathic manipulative treatment, which would most effectively support the patient's homeostatic mechanisms and/or the medical and/or surgical treatment planned for the patient. Osteopathic manipulation has the following benefits:

It is administered for the patient

It supports the body's homeostatic mechanisms

It removes somatic input to facilitated spinal cord segments

It makes the patient more comfortable during workup and treatment

It promotes a more comprehensive and efficient treatment

It encourages recovery that would be expected to be longer-lasting

DIAGNOSIS

Patient History

Consideration of the type of onset, duration, and progression of a complaint is important to arrive at a more accurate working diagnosis. A sudden onset with severe tearing abdominal pain, associated with the findings of an abdominal mass and a bruit, indicates the likelihood of an abdominal aneurysm. If there were no mass or bruit, and the patient had some distal progressive numbness of the lower extremity or extremities, and especially if there were bladder and/or bowel sphincter weakness, this same presentation of sudden onset abdominal tearing pain would more strongly indicate a cauda equina syndrome. In either case, an immediate surgical consult is indicated.

Take an inventory by systems when taking the history, and especially explore those systems that could be related to the lumbar complaints. Combine the positive clues obtained from

the history with a functional anatomical approach in the physical examination. This yields a more organized total picture of the possible causes for the problems.

This approach also permits questioning about dysfunctions in areas not included or considered important enough for the patient to mention in the history. For example, if a patient complained of lumbar dysfunction, include questions about the patient's bowel and bladder function, any dribbling, whether the urinary stream is full and forceful, and whether there is any pain or burning on urination. If the patient complained of acute tenderness when the iliotibial bands were palpated, ask questions about bowel habits and function or about menses and pelvic pain. Ask if chilling increases the symptoms, as it might if myofascial trigger points were a factor.

Ask about accidents, including a history of "pratfalls." Most people forget about these because they think "I didn't break anything when I fell; I recovered; therefore, it is not important to the doctor" or "I almost fell, but I caught myself."

Ask them about any choking feelings (thyroid) and breast changes or masses (breast tumors). These simple questions explore the possibility of cancer of the organs that usually metastasize to bone and/or that refer pain to the back region. The patient's answers may also give clues about back pain from myofascial triggers (chilling), infection of the genitourinary tract (frequency and burning), colon dysfunction (blood in stool, changes in bowel habit or function), nonphysiologic shear somatic dysfunction (pratfalls), etc.

Physical Examination

A complete physical examination is performed with special emphasis on regions that are spotlighted by the history or that might have functional association with the symptoms expressed by the patient. In this chapter, only the more important points as related to a patient with lumbar complaints are described.

Observation

What is the patient's appearance? Observation of posture and activity often provide the first clue to dysfunction. Posture often mimics patients' inner selves more than their complaints or their responses to direct questioning, as seen in the slumped posture of the depressed patient. Is there symmetry of the body as a whole? Could there be sacral base unleveling? Clues to lumbar dysfunction may be indicated by observing a difference in the space between the arms and the hip/waist on each side of the body. A discrepancy may indicate scoliosis, strain from sacral base unleveling, or a unilateral muscle spasm. If the patient is leaning forward, consider bilateral psoas muscle spasm with mechanical or visceral etiology, or a condition that is putting pressure on lumbar nerves in the intervertebral foramen. If the patient is leaning forward to one side and has the ipsilateral foot everted when standing or walking, think of a unilateral psoas spasm. If this develops into a full psoas syndrome on one side, there may also be complaints of pain in the contralateral hip and leg, rarely past the knee (Fig. 48.23). If the patient stands very erect and dislikes bending forward, think of a herniated disc or spinal stenosis, especially if there are other symptoms such as weakness, reflex changes, or atrophy.

If the patient has leg pain or paresthesia, ask the patient to show exactly where it is located. Then test and interpret if the pattern is dermatomal or radicular. A radicular pattern would alert you to the fact that this is a nerve root pressure, perhaps caused by a herniated disc or a tumor in the cauda equina. If it fits neither of these, you must then consider that it could be pain referred from a myofascial trigger point or pain from a sclerodermal or myodermal pattern of pain. Sclerotomes and myotomes have been mapped and are important but often overlooked pain patterns. This pain is referred to areas of the

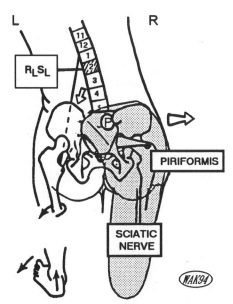

Figure 48.23. Psoas syndrome. *White arrow* under the R$_L$S$_L$ box (indicating key lesion at L2) is in psoas muscle and indicates that pull on left psoas produces rotation and side-bending left. *White arrow* to side of right hip indicates side-shift of pelvis to right. *Black line arrow* around shaft of femur indicates external rotation of leg. *Black arrows* on left foot indicate shortening of left leg and eversion of left food due to psoas muscle pull.

body that are neurologically or embryologically associated with bony or muscular embryologic causes.

Auscultation

Auscultate the four quadrants of the abdomen to determine the presence, location, frequency, and pitch of peristaltic waves. This could reveal the intermittent low, occasional slow gurgle that is normal, or the high-pitched, tinkling sounds of developing obstruction. Bowel sounds may be absent, indicating possible paralytic ileus. The midline of the abdomen between the xiphoid process and the umbilicus is auscultated for bruits. These could indicate an aneurysm and/or renal stenosis. Auscultate the periumbilical region and the junction between the middle and outer two-thirds of the inguinal region for a bruit that could be associated with a significant atherosclerosis of the common iliac or femoral artery. Other physical examination tests for the abdomen are not covered in this chapter.

Palpation and Motion Testing

Palpate for tender anterior Chapman's points (Fig. 48.24) as an indication to specific visceral irritation. Since a specific intercostal space is identified accurately by finding the sternal angle and counting down from rib 2, most osteopathic physicians begin palpation in the second intercostal space. Abdominal viscera, because of their innervations, have their first Chapman's points at the level of the fifth intercostal spaces. If an anterior Chapman's point is tender, ask the patient questions relating to dysfunction of the organ most likely to reflexly produce that tender point. A positive response helps to further rank the clue according to its possible importance. Palpate the abdomen for masses. This palpation is aided by mentally visualizing the location of the liver, the kidneys, the stomach, the small intestines, and the colon as you palpate. Palpate the midline region between the xiphoid and the umbilicus for any pulsating tumor (abdominal aneurysm). A normal abdominal aorta in an adult should not be wider than 1 inch. Pulsations occurring anteriorly are normal, but lateral pulsations from the aorta suggest a weak vessel wall or aneurysm. Palpate the inguinal area for a good pulse and compare the right and left sides. If decreased pulse is found on one or both sides, ask the patient about claudication and then palpate and evaluate the pulse of the popliteal, posterior tibial, and dorsal pedis arteries in that leg, and compare them to the pulses in the opposite side.

Screen the lumbar spine for rotation, which mainly occurs at the lumbar and thoracolumbar regions in this region of the spine. With the patient sitting with arms crossed over the chest, passively and/or actively rotate the body right and left. Normal rotation is about 90° in both directions. Failure to rotate as far in one direction as in the other is a positive screening test suggestive of a problem in rotation somewhere in the lumbar and/or lumbothoracic region.

Side-bending for the lumbar region is screened with a hip drop test. Ask the patient to stand on one leg and take the

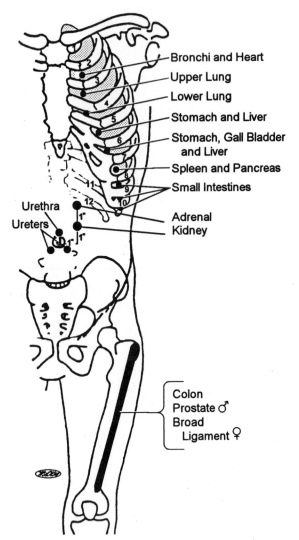

Figure 48.24. Anterior Chapman points commonly used.

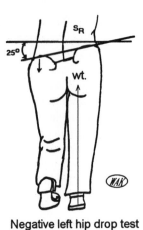

Negative left hip drop test

Figure 48.25. Negative standing flexion test.

position must be used for the examination. Note the level of tissue texture abnormality and make an attempt to relate this to a spinal level(s) of sympathetic innervation of the kidney, colon, or pelvic organs (T10-L2). Use anterior pressure on the transverse processes to test for rotation preference right or left. If rotational preference is found, this same region must also have side-bending preference, because rotation and side-bending occur together. If one vertebral unit is found to be rotated and side-bent to the same side, a nonneutral somatic dysfunction, the preference for flexion or extension is also determined at that segment. Nonneutral somatic dysfunctions are more likely to produce significant disability and be related to visceral dysfunction at the same level of sympathetic innervation from the spinal cord. Clinically, the dysfunctional organ is often found to be on the side of the rotational preference.

Chronic or subacute psoas muscle shortening may become evident if you have the patient flex one leg against the chest while the other leg remains extended. The extended leg flexes and lifts off the table if the psoas muscle on that side is shortened. Another way of testing chronic shortening of the psoas muscle is to have the patient prone on the table. Have the patient flex the knee to 90°. Grasp the thigh just above the knee and extend the hip to see if the psoas permits extension of the leg. If the leg cannot be extended, there is significant shortening of the psoas. If the leg can be extended to its limit of the muscular restrainer (barrier), compare the extension and the end-feel of the barrier of one leg with the extension and end-feel of the opposite one.

Lumbar rotational preference can be segmentally determined by having the patient prone or supine, identifying a lumbar spine that failed a motion screening test, and then evaluating the area 1 inch directly lateral to the spinous process. At this point you are over the lateral end of the transverse process of that lumbar vertebra. Anterior pressure evaluates resistance or ease of rotation of that vertebra. This rotation test is efficient and more sensitive than screening by springing in the sagittal plane, performing a hip drop test, or performing a

weight off the other leg, letting the hip drop on the side of non-weight bearing. If the hip on the unsupported side drops 20–25°, it is a negative test (Fig. 48.25). If the iliac crest does not drop 20–25° on the non-weight-bearing side (especially if this is related to a poor curve of the lumbar spine to the opposite side), the hip drop test is called "positive" on the hip drop (non-weight-bearing) side. This indicates that the lumbar and thoracolumbar spine has a problem side-bending to the side opposite the positive test. Since rotation and side-bending are linked motions, the physician may elect to use only one of these two screening tests. Neither test is as sensitive as segmental palpation, but either, properly performed, can identify gross motion restriction.

Palpate the paraspinal lumbar area for tissue texture abnormality. If the patient can tolerate it, the prone position relaxes the postural muscles and makes palpation of deep paraspinal muscles easier. A patient with an acute psoas muscle spasm may not be able to assume the prone position, and another seated rotational regional screen. This test can be used as a screen itself and is also faster since there are only five lumbar vertebrae to test.

Test side-bending in areas that resisted rotation, because rotation and side-bending are linked. This is performed in the lumbar spine by finding the interspinous ligament between the spinous processes of two successive vertebrae and then moving the thumbs out about 1 inch on each side of this interspace. The thumbs or a combination of the hands and thumbs are used to translate that unit right or left to determine side-bending ease or restriction. For example, translation left tests for right side-bending.

Once somatic dysfunction is identified by restriction in rotation and/or side-bending, it is likely that a sagittal plane preference exists as well. This plane must be determined if the somatic dysfunction is rotated and side-bent to the same side, that is, nonneutral. Nonneutral mechanics can occur with flexion or extreme extension of the lumbar spine. The sagittal plane preference to motion can be determined by anterior pressure on the spinous and interspinous regions of the lumbar spine. If the lumbar spine has somatic dysfunction and springing occurs with anterior pressure over the spine, the spine prefers extension and is restricted in flexion. If anterior pressure is resisted, the lumbar spine prefers flexion and is restricted in extension. The patient's sagittal plane motion can also be tested by having the patient assume a lateral recumbent position and then flexing and extending the knees and hips with one arm while palpating the lumbar interspinous spaces with the other hand.

An alternative method of testing lumbar segmental rotation with the patient in the prone position is to grasp the lower torso with both hands, thumbs contacting the transverse processes. Rotation is then tested by attempting to rotate the body at that region rather than just pushing anteriorly on a transverse process.

The stability of the patient in the prone position may actually interfere with motion testing. It is possible to evaluate group and segmental motion of the lumbar spine with the patient seated. For example, stand behind the seated patient. Place your left arm in front of the patient and your left hand over the patient's right shoulder. You should be able to rotate, side-bend, flex, and extend the lumbar spine with force applied to the patient's upper torso. Your right hand monitors the motion of the lumbar spine or assists in moving the spine. It is necessary to switch hands to move the patient in the other direction. During these tests you may have the patient's arms crossed over his or her chest.

Flexion and extension can be tested at the segmental level. In a flexed somatic dysfunction, flexion would be free, and extension would be restricted. Sometimes you may perceive that backward bending seems too free. This can be especially true at L5. This finding suggests hypermobility or instability of that vertebral unit. Hypermobility is a relative contraindication for the use of thrust-type activation to treat somatic dysfunctions in that region; it indicates that indirect or easy muscle energy procedures should be used. This area may need to be retested after it is treated for its somatic dysfunction and before exercises are given to strengthen the region. Interestingly, areas of hypermobility may resolve when adjacent areas of somatic dysfunction (hypomobile segments) are treated; in those cases, the hypermobility was a compensatory consequence of the adjacent dysfunction.

To record results from this method of testing, assess motion of the vertebral unit, noting that motion is springier in the "end-feel" of all planes of preference and stops abruptly in planes of restriction. Naming the dysfunction can be facilitated by remembering the phrase: "somatic dysfunction does." For example, if a somatic dysfunction is flexed, the motion of the other planes is freer if the patient is in a flexed position when the motions are tested. The same motion tests performed with the patient in an extended position are restricted. If L3 were flexed, side-bent right, and rotated right, rotation (and side-bending in this example) would be freer with the patient flexed than with the patient in the extended position.

The multifidi next to the spines, the quadratus lumborum muscle, and the gluteus medius attaching to the lateral iliac crest are palpated for Travell tender points. Iliopsoas tender points are also tested by palpation on the anterior side of the body, about 1 inch medial to each ASIS. These tender points are deep, not superficial abdominal wall tender points. Anterior Chapman's points may be tested to obtain clues to visceral dysfunctions (Fig. 48.24). Tender points found around the umbilicus may be related to the bladder, kidney, or adrenal glands; those near the symphysis may relate to the ovaries or uterus; and tenderness of the iliotibial bands on the lateral side of each thigh may relate to prostate or broad ligament and/or colon dysfunction. If Chapman myofascial tender points are to be tested, palpate them early in the examination because motion of the myofascial tissues in their area decreases their sensitivity. In this case, their diagnostic clue, tenderness with palpation, may not be evident. If a tender point is found in the left fifth interspace, for example, ask the patient about symptoms related to stomach or duodenal dysfunction to see if the history and the rest of the physical examination should be performed considering an upper gastrointestinal dysfunction.

With the patient supine, test the fascial preference of the entire thoracolumbar transitional junction by grasping the lower rib cage and testing for preference of its rotation. Test the fascial rotational preference of the lumbopelvic transition area by lifting one hip and then comparing that with the ease of lifting the other hip. Side-bending preference permitted by the thoracolumbar fascias is tested by translating this region of the body to the right and the left or attempting to rotate the region to the right or the left. Freedom of movement in both directions is normal. If somatic dysfunction is present, determine the direction of ease and restriction. These findings are then considered with the rotational preferences found at the occipitoatlantal (OA), the cervicothoracic, and the lumbosacral regions to determine if the fascial pattern of the patient is compensated or uncompensated (see Chapter 68, "Lymphatic System").

REFLEXES AND MUSCLE STRENGTH

The following reflexes and muscle tests are useful in the lumbar area. Deep tendon reflexes are the patellar reflex, which mainly tests integrity of the L4 nerve root (Fig. 48.26), and the Achilles reflex, which tests primarily the S1 nerve root. The cremasteric reflex, which is infrequently used, tests L1 and L2 somatic innervation. This latter test is not usually performed unless there is a specific history and/or physical findings that indicate this cord level may be in trouble. The muscle strength of representative muscles can also be tested: quadriceps and anterior tibialis muscles innervated predominantly by L4 (Fig. 48.26); the extensor digitorum longus, brevis, and hallucis longus innervated predominantly by the L5 nerve root (Fig. 48.27); and the gastrocnemius–soleus complex and intrinsic foot muscles innervated predominantly by the S1 nerve root. A screening test for the L5 and S1 nerve roots often involves asking the patient to walk on the heels (L5 muscle strength) and then on the toes (S1 muscle strength).

TREATMENT

Postural Stress or Decompensation

This is a commonly overlooked cause of lumbar and lumbopelvic pain. Usually tenderness of the iliolumbar ligament is the first sign of the decompensation and may be first evident to the patient when the physician, suspecting postural decom-

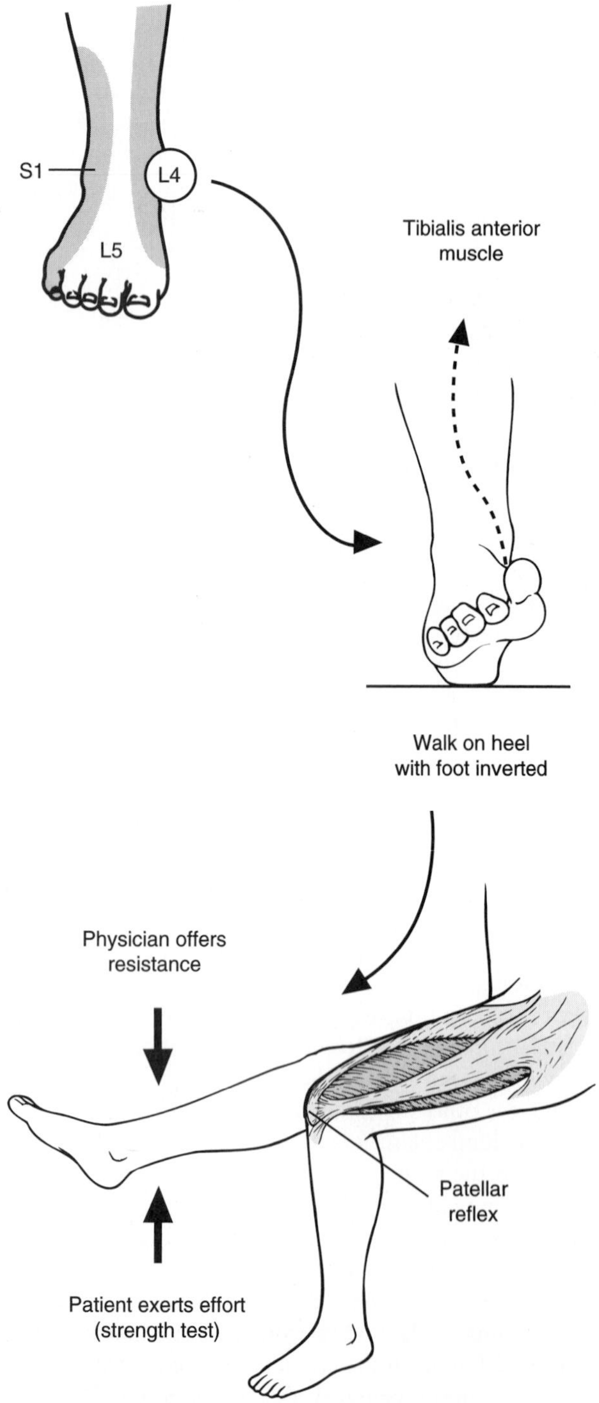

Figure 48.26. Tests for L4 nerve dysfunction.

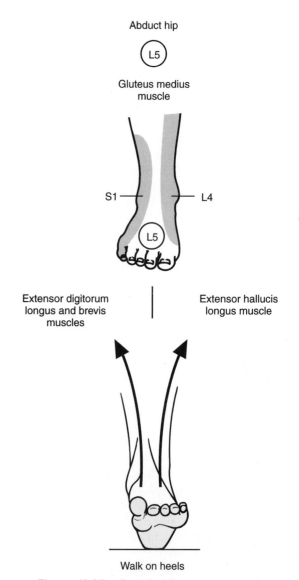

Figure 48.27. Tests for L5 nerve dysfunction.

pensation, palpates the ligament. Postural stress can be due to factors such as:

Problems that unlevel the coronal, sagittal, or horizontal planes of the body
Muscle imbalance
Neurologic and metabolic diseases
Compensation for unresolved somatic dysfunctions
Emotional disturbances
Other somatic expressions of the psyche

Spondylolisthesis and retrolisthesis are structural conditions that have significant postural components and that are capable of predisposing to low back pain.

Treatment of postural stress includes removing the causes, correcting deficiencies, and enhancing the body's homeostatic processes. Rehabilitation is accomplished with carefully designed exercises, ranging from resting fatigued muscles with a short period of bed rest or the use of supports, to muscle stretching and muscle strengthening. Sometimes this must be supplemented with orthotics such as braces for atrophic muscles, heel lifts for an unlevel sacral base, the Levitor for sagittal plane problems, and rarely, surgery. Specific proprioceptive and neuromuscular reeducation is possible with a number of modalities, including OMT, spray and stretch with vapocoolant spray, and various physical therapy modalities. Generalized proprioceptive and neuromuscular reeducation is often achieved through balance exercises.

Psoas Syndrome

"The iliopsoas muscle is the hidden prankster in the sense that it serves many critically important functions, often causes pain, and is relatively inaccessible."[1(p.89)] This condition is usually initiated by positions that shorten the origin and insertion of the psoas muscle for some significant length of time. This includes sitting in a soft easy chair or recliner, or bending over from the waist for a long period of time, working at a desk or weeding, and then suddenly getting up to the normal upright position. The condition can also be precipitated by doing sit-ups with the lower extremities fully extended. Apparently some neuromuscular imbalance produces psoas muscle lumbar spasm and somatic dysfunction of the lumbar spine. There are also organic causes for psoas spasm that must be ruled out by history and/ or physical examination and special tests. These include:

Femoral bursitis
Arthritis of the hip
Diverticulosis of the colon
Ureteral calculi
Prostatitis
Cancer of the descending or sigmoid colon
Salpingitis

The key problem that sets the patient up for development of a psoas syndrome is believed to be a nonneutral type somatic dysfunction that is $F R_x S_x$, usually occurring at the L1 or L2 vertebral unit. If this key somatic dysfunction remains, the patient's symptoms may progress to a full-blown syndrome that includes:

The nonneutral somatic dysfunction of L1 or L2
Sacral somatic dysfunction on an oblique axis
Pelvic shift to the opposite side
Spasm of the opposite piriformis muscle
Sciatic nerve irritation on the side of the piriformis spasm
Gluteal muscular and posterior thigh pain that does not go past the knee (Fig. 48.23)

These are all seen on the side opposite the psoas with the most spasm.

Treatment is preceded by clinically ruling out psoas spasm caused by one of the organic causes listed above. Treatment of the "key" somatic dysfunction, usually found at L1 or L2, is essential for the patient's comfort and efficacy of treatment regardless of other indications for medicines, chemotherapy, radiation, or surgery. Removing somatic dysfunction wherever it occurs in the body helps to quiet down the cord's facilitated segments and makes the patient more comfortable while supporting the body's homeostatic and defense mechanisms and hastening the patient's recovery.

Postfracture or Postoperative Ileus

Fractures of the lumbar or thoracic spine and abdominal surgeries are associated with a definite incidence of ileus of the intestines. Ileus is an absence (paralysis) of intestinal peristalsis. This condition can last from 1 to 3 days, to a week or longer, and can be mild or life threatening in its effects and results.

The best treatment is prevention. Experience has shown that inhibitory paraspinal treatment and/or rib raising in the splanchnic region before surgery may reduce the incidence of ileus. Although there have been clinical studies[10] on the good effects of paraspinal inhibition and/or rib raising in patients with postoperative ileus (and increased incidence of ileus without this treatment), to date there have not been any large-scale studies.

Osteopathic manipulative treatment to prevent or treat ileus consists of paraspinal inhibition through compression of the erector spinae mass, with the patient in the supine position. The treatment usually takes 30 seconds to 1–2 minutes and is completed when the paraspinal muscles relax and the lumbar hyperextension is reduced. If this treatment is given after ileus is diagnosed, it seems to speed the patient's recovery. Clinically, it often auscultates peristalsis immediately after treatment. There are no known side effects from this treatment other than occasionally some patient discomfort related to a slight increased lumbar extension as the inhibition treatment is applied.

The medical treatment for ileus consists of:

1. Having the patient receiving nothing per mouth (NPO)
2. Administering intramuscular analgesics and narcotics for pain
3. Injecting medications to stimulate peristalsis
4. Applying warm applications to the abdomen
5. Reducing as much stress on the patient as possible

Unfortunately, narcotics given to relax the patient and relieve discomfort tend to depress peristaltic action to varying degrees.

Radiculopathy

Radiculopathy is pain that follows the distribution of a nerve root. It is due to pressure, inflammation (radiculitis), or other irritation on that nerve root. The lumbar spine is a common site for this condition.

Causes for radiculopathy are multiple, and diagnosis can be confusing. Causes may be a ruptured disk pressing on the nerve root, cord or bone tumors, exostoses, spinal stenosis, or infections. Often radiculopathy is precipitated or aggravated by acute somatic dysfunction, especially when the intervertebral foramen and/or the spinal cord is already compromised by some other chronic process.

A ruptured and protruding disc producing pressure on the nerve root may be the first condition one considers when a patient has pain in a leg. As mentioned in the skeletal section of this chapter, L4 and L5 discs are at greatest risk for rupture. This is because this region of the lumbar spine has the most motion and the posterior longitudinal ligament is also narrower (deficient) at those segmental levels. The width of this ligament at L4 and L5 is only one-half the width it was at L1, producing a posterolateral weakness of the intervertebral disc at each of these sites.

Because the pedicle of a lumbar vertebra is located on the superolateral one-third of the lumbar vertebral body, a lumbar nerve winds around the pedicle and leaves its foramen, often without passing over the disc of its number (Fig. 48.5). It is much more common to see the L5 nerve irritated by pressure of a ruptured L4 disc and the S1 nerve root irritated by pressure by a ruptured L5 intervertebral disc.

Lumbar radiculopathy produces paresthesias in dermatomal patterns located on the anterior thigh, leg, and foot (Fig. 48.16). It may also produce decreased or absent deep tendon reflexes (DTRs) and weakness in the muscles associated with the level of the ruptured disk (Figs. 48.26 and 48.27). If any one of these three effects is seen, conservative care with adequate follow-up visits is indicated. If conservative care does not help reverse and resolve these effects in 8–10 weeks, and especially if this resistance is associated with two or three of the symptoms mentioned above, surgical (orthopaedic and/or neurologic) consultation and special tests must be performed. This course is required to determine if more aggressive care is indicated to prevent permanent weakness or loss of leg function.

Conservative care for a patient with radiculopathy consists of specific treatment of postural imbalance and somatic dysfunctions, medical treatment of contributing or primary factors, and reduction of other mechanical, structural, and psychological stresses to the patient. As a patient gets older, several infirmities can compromise the areas of the intervertebral foramen and disc:

Arthritis
Ligament hypertrophy   .

Disuse atrophy
Disc degeneration
Muscle imbalance
Inherent tissue qualities
Somatic dysfunctions

The contents of the intervertebral foramen take up only about one-third of the cross-section of the foramen. Removal of a somatic dysfunction may be just enough to make the patient comfortable or asymptomatic. Remember, 90% of low back ache is due to mechanical causes; studies have shown that probably only 5% of patients with ruptured discs require surgery.[11] Osteopathic manipulation is effective in improving biomechanical function and is a primary treatment for radiculopathy due to functional causes. Even in the 10% with medical or surgical problems, manipulation allows the patient to be more comfortable while the specific care is being administered or the patient is healing from a surgical treatment. It should also be realized that mere physician frustration about poor results from the use of some type of conservative treatment is not an indication for recommending surgery on a patient with back pain.

Adequate pain relief is necessary to prevent reflex muscle spasm and guarding. Failure to adequately control pain usually leads to increased disability and morbidity. Muscle relaxants and physical therapy treatments are helpful adjuncts in conservative care. The physician should expect that effective conservative treatment is accompanied by progressive subjective and objective signs of improvement in the patient during the course of the treatment. It is unreasonable to expect the patient to suddenly get better after a specific period of conservative treatment. The key to good results with conservative treatment is to provide all of the forms of conservative treatment that are indicated, to monitor progress, and to modify the treatment plan as clinically indicated.

Quadratus Lumborum Myofascial Triggers

This muscle acts as a lumbar extension of the abdominal diaphragm. Practitioners who understand trigger point examination and treatment consider the quadratus lumborum muscle the most frequent muscular cause of low back pain.[11(p.28)] This muscle can produce so much trouble, the patient may be unable to stand, walk, or even turn over in bed.

It is often overlooked as a cause of low back pain. Referred pain from myofascial trigger points in this muscle may extend into the gluteal region, just above the greater trochanter, into the inguinal region (Fig. 48.22) or the lower abdomen just above the inguinal ligament, and sometimes into the testicle and inner thigh. This is why patients with quadratus lumborum triggers may believe that they have a kidney stone, kidney disease, a hernia, or a testicular pathology. Its pain patterns are also similar to the pattern seen with iliolumbar ligament syndrome (the iliolumbar ligament is believed to be derived from the quadratus lumborum muscle). Tender trigger points in the quadratus lumborum muscle are palpable just below the 12th rib, just above the crest of the ilium, or deep in the muscle belly next to the spine. They are easier to find if this muscle is slightly stretched.

Treatment consists of manipulation to remove somatic dysfunctions affecting its attachments. Manipulate to treat lumbar, twelfth rib, or innominate somatic dysfunctions. Provide some method of removing the myofascial triggers, using:

Spray and stretch with a refrigerant spray
Ice stroke and stretching
Inhibitory pressure
Muscle energy OMT
Injection with a local anesthetic

Evaluate the patient's posture and clinically determine if there is any sacral base unleveling. The pain pattern described helps you to understand why these patients may believe that they have a kidney stone, kidney disease, a hernia, or testicular pathological condition resulting in symptom of a spasm in this muscle.

CONCLUSION

Despite the fact that mechanical problems, including somatic dysfunction, are responsible for most of the complaints of backache, the physician must always consider the functional connections of the back. The lumbar and pelvic regions are a frequent site of strain, pain, and disability. There are many lumbar and abdominal myofascial and neural interconnections with other regions of the body. The treatment offered must be directed toward the primary cause and not merely at the symptom of a backache or a back problem.

REFERENCES

1. Borenstein DG, Wiesel SW. *Low Back Pain: Medical Diagnosis and Comprehensive Management.* Philadelphia, Pa: WB Saunders Co; 1989.
2. Williams PL, Warwick RW, Dyson M, Bannister L. *Gray's Anatomy.* 37th ed. Edinburgh: Churchill Livingstone; 1989.
3. Lockhardt RD, Hamilton GF, Fyfe FW. *Anatomy of the Human Body.* Philadelphia, Pa: JB Lippincott Co; 1959:181.
4. Williams PL, Warwick RW, Dyson M, Bannister L. *Gray's Anatomy.* 35th ed. Edinburgh: Churchill Livingstone; 1978.
5. Borenstein DJ, Wiesel SW. *Low Back Pain.* Philadelphia, Pa: WB Saunders Co; 1989:310. (From Regato JA. *Pathways of Metastatic Spread of Malignant Tumors. Semin Oncol.* 1977;4:33.)
6. Hoppenfeld S. *Orthopaedic Neurology; A Diagnostic Guide to Neurologic Levels.* Philadelphia, Pa: JB Lippincott Co; 1977:49, 51.
7. The Glossary Review Committee of the Educational Council on Osteopathic Principles. In: Allen TW, ed. Glossary of osteopathic terminology. *AOA Yearbook and Directory of Osteopathic Physicians.* Chicago, Ill: American Osteopathic Association; 1993.
8. Travell JG, Simon DG. *Myofascial Pain and Dysfunction: The Trigger Point Manual. The Lower Extremities.* Vol. II. Baltimore, Md: Williams & Wilkins; 1992.
9. Travell JG, Simon DG. *Myofascial Pain and Dysfunction: The Trigger Point Manual.* Vol. I. Baltimore, Md: Williams & Wilkins; 1983:305–319, 636–656.
10. Herrmann E. *The DO.* October 1965:163–164.
11. Nachemson A. The lumbar spine—an orthopaedic challenge. *Spine J.* 1976;I:59.

49. Pelvis and Sacrum

KURT HEINKING, JOHN M. JONES III, AND ROBERT E. KAPPLER

Key Concepts

- **Functional anatomy of the pelvic girdle**

- **Motion and dysfunction of innominates, pubes, and sacrum**

- **Diagnosis and history of pelvic region**

- **Motion testing of pelvic region, including special tests**

- **Pelvic diagnoses and causes of sacroiliac dysfunction**

Accurate and efficient diagnosis of the pelvic girdle is of great importance to practitioners of manual medicine. The pelvis holds a central role in coupling the mechanical forces of the lower extremities with the axial skeleton above, as it is the foundation for body support and locomotion. Alterations and restrictions of motions in the pelvic girdle may have a profound effect on vertebral function, the thoracoabdominal diaphragm, and the urogenital diaphragm. Alterations in the biomechanical function of the pelvic girdle can also influence the craniosacral mechanism and vice versa. The pelvis functions in reproduction and elimination of wastes and is the site of parasympathetic innervation to the left colon and pelvic organs. Somatic dysfunction of the pelvic girdle may be causative, contributory, or diagnostic for a wide range of patient complaints. Such complaints may be somatic, visceral, or emotional in nature. The role of manual medicine in the management of the pelvic girdle is the restoration of functional symmetry between the arthrodial, vascular, lymphatic, and connective tissue elements.

FUNCTIONAL ANATOMY

Skeletal/Ligamentous Anatomy

The pelvis consists of three bones and three joints forming an open ring shape. The false pelvis is a part of the lower abdomen and is walled laterally by ilia. The true pelvis is located inferior and posterior to the abdomen. It begins at the level of the sacral promontory, arcuate line, pectinate line, and pubic bones, ending with the inferior fascia of the pelvic diaphragm.

In the past the hip bones were referred to as the innominate bones because each was composed of three bones joined together at the acetabular notch. Initially there was a single car-tilaginous model for the entire element, and the ischium, ilium, and pubis are the primary ossification centers before birth. Epiphyseal centers form in the cartilaginous iliac crest, anterior superior iliac spine, and ischial tuberosity (at puberty) and eventually fuse in the late teens or early twenties. The only remnants of the original cartilaginous model are the bilateral sacroiliac joints.

The three joints of the pelvis include the symphysis pubis and the two sacroiliac joints. The sacrum is attached to the lumbar vertebrae by a lumbosacral disk, two lumbosacral synovial joints, and ligaments. Anomalous development commonly results in asymmetric lumbosacral facets (facet tropism) and, less commonly, incomplete separation and differentiation of the fifth lumbar vertebrae (sacralization). When the transverse processes of the fifth lumbar vertebrae are atypically large, a pseudoarthrosis may occur with the sacrum or ilia(um). When this occurs bilaterally, it is termed a bat-wing deformity.

The acetabulum occupies the lateral aspect of the ilium and articulates with the head of the femur to create the hip joint. The two innominates are joined anteriorly by the symphysis pubis and cephalically with the sacrum via the bilateral sacroiliac joints. The female pelvis is less robust than the male pelvis, with smaller weight-bearing areas and less height. The female pelvis grows more rapidly in transverse dimensions during adolescence. This growth leads to a larger, more rounded pelvic inlet and outlet, a larger infrapubic angle, and a greater distance between the ischial tuberosities and the coccyx. Functionally, each innominate can be viewed as a lower extremity bone; and the sacrum, as a component part of the vertebral axis.

The pubic symphysis is a fibrocartilaginous joint that has motion determined by its anatomical shape, ligaments, and muscular attachments. Muscular forces acting on each pubic ramus can cause rotation upon each other at the symphysis, about a transverse axis.

The sacrum is shaped like an inverted triangle with the superior aspect being the base and the inferior aspect being the apex. The most anterior and superior portion of the first sacral vertebral body is called the sacral promontory. The anterior surface is concave, and the posterior surface is convex with palpable spinous tubercles. The medial row of tubercles is formed by fusion of the sacral articular processes. The lateral row is formed by the fusion of sacral transverse processes and inferiorly ends in a curve of the bone called the inferolateral angle. The sacrum contains the sacral canal and four bilateral sacral foramina for the passage of the ventral and dorsal rami of the first four sacral spinal nerves. The sacral hiatus is a defect near the apex, formed by a failure of laminal closure of the 5th sacral vertebrae. It is at this location that sacral epidural nerve blocks are performed. The coccyx attaches to the sacral apex via the sacrococcygeal joint. The ganglion impar (where the right and left sympathetic chains join) rests on the anterior surface of the coccyx.

The sacroiliac joints have been described as L- or C-shaped and are contoured with a shorter upper arm and longer lower arm with the junction occurring approximately at S2. The apex, or junction of the two arms of the sacroiliac joint, points anteriorly. The sacroiliac articulation is typically convex at the upper arm and concave at the lower arm. The sacroiliac joints converge inferiorly and posteriorly. The lumbosacral facets are predominantly coronal with the surface of the inferior lumbar facet slanting posteriorly. The sacral sulcus (Fig. 49.1) is a palpable groove just medial to the posterior superior iliac spine. Much variation exists between anatomic description and individual patient's anatomy. Weisl's work[1] demonstrates the varying contours of the articular surfaces of the sacrum and the ilia at their articulation with each other.

The sacrum is suspended between the innominate bones by three true and three accessory ligaments. The true pelvic ligaments include the anterior sacroiliac ligaments, interosseous sacroiliac ligaments, and posterior sacroiliac ligaments. The accessory pelvic ligaments include the sacrotuberous, sacrospinous, and iliolumbar ligaments. The iliolumbar ligaments attach from the anterior surface of the iliac crest and the anterior surface of the sacral base to the transverse processes of L4 and L5 (Fig. 49.2). The lower fibers blend in with the anterior sacroiliac ligament, thus integrating sacroiliac mechanics with the lumbar spine. There are anterior and posterior portions to the sacroiliac ligaments. The anterior ligaments are flat bands, while the posterior ligaments are thicker with multiple layers.[2] The bilateral sacrotuberous ligaments run from the inferior medial border of the sacrum and insert on the ischial tuberosities and the posterior margins of the sciatic notches. The bilateral sacrospinous ligaments lie anterior to the sacrotuberous ligaments and attach to the ischial spines, dividing this space into a greater and a lesser sciatic foramen (Fig. 49.2).

Anterior movement of the sacrum within the pelvic bones is restrained by the sacrospinous and sacrotuberous ligaments. Posterior, lateral, and axial rotation movements are restrained by the anterior, posterior, and interosseous ligaments. No muscles are specific for the movement of the sacroiliac joints. Motion at the sacroiliac joints results from actions of muscles that function to move the back or legs.[3]

In the weight-bearing position, without strong pelvic ligaments, the sacral base would tend to rock anteriorly. The downward effects of gravity, combined with environmental and genetic factors, can stress the tensile strength of these ligaments. These ligamentous stresses can create lumbosacral imbalance, chronic back pain, and joint degeneration. The iliolumbar ligament is prone to irritation by lumbosacral instability. When an iliolumbar ligament becomes irritated, its attachments to the crest and transverse processes of L4-L5 become tender to palpation. Pain may be referred to the groin via the ilioinguinal nerve, mimicking the pain felt in an inguinal hernia. Palpatory diagnosis should therefore always include ligamentous attachments (Fig. 49.3).

Muscles and Connective Tissue

Muscles and connective tissue of the thoracoabdominal wall aid in coordinating movements and pressures between the thoracic cage and the pelvic girdle. Muscles acting on or through the pelvis can be classified as primary (intrinsic muscles of the pelvic diaphragm) and secondary (muscles considered to have partial attachment to the true pelvis).

PRIMARY MUSCLES

Primary muscles and connective tissue intrinsic to the pelvic girdle include the pelvic and urogenital diaphragms. The pelvic diaphragm consists of the levator ani and coccygeus muscles,

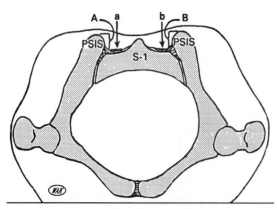

Figure 49.1. Cross-section of pelvis. Differential static landmarks for determining sacral sulcus depth (A and B) versus sacral base anterior or posterior (a and b). (Illustration by W.A. Kuchera.)

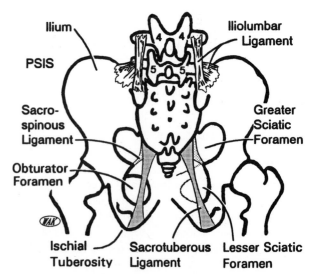

Figure 49.2. Pelvic ligaments and foramen. (Modified from Kuchera WA, Kuchera ML. *Osteopathic Principles in Practice.* 2nd ed. rev. Columbus, Ohio: Greyden Press; 1994.)

which form a basin, supporting the pelvic viscera and closing the pelvic outlet. The urogenital diaphragm spans the area between the ischiopubic rami and is formed by the deep transverse perineal and sphincter urethrae muscles and their fascias. The pelvic diaphragm slants downward from the lateral wall to the midline perineal structures while the urogenital diaphragm is rather level. This creates a small potential fingerlike space (ischiorectal fossa) on either side superior to the urogenital diaphragm and inferior to the pelvic diaphragm, which may provide an anterior avenue for the spread of perineal infections.

SECONDARY MUSCLES

Secondary muscles include:

Rectus abdominis
Transverse abdominis
Internal and external oblique
Quadratus lumborum

The external abdominal oblique forms the inguinal ligament as it courses between the anterior superior iliac spine and the pubic tubercle.

The lower extremity may influence the pelvic girdle through its musculature and connective tissue. The anterior and medial compartments of the thigh may affect iliac and pubic motion and contain the following muscles:

Quadriceps femoris
Sartorius
Gracilis
Adductor group

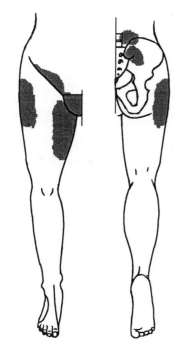

Figure 49.3. Pain referral pattern from iliolumbar ligament. (Modified from George S. Hackett, M.D.)

The iliopsoas may also be considered with this group. The deep fascia of the thigh (fascia lata) is continuous with the superficial thoracolumbar fascia of the thorax and splits to form the compartments of the lower extremity. Dysfunction of muscles or fascia of the posterior compartment or gluteal region may affect function of the pelvic girdle. These muscles include:

Gluteus maximus, medius, and minimus
Piriformis
Obturator externus
Superior and inferior gemellus
Biceps femoris
Semimembranosus
Semitendinosus

Collectively, the muscles of the gluteal region, the quadratus femoris and the iliopsoas, comprise the rotator cuff of the hip (Fig. 49.4).

The structure of the pelvic girdle and its function are intimately interrelated. The true pelvis is situated like a cul-de-sac or diverticulum off from the false pelvis and is not in the main stream of lymphatic flow from the legs to the abdomen. The pelvic diaphragm does not rhythmically contract, but when relaxed, it works synchronously with the abdominal diaphragm. This synchronous movement with the abdominal diaphragm preserves interstitial fluid homeostasis in the true pelvic region. A relaxed pelvic diaphragm is absolutely necessary for the efficient movement of lymphatic fluids away from the pelvis and perineal tissues.

Somatic dysfunction of the symphysis pubis or disturbed ilioilial mechanics (asymmetry of the relationship between the two innominates) can place asymmetric tensions on the pelvic and urogenital diaphragms. These tensions may result in tension myalgia of the pelvic floor, low back pain, dyspareunia, and painful defecation with associated constipation.[4] Appropriate pelvic musculoskeletal performance is essential for adequate bladder functioning. Tension on the pubovesicular and puboprostatic fascia from innominate dysfunction (especially pubic shears and compressions) may produce urinary tract symptoms such as burning, frequency, fullness, and a weak stream. Such tensions on the inguinal ligament from disturbed ilioiliac mechanics can affect the lateral femoral cutaneous nerve, resulting in anterior thigh pain.

Dysfunction of any of the abdominal muscles or their fascias may disturb respiratory excursion, compromising the intraabdominal pressure changes that promote lymphatic and venous return. The thoracolumbar and lumbosacral fascias contribute to the origin of the internal abdominal oblique and the transverse abdominis muscles. Fascial restrictions in these areas can restrict both thoracolumbar and sacral motion. The inner membranous layer of the superficial thoracolumbar fascia (Scarpa's) attaches to the iliac crest and pubic symphysis. It is continuous with the fascia of the thigh inferior to the inguinal ligament (fascia lata), the posterior perineal membrane, and the tunica dartos scrota. Fascial restrictions along its course may effect the thigh, perineum, or abdomen, as fluid collections can traverse along these planes.

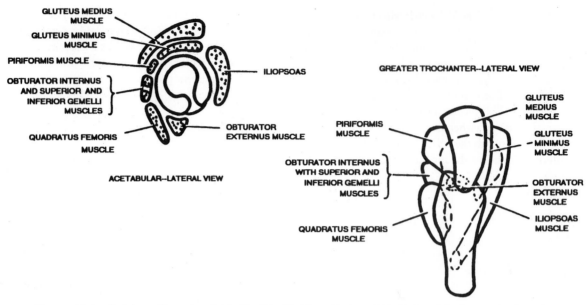

Figure 49.4.   Rotator cuff muscles of right hip. (Modified from Kuchera WA, Kuchera ML. *Osteopathic Principles in Practice.* 2nd ed. rev. Columbus, Ohio: Greyden Press; 1994.)

Dysfunction of the rectus femoris and the ipsilateral adductor group may cause an anterior rotation of the innominate and inferior shear at the pubes. Adductor dysfunction may be related to reflex changes at the ipsilateral iliolumbar ligament, while a pubic shear may affect the pelvic and urogenital diaphragms. Gait may be affected by lumbosacral somatic dysfunction, affecting the superior gluteal nerve (L4,5,S1) and the gluteus medius and minimus. Piriformis hypertonicity related to sacral somatic dysfunction may produce benign sciatica. Hamstring tension may cause a posterior rotation of the innominate and affect pelvic mechanics. Female patients under the influence of hormonal and structural changes during pregnancy, which shifts the center of gravity, are prone to pelvic somatic dysfunction.

Vascular/Lymphatic Anatomy

Following the bifurcation of the abdominal aorta at the approximate level of the umbilicus, the right and left common iliac arteries diverge and descend to the lumbosacral junction. Here they divide into the internal and external iliac arteries. The internal iliac arteries have two trunks that supply the pelvic viscera, perineum, and gluteal region. The proximal anterior trunk supplies the urinary bladder, uterus, vagina, and rectum. Distally the artery branches into the internal pudendal artery, supplying the genitalia and perineum, and the inferior gluteal artery, supplying the gluteal region. The posterior trunk contains the iliolumbar, lateral sacral, and superior gluteal arteries collectively supplying the intrinsic muscles of the pelvis, the sacrum, and the superior gluteal region.

Veins of the pelvic girdle form venous plexuses encircling the pelvic organs and the sacrum and generally following the arterial distribution. The rectal venous plexus communicates with the portal system via the superior rectal vein, which is valveless (Fig. 49.5).

Lymphatic drainage from the pelvic girdle generally follows the corresponding arteries. Lymphatic flow from the lower extremities and pelvic viscera (apart from the gut) passes through the pelvic girdle, terminating ultimately in the lateral aortic groups. Organs and tissues drained by these groups include:

Testes
Ovaries
Fallopian tubes
Uterus
Kidneys
Ureters
Posterior abdominal, pelvic, and perineal walls

Lymph from the remaining viscera (bladder) and gluteal region passes initially to regional nodes along the internal iliac arteries. The external genitalia drain to the inguinal nodes and then deeper into the external iliac and the intermediary lumbar groups.

Lymphatic drainage of the rectum and anal canal is unique in that above the pectinate line lymph follows a deep course to the internal iliac nodes and preaortic nodes. Below the pectinate line, the lymph drains superficially to the inguinal nodes. As lymph flows through a number of intermediary groups in the lumbar region, on up to the cisterna chyli and thoracic duct, the diameter of the thoracic duct and lymphatic channels is under sympathetic control similar to blood vessels. Hypersympathetic activity can reduce lymphatic flow capacity. Ac-

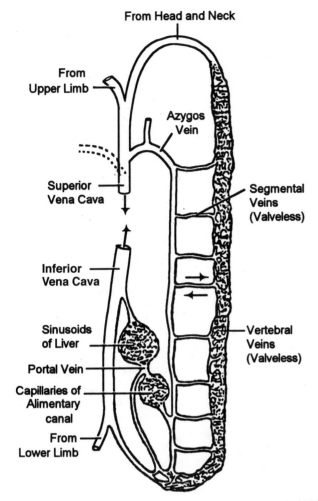

Figure 49.5. Valveless vertebral venous plexus. (Illustration by W.A. Kuchera; adapted from G. Zink.)

cumulation of pelvic lymph may occur in the preaortic, lateral aortic, or retroaortic lymph node groups. Peripherally compromised lymphatic drainage has been linked to the pathogenesis of atherosclerosis and to the development of hypertension.[5] Correction of pelvic girdle dysfunction may allow improved lymphaticovenous return, blood flow, and gait for a patient whose activities of daily living are already compromised by a cardiovascular condition.

Nerves

The nervous system may influence the pelvic girdle through one of four areas. These include the:

Lumbar plexus
Sacral plexus
Coccygeal plexus
Autonomic nerves of the pelvis

The lumbar plexus lies between the anterior and posterior masses of the psoas major, anterior to the transverse processes

of the lumbar vertebrae. The plexus is formed by the contributions of the ventral rami from T12 to L4 with only partial contributions from T12. The lumbar plexus gives motor supply to muscles in the abdomen and thigh, which act on the pelvic girdle. These muscles include the:

Psoas major and minor
Iliacus
Pectineus
Internal abdominal oblique
Transverse abdominis
Quadriceps group
Adductor group
Sartorius
Gracilis

The lumbar plexus also supplies sensation to the thigh, buttocks, lower abdomen, and pubic area.

The sacrum contains sacral foramen for passage of the sacral nerve roots, which exit anteriorly and posteriorly. The sacral plexus is formed by the lumbosacral trunk (ventral rami of L4 and L5), the first three sacral ventral rami, and a portion of the fourth. The ventral rami divide into anterior and posterior branches. The anterior branch forms anterior nerves that innervate the flexors and adductors; the posterior branch forms posterior nerves that innervate the extensors and abductors. The sacral plexus also has motor and sensory innervations in the pelvis and lower extremity and contains parasympathetic fibers (S2, S3, S4) for innervation of the left colon and pelvic organs. The muscular branches include the:

Sciatic
Pudendal
Superior gluteal
Inferior gluteal
Smaller muscular branches

The cutaneous innervation is through the posterior femoral cutaneous nerve.

The sciatic nerve is a muscular branch of the sacral plexus composed of fibers from the ventral rami of L4-S3. Pathology at the L4-5 or L5-S1 level is the usual cause of nerve root compression, as it is uncommon within the sacrum. The sciatic nerve is closely associated with the piriformis muscle. Eighty-five percent of the time the sciatic nerve passes through the greater sciatic notch just inferior to the piriformis; it passes through the muscle in less than 1% of the population. Since injections are sometimes given in myofascial trigger points when the muscle is spastic, it is important to realize that more than 10% of the time the peroneal portion of the sciatic nerve passes through the muscle, and in 2–3% it exits above the piriformis and passes posterior of the piriformis muscle[6] (Fig. 49.6). Piriformis hypertonicity can cause sciatica. There is evidence that this may not be due to pressure but to a chemical reaction that irritates peroneal fibers of the sciatic nerve. For this reason there is referred pain down the posterior thigh but not past the knee.

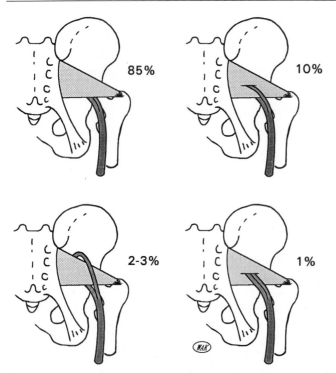

Figure 49.6. Position of sciatic nerve in relationship to the piriformis muscle. (Adapted from Beaton LE, Anson BJ. The sciatic nerve and the piriformis muscles: their interrelation as a possible cause of coccygodynia. *J Bone Joint Surg Br.* 1938;20:686–688.)

The coccygeal plexus is located on the pelvic surface of the coccygeus muscle and formed by the coccygeal nerve with contributions from S4 and S5. This plexus gives rise to the anococcygeal nerve that pierces the sacrotuberous ligament to supply the skin over the coccyx. The autonomic nerves of the pelvis include the sacral sympathetic trunks, the parasympathetic nerves of the pelvic splanchnics, and the inferior hypogastric plexus. The right and left sacral sympathetic trunks are extensions of the lumbar sympathetic chain ganglia and are located on the ventral surface of the sacrum medial to the sacral foramina. They contain four or five ganglia and eventually fuse over the coccyx to form the single ganglion impar. The sacral sympathetic trunks have gray rami communicantes that follow the sacral and coccygeal nerves for innervation of blood vessels and sweat glands in the body wall and extremities. Because the sacral and coccygeal nerves do not have white rami, visceral afferent impulses returning from sites of sympathetic innervation by the sacrum and coccyx refer viscerosomatic symptoms to the thoracolumbar region of the body. Examples include anterior lower thoracic or sacral exostoses and anterior disk protrusions or ruptures. Contractions of the uterus refer pain to the thoracolumbar region, as the visceral afferent nerves travel to this level from the uterine body.

Sacral splanchnics come off the chain and contribute to the formation of the inferior hypogastric plexus. The pelvic

splanchnics arise directly off the ventral rami of S2-S4 and supply parasympathetic innervation to the left colon and inferior hypogastric plexus for pelvic viscera. Visceral afferent nerves following parasympathetic nerve pathways produce viscerosomatic symptoms in the sacrum. An example is sacral pain and pressure from uterine contractions.

The inferior hypogastric plexus contains both sympathetic and parasympathetic fibers; it gives rise to smaller plexuses to the rectum, bladder, prostate, uterus, and vagina.

Somatic dysfunction of the lumbar spine may affect the lumbar plexus and produce symptoms in both the pelvis and lower extremity. Dysfunction of the quadratus lumborum may produce symptoms similar to a groin pull or hernia, by irritating the ilioinguinal and iliohypogastric nerves (L1) as they pass just anterior to this muscle. Dysfunction of the piriformis, or sacrum, can affect the sciatic nerve and cause signs and symptoms of sciatica.

Many visceral complaints are related to an imbalance in the autonomic control of the pelvic viscera. When irritable bowel syndrome is dominated by parasympathetic hyperactivity (headache, nausea, diarrhea, and cramps), relaxation of the pelvic diaphragm through ischiorectal fossa techniques relieves the congestion and pain by influencing the pelvic parasympathetic (S2, S3, S4). Primary dysmenorrhea may be treated by normalizing parasympathetic tone and encouraging venous and lymphatic return with firm continuous pressure over the sacral base.

MOTION AND DYSFUNCTION

The pelvic girdle holds a central role in coupling the mechanical forces from the lower extremities to the axial skeleton. An analysis of the mechanics and motions occurring in the lumbar spine and pelvis during walking demonstrates physiologic motions occurring around various axes of the pelvic girdle. Somatic dysfunction affecting any of these axes hinders gait, requires compensatory changes, and increases energy expenditure. Somatic dysfunction of the pelvis occurs when there are motion preferences during activity that become restricted when activity is completed and the joint has returned to a resting position. Shears are somatic dysfunctions that do not follow an axis.

Individual axes of the pelvic bones are described below, as well as the motion about or around those axes, followed by the integration of coupled movements during the motion cycle of walking.

Innominates

The innominates rotate anteriorly and posteriorly about the inferior transverse axis of the sacrum. The innominates may also be considered to rotate posturally around an axis passing through the greater trochanters of the femur. By virtue of their construction, a lower extremity, including the innominate attached, is likely to displace superiorly or inferiorly rather than have true pelvic rotation around an anteroposterior axis.

Reynolds[7] demonstrated that there was multiple varying instantaneous axes of rotation of the ilium about the sacrum when the thigh was used to introduce motion at the sacroiliac joint.

Pubes

The pubic bones may rotate about a transverse axis. Pubic somatic dysfunctions may occur where iliac movement is maximal and pubic shear is minimal. They may also be sheared (subluxed) superiorly or inferiorly along with the rest of the respective innominate. Anterior and posterior shears can also occur. These are rare and usually result from a significant traumatic event.

Sacrum

Ordinarily, sacroiliac motion is a result of mechanical forces acting on the sacrum. These forces can come from above, associated with changes of position or center of gravity within the torso, or from below, as in walking. While muscles are attached to the sacrum, sacral motion is not caused by sacral flexors, extensors, lateral flexors, and rotators.[3] Describing motion of the sacrum about certain axes is a model by which we explain how the sacrum seems to work as a result of the forces acting upon it. We are also able to gather palpatory information, use this model, and describe the motion present and motion restricted. This becomes objective evidence of sacroiliac motion disturbances. We can then design methods of manipulative treatment to remove the dysfunctions. By palpating landmarks and motion testing after manipulation we are able to evaluate the effectiveness of treatment.

AXES OF MOTION

Mitchell[3] describes three transverse axes. The superior transverse axis is at the level of the second sacral segment, posterior to the sacroiliac joint, in the spinous process area. This is the respiratory axis where flexion and extension associated with respiration occur, as well as nutation and counternutation in craniosacral mechanics. The middle transverse axis is located at the anterior convexity of the upper and lower limbs of the sacroiliac joint. Sacral postural flexion and extension occur about this axis. The inferior transverse axis is located at the posteroinferior part of the inferior limb of the sacroiliac joint and is the axis about which innominate (ilial) rotation occurs.

There are two oblique axes of the sacrum, named according to the side of the body toward which the superior end of the oblique axis is located. Motion about an oblique axis may actually result through motions occurring about a vertical and transverse sacral axis (combination of rotation and sidebending). Sacral movement can occur around an individual axis or simultaneously around multiple axes. Cadaveric studies of sacral/pelvic motion document movement of the sacroiliac joint and movement of the ilia in relation to the sacrum.[8]

TYPES OF SACRAL MOTION

Considering these principles, four types of sacral motion can be described. These include:

Postural
Respiratory
Inherent
Dynamic

Postural Motion

Postural motion of the sacrum occurs with flexion and extension of the torso in the standing or seated patient. Flexion and extension of the sacrum correspond to anatomic nomenclature, with a reference point at the anterior portion of the sacral base. Flexion (forward bending) occurs when the sacral base is moving forward or anteriorly. Extension is backward bending of the sacral base. Terminology for sacral motion uses the same reference point as terminology for spinal motion, the most anterior superior part of the body (in the case of the sacrum, the sacral base). Postural flexion/extension of the sacrum is sometimes referred to as sacral base anterior (for flexion) or posterior (for extension). This prevents confusion of understanding sacral motion that occurs during flexion and extension of the sphenobasilar joint during craniosacral motion (see the "Inherent Motion" section below). When a person is seated and the torso is forward bent, the sacral base moves anteriorly. When a person is standing and begins forward bending, the sacral base begins to move anteriorly, tightening the sacrotuberous ligaments. As forward bending continues, the pelvis moves posteriorly in relation to the feet. This shift in the base of support causes the sacral base to move posteriorly.

Respiratory Motion

Respiratory motion also effects the sacrum, partially because the diaphragm is attached to the top three lumbar vertebrae (L1-2 on the left and L1-3 on the right). Mitchell and Pruzzo[9] showed that the sacrum moves in response to respiration along a transverse axis. As inhalation occurs, the lumbar lordotic curve decreases, and therefore the sacral base moves posteriorly. As we exhale, the lumbar lordosis increases and the base of the sacrum moves slightly forward.

Inherent Motion

Inherent motion of the sacrum is considered in Chapter 64. Older osteopathic literature regarding the craniosacral mechanism reversed the terms flexion and extension in relating sacral inherent motion to palpated motion of the cranium about the sphenobasilar synchondrosis. However, when the sphenobasilar synchondrosis is in (craniosacral) flexion, the sacrum extends (by postural and respiratory terminology). Because of this confusion, the Educational Council on Osteopathic Principles has encouraged the use of the terms nutation and counternutation to describe sacral movement in the cranial cycle of flexion/extension. Nutation means nodding forward, referring to anterior motion at the sacral base. During the flexion phase of craniosacral inherent motion, the sacrum counternutates. During the extension phase, the sacrum nutates.

Dynamic Motion

Dynamic motion of the sacrum and pelvis occurs during walking. As weight bearing shifts to one leg, unilateral lumbar sidebending engages the ipsilateral oblique axis by shifting weight to that sacroiliac joint. The sacrum now rotates forward on the opposite side, creating a deep sacral sulcus. With the next step, this processes reverses as weight bearing changes to the other leg. The sacral base is constantly moving forward on one side, then the other, about oblique axes. As this occurs, the two innominates are rotating in opposite directions to each other about the inferior transverse sacral axis. One side rotates anteriorly as the other side rotates posteriorly. With the next step, this process reverses as the anteriorly rotated hip bone moves into posterior rotation.

Interacting with the bony and ligamentous structure during this motion are the viscera, the weight of the upper body, the muscles of locomotion and balance, and the pelvic diaphragm, all revolving around the constantly changing axes at the pelvis.

NORMAL MOTION OF WALK CYCLE

In the following passage from his paper, "Structural Pelvic Function," Mitchell[3] described this interplay of locomotion and balance as being *"the walking cycle"*:

The cycle of movement of the pelvis in walking will be described in sequence as though the patient were starting to walk forward by moving the right foot out first.

To permit the body to move forward on the right, trunk rotation in the thoracic area occurs to the left accompanied by lateral flexion to the left in the lumbar with movement of the lumbar vertebrae into the forming convexity to the right. There is a torsional locking at the lumbosacral junction as the body of the sacrum is moving to the left, thus shifting the weight to the left foot to allow lifting of the right foot. The shifting vertical center of gravity moves to the superior pole of the left sacroiliac, locking the mechanism into mechanical position to establish movement of the sacrum on the left oblique axis. This sets the pattern so the sacrum can torsionally turn to the left, thereby the sacral base moves down on the right to conform to the lumbar C curve that is formed to the right.

When the right foot moves forward there is a tensing of the quadriceps group of muscles and accumulating tension at the inferior pole of the right sacroiliac at the junction of the left oblique axis and the inferior transverse axis, which eventually locks as the weight swings forward allowing slight anterior movement of the innominate on the inferior transverse axis. The movement is increased by the backward thrust of the restraining ground, tension on the hamstrings begins; as the weight swings upward to the crest of the femoral support, there is a slight posterior movement of the

right innominate on the inferior transverse axis. The movement is also increased by the forward thrust of the propelling leg action. This iliac movement is also being influenced, directed and stabilized by the torsional movement on the transverse axis at the symphysis. From the standpoint of total pelvic movement one might consider the symphyseal axis as the postural axis of rotation for the entire pelvis.

As the right heel strikes the ground and trunk torsion and accommodation begin to reverse themselves, and as the left foot passes the right foot and weight passes over the crest of the femoral support, and the accumulating force from above moves to the right, the sacrum changes its axis to the right oblique axis and the sacral base moves forward on the left and torsionally turns to the right.

The cycle on the left is repeated identically to the right half movements. The shifting vertical center of gravity moves to the superior pole of the left sacroiliac locking the mechanism into mechanical position to establish movement of the sacrum on the left oblique axis.

Somatic dysfunctions may accentuate and retain portions of the motion described above. These are called physiologic somatic dysfunctions, because the muscles, connective tissue, and joints remain in positions that are normally a part of physiologic motion but are dysfunctional when the body should have returned to a neutral position but did not do so. Nonphysiologic somatic dysfunction is generally induced by trauma. It is evidenced by the joint, muscle, and connective tissue elements being in positions and/or relationships that are not part of the physiologic range of motion and do not involve the physiologic axes of motion. Examples include sacral, innominate, and pubic shears.

HISTORY AND PHYSICAL EXAMINATION

Motion restriction is palpated as part of the osteopathic screening examination. Motion testing is active, passive, regional, and segmental. Active motion testing is part of the observation or inspection. The physician asks the patient to move in a directed fashion. This is often done in cases of trauma before the physician tests for passive motion, allowing the physician to see whether there is a significant problem prior to inducing motion to potentially damaged structures.

A patient may have compensatory motion patterns that cover dysfunction but are revealed by careful inspection of focal areas in an overall pattern of satisfactory motion. Passive motion testing allows the physician to assess the quality and quantity of motion. Motion may be limited by pain rather than by the tightness of muscles. Left and right sides are compared for asymmetry, restriction in motion, and changes in tissue texture. Tenderness is assessed.

The sacral and pelvic regions are examined as part of the screening examination. If the screen is positive, the regions are examined joint by joint, as well as by muscle groups. If indicated, individual muscles, fascial restrictions, and pulses are assessed.

Diagnosis by History and Physical Examination

HISTORY

In the diagnosis of pelvic girdle dysfunction, taking a complete history and performing an in-depth physical examination cannot be overemphasized. The osteopathic examination is not a traditional history and physical with a palpatory examination added to it. An osteopathic examination strives to provide a time- and cost-effective diagnosis while encompassing the interrelationship between structure and function. Integration of the physical findings with the emotional, environmental, and genetic factors allows the osteopathic physician to understand their impact on body unity. In this fashion an osteopathic physician examines the homeostatic reserve of each patient, an area crucial in determining prognosis, treatment design, and prevention. *"To find health is the object of the physician, anyone can find disease."*[10]

A history is not just the complaint, the symptoms, and the history of the disease, but it is the history of the patient who has the disease. If the physician listens carefully, the patient's history usually reveals the diagnosis.[11]

In patients with pelvic girdle complaints, physicians should always be aware of their expressions, remarks, and gestures. A diseased organ does not walk into the physician's office, but an anxious and fearful patient does, who may misinterpret or be sensitive to the issues at hand.

A physician should never assume that a patient's low back or pelvic pain has a solely muscular cause. The history should always clarify if a visceral or an emotional cause exists.

Because the pelvic region includes the sexual organs, the patient's sexual history needs to be obtained when the patient presents with a complaint in the pelvic region. Considerations of the chief complaint should include[12] several questions. Tables 49.1 and 49.2 show the two mnemonics that are widely used. In addition, ask the following questions:

Are there any associated symptoms?
Is there a relationship to bodily functions and activities?
Have there been any changes in bowel or bladder habits?
Was there any previous medical care for a similar condition?
What was the treatment outcome?
Is the patient currently on any medications, including over-the-counter medications?
Are there any allergies?

Even when pain is the primary complaint and clinical suspicion centers on musculoskeletal causes, the physician remembers that "pain is a liar" and should address the contributory topics listed in Table 49.3.

PHYSICAL EXAMINATION

The physical examination of the pelvic girdle begins the moment the patient enters the room. Observe the patient's gait, structure, body habitus, and nutritional status. Ask permission to perform a genital or rectal examination. For female patients, a male physician may require a female health care provider to be in the same room during the examination.

Along with general observation, the osteopathic structural examination includes analysis of:

Gait
Structural asymmetry
Curvature of the spine
Postural balance

A screening structural examination is done to indicate whether a region has problems requiring a more in-depth or segmental examination. A palpatory examination is essential; the two forms of examination, observation and palpation, focus on the four criteria for identifying somatic dysfunction. The mnemonic TART (Table 49.4) helps to recall these.

PALPATORY EXAMINATION

The palpatory examination begins with the structural examination as bony anatomic landmarks are found. In the pelvic region, these should include:

Anterior superior iliac spines (ASIS)
Pubic symphysis
Posterior superior iliac spines (PSIS)
Sacral sulci
Sacral base
Inferior lateral angles of the sacrum
Ischial tuberosities
Iliac crests
Greater trochanters

Ligamentous structures to be palpated include the iliolumbar, posterior sacroiliac, and sacrotuberous ligaments. Soft tissue palpation should include:

Table 49.1
PQRST Mnemonic for Investigating Pain

Position, **P**alliation	Is it related to a particular position? Does anything make it better or worse?
Quality	What is it like? Sharp, stabbing, dull ache, burning, or electric?
Radiation	Where is the pain? Does it go anywhere else?
Severity	On a scale of 1–10, with 10 being worst, how bad is it?
Time	When did it start? How long does it last?

Table 49.2
COLDER Mnemonic for Investigating Pain

Condition, **C**haracter	What does it feel like (character or quality)?
Onset	When did it start? What were the circumstances?
Location	Where is it located? Does it radiate anywhere else?
Duration	How long does it last?
Exacerbation	Does anything make it worse?
Remission	Does anything make it better?

Table 49.3
Considerations for Complaints of Pain

In Male and Female Patients	In the Female Patient	In the Male Patient[16]
Employment risks	Menstrual history	Difficulty maintaining or achieving erection
Exercise risks/contact sports	Obstetric history	Difficulty with ejaculation
Hernia	Cleansing routines	Discharge or penile lesion
Past genitourinary surgeries	Douching history	Infertility
Cancer of the genitourinary tract	Abnormal vaginal bleeding	Urinary symptomatology
Chronic illness	Vaginal discharge	Urinary stream, good or poor
Family history	Date of last pelvic examination	Enlargement of the inguinal area
Psychiatric history	Date of last Pap smear and results	Testicular pain or mass
Medications, including contraceptive use	Past gynecologic procedures or surgery	Testicular self-examination practices
Sexual activity history		
Sexual orientation		
Sexually transmitted diseases		
Cancer of the reproductive organs		
Infertility		
Significant and related medical history (i.e., diabetes)		
Urinary tract symptoms		

Table 49.4
TART Criteria for Identifying Somatic Dysfunction

Tissue texture abnormalities	How the tissue feels to the palpating hand	Classify as acute or chronic
Asymmetry	Apparent relationship of landmarks and tissues	Made by observation, not palpation; is generally static positional asymmetry
Restriction of motion	How the tissue moves	Arthrodial, muscular, or fascial elements
Tenderness	Pain elicited by palpation	Generalized as in traumatic tissue damage, such as contusion, or specific for individual muscles or sclerotomal levels, as in tender point diagnosis

Rotator cuff muscles of the hip
Thoracolumbar and lumbosacral fascias
Lumbar paraspinal muscles
Trochanteric bursa
Piriformis and location of the sciatic nerve
Abdominal wall
Pelvic diaphragm

Palpation of the lower extremity may be indicated, if the hamstrings or iliopsoas are of unequal length when motion tested.

In addition to generalized changes in the pelvic girdle tissues, the physician may detect small myofascial tender points. Such areas may be characterized by a small, palpable, circumscribed thickening of tissue that is tender with moderate to deep palpation. These tender points may be associated with autonomic dysfunction or refer pain to a neurologic distribution. Muscles containing tender points reveal pain with active or passive range of motion. There may be areas of "patchy"

weakness in the range of motion of muscles containing painful tender points. Joints controlled by muscles with tender points may have a diminished range of motion. The pelvic girdle contains many of these myofascial tender points because myofascial structures are constantly working to maintain postural balance. Numerous authors[13,14] have indicated continuous postural strain as the cause of precipitating and/or perpetuating myofascial tender points.

Osteopathic physicians may discover paraspinal tissue texture changes that have characteristic palpatory qualities and conclude that these changes are due to visceral disturbances. These tissue texture changes are caused more by changes of the spine, subcutaneous tissue, and superficial and deep fascia rather than pinpoint tissues and muscle. The maximum intensity is at the costotransverse area in the thoracic spine and the region of the transverse processes in the lumbar spine. The quality of motion is a reluctance to move rather than an absolute restriction with loss of range. The skin and subcutaneous tissue findings exceed the muscle–bone–joint findings. In chronic viscerosomatic problems, they take on the characteristics of any chronic somatic dysfunction. Sometimes they present as an acute exacerbation of a chronic problem with the superficial puffiness of acute change and the motion restriction of chronic somatic dysfunction.

Skilled osteopathic physicians are able to palpate inherent motion of the human body. This motion has been described as a cyclic, rhythmic wave of motion; Sutherland referred to it as the primary respiratory mechanism.[15] This motion has been demonstrated in numerous studies, and there are various theories as to its origin. This motion continues even when the patient holds his or her breath. Physicians trained in craniosacral diagnosis can palpate this motion in the sacrum as the craniosacral mechanism moves the sacrum between the two ilia. Clinical significance of this motion is discussed in Chapter 64.

The palpatory examination should include an assessment of the patient's cardiovascular status. Pulses should be palpated and auscultated for bruits bilaterally. An abdominal pulse should be identified, classified, and auscultated. Peripheral edema, sacral edema, and trophic changes in the skin should be evaluated.

In addition to the auscultation over arteries in the periphery, auscultation of the heart, lungs, and abdomen should accompany any patient evaluation. If atheromatous disease is suspected, auscultation over the carotid and femoral arteries is imperative, and the diameter of the abdominal aorta is evaluated carefully.

For evaluation of the pelvic girdle, a complete examination of the abdomen is required. Following inspection, auscultation, and palpation, the physician can percuss the liver, spleen, and stomach, and palpate for any pelvic masses. Diaphragmatic excursion can be percussed posteriorly to evaluate respiratory dysfunction. A rectal examination, a pelvic examination in the female, and a prostatic examination in the male should be a part of a complete examination of the pelvic/sacral region.

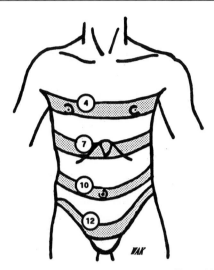

Figure 49.7. Anterior thoracic dermatomes. (From Kuchera WA, Kuchera ML. *Osteopathic Principles in Practice*. 2nd ed. rev. Columbus, Ohio: Greyden Press; 1994.)

Neurologic Examination of Pelvic Region

The neurologic examination of the pelvis and hip centers on muscle testing and sensation.[3]

MUSCLE TESTING

Muscles of the lower extremity and buttocks require assessment when evaluating the pelvis and hip. Descriptions of the innervation, functional anatomy, and dysfunction are discussed in Chapter 50, "Lower Extremities." Primary intrinsic muscles of the pelvis, although not tested for strength, may be palpated for tension, tissue texture changes, and tender points. Lumbar and pelvic muscles that may have trigger points referring pain to the pelvis should also be investigated.

SENSATION TESTING

The dermatomal distribution of sensory nerves to the pelvic girdle ranges from T10 to S5, involving nerve roots from the thoracic, lumbar, and sacral regions (Fig. 49.7). Dermatomes of the anterior abdominal wall run in transverse and oblique bands. These dermatomes begin at the umbilicus with the T10 strip followed inferiorly by the T11 strip. The T12 strip lies just superior to the inguinal ligament, while L1 lies just inferior to it. Inferior to the L1 dermatome lie the L2 and L3 strips covering the anterior thigh and ending at the patella. The buttocks, posterior superior iliac spines, and iliac crest are supplied by the cluneal nerves[16] (posterior primary divisions of L1, L2, L3). The posterior femoral cutaneous nerve (S2) supplies sensation to a longitudinal band traversing the posterior thigh. The lateral femoral cutaneous nerve (S3) supplies sensation to the lateral thigh. The cutaneous innervation of the perineum is arranged in concentric rings around the anus: the outermost (S2), middle (S3, S4), and innermost (S5).

MOTION TESTING PELVIC REGION

There are multiple methods for motion testing, which is customarily done in an integrated fashion with examination of the anatomic landmarks. The immediate objective of manipulative treatment is to improve motion. An initial diagnosis is made and treatment is begun; repeated integral motion testing and treatment follow. Movement of tissues is continuously assessed, determining freedom of, or resistance, to motion testing.

Anatomic Landmarks Used to Assess Pelvis

To assess static positional relationships and perform motion testing, the physician should be able to correctly locate (in the following positions) several landmarks:

Patient standing
    Level of iliac crests
    PSIS
    Greater trochanters of the femurs
Patient supine
    ASIS
    Pubic symphysis
    Pubic tubercles
    Medial malleoli
    Sacrum
Patient prone
    PSIS
    Sacral sulcus
    Sacral base
    Inferior lateral angle (ILA)
    Sacrotuberous ligament
    Ischial tuberosity
    Iliac crest
    Piriformis muscle
    Iliolumbar ligament insertion on ilium

Motion Testing Sequence

An example of a motion testing sequence follows:

Patient standing
    Trendelenburg test
    Iliac crests
    PSIS
    Standing flexion test
    Pelvic side-shift
Patient seated
    Seated flexion test
    Lateral translation sacroiliac motion test
    Upper lumbar for flexed somatic dysfunction and psoas
Patient supine:
    ASIS
    Pubes
    Medial malleoli
    Hamstrings
    Sacrum (for cranial rhythmic impulse)
Patient prone
    PSIS
    Sacral sulci
    Sacral base
    ILA
    Sacrotuberous ligaments
    Spring test
    Backward bending test
    Prone sacral motion tests
    Hamstring palpation for tension

Special Tests of Pelvis

TRENDELENBURG TEST

This test determines the strength of the gluteus medius muscle. During gait, the gluteus medius acts as a stabilizer, preventing the unsupported hip from dropping during the swing phase.

1. Stand behind the patient and observe the sacral dimples. With equal weight distribution over both legs, these dimples should be level.
2. Now have the patient stand on one leg. The opposing gluteus medius should contract, elevating the pelvis on the unsupported side and indicating a negative test. If the muscle is weak, the pelvis on the unsupported side stays level or drops, indicating a positive test.

Conditions that could cause a weakening or paralysis of the gluteus medius include:

Fractures of the greater trochanter
Slipped capital femoral epiphysis
Coxa vera
Poliomyelitis
Meningomyelocele
Nerve root lesions
Lumbar somatic dysfunction
Disturbed ilioiliac mechanics

ILIAC CREST LEVELNESS

Place your index fingers over the iliac crests, and maintain a position so that your eyes are level with the crests. Inspect to see whether the crests are at equal heights.

POSTERIOR SUPERIOR ILIAC SPINES LEVELNESS

Place your thumbs on the inferior slopes of the PSIS and note whether they are level. If one is more cephalad or caudad at the beginning of the standing flexion test, be sure that you include the difference in your end-point estimate before calling the test positive.

STANDING FLEXION TEST

The standing flexion test identifies the side of iliosacral dysfunction. It does not identify the specific type of dysfunction, only which side to treat. Mechanical forces from the lower extremity may influence this test.

A positive standing flexion test indicates three possibilities:

1. Iliosacral dysfunction
2. Contralateral tight hamstrings
3. Carryover from the seated flexion test

False-positive and false-negative test results do exist. A false-negative standing flexion test may be caused by ipsilateral hamstring shortness, but since hamstring tension can cause a false-negative result on the ipsilateral side, or a false-positive result on the contralateral side, testing for hamstring length identifies a hamstring cause for false-negative or false-positive standing flexion tests. If there are unilaterally tight hamstrings, the dysfunctional side should be treated so that both sides are equal, and the standing flexion test repeated. When the sacroiliac dysfunction is treated, the standing flexion test may become negative.

Some physicians feel that if a patient has unequal iliac crest heights, a false-negative test result may exist unless shimming is done to level the iliac crests prior to performing the test.

Patient Position

Standing with shoes removed, heels on a line and feet under the hips.

Physician Position

Kneeling or standing behind the patient, eyes level with the PSIS.

Procedure

1. Place your thumbs on the inferior slopes of the PSIS, and your fingers on the superolateral surface of the iliac crests. Obtain firm pressure on the PSIS to follow bony landmark motion rather than skin motion.
2. Ask the patient to bend forward, touching the floor if possible, but stopping short of pain.
3. Let your thumbs follow the motion of the PSIS. As the patient

bends forward, allow the pelvis to come back toward you. If you do not, the patient will fall forward.

4. Your eyes should be level with the PSIS at all times, so that, as the patient bends forward, you rise from a kneeling position to one where you are standing over the PSIS.

5. If one PSIS moves more cephalad at the end range of motion, the test is positive on that side. (Do not count the side that moves superior first as the positive side. Fascial drag can cause the positive side to end up inferior to the negative side at the completion of the test. If both sides are equal, the test is usually interpreted as negative.)

SEATED FLEXION TEST (SEATED FORWARD BENDING TEST)

A positive seated flexion test indicates sacroiliac dysfunction. In the seated position, mechanics of the lower extremity are not influencing the pelvis. A positive test indicates the dysfunctional side but not the specific type of dysfunction.

Patient Position

Seated, with both feet flat on the floor, or on the rung of a bench, shoulder width apart, and with the popliteal fossa against the edge of the table.

Physician Position

Kneeling or standing behind the patient, with eyes level with the PSIS.

Procedure

1. Place your thumbs on the inferior slopes of the PSIS.
2. Have the patient cross the arms in front of the chest.
3. Ask the patient to bend forward, as far as possible without pain.
4. Note the movement of the PSIS. If one side has moved cephalad at the endpoint of forward bending, the seated flexion test is positive for that side. If the PSIS remain equal, the test is negative.

INTERPRETATION OF STANDING/SEATED TEST RESULTS

If both tests are negative, there is no problem in the sacrum/pelvis. A true positive standing or seated test indicates a problem on that side. If positive, the tests should become negative after proper treatment.

Supine

ALIGN PELVIS ON TABLE

This is sometimes called a "hip flop." The purpose of this maneuver is to reset the pelvis so that the least effect of postural muscles is present. This should also be a comfortable position for the patient.

Procedure

1. Ask your supine patient to raise the knees while keeping the feet on the table.

2. Ask the patient to raise the buttocks slightly, so they are off the table.

3. Now have the patient drop the buttocks to the table and then lower the knees.

4. Continue your assessment with the following tests.

MEDIAL MALLEOLI LEVELNESS

The levelness of the medial malleoli used to be correlated with the findings of the standing structural examination, innominate rotations, and pelvic shears. Medial malleoli levelness is not very reliable for making a diagnosis of innominate dysfunction, as it may not fit the result expected. This is because the ankle, the knee, the hip, and all the fascias and muscles between the malleoli and the pelvis can affect the levelness of the malleoli. However, when the planes between the malleoli are unlevel, you are alerted to leg, hip, and ankle stress; this increases general body stress.

A patient with a short leg is similar to a building with the foundation slightly lower on one side. The body must adapt by seeking a new balance, and this produces tensions in all of the postural muscles. A short leg also places additional stress on the joints of the longer lower extremity. As the body seeks a new level of balance, there is generally a slight scoliotic curve in the lumbar region with the convexity on the short leg side and side-bent toward the long leg side. This is usually then compensated with additional curve(s) in the superior portions of the spine. The cause of a short leg may be anatomical (for example, the patient had a fractured tibia as a child and growth was slightly shortened) or functional (for example, the patient has a posteriorly rotated ilium, sacral torsion, or lumbar curve, causing one leg to be apparently shortened by its displacement in three planes).

Procedure

1. With the patient supine, place your thumbs on the inferior surfaces of the medial malleoli, with your fingers curved around the anterolateral aspect of the ankles.
2. Put slight traction, equal on both sides, on the legs.
3. Note whether one malleolus is more cephalad than the other, and if so, record the difference in length of the short leg.

HAMSTRING TEST

Patient Position

Supine.

Physician Position

Standing at the side of the table, facing the patient.

Procedure

1. Place your cephalad hand on the patient's opposite ASIS.
2. Place your other hand under the ankle of the leg on your side of the table.

3. Slowly lift the leg until you feel slight motion at the opposite ASIS. This occurs after the hamstrings on your side are tight enough to begin rotating the whole pelvis, which is when you feel the motion in your monitoring hand.
4. Note the angle at which this occurs.
5. Perform the same test on the opposite leg (from the opposite side of the table).
6. Mentally compare the angles at which you felt motion at the ASIS. If the leg angles are equal and about 85–90°, the test is considered negative. If you felt the motion sooner on one side, that side has restricted (tight) hamstrings.

Note: The hamstrings can be palpated directly for tension with the patient in the prone position. This is a good screening test but does not directly measure hamstring shortness.

ANTERIOR SUPERIOR ILIAC SPINES LEVELNESS

Procedure

1. Place your thumbs on the inferior surface of the ASIS.
2. Note whether one side is more inferior or superior.
3. Note whether one side or the other is more medial or lateral. Integrate this information with the rest of your diagnostics to make an iliosacral diagnosis.

Note: The innominates may be motion tested at this time. Normally, motion is freer in the direction of positional change. With a left posterior innominate, a posterior and superior direction motion to the supine patient's left ASIS is more free. With a left anterior innominate, a posterior- and superior-directed motion to the supine patient's left ASIS is restricted.

PUBIC SYMPHYSEAL LEVELNESS

Procedure

1. Inform the patient that you will be palpating the pubic symphysis and ask if that is all right.
2. Place the heel of your hand at about the level of the umbilicus. With slight pressure, slide it down the patient's abdomen until you reach the pubic symphysis.
3. Place your thumbs or fingers at the superior aspect of the pubic symphysis and move them slightly medial, slightly lateral.
4. Note whether one side is more caudad, the other more cephalad. Note also any tenderness or tissue texture abnormalities. Integrate this information with that from the rest of your diagnostic tests to make an iliosacral diagnosis.

Sacrum: Indirect Diagnosis

This assessment is often made after gross level motion dysfunctions have been treated with muscle energy, high-velocity low-amplitude (HVLA), strain/counterstrain, or other techniques.

PATIENT POSITION

Supine.

PHYSICIAN POSITION

Sitting at the side of the table facing the patient.

PROCEDURE

1. Ask the patient to raise the opposite knee, with the foot on the table, and to roll the opposite hip toward you.
2. Start with hand lateral to the raised hip and place it between the patient's sacrum and the table.
3. Have the patient roll the hip back to regain the supine position, and lower the knee.
4. Assess sacral motion for both respiratory effects and the cranial rhythmic impulse.

Posterior Superior Iliac Spines

PROCEDURE

1. Place your thumbs on the inferior surface of the PSIS.
2. Note whether one side is more inferior or superior than the other.
3. Integrate this information with the results of the rest of your diagnostic tests to make an iliosacral diagnosis.

Note: The innominates may be motion tested at this time. Normally, motion is freer in the direction of positional change.

Sacral Base

PATIENT POSITION

Prone.

PHYSICIAN POSITION

Standing at the side of the table, dominant eye centered.

PROCEDURE

1. Place your thumb pads about 1/2 inch above where you tested levelness of the PSIS and curl your thumbs from the iliac crest into the sacral sulcus at the base of the sacrum (Fig. 49.1).
2. Evaluate depth of the sacral sulci as an indication of sacral base position. Are both sides the same? Is the sacral sulcus depth normal? Is one side deep? Is one side shallow?
3. Push forward on one side of the sacral base, then the other. Note which side moves more easily. Motion should be freer on the deep side.
4. Mentally record the position of the sacral base and continue the examination.

Note: at this time, palpation of the sacral sulci for tissue texture abnormality is appropriate.

Sacral Inferolateral Angles

PATIENT POSITION

Prone.

PHYSICIAN POSITION

Standing at the side of the table, dominant eye centered.

PROCEDURE

1. Place your thumb pads on the inferolateral angles of the sacrum.
2. By inspection, note which side appears (a) anterior/posterior and (b) superior/inferior.
3. Mentally record which side is anterior/posterior and which is superior/inferior from your motion testing and continue the examination.

Note:

The ILA may be equal anteriorly/posteriorly; equal superiorly/inferiorly

One side may be anterior or posterior but level superiorly/inferiorly.

One side is anterior and superior; or one side is posterior and inferior.

Motion Test about Transverse Axis

PATIENT POSITION

Prone.

PHYSICIAN POSITION

Standing at side of table at hip level with palpating hand over sacrum, fingers pointing cephalad.

PROCEDURE

Place your hand over the sacrum with your fingers pointing cephalad. Alternatively apply pressure with the tips of your fingers, then with the heel of your hand in a gentle, slow, rocking motion. This introduces anatomic flexion and extension about a transverse axis. Assess the quality and quantity of motion and note which movement is freer.

Motion Test about Oblique Axis

PATIENT POSITION

Prone.

PHYSICIAN POSITION

Standing at the side of the patient at hip level.

PROCEDURE

Place the pads of the index and middle fingers of your monitoring hand so that one finger contacts the PSIS and the other finger rests in the sacral base. Place the heel of your active hand in contact with the inferior lateral angle on the contralateral side. With your active hand, apply downward (anterior) pressure on the ILA of the sacrum about an oblique axis. Note

freedom or restriction of motion, and with your monitoring hand appreciate anterior or posterior motion of the sacral base. Assess both quality and quantity of movement as the forces are slowly introduced. Evaluate motion on both left and right oblique axes. If the sacral base has rotated forward and become restricted, posterior motion of the sacral base at the sulcus is restricted. Palpatory examination typically finds the restriction; however, somatic dysfunction is named for the freedom of motion.

Test for Posterior Sacrum

This tests for restriction of lower limbs of "L" ("C").

PATIENT POSITION

Prone.

PHYSICIAN POSITION

Standing at the side of the patient at hip level.

PROCEDURE

Bilaterally contact the inferior portion of sacrum somewhere between the caudal border of the inferolateral angle and where you tested for levelness of the PSIS. Apply a cephalad, downward force. The inferior arms of the sacroiliac joints run anterior and superior, and their posterior borders are about 1 inch inferior to the caudal border of the PSIS. If there is restriction of the lower limb of the sacroiliac joints, this downward, cephalic pressure meets with resistance.

Lumbosacral Spring Test

This test may determine if an increased or decreased lumbar lordosis is present, as well as whether or not the sacrum is tilted forward at the base. If there is increased lumbar lordosis and/or the sacral base is forward, there is increased mechanical stress at the lumbosacral joint and in the articular structures of the lumbosacral region. This comes about because of changes in the postural line of the body. If the sacral base is able to move anteriorly, there is good spring (a negative spring test). If the sacral base is posterior, spring provides poor or nonexistent motion at the sacral base (a positive test).

PATIENT POSITION

Prone.

PHYSICIAN POSITION

Standing at the side of the table.

PROCEDURE

1. Place the heel of one hand over the lumbosacral junction, and the heel of the other hand on top of it.

2. Apply a gentle but rapid downward pressure on the lumbo-sacral junction, in a repeated fashion, two or three times.
3. If there is good springing motion, it is a negative test. If there is poor spring or no spring, it is a positive spring test.

Backward Bending Test

This test helps the examiner evaluate sacral somatic dysfunction at the upper arm of the sacroiliac joint. If the sacral base is anterior on one side, it continues to move anteriorly with the patient propped up on his or her elbows. The opposite side of the sacral base also moves anteriorly; the sacral base moves anteriorly (sacral flexion) on both sides, reducing asymmetry at the sacral base. The sacral sulci and ILAs are more equal in position if the lumbar spine is backward bent. If the sacral base is posterior on one side with a shallow sulcus (as with backward torsions), and the lumbar spine is backward bent by having the patient propped up on elbows, the sacral base posterior side (shallow sulcus side) resists anterior movement of the sacral base, while the other side of the sacral base moves anteriorly. This increases the asymmetry, making the sacral base, sacral sulci, and ILAs less equal in position.

PATIENT POSITION

Prone.

PHYSICIAN POSITION

Standing at the side of the table, dominant eye centered.

PROCEDURE

1. Place your thumbs in the sacral sulci or on the ILAs.
2. Ask the patient to take a position propped up on elbows, and then to relax the low back.
3. Examine the sacral sulci and ILAs. Note with each whether one side is deeper or more shallow than the other. Test with motion (anterior pressure) on one side, then on the other, to see in which direction the sulcus or ILA moves most easily.
4. Mentally record whether the patient improved (position and motion were more symmetrical and appropriate) or got worse in this position.

On a forward torsion, the asymmetry of the sacral base, sacral sulci, and ILAs decreases. On backward torsions, the asymmetry increases.

ASIS Compression Test

This is a test for lateralization of somatic dysfunction of the sacrum, innominate, or pubic symphysis (Fig. 49.8). It can be used to confirm the findings of the seated flexion test or to help localize to one side or another or to both sides when the standing or seated flexion test results are equivocal.

PATIENT POSITION

Prone.

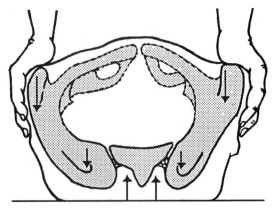

Figure 49.8. ASIS compression test. (Modified from Kuchera WA, Kuchera ML. *Osteopathic Principles in Practice.* 2nd ed. rev. Columbus, Ohio: Greyden Press; 1994.)

PHYSICIAN POSITION

Standing at side of patient, facing the head.

PROCEDURE

Contact the ASIS; apply a posterior compression on one ASIS while stabilizing the other. Test both sides. A posterior compression normally produces a palpatory sense of give or resilience as the innominate glides slightly posterior at the sacroiliac joint on that side. Somatic dysfunction of the pelvis on the side of compression produces resistance to the test. This is interpreted as a positive ASIS compression test.

Bilateral pelvic somatic dysfunction would produce similar findings on both sides and may be interpreted as negative. However, none of the normal resiliency would be found on either side.

Fascial Restrictions of Pelvis

The physician should be able to determine the direction of freer or restricted motion of a fascial plane through palpatory assessment. The direction of the fascia determined by this palpation often is a vector in three planes. Fascial assessment is more than an active, doing process. The hands must listen to the tissues and detect change. This is a sensomotor skill, one in which the physician must read or listen to the tissues and respond to the palpatory messages received.

A common fascial restriction of the pelvis exists between the two innominates. Positional asymmetry and motion disturbance between the two innominates may be related to fascia as well as to disturbance within the sacroiliac joints.

PATIENT POSITION

Supine.

PHYSICIAN POSITION

Standing at the side of the table, facing the head and dominant eye centered.

PROCEDURE

1. Place your hands on the anterior superior iliac spines and adjoining crests.
2. Apply downward pressure in a posterior superior direction alternatively to each side, monitoring for resistance or freedom of motion.

Freer motion is in the direction of positional change and is how somatic dysfunction is ordinarily named. This dysfunction can be treated using fascial release technique.

PELVIC DIAGNOSES

Mitchell divided pelvic and sacral diagnoses into iliosacral dysfunctions (including innominate and pubic dysfunctions) and sacroiliac dysfunctions (sacral diagnoses). The sacroiliac joint is composed of two bones with a joint separating them. One bone is the sacrum, and the other is the ilium. You can't have a disturbance in one without affecting the other. Innominate disturbances may sometimes be primarily a disturbed relationship between the two sides, maintained by muscle and fascial alterations. Within the 10 regions of somatic dysfunction (ICD-9), iliosacral diagnoses are listed as pelvic diagnoses. In the Mitchell muscle energy model of diagnosis, two assumptions are made when determining an iliosacral diagnosis. The first is that the dysfunction is due to neuromuscular imbalance, with the muscle(s) on one side being hypertonic and their opposites being hypotonic. The second is that the side of dysfunction is the side of the positive standing flexion test.

Iliosacral Somatic Dysfunctions

Iliosacral somatic dysfunctions include:

Innominate rotations, anterior and posterior
Innominate subluxations (shears), superior and inferior
Innominate flares (inflares and outflares)
Pubic shears (subluxations), superior and inferior
Unequal hamstring length
Unequal iliopsoas length

ANTERIOR INNOMINATE ROTATION

This exists when the dysfunctional side has the following characteristics:

Entire innominate appears to be rotated in a direction anterior to the other hip bone
ASIS is more inferior (caudad)
PSIS is more superior (cephalad)

Subjective complaints may include ipsilateral hamstring tightness and spasm, and sciatica (secondary to piriformis dysfunction). Palpatory findings may include tissue texture changes at the ipsilateral ILA of the sacrum, as well as iliolumbar ligament tenderness. Motion characteristics should indicate freedom of anterior rotation, about a low transverse axis, on supine motion testing, and resistance to posterior rotation.

POSTERIOR INNOMINATE ROTATION

This exists when the dysfunctional side has the following characteristics:

Entire innominate appears to be rotated in a direction posterior to the other hip bone
ASIS is more superior (cephalad)
PSIS is more inferior (caudad)

Subjective complaints may include inguinal/groin pain (secondary to rectus femoris dysfunction) and/or medial knee pain (secondary to sartorius dysfunction). Palpatory findings may include inguinal tenderness as well as tissue texture change at the ipsilateral sacral sulcus. Motion characteristics include freedom of posterior rotation about a low transverse axis on supine motion testing, and resistance to anterior rotation.

SUPERIOR INNOMINATE SHEAR (SUBLUXATION)

This exists when the dysfunctional side has the following characteristics:

ASIS is more superior (cephalad)
PSIS is more superior (cephalad)
Pubic ramus may be more superior (cephalad)

Note: The reciprocal positioning of the ASIS and PSIS exists only if there is a pure superior shear without any rotation of the innominate.

The two innominates appear to be sheared so that the one hip bone is subluxed superiorly to the other.

Subjective complaints may include pelvic pain. Palpatory findings may include tissue texture changes at the ipsilateral sacroiliac joint and ipsilateral pubes. Motion characteristics include freedom of superior translation.

INFERIOR INNOMINATE SHEAR (SUBLUXATION)

This condition exists when the dysfunctional side has the following characteristics:

ASIS is more inferior (caudad)
PSIS is more inferior (caudad)
Pubic ramus may be more inferior

The two innominates appear to be sheared so that the one hip bone is subluxed inferiorly to the other. This condition is rare, and walking tends to reduce it.

Subjective complaints may include pelvic pain. Palpatory findings may include tissue texture changes at the ipsilateral sacroiliac joint and ipsilateral pubes. Motion characteristics include freedom of inferior translation.

INNOMINATE FLARES

This condition is a positional change of an innominate in which the ASIS is medial or lateral to its usual position. This may be thought of as rotation of an innominate in relation to a vertical axis.

Flares are determined by imagining a transverse line going through the ASIS. Visually connect this line between the ASIS. Then connect a line from each ASIS to the umbilicus, forming a triangle. Bisect this triangle by visually connecting a line from the umbilicus to the pubic symphysis, dividing the triangle into two triangles. Examine the length of the bisected transverse line between the two anterior superior iliac spines, and determine which ASIS is more medial or lateral. If the ASIS is more lateral on the dysfunctional side, the patient has an innominate outflare. If the ASIS is more medial on the dysfunctional side, the patient has an innominate inflare.

Subjective complaints may include pelvic or sacroiliac pain. Palpatory findings may indicate greater laxity in the muscles on the side that is more lateral, and more tautness on the side that is more medial.

VERTICAL PUBIC SHEARS

Vertical pubic shears (subluxations) may or may not actually exist. They may be evidence of a rotation or subluxation that is difficult to diagnose. However, there are times when the ASIS appear to be equal, the PSIS appear to be equal, and yet the pubes are definitely displaced so that one is detectably superior and the other inferior. Since the ASIS and PSIS are equal, it does not appear that the hip bone is rotated or sheared. When the dysfunctional side is superior, it is said to be a superior pubic shear; if the dysfunctional side is inferior, it is an inferior pubic shear. Anterior pubic shears are uncommon but possible and are usually associated with trauma. In these cases, one side of the symphysis is anterior to the other.

PUBIC SYMPHYSIS COMPRESSIONS

Pubic symphysis compressions occur, evidenced by bilateral tenderness. These can be reduced by using the adductor muscles of the thigh in a muscle energy technique.

The L5 anterior counterstrain point is also located on the pubes. Treatment of this tender point with counterstrain technique may be appropriate and necessary in treating pubic symphysis symptoms because what appears to be a pubic dysfunction may actually be reflexive evidence of L5 dysfunction.

UNEQUAL HAMSTRING LENGTH

Unequal hamstring length can be considered either a pelvic or a lower extremity somatic dysfunction because the hamstrings are attached to both the pelvis and the lower extremity.

If the hamstrings are of unequal length, standing flexion test results may be either falsely positive or negative. Therefore, it is imperative to treat the hamstrings and retest. If the standing flexion test and pelvic landmark positions normalize, the dysfunctional hamstrings were the problem. Otherwise, treat as indicated by the second diagnosis.

UNEQUAL ILIOPSOAS LENGTH

Unequal psoas length may be suspected when pelvic side-shift is present, when the upper lumbar lordotic curve is flattened, or when seated or prone evaluation suggests upper lumbar flexed somatic dysfunction.

To test the ability of the psoas muscle to lengthen, place the patient in a prone position. Stand at the side of the table. Grasp the thigh just above the knee and extend the hip until the ASIS begins to raise off the table. Note the ease and degrees (quality and quantity) of hip extension on both sides. Also, on the tighter side the leg appears heavier. Compare the two sides.

DIAGNOSIS OF SACROILIAC DYSFUNCTION

The most common and standard diagnoses of sacroiliac somatic dysfunction include (but are not limited to):

> Sacrum anterior
> Sacrum posterior
> Forward torsions (rotation of the sacrum on the same oblique axis):
>> Left rotation on left oblique axis
>> Right rotation on right oblique axis
> Backward torsions (rotation of the sacrum on the opposite oblique axis):
>> Right rotation on left oblique axis
>> Left rotation on right oblique axis
> Bilateral sacral flexion
> Bilateral sacral extension
> Unilateral sacral flexion (sacral shear)
> Unilateral sacral extension (sacral shear)

In the osteopathic profession, several models of sacroiliac dysfunction have been described. Two systems of nomenclature currently used to define sacropelvic mechanics are those described by Strachan (HVLA) and Mitchell (muscle energy). The HVLA system is described in Walton's text *Osteopathic Diagnosis and Technique.*[17] Both models describe similar events, but from differing points of reference. Both systems are based on physiologic motion of the sacrum, pelvis, and lumbar spine. However, the Strachan model does not describe or identify what the Mitchell system refers to as backward sacral torsions, just as the Mitchell system has no equivalent for Strachan's posterior sacrum.

The following section describes sacroiliac dysfunction using the most consistent criteria of both systems. To integrate the following information into the clinical arena, the physician must consider three questions:

1. Is the sacrum "in trouble"?
2. Why is the sacrum restricted?
3. What are we going to do for the patient?

The information in Table 49.5 can be used clinically in a four-step process using four patient positions. This step-by-step approach can lead to the diagnosis of any somatic dysfunction of the sacroiliac articulation.

Collectively, these four steps integrate information in a logical and time-efficient way of approaching sacroiliac problems. Diagnosing these syndromes is complex, because they may occur in combination, jointly producing symptoms. For this rea-

Table 49.5
Examination for Somatic Dysfunction of Sacroiliac Articulation

Position	Examination	Results
Step 1. Patient standing	Evaluate anatomic landmarks, standing flexion test	A positive standing flexion test means dysfunction in the leg and/or pelvis on that side
Step 2. Patient seated	Perform seated flexion test	Will specifically determine whether there is a sacroiliac dysfunction, and if so, which side (but not which arm) of the sacroiliac joint is dysfunctional
Step 3. Patient supine	Positional assessment of ASISs, pubic tubercles, and medial malleoli	Helps determine the etiology of the problem and whether it is purely sacral or a "mixed" problem, incorporating iliac and pubic dysfunction
Step 4. Patient prone	Palpate for tissue texture changes, motion testing of the sacrum, motion testing of L5, ligamentous tension testing	Helps the physician discover which axis is involved, find what portion of the sacroiliac joint is restricted, determine L5 motion and position, and evaluate pelvic ligamentous tensions

son, many experienced osteopathic physicians repetitively diagnose during treatment to evaluate the efficacy of their therapeutic decision.

Positional terminology, such as Strachan's, was historically used in naming most somatic dysfunctions, although this did not imply that diagnosis was based on positional observation alone. The glossary of osteopathic terminology states that somatic dysfunction can be named in three ways:

1. Position of body part
2. Direction of freer motion
3. Direction of restriction

Strachan's model describes sacral dysfunction in relation to the ilium rather than to L5. Historically, prior to Mitchell's paper in 1958 on structural pelvic function,[3] sacroiliac problems were described as the sacrum in relation to the ilium, or the ilium in relation to the sacrum. Dysfunctions include anterior sacrum and posterior sacrum. Sacral movement is around an oblique axis: motion may be restricted at either the upper or lower arm of the L- (C-)shaped sacroiliac joint. Note that the ILA is not the lower arm of the joint, but a portion of the sacrum used for palpation and positional reference. The sacrum is diagnosed as either anterior or posterior to the ipsilateral ilium.

Anterior Sacrum

An anterior sacrum is a positional term describing a somatic dysfunction in which the sacral base has rotated forward and side-bent to the side opposite the rotation. The upper limb of the sacroiliac joint has restricted motion, and the dysfunction

is named for the side on which forward rotation occurs. An anterior sacrum is probably one type of Mitchell's forward torsion. For example, anterior sacrum left describes a condition in which the sacrum is rotated right and side-bent to the left, the directions of ease of motion. There is restriction of left rotation and right side-bending. The sacral sulcus is deep on the left, with tenderness and tissue texture abnormality in the left sulcus. When downward pressure is applied over the right ILA, attempting to rotate the sacrum about the right oblique axis, the left superior portion of the sacrum resists moving posteriorly, toward the ilium.

Posterior Sacrum

A posterior sacrum is diagnosed when the sacrum has rotated backward and side-bent to the side opposite of rotation and is named for the side of the backward or posterior rotation. This rotation—side-bending to the opposite sides—could be considered rotation about an oblique axis. The posterior sacrum is on the side opposite the deep sulcus at the inferior pole of the joint. The patient experiences discomfort at the inferior arm of the sacroiliac joint and possibly sciatic pain. There is a pelvic side-shift to the side of dysfunction, spinal asymmetry, and postural imbalance. There is a positive seated flexion test on the side of dysfunction, as well as ipsilateral piriformis tension, and the ipsilateral ILA is posterior and inferior. There may be contralateral psoas tension, and there is generally a contralateral short leg. For example, a posterior sacrum right has rotated right and side-bent left, the directions of ease of motion; rotation left and side-bending right are restricted. A posterior sacrum involves restriction of motion at the lower limb of the sacroiliac articulation. Tissue texture abnormality and tenderness are located over the inferior portion of the dysfunctional sacroiliac joint; in this example, the tenderness is on the right. The rotation, in this case, is in relation to the right oblique axis. A posterior sacrum is probably a form of forward torsion in which the major joint motion restriction is on the side opposite the deep sulcus. A motion test for lower pole (lower limb of the L) restriction (for example, posterior sacrum right) is to contact the inferior borders of the sacrum with both thumbs and apply a cephalad/anterior force, attempting to glide the sacrum in the direction of the lower limb of the joint. Restriction is felt on the posterior sacral side. Although there are similarities between the posterior sacrum and the forward torsion, there is no true Mitchell equivalent to Strachan's posterior sacrum. A posterior sacrum should not be confused with a backward torsion, a posterior sacral base, or an extension of the sacrum.

The Mitchell system, based on the cycle of walking (as previously detailed), describes sacral motion relative to L5. The sacrum can move forward or backward about left and right oblique axes depending on the individual's center of gravity and gait, can flex or extend around a transverse axis, or can shift in the L- (C-)shaped articulation, causing a shear. Mitchell's dysfunctions include sacral torsions, shears, flexion, and extension.

SACRAL TORSIONS

Sacral torsions refer to motion at the lumbosacral junction where the sacrum and L5 are rotating in opposite directions. Rotation of the sacrum is movement about an oblique axis or diagonal axis. Sacral torsion does not describe a relationship between the sacrum and the ilium.

FORWARD TORSIONS

Forward torsions occur when the lumbar spine is in neutral. In this example, side-bending of the lumbar spine to the left (during the motion cycle of walking) engages the left oblique axis. The lumbar spine, in neutral, rotates right with left side-bending. Since the left oblique axis is engaged, the sacrum rotates left about the left oblique axis, producing a deep sacral sulcus on the right. Torsion implies that the sacrum has rotated left, while the lumbar spine has rotated right. (Note that, with neutral lumbar mechanics, left side-bending produces rotation right.) The term "forward torsion" is derived from the observation that, in the erect posture, the sacrum is in a flexed forward position (45–55° from the vertical, or 35–45° from the horizontal). Ferguson's lumbosacral angle is measured from the horizontal. There are two forward torsions: left rotation on a left oblique axis (left on left), and right rotation about the right oblique axis (right on right). Positional findings with each of the two forward torsions include those shown in Table 49.6.

In the normal motion cycle of walking, the sacrum rotates from side to side. Dysfunction in the form of a forward torsion occurs when the sacral base rotates forward, becomes restricted, and does not rotate back as far as it should. The forward sacral torsion and anterior sacrum have several findings in common. Subjective complaints include sacroiliac, inguinal, or groin discomfort and low back pain. Objective findings include freedom of rotation anteriorly about an oblique axis, with sacral side-bending and rotation in opposite directions. There is an increased lordotic curve. Spinal asymmetry and postural imbalance are noted: The sacrum has rotated in a direction opposite to the supported lumbars. There is an ipsilateral positive seated flexion test, deep sacral sulcus with tissue texture abnormality, possible psoas tension, and short leg. Neutral mechanics apply to L5, with side-bending and rotation to the opposite side. However, rotation of L5 is also in a direction opposite to that of the sacrum.

BACKWARD TORSIONS

Backward torsions (nonneutral) occur when the lumbar spine is in nonneutral (flexion or, where the curve exceeds normal lordosis, extension) and the sacral base rotates posteriorly about the opposite oblique axis. While they do not occur within the cycle of walking, they are associated with physiologic motion when a person forward bends and then side-bends. Consider a patient in the standing position who bends forward. The sacrum actually extends or backward bends at this time. The lumbar spine is flexed to a point where any multiple plane motion results in nonneutral multiple plane motion. The patient reaches sideways to pick up an object. The lumbar spine side-bends to the right from the nonneutral sagittal plane position. The right oblique axis is engaged as a result of the right side-bending. L5 rotates right according to nonneutral lumbar mechanics. The sacral base moves posteriorly at the left base as the sacrum rotates to the left according to sacral nonneutral mechanics. This example is called left on right (left rotation about the right oblique axis). There are two types of backward sacral torsions: right rotation on a left oblique axis (right on left), and left rotation on a right oblique axis (left on right). Positional findings with each of the two backward torsions include those shown in Table 49.7.

A backward torsion is not the same as a posterior sacrum. A posterior sacrum is a type of forward torsion in which the inferior portion of the sacrum is posterior. In a backward torsion, the posterior portion is at the sacral base (the shallow sulcus).

Subjective complaints include low back pain or sacroiliac discomfort that gets worse when bending forward or walking. Objective findings include those listed above, plus a decreased lordotic curve. Palpatory findings include tissue texture abnormality and a shallow sacral sulcus on the side of the dysfunction, with tissue texture abnormality at L5. Nonneutral mechanics apply to L5, with rotation and side-bending occurring to the same side and opposite the side of the sacrum's rotation.

BILATERAL SACRAL FLEXION

If the sacrum is flexed forward, with the sacral base anterior, the lumbar lordosis appears to be increased, the seated flexion

Table 49.6
Position Findings for Two Forward Torsions

Sacral Rotation on Same Oblique Axis	Left Rotation on Left Oblique Axis	Right Rotation on Right Oblique Axis
Sacral base anterior, deep sacral sulcus	Right	Left
Posterior, inferior ILA	Left	Right
Lumbar curve convex to	Right	Left
L5 rotated to	Right	Left

Table 49.7
Positional Findings for Two Backward Torsions

Sacral Rotation on Opposite Oblique Axis	Right Rotation on Left Oblique Axis	Left Rotation on Right Oblique Axis
Sacral base anterior, deep sacral sulcus	Left (tender right)	Right (tender left)
Posterior, inferior ILA	Right	Left
Lumbar curve convex to	Right	Left
L5 rotated to	Left	Right

test is negative, the sacral sulci are bilaterally deep, and the ILAs are posterior. It is postulated that this motion occurs about a middle transverse axis of the sacrum. This is called a bilateral sacral flexion. When the lumbosacral spring test is performed, there is good spring (a negative test), because the sacral base, already anterior, moves forward easily. If the backward bending test is done, the sacral sulci is still deep (if not deeper), and the ILAs still posterior (or more posterior), because the base of the sacrum normally moves forward and the apex moves posteriorly during backward bending of the lumbar region.

This is an extremely common dysfunction in the postpartum female because of birth mechanics (see Chapter 29, "Obstetrics").

Subjectively, the patient complains of low back pain, worse when bending backward. Objective findings include:

Increased lumbar curve
Deep bilateral sacral sulci with tissue texture changes
Bilateral ILAs posterior
Negative lumbar spring test
No change with the hyperextension test

Motion characteristics include resistance to posterior rotation of the base of the sacrum if pressure is placed on the apex.

BILATERAL SACRAL EXTENSION

In some cases, the patient does not have a positive seated flexion test, yet complains of low back pain, and the sacrum seems to be at the center of the problem. At that time, the sacral sulci should be examined, the ILAs checked, the spring test and backward bending test performed, and a careful analysis made of the relationship of the sacrum to the lumbar spine. The lordotic curve may be increased or decreased. With postural flexion at the lumbar spine (forward bending), the sacrum extends (the base moves posterior), and there is a decrease in the lumbar lordotic curve. If the lordotic curve seems to be decreased, it may be that there is a posterior sacral base. In a bilateral extension, the sacrum is held in a backward bent position and does not easily bend forward. The lumbosacral spring test is therefore positive, meaning there is either poor spring or no spring. Sacral sulci and ILAs should appear symmetrical in either prone or backward bending position, and, if there is any difference on the backward bending test, the sulci look more shallow, and the ILAs anterior.

Subjectively, the patient complains of low back pain or fatigue, worse with forward bending. Objective findings include:

Decreased lumbar curve
ILAs equal and perhaps anterior
Positive lumbar spring test
ILAs stay equal during hyperextension test (superior/inferior)
Sacral sulci bilaterally shallow, with tissue texture changes
Sacrum resists posteroanterior pressure at base, but yields to
    posteroanterior pressure on apex

SACRAL SHEARS

The sacrum can appear as if it has slipped anteriorly or posteriorly around a transverse axis that allows it to shift within the L- (C-)shaped sacroiliac joint. If it slips forward, it produces a finding called a sacral shear or unilateral sacral flexions and extensions.

Unilateral Sacral Flexion

If there is a positive seated flexion test, with the base of the sacrum anterior on the dysfunctional side (sacral sulcus deep on that side) and the ipsilateral ILA is posterior, the patient has a unilateral sacral flexion. The ipsilateral medial malleolus is more inferior, and the transverse process of L5 is more posterior on the dysfunctional side. Both sides of the sacral base move anteriorly with exhalation but do not move easily in a posterior direction with inhalation. The spring test should be negative, since the base of the sacrum moves anteriorly easily when it is flexed. The backward bending test should show improvement because, while the one side is flexed forward, making the sacral sulcus deep, when the patient bends backward the other side of the sacral base should be pulled forward, increasing symmetry.

Unilateral Sacral Extension

If there is a positive seated flexion test, with the base of the sacrum posterior on the dysfunctional side (sacral sulcus shallow), and the ipsilateral ILA is anterior, the patient has a unilateral sacral extension. To confirm this, test the patient with the spring test and the backward bending test. The spring test should be positive, since the base of the sacrum does not move anteriorly easily when the sacrum is held in an extension position. On the backward bending test, the sulci and ILAs should look even less symmetrical because, while the one side is held backward, making the sacral sulcus shallow, when the patient bends backward, the other side of the sacral base should be pulled forward, so the results look worse.

CAUSES OF SACROILIAC DYSFUNCTION

Psoas

Psoas muscle hyperactivity compresses the lumbosacral area. To test for psoas muscle tension with the patient prone, extend the thigh (hip). Psoas problems also have a flexed upper lumbar somatic dysfunction with restriction of extension. Ordinarily, L1 or L2 is flexed, rotated, and side-bent to the side of the shorter psoas.

Short Leg Syndrome

The first symptoms are usually sacroiliac discomfort or pain. Symptoms are worse with excessive walking or running. Examination of the sacrum usually reveals a deep sacral sulcus on the short leg side with significant tissue texture abnormality and tenderness.

Postural Imbalance

Spinal asymmetry, lateral curves, and repetitive asymmetric activity can produce sacroiliac dysfunction.

L5 Problems

L5 problems such as spondylolysis, spondylolisthesis, and congenital anomalies predispose to sacroiliac dysfunction.

Disc

Disc problems at L4 or L5, in the early stages, radiate pain into the buttock region that is interpreted as sacroiliac pain. Often the sacrum is restricted from secondary muscle hypertonicity. In these cases, treating the sacroiliac restriction is not associated with the relief of pain.

Simple Traumatic Sacral Somatic Dysfunction

These patients usually limp in, leap out, and are forever grateful for the one treatment cure.

Reflex Causes

Reflex causes such as viscerosomatic reflexes from pelvis or unilateral sympathetic nervous system dysfunction are causes of sacroiliac pain. Viscerosomatic reflexes are associated with tissue texture abnormality along the sacroiliac joint, which is puffy and warm. This is similar to acute tissue texture abnormality found in the thoracic area from abdominal or thoracic visceral problems.

Clinical Pearls on Low Back Pain

1. L5 is a frequent site of pain and may be unstable as well as painful. Plan: Mobilize adjacent segments that are restricted. Avoid excessive HVLA to unstable joints.
2. Treat short hypertonic psoas.
3. Sacroiliac pain may be caused by L5 problems. In these cases, mobilization of the sacroiliac joint does not relieve the pain.
4. Iliolumbar ligament insertion on ilium may be very tender. Causes include ipsilateral lumbothoracic irritability, anterior rotation of L5, and pelvic side-shift to that side. This may be the first ligament to be strained with postural decompensation.
5. Nociceptive activity at lumbosacral junction causes lumbothoracic irritability with increased sympathetic tone.
6. Active exercises are essential to strengthen and stabilize a back. OMT can create an environment that allows exercises to work and compensations to occur. The primary rule for exercise is to stop short of pain.

CONCLUSION

Manual medicine can restore functional symmetry between the arthrodial, vascular, lymphatic, and connective tissue elements of the pelvic girdle. It can relieve a wide range of somatic, visceral, and emotional patient complaints and contribute to the health of vertebral function, the thoracoabdominal diaphragm, and the urogenital area.

REFERENCES

1. Weisl H. The articular surfaces of the sacroiliac joint and their relationship to the movements of the sacrum. *Acta Anat.* 1954;22:1–14.
2. Greenman PE. *Principles of Manual Medicine.* Baltimore, Md: Williams & Wilkins; 1989:226–227.
3. Mitchell FL. Structural pelvic function. In: *American Academy of Osteopathy Yearbook.* Indianapolis, Ind: American Academy of Osteopathy; 1967.
4. Thiele GH. Coccygodynia: cause and treatment. *Dis Colon Rectum.* 1963;6:422–436.
5. Korr IM. Sustained sympathicotonia as a factor in disease. In: *The Collected Papers of Irvin M. Korr.* Newark, Ohio: American Academy of Osteopathy; 1979:77–89.
6. Beaton LE, Anson BJ. The sciatic nerve and the piriformis muscle: their interrelationship as a possible cause of coccygodynia. *J Bone Joint Surg Br.* 1938;20:686–688.
7. Reynolds HM. Three dimensional kinematics in the pelvic girdle. *JAOA.* December 1980;80:277–280.
8. Strachan WF, et al. A study of the mechanics of the sacroiliac joint. *JAOA.* August 1938;43(12):576–578.
9. Mitchell FL, Pruzzo NA. Investigation of voluntary and primary respiratory mechanism. *JAOA.* June 1971;70:1109–1112.
10. Truhlar RE. *Doctor A.T. Still in the Living.* Privately published, Cleveland, Ohio: 1950. Distributed, Indianapolis, Ind: American Academy of Osteopathy; p 62.
11. Kuchera WA, Kuchera ML. *Osteopathic Principles in Practice.* 2nd ed. rev. Columbus, Ohio: Greyden Press; 1994.
12. Seidel HM, Ball JW, Dains JE, Benedict GW. *Mosby's Guide to Physical Examination.* St. Louis, Mo: CV Mosby Co; 1987.
13. Travell JG, Simons DG. *Myofascial Pain and Dysfunction: The Trigger Point Manual.* Vol. 1. Baltimore, Md: Williams & Wilkins; 1983.
14. Kuchera WA, Kuchera ML. *The Kuchera Manual: Osteopathic Principles in Practice.* Kirksville, Mo: KCOM Press; 1991.
15. Sutherland AS, Wales AL. *Collected Writings of William Garner Sutherland, D.O., D.Sc. (Hon.).* Produced under auspices of the Sutherland Cranial Teaching Foundation, 1967.
16. Hoppenfeld S. *Physical Examination of the Spine and Extremities.* Norwalk, Conn: Appleton & Lange; 1976:151–152, 164.
17. Walton WJ. *Osteopathic Diagnosis and Technique, Sacroiliac Diagnosis.* 1st ed. St. Louis, Mo: Matthews Book Co; 1966:187–197. Distributed, Colorado Springs, Colo: American Academy of Osteopathy. Reprinted, 1970.

50. Lower Extremities

MICHAEL L. KUCHERA AND JOHN P. GOODRIDGE

Key Concepts

- **Anatomy of lower extremity and hip**
- **Classification of ligamentous sprains**
- **Structures and factors influencing motion of hip**
- **Anatomy and function of knee, its major and minor motions, and structures and factors influencing its motion and function**
- **Meaning of genus, varus, and valgus**
- **Motions of fibular head and how motions of ankle affect fibular head motion**
- **Anatomy and function of ankle and what joints make up functional unit known as ankle**
- **Most common sprains in ankle and how they occur**
- **Anatomy and motions of foot**
- **Bony and ligamentous support of foot and ankle**
- **Effect of neuromuscular, vascular, and lymphatic structures on structure and function of lower extremity**
- **Neuromuscular imbalance and myofascial trigger points**

The lower extremities provide for support and locomotion with strong bones and powerful muscles. While many clinicians consider the pelvis to be the foundation on which the spine balances, the lower extremities form the final common platform for postural alignment. Somatic dysfunction in the lower extremities has systemic implications.

The lower extremities are often the site of referred pain from somatic structures in the lumbar and pelvic regions and/or from certain abdominopelvic viscera. While these relationships are mentioned in this chapter, see also the chapters associated with the primary problem. Clinical considerations discussed here include:

Ankle sprains
Pes planus
Plantar fasciitis
Chondromalacia patellae
Genu valgus

Screening of the lower extremity includes observation of gait; palpation; assessment of range of motion of each joint; and assessment of muscle strength, stability, and flexibility. Perform specific screening tests for neural, lymphatic, and vascular functions. This chapter reviews the functional anatomy and basic examination of the lower extremity in three sections:

1. Skeletal, arthrodial, and ligamentous structure and function
2. Neuromuscular structure and function
3. Vascular and lymphatic structure and function

SKELETAL, ARTHRODIAL, AND LIGAMENTOUS STRUCTURES AND FUNCTION

The bones of each lower limb include the (Fig. 50.1):

Innominate (pelvic bone)
Femur
Tibia
Fibula
7 tarsal bones (including the talus, calcaneus, navicular, cuboid, and three cuneiforms)
5 metatarsal bones
14 phalanges

Functionally, the lower extremity includes:

Hip (femoroacetabular joint)
Knee (femorotibial, proximal tibiofibular, and patellar joints)
Distal tibiofibular joint
Ankle (tibiotalar joint)
Subtalar (talocalcaneal joint)
Several intertarsal joints (including the talonavicular, the cuboidocalcaneal, and two small talocalcaneal joints) collectively called Chopart's joint
Numerous tarsometatarsal, metatarsal–phalangeal, and interphalangeal joints in the foot

Each of these joints is stabilized by ligaments, which limit joint motions and are a part of the normal end-feel sensed when palpating joint motion. The innominate are described in Chapter 49.

Ligamentous sprains are generally classified by degree. A first degree sprain assumes that the integrity of the ligament is un-

623

disturbed, resulting in generally intact tensile strength. Some label this degree of injury a strain, while others reserve the term strain for muscle injuries. A first degree sprain, while tender to specific palpation and painful when stressed, is generally stable to most orthopaedic ligamentous tests. A first degree sprain responds well to conservative osteopathic care and recovers with normal function and no ligamentous laxity. A third degree

sprain (also known as a grade III sprain) indicates complete disruption of the ligament with no remaining tensile strength. Orthopaedic testing indicates the sloppy end-feel of complete instability. Good splinting and early surgery may offer the best prognosis when dealing with third degree ligamentous sprains around the structurally unstable knee; with ligaments of the inherently more stable ankle joint, surgery may be delayed or unnecessary to reestablish stability.

Second degree sprains make up the ligamentous injuries in between these two diagnoses. Second degree sprains may be divided into grade I (partial tearing with slight laxity) and grade II (more complete tearing and moderate laxity) sprains. Second degree sprains, even grade II, do not usually require surgical repair if they are appropriately immobilized for a time appropriate to the amount of structural damage.

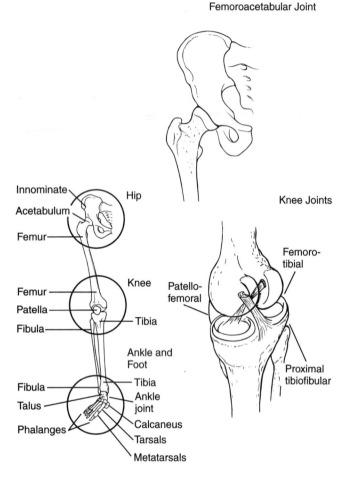

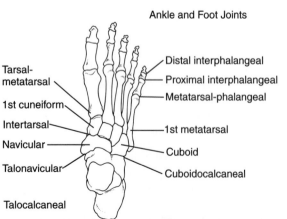

Figure 50.1. Bones and joints of the lower extremity.

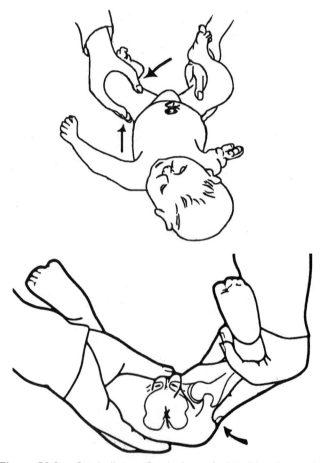

Figure 50.2. Ortolani's test. Ortolani's test for hip dislocation can be used in the first few weeks of life. In a subluxated hip, this maneuver creates resistance felt at 45–60°. A positive sign is a palpable "click" (not heard) when resistance is overcome and the femoral head reduces. (*Top*, From Kuchera ML, Kuchera WA. *Osteopathic Principles in Practice*. 2nd ed. rev. Columbus, Ohio: Greyden Press; 1994:636. (Illustration by W.A. Kuchera.) *Bottom*, Modified from Burnside JW. *Physical Diagnosis: An Introduction to Clinical Medicine*. 16th ed. Baltimore, Md: Williams & Wilkins; 1981:246.)

Hip

The hip, or coxa, is a term used loosely to indicate the articulation of the head of the femur with the acetabular socket of the innominate bone. The innominate is made up of portions of the ilium, ischium, and pubic bones. This is a ball-and-socket synovial joint with a socket deeper than the glenoid fossa of the shoulder, reflecting the stability characteristic of the joint. In the newborn with a congenitally shallow acetabulum, this lack of stability can be tested using Ortolani's test (Fig. 50.2) for dislocation and Barlow's test (Fig. 50.3) for reduction. Early discovery permits satisfactory results with triple diapering or conservative brace management. Failure to perform a satisfactory examination risks a late diagnosis and the necessity for surgical correction.

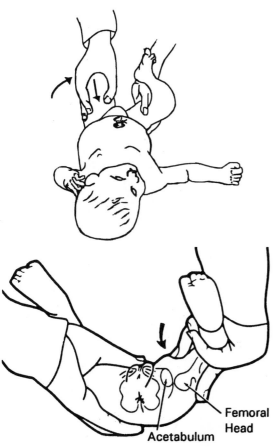

Figure 50.3. Barlow's test. Barlow's test for hip reduction is a modification of Ortolani's test used to identify an unstable hip in infants up to 6 months of age. To perform Barlow's test, Ortolani's test is first performed followed by a posterolateral pressure over the inner thigh. If the femoral head slips out over the posterior lip of the acetabulum and reduces spontaneously when the pressure is released, then the joint is not dislocated but is unstable. (*Top,* From Kuchera ML, Kuchera WA. *Osteopathic Principles in Practice.* 2nd ed. rev. Columbus, Ohio: Greyden Press; 1994:636. (Illustration by W.A. Kuchera.) *Bottom,* Modified from Burnside JW. *Physical Diagnosis: An Introduction to Clinical Medicine.* 16th ed. Baltimore, Md: Williams & Wilkins; 1981:246.)

Major motions of the hip joint are flexion–extension and abduction–adduction. Minor motions are anterior glide occurring with external rotation and posterior glide occurring with internal rotation.

LIGAMENTS

The iliofemoral ligament on the anterior aspect of the hip joint is the strongest ligament in the body. Because it is shaped like a Y it is also called the Y-ligament of Bigelow. This ligament tenses with full hip extension. It helps to maintain posture in the military at-ease position with minimal muscle activity. On the posterior side, the ischiofemoral ligament attaches to the ischial portion of the acetabular rim and wraps over the posterior and superior part of the hip joint to attach just medially to the base of the greater trochanter of the femur. This important anatomic configuration tends to screw the femoral head into the acetabulum with extension, thereby preventing hyperextension. Normal extension is limited to about 35° (Fig. 50.4).

FLEXION

Flexion of the hip is limited more by the muscles and soft tissues than by ligaments. Straight leg raising at the hip around

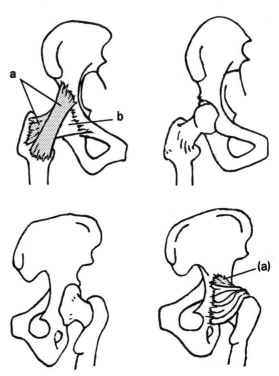

Figure 50.4. *Top,* Bones and ligaments of the right hip (anterior view). *a,* iliofemoral ligament (Y-ligament of Bigelow); *b,* pubofemoral ligament. The iliofemoral ligament on the anterior aspect of the joint is the strongest ligament in the body. *Bottom,* Bones and ligaments of the right hip (posterior view). The ischiofemoral ligament on the posterior side of the joint limits extension to 35°. (Illustration by W.A. Kuchera.)

a transverse axis is limited by the hamstring muscles to 85–90°. If the knee is bent to remove the hamstring influence, the thigh can normally be flexed 135° at the hip. Around an anteroposterior (AP) axis through the femoral head the hip can abduct 55° and adduct 35°. The major motions of the femoroacetabular (hip) joint are:

Flexion
Extension
Abduction
Adduction

FEMUR

The femur is the longest and heaviest bone in the body, attaining a length about one-fourth the height of an adult.[1] This fact allows the forensic pathologist or archaeologist to estimate

an individual's height. The angle formed by the intersection of the anatomical axis of the shaft of the femur and the longitudinal axis of the neck of the femur is called the angle of inclination. This angle normally measures 120–135°. If the angle of inclination is larger than 135°, the condition is referred to as coxa valgus. If it measures less than 120°, the condition is called coxa varus (Fig. 50.5). The femoral shaft is twisted so that the condyles of the distal femur are in a transverse plane even though the femoral neck angles forward 12–15°. This is called the angle of anteversion.

LONGITUDINAL AXIS

The anatomical longitudinal axis running down the shaft of the femur is not its functional axis. The functional longitudinal axis of the femur runs from the femoral head distally to a point

Figure 50.5. Angle of inclination in coxa varus (<120°) and coxa valgus (>135°). (Illustration by W.A. Kuchera.)

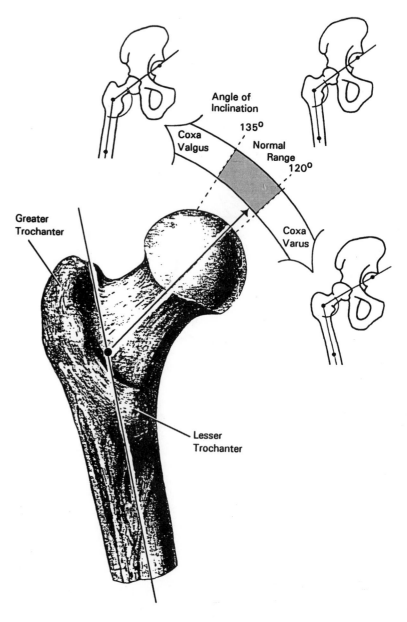

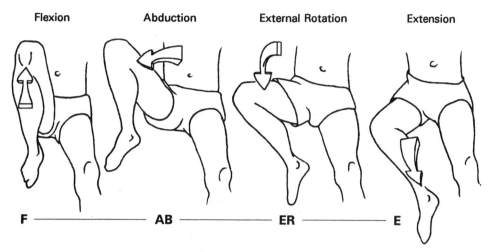

Figure 50.6. Patrick's FABERE test of the hip. (Illustration by W.A. Kuchera.)

midway between the condyles. With internal rotation at the hip on this functional axis, the femoral head glides posteriorly. With external rotation, the femoral head glides anteriorly. Internal rotation with posterior glide and external rotation with anterior glide are minor motions of the femoroacetabular joint. Arthritic change most often occurs first in the minor motions of the joint. An effective screening test for osteoarthritic changes in the hip is Patrick's test (Fig. 50.6). The acronym FABERE is often used (Patrick's FABERE test) to describe the order in which the test is performed:

Flexion
Abduction
External **R**otation
Extension

Arthritic change progresses from functional demand accentuated by biomechanical stress to pathophysiologic response to structural change. The biomechanical stress placed on the hip joint by a short lower extremity results in a higher incidence of greater trochanteric bursitis and of osteoarthritis,[2,3] both on the long leg side.

Knee

While this section also covers the patellofemoral joint, the true knee, genu, or femorotibial joint is a double condylar complex synovial joint formed by the femoral condyles and the tibial plateau (Fig. 50.7). This joint contains medial and lateral semilunar cartilages to provide some stability, smoothness, and resilience to pressure. The major motions of this joint are flexion and extension. Because of the irregular shape of the joint surfaces, these two motions are combined with some minor involuntary glides, rolling, and rotational motions. Minor motions of the tibial plateau at the knee include:

Anterior and posterior glides
Medial and lateral glides

Internal rotation with anteromedial glide
External rotation with posterolateral glide

Abduction of the tibia produces a lateral glide (and often slight internal rotation) of the tibia. Adduction of the tibia produces a medial glide (and often slight external rotation) of the tibia.

In the osteopathic examination of the knee, gather orthopaedic information about the stability of the knee structure with the same tests used to test for somatic dysfunction. In general during testing, if the end-feel of the test is too loose, there is an orthopaedic diagnosis. If motion ends too abruptly, without the normal physiologic barrier, it indicates somatic dysfunction. Interpreting each test for the available dual structure–function information provides twice the diagnostic information in the same amount of time usually spent in examining the knee structure alone.

Q-ANGLE

The angle formed by the intersection of the functional longitudinal axis of the femur and the tibial longitudinal axis is referred to as the Q-angle. Normally the Q-angle measures 10–12° (Fig. 50.8) An angle of 20° or more is abnormal. Here the enlarged Q-angle may be associated with symptoms of patellar pain due to ligamentous strain at the knee or abnormal patellar tracking mechanics. As the Q-angle increases, the patient appears more knock-kneed, a condition referred to as genu valgus. A bowlegged appearance is known as genu varus. Biomechanically, coxa varus increases the Q-angle, as does a pronated foot. Each enhances the possibility of genu valgus.

PATELLA

The Q-angle has a major effect on the tracking of the patella, a sesamoid bone in the tendon of the quadriceps femoris muscle group, and the femur. The patella may even sublux laterally with these biomechanical forces, especially with dysfunction or weakness of the vastus medialis muscle. Patellofemoral joint

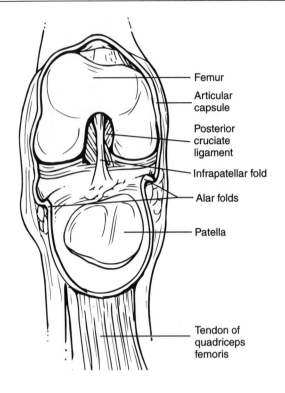

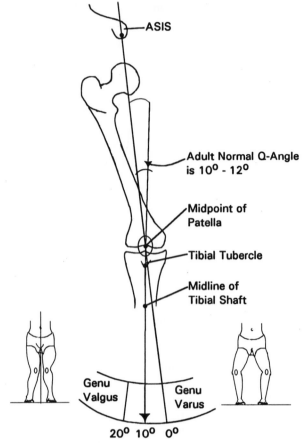

Figure 50.8. Q-angle (quadriceps angle) normally measures 10–12°. Key landmarks for establishing the Q-angle are the ASIS, the patella, and the tibial tuberosity. Note the change in the Q-angle in genu valgus and varus.

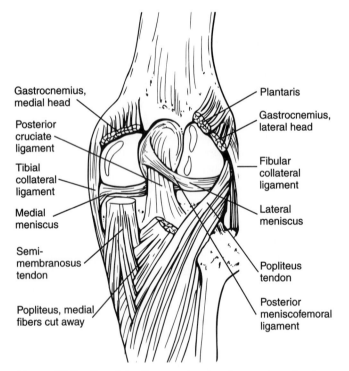

Figure 50.7. Knee joint. *Top,* anterior view. *Bottom,* posterior view.

dysfunction often arises from abnormal tracking of, or pressure on, the patella. Prolonged patellofemoral dysfunction, as with an increased Q-angle, predisposes to structural change such as irregular or accelerated wearing or roughening of the articular surface on the posterior surface of the patella. This coexistence of structural and functional disorders must be considered and

appropriately diagnosed and treated to encourage optimum healing.

Patellar structural problems such as chondromalacia patellae also arise from:

Patellar dislocation
Chronic or direct patellar trauma
Fracture of the lower extremity

Structural problems of the patella are evaluated, in part, by palpating over and around the patella. Look for subpatellar tenderness with compression against the underlying femur or when gliding the patella:

Medially
Laterally
Superiorly
Inferiorly

Effusion within the knee joint and/or crepitus with or without pain when actively contracting the quadriceps muscles also strongly suggests structural change. Careful palpation gliding the patella in all four directions, feeling for this crepitus, grinding, or clicking, provides an excellent structural assessment.

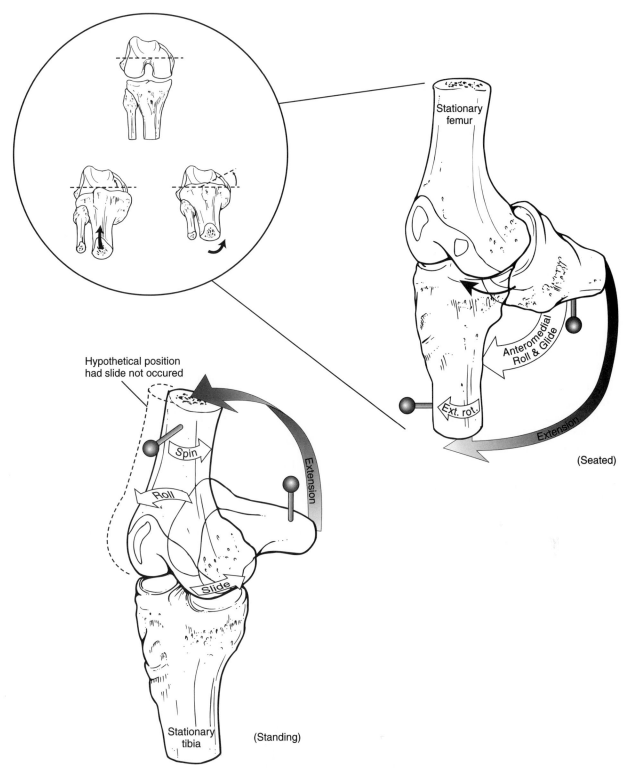

Figure 50.9. Structure–function relationship of the medial condyle. In knee extension, the medial but not the lateral femoral condyle will continue to track posteriorly, resulting in internal rotation of the femur (if the tibia is stationary) or external rotation (*Ext. rot.*) of the tibia (if the femur is held stationary). The condylar glide occurring with external rotation of the tibia is named anteromedial glide.

Locking of the patella strongly suggests myofascial trigger points in the vastus lateralis muscle. Complete locking of the patella immobilizes the knee joint in slight flexion, while partial locking causes difficulty in straightening the knee after sitting in a chair.

As a consequence of secondary bony alignment and muscular imbalance, patellar tracking difficulties may also be the presenting symptom of short leg syndrome.

EXTENSION

The knee should move into full extension with locking, freely and without restriction. Test this by grasping the foot of the supine patient with one hand and raising that lower extremity just off the table. With the other hand, flex the knee slightly. Release the slightly flexed knee, allowing it to extend. A normal knee drops freely into extension and "bounces" off the ligaments. Structural injuries, especially medial meniscal tears, may result in inability to extend fully, or guarding on extension. The hyperextended knee is referred to as genu recurvatum.

GLIDING

The medial condyle of the knee is longer than the articular surface of the lateral condyle (Fig. 50.9). This structural configuration affects joint function. With extension of the knee, the lateral condyle reaches its physiologic limit of motion while the medial condyle of the femur continues to track posteriorly on the tibial plateau. This results in posterolateral glide of the tibia with full extension of the knee. Full extension locking requires this minor rotational glide. The opposite (anteromedial glide) occurs with full flexion of the knee. Check these minor motions of the joint for somatic dysfunction by adding an anteromedial glide while inducing external rotation of the tibial plateau and a posterolateral glide while inducing internal rotation of the tibial plateau (Fig. 50.10).

LIGAMENTS AND CARTILAGE

Lateral and medial collateral ligaments placed to limit lateral glide of the tibia with adduction and medial glide of the tibia with abduction stabilize the true knee joint. The lateral (fibular) collateral ligament does not attach to the lateral semilunar cartilage (meniscus), while the medial (tibial) collateral ligament does attach to the medial semilunar cartilage (meniscus) (Fig. 50.11). This anatomic arrangement makes the medial cartilage more susceptible to injury. It also predisposes to displacement, especially from a blow to the knee which comes through the knee from the lateral to the medial side, or to twisting injuries of the knee. Valgus stress testing of the knee at 30° (Fig. 50.12A) induces abduction of the tibia with medial glide and provides information on stability of the medial collateral ligament. Varus stress testing at 30° (Fig. 50.12B) in-

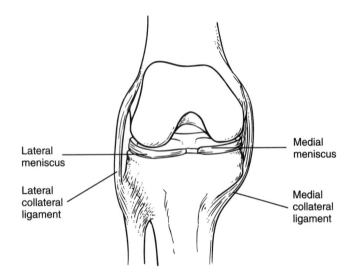

Figure 50.11. Relationship of collateral ligaments to knee cartilage (anterior view).

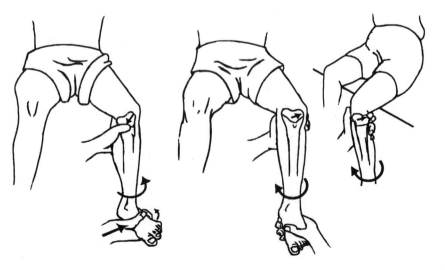

Figure 50.10. Physical examination of anteromedial glide with external rotation (**A**) and posterolateral glide with internal rotation (**B**) of the knee. (Illustration by W.A. Kuchera.)

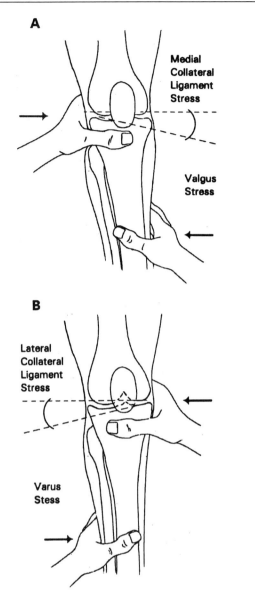

Figure 50.12. Tests for collateral ligament injury at the knee. Tibial abduction or genu valgus stress (**A**) tests for medial collateral ligament stability. Tibial adduction or genu varus stress (**B**) tests for lateral collateral ligament stability. (Illustration by W.A. Kuchera.)

duces adduction of the tibia with lateral glide and provides information on stability of the lateral collateral ligament. A palpable click accompanied by pain while performing McMurray's meniscal tests (Fig. 50.13) strongly suggests a meniscal tear.

The cruciate ligaments run between the tibia and femur and are named according to their tibial attachments. The posterior cruciate ligament attaches to the posterior part of the tibia and prevents excessive posterior glide of the tibia. The anterior cruciate ligament attaches to the anterior part of the tibia and prevents excessive anterior glide of the tibia at the knee joint. Check stability of the anterior cruciate ligament (Fig. 50.14*A*) with an anterior drawer test or, even more specifically, a Lachman's test. Check stability of the posterior cruciate ligament with a posterior drawer test (Fig. 50.14*B*).

The combination of torn anterior cruciate and medial collateral ligaments along with a torn medial meniscus occurs predictably from certain traumas featuring valgus stress forces (such as a tackle to the outside of the knee with the knee extended fully and the foot fixed). Because this injury causes significant knee instability, historically many clinicians referred to this constellation as the terrible triad, or O'Donaghue's Triad.

Fibular Motion

The proximal tibiofibular joint is a separate synovial joint at the knee (Fig. 50.15). While the angulation of the articulation actually permits the minor motions of anterolateral and posteromedial glide of the fibular head, clinicians report fibular head glide as anterior or posterior. The fibular head lies in the same horizontal plane as the tibial plateau. Be careful in grasping the fibular head not to cause undue pressure on the peroneal nerve, which lies directly posterior to this structure.

The distal tibiofibular articulation is a syndesmosis. This joint allows the fibula to move laterally from the tibia to accommodate the increased width of the talus presented during dorsiflexion. Restricted dorsiflexion of the ankle warrants examination and treatment of this syndesmosis.

When the fibular head glides anteriorly, reciprocal motion is initiated at the distal fibula (lateral malleolus), which glides posteriorly. Posterior fibular head motion is accompanied by anterior motion at the distal fibula.

EXTERNAL ROTATION

External rotation of the tibia and ankle carry the distal fibula posteriorly and elevate and glide the proximal fibular head anteriorly. The opposite occurs with internal rotation of the tibia and ankle (Fig. 50.16).

FIBULAR HEAD DYSFUNCTION

In recurrent ankle sprains, examine for fibular head dysfunction. It occurs frequently and responds well to manipulative procedures.[4] Be sure to check for reciprocal motion, because with trauma the physiologic, reciprocal motion described ear-

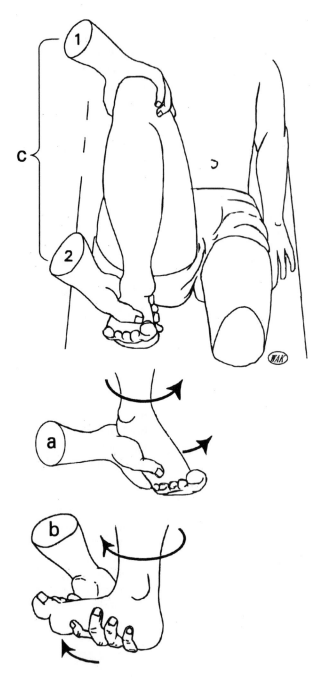

Figure 50.13. McMurray test for medial and lateral meniscal injury. The knee is fully flexed. One hand (*1*) palpates the knee at the medial and lateral joint line. The other hand (*2*) holds the foot to control internal (*a*) and external (*b*) rotation of the foot and tibia. *A test for lateral meniscus injury:* The foot and tibia are internally rotated (*a*), the two hands (*c*) place the tibia into adduction (genu varus), and while holding this positioning, the leg is extended. *A test for medial meniscus injury:* The foot and tibia are externally rotated (*b*), the two hands (*c*) place the tibia into abduction (genu valgus), and while holding this positioning, the leg is extended. (Illustration by W.A. Kuchera.)

lier may not occur. Palpation and manipulative treatment of tibiofibular interosseous membrane strain may help in treating patients who have incurred an ankle sprain.

GLIDING

With pronation of the foot, the distal talofibular joint glides posteriorly and the head of the fibula glides anteriorly. In the more common ankle sprain in which the foot tends to supinate, the distal fibula is often found to be anterior and the fibular head is posterior.

SOMATIC DYSFUNCTION

Posterior fibular head somatic dysfunction may cause symptoms related to entrapment neuropathy or compression of the common peroneal nerve.

Ankle

Inman and others have stated that the ankle has two joints, an upper and a lower; Inman would have them considered together as a functional unit.[5] The upper joint is the talocrural (tibiotalar) joint and the lower is the subtalar (talocalcaneal) joint. As the patient walks forward and bears weight on the foot, there is a visible medial rotation of the tibia with increasing dorsiflexion at the ankle. Inman and Mann[6] calculated the amount of medial rotation of the tibia (described by Levens et al.)[7] to be greater than could be attributed to movement only at the talocrural joint. Inman then studied the axis of the subtalar joint and attributed the increased medial rotation to coincide with a relative calcaneal eversion about the subtalar axis. As the stance phase of the walking cycle continues to the toe-off interval, the tibia externally rotates with simultaneous calcaneal inversion about the subtalar axis.

TALOCRURAL JOINT

The talocrural or tibiotalar joint involves the talus moving in the ankle mortise. Until the publication of Inman's studies, the axis of the talocrural joint was thought, and described in anatomic textbooks, to be a horizontal axis that corresponded with the articular surfaces of the joint. Inman demonstrated that a single empirical (functional) axis in 80% of his specimens was not horizontal. He described an oblique axis directed laterally and downward (average 8°) on a coronal plane and laterally and posteriorly (average 6°) on a transverse plane. Still, the major motions of this joint are described as dorsiflexion and plantar flexion. Minor motions occur with each, posterior glide with dorsiflexion and anterior glide with plantar flexion. Dorsiflexion is functionally the more stable of the two positions because the talus is structurally wider anteriorly and fits more securely with the posterior glide component (Fig. 50.17).

Position

Since the talocrural axis passes distally to the tip of each malleolus, its position may be estimated by placing the tips of your

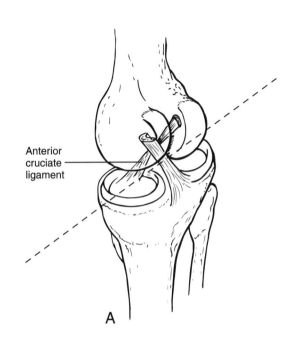

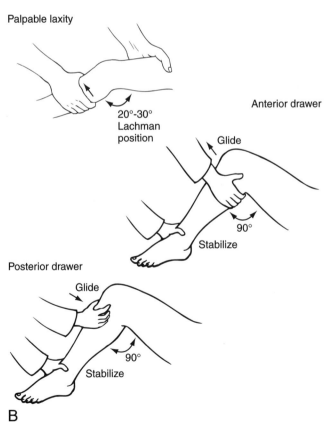

Figure 50.14. Structure–function tests of the anterior (**A**) and posterior (**B**) cruciate ligaments using the Lachman and drawer tests.

Figure 50.15. Proximal tibiofibular joint. Note that the fibular head and the tibial tuberosity are on the same horizontal plane.

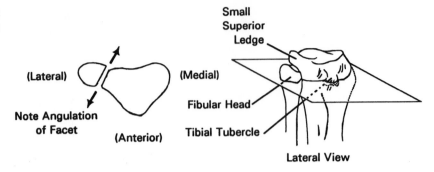

Figure 50.16. External rotation of the tibia (C) moves the distal fibula posteriorly (B) and reciprocally is associated with the fibular head moving anteriorly (B1). The opposite is true (A, A1) with internal rotation (D) of the lower leg. (Illustration by W.A. Kuchera.)

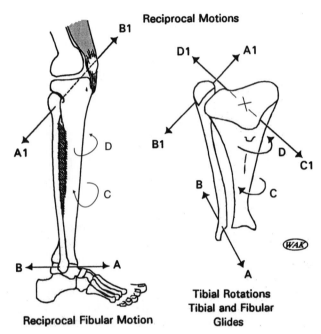

fingers at the most distal ends of the malleoli. At this position the fingers would be over the transverse axis of the talocrural joint.

Toeing

Since the axis is oblique rather than horizontal, toeing out of the free foot occurs with dorsiflexion; and toeing in, with plantar flexion. This is important to remember when setting up direct manipulative techniques addressing this joint.

PLANTAR FLEXION

Plantar flexion is accompanied by adduction and some supination of the foot. This motion also carries the lateral malleolus anteriorly. Through reciprocal action of the fibula, the proximal fibular head also glides posteriorly and inferiorly. The talus

glides anteriorly, placing the narrow portion of the talus in the ankle mortise, a less stable position. Ankle sprains, more likely to occur when the tibiotalar joint is plantar flexed, are discussed with supination in the later section on the foot.

Dorsiflexion

Dorsiflexion is accompanied by abduction and some pronation of the foot. This type of motion also carries the lateral malleolus posteriorly, and through reciprocal action glides the fibular head anteriorly and superiorly. The talus glides posteriorly, placing the wider portion in the ankle mortise, a more stable position. This stability is the reason taping in the treatment or prevention of ankle sprains usually emphasizes a dorsiflexion component.

SUBTALAR JOINT

The subtalar or talocalcaneal joint (Fig. 50.18) has been called the main shock-absorber joint.[8(p.657)] It earned this designation because, in coordination with the intertarsal joints, it determines the distribution of forces upon the skeleton and soft tissues of the foot. The strong talocalcaneal ligament stabilizes it. It is a synovial joint with a single oblique axis that declines backward and laterally. This joint acts like a mitered hinge so that movement of the calcaneus produces leg rotation. Inversion of the calcaneus produces external rotation of the tibia, and the talus glides posterolaterally over the calcaneus. Eversion of the calcaneus produces medial rotation of the tibia and anteromedial glide of the talus on the calcaneus.

Gliding

Clinically, these mechanics seem to explain the palpable talocalcaneal motions: posterolateral glide of the talus when the ankle is supinated and the anteromedial glide at the talocalcaneal joint when the ankle is pronated.

Subtalar Axis

Inman and Inman found the average inclination of the subtalar axis from the horizontal plane on the sagittal plane to be 42° (ranging from 20 to 68°). If the inclination of the axis is 45°, rotation of the tibia and calcaneus has a one-to-one relation-

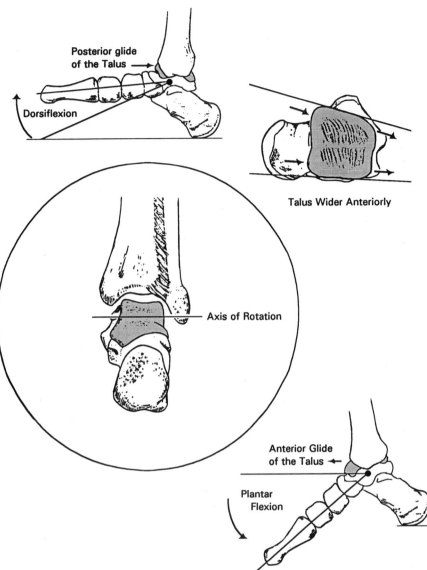

Figure 50.17. Ankle major and minor motions. Dorsiflexion with posterior glide is the most stable joint position because the wedge-shaped talus is engaged. (Illustration by W.A. Kuchera.)

ship. The more horizontal the axis, the more the calcaneus rotates and the less the leg rotates. This calcaneal rotation is not very obvious during walking because the metatarsals of the forefoot appear to remain stationary. Inman and Inman's studies concluded that approximately half of the population has some linear displacement of the talus along the axis with movement in the subtalar joint.

Pes Planus

Persons with pes planus (flat foot) have the more horizontal axis and greater motion in their feet. This explains why they break down their shoes quickly and prefer to go barefoot.

Pes Cavus

Persons with pes cavus (high arch) have a more vertical angle and a more rigid foot.

Movement

Hicks reported that without movement at the subtalar joint it would be difficult for a person to balance his or her body over one lower limb.[9]

Foot

The movement of the foot or pes is a composite movement of the talocalcaneal joint of the hind foot and movement of the forefoot about the talonavicular and calcaneocuboid joints. Inversion is that movement in which the heel (calcaneus) faces medially as the inside edge of the foot is lifted. Eversion occurs when the heel faces laterally as the outside edge of the foot is lifted. In the non-weight-bearing foot, inversion and eversion can be applied to the forefoot as it moves more medially or more laterally, respectively (Fig. 50.19).

In the upper extremity, pronation and supination are movements of the forearm and muscles of the forearm produced by supinator and pronator muscles. Supination means that the palm is up, such as when holding your hand out waiting for someone to put something into it. In the foot, however, there are no muscles anatomically labeled as pronators or supinators. An active attempt to supinate the foot results in a combination of adduction, plantar flexion, and inversion of the foot. Likewise, an attempt to pronate the foot results in abduction, dorsiflexion, and eversion. *Gray's Anatomy* has described pronation and supination in the foot as movements of the forefoot not including movement of the calcaneus. This is not true with weight bearing and active motion. With weight bearing, supination of the foot is accompanied by eversion of the calcaneus and posterolateral glide of the talus with respect to the navicular at the talocalcaneal joint. While providing less sta-

bility at the ankle, supination locks the foot, allowing stabilization at heel strike and propulsion at toe-off. Pronation during weight bearing stabilizes the ankle, creates eversion of the calcaneus with anterolateral glide of the talocalcaneal joint, and unlocks the foot for surface adaptation and shock absorption during running.

STABILIZING LIGAMENTS

Ankle sprains are very common in a general practice. The supination position, which includes the less stable plantar flexion position, predisposes the ankle to such injuries. Approximately 80% of all sprains are of the supination type.[10] These traumatize the lateral stabilizing ligaments of the ankle. Additionally, somatic dysfunction occurs during the mechanism of injury, which extends well beyond the local ligamentous stress (Fig. 50.20). In a supination sprain, there is eversion of the calcaneus and posterolateral glide at the talocalcaneal joint. Stretching and potential trigger point development in the peroneus (Fig. 50.21) as well as other lateral and anterior compartment muscles typically occur.[8(p.683–691)] The distal fibula may be drawn anteriorly with reciprocal posterior glide of the fibular head or, if the anterior talofibular ligament is torn, the distal fibula may move posteriorly with anterior glide of the fibular head. (Recall that sprains are traumatically induced, and therefore somatic dysfunction may not follow simple biomechanical predictions).

Somatic dysfunction does not stop here. The tibia often externally rotates with an anteromedial glide of the tibial plateau. The femur internally rotates. Myofascial forces (postural forces) then continue upward into the pelvis and spine. Failure

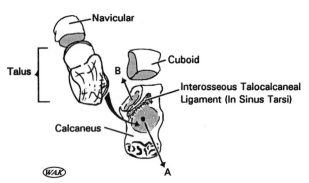

Figure 50.18. Subtalar joint. Persons with flat feet have a more horizontal axis and greater foot motion. Those with a more vertical axis have a more rigid, pes cavus foot. *A*, posterolateral glide; *B*, anteromedial glide.

Figure 50.19. Inversion, eversion, supination, and pronation of the left foot.

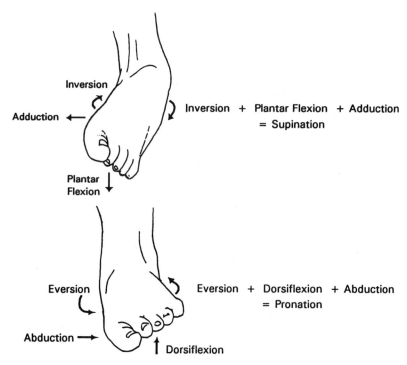

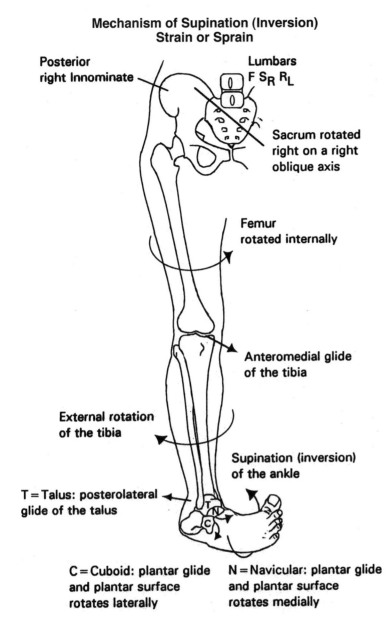

Mechanism of Supination (Inversion) Strain or Sprain

Posterior right Innominate

Lumbars F S$_R$ R$_L$

Sacrum rotated right on a right oblique axis

Femur rotated internally

Anteromedial glide of the tibia

External rotation of the tibia

Supination (inversion) of the ankle

T = Talus: posterolateral glide of the talus

C = Cuboid: plantar glide and plantar surface rotates laterally

N = Navicular: plantar glide and plantar surface rotates medially

Figure 50.20. Somatic dysfunctions and structural stress occurring in the more common supination ankle sprain.

to diagnose and treat or rehabilitate beyond the ankle itself increases recurrence rates and prolongs the healing and rehabilitation process. It also increases complaints in distant sites due to the patient's involuntary attempts to compensate for continued dysfunction.

There are really three separate ligaments stabilizing the lateral side of the ankle (Fig. 50.22). From anterior to posterior, these are the:

Anterior talofibular ligament
Calcaneofibular ligament
Posterior talofibular ligament

Because the biomechanical stresses associated with a supination strain progress from anterior to posterior, ankle sprains are often named by type according to the extent of ligamentous involvement:

1. Type 1: Involves anterior talofibular ligament only.
2. Type 2: Involves the anterior talofibular and calcaneofibular ligaments.
3. Type 3: Involves all three lateral supporting ligaments.

A pure inversion sprain can result in sprain of the calcaneofibular ligament alone. This can occur during rebounding in which basketball players land directly on the lateral aspect of the foot (without any plantar flexion). An understanding of the biomechanics of the foot and ankle explains why this is an uncommon ankle sprain.

DELTOID LIGAMENT

The deltoid ligament (Fig. 50.23) stabilizing the medial side of the ankle is so strong that trauma stressing this structure is more likely to fracture a piece of medial malleolus than tear

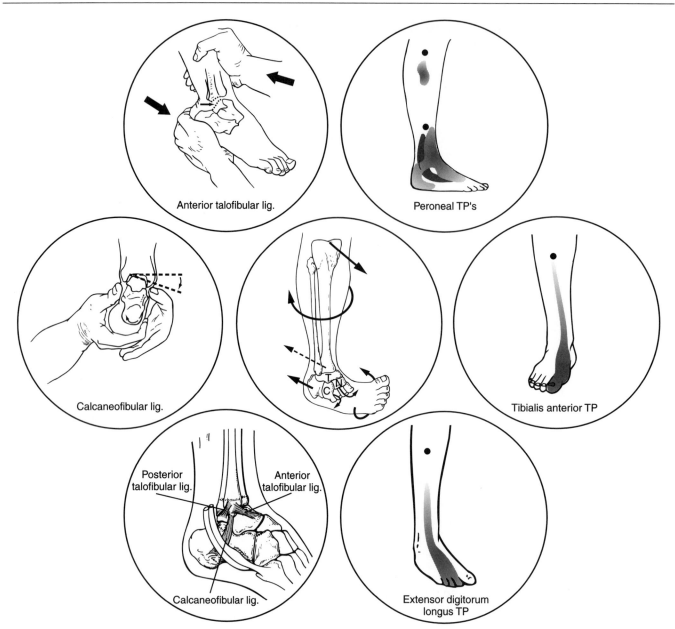

Figure 50.21. Trigger points (*TPs*) and ligamentous strain are somatic sources of pain in the more common supination ankle sprain. Muscles placed on stress are (in order): peroneus, tibialis anterior, and extensor digitorum longus. Ligaments (*lig.*) stressed are (in order): anterior talofibular, calcaneofibular, and anterior tibiotalar. *T,* talus; *N,* navicular; *C,* cuboid.

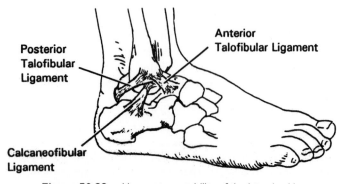

Figure 50.22. Ligamentous stability of the lateral ankle.

the ligament. Pronation sprains are uncommon. This is due both to the strength of the deltoid ligament and the stability imparted by gliding the wide portion of the talus into the tibiotalar joint during dorsiflexion.

The two main arches of the foot are the longitudinal and transverse arches. They are maintained by:

Interlocking articular facets of the bones
Interosseous ligaments
Special fascial sheaths
Plantar ligaments
Muscles and muscle tendons

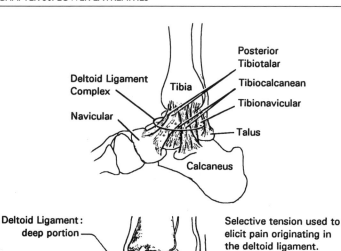

Figure 50.23. Deltoid ligament.

LONGITUDINAL ARCH

The longitudinal arch is divided into medial and lateral components. It is supported by the tibialis posterior muscle. Its tendon attaches to the navicular, first cuneiform, and bases of the second, third, and fourth metatarsals. The bony lateral longitudinal arch is the calcaneus, the cuboid, and the fourth and fifth metatarsals. The bony medial longitudinal arch consists of the talus, navicular, the three cuneiforms, and the first three metatarsals (Fig. 50.24).

TRANSVERSE ARCH

The transverse arch is composed of the cuboid, the navicular, the three cuneiforms, and the proximal ends of the metatarsals. This arch is supported by the peroneus longus muscle inferiorly and by the tibialis anterior muscle, which attaches to the medial and undersurface of the first cuneiform and proximal first metatarsal (Fig. 50.25).

PLANTAR LIGAMENTS

The plantar aponeurosis (Fig. 50.26) extends from the calcaneus to the phalanges and encompasses the sesamoid bones under the great toe. Functional demand causes chronic stress on this structure. Irritation caused by either excessive pronation or a high-arched cavus foot may result in plantar fasciitis. With time, calcium is laid down along lines of stress, leading to formation of a calcaneal heel spur. Correction of the underlying biomechanical dysfunction is the treatment of choice. Surgery is rarely necessary.

The long plantar ligament runs from the calcaneus to the lateral three metatarsals. It forms a tunnel for the passage of the peroneus longus muscle as that tendon passes under the foot to the first cuneiform and first metatarsal. The short plantar ligament is short. It lies medial to the lateral longitudinal arch and is attached between the calcaneus and the proximal end of the cuboid.

The spring ligament (calcaneonavicular) runs from the sustentaculum tali of the calcaneus to the navicular. The spring ligament strengthens the medial longitudinal arch.

TRANSVERSE TARSAL JOINT

The transverse tarsal joint contains the talonavicular and calcaneocuboid articulations, which are separate joints but which act together as a functional unit. It has its greatest influence during the stance phase of the walking cycle because it responds to eversion or inversion of the heel. The talonavicular and calcaneocuboid joints plus the two small talocalcaneal joints are collectively called Chopart's joint. The articulations of Chopart's joint are followed by a surgeon when amputating a foot. Between the intertarsal joints and the subtalar joint is a groove called the sinus tarsi. Attached along this groove is the very strong interosseous talocalcaneal ligament that provides stability for the subtalar and intertarsal joints.

With internal rotation of the leg and inversion of the heel, the lines of the talonavicular and calcaneocuboid axes coincide. This produces enough freedom in the transverse tarsal joint so that the forefoot can evert or invert to accommodate for an uneven terrain.

When the leg rotates laterally and inverts the heel on a weight-bearing forefoot, the transverse tarsal joint appears to become more rigid. This is because the two axes do not coincide. The forefoot can no longer accommodate for an uneven terrain in this position.

As the heel rises in plantar flexion, the transverse tarsal joint

Figure 50.24. Supports of the longitudinal arch of the foot. *1,* plantar aponeurosis, abductor digiti minimi, and flexor digitorum brevis IV and V; *2,* long plantar ligament; *3,* short plantar ligament; *P,* phalanges. (From Hamilton JJ, Ziemer LK. *Functional Anatomy of the Human Ankle and Foot. AAOS Symposium on Foot and Ankle.* St Louis, Mo: CV Mosby; 1983:13.)

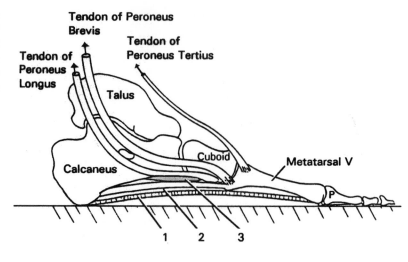

Figure 50.25. Supports of the transverse arch of the foot. *Stippled tube* represents tendon of tibialis posterior; *black areas* represent oblique head of adductor hallucis. (From Hamilton JJ, Ziemer LK. *Functional Anatomy of the Human Ankle and Foot. AAOS Symposium on Foot and Ankle.* St Louis, Mo: CV Mosby; 1983:13.)

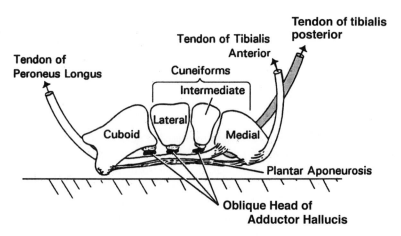

must follow the movement about the subtalar axis and invert with the heel to assist the toe-off interval.

SOMATIC DYSFUNCTION

Somatic dysfunction of the tarsal bones is relatively common. In middle- and long-distance runners these bones may even sublux. Somatic dysfunction of the cuboid involves the edge nearest the middle of the foot. This edge glides toward the plantar surface of the foot and rotates laterally around its AP axis. Somatic dysfunction of the navicular involves the edge nearest the middle of the foot gliding toward the plantar surface and rotating medially around its AP axis (Fig. 50.27). Cuneiform somatic dysfunction is usually manifested by the second cuneiform gliding directly toward the plantar. Somatic dysfunction of these tarsal bones can be diagnosed by the combination of tenderness and increased tissue tension over the plantar surface of each of these bones. Osteopathic manipulative treatment (OMT) is effective, although some patients find orthotics to modify predisposing biomechanical factors useful.

There are five metatarsal–phalangeal joints. As the forefoot inverts with plantar flexion, the body weight is transferred to

these articulations for push-off. Foot structure provides two functional axes for push-off: an oblique axis that passes through the heads of the second through fifth metatarsals, and a transverse axis that passes through the heads of the first and second metatarsals. Structurally, a Morton's foot is characterized by a short first metatarsal that is not designed to accept the normal weight-bearing function involved in the push-off portion of gait. A callus develops under the second and third metatarsal heads as they assume the weight-bearing function. Increased functional demand remodels bone. This results in thickening of the second metatarsal; the thickening is evident on x-ray films. Treatment consists of orthotics to modify the structure–function relationships (Fig. 50.28) and OMT to permit realignment.

SOMATIC DYSFUNCTION

Hallux valgus and bunions have a significant hereditary component. Hammer toes are acquired.

Hallus Valgus

Hallux valgus is a structural deformity resulting from contracture of various periarticular structures of the first metatarsal–phalangeal joint. It is progressive.

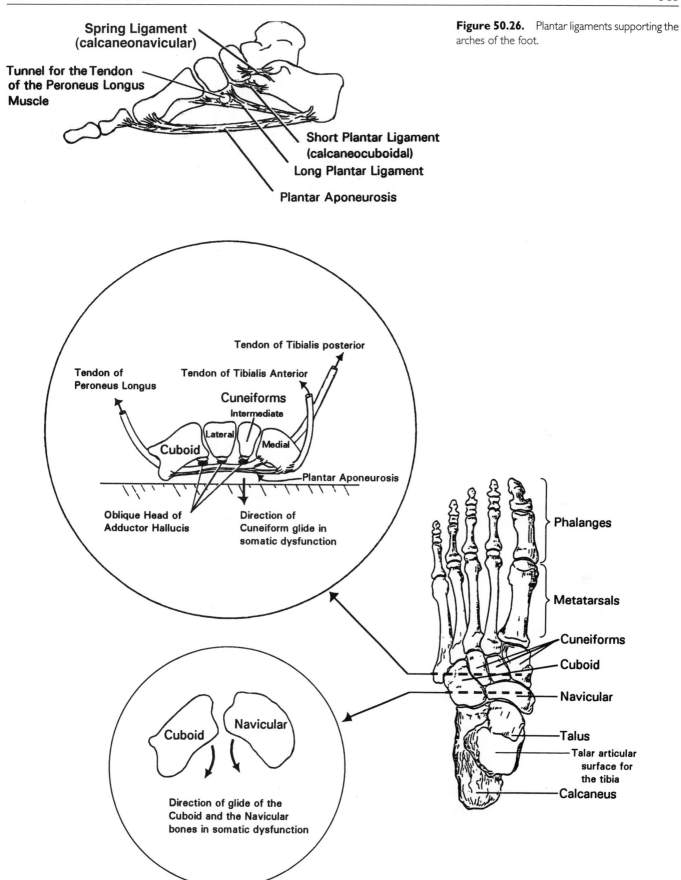

Figure 50.26. Plantar ligaments supporting the arches of the foot.

Spring Ligament
(calcaneonavicular)

Tunnel for the Tendon
of the Peroneus Longus
Muscle

Short Plantar Ligament
(calcaneocuboidal)

Long Plantar Ligament

Plantar Aponeurosis

Tendon of Tibialis posterior

Tendon of
Peroneus Longus

Tendon of Tibialis Anterior

Cuneiforms

Intermediate

Lateral

Cuboid

Medial

Plantar Aponeurosis

Oblique Head of
Adductor Hallucis

Direction of
Cuneiform glide in
somatic dysfunction

Phalanges

Metatarsals

Cuneiforms

Cuboid

Navicular

Talus

Talar articular
surface for
the tibia

Calcaneus

Cuboid

Navicular

Direction of glide of the
Cuboid and the Navicular
bones in somatic dysfunction

Figure 50.27. Navicular, cuboid, and cuneiform somatic dysfunction.

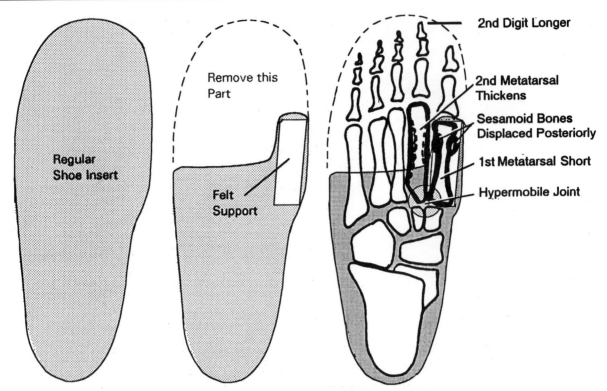

Figure 50.28. Orthotic used for Morton's foot to modify structure–function relationships. Toe portion of the sole insert is removed so support is under only the first metatarsal head. Lateral side of the support must not extend under second metatarsal head. Insert should reach to the distal end of the first metatarsal.

Bunions

Bunion protrusion is accentuated by varus deviation of the first metatarsal. Muscle imbalance aggravates symptoms, but surgical intervention of the structure is often required for symptomatic relief.

Hammer Toes

Hammer toes are often functional and may be associated with myofascial trigger points in the dorsal interossei. Deformation may disappear after treatment of this somatic dysfunction.[11(p.530)]

Somatic dysfunction of the tarsometatarsal, metatarsal–phalangeal, and interphalangeal joints involves their minor motions:

Plantar or dorsal glide
Internal or external rotation
Lateral or medial glide

It also involves compression or, less commonly, traction. Indirect stacking osteopathic manipulative techniques are especially helpful in jammed toes. A stacking technique is one where the physician moves a joint in the direction of preference in all of its planes, stacking one motion upon the other. Compression or traction is then applied to that combined position. The technique may require holding that position of ease for 90 seconds or until the joint tensions relax. The joint is then slowly returned to a neutral position and rechecked for motion.

NEUROMUSCULAR STRUCTURES AND FUNCTION

Neurological Examination

Early in the neuromuscular examination of the lower extremity, perform a traditional neurological examination to rule out associated neurological disease or a structural problem affecting the nervous system. Upper motor neuron disorders are characterized by hyperreflexia, often with pathologic reflexes such as ankle clonus or Babinski up-going toe reflex. Lower extremity muscles demonstrate spasticity or rigidity. Lower motor neuron disorders are generally characterized by hyporeflexia accompanying muscle weakness and/or flaccidity. Dermatomal patterns of pain and/or dysesthesia associated with radicular (nerve root) problems in the lower extremity follow general patterns as depicted in Figure 50.29. Review of the lumbar region is necessary to thoroughly understand neuromuscular problems affecting the lower extremities.

PATELLAR DEEP TENDON REFLEX

Suspect L4 radiculopathy when there is reduction of the patellar deep tendon reflex, dysesthesia in the L4 distribution, and weakness and cramping in those muscles innervated by the L4 nerve root such as the quadriceps and tibialis anterior.

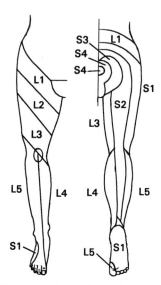

Figure 50.29. Dermatomal or radicular (nerve root) patterns. (Illustration by W.A. Kuchera.)

FOOT DROP

L5 radiculopathy has no abnormal deep tendon reflex; suspect it with dysesthesia in the L5 distribution and weakness and cramping in gluteus medius and ankle dorsiflexors such as tibialis anterior, extensor hallucis, and extensor digitorum brevis. Often this patient may complain of tripping over carpets or small cracks in the sidewalk because of a foot drop.

ACHILLES DEEP TENDON REFLEX

Suspect S1 radiculopathy with reduction of the Achilles deep tendon reflex, dysesthesia in the S1 distribution, and weakness and cramping of intrinsic foot muscles, the gastrocnemius–soleus complex, and the buttock/gluteal muscles. This is the most common radiculopathy, often resulting from a herniated disc between L5 and S1.

Referred Pain

Pain and dysesthesia are not limited to a nerve root or dermatomal pattern. Pain patterns referred from the facet joints of the lumbar spine overlap myofascial trigger point pain arising from the following muscles:[11(p.26)]

Multifidi
Quadratus lumborum
Glutei
Piriformis
Obturator internus

Myotomal referral often results in a "charley horse" or a crampy sensation. A myotomal distribution is associated with the location of muscles that share the neural (root, plexus, or peripheral nerve) innervation. Review the muscle innervations

provided in Tables 50.1 and 50.2. Sclerotomal referral is a deep, achy sensation that is toothachelike in quality. Sclerotomal (bony/ligamentous) distribution has also been mapped out (Fig. 50.30) but is frequently overlooked. Patients may dismiss it as arthritic pain. Notice that the knee and the hip joints share the same L3 sclerotome.

Referred pain in general is reproducible. An understanding of the patterns associated with each referral improves patient diagnosis and treatment design. Failure to appreciate nondermatomal patterns may lead a practitioner to incorrectly consider a patient with legitimate symptoms a malingerer.

LUMBAR AREA

Structures in the lumbar region often refer pain to the inguinal area and/or hip. This is the case with the iliolumbar ligament, the quadratus lumborum muscle, and a urinary tract stone passing down the ureter.

HIP AREA

Structures in the hip region often refer pain to the knee. An adolescent male with knee pain and no sign of knee dysfunction or structural abnormality should have a hip x-ray to rule out a slipped capital epiphysis or other hip joint pathological conditions.

MYOFASCIAL TRIGGER POINTS

Myofascial trigger points as described by Travell and Simons[11,12] also have predictable referral patterns not associated with dermatomes. See Figure 66.12 for a synopsis of representative trigger points associated with the lower extremity.

Somatic Dysfunction

Somatic dysfunction of lower extremity muscular structures is characterized by neuromuscular imbalance and/or myofascial trigger points. In neuromuscular imbalance, some muscles exhibit increased irritability (short and tight) while their antagonists demonstrate inhibition (weak and atrophic) (Fig. 50.31).[13] When stressed, the iliopsoas, piriformis, rectus femoris, and tensor fasciae latae all tend to tighten while the vasti (especially the vastus medialis), peroneus, and tibialis anterior all tend to be inhibited and weak. An understanding of the myotatic unit, muscle agonists and antagonists, and patterns of use is necessary for efficient diagnostic and therapeutic approaches in the neuromuscular system.

MUSCLES OF HIP

Muscles of the hip are generally large and powerful. They can be grouped according to their functional role (Table 50.1). Dysfunction leads to a number of patient symptoms that respond readily to a variety of osteopathic manipulative techniques, especially muscle energy and counterstrain activating

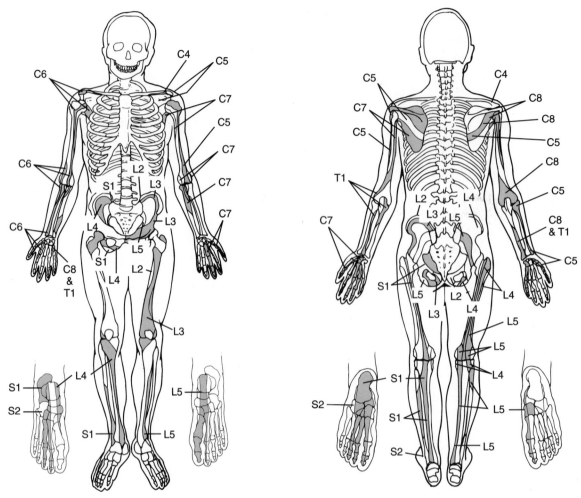

Figure 50.30. Sclerotomal pain patterns.

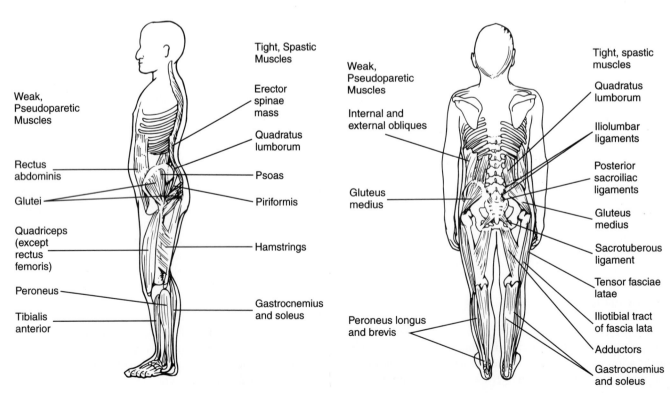

Figure 50.31. Muscle imbalance caused by biomechanical stressors.

Table 50.1
Functional Muscle Chart for the Hip

Muscle Innervation	Functional Anatomic Features	Dysfunction
Hip flexors		
Iliopsoas (L2–4)	Strongest flexor of thigh	Psoas posturing and psoas syndrome
	Postural significance: extension of spine while standing (lumbar lordosis); flexion of spine with bending	Activated by sit-ups or bending over a low table
		Aggravated by weight bearing; relief recumbent with knees bent
	Psoas attaches to T12–L5 vertebral bodies and associated intervertebral discs	Referral back and anterior groin
	Psoas crosses lumbar intervertebral, lumbosacral, sacroiliac, and hip joints	Positive Thomas test = iliopsoas contracture
		Usually develops spasm when stressed
Rectus femoris (L2–4; femoral n.)	Crosses both hip and knee	Referral patellar and deep knee pain
	Primarily an extender of the knee; only causes hip flexion when knee extended	Usually develops spasm when stressed
Pectineus	Flexion and adduction of thigh at hip	Referral deep-seated groin ache
	Designed for power not speed	
Also sartorius thigh adductors, t. fascia latae	Contribute to hip flexion	
Hip extensors		
Gluteus maximus (L5–S2; superior gluteal)	Type I (slow twitch) muscle fibers suited for continuous use	Decreases hip flexion
		Restlessness, pain on sitting or walking uphill
	Location and size unique providing anatomic basis for upright posture	Antalgic gait
		Referral to buttock
	Most powerful extensor	Usually becomes inhibited when stressed
Hamstrings (L5–S2; sciatic n.)	Restrains hip flexion produced by body weight during stance phase of walking; extension during walking	Decreased hip flexion with straight leg raising test
		Pain sitting and walking; disturbs sleep
		Perpetuated by chair pressure under thighs
		Referral posterior thigh
		Usually develops spasm when stressed
Adductor magnus (ischiocondylar portion: L4–S1 sciatic n.)	Only portion of adductor magnus assisting flexion and then only when the femur is flexed more than 70°	Referral to inner thigh
		Usually develops spasm when stressed
Hip abductors		
Gluteus medius (L4–S1; inferior gluteal)	Stabilizes pelvis during single limb stance (prevents nonstance innominate from falling inferior—negative Trendelenburg test)	TPs aggravated by walking, slouching in chair, or lying on back
		Referral to posterior iliac crest, SI joint, sacrum, and minor to buttock
		Positive Trendelenburg test = weakness in hip abductors
		Usually becomes inhibited when stressed
Gluteus minimus (L4–S1)	Stabilizes pelvis during single limb stance (prevents nonstance innominate from falling inferior—negative Trendelenburg test)	Travell calls TPs in this muscle "pseudosciatica"
		Characteristic pain arising from chair or walking; can be constant and excruciating
		Mistaken for L5 or S1 radiculopathy (but may coexist)
		Antalgic gait
		Referral buttock, lateral and posterior thigh
		Positive Trendelenburg test = weakness in hip abductors
		Usually becomes inhibited when stressed
Piriformis (S1–2)	Acts as abductor when thigh flexed	May entrap peroneal portion of sciatic nerve or cause sciatica
		Perpetuated by sacroiliac somatic dysfunction or irritation (especially sacral shear) and sitting on billfold
		Associated with pelvic floor dysfunction, dyspareunia, prostatodynia
		Usually develops spasm when stressed

Table 50.1—*continued*

Muscle Innervation	Functional Anatomic Features	Dysfunction
Also to lesser extent: sartorius, gluteus maximus, iliopsoas		
Hip adductors		
Adductor longus, brevis and magnus (L2–4; obturator n.)	Early in swing phase, these muscles pull limb toward midline	Referral distal to inguinal ligament, inner thigh, and upper medial knee
		Usually develops spasm when stressed
External rotators of the hip (L5–S2)		
Obturator internus (L5–S2)	When the thigh is extended, cause external rotation; when flexed, cause abduction	Responsible for pelvic floor symptoms (fullness in rectum)
		Referral to anococcygeal region (some to posterior thigh)
Internal rotators of the hip		
Gluteus medius and minimus (L4–S1)	(See hip abductors above)	(See hip abductors above)
Also from: gemelli and quadratus femoris (L4–S1). Less from piriformis	Piriformis only involved with external rotation when the femor is extended	

forces. They also respond to a number of manipulative techniques that address the muscles. These techniques include:

Soft tissue OMT
Myofascial spray and stretch
Injection
Dry needling

Often the joints between muscle origin and insertion need treatment. Also consider viscerosomatic referral as a primary source of secondary muscle dysfunction. Because crosstalk between the viscera and the soma tends to take place in the spinal cord, innervation of each muscle becomes clinically relevant for more than just the recognition of nerve root pathophysiology.

NERVE SUPPLY IN BUTTOCK AND THIGH

Nerve supply in the buttock and/or thigh may be functionally affected by the piriformis muscle. Biochemical irritation of the sciatic nerve is possible with irritation of the piriformis because of the close anatomic relationship between the two (Fig. 50.32). In approximately 10% of the U.S. population, the peroneal portion of the sciatic nerve actually passes through the piriformis muscle; this occurs in one-third of patients of Asian descent. In the presence of this anatomic variation, peroneal entrapment is likely. Because of this variant anatomy, therapeutic injections into the piriformis muscle should be approached with caution to avoid permanent nerve injury.

The sciatic nerve divides into a posterior tibial and common peroneal nerve in the thigh. Other thigh muscles are innervated by the obturator and femoral nerves. The gluteal muscles are innervated by gluteal nerves.

MUSCLES OF THIGH AND LEG

Muscles of the thigh and leg include those affecting knee, ankle, and foot function (Table 50.2 and Fig. 50.33). Several thigh muscles have already been described in relation to their effect at the hip. These include the:

Hamstrings
Rectus femoris
Tensor fasciae latae

The hamstrings and the short head of the biceps femoris are the chief flexors of the knee. The hamstrings, by definition muscles that attach to the ischial tuberosity, attach to the leg below the knee and are supplied by the tibial division of the sciatic nerve.[14] The head of the biceps femoris crosses the knee and is innervated by the peroneal portion of the sciatic nerve. Both heads of the biceps femoris also cause external rotation of the knee while the remaining hamstrings cause internal rotation.

NERVE SUPPLY IN THIGH, LEG, AND FOOT

Nerve supply in the thigh, leg, and foot divide off the posterior tibial and common peroneal nerves (Fig. 50.34). The tibial nerve supplies the posterior compartment of the leg and the muscles of the foot. The deep peroneal nerve supplies the anterior compartment of the leg with sensation to the webbing between the first and second toes. The superficial peroneal nerve supplies the lateral compartment of the leg as well as the skin on the anterolateral side of the leg and the dorsum of the foot.

VASCULAR AND LYMPHATIC STRUCTURES AND FUNCTION

The inferior margin of the acetabulum is incomplete, forming an acetabular notch through which the hip joint receives its blood vessels (Fig. 50.35). These vessels are easily disrupted by a femoral neck fracture, which creates the possibility of delayed healing or nonunion. The femoral artery is the major vessel supplying the lower extremity. This artery, easily located in the

Table 50.2
Functional Muscle Chart for the Thigh and Leg

Muscle Innervation	Functional Anatomic Features	Dysfunction
Knee flexors		
Biceps femoris (L5–S2; sciatic n. long head = tibial portion; short head = peroneal portion)	Long head crosses both hip and knee Short head crosses only knee Both heads plus semimembranosus establish a tripartite anchor on the fibular head Short head active in knee flexion for toe clearance during walking Active contraction also induces some external rotation of the knee	Pain referral is distalward from trigger points in the posterior thigh to the back of the knee or to the region of the fibular head Often wakes patient at night
Semimembranosus and semitendinosus (L5–S2; sciatic n. tibial portion)	Also hip extensors Hamstrings are not consistently active for knee flexion during walking (passive knee motion when the hip is flexed is more common) Active contraction also induces some internal rotation of the knee	Pain referral proximally to lower buttock; aggravated by walking often causing limp TPs often misdiagnosed as "sciatica" or "osteoarthritis of the knee" or "growing pains"[a] TPs remaining post-op often cause of "postlaminectomy syndrome"[b] Tightness in the hamstrings is associated with inhibition and laxity of the gluteal muscles
Also popliteus and gastrocnemius	Contribute somewhat to knee flexion Popliteus initiates flexion from fully extended position before hamstrings act	
Knee extensors		
Quadriceps (L2–4; femoral n.)	Rectus femoris crosses both hip and knee joints (proximal attachment to ASIS); also a hip flexor Three vasti cross only knee joint All 4 tendons unite into patellar tendon with patella anchored to tibial tuberosity by patellar ligament Q-angle is the quadriceps angle measured from ASIS to midpatella to tibial tuberosity (Fig. 50.5)	Thigh and knee pain and weakness of knee extension especially going up stairs Anterior knee pain is referred from vastus medialis and rectus femoris; may interrupt sleep Posterior knee pain and pain anywhere along the lateral thigh to the iliac crest are referred from vastus lateralis TPs in v. medialis cause "buckling knee"[c] and may cause patient to fall TPs in v. lateralis may restrict motion of the patella; pain with walking TPs in v. intermedius have difficulty straightening knee after prolonged sitting Imbalance in quadriceps with one another or with the hamstrings predispose to chondromalacia patellae as does an increased Q-angle Direct trauma to the quadriceps should be observed for myositis ossificans Usually becomes inhibited when stressed
Knee external rotator		
Biceps femoris	Also a knee flexor	See description with Knee Flexors above
Knee internal rotators		
Popliteus (L4–S1; tibial n.)	Unlocks knee at the start of weight bearing by "externally rotating the thigh on the fixed tibia"; internally rotates tibia when thigh is fixed Prevents posterior glide of tibia relative to femur while crouching	Pain behind the knee when crouching, walking down stairs or running downhill Aggravated by braking forward motions during twists (e.g., skiing), high heels by excessive foot pronation,[d] and by training on uneven ground Mimics symptoms of Baker's cyst but no associated swelling in the region
Semimembranosus and semitendinosus	Also knee flexors (primary)	See description under Knee Flexors above
Also sartorius (L2–3; femoral nerve) and gracilis (L2–3; obturator n.)	Sartorius is the longest muscle in the body crossing both hip and knee; it is a hip flexor and knee internal rotator Gracilis is the second longest muscle in the body crossing hip and knee	Pain from the sartorius in the anterior thigh is superficial and described as tingling or sharp; may exhibit symptoms of meralgia paresthetica (entrapment of lateral femoral cutaneous nerve)[e] Pain from gracilis is a hot stinging, superficial pain in the medial thigh; it may be relieved by walking

Table 50.2—*continued*

Muscle Innervation	Functional Anatomic Features	Dysfunction
Ankle dorsiflexors		
Tibialis anterior (L4–S1; deep peroneal n.)	An anterior compartment muscle A dorsiflexor at the taloitibial joint Also supinates foot at the talocalcaneal and transverse tarsal joints	Pain and tenderness referred into great toe and anteromedial ankle Weakness leads to varying degrees of foot drop; patients may complain of tripping over carpets, dragging foot, or "foot slap" Weakness in muscle may be caused by L5 radiculopathy, peroneal mononeuropathy, the habit of crossing the legs at the knee, or posterior fibular head somatic dysfunction
Extensor digitorium longus (L4–S1; deep peroneal n.)	Also everts the foot balancing inversion of tibialis anterior Helps prevent posterior postural sway	Pain pattern over dorsum of foot and ankle Dysfunction often results in foot slap after heel strike TPs may entrap fibers of the deep peroneal nerve Muscle imbalance may lead to formation of hammer toes
Peroneus tertitus (L5–S1; deep peroneal n.)	An anterior compartment muscle A dorsiflexor at the talotibial joint Also everts foot Tendon passes in front of lateral malleolus to insert on proximal 5th metatarsal	Pain referred along anterolateral ankle and sometimes to lateral heel; failure to identify and treat TPs post ankle sprain can prolong rehabilitation process Weakness in ankle dorsiflexion predisposing to ankle instability and repeat sprains May be mistaken for ankle arthritis[f] Weakness in muscle may be caused by L5 radiculopathy, peroneal mononeuropathy, the habit of crossing the legs at the knee, posterior fibular head somatic dysfunction or prolonged immobilization (as in an ankle cast)
Ankle plantar flexors		
Gastrocnemius (L5–S2; posterior tibial n.)	Gastrocnemius-soleus complex referred to as triceps surae; constitute close functional unit; share Achilles tendon attachment to calcaneus	Dysfunction often results in nocturnal leg cramps TP pain may be referred to upper posterior calf and/or to instep "Tennis leg" is a partial tearing of the gastrocnemius; symptoms include a sudden intense calf pain, as if kicked, followed by swelling and local tenderness; failure to recognize may lead to a posterior compartment syndrome
Soleus (S1–2; tibial n.)	Gastrocnemius-soleus complex constitute close functional unit; share Achilles attachment to calcaneus Soleus function during gait is to add to knee and ankle stability Acts as "second heart"[g] in moving venous and lymphatic fluid from lower extremity (e.g., fainting with military "attention" position Also aids in inversion of foot and extension of knee	Heel pain with TPs in this muscle and/or may refer proximally to sacroiliac joint or even temporomandibular joint May restrict dorsiflexion at ankle; pain severe walking up hill or stairs May be cause of growing pains in children Soleus TPs easily mistaken for Baker's cyst, thrombophlebitis, and/or Achilles tendinitis
Peroneus longus and brevis (L4–S1; superficial peroneal n.)	Lateral compartment muscles Plantar flex and pronate foot p. longus attaches to fibular head and to upper 2/3 of lateral fibula, crosses behind the lateral malleolus over the cuboid, and divides to attach to the 1st cuneiform and the base of the 1st metatarsal p. brevis travels with p. longus but inserts on the lateral aspect of the 5th metatarsal	Pain and tenderness projected to lateral malleolus and some of lateral leg TPs initiated by inversion twisting of ankle or prolonged immobilization in ankle cast Predispose to weak ankles and recurrent sprains May have deep peroneal nerve entrapment with some foot drop p. longus and brevis aggravated by Morton's foot structure Pain easily mistaken for arthritis in ankle[b] TPs in p. longus can entrap the common peroneal nerve and weaken both anterior and lateral compartment muscles; numbness often noted in web of great toe

Table 50.2—*continued*

Muscle Innervation	Functional Anatomic Features	Dysfunction
Foot supinators		
Tibialis anterior (L5–S1; deep peroneal n.)	An anterior compartment muscle Supinates foot at talocalcaneal and transverse tarsal joints Also dorsiflexes at the talotibial joint	Pain and tenderness referred into great toe and anteromedial ankle Weakness leads to varying degrees of foot drop; patients may complain of tripping over carpets, dragging foot, or "foot slap" Weakness in muscle may be caused by L5 radiculopathy, peroneal mononeuropathy, the habit of crossing the legs at the knee, or posterior fibular head somatic dysfunction
Foot pronators		
Peroneal muscles (L5–S1; deep peroneal n.)	Lateral compartment muscles are p. longus and brevis; p. tertius is an anterior compartment muscle Pronate the foot (eversion and abduction) p. tertius also dorsiflexes at the talotibial joint; p. brevis and longus also plantar flex Tendon passes in front of lateral malleolus to insert on proximal 5th metatarsal	Pain referred along lateral ankle and foot; sometimes to lateral heel; failure to identify and treat TPs post ankle sprain can prolong rehabilitation process Weakness in ankle dorsiflexion predisposing to ankle instability and repeat sprains May be mistaken for ankle arthritis[i] Weakness in muscle may be caused by L5 radiculopathy, peroneal mononeuropathy, the habit of crossing the legs at the knee, posterior fibular head somatic dysfunction or prolonged immobilization (as in an ankle cast)
Foot and/or toe flexors		
Flexor digitorum longus (L5–S1; tibial n.)		TP pain referred to sole of foot; worse with walking TP perpetuation by Morton's foot, running on uneven ground, or barefoot in the sand
Flexor hallucis longus (L5–S2; tibial n.)		TP pain referred to plantar surface of great toe and first metatarsal head TP perpetuation by Morton's foot, running on uneven ground, or barefoot in the sand
Also intrinsic foot muscles		Intolerably sore feet, limited walking range, limp
Foot and/or toe extensors		
Extensor digitorum longus (L4–S1; deep peroneal n.)	(See above under Ankle Dorsiflexors)	
Extensor hallucis longus (L4–S1; deep peroneal n.)		Dysfunction makes foot less adaptable to the ground while walking TP referred pain to dorsum of foot at the base of the great toe TPs may be perpetuated by L4–5 radiculopathy; often follow anterior compartment syndrome, prolonged jogging, or dorsiflexed ankle position during sleep
Also intrinsic foot muscles		Intolerably sore feet, limited walking range, limp

[a]Travell JG, Simons DG. *Myofascial Pain and Dysfunction: The Trigger Point Manual* (Vol II). Baltimore, Md: Williams & Wilkins; 1992:324.

[b]Travell JG, Simons DG. *Myofascial Pain and Dysfunction: The Trigger Point Manual* (Vol II). Baltimore, Md: Williams & Wilkins; 1992:324.

[c]Travell JG, Simons DG. *Myofascial Pain and Dysfunction: The Trigger Point Manual* (Vol II). Baltimore, Md: Williams & Wilkins; 1992:250.

[d]Brody DM. Running Injuries. *CIBA Clin Symp.* 1980;32(4):15–16.

[e]Travell JG, Simons DG. *Myofascial Pain and Dysfunction: The Trigger Point Manual* (Vol II). Baltimore, Md: Williams & Wilkins; 1992:229–232.

[f]Travell JG, Simons DG. *Myofascial Pain and Dysfunction: The Trigger Point Manual* (Vol II). Baltimore, Md: Williams & Wilkins; 1992:377.

[g]Travell JG, Simons DG. *Myofascial Pain and Dysfunction: The Trigger Point Manual* (Vol II). Baltimore, Md: Williams & Wilkins; 1992:427.

[h]Reynolds MD. Myofascial trigger point syndromes in the practice of rheumatology. *Arch Phys Med Rehabil.* 1981;62:111–114.

[i]Travell JG, Simons DG. *Myofascial Pain and Dysfunction: The Trigger Point Manual* (Vol II). Baltimore, Md: Williams & Wilkins; 1992:377.

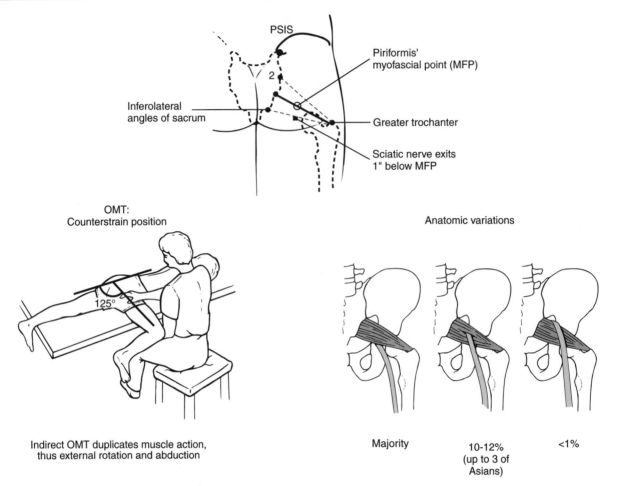

Figure 50.32. Piriformis structure–function relationships.

femoral triangle, is bounded by the sartorius and adductor muscles and the inguinal ligament. The mnemonic NAVEL provides a reminder of the order from lateral to medial of the structures in the femoral triangle:

Nerve
Artery
Vein
Empty space
Lymphatics

Evidence of terminal lymphatic drainage dysfunction for the lower extremities may be palpated just inferior to the inguinal ligament. Dysfunctional drainage results in tissues that are tight, tender, and/or ticklish in this region.

Knee

The vascular supply is very poor to the menisci in the knees (especially the central section) and to the synovial joint tissues in general. In large part, nutrition to the joints depends on good blood flow to the region and then diffusion into the synovial fluids. Metabolic waste products out of the arthrodial

tissues likewise diffuse into the synovial fluid. Intermittent compression of the joints provides for fluid movement and may aid in the exchange of nutrients into and waste products out of the arthrodial structures. In rheumatoid arthritis the synovial membrane thickens, and diffusion is impeded while oxygen demands in that joint increase.[15]

Lower Leg

The lower leg is divided into three compartments (Fig. 50.36):

Anterior osseofibrous compartment
Lateral osseofibrous compartment
Two posterior osseofibrous compartments—deep and superficial

Clinically, a compartment syndrome can arise from trauma or vigorous overuse, leading to a rise in intracompartmental pressure. This in turn compromises the circulation within that compartment, including venous return. Manage recurrent mild compartment symptoms with ice and OMT. Ice decreases pain and metabolic demand after activity. OMT also decreases pain and improves venous and lymphatic return. Management of

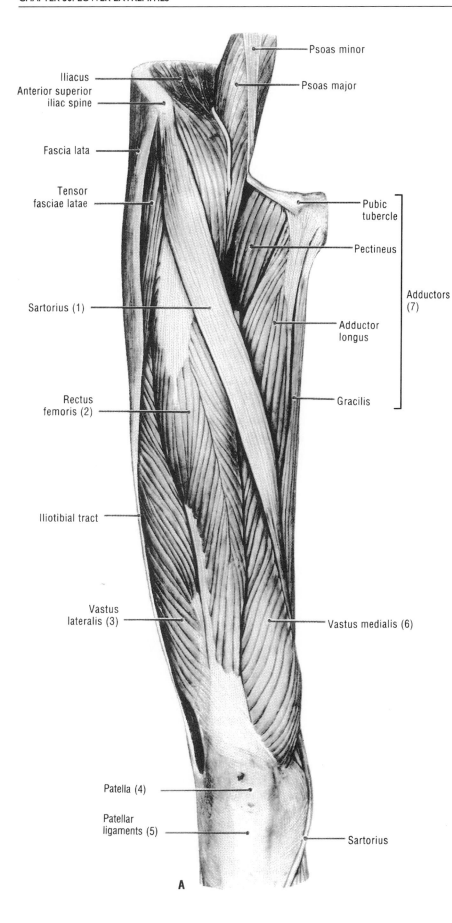

Iliacus

Anterior superior iliac spine

Fascia lata

Tensor fasciae latae

Sartorius (1)

Rectus femoris (2)

Iliotibial tract

Vastus lateralis (3)

Patella (4)

Patellar ligaments (5)

Psoas minor

Psoas major

Pubic tubercle

Pectineus

Adductor longus

Gracilis

Adductors (7)

Vastus medialis (6)

Sartorius

A

Figure 50.33. Muscles of thigh (**A**) and leg (**B**). (From Moore KL. *Clinically Oriented Anatomy.* 3rd ed. Baltimore, Md: Williams & Wilkins; 1992:394, 395, 442, 453.)

Figure 50.33—*continued*

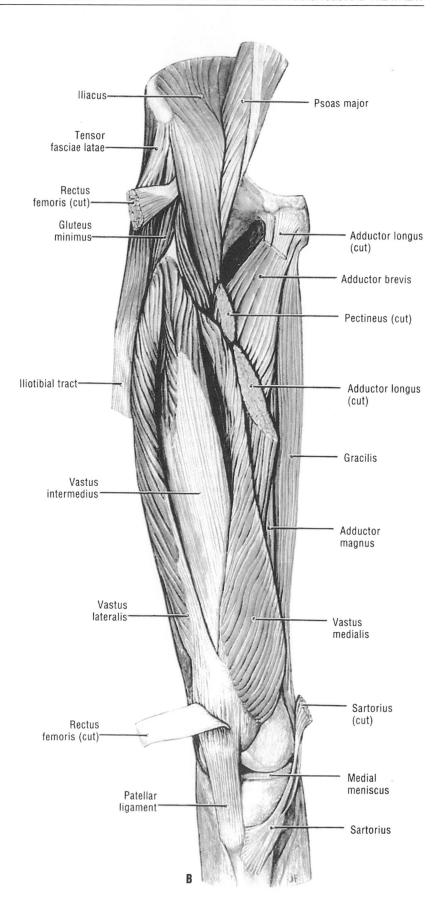

Figure 50.33—*continued*

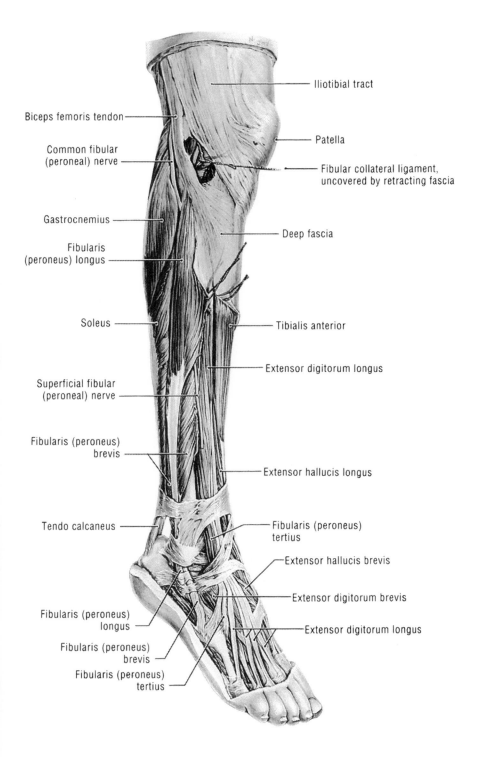

Iliotibial tract

Biceps femoris tendon

Patella

Common fibular (peroneal) nerve

Fibular collateral ligament, uncovered by retracting fascia

Gastrocnemius

Deep fascia

Fibularis (peroneus) longus

Soleus

Tibialis anterior

Extensor digitorum longus

Superficial fibular (peroneal) nerve

Fibularis (peroneus) brevis

Extensor hallucis longus

Tendo calcaneus

Fibularis (peroneus) tertius

Extensor hallucis brevis

Extensor digitorum brevis

Fibularis (peroneus) longus

Extensor digitorum longus

Fibularis (peroneus) brevis

Fibularis (peroneus) tertius

Figure 50.33.—*continued*

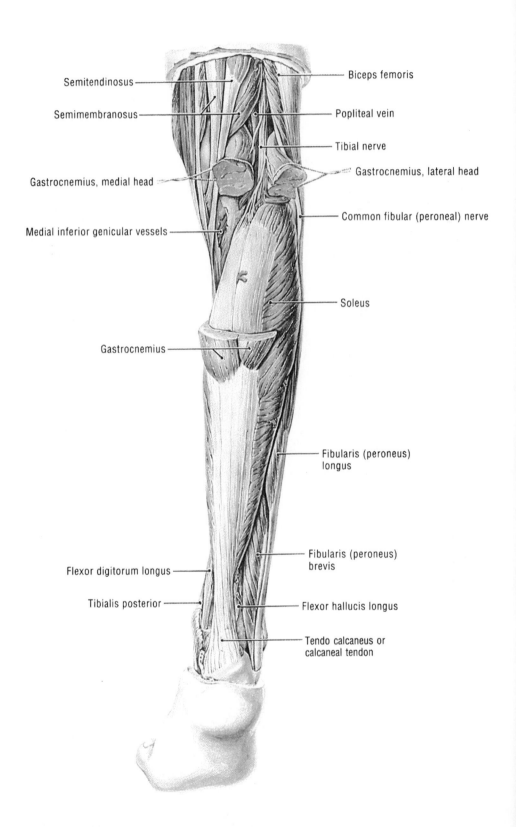

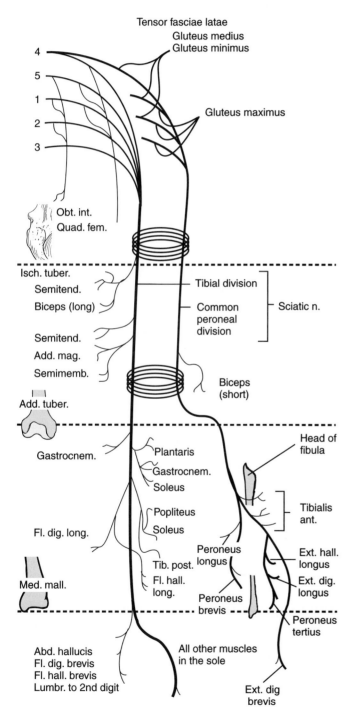

Tensor fasciae latae
Gluteus medius
Gluteus minimus

Gluteus maximus

4
5
1
2
3

Obt. int.
Quad. fem.

Isch. tuber.
Semitend.
Biceps (long)

Tibial division

Common
peroneal
division

Sciatic n.

Semitend.
Add. mag.
Semimemb.

Add. tuber.

Biceps
(short)

Gastrocnem.

Plantaris
Gastrocnem.
Soleus
Popliteus
Soleus

Head of
fibula

Tibialis
ant.

Fl. dig. long.

Tib. post.
Fl. hall.
long.

Peroneus
longus

Peroneus
brevis

Ext. hall.
longus

Ext. dig.
longus

Med. mall.

Peroneus
tertius

Abd. hallucis
Fl. dig. brevis
Fl. hall. brevis
Lumbr. to 2nd digit

All other muscles
in the sole

Ext. dig
brevis

Figure 50.34. Nerve supply of the lower extremity arising from the sciatic nerve and its branches.

coexisting trigger points is also helpful but not with injections; they would increase pressure in an already tight compartment. Modification of the running surface or the running shoe may also be required to prevent recurrent compartment syndromes.

ANTERIOR COMPARTMENT

The anterior compartment is covered anteriorly by a relatively nonexpansile fascia. Structurally, this creates the potential for development of an anterior compartment syndrome. Bleeding into this compartment from a fracture or other trauma creates increased pressure in this enclosed space. For runners, sometimes muscle swelling impairs venous outflow, resulting in a rise in intracompartmental pressure. If intracompartmental pressure becomes great enough, arterial circulation is reduced, and ischemia with potential necrosis of muscle in the compartment can occur. An acute compartment compression is a surgical emergency requiring fasciotomy. Such a situation is more likely to occur in the anterior compartment than in other divisions of the leg. The acute compartment compression may occur in runners where symptoms of intense pain develop during the run but do not subside afterwards.

Palpation reveals the entire tibialis anterior muscle to be hard and tender. Anterior compartment muscles may also exhibit weakness upon testing. Peripheral pulses are usually present. There is often decreased sensation between the first and second toes as a result of entrapment of the deep peroneal nerve. While primarily a clinical diagnosis, intracompartmental pressure can be measured with a wick catheter.[11(p.362)] Because of the location of the pain on the anterolateral side of the leg, recurrent anterior compartment syndrome is also called anterior shin splints.

LATERAL COMPARTMENT

In the lateral compartment syndrome, pain is located diffusely along the lateral aspect of the lower leg. It recurs in runners with excessive pronation of the foot or may result from rupture of the peroneus longus muscle.

POSTERIOR COMPARTMENT

The posterior compartment syndromes typically refer pain anteromedially. While some reserve the term shin splints only for periostitis along the line of attachment of a repeatedly overloaded muscle,[11(p.443)] others include posterior compartment syndrome in the differential diagnosis along with stress fractures of the tibia and chronic periostitis (the soleus syndrome). Posterior compartment syndromes are often bilateral and difficult to manage conservatively.

Bursitis

There are a number of bursae around the hip, knee, and ankle that may swell as a response to direct trauma or stresses placed on the joints of the lower extremity (Fig. 50.37). Bursitis is

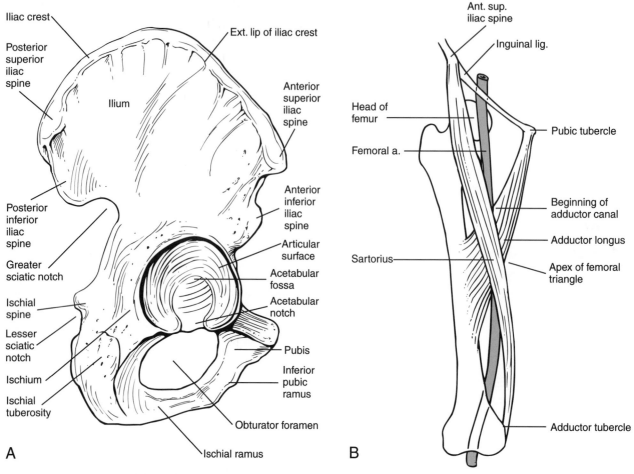

Figure 50.35. Anatomy of the acetabular notch (**A**) and femoral triangle (**B**).

inflammation of a bursa. There is palpable swelling that can be defined and that is sensitive to deep pressure. Pain alone in the region of the bursa frequently leads to misdiagnosis.

TROCHANTERIC

In the hip region, trochanteric bursitis is a common clinical diagnosis or, in many cases, a misdiagnosis. The subgluteus maximus (trochanteric) bursa lies at the root of the iliotibial tract. Here it separates the greater trochanter of the femur from the converging fibers of the gluteus maximus and the tensor fasciae latae. The bursa also separates these fibers from the origin of the vastus lateralis muscle. Trigger points in any of these muscles can refer pain to this site and are commonly misdiagnosed as a trochanteric bursitis. This is also the case in quadratus lumborum trigger points and in the ligamentous pain referral from iliolumbar ligament.

True inflammation and swelling of the trochanteric bursa (trochanteric bursitis) causes intense pain over the bursal location with radiation into the lateral thigh. Palpation of the bursa just below the greater trochanter reveals the swelling and

heat. Pressure here increases the pain. Walking, hip abduction, and internally rotating the hip aggravate the pain. Injection of the bursa with a local anesthetic with or without accompanying steroids quickly and significantly reduces pain. There is a higher incidence of trochanteric bursitis on the long leg side of individuals with unequal leg length.[3]

PATELLAR

The knee is a common site for trauma to the bursa designed to protect the relatively exposed superficial structures from injury against those underlying them. A large prepatellar bursa separates the patella from the skin anterior to it. Inflammation of this bursa from long-term kneeling or from other trauma results in housemaid's knee.

The suprapatellar bursa connects to the synovial cavity of the knee joint and can be used in physical diagnosis to determine if knee trauma has caused significant swelling. First, milk any fluid in this bursa from medial to lateral. By then palpating anteromedially for a fluid wave initiated by a gentle squeeze

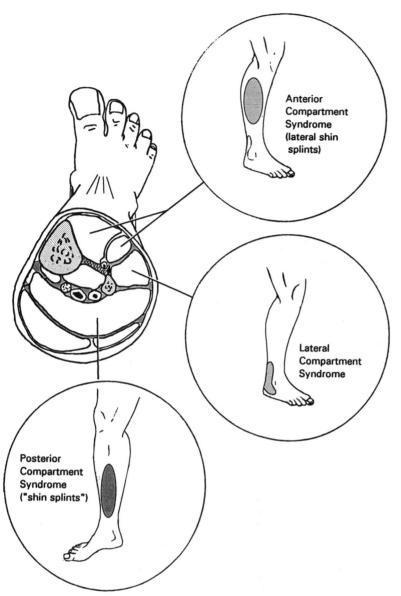

Figure 50.36. Fascial compartments of the lower extremity.

Anterior Compartment Syndrome (lateral shin splints)

Lateral Compartment Syndrome

Posterior Compartment Syndrome ("shin splints")

from the anterolateral side of the suprapatellar tendon, it is possible to detect 10–15 mL of effusion in the knee. This bulge test is used for small effusions (Fig. 50.38A). If the effusion is so large that the tissues become turgid, a fluid pulse may not be able to create a bulge and the test may provide a false-negative result. Large effusions are more accurately diagnosed with a ballottement test (Fig. 50.38B) in which the knee cap is tapped gently (ballotted). A palpable transmission of bony contact is palpated if the effusion is large enough to have distanced the patella from the bone behind it.

The superficial and deep infrapatellar bursae are less frequently involved in clinical problems.

A Baker's cyst arises from enlargement of either the semimembranosus bursa or the bursa behind the medial head of the gastrocnemius (Fig. 50.39). The swollen cyst is often painful, especially with flexion of the knee. The swelling is more prominent in the standing position. Both of these bursae commonly communicate with the synovial cavity of the knee. For this reason, knee trauma such as a meniscal tear, or disease such as rheumatoid arthritis, can initiate the cyst. Rupture of the Baker's cyst may be misdiagnosed as thrombophlebitis.

ACHILLES TENDON

In the ankle region, the superficial bursa of the Achilles tendon may be irritated by poorly fitting shoes and may swell. This results in a tender pump bump.

Treatment of vascular and lymphatic dysfunction of the

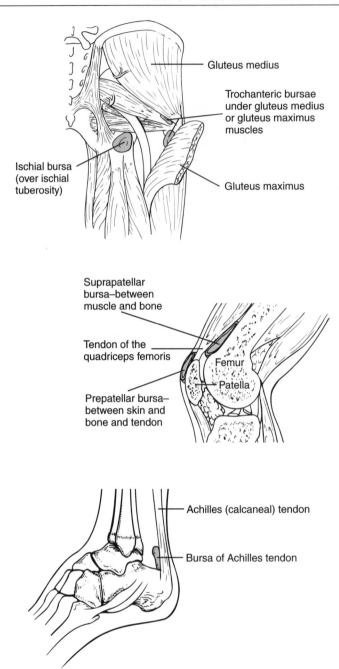

Figure 50.37. Bursae of the lower extremity.

lower extremities can be enhanced by understanding the influence of somatic dysfunction on neural, vascular, and lymphatic elements (Fig. 50.40). Treatment of somatic dysfunction can improve blood delivery by reducing hypersympathetic activity. This is important for nutrition of the tissues in the lower extremity. It is also important for delivering medications such as nonsteroidal antiinflammatory drugs to target tissues in the lower extremity where pharmacologic effectiveness is proportionate to tissue or synovial concentration of the drug. Open-

ing fascial pathways and eliminating myofascial trigger points can improve venous and lymphatic drainage of the extremities. Drainage can be enhanced using a variety of lymphatic pump techniques. This is especially true of the pedal pump techniques described in other chapters. Lymphaticovenous return is also enhanced by improving the mechanical lymphatic pumping, produced by muscular contraction, and maximal pressure gradients between the thorax and abdomen, produced by improving respiratory efficacy.

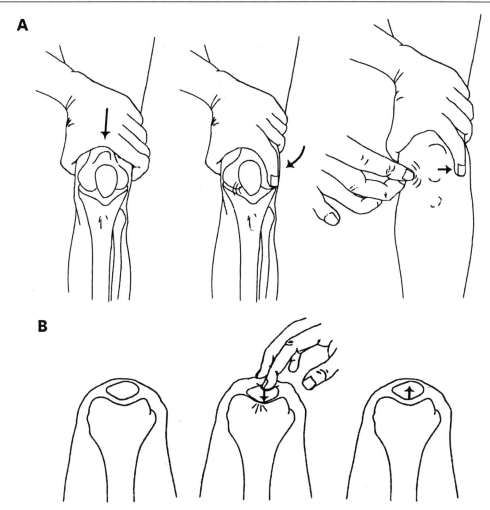

Figure 50.38. Tests for effusion in the knee. The bulge test (**A**) is useful for finding a minimal amount of effusion in the knee. The ballottement test (**B**) is positive if there is a large amount of effusion present. (Illustration by W.A. Kuchera.)

CONCLUSION

A thorough understanding of the functional anatomy of the lower extremity establishes a foundation for the osteopathic approach to this region and its effect on the body unit. The osteopathic physician seeks to improve function and balance to influence a wide range of patient encounters. From a sports medicine approach to the care of patients with deep vein thrombosis in an internal medicine practice, the osteopathic approach offers an effective approach to diagnosis, prevention, and/or treatment.

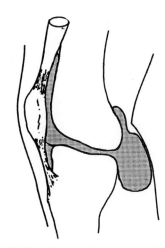

Figure 50.39. Bursae of the knee and Baker's cyst.

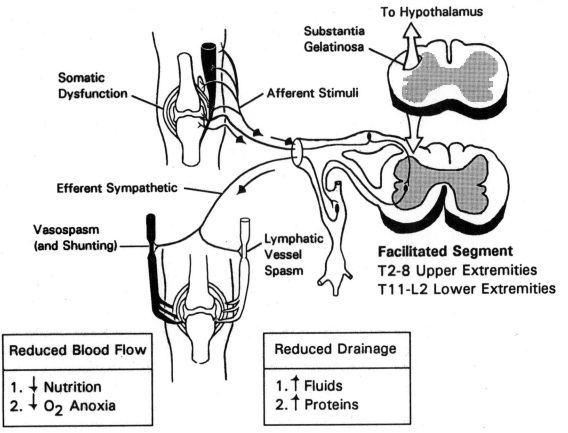

Figure 50.40. Influence of somatic dysfunction on normal vascular and lymphatic elements of the lower extremity. (Reprinted with permission from Kuchera ML, Kuchera WA. *Osteopathic Considerations in Systemic Dysfunction.* 2nd ed. rev. Columbus, Ohio: Greyden Press; 1994.)

REFERENCES

1. Moore KL. *Clinically Oriented Anatomy.* 2nd ed. Baltimore, Md: Williams & Wilkins; 1985:403.
2. Gofton JP, Trueman GE. Studies in osteoarthritis of the hip, Part II: osteoarthritis of the hip and leg-length disparity. *Can Med Assoc J.* 1971;104:791–799.
3. Brody DM. Running injuries. *CIBA Clin Symp.* 1980;32(4):25.
4. Blood SD. Treatment of the sprained ankle. *JAOA.* July 1980; 79:680–692.
5. Inman VT. *Joints of the Ankle.* Baltimore, Md: Williams & Wilkins; 1976:42.
6. Inman VT, Mann RA. Biomechanics of the foot and ankle. *DuVries' Surgery of the Foot.* 3rd ed. St. Louis, Mo: 1973:17.
7. Levens SA, et al. Transverse rotation of the segments of the lower extremity in locomotion. *J Bone Joint Surg.* October 1948;30A:859–872.
8. Kuchera WA, Kuchera ML. *Osteopathic Principles in Practice.* 2nd ed. rev. Columbus, Ohio: Greyden Press; 1994.
9. Hicks JH. The mechanics of the foot, I: the joints. *J Anat.* 1953; 87:345–357.
10. Roy S, Irvin R. *Sports Medicine: Prevention, Evaluation, Management, and Rehabilitation.* Englewood Cliffs, NJ: Prentice-Hall; 1983:380.
11. Travell JG, Simons DG. *Myofascial Pain and Dysfunction: The Trigger Point Manual. The Lower Extremities.* Vol. II. Baltimore, Md: Williams & Wilkins; 1992:530.
12. Travell JG, Simons DG. *Myofascial Pain and Dysfunction: The Trigger Point Manual, The Upper Extremities.* Vol. I. Baltimore, Md: Williams & Wilkins; 1983.
13. Janda V. Muscle weakness and inhibition (pseudoparesis) in back pain syndromes. In: Grieve GP, ed. *Modern Medicine Therapy of the Vertebral Column.* Edinburgh: Churchill Livingstone; 1986:197–200.
14. Basmajian JV. *Grant's Method of Anatomy.* 9th ed. Baltimore, Md: Williams & Wilkins; 1975:327–328.
15. Kuchera ML, Kuchera WA. *Osteopathic Considerations in Systemic Dysfunction.* 2nd ed. rev. Columbus, Ohio: Greyden Press; 1994:159–167.

51. **Thrust Techniques**

AN INTRODUCTION

ROBERT E. KAPPLER

> ## Key Concepts
>
> - **Definition and development of thrust technique**
> - **Indications and uses for thrust technique**
> - **Quantity and quality of motion loss with somatic dysfunction**
> - **End feel at restrictive barrier, and barrier engagement**
> - **Accumulation of force, and corrective force velocity and amplitude**
> - **Patient relaxation**
> - **Exaggeration technique**
> - **Mechanism of thrust technique action**
> - **Effect of technique on unstable hypermobile joint**
> - **Dose, precautions, and contraindications for thrust technique**
> - **Guidelines for safety, and benefits of technique**

Thrust technique is defined in the *Glossary of Osteopathic Terminology* as a type of direct technique that uses high-velocity low-amplitude forces.[1] The term "direct" refers specifically to positioning the restricted joint(s) toward the restrictive barrier. Simply stated, you move the restricted joint in the direction it won't move. After precise positioning against the restrictive barrier, the final force is a short (low-amplitude) quick (high-velocity) thrust. Philip Greenman, DO, has described the force as "impulse."[2] Ordinarily, a click or pop is heard at the time the force is applied. There is an immediate increase in the range of motion and the freedom of motion.

HISTORICAL PERSPECTIVE

Thrust technique has been the major type of technique taught in colleges of osteopathic medicine and has been practiced by osteopathic physicians for years. In the 1970s, the osteopathic medical school curricula began include other types of techniques. Until recently, however, osteopathic manipulation and high-velocity technique were essentially synonymous. Graduates are now exposed to a complete spectrum of direct and indirect techniques, and therefore osteopathic manipulation is no longer synonymous with "thrust technique."

A.T. Still used very little thrust technique. Instead, he used what we now describe as myofascial release and indirect techniques. It is interesting to speculate why osteopathic manipulative techniques as taught in the colleges evolved into the exclusive domain of thrust techniques and remained that way for so many years. Faculty may have been responsible for the change. Thrust techniques can be taught by precisely describing the nature of the restriction and providing techniques for treating the dysfunction. These techniques can be practiced. In contrast, fascial release and indirect techniques require skill in assessing motion patterns in the tissues. The technique is difficult to describe, because the physician is responding to tactile and proprioceptive input from his or her hands. Faculty find release techniques difficult to teach, and students may perceive them as abstractions. Thrust techniques are easier to teach and to learn. However, while thrust techniques can be described in a precise manner, the motor coordination necessary to use these techniques effectively requires extensive practice and experience.

INDICATIONS AND USES

Thrust technique is a method of specific joint mobilization. Proper use of thrust technique requires an assessment of restriction of joint motion along with the conclusion that treatment of this joint restriction will benefit the patient (for example, reduce pain, free motion, improve biomechanical function, reduce somatovisceral reflex).

The performance of thrust techniques requires an understanding of somatic dysfunction and the barrier concept. Thrust technique is indicated for treatment of motion loss in

Figure 51.1. Somatic dysfunction: quantity and quality of joint motion.

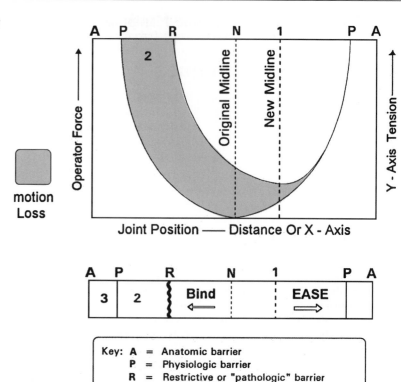

Key: A = Anatomic barrier
     P = Physiologic barrier
     R = Restrictive or "pathologic" barrier
     N = Midline or original neutral point of motion
     1 = New midline in plane with somatic dysfunction
     2 = Motion loss in somatic dysfunction
     3 = Range between physiologic and anatomic barriers

somatic dysfunction. Thrust technique is ordinarily not indicated for treatment of joint restriction due to anatomic/pathologic changes such as traumatic contracture, advanced degenerative joint disease, or ankylosis.

MOTION LOSS WITH SOMATIC DYSFUNCTION

Somatic dysfunction is impaired or altered function of related components of the somatic system:[1]

> Skeletal
> Arthrodial structures
> Myofascial structures
> Related vascular lymphatic and neural elements

Diagnostic tests for somatic dysfunction include TART:

> T: Tissue texture change *(feel)*
> A: Asymmetry or positional change *(look)*
> R: Restriction of motion *(move)*
> T: Tenderness

Somatic dysfunction exhibits a change in quantity and quality of motion.

Quantity of Motion

The quantity of motion involves the following general principles:

1. Motion beyond the anatomic barrier damages anatomic structures. It is also the endpoint of permitted passive motion.
2. The range of normal active motion occurs between the physiologic barriers.
3. With motion loss in somatic dysfunction, the restrictive or pathologic barrier is the endpoint of permitted motion.
4. A normal joint has a midline or neutral point within its range of motion.
5. In somatic dysfunction, there is frequently a positional change (or asymmetry) in the joint that shifts its "neutral" to a new midline.
6. Motion loss occurs in the range of normal physiologic motion.
7. The range between the physiologic barrier and the anatomic barrier is not as finite as the illustration depicts. There is some flexibility of the boundaries.

These principles describe motion loss in somatic dysfunction and a new position that is identified on examination as asymmetry or positional change. Inappropriate lay terminology is sometimes used to describe this positional change, for example, "out of place." This kind of term may lead to a misunderstanding of the nature of motion loss in somatic dysfunction and the positional change associated with this motion loss. Inappropriate lay terms to describe treatment as an "adjustment" (of position) or "putting it back" further complicate understanding. Thrust technique is designed to remove motion loss in somatic dysfunction. A positional change from the somatic dysfunction position (Fig. 51.1, *I*) to the normal neutral or midline (Fig. 51.1, *N*) is the result of effective treatment. Treatment involves the dynamics of motion, and not static positional change.

Quality of Motion

Somatic dysfunction exhibits qualitative as well as quantitative changes. To the experienced examiner, these qualitative changes are the clue to evaluating motion characteristics of somatic dysfunction. Motion is asymmetric, with restriction in one direction and freer motion in the other direction. The terms "ease" and "bind" are sometimes used to describe the asymmetric motion. Movement toward the restrictive barrier exhibits bind, while moving away from the barrier exhibits ease.

The qualitative aspects of motion can be depicted on the same graph (Fig. 51.1), with the *x* axis defining joint position and the *y* axis defining operator force to move the joint through a range of motion.

Figure 51.1 depicts the asymmetric quality of motion in somatic dysfunction. If the *y* axis of the graph is changed to "tension" rather than "force," it emphasizes a different component of motion in somatic dysfunction. There is increased tension in the dysfunctional joint as if both agonist and antagonist are too tight. Motion in a direction of balanced tension is the basis of functional technique, described elsewhere.[3]

Motion characteristics in somatic dysfunction can be described in three ways:

1. Where is it? (position)
2. What will it do?
3. What won't it do?

Using an example of rotational restriction of the atlas, this can be described as:

1. Rotated right (position)
2. Freer rotation right
3. Restriction of left rotation

DIRECT TECHNIQUE

End Feel at Restrictive Barrier

The use of direct technique requires engaging the barrier. The final activating force is a physician force: high-velocity low-amplitude (HVLA).

Figure 51.1, depicting the force necessary to move a joint to the barrier, is a graphic illustration of end feel. As the barrier is engaged, increasing amounts of force are necessary and the distance decreases. The term "barrier" may be misleading if it is interpreted as a wall or rigid obstacle to be overcome with a "push." As the joint reaches the barrier, restraints in the form of tight muscles and fascia serve to inhibit further motion. We are pulling against restraints rather than pushing against some anatomic structure.

The barrier involves a three-dimensional matrix, not just a single plane of motion. We can define motion in the three cardinal planes as flexion–extension, rotation, and side-bending. To be complete, there are components of translatory motion that should be considered. These are fore–aft translation, side-to-side translation, and compression–distraction. All of these single motions are combined into a single force vector when executing the technique. However, for purposes of diagnosis, each of these components can be tested separately.

For a high-velocity technique to be effective, the barrier must feel solid. If the barrier feels rubbery and indistinct, thrust technique may be ineffective.

Barrier Engagement

Experienced physicians develop skills to engage the barrier quickly. They sense how the tissues are responding to the force being applied and make subtle alterations in the direction of force to effectively engage the barrier in all planes. The novice takes more time by engaging one plane at a time. Being able to engage the barrier with accuracy and confidence is a skill acquired with practice and experience.

Accumulation of Force at Restriction

With a proper diagnosis, initial positioning engages the barrier. Forces must be applied so that they accumulate at the restricted joints. In the spinal area, the reference is a vertebral unit: two bones and the connections (joints) between them. Forces applied from above to the superior vertebra meet forces applied to the inferior vertebra. Forces from above and from below meet at the restricted joint.

Depending on the technique, force may be applied at one site; the opposing counterforce is resistance of inertia of body mass, resistance of the table, or other resistance. In all cases, direct the force at the restriction. Specificity of a technique is a measure of how accurately the force accumulates at the restriction. Force that does not accumulate at the lesion is dissipated through other parts of the patient's body. This could result in iatrogenic side effect. The greater the specificity, the lesser the force needed, and the potential for untoward side effects is minimized.

Final Corrective Force Velocity and Amplitude

HVLA thrust techniques use a short, quick thrust. High velocity does not mean high force, and it does not mean high amplitude. Once the barrier is engaged, the final force is applied from that position. Do not back off before delivering the corrective thrust. Likewise, do not carry the force through a great distance. Amplitude means distance. The amplitude is low, a small fraction of an inch. High amplitude defeats proper localization of force and decreases the likelihood of achieving the desired effect.

Do not be overly tentative and apply a low-velocity force, with an increase of force as well as amplitude. These efforts are often unsuccessful. The proper application has been described as a tack hammer blow, sudden but not forceful. The term "impulse" applied to HVLA technique recognizes that the force is a sudden acceleration and deceleration. Experience and practice are very helpful in knowing how to apply the force.

Some thrust techniques are not executed at high velocity. Consider an experience where you set up the patient to treat a joint restriction, the joint goes "click," and the restriction is released as you are positioning the patient and localizing forces. Sometimes you "tease" a joint with carefully and slowly applied forces. Again, experience is very beneficial in applying the proper force. While we describe HVLA thrust technique, the actual force may be modified to fit the patient's needs.

Patient Relaxation during Thrust Technique

Have the patient as relaxed as possible when applying the corrective force. The more tense the patient, the greater the force necessary, and the greater the risk of side effect or failure to overcome the motion restriction. If the patient feels comfortable and secure with the physician's hands, relaxation is not a problem. If the patient feels insecure, muscles will be tight rather than relaxed. If the technique is hurting the patient, muscles will involuntarily tighten. Nonverbal clues such as a facial grimace can alert the physician to a problem. A skilled physician senses when the patient is relaxed, and when not. The exhalation phase of respiration is the relaxation phase, and the final force is often applied during exhalation.

When using a thrust technique to treat cervical somatic dysfunction, some practitioners divert attention by instructing the patient to cross his or her legs. This may help in some cases, but it is not an adequate substitute for the physician's hands transmitting a sense of control, comfort, and confidence. This skill comes with practice and experience. It is possible to distract a patient and apply a corrective force when the patient does not anticipate it. However, if the technique is applied too quickly, forces may not be properly localized. A patient who has experienced a painful thrust in the past cannot be fooled.

Exaggeration Thrust Technique

Some practitioners of manual medicine use a form of thrust technique in which the direction of force is away from the restrictive barrier. For example, if T3 is extended, extension is free and flexion is restricted. The barrier is engaged by flexing T3. Exaggeration technique involves thrusting on T3 to extend it suddenly and forcibly.

Mechanism of Thrust Technique Action

The answer to the question of what maintains restriction of joint motion has been and is being explored by osteopathic physicians and scientists. In some cases, a joint gets stuck the same way an old loose window or drawer may get stuck, half open and half closed, in a position no longer parallel to the track. The sacroiliac joint is a good example of this type of restriction. A properly directed mechanical force frees the joint.

As with the stuck drawer, the proper force is not directly in or out, which is the major motion of the drawer. The proper force is an oblique or side force. Remember this in extremity techniques, where the minor motions or restoration of joint play is the object, not a direct force against the major motion of a joint. For example, if a wrist is restricted in extension, treatment might involve anterior or posterior translation of the carpal bones.

For mechanisms maintaining joint restriction, abnormal muscle activity is usually involved. Muscles maintain joint restriction. The palpatory findings in somatic dysfunction include tissue texture abnormality. Muscles are hypertonic and sometimes boggy and stringy. When the joint restriction is treated, there is an immediate change in the muscles and an immediate change in quality and quantity of motion. This change means an immediate change in neural activity. How does the thrust change neural activity? A likely answer lies in the mechanoreceptor in the joint capsule. A sudden stretch or change of position of the joint alters the afferent output of these mechanoreceptors, resulting in release of muscle hypertonicity. This is discussed in articles in the osteopathic and scientific literature on proprioceptors and somatic dysfunction.[4–8]

Pop or Click

Numerous studies have focused on the pop. One widely held hypothesis states that the sudden distraction of joint surfaces produces a nitrogen bubble, along with noise, and increased freedom of motion.[9] Osteopathic physicians prefer to focus on joint function and dysfunction and not on the noise. The objective of thrust technique is to overcome joint restriction. Always retest motion after the treatment. While the pop or click is usually indicative of success, it is possible that an unrelated joint made the noise and the restricted joint remained unaltered. It is also possible to have a successful treatment without any noise. Keep your focus on the patient and the joint restriction.

Unstable Hypermobile Joint

Some joints are unstable and hypermobile. Within the numerous joints of the spine, a pattern of alternating hypomobility and hypermobility may exist. The loose, hypermobile joints are overworked, while the stiff hypomobile joints escape excess motion.

A normal physiological reaction to a painful hypermobile joint is for muscles surrounding the joint to splint the joint and protect it from excess motion. Physical examination reveals restriction of motion. Underneath that protective muscle splitting is an unstable joint.

A high-velocity thrust technique may work, as evidenced by a decrease in pain and improvement in motion. Unfortunately, the treatment contributes to the joint instability. The more HVLA technique is used, the looser the joint becomes.

There are some spinal joints that tend to be loose. C5 and C6 become hypermobile (and arthritic). This process is maintained by a stiff flexed upper thoracic spine requiring a compensatory cervical lordosis. In the lumbar spine, the lumbosacral (LS) region tends to become hypermobile. A flexed upper lumbar associated with chronic psoas tension maintains LS dysfunction.[10]

Be aware of the possibility of unstable joints. Reevaluation of motion following treatment will reveal excess freedom of motion. Management involves modifying patient activity that contributes to instability, mobilizing adjacent hypomobile joints, and prescribing active rehabilitation exercises.

Dose of Thrust Technique

The compassionate physician may err on the side of overdose. Give the patient time to respond to the treatment. The sicker the patient, the less the dose. Older patients respond more slowly; young patients respond more quickly.[11]

For hospitalized patients, daily OMT may be appropriate, but daily thrust technique may be an overdose. Larson (N.J. Larson, personal communication, 1967–1978), when treating hospital patients on a daily basis, would vary the technique so he did not repeat the same technique on a given area. With the spectrum of techniques available, there should be no reason to overdose a patient on high-velocity technique. The more specific and precise the technique, the less iatrogenic the side effect.

Precautions and Contraindications

Most of the published precautions about OMT imply forceful HVLA thrust. Instead of presenting a list of absolutes, think in terms of risk/benefit relationships. If the risk of harming the patient exceeds the potential therapeutic benefit, the technique is not indicated. Risk also relates to the skill of the physician. There is more risk with an unskilled physician. While forceful direct techniques may harm the patient, gentle indirect release techniques might be safe.

Neurologic complications from thrust manipulation can be fatal or result in permanent neurologic impairment. Cervical manipulation has been associated with vertebral basilar thrombosis.[12] Dislocation of the dens associated with rupture or laxity of the transverse ligament of the atlas can cause death or quadriplegia. In the low back, massive protrusion of a disc can produce cauda equina syndrome with loss of bowel, bladder, and sexual function.

Pathologic fractures can result from osteoporotic or metastatic bone. Excess force may injure fragile tissues. Joints could be sprained. Arthritic spurs could be broken off.

There may be psychological contraindications to the use of HVLA. Apprehension on the part of the patient is a relative contraindication. Make sure the patient understands what is expected during and after treatment.

Guidelines for Safety

1. Be aware of possible complications.
2. Make a diagnosis.
3. A palpatory examination is a prerequisite for treatment.
4. Listen with your hands and fingers. If it doesn't feel right, back off and get more data.
5. If the barrier doesn't feel right, don't thrust, but select an alternate technique.
6. Emphasize specificity, not force.
7. Ask permission to treat.
8. If response to treatment does not meet your expectations, reevaluate the patient.
9. Somatic dysfunction with joint restriction is the indication. Pain is not an indication for high-velocity manipulation.
10. Somatic dysfunction often coexists with "orthopaedic disease" (spondylosis, disc degeneration, spondylolysis).
11. Be aware of the total picture.

Beneficial Use of HVLA Thrust Technique

Thrust technique is a very efficient use of physician's time in treating a patient, as long as the physician has met the prerequisite of an effective skill level. When a patient is able to tolerate thrust technique, the results are long lasting rather than temporary. The patient usually experiences immediate relief, with decreased pain and increased freedom of motion. For years, osteopathic physicians have treated patients using thrust techniques; these patients continue to seek the services of an osteopathic physician.

CONCLUSION

The principles of HVLA thrust technique are to:

1. Identify the motion restriction of somatic dysfunction.
2. Engage the barrier.
3. Apply the activating force, an HVLA thrust.
4. Reevaluate.

The ultimate effective use of these techniques demands considerable knowledge, skill, and experience.

REFERENCES

1. The Glossary Review Committee of the Educational Council on Osteopathic Principles. Glossary of Osteopathic Terminology. In: Allen TW, ed. *AOA Yearbook and Directory of Osteopathic Physicians.* Chicago, Ill: American Osteopathic Association; 1994.
2. Greenman PE. *Principles of Manual Medicine.* Baltimore, Md: Williams & Wilkins; 1989:94.
3. Bowles CH. Functional technique: a modern perspective. In: Beal MC, ed. *The Principles of Palpatory Diagnosis and Manipulative Technique.* Newark, Ohio: American Academy of Osteopathy; 1992:174–178.
4. Korr IM. *The Collected Papers of Irwin Korr.* Colorado Springs, Colo: American Academy of Osteopathy; 1979.
5. Korr IM. Proprioceptors and somatic dysfunction. *JAOA.* March 1975;74:638–650.
6. Patterson M. A theoretical neurophysiologic mechanism for facilitated segment. *J Am Osteopath Assoc.* January 1978;77(5):399.
7. Patterson M. A model mechanism for spinal segmental facilitation. *J Am Osteopath Assoc.* September 1976;(1):62–72.

8. Van Buskirk R. Nociceptive reflexes and the somatic dysfunction: a model. *JAOA.* September 1990;(9):792–809.

9. Hargrove-Wilson. Symposium: manipulative treatment. *Med J Aust.* June 1967;24:274–280.

10. Kappler R. Role of psoas mechanism in low back pain. *JAOA.* April 1973;72.

11. Kimberly PE. Formulating a prescription of osteopathic manipula-tive treatment. In: Beal MC, ed. *The Principles of Palpatory Diagnosis and Manipulative Technique.* Newark, Ohio: American Academy of Osteopathy; 1992:146–152.

12. Hamann G, Haass A, Kujat D, Felber S, Strittmatter M, Schimrigk K, et al. Cervicocephalic artery dissection and chiropractic manip-ulation. *Lancet.* March 1993;20:34(8847):764–765. Letter.

52. High-Velocity Low-Amplitude Thrust Techniques

ROBERT E. KAPPLER AND JOHN M. JONES III

Key Concepts

- **Methods for carrying out high-velocity low-amplitude thrust techniques, including identifying positional diagnosis, restriction, objective, range, patient position, and procedure in the following areas:**
    - **—Cervicals**
    - **—Thoracics**
    - **—Ribs**
    - **—Thoracolumbar area**
    - **—Pelvis**
    - **—Upper extremity**
    - **—Lower extremity**

This chapter describes high-velocity low-amplitude thrust techniques (HVLA) for areas and diagnoses throughout the body.

CERVICALS

Occipitoatlantal: Side-bending Focus

POSITIONAL DIAGNOSIS

Occipitoatlantal (OA) $S_R R_L$ or C0 $S_R R_L$. The occiput is side-bent right, rotated left in relationship to the atlas (posterior occiput left).

RESTRICTION

Left side-bending and right rotation.

OBJECTIVE

Restore physiologic range of motion to the OA joint so that, in resetting itself, appropriate physiologic motion is restored.

PATIENT POSITION

Supine.

PROCEDURE

After making a diagnosis and using soft tissue preparation:

1. Stand to the left of the patient, at the head of the table (Fig 52.1).
2. With your right hand, cup the patient's chin, palm at the zygomatic process.

3. Place the metacarpophalangeal (MP) or proximal interphalangeal (PIP) joint of your left index finger on the bony calaverium (left occiput: avoid the mastoid portion of the temporal bone).
4. Add a mild extension component, making sure that the extension is limited to the OA joint. Be cautious to avoid hyperextension.
5. Rotate the head gently to the right.
6. Side-bend to the left, by using translation downward (caudad) with the left MP (or PIP) joint and slightly upward with the right hand.
7. Approach the barrier (left side-bending, right rotation).
8. Have the patient breathe in and exhale.
9. At end of exhalation, apply a high-velocity thrust by increasing the side-bending component with translation through the left MP (or PIP) joint, directing the force toward the right eye.
10. Retest the range of motion.

Atlantoaxial: Neutral

POSITIONAL DIAGNOSIS

Atlantoaxial (AA) R_R. The atlas is rotated right in relationship to the axis and moves more easily in this direction.

RESTRICTION

Left rotation.

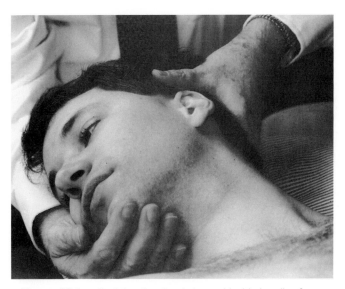

Figure 52.1. Occipitoatlantal technique with side-bending focus.

OBJECTIVE

Restore physiologic range of motion to the AA joint so that, in resetting itself, there is a physiologic increase in left rotation.

PATIENT POSITION

Supine.

PROCEDURE

After diagnosis and soft tissue preparation:

1. Stand to the right of the patient, at the head of the table (Fig. 52.2).
2. Grasp the chin with your left palm and fingers, with the heel of your palm or your forearm at the patient's left zygomatic process.
3. Place your right index finger proximal phalanx by the soft tissue next to the AA joint, and your thumb contacting the lateral aspect of the patient's face in the region of the right zygomatic process (avoid the mandible).
4. Rotate the patient's head to the left, with just enough flexion–extension and/or side-bending to engage the restrictive barrier. Note the resilience of the end feel.
5. Have the patient breathe in and exhale.
6. Apply a high-velocity low-amplitude thrust in a left rotational pattern, focusing the force at the same time by using your right index finger as a fulcrum.
7. Retest the range of motion.

Typical Cervicals (C2-C7): Side-bending Focus

POSITIONAL DIAGNOSIS

C3 FS$_L$R$_L$. C3 is flexed, side-bent left and rotated left in relationship to C4, and moves more easily in these directions.

RESTRICTION

Right side-bending and right rotation of C3 when the patient is examined in extension.

OBJECTIVE

Restore physiologic range of motion to the C3/C4 joint so that, in resetting itself, appropriate physiologic motion is restored.

PATIENT POSITION

Supine.

PROCEDURE

After diagnosis and soft tissue preparation:

1. Stand to the right side of the supine patient at the head of the table (Fig. 52.3).
2. Cup the chin with your left palm, with your palm or left forearm supporting the patient's head in the area of the zygomatic process.
3. Place your right index finger MP or PIP joint at the soft tissue next to the articular pillar of C3.
4. Flex the patient down to and including the C3/C4 joint space. Induce mild extension by a small amount of anterior translation of C3 at your fulcrum, to address the sagittal plane restriction.
5. Side-bend the patient's head to the right over your fulcrum (your index finger) until you feel localization at the C3/C4 joint space.
6. Then rotate the patient's head and neck to the left down to the C3, obtaining facet locking down to the somatic dysfunction; continually adjust the side-bending and extension to localize at C3.
7. Apply a high-velocity low-amplitude right side-bending thrust by translatory motion toward the left through the right index finger MP or PIP joint. Aim the thrust in a vector toward the opposite shoulder.
8. Retest the range of motion.

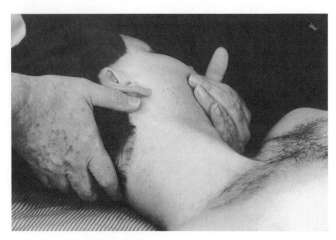

Figure 52.2. Atlantoaxial technique.

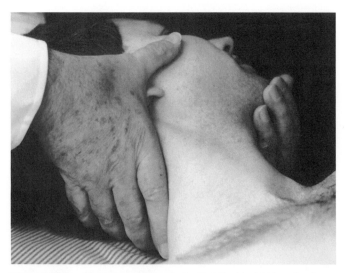

Figure 52.3. Technique for cervicals C2-C7 with side-bending focus.

All of the typical cervicals are treated in essentially the same manner. However, as you treat lower cervical levels, gradually alter the angle of the thrust to match the changing angle of the facets. The direction of the thrust by the time you are down to C6-C7 is aimed more in the direction of the opposite nipple.

Typical Cervicals (C2-C7): Rotational Focus

POSITIONAL DIAGNOSIS

C6 FS$_R$R$_R$. C6 is flexed, side-bent right, and rotated right in relationship to C7, and moves more easily in these directions.

RESTRICTION

Left side-bending and left rotation of C6 when the patient is examined in extension.

OBJECTIVE

Restore physiologic range of motion to the C6/C7 joint so that in resetting itself, appropriate physiologic motion is restored.

PATIENT POSITION

Supine.

PROCEDURE

After diagnosis and soft tissue preparation:

1. Stand to the right side of the head of the table (Fig. 52.4).
2. Cup the chin with your left palm, with your palm and forearm supporting the patient's head in the area of the zygomatic process.
3. Place your right index finger MP or PIP joint at the soft tissue next to the articular pillar of C6.
4. Flex the patient down to C6; then induce mild extension by a small amount of anterior translation of C6 at your fulcrum (index fingers).

5. Side-bend the patient's neck to the right over your fulcrum to lock the upper joint facets down to C6.
6. Then segmentally rotate the patient's neck to the left at C6, to the restrictive barrier of rotation.
7. Apply a high-velocity low-amplitude left rotational thrust, using your right MP or PIP joint as a fulcrum. Aim the thrust at the opposite eye.
8. Retest the range of motion.

THORACICS

Single Plane: Flexion, Supine

POSITIONAL DIAGNOSIS

T6 F. T6 is in a flexed position relative to T7 and flexes more easily.

RESTRICTION

Extension of T6.

OBJECTIVE

Restore physiologic range of motion to the T6/T7 joint so that, in resetting itself, appropriate physiologic extension is restored.

PATIENT POSITION

Supine.

PROCEDURE

After diagnosis and soft tissue preparation:

1. Stand on either side of the patient, facing the head (Fig. 52.5).
2. Have patient cross arms over the chest, grasping the lateral portion of each shoulder, with the arm on your opposite side superior.
3. Use a bilateral fulcrum (thenar eminence and flexed middle

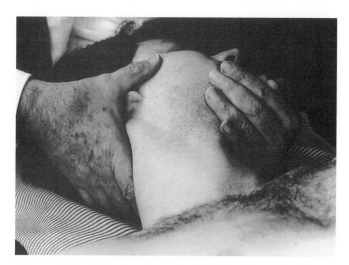

Figure 52.4. Technique for cervicals C2-C7 with rotational focus.

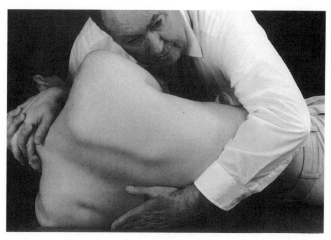

Figure 52.5. Hand placement for thoracic supine techniques.

phalanges), to contact the soft tissues overlying the transverse processes of the dysfunctional vertebra.[a]

4. Support the patient's head and neck with the cephalad hand as you flex the patient to a point where you can palpate motion at the dysfunctional vertebra and the joint space below it.
5. Contact the patient's elbows with your epigastric area (or use a small pillow between the elbows and your epigastric area). Localize your force to the midline by transferring a portion of your body weight so you can feel motion focused at your other hand, which serves as a fulcrum.
6. Have the patient breathe in and exhale, localizing your force during exhalation.
7. Apply a high-velocity low-amplitude thrust by momentarily dropping your body weight as you bend your knees, producing a force with a vector straight down toward your fulcrum (usually straight down toward the floor).
8. Retest the range of motion.

Single Plane: Extension, Supine

POSITIONAL DIAGNOSIS

T6 E. T6 is in an extension position relative to T7 and extends more easily.

RESTRICTION

Flexion of T6.

OBJECTIVE

Restore physiologic range of motion to the T6/T7 joint so that, in resetting itself, appropriate physiologic flexion is restored.

PATIENT POSITION

Supine.

PROCEDURE

After diagnosis and soft tissue preparation:

1. Stand on either side of the patient, facing the head.
2. Have patient cross arms over the chest, grasping the lateral portion of each shoulder, with the arm on the opposite side of the physician superior.
3. Use a bilateral fulcrum (thenar eminence and flexed middle phalanges) to contact the soft tissues overlying the transverse processes of the vertebra (T7) below the dysfunctional segment.

---

[a]Use of the hand as a fulcrum (at spinal segment level) depends on the thrust itself. In a flexion somatic dysfunction, some physicians will have the bilateral fulcrum at the level of the dysfunctional segment. This places the effective fulcrum at the level of the joint space as they ''roll'' the patient over it during the thrust maneuver. Other physicians will stabilize the segment below the dysfunctional vertebra and obtain the same effect with their thrust by less cephalad motion during the roll. Either way, the biomechanics of the thrust necessitate a confrontation of the barrier, with a gapping action at the dysfunctional joint level, reestablishing normal motion.

4. Support the patient's head and neck with your cephalad hand as you flex the patient to a point where you can palpate motion at the joint space below the dysfunctional vertebra.
5. Contact the patient's elbows with your epigastric area (or use a small pillow between the elbows and your epigastric area). Use a portion of your body weight to localize your force so you can feel it focused over your caudad hand, which serves as a fulcrum.
6. Have the patient breathe in and exhale, localizing your force during exhalation.
7. Apply a high-velocity low-amplitude thrust by momentarily dropping your body weight as you bend your knees, producing a force with a vector approximately 45° cephalad and posterior.
9. Retest the range of motion.

Multiple Plane: Type I, Supine

POSITIONAL DIAGNOSIS

T7 NS_RR_L. A levoscoliotic curve (left convexity) with right side-bending and left rotation. T7 is at the apex of the curve, side-bent right and rotated left in relationship to T8, and moves more easily in these directions.

RESTRICTION

Left side-bending and right rotation.

OBJECTIVE

Restore physiologic range of motion to the T7/T8 joint.

PATIENT POSITION

Supine.

PROCEDURE

After diagnosis and soft tissue preparation:

1. Stand on the right side of the patient (the side opposite the posterior transverse process, Figure 52.6).
2. Have the patient cross arms over the chest, grasping the outside portion of each shoulder, with the arm opposite to you superior to the other.
3. Use your cephalad hand to rotate the patient's opposite shoulder and thorax toward you.
4. Reach across and under the patient to contact the (left) T7 posterior transverse process, using your (caudad) thenar eminence as a fulcrum.
5. Support the patient's head, neck, and shoulders with your cephalad hand. Flex the patient through T7 to the dysfunctional joint space (T7/T8).
6. Side-bend the patient's spine down to the T7 to T8 junction.
7. Localize your force over the fulcrum (thenar eminence) by adjusting your weight over the patient's elbows through your epigastric region.
8. Have the patient take a deep breath and increase your localization as he or she exhales.

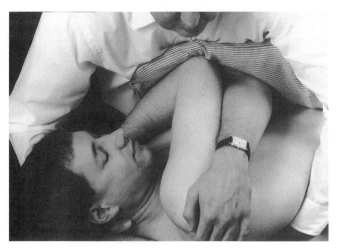

Figure 52.6. Thoracic multiple plane technique, type I.

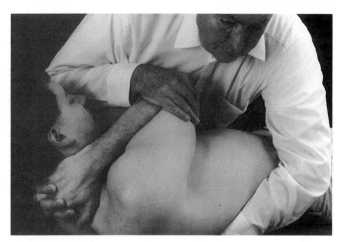

Figure 52.7. Thoracic multiple plane technique, type II, flexion.

9. Apply a high-velocity low-amplitude thrust at the end of exhalation through the patient's thorax. The thrust is in a vector aimed straight down toward your fulcrum (usually straight down toward the floor), produced more by a momentary drop of your body weight than by squeezing or compression of the patient.
10. Retest the range of motion.

These techniques have sometimes been referred to by their colloquial name, the "Kirksville Krunch."

Multiple Plane: Type II, Flexion

POSITIONAL DIAGNOSIS

T5 FS$_R$R$_R$. T5 is flexed, side-bent right, and rotated right in relationship to T6, and moves more easily in these directions.

RESTRICTION

Extension, left side-bending, and left rotation.

OBJECTIVE

Restore physiologic range of motion to the T5/T6 joint.

PATIENT POSITION

Supine.

PROCEDURE

After diagnosis and soft tissue preparation:

1. Stand on the left side of the patient (the side opposite the posterior transverse process, Figure 52.7).
2. Have the patient cross arms over the chest, grasping the outside portion of each shoulder, with the arm opposite to you superior to the other. (This can also be done with hands interlaced behind the neck).
3. Use your cephalad hand to rotate the patient's opposite shoulder and thorax toward you.

4. Reach across and under the patient to contact the (right) T5 posterior transverse process, using your (caudad) thenar eminence as a fulcrum.
5. Support the patient's head, neck, and shoulders with your cephalad hand. Flex down through T5 to the dysfunctional joint space (T5-T6).
6. Localize your force over your fulcrum (thenar eminence) by adjusting your weight over the patient's elbows through your epigastric region.
7. Use your cephalad hand under the neck and cervicothoracic junction to induce a component of left side-bending at the T5/T6 joint space.
8. Have the patient take a deep breath and increase your localization as he or she exhales.
9. Apply a high-velocity low-amplitude thrust straight down toward your fulcrum at the end of exhalation (usually straight down toward the floor), produced more by a momentary drop of your body weight than by squeezing or compression of the patient.
10. Retest the range of motion.

Multiple Plane: Type II, Extension

POSITIONAL DIAGNOSIS

T7 ES$_L$R$_L$. T7 is extended, side-bent left, and rotated left in relationship to T8, and moves more easily in these directions.

RESTRICTION

Flexion, right side-bending, and right rotation.

OBJECTIVE

Restore physiologic range of motion to the T7/T8 joint.

PATIENT POSITION

Supine.

PROCEDURE

After diagnosis and soft tissue preparation:

1. Stand on the right side of the patient (the side opposite the posterior transverse process, Figure 52.8).
2. Have the patient interlace hands behind the neck. (This can also be done with the arms crossed over the chest.)
3. Use your cephalad hand to rotate the opposite shoulder and thorax toward you.
4. Reach across and under the patient to contact the right transverse process of T8, using your (caudad) thenar eminence as a fulcrum. Note that this is the transverse process of the segment below the dysfunctional joint space, on the side opposite the malrotation.
5. Support the patient's head, neck, and shoulders with your cephalad hand. Flex down through T7 to the dysfunctional joint space (T7/T8).
6. Localize your force over your fulcrum (thenar eminence) by adjusting your weight over the patient's elbows through your epigastric region.
7. Use your cephalad hand under the neck and cervicothoracic junction to induce a component of right side-bending at the T7/T8 joint space.
8. Have the patient take a deep breath and increase your localization upon exhalation.
9. Apply a high-velocity low-amplitude thrust toward your fulcrum at the end of exhalation. The thrust is in a vector aimed 45° between the floor and the patient's head, produced more by a momentary drop of your body weight than by squeezing or compression of the patient.
10. Retest the range of motion.

Prone, Crossed Hand

POSITIONAL DIAGNOSIS

T8 FS_RR_R. T8 is flexed, side-bent right, and rotated right in relationship to T9, and moves more easily in these directions.

RESTRICTION

Extension, left side-bending, and left rotation.

OBJECTIVE

Restore physiologic range of motion to the T8/T9 joint.

RANGE

Midthoracic.

PATIENT POSITION

Prone.

PROCEDURE

After diagnosis and soft tissue preparation:

1. Stand on the right side of the patient (the side of the posterior transverse process, Figure 52.9). You may put a pillow under the thorax to increase thoracic kyphosis.
2. Have patient turn head toward you and place arms at the sides.
3. Contact the posterior transverse process (T8) with the hypothenar eminence or pisiform region of your caudad hand, which now moves into a more cephalad position. Your fingers point toward the patient's head.
4. Contact the opposite transverse process of the segment below the dysfunctional joint space (T9) with the thenar eminence of your cephalad hand, which now becomes caudad in position, as this is a crossed-arm technique. Your fingers point toward the patient's feet.
5. Have the patient inhale, then exhale, through more than one cycle as you localize your forces. Pressure through the hand over the posterior transverse process is in a cephalad and downward (toward the floor) direction. Pressure through the T9 hand is caudad and downward (toward the floor). Rotation is induced by the posteroanterior forces. A translatory force is also induced to the entire region, moving the hands toward you and therefore decreasing the dysfunctional side-bending.

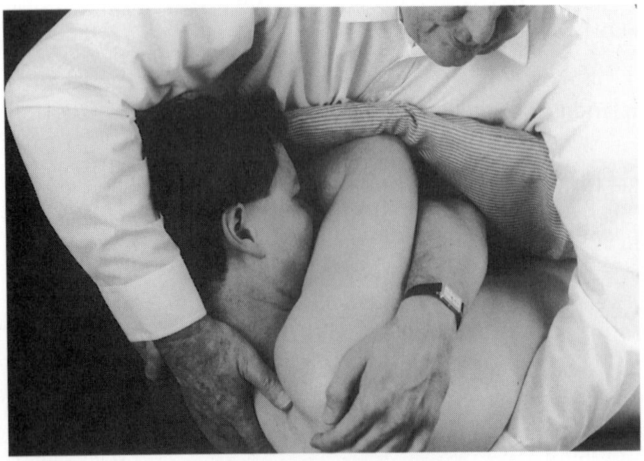

Figure 52.8. Thoracic multiple plane technique, type II, extension.

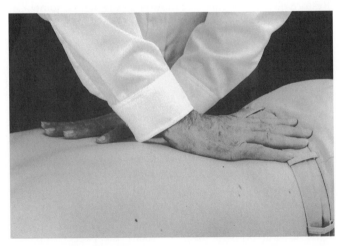

Figure 52.9. Thoracic technique with crossed hand.

6. Apply a high-velocity low-amplitude thrust in the directions already specified, using a momentary drop of your body weight to transmit the force through wrists and elbows held rigid.
7. Retest the range of motion.

This commonly used thoracic technique has earned the sobriquet the "Texas Twist."

Upper Thoracic: Prone, Crossed Hand

POSITIONAL DIAGNOSIS

T1 FS_LR_L. T1 is flexed, side-bent left, and rotated left in relationship to T2, and moves more easily in these directions.

RESTRICTION

Extension, right side-bending, and right rotation.

OBJECTIVE

Restore physiologic range of motion to the T1/T2 joint.

RANGE

T1-T4.

PATIENT POSITION

Prone.

PROCEDURE

After diagnosis and soft tissue preparation:

1. Stand on the left side at the head of the table (Fig. 52.10).
2. Place the patient's chin on the table. Side-bend neck to the right (side of restricted side-bending), through the level of T1 to the dysfunctional joint space.
3. Rotate the head to the left slightly, to obtain ligamentous tension locking.
4. Place your right hand on the side of the patient's head.

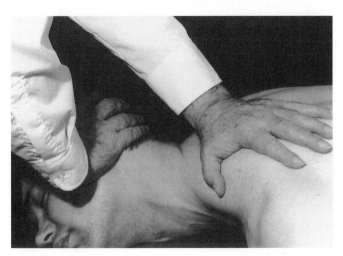

Figure 52.10. Upper thoracic technique with crossed hand.

5. Place the hypothenar eminence (pisiform region) or thenar eminence of your left hand over the left T1 transverse process.
6. Have the patient breathe in and exhale several times as you take up the tissue slack, localizing your forces.
7. Use a high-velocity low-amplitude thrust through the pisiform in a lateral, posteroanterior (toward the floor) and caudad direction. This side-bends the patient in a direction opposite the dysfunctional side-bending. Use the hand on the head to stabilize it as your force is transmitted through the T1 transverse process. The posteroanterior force on the left transverse process of T1 induces right rotation while the stabilizing hand on the head effects a slight relative rotation in an opposite direction.
8. Retest the range of motion.

Multiple Plane, Flexion: Seated, with Pillow Fulcrum

POSITIONAL DIAGNOSIS

T4 FS_RR_R. T4 is flexed, side-bent right, and rotated right in relationship to T5, and moves more easily in these directions.

RESTRICTION

Extension, left side-bending, and left rotation.

OBJECTIVE

Restore physiologic range of motion to the T4/T5 joint.

PATIENT POSITION

Seated.

PROCEDURE

After diagnosis and soft tissue preparation:

1. Stand behind the patient (Fig. 52.11).
2. Place a small pillow between your epigastric region (or chest) and the right transverse process of T4.
3. Induce extension down to and including T4, using your epigastric region and the pillow as your fulcrum.
4. Have the patient put hands behind the neck, with the fingers interlaced.
5. Put your arms through the axillae and contact the dorsal aspect of the patient's wrists. Do not use them to pull down and induce flexion.
6. Induce left side-bending through right translatory motion at the level of your fulcrum. The pillow itself will direct rotation to the left.
7. Have the patient take a breath and exhale, and relax the shoulders and back.
8. At end of expiration, ask the patient to bring the elbows together. As you feel localization occur in the tissues, use an anterior high-velocity low-amplitude thrust through your epigastrium and the pillow. Simultaneously induce superior traction through your arms and the epigastrium (a lifting motion).
9. Retest the range of motion.

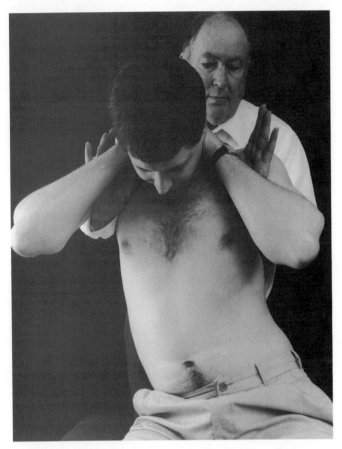

Figure 52.11. Thoracic multiple plane technique, flexion.

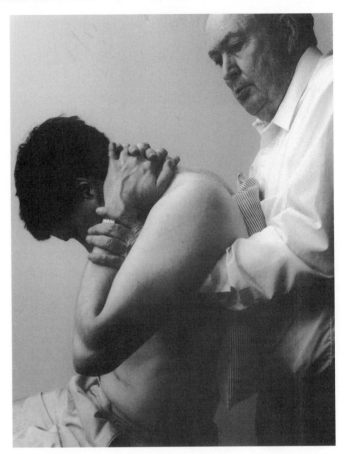

Figure 52.12. Thoracic multiple plane technique, extension.

Multiple Plane, Extension: Seated, with Pillow Fulcrum

POSITIONAL DIAGNOSIS

T6 ES_LR_L. T6 is extended, side-bent left, and rotated left in relationship to T7, and moves more easily in these directions.

RESTRICTION

Flexion, right side-bending, and right rotation.

OBJECTIVE

Restore physiologic range of motion to the T6/T7 joint.

PATIENT POSITION

Seated.

PROCEDURE

After diagnosis and soft tissue preparation:

1. Stand behind the patient (Fig. 52.12).
2. Place a small pillow between your epigastric region (or chest) and the segment to be treated.

3. Have the patient put hands behind the neck, with the fingers interlaced.
4. Put your arms through the axillae and contact the dorsal aspect of the patient's wrists.
5. Induce flexion by posterior translation at T6. This is accomplished by having the patient slump forward and pulling the upper body back toward you over your fulcrum.
6. Induce right side-bending through left translatory motion at T6. The pillow itself induces right rotation.
7. Have the patient take a breath and exhale, and relax the shoulders and back.
8. At end expiration, ask the patient to bring the elbows together. As you feel localization occur in the tissues, use an anterior high-velocity low-amplitude thrust through your epigastrium and the pillow. Simultaneously induce superior traction through your arms and the epigastrium (a lifting motion).
9. Retest the range of motion.

RIBS

Rib 1: Prone

POSITIONAL DIAGNOSIS

Rib 1 elevated on the left (superior shear, superior translation). Posterior portion (tubercle) of left rib 1 appears ele-

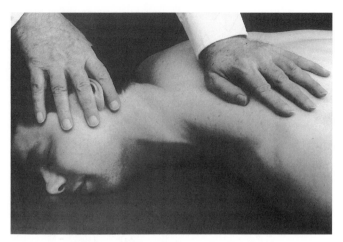

Figure 52.13. Rib 1 technique, prone.

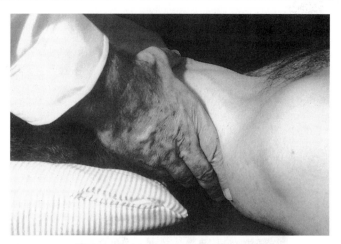

Figure 52.14. Rib 1 technique, supine.

vated, with surrounding tissue texture changes and tenderness. Cervicothoracic junction is usually side-bent right.[b]

RESTRICTION

Caudad motion of left rib 1 tubercle when pressure is applied.

OBJECTIVE

Restore physiologic range of motion to the T1/rib 1 costovertebral joint.

PATIENT POSITION

Prone.

PROCEDURE

After diagnosis and soft tissue preparation:

1. Stand on the right side of your prone patient, at the head of the table (Fig. 52.13).
2. Side-bend the head and neck to the right, through the level of T1 to the dysfunctional joint space.
3. Using the chin as a pivot, rotate the head to the left, to obtain ligamentous tension locking.
4. Place your right hand on the left side of the patient's head.
5. Place the thenar eminence or hypothenar eminence (pisiform region) of your left hand over the tubercle of the left rib 1. Your arms are crossed, with the right arm superior.
6. Have the patient breathe in and exhale several times as you take up the tissue slack, localizing your forces.
7. Use a high-velocity low-amplitude thrust through the thenar eminence in a posteroanterior and caudad direction. Use the hand on the head to stabilize it as your force is transmitted through the tubercle of rib 1. Induce a small amount of left rotation to T1 by slight opposite rotatory motions, through

the pisiform or thenar eminence on the right transverse process of T1, while the hand on the head induces slight rotation in an opposite direction.
8. Retest the range of motion.

Rib 1: Supine

POSITIONAL DIAGNOSIS

Rib 1 elevated on the right (superior shear, superior translation). Posterior portion (tubercle) of left rib 1 appears elevated, with surrounding tissue texture changes and tenderness. Cervicothoracic junction is usually side-bent left.[c]

RESTRICTION

Caudad motion of right rib 1 tubercle when pressure is applied.

OBJECTIVE

Restore physiologic range of motion to the T1/rib 1 costovertebral joint.

PATIENT POSITION

Supine.

PROCEDURE

After diagnosis and soft tissue preparation:

1. Stand at the right side of your supine patient, at the head of the table (Fig. 52.14).
2. Place the MP or PIP joint of your right index finger on the upper surface of the tubercle of the left first rib.
3. Place your left hand on the left side of the patient's head.
4. Rotate the head and neck to the left, to the level of the T1/rib 1 joint space.

---

[b]These same findings are also present with a fascial dysfunction involving presence of left side-bending and rotation at the cervicothoracic junction (thoracic inlet).

[c]These same findings are also present with a fascial dysfunction involving presence of right side-bending and rotation at the cervicothoracic junction (thoracic inlet).

5. Side-bend the head and neck right, to the level of the tubercle.
6. Flex the head and neck to the level of T1.
7. Have the patient breathe in and exhale, localizing your forces with exhalation.
8. Use a high-velocity low-amplitude thrust, directed medially, inferior and posterior. Your index finger is the fulcrum as you side-bend the head/neck to the right, using a component of flexion and slight rotation to the left.
9. Retest the range of motion.

Rib 1: Seated

POSITIONAL DIAGNOSIS

Rib 1 elevated on the right (superior shear, superior translation). Posterior portion (tubercle) of right rib 1 appears elevated, with surrounding tissue texture changes and tenderness. Cervicothoracic junction is usually side-bent left.[a]

RESTRICTION

Caudad motion of right rib 1 tubercle when pressure is applied.

OBJECTIVE

Restore physiologic range of motion to the T1/rib 1 costovertebral joint.

PATIENT POSITION

Seated.

PROCEDURE

After diagnosis and soft tissue preparation:

1. Stand behind your seated patient (Fig. 52.15).
2. Place your left foot on the table, and drape the patient's left arm over a pillow on your left knee or thigh.
3. Place your left elbow in front of the patient's shoulder, with your forearm contacting the left side of the face, and your hand over the top of the head.
4. Place your right palm on the patient's right shoulder, with the first metacarpophalangeal joint contacting the tubercle of rib 1.
5. Slowly rotate and side-bend the head and neck to the right, to the level of the rib, with simultaneous downward pressure on the rib. A slight movement of the patient to the left and posteriorly (using your left knee) may aid in localization.
6. Have the patient breathe in and exhale, localizing your force on exhalation. Sometimes a slight rotation of the head and neck to the left may further free the first rib head.
7. Perform a high-velocity low-amplitude thrust through the right MP joint, posteroinferior and medial, while slightly increasing the right side-bending/rotation of the neck.
8. Retest the range of motion.

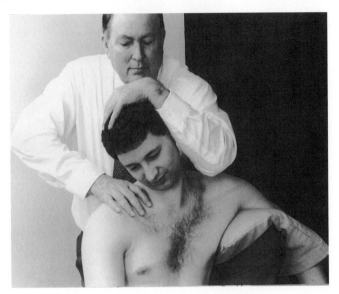

Figure 52.15.   Rib 1 technique, seated.

Rib 2: Seated

POSITIONAL DIAGNOSIS

Rib 2 elevated on the right. Posterior portion (tubercle) of right rib 2 appears elevated, with surrounding tissue texture changes and tenderness.

RESTRICTION

Caudad motion of right rib 2 tubercle when pressure is applied.

OBJECTIVE

Restore physiologic range of motion to the rib 2 costotransverse joint.

PATIENT POSITION

Seated.

PROCEDURE

After diagnosis and soft tissue preparation:

1. Stand behind your seated patient (Fig. 52.16).
2. Place your left foot on the table, and drape the patient's left arm over a pillow on your left knee or thigh.
3. Place your left elbow in front of the patient's shoulder, with your forearm contacting the left side of the face and your hand over the top of the head.
4. Place your right hand (dorsum up) on the patient's right shoulder, with the thumb contacting the tubercle of rib 2.
5. Slowly rotate the head and neck to the left, disengaging the rib head as T1 rotates away from it. Side-bend the region to the right to the level of the rib (reducing influence of the scalenes), exerting simultaneous downward pressure on the rib

---

[a]These same findings are also present with a fascial dysfunction involving presence of left side-bending and rotation at the cervicothoracic junction (thoracic inlet).

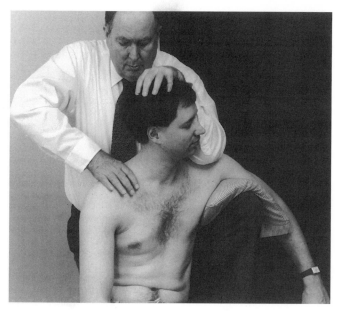

Figure 52.16. Rib 2 technique, seated.

with your fulcrum. Cease rotation when the rib exhibits less resistance to this downward pressure.

6. Have the patient breathe in and exhale, localizing your force on exhalation.
7. Perform a high-velocity low-amplitude thrust through the right MP joint, inferior and medial with a small posterior vector.
8. Retest the range of motion.

Ribs 2-10, Inhalation and Exhalation: Supine

POSITIONAL DIAGNOSIS

Exhalation lesion: the posterior inferior border of the rib angle is more prominent.

Inhalation lesion: the posterior superior border of the rib angle is more prominent.

RESTRICTION

If an exhalation lesion, inhalation motion is restricted. If an inhalation lesion, exhalation motion is restricted.

OBJECTIVE

Restore physiologic range of motion to the costovertebral joint.

PATIENT POSITION

Supine.

PROCEDURE

After diagnosis and soft tissue preparation:

1. Stand on the opposite side of the patient's dysfunctional rib.
2. Have the patient cross arms with the opposite arm superior and the hands on the lateral aspects of the shoulders. (This can also be accomplished with the hands interlaced behind the neck.)
3. Use your cephalad hand to rotate the opposite shoulder and thorax toward you.
4. Reach across and under the patient with the thenar eminence of your caudad hand to contact the dysfunctional rib at its posterior angle.[e]
5. Support the patient's head, neck, and shoulders with your cephalad hand. Flex to and slightly side-bend away from the dysfunctional rib.
6. Localize your forces by rolling the patient's body over the fulcrum, past the midline, focusing your weight between the epigastrium and the thenar eminence. Use a pillow between your epigastric region and the elbows if desired.
7. Have the patient take a deep breath and increase your localization during exhalation.
8. Apply a high-velocity low-amplitude thrust at the end of exhalation, through your epigastrium and the patient's thorax. The thrust is in a vector straight down, produced more by a momentary drop of your body weight than by squeezing or compression of the patient.
9. Retest the rib angle for tenderness and for motion during breathing.

Ribs 2-10: Prone, Crossed Hand

POSITIONAL DIAGNOSIS

Rib 8 on the right is held in exhalation.

RESTRICTION

Lateral or anterior elevation (during inhalation) in comparison with the corresponding contralateral rib (rib 8 major motion: bucket-handle mechanics; minor motion: pump-handle mechanics).

OBJECTIVE

Restore physiologic range of motion to the rib at the costovertebral articulation, allowing free lateral and anterior elevation during the inhalation phase.

PATIENT POSITION

Prone.

---

[e]The actual contact and vector of force applied to this portion of the rib to engage the barrier benefits from applying "pump-handle" mechanics (where in inhalation, the anterior portion of the rib is elevated, while it is depressed in back). Apply your contact in a manner that takes the slack out of the soft tissues and posterior costal articulations, drawing inferiorly on the superior rib border for exhalation somatic dysfunction, or pushing superiorly on the inferior border for inhalation somatic dysfunction.

PROCEDURE

After diagnosis and soft tissue preparation:

1. Stand on the side of the prone patient's dysfunctional rib (right, Figure 52.17).
2. Have patient turn head away from you and place arms at the sides.
3. Move the patient's torso and, if necessary, hips to induce left side-bending with the apex at the level of the dysfunctional rib.
4. Contact the posterior rib with your hypothenar eminence or pisiform region of your caudad hand on the superior border of the rib.
5. Contact the paravertebral area over the opposite rib with the palmar surface of your cephalad hand, which will serve as a stabilizing force. (This is a crossed-arm technique.) Your fingers point toward the patient's head.
6. Have the patient inhale, then exhale, through more than one cycle as you localize your forces. Pressure through the hand over the rib is in a caudad and anterior vector. Pressure through the opposite paravertebral area is toward the floor.
7. At end of exhalation, apply a high-velocity low-amplitude thrust in a caudad/anterior vector.
8. Retest the range of motion.

Ribs 11-12: Prone

POSITIONAL DIAGNOSIS

Rib 11 on the right is held in inhalation. Its position is more posterior than that of the opposite rib. The tenth intercostal space is decreased in comparison to the contralateral side.

RESTRICTION

Anterior caliper motion on exhalation (but it will rotate backward on inspiration) and decreased lowering during exhalation (bucket-handle motion).

OBJECTIVE

Restore physiologic range of motion to the rib at its costovertebral articulation so that it will exhibit both anterior and posterior rotatory caliper motion and increased lateral depression (bucket handle) during exhalation.

PATIENT POSITION

Prone.

PROCEDURE

After diagnosis and soft tissue preparation:

1. Stand to the left side (opposite the dysfunctional rib) of the patient, at the level of the hip (Fig. 52.18).
2. Induce a left side-bending curve in the patient's thorax by pulling first the feet, then the shoulders, to the left. The convexity has its apex at the dysfunctional rib.
3. The patient's right arm is at the side. Note: In a rib held in exhalation, the arm is hyperabducted to the side of the patient's head.
4. Contact the most medial aspect of the patient's right rib 11 with the thenar eminence of the cephalad hand.
5. Grasp the opposite anterior superior iliac spine with the caudad hand.
6. Apply a longitudinal stretch between the hand contacts sufficient to take the slack out of the tissues. This will usually lift the hip off the table by a few inches.
7. With your cephalad hand, push the rib anterior, lateral, and superior, localizing your disengagement force on the rib.
8. Have the patient inhale and then exhale as you localize your force further.
9. At end of exhalation, apply a high-velocity low-amplitude thrust through the thenar eminence of your cephalad hand, with a vector anterior, lateral, and superior. Alternatively, have the patient cough instead of applying the thrust.
10. Retest the range of motion.

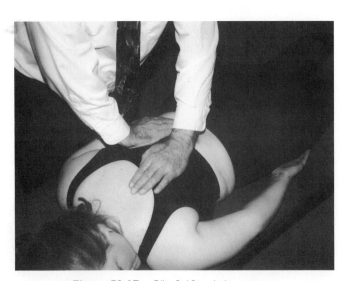

Figure 52.17. Ribs 2-10 technique, prone.

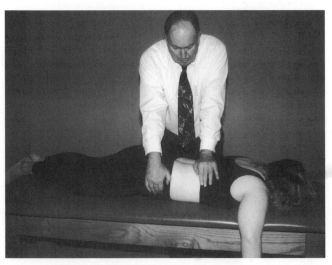

Figure 52.18. Ribs 11-12 technique, prone.

Note: The hip is used to pull the lateral aspect of the rib posteroinferiorly through stretch of the quadratus lumborum muscle and associated fascia. The cephalad hand's superior thrust will torque the medial aspect of the rib around an effective fulcrum, which is slightly lateral to your hand.

THORACOLUMBAR REGION

Type I: Lateral Recumbent (Posterior Transverse Process Down)

POSITIONAL DIAGNOSIS

L3 NS_LR_R. L3 is at the apex of a left side-bending group curve (dextrorotoscoliosis) and is side-bent left, rotated right in relationship to L4. It moves more easily in these directions.

RESTRICTION

Right side-bending and left rotation with the patient in (sagittal) neutral position.

OBJECTIVE

Restore physiologic range of motion to the L3/L4 joint.

RANGE

T10-L5.

PATIENT POSITION

Lateral recumbent, posterior transverse process down.

PROCEDURE

After diagnosis and soft tissue preparation:

1. Stand in front of the patient (Fig. 52.19).
2. Flex the legs until you palpate motion at the L3/L4 joint space.
3. Straighten the inferior leg.
4. Rotate the patient's torso anteriorly by pulling anteriorly on the right (lower) arm until you palpate rotation at L3.
5. Pull the arm caudad to induce right side-bending down to the L3/L4 joint space.
6. Place your caudad forearm over the area inferior to the iliac crest.
7. Put your cephalad forearm in the patient's uppermost axilla.
8. Your fingers monitor the forces localized at the L3/L4 articulation.
9. Have the patient breathe in and exhale, taking up tissue slack and localizing your forces on end exhalation.
10. Observe the direction in which the pelvis moves with exhalation. The structure of the patient's facets determines the optimal direction of thrust. If the primary motion you observe is rotation, then your thrust will have more of a rotatory component. If the primary motion is side-bending, then your thrust should have more of a side-bending component.
11. Perform a high-velocity low-amplitude thrust with your caudad forearm toward your knees by momentarily dropping

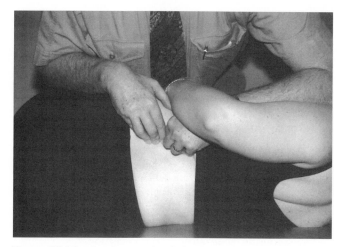

Figure 52.19. Lumbar type I technique, posterior transverse process down.

your body weight, thereby rotating the lumbar region left and side-bending right up through L3. Although your cephalad arm mainly serves as a stabilizing force, it may simultaneously add a small component of left rotation and right side-bending.
12. Retest the range of motion.

Type I: Lateral Recumbent (Posterior Transverse Process Up)

POSITIONAL DIAGNOSIS

L3 NS_LR_R. L3 is at the apex of a left side-bending group curve (dextrorotoscoliosis) and is side-bent left, rotated right in relationship to L4, and moves more easily in these directions.

RESTRICTION

Right side-bending and left rotation with the patient in (sagittal) neutral position.

OBJECTIVE

Restore physiologic range of motion to the L3/L4 joint.

RANGE

T10-L5.

PATIENT POSITION

Lateral recumbent, posterior transverse process up.

PROCEDURE

After diagnosis and soft tissue preparation:

1. Stand in front of the patient (Fig. 52.20).
2. Flex the patient's legs until you palpate motion at the L3/L4 joint space.
3. Straighten the inferior leg.

4. Pull the left arm superiorly and slightly forward to reduce the left side-bending (and/or induce right side-bending).
5. Place your caudad forearm over the area inferior to the iliac crest.
6. Put your cephalad forearm in the patient's uppermost axilla.
7. Your fingers monitor the motion at the L3/L4 articulation.
8. Using slight anterosuperior pressure through your caudad forearm, rotate the patient's hips and lumbar spine to the left, to the point where you palpate rotation at L4. Simultaneously, you rotate the thoracolumbar spine to the right by light pressure through your axillary forearm.
9. Rotate the patient slightly toward you while maintaining your localization (side-bending, flexion, rotation).
10. Have the patient breathe in and exhale, taking up tissue slack and localizing your forces on end exhalation.
11. Perform a high-velocity low-amplitude thrust with your caudad forearm toward the table by momentarily dropping your body weight, thereby side-bending the lumbar region right. Your cephalad arm is mainly stabilizing the torso, although a slight simultaneous component of left rotation and right side-bending may occur.
12. Retest the range of motion.

Type II, Extension: Lateral Recumbent (Posterior Transverse Process Up)

POSITIONAL DIAGNOSIS

L3 ES$_R$R$_R$. L3 is extended, side-bent right, and rotated right in relationship to L4, and moves more easily in these directions.

RESTRICTION

Left side-bending and left rotation with the patient in flexion.

OBJECTIVE

Restore physiologic range of motion to the L3/L4 joint.

RANGE

T10-L5.

PATIENT POSITION

Left lateral recumbent (posterior transverse process up).

PROCEDURE

After diagnosis and soft tissue preparation:

1. Stand in front of the patient (Fig. 52.21).
2. Flex the patient's legs until you palpate motion at the dysfunctional transverse process.
3. Straighten the inferior leg.
4. Hook the patient's uppermost foot in the lower popliteal fossa.
5. Rotate the patient's torso (by pulling the left arm) down to but not including the dysfunctional vertebral segment. Use your caudad hand to monitor the posteriorly rotated transverse process throughout the procedure.
6. Place your caudad forearm on the iliac crest, just superior to the posterosuperior iliac spines (PSIS). Continue monitoring the dysfunctional segment with at least one finger.
7. Place your cephalad arm in the axilla, beneath the patient's upper arm, to stabilize the thorax.
8. Rotate the patient slightly toward you while maintaining your localization (side-bending, flexion, rotation).
9. Have the patient breathe in and exhale, taking up tissue slack and localizing your forces on end exhalation.
10. Perform a high-velocity low-amplitude thrust with your caudad forearm toward the table by momentarily dropping your body weight, thereby side-bending the lumbar region left. Your cephalad arm is mainly stabilizing the torso, although a slight simultaneous component of right rotation and right side-bending may occur.
11. Retest the range of motion.

Type II, Extension: Lateral Recumbent (Posterior Transverse Process Down)

POSITIONAL DIAGNOSIS

L3 ES$_R$R$_R$. L3 is extended, side-bent right, and rotated right in relationship to L4, and moves more easily in these directions.

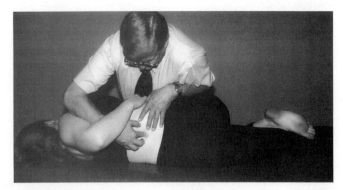

Figure 52.20. Lumbar type I technique, posterior transverse process up.

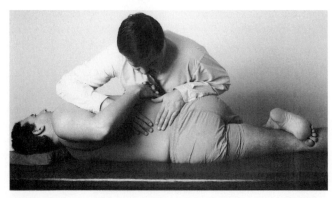

Figure 52.21. Thoracolumbar type II technique, posterior transverse process up.

RESTRICTION

Left side-bending and left rotation with the patient in flexion.

OBJECTIVE

Restore physiologic range of motion to the L3/L4 joint.

RANGE

T10-L5.

PATIENT POSITION

Right lateral recumbent (posterior transverse process down).

PROCEDURE

After diagnosis and soft tissue preparation:

1. Stand in front of the patient (Fig. 52.22)
2. Flex the patient's legs until you palpate motion at the L3/L4 joint space.
3. Straighten the inferior leg.
4. Now pull the right arm cephalad and upward to induce left side-bending to the L3/L4 joint space. If additional flexion is desired, the thoracic area may be brought anteriorly through a pull on the shoulder.
5. Place your caudad forearm inferior to the iliac crest.
6. Put your cephalad forearm in the patient's uppermost axilla.
7. Have the patient breathe in and exhale, taking up tissue slack and localizing your forces on end exhalation.
8. Your fingers monitor the motion at the L3/L4 articulation.
9. Perform a high-velocity low-amplitude thrust with your caudad forearm with a vector toward the patient's head and downward to encourage side-bending. Your cephalad arm functions as a stabilizer of the upper torso.
10. Retest the range of motion.

Note: This produces side-bending left and rotation of the pelvis toward you (right). The rotation of the pelvis is transmitted through L4, giving a relative left rotation to L3. Re-member, however, that there is approximately 1° of rotation at any lumbar segment.

Type II, Flexion: Lateral Recumbent (Posterior Transverse Process Down)

POSITIONAL DIAGNOSIS

L1 $FS_R R_R$. L1 is side-bent right, rotated right in relationship to L2, and moves more easily in these directions.

RESTRICTION

Left side-bending and left rotation with the patient in extension.

OBJECTIVE

Restore physiologic range of motion to the L1/L2 joint.

RANGE

T10-L5.

PATIENT POSITION

Right lateral recumbent (posterior transverse process down).

PROCEDURE

After diagnosis and soft tissue preparation:

1. Stand in front of the patient (Fig. 52.23).
2. Flex the patient's legs until you palpate motion at the L1/L2 joint space. This "locks" the lower lumbar facets.
3. Straighten the inferior leg.
4. Induce extension to the L1/L2 joint space by pushing the inferior elbow in a posterior direction with your cephalad hand while you palpate the L1 area with your caudad hand.
5. Now pull the right arm cephalad and upward to induce left side-bending and rotation down to the L1/L2 joint space. Be sure you do not rotate below L1.
6. Place your caudad forearm inferior to the iliac crest.

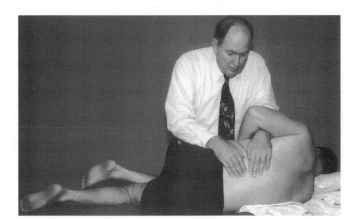

Figure 52.22. Thoracolumbar type II technique, posterior transverse process down.

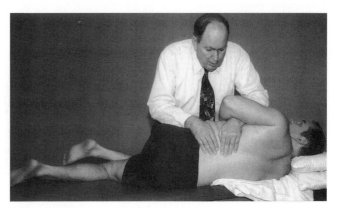

Figure 52.23. Lumbar type II technique, flexed: posterior transverse process down.

7. Put your cephalad forearm in the patient's uppermost axilla.

8. Ask patient to rotate the head to the left to rotate the neck and trunk to the left.

9. Have the patient breathe in and exhale, taking up tissue slack and localizing your forces on end exhalation.

10. Perform a high-velocity low-amplitude thrust with your caudad forearm with a vector toward the patient's head and downward. This rotates the patient's pelvis toward you, producing left lumbar side-bending and right rotation of the pelvis. The rotation of the pelvis is transmitted through L2, giving a relative left rotation to L1. Your cephalad arm functions as a stabilizer of the upper torso.

11. Retest the range of motion.

PELVIS

Anterior Sacrum, Right (Left Rotation on Left Oblique Axis)

DIAGNOSIS

The sacral sulcus is deep on the right, with associated tissue texture changes and tenderness. The left inferolateral angle is posterior. (The sacrum is effectively rotated left, side-bent right.)

RESTRICTION

Posterior motion by the right sacral sulcus when anterior pressure is applied to the left inferolateral angle.

OBJECTIVE

Restore physiologic range of motion to the sacroiliac joint.

PATIENT POSITION

Left lateral recumbent.

PROCEDURE

After diagnosis and soft tissue preparation:

1. Stand in front of the patient (Fig. 52.24).
2. Flex the hips (with bent knees) to the point where you feel motion at the right sacral sulcus.
3. Drop the upper leg and foot off the side of the table to induce left side-bending.
4. Place the flexor surface of your caudad forearm parallel to the lower spine, posterior to and crossing the iliac crest. This will brace the pelvis.
5. Put your cephalad forearm through the uppermost axilla, with the hand posterior and inferior to the shoulder and the elbow braced against the anterior shoulder. Rotate the shoulder posteriorly to stabilize the patient.
6. Have the patient breathe in and exhale, monitoring the localization of forces at the end of the patient's exhalation.
7. Perform a high-velocity low-amplitude thrust with the caudad

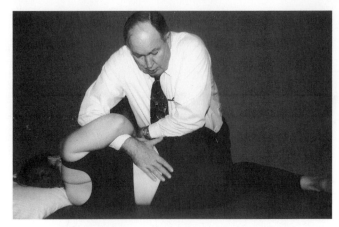

Figure 52.24.   Anterior sacrum right technique.

arm, following a circular motion with the ilium, rotating it anteriorly from behind.

8. Retest the range of motion.

Posterior Sacrum, Left (Left Rotation on Left Oblique Axis)

DIAGNOSIS

Tissue texture change and tenderness at the left inferior pole of the SI joint. The sacral sulcus is deep on the right. The left inferolateral angle is posterior. (The sacrum is effectively rotated left, side-bent right.)

RESTRICTION

Cephalad and downward motion at the left inferior pole of the SI joint when anterior pressure is applied to the left inferolateral angle.

OBJECTIVE

Rotate the sacrum right and side-bend it left by applying force from above down through the sacrum, with a counterforce on the left ilium, localizing force to the left sacroiliac joint.

PATIENT POSITION

Supine.

PROCEDURE

After diagnosis and soft tissue preparation:

1. Stand on the right side of the patient (Figs. 52.25 and 52.26).
2. Move the shoulders so that the upper torso is side-bent left and the shoulder closest to you is in the middle of the table.
3. Have patient interlace fingers behind the neck.
4. Insert your cephalad hand through the posterior aspect of the opposite axilla so that the dorsum of the hand is contacting the sternum.
5. Introduce right rotation through your cephalad arm, pivoting

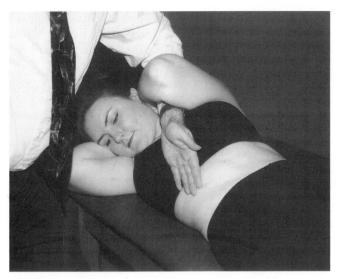

Figure 52.25. Posterior sacrum left technique.

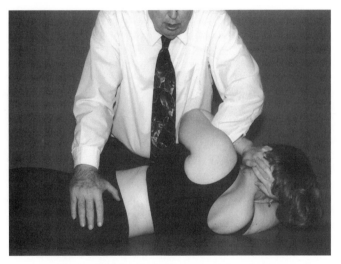

Figure 52.26. Posterior sacrum left technique.

around the shoulder closest to you. Do not flex the patient. You may need to use your caudad hand to stabilize the shoulder during this rotation in order to avoid flexing.
6. Place your caudad hand over the left iliac crest.
7. Continue your right rotation from above until the force is felt to accumulate at the left iliac crest.
8. Perform a high-velocity low-amplitude rotatory thrust with the cephalad arm, rotating the opposite shoulder anteriorly from behind, while you exert a small counterforce on the far ilium through your caudad hand. Note: increased force at the ilium will rarely increase the effectiveness of this technique.
9. Retest the range of motion.

A posterior sacrum (right) has the same motion description as an anterior sacrum (left) (rotated right, side-bent left), but the restriction and tissue change is dominant on the posterior

sacrum side. The technique localizes force to the posterior sacrum side.

Anteriorly Rotated Ilium (Innominate)

POSITIONAL DIAGNOSIS

Standing flexion test is positive on the side of dysfunction. The anterosuperior iliac spine (ASIS) is more caudad on the dysfunctional side. The ipsilateral pubic ramus is more caudad (not always detectable). The ipsilateral posterosuperior iliac spine (PSIS) is more cephalad.

RESTRICTION

Backward rotation of the ilium about a transverse axis.

OBJECTIVE

Mobilize the ilium in a posterior rotatory fashion to eliminate the restriction of motion.

PATIENT POSITION

Lateral recumbent, dysfunctional ilium up.

PROCEDURE

After diagnosis and soft tissue preparation:

1. Stand facing the patient (Fig. 52.27).
2. Flex the hips and knees to 90°, and then drop the upper leg off the table in front of the lower leg.
3. Contact the ilium with your caudad forearm on a line between the PSIS and the greater trochanter; place the thenar eminence of your cephalad hand on the anterior surface of the ASIS.
4. Apply firm pressure in a direction to follow the line of the upper femur. You should feel as though this force is posteriorly rotating the entire innominate (i.e., backward rotation on the transverse axis).
5. With your cephalad hand, place a force on the upper shoulder,

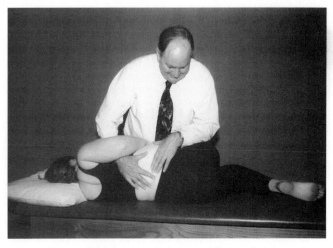

Figure 52.27. Anteriorly rotated ilium technique.

carrying the shoulder backward until force is localized to the sacroiliac (SI) joint.

6. Have the patient breathe in and exhale, localizing your forces on exhalation.

7. At end exhalation, apply a high-velocity low-amplitude anterior rotatory thrust directed down the shaft of the femur. Since you are below the axis of rotation, this rotates the ilium posteriorly.

8. Retest the position and range of motion.

Posteriorly Rotated Ilium (Innominate)

POSITIONAL DIAGNOSIS

Standing flexion test is positive on the side of dysfunction. The ASIS is more cephalad. The ipsilateral pubic ramus is more cephalad (may not be detectable). The ipsilateral PSIS is more caudad.

RESTRICTION

Anterior rotation of the ilium about a transverse axis.

OBJECTIVE

Mobilize the ilium in a forward rotatory fashion to eliminate the restriction of motion.

PATIENT POSITION

Lateral recumbent, dysfunctional side up.

PROCEDURE

After diagnosis and soft tissue preparation:

1. Stand facing the patient (Fig. 52.28).
2. Straighten the lower leg; flex the hip and knee of the upper leg and place the foot in the popliteal fossa of the lower leg.
3. Contact the posterior superior iliac spine of the upper ilium with the palmar surface of your caudad forearm (or thenar eminence).

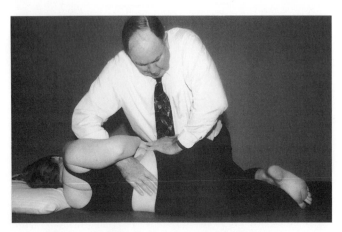

Figure 52.28. Posteriorly rotated ilium technique.

4. Apply firm pressure on the PSIS, directed toward the umbilicus. You should feel as though this force is anteriorly rotating the entire innominate (i.e., forward rotation on the transverse axis).

5. Place your cephalad hand or forearm on the upper shoulder to stabilize the patient.

6. Have patient breathe in, then exhale. Localize your forces on exhalation.

7. At end of exhalation, apply a high-velocity low-amplitude anterior rotatory thrust directed toward the umbilicus.

8. Retest the position and range of motion.

Superior Ilial Shear (Upslipped Innominate)

POSITIONAL DIAGNOSIS

The standing flexion test is positive on the dysfunctional side. The ASIS, pubic ramus and PSIS are all superior on the dysfunctional side.

RESTRICTION

Downward motion of the innominate.

OBJECTIVE

Mobilize the sacroiliac joint so that increased downward motion is possible.

PATIENT POSITION

Supine.

PROCEDURE

After diagnosis and soft tissue preparation:

1. Stand at the feet of the patient (Figs. 52.29 and 52.30).

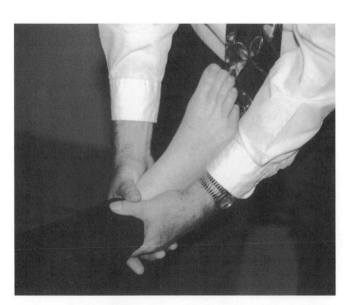

Figure 52.29. Superior ilial shear technique.

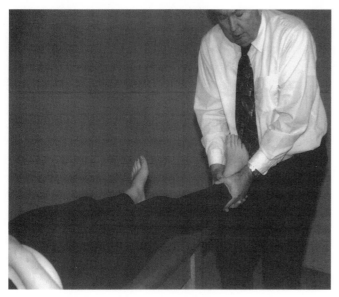

Figure 52.30. Superior ilial shear technique.

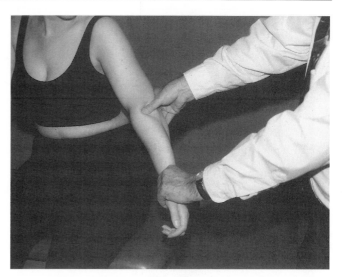

Figure 52.31. Posterior radial head technique.

2. Grasp the leg superior to the ankle on the dysfunctional side.
3. Flex the hip slightly, and apply traction and internal rotation to the leg.
4. Ask the patient to relax the knee, then the hip. Have the patient breathe in and out as you localize your forces to the ilium.
5. On end exhalation, apply a high-velocity low-amplitude tractional force to the leg.
6. Retest the range of motion.

UPPER EXTREMITY

Posterior Radial Head

POSITIONAL DIAGNOSIS

Tenderness over the radial head. Posterior glide of the radial head is free.

RESTRICTION

Anterior glide of the radial head is restricted.

OBJECTIVE

Increase the range of anterior glide.

PATIENT POSITION

Seated.

PROCEDURE

After diagnosis and soft tissue preparation:

1. Stand on the dysfunctional side of your seated patient (Fig. 52.31).
2. Grasp the patient's flexed elbow with one hand, placing your thumb over the posterolateral aspect of the radial head.

3. Grasp the wrist with your other hand, so that your thumb is over the dorsum of the distal ulna.
4. Supinate the wrist with your distal hand while extending the elbow with your proximal hand.
5. Just before reaching complete extension, apply a high-velocity low-amplitude thrust through your thumb on the radial head in a ventral direction, with simultaneous slight increase in supination by your distal hand.
6. Retest the range of motion.

Alternate method: If the radial head restriction is greater in pronation, treat with the forearm pronated.

Abducted Elbow (Humeroulnar)

POSITIONAL DIAGNOSIS

The angle between the ulna and humerus is increased (increased carrying angle). Abduction places pressure on the proximal radius, forcing it distally in relation to the ulna.

RESTRICTION

Adduction of the elbow, and radiocarpal abduction.

OBJECTIVE

Increase adduction of the elbow and radiocarpal abduction.

PATIENT POSITION

Seated. Note: Elbow restriction should be treated before wrist restrictions.

PROCEDURE

After diagnosis and soft tissue preparation:

1. Stand on the dysfunctional side in front of the patient (Fig. 52.32).

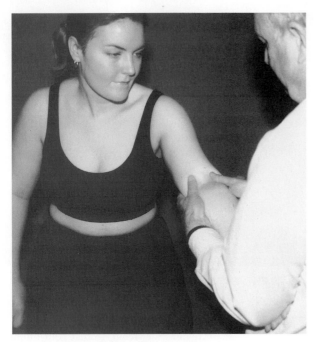

Figure 52.32. Abducted elbow technique.

2. Place the wrist of the dysfunctional extremity between your arm and lateral chest wall.
3. Grasp the elbow with both hands, with your thumbs in the antecubital region over the proximal radius and ulna. (Avoid direct pressure by the fingers over the ulnar nerve).
4. With the elbow close to full extension (slight flexion is required to avoid extension locking), apply a lateral translatory force to take the ulna into adduction (a varus force).
5. Apply a high-velocity low-amplitude thrust in the same vector when you have reached the restrictive barrier.
6. Retest the range of motion.

Wrist

POSITIONAL DIAGNOSIS

Increased adduction, abduction, flexion, or extension of the wrist. The position of the involved bones may not be altered demonstrably, but motion will be more free in one direction and restricted if attempted in the opposite direction.

RESTRICTION

Motion opposite to the increased or free motion.

OBJECTIVE

Restore physiologic range of motion to the radiocarpal joint.

PATIENT POSITION

Seated or supine. Note: Elbow restriction should be treated before wrist restrictions.

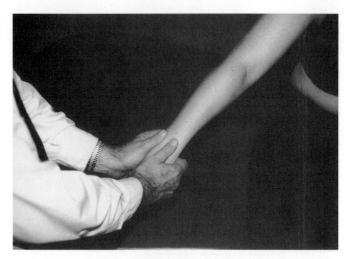

Figure 52.33. Wrist technique.

PROCEDURE

After diagnosis and soft tissue preparation:

1. Face the patient (Fig. 52.33).
2. Grasp the patient's dysfunctional wrist in both hands, with your fingers under the palm of the hand on the medial and lateral sides.
3. Place your thumbs on the dorsal surface of the hand, with the pads over the dorsal surface of the carpal bones.
4. Circumduct the wrist as you put traction on the upper extremity through the level of the wrist.
5. Complete your motion by dorsiflexing the wrist as your thumbs press firmly downward.
6. Retest the range of motion.

Note: This is actually an articulatory technique. If the physician feels it is necessary, a thrust with minimal force can be added as the restrictive barrier is reached. This technique may be modified to treat restrictions of motion of individual carpal bones by superimposing the thumbs over the involved carpal bone.

LOWER EXTREMITY

Posterior Fibular Head

DIAGNOSIS

Palpable muscle/connective tissue tension in the interosseous region between the tibia and fibula. Possible posterior displacement of the fibular head; posterior glide is free.

RESTRICTION

Anterior glide of the fibular head.

OBJECTIVE

Increase the anterior glide of the fibular head.

PATIENT POSITION

Supine.

PROCEDURE

After diagnosis and soft tissue preparation:

1. Stand on the dysfunctional side of the patient (Fig. 52.34).
2. Flex the hip and knee.
3. Place your cephalad hand in the popliteal space, palm upward, with your first MP joint posterior to the fibular head. (Avoid direct pressure over the common peroneal nerve.)
4. Grasp the patient's leg proximal to the ankle with your caudad hand.
5. Flex the knee to the point where you feel pressure of the fibular head on your first MP joint, simultaneously externally rotating the ankle.
6. Apply a high-velocity low-amplitude thrust by flexing the leg with your caudad hand, while you apply an anterior counterforce to the fibular head with your first MP joint.
7. Retest the range of motion.

This technique can be done in a prone position with slight modifications.

Anterior Fibular Head

DIAGNOSIS

Palpable muscle/connective tissue tension in the interosseous region between the tibia and fibula. Possible anterior displacement of the fibular head; anterior glide is free.

RESTRICTION

Posterior glide of the fibular head.

OBJECTIVE

Increase the posterior glide of the fibular head.

PATIENT POSITION

Supine.

PROCEDURE

After diagnosis and soft tissue preparation:

1. Stand at the foot of the table on the side opposite the dysfunction (Fig. 52.35).
2. Place a pillow below the knee to avoid locking it in extension.
3. Grasp the leg immediately proximal to the ankle with your caudad hand.
4. Place the thenar eminence of your cephalad hand on the anterior aspect of the fibular head.
5. Internally rotate the ankle to draw the distal fibula anteriorly.
6. Apply a high-velocity low-amplitude thrust in a posterolateral vector to the fibular head, while simultaneously applying a slight internal rotation counterforce to the ankle.
7. Retest the range of motion.

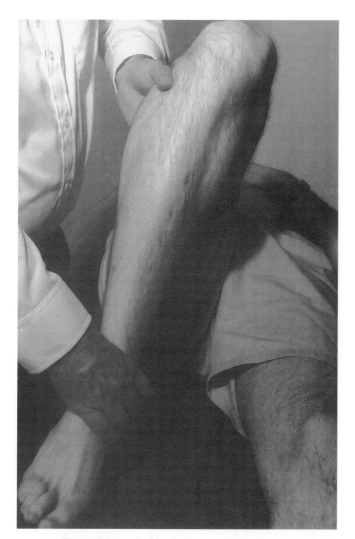

Figure 52.34. Posterior fibular head technique.

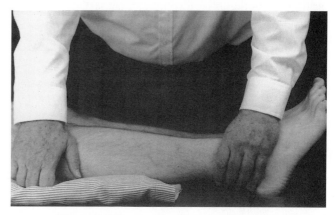

Figure 52.35. Anterior fibular head technique.

Anterior Lateral Malleolus

DIAGNOSIS

The lateral malleolus (distal fibula) has free anterior glide relative to the distal tibia. The distal medial border of the talus is more prominent.

RESTRICTION

Posterior glide of the lateral malleolus.

OBJECTIVE

Increase posterior motion of the lateral malleolus.

PATIENT POSITION

Supine.

PROCEDURE

After diagnosis and soft tissue preparation:

1. Stand at the foot of the table (Fig. 52.36).
2. Grasp the heel with the cupped fingers of your lateral hand.

Your palm is on the lateral aspect of the heel, and your thumb is in contact with the anterior surface of the lateral malleolus.
3. Grasp the medial side of the ankle with your other hand, reinforcing your first thumb by placing your other thumb on top of it.
4. Accumulate a posterior force on the lateral malleolus by dorsiflexing the foot and applying posterior pressure with the thumbs.
5. Prior to full dorsiflexion, apply a high-velocity low-amplitude thrust through your thumbs to the lateral malleolus in a posterior vector.
6. Retest the range of motion.

Posterior Lateral Malleolus

DIAGNOSIS

The lateral malleolus (distal fibula) has free posterior glide relative to the distal tibia. The anterior portion of the talus is displaced in a lateral direction.

RESTRICTION

Anterior glide of the lateral malleolus.

OBJECTIVE

Increase anterior glide of the lateral malleolus.

PATIENT POSITION

Prone.

PROCEDURE

After diagnosis and soft tissue preparation:

1. Stand at the foot of the table (Fig. 52.37).
2. Grasp the dorsum of the foot with the cupped fingers of your lateral hand. Your thumb is in contact with the posterior surface of the lateral malleolus.

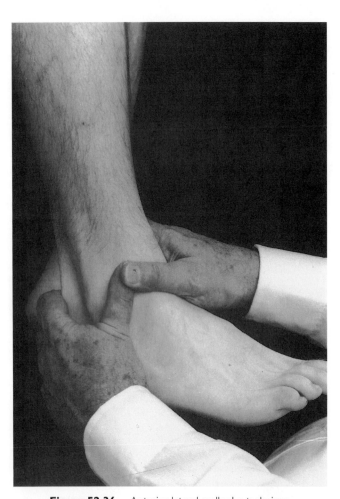

Figure 52.36. Anterior lateral malleolus technique.

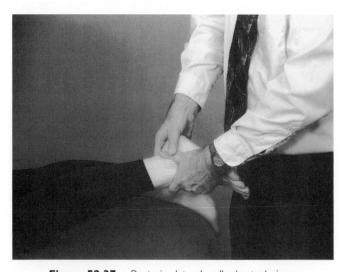

Figure 52.37. Posterior lateral malleolus technique.

3. Grasp the medial side of the ankle with your other hand, reinforcing your first thumb by placing your other thumb on top of it.
4. Accumulate an anterior force on the lateral malleolus by plantar-flexing the foot and applying anterior pressure with the thumbs.
5. Prior to full plantar flexion, apply a high-velocity low-amplitude thrust through your thumbs to the lateral malleolus in an anterior vector.
6. Retest the range of motion.

Talotibial Joint: Anterior Tibia on Talus

POSITIONAL DIAGNOSIS

Tibia is anterior on the talus. The ankle prefers dorsiflexion.

RESTRICTION

Tibia is restricted in gliding posteriorly on the talus. The ankle is restricted in plantar flexion.

OBJECTIVE

Restore physiologic range of motion to the tibiotalar joint (true ankle), specifically to restore full plantar flexion of the ankle (posterior glide of the tibia over the talus).

PATIENT POSITION

Supine.

PROCEDURE

After diagnosis:

1. Stand at the foot of the table to the side of somatic dysfunction (Fig. 52.38).
2. Grasp the patient's heel and apply traction to it, dorsiflexing the ankle.
3. Grasp the distal end of the tibia with your other hand, palm over its anterior surface near the talotibial joint, and apply posterior pressure (down toward the table).
4. Apply a high-velocity low-amplitude thrust posteriorly through the distal tibia as the foot is dorsiflexed with the other hand on the heel.
5. Retest the range of talotibial motion.

Talus in Plantar Flexion: Ankle Tug

POSITIONAL DIAGNOSIS

Tibia is posterior on the talus. The ankle prefers plantar flexion.

RESTRICTION

Tibia is restricted in gliding anteriorly on the talus. The ankle is restricted in dorsiflexion.

OBJECTIVE

Restore physiologic range of motion to the tibiotalar joint (true ankle), specifically to restore full dorsiflexion of the ankle (anterior glide of the tibia over the talus).

PATIENT POSITION

Supine.

PROCEDURE

After diagnosis:

1. Stand or sit at the foot of the table (Fig. 52.39).
2. Grasp the patient's foot, curling your 5th or 4th finger over the dorsal surface of the head of the talus. Also grasp the foot with your other hand and clasp your fingers so that the 5th or 4th finger supports the same finger of the opposite hand (over the talar head).
3. Place your thumbs over the ball of the foot and dorsiflex the foot at the ankle. This dorsiflexion of the ankle is maintained throughout this technique.

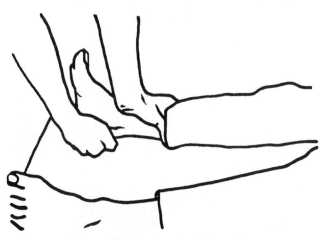

Figure 52.38. Anterior tibia on talus.

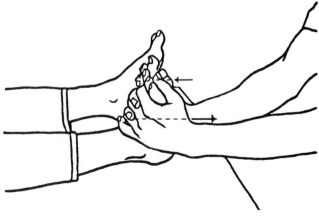

Figure 52.39. Inverted talus (plantar flexion of talus).

4. Apply traction, with continued dorsiflexion and slight eversion at the ankle, until all joint play is out of the ankle joint.
5. Apply a high-velocity low-amplitude tug to reseat the talus in the mortise of the ankle.
6. Retest the range of talotibial motion.

Note: This type of somatic dysfunction may be accompanied by tissue congestion and spasm of the peroneus muscles and/or fibular head somatic dysfunction.

Hiss Plantar Whip: Cuboid

POSITIONAL DIAGNOSIS

The cuboid is displaced inferiorly, with the medial edge gliding laterally, flattening the lateral longitudinal arch. There is palpable tenderness on the plantar surface of the cuboid.

RESTRICTION

Motion toward the dorsal surface of the foot.

OBJECTIVE

Restore the cuboid to its appropriate position.

PATIENT POSITION

Prone.

PROCEDURE

After diagnosis and soft tissue preparation:

1. Stand at the foot of the table (Fig. 52.40).
2. The dysfunctional leg is off the table.
3. Grasp the foot so that the thumb of your lateral hand is contacting the soft tissue over the medial plantar surface of the cuboid.
4. Grasp the foot on the medial side with your medial hand, placing your second thumb over the first.
5. Induce a series of oscillating motions, swinging the foot to produce plantar flexion.
6. Apply a high-velocity low-amplitude thrust by performing a whiplike motion in the same direction as above (i.e., as you pull the foot toward you in the final motion, your thumbs

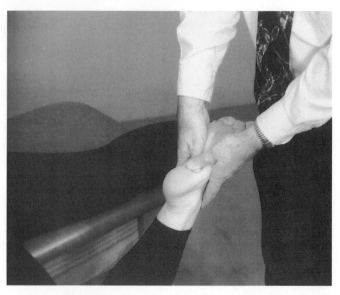

Figure 52.40.   Hiss plantar whip technique.

impart a sudden downward and lateral motion, thrusting the cuboid toward the dorsolateral surface of the foot).
7. Retest the range of motion.

This same technique may be used with variations for other somatic dysfunctions of the foot (navicular, cuneiforms, metatarsal bases), as follows.

NAVICULAR

Place your thumb on the lateral margin of the plantar surface of the navicular bone. With your thrust straight down, your thumb will direct the force medially.

CUNEIFORMS

Put your thumb on the plantar surface of the appropriate cuneiform.

CONCLUSION

Careful execution of high-velocity low-amplitude thrust techniques in the areas presented can help patients and bring them healing of dysfunction.

53. Muscle Energy Technique Procedures

JOHN P. GOODRIDGE

Key Concepts

- **History of muscle energy technique**

- **Uses of muscle energy technique, including joint mobilization, strengthening and stretching of muscles, improving circulation, and balancing neuromuscular relationships**

- **Procedures to diagnose asymmetry, motion, and tissue texture changes**

- **Types of muscle contractions**

- **Physiological principles of muscle energy**

- **Steps of muscle energy treatment**

- **Efficiency factors and contraindications to muscle energy technique**

Muscle energy is an osteopathic technique with roots extending back to Andrew Taylor Still. Still did not record the way that he treated, preferring to insist that his students conduct an exhaustive study of anatomy while absorbing the osteopathic philosophy. He told students that, if they knew anatomy and understood osteopathic philosophy, they would know what to do. As the osteopathic profession sought to increase the efficiency of teaching students how to treat patients, certain key individuals made contributions by developing a particular type of technique into a plan. Fred Mitchell, Sr. contributed by developing a plan of diagnosis and treatment that he called muscle energy because of its reliance on active patient effort through muscular contraction.

Mitchell[1] credited Kettler as *"the first to focus (his) attention on the importance of the vast amount of tissue involved between joints, muscle and fascia, and the changes it undergoes in the lesioning process."* Kettler also emphasized that *"without establishing bilateral myofascial harmony, the lesion pattern is not obliterated and returns again and again."* Mitchell quoted A.T. Still also, showing that he knew about this: *"The attempt to restore joint integrity before soothingly restoring muscle and ligamentous normality was putting the cart before the horse."*[1]

Some sources allege that muscle energy techniques are an outgrowth of a method developed by T.J. Ruddy,[2] called "resistive duction." In Ruddy's method the physician offers resistance to the patient's active movement, but the patient is required to move quickly, often at a rate of 60 excursions per minute, or equal to the patient's pulse rate. Ruddy's purpose in having the patient contract muscle quickly and repetitively was twofold:

1. To increase blood (and other tissue fluid) movement to remove metabolic waste products from the cells and circulate oxygen
2. To tone inactive muscles that might be weak

Mitchell and Kettler must have been unaware of the proprioceptive neuromuscular facilitation (PNF) techniques developed by Kabat, Knott, and Voss at the Kabat-Kaiser Institute during the late 1940s. These techniques were not widely known. PNF uses skills to reeducate muscle for several reasons:[3]

> *"To gain inhibition in muscles which may be in a protective spasm"*
> *"To improve range (of motion) at an intervertebral level."*

Mitchell first published his work in the *Yearbook of the American Academy of Osteopathy* in 1958, after receiving requests for a written description of the work he had developed in the 1940s and 1950s. He described *"one method of correction"* that used the effort of an extrinsic guiding operator as the activating force plus the intrinsic respiratory and muscular cooperation of the patient. He wrote about the direct method treatments of soft tissues (with attention to fascias) and treatment using Neidner's fascial release prior to articular correction. *"Muscular energy technique,"* he wrote, *"with its many ramifications, is a most useful tool in preparation of the soft tissues. Ligamentous stretching may also be of use before articular correction is attempted."*[1]

Lewit and Simons (1984) wrote that, *"the use of post-isometric relaxation was pioneered by Fred Mitchell Sr. and clearly described by F.L. Mitchell Jr. as a mobilization technique that applies gentle force to improve 'articulation' and thereby restore previously restricted movement".*[4] Later authors believed that Mitchell's muscle energy approach did this more quickly than PNF techniques. Probably because Mitchell's work was not recorded in indexed allopathic literature, Travell and Simons credited Lewit in their text by stating, *"the concept of applying post-isometric relaxation in the treatment of myofascial pain was presented for the first time in a North American Journal in 1984."*[5]

Mitchell taught his techniques in tutorials to numerous physicians. The first 5-day Mitchell Tutorial was held in Fort Dodge, Iowa in 1970 and attended by John Goodridge, Philip Greenman, Rolland Miller, Devota Nowland, Edward Stiles, and Sara Sutton—all osteopathic physicians. Several tutorials

691

followed across the country. In 1972, Mitchell's examination and treatment procedures were videotaped at Michigan State University's College of Osteopathic Medicine. Following Mitchell's death in 1974, the American Academy of Osteopathy organized a committee of physicians who had taken a tutorial with Mitchell and developed a manual for the presentation of 5-day courses to familiarize others with Mitchell's work. Additional tutorials were conducted for new faculty at the newly established colleges of osteopathic medicine from 1977 to 1981. The five earlier established osteopathic colleges began to integrate muscle energy procedures into their curriculum. In 1979, Mitchell Jr., Moran, and Pruzzo[6] published the manual that was and still is used as a reference in most osteopathic medical colleges. Muscle energy diagnostic and treatment procedures developed by Fred Mitchell, Sr. are currently a standard part of the osteopathic manipulative medicine curriculum and are also used by many physical therapists.

DEFINITION

Muscle energy technique has been defined as a form of osteopathic manipulative treatment in which the patient's muscles are actively used on request, from a precisely controlled position, in a specific direction, and against a distinctly executed counterforce. Muscle energy techniques are used to:

Mobilize joints in which movement is restricted
Stretch tight muscles and fascia
Improve local circulation
Balance neuromuscular relationships to alter muscle tone

Muscle energy techniques involve the patient's active cooperation, to contract a muscle or muscles, inhale or exhale, or move one bone of a joint in a specific direction relative to the adjacent bone. For these reasons, muscle energy can not be used if the patient is in a coma, uncooperative, or unresponsive.[7]

DIAGNOSIS

Before a therapeutic procedure is performed, obtain a working diagnosis and develop a visual image of the dysfunction and the direction of therapeutic forces. Examine the patient for asymmetry of muscle tone, quality and range of motion, and tissue texture changes. Localized tenderness in muscle and connective tissue elements may also provide valuable diagnostic information.

Some positional asymmetries in the static state suggest asymmetrical movements. Use functional assessments to confirm the static suggestion and indicate the true direction of force required to balance the tone or increase the range of motion. More often than not, the movement of the bones at a joint is restrained rather than impeded by obstacles in its path.

Procedures

Any one of the following procedures is acceptable for determining asymmetry of range and quality of movement. Although movement of the femur at the femoroacetabular joint is used as an example of range and quality of movement, the principles underlying this examination apply to examination of any part of the body using movements such as:

Flexion
Extension
Side-bending right and left
Rotation right and left
Internal or external rotation right versus left side (see Chapters 43–50 on "Regional Examination and Treatment.")

For the purpose of discussion, the patient is supine.

1. One could forcefully carry the femur toward its anatomical limit of motion and compare abduction to the left with abduction to the right. Resistance perceived this way is analogous to that of meeting a wedge or steel barrier (endpoint).
2. One may abduct the femur slowly and carefully, noting a sense of increased tension long before the anatomic limit is reached. The sensation perceived by this second method might be likened to that of reaching the end of a restraining rope within the range of movement, like that of a dog reaching the end of a leash or tether.
3. One may initiate abduction of the femur even more slowly to perceive an even earlier beginning of the tension increase, acutely perceiving even a more subtle resistance more easily detected on either the left or right side. This third procedure is similar to sensing the initial illumination of a rheostat-controlled light switch.

Any of these three ways for determining restriction or ease of motion may be used to perceive the quality of resistance, but when the two sides are compared, use the same method for each side to make a valid comparison. If an abducted right femur reaches resistance sooner than the left, the range of abduction to the right is less than the range of abduction to the left. Note quality: Is the resistance soft and rubbery or abrupt and firm?

The sense of resistance might be more realistic if you visualize a gate that is open, another that is partially closed, and another that is closed (Figs. 53.1–53.3). The striking bar on a gatepost represents an end point much like that of a bony ridge in the body's skeletal system on the gate that closes completely. A wet rope attached to that gate might restrain its range of motion and prevent it from closing completely. On another gate is a rope that has dried and is shortened; it offers further restraint to motion, somewhat resembling that of a muscle that is shortened. If the gate has spring-type hinges, they produce greater initial resistance than ordinary hinges, requiring more initial force to overcome the spring resistance before the gate is moved. A similar proprioceptive sensation may be perceived in human tissue; the restrainers may be muscular or ligamentous and may be maintained by voluntary or involuntary mechanisms.

Palpatory Exercise in Diagnosis

The following exercise in diagnosis develops a sense of the beginning of resistance.

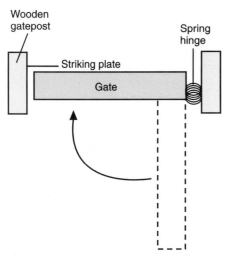

Figure 53.1. Resistance: the gate fully open. (From Goodridge JP. Muscle energy technique: definition, explanation, methods of procedure. *JAOA*. 1981;81:249–254.)

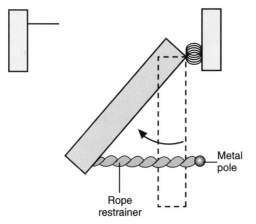

Figure 53.2. Resistance: the gate partially open. (From Goodridge JP. Muscle energy technique: definition, explanation, methods of procedure. *JAOA*. 1981;81:249–254.)

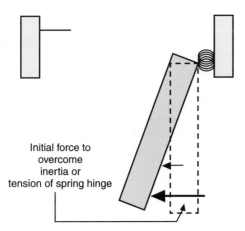

Figure 53.3. Resistance: the gate closed. (From Goodridge JP. Muscle energy technique: methods of procedure. *JAOA*. 1981;81:249–254.)

1. With one hand, grasp the foot and ankle of a supine patient to abduct the lower extremity. Close your eyes to enhance your focus. Rather than using your eyes, sense through the hand, forearm, and upper arm of the hand that is abducting.
2. Take the limb into abduction slowly, carefully sensing when resistance first occurs.
3. Open your eyes when you first feel resistance, observing how many degrees of an arc the patient's limb has negotiated.
4. Perform the same evaluation on the other leg and compare to see which had resistance occurring sooner, as indicated by the lesser of the two arcs.

TECHNICAL PRINCIPLES IN MUSCLE ENERGY TREATMENT

Muscle energy procedures attempt to shorten or lengthen the distance between the origin and insertion of certain muscles, depending on how they are applied. The goals are to:

Strengthen the weaker side of an asymmetry
Decrease hypertonicity
Lengthen muscle fibers
Reduce the restraint of movement
Alter related respiratory and circulatory function

Muscle contractions are classified as isometric, isotonic concentric, and isotonic eccentric. The term "isolytic" has been coined to describe procedures that increase the distance between the origin and insertion of a muscle while the patient actively resists. Because it is not a physiologic category of muscle contraction, and its use interferes with communication across disciplines, this term is used less often.

Isometric Contraction

The distance between the origin and the insertion of the muscle remains the same as the muscle contracts. Neither the patient's effort nor the physician's resistance wins. This apparently resets the muscle proprioceptors as the tight muscle lengthens.

Isotonic Concentric Contraction

The overall length of the muscle shortens, approximating the origin and the insertion. Physiologically, this is like the work of the biceps lifting a glass of water from a table to one's mouth. The patient's effort exceeds the physician's resistance. This method is helpful in building muscle strength.

Isotonic Eccentric Contraction

The distance between the origin and insertion is increased. This type of contraction occurs when the biceps lowers a glass of water to the table without spilling it. In the treatment mode, this type of muscle contraction occurs *"when a given resistance overcomes the muscle tension so that the muscle actually lengthens."*[8]

PHYSIOLOGICAL PRINCIPLES OF MUSCLE ENERGY

Postisometric Relaxation

Mitchell Jr.[9] postulated that *"immediately following (an isometric) contraction, the neuromuscular apparatus is in a refractory state during which passive stretching may be performed without encountering strong myotatic reflex opposition. All the operator needs to do is resist the contraction and then take up the slack in the fascias during the relaxed refractory period."* With muscle contraction, there also may be increased tension on the Golgi organ proprioceptors in the tendons; this inhibits the active muscle's contraction.

Reciprocal Inhibition

Another less common muscle energy activation utilizes the reflex mechanism of reciprocal inhibition when antagonistic muscles are contracted. A natural physiologic example of this reflex is the relaxation of the triceps muscle when the biceps contracts, and vice versa. In this method, the physician isometrically resists the patient's effort to flex the arm at the elbow.

ACTIVATING FORCES

Activating forces make techniques work. They can be classified as extrinsic and intrinsic.[10] Extrinsic forces come from outside the patient. Examples include physician effort such as guiding or thrusts and traction. Intrinsic forces come from within the patient and include active muscle contraction by the patient, active patient positioning, and respiratory cooperation.

In muscle energy technique, the physician offers stabilizing forces as the patient uses active muscle force. The physician usually positions the patient's tissues at the initial point of resistance to a specific movement and then offers resistance or counterforce to the patient's contractile force (of the tight muscle). This is not an all-or-nothing phenomenon. It is most effective when activation and equal counterforce are directed toward a group of muscle fibers that precisely move the body part in the direction desired. Muscle energy techniques are carried out within a range of movement against a sense of increased tension or resistance.

Lengthening a Shortened Muscle

There are several ways to lengthen shortened muscles by muscle energy procedures. An isometric muscle energy technique can be set up so that the activating muscle contraction attempts to pull in the restricted direction or away from the restricted direction. Some say the restricted direction is a restrictive barrier. In that case, the contraction would be to pull toward or away from the restrictive barrier.

Treatment of a patient with an acute right torticollis illustrates two ways to use muscle energy technique. The patient presents with the neck held close to his or her right shoulder with passive left side-bending (lateral flexion) restricted and painful. The patient's neck (from a probable side-bent right position) is side-bent in a left direction to the initial point of its restriction in motion. At that point, the patient is instructed to produce a contraction toward the right, away from the resisted motion. The tight right cervical musculature lengthens as the isometric contraction activates a Golgi tendon body reflex. This is the most common way to use muscle energy.

A less common way of using muscle energy activation is to position the patient's neck at the initial point of resistance. The patient is instructed to attempt side-bending of the neck toward the left by contracting the stretched muscles. This form of muscle energy activation is also effective in relaxing the tight right cervical muscles, but this time by activating the reciprocal inhibition reflex.

Clinically, the patient may find active right side-bending (lateral flexion) against the physician's counterforce painful and active left side-bending (lateral flexion) against a counterforce not painful. Muscles that have painful contractions do not contract well.[11]

In the case of the hip, if the range of abduction to the right is restricted, the goal is to lengthen the shortened right adductor muscles. First, the patient's limb is positioned in abduction at the point where resistance was first perceived. Then the physician employs a muscle energy contraction (activation) to decrease restriction and increase the range of the limb or tissue movement. Lengthening of the restricted muscle(s) may be accomplished by any of the following techniques.

ISOMETRIC CONTRACTION USING ADDUCTOR MUSCLE

With the limb at the position of initial resistance, the patient contracts the right adductor muscle group, and the physician applies an isometric force counter to and equaling the patient's muscle effort (isometric force). After a slow, balanced cessation of both forces, the adductor muscle group may be longer, permitting a greater range of abduction.

ISOMETRIC CONTRACTION USING ABDUCTOR MUSCLE

With the limb at the position of initial resistance, the patient contracts the right abductor muscle group as the physician applies force counter to and equaling the patient's muscle effort (isometric force). After a slow, balanced cessation of both forces, the adductor muscle group may relax and be longer, permitting a greater range of abduction (the result of a reciprocal inhibition reflex).

ISOTONIC ECCENTRIC TREATMENT (ISOLYTIC)

The patient contracts the right adductor group, and the physician applies a force counter to and greater than the patient's muscular effort, so that the right adductor group lengthens eccentrically as the result of Golgi receptor reflexes. Use this method to lengthen a muscle and to break down adhesions in the muscles or tissues. It has the potential of injuring muscle tissue.

SEQUENTIAL STEPS OF MUSCLE ENERGY TREATMENT

Diagnosis

Never give a form of treatment without first having an accurate diagnosis. Although diagnoses of somatic dysfunction from the muscle energy perspective has some unique elements, they are well described in the chapters on regional examination of the body. The reader is referred to those chapters to learn the appropriate diagnostic techniques.

Sequence

Based on an accurate diagnosis, a muscle energy procedure to lengthen shortened muscles and/or fascial elements follows these principles:

1. The physician positions the bone, joint, or body part appropriately at the position of initial resistance.
2. The physician instructs the patient about his or her participation and helps the patient to obtain an effective direction of movement for the limb, trunk, or head. The patient is instructed in the intensity of contraction and the duration of contraction (3–5 seconds or whatever is necessary to get a good contraction).
3. The physician directs the patient to contract the appropriate muscle(s) or muscle group.
4. The physician uses counterforce in opposition to and equal to the patient's muscle contraction.
5. The physician maintains forces until an appropriate patient contraction is perceived at the critical articulation or area. This generally takes 3–5 seconds, but the duration varies with the size of the muscle being treated.
6. The patient is directed to gently cease contraction, while the physician simultaneously matches the decrease in patient force.
7. The physician allows the patient to relax and senses the tissue relaxation with his or her own proprioceptors.
8. The physician takes up the slack permitted by the procedure. The slack is allowed by the decreased tension in the tight muscle, allowing it to be passively lengthened. Increased range of motion is noted by the physician.
9. Steps one to eight are repeated two to four times until the best possible increase in motion is obtained. The quality of response often peaks at the third excursion, with diminishing return thereafter.
10. The physician reevaluates the original dysfunction.

EFFICIENCY FACTORS

Good results depend on accurate diagnosis, appropriate levels of force, and sufficient localization. Poor results are most often caused by inaccurate diagnosis, improperly localized forces, or forces that are too strong.

Diagnosis

An inaccurate diagnosis may lead to inappropriate treatment and does not achieve the desired improvement in the patient's condition. Even if a segmental diagnosis is accurate, complicating factors and the entire clinical picture of the patient need to be considered. For example, a careful diagnosis may indicate that side-bending is restricted at a segment superior to the one identified for treatment; this then interferes with the localization required, and the superior segment may need to be treated before the inferior segment.

Amount of Force

Muscle energy technique is not a wrestling match. The amounts of force and counterforce are governed by the length and strength of the muscle group involved, the ability of the patient to accurately pull the body part in the direction you desire it to move, and the patient's symptoms. To affect a large muscle requires a stronger force than that required by a small or short muscle. A small amount of force should be used at first, with increases as necessary. This is much more productive than beginning with too much force. Care must be taken to limit counterforce, because the patient will work to equal it. Kilograms of force may be considered in dealing with large muscles such as the hip, while only grams of force might be very adequate when weaker, shorter, and smaller muscles (such as in the cervical region) are being treated. In the upper cervical region especially, even the movement of the eyes in a certain direction with isometric resistance of the cervical tension automatically generates enough force to treat a cervical somatic dysfunction effectively.

Localization

The localization of force is more important than the intensity of force. Localization depends on the physician's palpatory perception of movement (or resistance to movement) at or about a specific articulation. Such perception enables the physician to make subtle assessments about a dysfunction and create variations of suggested treatment procedures.

Monitoring the localization of forces and confining the direction of force by the diagnosed muscle group to the level of somatic dysfunction are important to achieve desired results. When the physician introduces motion into an articulation that is a segment or two below the dysfunctional one, the probability of success greatly decreases because the forces have been directed to the wrong muscles.

Asymmetrical Muscle Strength

Where asymmetry of range of motion occurs, consider and test the possibility of asymmetrical strength. Some ranges of motion may be asymmetrical because of weakness of a group of muscles rather than the shortness of the antagonist group. If asymmetry of muscle strength is present, employ a method to increase the strength of the weak muscle group. Progressive resistance exercises are used to strengthen weakened groups of muscles. If weakness and shortness occur in different muscle groups but on the same side, attend to the shortness first. Jull and Janda feel the agonists spontaneously increase their strength if the shortened or hypertonic fibers are lengthened.[11]

CONTRAINDICATIONS

Muscle energy procedures should not be requested of a painful muscle or muscle group. They should not be requested of a patient with low vitality who could further be compromised by adding active muscular exertion. Examples include a post-surgical patient or a patient on a monitor and in an intensive care unit who is experiencing a myocardial infarction.

CONCLUSION

Muscle energy techniques are helpful in preparing the soft tissue about an articulation before using a high-velocity low-amplitude (HVLA) technique. After using the muscle energy procedure, it is common to find that the somatic dysfunction has cleared and the HVLA is not needed. Muscle energy procedures are also used to increase coordination of musculoskeletal tissues or to lengthen muscles that are short and inappropriately contracted (hypertonic). The procedures can also be used to strengthen muscles that are weak (hypotonic) and thereby reduce pain, improve symmetry of articular mobility, and enhance a more appropriate circulation of body fluids.

REFERENCES

1. Mitchell FL Sr. Structural pelvic function. In: Barnes MW, ed. *Yearbook of the Academy of Applied Osteopathy*. Indianapolis, Ind: American Academy of Osteopathy; 1958:79.

2. Ruddy TJ. Osteopathic rhythmic resistive duction therapy. In: Barnes MW, ed. *Yearbook of Academy of Applied Osteopathy*. Indianapolis, Ind: American Academy of Osteopathy; 1961:58.

3. Guyer AF. Proprioceptive neuromuscular facilitation for vertebral joint conditions. In: Grieve GP, ed. *Modern Manual Therapy of the Vertebral Column*. New York, NY: Churchill Livingstone; 1986:626.

4. Lewit K, Simons DG. Myofascial pain: relief by post-isometric relaxation. *Arch Phys Med Rehabil*. 1984;65:453–456.

5. Travell JG, Simons DG. *Myofascial Pain and Dysfunction: The Trigger Point Manual*. Vol. 2. Baltimore, Md: Williams & Wilkins; 1992:10.

6. Mitchell Jr FL, Moran PS, Pruzzo NA. *An Evaluation and Treatment Manual of Osteopathic Muscle Energy Procedures*. Valley Park, Mo: Mitchell, Moran, and Pruzzo; 1979.

7. Goodridge JP. Muscle energy technique: definition, explanation, methods of procedures. *JAOA*. 1981;81:249–254.

8. Rash PJ, Burke RK: *Kinesiology and Applied Anatomy. The Science of Human Movement*. 6th ed. Philadelphia, Pa: Lea & Febiger; 1979.

9. Mitchell Jr FL, Moran PS, Pruzzo NA. *An Evaluation and Treatment Manual of Osteopathic Manipulative Procedure*. 2nd ed. Kansas City, Mo: Institute for Continuing Education in Osteopathic Principles, Inc; 1973:325.

10. Kuchera WA, Kuchera ML. *Osteopathic Principles in Practice*. 2nd ed. rev. Columbus, Ohio: Greyden Press; 1994:301.

11. Jull GA, Janda V. Muscles and motor control in low back pain; assessment and management. In: Twomaey LT, Taylor JR, eds. *Physical Therapy for the Low Back*. New York: Churchill Livingstone; 1987:272.

54. **Muscle Energy Treatment Techniques for Specific Areas**

JOHN P. GOODRIDGE AND WILLIAM A. KUCHERA

Key Concepts

- **Muscle energy techniques for axial skeleton, upper and lower extremities, and nonarticular surfaces**

- **Positional diagnosis and restricted motion descriptions of dysfunctions**

- **Procedures using resistance and localization of force**

This chapter presents muscle energy techniques for the axial skeleton, the upper and lower extremity, and some nonarticular structures. The axial skeleton is divided into regions according to segments that may be manipulated in a similar manner or that have special considerations for treatment. These are:

Occipitoatlantal (OA) region
Atlantoaxial (AA) region
Typical cervical region (C2-C7)
Upper thoracic region (T1-T4)
Lower thoracic region (T5-T10)
Lumbar region (T11-L5)
Pelvis (pelvic bones, sacrum, and pubes)

Muscle energy treatment for somatic dysfunction of the upper and lower extremities is presented.

Before a therapeutic procedure is performed, a working diagnosis must be postulated and a visual image of the dysfunction and the direction of therapeutic forces developed. In the following examples of treatment procedures, somatic dysfunctions are described as a positional (static) diagnosis and then as the motion that is restricted. For the extremities, the diagnoses are described only as restriction of motion without a positional diagnosis. Only examples of muscle energy techniques are presented. You may wish to use a modification of an example or design a procedure of your own that adheres to the principles and still achieves the objective.

Terms and their meanings include:

Flexion (F) means forward bending
Extension (E) means backward bending
(S) means side-bending
(R) means rotation

Each is followed by subscript R for right or L for left. Rotation and side-bending movements in the vertebral column are cou-

pled motions. Activation of either the rotation or the side-bending preference automatically produces the other plane of motion.

Descriptions include the phrase "to initial resistance," which means the beginning increase of resistance. Fred Mitchell, Sr. described this as the feather edge of resistance. It must be emphasized that the more localized the contractile force of the muscle fibers when using muscle energy activation, the more effective the treatment and the less intrinsic forces needed. The intrinsic force (patient effort) is balanced by extrinsic force (physician resistance).

After a sufficient muscular effort by the patient is equally balanced by the resistance of the physician, the physician asks the patient to relax. The physician relaxes resistive force simultaneously with the patient and tries very hard not to push into the resistance as the patient relaxes. To take up slack means to move to the next initial resistance after the isometric procedure has changed the tissue resistance and moved the restrictive barrier closer to the physiologic barrier.

When rib dysfunction is present, there is tenderness to palpation. A first rib somatic dysfunction is tender over the very posterior aspect of the rib near the rib head. Ribs 2-10 tend to have tenderness to palpation over the posterior angles when somatic dysfunction is present. Pump-handle somatic dysfunction often also produces subjective pain anteriorly in the area of the costochondral junction[1] or midclavicular line; bucket-handle somatic dysfunction also produces subjective pain at the midaxillary line.[1]

When nonneutral somatic dysfunction occurs in the thoracic or lumbar spine (i.e., in flexion or extension), it usually involves a single segment, for example, T8 E $S_R R_R$.

The following steps present the principle of a muscle energy procedure to lengthen shortened or hypertonic muscles and/or fascia. The last several steps are repeated for each procedure. This format was adopted to assist anyone looking in the book for one specific procedure.

1. Make an accurate diagnosis.
2. Move the body part to initial resistance of a specific motion.
3. While holding this position, instruct the patient to exert a gentle muscular effort against your counterforce. Explain the direction in which the patient is to move the limb, trunk, or head; the intensity of contraction; and the duration of contraction. The patient's contraction must be perceived by the physician as firm and sustained. This usually requires only a few (3–5) seconds.
4. Direct the patient to gently ease the isometric contraction as you simultaneously reduce your counterforce.

5. Maintain your support and wait until the monitoring hand or finger senses the relaxation of area tissues before you move the body part to the next initial resistance.

6. Repeat the above steps until there is no further increase in the range of motion obtained after the patient relaxes. The quality of response often peaks by the third excursion and decreases thereafter.

7. Reevaluate for change in the original dysfunction (retest).

Localization of your force is more important than intensity of force. Localization depends on your palpatory proprioceptive perception of movement (or resistance to movement) at or about a specific articulation. Such perception enables you to make subtle assessments about a dysfunction and to create variations of suggested treatment procedures.

Monitoring and confining forces to the muscle group or level of somatic dysfunction involved are important for achieving desirable changes. Poor results are most often due to improperly localized forces, often with excessive patient effort. When your muscle energy activation introduces motion a segment or two below the dysfunctional one, the chance for success is diminished because the forces have been misdirected, almost as if they had been dissipated. Poor results may also be due to the presence of another somatic dysfunction that interferes with your present treatment. An example is if the presence of a restriction in side-bending at a segment superior to the one identified for treatment interferes with the localization of the muscle fibers at the inferior level. In this example, the superior segment needs treatment first.

CERVICAL SOMATIC DYSFUNCTION

Occipitoatlantal Joint

SINGLE PLANE

Positional Diagnosis

OA E; OA extended; occiput (C0) is extended on the atlas (C1); O E.

Restriction

OA restricted F; OA restriction of flexion; occipital (C0) restriction of flexion on the atlas (C1).

Objective

Increase occipital (C0) flexion on the atlas (C1).

Position

Supine (Fig. 54.1).

Procedure

1. Sit at the head of the table.
2. Place one hand at the external occipital protuberance and the

fingers of the other hand on the forehead over the metopic suture.

3. Forward bend the occiput to initial resistance of the occiput on the atlas.

4. Direct the patient to "Lift chin toward the ceiling," extending the occiput in relation to the atlas (or have the patient look hard toward the top of his or her head). This action needs to generate only a few ounces of force.

5. Exert an equal amount of counterforce through your hand and fingers.

6. Maintain these forces long enough to sense the patient's contractile force at the localized segment or area (usually 3–5 seconds).

7. Direct the patient to relax the muscular effort; simultaneously cease your counterforce.

8. Wait 2 seconds for the tissues to relax, then take up the slack to the new point of initial resistance.

9. Repeat until the best possible increase of motion is obtained.

10. Retest.

Positional Diagnosis

OA F; OA flexed; occiput (C0) is flexed on the atlas (C1); O F.

Restriction

OA restricted E; OA restriction of extension; occiput (C0) restriction of extension on the atlas (C1).

Objective

Increase occipital (C0) extension on the atlas (C1).

Position

Supine (Fig. 54.2).

Procedure

1. Sit at the head of the table.
2. Place one hand at the external occipital protuberance and other hand with your fingers on the patient's forehead.
3. Backward bend to initial resistance of occipital extension. This is localization.
4. Direct the patient to "Tuck your chin toward your throat" (or "Look hard toward your feet").
5. Exert an equal amount of counterforce through the hand and fingers.
6. Maintain the forces long enough to sense the patient's contractile force at the localized segment or area (usually 3–5 seconds). This is monitoring.
7. Direct the patient to gently cease the directive force; cease your counterforce gently; do these simultaneously.
8. Wait 2 seconds for the tissues to relax, then take up the slack to the new point of initial resistance.
9. Repeat until the best possible increase of motion is obtained.
10. Retest.

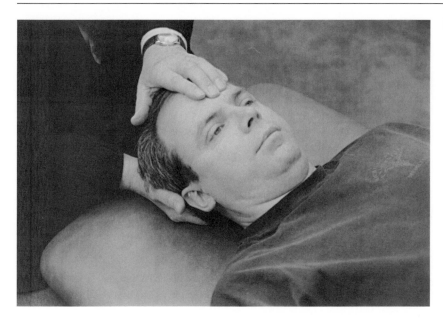

Figure 54.1. Treatment for occiput extended.

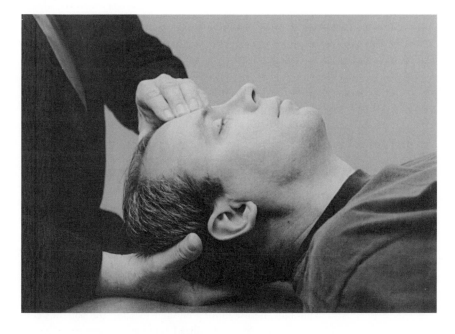

Figure 54.2. Treatment for occiput flexed.

MULTIPLE PLANE

Positional Diagnosis

OA S_L R_R; occiput (C0) is side-bent left and rotated right on the atlas (C1);O (C0) S_L R_R.

Restriction

OA restricted S_R R_L; occipital (C0) restriction of side-bending right and rotating left on atlas (C1).

Objective

Increase occipital (C0) right side-bending and left rotation on the atlas (C1). In this example, emphasis is on the side-bending.

Position

Supine (Fig. 54.3).

Figure 54.3.   Treatment for side-bent left, rotated right.

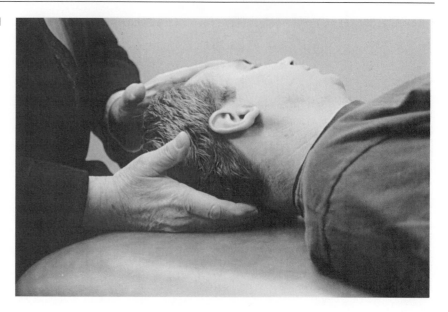

Procedure

1. Stand or sit at the head of the table.
2. Place the distal pad of one finger (index or middle finger) of right hand against the posterolateral portion of the patient's right OA joint to monitor tissue response and movement at that area.
3. Place the palmar surface of the left hand and fingers against the left side of the patient's head.
4. Begin side-bending right from a negative degree of side-bending left. Start your right side-bending from left of the midline, so you are certain to feel the beginning of the resistance. This is localization.
5. Monitor with the finger of your right hand for beginning tension at the right OA joint.
6. Direct the patient to use a small amount of force to side-bend the head toward your left hand while you exert an equal amount of counterforce. (Instruct the patient, "Move your left ear toward your left shoulder.")
7. Maintain the forces long enough to sense the patient's contractile force at the localized segment or area (usually 3–5 seconds). This is monitoring.
8. Direct the patient to gently cease the directive force; cease your counterforce gently; do these simultaneously.
9. Wait 2 seconds for the tissues to relax, and then take up the slack to the new point of initial resistance.
10. Repeat until the best possible increase of motion is obtained.
11. Retest.

Objective

Increase occipital (C0) right side-bending and left rotation on the atlas (C1). In this example, emphasis is on the rotation, using the oculocephalogyric reflex.[2]

Position

Supine (Fig. 54.4).

Procedure

1. Stand or sit at the head of the table.
2. Place the distal pad of one finger (index or middle finger) of the right hand against the posterolateral portion of the patient's right OA joint to monitor tissue response and movement at that area.
3. Place the palmar surface of the left hand and fingers against the left side of the patient's head.
4. From a left side-bending position, translate the head slightly to the left to introduce right side-bending. This permits you to better feel the beginning of the resistance to right side-bending.
5. Rotate the occiput left to initial resistance. This is localization.
6. Direct the patient, "Look hard to the right with your eyes," while equally countering this effort with your right hand.
7. Maintain the forces long enough to sense the patient's contractile force at the localized segment or area (usually 3–5 seconds). This is monitoring.
8. Direct the patient to gently cease the directive force; cease your counterforce gently; do these simultaneously.
9. Wait 2 seconds for the tissues to relax, then take up the slack to the new point of initial resistance.
10. Repeat until the best possible increase of motion is obtained.
11. Retest.

Atlantoaxial Joint

POSITIONAL DIAGNOSIS

AA R_R; C1 R_R; atlas (C1) is rotated right on the axis (C2).

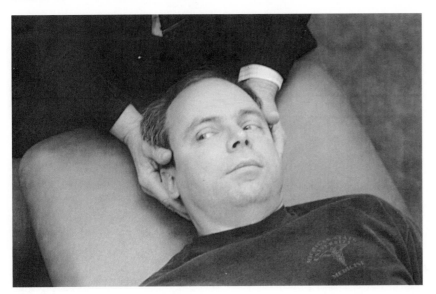

Figure 54.4. Treatment for occiput side-bent left, rotated right using the oculocephalogyric reflex.

RESTRICTION

AA restricted R_L; atlas (C1) is restricted in rotation left on the axis (C2).

Objective

Increase left rotation of the atlas (C1) on the axis (C2). In this example, the neck is at neutral and emphasis is on neck rotation.

Position

Supine (Fig. 54.5).

Procedure

1. Sit at the head of the table.
2. Cradle the occiput in your hands and flex the patient's cervical spine enough to straighten the cervical curve.
3. Place the first two fingers of each hand behind the AA joint.
4. Maintain position of the fingers while letting the patient's head backward bend to the level of the AA joint. This relative extension aids in localization.
5. Rotate the atlas to the left to the point of initial resistance and hold. This is localization.
6. Direct the patient, "Gently rotate your head to the right," while equally exerting counterforce through the fingers and hands.
7. Maintain the forces long enough to sense the patient's contractile force localize at the segment or area (usually 3–5 seconds). This is monitoring.
8. Direct the patient to gently cease the directive force; cease your counterforce gently; do these simultaneously.
9. Wait 2 seconds for the tissues to relax, then take up the slack to the new point of initial resistance.

10. Repeat until the best possible increase of motion is obtained.
11. Retest.

Objective

Increase left rotation of the atlas (C1) on the axis (C2). Use the oculocephalogyric reflex for activation by having the patient move the eyes in multiple directions.

Position

Supine (Fig. 54.6).

Procedure

1. Sit at the head of the table.
2. Cradle the occiput in your hands and flex the patient's cervical spine enough to straighten the cervical curve.
3. Place the first two fingers of each hand behind the AA joint.
4. Maintain position of the fingers while letting the patient's head backward bend to the AA joint.
5. Rotate the atlas to the left to initial resistance and hold. This is localization.
6. Direct the patient, "Look hard to the right with your eyes," while equally exerting counterforce through the fingers and hands.
7. Maintain the forces long enough to sense the patient's contractile force at the localized segment or area (usually 3–5 seconds). This is monitoring.
8. Direct patient, "Now look forward," and also cease your counterforce gently; do these simultaneously.
9. Wait 2 seconds for the tissues to relax, then take up the slack to the new point of initial resistance.
10. Repeat until the best possible increase of motion is obtained.
11. Retest.

Figure 54.5.   Treatment for atlas rotated right.

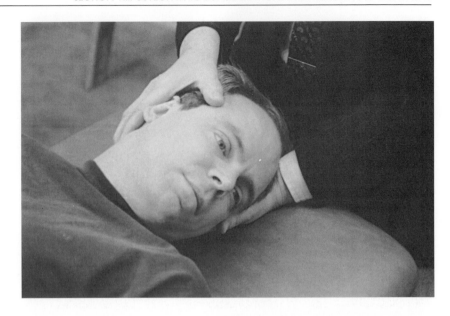

Figure 54.6.   Treatment for atlas rotated right using oculocephalogyric reflex.

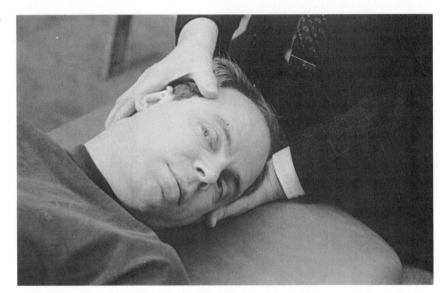

Objective

Increase left rotation of the atlas (C1) on the axis (C2). The entire neck is forward bent and emphasis is on the rotation of the neck.

Position

Supine (Fig. 54.7).

Procedure

1. Stand or sit at the head of the table.
2. Hold the patient's head with both hands, flex the patient's neck to its limit during this technique. This locks out lower cervical motion.
3. Rotate the patient's head left to initial resistance. This is localization.
4. Support the patient's head with your left hand (the posterior hand).
5. Place the right hand (anterior hand) on the anterior presenting side of the patient's face with the thumb along the forehead.
6. Direct the patient to use a small amount of force to rotate head right toward your right hand (hand on the patient's face) and offer equal counterforce.
7. Maintain these forces long enough to sense the patient's contractile force at the localized segment or area (usually 3–5 seconds). This is monitoring.
8. Direct the patient to gently cease the directive force; cease your counterforce gently; do these simultaneously.
9. Wait 2 seconds for the tissues to relax, then take up the slack to the new point of initial resistance.
10. Repeat until the best possible increase of motion is obtained.
11. Retest.

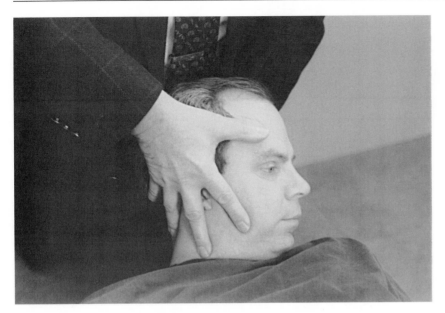

Figure 54.7. Treatment for atlas rotated left with neck flexed.

Typical Cervicals

MULTIPLE PLANE

The typical cervical spine has been arbitrarily divided to include C2-6 because C7 tends to act more like an upper thoracic segment. The inferior facets of C7 are more like the facets of the upper thoracic vertebrae.

Positional Diagnosis

C5 S_LR_L; C5 is side-bent and rotated left.

Restriction

C5 restricted S_RR_R; right rotation and right side-bending is restricted at C5.

Note: If the resistance to translation is greatest when the segment is extended, extension should be introduced, localized at that segment, and treated at that position to increase side-bending and rotation to the same side.

If resistance is greatest when the segment is flexed, flexion should be introduced, localized at that segment, and treated at that position to increase side-bending and rotation to the same side.

Objective

Increase right rotation, right side-bending, and extension of C5. Use oculocephalogyric reflex for activation.

Position

Supine (Fig. 54.8).

Procedure

1. Stand at the head of the table.

2. Cradle the head and neck in both hands and flex the neck to straighten the cervical curve.
3. Place the first two fingers of each hand on the C5 joint.
4. Let the head extend in a controlled manner to backward bend the cervical spine down to the fingers at the C5 joint. This aids in localization at C5.
5. Rotate C5 right to its initial resistance and hold to monitor. (The left hand is more supportive to head and neck as the right hand monitors motion over the right C5 joint at the articular column.) This is localization.
6. Direct the patient, "Look sharply to the left with your eyes."
7. Exert equal counterforce through the fingers and hands.
8. Maintain the forces long enough to sense the patient's contractile force at the localized segment or area (usually 3–5 seconds). This is monitoring.
9. Direct the patient to "look forward"; cease your counterforce gently; do these simultaneously.
10. Wait 2 seconds for the tissues to relax, then take up the slack to the new point of initial resistance.
11. Repeat until the best possible increase of motion is obtained.
12. Retest.

Objective

Increase right side-bending and rotation of C5. Patient side-bends or rotates the neck.

Position

Supine (Fig. 54.9).

Procedure

1. Stand or sit at the head of the table.
2. Place the finger of the right hand on the posterolateral area

Figure 54.8. Treatment for C5 flexed rotated and side-bent right using oculocephalogyric reflex.

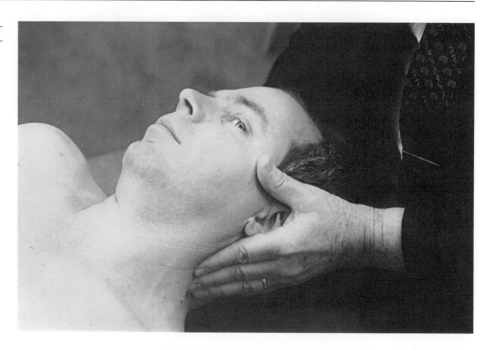

Figure 54.9. Treatment for C5 flexed rotated and side-bent left.

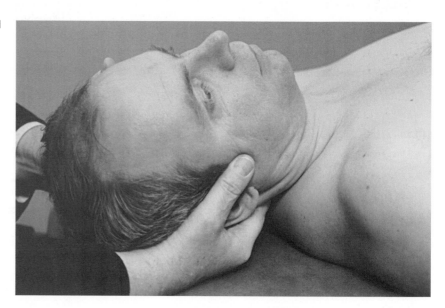

of the right articular pillar of C5 and to the superior tip of the pillar of C6 to monitor tissue response and movement.

3. Place the left hand on the left side of the patient's head to introduce side-bending right and rotation right to the point of its initial resistance. This is localization.

4. Direct the patient to make a small side-bending and/or rotation effort against your left hand or fingers.

5. Offer a counterforce equal to patient's force.

6. Maintain the forces long enough to sense the patient's contractile force at the localized segment or area (usually 3–5 seconds). This is monitoring.

7. Direct the patient to gently cease the directive force; cease your counterforce gently; do these simultaneously.

8. Wait 2 seconds for the tissues to relax, then take up the slack to the new point of initial resistance.

9. Repeat until the best possible increase of motion is obtained.

10. Retest.

THORACIC SOMATIC DYSFUNCTION

Upper Thoracic Spine

MULTIPLE PLANE

Positional Diagnosis

T3 E S_LR_L; T3 is extended, side-bent left, and rotated left.

Restriction

T3 restricted F S_R R_R; there is restriction of flexion, side-bending right, and rotation right at T3.

Objective

Increase the flexion, side-bending right, and rotation right of T3 on T4.

Position

Seated (Fig. 54.10).

Procedure

1. Stand behind or to the right of the patient.
2. Place the middle finger of your left hand between the spinous processes of T3-T4; index finger is between T2 and T3, and the third finger is between T4 and T5. (This is a good contact to appreciate localization of forces; you may prefer to place your fingers to the left or both sides of the T3 spinous process.)
3. Place your right hand on top of the patient's head to passively produce flexion, right side-bending, and right rotation of T3 to the point of initial resistance. This is localization.
4. Direct the patient to extend the lower cervical and upper thoracic areas to include T3.[a]
5. Offer counterforce equal to patient's force (of about 3 pounds).
6. Maintain the forces long enough to sense the patient's contractile force at the localized segment or area (usually 3–5 seconds). This is monitoring.
7. Direct the patient to gently cease the directive force; cease your counterforce gently; do these simultaneously.
8. Wait 2 seconds for the tissues to relax, then take up the slack to the new point of initial resistance.
9. Repeat until the best possible increase of motion is obtained.
10. Retest.

Positional Diagnosis

T3 F S_L R_L; T3 is flexed side-bent left and rotated left.

Restriction

T3 restricted E S_R R_R; there is restriction of extension, side-bending right, and rotation right of T3 on T4.

---

[a]Note: From the specific position created prior to activating forces, a patient's extension movement may be directed along a coordinated vector of forces so that it also affects rotation and side-bending; when the patient relaxes this vector of force, a recheck determines that it has produced the desired slack (lengthening or relaxation); if not, then each separate motion may be positioned and activated separately, using the above commands.

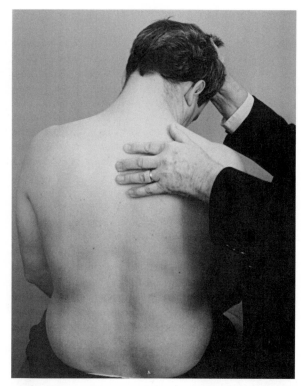

Figure 54.10. Treatment for T3 extended, rotated, and side-bent left.

Objective

Increase extension, right side-bending, and right rotation of T3 on T4 (Fig. 54.11).

Note: The procedure for this diagnosis is like the last procedure. To resolve restriction of extension, position to initial resistance of extension, right side-bending, and right rotation, and then ask the patient to flex the neck and upper thoracic area against your equal counterforce. This procedure may be used to resolve somatic dysfunctions of the lower cervical spine.

Position

T3 N S_L R_R (there is a neutral group curve that is convex right and the apex is at T3); a neutral group curve is side-bent left and its apex at T3 is rotated right.

Restriction

T3 N restricted S_R R_L; T3 is at the apex of a neutral group curve and is found to have restriction of side-bending right and rotating left.

Objective

Increase right side-bending and left rotation of T3 on T4.

Position

Left lateral recumbent (Fig. 54.12).

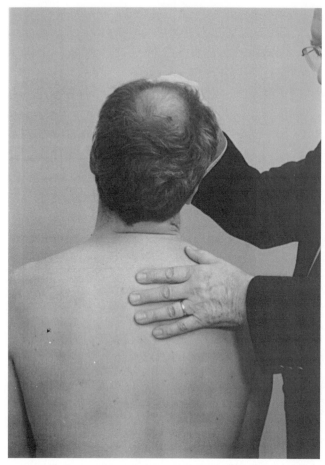

Figure 54.11. Treatment for T3 flexed, rotated, and side-bent left.

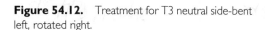

Figure 54.12. Treatment for T3 neutral side-bent left, rotated right.

Procedure

1. Stand facing the patient.
2. Cradle the head and neck in your right arm so you can control the neck in side-bending and the head into rotation.
3. Place the fingers of your left hand at the T3 interspinous ligament.
4. Extend, or flex, the spine down to localize forces at T3.
5. Place the thumb or first two fingers of your left hand on the left transverse process of T3 to monitor motion.
6. With your right arm, side-bend the patient's head to the right and rotate it to the left down to T3.
7. Direct the patient, "Gently pull your head and neck toward the table." You equally resist this effort with gentle counterforce through your right arm.
8. Maintain the forces long enough to sense the patient's contractile force at the localized segment or area (usually 3–5 seconds). This is monitoring.
9. Direct the patient to gently cease the directive force; cease your counterforce gently; do these simultaneously.
10. Wait 2 seconds for the tissues to relax, then take up the slack to the new point of initial resistance.
11. Repeat until the best possible increase of motion is obtained.
12. Retest.

Lower Thoracic Spine

Note: The lower thoracic region has been arbitrarily divided into the T4-T10 segments. It may extend from T3 or down to T11.

SINGLE PLANE

Positional Diagnosis

T5 E; T5 extended; T5 backward bent.

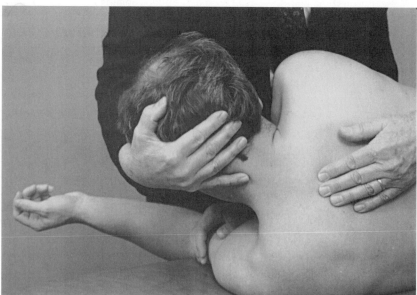

Restriction

T5 restricted F; T5 restriction of flexion; T5 restricted of forward bending.

Objective

Increase forward bending of T5 on T6.

Position

Seated (Fig. 54.13).

Procedure

1. Stand behind the patient.
2. Palpate the spine of T6 (one spine below the involved vertebral segment) with one hand.
3. With your other hand above the vertebral segment with the somatic dysfunction, guide the patient into forward bending to initial resistance (until tension is palpated at the T6 segment with the palpating hand). This is localization.
4. With one of your hands a few segments above T5 and the other a few segments below T5, guide the patient to "bend backwards, right here" at the T5-T6 interspinous area and resist this effort with equal counterforce.
5. Maintain the forces long enough to sense the patient's contractile force at the localized segment or area (usually 3–5 seconds). This is monitoring.
6. Direct the patient to gently cease the directive force; cease your counterforce gently; do these simultaneously.
7. Wait 2 seconds for the tissues to relax, then take up the slack to the new point of initial resistance.
8. Repeat until the best possible increase of motion is obtained.
9. Retest.

Positional Diagnosis

T5 F; T5 flexed; T5 forward bends.

Restriction

T5 restricted E; restriction of backward bending at T5, T5 restriction of extension.

Objective

Increase backward bending (extension) of T5 on T6.

Position

Seated (Fig. 54.14).

Procedure

1. Stand behind the patient.
2. Palpate the T5-T6 interspace with your caudad hand.
3. Place your cephalic hand on the patient's upper sternum.
4. Extend the patient's upper thoracics until motion is palpated at the T5 interspinous ligament. This is localization.

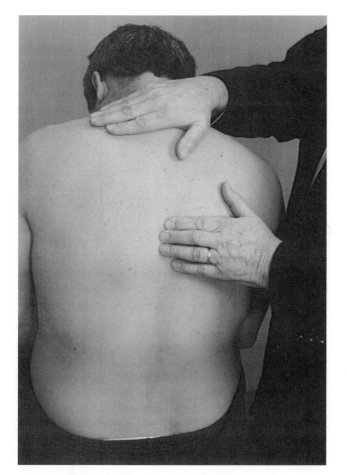

Figure 54.13. Treatment for T5 extended.

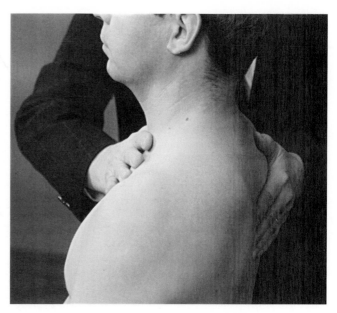

Figure 54.14. Treatment for T5 flexed.

5. Direct the patient to forward bend against the equal counterforce provided through your cephalic hand.

6. Maintain the forces long enough to sense the patient's contractile force at the localized segment or area (usually 3–5 seconds). This is monitoring.

7. Direct the patient to gently cease the directive force and cease your counterforce gently; do these simultaneously.

8. Wait 2 seconds for the tissues to relax, then take up the slack to the new point of initial resistance.

9. Repeat until the best possible increase of motion is obtained.

10. Retest.

MULTIPLE PLANE

Note: Dysfunctions involving multiple segments of the thoracic spine are usually treated at the apex of the curve where there is the greatest side-bending in one direction and rotation in the other direction as diagnosed by motion testing.

Positional Diagnosis

T6 N S_L R_R; a neutral group curve is convex to the right with its apex at T6, where T6 is side-bent left and rotated right.

Restriction

T6 N restricted S_R R_L; T6 is at the apex of a neutral group curve and is found to have restriction of side-bending right and rotating left.

Objective

Increase right side-bending and left rotation of T6 on T7. This examples shows rotation activation.

Position

Seated (Figs. 54.15 and 54.16).

Procedure

1. Stand or sit behind the patient.

2. Instruct the patient, "Put your left hand behind your neck and your right hand on your left elbow."

3. Put your left arm under the patient's left arm and your left hand on the patient's right biceps area to control, position, and balance the patient.

4. Place the fingers of your right hand on the patient's spine at the T6-7 interspinous area.

5. Have the patient sit up straight until there is motion palpated at the T6 interspinous area.

6. Adjust the sagittal plane to maintain localization while side-bending the patient to the right down to the T6 level.

7. Move your right hand to place the thenar/hypothenar eminence on the right transverse process of T6.

8. Maintaining the side-bending motions localized at T6, rotate T6 to the left to initial resistance.

9. Instruct the patient, "Rotate to the right against my hand," as your right hand exerts an equal amount of counterforce,

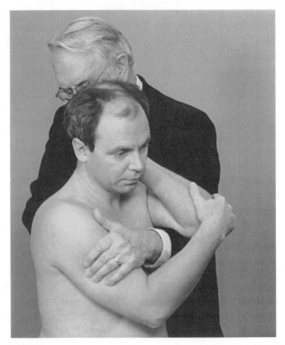

Figure 54.15. Treatment for T6 neutral, side-bent left, rotated right; anterior view.

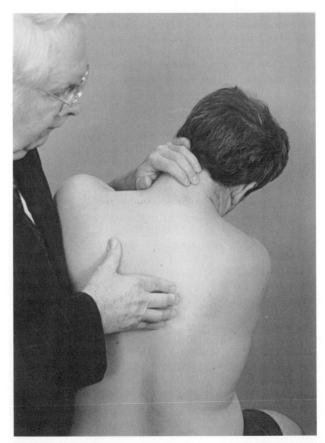

Figure 54.16. Treatment for T6 neutral, side-bent left, rotated right; posterior view.

or, "Side-bend your back to the left," as you exert an equal amount of counterforce through your left arm and shoulder.

10. Maintain the forces long enough to sense the patient's contractile force at the localized segment or area (usually 3–5 seconds). This is monitoring.
11. Direct the patient to gently cease the directive force and cease your counterforce gently; do these simultaneously.
12. Wait 2 seconds for the tissues to relax, then take up the slack to the new point of initial resistance.
13. Repeat until the best possible increase of motion is obtained.
14. Retest.

Objective

Increase side-bending right and rotation left of T6 on T7. This example shows side-bending activation.

Position

Supine.

Procedure

1. Sit at the right side of the patient.
2. Side-bend the patient down to T6 by cradling the head, neck, and shoulders with the left arm.
3. Pass the right arm under the patient's spine at T6; with the fingers of your right hand, pull the T6 spinous process toward you to encourage rotation of T6 to the left. This is also localization.
4. Direct the patient to side-bend the shoulders (or the hips) toward the left as you maintain equal counterforce through the shoulders (or hips).
5. Maintain the forces long enough to sense the patient's contractile force at the localized segment or area (usually 3–5 seconds). This is monitoring.
6. Direct the patient to gently cease the directive force; cease your counterforce gently; do these simultaneously.
7. Wait 2 seconds for the tissues to relax, then take up the slack to the new point of initial resistance. Repeat until the best possible increase of motion is obtained.
8. Retest.

Positional Diagnosis

T7 E S_L R_L; T7 extended, side-bent left, and rotated left.

Restriction

T7 restricted F S_R R_R; restriction of flexion, side-bending right, and rotating right of T7 on T8.

Objective

Increase flexion, side-bending right, and rotation right of T6 on T7.

Position

Seated

Procedure

1. Stand behind and to the right side of the patient.
2. Place your right axilla superior to the patient's right acromioclavicular joint (to induce right side-bending).
3. Place your right forearm across the patient's upper anterior chest.
4. With your right hand, hold the patient's left shoulder (to induce right rotation).
5. Monitor at the T7-T8 interspinous space with the fingers of your left hand.
6. Position T7 to initial resistance of flexion, right rotation, and right side-bending.
7. Localize by monitoring the movement response at T7 with your left hand.
8. Direct the patient, "Turn to the left."
9. Offer counterforce equal to patient's directed force (about 3 pounds).
10. Maintain the forces long enough to sense the patient's contractile force at the localized segment or area (usually 3–5 seconds). This is monitoring.
11. Direct the patient to gently cease the directive force; cease your counterforce gently; do these simultaneously.
12. Wait 2 seconds for the tissues to relax, then take up the slack to the new point of initial resistance.
13. Repeat until the best possible increase of motion is obtained.
14. Retest.

Positional Diagnosis

T9 F $R_L S_L$; T9 flexed, rotated left, side-bent left.

Restriction

T9 restricted E $R_R S_R$; T9 is restricted in extension, side-bending right, and rotating right.

Objective

Increase T9 extending, side-bending right, and rotating right.

Position

Seated (Fig. 54.17).

Procedure

1. Stand to the right side of the patient.
2. Drape your right forearm over the posterior aspect of the patient's shoulder and place your left hand at the T9 interspace of the patient.
3. Direct the patient to backward bend until extension at T9 is palpated by your left hand.
4. Passively rotate right, and right side-bend the patient down to the T9 segment, to the point of initial tissue resistance. This is localization.
5. Direct the patient to rotate to the left as you equally resist the effort with your right hand (on the patient's shoulders).

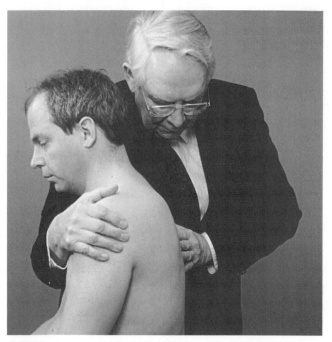

Figure 54.17.   Treatment for T9 flexed, rotated left, side-bent left.

6. Maintain the forces long enough to sense the patient's contractile force at the localized segment or area (usually 3–5 seconds). This is monitoring.
7. Direct the patient to gently cease the directive force; cease your counterforce gently; do these simultaneously.
8. Wait 2 seconds for the tissues to relax, then take up the slack to the new point of initial resistance.
9. Repeat until the best possible increase of motion is obtained.
10. Retest.

RIB SOMATIC DYSFUNCTIONS

Rib somatic dysfunctions are divided into two groups according to the similarity of manipulative treatment methods for each group. These two groups are ribs 2-10 and ribs 1, 11, and 12. Rib 1 is attached to the sternum through a synchondrosis and so is very stable. It elevates and depresses and does not have the pump-handle or bucket-handle motions of ribs 2-10. Ribs 2-10 have varying proportions of motion about two functional axes, depending upon their location in the rib cage. Motion about a rib's "transverse" axis produces a pump-handle-like motion with the greatest motion occurring at the anterior midclavicular line; there is a lesser arc of motion in the opposite direction at the posterior part of the rib. Motion about a rib's "longitudinal" axis results in a bucket-handle-like motion with the most motion occurring at the mid-axillary line. The upper ribs (2-7) tend to have more pump-handle motion, and the lower ribs (8-10) tend to have more bucket handle motion. Ribs 2-10 are all believed to have some element of each motion. Ribs 11 and 12 have no anterior connection to cartilage or bone, and their motion characteristics are different from the other ribs. They have caliper or pincer motion, which is characterized by a slight elevation and

lateral spread of their distal ends during inhalation and a depression and approximation with exhalation.

A group of ribs held in inhalation may respond to manipulative treatment of the lowest rib in the group. A group of ribs held in exhalation may respond to successful manipulation of the most superior rib in the group. As a general rule, ribs with pump-handle somatic dysfunctions tend to occur in groups, and bucket-handle rib somatic dysfunctions tend to be single. Rib somatic dysfunctions are also found secondary to a primary somatic dysfunction of their related thoracic vertebrae.

A functional anatomic point of clinical importance is that each of the sympathetic chain ganglia of nerves T1-12 lie in the prevertebral fascia which also incorporates the rib head. This provides a functional link between visceral hypersympathetic activity present in disease processes and the therapeutic clinical effects observed following rib raising manipulative treatment.

Typical Ribs

INHALATION

Positional Diagnosis

Inhalation left 6th rib; L rib 6 ↑ ; left 6th rib moves fully in inhalation; left 6th rib is held in inhalation.

Restriction

Left 6th rib restriction of exhalation; left 6th rib stops early in exhalation; extent and duration of exhalation movement of the 6th rib is decreased.

Note: The intercostal muscles are considered to influence the inhalation and exhalation dysfunctions and are also affected by the muscle energy treatment.

Objective

Increase movement of the left 6th rib during exhalation. This technique can be modified for treating either bucket-handle or pump-handle rib somatic dysfunction.

Position

Supine (Fig. 54.18).

Procedure

1. Stand at the head of the table and slightly to left side.
2. Place the thumb and thenar eminence of your left hand on the lateral or anterior portion of the rib cage, whichever has the most motion, i.e., on the side of the rib cage for ribs that have more bucket-handle motion and at anterior clavicular line to treat a rib exhibiting more pump-handle motion.
   a. Position for pump handle: Place your left thumb superior to the left rib 6 at the anterior midclavicular line. With your right hand, flex the patient's head, neck, and upper thoracic vertebrae until your left thumb feels movement at rib 6.

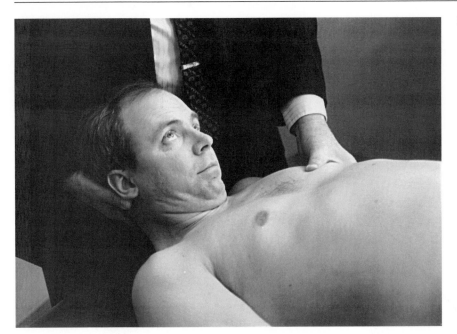

Figure 54.18. Treatment for left 6th inhaled rib.

b. Position for bucket handle: Place your left thumb superior to left rib 6 at the midaxillary line.

3. Direct the patient to reach the left arm along the table toward the left knee, or with your right forearm under the upper thoracic vertebrae, side-bend the area to the left until you feel movement at rib 6.

4. Instruct the patient, "Take a deep breath in and out through the mouth."

5. Follow the 6th rib into its caudal movement during exhalation. During this exhalation you might also instruct the patient, "Reach with your left arm toward your feet."

6. Hold the rib at its new position as the patient inhales deeply; resist the movement of the rib with inhalation.

7. Follow the 6th rib in its further caudal movement during the next exhalation and hold.

8. Repeat until the best possible increase of motion is obtained.

9. Retest.

EXHALATION

Note: The intercostal muscles are considered to influence inhalation and exhalation rib dysfunctions and are affected by muscle energy activation. Other muscles are recruited for muscle energy treatment of the ribs. Proper positioning of the patient improves the effectiveness of muscle energy activation. This "positioning" might include side-bending to the opposite side or placing the arm or forearm on the side of the exhalation rib above the head or on the forehead. Tables 54.1 and 54.2 list the muscles that are used in muscle energy activation of techniques designed to elevate depressed ribs.

Positional Diagnosis

Exhalation rib; rib ↓ ; rib moves fully in exhalation; rib held in exhalation.

Table 54.1
Muscles Used to Elevate Ribs with Exhalation Somatic Dysfunction

Muscles Activated	Ribs Affected
Anterior and medial scalenes	Rib 1
Posterior scalene	Rib 2
Pectoralis minor	Ribs 3–5
Serratus anterior	Ribs 6–9
Latissimus dorsi	Ribs 10–12

Restriction

Rib restricted of inhalation; rib stops early in inhalation; movement during inhalation is decreased.

Objective

Increase the duration of the superior movement of a rib during inhalation.

Position

Supine (Fig. 54.19).

Procedure

1. Stand at side opposite the rib dysfunction, and face the patient.

2. Pass your caudal arm across the patient's anterior chest and then posterior to the chest to contact and pull caudad and laterally on the posterior angle of the rib being treated.

3. Place the patient's arm in a position that localizes an effective muscular pull on the rib being treated (Table 54.1.)

4. Instruct the patient to move the head (for ribs 1 or 2) or the arm (for ribs 3-10) as needed to activate the proper muscle

Table 54.2
Positioning of the Patient's Arm for the Most Effective Muscle Pull during Muscle Energy Activation

Muscle	Patient Position	Isometric Contraction
Anterior and medial scalenes	Arm flexed, placed on forehead, head turned away	Patient attempts to forward bend the head and neck
Posterior scalene	Arm flexed, on forehead, head turned away	Patient presses head and elbow anteriorly
Pectoralis minor	Arm flexed and along side of head	Patient presses elbow toward the sternum
Serratus anterior	With dorsum of hand on forehead, elbow flexed	Patient presses anteriorly
Latissimus dorsi	Arm, with elbow flexed, abducted from 90 to 130° depending on rib being treated	Patient abducts the arm

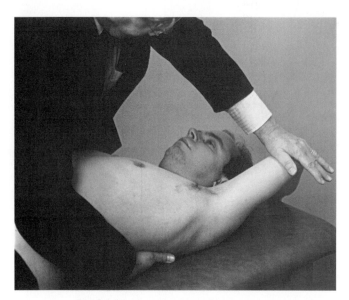

Figure 54.19.   Treatment for exhaled rib.

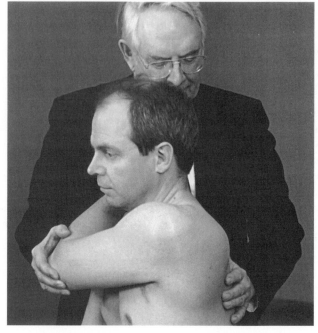

Figure 54.20.   Treatment for left anterior 4th rib.

(see charts above); offer equal counterforce to the patient's effort with your cephalic hand.

5. Maintain the forces long enough to sense the patient's contractile force at the localized segment or area (usually 3–5 seconds). This is monitoring.
6. Direct the patient to gently cease the directive force; cease your counterforce gently; do these simultaneously.
7. Wait 2 seconds for the tissues to relax, then take up the slack to the new point of initial resistance.
8. Repeat until the best possible increase of motion is obtained.
9. Retest.

Anterior Rib

The anatomical concept of a rib anterior visualizes that the head of the rib (ribs 2-9) has moved slightly anteriorly within the demifacets of the costovertebral joint formed by its related two adjacent thoracic vertebrae. Thus, the angle of the rib has moved slightly medial relative to the angles of the ribs superior and inferior to it; and this is obvious to palpation in a sagittal plane medial to the angles of the remaining ribs.

POSITIONAL DIAGNOSIS

Left anterior 4th rib; anterior 4th left rib; rib 4 left anterior.

RESTRICTION

Left 4th rib 4 resists moving posteriorly.

Objective

Move the left 4th rib posteriorly relative to bodies of T4 and T5.

Position

Patient seated (Fig. 54.20).

Procedure

1. Stand behind the patient.
2. Have the patient place the left hand on the right shoulder; left arm bent at elbow and adducted in front of the chest.
3. Place your right hand on patient's left elbow, your left thumb medial to the rib angle of left rib 4.
4. Use your right hand to pull the patient's left elbow to the right in a horizontal plane to the point of initial resistance; your right hand raises or lowers the patient's left elbow until your left thumb feels forces localized at rib 4.

5. Use your left thumb to follow the angle of rib 4 laterally to initial resistance.
6. Direct the patient to press elbow to the left against equal counterforce of your right hand.
7. Maintain the forces long enough to sense the patient's contractile force at the localized segment or area (usually 3–5 seconds). This is monitoring.
8. Direct the patient to gently cease the directive force; cease your counterforce gently; do these simultaneously.
9. Wait 2 seconds for the tissues to relax, then take up the slack to the new point of initial resistance.
10. Repeat until the best possible increase of motion is obtained.
11. Retest.

Atypical Ribs

Though the sternum moves superiorly during deep inhalation, it is clinically observed that the first rib has most of its motion at its posterior end; this may be because its anterior synchondrosis with the sternum permits minimal joint motion. The first rib's primary function seems to be to anchor the upper end of the chest cage during inhalation. With this anchor, the motions of the other ribs is much more effective. For these reasons, the posterior end of the rib near its costotransverse articulation elevates and depresses (slightly) during the breathing cycle. An elevated rib is most common because of the activity of the anterior and medial scalenes during forced inhalation and during normal active motions of the head and arms.

RIB I

Positional Diagnosis

Elevated right first rib; the right first rib elevates fully when the shoulders are depressed (when the patient drops the shoulders) or the patient takes a deep breath.

Restriction

The right first rib stops early or does not move inferiorly when shoulders are shrugged superiorly or the patient exhales completely.

Objective

Move the elevated right first rib inferiorly.

Position

Seated (Fig. 54.21).

Procedure

1. Stand behind the patient with your left foot on the table or stool so the patient's left axilla can be supported by your left knee or thigh.
2. Place your right index finger's metacarpophalangeal joint superiorly against the first rib's tubercle.

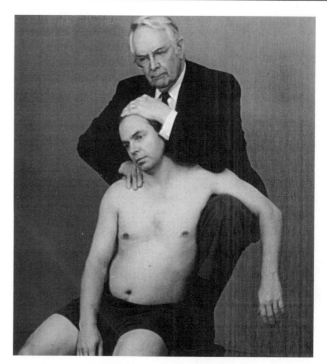

Figure 54.21. Treatment for elevated right first rib.

3. Place the left hand to the left side of the patient's head with your elbow anterior to the patient's left shoulder.
4. Move your left thigh and knee to the left to provide the best support for the patient's trunk.
5. Move the left hand to increase right side-bending and left rotation of T1 so its transverse process moves relatively anterior to the tubercle of the right rib and permit the right rib to slide inferiorly (releasing the rib costovertebral articulation).
6. Use your right metacarpophalangeal joint to take up the slack as the rib moves inferiorly.
7. Direct the patient, "Press your head left against my hand."
8. Offer counterforce with your left hand equal to the patient's force.
9. Maintain the forces long enough to sense the patient's contractile force at the localized segment or area (usually 3–5 seconds). This is monitoring.
10. Direct the patient to gently cease the directive force; cease your counterforce gently; do these simultaneously.
11. Wait 2 seconds for the tissues to relax, then take up the slack to the new point of initial resistance.
12. Repeat until the best possible increase of motion is obtained.
13. Retest.

RIBS 11 AND 12

These ribs also have special movement during breathing. With inhalation they open up in a pincerlike motion, and during exhalation they close. The tips of these ribs elevate and separate from each other during inhalation, and the motion is reversed during exhalation. They lack the axes of motion that are present in the typical ribs, and they do not have anterior attachments to the sternum or the chondral masses. Their somatic dysfunctions are diagnosed as: inhalation 11th (or 12th) rib; and exhalation 11th (or 12th) rib, pincer motion.

Positional Diagnosis

Inhalation left 12th rib; left 12th rib moves fully during inhalation; left rib 12 held in inhalation; L rib 12 ↑ .

Restriction

Left rib 12 has restriction of exhalation; the motion of the left 12th rib stops early during exhalation.

Objective

Move the left 12th rib inferiorly during exhalation.

Position

Prone (Fig. 54.22).

Procedure

1. Stand beside the patient, opposite the side of the affected rib.
2. Place the thumb or thenar eminence of your right hand against the inferior surface of the left 12th rib near its proximal or posterior end (near the vertebra).
3. Reach across the back of the pelvis and contact the patient's left anterior superior iliac spines (ASIS) with your left hand.
4. Apply anterosuperior pressure at the contact point on the posterior end of the 12th rib, and instruct the patient "Exhale; hold your breath; and now pull your left hip toward the table."
5. Maintain the forces long enough to sense the patient's contractile force at the localized segment or area (usually 3–5 seconds). This is monitoring.
6. Direct the patient to gently cease the directive force; cease your counterforce gently; do these simultaneously.

7. Wait 2 seconds for the tissues to relax, then take up the slack to the new point of initial resistance.
8. Repeat until the best possible increase of motion is obtained.
9. Retest.

Positional Diagnosis

Inhalation left 11th rib; left rib moves fully during inhalation; left rib 11 held in inhalation; L rib 11 ↑ .

Restriction

Left rib 11 has restriction of exhalation; the movement of the 11th left rib stops early during exhalation; the extent and duration of its movement during exhalation is decreased.

This procedure is similar to the one used for the inhalation 12th rib except the contraction of the quadratus lumborum muscle pulls on the 12th rib and the intercostal muscle between rib 12 and 11 to encourage the 11th rib to move inferiorly toward an exhalation position. The "right finger fulcrum" is the right thumb pressing anterosuperiorly and slightly laterally at the proximal end of the 11th rib.

Positional Diagnosis

Exhalation left 12th rib; L rib 12 ↓ ; left 12th rib moves fully during exhalation.

Restriction

Left rib 12 has restriction of inhalation; the left 12th rib stops movement early during inhalation; the extent and duration of movement during inhalation is decreased.

Objective

Increase excursion and duration of movement of the left 12th rib during inhalation.

Figure 54.22. Treatment for inhalation left 12th rib.

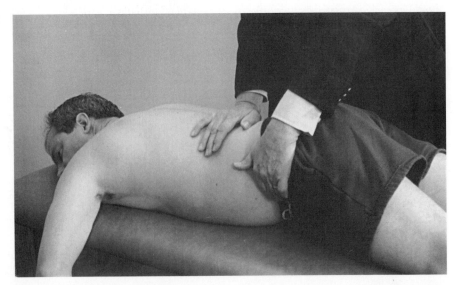

Position

Prone (Fig. 54.23).

Procedure

1. Stand beside the patient opposite to the side of the affected rib.
2. Place the thumb or thenar eminence of your right hand against the shaft of the 12th rib.
3. Use your left hand to reach across and under the left pelvic bone to contact the patient's left ASIS.
4. Hold anterosuperior pressure at the contact point on the 12th rib and ask the patient to, "Take a deep breath in; now exhale deeply and hold it."
5. While the patient holds in exhalation, pull the patient's left innominate posterior and hold.
6. Have the patient pull the left hip toward the table while you offer equal counterforce through your left arm and its hand contact with the ASIS.
7. Maintain the left rotation of the hip and the anterosuperior contact with your right hand while the patient breathes in and then out deeply.
8. Maintain the forces long enough to sense the patient's contractile force at the localized segment or area (usually 3–5 seconds). This is monitoring.
9. Direct the patient to gently cease the directive force; cease your counterforce gently; do these simultaneously.
10. Wait 2 seconds for the tissues to relax, then take up the slack to the new point of initial resistance.
11. Repeat until the best possible increase of motion is obtained.
12. Retest.

Positional Diagnosis

Exhalation 11th left rib; L rib 11 ↓ ; left rib moves fully during exhalation; left 11th rib is held in exhalation.

Restriction

Left rib 11 has restriction of inhalation; excursion during inhalation is decreased.

Objective

Increase excursion of left 11th rib during inhalation.

Position

Prone (Fig. 54.24).

Procedure

1. Stand next to the left side of the patient, facing slightly toward the patient's feet.
2. Instruct the patient to extend the left arm over the head and place your left hand at the patient's left elbow.
3. Find the shaft of the 11th rib with the fingers of your right hand and pull it superiorly to initial resistance.
4. Instruct the patient, "Take in a deep breathe and hold it"; follow the elevation of the rib during inhalation and hold it with the fingers of your right hand, guide the patient into pulling the arm laterally (in an arc) toward the hip. (The isometric contraction of the left latissimus dorsi muscle assists in further elevation of the 11th rib.)
5. Maintain the forces long enough to sense the patient's contractile force at the localized segment or area (usually 3–5 seconds). This is monitoring.
6. Direct the patient to gently cease the directive force; cease your counterforce gently; do these simultaneously.
7. Wait 2 seconds for the tissues to relax, then take up the slack to the new point of initial resistance.
8. Repeat until the best possible increase of motion is obtained.
9. Retest.

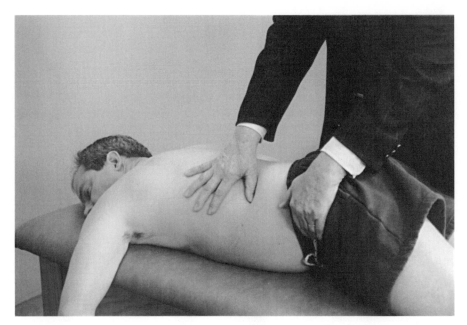

Figure 54.23. Treatment for exhalation left 12th rib.

Figure 54.24. Treatment for exhalation left 11th rib.

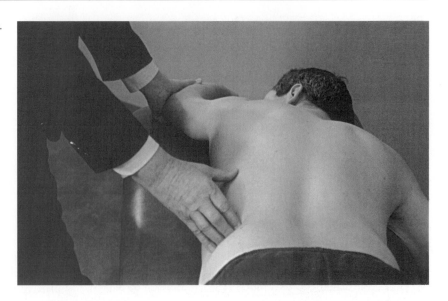

LUMBAR SPINE SOMATIC DYSFUNCTION

Note: The lumbar region has been arbitrarily divided into the T11-L5 segments. It may extend from T10 down to L5.

Single Plane

POSITIONAL DIAGNOSIS

L3 F; L3 flexed; L3 forward bent.

RESTRICTION

L3 restricted E; L3 has restriction of extension; L3 has restriction of backward bending.

Objective

Increase the extension of L3 on L4.

Position

Supine with legs extended (Fig. 54.25).

Procedure

1. Sit beside the patient.
2. Slide one hand under the patient so your fingers can contact the L3 segment; reinforce this hand with your other hand.
3. Apply an anteriorly directed force with the fingers of your hands until extension at L3 is palpated.
4. Instruct the patient, "Flatten (or arch) your back against my hands and the table."
5. Maintain the forces long enough to sense the patient's contractile force at the localized segment or area (usually 3–5 seconds). This is monitoring.
6. Direct the patient to gently cease the directive force; cease your counterforce gently; do these simultaneously.
7. Wait 2 seconds for the tissues to relax, then take up the slack to the new point of initial resistance.

8. Repeat until the best possible increase of motion is obtained.
9. Retest.

POSITIONAL DIAGNOSIS

L3 E; L3 extended; L3 is backward bent.

RESTRICTION

L3 restricted F; L3 has restriction of forward bending.

Objective

Increase the flexion of L3 on L4.

Position

Supine (Fig. 54.26).

Procedure

1. Stand beside the patient.
2. Direct the patient to flex the knees and hips.
3. Pass your caudal arm over the legs to the paraspinal area on the far side of L3 and slide your other hand under the patient to the paraspinal area on the near side of L3.
4. Rest the patient's knees against your chest without inducing any side-bending or rotation, and flex the spine to the L3 area.
5. Guide the patient into gently pushing the knees against your chest in such a way that posterior tension is sensed by your monitoring fingers at the L3 paraspinal area. Equally counter the patient's effort.
6. Maintain and monitor the forces long enough to sense the patient's contractile force at the localized segment or area, usually 3–5 seconds.
7. Direct the patient to gently release the directive force as you gently and simultaneously release your counterforce.

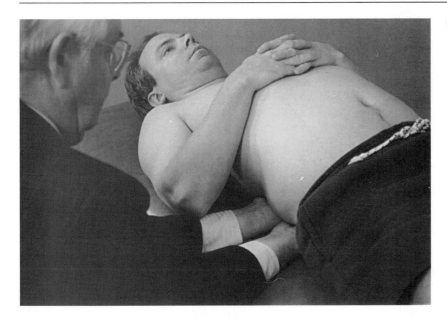

Figure 54.25. Treatment for L3 flexed.

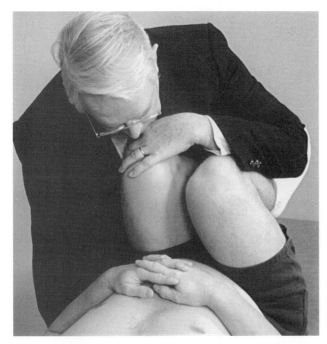

Figure 54.26. Treatment for L3 extended.

8. Wait a few seconds for the tissues to relax, then take up the slack to the new point of initial resistance, i.e., the first indication of a new barrier.
9. Repeat until the best possible increase of motion is obtained.
10. Retest.

Multiple Plane

POSITIONAL DIAGNOSIS

L3 N $S_L R_R$; L3 is at the apex of a neutral group curve and is side-bent left and rotated right.

RESTRICTION

L3 restricted to side-bend right and rotate left.

Objective

Increase right side-bending and left rotation of L3 on L4.

Position

Seated (Fig. 54.27).

Procedure

1. Stand behind the patient.
2. Direct the patient to put the left hand behind the neck and the right hand on the left elbow.
3. Place your left arm under the patient's left arm and place your left hand on patient's right biceps area to control the patient's motion and balance.
4. Place the fingers of your right hand over the interspinous area of L3 to L4.
5. Localize the sagittal plane by having the patient relax into forward bending (slouch or slump) until there motion is felt at the L3-L4 interspinous ligament.
6. Side-bend the patient to the right down to the L3 vertebra. (Note: Some degree of left translation is necessary so that the patient remains balanced over the pelvis as side-bending progresses downward.)
7. Shift your right hand position so that your fingers are over the right transverse process of the L3 vertebra.
8. Rotate L3 to initial resistance of its left rotation and hold it there.
9. Instruct the patient to rotate to the right against your right hand and exert an equal amount of counterforce through

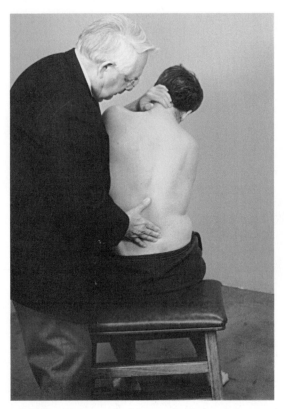

Figure 54.27. Treatment for L3 neutral, side-bent left, rotated right.

your left and right hands. (You could also use instruction to have the patient "Side-bend to the left" against your left arm and shoulder and equally resist that effort.)

10. Maintain and monitor the forces long enough to sense the patient's contractile force at the localized segment or area, usually 3–5 seconds.
11. Direct the patient to gently release the directive force as you gently and simultaneously release your counterforce.
12. Wait a few seconds for the tissues to relax, then take up the slack to the new point of initial resistance, i.e., the first indication of a new barrier.
13. Repeat until the best possible increase of motion is obtained.
14. Retest.

POSITIONAL DIAGNOSIS

L3 N $S_L R_R$; L3 is at the apex of a neutral group curve (convex right) and is side-bent left and rotated right.

RESTRICTION

L3 restricted to side-bend right and rotate left.

Objective

Increase right side-bending and left rotation of L3 on L4.

Position

Supine (Fig. 54.28).

Procedure

1. Sit next to the right side of the patient, facing toward the patient's head. The patient's hips are flexed to about 90°.
2. Pass your left hand under the patient's lumbar spine to induce slight extension and to pull the spine of L3 toward the right, inducing left rotation; this is monitored at the L3 vertebral unit.
3. Use your right arm and hand to slide the patient's feet and hips to the right on the table (to side-bend the lumbar spine to the right) to the point where side-bending motion is palpated with your left hand at the L3 level.
4. Direct the patient to "Slide feet to the left," and equally resist that effort with your right arm.
5. Maintain and monitor the forces long enough to sense the patient's contractile force at the localized segment or area, usually 3–5 seconds.
6. Direct the patient to gently release the directive force as you gently and simultaneously release your counterforce.
7. Wait a few seconds for the tissues to relax, then take up the slack to the new point of initial resistance, i.e., the first indication of a new barrier.
8. Repeat until the best possible increase of motion is obtained.
9. Retest.

POSITIONAL DIAGNOSIS

T11 F $S_L R_L$; T11 flexed, side-bent left, and rotated left; (T11 is nonneutral and side-bent to the left).

RESTRICTION

T11 E $S_R R_R$; T11 has restriction of extension, side-bending right, and rotation right.

Objective

Increase extension, right side-bending, and right rotation of T11 on T12.

Position

Seated (Fig. 54.29).

Procedure

1. Sit on a stool or chair behind the patient; the patient is seated on a stool so the feet are on the floor, knees and hips flexed to 90°, left hand and arm in the lap, and the right hand lateral to the right hip.
2. Place your right hand superior and anterior to the patient's right shoulder at the lateral end of the clavicle.
3. Monitor the posterior and inferior movement of the right transverse process of T11 with the finger or thumb of your left hand at the T11-T12 interspinous space, or at the right T12 transverse process.
4. Using your right hand, side-bend the patient to the right and translate the vertebral column left from above downward to include T11 but not T12.

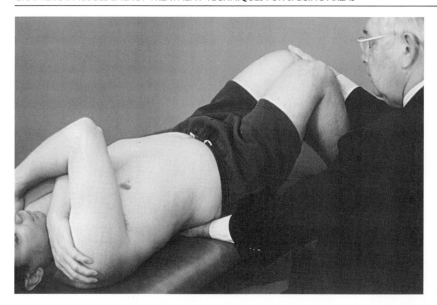

Figure 54.28. Treatment for L3 neutral side-bent left, rotated right, patient supine.

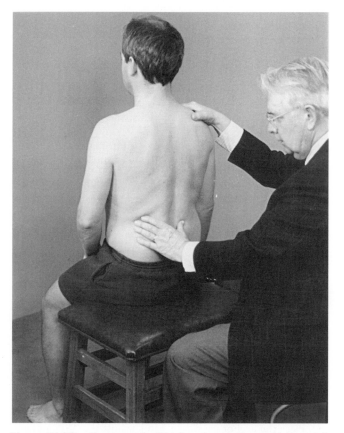

Figure 54.29. Treatment for T11 flexed, rotated, and side-bent left.

5. Rotate the patient's shoulder and trunk to the right to rotate the vertebral column from above down to include T11 but not T12. Apply posterior pressure through the patient's shoulder and/or guide the patient into sitting up straighter to localize extension at T11. Perform fine adjustments to localize initial resistance at T11 in all three planes of motion.

6. Direct the patient to rotate the spine to the left.
7. Offer counterforce equal to the patient's force (about 3 pounds).
8. Maintain and monitor the forces long enough to sense the patient's contractile force at the localized segment or area, usually 3–5 seconds.
9. Direct the patient to gently release the directive force as you gently and simultaneously release your counterforce.
10. Wait a few seconds for the tissues to relax, then take up the slack to the new point of initial resistance, i.e., the first indication of a new barrier.
11. Repeat until the best possible increase of motion is obtained.
12. Retest.

Note: With this technique you can ask the patient to backward bend over your left thumb (which is on the patient's right side). If patient extends and lateral bends to the right over your thumb along the proper vector, the desired combination of movements can occurred with a single muscular activation.

POSITIONAL DIAGNOSIS

L2 E $S_L R_L$; L2 is extended, side-bent left, and rotated left.

RESTRICTION

L2 F $S_R R_R$; L2 has restricted of flexion, side-bending right, and rotating right.

Objective

Increase flexion, side-bending right, and rotation right of L2 on L3.

Position

Seated (Fig. 54.30).

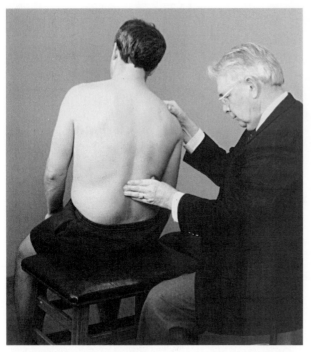

Figure 54.30.   Treatment for L2 extended, rotated, and side-bent left.

Procedure

1. Sit on a stool behind the patient.
2. Place your right hand anterior to patient's right acromioclavicular joint.
3. Place the fingers of your left hand at one of the following:
   a. the L2-3 interspinous space
   b. bilaterally at spinous process of L2
   c. posterior to left transverse process of L2
4. Direct the patient to slouch, or flex, to include L2 but not L3.
5. Side-bend the patient to the right to include L2.
6. Rotate the patient to the right. Fine tune the motions at L2, to localize initial resistance in all three planes of motion.
7. Direct the patient to rotate the trunk to left.
8. Offer equal counterforce (about 3 pounds).
9. Maintain and monitor the forces long enough to sense the patient's contractile force at the localized segment or area, usually 3–5 seconds.
10. Direct the patient to gently release the directive force as you gently and simultaneously release your counterforce.
11. Wait a few seconds for the tissues to relax, then take up the slack to the new point of initial resistance, i.e., the first indication of a new barrier.
12. Repeat until the best possible increase of motion is obtained.
13. Retest.

PELVIS

Innominate

POSITIONAL DIAGNOSIS

Right innominate anterior; right pelvic bone anterior; the right innominate moves anteriorly.

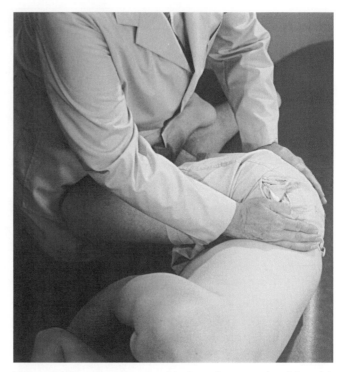

Figure 54.31.   Treatment for right innominate anterior; right pelvic bone anterior (hand placement).

RESTRICTION

Right innominate has restriction of posterior rotation; right innominate restricted from moving posteriorly.

Objective

Increase the posterior rotation of the right innominate.
   Example 1:

Position

Left lateral recumbent (Figs. 54.31 and 54.32).

Procedure

1. Stand facing the patient.
2. Use your left hand to position the patient's right hip in flexion.
3. Place the patient's right knee against your thigh in a comfortable position.
4. Place the heel of your right hand against the ASIS and your left hand on the ischial tuberosity of the patient's right innominate to encourage posterior rotation.
5. Direct the patient to push the right knee against your leg, as you resist the effort with equal counterforce.
6. Maintain and monitor the forces long enough to sense the patient's contractile force at the localized segment or area, usually 3–5 seconds.
7. Direct the patient to gently release the directive force as you gently and simultaneously release your counterforce.
8. Wait a few seconds for the tissues to relax, then take up the

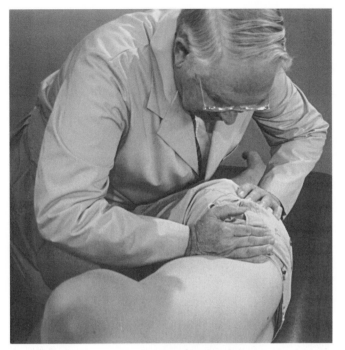

Figure 54.32. Treatment for right innominate anterior; right pelvic bone anterior (treatment position).

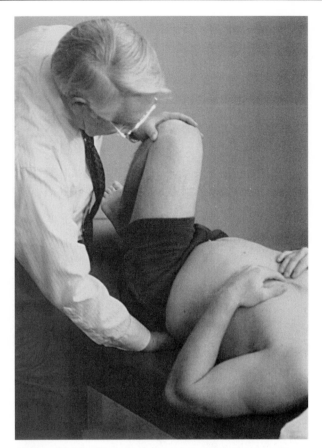

Figure 54.33. Treatment for supine rotation left innominate.

slack to the new point of initial resistance, i.e., the first indication of a new barrier.
9. Repeat until the best possible increase of motion is obtained.
10. Retest.

Objective

Increase posterior rotation of the right innominate

Position

Supine (Fig. 54.33).

Procedure

1. Stand on the right side of the patient.
2. The fingers of your left hand monitor the movement of the posterior portion of the right innominate in relation to the right sacroiliac joint.
3. Use your right hand at the patient's right knee to introduce flexion of the right hip as the left hand is monitoring the right sacroiliac joint.
4. Your right hand at knee introduces slight abduction or adduction to produce a sense of decreased resistance at the sacroiliac joint.
5. Direct the patient, "Press your right knee against my hand."
6. Offer counterforce equal to the patient's force.
7. Maintain and monitor the forces long enough to sense the patient's contractile force at the localized segment or area, usually 3–5 seconds.
8. Direct the patient to gently release the directive force as you gently and simultaneously release your counterforce.

9. Wait a few seconds for the tissues to relax, then take up the slack to the new point of initial resistance, i.e., the first indication of a new barrier.
10. Repeat until the best possible increase of motion is obtained.
11. Retest.

POSITIONAL DIAGNOSIS

Right innominate posterior.

RESTRICTION

Right innominate restriction of anterior rotation; the right innominate is restricted in its ability to rotate anteriorly.

Objective

Increase anterior movement of the right innominate.

Position

Prone (Fig. 54.34).

Procedure

1. Stand on the left side of the patient. Place the heel of your left hand on patient's right iliac crest, superior to the PSIS.
2. Hold the patient's right thigh with your right hand proximal

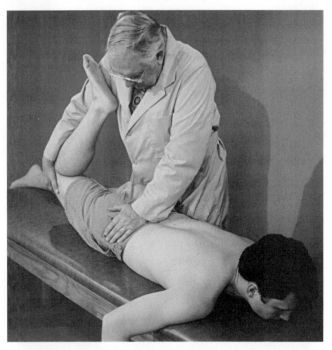

Figure 54.34.   Treatment for right innominate posterior.

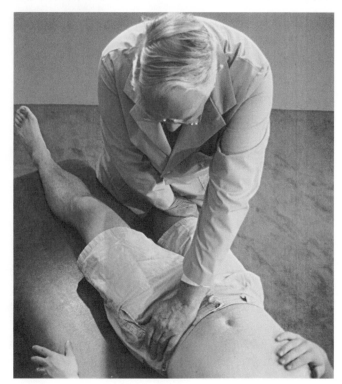

Figure 54.35.   Treatment for anterior rotation right innominate.

to the flexed knee and extend the patient's right thigh to the point of initial resistance.

3. Direct the patient, "Press your right knee toward table." Offer counterforce equal to the patient's force.
4. Maintain and monitor the forces long enough to sense the patient's contractile force at the localized segment or area, usually 3–5 seconds.
5. Direct the patient to gently release the directive force as you gently and simultaneously release your counterforce.
6. Wait a few seconds for the tissues to relax, then take up the slack to the new point of initial resistance, i.e., the first indication of a new barrier.
7. Repeat until the best possible increase of motion is obtained.
8. Retest.

Objective

Increase anterior rotation of the right innominate.

Position

Supine (Fig. 54.35).

Procedure

1. Stand to the right side of the patient (the side of the pelvic bone somatic dysfunction).
2. Move the patient to extend the right leg off the side of the table, with very little abduction of the leg. Make sure that the patient is stable on the table.
3. Place your right hand on the patient's right knee.
4. Place your left hand on the patient's left ASIS area to stabilize the patient.

5. Direct the patient, "Lift your knee toward the ceiling," while you equally balance this effort with the counterforce of your right hand on the patient's right knee.
6. Maintain and monitor the forces long enough to sense the patient's contractile force at the localized segment or area, usually 3–5 seconds.
7. Direct the patient to gently release the directive force as you gently and simultaneously release your counterforce.
8. Wait a few seconds for the tissues to relax, then take up the slack to the new point of initial resistance, i.e., the first indication of a new barrier.
9. Repeat until the best possible increase of motion is obtained.
10. Retest.

Pubic Bone

POSITIONAL DIAGNOSIS

Right inferior pubic shear; right pubis inferior; right pubic ramus sheared inferiorly (inferior subluxation); right pubic ramus is inferior to the left pubic ramus at the pubic symphysis.

RESTRICTION

Right pubic bone resists superior glide to obtain symmetry with the left pubic bone at the pubic symphysis.

Objective

Move right pubic ramus superiorly to obtain symmetry with left pubic bone at the symphysis.

Position

Supine.

Procedure

1. Stand on the right side (can be either) of the patient.
2. Place the palm of your right hand against the patient's right ischial tuberosity; the thigh is flexed 70–90° (from 70 to 90° the adductor magnus acts as an additional extensor of the thigh); your forearm may be lateral or medial to the patient's thigh.
3. Slightly abduct the patient's right thigh to gap the pubic symphysis.
4. Place your left axilla or left hand against the patient's right knee and take up slack to the limit of thigh flexion, but not more than 90°.
5. Direct the patient to press the right knee toward the foot of the table.
6. Offer isometric counterforce equal to the patient's force.
7. Maintain the force long enough to sense the patient's contractile forces at the localized segment or area. This monitoring usually takes 3–5 seconds.
8. Direct the patient to gently let up on the force as you gently and simultaneously release the counterforce.
9. Wait a few seconds for the tissues to relax, then take up the slack to the new point of initial resistance, i.e., the first hint of a barrier.
10. Repeat until the best possible increase of motion is obtained.
11. Retest.

Objective

To move the right pubic ramus superiorly to obtain symmetry with the left.

Position

Left lateral recumbent (Figs. 54.31 and 54.32).

Procedure

1. Stand facing the patient.
2. Flex the patient's right knee to 90° and place the knee against your left thigh for control.
3. Place your left hand on the right ischial tuberosity, and the right hand on the crest of the patient's right pelvic bone.
4. Have the patient push the right knee toward the end of the table as you maintain equal counterforce through your left thigh.
5. Maintain and monitor the forces long enough to sense the patient's contractile force at the localized segment or area, usually 3–5 seconds.
6. Direct the patient to gently release the directive force as you gently and simultaneously release your counterforce.
7. Wait a few seconds for the tissues to relax, then take up the slack to the new point of initial resistance, i.e., the first indications of a new barrier.

8. Repeat until the best possible increase of motion is obtained.
9. Retest.

POSITIONAL DIAGNOSIS

Right superior pubic shear; right pubis superior; superior pubic shear on the right; right pubic subluxation; the right pubic ramus is superior to the left at the pubic symphysis.

RESTRICTION

The right pubic ramus is superior to the left pubic ramus at the pubic symphysis; the right pubic ramus resists movement inferiorly to obtain symmetry with left pubic ramus at the pubic symphysis.

Objective

Move the right pubis inferiorly to obtain symmetry with the left pubic ramus at the pubic symphysis.

Position

Supine (Fig. 54.33).

Procedure

1. Stand at the right side of the patient, facing toward the patient's head.
2. Abduct and extend the patient's right thigh by letting the right leg drop off the table. (It is more comfortable for the patient if you support the leg with your foot under the patient's heel.)
3. Stabilize the patient's pelvis by placing your right hand against the patient's left ASIS.
4. Place your left hand proximal to the patient's right knee and press the extended limb toward the floor to the point of initial resistance.
5. Direct the patient, "Keep your knee straight and raise your right knee and foot toward ceiling."
6. Offer counterforce equal to the patient's force.
7. Maintain and monitor the forces long enough to sense the patient's contractile force at the localized segment or area, usually 3–5 seconds.
8. Direct the patient to gently release the directive force as you simultaneously and gently release your counterforce.
9. Wait a few seconds for the tissues to relax, then take up the slack to the new point of initial resistance, i.e., the first indication of a barrier.
10. Repeat until the best possible increase of motion is obtained.
11. Retest.

POSITIONAL DIAGNOSIS

Pubes compressed.

RESTRICTION

Normal pubic motion is restricted and there is no evidence of pubic shear (the pubic symphysis is usually tender bilaterally).

Objective

Decompress the pubic symphysis.

Position

Supine (Figs. 54.36 and 54.37).

Procedure

1. Stand beside the patient.
2. Have the patient flex the hips and knees and place the feet about 4 inches apart on the table.
3. Hold both knees about 4 inches apart.
4. Instruct the patient to forcibly approximate the knees as you resist the effort with equal counterforce from each hand. Alternately, you can place one elbow, forearm, wrist, and hand between the knees as the patient contracts isometrically.
5. Maintain and monitor the forces long enough to sense the patient's contractile force at the localized segment or area, usually 3–5 seconds.
6. Direct the patient to gently release the directive force as you simultaneously and gently release your counterforce.
7. Wait a few seconds for the tissues to relax, then take up the slack to the new point of initial resistance, i.e., the first indications of a barrier.
8. Repeat until the best possible increase of motion is obtained.
9. Retest.

Note: Force into the pubic area tends to produce compression of the pubic symphysis. Some compression is believed to be present in any dysfunction of the pubic symphysis. It is the pull of the adductor muscles of the thigh that decompresses the pubic symphysis in the above technique. Fascial and mus-

cular attachments to the pelvic diaphragm and bladder are disturbed by pubic compression and/or a pubic shear. This disturbed function has been observed as an etiologic explanation for genitourinary symptomatology (frequency, burning, vaginismus, prostatic spasms, etc.) presented subjectively and without the usual supporting clinical evidence of an infective process. Often treatment for a pubic compression results in the simultaneous removal of a pubic shear.

Sacrum

The following are criteria of a positional diagnosis of a left sacral torsion:

> L5 transverse process posterior right; L5 rotated right
> Right sacral sulcus deeper than left
> Left inferior lateral angle (ILA) of sacrum more posterior than the right ILA
> Left medial malleolus may appear to be more superior than right because often the right innominate rotates anteriorly with the right sacral base, making the right leg appear to be longer.

Clinical methods of locating the oblique axis include:

1. Spring test (Fig. 54.38): anteriorly directed pressure at L-S and look for resistance:

> Much resistance suggests backward torsion (opposite axis)
> Little resistance suggests forward torsion (same axis)

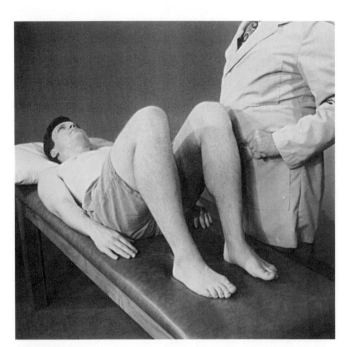

Figure 54.36. Treatment for pubes compressed, showing position of feet and knees.

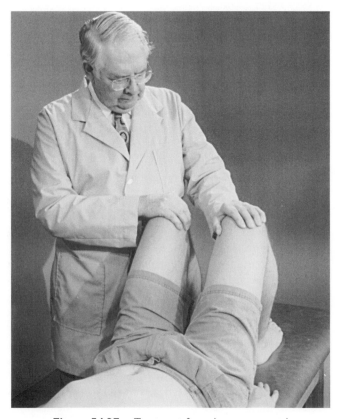

Figure 54.37. Treatment for pubes compressed.

Figure 54.38. Spring test.

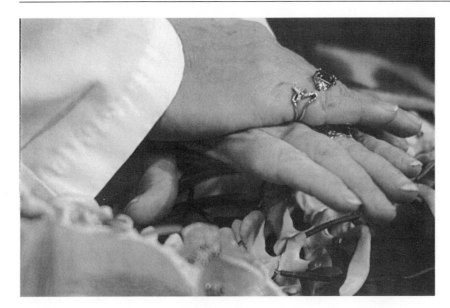

Figure 54.39. Test for lumbopelvic hypertension.

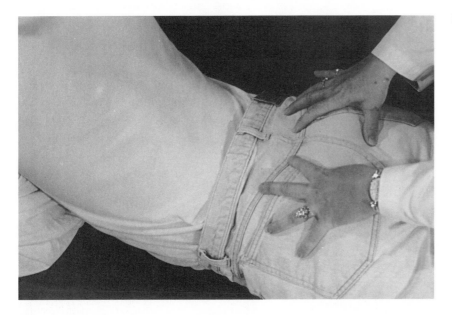

2. Lumbopelvic hyperextension (Fig. 54.39), the sphinx test, looking for asymmetrical findings at the sacral base:

Increased sacral base asymmetry signals a backward sacral torsion, such as right sacral torsion on a left oblique axis, i.e., the torsion is opposite to the oblique axis.

Decreased sacral base asymmetry (it feels more symmetrical), signals a forward sacral torsion on the same axis, such as a left sacral torsion on a left oblique axis. The torsion is in the same direction as the oblique axis.

3. Four-digit contact on the sacrum (Figs. 54.40 (cephalic view) and 54.41 (caudal view)) while monitoring respiration and interpreting motions:

Movement under digits indicates motion is present and suggests the oblique axis

4. Seated assessment of inferior lateral angle symmetry during

sagittal plane lumbar flexion (Figs. 54.42 (at starting position) dand 54.43 (at end of flexion)):

Asymmetry decreases with backward torsions (opposite axis)

Asymmetry remains the same with forward torsions (same axis)

FORWARD SACRAL TORSIONS

See Chapter 49, "Regional Examination of the Pelvis and Sacrum."

Positional Diagnosis

Left sacral torsion on a left oblique axis; L on L (the first L is for direction of torsion; the second L designates the axis); to

Figure 54.40. Test for four-digit contact on sacrum (cephalic view).

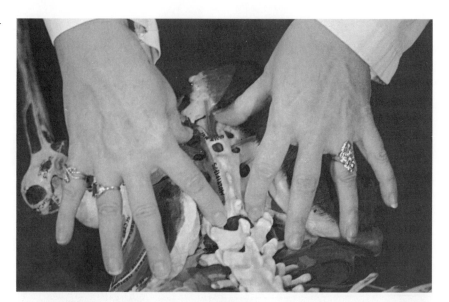

Figure 54.41. Test for four-digit contact on sacrum (caudal view).

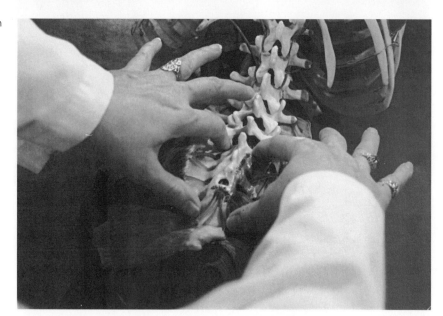

Figure 54.42. Test for inferior lateral angle symmetry (at starting position).

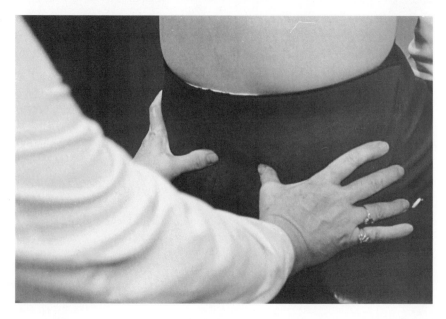

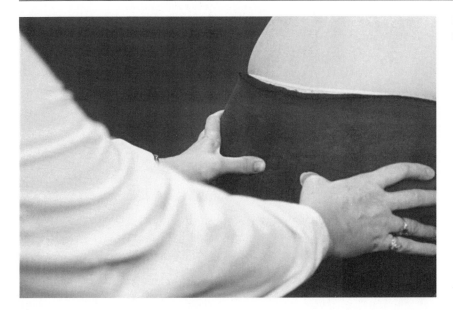

Figure 54.43. Test for inferior lateral angle symmetry (at end of flexion).

qualify as a left anterior torsion, the lumbars must be in neutral, that is, facets are not engaged, side-bent left and rotated right.

Restriction

The oblique axis is not free to swing from side to side during walking; the sacrum has restriction of movement about the right oblique axis; L5 restricted $S_R R_L$ is also found when an anterior sacral base rotation is termed a left torsion of the sacrum.

Objective

By Method 1: Rotate L5 to the left and activate the right piriformis to free the left oblique axis. Effective treatment of torsions about oblique or diagonal axes with this method requires a positioning of the patient that focuses on derotation of L5 and active contraction of the piriformis muscle. The latter is used to derotate the sacrum. When the thigh is flexed, the piriformis muscle acts more as an abductor of the thigh than an external rotator. Since the sacral attachments of the piriformis lie in a plane parallel to the diagonal axes of the sacrum, right piriformis isometric or isotonic contraction and postisometric relaxation can do one or either of two things, for example: pull the left sacral base laterally to the right, away from the left ilium, or decrease right sacral base and right sacroiliac close packing by reducing resting tone in the hypertonic right piriformis, which may release the right superior limb of the sacrum from the ilium.

Position

Left lateral Sims' position (Figs. 54.44 and 54.45).

Procedure

1. Flex both thighs until the lumbosacral joint is at neutral. Then let the legs drop free of table left lumbar side-bending.

2. Sit on the table to the patient's flexed hips and thighs.
3. Lift the flexed thighs over your left thigh. You may wish to support your left foot on a chair or stool rung to reduce compression on your left thigh.
4. Monitor ranges of sacral base and lumbosacral joint flexion and extension with the fingers of your left hand.
5. Flex and extend the lumbosacral joint to a freely moving position. Some refer to this as an idling state. To achieve this, you may need to flex the thighs more or less by sliding forward and backward on the table.
6. Ask the patient to reach the right hand toward the floor as your left hand monitors the left rotation of L5, which typically occurs with this set of findings.
7. By placing your left thigh under the patient's thighs, the pelvis and sacrum rotate to the right.
8. Direct the patient to lift the right leg upward toward the ceiling as you offer counterforce below the knee. This move induces the piriformis strain and stress discussed above.
9. Maintain and monitor the forces long enough to sense the patient's contractile force at the localized segment or area, usually 3–5 seconds.
10. Direct the patient to gently release the directive force as you gently and simultaneously release your counterforce.
11. Wait a few seconds for the tissues to relax, then take up the slack to the new point of initial resistance, i.e., the first indication of a new barrier.
12. Repeat until the best possible increase of motion is obtained.
13. Retest.

Positional Diagnosis

Same diagnosis as above: Left sacral torsion on a left oblique axis; L on L (the first L is for direction of torsion; the second L designates the axis); to qualify as a left anterior torsion, the lumbars must be neutral, side-bent left, and rotated right.

Figure 54.44. Treatment for forward sacral torsion, left lateral Sims' position.

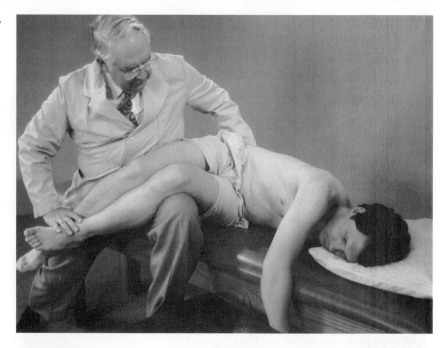

Figure 54.45. Treatment for forward sacral torsion, left lateral Sims' position.

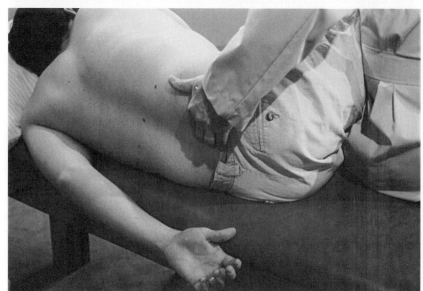

Restriction

The oblique axis is not free to swing from side to side during walking; sacral movement is restricted about a right oblique axis; L5 is restricted $S_R R_L$.

Objective

Establish side-bending left and nonneutral mechanics at the lumbosacral junction, i.e., F $R_L S_L$. First you maintain the left oblique axis; establish nonneutral positioning at the lumbosacral junction, which has side-bending to the left; and then use isometric–isotonic muscle energy activation to create lumbosacral and pelvic movement. In this position, the right sacral base moves to the right, thereby removing the sacral rotation to the left on a left oblique axis.

Position

Left lateral recumbent position (Figs. 54.46 and 54.47).

Procedure

1. Stand in front of the patient.
2. Flex the patient's knees to about 90°.
3. The patient is instructed to leave the hips and legs on the table, rotate the upper body to the left and place the chest on the table.
4. Place your right hand on the spine of L5 or monitor the sacroiliac joint.
5. Drop the patient's legs off the table and support the thigh on your knee (to protect it from pressure by the side of the

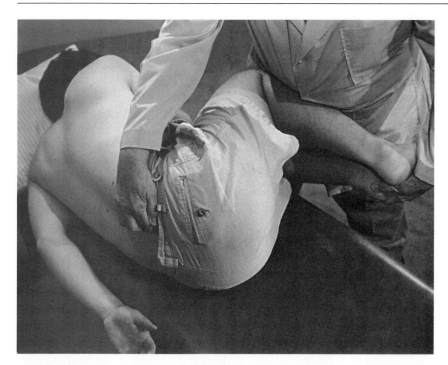

Figure 54.46. Treatment for forward sacral torsion.

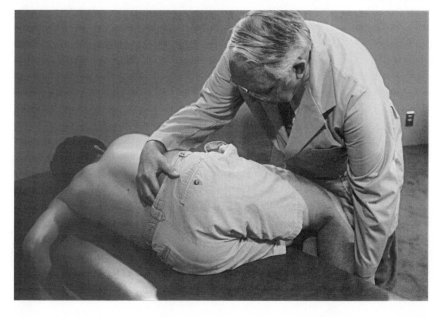

Figure 54.47. Treatment for forward sacral torsion.

table). This maneuver engages the left oblique sacral axis (LOA).

6. Activate to make the sacrum work in this position: With the lumbosacral flexed to about 90°, side-bent and rotated right, any stimulus to move the sacrum physiologically causes the sacrum to rotate to the right on its left oblique axis (R on LOA) and reverse the rotation found in the somatic dysfunction (L on LOA). The isometric contraction of the piriformis produces the sacral motion and probably helps to free the restrictions that produced the opposite oblique axis.

7. Activating forces available to use singly or in combination are:

a. *To affect the sacrum:* Instruct the patient to "Lift your feet and knees to the ceiling" while you isometrically resist this effort with your right hand on the patient's ankle.
b. *To affect the sacrum:* Spring the legs toward the floor.
c. *To affect L5:* Use your left hand to pull the patient's L5 spinous process to the right. This increases the left rotation of L5 and secures the nonneutral positioning (F R_L S_L) of the lumbosacral junction.
d. *To affect L5:* Instruct the patient, "Reach for the floor with your right hand." This increases lumbar rotation to the left.

8. Maintain the forces long enough to sense the patient's con-

tractile force at the localized segment or area (usually 3–5 seconds). This is monitoring.

9. Direct the patient to gently cease the directive force; cease your counterforce gently; do these simultaneously.

10. Wait 2 seconds for the tissues to relax, then take up the slack to the new point of initial resistance.

11. Repeat until the best possible increase of motion is obtained.

12. Retest.

Position

Right lateral recumbent position, side of the deeper sulcus (Figs. 54.48 and 54.49). (This position does not require the patient to drop the legs off the table.)

Procedure

1. Stand in front of the patient. Hold the patient's legs with your right hand while palpating the lumbosacral junction with your left hand.

2. Flex the patient's hips until motion is palpated at the lumbosacral junction.

3. Instruct the patient to rotate the left shoulder posteriorly until you sense initial resistance of rotational motion at the lumbosacral junction. This rotates L5 to the left.

4. Raise the patient's feet and legs toward the ceiling until you palpate initial resistance of movement at the lumbosacral junction. This engages the left oblique sacral axis.

5. Direct the patient, "Press your feet and knees toward the floor," while you offer an equal counterforce with your right hand.

6. Maintain the forces long enough to sense the patient's contractile force at the localized segment or area (3–5 seconds). This is monitoring.

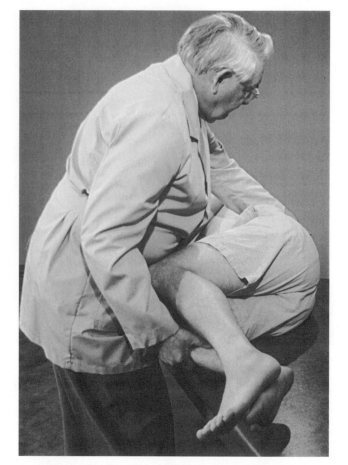

Figure 54.48. Treatment for forward sacral torsion.

Figure 54.49. Treatment for forward sacral torsion.

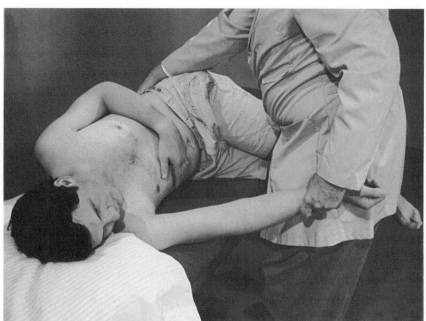

7. Direct the patient to gently cease the directive force; cease your counterforce gently; do these simultaneously.
8. Wait 2 seconds for the tissues to relax, then take up the slack to the new point of initial resistance.
9. Repeat until the best possible increase of motion is obtained.
10. Retest.

Positional Diagnosis

Right sacral torsion on a right oblique axis; R on R.

Criteria and treatment procedures for this diagnosis are the mirror images of those described for the left torsion about a left oblique axis.

BACKWARD SACRAL TORSIONS

See description in Chapter 49.

Positional Diagnosis

Left sacral torsion on a right oblique axis; L on right oblique axis (ROA); L on R (the first letter, L, designates the direction of sacral base rotation; the second letter, R, designates the right oblique axis); to qualify as a backward sacral torsion, the lumbars must be side-bent right and rotated right. The sacrum has rotated to the left about a right oblique axis so the left sacral base is posterior and resists anterior rotation; the right inferior angle has moved anteriorly and slightly superiorly and is restricted to move posteriorly and inferiorly.

Restriction

The oblique axis is not free to swing from side to side during walking; the sacrum has restriction of movement about the left oblique axis; L5 is restricted in side-bending left and rotating left when the sacral base rotation is termed a backward torsion.

Objective

Rotate L5 to left and activate left piriformis to free the right oblique axis.

Method 2.

Position

Right lateral recumbent position (Figs. 54.50 and 54.51).

Procedure

1. Stand in front of the patient.

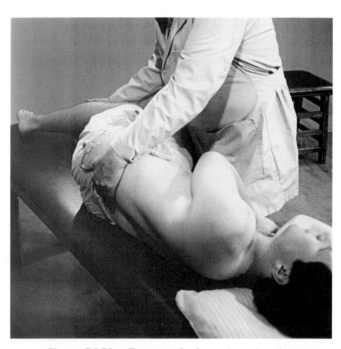

Figure 54.50. Treatment for forward sacral torsion.

Figure 54.51. Treatment for backward sacral torsion.

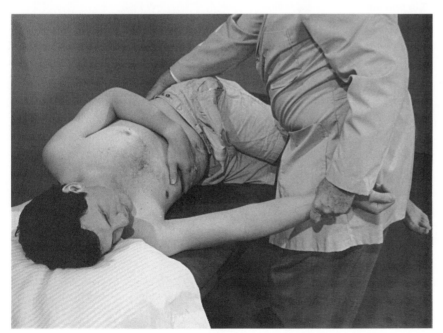

2. Flex the patient's hips and knees to about 10–20°.

3. The patient is instructed to leave the hips and knees where they are; introduce left rotation of the trunk to include L5 by pulling the patient's right arm toward you. This rotates the lumbosacral junction to the left.

4. Drop the patient's legs off the table and support the thighs or your knee (to protect it from pressure by the side of the table). This engages the right oblique sacral axis.

5. Activate to make the sacrum work in this position. These activating forces may be used singly or in combination:

    Instruct the patient to "Lift your feet and knees to the ceiling" while you isometrically resist this effort with your left hand on the patient's lower leg.

    Spring the leg toward the floor (to affect the sacrum).

    Pull the patient's L5 transverse process to the left (to affect L5).

    Have the patient rotate the left shoulder backward (to affect L5)

    Have the patient exhale deeply

    With the lumbosacral junction in this position (flexed very little (much less than 90°), side-bent right and rotated left) and a right oblique axis of the sacrum maintained, any action affecting the sacrum physiologically induces the sacrum to rotate to the right on its right oblique axis and reverse the rotation found in the somatic dysfunction. The isometric contraction of the left piriformis produces the sacral motion and probably helps to free restrictions of the right oblique axis.

6. Maintain the forces long enough to sense the patient's contractile force at the localized segment or area (usually 3–5 seconds). This is monitoring.

7. Direct the patient to gently cease the directive force; cease your counterforce gently; do these simultaneously.

8. Wait 2 seconds for the tissues to relax, then take up the slack to the new point of initial resistance.

9. Repeat until the best possible increase of motion is obtained.

10. Retest.

Positional Diagnosis

Left sacral torsion on a right oblique axis; L on ROA; L on R (The first letter, L, designates the direction of sacral base rotation; the second letter, R, designates the right oblique axis); to qualify as a backward sacral torsion, the lumbars must be side-bent right and rotated right.

Objective

Rotate L5 to the left and activate the piriformis muscle to free the right oblique axis. Flex and/or extend lumbosacral joint to idling state; rotate L5 to left to initial resistance; keep sacrum from rotating left with L5 by dropping left leg off the table toward the floor; contract left piriformis muscle, which is at the inferior end of the right oblique axis.

Position

Right lateral recumbent position (Figs. 54.50–54.53).

Procedure

1. Stand facing the patient.

2. Place the fingers of your left hand at the lumbosacral interspinous area to monitor movements at the lumbosacral joint.

3. Hold the patient's right knee with your right hand (the patient's left knee is resting on the right knee). Flex and extend the lumbosacral junction to the neutral position.

4. Move left knee superior and anterior to right knee while maintaining idling at L-S.

5. Hold patient's right forearm to rotate upper torso to left until left rotation is perceived at L5; patient may use deep inhalations to assist this rotation.

6. Direct the patient, "Drop your left foot and ankle off the table toward the floor," while you hold the right hip with your right forearm so the sacrum doesn't follow L5 rotation to left. This engages the right oblique sacral axis.

7. Direct the patient, "Lift your left leg toward the ceiling"; the left thigh should be flexed so the left piriformis can act as an abductor.

8. Offer counterforce equal to the patient's force.

9. Maintain the forces long enough to sense the patient's contractile force at the localized segment or area (usually 3–5 seconds). This is monitoring.

10. Direct the patient to gently cease the directive force; cease your counterforce gently; do these simultaneously.

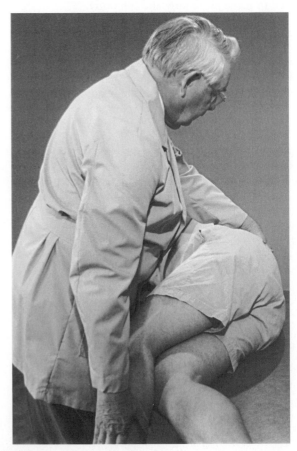

Figure 54.52. Treatment for backward sacral torsion.

11. Wait 2 seconds for the tissues to relax, then take up the slack to the new point of initial resistance.
12. Repeat until the best possible increase of motion is obtained.
13. Retest.

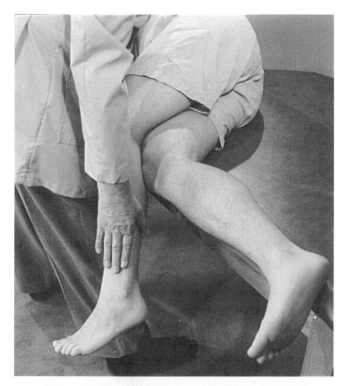

Figure 54.53. Treatment for backward sacral torsion.

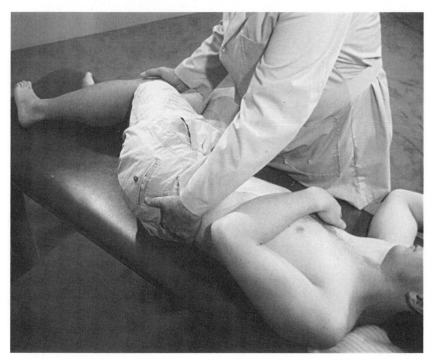

Positional Diagnosis

Left sacral torsion on a right oblique axis L on ROA (right oblique axis); L on R (the first letter, L, designates the direction of sacral base rotation; the second letter, R, designates the right oblique axis); to qualify as a backward sacral torsion, the lumbars must be side-bent right and rotated right.

Position

Right lateral recumbent position; side of deeper sulcus (Fig. 54.54).

Procedure

1. Extend the patient's hips until motion is palpated at the lumbosacral junction.
2. While palpating the lumbosacral junction, rotate the patient's left shoulder posteriorly until you sense initial resistance of motion at the lumbosacral junction.
3. Hold the patient's left leg and flex it slightly at the hip and knee. Apply downward (toward the floor) pressure on the left knee until you sense initial resistance of motion at the lumbosacral junction.
4. Direct the patient, "Press the knee toward the ceiling," while you offer an equal counterforce.
5. Maintain the forces long enough to sense the patient's contractile force at the localized segment or area (3–5 seconds). This is monitoring.
6. Direct the patient to gently cease the directive force; cease your counterforce gently; do these simultaneously.
7. Wait 2 seconds for the tissues to relax, then take up the slack to the new point of initial resistance.

Figure 54.54. Treatment for backward sacral torsion.

8. Repeat until the best possible increase of motion is obtained.
9. Retest.

Positional Diagnosis

Right sacral torsion on a left oblique axis; R on LOA; R on L.
   Criteria and treatment procedures for this diagnosis are the mirror image of the same for a left torsion on a right oblique axis.

Positional Diagnosis

Left sacral shear; left unilaterally sacral flexion.

Restriction

Left sacral base is restricted from moving posteriorly with inhalation and the left ILA resists anterior motion.

Objective

Restore posterior movement of sacrum on superior arm (cranial limb) of the left sacroiliac joint, i.e., extend the sacrum on the left.

Position

Prone (Figs. 54.55–54.57).

Procedure

1. Stand to the left side of the patient.
2. Place a finger of your left hand posterior to the left sacral base (in sacral sulcus), contacting tissue posterior to the left sacroiliac joint.

3. With your right hand and arm holding the patient's left lower limb, abduct and adduct it, sensing for the position that permits the least tension under the fingers of your left hand (at the left sacroiliac joint).
4. Place the hypothenar eminence of your right hand over the sacrum, posterior to the left ILA; lean over and on the patient, with your right arm extended at the elbow.
5. Move your shoulder from left to right in a transverse plane to find the least tension at the patient's left sacroiliac joint, and position your shoulder at that optimum location.
6. Move your shoulder in a superoinferior direction in the sagittal plane to find the least tension at the left S-I joint, and position your shoulder at that location.
7. Direct the patient to inhale deeply and hold the breath until directed to exhale.
8. Follow any movement of the left ILA in an anterosuperior arc with your right hypothenar eminence, and hold it there as the patient exhales.
9. Repeat steps 5 through 8 until the best possible increase of motion is obtained.
10. Retest.

UPPER EXTREMITY SOMATIC DYSFUNCTIONS

Somatic dysfunctions of the extremities are presented as restrictions in motion. Terminology includes

   Vertical flexion or vertical extension, meaning these movements in the sagittal plane
   Horizontal flexion or extension, meaning these movements in the transverse plane

Figure 54.55. Treatment for backward sacral torsion.

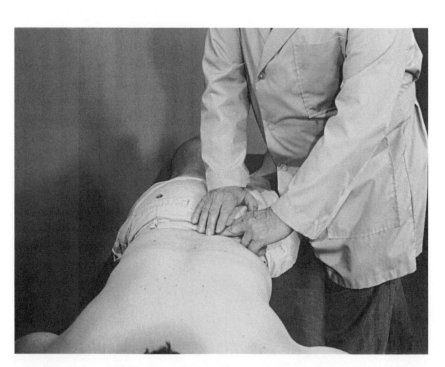

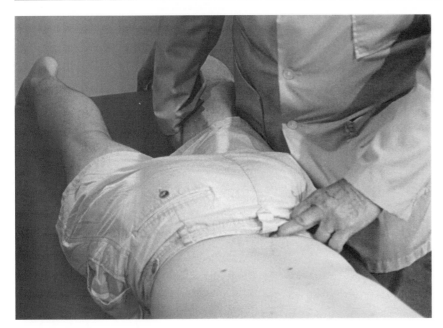

Figure 54.56. Treatment for backward sacral torsion.

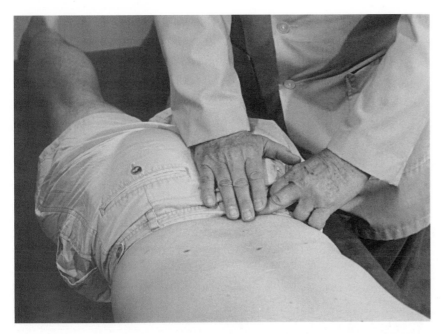

Figure 54.57. Treatment for backward sacral torsion.

Glenohumeral Joint

RESTRICTION

Right humerus has restriction of flexion; the right humerus has restriction of vertically flexing the arm; restriction of moving the humerus anteriorly in the sagittal plane.

Objective

Increase the range of flexion of the arm at the glenohumeral joint.

Position

Left lateral recumbent (or seated).

Procedure

1. Stand in front of the patient.
2. Place your right hand over the top of the patient's shoulder (and superior part of scapula) and cup the glenohumeral joint to palpate for motion. The right hand also restricts shoulder girdle motion (scapulothoracic and clavicular) and ensures that all forces localize to the glenohumeral joint and the musculo-tendinous cuff.

3. Use your left hand and forearm to support the patient's flexed right elbow and flex the humerus at the glenohumeral joint and in the sagittal plane to the initial point of resistance.

4. Direct the patient to extend the elbow (draw the elbow posteriorly, "vertical extension") against your equal counterforce at elbow.

5. Maintain the forces long enough to sense the patient's contractile force at the localized segment or area (usually 3–5 seconds). This is monitoring.

6. Direct the patient to gently cease the directive force; cease your counterforce gently; do these simultaneously.

7. Wait 2 seconds for the tissues to relax, then take up the slack to the new point of initial resistance.

8. Repeat until the best possible increase of motion is obtained.

9. Retest.

RESTRICTION

Right humerus has restriction of extension; vertical extension is extension in the sagittal plane.

Objective

Increase the range of extension of the glenohumeral joint.

Position

Left lateral recumbent (Fig. 54.58).

Procedure

1. Stand in front of the patient.

2. Place your right hand over the top of the patient's shoulder at the superior part of the scapula, and cup the glenohumeral joint to palpate for motion.

3. Use your left hand to support the patient's flexed right elbow; your thumb is in the cubital fossa and your fingers are posterior to the humerus. The patient's arm is extended in the sagittal plane to the point of initial resistance.

4. Direct the patient to push the elbow anteriorly (vertical flexion) against your equal counterforce at the elbow.

5. Maintain the forces long enough to sense the patient's contractile force at the localized segment or area (usually 3–5 seconds). This is monitoring.

6. Direct the patient to gently cease the directive force; cease your counterforce gently; do these simultaneously.

7. Wait 2 seconds for the tissues to relax, then take up the slack to the new point of initial resistance.

8. Repeat until the best possible increase of motion is obtained.

9. Retest.

RESTRICTION

The right humerus has a restriction of abduction.

Objective

Increase the range of abduction of the right glenohumeral joint.

Position

Left lateral recumbent (or seated) (Fig. 54.59).

Procedure

1. Stand in front of the patient.

2. Place your right hand over the superior part of the patient's shoulder and scapula. Cup the glenohumeral joint to palpate for motion.

Figure 54.58. Treatment for right glenohumeral joint restriction of extension.

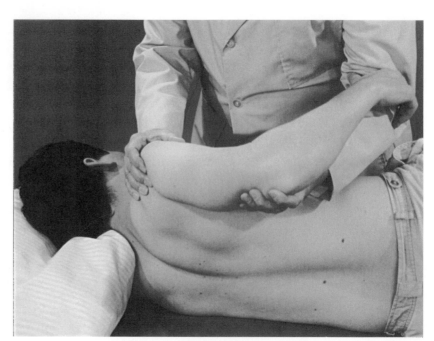

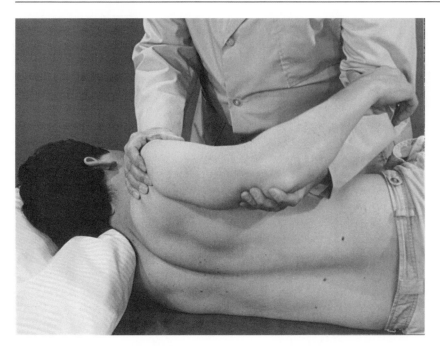

Figure 54.59. Treatment for right glenohumeral joint restriction of abduction.

3. Hold the patient's flexed right elbow with your left hand and abduct the arm to initial resistance.
4. Direct the patient to press the elbow toward the body (adduct) against equal counterforce at the elbow.
5. Maintain the forces long enough to sense the patient's contractile force at the localized segment or area (usually 3–5 seconds). This is monitoring.
6. Direct the patient to gently cease the directive force; cease your counterforce gently; do these simultaneously.
7. Wait 2 seconds for the tissues to relax, then take up the slack to the new point of initial resistance.
8. Repeat until the best possible increase of motion is obtained.
9. Retest.

RESTRICTION

The right glenohumeral joint has restriction of internal rotation (medial rotation).

Objective

Increase the internal rotation of the right humerus.

Position

Left lateral recumbent (or seated) (Fig. 54.60).

Procedure

1. Stand facing the patient.
2. Carefully place the dorsum of the patient's right hand against the patient's back (if possible); do this within the range of comfort.
3. Place your right hand over the top of the shoulder and superior part of the scapula with your fingers pointing poste-

riorly and your right palm protecting the anterior side of the shoulder capsule. Cup the patient's right glenohumeral joint to palpate for motion.
4. Place the finger of your left hand posterior to the patient's flexed right elbow and gently pull anteriorly to internally rotate the humerus to initial resistance.
5. Direct the patient, "Press your right elbow against my fingers"; this attempts to produce lateral, or external, rotation of the humerus at the glenoid fossa; maintain an equal counterforce with your left hand.
6. Maintain the forces long enough to sense the patient's contractile force at the localized segment or area (usually 3–5 seconds). This is monitoring.
7. Direct the patient to gently cease the directive force; cease your counterforce gently; do these simultaneously.
8. Wait 2 seconds for the tissues to relax, then take up the slack to the new point of initial resistance.
9. Repeat until the best possible increase of motion is obtained.
10. Retest.

RESTRICTION

Right humerus restriction of external rotation (lateral rotation).

Objective

Increase external rotation of the humerus at the shoulder joint.

Position

Left lateral recumbent (or seated) (Fig. 54.61).

Procedure

1. Stand behind the patient.

Figure 54.60. Treatment for right glenohumeral joint restriction of internal rotation.

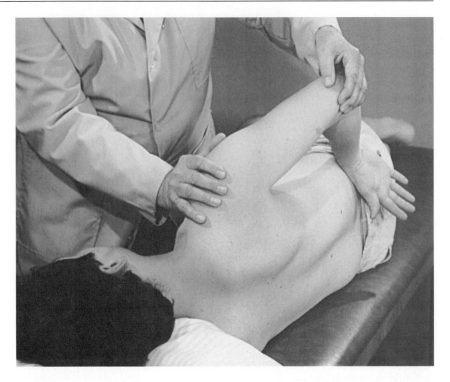

Figure 54.61. Treatment for right humerus restriction of external rotation.

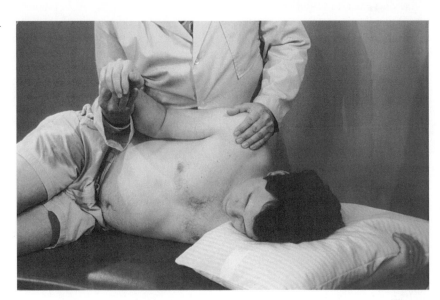

2. Place your left hand superior to the patient's glenohumeral joint.
3. Place your right forearm medial to the patient's flexed right forearm, with your right hand supporting the patient's right hand and wrist; hold the elbow close to the patient's body. Externally rotate the patient's arm to initial resistance.
4. Direct the patient to attempt to internally rotate the arm by pressing the right hand against the equal counterforce of your right hand; the patient's elbow is the pivot point.
5. Maintain the forces long enough to sense the patient's contractile force at the localized segment or area (usually 3–5 seconds). This is monitoring.

6. Direct the patient to gently cease the directive force; cease your counterforce gently; do these simultaneously.
7. Wait 2 seconds for the tissues to relax, then take up the slack to the new point of initial resistance.
8. Repeat until the best possible increase of motion is obtained.
9. Retest.

Sternoclavicular Joint

POSITIONAL DIAGNOSIS

"Superior clavicle"; the medial end of the clavicle moves superiorly on the sternum.

RESTRICTION

The right medial end of the clavicle does not move inferiorly on the sternum.

Objective

Move the medial end of the clavicle inferiorly on the sternum.

Position

Supine (Figs. 54.62 and 54.63).

Procedure

1. Stand to the right side of the patient.
2. Take the patient's right arm, abduct it 45°, and let it hang off the table.
3. Palpate the sternoclavicular joint with your right hand.
4. Grasp the patient's extended right wrist; externally rotate the arm and gently press it toward the floor to the point of initial resistance.
5. Direct the patient, "Lift your arm toward the ceiling"; the patient attempts to lift the extended arm against your equal counterforce. In this instance (which might be called an iso-

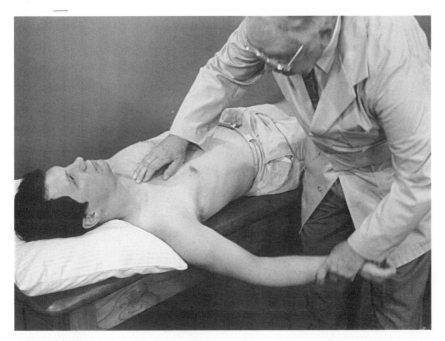

Figure 54.62. Treatment for superior clavicle.

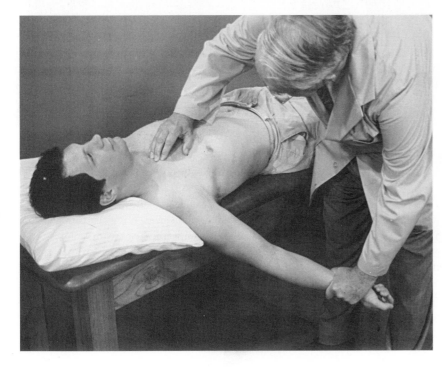

Figure 54.63. Treatment for superior clavicle.

tonic concentric contraction), the pectoralis muscles pull the medial end of the clavicle inferiorly on the sternum.

6. Maintain the forces long enough to sense the patient's contractile force at the localized segment or area (usually 3–5 seconds). This is monitoring.
7. Direct the patient to gently cease the directive force; cease your counterforce gently; do these simultaneously.
8. Wait 2 seconds for the tissues to relax, then take up the slack to the new point of initial resistance.
9. Repeat until the best possible increase in motion is obtained.
10. Retest.

RESTRICTION

The right clavicle has restriction of rotating posteriorly on the sternum.

Objective

Increase posterior rotation of the right clavicle on the sternum.

Position

Seated (Fig. 54.64).

Procedure

1. Stand behind and slightly to the right of the patient.

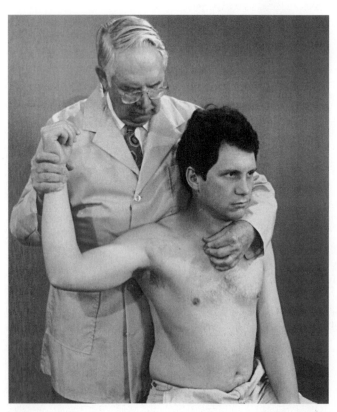

Figure 54.64. Treatment for right clavicle restriction posterior rotation.

2. Use your left thumb and index finger to monitor the right sternoclavicular joint.
3. Hold the patient's right wrist with your right hand; abduct the patient's arm to 90° and flex the elbow to 90°. (If the patient is sitting on a treatment table, putting your foot on the table and supporting the patient's elbow on your right knee assists you.)
4. Rotate the patient's arm posteriorly so the arm is externally rotated to initial resistance.
5. Direct the patient, "Gently press the wrist forward and toward the floor," (anteriorly and inferiorly toward the floor in a rotary arc with the elbow as the pivot point); this effort is applied against an equal counterforce provided through your right hand.
6. Maintain the forces long enough to sense the patient's contractile force at the localized segment or area (usually 3–5 seconds). This is monitoring.
7. Direct the patient to gently cease the directive force; cease your counterforce gently; do these simultaneously.
8. Wait 2 seconds for the tissues to relax, then take up the slack to the new point of initial resistance.
9. Repeat until the best possible increase of motion is obtained.
10. Retest.

Humeroulnar Joint (Elbow)

RESTRICTION

Right ulna has restriction of extension at elbow.

OBJECTIVE

Increase ulnar extension at elbow.

Position

Seated (Fig. 54.65).

Procedure

1. Stand to the right side, facing the patient.
2. Support the patient's flexed right elbow with your left hand (the patient's forearm is in the neutral position).
3. Place your right hand at patient's right wrist; extend the ulna at the elbow to the point of initial resistance.
4. Direct the patient to gently pull the wrist toward the right shoulder (flex the biceps muscle) against an equal counterforce applied with your right hand.
5. Maintain the forces long enough to sense the patient's contractile force at the localized segment or area (usually 3–5 seconds). This is monitoring.
6. Direct the patient to gently cease the directive force; cease your counterforce gently; do these simultaneously.
7. Wait 2 seconds for the tissues to relax, then take up the slack to the new point of initial resistance.
8. Repeat until the best possible increase of motion is obtained.
9. Retest.

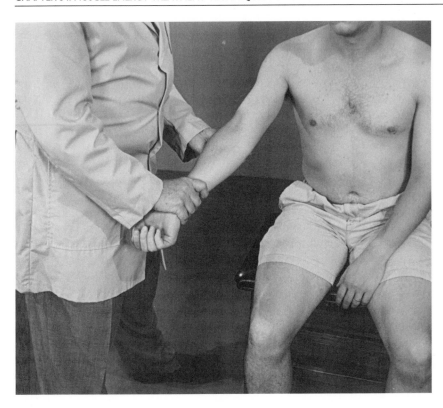

Figure 54.65. Treatment for right ulna restriction of extension.

RESTRICTION

The right ulna has restriction of flexion at elbow.

Objective

Increase flexion of the ulna at elbow.

Position

Seated (Fig. 54.66).

Procedure

1. Stand to the right side, facing the patient.
2. Support the patient's flexed right elbow with your left hand (the patient's forearm is in neutral position).
3. Place your right hand at the ulnar side of the patient's right wrist. Flex the ulna to the point of initial resistance.
4. Direct the patient to gently press the hand and wrist against your right hand (extend the arm); offer an equal counterforce to this effort.
5. Maintain the forces long enough to sense the patient's contractile force at the localized segment or area (usually 3–5 seconds). This is monitoring.
6. Direct the patient to gently cease the directive force; cease your counterforce gently; do these simultaneously.
7. Wait 2 seconds for the tissues to relax, then take up the slack to the new point of initial resistance.
8. Repeat until the best possible increase of motion is obtained.
9. Retest.

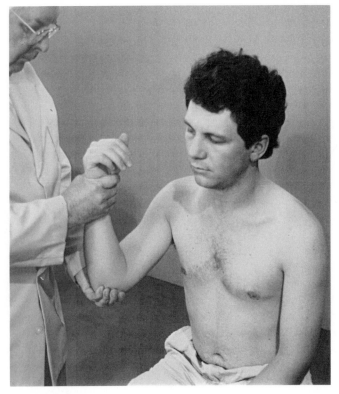

Figure 54.66. Treatment for right ulna restriction of extension.

RESTRICTION

Right forearm has restriction of supination.

Objective

Increase supination of the right forearm.

Position

Seated (Fig. 54.67).

Procedure

1. Stand facing the patient.
2. Support the patient's right elbow with your left hand.
3. Place your right hand at the distal end of the patient's right forearm and supinate it to initial resistance.
4. Direct the patient to pronate the right forearm against equal resistance supplied through your right hand.
5. Maintain the forces long enough to sense the patient's contractile force at the localized segment or area (usually 3–5 seconds). This is monitoring.
6. Direct the patient to gently cease the directive force; cease your counterforce gently; do these simultaneously.
7. Wait 2 seconds for the tissues to relax, then take up the slack to the new point of initial resistance.
8. Repeat until the best possible increase of motion is obtained.
9. Retest.

RESTRICTION

The right forearm has restriction of pronation.

Objective

Increase the pronation of the right forearm.

Position

Seated (Fig. 54.68).

Procedure

1. Stand facing the patient.
2. Support the patient's right elbow with your left hand.
3. Place your right hand at the distal end of the patient's right forearm and pronate it to initial resistance.
4. Direct the patient to supinate the right forearm against an equal counterforce supplied through your right hand.
5. Maintain the forces long enough to sense the patient's contractile force at the localized segment or area (usually 3–5 seconds). This is monitoring.
6. Direct the patient to gently cease the directive force; cease your counterforce gently; do these simultaneously.
7. Wait 2 seconds for the tissues to relax, then take up the slack to the new point of initial resistance.
8. Repeat until the best possible increase of motion is obtained.
9. Retest.

Radiocarpal Joint (Wrist)

RESTRICTION

The right wrist has restriction of flexion.

Objective

Increase flexion of the right wrist.

Figure 54.67. Treatment for right forearm restriction of supination.

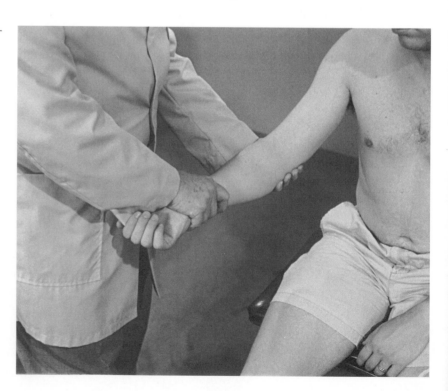

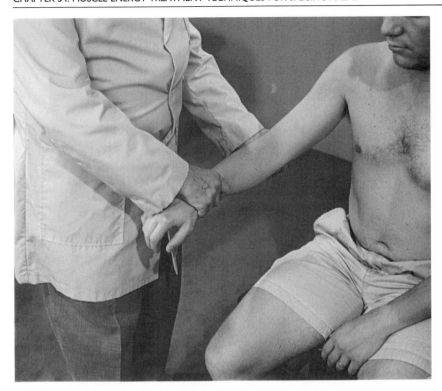

Figure 54.68. Treatment for right forearm restriction of pronation.

Position

Seated (or standing) (Fig. 54.69).

Procedure

1. Stand or sit facing the patient.
2. Support the distal end of the patient's right forearm with your left hand.
3. Place your right hand over the dorsum of the patient's right hand. Flex the hand at the wrist to the point of initial resistance.
4. Direct the patient to gently press the right hand against your right hand as you offer equal counterforce.
5. Maintain the forces long enough to sense the patient's contractile force at the localized segment or area (usually 3–5 seconds). This is monitoring.
6. Direct the patient to gently cease the directive force; cease your counterforce gently; do these simultaneously.
7. Wait 2 seconds for the tissues to relax, then take up the slack to the new point of initial resistance.
8. Repeat until the best possible increase of motion is obtained.
9. Retest.

RESTRICTION

The left wrist has restriction of extension.

Objective

Increase extension of the left wrist.

Position

Seated (Fig. 54.70).

Procedure

(All steps are the same as listed for the technique used to increase flexion except for steps 3 and 4.)

1. Stand or sit facing the patient.
2. Support the distal end of the patient's left forearm with your left hand.
3. Place the heel of your right hand against the distal palm of the patient's left hand and extend the hand at the wrist to initial resistance.
4. Direct the patient to flex the hand at the wrist against an equal counterforce offered by your left hand.
5. Maintain the forces long enough to sense the patient's contractile force at the localized segment or area (usually 3–5 seconds). This is monitoring.
6. Direct the patient to gently cease the directive force; cease your counterforce gently; do these simultaneously.
7. Wait 2 seconds for the tissues to relax, then take up the slack to the new point of initial resistance.
8. Repeat until the best possible increase of motion is obtained.
9. Retest.

POSITIONAL DIAGNOSIS

Right wrist is deviated toward the ulnar side. The hand is adducted.

Figure 54.69.   Treatment for right wrist restriction of flexion.

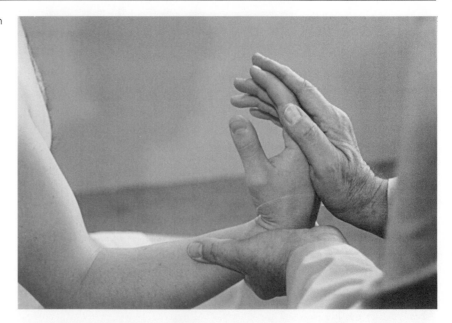

Figure 54.70.   Treatment for right wrist restriction of extension.

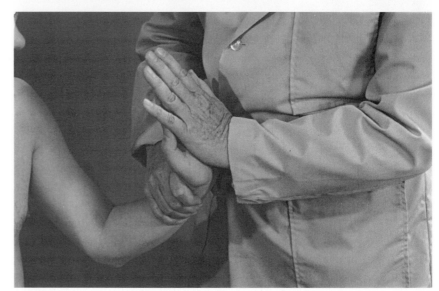

RESTRICTION

The right hand has restriction of abduction at wrist.

Objective

Increase abduction of the right hand at wrist.

Position

Seated or standing (Fig. 54.71).

Procedure

1. Stand or sit facing the standing or seated patient.
2. Use your left hand to support the distal end of the patient's supinated forearm.
3. Place your right hand at the medial (ulnar) side of the patient's hand and abduct the hand at the wrist to initial resistance.

4. Direct the patient to gently press the hand against your right hand which offers an equal counterforce.
5. Maintain the forces long enough to sense the patient's contractile force at the localized segment or area (usually 3–5 seconds). This is monitoring.
6. Direct the patient to gently cease the directive force; cease your counterforce gently; do these simultaneously.
7. Wait 2 seconds for the tissues to relax, then take up the slack to the new point of initial resistance.
8. Repeat until the best possible increase of motion is obtained.
9. Retest.

POSITIONAL DIAGNOSIS

The right hand is abducted at the wrist. The right hand is deviated toward the radial side.

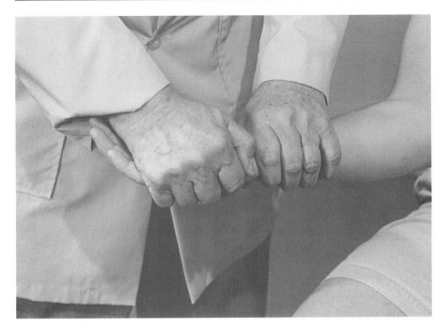

Figure 54.71. Treatment for right wrist deviated to ulnar side.

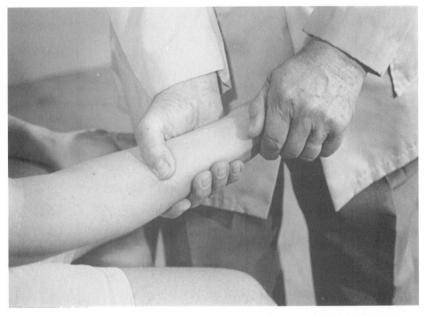

Figure 54.72. Treatment for right hand abducted at wrist.

RESTRICTION

The right hand has restriction of adduction at the wrist.

Objective

Increase right hand adduction at the wrist.

Position

Seated or standing (Fig. 54.72).

Procedure

Same as for treatment of restricted abduction except steps 2, 3, and 4.

1. Stand or sit facing the standing or seated patient.
2. Use your right hand to hold the patient's supinated forearm at the distal end.
3. Place your left hand at the radial side of the hand and adduct to initial resistance.
4. Direct the patient to abduct the hand against your equal counterforce.
5. Maintain the forces long enough to sense the patient's contractile force at the localized segment or area (usually 3–5 seconds). This is monitoring.
6. Direct the patient to gently cease the directive force; cease your counterforce gently; do these simultaneously.
7. Wait 2 seconds for the tissues to relax, then take up the slack to the new point of initial resistance.

8. Repeat until the best possible increase of motion is obtained.
9. Retest.

LOWER EXTREMITY SOMATIC DYSFUNCTIONS

Muscle energy does not depend on an "all-or-none" contraction of the muscle. The well-directed pull of muscle fibers with isometric resistance effectively removes restrictions or restraints of joint motion; this is called isometric muscle contraction.

When muscle energy procedures are used to strengthen muscle groups, a counterforce that is less than the maximum contraction that the patient produces to move an appendage through its full range of motion is used; this is called isotonic or eccentric muscle contraction.

Hip Joint

RESTRICTION

The right femur has restriction of abduction at the hip.

Objective

Increase abduction of the right femur.

Position

Supine (Figure 54.73).

Procedure

1. Stand at the foot of the supine patient.
2. Place your left hand at the distal end of right leg; lift and

abduct the right lower limb at the hip joint to the point of initial resistance.
3. Step between the patient's right limb and table and press your thigh against the medial side of the right limb.
4. Direct the patient to press the right limb against your thigh (attempting adduction) while your offer an equal counterforce.
5. Maintain the forces long enough to sense the patient's contractile force at the localized segment or area (usually 3–5 seconds). This is monitoring.
6. Direct the patient to gently cease the directive force; cease your counterforce gently; do these simultaneously.
7. Wait 2 seconds for the tissues to relax, then take up the slack to the new point of initial resistance.
8. Repeat until the best possible increase of motion is obtained.
9. Retest.

RESTRICTION

The right femur has restriction of adduction at hip.

Objective

Increase adduction of the right femur.

Position

Supine (Fig. 54.74).

Procedure

1. Stand at the foot of the table.
2. With your left hand at the distal end of right leg; lift and adduct the right lower limb at the hip joint to the point of initial resistance.

Figure 54.73. Treatment for right femur restriction of abduction at hip.

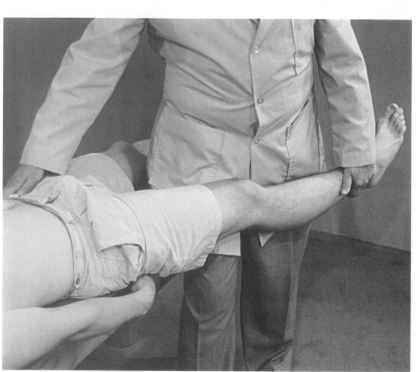

3. Direct the patient to press the right limb against your left hand (attempt to abduct the femur) as you offer an equal counterforce.

4. Maintain the forces long enough to sense the patient's contractile force at the localized segment or area (usually 3–5 seconds). This is monitoring.

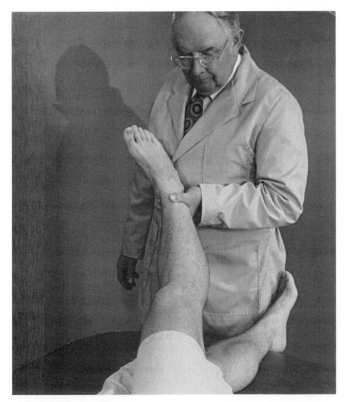

Figure 54.74. Treatment for right femur restriction of abduction at

5. Direct the patient to gently cease the directive force; cease your counterforce gently; do these simultaneously.

6. Wait 2 seconds for the tissues to relax, then take up the slack to the new point of initial resistance.

7. Repeat until the best possible increase of motion is obtained.

8. Retest.

RESTRICTION

The right femur has restriction of extension caused by a shortened right iliopsoas muscle.

Objective

Lengthen the right iliopsoas muscle to increase extension of the right femur at the hip.

Position

Supine (Figs. 54.75 and 54.76). See also Figure 54.77, alternative handhold for physician.

Procedure

1. Treatment is contraindicated if the patient has low back pain and restricted motion in the lumbar area.

2. Stand to the right of the supine patient.

3. Direct the patient to flex both thighs to abdomen, which also flattens lumbar lordosis.

4. Lower the right limb to the table as the patient's arms hold the left thigh flexed tightly against the abdomen. If the iliopsoas is short, the posterior thigh does not touch the table.

5. Gently place your right hand on patient's right thigh just proximal to the extended knee.

Figure 54.75. Treatment for right femur restriction of extension (shortened right iliopsoas muscle).

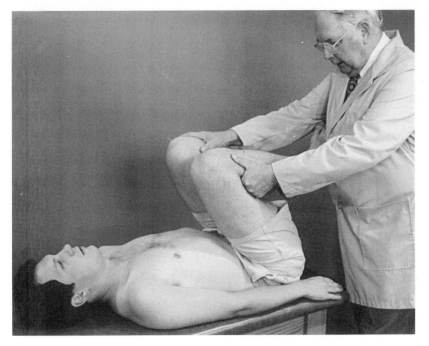

Figure 54.76. Treatment for right femur restriction of extension (shortened right iliopsoas).

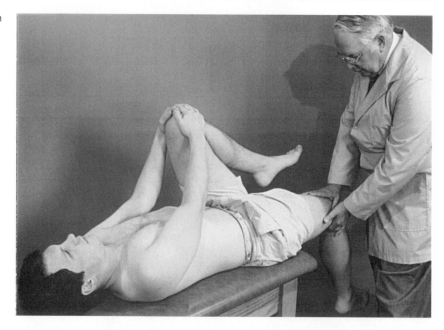

Figure 54.77. Treatment for right femur restriction of extension (shortened right iliopsoas).

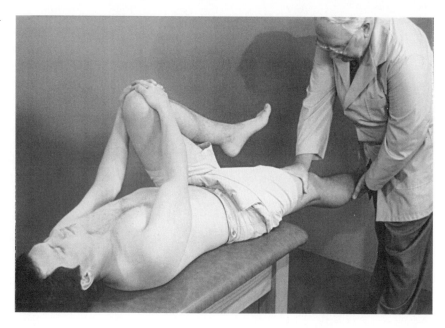

6. Direct the patient to press the right thigh toward the ceiling and against your right hand, which offers an equal counterforce.
7. Maintain the forces long enough to sense the patient's contractile force at the localized segment or area (usually 3–5 seconds). This is monitoring.
8. Direct the patient to gently cease the directive force; cease your counterforce gently; do these simultaneously.
9. Wait 2 seconds for the tissues to relax, then take up the slack to the new point of initial resistance.
10. Repeat until the best possible increase of motion is obtained.
11. Retest.

RESTRICTION

Restriction of flexion of the right hip (restriction of right straight leg raising) attributed to a short hypertonic hamstring muscles.

Objective

Increase the range of right straight leg raising (flexion of the hip) by lengthening the right hamstring muscle.

Position

Supine (Figs. 54.78 and 54.79).

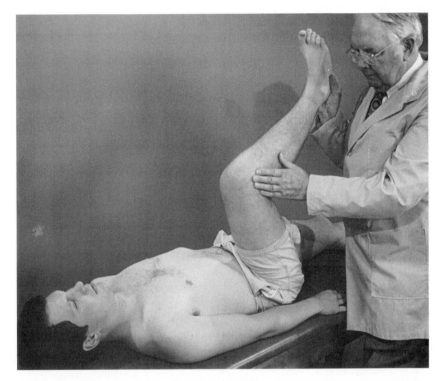

Figure 54.78. Treatment for restriction of flexion of right hip.

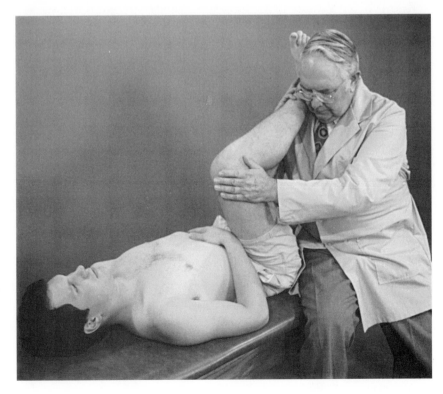

Figure 54.79. Treatment for restriction of flexion of right hip.

Procedure

1. Stand at the right side of the patient.
2. Use your right hand to cup the patient's right heel and raise the patient's right limb toward the ceiling. Allow some flexion at knee to avoid hyperextension. Raise the extremity to initial resistance.
3. Direct the patient to press the right heel into your right hand while offering equal counterforce. An alternative to cupping the patient's heel with your hand is to place the right heel on your right shoulder. Initially you can sit on the table, and with subsequent excursions you can stand. Your left hand may be placed anterior to the patient's knee to encourage increased extension. Remember to avoid hyperextension of the knee.
4. Maintain the forces long enough to sense the patient's contractile force at the localized segment or area (usually 3–5 seconds). This is monitoring.
5. Direct the patient to gently cease the directive force; cease your counterforce gently; do these simultaneously.
6. Wait 2 seconds for the tissues to relax, then take up the slack to the new point of initial resistance.
7. Repeat until the best possible increase of motion is obtained.
8. Retest.

RESTRICTION

Restriction of external rotation of the right femur at the hip when the femur is flexed 90° at the hip (restriction of lateral rotation of the femur).

Objective

To increase external rotation of the femur when the hip is flexed 90° at the hip.

Position

Supine (Figs. 54.80 and 54.81).

Procedure

1. Stand at the right side of the supine patient.
2. Maintain 90° of flexion at the patient's right hip.
3. Use your right hand to cup the heel of the patient's right foot.
4. Use your left hand to stabilize the right knee in the sagittal plane.
5. Use your right hand to move the patient's right foot medially in an arc about a pivot point at the knee. As the foot moves medially, a point on the shaft of the femur is rotating laterally. Move to initial resistance.
6. Direct the patient to push the foot laterally in an arc (shaft of femur is rotating medially) against your right hand, which offers an equal counterforce.
7. Maintain the forces long enough to sense the patient's contractile force at the localized segment or area (usually 3–5 seconds). This is monitoring.
8. Direct the patient to gently cease the directive force; cease your counterforce gently; do these simultaneously.

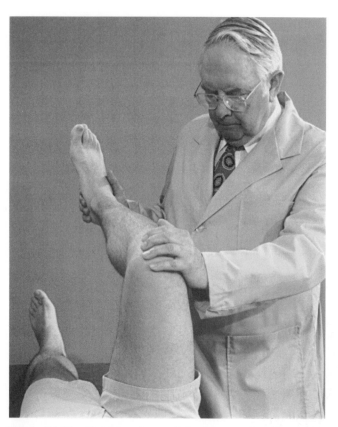

Figure 54.80. Treatment for restriction of external rotation of right femur at hip.

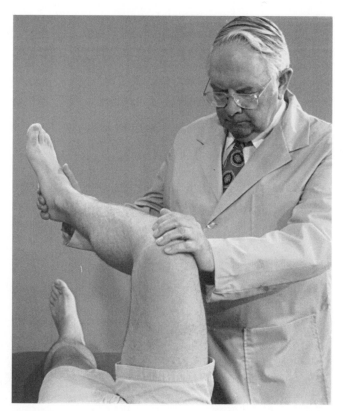

Figure 54.81. Treatment for restriction of external rotation of right femur at hip.

9. Wait 2 seconds for the tissues to relax, then take up the slack to the new point of initial resistance.
10. Repeat until the best possible increase of motion is obtained.
11. Retest.

RESTRICTION

The right femur has restriction of external rotation (lateral rotation).

Objective

Increase the external rotation of the right femur.

Position

Prone (Figs. 54.82 and 54.83).

Procedure

1. Stand next to the right side of the patient whose right leg is flexed 90° at the knee.
2. Use your left hand to hold the sole of the patient's right foot and your right hand to stabilize the right knee. Maintain the hip on the table and move the right foot medially in an arc, to the point of initial resistance.

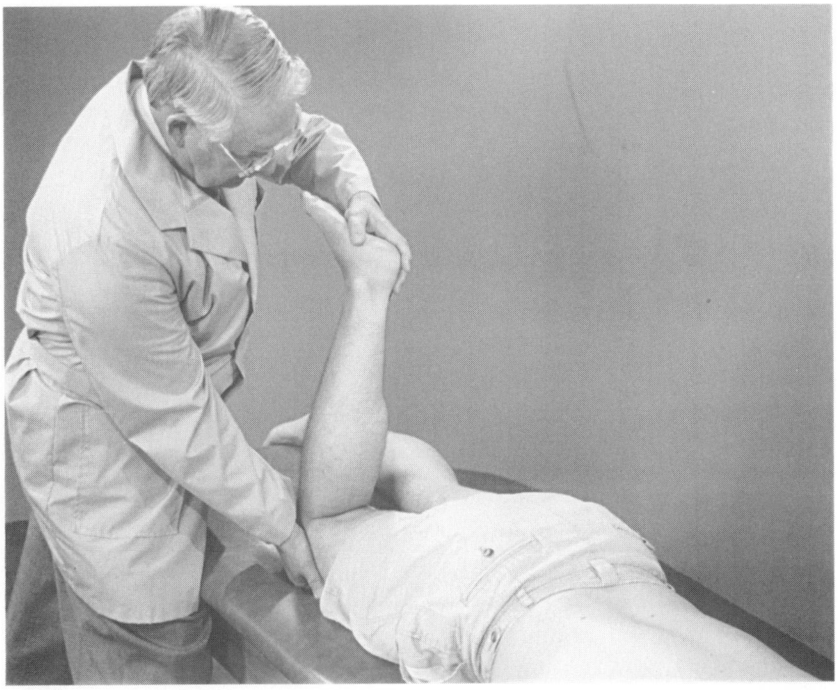

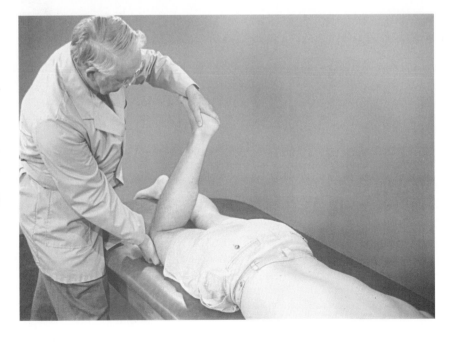

Figure 54.82. Treatment for right femur restriction of external rotation.

Figure 54.83. Treatment for right femur restriction of external rotation.

3. Direct the patient to move the right foot in an arc laterally against your left hand while offering an equal counterforce.
4. Maintain the forces long enough to sense the patient's contractile force at the localized segment or area (usually 3–5 seconds). This is monitoring.
5. Direct the patient to gently cease the directive force; cease your counterforce gently; do these simultaneously.
6. Wait 2 seconds for the tissues to relax, then take up the slack to the new point of initial resistance.
7. Repeat until the best possible increase of motion is obtained.
8. Retest.

RESTRICTION

The right femur has restriction of internal rotation (medial rotation).

Objective

Increase internal rotation of the right femur.

Position

Prone (Figs. 54.84 and 54.85).

Figure 54.84. Treatment for right femur restriction of internal rotation.

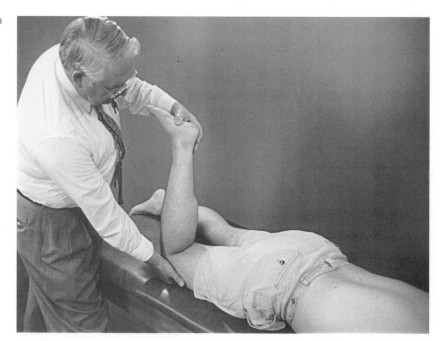

Figure 54.85. Treatment for right femur restriction of internal rotation.

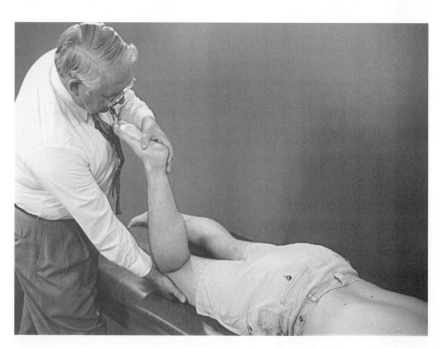

Procedure

1. Stand next to the right side of the prone patient; the patient's knee is flexed 90°.
2. Use your left hand to hold the sole of the patient's right foot, and your right hand to stabilizing the right knee. Maintain the hip on the table and move the right foot laterally in an arc, to the point of initial resistance.
3. Instruct the patient to push the right foot in an arc, medially against your left hand, while you offer an equal counterforce.
4. Maintain the forces long enough to sense the patient's contractile force at the localized segment or area (usually 3–5 seconds). This is monitoring.
5. Direct the patient to gently cease the directive force; cease your counterforce gently; do these simultaneously.
6. Wait 2 seconds for the tissues to relax, then take up the slack to the new point of initial resistance.
7. Repeat until the best possible increase of motion is obtained.
8. Retest.

Knee Joint

RESTRICTION

The right knee has restriction of flexion.

Objective

Increase flexion at the right knee.

Position

Prone (Figs. 54.86 and 54.87).

Procedure

1. Stand next to the patient's right side at the level of the knee.
2. Place your right hand (palm up) under the anterior distal end of the right leg. Use your left hand to stabilize the right knee. Passively flex the knee to initial resistance.
3. Direct the patient to extend the right leg (using quadriceps femoris) against your left hand, which offers equal counterforce.
4. Maintain the forces long enough to sense the patient's contractile force at the localized segment or area (usually 3–5 seconds). This is monitoring.
5. Direct the patient to gently cease the directive force; cease your counterforce gently; do these simultaneously.
6. Wait 2 seconds for the tissues to relax, then take up the slack to the new point of initial resistance.
7. Repeat until the best possible increase of motion is obtained.
8. Retest.

Proximal Tibiofibular Joint

POSITIONAL DIAGNOSIS

The right proximal fibula glides anteriorly; the proximal fibula is anterior along the tibial articular surface.

RESTRICTION

The right proximal fibula has restriction of gliding posteriorly.

Objective

Glide the proximal head of the right fibula posteriorly along the articular surface of the tibia.

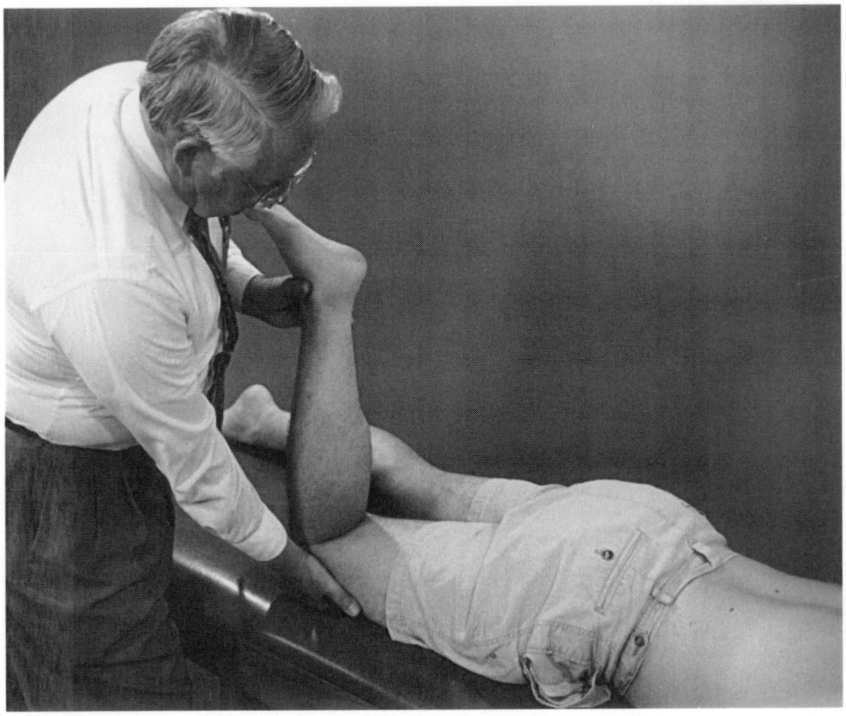

Figure 54.86. Treatment for right knee restriction of flexion.

Figure 54.87. Treatment for right knee restriction of flexion.

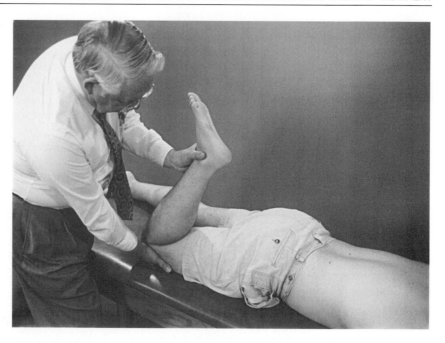

Figure 54.88. Treatment for right proximal fibula restriction of gliding.

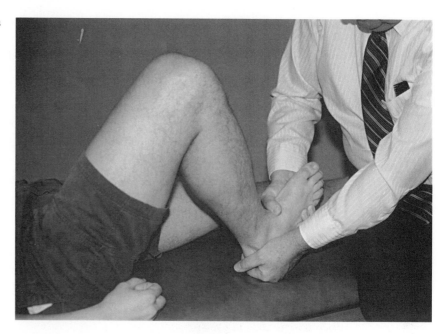

Position

Supine with right hip and knee flexed and the right foot on the table; left leg hangs off the end of the table (Fig. 54.88).

Procedure

1. Stand at the foot of the table, facing the patient's head.
2. Place your left hand on the lateral side of patient's foot. Your thumb should be pointing posteriorly and your fingers wrapped around the sole of the foot.

3. Invert the patient's foot to initial resistance.
4. Place the heel of your right hand against the metatarsal heads of the patient's right foot and dorsiflex to initial resistance.
5. Direct the patient to evert the foot against counterforce offered by the thenar eminence of your left hand (this is thought to isotonically contract the peroneus longus and draw the fibula laterally from the tibia, making posterior gliding easier), and direct the patient to plantar flex the right foot against the heel of your right hand, which offers an equal counterforce (this is thought to isotonically contract the soleus and draw the fibula

posteriorly along the tibial articular surface). Counterforce may also be offered by placing your right knee against the sole of the patient's right foot.

6. Direct the patient to gently cease the directive force; cease your counterforce gently; do these simultaneously.
7. Wait 2 seconds for the tissues to relax, then take up the slack to the new point of initial resistance.
8. Repeat until the best possible increase of motion is obtained.
9. Retest.

POSITIONAL DIAGNOSIS

Right fibular head posterior; right proximal fibula posterior.

RESTRICTION

The right proximal fibula has restriction of anterior glide.

Objective

Increase anterior glide of the right proximal fibula along the tibial articular surface.

Position

Supine with right hip and knee flexed and the right foot on the table (Fig. 54.89).

Procedure

1. Stand at the foot of the table, facing the patient's head.
2. Place your right hand on the dorsum of the patient's right foot with your thumb pointing posteriorly along the lateral surface of the foot and the remaining fingers wrapped around the medial side of the foot. Plantar flex the foot to initial resistance.

3. Place your left hand over the lateral side of the patient's foot, your thumb pointing posteriorly and your fingers wrapped around the sole of the foot. Invert the patient's right foot to initial resistance.
4. Direct the patient to evert the foot against your left thenar eminence, which offers equal counterforce; direct the patient to dorsiflex the foot against counterforce of your right palm on the dorsum of the foot. (This is thought to contract the extensor digitorum longus, which attaches to the lateral condyle of the tibia and the upper three-fourths of the medial surface of the fibula, and the tibialis anterior muscle, which attaches to the lateral surface of the tibia and the anterior surface of the interosseus membrane between the tibia and fibula. The actions of these muscles draw the fibula anteriorly along the tibial articular surface.)
5. Direct the patient to gently cease the directive force; cease your counterforce gently; do these simultaneously.
6. Wait 2 seconds for the tissues to relax, then take up the slack to the new point of initial resistance.
7. Repeat until the best possible increase of motion is obtained.
8. Retest.

Ankle Joint

RESTRICTION

The right ankle has restriction of dorsiflexion.

Objective

Increase the range of dorsiflexion of the right ankle.

Position

Supine with right hip and knee extended (Fig. 54.90).

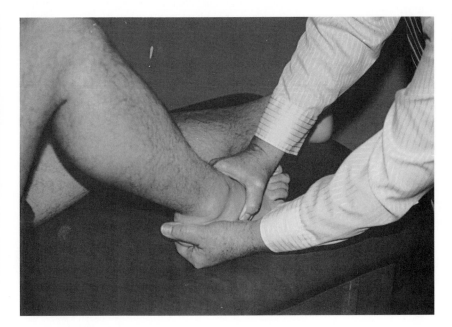

Figure 54.89. Treatment for right proximal fibula restriction anterior glide.

Figure 54.90.   Treatment for right ankle restriction dorsiflexion.

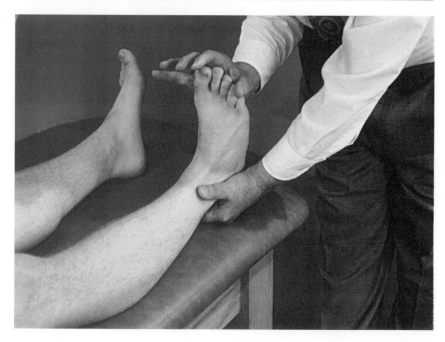

Procedure

1. Stand next to the right side of the patient's foot.
2. Cup the heel of the patient's right foot in the palm of your left hand. Place the heel of your right hand against the metatarsal heads of the patient's right foot. Dorsiflex the right ankle to the point of initial resistance.
3. Direct the patient, "Push the 'ball' of your right foot against my hand," (to attempt plantar flexion of the right foot). Offer equal counterforce.
4. Maintain the forces long enough to sense the patient's contractile force at the localized segment or area (3–5 seconds). This is monitoring.
5. Direct the patient to gently cease the directive force; cease your counterforce gently; do these simultaneously.
6. Wait 2 seconds for the tissues to relax, then take up the slack to the new point of initial resistance.
7. Repeat until the best possible increase of motion is obtained.
8. Retest.

RESTRICTION

The right ankle has restriction of plantar flexion.

Objective

Increase plantar flexion of the right ankle.

Position

Supine with right hip and knee extended (Figs. 54.91 and 54.92).

Procedure

1. Stand at the foot of the table and lateral to the patient's right foot.

2. Cup the heel of the patient's right foot in the palm of your left hand. Place the palm of your right hand over the dorsal surface of the patient's right foot. Plantar flex the right ankle to the point of initial resistance.
3. Direct the patient, "Pull your toes and the top of your foot upward toward your knee to flex your right ankle." Offer equal counterforce through your right palm.
4. Maintain the forces long enough to sense the patient's contractile force at the localized segment or area (usually 3–5 seconds). This is monitoring.
5. Direct the patient to gently cease the directive force; cease your counterforce gently; do these simultaneously.
6. Wait 2 seconds for the tissues to relax, then take up the slack to the new point of initial resistance.
7. Repeat until the best possible increase of motion is obtained.
8. Retest.

NONARTICULAR SOMATIC DYSFUNCTION

Thoracoabdominal Diaphragm

The chest cage and the abdominal wall act like a cylinder, which is separated by the thoracoabdominal diaphragm. The fibromuscular thoracoabdominal diaphragm closes the inferior thoracic aperture. It is attached to the xiphoid process, the lower six ribs, and by crura to the upper three lumbar vertebrae on the right and the upper two lumbar on the left. Diaphragmatic tension may be produced by specific joint somatic dysfunctions and also by fascial pull or torsion at the thoracolumbar junction. These tensions may be related to asymmetries and dysfunctions of one or both sides of the thoracoabdominal diaphragm and reduce the efficiency of its function.

This is one of a variety of ways to diagnose asymmetrical motion of the diaphragm.

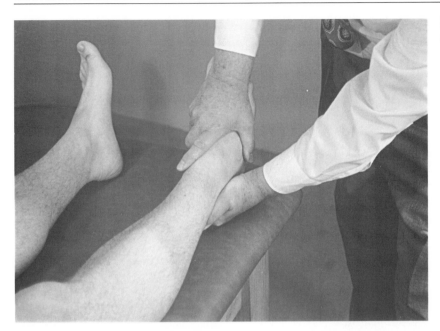

Figure 54.91. Treatment for right ankle restriction of plantar flexion (anterolateral view).

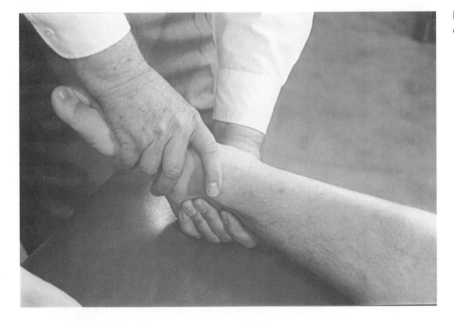

Figure 54.92. Treatment for right ankle restriction of plantar flexion (medial view).

EXAMINATION

Procedure

1. Stand at the side of your supine patient, facing the head of the table.
2. Hold the lateral sides of the lower chest cage with the palms of your hands.
3. Rotate the lower thoracic "cylinder" (thoracolumbar junction) toward the right and then the left. Sense any asymmetry in fascial and gross motion.
4. Translate cylinder right and left to determine any preference in side-bending in this area. Record the preference. The thoracolumbar fascia usually prefers to rotate in one direction and side-bend in the other.

When both sides of the chest are palpated to have good excursion during inhalation, both sides of the diaphragm are effectively working.

POSITIONAL DIAGNOSIS

Fascias of the thoracolumbar junction permit this region to be rotated to the left and side-bent right.

RESTRICTION

The fascias of the thoracolumbar junction resist this region's rotation right and side-bending left. (Bilateral palpation of the thoracolumbar junction while the patient deeply inhales and exhales, usually detects asymmetrical contraction of the abdominal diaphragm.)

Objective

Establish symmetrical excursion of the thoracoabdominal diaphragm by rotating the myofascial tissues of the thoracolumbar cylinder to the right and translating them to the right. (This is a direct method treatment, using a myofascial technique and patient respiratory cooperation.) Holding the chest in this position and asking the patient to take three or four deep breaths allows the diaphragm to redome itself and become more effec-

tive in the processes of respiration and as an extrinsic pump for the lymphatic system.

Position

Supine (Figs. 54.93 and 54.94).

Procedure

1. Stand by the side of the patient, facing the head of the table.
2. Place your hands and fingers on the lower thoracic cage in the same position used to check fascial preference. Rotate the lower rib cage to the right until a moderate firm resistance is sensed,

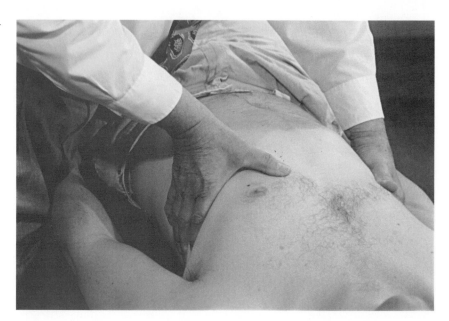

Figure 54.93. Treatment for fascias of thoracolumbar junction, rotate left, side-bent right.

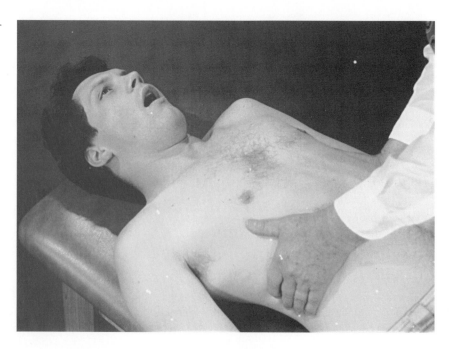

Figure 54.94. Treatment for fascias of thoracolumbar junction, rotate left, side-bent right.

and hold it.

3. Ask the patient, "Open your mouth wide and take in a deep breath and then exhale."

4. Usually, at this point the right side moves well laterally and the left side has little or no motion.

5. Maintain the right rotation and induce superior translation with your left hand and inferior translation with your right hand (this tends to side-bend the region to the left). Have the patient take another deep breath in and out. If at this position symmetrical lateral expansion of the lower thoracic cage is not felt, reverse the direction of the translations but maintain the position of right rotation. Repeat the patient's deep inhalation and exhalation.

6. Hold the chest cage in the position of greatest motion during deep breaths; have the patient take 3 or 4 deep breaths while you continue to hold (the action of the diaphragmatic contraction domes the diaphragm).

7. Return the patient to neutral and recheck movement of the lower chest cage with deep inhalation and exhalation.

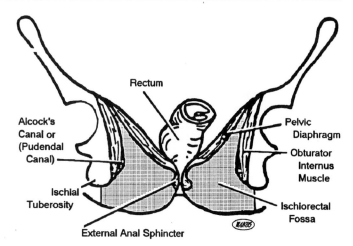

Figure 54.95. Treatment for coronal section of ischiorectal fossa.

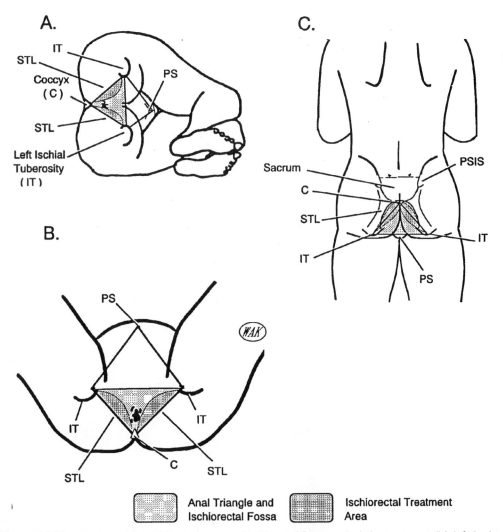

Figure 54.96. Landmarks for pelvic diaphragm and ischiorectal fossa manipulative treatment. *ILA*, inferior lateral angles; *IT*, ischial tuberosities; *STL*, sacrotuberous ligament; *C*, coccyx; *PS*, pubic symphysis.

Ischiorectal Fossa

It is very important to understand the exact anatomical landmarks so that treatment to relax the pelvic diaphragm is effective (Fig. 54.95).

Bilateral relaxation of this diaphragm permits it to work efficiently in concert with the thoracoabdominal diaphragm. Parallel motion of these diaphragms improves lymphatic flow from the pelvic organs in particular, and the flow of lymph through the thoracic duct in general. Asymmetry in tension and motion of the pelvic diaphragm can be associated with such conditions as prostatic spasm, vaginismus, bladder symptomatology without infection, etc.

EXAMINATION

Pelvic diaphragm tension is palpated by inserting extended fingers along the lateral wall of the ischiorectal fossa. This is facilitated by having the patient breathe in and then out. During exhalation the diaphragm relaxes. Asymmetry in the tension of the right and left sides is a positive sign for dysfunction. (Tension could also be evaluated during a vaginal or rectal examination by sensing the tension of the right and left halves of the pelvic diaphragm located lateral to these structures.) It is important to know the pelvic landmarks of the fossa to avoid palpation of the area of the genital triangle (Fig. 54.96, A–C).

TREATMENT

Objective

Reduce the myofascial tension of the pelvic diaphragm.

Position

Left lateral recumbent position with knees and hips flexed (Figs. 54.97 and see also Fig. 54.96A).

Procedure

1. Stand behind the patient.
2. Instruct the patient, "Relax the muscles of the buttocks region." (Relax the perineal muscles.)
3. Place the extended fingers of your right hand near the lateral end of an imaginary line between the tip of the coccyx and the patient's right ischial tuberosity.
4. Gently insert the extended fingers along the lateral wall of the ischiorectal fossa, contacting the medial surface of the ischium and the obturator internus muscle; continue insertion of the fingers until tension is experienced. Have the patient breathe in and then out. During exhalation, follow the pelvic diaphragm cephalad as it relaxes and allows your fingers to extend farther into the ischiorectal fossa.
5. When no further extension is comfortably possible, have the patient cough and sense the pelvic diaphragm as it pushes and stretches against your fingers.

This procedure is both a diagnostic test (how tense is this half of the pelvic diaphragm?) and a treatment (inhibition and stretching of the diaphragm).

Position

Lithotomy position (Fig. 54.98 and see also Fig. 54.96B).

Procedure

The only difference between this and the technique described with the patient in lateral recumbent position is that the patient is in the lithotomy position. It may be more difficult to place the fingers in the correct position when the patient is in this position. In general, you would use the extended fingers of the right hand to treat the patient's right ischiorectal fossa and the fingers of your left hand to treat the left ischiorectal fossa.

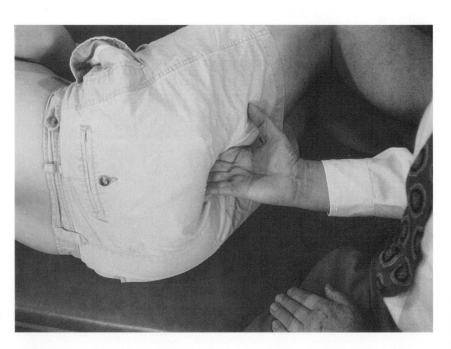

Figure 54.97. Treatment for myofascial tension pelvic diaphragm.

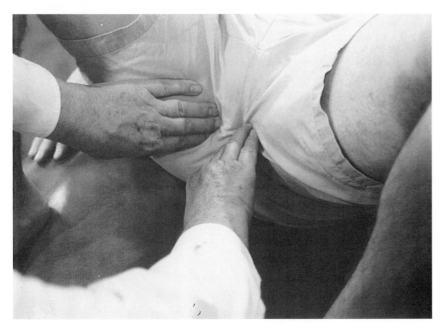

Figure 54.98. Treatment for myofascial tension pelvic diaphragm.

The fingers are always posterior to an imaginary line that connects the ischial tuberosities. This insures that the fingers are not in the genital triangle (see diagrams of the posterior anal triangles in Fig. 54.98, *A–C*).

Position

Prone position (Fig. 54.96 *C*).

Procedure

1. Stand to the side of the prone patient.
2. Identify the coccyx and the ischial tuberosities.
3. Place your thumbs pointing toward the table and about 1 to 1½ inches apart. Place them on the inferior surface of the inferior lateral angles, press laterally and superiorly and ask the patient to cough.
4. Now insert your thumbs into the ischiorectal fossa medial to the midpoint of the sacrotuberous ligaments until they meet initial resistance. Determine if there is asymmetry of tension on the right and left sides. Press laterally against the sacrotuberous ligaments, hold and ask the patient to cough.
5. Then place your fingers on the medial edges of the ischial tuberosities and press laterally. Have the patient cough again.

CONCLUSION

Muscle energy techniques, when used according to these procedures, can aid in the resolution and healing of somatic dysfunction.

REFERENCES

1. Kimberly PE. *Somatic Dysfunction Principles of Manipulative Treatment: Illustrative Procedures for Specific Joint Mobilization.* 2nd ed. Kirksville, Mo: KCOM Press; 1980.
2. *Stedman's Medical Dictionary.* 24th ed. Baltimore, Md: Williams & Wilkins; 1982.

55. Articulatory Techniques

DAVID A. PATRIQUIN AND JOHN M. JONES III

Key Concepts

- **Design of articulatory, or springing, technique**
- **Uses of and additions to articulatory activation**
- **Diagnostic findings suggesting use of articulating technique**
- **Special cases suitable for application of technique**
- **Contraindications**
- **General instructions of design of technique**
- **Rib raising and Spencer techniques**
- **Specific articulatory techniques by region, including cervical, cervicothoracic, thoracic, costal, lumbar, pelvic, and extremities**

Articulatory technique, also called "springing" technique, is a direct technique. The physician gently and repetitively forces the part of the body being treated against the restrictive barrier (generally maintained by tight muscles and connective tissues acting as restrainers), intending to reduce that barrier and improve physiologic motion. This form of osteopathic treatment is called low-velocity moderate- to high-amplitude, or long-lever, technique. "Rib raising" with the patient in the supine position, or the Spencer series of techniques for articulating all ranges of motion of the dysfunctional shoulder, are examples of articulatory technique.

DESIGN AND USE OF ARTICULATING ACTIVATION

Articulating activation can be designed and applied to resolve either a simple problem with a single restrictive barrier or a complex problem with multiple joint and tissue restrictive barriers. This type of technique is particularly useful where the application of low, gentle, controlled movements is indicated. Postoperative patients and elderly patients suffering from arthritis or osteopenia find this type of direct treatment more acceptable than the vigorous types, because in most settings the articulating forces are gentle.

Respiratory cooperation (inhalation to accumulate tissue tension or exhalation to induce relaxation) and active muscle contraction or relaxation are frequently added. These additions enhance the effect of passive articulating motion by resisting it (inhalation or muscle contraction) or permitting increased range of motion (exhalation or muscle relaxation). The appropriate modification is selected to increase the range of motion while limiting the amount of discomfort induced by the procedure.

As an example, a direct articulating treatment can be applied to a vertebral unit restricted in right rotation. Make repeated attempts to increase right rotation of the vertebra by slowly, gently encouraging the affected vertebra into right rotation against the restrictive motion barrier. Slightly increase the force or induce a wider range of motion on each cycle. Finally, once the barrier to motion is firmly engaged, instruct the patient to take a deep breath—as deep as is comfortable. The intrinsic force generated by this action markedly augments the stretching, mobilizing forces applied by the physician. The intrinsic force generated by deep inspiration opposes those forces the operator already induced. The combination of operator and intrinsic forces results in more tension in soft tissues and produces greater stretching and lengthening in them than would operator force alone.

The repetitive application of gentle force may be directed to the reduction of one barrier at a time, in successive steps, or the physician may attempt to engage two or more barriers with one movement. While the same principles of technique design apply in the case of motion restriction in multiple planes, the actual directions and forces used may be so complex as to defy description. There are many possible combinations of vectors of motion and sequence during one treatment when applying this type of manipulation to multiple plane restrictions in a single treatment. Simple passive efforts strongly reinforce the addition of intrinsic forces such as respiratory cooperation or isometric muscle energy activity.

COMMON QUESTIONS

Diagnosis

What diagnostic findings suggest the therapeutic use of articulating technique? The cardinal clinical indicator for applying an articulating technique is limited or lost articular motion. The most common cause for this loss of articular motion is a dysfunction in the local (periarticular) supporting tissues or in the longer muscles or ligaments associated with the articulation. There are secondary indicators for the application of an articulatory technique. These include a need to increase the frequency or amplitude of motion in a body region. An example of this is the need to increase the frequency and amplitude of motion in the chest of a person with respiratory disease. Accomplish this by applying thoracic lymphatic pump treatment. Expect increased amplitude and efficiency of chest motion to follow this treatment.

Special Cases

Are there special cases most suitable for the application of articulating technique? Very young and elderly patients respond well to this type of treatment. They also suffer less reaction in terms of discomfort and posttreatment stiffness than if a high-velocity low-amplitude technique is employed. Articulating technique permits accurate dosage of force and duration of treatment. It also permits careful and accurate localization of forces. The amount and direction of force can be altered during the course of treatment because movements are slow, deliberate, repeated, and constantly monitored by palpation through the physician's hands. Because the treatment is applied slowly, adjustments can be made immediately, responding to any discomfort reported by the patient in the course of the treatment.

Contraindications

Are there contraindications to the use of articulating technique? There are general cautions that apply to the use of any manual procedure in the treatment of a patient (see Chapter 73, "Efficacy and Complications"). Because articulating technique consists of repetitive applications of force, it can be quickly modified between applications of force, in response to the reaction of the patient. In the upper cervical region, it is wise to avoid simultaneous hyperrotation and extension. Repeated application of force to the upper cervical area positioned in extension and hyperrotation may damage the vertebral arteries. It is also not appropriate to use repetitive motion on an acutely inflamed joint, especially one where the cause of inflammation may be infection or reaction to a fracture.

Instructions for Design

What are the general instructions for the design of an articulating technique?

PATIENT POSITION

Use any comfortable position that permits the problem area to be passively moved completely through the affected range of motion.

PHYSICIAN POSITION

Use a comfortable position that permits the application of passive motion through the complete range of motion of the affected articulation.

PROCEDURE

Move the affected joint to the limit of all ranges of motion. As the restrictive barrier is reached, slowly and firmly continue to apply gentle force against it to the limit of tissue motion or the patient's tolerance to pain or fatigue. Then return the articulation slowly toward the neutral portion of its motion. Repeat this process several times, each time gaining range and improved quality of motion. Cease repetition of motion when no further response is achieved.

ENHANCEMENT

Intrinsic forces such as respiratory assistance or a muscle energy technique may be added once maximum range of motion has been achieved by positioning alone. Similar modifications can measurably increase motion range and quality.

SAMPLE CLINICAL APPLICATION

Rib Raising

DIAGNOSIS AND FINDINGS

A patient has viral pneumonia with a resistant or noncompliant chest wall in which the motion of all ribs is reduced in both inspiration and expiration. There is paraspinal soft tissue tenderness to light pressure, with decreased rib motion and accompanying increased soft tissue tightness (tension/tone) throughout the posterior thorax, especially at the level of the upper five thoracic vertebrae and ribs.

PATIENT POSITION

Supine, with the thorax and head slightly elevated as necessary for patient comfort.

PROCEDURE

1. Stand at the head of the treating table, facing the patient.
2. Reach under the patient's back, extending the forearms and hands palms upward, so that the finger tips can, on flexion, engage paired upper ribs near their angles on each side of the midline. This is a bilateral treatment technique.
3. Gently pull cephalad. This attempts to mobilize the costotransverse and costovertebral articulations and stretch the intercostal and more superficial thoracic tissues.
4. Hold the tension for 5–10 seconds, then slowly release.
5. Rib raising (articulatory) technique is markedly augmented when the patient exhales deeply, once full cephalad tension is applied to the ribs.
6. When repetition of this treatment no longer produces increased range of motion at this level, move your hands to the next inferior group of ribs and repeat the articulating treatment process. Treat groups of two to four ribs progressively, from above downward, until all ribs on both sides are moving freely.
7. Then move to the side of the table, beside the patient's hips, and face toward the head of the table.

8. Extend your forearm and hand, placing them under the upper thorax of the patient, with your finger tips engaging the superior surface of the upper ribs at their angles. (This is a unilateral rib articulating procedure.)

9. Pull caudally, attempting to move the ribs inferiorly in relation to other thoracic structures.

10. Repeat the process until there is no increase in motion. Treat successive lower groups of ribs in the same fashion.

11. Rib raising (articulatory) technique is markedly augmented in this phase of treatment by the addition of a deep inhalation by the patient once full caudad tension is applied to the ribs.

Alternate Technique

PATIENT POSITION

Supine.

PROCEDURE

1. Stand facing the foot of the treatment table, at the level of the patient's shoulder on the side of the rib cage to be treated.

2. Hold the patient's forearm between your arm and chest while grasping the patient's midarm with your hand.

3. Place your other arm obliquely downward under the patient's rib cage. Flex your fingers so that the fingertips engage the caudad edges of the angles of the ribs.

4. Pull cephalad on the rib angles with your fingers, reinforced by an augmenting pull on the patient's arm (generated by a cephalad sway of your entire upper body).

5. Hold the tension for 5–10 seconds before releasing. After a few seconds of rest, repeat the process, hold 5–10 seconds, and release.

6. Repeat this cycle until free motion results or patient fatigue or discomfort suggests termination.

7. When repetition of this treatment no longer produces increased range of motion at this level, move your hands to the next inferior group of ribs and repeat the articulating treatment process. Treat groups of two to four ribs progressively, from above downward, until all ribs on both sides are moving freely.

This technique may be modified by adding the patient's inspiratory effort to produce more tension and therefore induce increased range of motion. Direct the patient to take a deep breath, once you have generated maximum tension. When you are ready to release the external traction, instruct the patient to exhale and relax as the tensions diminish.

Note: The above techniques may be modified by starting on the lower ribs and progressing cephalad, rather than starting on the upper ribs and progressing downward.

SHOULDER TREATMENT: SPENCER TECHNIQUE

This is a classical clinical application of stepwise articulating technique. Seven different but related articulating procedures are carried out in sequence in this treatment. Separate ranges of motion are consecutively engaged, beginning with those least likely to be disturbed (flexion/extension) and progressing

to those most commonly restricted (internal/external rotation). It is easy to perform an articulatory technique to increase one or more ranges of shoulder joint motion, using the arm as a long lever against a shoulder girdle fixed to the patient's thorax by the other hand of the physician. Each step of the treatment may be enhanced by the addition of muscle energy activation and/or respiratory force, once the barrier has been engaged.

For example, once the lateral traction, stretching, and "fluid pumping" of the initiating stage of Spencer have been completed, carry the patient's arm, flexed at the elbow, slowly but firmly into extension against the resistance of a fixed scapula and clavicle. After release of the tension repeat the process until no increase in motion results from application of this phase of the treatment.

ARTICULATORY TECHNIQUES BY REGION

Reminders

1. An articulatory technique may be used to increase motion generally in all joints in that region, or it may be used more specifically at a particular joint by repetitively engaging a specific motion restriction. Most of the force used is at the end-range of motion.

2. Articulatory techniques use passive, smooth, rhythmic motions designed to stretch contracted muscles, ligaments, and capsules.

3. Articulatory techniques decrease tissue tension, enhance lymphatic flow, and stimulate increased joint circulation.

4. Articulatory techniques are especially useful in treating transitional zones, such as cervicothoracic, thoracolumbar, and lumbosacral.

5. Articulatory techniques may be used as preparation for high-velocity low-amplitude (HVLA) techniques.

6. Discomfort during treatment is acceptable. Pain is not.

7. Although the treatment is directed to a restriction on one side, some physicians prefer to do these treatments bilaterally, so as not to induce an imbalance in the tonicity of the musculature.

Indications

1. Restriction of joint motion
2. Myofascial shortening
3. Bilateral or unilateral somatic dysfunction in a region or at a segmental level
4. Preparation for HVLA specific thrust

Contraindications

1. Advanced bone-wasting diseases
2. Fractures
3. Acute local inflammatory condition
4. Acute localized infection
5. Neurologic signs elicited during pretest or treatment means that you must *stop* your treatment by this method.

Cervical Techniques

FLEXION

Diagnosis

Reduced cervical flexion.

Objective

Increase cervical flexion.

Patient Position

Supine.

Procedure

1. Sit behind the head of the patient (Fig. 55.1).
2. Place one hand on the patient's shoulder.
3. Place the other hand cradling the occipital region.
4. Lift the head until full flexion is obtained.
5. Hold in full flexion for 3–5 seconds, then return toward neutral.
6. Repeat slowly in a smooth, rhythmic fashion, until there is improved motion (or to the tolerance of the patient).

Alternative Procedure

1. Cross both forearms and place your hands on the patient's shoulders to support the head.
2. Use your arms to flex the head and neck.

EXTENSION

Diagnosis

Decreased cervical extension.

Objective

Increase cervical extension.

Patient Position

Supine.
    Caution: Do not perform this technique on a patient with neurological signs on cervical extension or a patient who reports symptoms of vertebrobasilar insufficiency.

Procedure

1. Sit behind the head of the patient (Fig. 55.2).
2. Place one hand under the patient's neck.
3. Use your thumb and forefinger as a fulcrum by pressing them against the posterior aspects of a vertebra.
4. Grasp the patient's chin with your other hand and lift the chin to extend the neck. In patients with temporomandibular joint (TMJ) dysfunction, grasp the patient's forehead instead of chin.
5. Using smooth, rhythmic motion, repeat several times.
6. Shift your fulcrum to another vertebra and repeat until you have treated all of the cervicals.

ROTATION

Diagnosis

Decreased cervical rotation.

Objective

Increase cervical rotation.

Patient Position

Supine.
    Caution: Do not perform this technique on a patient with

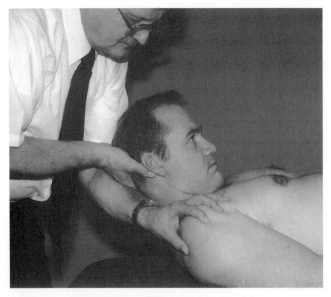

Figure 55.1. Cervical flexion technique.

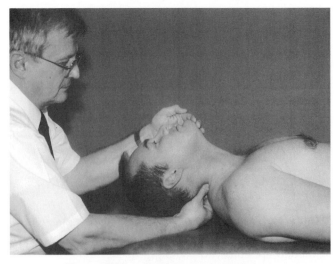

Figure 55.2. Cervical extension technique.

neurological signs upon cervical rotation or a patient who reports symptoms of vertebrobasilar insufficiency.

Procedure

1. Sit behind the head of the patient.
2. Grasp the patient's chin with your hand, with your forearm contacting the patient's zygoma.
3. Cup the patient's occiput with your other hand.
4. Rotate the head toward the side of decreased motion.
5. Hold for 3–5 seconds, then return toward neutral.
6. Repeat slowly in a smooth, rhythmic fashion until there is improved motion (or to the tolerance of the patient).

Alternative Procedure

1. You may rotate one direction, go through neutral, and rotate the other direction if you are treating a patient with bilateral decrease due to myofascial shortening. (This may require change in hand position.)
2. You may also do this in flexion.
3. Do not do it in extension.

REGIONAL SIDE-BENDING

Diagnosis

Decreased cervical side-bending (lateral flexion).

Objective

Increase cervical side-bending.

Patient Position

Supine.

Procedure

1. Sit behind the head of the patient (Fig. 55.3).
2. Place one hand on the shoulder, using the other hand to cradle the occipital region.
3. Firmly side-bend the neck toward the shoulder on the unrestricted side. You may reinforce this lateral movement by gently leaning against the head (with your abdomen). Do not use inferior vertical pressure on the vertex, especially if the patient has any signs of nerve root compression.
4. Hold for 3–5 seconds, then return toward neutral.
5. Repeat slowly in a smooth, rhythmic fashion until there is improved motion (or to the tolerance of the patient).

SEGMENTAL SIDE-BENDING

Procedure

1. Place the medial aspect of the middle phalanx or the pad of the distal phalanx against a specific joint level, as a fulcrum. This should be done on the side of restriction.
2. Grasp the posterior aspect of the head with the palm and fingers of your opposite hand.

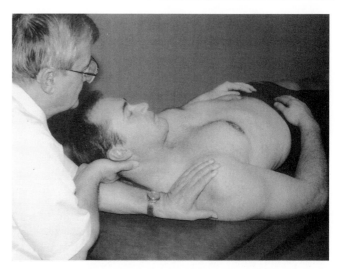

Figure 55.3. Cervical regional side-bending technique.

3. Use lateral translation to induce side-bending with your localized digit. At the same time, use lateral translation of the head in the opposite direction, achieving side-bending around the fulcrum.
4. Hold for 3–5 seconds, then return toward neutral.
5. Repeat slowly in a smooth, rhythmic fashion until there is improved motion (or to the tolerance of the patient).

Cervicothoracic Technique

FLEXION, EXTENSION, SIDE-BENDING

Diagnosis

Decreased regional flexion, extension, side-bending (lateral flexion), or rotation.

Objective

Introduce motion where it has been inappropriately restricted.

Patient Position

Lateral recumbent (restricted side up).

Procedure

1. Stand in front of the patient (Fig. 55.4).
2. Support the patient's head and neck with your hand and forearm. The patient's arm nearest the table should be flexed at the shoulder and elbow, while the opposite arm is adducted on the lateral thorax and hip area.
3. Grasp the spinous process of T1 with your caudal hand, to stabilize it against forces applied from above.
4. Use your other hand to extend, side-bend, or rotate the head and neck to the restriction of motion at the joint level you are treating (C7/T1).
5. Hold for 3–5 seconds, then return toward neutral.
6. Repeat slowly in a smooth, rhythmic fashion, until there is improved motion (or to the tolerance of the patient).

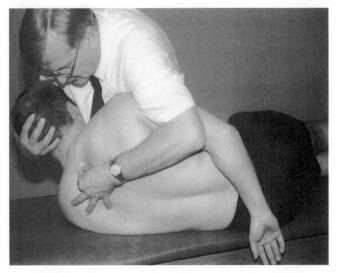

Figure 55.4. Cervicothoracic side-bending technique.

7. Move sequentially to the next inferior joint and repeat the process.

Thoracic Techniques

FLEXION

Diagnosis

Decreased flexion.

Objective

Increase thoracic flexion.

Patient Position

Seated.

Procedure

1. Stand behind the patient (Fig. 55.5).
2. Put your arm over the patient's shoulder across his or her chest and place your hand on the patient's opposite shoulder. The patient hooks his or her hands over your arm.
3. Stabilize the lower of the two vertebrae being treated by grasping and fixing the spinous process with your fingers and thumb.
4. Use your other arm to flex the upper thorax of the patient to the level of your stabilizing hand, achieving maximal flexion stretch at the joint space above.
5. Hold for 3–5 seconds, then return toward neutral.
6. Repeat slowly in a smooth, rhythmic fashion, until there is improved motion (or to the tolerance of the patient).
7. Move your stabilizing hand to the next inferior vertebra and repeat the process until you have treated all the involved segments.

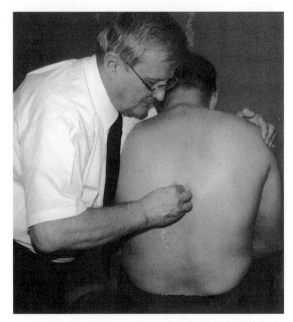

Figure 55.5. Thoracic flexion technique.

EXTENSION

Diagnosis

Decreased thoracic extension.

Objective

Increase thoracic extension.

Patient Position

Seated.

Procedure

1. Stand behind the patient.
2. Put your arm over the patient's shoulder across his or her chest and place your hand on the patient's opposite shoulder. The patient hooks his or her hands over your arm.
3. Stabilize the lower of two vertebrae with the thenar eminence of your other hand or by grasping and fixating the spinous process with your fingers and thumb. You also use this hand as a fulcrum.
4. Introduce extension by anterior translation of your stabilizing hand, as your other arm bends the upper thorax backward around the fulcrum, achieving maximal extension stretch at the joint space above.
5. Hold for 3–5 seconds, then return toward neutral.
6. Repeat slowly in a smooth, rhythmic fashion, until there is improved motion (or to the tolerance of the patient).
7. Move your stabilizing hand to the next inferior vertebra, and repeat the process until you have treated all the involved segments.

Note: This technique is contraindicated in a patient with facet arthritis, because increased pressure exerted on the facets by the use of extension can aggravate that problem.

ROTATION

Diagnosis

Decreased thoracic rotation.

Objective

Increase thoracic rotation.

Patient Position

Seated.

Procedure

1. Stand to the right, behind the patient, and pass your right hand under the patient's right axilla, grasping the anterior right shoulder (Fig. 55.6).
2. Place your thumb and fingers on both sides of the spinous processes to stabilize the vertebra below the restricted segment.
3. Use your hand on the shoulder to induce rotation to the right, to the point that you feel the rotation at the joint space above your stabilizing hand.
4. Hold for 3–5 seconds, then return toward neutral.
5. Repeat slowly in a smooth, rhythmic fashion until there is improved motion (or to the tolerance of the patient).
6. Move your stabilizing fingers to the next inferior vertebra, and repeat the process until you have treated all the segments desired.

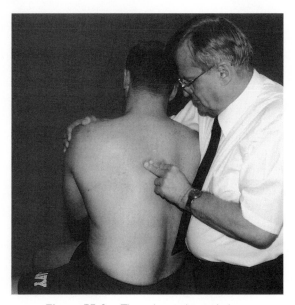

Figure 55.6. Thoracic rotation technique.

SIDE-BENDING

Diagnosis

Decreased thoracic side-bending.

Objective

Increase thoracic side-bending.

Patient Position

Seated.

Procedure

1. Stand to the right behind the patient, who is seated with arms folded across his or her chest.
2. Pass your right arm over the patient's right shoulder and across the chest and put your hand into the left axilla, palm against the thoracic wall.
3. Apply a stabilizing pressure with your index and long fingers and thumb on the sides of the spinous process at the vertebra below the segment you wish to treat. An alternative is to use the thenar eminence, placed against the side of the spinous process, as a fulcrum.
4. Introduce right side-bending by applying a downward pressure through your axilla on the patient's right shoulder and an upward lift of the patient's left shoulder with your right hand. This forms a convexity on the left, side-bending the spine to the right. You should feel maximal stretch at the joint space above your stabilizing hand (fulcrum).
5. Hold for 3–5 seconds, then return toward neutral.
6. Repeat slowly in a smooth, rhythmic fashion, until there is improved motion (or to the tolerance of the patient).
7. Move your stabilizing hand to the next inferior vertebra, and repeat the process until you have treated all the involved segments.

Costal Articulatory Techniques

Reminder: For a patient who has difficulty breathing, whether because of chronic obstructive pulmonary disease or any other reason, you may need to adjust the timing of these techniques to minimize interference with the already limited breathing cycle. It is generally best to treat the ribs on both sides, even if restriction is most apparent on one side.

ANTERIOR APPROACH

Diagnosis

Decreased costal motion during breathing cycle.

Objective

Enhance or optimize costal motion.

Patient Position

Supine.

Procedure

1. Stand on the restricted (right, in this example) side of the supine patient (Fig. 55.7). Grasp his or her right wrist with your cephalad hand. Stretch the patient's arm upwards and to the point where it is fully extended at the elbow and flexed at the shoulder superior to the head.
2. Stabilize the anterior right ribs with your caudad hand. Use either the hypothenar eminence and little finger, the thumb and thenar eminence, or group the fingertips in a row along the superior border to stabilize the lower of the two ribs being treated.
3. Use the patient's right arm to stretch soft tissues in the intercostal space superior to your stabilizing hand. Have the patient breathe in deeply, synchronizing your stretch with full inspiration.
4. Hold for 3–5 seconds, then return toward neutral.
5. Repeat slowly in a smooth, rhythmic fashion until there is improved motion (or to the tolerance of the patient).
6. Move your stabilizing hand to the next superior costal border, and repeat the process until you have treated all the ribs desired.

POSTERIOR APPROACH

Diagnosis

Decreased costal motion during breathing cycle.

Objective

Enhance or optimize costal respiratory motion.

Patient Position

Prone.

Procedure

1. Have the patient lie prone with head facing to the left (Fig. 55.8). Stand to the left at the head of the table and use your right hand to grasp the patient's left arm just proximal to the elbow, stretching the arm into full abduction with a slight backward angle and external rotation.
2. Stabilize the inferior of the two ribs being treated with your left thumb and thenar eminence at the superior border of the lower rib near the angle.
3. Achieve a stretch of the latissimus dorsi and the intercostal muscles by using the arm as a long lever (with abduction/extension) at the same time that you stabilize the inferior rib.
4. Hold for 3–5 seconds, then return toward neutral.
5. Repeat slowly in a smooth, rhythmic fashion until there is improved motion (or to the tolerance of the patient).
6. Move your stabilizing hand to the next superior rib and repeat the process until you have treated all the ribs desired.

LATERAL RECUMBENT

Diagnosis

Decreased bucket-handle excursion during breathing cycle.

Objective

Enhance or optimize costal respiratory motion.

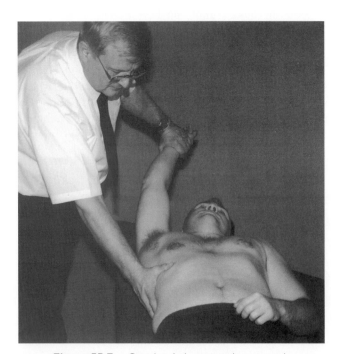

Figure 55.7. Costal technique, anterior approach.

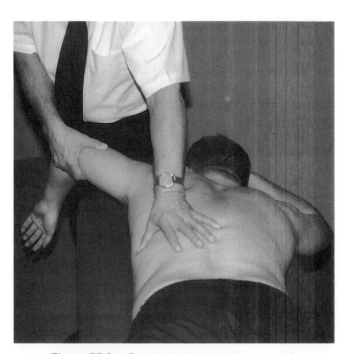

Figure 55.8. Costal technique, posterior approach.

Patient Position

Lateral recumbent (restricted side up; left, in this example).

Procedure

1. Stand in front of your right lateral recumbent patient (Fig. 55.9). The patient's left elbow should be flexed.
2. Grasp the patient's left elbow with your left arm and place the shoulder in full abduction.
3. Stabilize the inferior of the two ribs being treated in the mid-axillary line with your right thumb and thenar eminence.
4. Achieve a stretch/separation of the soft tissues between the ribs by abducting the arm as a long lever at the same time that you stabilize the inferior rib. Synchronize this with the patient's full inspiration.
5. Hold for 3–5 seconds, then return toward neutral.
6. Repeat slowly in a smooth, rhythmic fashion until there is improved motion (or to the tolerance of the patient).
7. Move your stabilizing hand to the next superior rib. Repeat the process until you have treated all the involved ribs.

POSTERIOR RIB RAISING

Diagnosis

Decreased costal motion during breathing cycle.

Objective

Enhance or optimize costal respiratory motion.

Patient Position

Supine.

Procedure

1. Stand on the restricted side of your supine patient (Fig. 55.10).
2. Place the patient's arm into full abduction, holding the wrist firmly in your cephalad axilla.

3. Place your caudal hand under the patient's thorax. Press the tips of your fingers firmly against the inferior surface of the angles of the patient's ribs and at the same time extend and abduct the patient's arm (long lever stretch). Synchronize this with the patient's full inspiration. You may need to bend your knees slightly to do this comfortably.
4. Hold for 3–5 seconds, then return toward neutral.
5. Repeat slowly in a smooth, rhythmic fashion until there is improved motion (or to the tolerance of the patient).
6. Move your (fulcrum) hand to the inferior border of the angle of the next inferior rib and repeat the process until you have treated all the involved ribs.

Lumbar Articulatory Techniques

FLEXION

Diagnosis

Decreased lumbar flexion.

Objective

Increase lumbar flexion.

Patient Position

Seated.

Procedure

1. Stand behind and to the side of your patient, who is seated on or straddling the table (Figs. 55.11 and 55.12).
2. Put one arm over his or her near shoulder across his or her

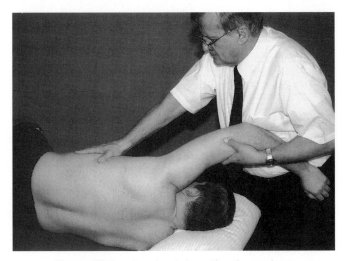

Figure 55.9. Costal technique, lateral recumbent.

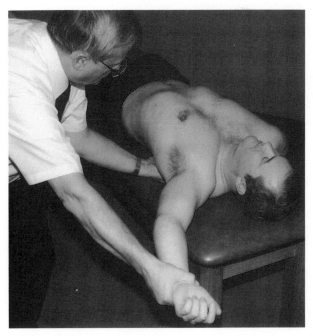

Figure 55.10. Costal technique, posterior rib raising.

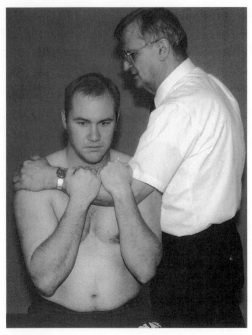

Figure 55.11. Lumbar flexion technique, anterior view.

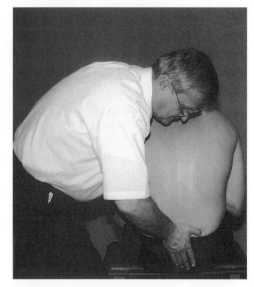

Figure 55.12. Lumbar flexion technique, posterior view.

chest with your hand on the opposite shoulder. The patient hooks his or her hands over your arm.

3. With the thenar eminence of your other hand, stabilize one vertebra in the lumbar spine. With your forearm against the patient's sternum, direct the force of flexion straight through the patient toward your stabilizing hand, gapping the joint above it.
4. Hold for 3–5 seconds, then return toward neutral.
5. Repeat slowly in a smooth, rhythmic fashion until there is improved motion (or to the tolerance of the patient).
6. Move your stabilizing hand to the next inferior vertebra and repeat the process until you have treated all the involved segments.

FLEXION (Lateral Recumbent)

Diagnosis

Decreased lumbar flexion.

Objective

Increase lumbar flexion.

Patient Position

Lateral recumbent.

Procedure

1. Stand in front of the patient.
2. Face him or her. Flex the patient's knees and rest them together against your thigh or inguinal area.
3. Bend forward at the waist and flex your own knees. Gently

flex your patient's lumbar spine by swinging your pelvis toward the head of the table area.

4. Use your caudal hand to pull the inferior lumbar vertebra in a caudal direction as you induce flexion to the joint space above it. Your cephalad hand should stabilize the superior lumbar vertebra.
5. Hold for 3–5 seconds, then return toward neutral.
6. Repeat slowly in a smooth, rhythmic fashion until there is improved motion (or to the tolerance of the patient).
7. Move your stabilizing hand to the next inferior vertebra and repeat the process until you have treated all the involved segments.

FLEXION (SUPINE)

Diagnosis

Decreased lumbar flexion.

Objective

Increase lumbar flexion.

Patient Position

Supine.

Procedure

1. Stand to the side of your supine patient and flex his or her hips and knees. Resting your pectoral area on the knees, place your hands below the patient's lumbar region, one on each side of the spine.
2. Press toward the table through the patient's knees and thighs, in a superior anteroposterior fashion to "spring" the lumbar joint space in flexion. Use your hands to pull caudally, stretching the joint space above.
3. Hold for 3–5 seconds, then return toward neutral.

4. Repeat slowly in a smooth, rhythmic fashion until there is improved motion (or to the tolerance of the patient).
5. Move your stabilizing hand to the next inferior vertebra and repeat the process until you have treated all the involved segments.

EXTENSION (SEATED)

Diagnosis

Decreased lumbar extension.

Objective

Increase lumbar extension.

Patient Position

Seated.

Procedure

1. Stand behind and to the right side of your patient, who is straddling the table (Fig. 55.13). Have the patient cross arms in front, with each hand grasping the opposite shoulder. As the patient leans forward slightly, place your right arm under his or her arms, with your hand under the opposite axilla.
2. Place your left thenar eminence against the spinous process of a lumbar segment as a fulcrum around which you extend the lumbar spine.
3. Use your right hand or arm to lift the patient's elbows, introducing thoracolumbar extension to the joint space/segment above your fulcrum. Accentuate this extension with your left thenar eminence, applying an anterior translatory force at the segment level.
4. Hold for 3–5 seconds, then return toward neutral.

5. Repeat slowly in a smooth, rhythmic fashion until there is improved motion (or to the tolerance of the patient).
6. Move your stabilizing hand to the next inferior vertebra and repeat the process until you have treated all the involved segments.

EXTENSION (LATERAL RECUMBENT)

Diagnosis

Decreased lumbar extension.

Objective

Increase lumbar extension.

Patient Position

Lateral recumbent.

Procedure

1. Stand in front of and facing the patient in the right lateral recumbent position (Fig. 55.14). Flex the patient's knees and hips to 90°, resting the knees against your thigh or inguinal area.
2. Place your hands posterior to two adjacent lumbar vertebral segments, so that your fingertips meet at the joint space.
3. Bend forward at the waist and flex your own knees. By inducing posterior and caudad motion through the patient's knees, extend your patient's lumbar spine. Localize motion to the joint space at which your fingers meet. Pull the inferior lumbar vertebra in an inferoanterior direction, as your cephalad hand pulls the superior vertebra in a superoanterior direction.
4. Hold for 3–5 seconds, then return toward neutral.
5. Repeat slowly in a smooth, rhythmic fashion until there is improved motion (or to the tolerance of the patient).
6. Move your stabilizing hand to the next inferior vertebra and repeat the process until you have treated all the involved segments.

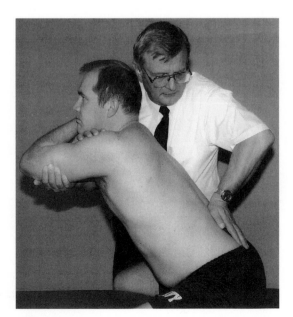

Figure 55.13. Lumbar extension technique, seated.

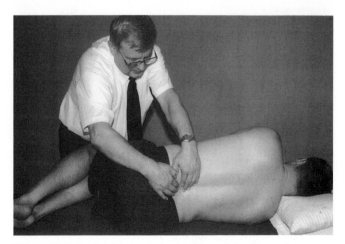

Figure 55.14. Lumbar extension technique, lateral recumbent.

SIDE-BENDING (SEATED)

Diagnosis

Decreased lumbar side-bending (lateral flexion).

Objective

Increase lumbar side-bending (lateral flexion).

Patient Position

Seated.

Procedure

1. Stand behind and to the right side of your seated patient (Fig. 55.15). Your right axilla overlies the patient's right shoulder, and your right hand grasps the opposite shoulder or axilla.
2. Place your left hand (thenar eminence, or the pads of several fingers) on the right side of a vertebra in the patient's lumbar spine, just lateral to the spinous process.
3. Use your left hand as a fulcrum, inducing left lateral translatory force as you create right side-bending by depressing the patient's right shoulder. Repeat in a rhythmic manner to all segments, side-bending more for the lower lumbar segments.
4. Introduce right side-bending by applying a downward pressure through your right axilla on the patient's shoulder and an upward lift of the patient's left shoulder with your right hand. This forms a convexity on the left, side-bending the spine to the right. You should feel maximal stretch at the joint space above your stabilizing (fulcrum) hand.
5. Hold for 3–5 seconds, then return toward neutral.
6. Repeat slowly in a smooth, rhythmic fashion until there is improved motion (or to the tolerance of the patient).
7. Move your stabilizing hand to the next inferior vertebra and

repeat the process until you have treated all the involved segments.

SIDE-BENDING (LATERAL RECUMBENT)

Diagnosis

Decreased left lumbar side-bending (lateral flexion).

Objective

Increase left lumbar side-bending (lateral flexion).

Patient Position

Right lateral recumbent (right side down).

Procedure

1. Stand at the side of the table, in front of and facing the patient (Fig. 55.16).
2. Flex his or her knees and hips to approximately 90°.
3. Place your left hand so that your fingers are palpating the spinous processes of the lumbar spine.
4. Place your right hand and forearm under the patient's ankles and lift them toward the ceiling until your left hand palpates that you have introduced left side-bending in the lumbar region at the desired level.
5. Hold this stretch for 3–5 seconds, then return toward neutral.
6. Repeat slowly in a smooth, rhythmic fashion until there is improved motion (or to the tolerance of the patient).
7. If you are performing this as a regional motion, complete the treatment by treating the other side in the same manner.
8. If you are attempting to induce more specific articulatory treatment to a particular segmental level, your left hand placement is such that your thumb and fingers hold the spinous process

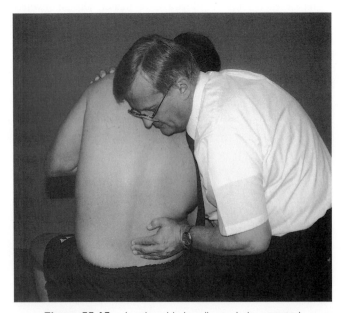

Figure 55.15. Lumbar side-bending technique, seated.

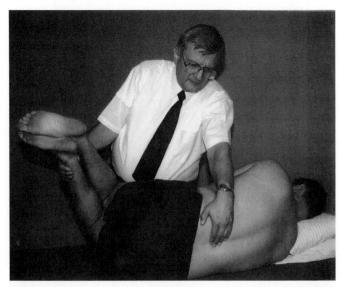

Figure 55.16. Lumbar side-bending technique, lateral recumbent.

of a particular vertebra, stabilizing it as you induce side-bending to the joint below via the long lever moved by your right hand. When you have achieved the desired effect at a particular level, move to the next superior level to be treated.

ROTATION (SEATED)

Diagnosis

Decreased right lumbar rotation.

Objective

Increase right lumbar rotation.

Patient Position

Seated.

Procedure

1. Stand behind and to the right of the patient, who is straddling or sitting on the table (Fig. 55.17). Your right axilla overlies the patient's right shoulder, and your right hand grasps the opposite shoulder or axilla. The patient hooks his or her hands over your arm.
2. Regional: Place your left hand just to the right of the spinous processes and encourage right rotation by applying a left lateral force to the spinous processes.
3. Segmental: If you want to be more specific in your treatment, stabilize a particular spinous process with your thumb and fingers, and resist the rotation you induce with the other hand or arm, confining the stretching, rotational forces to the joint above the segment you are stabilizing.
4. Induce right rotation to the lumbar spine by rotating the patient's thorax to the right with your right arm and hand.
5. Hold for 3–5 seconds, then return toward neutral.

6. Repeat slowly in a smooth, rhythmic fashion until there is improved motion (or to the tolerance of the patient).
7. Move your stabilizing hand to the next inferior lumbar region or segment, and repeat the process until you have treated the lumbar region or the specific involved segments.

Note: For decreased left lumbar rotation, make the appropriate adjustments to treat the other side.

Pelvic Articulatory Techniques

ANTERIOR ROTATION TO INNOMINATE

Diagnosis

Posteriorly rotated innominate.

Objective

Normalize innominate position and motion.

Patient Position

Supine, with the leg of the posteriorly rotated innominate hanging over the side of the table, inducing hip extension.

Procedure

1. Stand on the dysfunctional side (Fig. 55.18).
2. Place your cephalad hand behind the posterior superior iliac spine (PSIS), cupping it.
3. Place your caudad hand on the distal thigh, to induce further hip extension.
4. Induce further hip extension by pressing down on the distal thigh, while simultaneously pulling the PSIS anteriorly, inducing anterior rotation to the innominate.
5. Hold for 3–5 seconds at the endpoint, then return toward neutral.
6. Repeat slowly in a smooth, rhythmic fashion until there is improved motion (or to the tolerance of the patient).

Note: This technique can easily be adapted to the lateral recumbent position, with the physician standing behind the patient and treating the upper hemipelvis.

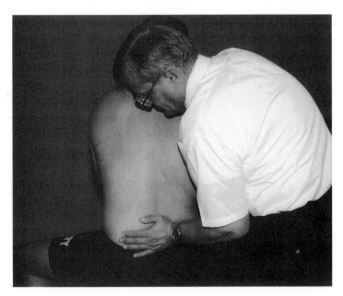

Figure 55.17. Lumbar rotation technique, seated.

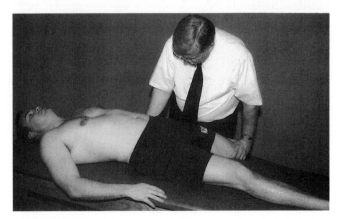

Figure 55.18. Pelvis technique, anterior rotation of innominate.

POSTERIOR ROTATION TO INNOMINATE

Diagnosis

Anteriorly rotated innominate.

Objective

Normalize innominate position and motion.

Patient Position

Supine.

Procedure

1. Stand at the side of your patient's anteriorly rotated innominate (dysfunctional side), facing toward the patient's head (Fig. 55.19).
2. Flex the patient's knee and hip, grasping the knee between your caudal arm and pectoral area.
3. Place your cephalad hand on the anterosuperior iliac spine (ASIS).
4. Use your caudad hand to grasp the ischial tuberosity.
5. Apply a posterior rotational torque with both hands by exerting downward pressure on the ASIS while pulling upward on the ischial tuberosity. You may slightly adduct the thigh, to gap the sacroiliac (SI) joint.
6. Hold for 3–5 seconds at the endpoint, then return toward neutral.
7. Repeat slowly in a smooth, rhythmic fashion until there is improved motion (or to the tolerance of the patient).

Note: This technique can easily be adapted to the lateral recumbent position, with the physician standing behind the patient and treating the upper hemipelvis.

SACROILIAC JOINT GAPPING

Diagnosis

Innominate outflare or inflare.

Objective

Normalize innominate position and motion.

Patient Position

Supine.

Procedure

1. Stand at the patient's dysfunctional side (Figs. 55.20 and 55.21).
2. Grasp the patient's flexed knee with your caudal hand.
3. Grasp the patient's ASIS (inflare) or PSIS (outflare) with your cephalad hand.
4. Inflare: Pull the ASIS laterally and toward the table as you abduct the hip by pulling laterally on the knee.
5. Outflare: Pull laterally on the PSIS as you adduct the hip by pushing medially on the knee.
6. Hold for 3–5 seconds at the end range, then return toward neutral.

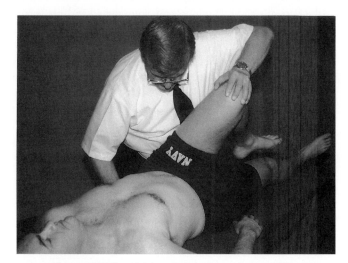

Figure 55.20.   Pelvis technique, innominate outflare.

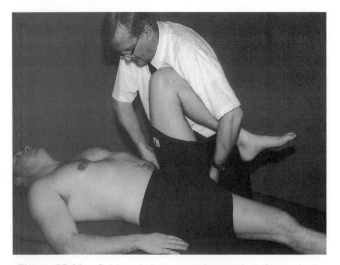

Figure 55.19.   Pelvis technique, posterior rotation of innominate.

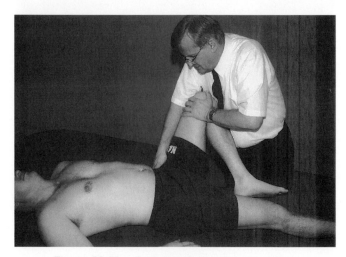

Figure 55.21.   Pelvis technique, innominate inflare.

7. Repeat slowly in a smooth, rhythmic fashion until there is improved motion (or to the tolerance of the patient).

Articulatory Techniques in Extremities

The same principles that apply to the spinal segments can be used to treat the extremities. In the extremities, the techniques are particularly useful when a degree of restriction or fibrosis has developed in the surrounding soft tissues during a period of inactivity following injury. This problem often follows a capsular tear, subsequently healed, or immobilization in a cast. These techniques should be used with caution and gentleness on patients who have tissue contractures. Remember to inform your patients that discomfort during treatment is acceptable. With that knowledge, they can give you the feedback you need to adjust the force applied in these techniques.

An example of extremity treatment using articulatory technique is the treatment of the shoulder with "Spencer techniques," described and improved by H. Spencer.[1-3] They are useful in diagnosing and treating musculoskeletal dysfunctions of the shoulder and are outlined here as they are presently being taught in most osteopathic colleges.

Spencer's original techniques have undergone some modification with use. An important modification is the addition of muscle energy and the use of compression or traction to evaluate joint articular cartilage and capsule.

STAGE I: EXTENSION WITH ELBOW FLEXED (Fig. 55.22)

Patient Position

Lateral recumbent (affected shoulder up).

1. Neutral position of the patient's arm with the elbow flexed (operator to side of table facing the patient). Grasp the patient's elbow using the caudal hand; the cephalic hand compresses the scapula and clavicle (shoulder girdle) against the thorax (a critical component).

2. Move the patient's arm into extension in the horizontal plane while holding the shoulder girdle firmly against the superior thorax; move slowly, sensing any resistance, and repeat until no further range of motion (ROM) is achieved.

3. Muscle energy activation: At the first sign of resistance (barrier engagement), instruct the patient, "Push your elbow toward your feet." Resist isometrically until effective contraction is localized at the shoulder. At that point, ask the patient to relax the muscular contraction and simultaneously and slowly release the isometric resistance.

4. Take the elbow to its new position of resistance to extension, and repeat step 3 until no further ROM is achieved.

STAGE 2: FLEXION WITH ELBOW EXTENDED (Fig. 55.23)

1. Neutral position of the patient's arm with elbow flexed. Grasp the patient's forearm using the cephalic hand; the caudal hand compresses the scapula and clavicle against the thorax.

2. Move the patient's arm into flexion in the horizontal plane while holding the shoulder girdle firmly against the superior thorax; move slowly and sense any resistance; repeat until no further ROM is achieved.

3. Muscle energy activation: At the first sign of resistance (barrier engagement), instruct the patient, "Pull your elbow toward your feet." Resist isometrically until effective contraction is localized at the shoulder. At that point, ask the patient to relax the muscular contraction, and simultaneously and slowly release the isometric resistance.

4. Take the arm to its new position of resistance to flexion, and repeat steps 3 and 4 until no further ROM is achieved.

STAGE 3: CIRCUMDUCTION WITH SLIGHT COMPRESSION AND ELBOW FLEXED (Fig. 55.24)

1. The patient's arm with elbow flexed is abducted to 90°. Grasp the patient's elbow with caudal hand; the cephalic hand compresses the scapula and clavicle (shoulder girdle) against the thorax.

2. Move the patient's arm through full clockwise circumduction

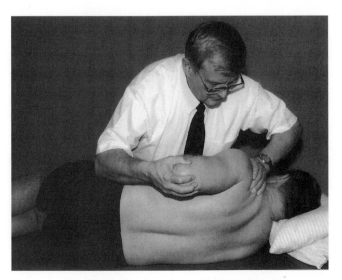

Figure 55.22. Extension with elbow flexed.

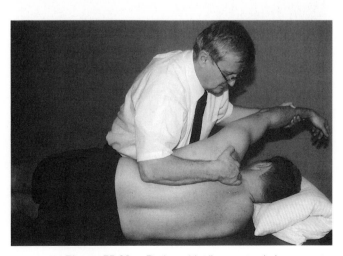

Figure 55.23. Flexion with elbow extended.

with slight compression; move slowly and firmly; repeat several times to gain ROM. This step evaluates circumduction ROM with the elbow flexed and also assesses the comfort of moving the articular surface of the humeral head over the articular surface of the glenoid fossa.
3. Then move the patient's arm through full counterclockwise circumduction; move slowly and firmly, repeating several times to gain ROM.
4. A muscle energy activation does not apply in this step.

STAGE 4: CIRCUMDUCTION WITH TRACTION WITH ELBOW EXTENDED (Fig. 55.25)

1. The patient's arm with elbow extended is abducted to 90°. With the caudal hand grasp the patient's forearm; the cephalic hand compresses the scapula and clavicle (shoulder girdle) against the thorax.
2. Move the patient's arm through full clockwise circumduction with slight traction; move slowly; repeat several times to gain ROM. This step evaluates circumduction ROM with the arm extended and also assesses the comfort of applying tension to the capsule of the glenohumeral joint.
3. Then move the patient's arm through full counterclockwise circumduction with traction; move slowly; repeat several times to gain ROM.
4. A muscle energy activation does not apply in this step.

STAGE 5: ABDUCTION AND INTERNAL ROTATION WITH ELBOW FLEXED

1. Neutral position of the patient's arm with elbow flexed. With the caudal hand grasp the patient's elbow; the cephalic hand compresses the scapula and clavicle (shoulder girdle) against the patient's thorax; the patient's hand (of the arm being treated) is resting on the wrist of your cephalic hand to stabilize the patient's arm.

2. With your caudal hand, move the patient's elbow in an arc toward the patient's head; this abduction is accompanied by internal rotation.
3. Muscle energy activation: At the first sign of resistance (barrier engagement), instruct the patient, "Pull your elbow toward your waist." Resist isometrically until effective contraction is localized at the shoulder. At that point, ask the patient to relax the muscular contraction, and simultaneously release the isometric resistance.
4. Move the elbow to its new resistance to abduction, and repeat steps 3 and 4 until no further ROM is achieved.

STAGE 5A: ADDUCTION AND EXTERNAL ROTATION WITH ELBOW FLEXED (Fig. 55.26)

1. Neutral position of the patient's arm with elbow flexed. With the caudal hand grasp the patient's elbow; the cephalic hand

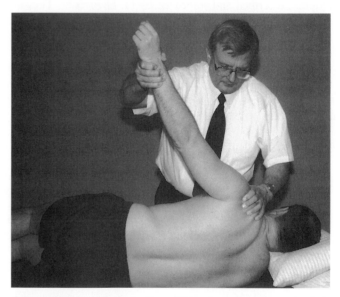

Figure 55.25. Circumduction with traction with elbow extended.

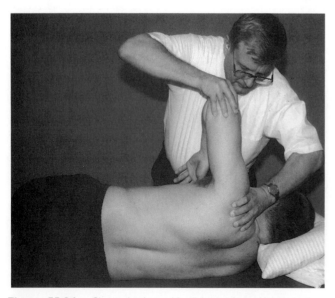

Figure 55.24. Circumduction with slight compression and elbow flexed.

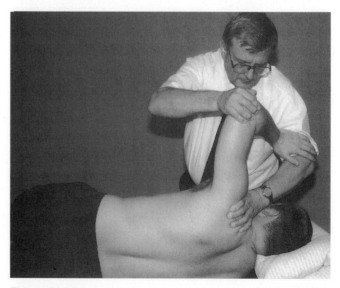

Figure 55.26. Adduction with external rotation with elbow flexed.

compresses the scapula and clavicle (shoulder girdle) against the patient's thorax; the patient's hand (of the arm being treated) is resting on the wrist of your cephalic hand to stabilize the patient's arm.

2. With your caudal hand, move the patient's elbow in an arc toward his or her face and toward the floor; this produces adduction and external rotation at the shoulder.

3. Muscle energy activation: At the first sign of resistance (barrier engagement), instruct the patient, "Pull your elbow toward the ceiling." Resist isometrically until effective contraction is localized at the shoulder. At that point, ask the patient to relax the muscular contraction, and simultaneously release the isometric resistance.

4. Move the elbow to its new position of resistance to adduction and external rotation, and repeat steps 3 and 4 until no further ROM is achieved.

STAGE 6: ABDUCTION AND INTERNAL ROTATION WITH THE ARM BEHIND THE BACK (Fig. 55.27)

1. Position the patient's hand behind the back (to the extent permitted by the patient's comfort with this positioning), observing if the dorsal surface of the hand can be placed against the dorsal surface of the ipsilateral flank area.

2. Grasp the patient's elbow (or place your index and middle fingers around the elbow) and slowly move the elbow ventrally (toward you); repeat to gain ROM.

3. Muscle energy activation: At the first sign of resistance (barrier engagement), instruct the patient, "Pull your elbow away from me." Resist isometrically until effective contraction is localized at the shoulder. At that point, ask the patient to relax the muscular contraction, and simultaneously and slowly release the isometric resistance.

4. Move the elbow to its new position of resistance to abduction and internal rotation, and repeat steps 3 and 4 until no further ROM is achieved.

STAGE 7: STRETCHING TISSUES AND PUMPING FLUIDS WITH THE ARM EXTENDED (Fig. 55.28)

Note: This technique is often performed before Stage 1 to "pump fluids and stretch tissues."

1. Position the patient's arm on your shoulder, elbow extended (an alternate patient positioning and hold is shown in Figure 55.7).

2. Grasp the patient's proximal humeral area with both hands.

3. Pull the patient's humerus toward you (traction), gently and slowly, holding tension on the periarticular tissues. Do not press on the neurovascular bundle with your thumbs. Release traction force slowly.

4. Compress articular area (shoulder) by guiding the humerus toward the glenoid fossa with both hands. Release compression. The traction and compression can be done rhythmically or in a random on-and-off manner.

5. Repeat steps 3 and 4 in sequence until motions are freer.

6. Move patient's shoulder in translatory directions—anterior/posterior, cephalad/caudal—to limits of motion. Hold, release forces, and repeat until motions are freer.

COMMENTS ON SPENCER SHOULDER TECHNIQUES

Spencer used his shoulder treatment program for pumping fluids and stretching tissues around the shoulder. He advised that stage 7 be duplicated, that is, used before the treatment sequence started, to prepare the shoulder tissues for the sequence. In that case he would still repeat the step as "step 7" at the end of his sequence. Spencer is also reported to have repeated steps 1 and 2. The first time he would treat the patient with the elbow flexed and then repeat the stage with the arm extended. He stated that in this way the lever arm was short for initial testing and treatment and was then increased by arm extension. The modified Spencer motion techniques add com-

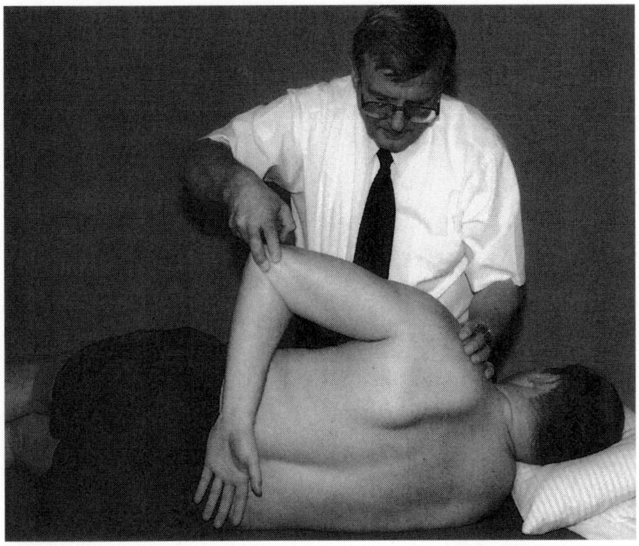

Figure 55.27. Abduction and internal rotation with the arm behind the back.

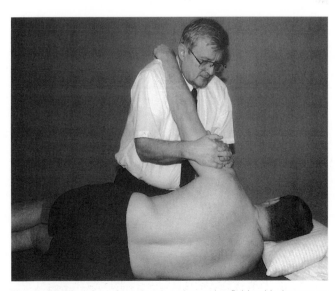

Figure 55.28. Stretching tissues and pumping fluids with the arm extended; stretching tissues and pumping fluids with the extremity extended and elbow flexed.

pression and traction to steps 3 and 4. They also add muscle energy to the applicable steps to enhance treatment possibilities, that is, steps 1 and 2, and 5 and 6. Experienced physicians report that the Spencer techniques do not seem to have rapid results in patients with metabolic or other debilitating disease.

Treatment of the shoulder using "the 7 motions of Spencer"[2,3] in their original form or in their modified form provides objective diagnostic tests and articulatory treatment for soft tissue restrictions and gives objective evidence supporting the clinical prognosis of a patient undergoing treatment for shoulder dysfunction.

CONCLUSION

Articulatory technique consists of movements against a diagnosed barrier to (limitation of) motion in an articular structure. These movements are:

Controlled
Slow
Repetitive
Passive

Pressure against the resistant barrier is held long enough in each cycle to allow a stretching of the tissues controlling and limiting the motion of the joint. These techniques are designed to deal with one or several ranges of motion as indicated by the diagnosis and the nature of the articulation being treated. Passive force against the barrier may be augmented by incorporating patient generated (intrinsic) force such as that found in the final stage of muscle energy technique.

Articulatory technique may be the principal component of a treatment program. It is also used to prepare an articular area for other forms of manipulative treatment. It may be preferred to high velocity treatment in infants, postoperative patients, compromised or debilitated patients, and elderly patients. Articulating technique is often applied to support general body functions, such as respiratory efficiency.

REFERENCES

1. Spencer H. Shoulder technique. *JAOA.* 1916;15:2118–2220.
2. Spencer H. Treatment of bursitis and tendinitis. *JAOA.* 1926;25:528–529.
3. Patriquin DA. The evolution of osteopathic manipulative technique: the Spencer technique. *JAOA.* 1992;92:1134–1146.

56. Soft Tissue Techniques

WALTER C. EHRENFEUCHTER, DAVID HEILIG, AND ALEXANDER S. NICHOLAS

Key Concepts

- **Soft tissue techniques and classification as direct or indirect techniques**
- **Goals attainable with soft tissue techniques**
- **Three basic mechanisms used in soft tissue techniques**
- **Manner in which soft tissue techniques can be used alone or in combination with other manipulative techniques**
- **Objective, patient positioning, physician positioning, and implementation of soft tissue techniques for following regions:**
  - **—Cervical**
  - **—Thoracic**
  - **—Lumbar**
  - **—Sacrum**
  - **—Upper extremity**
  - **—Lower extremity**

Soft tissue techniques are defined as direct techniques that address the muscular and fascial structures of the body and associated neural and vascular elements. Soft tissue techniques may be applied in a number of different ways to:

1. Relax hypertonic muscles
2. Stretch passive fascial structures
3. Enhance circulation to the local myofascial structures
4. Improve local tissue nutrition, oxygenation, and removal of metabolic wastes
5. Improve abnormal somatosomatic and somatovisceral reflex activity
6. Identify areas of somatic dysfunction
7. Observe tissue response to the application of manipulative technique
8. Improve local and systemic immune responsiveness
9. Provide a general state of relaxation
10. Provide a general state of tonic stimulation

The choice of technique is based on the treatment goals. There are three basic mechanisms used in applying soft tissue technique to muscular structures and their associated fascial elements:

1. Tractional technique, also called stretching, in which the origin and insertion of the myofascial structures being treated are longitudinally separated
2. Kneading, a rhythmic, lateral stretching of a myofascial structure, in which origin and insertion are held stationary and the central portion of the structure is stretched like a bowstring
3. Inhibition, sustained deep pressure over a hypertonic myofascial structure

Other mechanisms used on more superficial fascial structures include variants on techniques developed in the European massage movement:

Effleurage
Pétrissage
Tapotement
Skin rolling

Soft tissue techniques may be used alone or in combination with any other manipulative technique. Many of the positions used for soft tissue techniques readily lend themselves to conversion to other techniques such as the following:

Articulatory
Muscle energy
Counterstrain
Functional
Cranial
High-velocity low-amplitude (HVLA) thrusting

CERVICAL TECHNIQUES

Suboccipital Inhibition

OBJECTIVE

Suboccipital inhibition, decrease in suboccipital muscle tone.

POSITION

Supine (Fig. 56.1).

PROCEDURE

1. Sit at the head of the table.
2. Place the pads of your fingers just inferior to the superior nuchal line in the suboccipital tissues.
3. Lift the head so that the patient's weight is entirely supported on the pads of your fingers. The head is slightly above, but not resting on, your palms.
4. Maintain this position until you achieve the desired relaxation of the suboccipital soft tissues.

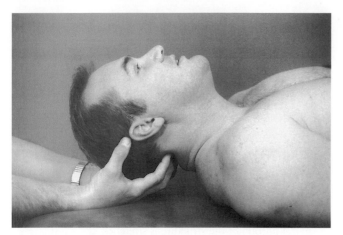

Figure 56.1. Suboccipital inhibition.

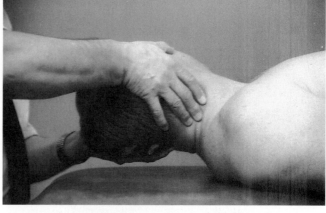

Figure 56.2. Cervical rotation.

Note: This technique is similar in position to the method used by A.T. Still when he created a rope sling to relieve his own headaches.

Rotation

OBJECTIVE

Increase cervical rotation.

POSITION

Supine (Fig. 56.2).

PROCEDURE

1. Sit at the head of the table.
2. Use your hands to cradle the head, taking care not to occlude the ear canals.
3. Rotate the patient's head away from you slowly until tissue tension restricts you from further motion.
4. Gently increase the tension by rotating into the restrictive barrier, hold the tension for 1–2 seconds, and then slowly release it.
5. Repeat as many times as necessary to achieve the desired effect.

Note: This neck position allows for conversion to a muscle energy cervical range of motion technique or for an HVLA thrust for atlantoaxial segmental dysfunction.

Traction

OBJECTIVE

Stretch paravertebral muscles.

POSITION

Supine.

PROCEDURE

1. Sit behind the patient at the head of the table.

2. Place one hand cradling the occiput between the thumb and index finger. Place your other hand across the patient's forehead.
3. Exert a gentle axial traction with your occipital hand.
4. Use your hand on the forehead to prevent forward tilt of the patient's head, also applying slight traction.
5. Apply the tractional force slowly; release it slowly.
6. Repeat as many times as necessary to achieve the desired effect.

Forward Bending

OBJECTIVE

Stretch posterior cervical soft tissues.

POSITION

Supine (Fig. 56.3).

PROCEDURE

1. Sit or stand at the head of the table.
2. Cross your forearms and place them behind the patient's head with your hands on the patient's shoulders.
3. Exert a slow, forward bending stretch until a restrictive barrier is engaged.
4. Gently, slowly increase the stretch, then release it just as slowly.
5. Repeat as many times as necessary to achieve the desired effect.

Note: This position allows use of a range-of-motion muscle energy technique, and it may also be used to treat anterior counterstrain tender points.

Contralateral Traction

OBJECTIVE

Relax the cervical paravertebral muscles.

POSITION

Supine.

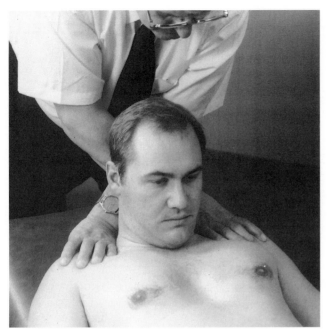

Figure 56.3. Cervical forward bending.

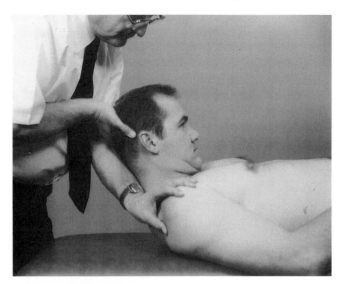

Figure 56.4. Cervical contralateral traction.

PROCEDURE

1. Stand at the side of the head of the table.
2. With your caudad hand, reach across the patient and under the opposite side of the neck to grasp the paravertebral muscles with the pads of your fingers.
3. Grasp the forehead lightly with your cephalad hand.
4. With your caudad hand, draw the paravertebral muscles laterally and anteriorly until you reach the initial restrictive barrier.
5. Increase the anterolateral traction slightly to take the tissues slightly beyond the barrier.
6. Repeat as many times as necessary to achieve the desired effect.

Note: By increasing the rotational force, this technique may be converted to a deep articulatory technique. By adding more of a milking motion, it may be used to enhance lymphatic drainage in the cervical lymph node chains.

Longitudinal Traction

OBJECTIVE

Relax the cervical paravertebral muscles.

POSITION

Supine (Fig. 56.4).

PROCEDURE

1. Sit at the head of the table.
2. Bring the palmar surfaces of the fingers of both hands under the neck near the spinous processes.

3. Lift the cervical paravertebral musculature and draw it cephalad.
4. Slowly releasing the musculature, carry the hands caudally.
5. Repeat as many times as necessary to achieve the desired effect, shifting position along the length of the cervical spine.

THORACIC

Prone Pressure

OBJECTIVE

Relax the thoracic paravertebral muscles.

POSITION

Prone (Figs. 56.5 and 56.6).

PROCEDURE

1. Stand at the side of your patient, who has his or her head turned away from the side to be treated.
2. Place your thumb and thenar eminence of one hand on the far side of the thoracic spine, between the spinous and transverse processes.
3. Place your other hand reinforcing the first or working in tandem with it along the spine.
4. Exert an anterolateral pressure on the soft tissues, directed away from the spine.
5. You may maintain the pressure as a sustained, inhibitory pressure or use it in an intermittent kneading fashion.
6. Repeat as many times as necessary at various levels to achieve the desired effect.

Note: Additional downward vertical pressure converts this into a deep articulatory technique.

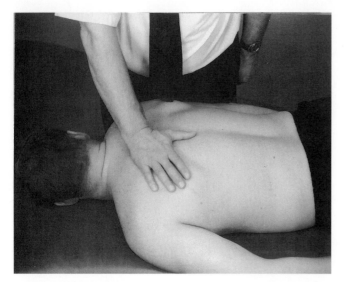

Figure 56.5. Placement of thumb for thoracic thumb pressure.

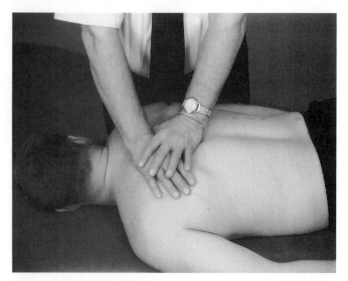

Figure 56.6. Caudad hand reinforcing thumb pressure for thoracic thumb pressure.

Prone Thumb Pressure

OBJECTIVE

Decrease paravertebral muscle hypertonicity.

POSITION

Prone.

PROCEDURE

1. Stand at the head of the table.
2. Place the thumbs of both hands just lateral to the spinous processes, on the paravertebral muscles, with your fingers fanned out.
3. Exert a caudad, anterior pressure, allowing muscle to relax and stretch, finishing with a lateral sweeping motion.
4. A kneading motion or inhibitory pressure may be used.
5. The technique is repeated at as many spinal levels as is desired, as many times as necessary to achieve the desired effect.

Prone Pressure with Counterpressure

OBJECTIVE

Relax deep intrinsic spinal muscles.

POSITION

Prone.

PROCEDURE

1. Stand at the side of the table.
2. Have the patient turn his or her head toward you.
3. Place one hand on the far side of the spine over the transverse processes with your fingers pointing cephalad.

4. Place your other hand on the near side of the spine with your fingers pointing caudad.
5. Exert simultaneous longitudinal and anterior pressure with both hands, imparting a side-bending motion to the thoracic segments under the treating hands. The degree of vertical pressure exerted is varied according to the patient's condition and the degree of vertebral and costal articulation desired.
6. Use a repetitive kneading motion.
7. Repeat as many times as necessary to achieve the desired effect.

Note: This technique can be used as a deep articulatory technique or can readily be converted to a thrust technique directed at thoracic segmental dysfunction.

Upper Thoracic: Lateral Recumbent

OBJECTIVE

Relax upper thoracic paravertebral muscles.

POSITION

Lateral recumbent (Fig. 56.7).

PROCEDURE

1. Stand at the side of the table facing the patient.
2. Pass your caudad hand under the patient's arm, grasping the upper side paravertebral muscles just lateral to the spinous processes with the pads of your fingers.
3. Contact the anterior portion of the shoulder with your cephalad hand to provide an effective counterforce.
4. Draw the paravertebral muscles laterally away from the spine until restriction is palpated.

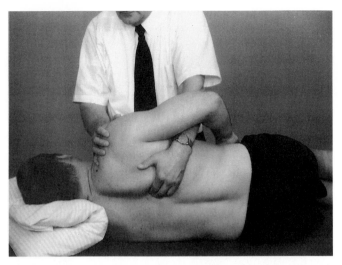

Figure 56.7. Lateral recumbent position for upper thoracic technique.

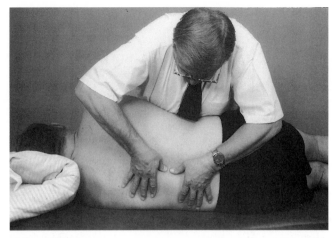

Figure 56.8. Lateral recumbent thumb pressure for thoracic technique.

5. Continue to apply lateral traction until the tissues relax, soften, and lengthen. The lateral traction is then slowly released.
6. Work your way up and down the spinal column from the cervicothoracic junction to about the midthoracics.
7. Repeat as many times as necessary to achieve the desired effect.

Lower Thoracic: Lateral Recumbent

OBJECTIVE

Relax the lower thoracic paravertebral muscles.

POSITION

Lateral recumbent, treatment side up.

PROCEDURE

1. Stand at the side of the table.
2. Reach both hands under the patient's arm, contacting the para--vertebral muscles just lateral to the spinous processes with the pads of your fingers.
3. Pull the pads of your fingers toward the center of the body, drawing the musculature laterally like a bowstring.
4. Slowly release this lateral traction, and reposition your hands along the spine to treat other levels as desired.
5. Repeat as many times as necessary to achieve the desired effect.

Lateral Recumbent Thumb Pressure

OBJECTIVE

Relax the thoracic paravertebral muscles.

POSITION

Lateral recumbent, treatment side down (Fig. 56.8)

PROCEDURE

1. Stand at the side of the table, facing the patient.

2. Reach across the back of the patient until your thumbs are contacting the paravertebral tissues just lateral to the far side of the spinous processes.
3. Exert pressure with your thumbs toward the center of the body and down toward the table.
4. You may use an intermittent kneading or sustained inhibitory pressure.
5. Repeat as many times as necessary to achieve the desired effect.

Side Leverage

OBJECTIVE

Relax thoracic paravertebral muscles.

POSITION

Lateral recumbent, treatment side down (Fig. 56.9).

PROCEDURE

1. Sit at the side of the table, facing the patient.
2. Position your caudad arm so that the patient's shoulder is in your axilla, with your thumb medial to the paravertebral muscles on the far side of the spine.
3. Lift the patient's head away from the table, introducing a cervical and upper thoracic side-bending force.
4. Simultaneously, your caudad thumb exerts a downward pressure on the upper thoracic paravertebral musculature. This may be applied as a combination of intermittent traction and kneading or with a sustained inhibitory pressure.
5. Repeat as many times as necessary to achieve the desired effect.

Note: This technique can be converted to either a deep articulatory technique or an HVLA thrust with minimal repositioning of the physician's caudad hand.

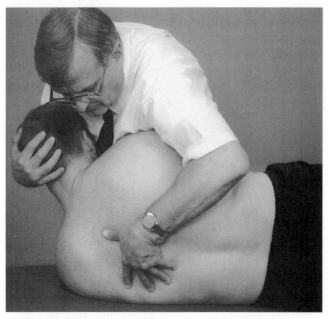

Figure 56.9.   Side leverage for thoracic technique.

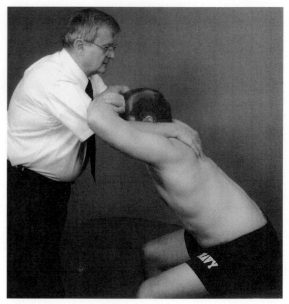

Figure 56.10.   Seated position using over/under method for thoracic technique.

Seated, Over/Under

OBJECTIVE

Relax upper thoracic paravertebral muscles.

POSITION

Seated (Fig. 56.10).

PROCEDURE

1. Stand facing your patient. Have your patient cross his or her arms, hooking the patient's thumbs in the antecubital fossae.
2. Reach under the patient's forearms and over his or her shoulders.
3. Contact the paravertebral tissues over the upper thoracic transverse processes with your finger pads.
4. Lean back, drawing the patient toward you as you simultaneously exert an upward leverage on the forearms.
5. Exert a downward pressure into the soft tissues with the pads of your fingers, then draw them cephalad with a kneading motion.
6. Repeat as many times as necessary to achieve the desired effect.

Note: This technique may converted to a deep articulatory technique by increasing the amount of inward pressure on the pads of the fingers, producing thoracic backward bending.

Supine Extension

OBJECTIVE

Relax the thoracic paravertebral muscles.

POSITION

Supine (Fig. 56.11).

PROCEDURE

1. Sit at the side of the table.
2. Slide your hands under the patient until the pads of your fingers contact the paravertebral soft tissues on the near side.
3. By leaning down onto the elbows, you create a fulcrum, transmitting pressure upward into the paravertebral soft tissues.
4. Simultaneously draw your finger pads toward you.
5. This may be performed in a kneading fashion or with deep inhibitory pressure.
6. Repeat as many times as necessary to achieve the desired effect.

Note: This technique is commonly used in the postoperative setting to prevent and/or treat postoperative paralytic ileus. In this setting, the technique has been referred to as rib raising.

Midthoracic Extension

OBJECTIVE

Relax the midthoracic paravertebral muscles.

POSITION

Seated (Fig. 56.12).

PROCEDURE

1. Stand behind the patient, and have the patient clasp hands behind the neck.
2. Grasp the patient's arms under the elbows.

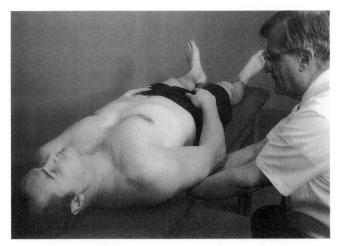

Figure 56.11. Thoracic extension in supine position.

3. Place your other hand so that it is straddling the spine, with fingers pointed cephalad.
4. Elevate the patient's elbows, applying tractional force as you simultaneously press forward with the hand straddling the spine.
5. Repeat as many times as necessary to achieve the desired effect.

Note: This technique may be converted to a deep articulatory technique by varying the amount of anterior pressure applied through your posterior hand.

LUMBAR

Supine Flexion

OBJECTIVE

Relax the lumbar paravertebral muscles.

POSITION

Supine.

PROCEDURE

1. Stand at the side of the table.
2. Have the patient flex both hips, drawing the knees up toward the chest.
3. Grasp the patient's knees, further flexing the hips until the pelvis begins to follow, exerting a tractional force on the lumbar paravertebral muscles.
4. Continue the tractional stretch in an intermittent or continuous fashion.
5. Additional traction may be brought to bear on either side of the spine by adding side-bending away from the side to be treated.
6. Repeat as many times as necessary to achieve the desired effect.

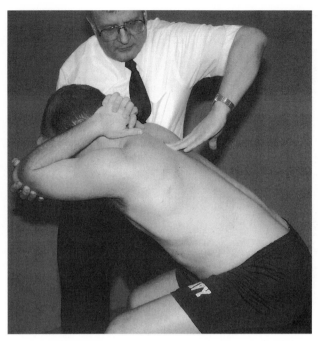

Figure 56.12. Seated position for midthoracic extension.

Supine Rotation with Counterleverage

OBJECTIVE

Relax lumbar paravertebral muscles.

POSITION

Supine (Fig. 56.13).

PROCEDURE

1. Stand at the side of the table and have your patient flex the knees and hips.
2. Draw the patient's knees toward you with your caudad hand, while the cephalad hand reaches under the lumbar region to grasp the paravertebral tissues with your finger pads.
3. Pull your cephalad hand upward toward the ceiling.
4. Produce a rotational counterforce by simultaneously pushing the knees away from you.
5. Apply the technique in either a kneading manner or with deep inhibitory pressure.
6. Repeat as many times as necessary to achieve the desired effect.

Prone Pressure with Counterleverage

OBJECTIVE

Relax lumbar paravertebral muscles.

POSITION

Prone (Fig. 56.14).

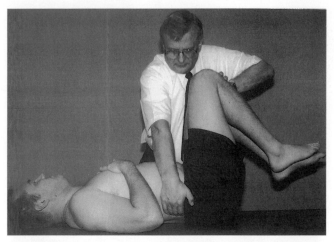

Figure 56.13. Supine rotation with counterleverage for lumbar technique.

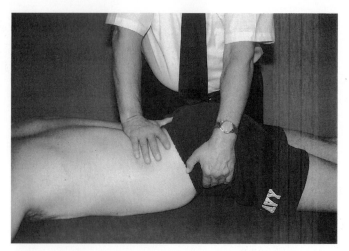

Figure 56.14. Prone pressure with counterleverage for lumbar technique.

PROCEDURE

1. Stand at the side of the table.
2. Contact the lumbar paravertebral musculature on the opposite side of the spine with the heel of your cephalad hand.
3. Grasp the anterior superior iliac spine (ASIS) with your caudad hand, pulling upward toward the ceiling.
4. Apply a simultaneous anterior and lateral force, stretching the lumbar paravertebral tissues like a bowstring.
5. Use either a kneading motion, or deep inhibitory pressure.
6. Repeat as many times as necessary to achieve the desired effect.

Prone Scissors Technique

OBJECTIVE

Relax lumbar paravertebral muscles.

POSITION

Prone (Fig. 56.15).

PROCEDURE

1. Stand at the side of the table.
2. Grasp the patient's opposite leg just above the knee with your caudad hand, lifting the leg far enough to cross it behind the nearer leg. Your hand is now between the patient's knees.
3. Contact the lumbar paravertebral muscles (on the far side) with the heel of your cephalad hand.
4. Apply an anterior and lateral pressure with the cephalad hand, while simultaneously increasing the amount of scissoring with the legs.
5. Use an intermittent kneading motion, or sustained inhibitory pressure.
6. Repeat as many times as necessary to achieve the desired effect.

Prone Traction

OBJECTIVE

Relax lumbar paravertebral muscles.

POSITION

Prone (Fig. 56.16).

PROCEDURE

1. Stand at the side of the table.
2. Place your cephalad hand over the base of the sacrum, with the fingers pointing toward the coccyx.
3. Place your other palm straddling the spinous processes of the lumbar vertebrae, with your fingers pointing cephalad.
4. Exert a separating tractional force in the directions in which the fingers point.
5. Use either intermittent traction or sustained inhibition.
6. The position of the caudad hand may be altered by placing it to one side of the spine, thus bringing more force to bear on the paravertebral soft tissues on that side.
7. Repeat as many times as necessary to achieve the desired effect.

Bilateral Thumb Pressure

OBJECTIVE

Relax lumbar paravertebral muscles.

POSITION

Prone.

PROCEDURE

1. Stand at the side of the table, near the patient's knees.
2. Place the thumbs of both hands on the paravertebral muscles overlying the transverse processes, with the fingers fanned out over the lateral abdominal muscles.

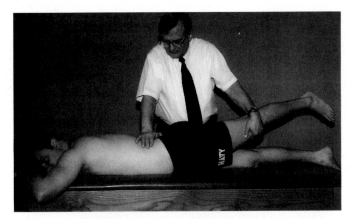

Figure 56.15. Prone scissors technique.

3. Apply bilateral pressure anteriorly and cephalad until the limits of tissue motion are reached.
4. Sweep your thumbs in a lateral direction.
5. Reposition your thumbs at a different lumbar segment.
6. Repeat steps 4 and 5 in a kneading fashion, as many times as necessary to achieve the desired effect.

Supine

OBJECTIVE

Relax lumbar paravertebral muscles.

POSITION

Supine.

PROCEDURE

1. Sit at the side of the table.
2. Reach under the lumbar region with both hands, contacting the ipsilateral paravertebral tissues overlying the transverse processes with the pads of your fingers.
3. Lean down into the elbows, producing an upward leverage at the wrists and hands, simultaneously drawing your hands toward you.
4. Use either a kneading motion or sustained inhibitory pressure.
5. Repeat as many times as necessary to achieve the desired effect.

Lateral Recumbent

OBJECTIVE

Relax lumbar paravertebral muscles.

POSITION

Lateral recumbent, treatment side up (Fig. 56.17).

PROCEDURE

1. Stand at the side of the table.
2. Have your patient flex the hips and knees; place your thigh against the infrapatellar region.

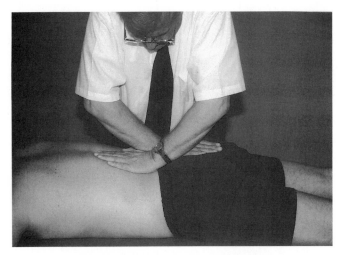

Figure 56.16. Prone traction technique.

3. Reach over the back and grasp the paravertebral muscles of the lumbar region, drawing them toward you and away from the spine simultaneously.
4. Your thighs against the patient's knees may simply be used for bracing or they may also be simultaneously flexed to provide a combined bowstring and longitudinal traction force on the paravertebral musculature.
5. Use either a kneading motion or sustained inhibitory pressure.
6. Repeat as many times as necessary to achieve the desired effect.

Seated

OBJECTIVE

Relax lumbar paravertebral muscles.

POSITION

Seated (Fig. 56.18).

PROCEDURE

1. Stand behind the patient, opposite the treatment side.
2. Have the patient place his or her hand on the side to be treated behind the neck. The opposite hand grasps the elbow of the first hand.
3. Reach under the near axilla, grasping the far arm just proximal to the elbow.
4. Place the heel of your posterior hand over the paravertebral tissues on the far side of the spine.
5. Have the patient allow his or her weight to drop forward onto your arm.
6. Rotate the patient toward you with your anterior hand.
7. Your posterior hand provides a lateral force on the lumbar paravertebral muscles, away from the spine.
8. Repeat as many times as necessary to achieve the desired effect.

Note: This technique may also be used for deep articulation. It is also readily converted to muscle energy and HVLA thrust techniques.

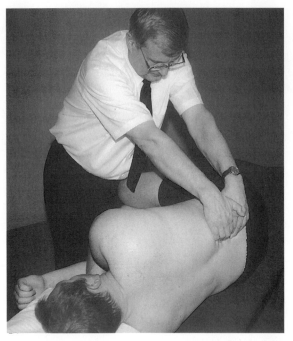

Figure 56.17. Lateral recumbent position for lumbar technique.

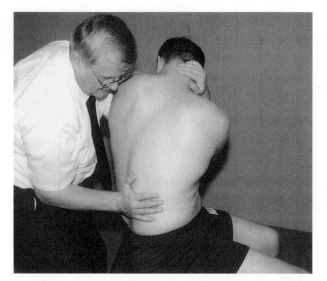

Figure 56.18. Seated position for lumbar technique.

SACRUM

Sacral Rock

OBJECTIVE

Relax the muscles at the lumbosacral junction.

POSITION

Prone (Fig. 56.19).

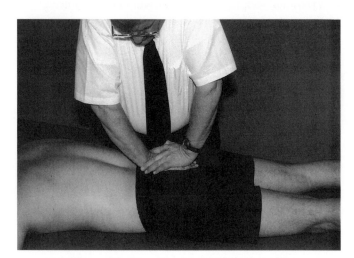

Figure 56.19. Prone position for sacral rock.

PROCEDURE

1. Stand at the side of the patient's pelvis.
2. Place the heel of your cephalad hand on the sacral base, with your fingers pointing toward the coccyx.
3. Place your caudad hand on top of the first hand, with your fingers pointing in the opposite direction.
4. Exert a gentle pressure straight down toward the table.
5. Alternate the direction of your pressure to synchronize it with and augment the natural motion accompanying respiration, "rocking" the sacrum into flexion and extension.
6. Repeat as many times as necessary to achieve the desired effect.

Note: This technique may be converted to a craniosacral technique by following the cranial rhythmic impulse rather than pulmonary respiration.

Sacral Inhibition

OBJECTIVE

Inhibit sacral motion, altering parasympathetic nervous system balance.

POSITION

Prone.

PROCEDURE

1. Stand at the side of the patient's pelvis.
2. Place the heel of your cephalad hand on the sacral base, with your fingers pointing toward the coccyx.
3. Place your caudad hand on top of your other hand, with fingers pointing in the opposite direction.
4. Direct deep pressure straight down toward the table.
5. Maintain this pressure (without rocking motion) for 30 seconds to 2 minutes.

Note: This technique may be converted to a craniosacral technique by following the cranial rhythmic impulse to a still point. This is sometimes referred to as a sacral CV4.

UPPER EXTREMITY

Pectoral Traction

OBJECTIVE

Relax the anterior muscular attachments of the upper extremity.

POSITION

Supine (Fig. 56.20).

PROCEDURE

1. Stand at the head of the table.
2. Hook the pads of your fingers into both anterior axillary folds.
3. Apply a cephalad anterior traction.
4. Have your patient inhale.
5. With inhalation, increase your cephalad and anterior traction, and maintain it as the patient exhales.
6. This cycle of inhalation/traction/resisted exhalation may be repeated until no further stretch of the pectoral muscles or expansion of the rib cage is noted or until you achieve the desired effect.

Note: This technique is frequently applied following thoracic pump technique to relieve a patient's sense of chest compression. It may also be used as a lymphatic pump by increasing inhalation excursion of the upper seven ribs, thus increasing inhalation negative pressure.

Posterior Axillary Folds

OBJECTIVE

Relax the posterior muscle attachments to the upper extremity.

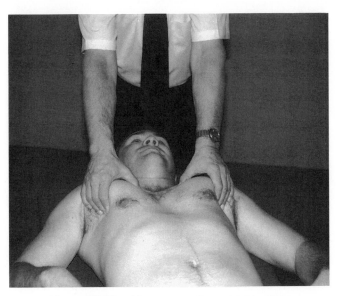

Figure 56.20. Upper extremity pectoral traction.

POSITION

Supine, treatment arm palm down on abdomen (Fig. 56.21).

PROCEDURE

1. Sit at the side of the table, facing the patient's head.
2. Using the hand closest to the patient, grasp the posterior axillary fold between your thumb and fingers.
3. Starting near the trunk, apply a milking motion, rolling along the fold toward the thorax.
4. Gradually, as the muscle softens, work your way away from the trunk, including more of the posterior axillary fold in the sequential rolling motion until the entire fold has been treated.

Note: A similar approach may be applied to the anterior axillary fold.

Interosseous Membrane of Forearm

OBJECTIVE

Relax the interosseous membrane and soft tissues of the forearm.

POSITION

Seated.

PROCEDURE

1. Stand facing your patient.
2. Grasp the hand of the arm to be treated, as if to shake hands.
3. Wrap your other hand over the top of the forearm.
4. Slowly induce pronation through the patient's hand.
5. Use your other hand to apply a gentle, opposing wringing motion to the soft tissues of the forearm, stretching and relaxing the muscles.
6. Apply similar treatment in the opposite direction, inducing supination to stretch and relax the muscles.
7. Repeat as many times as necessary to achieve the desired effect.

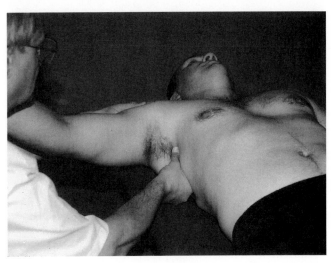

Figure 56.21. Upper extremity posterior axillary folds technique.

Rhomboids

OBJECTIVE

Relax the rhomboid muscles.

POSITION

Lateral recumbent, treatment side up (Fig. 56.22).

PROCEDURE

1. Stand at the side of the table, facing your patient.
2. Grasp the shoulder with your cephalad hand to control tension in the rhomboid and trapezius musculature.
3. Grasp the rhomboid muscles with your caudad hand, just medial to the vertebral border of the scapula.
4. Gently pull up toward the scapula, drawing the scapula slightly away from the ribs.
5. Use either a kneading motion or sustained inhibitory pressure.
6. Repeat as many times as necessary to achieve the desired effect.

LOWER EXTREMITY

Fascia Lata (Method 1)

OBJECTIVE

Relax the fascia lata.

POSITION

Prone (Fig. 56.23).

PROCEDURE

1. Stand at the side of your patient, opposite the side to be treated.
2. With your caudad hand, grasp the leg to be treated just above the knee.

3. Anchor the pelvis against the table with your cephalad hand.
4. Extend the hip of the leg being treated and adduct the hip across the midline until the desired tension is developed in the lateral soft tissues of the thigh.
5. Apply either intermittent or sustained traction as in a direct myofascial release technique.
6. Repeat as many times as necessary to achieve the desired effect.

Fascia Lata (Method 2)

OBJECTIVE

Relax the lateral soft tissues of the thigh.

POSITION

Lateral recumbent, treatment side up (Fig. 56.24).

PROCEDURE

1. Sit on the side of the table behind the patient's knees.
2. Place the thigh to be treated just in front of the other leg with the foot on the table, so that there is a downward slope to the thigh.

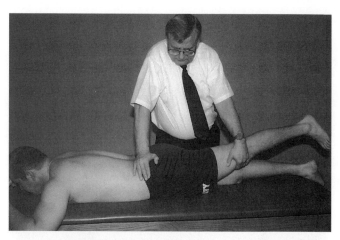

Figure 56.23.   Lower extremity fascia lata technique.

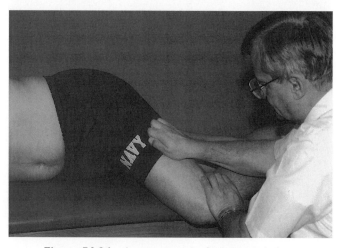

Figure 56.24.   Lower extremity fascia lata technique.

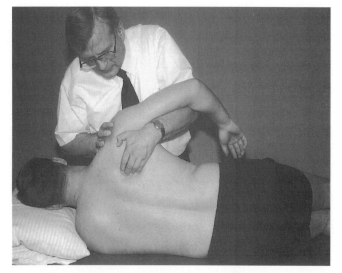

Figure 56.22.   Upper extremity rhomboids technique.

3. Apply pressure against the iliotibial band just caudad to the greater trochanter, using the flats of the middle phalanges of your closed fist.

4. Maintaining this inward pressure, drag your fist down the length of the iliotibial band to the level of the knee.

5. Repeat as many times as necessary to achieve the desired effect, that is, stretch in the lateral fascial structures of the thigh.

Fascia Lata (Method 3)

OBJECTIVE

Relax and stretch the iliotibial band.

POSITION

Prone (Fig. 56.25).

PROCEDURE

1. Stand at the side of the table, opposite the thigh to be treated.

2. Flex the patient's knee to 90° and grasp it with your caudad hand.

3. Use the pads of the fingers on your cephalad hand to hook the iliotibial band and pull upward toward yourself.

4. Simultaneously carry the foot of the same leg away from the midline, increasing the tension on the iliotibial band.

5. Continue with a kneading motion.

6. Repeat as many times as necessary to achieve the desired effect.

Piriformis

OBJECTIVE

Relax the piriformis muscle.

POSITION

Prone (Fig. 56.26).

PROCEDURE

1. Stand at the side of the table, opposite the muscle dysfunction.

2. Beginning near the sacrum, apply double thumb pressure into the piriformis muscle, rolling toward the trochanteric insertion. (The piriformis muscle may be accessed on a line beginning midway between the posterior superior iliac spine and the inferior lateral angle of the sacrum, extending to the postero-superior pole of the greater trochanter.

3. Move sequentially along the muscle toward the trochanter, taking care not to exert too much pressure directly over the sciatic nerve.

4. For heavier patients, you may use your elbow rather than double thumb pressure.

5. Use either a kneading motion or sustained inhibitory pressure.

6. Repeat as many times as necessary to achieve the desired effect.

Plantar Fascia

OBJECTIVE

Relax and stretch the plantar fascia.

POSITION

Supine (Fig. 56.27).

PROCEDURE

1. Sit at the foot of the table.

2. Use the proximal phalanges of your closed fist to contact the sole of the patient's foot just posterior to the metatarsal heads.

3. While applying pressure toward the dorsum of the foot, drag your fist over the plantar fascia toward the heel.

4. Repeat as many times as necessary (toes to heel) to achieve the desired effect.

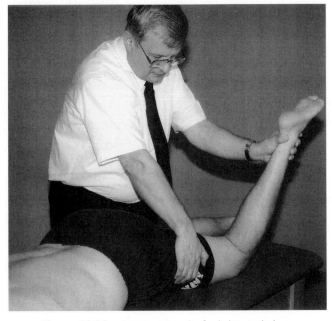

Figure 56.25. Lower extremity fascia lata technique.

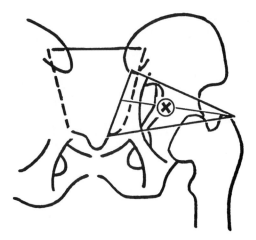

Figure 56.26. Location of piriformis tender point.

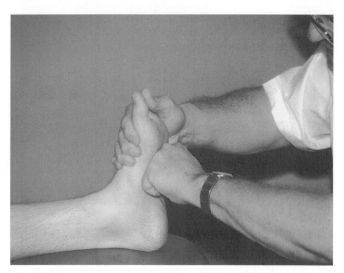

Figure 56.27. Lower extremity plantar fascia technique.

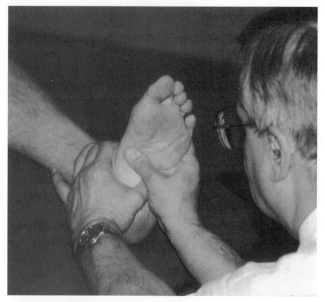

Figure 56.28. Lower extremity arch springing technique.

Arch Springing

OBJECTIVE

Relaxation of the muscles of the arch of the foot.

POSITION

Supine (Fig. 56.28).

PROCEDURE

1. Sit at the foot of the table.
2. Grasp the foot with both hands, with your thumbs under the arch and fingers on the dorsum of the foot.
3. Move the midfoot toward supination, using your proximal hand, while simultaneously moving the forefoot toward pronation with your distal hand. (This "wringing" motion tends to stretch the fascias of the foot toward a position of reestablishing the longitudinal arch of the foot.)
4. Repeat as a kneading type of motion, as many times as necessary to achieve the desired effect.

Note: This could also be considered a deep articulatory technique for the arch.

CONCLUSION

Soft tissue direct techniques address the muscular and fascial structures of the body and associated neural and vascular elements. They can relax and stretch structures and muscles, enhance circulation and nutrition, improve reflex activity and immune response, identify areas of change or dysfunction, and provide a state of relaxation and tonic stimulation.

BIBLIOGRAPHY

Nicholas NS. *Atlas of Osteopathic Techniques.* Philadelphia, Pa: Philadelphia College of Osteopathic Medicine; 1981.

Rubinstein S, Eimerbrink JH, Heilig D, Pratt W. *Osteopathic Techniques.* Philadelphia, Pa: Osteopathic Publications; 1949.

Zink JG. Holistic approach to homeostasis. In: Barnes MW, ed. *American Academy of Osteopathy Yearbook.* Indianapolis, Ind: American Academy of Osteopathy; 1973.

57. Functional Technique

AN INDIRECT METHOD

WILLIAM L. JOHNSTON

Key Concepts

- **History of indirect technique**
- **Historic principles behind indirect technique**
- **Motion–function test pattern**
- **Palpable motor dysfunction: descriptive research**
- **Functional technique as an indirect method**
- **Diagnosis in functional technique, including tissue compression and motion testing stages**
- **Treatment involved in functional technique**
- **Guidelines for application of an indirect manipulative method**
- **"Response information" guides indirect technique**
- **Conceptual basis of functional technique**
- **Practical application of functional technique for the body, including thoracic, lumbar, and sacral regions, cervical region, innominate, appendicular regions, and thoracic cage**

In the history of osteopathy, information derived from palpatory examination has led to the development of a method of manipulation. The terms *direct* and *indirect* have been used as descriptions in classifying methods of osteopathic manipulation. A brief look at 100 years of professional history indicates a significant struggle regarding terminology. This involves two areas:

Verbalizing palpatory findings in the musculoskeletal system

Conceptualizing models, for example, bony malposition at a joint, to depict a local area of somatic dysfunction (referred to in the past as a lesion, the Still lesion, or osteopathic lesion)

Difficulties with terminology are the reason there is a problem communicating clinical signs of musculoskeletal dysfunctions. Although the conceptual model of bony malposition is rela-

tively more easy to teach, it is narrow and limiting in its application to manipulative procedures and to the development of palpatory skills. Initial concepts of somatic dysfunction focused on a joint and the malposition of one bone on the bone below. Joint restriction and direct forces to encounter and overcome restriction described a direct manipulative technique; this fit the layperson's concept of "putting the bone back in place."

Other techniques did not directly encounter the restriction yet still overcame restricted movement. These did not fit the direct method model. These manipulative techniques effectively used motion and maneuvers in the opposite direction of the restriction and were termed indirect methods. Because they defied positional relationships and joint concepts, they presented a special challenge to instruction using the models of thought of those times.

Several early osteopathic practitioners addressed this issue. Edythe Ashmore, an early faculty member at the Kirksville College, wrote the first textbook on the mechanics of osteopathy in 1915. She stated,[1]

There are two methods commonly employed by osteopathists in the correction of lesions the older of which is the traction method, the later the direct method or thrust.[a] Those who employ the traction method secure the relaxation of the tissues about the articulation by what has been termed exaggeration of the lesion, a motion in the direction of the forcible movement which produced the lesion, as if its purpose were to increase the deformity. . . . The exaggeration is held, traction made upon the joint, replacement initiated and then completed by reversal of the forces.[b]

The direct method consists in the application of a precisely directed force toward a bony prominence during the process of putting the articulation or lesion through the spinal movement which is the reversal of that which produced the lesion.

---

[a] *The term "direct" is preferred for the reason that the imitators of osteopathy have given the word "thrust" an objectionable meaning of harshness.* [b] *This [traction] method is the more difficult of the two and for the instruction of students does not find favor with the author.*

Ashmore's footnotes about terminology and instructional problems are particularly illuminating. The limited concepts implied by the expressions *"exaggerating the lesion"* and *"reversal of that* [movement] *which produced the lesion"* remained in use for many years. The direction of restricted movement was even then becoming a determinant for methods of manipulative technique and their classification as direct and indirect.

Another osteopathic pioneer who actively contributed to osteopathic literature from 1905 to 1938 was Carl P. McConnell, D.O. He commented,

So, striving to get the bones in normal position, per se, or perhaps to keep them in position, is simply hopeless. In this regard, the bony item is simply an idol, and a similar idol could be made of the muscles, and so forth.[2]

Precision of method follows definiteness of diagnosis. It is evident that there are many ways of applying the same mechanical principles. But ease and effectiveness should be the goal of operative activity. In adjusting lesions it is obvious that a method which retraces the path of the lesion with a minimum of irritation is highly desirable.[3]

McConnell's orientation was still on *"the path of the lesion,"* but this was tempered by a growing discomfort with using bony position or any single anatomic structure as the key to conceptualizing about areas of musculoskeletal dysfunction.

By 1923, in *Principles and Practice of Osteopathy,* C. Harrison Downing[4] goes a step further in describing restriction at a lesioned segment. He refers to the fact that, when testing a physiologic motion, the lesioned segment becomes more restricted going in one direction. He adds that the restriction decreases in the opposite direction, and *"apparently disappears."* Keeping his motion testing procedure as a frame of reference, Downing provides palpatory information about the restriction *decreasing* in a direction opposite to the direction of restricted motion. These new facts sometimes supported the concepts centered on the joint and bony description of malposition, and sometimes did not.

By 1949, Howard A. Lippincott reported on the osteopathic technique of William G. Sutherland as follows:

The articulation is carried in the direction of the lesion, exaggerating the lesion position as far as is necessary to cause the tension of the weakened elements of the ligamentous structure to be equal to or slightly in excess of the tension of those that were not strained. This is the point of balanced tension.... When the tension is properly balanced, the respiratory or muscular cooperation of the patient is employed to overcome the resistance of the defense mechanism of the body to the release of the lesion.[5]

This described an indirect method of treatment, but the anatomic construct was more *"ligamentous."* The *"point of balanced tension"* (also referred to as *"the point of balanced ligamentous tension"*) became the significant phrase used to describe techniques where the physician palpated throughout the procedure and continually adjusted treatment to the changing tissue tensions. Descriptive terminology still relied mainly on a positional orientation to express this important feedback of palpable information during motion. "Balance and hold" became another phrase to describe indirect techniques, but this phrase fails to point out the continued balancing carried out by the physician in response to the tissues changing.

In the early 1940s at the Chicago College of Osteopathy, indirect techniques were not a part of students' formal training.

However, preparatory steps in this direction involved instructing them regarding the diagnosis of directions of motion that would initially relax the tissues. In Boston, in 1944, indirect techniques were already practiced by some very prominent physician teachers in the New England area; however, the difficulty in communicating these skills was still a problem.

In the 1940s, the Academy of Applied Osteopathy (now known as the American Academy of Osteopathy) initiated a national program of education[6] to improve *"the concepts and abilities of physicians ... to the proficiency in practice attainable only by those who constantly apply these principles [of Still]."* This was done through the implementation of postgraduate instruction. Harold Hoover was a part of this effort. His classification of direct and indirect manipulative techniques included the following:

1. Direct technique: the method of moving one bone or segment of the articular lesion directly to a normal relationship with its neighbor. This is accomplished against the resistance of tissues and fluids maintaining the abnormal relationship.... Direct technique is the most commonly taught and used type of corrective treatment.
2. Indirect technique: the method of moving one bone or segment slightly in the direction away from the direction of correction until the resistance of holding tissues and fluids is partially overcome and the tensions are bilaterally balanced, then allowing the released ligaments and muscles themselves to aid in pulling the part toward normal. Other body forces, including that of respiration may be employed.[7]

Hoover recognized that *motor function* had a broader conceptual framework than just bony relationships. He reported on palpatory tests, palpable findings, and manipulative procedures, especially those of the clinically effective indirect method. He frequently introduced his functional approaches in seminars. His presentation in New England in 1951 initiated an era of development in the New England Academy of Osteopathy. Biyearly study sessions, led by Charles Bowles, resulted in a series of three publications entitled, "A Functional Orientation for Technic."

In his initial report, Bowles wrote:

This was not the birth of a new entity in osteopathy, but simply a new type of measuring stick for evaluating the Still lesion as a process of aberrated function ... our functional investigation had become formalized by using the pattern of a demand–response transaction, instituting motion demands (which could be named) with a motive hand, down to, and through a given segment, while assessing the motion response of this given segment through a palpatory listening hand.... To best understand, follow, and control this demand–response transaction therapeutically at a segmental level, certain specific insights seem necessary, namely:
1. An understanding of typical motion–demands and a system of annotation that makes them easily communicable between operators,
2. An understanding of responses which allows an accurate reporting and a useful evaluation of the specific demand–response

transaction taking place currently under the fingertips of the palpating or "listening" hand during manipulation, and

3. An understanding of criteria for lesioned and non-lesioned performance, i.e., in terms of functional adequacy.

Thus the significant functional information about vertebral motion or restriction is not so much that there is motion or restriction, but rather how these motions and restrictions change, and under what circumstances, and in response to what demands.

It is . . . the response information that eventually guides functional technic[8]

(This is in contrast to guides based on anatomic concepts: bony, muscular, or ligamentous.)

By 1961, Lippincott was expressing educational concerns similar to those of Ashmore. He reported student confusion, as well as practice trends, that were leading him to analyze and clarify the various methods of correcting lesions. In "Basic Principles of Osteopathic Technique," he reports,

It is evident that Dr. Still treated his patients carefully, with due consideration for the delicacy and the welfare of the tissues beneath his fingers. It is also evident that he imparted to the students who came under his supervision this wholesome respect for the tissues, the structures, and their functioning. Then, after the turn of the century, it became popular with many of the vigorous and enthusiastic young doctors to treat with vigor and enthusiasm. They developed techniques that would produce a "pop" regardless of the force required to produce it. This gave them a sense of accomplishment but it also gave osteopathy a reputation for being rough, painful, and even dangerous, a stigma that still persists among the uninformed. Within a decade or two the trend turned back toward more careful and intelligent, but perhaps less spectacular methods. . . . The result is a wealth of technical procedures representing varied approaches to the correction of osteopathic lesions. It is a decided advantage for the physician to have at his command a variety of methods whereby he can meet the needs of each individual patient.[9]

During the 1960s and 1970s, the steadfastness of positional concepts continued to be reflected in the development of new techniques. In 1964 Lawrence H. Jones published his original article, "Spontaneous Release by Positioning," introducing the method of treatment called strain/counterstrain. Dr. Jones questioned,

Is the muscular tension arranged so as to splint this joint, to prevent it from moving back into its eccentric position? No! The muscular tension resists any position away from the extreme position in which the lesioning occurred. Even the severest lesions will readily tolerate being returned to the position in which lesion formation originally occurred, and only to this position. When the joint is returned to this position (indirect), the muscles promptly and gratefully relax.[10]

Since 1969, and possibly starting during the Bowles initiative in New England in 1955, there has been a growing interest in motor function. A test pattern of passive gross motions was standardized relevant to the six elementary directions of the body's movement (Figs. 57.1 and 57.2). These are:

Flexion/extension
Side-bending
Rotation
Translation from side to side
Translation anteriorly/posteriorly
Translation cephalad/caudad (traction/compression)

This test pattern allows implementation of an organized diagnostic process for describing neuromusculoskeletal dys-

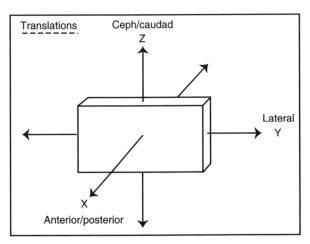

Figure 57.1. Coordinate system to illustrate straight-line directions of movement, used to describe translatory motion tests. (Reproduced with permission from Johnston WL. Segmental definition, Part I: a focal point for diagnosis of somatic dysfunction. *JAOA.* 1988;88:99–105).

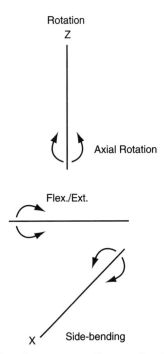

Figure 57.2. Coordinate system to illustrate directions of movement about axes, used to describe rotary motion tests. (Reproduced with permission from Johnston WL. Segmental definition, Part I: a focal point for diagnosis of somatic dysfunction. *JAOA.* 1988;88:99–105).

functions. Investigations[11] using this test pattern advanced our knowledge about motor aspects of both regional and segmental somatic dysfunction in the following ways.

1. Passive gross motion tests are used for gathering a sequence of palpatory information:

   Examining regional motor performance[12]
   Locating segmental motor defects[13,14]
   Characterizing the specifics of a segment's motor dysfunction as a basis for designing manipulative interventions to address somatic dysfunction[15–17]

2. Segmental somatic dysfunction is a complete asymmetry of all of its elementary motor functions: three rotary, three straight-line translatory, and respiratory[18] (respiratory was the seventh function, and takes under consideration the effects of inhalation/exhalation). Palpable recordable cues evident in response to these motion tests provide seven possible descriptors for the motion characteristics of each motor defect.

3. A fundamental unit of segmental somatic dysfunction[16,19] consists of a *three-segment complex*, as illustrated in Figure 57.3. A central asymmetric segment is the primary defect. Mirror-image (opposing) motion asymmetries are present at the adjacent segments, above and below. (These are secondary and adaptive, implying a basis in somatosomatic reflex activity.)

4. A different organizational principle operates when primary defects are identified at a midline vertebra and an adjacent rib at the same spinal level with *similar* motor asymmetries, a complete contrast to mirror images.[20] An example is illustrated in Figure 57.4 at T2 and left rib 2. Present in this defective area

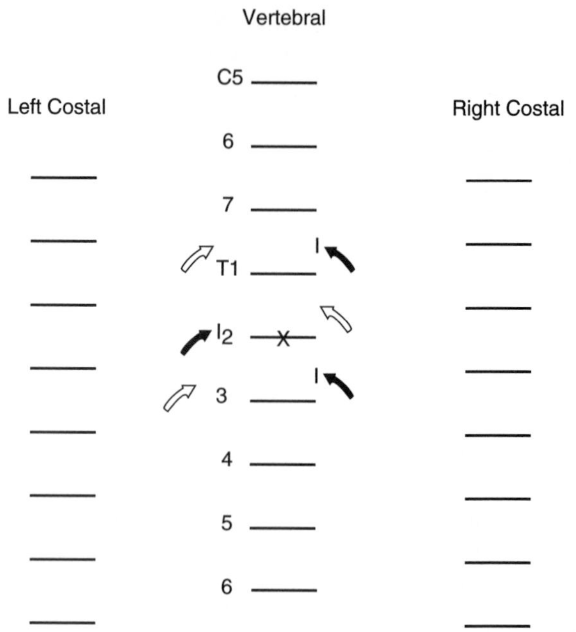

Figure 57.3. Schematic representation of three mobile columns in thoracic region, with a three-segment unit of dysfunction in vertebral column. *X*, location of primary functional defect at T2, with resistance to shoulder/trunk rotation to right (*short, solid arrow, with bar* representing sense of resistance). In adjacent T1 and T3 segments, mirror-image resistance to left rotation is secondary (*short, solid arrows with bars*). *Longer, open arrows without bars* at each level represent sense of compliance with motion and a greater range of motion in directions opposite to directions of limited mobility. (Reproduced with permission from Johnston WL. Somatic manifestations in renal disease: a clinical research study. *JAOA.* 1987;87:22–35.)

Figure 57.4. Schematic representation of two primary motor asymmetries at T2 spinal level, indicated by *X* in vertebral and adjacent left costal columns. *Arrows with bars* at T2 spinal level indicate resistance in both columns to right rotation of shoulders/trunk. Secondary mirror-image asymmetries of restricted motor function are indicated at T1 and T3 spinal levels by *bars on arrows* for left rotation that is (again) present in both columns.

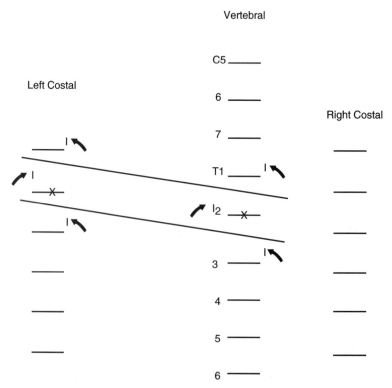

are the mirror-image asymmetries at adjacent segments above and below in both the midline vertebral and left costal columns. Clinical research[21] has supported the premise that visceral afferents contribute to this characteristic configuration of two motor units *linked* in similar primary motor asymmetries at the same spinal level.

This historical perspective resembles the classic tale of the blind men and the elephant, with each man describing the elephant according to the part being touched. From clinical palpatory experience, asymmetry (A) of joint position, restriction (R) of motion, and changes in tissue texture (T) are expressed in the mnemonic acronym ART. Tenderness (T) has recently been added to the acronym, making it TART, with the first "T" representing tissue texture change. Each of the first three has emerged as a palpable sign of segmental somatic dysfunction, where motor function is asymmetric, and manifestations are present in structure, motion, and tissue. The functional characteristics of motor asymmetry emerge primarily from motion tests. These characteristics provide the detailed descriptors for the purpose of differential diagnosis and also establish the basis for a classification of methods of manipulation as direct and indirect.

FUNCTIONAL TECHNIQUE

The term "functional technique" has been used to describe osteopathic manipulative procedures that apply palpatory information gained from tests for motor function. Passive gross motion testing identifies a disturbance of motor (motion) symmetry at an individual mobile segment. Temporarily set aside palpatory information about static position of joints. Apply criteria for determining a mobile segment's resistance to or compliance with opposing directions of specifically induced motion tests. Figure 57.5 demonstrates a single axial motion test introduced through the shoulders and trunk in rotation to the right. With patient seated and arms folded, right rotation of shoulders and trunk is introduced by the physician's right hand at the patient's right elbow. The fingers of the left hand bilaterally monitor the *initial response* of paravertebral tissues overlying transverse processes at the midthoracic mobile segment. For rotation to the left, the operator stands to the left and the hand positions are reversed.

Figure 57.6 illustrates the palpable symmetry in the segment's initial compliance to move right and left. The tone scale registers changes in tension in underlying segmental soft tissues. Also indicated is the normally increasing resistance to the range of motion in a nonlesioned segment as it approaches a physiologic and an anatomic barrier. The initial resting level of minimal muscle tone or tension at X is perceived by the palpable resistance that the operator's fingers sense as they lightly contact the tissues overlying the bony segment at rest.

Start with a compression test. The compression test is the application of pressure through the fingers to sense any increased tissue tension at one segment compared with adjacent segments. Even at rest, a compression test of a *dysfunctional*

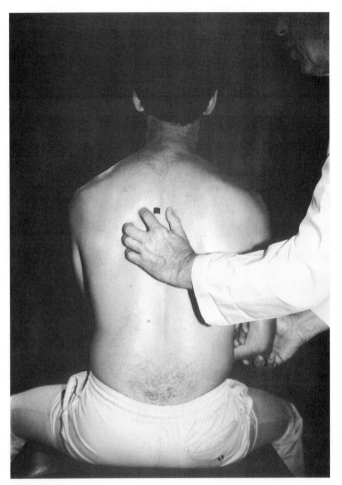

Figure 57.5. Single axial motion test of shoulders and trunk in rotation to right. (Reproduced with permission from Johnston WL. Segmental definition, Part I: a focal point for diagnosis of somatic dysfunction. *JAOA.* 1988;88:99–105).

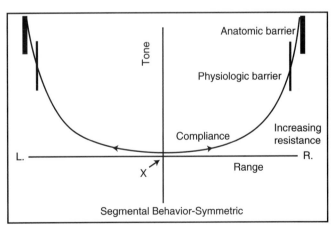

Figure 57.6. Symmetric response to motion at a nonlesioned thoracic segment where only axial rotation is represented. Shown are equal initial compliance to right (R) and left (L), and then increasing resistance toward equidistant final anatomic endpoint. (Reproduced with permission from Johnston WL. Segmental definition, Part I: a focal point for diagnosis of somatic dysfunction. *JAOA.* 1988;88:99–105).

segment will register the local increased resistance of that segment's deep musculature; this can be illustrated as an elevation to "X1" on a tone scale (Fig. 57.7). The fingertips mark the site of the initial palpatory contact.

The segment's tissues in the marked area change during motion testing. This provides a palpable measure of the degree of disturbed motor function. The way this measure changes throughout the treatment provides a guide both for treatment and for judging its effectiveness. During motion testing, palpatory cues of increasing resistance in one direction (in this example, to the right) are sensed *immediately*, along with an immediate sense of decreasing resistance (increasing ease) in the opposing direction. Treatment with functional technique is an indirect method of manipulation. Specific directions of passive motion are combined in their *initial stages of increasing ease*. A specific phase of active respiration also increases this sense of ease in movement. Summing up each of these elementary directions of increasing ease response signals a rapidly improving motor function palpable at the fingertips.

Guidelines

Certain procedural aspects of functional technique help to ensure success in the application of an indirect method of manipulation.[22]

1. The initial introduction of motion in any one elementary direction is small (not range), with minimal forces applied.
2. Motion directions are toward a sense of immediately increasing ease. This response is manifested by a decreasing sense of resistance-to-pressure at fingers monitoring response at the tense dysfunctional segment (at the same time, motions are away from the opposing direction in which increasing resistance is encountered).
3. Single elements of rotary and translatory directions are combined, effecting the control of an eventual smooth torsion arc for body movement. The order of introduction of these elements is not important.

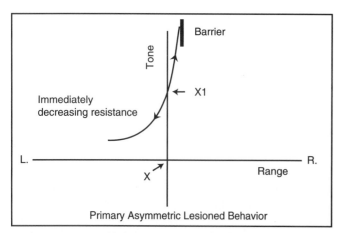

Figure 57.7. Asymmetric behavior at a dysfunctional (lesioned) segment. (Reproduced with permission from Johnston WL. Segmental definition, Part I: a focal point for diagnosis of somatic dysfunction. *JAOA*. 1988;88:99–105).

4. The final step of the functional procedure involves request for a specific direction of active respiration, whichever direction (inhalation or exhalation) contributes further to the increasing ease. For example, if inhalation, the request is for the subject to take a deep breath *slowly* and hold briefly.
5. This respiratory interval, adding to a continuous feedback of decreasing resistance, allows the operator to combine the appropriate translatory and rotary directions. The objective is to reach a sense of release of tissue tension at the fingertips, which are monitoring the dysfunctional segment.
6. The release of restraint in the motor mechanism allows a return to midline resting, unobstructed by any sense of the resistance previously encountered in the return direction.

A successful outcome is signaled by a sensed release of the segmental tissues' holding forces, which then allows a free return to a resting position. The segment's new functional symmetry is evident in the responses to further motion retesting. The segment fails to encounter any further palpable sense of immediately increasing resistance.

Examples of applying this functional method of treatment are presented in the technique section. To copy any technique as a "technique procedure" would be inappropriate and probably clinically ineffective. Bowles[23] stated, *"It is . . . the response information that eventually guides functional technic."* Therefore, focus attention on the following:

1. The criteria for lesioned and nonlesioned motor function
2. The orientation of motor testing to the palpable findings
3. The way, through your fingertips, diagnostic tests guide the development of each individual manipulative procedure

Conceptual Basis

The following phrases reveal the static positional concepts that emerged during osteopathy's early professional history:

Describing the lesion as a bone out of place
Exaggerating the lesion position
Retracing the path of the lesion
Noting the position in which the lesion occurred
Stacking positions to balance the tension

Comments about demand/response transactions and the motor coordination necessary for each bone to be in the right place at the right time during demands for body movement strongly indicate that Bowles was moving away from static positional concepts. Bowles' conceptual bias for motor function called for the recognition of a mobile system and mobile segments that acted in concert with one another to:

1. Maintain postural position
2. Carry out active movements
3. Allow passive movement

For Bowles, functional diagnosis and technique were *"unique in accuracy and universal in nontraumatic application."*[24]

Currently there is widespread recognition, but still limited understanding, of the neural control of these motor dynamics.

In 1978, Stein[25] reviewed principles emerging from studies of the properties of interneurons and their application to the organization of the body's motor patterns. Fundamental concepts of command neurons and pattern generators furnished a baseline for continuing research in this field. This growing knowledge about neural networks and motor control systems has recently been reviewed by Getting.[26] Atsuta et al.'s research presents an ongoing example.[27] In areas where motion tests detect signs of segmental motor asymmetry, somatic proprioceptive and nociceptive afferents (sensory impulses) acting through feedback loops effect adaptive changes in motor patterns. These are palpable as a three-segment unit of segmental dysfunction, which describes a basic unit of defective and adapted function.

During functional technique, the release of holding forces (using minimal force) and the return to motor symmetry have been expressed as follows:[28]

At the moment when the release of resistance forces is sensed, the response (conceptually) appears to be the result of a matching in movement function, in which the local segmental control becomes appropriate to the current, overall movement—a matching of adequacy in physiologic response to specific motion demand. The return to local controlled compliance of the mobile segment within the whole complex movement restores the opportunity for adequate part-to-whole functional relations of this segment within the mobile system.

Basic knowledge about proprioceptor and nociceptor stimuli as a source of reflex communication from somatic tissues to other somatic tissues is well established.[29] Even at rest, in response to only gravity and positional demands, the palpable findings of bony irregularity and increased resistance of muscular tissue to pressure at dysfunctional segments reflect ongoing stimulation of proprioceptor sensors. During movement, these palpable cues to the traffic on afferent pathways are highly erratic, since in some directions of ease they decrease whereas in opposing directions of resistance they increase.

The sheer immediacy of the changes palpated during motion testing and treatment suggests the movement-to-moment afferent monitoring by numerous muscle spindle stretch receptors and the resulting efferent control of muscle contraction/relaxation as a physiologic basis for interpreting the response to osteopathic manipulation being reported here.[28]

The stress of daily demands for movement and positioning accounts for a major increase in somatic sensory afferent impulses reaching the spinal cord at levels where segmental motion asymmetry is present.[30] A concept of *afferent reduction* has application where the palpable sense of decreasing resistance, followed throughout a functional manipulative procedure, successfully restores symmetric motor function.

Examples of Functional Technique

THORACIC, LUMBAR, AND SACRAL REGIONS

The method described in the following example of functional technique[17] applies effectively to thoracic, lumbar, or sacral spinal regions.

Findings

This patient has a dysfunctional T6 segment, with resistance to rotation of shoulders and trunk to the right. Additional findings on shoulder/trunk rotation tests indicate that the increasing ease in rotation left at T6 is accompanied by resistance to rotation left at T5 and T7. Other rotary motion tests reveal initial increasing ease at T6 to side-bending left and to extension, and to initial *inhalation* on respiratory testing. These directions are resisted at T5 and T7. In the next test (Fig. 57.8A), the physician initiates right side-bending of the trunk with moderate caudally directed force through the right hand, which is at the patient's right shoulder. Response at T6 is monitored by the physician's left hand. In the second test (Fig. 57.8B), trunk flexion and extension are initiated, being careful not to introduce translatory aspects of movement, e.g., the patient is maintained in midline of the intersection of midcoronal and sagittal planes. Slightly relaxed slumping supported by the physician's left arm initiates flexion. Reversal of this rotary direction (about the *y* axis of Figure 57.2) initiates extension. The physician's right fingers compare responses to these opposing directions of motion.

Position

The patient is in the seated position. As indicated in Figure 57.9, the physician's left arm is over the left and under the right shoulder of the patient to allow easy introduction of side-bending left and rotation left in the following functional application of an indirect method of manipulation.

Procedure

1. Hold the patient to provide control in side-bending left, rotation left, and extension, in a smooth torsional arc. Each of these directions will begin to diminish the local tissue resistance being monitored at T6 during the manipulative procedure.
2. Using slight shifting of postural forces to control movement of the patient's body, three translatory tests can be completed. In Figure 57.10A, with patient's hips relatively fixed by sitting position, a slight shift in the physician's body weight to right and then to left allows comparison of response of T6 to lateral translations of patient's trunk. In Figure 57.10B, a slight shift in the physician's weight controls patient's shoulders and trunk to initiate anterior and then posterior motion testing at T6. In Figure 57.10C, for testing cephalad/caudad directions, the physician initiates slight lifting cephalad through the patient's shoulders and trunk, and then caudad by applying mild body compression; the segment's responses to opposing directions are monitored by the physician's right hand.

    In this example, movements are added with increasing ease in translations to the left, anterior, and cephalad. Testing had indicated increasing resistance in each opposing translatory direction. Initial introduction of each appropriate direction is more important than extent of range in any one alone.
3. The final component is to direct a slow inhalation by the patient. The additional element of increasing ease promotes a

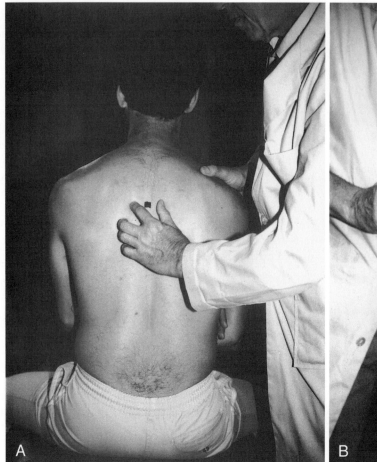 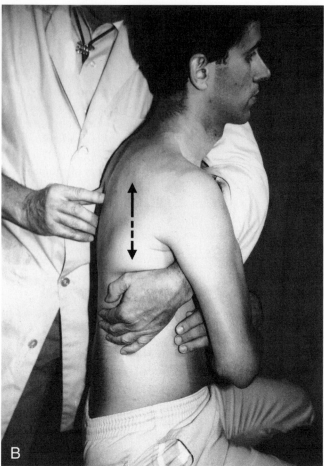

Figure 57.8. Additional rotary motion tests. **A.** Physician initiates right side-bending of trunk. **B.** Trunk flexion and extension. (Reproduced with permission from Johnston WL. Segmental definition, Part II: application of an indirect method in osteopathic manipulative treatment. *JAOA*. 1988; 88:211–217.)

release of the holding tensions at the dysfunctional segment. The release allows return to a central resting position without encountering the previous resistance in these opposing directions.

4. Following successful release, retesting confirms a return to compliance and symmetry in response throughout the T5-T7 area.

CERVICAL REGION

In this example, the cervical region is examined initially in the seated position, followed by treatment in the supine position.

Findings

The first cervical vertebra (atlas) is limited in head and neck rotation left.

Position No. 1

The patient is seated; stand behind the patient.

Procedure

1. With the left hand, contact the frontoparietal region, palm frontal, with finger pads at the right, thumb at the left.
2. Introduce a motion test with the left hand. The right hand monitors for restricted motion response to the rotation left, with the third finger pad of the right hand at the right, thumb at the left, and overlying the facet processes. (Hand placements are reversed to monitor the associated limitations in rotation right at occiput and at C2.)

Position No. 2

The patient is supine; sit at the head of the table as in Figure 57.11. Positioning of the physician's arms with elbows supported on the knees provides comfortable support of the patient's occiput in the palms of the physician, who then monitors response to introduced motion. The third fingertips overlie cervical articular facets at C1 bilaterally to monitor response.

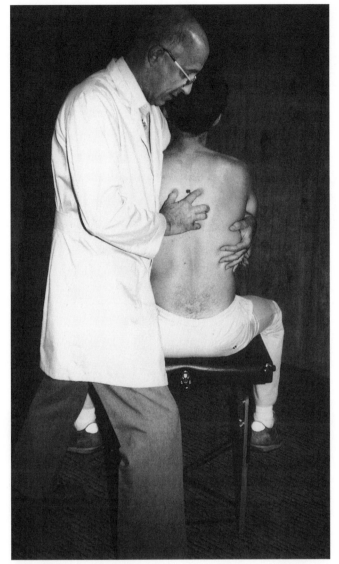

Figure 57.9. Positioning of patient and physician to facilitate initial introduction of combined three rotary components toward a sense of increasing compliance (ease) in extension, left side-bending, and left rotation. (Reproduced with permission from Johnston WL. Segmental definition, Part II: application of an indirect method in osteopathic manipulative treatment. *JAOA*. 1988;88:211–217.)

Procedure

1. Continuing rotary motion tests, C1 responds with initial increasing ease in side-bending right and flexion. During respiration, exhalation is easier.
2. To small amounts of each of the three directions of rotary ease, add translatory components in straight-line directions of increasing ease to the left, posterior, and caudal approximation. (Translatory testing in this example has indicated increasing resistance in each opposing direction.)
3. The increasing ease accumulating at C1 during the initial introduction of these six specific elements of motion is enhanced during a directed exhalation.

4. The smooth torsion pathway for final release of tissue tension allows an easy return to a central resting position.
5. Reexamination in the seated position should reveal a return to symmetry in response to head/neck rotation tests including the occiput, C1, and C2.

INNOMINATE

The patient has an elementary pelvic dysfunction, with palpatory findings localized to one side of the pelvis, here at the left, with asymmetric response just to motion tests introduced through the ipsilateral limb.

Findings

There is a tissue texture abnormality (TTA) and limited mobility at the left ilium/gluteal region (at the level of S2). There is palpable resistance at the left innominate to external rotation (eversion) of the left limb, introduced by the physician's left hand at the left knee.

Position No. 1

The patient is supine, with the left knee semiflexed and the foot resting on the table; stand at the patient's left.

Procedure

1. Locate with the right hand the area of TTA and limited mobility at the left ilium/gluteal region, at the S2 level, and maintain contact throughout the procedure.
2. With the left hand at the patient's left knee, initiate internal and external rotation (moving knee toward right, then left), revealing resistance palpated at the right hand to the initiation of external rotation (eversion).
3. Introduce similar comparison of internal and external rotation tests through the right semiflexed limb, but monitor it at the right hand, revealing left innominate compliance to both directions of the test.

Position No. 2

The patient is positioned in a right lateral recumbent position; stand in front of the patient (Fig. 57.12). The left hand now monitors at the innominate contact (level S2).

Procedure

1. Position the patient's pelvis in a slight anterior translated position relative to the shoulders, as long as this direction decreases tension at the S2 level, compared with posterior translation.
2. Introduce flexion through both legs together, to localize action at the S2 sacral level monitored by the left hand.
3. Support the left leg at the knee with the right hand/forearm to monitor (in this example) the increasing ease at your left

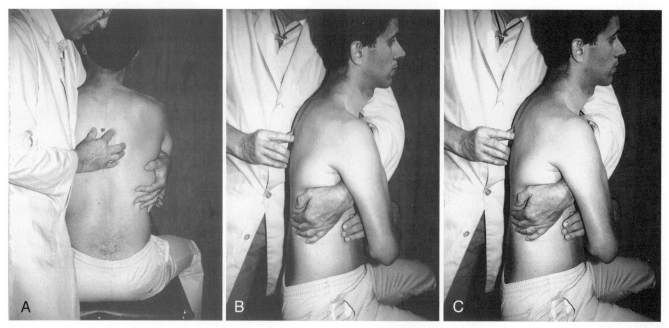

Figure 57.10. Translatory motion tests. **A.** Patient in sitting position for comparison of response of T6 to lateral translations of trunk. **B.** Shift in physician's weight initiates anterior and then posterior motion testing at T6. **C.** Testing cephalad/caudad directions. (Reproduced with permission from Johnston WL. Segmental definition, Part II: application of an indirect method in osteopathic manipulative treatment. *JAOA.* 1988; 88:211–217.)

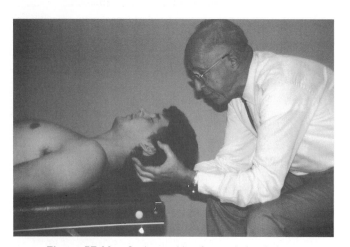

Figure 57.11. Supine position for cervical technique.

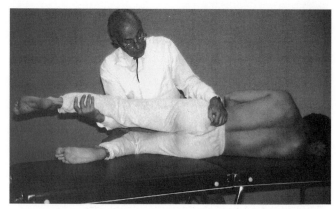

Figure 57.12. Right lateral recumbent position for left innominate technique.

hand in response to abduction of the limb (versus adduction), backward bending (versus flexion), and caudal traction (versus cephalad). Each of these components is combined during introduction of internal rotation (external rotation is resisted).

4. Direct the patient in inhalation (the direction of ease of the TTA).

5. During the final component of directed inhalation ease, combine these motion elements appropriately to achieve a palpable sense of release by the holding forces. Return the limb to its resting position with the patient lateral recumbent.

6. Reexamining the motion tests supine indicates a return to symmetry of response at the left innominate, with reduced tissue tension of the left gluteal musculature.

Variations in the findings from those described for this example simply require application of elementary motion testing procedures at a diagnosed focus of TTA, and restricted mobility, wherever these are evident on pelvic structural examination.[31] Then apply specific directions of positioning and motion in a controlled manner to the pelvic location diagnosed, to ease increasingly the holding forces of restricted function.

APPENDICULAR REGIONS

Note the continuing application of principle here, when the physician uses the six elementary motions, and respiration, as functional tools for testing and reducing specific dysfunction in an appendage.

Findings

In this example, the left knee fails to hyperextend. On examination in the supine position with the physician standing at the left side, the left knee lies slightly raised from the table surface when compared with the right. In this uncomfortable, slightly flexed position, it is more tense to palpation than the right and resists further passively introduced extension. A prominence is palpable at the anteromedial border of the joint interspace (tibiofemoral), indicating the edge of the medial semilunar cartilage.

Position

The patient is supine and the left knee is flexed; stand by the left side of the table.

Procedure

1. The right palm spans the patellar area with the thumb following the lateral aspect of the joint interspace. The third finger follows the medial aspect, as indicated in Figure 57.13. This hand is keyed sharply to the distorted sense of rigid binding resistance where it is most apparent. Keep the contact light enough to appreciate this palpable marker, yet firm enough in grasp to assist in the manipulative procedure.
2. The left hand firmly grasps above the left ankle to assist in slowly bringing the knee up into the freer direction of flexion.
3. Explore additional directions of motion test for the limb while it is supported in freedom from the table by both hands. The motions include rotatory aspects that are found to be more free in medial rotation and abduction. Introduce these motions with the left hand and monitor response with the right.

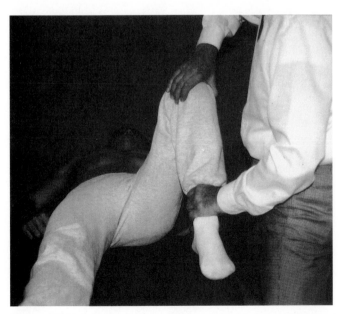

Figure 57.13. Appendicular example at the left knee: Right hand monitors and supports. Left hand introduces major motions in testing and treatment.

4. The motions of ease—flexion, medial rotation, and abduction—are now maintained.
5. Still monitoring at the knee, tests using translatory directions for the limb indicate increasing ease anterior, above the table (binding posterior), increasing ease to the left (compared with right), and cephalad (with binding in caudal traction). The respiratory test indicates easier response to inhalation.
6. In the final maneuver, the right hand contact at the knee guides the lifting support anteriorly to the left, while the left hand controls the amount of each rotary motion in a cephalad direction via the distal tibiofibular contact. There is a proportionately larger amount of flexion introduced, guided by the sense of continuing increasing ease. (This aspect of the knee's template of motion has the greatest range.)
7. Direct the patient to slowly exhale to promote the final release of holding forces. Mobility then allows an easier return into improved extension range as the leg is guided back down onto the table.

THORACIC CAGE

When diagnosing the motor functions of ribs, it is significant to recognize that their elementary function is respiratory. Ribs also function, however, within the context of gross body movements that involve the thoracic spine and cage. Rib function, therefore, can be examined with fingertip contact over the rib angle to monitor a rib's response to the spinal test pattern of elementary passive gross movements (rotations and translations), as well as active respiration. In principle, costal mobile units also function in movement of the upper extremities. Recognizing their intermediary role in so much of the body's movement suggests that costal dysfunctions may show more complex characteristics of motor asymmetry because they have one major motor function (inspiratory/expiratory) and two subsidiary motor roles active in trunk and appendicular movement.

This complexity becomes evident when the palpatory characteristics of costal motor asymmetries are identified. There appears to be an element of simplicity, however, in the manner in which that asymmetry is organized. The primary movement of the ribs occurs in inhalation and exhalation. It is this inhalation/exhalation primacy that appears to dictate the remaining characteristics of the total motor asymmetry when a rib becomes dysfunctional.

For example, if a primary costal defect is more free during exhalation and resists inhalation, it distinctively patterns the motor dysfunction of that rib. This will be revealed when tested through the shoulders and trunk, with the patient seated, and through the ipsilateral arm with the patient in the lateral recumbent position. If the dysfunctional rib is more free during inhalation and resists exhalation, the asymmetric pattern of this rib's motor function is largely reversed from that of the previous (exhalation) example.

Ribs are also involved in asymmetric motor function associated with afferent input from visceral disease. This distinctive category of a viscerosomatic component needs consideration separate from the two dysfunctions to be detailed here. They arise more strictly from the physical stresses incurred in this somatic region.

The following two examples illustrate the most common kinds of dysfunction in the rib cage (essentially somatic in origin, rather than visceral). One shows elementary limitation on exhalation; one is limited in inhalation. The predominance of bucket-handle or pump-handle motion during the inspiratory and expiratory function varies throughout the rib cage and is not considered in these examples. Instead, each example is concerned with monitoring a rib's response to specific demands for rotary and translatory aspects of passive motion tests. These are introduced through the shoulders and trunk of the seated patient and through the ipsilateral upper extremity when the patient is in the lateral recumbent position. Each example of treatment has two components, one seated and one side-lying.

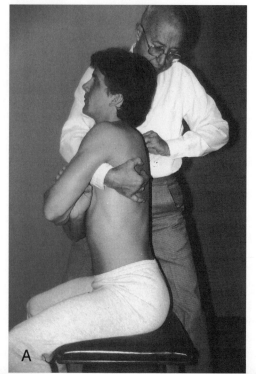

Findings in Example 1

The right rib 3 resists exhalation. It predictably resists shoulder/trunk rotation left and side-bending left, monitored with the right fingertips overlying the rib angle. Testing adjacent ribs above and below demonstrates mirror-image asymmetries if the 3rd right rib is the primary functional defect.

Position No. 1

The patient is seated. Stand at the right of the patient.

Procedure

1. Monitor directions of increasing ease of motion with the left fingers.
2. The right arm is over the patient's right shoulder and under the left to control initiation of motions through the shoulders and trunk during side-bending and rotation to the right (Fig. 57.14A).
3. Tissue tension and limited mobility continue to improve during initial introduction of backward bending and translations to the right and anterior. They worsen during flexion and translations to the left and posterior.
4. Direct the patient to inhale slowly and hold the inhalation phase momentarily as directions of motion are carefully combined in a smooth torsion arc of movement. This promotes a release and return to a central resting position.
5. Retest shoulder/trunk movements, seated, to assess return to symmetry of these motion components.

Position No. 2

The patient is in a left lateral recumbent position. Stand in front of the patient with the patient's right upper arm supported just cephalad to the elbow, as shown in Figure 57.14B, on the physician's left forearm. The patient's right hand hangs toward the floor.

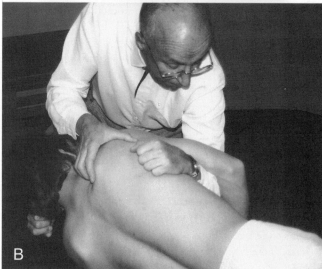

Figure 57.14. Example I: Right rib 3 resists exhalation. **A.** In seated position, motions introduced through the shoulder/trunk. **B.** In left side-lying position, motions introduced through the right arm.

Procedure

1. The right fingers monitor overlying tissue tension/restriction identified at the rib angle, to confirm continuing resistance to exhalation.
2. Palpate for response to motion tests introduced through the patient's right arm. Typical findings include resistance to external rotation (about the long axis of the humerus), abduction, and cephalad movements.

3. During the treatment procedure, increasing ease is monitored during internal rotation, adduction, and caudad movements.
4. The procedure is enhanced by directing the patient to take a prolonged inhalation.
5. Following a successful release, retest the arm motion components in the side-lying position.
6. Following successful release in each of these features of motor asymmetry at right rib 3 resisting exhalation, retesting throughout right ribs 2, 3, and 4 confirms return to functional symmetry in this area of the rib cage.

Findings in Example 2

Right rib 3 resists inhalation. During diagnostic testing, stand on the right to test rotation to the right, and on the left to rotate left. The right rib 3 resisting inhalation predictably resists shoulder/trunk rotation right and side-bending right. Monitor this with left fingertips overlying the rib angle. Testing adjacent ribs above and below demonstrates mirror-image motion asymmetries, if the right rib 3 is the site of the primary dysfunction.

Position No. 1

The patient is seated. Stand at the left of the patient during the treatment procedure.

Procedure

1. Directions of increasing ease of motion are monitored with the right fingers.
2. The left arm is over the patient's left shoulder and under the right to control initiation of motions through the shoulders and trunk during side-bending left and rotation to the left, as shown in Figure 57.15A.
3. Tissue tension and limited mobility continue to improve as you allow initial slouched flexion over the left arm support and translate to the right and posterior. They worsen during backward bending and translations to the left and anterior.
4. Direct the patient to exhale slowly and hold the exhalation phase momentarily as directions of motion are carefully combined in a smooth torsion arc of movement to promote a release and return to a central resting position.
5. Retest shoulder/trunk motions in the seated position.

Position No. 2

The patient is in a left lateral recumbent position. Stand in front of the patient. With the left forearm, support and introduce motion through the patient's right arm, having it relaxed and folded at the elbow as seen in Figure 57.15B.

Procedure

1. The right fingers monitor overlying tissue tension/restriction identified at the rib angle, to confirm continuing resistance to inhalation.

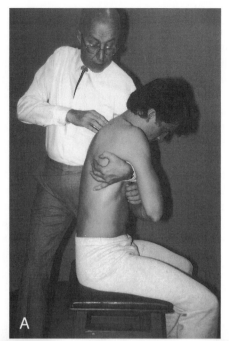
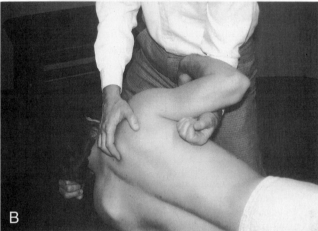

Figure 57.15. Example 2: Right rib 3 resists inhalation. **A.** In seated position. **B.** In left side-lying position.

2. Palpate for response to motion tests introduced through the patient's right arm. Typical findings include resistance to internal rotation (about the long axis of the humerus), adduction, and caudad movements.
3. During the treatment procedure, increasing ease is monitored during external rotation, abduction, and cephalad directions.
4. Enhance the procedure by directing the patient to take a prolonged exhalation.
5. Following release, retest arm motion components in the side-lying position and retest inhalation and exhalation throughout right ribs 2, 3, and 4.

Although the description of these two examples of rib technique (exhalation restriction and inhalation restriction) begin with the seated phase followed by the side-lying, the order is not necessarily important and can be optional.

The physician's approach in functional technique is important. Evaluate at its initial stage of motion each direction of motion that is introduced. Combine these minor ranges in each direction, as described, to produce a smooth torsion arc of motion during the appropriate respiratory phase. This complements the continually monitored response of increasing ease. The tension decreases to a release, and the patient is returned to a resting state. Although these aspects of rib technique are presented as specific directions patterned to inhalation or exhalation restrictions, they should not be applied as if to copy a technique procedure. Rather, test each direction to promote appropriate summation of increasing ease, and monitor decreasing tension throughout each manipulation.

CONCLUSION

The term functional technique applies to an indirect method of osteopathic manipulation in which the treatment procedure is organized around palpatory information gained from tests for motor function. The physician who pays attention to the feedback constantly monitored by the fingertips will experience improved psychomotor skill and proficiency in the use of this treatment method, and many other clinical procedures as well.

REFERENCES

1. Ashmore EF. *Osteopathic Mechanics.* Kirksville, Mo: Journal Printing Co; 1915:72.
2. McConnell CP. Osteopathic art, V. *JAOA.* 1935;34:369–374.
3. McConnell CP. Osteopathic studies, IV. *JAOA.* 1931;31:206–212.
4. Downing CH. *Principles and Practice of Osteopathy.* Kansas City, Mo: Williams Publishing Co; 1923:162.
5. Lippincott HA. The osteopathic technique of Wm. G. Sutherland, D.O. In: Northup TL, ed. *Yearbook of the Academy of Applied Osteopathy.* Ann Arbor, Mich: Edwards Brothers Inc; 1949:1–24.
6. Hoover HV. The Academy program of education. In: Page LE, ed. *Yearbook of the Academy of Applied Osteopathy.* Ann Arbor, Mich: Cushing-Malloy Inc; 1950:45–46.
7. Hoover HV. Fundamentals of technique. In: *Yearbook of the Academy of Applied Osteopathy.* Ann Arbor, Mich: Edwards Brothers Inc; 1949:25–41.
8. Bowles CH. A functional orientation for technic. In: Page LE, ed. *Yearbook of the Academy of Applied Osteopathy.* Carmel, Calif: Academy of Applied Osteopathy; Indianapolis, Ind: American Academy of Osteopathy; 1955:177–191.
9. Lippincott HA. Basic principles of osteopathic technique. In: Barnes MW, ed. *Yearbook of the Academy of Applied Osteopathy.* Carmel, Calif: Academy of Applied Osteopathy; Indianapolis, Ind: American Academy of Osteopathy; 1961:45–48.
10. Jones LH. Spontaneous release by positioning. *The DO.* 1964; 4:109–116.
11. Johnston WL. Interexaminer reliability studies. Spanning a gap in medical research. *JAOA.* 1982;81:819–829.
12. Johnston WL. Passive gross motion testing, Part 1: its role in physical examination. *JAOA.* 1982;81:298–303.
13. Johnston WL, Hill JL. Spinal segmental dysfunction: incidence in cervicothoracic region. *JAOA.* 1981;81:67–76.
14. Johnston WL, Kelso AF, Hollandsworth DL, Karrat J. Somatic manifestations in renal disease: a clinical research study. *JAOA.* 1987; 87:22–35.
15. Kelso AF, Grant RG, Johnston WL. Use of thermograms to support assessment of somatic dysfunction or effects of osteopathic manipulative treatment. *JAOA.* 1982;82:182–188.
16. Johnston WL. Segmental definition, Part I: a focal point for diagnosis of somatic dysfunction. *JAOA.* 1988;88:99–105.
17. Johnston WL. Segmental definition, Part II: application of an indirect method in osteopathic manipulative treatment. *JAOA.* 1988; 88:211–217.
18. Johnston WL. Segmental behavior during motions, 1: a palpatory study of somatic relations. *JAOA.* 1972;72:352–361.
19. Johnston WL, Hill JL. Spinal segmental dysfunction: incidence in cervicothoracic region. *JAOA.* 1981;81:22–28.
20. Johnston WL. Segmental definition, Part III: definitive basis for distinguishing somatic findings of visceral reflex origin. *JAOA.* 1988; 88:347–353.
21. Johnston WL, Kelso AF, Hollandsworth DL, Karrat J. Somatic manifestations in renal disease: a clinical research study. *JAOA.* 1987; 87:22–35.
22. Johnston WL, Friedman HD. *Functional Methods: A Manual for Palpatory Skill Development in Osteopathic Examination and Manipulation of Motor Function.* Indianapolis, Ind: American Academy of Osteopathy; 1995:44–45.
23. Bowles CH. A functional orientation for technic. In: Page LE, ed. *Yearbook of the Academy of Applied Osteopathy.* Carmel, Calif: Academy of Applied Osteopathy; 1955:177–191.
24. Bowles CH. Functional technique: a modern perspective. *JAOA.* 1981;80:326–331.
25. Stein PSG. Motor systems, with specific reference to the control of locomotion. *Annu Rev Neurosci.* 1978;1:61–81.
26. Getting PA. Emerging principles governing the operation of neural networks. *Annu Rev Neurosci.* 1989;12:185–204.
27. Atsuta Y, Garcia-Rill E, Skinner RD. Characteristics of electrically induced locomotion in rat in vitro brain stem–spinal cord preparation. *J Neurophysiol.* 1990;64:727–735.
28. Johnston WL. Segmental definition, Part II: application of an indirect method in osteopathic manipulative treatment. *JAOA.* 1988; 88:211–217.
29. Henneman E. Organization of the spinal cord and its reflexes. In: Mountcastle VB, ed. *Medical Physiology.* 14th ed. Vol. 1. St. Louis, Mo: CV Mosby; 1980:762–786.
30. Johnston WL. Osteopathic clinical aspects of somatovisceral interaction. In: Patterson MM, Howell JH, eds. *The Central Connection: Somatovisceral/Viscerosomatic Interaction.* Indianapolis, Ind: American Academy of Osteopathy; 1992.
31. Johnston WL, Friedman HD. *Functional Methods: A Manual for Palpatory Skill Development in Osteopathic Examination and Manipulation of Motor Function.* Indianapolis, Ind: The American Academy of Osteopathy; 1995:83–91.

58. Strain and Counterstrain Techniques

JOHN C. GLOVER AND HERBERT A. YATES

Key Concepts

- Origin of counterstrain and why the term is used

- Meaning of "spontaneous release by positioning"

- Nature of a strain

- Treatment sequence for applying counterstrain

- Importance of tender points in applying counterstrain and how to find and use them

- How to establish a tenderness scale with the patient

- How to find the position of optimal comfort when treating with counterstrain, and how much pain in the tender point should be reduced by placing the patient in that position

- Three purposes of feedback from the patient regarding tender points

- How to treat "maverick" when present

- How long to maintain the position of comfort and the importance of returning the patient to the neutral starting position

- Importance of rechecking the tender point and the reasons why there might be no lessening of tenderness in the point

- What will happen to the tender point if it was a result of a viscerosomatic reflex

- What may occur clinically after a counterstrain treatment

- Ability to apply selected counterstrain treatments

Counterstrain is an indirect technique in which the tissue being treated is positioned at a point of balance, or ease, away from the restrictive barrier. To treat the strain, the physician counters the strain by reintroducing the original strain, which is the position of ease. Counterstrain is based on identifying tender points and positioning the patient to eliminate the tenderness.

HISTORY

Counterstrain began in 1955 as a discovery in the rural Oregon office of Lawrence H. Jones, D.O. An athletic-looking young man entered the office bent forward and unable to stand erect. The young man reported no history of trauma. His problem, begun 2½ months earlier, had developed gradually. Since then he had received treatment by two chiropractic physicians with no substantial improvement. Jones treated the man several times over the course of 6 weeks with similar results.

After nearly 4 months of treatment, the man had difficulty sleeping due to pain. Jones decided to try something different. He helped the man maneuver himself into a position in which he was comfortable lying on a treatment table propped up with pillows. He left the young man in this position and departed from the room to treat another patient. He returned about 20 minutes later to find the young man still comfortable. Jones slowly assisted the young man to stand up. To their surprise, the patient stood erect for the first time in 4 months. Jones instructed the man on how to obtain the position at home when in bed so that he could rest more comfortably. Since he had been frustrated by his previous failure to help, Jones was powerfully impressed by the "spectacular cure" and was determined to understand what had happened.

Over the next several months, Jones experimented by treating patients with positions of comfort. He had frequent success. He also noticed that paravertebral areas that were sore and tender to palpation were relieved after placing the patient in a position of comfort and then slowly returning the person to a relaxed, neutral position.

Ninety seconds in a position of comfort proved to be the optimal time required to benefit the patient. Shorter periods of time did not yield lasting relief, and longer periods did not yield greater relief. The reason for this is not understood, but research has shown that learning at the spinal cord level requires 90 seconds. Thirty years of clinical practice by Jones and others trained in these techniques have demonstrated the technique's effectiveness.

Finding the position of comfort, maintaining the position for a time, and returning the patient slowly from the position of comfort were three essentials for these techniques to be effective. The presence of tender paravertebral areas in about half of the patients, and relief of the tenderness by using the three steps, intrigued Jones. Tender areas were almost always relieved by his treatment, but he could find posterior tender points in about half the patients.

A patient of Jones struck himself in the groin with a short-handled hoe while gardening. Fearing he may have "ruptured" himself, the man immediately came to see Jones. Examination revealed no inguinal hernia, but the area was tender. Jones placed him in a position of comfort. With the patient in the position, Jones palpated the injured area. To their mutual surprise, it was no longer tender. After he slowly returned the patient to a neutral position, the groin remained nontender.

Apparently there were anterior as well as posterior tender points. Jones began to search for tender points in the anterior tissues. The front is reciprocally connected to the back. This observation is consistent with osteopathic principles. The emphasis on spinal function and posterior biomechanics had eclipsed this connection. At that time, only Owens's discussion of Chapman's reflex points and some myofascial and Sutherland-type techniques emphasized the connection between anterior and posterior aspects of the body.

Both Jones and Janet Travell, M.D., developed diagnostic and treatment approaches that identified discrete areas of tense, tender tissue. Travell[1] used the term "trigger point," and initially Jones used the same term. In correspondence between the two physicians, they identified similarities and differences between their diagnostic and treatment approaches. Whereas Travell believed that the pathology of her tender point system was the trigger point, Jones believed that his trigger points were only a manifestation of a somatic dysfunction found elsewhere. Another characteristic of a trigger point is radiation of pain when the point is pressed. By contrast, Jones's points were found to be locally tender.

Treatment approaches also differed. Travell treated the tender points with injection, or spray and stretch. Jones treated the hypertonic muscle associated with the somatic dysfunction via counterstrain. As a result, colleagues of Jones suggested he use a term other than trigger point (Jones LH. Personal communication, 1993). The term suggested was "tender point." Many physicians use the terms "Jones' point" and "Travell's point" to distinguish the two tender point systems. There have been approximately 200 specific tender points (Jones' points) identified to date, and new tender points continue to be found.

Initially, Jones referred to his new treatment approach as spontaneous release by positioning. This describes the basic process involved in treatment, but because the term was cumbersome, Jones decided to use a shorter term, strain counterstrain. The phrase was derived from what Jones believed occurred when treating the somatic dysfunction. The initial injury produces a strain in a muscle. Counterstrain is an indirect technique, where the tissue being treated is positioned at a point of balance, or ease, away from the restrictive barrier. To treat the strain, the physician counters the strain by reintroducing the original strain, which is the position of ease. Other individuals have used other terms to describe the approach, but the term strain counterstrain, or simply counterstrain, is preferred by Jones.

Jones made two discoveries:

1. Tender points can be relieved by a position of comfort.
2. The anterior aspect of the patient must be evaluated as well as the posterior to effectively diagnose and treat somatic dysfunctions.

TREATMENT

Too often, medicine is oriented toward symptoms. One can become myopic, looking only at the area of chief complaint. As all medical practitioners know, this is a tendency that can lead to missing a diagnosis. This is especially true with tender point diagnosis. An important osteopathic principle is to treat the patient, not the complaint. Therefore, merely memorizing the location of tender points and finding them without evaluating the patient ignores this principle.

Counterstrain is based on identifying tender points and positioning the patient to eliminate the tenderness. Counterstrain is easy to understand and apply, but mastery requires time to learn the location of tender points and skill in fine-tuning the treatment position for maximum results.

Basic steps for treating with counterstrain are the following:

1. Find a significant tender point.
   a. Evaluate the patient to determine where tender points might occur.
   b. Palpate to locate specific points.
2. Place the patient in a position of optimal comfort.
   a. Find the approximate position, shown at the end of the chapter.
   b. Fine-tune through small arcs of motion.
3. Maintain the position of comfort for 90 seconds.
4. Slowly return the patient to neutral.
5. Recheck the tender point.

Significant Tender Point

DETERMINE TENDER POINT LOCATION

One method to determine where tender points occur is to perform a standard osteopathic structural examination and then palpate for the tender points associated with the dysfunctional segment. A second method is to evaluate the patient for variations from ideal posture and palpate those areas for tender points. For example, a patient presenting with flattening of the normal thoracic kyphotic curve is likely to have one or more posterior thoracic tender points associated with the extension in this region. A third is to scan a region for tender points based on clinical history and presenting complaints. By knowing the initial position of injury, the most likely places for significant tender points can be deduced.

Anyone who has a significant tender point attempts to obtain a position of comfort to alleviate distress. This is an unconscious attempt by the patient to shorten and relieve tense myofascial tissues. People tend to bend around tender points. That is, tender points tend to be at the apex or focal point of the concavity of the patient's position. If the patient is forward bent, tender points tend to be anterior. If a patient is extended, tender points tend to be posterior. Jones found patients who present side-bent to the right tend to have tender points on the left side of the spine or anteriorly. Conversely, patients side-bent to the left usually have tender points on the right or anteriorly (Jones LH. Personal communication, 1993).

As a rule, the closer tender points are to the midline, the more flexed or extended is the patient's presenting posture, and more flexion or extension is required for treatment. With tender points more distant from the midline, more side-bending and rotation are usually required for treatment. With relatively little practice, beginning practitioners can predict the general areas in which the most significant tender points occur simply by observing and palpating for the tender point around which the patient appears to be bending or folding the body.

Tender points are frequently found in areas other than those that are the basis of the patient's complaint of pain or discomfort. The primary or key strain may induce a secondary or compensatory strain elsewhere, which may be more symptomatic. Treatment of the primary tender point often alleviates symptoms reported elsewhere. For example, when the psoas muscle goes into spasm, patients seldom complain of abdominal or anterolateral hip pain. They complain instead of pain in the lumbosacral or sacroiliac regions due to the strain placed on those regions by the spasm. The tender points are frequently 180° around the body from the site of the pain. For example, in a patient with an acute psoas spasm, the tender point is usually in the anterior abdominal region, either immediately medial to the anterior superior iliac spine or in the periumbilical region, not in the area of pain.

PALPATE FOR SPECIFIC POINTS

Tender points are typically located near bony attachments of tendons, ligaments, or in the belly of some muscles. If the tender point is not directly associated with the dysfunctional muscle, it is found in the dermatome of the spinal nerve to that segment. Tender points are palpated as small, tense, edematous areas of tenderness about the size of a fingertip, although sometimes the soft tissue changes may be difficult to palpate. The area around the tender point becomes progressively more tense, peripherally to centrally, as the tender point is palpated.

The usual method for verifying the presence of a tender point is to ask, "Is this tender?" as the area where an expected tender point is palpated. Tenderness is a sign elicited by palpation. In contrast, pain is a symptom, a particular type of discomfort reported by the patient. If there are multiple tender points in a given area, ask, "Which is most tender?" Treat the most severe tender point first.

Palpate for a tender point with the pad of your finger or thumb. The pads of the fingers are profoundly more sensitive to tactile input and thus better at predicting the location of tender points. Avoid using the fingertips, especially if you have long fingernails. Fingertips are less sensitive and can elicit iatrogenic tenderness rather than an actual tender point. The angle of approach is often critical because superficial tissues need to be gently moved aside to press more directly on the tender point. Often the tender point is pressed against firm tissue such as bone.

Palpation should be firm but gentle. The pressure used to elicit a tender point is typically a few ounces. It does not cause tenderness in normal tissue. You do not injure a patient if you gradually increase pressure as you palpate the tender point. To determine if a tender point is clinically significant, check the same spot on the opposite side, and/or check the other tender points in the general area. Also check for any other pathology that might be inducing tenderness that is not related to neuromusculoskeletal tender points, for example:

Local areas of irritation
Infection
Inflammation
Viscerosomatic referred pain

Often the patient has no knowledge of the existence of a specific tender point and may react with surprise at your discovery. A patient may even accuse you of creating the point by your palpation. The pressure required to elicit a response is variable. Some patients react dramatically to only slight pressure; others may not report pain when you press a point you can easily identify by palpation. Typically, the better conditioned or more athletic the patient is, the more pressure must be applied to elicit tenderness.

Jones refers to patients who do not report significant discomfort when a tender point is palpated as "stoics" (Jones LH. Personal communication, 1993). Although stoics account for only 1% of presenting patients, they can be frustrating for practitioners. If a tender point is clearly palpated and consistent with the patient's history, it should be treated whether or not the patient reports discomfort.

Position of Optimal Comfort

Treatment is always in a position of comfort. This is one of the greatest advantages of counterstrain. The position of comfort is the same as the position of injury. If an adequate history can be elicited, frequently the position in which the patient needs to be treated can be deduced and used as the treatment position. For example, if the patient attempted to lift an object while bending forward at the waist and side-bending to the right, then the position of treatment is with the patient forward bent and side-bent to the right.

By placing a patient in a position of comfort, discomfort is avoided and injury is unlikely to occur. This is true of even the most frail patient. Counterstrain can be used with patients who have severe osteoporosis, metastatic bone cancer, or acute injuries, unless gently moving the patient into the specific treatment position is contraindicated. At times, technique modifications need to be made. The only absolute requirement is that the patient must be able and willing to relax his or her muscles.

Counterstrain techniques are very powerful, yet very tolerable. They can be used on almost all patients. Approximately 20–30% of patients experience generalized soreness or a flulike reaction 1–48 hours after treatment. This typically happens on the following morning and may last 2–4 days. The reaction usually happens only after the first treatment but may occur for as many as six treatments. Cause of the reaction is unclear, but the patient must be alerted to the possibility of a reaction. It also provides a reason for caution when using counterstrain to treat some severely ill patients. The reaction may be minimized by having the patient apply ice to the treated area for 20 minutes and take a nonsteroidal antiinflammatory drug like aspirin.

Continuous light contact with the tender point during treatment is important. Establish a means of monitoring the tenderness of the tender point with the patient. Ask the patient for the level of tenderness after pressing the tender point, then release the pressure and return to light contact.

Most practitioners establish a scale with the patient to enhance verbal feedback. Several scales have been used effectively. A 0-to-10 scale, with 10 being equal to the initial tenderness and 0 representing no pain, can be used. Some people prefer to use a 0-to-100 scale to differentiate more finely the level of tenderness. A variation of this scale is to ask the patient, "If you started out with one dollar of pain, how much change do you have left?". Other practitioners use percentages or fractions to indicate the amount of tenderness remaining. Some practitioners only ask the patient if the tenderness is better, worse, or the same until the tenderness is reduced by 70% or gone. The scale is important only in that it allows the patient to communicate changes in the tenderness. It should be emphasized that this is not acupressure or a form of massage. Firm pressure is applied only when trying to elicit tenderness.

As the treatment proceeds, the practitioner presses on the point several times and asks the patient the level of remaining tenderness to help establish the position of comfort. This feedback from the patient serves several purposes. First, it provides a means of gauging the effectiveness of the treatment position as the practitioner moves the patient toward the position of optimal comfort. Second, it helps the practitioner maintain the optimal treatment position once it has been achieved. Third, it involves the patient with the treatment and invests the patient in the outcome.

APPROXIMATE POSITION

Slowly move the patient toward the expected position of comfort, while monitoring the tender point for relaxation of the tissue. Obtain the patient's feedback about the level of tenderness. As you get close to the optimal position, a small change in position markedly reduces tenderness. The same amount of change away from the optimal position produces more tenderness or no improvement.

FINE-TUNE

When the patient is close to the optimal position of comfort, fine-tune the position through small arcs of motion (1–5°). Slow movements, constant light contact for monitoring, and retesting the tender point for reduction of tenderness with each

new position allow the practitioner to find the precise position of optimal comfort. If the optimal position is overshot, the level of tenderness increases. Fine-tune the position until the tenderness has been reduced by at least 70%, preferably 100%. The position of comfort must be at least 70% improved over the initial tenderness or the technique is ineffective. Jones recommended a reduction of at least two-thirds, whereas other practitioners have suggested three-fourths. An effort should be made to maximally reduce the tenderness. This increases the probability of success.

Suboptimal treatment (less than 70% tenderness reduction) can be used in the treatment of severely ill patients. For these patients, posttreatment reaction must be avoided. When treating a patient who has an acute, severe condition such as acute myocardial infarction, counterstrain must be used carefully to avoid posttreatment reaction. Stop at 50–60% improvement of tenderness by placing the patient in a suboptimal position of comfort. This is done knowing that the tender point will probably recur. However, the temporary relief can be of significant benefit to the patient. As the patient recovers, the tenderness remaining in the position of comfort can be reduced. Unwanted cardiac problems are typically associated with marked flexion producing a Valsalva effect, so this position should be avoided. Another approach is to reduce the tenderness by 100%, but treat only the most critical areas. Also treat any respiratory restrictions.

Occasionally the recommended or expected treatment position does not turn off a tender point, even with careful fine-tuning. Approximately 5% of tender points, called mavericks, fall into this category. These are treated by positioning the patient in a position opposite what would normally be used. Change the rotation and/or side-bending component first and the flexion or extension component last.

A common mistake is to maintain a constant firm pressure on the tender point throughout the treatment sequence. Instead, constant light contact should be maintained. Once the optimal treatment position has been determined, be sure to maintain only light contact with the tender point. There are three important reasons for maintaining contact:

1. The tissue changes that occur in the tender point can be monitored and can aid in determining the endpoint of treatment.
2. The tender point can continue to be intermittently fine-tuned to maintain the optimal position of comfort, because the position may change slightly during treatment.
3. Both the patient and the practitioner are sure of the location of the tender point.

The last reason may seem unimportant, but when contact with the tender point is lost, the patient may question whether the same point is being pressed. The practitioner may in fact have difficulty reestablishing contact with the point with enough confidence to allow an accurate recheck.

Another palpatory phenomenon may be felt, a pulsation, sometimes referred to as the "therapeutic pulse." Although its intensity may vary, it is often close to the intensity of the radial pulse. In fact, palpating the patient's radial artery with the other hand typically shows it to be synchronous with the therapeutic pulse. For this reason, it is postulated that the position of release results in a sympathetic vasodilation of the small arterioles of the tissue. At times, the therapeutic pulse can be palpated while attempting to find the optimal position of comfort, enabling the practitioner to establish the position more accurately. At other times, the therapeutic pulse cannot be palpated until the treatment position has been maintained for 90 seconds. In either case, the appearance of the therapeutic pulse can be used during treatment as an aid to obtain the optimal position of comfort or to determine the time needed to maintain the treatment position.

Maintain Position of Comfort

Once the position of comfort has been established, hold it for 90 seconds. The patient must remain relaxed. It may be necessary to remind the patient several times to relax during the 90 seconds, because often she or he contracts muscles unconsciously. Patients who are not comfortable will not be able to relax for the entire 90 seconds. If the practitioner is not comfortable, it is difficult to hold the patient in the treatment position for 90 seconds. Experiment to find the best way to remain comfortable during treatment; different patients and different clinical settings offer different challenges. It may be necessary to invent a new treatment position to enable you and the patient to remain comfortable.

Feel for tissue changes in the tender point and the surrounding tissues. As time in the treatment position increases, the tissue of the tender point relaxes, feeling like melting butter. The myofascial tissue around the tender point may begin to move in a seemingly random pattern. This sensation is due to the relaxation of myofascial tissue, and it is useful when learning myofascial release techniques. You may also feel the therapeutic pulse, indicating the patient has been in the treatment position long enough. When the therapeutic pulse has disappeared, fine-tune again and feel for its return. Once the therapeutic pulse does not return after fine-tuning several times, move back to the neutral starting position.

Return Patient to Neutral

After maintaining the position of comfort for 90 seconds, slowly return the patient to neutral.

Before starting to return the patient to neutral, ask the patient to remain relaxed and not try to help by actively moving. Many patients are concerned that the practitioner may be hurt while returning them to a neutral position. Other patients unconsciously help unless they are reminded their help is not needed.

The first few degrees of motion during return are the most critical. Return should be done slowly and carefully. If the patient starts to help or move, stop moving. Remind the patient not to help and that his or her cooperation is important to achieve the maximum effectiveness of the treatment. When the patient has relaxed, start moving again with a slower movement. If the return is too fast, the patient contracts muscles to stop the movement ("guard"), so watch for flinching and feel for muscle contraction. An apparent decrease in the patient's body weight or slight movement by the patient is an indication the patient is contracting muscles. Motion should be stopped and started again only after reminding the patient to remain relaxed.

Recheck Tender Point

Once the patient has been returned to a resting neutral position, recheck the tender point. No more than 30% of the original tenderness should remain. Ideally, all of the tenderness will have resolved. If tenderness remains, there are several possible reasons. The patient may not have been optimally positioned or may have moved during the 90-second holding time. Repeat the positioning with particular attention to obtaining and maintaining the optimal position.

Another cause for failure is that another tender point in the region is the primary problem, and the worst point was not treated. Evaluate the area around the tender point to see if another, more important, tender point is present. Consider the possibility that the primary tender point is distant from the area evaluated or on the opposite side of the body from the reported problem. A chronic tender point may not completely resolve. If the most significant point is treated, it is better when reexamined several days later. Also, lack of pain resolution does not necessarily mean that the tender point has not been effectively treated. Often a beginning practitioner is not careful to maintain the treatment position for the full 90 seconds. Although treatment time may not always be exactly 90 seconds, it is important to maintain the treatment position for 90 seconds when learning counterstrain.

After the palpatory changes that signal the end of treatment can be felt with confidence, watching the clock is not important. A common error when learning counterstrain is to return the patient to neutral too quickly. This can be avoided by watching the patient for flinching or guarding gestures and by palpating for muscle contraction. When the tender point resulted from a viscerosomatic reflex, tenderness returns within minutes or hours. When this happens, a review of medical history and more careful physical examination is recommended. Be sure all of the possible causes of the original tenderness have been considered. For more information about viscerosomatic reflexes, see Myron Beal's article.[2] This information is also important when treating patients in the hospital. Harold Schwartz[3] fully discusses treating hospital patients.

Recheck the original structural findings to evaluate effectiveness of the treatment. The importance of rechecking cannot be overstated. Remember, you are treating a somatic dysfunction, not a tender point. Motion restrictions disappear and tissue texture changes start to return to normal. With chronic somatic dysfunctions, the tissue changes are slower to return to normal.

A few other clinical tips help to understand the counterstrain approach to treatment. It is possible to have both anterior and posterior, or right and left, tender points associated with the same anatomical segmental level. This is because tender points are mediated through the nervous system and can result in points on both sides of the body. It does not mean a segment is both flexed and extended at the same time. Jones recommends no more than six tender points be treated at an appointment (Jones LH. Personal communication, 1993). This reduces the chances that a patient will have a treatment reaction. Jones also did not have a patient return for another treatment for at least 3 days.

STRAIN AND COUNTERSTRAIN TECHNIQUES

Cervical Spine

The cervical spine has the greatest number of maverick tender points. Be ready to look for treatment positions other than those presented here. Anterior tender points are typically located on the most lateral aspect of the lateral masses or slightly anterior on the lateral masses. Posterior tender points are found mostly associated with the tip of the spinous processes or on the lateral sides of the spinous processes. In addition to the typical examples given here, there are several tender points, mostly associated with the atypical cervical vertebra, found in locations other than the lateral masses and spinous processes. Several references on counterstrain describe specific locations and other considerations of the techniques.[4–13]

ANTERIOR FOURTH CERVICAL

Findings and Position

Tender point: AC4 (Fig. 58.1)
Location: Anterior lateral mass of C4
Patient position: Supine

Procedure

1. Sit at the head of the table.
2. Flex the patient's neck to the level of the tender point (sometimes extension).

3. Side-bend and rotate the patient's neck away from the side of the tender point to the position of optimal patient comfort.
4. Hold that position for 90 seconds.
5. Slowly return the patient to neutral.

POSTERIOR FOURTH CERVICAL

Findings and Position

Tender point: PC4 (Fig. 58.2)
Location: Spinous process of C4 or in the paraspinal muscle mass at that level
Patient position: Supine

Procedure

1. Sit at the head of the table.
2. Extend, side-bend (slightly), and rotate away from the side of the tender point to the position of optimal patient comfort.
3. Hold that position for 90 seconds.
4. Slowly return the patient to neutral.

Thoracic Spine

Anterior thoracic spine tender points are located in two major areas. The first group of tender points, AT1-6, are located midline on the sternum. They can be located by palpating for tense tissue overlying the sternum. The second group is located in the abdominal wall. Most are located in the rectus abdominis muscle about 1 inch lateral to midline on the right or left.

Several of the anterior tender points are found in locations other than those described here and are best described in a book devoted to counterstrain. Posterior thoracic tender points are found on two parts of each vertebra. One location is associated with the spinous process, typically on either side. The second location is on either transverse process.

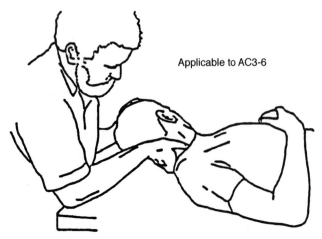

Applicable to AC3-6

Figure 58.1. Anterior fourth cervical (AC4).

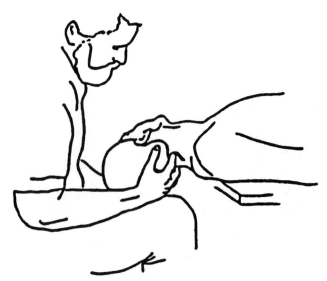

Figure 58.2. Posterior fourth cervical (PC4).

ANTERIOR FOURTH THORACIC

Findings and Position

Tender point: AT4 (Fig. 58.3)
Location: Midline of sternum about at the level of the attachment of the fourth ribs
Patient position: Supine

Procedure

1. Flex the patient and maintain the position by placing your knee under the patient's back.
2. Add a small amount of side-bending and rotation away from the side of the tender point, to fine-tune the position of optimal comfort for the patient.
3. Hold that position for 90 seconds.
4. Slowly return the patient to neutral.

POSTERIOR THIRD THORACIC

Findings and Position

Tender point: PT3 (Fig. 58.4)
Location: Spinous process or over the transverse process of T3
Patient position: Prone

Procedure

1. Stand on the same side as the tender point with your knee on the table supporting the patient's shoulder.
2. Extend, rotate away, and side-bend slightly away from the tender point to the position of optimal patient comfort.
3. Hold that position for 90 seconds.
4. Slowly return the patient to neutral.

Ribs

Anterior tender points correspond to anteriorly depressed ribs, while posterior tender points correspond to posteriorly depressed ribs. The anterior rib tender points start just below the medial end of the clavicle on the lateral edge of the sternum and move laterally. Most of the anterior rib tender points are on the ribs along the anterior axillary line. It is unusual to find tender points below the sixth rib. The posterior ribs are located on the angle of the ribs. Jones recommends maintaining rib treatment positions for 120 seconds instead of 90 seconds to allow the patient extra time to relax. This makes the treatment more effective.

ANTERIOR FOURTH RIB

Findings and Position

Tender point: AR4 (Fig. 58.5)
Location: On the fourth rib in the anterior axillary line
Patient position: Seated

Procedure

1. Instruct the patient to bring both legs onto the table on the same side as the tender point to induce side-bending and depression of the rib to that side.
2. Place one foot on the table on the side opposite the anterior tender point and support the patient's axilla on your knee to depress the anterior tender point. (If the patient cannot tolerate having both legs on the table at the same time, he or she can drape the leg on the side of the tender point over the other leg).

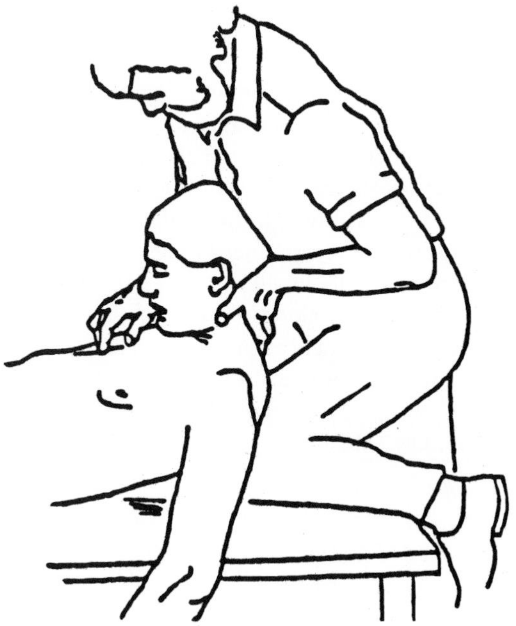

Figure 58.3. Anterior fourth thoracic (AT4).

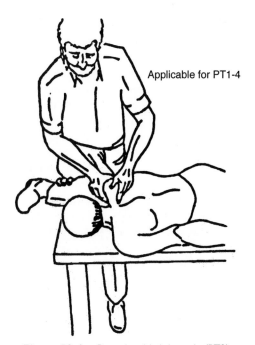

Applicable for PT1-4

Figure 58.4. Posterior third thoracic (PT3).

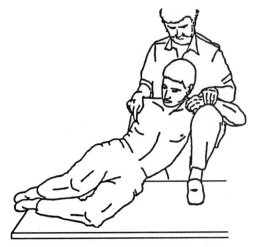

Figure 58.5.   Anterior fourth rib (AR4).

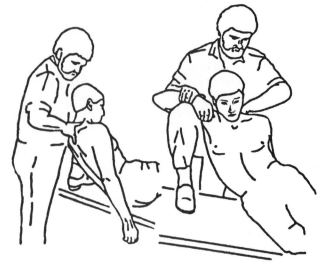

Figure 58.6.   Posterior fourth rib (PR4).

3. Encourage slight flexion with side-bending and rotation of the thoracic spine toward the tender point while instructing the patient: "Drop your arm (the one on the side of the tender point) off of the table behind you; relax and let me support your weight." Find the position of optimal patient comfort.
4. Hold that position for 90 seconds.
5. Slowly return the patient to neutral.

POSTERIOR FOURTH RIB

Findings and Position

>   Tender point: PR4 (Fig. 58.6)
>   Location: At the angle of the fourth rib
>   Patient position: Seated

Procedure

1. Instruct the patient to bring both legs onto the table on the same side as the tender point to induce side-bending and depression of the rib to that side.
2. Place one foot on the table on the side of the posterior tender point and support the patient's axilla on your knee to elevate the posterior aspect of the patient's rib. (If the patient cannot tolerate having both legs on the table at the same time, he or she can drape the leg on the side of the tender point over the other leg.)
3. Encourage slight flexion with side-bending and rotation of the thoracic spine away from the tender point while instructing the patient: "Drop your arm (the one on the side opposite the tender point) off of the table behind you; relax and let me support your weight." Find the position of optimal patient comfort.
4. Hold that position for 90 seconds.
5. Slowly return the patient to neutral.

Lumbar Spine

Anterior lumbar spine tender points are mostly located around the rim of the pelvis anteriorly. They can be found in associ-

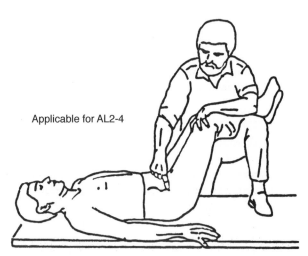

Applicable for AL2-4

Figure 58.7.   Anterior second lumbar (AL2).

ation with the anterior superior iliac spine (ASIS), anterior inferior iliac spine (AIIS), and anterior surface of the pubes. One anterior tender point is in the abdominal wall. Posterior lumbar tender points are found mostly in the same places as in the thoracic spine, although the tender points found on the tips of the transverse processes need to be approached by pressing anteromedially at about a 45° angle. Tender points for L3, L4, and L5 are located along the rim of the iliac crests and around the posterior superior iliac spines. These points are specifically identified in counterstrain books.

ANTERIOR SECOND LUMBAR

Findings and Position

>   Tender point: AL2 (Fig. 58.7)
>   Location: Medial surface of the AIIS
>   Patient position: Supine, knees and hips flexed, and markedly rotated away from the side of the tender point

Procedure

1. Stand on the side opposite the tender point and place your caudal foot up on the table.
2. Increase flexion of the patient's knees and markedly rotate the patient's knees and hips away by placing the patient's ankles on the knee of your caudal leg.
3. A small amount of side-bending away may need to be added.
4. Hold at the position of optimal comfort for 90 seconds.
5. Slowly return the patient to neutral.

POSTERIOR FIRST LUMBAR

Findings and Position

Tender point: PL1 (Fig. 58.8)
Location: Side of spinous process or over the transverse process of L4
Patient position: Prone

Procedure

1. Stand on the side opposite the tender point.
2. Lift the patient's ilium on the side of the tender point to induce extension and rotation toward the tender point.
3. Add a little side-bending away from the side of the tender point.
4. Hold at the position of optimal comfort for 90 seconds.
5. Slowly return the patient to neutral.

Pelvis

There are several anterior tender points and several posterior tender points useful for diagnosis and treatment of pelvic somatic dysfunctions. The anterior points require flexion and rotation of varying amounts and side-bending to a lesser degree. Posteriorly tender points are associated with sacral problems and muscles of the pelvis. Extension is the predominant motion associated with the posterior tender points, although three points may require some degree of flexion.

LOW ILIUM

Findings and Position

Tender point: LI (Fig. 58.9)
Location: On the superior surface of the lateral ramus of the pubic bone
Patient position: Supine

Procedure

1. Stand on the side of the tender point.
2. Grasp the patient's knee. Flex it 40–90° and slightly externally rotate it to the point of optimal patient comfort.
3. Hold at the position for 90 seconds.
4. Slowly return the patient to neutral.

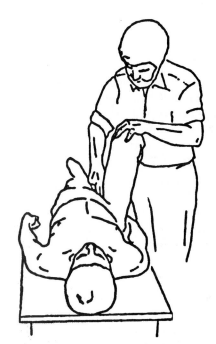

Figure 58.9. Low ilium (LI).

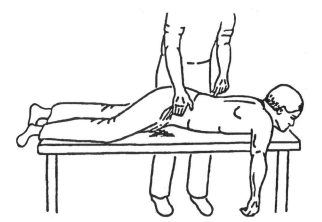

Figure 58.8. Posterior first lumbar (PL1).

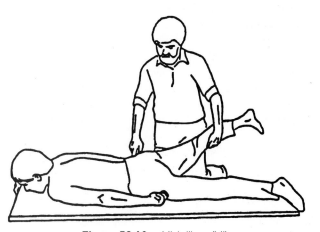

Figure 58.10. High ilium (HI).

HIGH ILIUM

Findings and Position

Tender point: HI (Fig. 58.10)
Location: 1½ inches lateral to the posterior superior iliac spine
Patient position: Prone

Procedure

1. Stand on the side of the tender point.
2. Extend and slightly abduct the patient's leg to the point of optimal patient comfort.
3. Hold that position of comfort for 90 seconds. (You may place your knee under the patient's extended thigh to help support the leg.)
4. Slowly return the patient to neutral.

CONCLUSION

The approach to healing developed by Jones addresses somatic dysfunction as revealed by tender points and is consistent with osteopathic principles. With an evaluation of the whole patient to identify tender points, and with counterstrain treatment using the position of comfort, patients can be returned to a state of health.

REFERENCES

1. Travell JG, Simons DG. *Myofascial Pain and Dysfunction: The Trigger Point Manual.* Vol. 1. Baltimore, Md: Williams & Wilkins; 1983.
2. Beal M. The central connection: somatovisceral/viscerosomatic interaction. *JAOA.* 1985;85(12):786–801.
3. Schwartz H. The use of counterstrain in an acutely ill in-hospital population. *JAOA.* 1986;86(7):433–442.
4. Jones LH. *Strain and Counterstrain.* Newark, Ohio: American Academy of Osteopathy; 1981.
5. Ramirez MA, Haman J, Worth L. Low back pain: diagnosis using six newly discovered sacral tender points and treatment with counterstrain. *JAOA.* 1989;89(7):905–913.
6. Jones LH. Spontaneous release by positioning. *The DO.* Jan 1964; 4:109–116.
7. Jones LH. Missed anterior spinal lesions. A preliminary report. *The DO.* Mar 1966;6:75–77.
8. Ask S, Ramirez AL, Schwartz H. Low back pain: treatment of forward and backward sacral torsions using counterstrain technique. *JAOA.* Mar 1991;91:255–259.
9. Groves PM, Thompson RF. Habituation: a dual-process theory. *Psychol Rev.* 1970;77(5):419–450.
10. Bailey M, Dick L: Nociceptive considerations in treating with counterstrain. *JAOA.* 1992;92(3):337–341.
11. Woolbright JL. An alternative method of teaching strain/counterstrain. *JAOA.* 1991;91(4):370, 373–376.
12. Brandt B, Jones L. Some methods of applying counterstrain. *JAOA.* May 1976;75:786–789.
13. Yaw ILK, Glover JC. *Counterstrain: A Handbook of Osteopathic Technique.* Tulsa, Okla: Y Knot Publishers; 1994.

59. Fascial–Ligamentous Release

INDIRECT APPROACH

ANTHONY G. CHILA

Key Concepts

- Relevance of osteopathic philosophy to the technique of fascial–ligamentous release

- Location and function of fascia (superficial, subserous, and deep), aponeurosis, and tendon

- Indirect techniques of functional release and strain/counterstrain as manipulative models, and how they are incorporated into the technique of fascial–ligamentous release

- Basic procedures involved in fascial–ligamentous release

- "Hysteresis" and "creep," how they allow for relaxation of tissues, and why the relaxation may be temporary

- How fascial–ligamentous release allows for sustained relaxation and resolution of chronic dysfunction via central nervous system desensitization

- Supine treatment model

- Three components of the doctor–patient relationship in making a diagnosis

- Benefits of using a fulcrum in treatment

- Positioning for the following areas: sacrum and pelvis, sacrum, iliosacrum, lower lumbar, abdominal fascia, upper lumbar, psoas muscle, liver, lower extremity (abduction phase, adduction phase, and foot), rib cage, lower and upper thorax, cervical, upper extremity (scapula, axilla, thoracic apertures, clavicle, radius, ulna, hand, and fingers), and occipitoatlantal joint basilar axes of the skull

Classic osteopathic thought has assigned importance to the role of the connective tissue system of the body in health and disease. In his writings, A.T. Still emphasized the connective tissue system in the diagnosis and treatment of dysfunction. Al-though manipulative approaches based on fascial–ligamentous considerations have enjoyed a reawakening in recent years, these tissues were manipulated by some of the oldest methods. This chapter offers a synthesis of the thoughts of various representative osteopathic authors on this subject. Other sources provide further detail about fascial–ligamentous release.[1–8]

PHILOSOPHY OF MANIPULATION

A philosophy of manipulation is central to, and not synonymous with, the practice of osteopathy. Osteopathic theory holds that when the anatomicophysiological tendency of a human being is toward a state of health, all functions of the body have an optimal performance capacity. Still made reference to a philosophy of manipulation that was based on absolute knowledge of form and function proceeding from a perfect image of the normal articulations. In Still's view, the adjustment of tissues of the body according to form, function, and image was the basis of treatment. Still indicated equally clearly that diseases could be regarded as effects occurring in regions of the body when optimal performance capacity became compromised.

FASCIA

Fascia of the human body can be described as a sheet of fibrous tissue that envelops the body beneath the skin; it also encloses muscles and groups of muscles, separating their several layers or groups. An aponeurosis is a fibrous sheet or expanded tendon that gives attachment to muscular fibers and serves as the means of origin or insertion of a flat muscle. It sometimes performs the office of a fascia for other muscles. A tendon is a fibrous cord or band that connects a muscle to bone or some other structures. It consists of fascicles of densely arranged collagenous fibers, tendon cells, and a minimum of ground substance.

In addition to extensive attachment for muscles, the fascia of the human body is provided with sensory nerve endings and is thought to be elastic as well as contractile. Fascia supports and stabilizes, helping to maintain balance. It assists in the production and control of motion and the interrelation of motion of related parts. Many of the body's fascial specializations have postural functions in which stress bands can be demonstrated. Finally, the dura mater is a special connective tissue surrounding the central nervous system. Bony anchors for this tissue exist in the skull and at the sacrum.

Fascia in the human body is described as being superficial, deep, or subserous. The superficial and deep layers are found everywhere in the body as complete ensheathments. The subserous layer lies innermost on the deep layer anywhere there is a body cavity. The deep layer of fascia is the most complicated of the three, being two-layered with intervening septa.

Clinically, it is possible to conceptualize such wrapping as being a "big bandage" of the body. Such an analogy is implied in osteopathic literature. One can find reference to the idea that the body retains form even if everything except the connective tissue framework is removed. If this is so, then it is also reasonable that form permits the consideration of motion. The continuity of this arrangement and considerations of structural–functional interrelationships make it possible to discuss biomechanical attributes of fascia in relation to manipulative treatment.

MANIPULATIVE MODELS

The study of the application of force in osteopathic manipulative treatment has led to the development of several manipulative models. In particular, those that seek to reduce the possibility of microtrauma to tissues and joints have built on considerations of fascial distribution and specialization. This is especially so in those models that require refinement of palpatory skills to appreciate subtleties of stress patterns and motion characteristics.

The corrective forces underlying these models are indirect techniques in which the dysfunctional component of resistance to motion is carried to a point of simultaneous balance and decreased tension. The focus of procedures in such models is on the quality of movement, particularly on initiation of motion. There is a reduced emphasis on the range of motion and the endpoint of motion. The correct gauging of force and velocity provides infinite variation in the delivery of technique. Control minimizes force. The effective physician should be able to vary the applications of force during a single manipulative treatment or over time for continuing manipulative management. Appropriate use of a fulcrum and leverage can refine the physician's diagnostic touch and treatment effectiveness.

The emphases peculiar to the various manipulative models can be selectively used in preparing the individual patient's manipulative prescription. Sequencing the diagnosis and treatment allows the physician to improve the quality of office records. The level of the patient's response to manipulative treatment can be better documented. Longitudinal assessment of the patient's progress is facilitated. In general, such models are hypothesized to reduce the flow of abnormal afferent impulses into the central nervous system by reprogramming for more normal function. There are several better known models of treatment.

Functional Release

In functional release, the manipulative procedure is guided by palpation at the dysfunctional segment (spinal or appendicular)

for continuous feedback information about the patient's physiologic response to motion. Operator-induced motion compares relative degrees of compliance or resistance of component parts. It does so in opposing directions. The motions introduced are those that lead to an increased sense of compliance (decreased resistance) of component parts.

Strain and Counterstrain

In strain and counterstrain, passive movement away from the area of resistance to motion is induced toward and into planes of increased motion, always searching for the position of greatest comfort. The body is folded around the tender point. A position of mild but asymptomatic strain is induced, which is thought to produce the most efficient reflex release of joint dysfunction within a prescribed period of time.

Fascial–Ligamentous Release

Elements of each of the preceding models are incorporated when using fascial–ligamentous release. The patient provides breath assistance and/or muscular assistance in the corrective procedure. The establishment of a fulcrum is sought within the physician's body to match or balance the fulcrum within the patient's body; this facilitates a continuum of reflex release from within the patient's body. Once local and regional dysfunction have been addressed by the establishment of an appropriate fulcrum, expanding leverage is achieved through torsion and traction applied to the extremities. It is the ongoing analysis of dysfunction within this continuum that makes possible the integration of a multiple manipulative approach through variable applications of force.

TREATMENT CONSIDERATIONS

In performing manipulative procedures, the body responds comprehensively to an externally applied force. From the moment of contact with the skin, avenues for the implementation of variations of force are provided by palpatory clues. In the sense of a body covering, the skin may be regarded as a mass adrenergic medium that is useful in the facilitation and amplification of proprioceptive interchange between unique persons, the patient and the physician.

Osteopathic diagnosis and treatment does not concern itself simply with the performance of a single manual procedure. The particular treatment as well as the construct of a management program often require variation in technical approaches. Visualization and synthesis of messages received through the fingers is the basis for clinical behavior. Conceptualization of anatomicophysiological dysfunction peculiar to a given patient is the key to maximizing manipulative responses. The sustained effective response following treatment is contingent on selective and controlled variation of force from an appropriate fulcrum. When these conditions are met, inherent neuroregulatory mechanisms acting in accordance with the capacity of the patient will facilitate the resolution of dysfunction.

Generally speaking, the body's connective tissues are under some degree of load and extension. The increase and subsequent reversal of extension produces a degree of tissue response less than the relatively unloaded state. This phenomenon is referred to as hysteresis. It implies the occurrence of some flow and dissipation of energy throughout the loaded tissue. Hysteresis occurs less with successive cycles of extension, indicating stabilization of response.

Connective tissues under sustained load will extend in response to the load. In biomechanical terms, this continued extension is referred to as "creep." An imposed constant load will result in "relaxation" as the extension remains constant. In either situation, the tissue displays less subsequent resistance to extension than in the original state.

Behaviors of connective tissues depend on previous mechanical history. Extension effects revert to their preextension responses. This observation may be useful in appreciating recurrence of dysfunctional complaints. The principle of timed release of tissues associated with the fascial–ligamentous release model of manipulative treatment considers these factors. The sequential and expanding progression of this approach permits the patient to tolerate central nervous system modulation. The lowering of afferent inputs is gradually facilitated. If the patient's capacity to respond is appropriate, the model seeks to ensure the significant reduction or elimination of sensitization. This view is attuned to the idea that central nervous system conditioning over time may be the vehicle for the retention as well as the reduction of dysfunctional states. The physician's role is that of a facilitator. By appropriate facilitation, the physician is able to observe the capacity for change while the patient is enabled to expand the power of the change. The standard for the successful outcome of this interchange is the motivation of the patient.

SUPINE TREATMENT

Observation and Palpation

With the patient lying in the supine position, observational and systemic palpatory findings help to establish a diagnosis related to the mechanical forces associated with body position. With the head unsupported and the legs fully extended, note effects on the cervical and lumbar lordotic curves. Compromised respiratory–circulatory effectiveness is the result of generalized fascial–ligamentous tension throughout the body. For that reason the character of respiration provides information about such tension. Observe four factors about respiration:

1. Type of respiration: diaphragmatic, costal, or mixed
2. Abdominal wall motion: visible to the level of the umbilicus; visible to the level of the symphysis pubes
3. Rate: slow, rapid; documented before and after treatment
4. Duration of cycle: inspiration and expiration equal, inspiration shorter in duration than expiration, inspiration longer in duration than expiration, dilation of the nares during respiration

Diagnostic Touch

Diagnosis is an important component in patient care. There are three central elements in an encounter between a physician and a patient:

1. The patient's ideas and beliefs of what the problem could be
2. The physician's concept of what the problem could be
3. That which the anatomicophysiological wholeness of the patient's body knows the problem to be

With respect to the last of these aspects, osteopathic manipulative treatment must allow the physiological function within to manifest its own potency rather than use blind external force and overpower its assistance. This is accomplished through the use of a fulcrum, which is the support or point of support on which a lever turns in raising or moving something.

The establishment of an appropriate fulcrum facilitates diagnostic touch. The placing of the hands and fingers on the tissues under examination is done with the idea that the fingers can mold themselves to the patient's body. The initiation of the pattern within the area of complaint is realized by a slight compression at the fulcrum points. The application of the principle of the fulcrum is as varied as the list of complaints brought to the physician's office. The use of this method is not a time-consuming process. Mechanisms already in action are used. It is necessary only to contact them and to sense them speaking for themselves. There are no techniques. The point or points are listening posts. Let the tissues tell the story; be quiet and listen. Biokinetic (dysfunctional) energies or forces are always at work in all physiological and pathological processes. With the appropriate use of diagnostic touch, the biodynamic (healing) intrinsic force within is allowed to manifest itself.

The findings noted on observation and palpation contribute to the evaluation that governs the administration of osteopathic manipulative treatment. The clinical diagnosis and the tolerance of the patient govern the application of forces in osteopathic manipulative treatment. Any sequence for treatment adopted by a physician should have two intentions:

1. The alleviation or elimination of effects of disease processes that have occurred or are occurring in the various regions of the body
2. The restoration of the patient's ability to resume command of the clinical situation

Positions for diagnostic touch of various areas of the body using the principle of fulcrum are outlined below.

Lower Body

The patient's knees are flexed, and the feet placed flat on the table. Lateralization of the feet, with inversion of the toes, helps to stabilize the pelvis.

SACRUM AND PELVIS

Mold with the patient's sacrum with one hand (Fig. 59.1). Place the fingertips of this hand at the level of the spinous

Figure 59.1. Sacrum and pelvis. One hand molds sacrum.

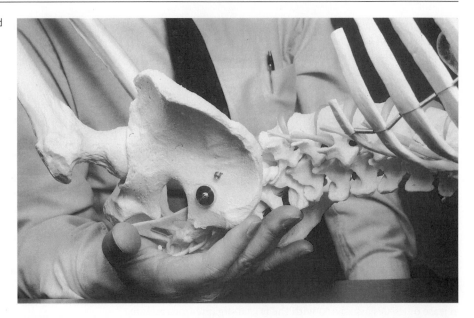

Figure 59.2. Sacrum and pelvis. Bridge anterior superior iliac spine.

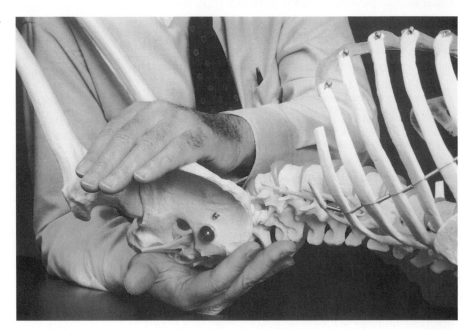

process of the fifth lumbar segment (L5). The opposite arm and hand bridge the anterior superior iliac spine (ASIS) on each side of the pelvis (Fig. 59.2). The fulcrum is established by the elbow, which is leaning on the treatment table.

SACRUM, ILIOSACRUM, LOWER LUMBAR

Mold with the patient's sacrum with one hand (Fig. 59.3). Place the opposite hand under the iliosacral articulation. The fingertips of this hand contact the spinous process of the lower lumbar segments (L3, L4, L5). Both elbows establish the fulcrum: one leaning on the treatment table (sacrum), and the other leaning on the physician's knee (iliosacrum; lower lumbar).

ABDOMINAL FASCIAL TENSION

Mold with the sacrum with one hand. The opposite hand accomplishes multiple assessments: the abdominal quadrants, costal margins and linea alba; tension of the inguinal ligaments; and shear dysfunctions at the pubic symphysis. Both elbows establish the fulcrum: one leaning on the treatment table (sacrum), and the other being the elbow of the exploring arm (abdomen).

UPPER LUMBAR, PSOAS MUSCLE

Place one hand under the upper lumbar area (Fig. 59.4). The opposite arm and hand bridge the flexed knees. The fulcrum is established by the elbow on the knee (upper lumbar area).

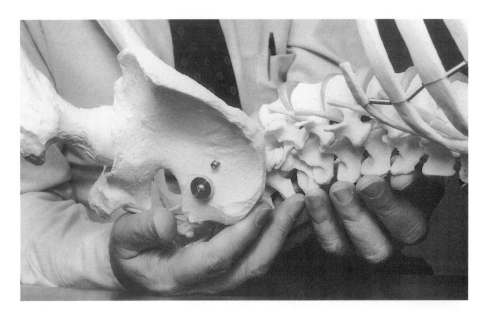

Figure 59.3. Sacrum, iliosacrum, lower lumbar.

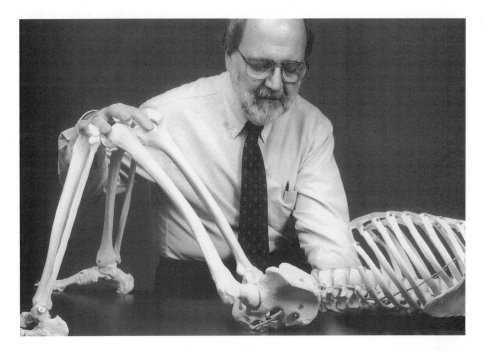

Figure 59.4. Upper lumbar, psoas muscle.

LIVER

Place one hand under the lower ribs beneath the liver. Place the opposite hand over the anterior surface of the liver. The fulcrum is established by the elbow on the knee (lower ribs).

LOWER EXTREMITY

Selectively employ torsion (rotation) and traction in two phases to release muscular, fascial, ligamentous, and articular dysfunction. The fulcrum is established by the elbows of the phys-

ician's arms in supporting the motions of the patient's foot, lower leg, and knee.

Abduction Phase (Lower Leg)

Invert the plantar surface of the foot (Fig. 59.5). Introduce torsion between the ankle and the knee. Advance the effect of torsion by slowly moving the knee across the lower abdomen, resulting in progressive abduction of the lower leg. The torsion will be felt in the lateral malleolar area, the medial compartmental area of the knee, the tensor fascia lata area, and the

Figure 59.5. Lower extremity, abduction phase.

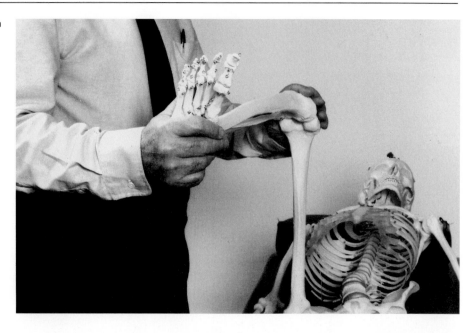

Figure 59.6. Lower extremity, adduction phase

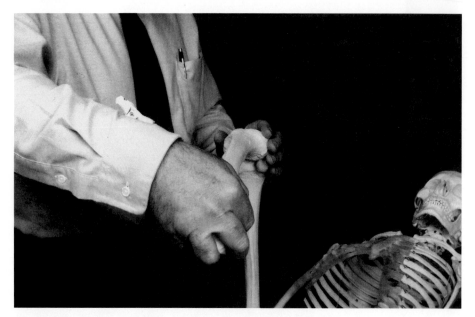

trochanter area. Upon completion of this phase, gradually extend the lower extremity and slowly return it to the tabletop.

Adduction Phase (Lower Leg)

Evert the plantar surface of the foot (Fig. 59.6). Introduce torsion between the ankle and the knee. Steadily advance the effect of torsion by slowly moving the knee away from the lower abdomen, resulting in progressive adduction of the lower leg. The torsion will be felt in the medial malleolar area, the lateral compartmental area of the knee, the medial thigh area, and the inguinal area. Upon completion of this phase, gradually extend the lower extremity and slowly return it to the tabletop.

Foot

Note tenderness to palpation in the plantar myofascial tissues. Give particular attention to such findings along the medial longitudinal arch. The contour of the foot can be analogized to the spinal complex:

The calcaneus represents the sacrum
The tarsal bones represent the lumbar region
The tarsometatarsal area represents the thoracolumbar junction
The metatarsal area represents the thoracic region
The metatarsophalangeal area represents the cervicothoracic junction
The phalangeal area represents the cervical region

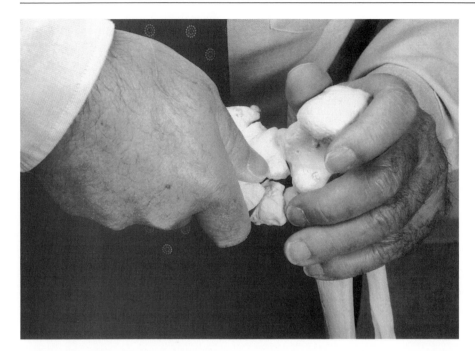

Figure 59.7. Foot.

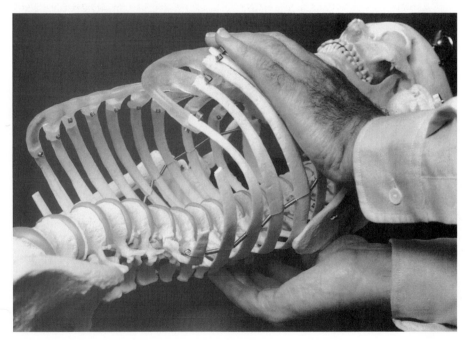

Figure 59.8. Rib cage.

Tender points can be analogized to the ipsilateral spinal level, including paraspinal tissues

Treatment is by increased plantar flexion of the foot about the point of greatest tenderness (Fig. 59.7). Perform articulatory release of the small joints of the toes in sequence, from the great toe to the small toe.

UPPER BODY

RIB CAGE

Place one hand beneath the rib cage, with the fingertips just beyond the spinous processes of the associated thoracic vertebrae (Fig. 59.8). Place the other hand on the anterior ends of the ribs. The fulcrum is established by the elbow on the knee.

LOWER THORAX

Place both hands beneath the patient at the level of the 12th thoracic segment (T12) (Fig. 59.9). This area corresponds to the level of the insertion of the trapezium muscles bilaterally. The fulcrum is established bilaterally by the elbows resting on the tabletop.

Figure 59.9.   Lower thoracic.

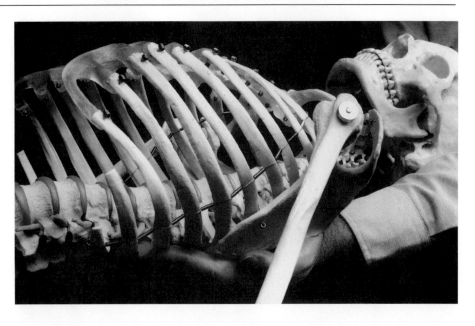

Figure 59.10.   Upper thoracic.

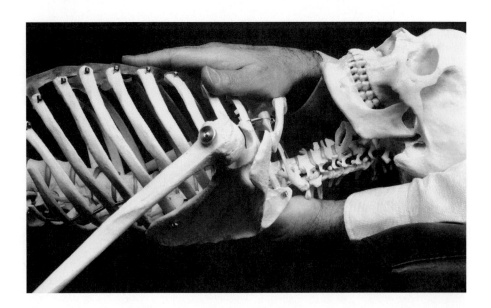

UPPER THORAX

The patient's head rests on a pillow. One hand and arm contact the upper thoracic spinous processes, with the fingers spread slightly to contact the ribs on each side (Fig. 59.10). Place the opposite hand on the sternum. The fulcrum is established by the elbow on the tabletop, beneath the patient's head.

CERVICAL AREA

Both hands bridge the entire cervical area from the base of the skull to the upper thorax (Fig. 59.11). The fulcrum is established bilaterally by the elbows and forearms resting on the tabletop.

UPPER EXTREMITY

Scapulofascial Release

Accomplish this by exploring ease and resistance to motion in several planes: cephalad, caudad, medially, laterally, clockwise, and counterclockwise (Fig. 59.12). Both hands are used to grasp the scapula completely, medially, and laterally.

Axillary Release

Accomplish this by manual decongestion of the posterior axillary tissues and the pectoral tissues.

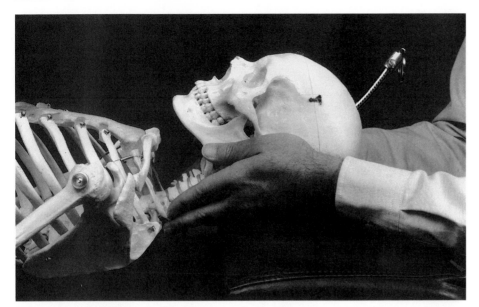

Figure 59.11. Cervical area.

Figure 59.12. Upper extremity, scapulofascial release.

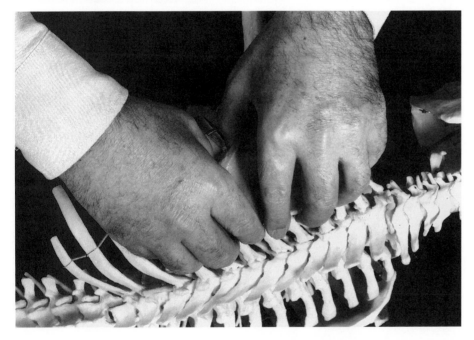

Expansion of the Inferior Thoracic Aperture

Accomplish this by supporting the elbow region with one hand and the wrist region with the other hand. For this and all subsequent procedures, the fulcrum is established by the elbows of the physician's body in support of the motions of the patient's upper extremity. Bring the extended upper extremity of the patient closer to the side of the body. Sustained supination as the upper extremity is carried toward the posterior thorax facilitates release of the thoracolumbar junction. Sustained pronation as the upper extremity is carried toward the xiphoid process facilitates musculofascial release along the cos-

tal. The cumulative effect of these forces contributes to ligamentous articular release of the elbow region.

Clavicular and Glenohumeral Release

Accomplish this by placing the extended upper extremity in a neutral position with respect to the side of the body, and abducting to the point where a continuum exists between the upper extremity and the position of the clavicle. Sustained pronation as the upper extremity is carried toward the manubrial region facilitates release of the manubrial area and the sterno-clavicular articulation. Sustained supination as the upper ex-

Figure 59.13. Upper extremity, radioulnar.

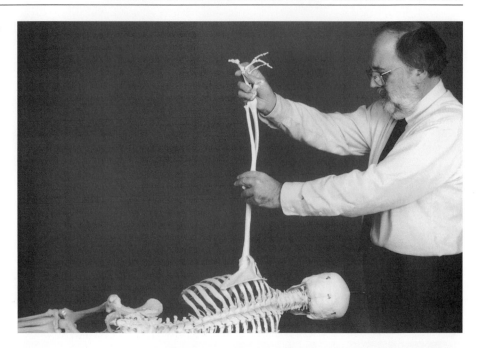

Figure 59.14. Upper extremity, wrist.

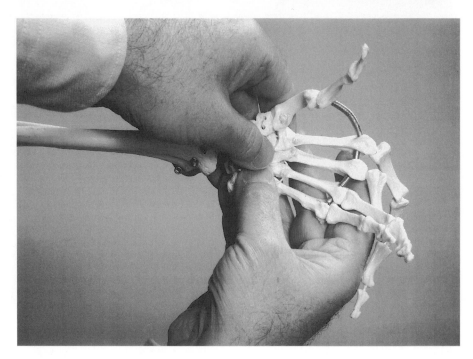

tremity is carried toward the posterior thorax facilitates release of the acromioclavicular articulation and the glenohumeral area.

Radioulnar, Wrist, Hand, and Fingers Release

Accomplish this by sustained alternating supination and pronation. This facilitates the release of fascial–ligamentous tension along the course of the interosseous membrane to the flexor retinaculum (Fig. 59.13). The addition of alternating flexion and extension of the wrist facilitates the release of articular dysfunctions of the carpal bones (Fig. 59.14). Fascial ligamentous release of the palmar area precedes articulatory release of the small joints of the fingers and thumb. The progress of the sequence is from the small finger to the thumb (Fig. 59.15).

Expansion of the Superior Thoracic Aperture

Accomplish this by grasping the deep webbing between the index finger and thumb of the patient's extended upper extremity. Sustained alternating supination and pronation facilitates the release of congestion in this area and contributes to release of the cervicothoracic junction.

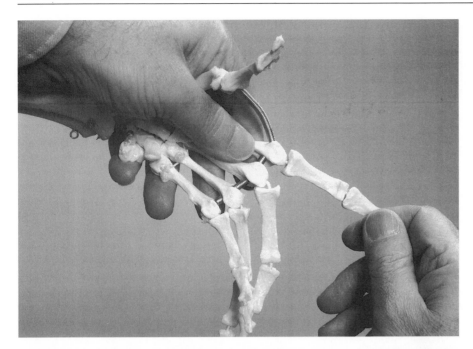

Figure 59.15. Upper extremity, hand and fingers.

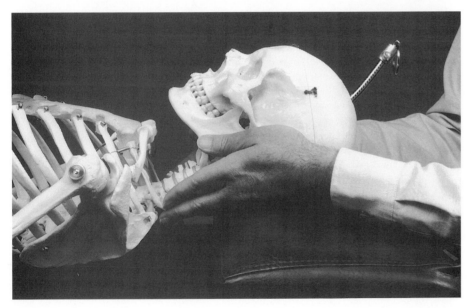

Figure 59.16. Occipitoatlantal articulation.

Cranium and Sacrum

OCCIPITOATLANTAL ARTICULATION

One hand contacts the posterior tubercle of the atlas (Fig. 59.16). The opposite hand contacts the vertex of the patient's head. The fulcrum is established by the placement of the elbow on the tabletop.

BASILAR AXES OF THE SKULL

The patient's head rests on the interlaced or overlapped fingers of the physician. The physician's thumbs extend above the ears toward the forepart of the head. The fulcrum is established by the placement of the elbows on the tabletop.

CONCLUSION

Osteopathic treatment does not concern itself simply with the performance of a single manual procedure. The particular treatment requires variation in technical approaches. Visualization and synthesis of messages received through the fingers is the basis for a keen clinical behavior. Conceptualization of anatomicophysiological dysfunction peculiar to a given patient is the key to maximizing manipulative responses. The sustained effective response following treatment is contingent upon selective and controlled variation of force from an appropriate fulcrum. When these conditions are met, inherent mechanisms acting in accordance with the capacity of the patient will lead to a state of health.

REFERENCES

1. Becker RE. Diagnostic touch—its principles and application. In: Barnes MW, ed. *Academy of Applied Osteopathy Yearbooks.* Indianapolis, Ind: American Academy of Osteopathy; Part I. 1963:32–40. Parts II and III. 1964:153–166. Part IV. 1965:165–177.

2. Becker RF. The meaning of fascia and fascial continuity. *Osteopathic Ann.* 1975;3(6):186/35.

3. Cathie AG. Fascia of the body in relation to function and manipulative therapy. *Academy of Applied Osteopathy Yearbook.* Barnes MW, ed. Indianapolis, Ind: American Academy of Osteopathy, 1960:74.

4. Greenman PE. *Principles of Manual Medicine.* Williams & Wilkins; Baltimore, Md: 1989.

5. Hubbard RP. Mechanical behavior of connective tissue. In: Greenman PE, ed. *Concepts and Mechanisms of Neuromuscular Functions.* New York, NY: Springer-Verlag; 1984:47–54.

6. Jones LH. *Strain and Counterstrain.* Colorado Springs, Colo: The American Academy of Osteopathy; 1981.

7. Lippincott HA. The osteopathic technic of Wm. G. Sutherland D.O. In: Northup TC, ed. *Academy of Applied Osteopathy Yearbook.* Indianapolis, Ind: American Academy of Osteopathy; 1949:1–24.

8. Zink JG, Lawson WB. An osteopathic structural examination and functional interpretation of the soma. *Osteopathic Ann.* 1979; 7(12):433–440.

60. Facilitated Positional Release

STANLEY SCHIOWITZ

Key Concepts

- Technique of facilitated positional release

- Possible mechanisms for effectiveness of facilitated positional release

- Benefits of using facilitated positional release

- History of facilitated positional release

- Diagnosis of any form used with this technique

- Two levels of facilitated positional release and treatment programs appropriate to each level

- Specific treatments for these tissue texture changes and intervertebral motion restrictions:
  —Cervical soft tissue
  —Cervical segmental somatic dysfunction
  —Thoracic, seated
  —Thoracic, supine
  —Thoracic, prone
  —First rib
  —Lumbar soft tissue
  —Lumbar extension somatic dysfunction
  —Lumbar flexion somatic dysfunction
  —Sacroiliac discogenic pain syndrome
  —Gluteal and hip soft tissue

Facilitated positional release (FPR) is an indirect method of treatment. The sagittal posture is modified by balancing between flexion and extension to approach the neutral position as defined by Fryette.[1] An activating force is then applied to facilitate an immediate release of tissue tension, joint motion restriction, or both. The goal of treatment is to decrease tissue hypertonicity but it can be modified to influence deep muscles involved in joint mobility.

The modality is easily applied, nontraumatic, and efficient. When properly performed, the patient reports immediate relief of point tenderness and restoration of function. If complete normalization is not achieved, it can be repeated, or other methods of treatment can be applied immediately.

THEORY OF EFFECTIVENESS

A neurophysiologic explanation that may explain the effectiveness of this method of treatment was first suggested by Korr.[2] He wrote that the behavior of the lesioned segment was initiated or maintained by an increased gain in gamma motor neuron activity of that segment. Subsequently, Bailey[3] proposed that an inappropriate high "gain-set" of the muscle spindle results in changes characteristic of somatic dysfunction.

When using facilitated positional release, the region of somatic dysfunction is first placed into its neutral position to unload the facets, which allows the area of dysfunction to respond easily and rapidly to the applied motion and force. A facilitating force (compression and/or torsion) is applied and maintained, followed by further positioning of the somatic dysfunction into all three planes of relative freedom. This method may result in an immediate effect on the muscle spindle-gamma loop, which allows the extrafusal muscle fibers to lengthen to their normal relaxed state.

Carew,[4] in discussing the feedback mechanism of the muscle spindle stretch reflex, stated that shortening the muscle *"more than intended"* caused a decrease in spindle output, lowering the afferent excitatory input to the spinal cord through the Ia fibers. This results in a decrease in gamma motor gain to the spindle, and by reflex action decreases tension of the extrafusal muscle fibers. As a result, hypertonicity of the muscle mass is reduced.

Joint motion asymmetry decreases after treatment with the facilitated positional release modality if its mobility was impaired by muscle hypertonicity. If the asymmetry of joint motion is caused by other factors, such as meniscoid or synovial impingement or degenerative arthritis, mobility is not restored; the joint remains restricted.

HISTORY

Many osteopathic physicians have contributed to the wealth of techniques available to today's practitioners. When the American School of Osteopathy was founded in 1892, Still was using techniques that he had not tried to describe to others, although he had probably taught a few to family members. He founded the college so that osteopathy would remain alive after his death, but instead of teaching techniques, he insisted that the students study anatomy and osteopathic philosophy, so that they would know how to develop their own treatments.

Because of my own busy practice and not enough time to provide time-intensive treatments, I sought methods for fast and effective relief for patients that were still soundly based on anatomical and physiological principles. Other practitioners had already used some of the techniques of facilitated positional release, which probably date back to the time of Dr. Still. In 1977 I was able to further develop and systematize the principles of this form of treatment. Over time, faculty members in many colleges of osteopathic medicine have added FPR to the curriculum.

DIAGNOSIS

Diagnosis has been described by many authors. Methods may consist of:

Skin rolling described by Mennell[5]
Testing for thoracic/lumbar rotoscoliosis in the method of Mitchell and colleagues[6]
Palpatory motion testing as described by Johnston[7]
Other direct or indirect tissue or motion testing procedures described in the literature

Diagnosis of somatic dysfunction is described in other chapters in this text. The use of FPR treatment procedures does not require special diagnostic tests unique to FPR. However, diagnosis is a prerequisite to treatment.

TREATMENT

Facilitated positional release treatments are classified as two kinds. One is directed at normalization of palpable abnormal tissue texture, and the other is modified to influence deep muscle involved in joint mobility. Sometimes it is difficult for the physician to make a clear diagnostic distinction as to which one of these is primarily involved in the somatic dysfunction.

If in doubt, the palpable tissue changes should be treated first. If motion restriction persists after this treatment, design and apply a technique to normalize the deep muscles involved in the specific joint motion restriction.

Tissue Texture Change Treatment

1. The physician places the patient (patient's musculature) in a relaxed position.
2. The anteroposterior spinal curve of the treatment area is flattened. This position places that region of the spine into its position of ease of motion, which shortens and softens associated muscle.
3. A facilitating force is applied. This may be compression, torsion, or a combination of the two.

4. The position is held for 3–4 seconds, then released.
5. Reevaluate the patient's condition.

Note: The order of the two steps, first placing the tissue into its position of ease and then applying the facilitating force, may be reversed.

Intervertebral Motion Restriction Treatment

The same procedures used for tissue changes are used to address intervertebral motion restrictions, with the additional requirement that the physician place the vertebra into a position that allows freedom of motion in all planes. In the following example, with a restriction at C3 ES_RR_R, the fourth cervical vertebra moves more easily into extension, right rotation, and right side-bending.

1. Place the third cervical vertebra into a position of extension, right lateral flexion, and right rotation with respect to the fourth cervical vertebra.
2. Apply a facilitating force: compression, torsion, or a combination.
3. Hold the position for 3–4 seconds; release should be palpable.
4. Reevaluate the patient.

CONCLUSION

Facilitated positional release is easily applied, nontraumatic, and efficient. When it is properly performed, the patient reports immediate relief of point tenderness and restoration of function. If complete normalization is not achieved, it can be repeated, or other methods of treatment can be applied immediately.

REFERENCES

1. Fryette HH. *Principles of Osteopathic Technic*. Carmel, Calif: Academy of Applied Osteopathy; 1980:19.
2. Korr IM. Proprioceptors and somatic dysfunction. *JAOA*. 1975; 75:638–650.
3. Bailey HW. Some problems in making osteopathic spinal manipulative therapy appropriate and specific. *JAOA*. 1976;75:486–499.
4. Carew TJ. The control of reflex action. In: Kandel ER, Schwartz JH, eds. *Principles of Neural Science*. 2nd ed. New York, NY: Elsevier Science Publishing Co Inc; 1985:464.
5. Mennell JM. *Back Pain: Diagnosis and Treatment Using Manipulative Techniques*. Boston, Mass: Little, Brown & Co; 1960:75.
6. Mitchell FL Jr, Moran PS, Pruzzo NA. *An Evaluation and Treatment Manual of Osteopathic Muscle Energy Procedures*. Valley Park, Mo: Mitchell, Moran & Pruzzo Assoc; 1979:229–253.
7. Johnston WL. Segmental definition, Part 1: a focal point for diagnosis of somatic dysfunction. *JAOA*. 1988;88:99–105.

61. Facilitated Positional Release Techniques

EILEEN L. DiGIOVANNA AND DENNIS J. DOWLING

Key Concepts

- **Patient positioning for facilitated positional release (FPR) techniques**
- **Physician positioning for FPR techniques**
- **Procedures for FPR techniques**

The treatment methods described in the following sections use positional release techniques.

CERVICAL

Soft Tissue Treatment

FINDINGS

Posterior cervical muscle hypertonicity (soft tissue texture abnormalities).

POSITION

Supine on the table; the patient's head is beyond the end of the table, resting on a pillow on the physician's lap (Fig. 61.1).

PROCEDURE

1. Sit at the head of the table.
2. Cup the patient's neck in the palm of your hand, with the pad of the index or long finger, acting as both monitoring finger and fulcrum, on the contralateral tense tissue to be treated. Your thumb rests on the other side of the neck.
3. Using your nonmonitoring hand on the top of the patient's head, straighten the cervical lordosis by slightly forward bending the neck.
4. Using the same hand, apply a compressive facilitating force to the neck, through the patient's head.
5. Maintaining the compressive force, introduce extension to the neck to the level of the monitoring finger. (If the tissues being treated are anterior rather than posterior, introduce flexion rather than extension.) This should cause a palpable softening of the tissue being treated.
6. Add side-bending and rotation, usually toward the side of the tense tissues, to the point that the tissues continue to soften.
7. Hold the tissue in this relaxed position for 3 seconds, and then return the neck slowly to a neutral position.
8. Reevaluate the tissue being treated.

Note: If tissue changes are found anteriorly, forward bending is usually required. Some muscles have a contralateral side-bending, a rotatory component, or both. Those muscles must be placed in their individual shortened positions determined by palpation and tissue response. Careful localization of the component motions of forward/backward bending, side-bending/rotation, and compression to the area of tissue texture change will result in faster and more efficient results.

Cervical Segmental Somatic Dysfunction

FINDINGS

C3 ES_LR_L.

POSITION

Supine, with the patient's head beyond the end of the table, resting on a pillow on the physician's lap (Fig. 61.2).

PROCEDURE

1. Sit at the head of the table.
2. Cup the patient's neck in the palm of your right hand, with the pad of the index or long finger on the left articular pillar of C3.
3. Using your left hand on the top of the patient's head, straighten the cervical lordosis by forward bending the neck to the monitoring finger on C3.
4. Add a compressive force through your left hand, directed through the head to the neck.
5. Extend the neck through the level of C3 while maintaining the compression.
6. Side-bend C3 to the left by adding a translatory force through your monitoring finger, pulling C3 to the right.
7. Add a slight rotation of the head and neck through the level of C3. This places C3 in all three planes of freedom of motion.
8. Hold this position for 3–4 seconds, then slowly return the neck to neutral.
9. Reevaluate C3 motion.

Note: If the diagnosis is flexion rather than extension (C3 FS_LR_L), step 4 is replaced by adding flexion through the level of C3 rather than adding extension. Similarly, if the diagnosis is one of right side-bending and right rotation, the appropriate adjustments should be made.

When applying this procedure to dysfunctions of the suboccipital area, or to the atlantooccipital articulation, localize the flexion/extension using a nodding motion to the skull and

Figure 61.1. Soft tissue technique.

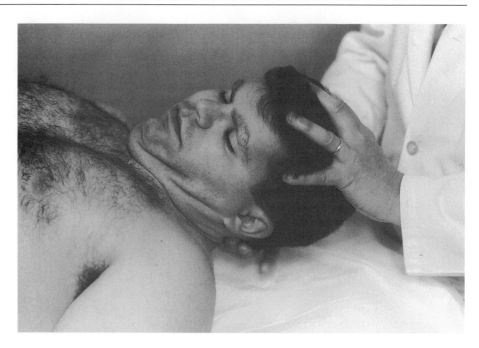

Figure 61.2. Typical cervical C3 ES$_L$R$_L$ technique.

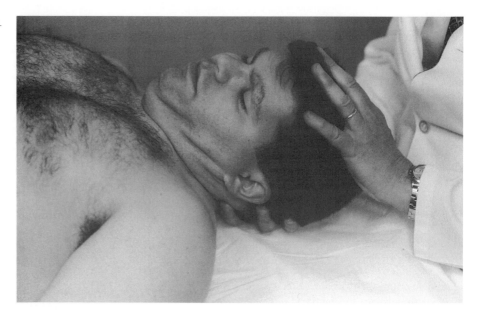

not total flexion/extension of the cervical spine. Also, the atlantooccipital joint lateral flexes in one direction and rotates in the opposite direction.

THORACIC

Thoracic Spine, Seated

FINDINGS

T6 FS$_L$R$_L$.

POSITION

Seated on the edge of the table (Fig. 61.3).

PROCEDURE

1. Stand behind and to the left of the patient.
2. Ask the patient to sit up as straight as possible and push his or her chest out toward the wall in front. This will straighten the thoracic kyphosis.
3. Monitor the transverse process of T6 with your right index or long finger.
4. Place your left axilla over the patient's left shoulder, with your forearm in front of the patient and your left hand in the patient's right axilla or grasping the patient's right shoulder.
5. Add a compressive force through your left axilla (toward the table), causing left side-bending down through the level of the monitoring finger at T6.

6. Add flexion to the level of T6 by pulling forward on the patient's shoulders while maintaining the side-bending.
7. Rotate the thoracic spine to the left down through the level of T6 by pushing or pulling the right shoulder back.
8. Hold this position for 3–4 seconds, and then slowly return the patient to a neutral position.
9. Reevaluate.

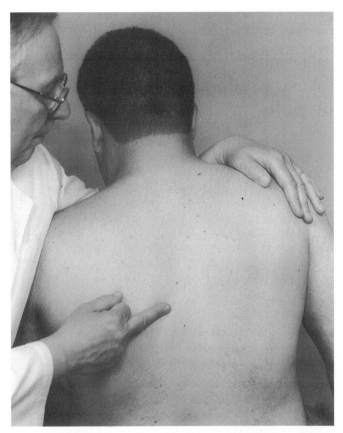

Figure 61.3. Thoracic spine T6 FS$_L$R$_L$ technique, seated.

Note: If the diagnosis is extension rather than flexion (T6 ES$_L$R$_L$), replace step 5 by creating extension through the level of T6, pulling back on the shoulders. Similarly, if the diagnosis is side-bending and rotation is to the right, make appropriate adjustments. If the somatic dysfunction is neutral, do not induce flexion or extension, and adjust so that side-bending and rotation are achieved in the appropriate directions.

Thoracic Spine, Prone

FINDINGS

T8 ES$_R$R$_R$.

POSITION

Prone, with pillows beneath the abdomen and head. The patient's arms are at the sides (Fig. 61.4).

PROCEDURE

1. Stand at the left side of the patient.
2. Palpate the T8 posterior transverse process (right) with the fingers of your left hand.
3. With your other hand, grasp the patient's right shoulder. The patient's entire shoulder should be held with your fingers directed cephalad.
4. Pull the patient's shoulder medially toward the spine (this flattens the spine in the anteroposterior plane), then toward the patient's feet (this compressive force creates right side-bending).
5. Extend the spine through the level of T8 by maintaining traction on the shoulder as you step further down the table, until motion can be palpated at the level of your monitoring fingers.
6. Stand up straighter, pulling the patient's shoulder posteriorly, creating right rotation down through the level of T8.

Figure 61.4. Thoracic spine T8 ES$_R$R$_R$ technique, prone.

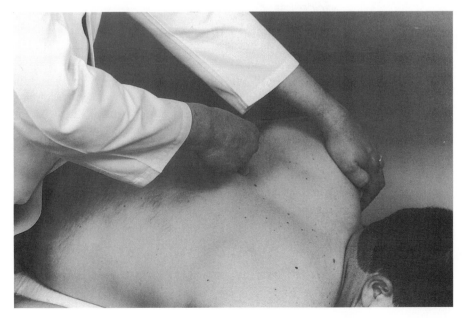

7. Hold this position for 3–4 seconds, and then slowly return to the neutral position.
8. Reevaluate T8 motion.

Note: If the diagnosis is flexion, rather than extension (T8 ES_RR_R), facilitated positional release is more easily accomplished with the patient in the seated position. However, it can be accomplished in the prone patient if you direct the facilitating force medially and toward the patient's feet as described above, without introducing truncal extension. Flexion is introduced by having the patient take and hold a deep breath until completion of the treatment (3–4 seconds).

FIRST RIB

Soft Tissue Treatment

FINDINGS

First rib elevated on left.

POSITION

Supine (Fig. 61.5).

PROCEDURE

1. Stand to the left of the patient, facing toward the head of the table.
2. Place the monitoring finger of your left hand over the posterior portion of the left first rib. The finger should contact the most tense tissue in this area.
3. With your right hand, grasp the patient's left elbow and flex and abduct the upper arm to the position in which the tissues soften maximally.
4. Create a compressive force through the left elbow, directed toward the monitoring finger.
5. Press the volar surface of your left forearm against the dorsal surface of your patient's left forearm, causing an internal rotation of the humerus.
6. Hold this position for 3–4 seconds.
7. Maintaining the compressive force and the internal rotation, adduct the upper arm and swing it down through a curving motion into a neutral position.
8. Reevaluate the motion of the first rib.

LUMBAR

Soft Tissue Treatment

FINDINGS

Hypertonic right paravertebral lumbar muscles.

POSITION

Prone, close to the right edge of the table, with a sufficient number of pillows beneath the abdomen to cause flattening of the lumbar lordosis (Fig. 61.6).

PROCEDURE

1. Stand at the right side of the table.
2. Monitor the tissue tension with a finger of the right hand.
3. Place your left knee on the table next to the patient's pelvis.
4. With your left hand, grasp the patient's left knee.
5. Pull the patient's legs toward you to induce right lumbar side-bending until you feel motion and/or softening at your monitoring finger.
6. Remove your knee from the table.
7. Cross the patient's legs by placing the left ankle over the right.
8. With your left hand, reach around the left thigh from behind it, so that your palm is on the anterior and medial left thigh.
9. Lift it slightly toward you, so that the dorsal surface of your left hand is against the back of the right thigh.
10. Do this by standing upright with your arm straight, using postural rather than arm muscles to protect your own muscles. (When you pull the left leg toward the dysfunctional side, you are adducting it and inducing external rotation, at the same time extending the lumbar region and inducing a relative rotation of the upper trunk toward the right.)
11. Hold this position for 3–4 seconds, and then slowly return the patient to the initial position.
12. Reevaluate the soft tissue.

Extension Somatic Dysfunction

FINDINGS

L3 ES_LR_L.

POSITION

Prone, close to the left edge of the table, with a sufficient number of pillows beneath the abdomen to cause flattening of the lumbar lordosis (Fig. 61.7).

PROCEDURE

1. Stand at the left side, facing the head of the table.
2. Monitor the posterior transverse process (left) with a finger of the right hand.
3. Place a small pillow between the patient's left thigh and the table. This will provide a fulcrum for the treatment while protecting the thigh from pressure from the table's edge.
4. Use your left hand to abduct the right leg, creating left lumbar side-bending, and stand between the table and the patient's abducted leg.
5. Grasp the patient's left lower leg or ankle and internally rotate the leg until you feel motion at the monitoring finger (this creates rotation).
6. Move the patient's abducted leg toward the floor (hip flexion) until you palpate motion at the monitoring finger. With the thigh pillow acting as a fulcrum, this induces lumbar extension.
7. Hold this position until there is a sudden release of the somatic

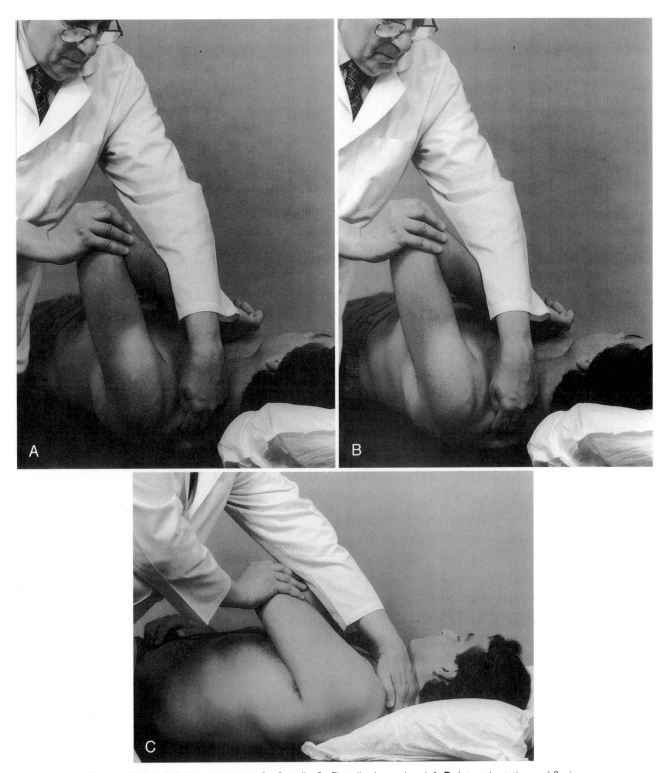

Figure 61.5. Soft tissue treatment for first rib. **A.** First rib elevated on left. **B.** Internal rotation and flexion introduced. **C.** Adduction and circumduction added.

Figure 61.6. Lumbar soft tissue technique.

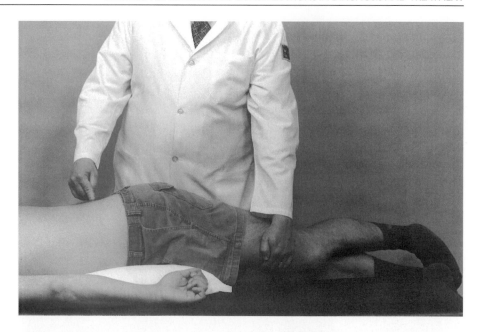

Figure 61.7. Lumbar extended L3 ES_LR_L technique.

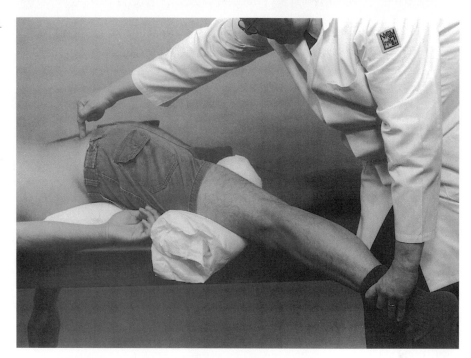

dysfunction (usually in about 3–4 seconds), and then slowly return the patient to a neutral position.

8. Reevaluate L3 motion.

Flexion Somatic Dysfunction

FINDINGS

L4 FS_LR_L.

POSITION

Prone, close to the left edge of the table, with a sufficient number of pillows beneath the abdomen to cause flattening of the lumbar lordosis (Fig. 61.8).

PROCEDURE

1. Sit on a rolling stool at the left side of table, with thighs parallel to the table, at the level of the patient's pelvis, facing the patient's head.
2. Monitor the posterior transverse process (left) with a finger of your right hand.
3. Flex the left leg at the knee and hip, with the lower leg coming to rest between your knees, to the point where you feel motion at your monitoring finger.
4. Use your left hand to grasp the left knee, adducting it toward and under the edge of the table until you feel motion at the monitoring finger. You will hold and support the knee during the rest of the technique. (This induces left rotation, as internal

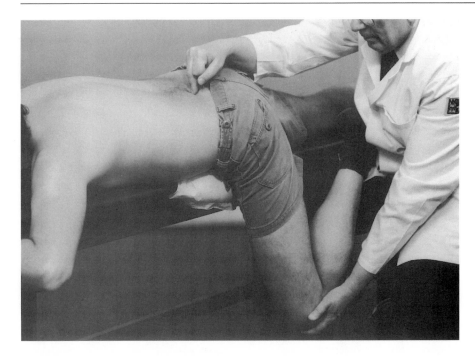

Figure 61.8. Lumbar flexed L4 FS$_L$R$_L$ technique.

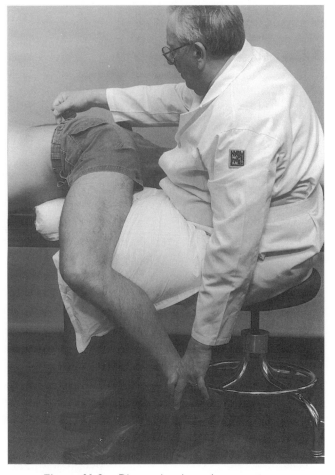

Figure 61.9. Discogenic pain syndrome treatment.

rotation of the leg causes pelvic rotation to the contralateral side, and relative lumbar rotation toward the posterior transverse process.)

5. Abduct the lower leg by shifting your own body and rotating your outermost shoulder anterior and toward the table, until you feel motion at your monitoring finger (this induces left side-bending).

6. Hold this position until there is a sudden release of the somatic dysfunction (usually in about 3–4 seconds), and then slowly return the patient to a neutral position.

7. Reevaluate L4 motion.

Discogenic Pain Syndrome Treatment

FINDINGS

Left lumbar disk bulge with left radiculitis.

POSITION

Prone, close to the left edge of the table, with a sufficient number of pillows beneath the abdomen to cause flattening of the lumbar lordosis (Fig. 61.9).

PROCEDURE

1. Sit on a rolling stool at the left side of table, with thighs parallel to the table, at the level of the patient's pelvis, facing the patient's head.

2. Use a finger of your right hand to monitor the area of disc bulge.

3. With your left hand, flex the patient's left hip and knee.

4. Place the upper leg across your anterior thighs, moving to create abduction and external rotation.

5. Localize motion to the involved segment by moving the patient's leg in a cephalad direction. It is easiest to do this by rolling the stool closer to the head of the table.

Figure 61.10. Motion restriction treatment for sacroiliac joint.

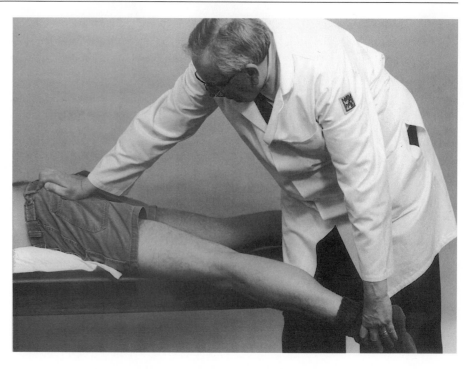

6. Raise your left knee by lifting your heel off the floor. Push the lateral part of your knee into the popliteal fossa of the patient's knee. Create a traction force that can be modified (as you further raise and move your knee laterally) until you palpate motion at your monitoring finger. Your knee is now at the medial surface of the popliteal fossa and the medial surface of the knee and acts as a fulcrum for the rest of the technique.

7. Using your left hand, push the left lower leg toward the floor until you palpate motion at your monitoring finger. You will note a slight amount of tension at the monitored location.

8. Maintain this position until a release is noted, generally in 3–4 seconds, and then slowly return the patient to a neutral position.

9. Reevaluate the lumbar region.

SACROILIAC JOINT

Motion Restriction Treatment

FINDINGS

Left sacroiliac motion restriction.

POSITION

Prone, with a sufficient number of pillows under the abdomen to flatten the lumbosacral junction (Fig. 61.10).

PROCEDURE

1. Stand to the left side of the table facing the head of the table.

2. Monitor the left sacroiliac (SI) joint with a finger of your right hand and place your right hypothenar eminence on the left inferior lateral angle (ILA) of the sacrum.

3. Using your left hand, abduct the left leg until the thigh is over the edge of the table.

4. Place a small pillow between the patient's left thigh and the table. This will provide a fulcrum for the treatment while protecting the thigh from pressure from the table's edge.

5. Using your left hand, press the left leg down toward the floor. Simultaneously press your hypothenar eminence down on the ILA to bend the base of the sacrum backward on the left. Apply an upward (cephalad) force to slide the sacral portion of the SI joint along the ilial portion.

6. Ask the patient to take a deep breath and hold it 3–4 seconds.

7. As the patient exhales, return the leg to a neutral position and release your pressure from the ILA.

8. Reevaluate motion of the SI joint.

GLUTEAL AND HIP

Soft Tissue Treatment

FINDINGS

Right hip muscles or gluteal musculature hypertonicity.

POSITION

Prone, close to the edge of the table, with a sufficient number of pillows under the abdomen to flatten the lumbar lordosis.

PROCEDURE

1. Sit on a rolling stool at the right side of table, with thighs parallel to the table, at the level of the patient's pelvis, facing the patient's head.

2. Monitor the soft tissue to be treated with a finger of your left hand.

3. Using your right hand, slightly abduct the patient's right leg, flexing the hip and knee until you feel motion at your monitoring finger. The patient's lower leg will come between your knees, and the ankle will rest on the your lap. Insert a small pillow between the patient's inner thigh and the table edge for comfort and to provide a fulcrum.

4. Push the patient's flexed knee into adduction beneath the table until you palpate motion at the monitored location.

5. Induce internal rotation of the thigh with your hand on the knee. This can be further accentuated by swiveling your own body and right shoulder forward, causing adduction of the lower leg.

6. Place your right palm and fingers so that they encompass the femoral condyles, upper tibia, and patella.

7. Direct a compressive force along the long axis of the femur, upward to the hip and gluteal region.

8. Maintain this position until a release is noted, generally in 3–4 seconds, then slowly return the patient to a neutral position.

9. Reevaluate the soft tissue.

CONCLUSION

Although primarily axial procedures have been described here, it is possible to use facilitated positional release for other regions of articular and soft tissue dysfunction. Rather than describe these in detail, it is left to the reader to apply these principles to the individual region.

62. Integrated Neuromusculoskeletal Release and Myofascial Release

AN INTRODUCTION TO DIAGNOSIS AND TREATMENT

ROBERT C. WARD

Key Concepts

- The meaning of the term "myofascial release" (MFR)

- The meaning of the term "integrated neuromusculoskeletal release" (INR)

- A theoretical basis for using MFR and INR concepts

- Some of the science that supports INR/MFR ideas

- How the neuromusculoskeletal system responds to mechanical forces

- How integrated peripheral and central neuroreflexive activities influence myofascial functions

- General INR and MFR applications

Integrated neuromuscular and myofascial release approaches and treatment processes are used to diagnose and modify altered reflex and mechanical patterns anywhere in the body. Applying this form of treatment depends on one's ability to palpate and interactively respond to shifting reflex and mechanical changes as they occur. Recognition of both local and general patterns are important elements in the process.

The key to clinical success is the development of the MAN acronym, a clear idea of the interdependent *m*echanical, *a*natomical, and *n*eurological relationships. As Viidik writes,

The structure of most biological materials (tissues) is to some extent influenced or modified by the in vivo generated mechanical forces which act upon them under physiologic . . . (and pathophysiologic) . . . conditions. The mechanical properties of all materials, living tissues as well as "dead" . . . are dependent on their structural configurations from the molecular level to the macroscopic.[1]

Mechanical and behavioral patterns affect neuroreflexive and neurovascular activities, and vice versa. Patterns arise from a variety of factors such as genetics; age; behavioral characteristics such as elation and depression; and lifestyle factors such as good health, effects of accidents, nutrition, drug use, and physical fitness. For neuromusculoskeletally oriented osteopathic physicians, the challenge is to understand the clinical effects of these interdependent factors.

Integrated neuromusculoskeletal release and myofascial release ideas have been a part of American osteopathic thinking from early in the profession's history. Until recently, they were commonly referred to as isometric–isotonic, fascial release, and functional techniques. Oral traditions over four or five generations suggest that A.T. Still himself used reflex-based stretch and relaxation procedures without referring to them as such. Whether this is actually true has not been documented. Unfortunately, his descriptions lack detail, but Still's writing gives heavy emphasis to both anatomy and mechanics.[2]

This author has been using combinations of isometric–isotonic, functional, and myofascial release concepts since the early 1950s. At that time, osteopathic medical students attending the Kansas City (Missouri) College of Osteopathy and Surgery were introduced to these procedures by Wilbur Cole and Esther Smoot. Dr. Cole taught preclinical osteopathic manipulative treatment (OMT) skills, neuroanatomy, and clinical neurology. He was also a neuroanatomy researcher and published two early papers dealing with motor end plates on striated muscles.[3,4] Dr. Smoot, with a full-time practice in the Osteopathic Hospital of Kansas City, said she learned her methods from several osteopathic pioneers but she never specifically described her experiences or teachers.

Along with Still and Smoot, William Neidner, who practiced in both Massachusetts and Michigan, was an early proponent of "fascial twist" maneuvers but wrote little about his work (F.L. Mitchell, personal communication, 1970; R. Hruby, personal communication, 1989). No doubt there were others.

DEFINITION

INR and MFR techniques are "combined procedures"[5] designed to stretch and reflexly release patterned soft tissue and joint-related restrictions. Both direct and indirect methods[5] are used interactively. (See *osteopathic manipulative treatment* in the Glossary.)

GOAL

Because neuromusculoskeletal movement patterns are determined by every aspect of biology and behavior, a fundamental treatment goal is to interactively assess and modify maladaptive patterns within the ability of the patient to adapt. This process is more effective when the operator uses simultaneously applied, two-handed palpation, much like playing a two-handed musical instrument.

By searching out tight and loose "end feels,"[5] patterned soft tissue and joint-related movements are assessed and treated simultaneously. As both static[5] and dynamic barriers[5] are encountered, they are released by mechanically loading areas of tightness using compression, traction, and twisting maneuvers. (Static barrier is defined as any soft tissue or bony impediment to passively induced motion by an operator. Dynamic barrier is defined as any soft tissue or bony impediment to inherent tissue motion.) By integrating patient-assisted release-enhancing maneuvers, the treatment process is accelerated. These reflexly modulated releases occur as varieties of direct and indirect maneuvers stress and strain the neuromusculoskeletal network from the skin to deep spinal joints. A working knowledge of musculoskeletal mechanics is essential (see Chapters 43–50). Additional discussion of neutral and nonneutral spinal mechanics including vertebral dysfunctions can be found in Greenman's text.[6(pp.65–74)]

FUNCTIONAL ANATOMY AND PROBLEM SOLVING

Osteopathic physicians are advised to learn functional relationships among groups of muscles, fascias, and ligaments from the floor to the top of the head. The time will be well spent.

The Tight–Loose Concept

Looking for three-dimensionally related tightness and looseness is essential to the process. For example, patterned three-dimensional changes can be sensed as large or small areas of myofascial and bony positional asymmetry that are tight and loose relative to one another. Tight–loose patterns always interactively involve superficial and deep, as well as large and small muscle groups, as well as the bony skeleton.

Examples include:

One shoulder commonly tight and the other loose
Tight left hip and sacroiliac mechanics, loose right
Tight left cervicothoracic junction, loose right
Tight right sternocleidomastoid, loose right scalenes
Tight right sternocleidomastoid, tight left scalenes

MECHANICS AND FORCES

Patterns can be mechanically understood by noting the effects of multidirectional forces on both local and distant joints and soft tissues. The following important definitions are from the American Academy of Orthopedic Surgeons.[7]

Motion segment: A vertebra, its disk, and associated ligaments.
Stress: Force normalized over the area on which it acts. Normal stress is perpendicular to the cross-section, and sheer stress is parallel to it.
Strain: Change in shape as a result of stress.
Stiffness: The ratio of a load to the deformation (strain) it causes (the tight concept).
Compliance: The inverse of stiffness (the loose concept).
Creep: The continued deformation (increasing strain) of a viscoelastic material with time under constant load. (Traction, compression, and twist create creep.)
Viscoelastic material: Any material that deforms in relation to the rate of loading and deformation. Mechanically related biological materials exhibit varying densities (viscosities). For example, tendons deform at different rates than muscle fibers and ligaments. Different viscosities create different time-dependent responses to applied forces, that is, extension (traction), compression, and twist.

Applied to clinical palpation, these time-dependent responses arise because both normal and angular stressing occur simultaneously; that is, they cannot be separated into component parts because of the inherent complexity.

All tissues are mechanically responsive and exhibit stress–strain responses. The body's mechanical system is composed of water-absorbing collagen and ground substances that include glycoproteins, glycosaminoglycans, and other low-molecular-weight substances. It is on this background that mechanical forces exert their effects.[1(p.258)] Mechanical principles, therefore, interdependently affect the body neurologically and anatomically, governed by the mechanical principles found in Wolff's law, Hooke's law, and Newton's third law. These laws may be interpreted as follows: Wolff's law is biologic systems deform in relation to lines of force placed upon them. This includes both soft and hard tissues.[8] Hooke's law is the strain (deformation) placed on an elastic body is in proportion to the stress (force) placed upon it.[8] Newton's third law is when two bodies interact, the force exerted by the first on the second is equal in magnitude and opposite in direction to the force exerted by the second on the first.[8]

Passive and Active Patterns

Mechanical patterns are both passive and active.

Passive external factors such as body conformation are easily recognizable. Passive internal factors, such as asymmetrical structural supports, muscle inhibition, and bony asymmetries, are less evident.

Active patterns, that is, those arising from neurally mediated activities, are superimposed on the passive system. Examples include:

Sitting
Standing
Walking
Sleeping
Working
Sporting activities

Figures 62.1–62.3 demonstrate a 1987 soft tissue dissection done by Frank George in the anatomy laboratories of Michigan State University. From this work, we learned that fascia and muscle are anatomically inseparable. Earlier authors like Cathie[9] and Becker[10] suggested that fascias move independently. George's work suggests that fascias probably move in response to complex muscle activities acting on not only bones and joints but also ligaments, tendons, and fascias.

This view is reinforced by other research highlighting the importance of fascia in maintaining general proprioception. Since proprioception is ultimately controlled by combined neural and muscular elements, both small and large inputs are needed to maintain postural balance. After joint and muscle spindle activity is accounted for, 75% of remaining proprioception occurs in fascial sheaths.[11] Such responses were actually demonstrated neurophysiologically in the 1960s by Earl[12] and Wilson[13] in their work dealing with muscles under stretch.

Palpation

Because palpation is the key to successful use of any manipulative method, one must spend considerable time developing these abilities. Some untrained observers occasionally suggest that the ability to palpate is inborn and difficult to teach. This may be true in a few instances, but all health care professionals are regularly challenged to develop palpation skills when performing physical examinations and myriad medical and surgical procedures.

Palpatory and manipulative treatment skills improve with practice. In an almost literal sense, skilled palpating hands learn

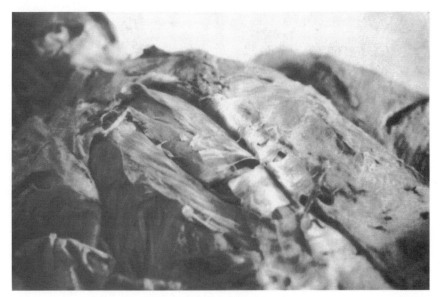

Figure 62.1. Fascia in gross dissection. (From Basmajian JV, Nyberg R. *Rational Manual Therapies.* Baltimore, Md: Williams & Wilkins; 1993:230.)

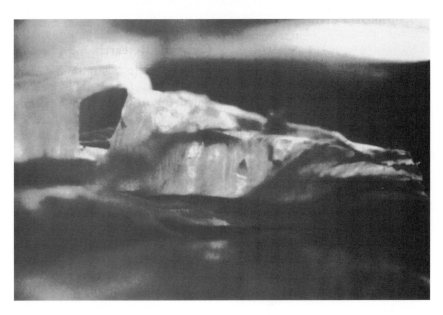

Figure 62.2. Closer view of fascia in gross dissection. (From Basmajian JV, Nyberg R. *Rational Manual Therapies.* Baltimore, Md: Williams & Wilkins; 1993:230.)

Figure 62.3. Sharp dissection difficulties resulting from muscle and fascia being inseparable. (From Basmajian JV, Nyberg R. *Rational Manual Therapies*. Baltimore, Md: Williams & Wilkins; 1993:231.)

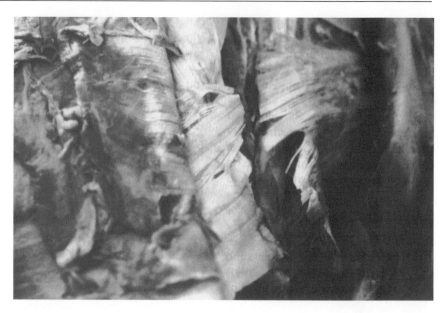

to see anatomical and mechanical detail, much like a blind person senses the environment. As improvements appear, expectations change as appreciation for new-found subtleties emerges and previously puzzling diagnostic and treatment details become less demanding.

Music and sports are good analogies. One can learn to appreciate and perform at many levels. Low-level and high-level skills are common to each. Admiring, being intimidated by, or even critical of another's skills and individual interpretations does not suggest we can or cannot perform similarly.

Sensing of Positional and Movement-Related Asymmetries

One key to success is identifying tethering effects that create and maintain asymmetries. Tightness suggests tethering, while looseness suggests joint and/or soft tissue laxity with or without neural inhibition. Sometimes tethering relates directly to changes in coupled vertebral motions and altered joint play, that is, the motion segment is altered. Knowing the difference between neutral and nonneutral vertebral mechanics is essential[7] (see Chapters 45, 47, and 48). Both local soft tissue and neuroreflexive–neurocirculatory changes, such as viscerosomatic reflex changes, are common contributors to tethering.

Tethering arises from many sources:

The spine, with altered coupled vertebral motions from any source
The synovial joints, with their influences on joint play
Altered soft tissue mechanics (Note: All tissues and motions are inherently asymmetrical.)
Asymmetric neural inputs arising from:
Multiple levels of the central nervous system, including cranial nerves, brainstem, midbrain, thalamus, and cortex
Limbic system and reticular activating system
Spinal cord itself

Peripheral nervous system in general
Viscerosomatic reflexes
Somatosomatic reflexes
Neurohumoral activities of all kinds
Lowered reflex, such as facilitated thresholds from specific sites, for example, sites of disease, injury, and degeneration
Biobehavioral and sociocultural factors

Awareness of one's personal perceptions and biases in relation to the patient's beliefs and biases is an essential exercise for both clinician and patient. One must always remember that help is commonly sought when environmental stressors trigger overwhelming psychoemotional events. Medicalization and encouragement of dependent behaviors, including requests for manipulative treatments, during these calls for help risk interfering with short-term recovery and long-term coping.

Monitoring Inherent Tissue Motion

Inherent tissue motions are palpably evident, asymmetrically patterned, neuroreflexive activities in the soft tissues. They move constantly but at variable rates. Palpation that focuses on these motions should identify asymmetrical tightness and looseness. Movements are easier in some directions, less so in others. Asymmetrically perceived end feels are commonly referred to as direct and indirect barriers. Myofascially, tightness–looseness identifies direct and indirect movement barriers that are both independent of and linked to joint mechanics.

TREATMENT SKILLS

Treatment skills improve as one learns to apply well-directed forces interactively against direct and indirect barriers, such as tightness and looseness. A common example is when restrictions involving one side of the pelvis frequently affect the:

Opposite lower limb
Lower costal cage

Opposite shoulder
Cervical spine
Cranial base

Links between Research and Treatment

In some cases, it is likely that successful treatments link as yet unclear intrinsic body movements of both the patient and operator at some level. How this occurs is unknown, but it is likely that both conscious and subconscious brain-mediated factors are at play. Experienced practitioners and patients often comment that, "This treatment went especially well," or "Things did not go well today." Some research indirectly suggests how this occurs.

Electroencephalography (EEG) was used as a means for studying silent communication patterns between two individuals. In 1989, Grinberg-Zylerbaum and Ramos reported on their studies of nontouching, silent communication between two or more individuals. Partners who reported feelings of being blended with one another altered their EEG patterns to the point of being virtually identical.[14] This author and others have repeatedly identified similar blending effects during myofascial release and craniosacral treatment encounters, in both the classroom and clinical settings. Whether these experiences are in any way similar to the Grinberg-Zylerbaum and Ramos work has not been investigated.

Other hypotheses and experiments point out subtle cranial bone movement changes that may be factors. In one instance, Norton hypothesized a model for quantitatively assessing pressure variations in soft tissues of both the subject and examiner. His study is completely theoretical, however, and lacks experimental data.[15] Adams et al., on the other hand, made parietal bone movement measurements in cats that suggest the presence of neurally generated wave forms that create 1- to 2-μm movements in cranial sutures.[16] Individual abilities to palpate such subtle changes have been carried out in a number of experiments.[17,18]

Tight–Loose Concept

An exercise illustrates the tight–loose concept. With the patient lying supine, the operator grasps the patient's wrists. By slowly and deliberately raising the upper limb toward full overhead extension, one gets a sense of shifting, three-dimensional tightness or looseness that begins at the wrists and eventually involves the whole body. By carefully attending to both the quality and amplitude of the passively induced operator forces, clearly defined mechanically asymmetrical sites of tightness and looseness become apparent.

As each limb is moved separately and together, tight–loose asymmetries vary considerably, and their end feels are different. Some are abrupt, almost like hitting a wall. Others are soft, like either falling into or fluffing a pillow. Importantly, these mechanically and neurally mediated tight–loose shifts rarely follow classic anatomical patterns. With practice, variable tensions and loads are readily sensed from the hands and wrists distally into the lumbodorsal fascia and pelvis.

Pain at Loose Sites

Painful sensations are common at loose sites, particularly in chronic cases. Typically, there is little muscle spasm or tightening; muscles are weak and inhibited. Some practitioners refer to these sites as hypermobile, implying that ligamentous laxity and joint instability are the fundamental problems. Neither hypothesis has been proven scientifically. An alternative idea concludes that loose, painful muscles are weak and inhibited over large, often ill-defined, areas, including vertebral mechanics.

From a clinical perspective, whole body effects are the rule rather than an exception. Loosened sites are often vulnerable to injury under relatively trivial circumstances. Repeated ankle and lumbosacral sprains, as well as neck and shoulder problems arising from altered lumbopelvic and lower limb mechanics, are common examples.

CLINICAL ASSESSMENT

Tightness and looseness should be evaluated from a patterned three-dimensional context that includes:

Skeletal and soft tissue configurations
Upper and lower motor neuron influences
Effects of mechanical modeling and remodeling of bones, joints, and soft tissues
Effects of general skeletal factors
Injury history
Effects of repetitive daily activities
Psychoemotional states
Limiting psychosocial factors

Locating direct and indirect barriers is a useful method for understanding tightness, looseness, and tethering effects. *Tightness* suggests tethering and direct barriers (see the Glossary). Whether tethers should be removed requires careful assessment.

Tight muscles are not always sources of pain and altered neuromusculoskeletal functioning. One form of tethering is *acute muscle spasm*, which is almost always self-limited. *True spasticity*, on the other hand, suggests upper motor neuron involvement, such as centrally mediated neural tethering.

Scar tissue implies the presence of passive, mechanical tethering that may actually stabilize an otherwise unstable site.

Acute localized muscle tension generally implies peripheral neural involvement with tethering associated with any of many musculoskeletal and behavioral factors.

Looseness generally occurs in association with indirect barriers. Muscle weakness and ligamentous and joint laxity are commonly associated.

THREE-DIMENSIONAL PATTERNS

Three-dimensional vertical, horizontal, and wraparound patterns are the rule and can be identified with some practice. Looking for three-dimensionally related areas of tightness and looseness is the key. For example, in the prone position, right hip extension should create left lumbar, latissimus dorsi, and shoulder movements, and vice versa. Well-conditioned individuals will extend the hip with minimum use of contralateral back extensors and shoulder groups. The pattern often changes when the head is sequentially changed from left to center to right.

A common prone wraparound pattern is as follows:

Tight posterior left hip, sacroiliac joint, lumbar erector spinae, and lower costal cage
Loose posteriorly on the right
Tight anterior and right lateral costal cage
Tight right upper anterior costal cage
Tight left thoracic inlet, posteriorly
Tight left craniocervical attachments, including jaw and facial mechanics

When the diagnosis is clarified, a specific treatment and exercise prescription can be developed.

TREATMENT GOALS

The general goal is to release tightness and restore three-dimensionally patterned functional symmetry to the extent possible without aggravating hypermobility. As forces against direct and indirect barriers are sequentially applied, an experienced operator can efficiently treat the whole body in a reasonably short time.

Direct and Indirect Techniques

Simultaneous direct and indirect two-handed techniques are used. With practice, direct and indirect maneuvers can be applied simultaneously, one hand doing direct release while the other does indirect.

Release Maneuvers and Integrated Neuromuscular Release

Starting from the skin and working inward, varieties of traction, twist, shear, and compression are applied three-dimensionally while inherent tissue and joint motions are simultaneously monitored for shifting tightness and looseness.

Direct Myofascial Release

Direct myofascial release maneuvers strain (deform) areas of tightness. Releases are triggered by holding firmly against the soft tissue resistance, that is, direct myofascial barriers. By making tightness tighter, releases occur rather quickly, often in multiple directions at the same time. When this happens, the tissues often feel as though they are quivering in multiple directions at the same time. The art lies in being able to palpate both single and multiple releases to follow the changing patterns. Unwinding techniques depend on these principles.

Indirect Myofascial Release

For every tightness, there is three-dimensionally related looseness. Commonly, the looseness is in exactly the opposite direction from the tightness. This concept is somewhat similar to the functional indirect methods described in Chapters 57 and 59. Experienced operators locate these interdependent relationships quite readily, finding it easier to follow gently behind releases as they occur in sequence.

Integrated Neuromuscular Release

Patient assistance with release-enhancing maneuvers helps speed the treatment process. A few are listed below:

1. Breath holding during phases of inhalation and exhalation changes both intrathoracic and intraabdominal pressures, which, in turn, alter costodiaphragmatic, shoulder girdle, and lumbopelvic asymmetries.
2. Prone and supine simulated swimming maneuvers use the arms and legs as the operator loads the system.
3. Right, center, and leftward head turning in any body position is often helpful.
4. Isometric limb and neck movements against the table or chair create postisometric muscle relaxations at various sites. For example, stubborn lumbopelvic problems often persist until proximal thoracolumbar and iliopsoas attachments are stressed by alternately forcing the knees, that is, hip flexors, into the table. This can be easily done both prone and supine. Efficiency increases as one learns the contributing roles of specific muscle groups.
5. For reasons as yet unclear, varieties of patient-invoked cranial nerve activities, such as eye, tongue, jaw, and oropharyngeal movements are also helpful. We assume that progressive cranial nerve activities create central and peripherally mediated neural distractions. We also think the maneuvers are similar to the Jendrassik maneuver used to enhance the patellar jerk reflex by isometrically separating the flexed fingers against each other.

POSTTREATMENT EVALUATION

Posttreatment evaluation is essential for a number of reasons:

1. To know whether appropriate and helpful changes have occurred
2. To help the patient understand what to expect
3. To help design an appropriate, individualized exercise program
4. To help develop an appropriate pharmacologic program, should it be necessary
5. To identify and accurately record changes for the medical record

POSTTREATMENT DISCOMFORT

Patients commonly experience a temporary worsening of discomfort following the first treatment or two. The possibility should be identified for them in advance. The phenomenon seems similar to postexercise muscle soreness, although no research has been done on it. Usually the experience occurs only once, but patients with immunologic disorders such as lupus erythematosus and fibromyalgia can experience repeated flare-ups, so one must be cautious.

ROLE OF EXERCISE IN MAINTAINING CHANGES

It is essential that a simple, time-efficient exercise program be worked out. The program should stretch areas of tightness without aggravating pain or instability. Restoring adequate proprioception by using one-leg standing activities is essential for long-term success. Looseness, or areas of inhibited individual and patterned muscle activities, requires strengthening and toning. For example, identification of weak, inhibited muscle groups, such as altered gluteus maximus and hamstring firing sequences, helps develop a clear focus for rehabilitation. In this example, back pain patients frequently fail to fire one or both gluteus maximus muscles during prone straight leg hip extensions.

CONCLUSION

This chapter introduces a few basic myofascial and integrated neuromusculoskeletal release concepts. Keys to diagnostic and treatment successes lie in the ability to sort out interdependent mechanical, anatomical, and neurologic problems that contribute to alternated three-dimensional movement patterns. Hallmarks for identifying these patterns lie in the ability to assess and treat interactive areas of tightness, looseness, and tethering. A well-designed, individualized, easy-to-follow exercise program is essential for long-term success. Chapters 16 and 76 in this text and Greenman[6(pp.449–523)] present a few useful techniques.

REFERENCES

1. Viidik A. Interdependence between structure and function in collagenous tissues. In: Viidik A, Vuust J, eds. *Biology of Collagen.* New York, NY: Academic Press; 1987:257.
2. Still AT. *Philosophy of Osteopathy.* Kirksville, Mo: Journal Printing Co; 1899.
3. Cole WV. Some histological aspects of the motor end plate. *J Osteop.* 51:7:18–20:44.
4. Cole WV. A gold chloride method for motor end plates. *Stain Technology.* 1946;21:23–25.
5. The Glossary Review Committee of the Educational Council on Osteopathic Principles. In: Allen TW, ed. Glossary of osteopathic terminology. *AOA Yearbook and Directory of Osteopathic Physicians.* Chicago, Ill: American Osteopathic Association; 1996.
6. Greenman PE. *Principles of Manual Medicine.* 2nd ed. Baltimore, Md: Williams & Wilkins; 1996:65–73, 449–523.
7. Woo S-L, An K-N, Arnoczky SP, Wayne JS, Fithian DC, Myers DS. Anatomy, biology, and biomechanics of tendon, ligament, and rotation. In: Simon SR, ed. *Orthopedic Basic Science.* American Academy of Orthopedic Surgeons; 1994:45–88.
8. *The New Lexicon Webster's Dictionary of the English Language.* New York, NY: Lexicon Publications; 1988.
9. Cathie AG. The fascia of the body in relation to function and manipulative therapy. In: *The American Academy of Osteopathy Yearbook.* Indianapolis, Ind: American Academy of Osteopathy; 1974:81–87.
10. Becker RF. The meaning of fascial and fascial continuity. *Osteopath Ann.* 1975;3:8–32.
11. Bonica JJ. *The Management of Pain.* 2nd ed. Philadelphia, Pa: Lea & Febiger; 1990:66.
12. Earl E. The dual sensory role of muscle spindles. *Phys Ther J.* 1965; 45:4.
13. Wilson VJ. Inhibition in the central nervous system. *Sci Am.* 1966; 5:102–108.
14. Grinberg-Zylerbaum J, Ramos J. Interpersonal communication: an experimental approach. *Int J Neurosci.* 1989;36:41–52.
15. Norton JN. A tissue pressure model for the palpatory perception of the cranial rhythmic impulse. *JAOA.* 1991;10:975–994.
16. Adams TA, Heisey RC, Briner BA. Parietal bone mobility in the anesthetized cat. *JAOA.* 1992;5:599–622.
17. Upledger JE. Reproducibility of craniosacral examination findings: a statistical analysis. *JAOA.* 1977;6:746.
18. Upledger JE, Karni Z. Mechanoelectric patterns during craniosacral osteopathic diagnosis and treatment. *JAOA.* 1978;11:782–791.

63. Integrated Neuromusculoskeletal Techniques for Specific Areas

ROBERT C. WARD

Key Concepts

- **To gain an understanding of and apply general myofascial release (MFR) and integrated neuromuscular release (INR) techniques**

There are many ways to approach neuromusculoskeletal problems manually. Many techniques look similar but are explained differently using the different terminology of the individual practitioner. This chapter is no exception. For the sake of practicality, descriptions are limited to a few methods that are applied with relative ease and have stood the test of time. Those familiar with muscle energy terminology and diagnosis will find that they can record and monitor INR/MFR processes by superimposing functional anatomy descriptors on bony positional changes such as unilateral left sacral flexion (also called sacral shear), left on right sacral torsion, and L4 nonneutral ERS-left.

LUMBOSACRAL SPINE AND PELVIS

The goal is to three-dimensionally balance lumbopelvic mechanics, keeping in mind that the costal cage and lower limbs play major roles in the patterning process.

Thoracolumbar Release (Figs. 63.1–63.8)

OBJECTIVE

To balance the thoracolumbar junction three-dimensionally in relation to both lumbopelvic and thoracocostal mechanics.

PROCEDURE

1. The patient's feet should be off the end of the table to minimize lower limb stresses in relation to the pelvis and low back (Figs. 63.1–63.3).
2. The patient's head should be turned to the most comfortable side. Holding it in the midline, as many wish to do, often obscures tight–loose effects at the thoracolumbar junction.
3. The hands and arms are comfortably placed either over the sides of the table, or on the table beside the hips and thighs.
4. Stand beside the patient's hip, facing cephalad (Fig. 63.3).
5. Place your hands at the thoracolumbar junction, covering

posteroinferior rib–trunk rotator–diaphragmatic sites (Figs. 63.4–63.7).

6. Place hands widely open with the thumbs pointed cephalad along either side of the spinous processes while the remainder of each hand spreads over the posteroinferior costodiaphragmatic areas.
7. Identify superficial and deep tightness and looseness patterns three-dimensionally.
8. Firmly separate the thumbs across the midline as the left hand creates clockwise and the right hand creates counterclockwise traction. The hands should not slide on the skin.
9. As the skin is stretched between the thumbs, it will initially blanch. As traction and twist are maintained, tissues begin to relax both reflexly and mechanically in accordance with principles discussed previously. After initial blanching, areas receiving major stressing commonly become reddened and warmer. This is the so-called blush phenomenon (Fig. 63.8).
10. Releases occur in three dimensions with sustained traction and twist, and they can be single or multiple. Unwinding phenomena often occur as shifting patterns of tightness and looseness alter three-dimensional relationships.
11. Treatment is complete when repetitive stressing of the site in question no longer creates asymmetrical tightening and loosening. With practice, one learns to feel deeply into the areas surrounding facet joints. Symmetrical segmental movements to passive stressing suggest that the procedure is complete.

Combined Sacroiliac, Sacral Base, and Lumbopelvic Releases (Figs. 63.9–63.16)

The goal is to establish symmetrical sacral nutation and counternutation movements in relation to the innominates, lumbar spine, and lower limbs. Nutation is anterior nodding (flexion) of the sacral base in relation to the lumbar lordosis; counternutation is posterior nodding (extension) of the sacral base in relation to the lumbar lordosis.

DIAGNOSIS

With practice, sacral torsions, flexions (also called sacral shears), and innominate positions become readily apparent.

PROCEDURE

1. The feet should be off the end of the table to minimize lower limb stresses in relation to the pelvis and low back.
2. The head should be turned to the most comfortable side.

Figure 63.1. Position for thoracolumbar release: head to most comfortable side with arms off table.

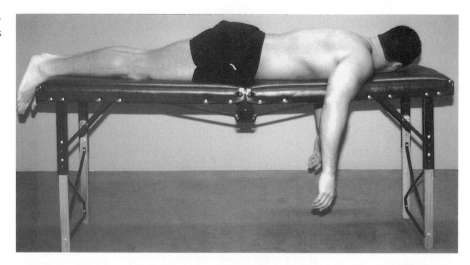

Figure 63.2. Position for thoracolumbar release: head to most comfortable side with arms on table.

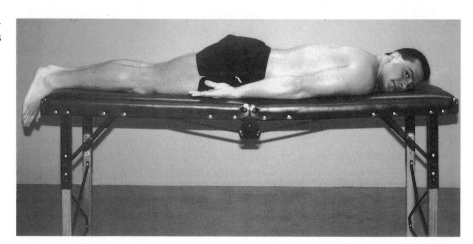

Figure 63.3. Position for thoracolumbar release: head comfortable, feet and arms off table.

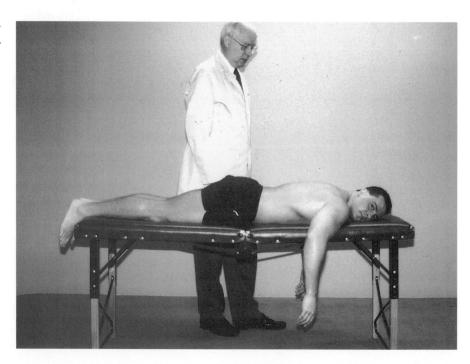

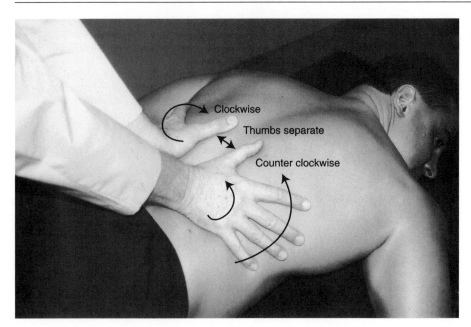

Figure 63.4. Operator stands beside patient's hip, with head to side.

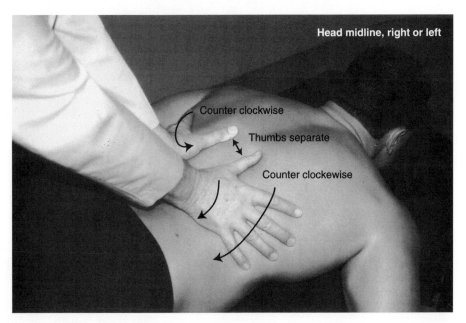

Figure 63.5. Hands placed at thoracolumbar junction, with head in midline.

Holding it in the midline, as many wish to do, often obscures tight–loose effects in the thoracolumbar regions.

3. The hands and arms are comfortably placed either over the sides of the table, or on the table beside the hips and thighs.

4. Stand at the patient's left shoulder facing caudad.

5. Place your proximal left hand longitudinally over the thoracolumbar junction, with the long finger covering the upper lumbar spinous processes. For best results, place the metatarsophalangeal joint of the long finger precisely at the T12-L1 junction (Fig. 63.9).

6. The distal right hand covers the sacrum between the two innominates with the index finger overlying the right sacroiliac joint and inferior lateral angle while the ring finger covers the left. The long finger will fall naturally over the sacral spines and sacral hiatus (Fig. 63.10).

7. Evaluate patterns of tightness and looseness:
   Proximally and distally by distracting the sacrum and lumbar spine in the long axis of the spine (Fig. 63.12)
   Circumferentially by transversely translating each hand in opposite directions across the lumbopelvic system (Figs. 63.13–63.16)

Figure 63.6. Head midline.

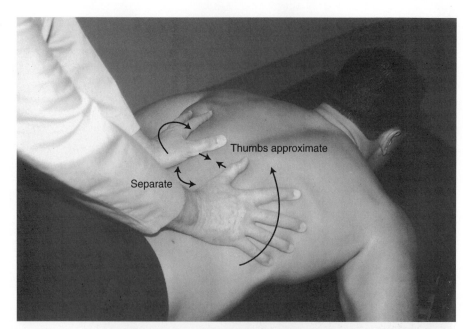

Figure 63.7. Head right.

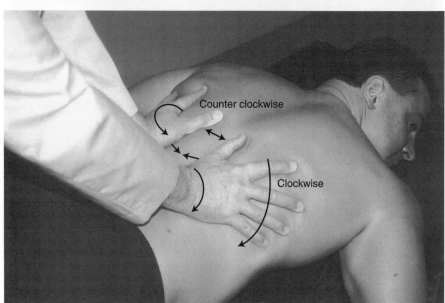

Figure 63.8. Blush sign. After blanching, areas receiving major stressing commonly become reddened and warmer.

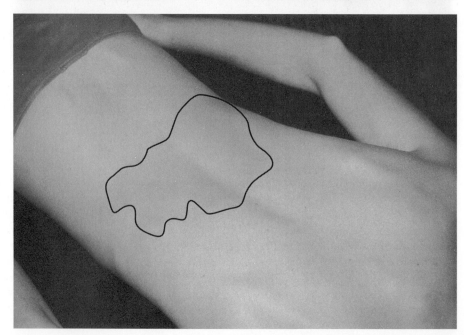

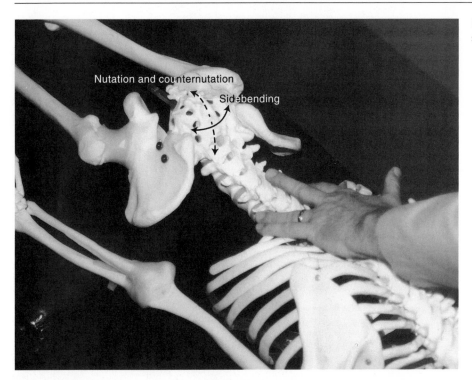

Figure 63.9. Position for combined sacroiliac, sacral base, and lumbopelvic releases.

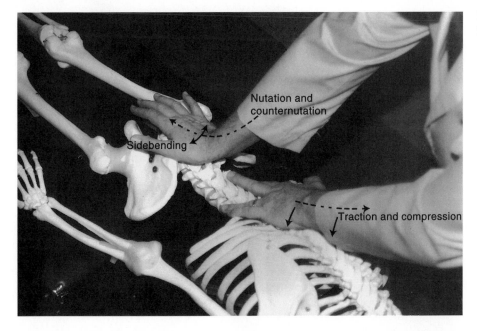

Figure 63.10. Position for combined sacro-iliac, sacral base, and lumbopelvic releases.

8. Induce lumbosacral distraction by assertively moving the left hand proximally and forcing the right hand distally up and over the natural curve of the sacrum (Fig. 63.12). Importantly, one must honor the sacral curve. Some are in a more or less straight-line relationship with the back, while others are acutely angled, demonstrating more or less perpendicular relationships with the spine and pelvis.

9. Both heavy-handed and, in some cases, light-handed loads mechanically induce reflexly controlled inherent tissue and sacral movements.

10. As loading develops, varieties of three-dimensional tightness and looseness become apparent. Sacral torsions, flexions (shears), innominate changes, and sacroiliac joint factors, such as close and loose packing, are diagnosed.

11. By using combinations of distraction and compression (Figs. 63.11 and 63.12) while monitoring inherent tissue movements, sacroiliac positional and movement changes commonly give way and become more symmetric. Sacral nutation and counternutation are more symmetric.

12. As the lumbopelvic complex drifts right and left, change the

Figure 63.11.

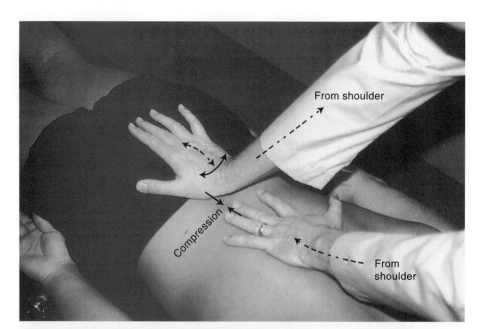

Figure 63.12.

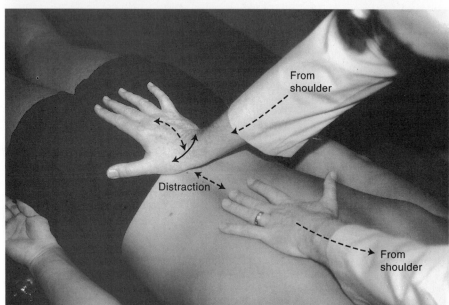

Figure 63.13.

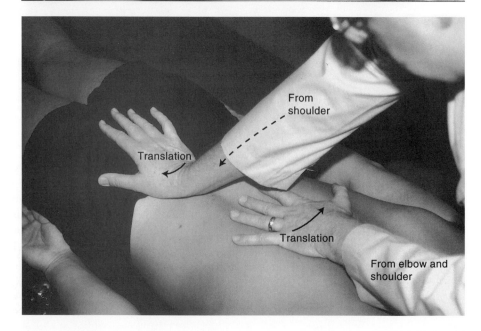

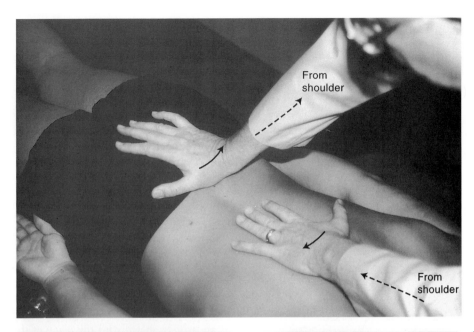

Figure 63.14.

From
shoulder

From
shoulder

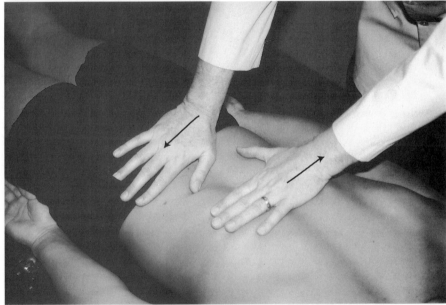

Figure 63.15.

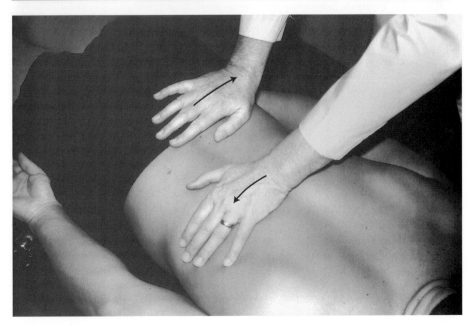

Figure 63.16.

hands 90° to induce further movement in a crosswise fashion (Figs. 63.15 and 63.16).

13. Treatment is complete when sacroiliac joint and general lumbar movements are as symmetrical as can reasonably be expected.

Focused Prone Sacral Base Release: Two-handed Technique (Figs. 63.17 and 63.18)

The goal is to balance the sacral base in relation to L4-L5 mechanics, the iliolumbar ligament, and innominate asymmetries.

DIAGNOSIS

See the section on sacroiliac release.

PROCEDURE

1. The feet should be off the end of the table to minimize lower limb stresses in relation to the pelvis and low back.
2. The head should be turned to the most comfortable side.
3. The hands and arms are comfortably placed either over the sides of the table or on the table beside the hips and thighs.
4. If right-handed, stand at the patient's left shoulder, facing caudad.
5. Place one hand horizontally, or transverse to the sacrum. It contacts the posterior superior iliac spine and medial gluteus maximus attachments bilaterally.
6. Place the other hand over the bottom hand and along the long axis of the sacrum between the two innominates, with the index finger overlying one sacroiliac joint and inferior lateral angle as the ring finger covers the other. By using this hand placement, the long finger falls naturally over the sacral spines and sacral hiatus.

7. Evaluate patterns of tightness and looseness by rocking the sacrum in multiple planes:

    Proximally and distally by distracting the sacrum and lumbar spine at the sacral base along the long axis of the spine;
    Circumferentially by transversely translating each hand in opposite directions across the lumbopelvic system.

8. Using a rocking motion, induce lumbosacral joint distraction by assertively separating the top hand toward the feet (Fig. 63.18). It is also helpful to passively induce sacral base nutation and counternutation during the distractive maneuver. Be sure to create the motion by moving the hand distally as well as up and over the natural curve of the sacrum. One must honor the sacral base curve and its functional geometry. Some are in a more or less straight-line relationship with the spine, while others are acutely angled with the plane of the sacral base virtually perpendicular to the flow.

9. Both light- and heavy-handed forces can be used, depending on your skill. A key to success is having the ability to monitor, induce, and enhance the subtle but powerful inherent tissue and cranially related sacral movements.

10. As differential loads are applied, both static and dynamic, that is, inherent tissue movement-related, tightness and looseness become apparent.

11. Give special attention to the sacral base in relation to L4/L5 mechanics, iliolumbar ligament anomalies, degenerative changes, and nonneutral vertebral mechanics.

12. Treatment is complete when L5 and sacral base mechanics and inherent motions are as symmetrical as can reasonably be expected.

Figure 63.17.

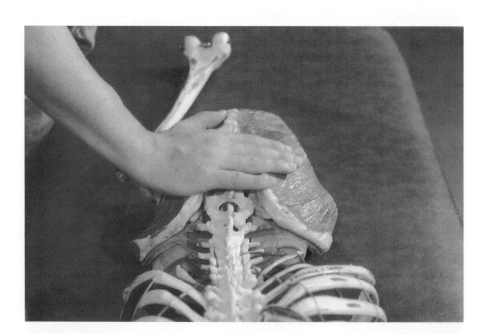

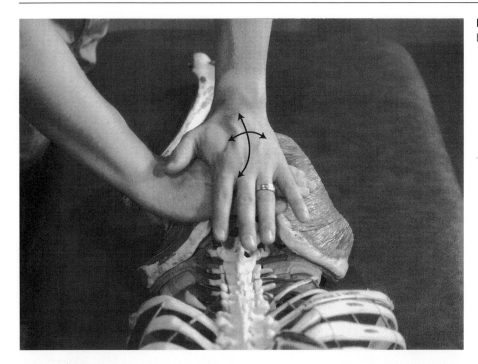

Figure 63.18. Using a rocking motion, induce lumbosacral joint distraction.

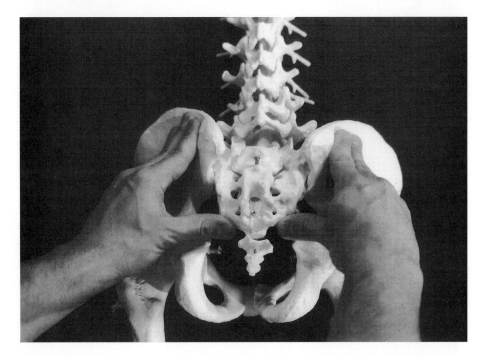

Figure 63.19. Inferior sacral surface.

Sacrotuberous Ligament Release: Prone

The goal is to balance sacrotuberous–sacrospinous ligament factors affecting lumbopelvic, lower limb, and pelvic diaphragm mechanics.

PROCEDURE

1. The patient's feet should be off the end of the table to minimize lower limb stresses in relation to the pelvis and lower limb.

2. The patient's head should be turned to the most comfortable side.

3. The hands and arms are comfortably placed either over the sides of the table, or on the table beside the hips and thighs.

4. Stand beside the patient's left knee, facing cephalad.

5. Identify inferior and posterior sacral surfaces near the apex (Figs. 63.19 and 63.20).

6. Identify the medial surface of the sacral tuberosity where the sacrotuberous–sacrospinous system attaches (Figs. 63.21 and 63.22).

7. With a firm grasp on each buttock, place the thumbs half way between the sacral apex and each sacral tuberosity, pressing firmly anteriorly and superiorly toward the symphysis pubis (Figs. 63.23 and 63.24). Identify tightness and looseness three-dimensionally.
8. Simultaneously press anteriorly and superiorly while turning the thumbs systematically against either tightness or looseness, as if turning a steering wheel. Tightness and looseness in both the ligaments and pelvic diaphragm become quickly apparent (Fig. 63.25).
9. Using each hand interactively, sequentially induce forces against tightness and looseness, stressing both direct and indirect barriers until releases occur.
10. Treatment is complete when sacrotuberous–pelvic diaphragm mechanics and inherent motions are as symmetrical as can reasonably be expected.

Supine Releases

Even after prone maneuvers have been successful, lumbopelvic mechanics are commonly asymmetrical when assessed with the patient supine. As a result, one should always be ready to release

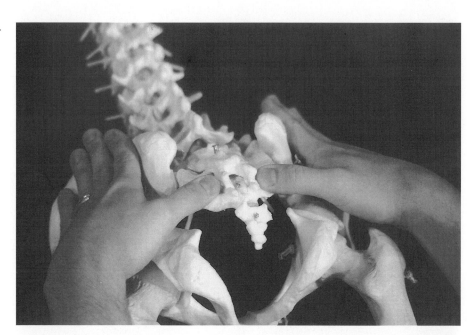

Figure 63.20. Posterior sacral surface.

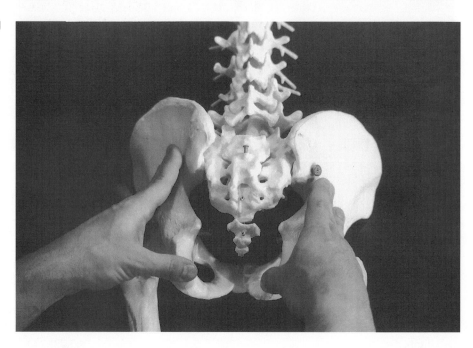

Figure 63.21. Medial surface of the sacral tuberosity.

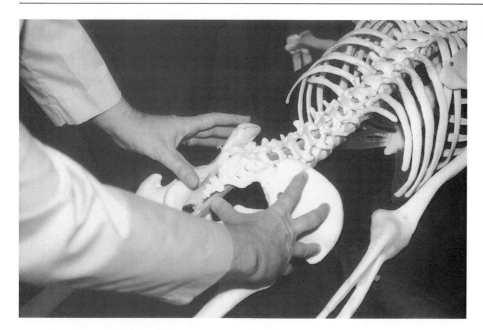

Figure 63.22. Medial surface of the sacral tuberosity.

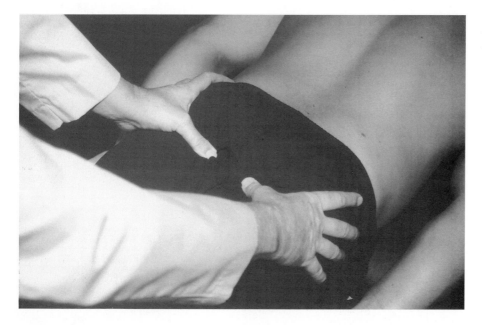

Figure 63.23. Place thumbs halfway between the sacral apex and each sacral tuberosity.

the lumbopelvic, diaphragmatic–trunk rotator–pelvic–hip rotator mechanics from this position.

The general goals are to release and restore functional symmetry to the lumbopelvic system, with primary focus on the sacrum, pelvis, trunk rotators, and thoracolumbar junction.

PUBIC SYMPHYSIS RELEASE

The goal is to restore symmetry to the pubic symphysis, paying particular attention to three-dimensional relationships among lower limb adductors, innominate asymmetries, and changes in rectus sheath attachments to the pubes.

Procedure

1. The patient lies supine with heels on the table and the arms comfortably at the sides. This more or less assures that unusual mechanical stresses transmitted through the Achilles tendons and ankles will be neutralized. For those patients with significant kyphoses, it is helpful to use a large pillow to minimize cervical and thoracolumbar problems.
2. Facing cephalad, sit or stand beside the patient's right thigh, near the knee.
3. First assess for symphyseal shear and positional asymmetry (Figs. 63.26 and 63.27). Tightness and looseness in the rectus

Figure 63.24. Place thumbs halfway between the sacral apex and each sacral tuberosity.

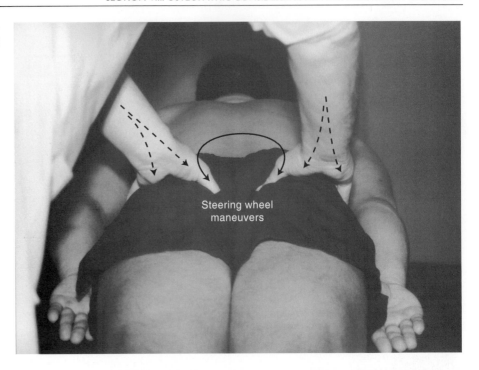

Figure 63.25. Press anteriorly and superiorly while turning thumbs systematically against either tightness or looseness.

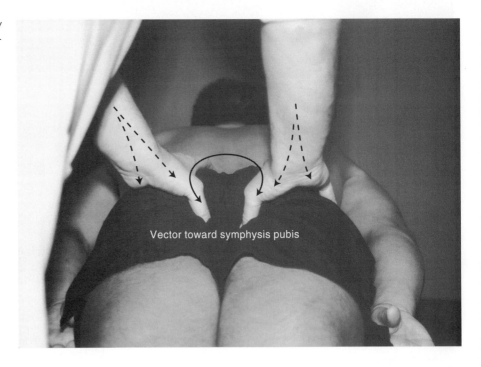

sheath often identifies the most problematic site. Sometimes tightness will be on the inferior side, sometimes superior. The area must be assessed to know for sure. Usually there are strong correlations with innominate positioning, but there are enough exceptions that one must be alert.

4. Place the thenar eminences on either side of the symphysis pubis, thumbs pointed superiorly and anteriorly. Proximal adductor and iliacus tendon attachments should be palpably evident (Figs. 63.28 and 63.29).

5. Induce firm, slow forces that initially either exaggerate (indirect barriers) or decrease (direct barriers) symphysis asymmetry. Direct rocking back and forth, similar to an articular maneuver, is often effective. Hold against the barriers until releases occur. Mild oscillations usually become evident as the

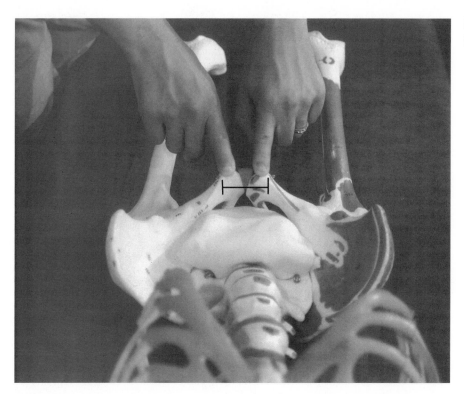

Figure 63.26. Assess for symphyseal shear and positional asymmetry.

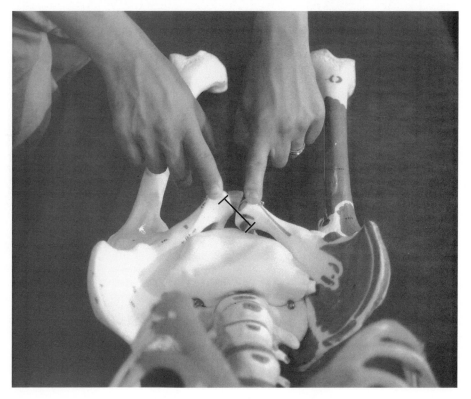

Figure 63.27. Assess for symphyseal shear and positional asymmetry.

Figure 63.28. Symphysis release. Thenar eminences are placed on either side of symphysis pubis, thumbs pointed superiorly and anteriorly.

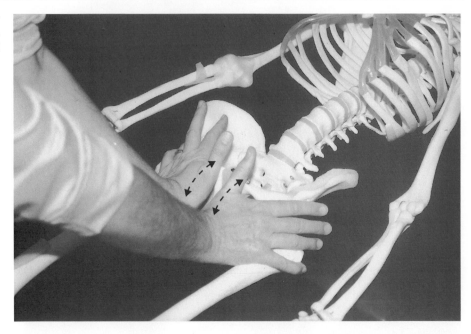

Figure 63.29. Thenar eminences are placed on either side of symphysis pubis, thumbs pointed superiorly and anteriorly.

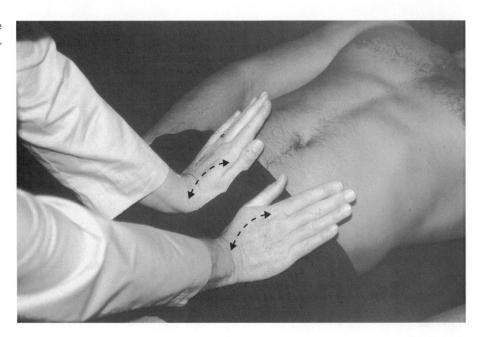

rectus fascias, pelvis, trunk rotators, and thigh adductors gradually become more symmetrical.

Anterior Pelvic–Innominate Release (Figs. 63.30–63.35)

The goal is to reduce obliquity of the two innominates in relation to one another.

PROCEDURE

1. The patient lies supine with heels on the table, arms comfortably at the sides. This more or less assures that unusual mechanical stresses transmitted through the Achilles tendons and ankles will be neutralized. For those patients with significant kyphoses, it is helpful to use a large pillow to minimize cervical and thoracolumbar problems.
2. Facing cephalad, stand beside the patient's right thigh.

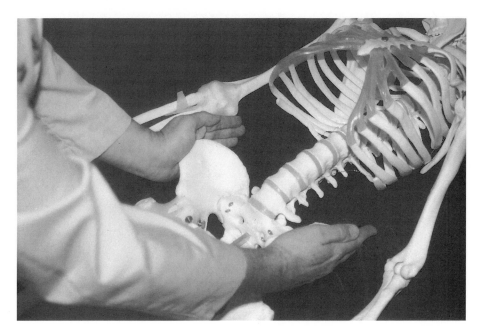

Figure 63.30.

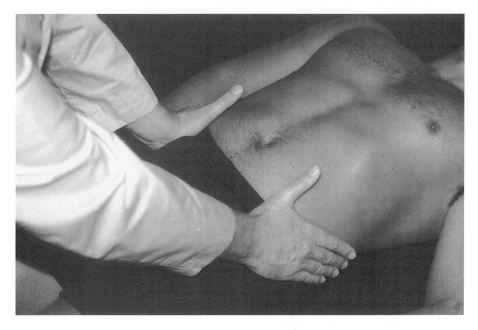

Figure 63.31.

3. Place your palms across the anterosuperior iliac spines, being sure to cover the inguinal ligament medially and the iliopsoas muscles as they past beneath the ligament toward their attachments on the lesser trochanter of the femur (Figs. 63.30 and 63.31).

4. Assess pelvic obliquity both positionally and functionally. Usually the right innominate is more anterior and resists posterior displacements against the direct barrier by the operator. In like manner, the left innominate is usually more posterior posi-

tionally and resists anterior displacements by the operator against the direct barrier. Indirect barrier displacements and assessments are done in directions opposite to those mentioned above (Figs. 63.32 and 63.33).

5. Barriers can be stressed both directly and indirectly at the same time by holding the innominates in each hand and exaggerating pelvic obliquity (Figs. 63.34 and 63.35). As barriers are approached, a sense of tension occurs, sudden firmness against direct barriers, and a softer pillowlike sensation against the

Figure 63.32.

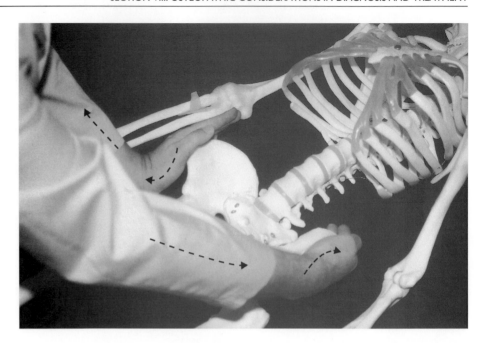

Figure 63.33.

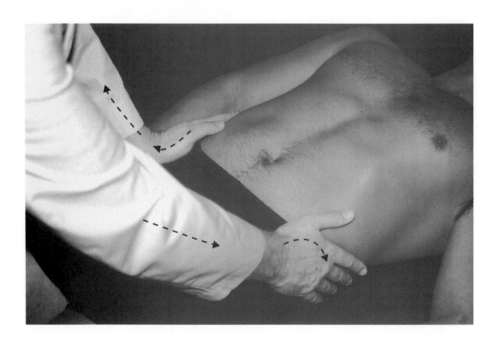

indirect barriers. Hold against the barriers until releases occur. Usually there are more than one. Also assess for sequential tight–loose changes in the ilioinguinal area as positional symmetry becomes more evident. Treatment is complete when positional and tight–loose asymmetries are resolved.

Sacroiliac Release: Supine (Figs. 63.36–63.43)

The goal is to create both positional and movement symmetry, nutation and counternutation, in the sacroiliac joints and at the sacral base.

PROCEDURE

1. The patient lies supine with heels on the table, arms comfortably at the sides. This more or less assures that unusual mechanical stresses transmitted through the Achilles tendons and ankles will be neutralized. For those patients with significant kyphoses, it is helpful to use a large pillow to minimize cervical and thoracolumbar problems.

2. Sit beside the patient's right knee.

3. Resting comfortably on the right forearm, place your right hand beneath the sacrum so that each sacroiliac joint is covered

Figure 63.34.

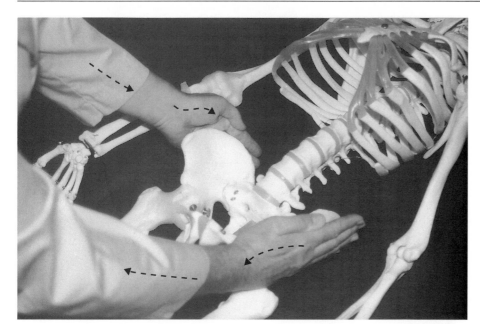

Figure 63.35.

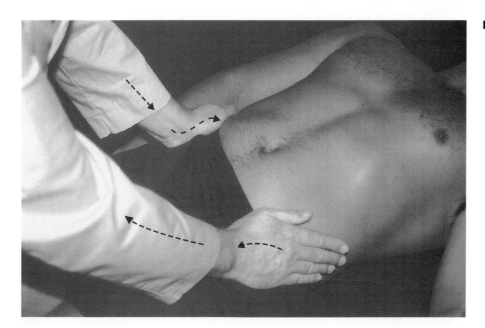

by the index and ring fingers while the apex covers the metatarsophalangeal joints (Fig. 63.36).

4. Identify the following:

Positional and movement asymmetries in relation to the innominates. With practice one can learn to identify sacral flexions and torsions as identified in muscle energy terminology.

General tight–loose active and passive movement asymmetries

Sacral nutation and counternutation, side-bending, and axial twist

Positional and movement asymmetries in relation to the pelvic diaphragm and lower limb

Sacral movements arising from craniosacral rhythm

5. With distraction, compression, and twisting movements simultaneously stress direct and indirect barriers (Figs. 63.37–63.43). Sustained forces invoke mechanical and neurological releases as preexisting tightness and looseness.

6. After myofascial and sacral balancing have occurred, monitor sacral nutation and counternutation (craniosacral flexion and extension) until the rhythm is smooth and symmetrical.

Figure 63.36. Hand position for sacroiliac release.

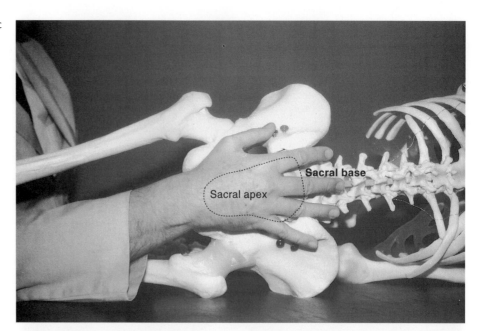

Figure 63.37. Hand position for sacroiliac release.

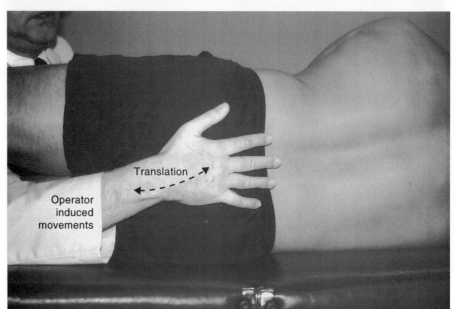

Figure 63.38.

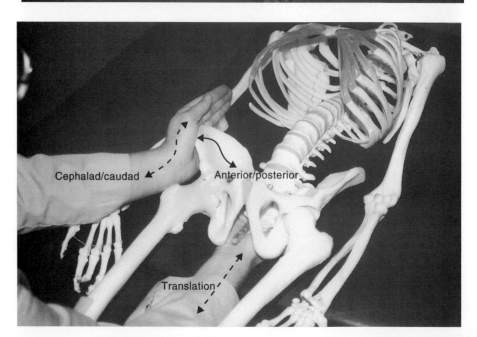

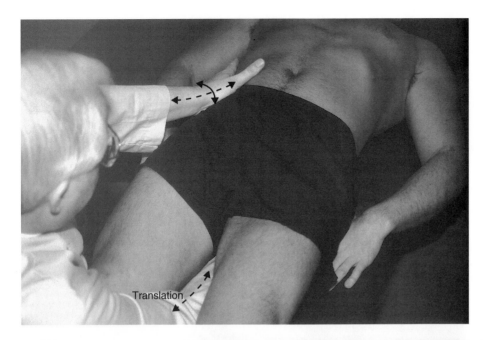

Figure 63.39.

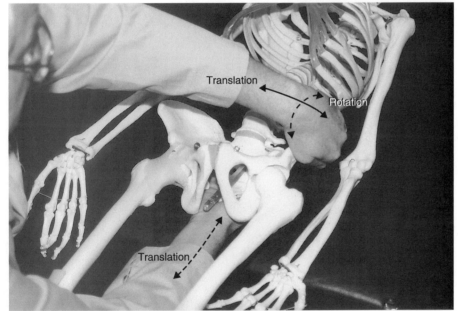

Figure 63.40.

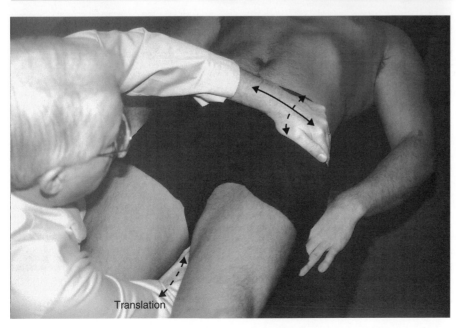

Figure 63.41.

Figure 63.42.

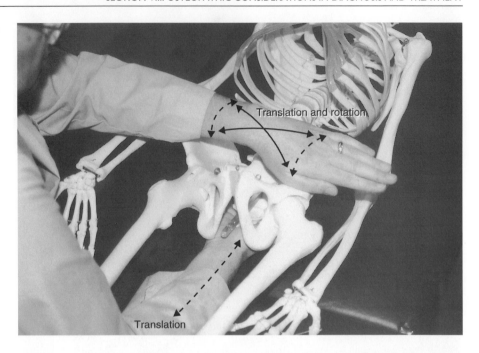

Figure 63.43.

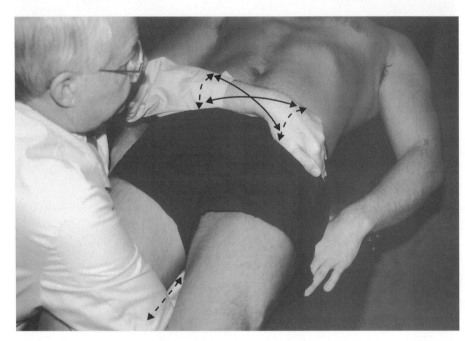

THORACIC CAGE, SPINE, AND DIAPHRAGM: PRONE

The goal is to three-dimensionally balance the thoracic cage and spine in relation to the upper limbs, diaphragm, trunk rotators, and lumbopelvic mechanics.

This technique is virtually identical to the prone basic thoracolumbar junction release described previously. The only difference is the movement of the hands cephaloward between the scapulae. The major differences are the tight–loose functional anatomical relationships associated with the trapezius, rhomboids, scapular mechanics, iliocostalis, and thoracic attachments of the cervical muscles, such as splenius cervicis.

Thoracic Cage, Spine, Diaphragm, and Lower Costal Cage: Supine (Figs. 63.44–63.50)

The goal is to three-dimensionally balance scapulothoracic, thoracic spine, and costodiaphragmatic relationships.

PROCEDURE

1. The patient lies supine with heels on the table, arms comfortably at the sides. This more or less assures that unusual mechanical stresses transmitted through the Achilles tendons and ankles will be neutralized. For those patients with sig-

Figure 63.44.

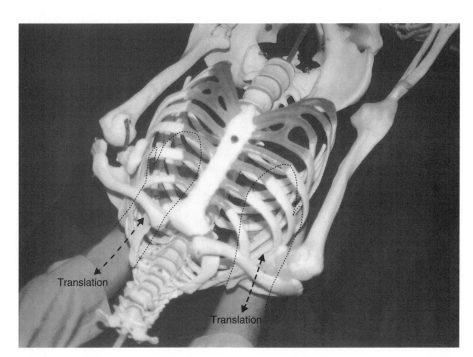

Translation

Translation

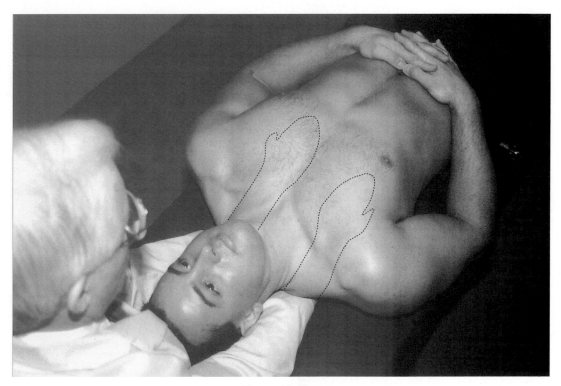

Figure 63.45.

nificant kyphoses, it is helpful to use a large pillow to minimize cervical and thoracolumbar problems.

2. Sit at the head of the table.

3. Reaching between the patient and the table, place the hands firmly against inferior costothoracic attachments on either side of the thoracic spine. Maintaining whole hand contact across the erector spinae and around the costal cage is essential (Figs. 63.44 and 63.45).

4. Both positional and tight–loose asymmetries will be readily apparent.

5. Additional tight–loose assessments focus on the following:

Diaphragmatic asymmetries, which are assessed by having the patient slowly but deeply inhale and exhale (Fig. 63.46)

Upper limb asymmetries, which are assessed by moving the upper limbs in a variety of directions (Figs. 63.47–63.50) both actively and passively

Thoracolumbar junction asymmetries, which are assessed by having the patient move the lower limbs in a variety of directions both actively and passively

Give particular attention to the proximal iliopsoas and other, more distal, lumbopelvic relationships.

6. By gently but firmly lifting the thoracolumbar attachments

Figure 63.46.

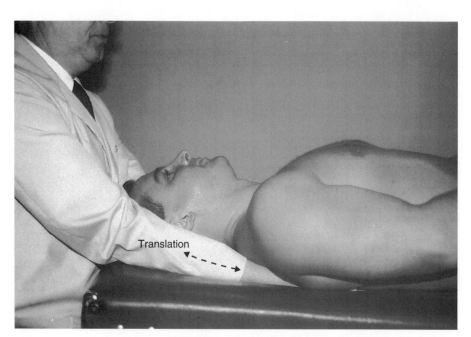

Figure 63.47.

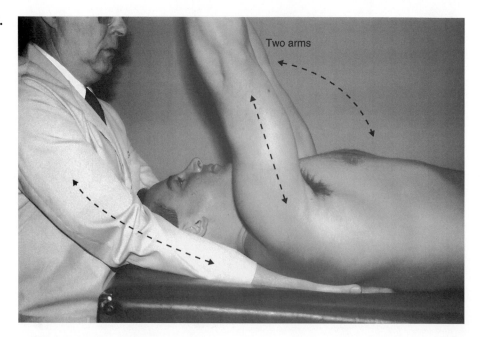

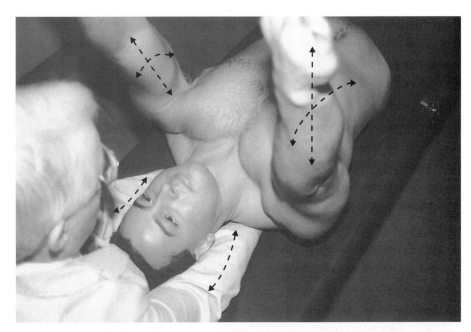

Figure 63.48.

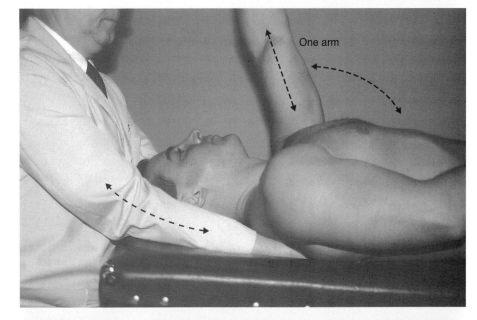

One arm

Figure 63.49.

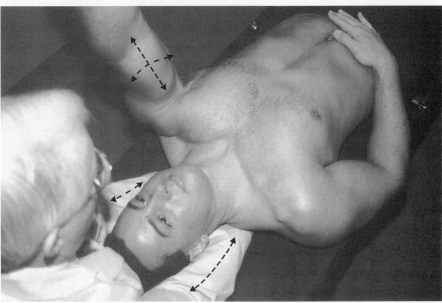

Figure 63.50.

anteriorly and laterally, tightness and looseness are balanced in relation to one another as inherent tissue movements become apparent. Sometimes considerable traction and twist are needed, but not often, because other techniques have been used first.

7. As tightness releases, varieties of upper and lower limb movements in all directions together with breath holding at neutral, deep inhalation, and deep exhalation, will enhance movements toward better symmetry.

8. Treatment is complete when thoracocostal movements are as functionally symmetrical as can be expected.

CRANIOCERVICAL SPINE

Seated Position (Figs. 63.51–63.54)

The goal is to increase general cervical–upper thoracic range of motion by focusing on both cervical and upper thoracic mechanics.

Procedure

1. The patient sits with relaxed posture.
2. Stand behind the patient.
3. With each hand, assess lateral, thoracic inlet, and posterior cervicothoracic mechanisms for tightness and looseness (Fig. 63.51). Using combinations of active and passive operator- and patient-induced neck movements in all ranges is essential (Figs. 63.52 and 63.53). Differences at the same sites with passive and active movements are frequent.
4. Commonly tightness occurs in upper and middle thoracic sites where cervical muscles attach to the upper and middle back.

For example, trapezius, splenius cervicis, levator scapulae, and semispinalis capitis frequently exhibit tightness as low as T6-7.

5. Tight–loose asymmetries involving deep cervical rotators and side-benders as well as sternocleidomastoids and scalenes factors are common.
6. Place the hands around lateral and posterior cervicothoracic attachments. Be prepared to move anteriorly and laterally as releases get under way. Cranial nerve and upper limb integrated release-enhancing maneuvers are particularly helpful (Fig. 63.54).
7. Bilateral, anteroinferior circumferential twist and stress is induced across and around the cervicothoracic junction against both direct and indirect barriers.
8. Releases generally begin fairly quickly. Once under way, inherent tissues movements can be followed until symmetry occurs across the cervicothoracic junction. It is particularly important to assess changes in conjunction with combined varieties of active and passive head, cervical spine, upper limb, and respiratory efforts.
9. Treatment is complete when three-dimensional symmetry has been established in relation to active and passive cervicothoracic, upper limb, respiratory, and costal cage mechanisms.

Supine (Figs. 63.55–63.61)

The goal is to establish three-dimensional movement symmetry in the cervical spine. Particular emphasis is placed on restoration of adequate side-bending and rotation, both generally and in relation to single segment mobility. This technique is usually more effective after lower cervical, cervicothoracic junction, and upper thoracic, upper limb factors have been released (Figs. 63.55–63.57).

Figure 63.51.

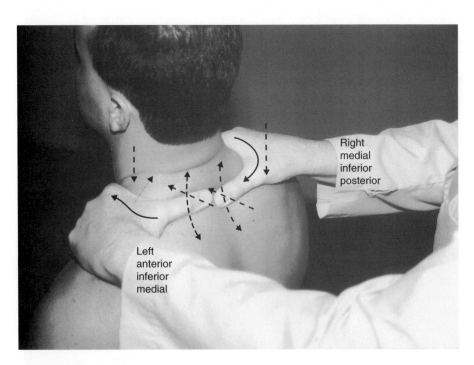

Right medial inferior posterior

Left anterior inferior medial

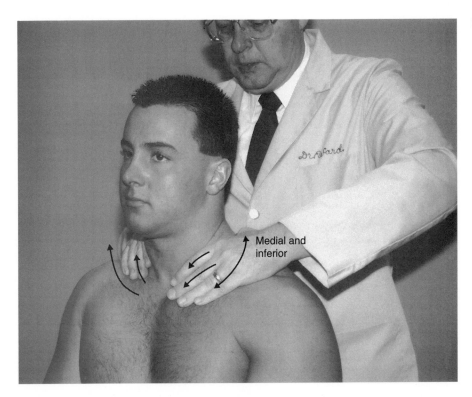

Figure 63.52.

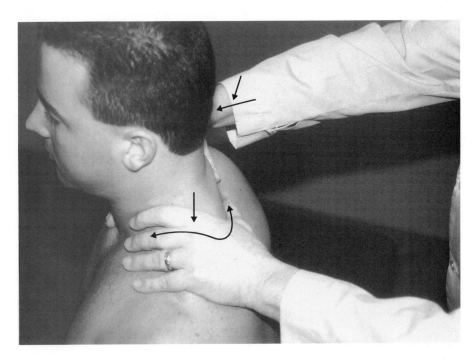

Figure 63.53.

Figure 63.54.

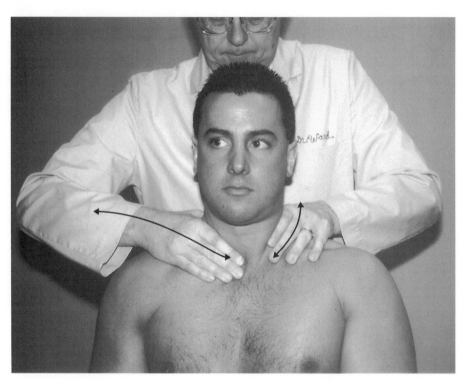

Figure 63.55.

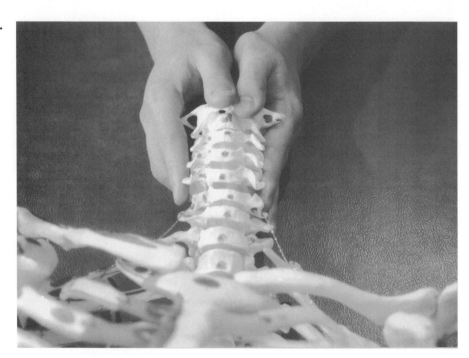

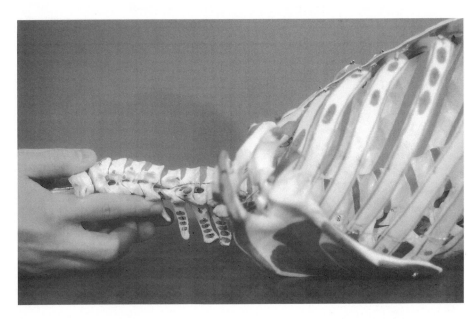

Figure 63.56.

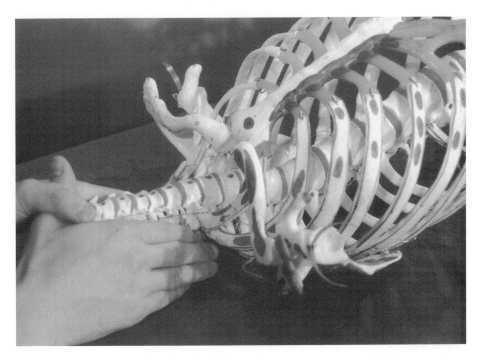

Figure 63.57.

Figure 63.58.

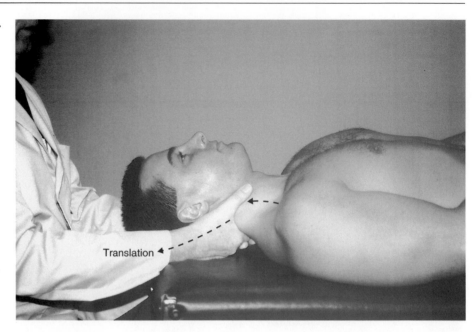

Figure 63.59.

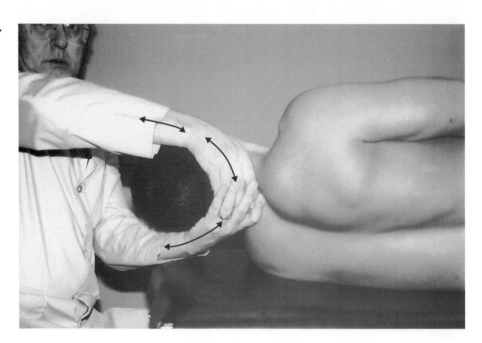

PROCEDURE

1. The patient lies supine with heels on the table, arms comfortably at the sides. This more or less assures that unusual mechanical stresses transmitted through the Achilles tendons and ankles will be neutralized. For those patients with significant kyphoses, it is helpful to use a large pillow to minimize cervical and thoracolumbar problems.

2. Sit at the patient's head.

3. Two hand positions, among many, are particularly useful:
   a. One hand overlapping the other so that generally applied, carefully controlled and focused, twist, traction, and side-bending maneuvers can be used both independently and together with patient cooperation (Figs. 63.58 and 63.59).
   b. Each hand grasping the basiocciput with the palms, leaving the fingers free to deal with both superficial and deep myofascial factors in relation to altered vertebral unit mechanisms (Figs. 63.60 and 63.61).

4. From either hand position, traction, turning and side-bending maneuvers assess myofascial and joint-related tightness and looseness. Pay particular attention to tightness, remembering that loose joints with surrounding inhibited muscle groups are common sources of pain and disability. In more acute situations, on the other hand, loose joints are usually

Figure 63.60.

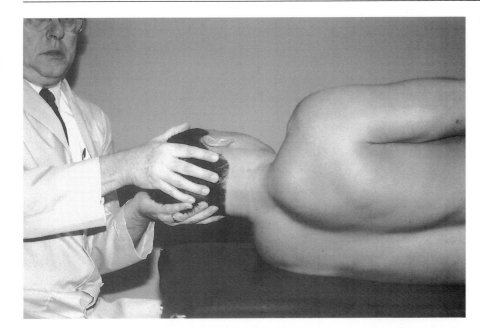

Figure 63.61.

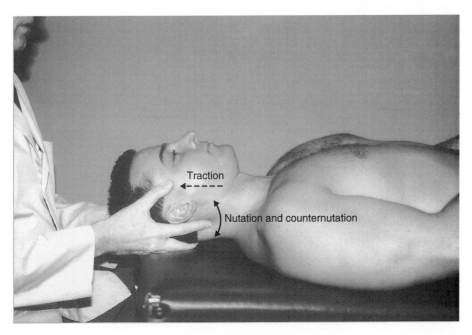

associated with tight muscles as they work to stabilize the system. The opposite findings are also common, such as tight joints with accompanying inhibition of overlying muscles.

5. Facet joints are often tight on one side, loose on the other. Side-to-side motion testing with only a little rotation will determine which facets are failing to effectively open or close.

The goal, once again, is to persistently, but carefully, apply well-focused stress against tight sites with and without patient assistance. INR cranial nerve and upper limb activities such as finger tapping and hand rolling are helpful.

Note: To protect the vertebral arteries, take particular cau-

tion to avoid simultaneous side-bending and extension maneuvers. While important for all age groups, most injuries have occurred under age 35.

6. Linking translatory maneuvers, for example, combinations of distraction and extension with flexion, extension, side-bending, and rotation, is particularly helpful.

7. Release deep upper cervical muscles by combining cranial nerve activities with occipitoatlantal nutation and counternutation, singly and together.

8. Atlantoaxial joints and surrounding attachments are carefully rotated against tightness.

9. Middle and lower cervical attachments are stressed with com-

binations of side-bending, flexion, and extension without a lot of rotation.

10. Treatment is complete when symmetrical movements are restored to facet joints and surrounding soft tissues within the ability of the patient to adapt.

LOWER LIMB (FIGS. 63.62–63.65)

The goal is to release each lower limb from lumbopelvic and hip rotator attachments to the foot and ankle.

Procedure

1. The patient's feet should be on the table to minimize lower limb stresses in relation to the pelvis and lower limb.
2. The patient's head and neck should be comfortable with minimal stress on the spine and pelvis.
3. The hands and arms are comfortably placed.
4. Sit or stand beside the patient.
5. Grasp each knee in sequence firmly across the distal femur and distal patellar attachments (Fig. 63.62) so that tightness

Figure 63.62.

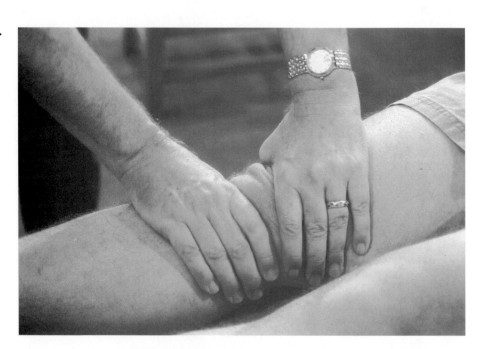

Figure 63.63.

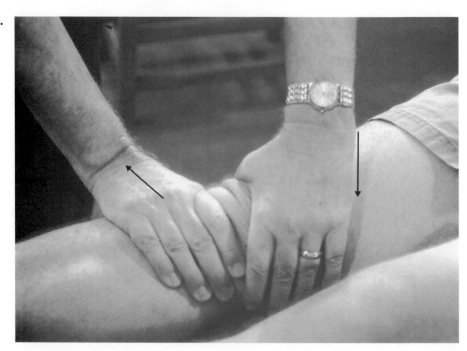

Figure 63.64.

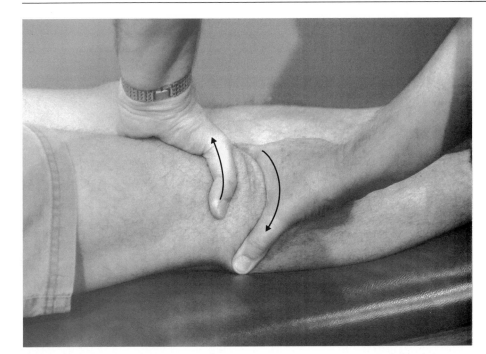

Figure 63.65.

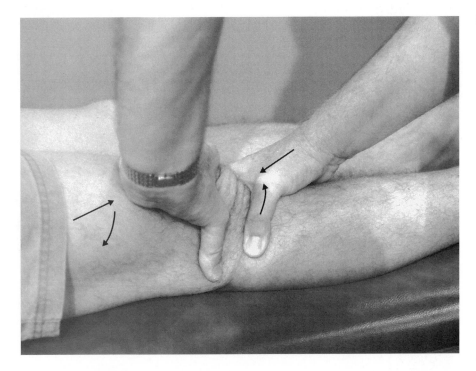

and looseness can be assessed during passively induced movements (Figs. 63.63–63.65) and during active muscle contractions.

Note: Myofascially, this is a fairly ambiguous area to assess and treat, so one must subjectively rely on tight–loose end feels, both quantitatively and qualitatively to a greater extent than at some other sites. This is because both lumbopelvic

and foot–ankle mechanics have such a great influence on this system. Specific knowledge of the underlying functional anatomy is particularly helpful.

6. Particular care is taken in assessing medial hamstring as well as lateral hamstring/iliotibial band/proximal fibular head tight–loose relationships.

7. Perform passive internal and external limb rotation.

8. Perform active internal and external rotation.

9. Three-dimensional motion qualities against tight and looseness are assessed with the knee in full extension and in varieties of flexion.

10. Assess hip function in the same way, with the leg in full extension and then with varieties of flexion, internal and external rotation, abduction, and adduction.

    Note: Remember to check for leg length inequalities and altered hip mechanics both prone and supine. It is common to find differences from prone to supine.

    For leg length inequalities to make a difference, the discrepancy typically is greater than 3 mm (1/8 inch) for genuine significance.

    For hip-related problems, in the absence of hip degenerative changes, adductor and medial hamstring problems are common areas of restriction.

11. It is common to find asymptomatic lateral knee/fibular head problems (tightness) in response to medial complaints where the knee is generally more mobile.

12. Remember that proximal sacroiliac joint and sacrotuberous–sacrospinous ligamentous factors are common sources of distal difficulties, and vice versa.

13. Grasp the knee firmly both proximally and distally, noting areas of tightness and looseness before passive movements are induced (Figs. 63.62–63.65).

14. Twist the passive knee in opposite directions (axial twist), being sure that the hand and fingers are firmly in contact with areas of maximum tightness. Usually maximum tightness is in two places:

    a. Laterally around distal iliotibial band attachments and proximal fibular head

    b. Medially and posteriorly near and around distal hamstring attachments

Alternative Treatment (Figs. 63.66–63.73)

With limb extended, focus on hip rotator–lumbopelvic factors.

After assessing and releasing knee mechanics, one commonly encounters proximal hip rotator/abductor/adductor tight–loose problems. Search out these elements by carrying the extended limb into varieties of rotation, abduction, and adduction. Holding against the barrier, either direct or indirect, while focusing on the underlying anatomy is particularly helpful.

Both soft tissue and joint tightness are released by three-dimensionally stressing specifically tight sites. Twist, traction, compression, and shear are used interactively as one follows inherent tissue motions.

Unwinding Maneuvers

From the foot of the table, long lever unwinding maneuvers use similar stressing to release the whole lower limb, including foot and ankle in relation to lumbopelvic mechanism (Figs. 63.66–63.73). With practice, one can learn to use the lower limbs to work through the whole body. This is a form of unwinding technique.

Unwinding is a term used to describe long lever bending and twisting maneuvers of the limbs that help reveal both rapid and slow-moving myofascial changes. Combinations of traction, compression, twisting, and bending are used to sequentially follow tight and loose inherent tissue movements. The

Figure 63.66.

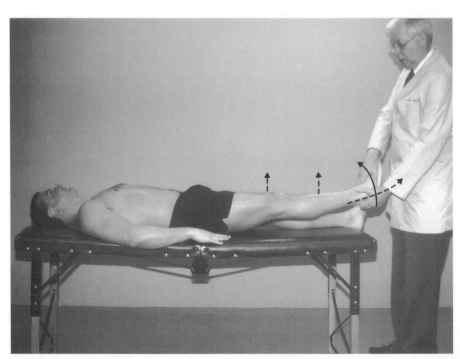

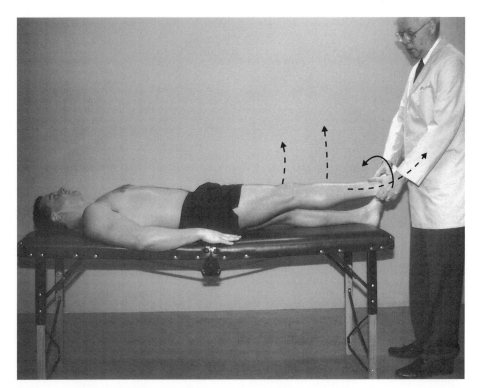

Figure 63.67.

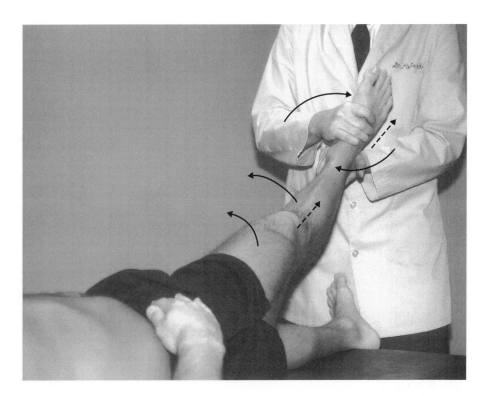

Figure 63.68.

Figure 63.69.

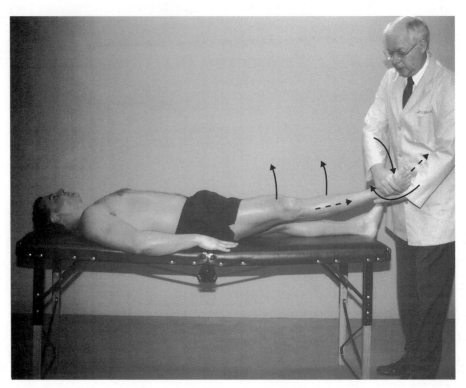

Figure 63.70.

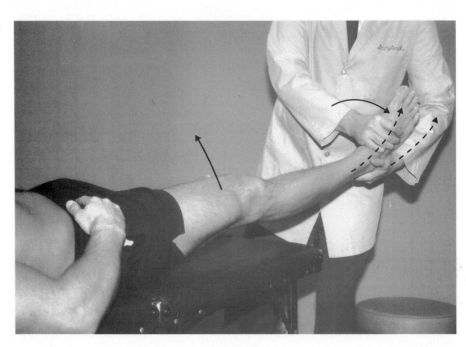

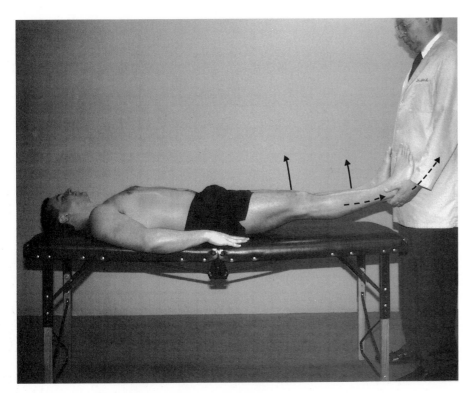

Figure 63.71.

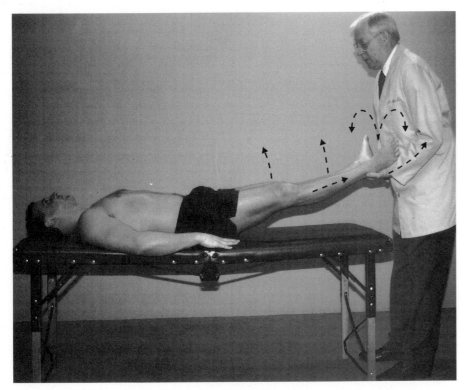

Figure 63.72.

Figure 63.73.

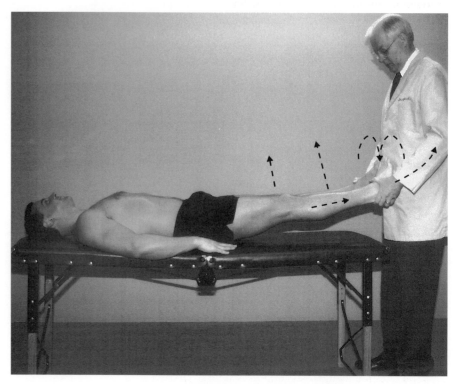

Figure 63.74.

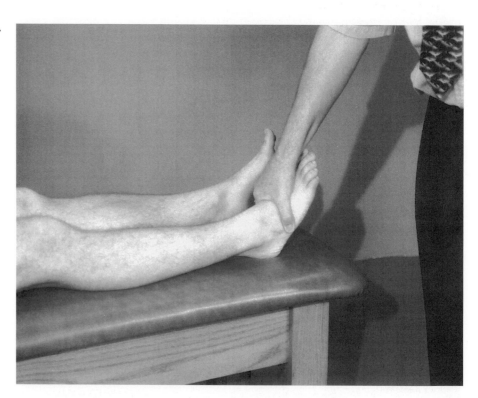

phenomenon occurs in both upper and lower limbs as well as throughout the body. Sometimes the limb moves rapidly, and sometimes slowly, as the operator feels and listens with highly developed palpatory skills. These events have been empirically described for decades by many osteopathic practitioners. The origin of the term, unwinding, is not clear.

Some describe unwinding movements using functional technique terminology as they describe combinations of ease and bind. Still others refer to balance and hold methods in areas of maximum ease.

Whatever the description, experienced practitioners are able to follow behind or move directly into and toward unwinding barriers. As the limb moves toward looseness (ease), tightness (bind), or balances at positions of maximum ease, the myofascial system commonly begins to move about in almost random ways. Sometimes movements are extremely slow; at other times, very rapid. When releases occur, movements temporarily cease. As operator skill improves, following the movements becomes increasingly easy.

Presumably, these different rates reflect differing central, peripheral, and specific muscle group electromechanical events. To date, satisfactory scientific descriptions are lacking.

Foot and Ankle

Treatment of the foot and ankle (Figs. 63.74–63.77) from this position is virtually identical to the treatment principles relating to the knee. It is always important to understand tight–loose factors and that symptomatic looseness, for example on the lateral aspect of the ankle, is commonly associated with medial foot tightness involving the deltoid ligament. Whether release of the tightness is helpful is a matter of clinical judgment.

UPPER LIMB AND SHOULDER

Prone (Figs. 63.78–63.82)

Most of the time this position is used to deal directly with compromised shoulder and scapulocostal mechanics. Direct stressing across the rotator cuff; acromioclavicular joint; distal glenohumeral attachments; and inferior subscapularis, latissimus dorsi, teres attachments is essential.

Frozen shoulder, in particular, is a self-limited problem, with most disappearing in 18–24 months no matter what is done.

PROCEDURE

1. The patient's feet should be off the end of the table to minimize lower limb stresses in relation to the pelvis and lower limb.
2. The patient's head should be turned to the most comfortable side. Note the effect of head turning on tightness and looseness across the shoulder in question. Proximal and superior cervical attachments are often compromised.
3. The hands and arms are comfortably placed either over the sides of the table or on the table beside the hips and thighs. If the hands are over the sides of the table, be sure to know the effect on scapulocostal gliding.
4. Sit on a rolling stool that allows moving in response to shifting tightness and looseness.
5. Hold the affected arm between your knees so the rolling stool can be used to guide movements in cooperation to shoulder stressing induced by the hands.
6. Initially, place your hands firmly around the glenohumeral attachments (Figs. 63.78–63.80).

Figure 63.75.

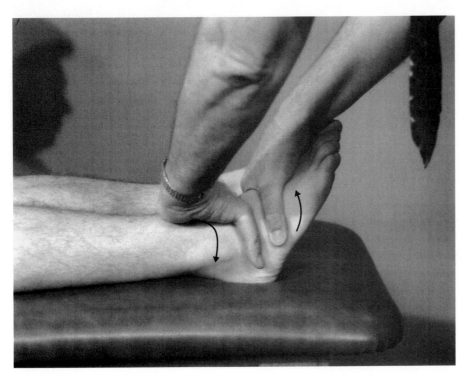

Figure 63.76.

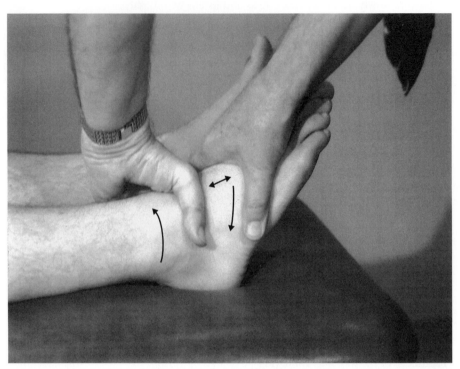

Figure 63.77.

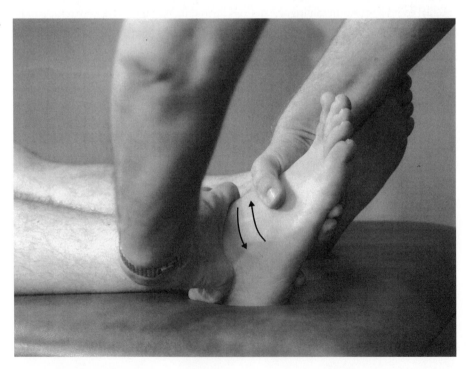

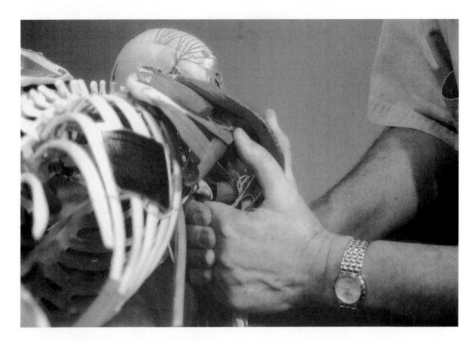

Figure 63.78.

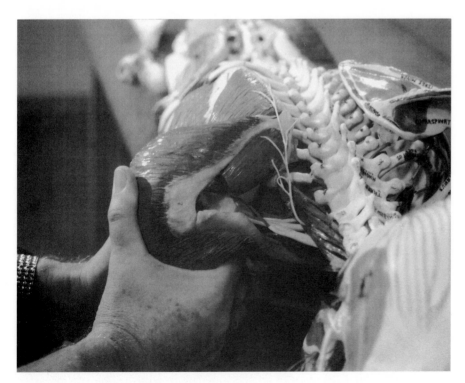

Figure 63.79.

Figure 63.80.

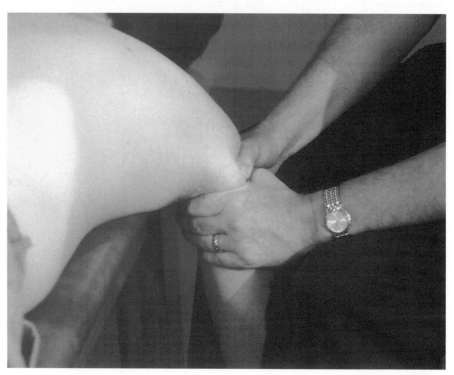

Figure 63.81.

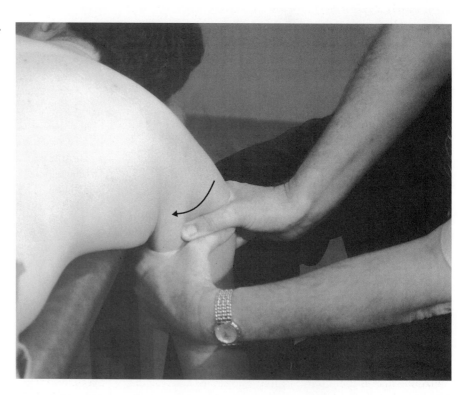

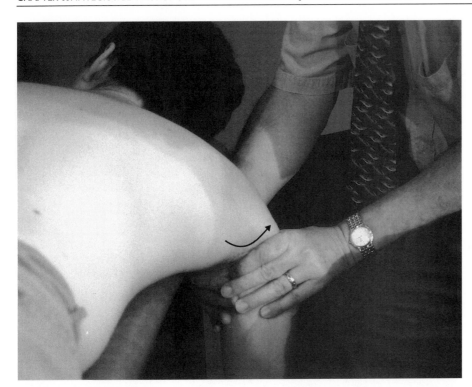

Figure 63.82.

Note: X-ray studies are essential, because one must know whether there are interfering joint changes of any kind. Remember also that cervical problems commonly interfere with shoulder and rotator cuff activities.

7. Assess tightness and looseness by three-dimensionally stressing the system using distraction, compression, twist, and shear (Figs. 63.81 and 63.82).

8. Direct and firm stressing against tightness gets the process under way. For example, 5–15 pounds of load are common before initial releases begin.

9. Following inherent tissue movements is sometimes successful, particularly in mild situations. Long-term problems, however, usually require firmly held movements that assertively stretch the area without interfering with neurocirculatory functions.

10. A well-organized home exercise and/or physical therapy program is usually needed to maintain and increase improvements.

11. Pay particular attention to posterior and inferior glenohumeral restrictions close to the scapula.

Supine (Figs. 63.83 and 63.84)

The goal is to generally mobilize the shoulder girdle in relation to both the cervical spine and thorax.

Note: this positioning is less helpful for frozen shoulder situations than is the prone position. The supine position can be particularly helpful for more general craniocervical–scapulocostal–upper limb problems.

PROCEDURE

1. The patient lies supine with heels on the table, arms comfortably at the sides. This more or less assures that unusual mechanical stresses transmitted through the Achilles tendons and ankles will be neutralized. For those patients with significant kyphoses, it is helpful to use a large pillow to minimize cervical and thoracolumbar problems.

2. Stand at either the side or head of the table. Choice of position is dictated by scapulocostal–glenohumeral range of motion, and tight–loose factors.

3. Grasp the patient's wrists.

4. Distraction, compression, and twist are used to mechanically and neurologically assess tight–loose range of motion capabilities (Figs. 63.84 and 63.85).

5. Direct stress against tight or loose (direct/indirect) barriers usually creates a series of unwinding activities that gradually increase shoulder range of motions if intrinsic joint mechanics are adequate.

FOREARM, ELBOW, AND WRIST RELEASE

Direct Technique, Transverse Approach (Figs. 63.85–63.88)

By way of a historical note, this was the first direct myofascial release technique developed in this system of treatment. It was designed in 1976 when having particular difficulty treating a patient who had scleroderma. Her skin was generally thickened

Figure 63.83.

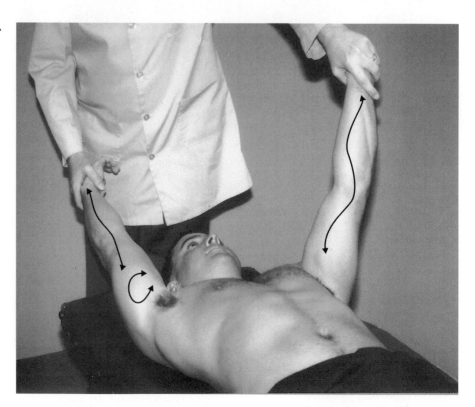

Figure 63.84.

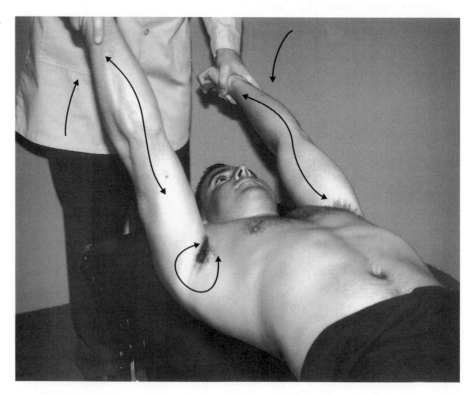

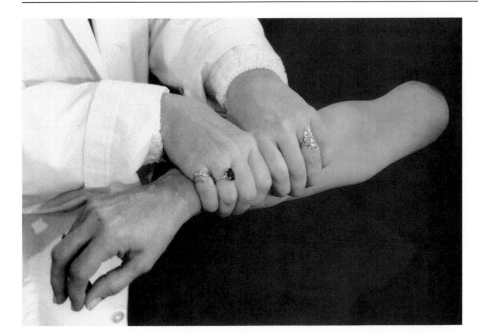

Figure 63.85.

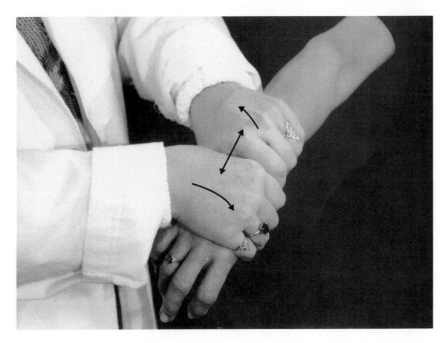

Figure 63.86. Forearm elbow wrist release, direct technique, transverse approach.

by pannus (inflammatory granulation tissue) that had severely restricted most of her available myofascial and joint movements about the head, neck, face, chest wall, and upper limbs. Facial restrictions were so marked, she could open her mouth about 1.5 cm rather than the expected 4–5 cm. Facial expressions were masklike and almost immobile—a source of major stress and frustration for her. There was also some anterior abdominal wall involvement. Swallowing was an increasing problem because of externally related factors. Fortunately, visceral involvement was minimal. Raynaud's phenomenon was severe, with marked flexion contractures of the palmar fascias

and finger flexors. She had previously been placed on penicillamine and had had physical therapy without substantial success.

After working with her for several visits, it was clear that standard osteopathic manipulative approaches were not helpful. Having had considerable experience with muscle energy techniques as well as fascial twisting maneuvers advocated by Ruddy and Neidner, it was asked if an assertive twist of the forearms, elbows, wrists, and hands could be performed. The patient readily agreed, and, surprisingly, the skin and underlying tissues gave way under the loads.

From this beginning, a series of assertive release maneuvers were designed to restore soft tissue resilience anywhere on the body. In this particular instance, family members were taught the maneuvers. They turned out to be of great help, and most of her flexibility was restored. This included the upper limbs, facial muscles, and craniomandibular mechanics. At the time of this writing, she was carrying on a normal lifestyle with minimal need for further attention.

The goal is to generally release the forearm, elbow, and wrist by transversely straining direct myofascial barriers along the forearm, elbow, and wrist in a stepwise fashion.

PROCEDURE

1. The patient is seated, standing, supine, or prone. Stand or sit comfortably for easy access.
2. Place hands transversely across the forearm, knuckles together, with a light hold on the skin (Fig. 63.85), then a transverse hold across wrist (Fig. 63.86).
3. Induce deformation against the direct barrier. Usually the tightness is more pronounced on the extensor surface. Induce deformation in the opposite directions (Figs. 63.87–63.88).
4. When barriers are encountered, hold firmly until they give way

Figure 63.87. Forearm elbow wrist release, direct technique, transverse approach.

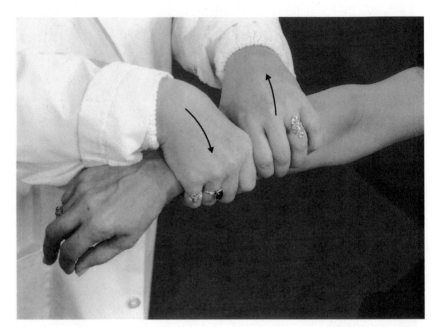

Figure 63.88. Forearm elbow wrist release, direct technique, transverse approach.

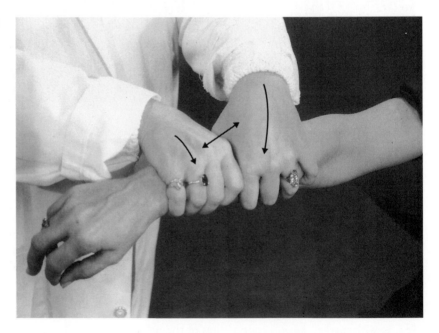

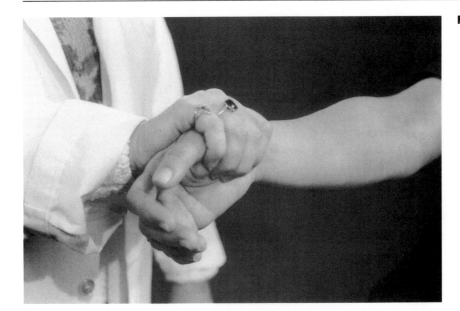

Figure 63.89.

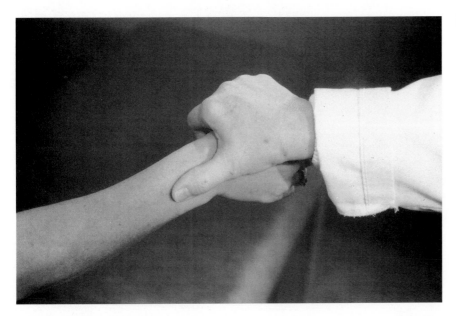

Figure 63.90.

against the load. Sometimes considerable force is needed to create a release, sometimes not.

5. Treatment is complete when as much soft tissue motion occurs as can be reasonably expected. Commonly, the tissues will spring back after a release. What this event represents is unknown, but it is assumed that the phenomenon represents a combination of viscoelastic rebound working together with a combination of peripheral and centrally controlled neurovascular changes.

Wrist–Forearm–Elbow

DIRECT TECHNIQUE, LONG AXIS APPROACH (FIGS. 63.89–63.93)

The goal is generally to release forearm flexors and extensors in relation to distal wrist–hand mechanics, and proximal lateral and medial elbow to shoulder mechanics. As the release process unfolds or unwinds, special attention is paid to sequential release processes affecting both superficial and deep muscle, reflex, and vascular mechanics.

Figure 63.91. Wrist forearm elbow, direct technique, long axis approach.

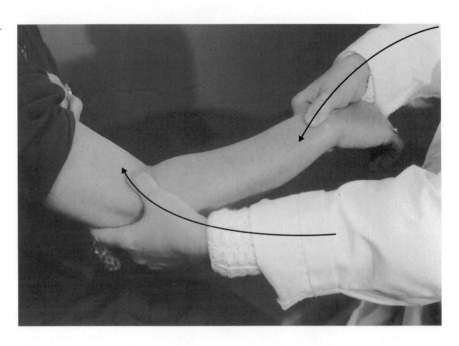

Figure 63.92. Wrist forearm elbow, direct technique, long axis approach.

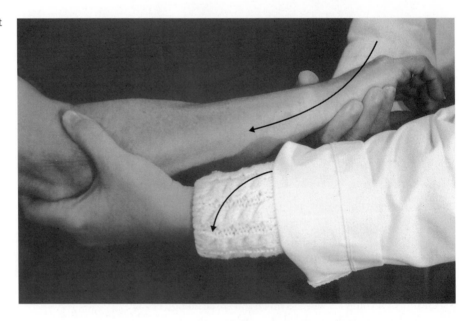

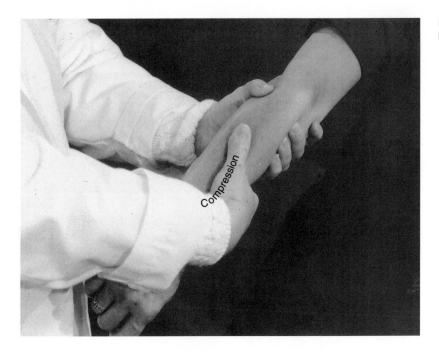

Figure 63.93. Wrist forearm elbow, direct technique, long axis approach.

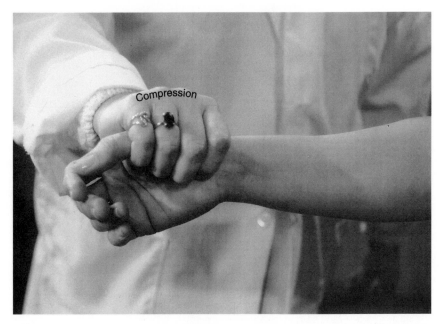

Figure 63.94. Wrist/carpal tunnel release.

Figure 63.95.

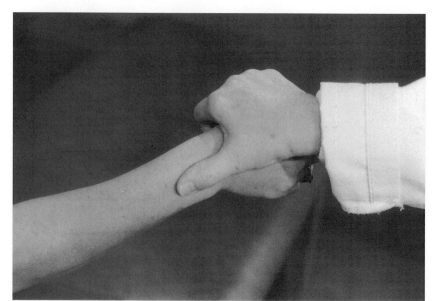

Figure 63.96. Wrist/carpal tunnel release.

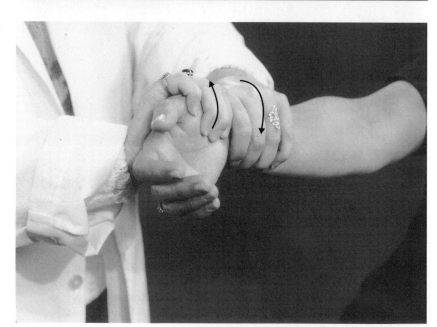

Figure 63.97. Wrist/carpal tunnel release.

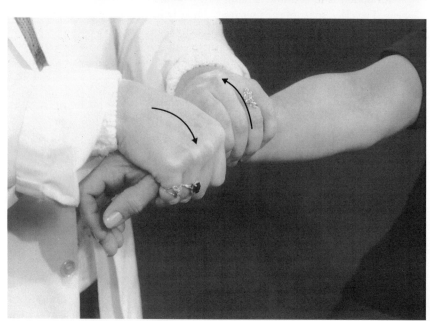

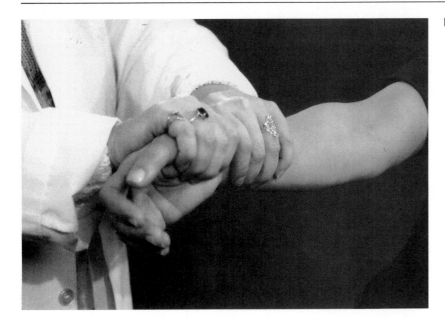

Figure 63.98.

Procedure

1. The patient is standing, seated, or supine. Take a general hand hold on thenar eminence (Fig. 63.89), with thumb placement along long axis of forearm over the wrist (Fig. 63.90). Figure 63.93 shows an alternative hand position.
2. Grasp forearm at elbow and wrist distally.
3. With elbow firmly held, turn the wrist until a tight barrier is noted at either side of the elbow, or within the mechanics of the wrist and hand. (Figure 63.91 shows twist in one direction, Figure 63.92 twist in opposite direction.)
4. Hold the tightness firmly for a few seconds until mechanical release is induced. At this point, the limb can be safely released and retested for soft tissue resilience and joint ranges of motion.

   An option is to continue holding firmly to see what happens. Typically, some of the muscles begin to writhe about in what can seem like random activities as described in the section on unwinding. Sometimes the movements are slow and arclike, involving the whole limb. At other times they are rapid, even jerky, like a spring suddenly uncoiling.
5. Treatment is complete when as much soft tissue motion occurs as can be reasonably expected.

Carpal and Palmar Tunnel Release

DIRECT TECHNIQUE, TRANSVERSE APPROACH (FIGS. 63.94–63.98)

The goal is to restore freedom of movement to the carpal and palmar tunnels by simultaneously releasing the soft tissues of the wrist, the carpal bones, and the palmar–carpal tunnel.

Procedure

1. The patient is seated, standing, or supine. Stand comfortably in front or beside the patient.
2. With distal hand, grasp the thenar–palmar tunnel attachments (Fig. 63.94). The distal hand thumb points along long axis of forearm (Fig. 63.95).
3. With proximal hand, grasp the wrist with specific attention to carpal–metacarpal and palmar tunnel–carpal tunnel tight-loose relationships.
4. Twist in supination until the myofascial barrier separates and opens the carpal tunnel (Fig. 63.96). Then twist in pronation to further release the radiocarpal attachments (Fig. 63.97).
5. Hold the tightness firmly for a few seconds until mechanical release is induced. At this point, the limb can be safely released and retested for soft tissue resilience and joint ranges of motion.

   A second option is to continue holding firmly to see what happens. Typically, some of the muscles will begin to writhe about in what can seem like random activities as described in the unwinding discussion above. Sometimes the movements are slow and arclike, involving the whole limb. At other times they are rapid, even jerky, like a spring suddenly uncoiling.
6. Treatment is complete when as much soft tissue motion occurs as can be reasonably expected.

CONCLUSION

These myofascial release and integrated neuromusculoskeletal techniques can help ease neuromusculoskeletal problems. They can be learned and applied with relative ease and have stood the test of time.

64. **Cranial Field**

EDNA M. LAY

During my years in practice as an osteopathic physician, there never has been one regret for having chosen this field for my life's work. Professional experience daily demonstrates the truth that the Science of Osteopathy includes the key to the great physiological chemical laboratory, the human body, unlocking the living potent forces that heal. To the student looking forward to a professional field of scientific research, and with the desire in his or her heart to render beneficial service to humanity, let me truly say: Osteopathy Provides The Golden Opportunity.

—W.G. SUTHERLAND, DO

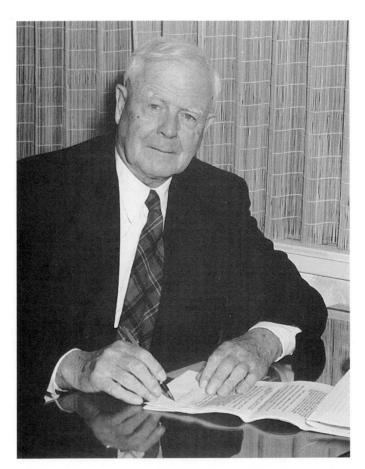

William G. Sutherland, DO, DSc (Hon)

Key Concepts

- **History of osteopathy in the cranial field, including the contribution of William G. Sutherland**

- **The primary respiratory mechanism**

- **The mechanics of physiologic motion**

- **Strains**

- **Diagnosis via history, observation, and palpation**

- **Clinical problems requiring treatment**

- **Principles of treatment**

Osteopathy is a philosophy, a science, and an art. The study of osteopathy in the cranial field offers a unique perspective on all three areas. Through persistent study of the intricate osseous armor that protects the brain and spinal cord, keen observation, and a compassionate dedication to relieve human suffering, William Garner Sutherland, DO, made an important discovery about the central nervous system that is important in osteopathy today.

HISTORY

William G. Sutherland, DO, DSci (Hon) (1873–1954) was an early student of Dr. A.T. Still. Sutherland graduated from the American School of Osteopathy in Kirksville, Missouri in 1899. While a student, he observed a mounted disarticulated skull. The sphenoid and the squamous portions of the temporal bones caught his attention, and he remembers:

As I stood looking and thinking in the channel of Dr. Still's philosophy, my attention was called to the beveled articular surfaces of the sphenoid bone. Suddenly there came a thought; I call it a guiding thought—beveled like the gills of a fish, indicating articular mobility for a respiratory mechanism.[1]

He dismissed the thought but it kept returning, as if goading him to study the details of the various articulations of the skull.

Sutherland was an original thinker, and his application of Still's philosophy is recognized as "one of the most innovative ideas to be advanced by a member of the osteopathic profession."[2] Even though anatomy books at that time stated that the sutures of the cranium were immovable, Sutherland's determination to understand why the articular surfaces have such a unique design drove him to persevere until he understood that the design was accommodative to the function of the central nervous system (CNS), cerebrospinal fluid (CSF), and dural membranes, all of which function as a unit. He named this functional unit the primary respiratory mechanism (PRM).

Sutherland established his practice in Minnesota and devoted 30 years to study, original research on himself, and observation of his patients before he began to share his discovery

with his colleagues. The remarkable results he obtained with patients aroused the interest of other physicians. They prevailed on him at his home to teach them his method of treatment. The classes and the interest grew, slowly but steadily, because those who were able to learn the concept and apply this method of osteopathic diagnosis and treatment had similar results of relieving patients of pain and distressful conditions when other forms of treatment failed to help.

As more physicians studied and practiced this method of osteopathic treatment, they formed an organization, the Osteopathic Cranial Association, for the purpose of joining together to promote further study, support research, and publish literature to help educate physicians and lay persons. This membership organization later changed its name to the Cranial Academy and became a component society of the American Academy of Osteopathy.

Dr. Sutherland, with Drs. C. Handy and H. Magoun, Sr, established the Sutherland Cranial Teaching Foundation, Inc., in 1953, for the purpose of continuing the teaching of the cranial concept. Dr. Sutherland had established that an accurate diagnosis and successful treatment required sensitive and proficient palpation that could not be learned from a book; expert instructors using hands-on teaching and repeated verification were needed.

Dr. Still's teachings also provided the basic principles:

The body functions as a unit
The body possesses self-regulatory mechanisms
Structure and function are reciprocally interrelated
Rational treatment is based on application of these three principles

Dr. Sutherland's discovery and teachings have supplied knowledge and methods that clarify and expand on the science of osteopathy. Prior to Dr. Sutherland's work, the body was treated as if the head was incapable of having somatic dysfunction. Osteopathy in the cranial field is osteopathy of the entire person because the inherent force that manifests from within the head region functions throughout the body; therefore, this form of diagnosis and treatment affects the whole person rather than being limited to the cranium.

The insights and techniques derived by Dr. Sutherland's expansion of basic osteopathic principles are increasingly integrated into osteopathic teaching and care.[3–5] The International Classification of Disease (ICD-9) delineates coding for somatic dysfunction of the cranium. Competency testing of osteopathic manipulative treatment (OMT) to treat this dysfunction is available to nonspecialists and specialists alike. In recent years, the American Osteopathic Association (AOA) has received numerous research grant proposals from both clinicians and basic scientists to study the mechanisms and/or efficacy of this approach; the AOA has funded several of these projects.[6–10]

PRIMARY RESPIRATORY MECHANISM

Primary refers to first in importance; Dr. Sutherland considered thoracic respiration secondary to the PRM. By this he meant that the physiologic centers that control and regulate pulmonary respiration, circulation, digestion, and elimination are located in the floor of the fourth ventricle and depend on the function of the CNS.[11(p34)] Respiratory refers to the exchange of gases and other metabolites at the cellular level. Mechanism implies an integrated machine, each part in working relationship to every other part. The PRM is described as having five anatomic-physiologic components, described in the following sections.

Inherent Motility of Brain and Spinal Cord

The inherent motion of the CNS is a subtle, slow, wormlike movement. It is rhythmic with a biphasic cycle. The entire CNS shortens and thickens during one phase and lengthens and thins during the other.[11(p35)] As the cerebral hemispheres develop in fetal life, they grow, lengthen, and curl or coil within the developing cranium in the shape of a pair of ram's horns. Some evidence suggests that the inherent nature of the neuroglial cells of the CNS causes them to move rhythmically, in unison, resulting in the biphasic cycle of PRM. Lassek described the brain as being *vibrantly alive . . . incessantly active . . . dynamic . . . highly mobile, able to move forward, backward, sideward, circumduct and to rotate.* He further stated:

The normal, human brain is a wondrous, enormously complex, master organ which can be only made by nature. There are probably approximately twenty billion neurons in the central nervous system of man and it runs on a mere 25 watts of electrical power.[11(p23)]

Fluctuation of Cerebrospinal Fluid

The CSF is formed by the choroid plexuses and circulates through the ventricles, over and around the surface of the brain and spinal cord through the subarachnoid spaces and cisternae. Thus, the CSF is inside and outside of the CNS, bathing, protecting, and nourishing it. Fluctuation is defined as "a wavelike motion of fluid in a natural or artificial cavity of the body observed by palpation or percussion."[12] As the CNS shortens and lengthens in a biphasic rhythmic motion, the ventricles of the brain change shape slightly and the fluid moves concurrently. Sutherland observed this subtle rhythmic activity by palpation and determined that its normal rate is 10–14 cycles per minute. This phenomenon is called the cranial rhythmic impulse or the CRI.

The combined motility of the CNS and the fluctuation of CSF manifests as a hydrodynamic activity as well as a bioelectric interchange throughout the body. Stated simply, they function both as a pump and as an electric generator.

Mobility of Intracranial and Intraspinal Membranes

The meninges surround, support, and protect the CNS. The dura mater—the outermost of the three coverings—is composed of two layers of tough fibrous tissue. The outer layer of dura mater lines the cranial cavity, forming a periosteal covering for the inner aspect of the bones, and extends through the sutures of the skull to become the periosteum on the outer surface of the skull.

The inner layer of dura mater covers the brain and spinal cord and has reduplications named the falx cerebri and the tentorium cerebelli. These sickle-shaped structures arise from a common origin along the straight sinus and invest the various bones of the cranium. The two layers of dura mater are blended or fused in certain areas and are separated in other areas, forming the intradural venous sinuses.

The dura mater extends down the spinal canal with firm attachment around the foramen magnum, to C2 and C3, and to the lower lumbar and sacrum at the level of the second segment. The falx cerebri arises from the straight sinus, attaching to the occiput, parietals, frontals, and the crista galli of the ethmoid. The two halves of the tentorium cerebelli arise or originate at the straight sinus and attach to the occiput, temporals, and sphenoid bone.

The spinal and cranial dura and its reduplications respond to the inherent motion of the CNS and fluctuation of CSF and move through the biphasic cycle, influencing the bones of the cranium and the sacrum. Sutherland named this functional anatomic unit, consisting of the dura mater within the cranium and spinal canal, the reciprocal tension membrane (RTM).[11(p30)] It has also been referred to as the core link [11(p33)] because it transmits forces by linking the cranium to the sacrum. Influences such as trauma and postural strains that affect one part of the mechanism have been clinically observed to affect the entire unit of function.

Articular Mobility of Cranial Bones

Detailed study of the cranial sutures by Pritchard, Scott, and Girgis[11(p13)] demonstrated four layers of investing membrane between the bones. The recent series of research studies by S. Heisey and T. Adams has demonstrated quantitatively in the animal model that cranial bones move relative to each other[6,13] and that this movement contributes to a homeostatic mechanism: cranial compliance.[14] Retzlaff and associates confirmed the finding of several layers of tissue and found nerve fibers and blood vessels in the intervening space between bones.[15] These and a number of studies strongly support Dr. Sutherland's hypothesis that the cranial sutures are movable (Fig. 64.1).

Careful study of the design of the various articulations of the cranium and face and the RTM and its influence on the bones led Sutherland to an understanding of the mechanical design and relationship of the inherent motility of the CNS and CSF. At birth, the cranial bones are smooth-edged osseous plates with membrane and/or cartilage between them. With growth and motion the edges of the plates develop sutures between them that develop in a way that allows for a minimal amount of motion and yet provides protection for the brain.

Involuntary Mobility of Sacrum Between Ilia

The cranial dura is continuous with the spinal dura; the spinal dura extends through the vertebral canal into the sacral canal, attaching at the level of some lumbar segments and the second

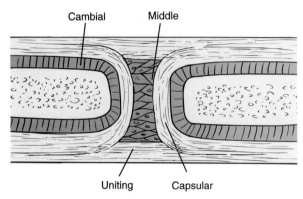

Cambial   Middle

Uniting   Capsular

Figure 64.1. Histology of cranial sutures. (Reprinted with permission from Magoun HI. *Osteopathy in the Cranial Field.* 2nd ed. Kirksville, Mo: Journal Printing Company; 1966.)

sacral segment. Careful study of the design of the articular surfaces reveals that the sacrum may move on one or several postural axes in relation to the ilia (pelvic bones). In addition to these voluntary or postural movements, the sacrum also responds to the inherent motility of the CNS, to the fluctuation of the CSF, and to the pull of the intracranial and intraspinal membranes with an involuntary movement that can be observed by palpation in the living body. This slight rocking motion occurs around a transverse axis (called the respiratory axis). Normally, the involuntary motion of the sacrum is synchronous with the involuntary motion of the occiput, each bone being influenced by the rhythmic pull of the spinal and cranial dura mater.

Try to visualize this physiologic unit of function with all five components moving slightly but steadily in the living body from before birth until death. Becker[16] summarized its influence on the total body economy thus:

Health requires that the PRM have the capacity to be an involuntary, rhythmic, automatic, shifting suspension mechanism for the intricate, integrated, dynamic interrelationships of its five elements. It is intimately related to the rest of the body through its fascial connections from the base of the skull through the cervical, thoracic, abdominal, pelvic, and appendicular areas of the body physiology. Since all of the involuntary and voluntary systems of the body, including the musculoskeletal system, are found in fascial envelopes, they, too, are subjected to the 10 to 14 cycle-per-minute rhythm of the craniosacral mechanism in addition to their own rhythms of involuntary and voluntary activity. The involuntary mobility of the craniosacral mechanism moves all the tissues of the body minutely into rhythmic flexion of the midline structures with external rotation of the bilateral structures and, in the opposite cycle, extension of the midline structures with internal rotation of the bilateral structures 10 to 14 times per minute throughout life.

MECHANICS OF PHYSIOLOGIC MOTION

The overall shape of the skull is that of a relative sphere with its inferior surface indented. The terminology used to describe the directions of motion of the various bones is similar to that

for the motions of the spine and extremities. Midline bones move through a flexion phase and an extension phase during their biphasic cycle. Paired bones move through external rotation and internal rotation during the cycle. The flexion phase of midline bones is simultaneous with external rotation of paired structures. The extension/internal rotation phase occurs reciprocally.

The sphenoid and occiput (midline bones) form the key articulation at the sphenobasilar symphysis (or synchondrosis) in the base of the skull. This is a cartilaginous union up to the age of 25 years and thereafter has the resiliency of cancellous bone.[17] This articulation is slightly convex on its superior surface. With flexion of this joint there is slight increase in this convexity. The motion of each midline bone occurs around a transverse axis. The other midline bones of the mechanism are the ethmoid, vomer, and sacrum. They are moved through the biphasic cycle in response to the pull or influence of the dural membranes that are influenced by the coiling and uncoiling of the CNS and the fluctuation of the CSF. The motion is initiated from within the living body and is referred to as inherent motion or involuntary motion.

The overall motion of the cranium is similar to the motion of the chest during respiration, but the two do not occur simultaneously. Thoracic respiration occurs 12–16 cycles per minute in adults and up to 44 cycles per minute in newborns[18]; motion of the PRM normally occurs 10–14 cycles per minute.[11(p25)] During flexion of the midline bones, palpation senses that the head widens slightly in its transverse diameter and shortens slightly in its anteroposterior diameter. The area where the coronal and sagittal sutures join, called bregma, descends. This widening occurs as the paired bones move toward external rotation.

With extension of the midline bones, the head narrows and lengthens slightly as the bregma ascends, and all paired bones move toward internal rotation. During the biphasic cycle, the osseous cranium changes shape slightly but its volume remains constant.

During flexion, the sacrum is influenced by the spinal dura and core link and moves posterosuperiorly at its base while the apex moves anteriorly toward the pubes. During extension, the base moves anteriorly and the apex moves posteriorly. This motion occurs around a transverse axis in the area of the second sacral segment posterior to the sacral canal and is called the respiratory axis of the sacrum. The other axes of sacral motion are postural axes (Fig. 64.2).

The inherent motion of the cranium is not visible but it is palpable. This motion is perceived as a subtle, soft, slight movement of fluid (CSF) and semifluid (CNS) inside an osseous case. The first attempts at this palpatory exercise may not reveal anything, or you may feel the subject's thoracic respiration transmitted through the neck to the head. If the breathing is a distraction, ask the patient to hold his or her breath for a moment. If you can still sense the rhythmic motion in the head, you know that the inherent motion is coming from within the cranium. With palpatory experience, you learn to distinguish between these different motions.

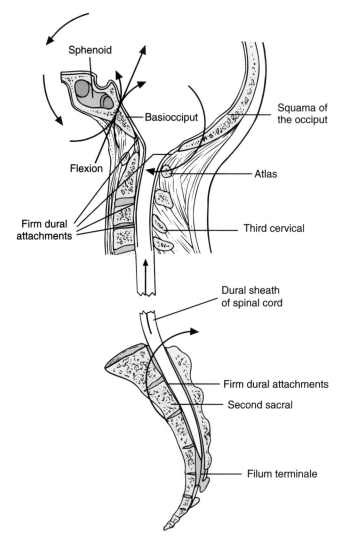

Figure 64.2. Craniosacral mechanism with arrows indicating direction of motion during flexion phase of physiologic motion. (Reprinted with permission from Magoun HI. *Osteopathy in the Cranial Field.* 2nd ed. Kirksville, Mo: Journal Printing Company; 1966.)

Follow these steps to palpate this rhythmic motion:

1. Position the patient supine, with the head 8–10 inches from the head of the table.
2. Sit comfortably at the head of the table with your forearms resting on the table and your hands placed on the sides of the patient's head. Have the patient move up or down on the table to comfortably accommodate to your relaxed posture.
3. Contact the patient's head lightly, allowing the fingers and part of the palms to gently conform to the curvature of the head. (It is essential that the palmar surface of all the fingers, not the thumbs, contact the head because the nerve endings that sense the subtle cranial motion are proprioceptors located in tendons and around joints. The numerous tactile sensors in the finger pads are not as receptive to this motion. Even though a gentle and light contact is essential, it is not a fingertip contact.)
4. Allow your mind to become quiet and direct your attention

to the space between your hands, allowing what is sensed by your proprioceptors to be perceived by your brain. (Continue to stay relaxed; do not try to feel something. If the patient's head has fairly normal motion, you may feel a slow, rhythmic "swelling" or widening followed by a "receding" or narrowing. This constitutes one cycle of inherent motion. This cycle is usually steadily repeated. The motion is so mild and subtle that it may actually feel as if the head is breathing.)

Subtle motion is easier for some physicians to palpate than for others. Some find this difficult to sense because they try too hard. Their intensity is so set, their effort so strong, that they block their own sensorium. It is essential to be relaxed, physically, mentally, and emotionally. Your attitude should be similar to one who is trying to hear a minor sound—complete attention is given to listening.

Keep the hand contact light. Pressure by the hands will suppress the inherent motion and/or distract the sensors (proprioceptors) in the hands. If excessive hand pressure is continued, the patient gets a headache.

If you have difficulty perceiving the motion in one patient, try other patients. The rate of this rhythmic motion and its amplitude (strength or power) usually varies from one individual to another.

The biphasic cycle of motion, the CRI, normally occurs 10–14 times per minute. When observing the rate, allow one full minute and count the number of cycles (one flexion phase plus one extension phase equals one complete cycle). Evaluating the amplitude of the CRI in patients who have clinical problems requires experience. After palpating 5 or 10 individuals, one can determine that the strength or vitality of the rhythm is stronger in one or two individuals, fair or medium in some, and weak or poor in others. With experience in palpation and clinical knowledge of the patient's history and symptoms, the rate and amplitude become an additional diagnostic indication of his or her state of health and is helpful in determining a prognosis.

The rate of CRI may be increased slightly:

Following vigorous physical exercise
With systemic fevers
Following effective OMT of the craniosacral mechanism

The rate may be decreased with:

Stress (mental, emotional, physical)
Chronic fatigue
Chronic infections
Mental depression and other psychiatric conditions[19]
Chronic poisoning
Other debilitating conditions

The CRI, originating within the PRM, is most evident to palpation in the head region but is palpable in every part of the body. The impulse moves longitudinally through the body and extremities, with midline structures moving through flexion/ extension and paired structures moving through external/internal rotation. Its presence or absence and its deviation from normal direction are useful diagnostic signs.

The body is subject to stresses and strains from before birth until death. Pressures and forces affect the developing fetus, the neonate during birth, and the individual through childhood, adolescence, and adulthood. These forces cause minor to major distortions of the cranium that result in strains of the sphenobasilar synchondrosis (SBS). With induced strain, the efficiency of the PRM is compromised. The compromise may be minor to major in its effect on the health of the individual.

STRAINS

There are several strains of the SBS.

Torsion occurs around an anterior-posterior (AP) axis of the skull that extends from nasion through the symphysis to opisthion (Fig. 64.3A). The sphenoid and related structures of the anterior cranium rotate in one direction about this axis; the occiput and related structures of the posterior cranium rotate in the opposite direction, producing a twist or torsion at the SBS. This strain is named for the side of the high wing of the sphenoid, right torsion (RT) or left torsion (LT).

Side-bending/rotation at the SBS occurs around an anteroposterior axis and around two parallel vertical axes, one through the body of the sphenoid and one through the foramen magnum, perpendicular to the physiologic transverse axes and the anteroposterior axis (Fig. 64.3B). This is a compound movement similar to physiologic motion in the spine when rotation and side-bending are concomitant movements. Because the sphenobasilar symphysis is slightly convex upwards, as the two bones side-bend away from each other (around the two parallel axes). both bones rotate inferiorly on the convex side (around the AP axis) and superiorly on the concave side. This strain pattern is named for the side of the convexity, SBR right (SBR_R) or SBR left (SBR_L). These four strain patterns (RT, LT, SBR_R, SBR_L) are common and are considered physiologic if their presence does not interfere with the flexion-extension motion of the mechanism.

Extreme or exaggerated flexion with decreased extension of the SBS is considered a strain pattern. Conversely, marked or exaggerated extension with decreased flexion is considered a strain pattern. Normally, the mechanism moves through the flexion and extension phases equally and fully.

Vertical and lateral strains or displacement occur at the SBS and can be superimposed on the above strains.

Vertical strain at the SBS is present when movement occurs in the same direction for the sphenoid and the occiput, around the two transverse axes (like flexion-extension) (Fig. 64.4A). This creates a superior or inferior strain at the SBS and disrupts normal flexion-extension. Vertical strain is named for the relative position of the basisphenoid, superior or inferior.

Lateral strain at SBS occurs when both bones rotate in the same direction, clockwise or counterclockwise, around two parallel vertical axes (Fig. 64.4B). Basisphenoid and basiocciput veer in opposite directions, producing a shearing type of resultant motion. When this strain occurs in utero or during

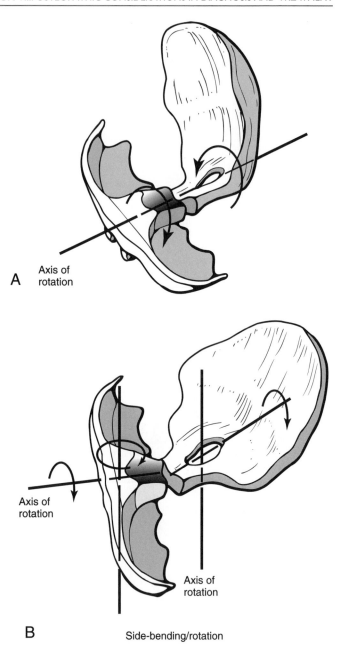

A Axis of rotation

B Side-bending/rotation

Torsion

Figure 64.3. Schematic patterns of sphenobasilar junction. In torsion and side-bending/rotation, sphenoid and occiput rotate in opposite directions about axes indicated. **A**, Torsion with great wing high on the right. Occiput is lower on the side of high great wing. **B**, Side-bending/rotation with convexity to the left. Both great wing of sphenoid and occiput are lower on the side of convexity. (Reprinted with permission from Sutherland WG, Wales AL. *Teachings in the Science of Osteopathy.* Portland, Oregon: Rudra Press; 1990.)

the birth process, it results in a parallelogram-shaped head in the infant. Lateral strain is named for the direction the basisphenoid shifts, right or left.

SBS compression is a strain in which the sphenoid and occiput have been forced together so that physiologic flexion-

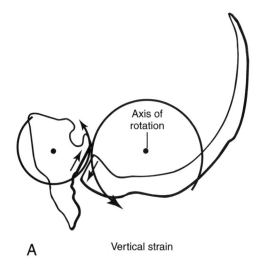

A   Vertical strain

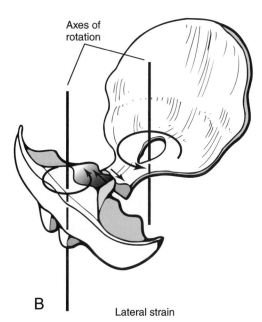

B   Lateral strain

Figure 64.4. Schematic patterns of sphenobasilar junction. In vertical and lateral strain patterns, sphenoid and occiput rotate in same direction around parallel axes. **A**, Superior vertical strain. As a result of bones' rotation, base of the sphenoid is relatively elevated with the base of occiput relatively depressed. **B**, Right lateral strain. As a result of bones' rotation, base of the sphenoid is relatively displaced to the right with the base of the occiput relatively displaced to the left. (Reprinted with permission from Sutherland WG, Wales AL. *Teachings in the Science of Osteopathy*. Portland, Oregon: Rudra Press; 1990.)

extension is impaired. Compression varies from mild to moderate to severe and occurs from a force to the back of the head, to the front of the head, or from a circumferential compression (as during birth) that exceeds the resiliency of the tissues.

Strains of the SBS involve the entire cranial and facial structure and influence the position and motion of the sacrum by way of the RTM. The midline bones and paired bones accommodate to the strain or strains in the base of the skull. Trauma

to the head, face, spine, sacrum, pelvis, or lower extremities is a common strain-producing factor. A strain in the base of the skull affects pelvic function or is accommodative to a strain in the pelvis. The body, including the head, truly functions as a unit.

PRINCIPLES OF DIAGNOSIS

The diagnosis of a pathologic condition or malfunction of the PRM is based on the history, observation, and palpation. Palpation by a well-trained and sensitive operator is the most reliable source of information.

Patient History

Taking the patient's history includes asking leading and pertinent questions to encourage the patient to recall relevant past events and to describe the complaint in some detail. In addition to the usual questions pertaining to heredity, childhood diseases, adult diseases, and surgeries, two other areas for questioning are pertinent to dysfunction of the craniosacral mechanism: trauma history and information about the delivery and newborn recovery period.

TRAUMA

Obtain the following information about trauma:

1. Age at which the trauma occurred; this includes birth trauma
2. Type of force as well as amount, velocity, direction, and the area of impact; vehicular accidents, blows to the face or head, and falls on the tail bone or buttocks are common
3. Dental history including extractions, orthodontia, malocclusion, bruxism, and temporomandibular joint problems
4. Fractures, concussions, inertial injuries, coma
5. Habitual head pressures such as sleeping positions, thumb sucking, ear phones, orthodontic head gear, new dentures, etc
6. Extremes of temperature: chilling of the face or head may precede Bell's palsy; heat stroke or sun stroke may be related to headache
7. Surgical procedures involving the head such as the mouth gag, the bite block, the bronchoscope or gastroscope, or the anesthetic mask held over the nose-mouth for prolonged periods with a tight headband to keep it in place
8. Changes in appearance or personality following severe trauma

Adult patients tend to recall only injuries of the recent past. They believe that injuries from infancy, childhood, or adolescence are of no importance and tend to forget past trauma. They may need leading questions to elicit this information. Some patients have amnesia related to trauma to the head and cannot relate accurate information. A family member may be able to give additional history.

HISTORY OF DELIVERY AND NEWBORN PERIOD

If the patient is an infant or child, a more detailed history from the parent(s) is essential. Questions concerning the health of the mother during pregnancy, the number and character of pregnancies, the details of the delivery, the appearance and action of the newborn, and the development of the infant should be asked. Signs and symptoms compatible with severe forces of labor and delivery are an indication for considering OMT in the care of these patients. These signs and symptoms include:

Distortion of the cranium
Excessive molding
Ridging or overriding along any suture
Difficulty in suckling or swallowing
Vomiting
Respiratory distress
Bradycardia
Tachycardia
Abnormal crying
Strabismus
Nystagmus
Spasticity or flaccidity of the limbs
Opisthotonos
Drowsiness
Cyanosis
Convulsions
Fever
Tremors

Abnormal habits such as lying with the head turned to one side only, head banging, or constant rubbing of the back of the head against the sheet are indicative of strains of the cranium.

Diagnosis by Observation

Look for symmetry or distortion of the osseous structure beneath the soft tissues. Observe the face and head: the shape and contours of the head and face show hereditary influences as well as the combined effect of the forces of labor on the bones. At birth the sphenoid, temporals, and occiput are made up of several osseous parts with cartilage between parts and between bones to allow for compression and molding of the head during birth. Strains within a bone may occur and are called intraosseous strains.

The flexion type of skull is round in shape with a wide transverse and a shortened AP diameter, with the temporals in relative external rotation (flared laterally). In this type of skull, the frontals are wide and sloping upward, the cheek bones are wide, and an open mouth view of the maxillary region of the hard palate reveals it to be wide and with a low arch to the vault. All paired structures are in a position of relative external rotation.

The extension type of skull is long and narrow with temporals in relative internal rotation, frontals narrow with the brow appearing more vertical, orbits and face narrow, and maxillae (hard palate) narrow with a high arched vault. All paired structures are in a position of relative internal rotation.

Note the positioning of the bones. The position of the sphenoid bone influences the position of the peripheral bones of the anterior cranium, which includes the frontals and all bones of the face except the mandible. The position of the occiput influences the position of the bones of the posterior cranium (the parietals and temporals) and in turn influences the position of the mandible.

With torsion and side-bending/rotation of the SBS, the facial structures tend to appear asymmetric as they assume a position of relative external rotation on the side of the high wing and a position of relative internal rotation on the low wing side. If the sphenoid is rotated on an AP axis, the eyes and orbits will appear unlevel. Compare the relative positions of the cheek bones and the maxillae.

Note the relative positioning of landmarks. It is sometimes difficult to determine if the occiput has rotated on the AP axis because it is hidden by hair. As the occiput tilts on this axis, it carries the temporals with it. The temporal on the low side of the occiput is positioned toward relative external rotation, and the temporal on the high side of the occiput is positioned toward relative internal rotation. Therefore, the relative position of the ears gives an indication of the tilt of the occiput. Compare right and left ear lobes to see if they are level; note flaring of the ears. A temporal positioned toward external rotation tends to be more flared; a temporal positioned toward internal rotation tends to be more flat. By combining the findings of the anterior and posterior cranium, the observer is able to arrive at a tentative or working diagnosis of torsion or side-bending/rotation of the SBS.

Viewing the midline of the face, noting the nose, mouth, and center of the chin, provides additional information. Nasal deviation may indicate the relative position of the maxillae and sphenoid or may indicate past trauma or fracture. The chin (mandible) tends to deviate to the side of the externally rotated temporal bone. Heredity also influences facial characteristics and is a significant consideration for establishing a prognosis.

Strains of the cranial base occur during birth or from trauma. If trauma is induced into a prior strain pattern, the findings of observation are not reliable for diagnosis.

Diagnosis by Palpation

To become expert at the art of palpation for diagnosis and treatment requires repeated experience, patience, and perseverance. These guidelines help improve palpatory skill:

1. Use a light hand contact. If your contact is stronger than the force of the inherent motion, you interfere with the mechanism you are attempting to diagnose or treat. Do not interject yourself into the patient's mechanism.
2. Have a clear visualization of the structure(s) beneath your hands. This requires a detailed study of the anatomy and physiologic motion of each of the bones of the body, including the cranium and face. The design of the articulations between bones and their mechanical and physiologic relationship is a complex study, but it is essential to providing accurate diagnosis and successful treatment. (Space does not permit such detailed study in this chapter.)
3. Understand that the job of the physician is to assist the patient

to obtain or maintain optimal health. The physician does not do the healing; healing comes from within the patient. With knowledge and experience, one learns to tune in to and be guided by the PRM of the patient to facilitate this healing process, assisting the patient's own inherent healing capacity to release biomechanical impediments. The automatic processes that promote healing are much more intelligent and efficient in the management of the health of the individual than any external force or person can be.

CLINICAL PROBLEMS REQUIRING OSTEOPATHIC MANIPULATIVE TREATMENT

Neonatal

OMT of infants and children can be a rewarding experience for the patient and the doctor. Children respond to treatment faster than do adults.

Compromised function of the PRM is a cumulative process beginning in utero or during birth, plus the various traumatic incidents of growing up, plus one or more traumatic events as an adult. The physician must keep this in mind when taking the history.

Consideration of the trauma of the birth process deserves further explanation. The base of the skull is formed in cartilage and the vault is formed in membrane. At birth, the sphenoid is in three parts, the temporal is in three parts, and the occiput is in four parts, with cartilage intervening between the osseous elements.[20(p107–111)] The frontal and mandible are in two parts and each maxilla is in two parts. This is nature's way of protecting the CNS and providing for compressibility of the head as it passes through the birth canal. The bones of the vault are osseous plates that overlap at the edges. The cartilaginous base tends to compress, bend, twist, or buckle depending on the amount and direction of compression and rotational forces of labor and birth. These various parts are vulnerable to misalignment; the brain, cranial nerves, and intracranial membranes are subject to possible injury or malfunction. One or more of the strain patterns of the SBS generally has its beginning during the birth process (Figs. 64.5 and 64.6).

The infant's first breath and subsequent crying with deep breathing, kicking, squirming, and suckling assist with decompression of the cranium, face, and pelvis.[20(p114–115)] If the activities of the neonate are not strong enough to open up the entire PRM to its optimal function, these neonates benefit from the assistance of an osteopathic physician trained in the cranial concept and in treatment procedures. Examination and treatment are best given during the first few days of life, at which time a great deal is accomplished by releasing the compressive forces of birth. If no treatment is provided, as time passes and growth progresses, the strains become more established. In time, the formative parts of the various bones of the base change from cartilage to osseous tissue. If overlapping of the osseous plates of the vault is allowed to remain, the plates grow together, forming a synostosis. When synostosis pervades the vault, the osseous case cannot grow and expand at the same rate as the brain inside, and the brain function of that individ-

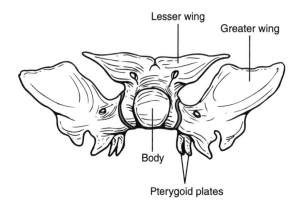

Figure 64.5. Sphenoid at birth in three parts. Cartilage intervenes between body-lesser wing unit and greater wing-pterygoid units. (Reprinted with permission from Sutherland WG, Wales AL. *Teachings in the Science of Osteopathy.* Portland, Oregon; Rudra Press; 1990.)

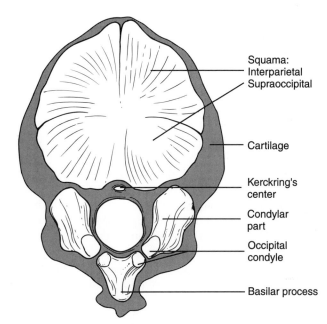

Figure 64.6. Occiput at birth in four parts within a cartilaginous matrix. Articular condyles receive contributions from both condylar and basilar parts of the occiput. (Reprinted with permission from Sutherland WG, Wales AL. *Teachings in the Science of Osteopathy.* Portland, Oregon; Rudra Press; 1990.)

ual is compromised. Expert treatment given early in the life of an individual can be one of the most important therapeutic measures in preventive medicine. Treatment given later is beneficial, but more can be accomplished in less time and with less effort and expense if treatment is given soon after the stresses and strains occur.

An example of disturbance of function directly related to the compressive forces of birth concerns the posterior part of the cranial base. The four parts of the developing occiput are the:

Basilar process
Two condylar parts along the lateral sides of foramen magnum
Squama extending from the posterior border of the foramen magnum to the lambdoid suture

The medulla oblongata rests on the basilar part, and the spinal cord extends through the space within the four parts. The ninth, tenth, and eleventh cranial nerves and the jugular veins pass through the jugular foramina at the anterolateral border of each condylar part. The twelfth cranial nerves pass through the anterior condylar canals located within the condylar parts near the junction between the condylar parts and basilar part. Compression with rotation of the posterior cranium during birth with distortion, displacement, and jamming of these four osseous plates and intervening cartilage is easily visualized (Fig. 64.6). The symptoms manifested in the newborn or young infant that indicate the presence of abnormal mechanical stress in this area include:

Respiratory distress
Excessive crying
Inability to suckle or weak suckling
Vomiting
Bradycardia
Tachycardia
Tremors
Spasticity or flaccidity of the limbs
Cyanosis
Torticollis

This abnormal mechanical stress on the brainstem, cranial nerves, and venous drainage is treated by gentle application of mild, sustained spreading of the formative parts of the base of the skull by a physician trained to apply OMT in this manner.

The relative position and motion of the temporal bones affect drainage from the middle ear through the pharyngotympanic tube; their somatic dysfunction is clinically capable of resulting in tinnitus, dizziness, and decreased hearing. Treatment is aimed at releasing membranous strains of the cranial base, temporal bones, and upper cervical spine to help reestablish equal and synchronous motion to the temporals as well as the entire mechanism. Consider these factors:

1. Without normal motion present, stasis of fluids and lack of oxygen provides an ideal medium for microorganisms
2. When the inherent motion throughout the cranium and face is optimal, the movement of fluids and mucus is enhanced (a provision of nature for emptying the ethmoid, sphenoid, and maxillary sinuses)
3. The autonomic nerve supply to the nasal mucosa by way of the sphenopalatine ganglion is vulnerable to impinging adnexa
4. Middle ear infections, sinusitis, pharyngitis, and other acute inflammatory processes are frequently associated with altered cranial functions[21]

Vascular Supply

Consider the vascular supply to the brain. The internal carotid arteries enter the petrous portions of the temporal bones, extend forward and medially within those bones, exit from the tips of the petrous, and turn superiorly along the sides of the basisphenoid to enter the cranial cavity. Disturbance in physiologic motion in which the petrous portion of the temporal articulates with the basiocciput and the basisphenoid compromises the optimal function of these arteries through related dural tension. The vascular interchange between the choroid plexus and the CSF (occurring within the ventricles of the brain) is affected by the widening and narrowing of the ventricles, which occurs with each rhythmic motion of the PRM.

The venous drainage from the brain is by way of the various intracranial veins emptying into the venous sinuses, which are channels between layers of dura mater. The great cerebral vein enters the straight sinus, which joins the transverse sinus to become the sigmoid sinus. That sinus becomes the jugular vein, which passes through the jugular foramen to exit the skull. The jugular foramen is an aperture between the occiput and temporal bones. Ninety-five percent of the venous blood from the brain exits the skull through these two apertures.[11(p20)] This area is extremely vulnerable to trauma to the back or side of the head. Impaired venous drainage leads to venous stasis. The movement of venous blood along the various venous sinuses directly depends on the biphasic motion of the RTM and the bones to which it attaches.[21(p129–131)] Consider venous stasis as a causative factor for headache, decreased cerebral function, and depression.

The pituitary body is located in the sella turcica on the superior surface of the sphenoid bone just anterior to the SBS. This neuroendocrine gland, an extension of the brain, secretes a number of hormones that affect all the glands of the endocrine system. A reduplication of dura, the diaphragma sella, encircles the stalk of the pituitary like a collar. The hormones secreted by the pituitary pass into the vascular plexus surrounding it. Pituitary function is compromised if the inherent motility of the CNS or the movement of blood through the cranial vascular system is impaired.[5(p36)]

The dura mater lines the skull and spinal canal, and extensions of it continue beyond the various apertures as the sheaths of the cranial and spinal nerves. Entrapment neuropathy describes the localized injury or irritation to nervous tissue from the mechanical effect of impinging adnexa. There are multiple examples[21–23] of entrapment of cranial and spinal nerves and their branches throughout the body, all of which are amenable to osteopathic treatment by releasing membranous and/or ligamentous articular strains.

The interstitial fluids of the entire body are constantly influenced by the biphasic rhythm of the PRM. This movement of fluids is slow, steady, and efficient even at the cellular level with the exchange of metabolites across the cell membrane. In that sense, the CNS functions as a pump. Sutherland compared this fluid motion in the body to the tide of the ocean.[11(pp31–34,172–174)] It is a major factor in the repair of damaged tissue from contusions, sprains, strains, and inflammatory processes.[11(pp35,188)] A knowledge of the PRM and its effects on the health of the total being broadens our understanding of the self-healing and self-regulatory mechanisms taught by Dr. Still.

Trauma

Trauma is by far the major cause of disruption and malfunction of the PRM. The force of the trauma is extreme in vehicular accidents. The force from a fall is transmitted from the feet or ischial tuberosities upward through the body into the base of the skull. The vector of force established through the body or head is palpable[24–25] and is an important diagnostic sign. The direction of motion of the CSF and CNS is disrupted, and the function of the PRM is mildly to severely impaired, depending on the severity of the trauma and the response of the patient.

Trauma to the PRM can occur from mild, sustained force such as wearing a spring type of headset or from orthodontic appliances on the teeth[26]; wearing a tight hat or swim cap will augment or create or alter existing patterns. Trauma occurs in various degrees and in innumerable forms.

The PRM functions as a unit; trauma to one area affects the entire RTM. The mechanism does its best to continue to function, but the quality of that function decreases with the passage of time and additional trauma. The rate and amplitude of the CRI is a most valuable diagnostic and prognostic indicator of the severity of the compromise and response to treatment.[27] A slow rate and a low amplitude are dependable indicators of a long-standing and/or overwhelming problem during which the patient's vitality has been depleted, indicating more treatment over a longer period of time will be required.[27] The reciprocal is also true. In the course of treatment, improvement is associated with a rate and amplitude increase toward normal.

Dentistry

Osteopathy in the cranial field is especially pertinent to the practice of complete dentistry.[28] Improperly directed forces of extraction, fillings, setting of crowns, and improperly fitted dentures alter the occlusion of maxillary and mandibular teeth and disturb the PRM.[29] Resultant symptoms include:

Headaches
Vertigo with its attendant gastrointestinal symptoms
Cervical syndromes
TMJ dysfunction syndrome

Clinical enigmas of the head and neck (such as atypical facial pain) require evaluation of dental problems and the effects of dental procedures and orthotics on the PRM.[30] Satisfactory therapeutic response depends on evaluation and treatment by both the dentist and the osteopathic physician.

PRINCIPLES OF TREATMENT

The aim of treatment, as with any osteopathic procedure, is to normalize structure and function. The optimal function of the PRM affects not only the CNS but also every cell and tissue

in the body. Regardless of which method or procedure a physician elects to use, this constant rhythmic motion is at work behind the scenes every minute of every hour of every day of every year of the life of the individual.

Goals of Treatment

The goals of treatment include:

Normalizing nerve function, including all cranial and spinal nerves as well as the autonomic nervous system
Counteracting stress-producing factors by normalizing function of the cerebrum, thalamus, hypothalamus, and pituitary body
Eliminating circulatory stasis by normalizing arterial, venous, and lymphatic channels
Normalizing CSF fluctuation
Releasing membranous tension
Correcting or resolving cranial articular strains
Modifying gross structural patterns

Some hindrances to treatment are myofascial strains from below the cranium or the sacrum, local or general infections, nutritional deficiencies, and organic poisons.[11(p99)] Removal of nonstructural hindrances must be addressed as well as OMT in the management of the patient's health problems. To use the power or potency of the inherent activity of the PRM within the patient to assist with the release of strains (somatic dysfunctions), it is necessary to understand balanced ligamentous tension and balanced membranous tension. Balanced ligamentous tension is used in treating any articulation supported and protected by ligaments. Balanced membranous tension refers to the dura mater (RTM) and is used to treat the articulations of the cranium, face, and sacrum.

The point of balanced membranous tension is defined as that point in the range of motion of an articulation where the membranes are poised between the normal tension present throughout the free range of motion and the increased tension preceding the strain or fixation that occurs as a joint is carried beyond its normal physiologic range.[11(p99)] Thus, it is the most neutral position possible under the influence of all the factors responsible for the existing pattern, all attendant tensions having been reduced to the absolute minimum.

This point is unique for each strain that occurs. It is the point at which the inherent force can move through the involved tissues at its maximum efficiency. The operator seeks to position the bones making up the articulation at the point of balanced membranous tension by keen, sensitive, knowledgeable palpation. Dr. Sutherland expressed this as palpating "with seeing, feeling, thinking, knowing fingers."

Figure 64.7 illustrates arriving at the point of balanced membranous tension by positioning the components. The squares indicate two bones making up an articulation, and the arrows represent the directions the operator employs for positioning.[11(p100–101)]

Figure 64.7A illustrates indirect action or exaggeration. This procedure is commonly employed from the age of 5 through

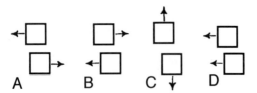

Figure 64.7. Methods for arriving at the point of balanced membranous tension. **A**, Indirect action (exaggeration). **B**, Direct action. **C**, Disengagement. **D**, Opposite physiologic motion. (Reprinted with permission from Magoun HI. *Osteopathy in the Cranial Field.* 2nd ed. Kirksville, Mo: Journal Printing Company; 1966.)

adulthood. It is not used in acute trauma to the head when exaggeration of misalignment may produce or increase intracranial hemorrhage. To employ this method, increase the abnormal relationship at the joint by moving the articulation slightly in the direction toward which it was lesioned.

Figure 64.7B illustrates direct action. This treatment method is employed when exaggeration is not desirable, as in acute trauma and in young children in whom the sutural pattern has not yet developed. This treatment is also used when there are overriding sutures. The components are gently guided back toward their normal position.

Figure 64.7C illustrates disengagement. This treatment method is used when the osseous components have become impacted by force or excessive membranous tension. Disengagement technique merely separates the opposing surfaces within the anatomic and physiologic limits of permitted motion.

Figure 64.7D illustrates opposite physiologic motion. This method is seldom used, but when needed it is employed to release a strain when a traumatic force has severely violated the physiologic pattern. One component is influenced by direct action; the other is influenced by indirect action.

The physician selects the method of choice according to the patient's age and history, as well as by palpatory diagnosis.

Respiratory cooperation may be used to enhance the effort of inherent motion. The patient is asked to hold his or her breath in full inhalation or exhalation after the physician has positioned the articulation at balanced ligamentous or membranous tension. Holding the breath at full inhalation is more commonly used, but if the articulation is held toward extension or internal rotation, holding the breath at full exhalation is more effective.

EXAMPLE ONE

An example of treatment follows.

Diagnosis

Somatic dysfunction of the midcervical spine (C4 E R_R S_R).

Treatment

Indirect method, using balanced ligamentous tension, exaggeration, and inherent force.

Procedure

1. Position the patient supine.
2. Sit at the head of the table.
3. Place the finger pads of the two index fingers at the lateral border of the articular pillars of C5, with the long (third) finger pads at the articular pillars of C4. This gives you optimum contact for precise positioning of the two bones and for maximum sensing of the soft tissues over the articulation.
4. Slowly and gently position the two segments so that C4 is sidebent right, rotated right, and slightly extended to the point of balanced ligamentous tension. Note that the tension on the involved muscles and ligaments eases, softens, and cannot be perceived as tension. The joint is not in physiologic neutral, but is in neutral for this ligamentous strain in all three planes.
5. Maintain this position and allow the inherent force to work. Keep your sensing apparatus alert so that it perceives the slow rhythmic movement of the PRM. This movement feels like a longitudinal ebb and flow or a subtle pumping effect up and down the spine.
6. Continue to maintain the positioning and to observe this rhythmic motion; the inherent force is working through the tissues that are maintaining the somatic dysfunction. As they accomplish their task for this articulation at this time, the amplitude of the inherent rhythm lessens and the pumping decreases, and the tissues beneath your palpating fingers seem to soften or melt.
7. At that time, cease to hold the articulation in the treatment position. Gently recheck the motion of the articulation to ascertain the therapeutic response. Physiologic motion is restored to varying degrees.

A strain of the cranial base can be treated using the inherent forces and positioning for balanced membranous tension of the reciprocal tension membranes. This technique is applicable for an uncomplicated strain of the SBS. If a strain of the cranial base is complicated by additional traumatic strains such as a frontosphenoidal or occipitomastoid strain, the technique as described will probably not be successful. The complicating strains from induced trauma are treated before treating the sphenobasilar strain.

EXAMPLE TWO

Diagnosis

Somatic dysfunction of the sphenobasilar symphysis is sidebending/rotation right (SBS is SBR_R).

The sphenoid and occiput have rotated on an AP axis so that the right side of the cranium is relatively inferior (caudad) and the left side relatively superior (cephalad). Concomitant with that position, the greater sphenoid wing and the lateral angle of the occiput on the right side are slightly spread and the greater sphenoid wing and the lateral angle of the left occiput are slightly approximated.

Treatment

Indirect method, balanced membranous tension, with exaggeration and inherent forces to balance the RTM.

Procedure

1. Position the patient supine.
2. Sit at the head of the table.
3. Place your hands on the lateral sides of the patient's head with the index fingers contacting the greater wings of the sphenoid and the little fingers contacting the lateral angles of the occiput (vault contact).
4. Gently palpate the rhythmic activity of the patient's PRM and RTM.
5. The right hand slowly moves slightly caudad with index and fifth fingers spreading slightly while the left hand moves slightly cephalad and fingers approximate slightly. This positioning is slight and must be accurate, being guided by the ease of tension in the membranes within the cranium. With the ease of membranous tension, the inherent forces begin to manifest with increased vigor. The amplitude of the CRI automatically increases.
6. Maintain the positioning and carefully and continuously observe the increased activity of the inherent forces at work within the patient's mechanism. As the inherent forces work through the membranous strain, they gradually cease the increased activity and become quiet. This cessation of the inherent rhythm is called a still point.[20]
7. After the still point occurs, cease to maintain the positioning of the bones and membranes and continue to observe the fluctuant activity by light palpation. The quiet period passes, the rhythmic fluctuation resumes, increasing slowly and steadily in amplitude until it has returned to a more normal flexion-extension of the SBS.
8. Gently remove your hands.

Treatment procedures of the cranium should be used only by physicians experienced with palpation of the subtle activity of the PRM. Guidance by a physician experienced with the function of the PRM and the inherent forces is essential to learning this technique.

CONCLUSION

Much research remains to demonstrate the exact mechanisms involved in craniosacral dysfunction and recovery. However, more than 50 years of clinical experience has indicated that the use of osteopathy in the cranial field has given relief to many patients in whom no other treatment was effective.

REFERENCES

1. Sutherland AS. *With Thinking Fingers.* Indianapolis, Ind: Cranial Academy. Originally printed by Journal Printing Company, Kirksville, Mo 1962:12–13.
2. Northrup GW, ed. *Osteopathic Research: Growth and Development.* Chicago, Ill: American Osteopathic Association; 1987:40.
3. DiGiovanna EL, Schiowitz S. *Osteopathic Approach to Diagnosis and Treatment.* New York, NY: JB Lippincott; 1991.
4. Greenman PE. *Principles of Manual Medicine.* Baltimore, Md: Williams & Wilkins; 1991.
5. Kuchera ML, Kuchera WA. *Osteopathic Considerations in Systemic Dysfunction.* 2nd ed; revised 1994. Columbus, Ohio: Greyden Press; 1994.
6. Heisey SR, Adams T. Effects of cranial bone mobility on cranial compliance. In Thirty-sixth annual AOA Research Conference Abstracts, 1992, part 2. *JAOA.* October 1992;92(9):1284.
7. Heisey SR, Adams T, Smith MC, Briner B. The role of cranial suture compliance in defining intracranial pressure. In: Thirty-seventh Annual AOA Research Conference Abstracts, 1993, part 2. *JAOA.* September 1993;93(9):951.
8. Norton JM, Sibley G, Broder-Oldach RE. Quantification of the cranial rhythmic impulse in human subjects. In: Thirty-sixth Annual AOA Research Conference Abstracts, 1992, part 2. *JAOA.* October 1992;92(9):1285.
9. Sibley G, Broder-Oldach E, Norton JM. Inter-examiner agreement in the characterization of the cranial rhythmic impulse. In: Thirty-sixth Annual AOA Research Conference Abstracts, 1992, part 2. *JAOA.* October 1992;92(9):1285.
10. Norton JM. Failure of a tissue pressure model to predict cranial rhythmic impulse frequency. In: Thirty-sixth Annual AOA Research Conference Abstracts, 1992, part 2. *JAOA.* October 1992; 92(9):1285.
11. Magoun HI. *Osteopathy In The Cranial Field.* 2nd ed. Kirksville, Mo: Journal Printing Company; 1966.
12. *Dorland's Illustrated Medical Dictionary.* 26th ed. Philadelphia, Penn: WB Saunders Company; 1981.
13. Adams T, Heisey SR, Smith MC, Briner BJ. Parietal bone mobility in the anesthetized cat. *JAOA.* 1992;92:599–622.
14. Heisey SR, Adams T. Role of cranial bone mobility in cranial compliance. *Neurosurgery.* 1993;33:869–877.
15. Retzlaff EW, Michael D, Roppel R, Mitchell F. The structures of cranial bone sutures. *JAOA.* 1976;75:607–608.
16. Becker RE. Craniosacral trauma in the adult. *Osteopath Ann.* 1976; 4:43–59.
17. Williams PL, Warwick R, Dyson M, Bannister LH. *Gray's Anatomy.* 37th ed. Edinburgh: Churchill Livingstone; 1988.
18. Bates B. *A Guide to Physical Examination.* 3rd ed. Philadelphia, Penn: JB Lippincott; 1983:149.
19. Woods RH. A physical finding related to psychiatric disorders. *JAOA.* August 1961;60:988–993.
20. Sutherland WG, Wales AL. *Teachings in the Science of Osteopathy.* Portland, Oregon: Rudra Press; 1990.
21. Magoun HI. Entrapment neuropathy in the cranium. *JAOA.* February 1968;67:643–652.
22. Magoun HI. Entrapment neuropathy of the central nervous system, Part II. *JAOA.* March 1968;67:779–787.
23. Magoun HI. Entrapment neuropathy of the central nervous system, Part III. *JAOA.* April 1968;67:889–899.
24. Magoun HI. Whiplash injury: A greater lesion complex. *JAOA.* February 1964;63:524–535.
25. Harakal JH. An osteopathically integrated approach to the whiplash complex. *JAOA.* June 1975;74:941–955.
26. Lay EM. In: Gelb H, ed. *Clinical Management of Head, Neck and TMJ Pain and Dysfunction.* Philadelphia, Penn: WB Saunders Company; 1977;17.
27. Becker RE. *Lecture: Sutherland Cranial Teaching Foundation Basic Course.* Colorado Springs; 1985.
28. Magoun HI. Dental equilibration and osteopathy. *JAOA.* June 1975; 74:981–991.
29. Magoun HI. Osteopathic approach to dental enigmas. *JAOA.* October 1962;62:110–118.
30. Magoun HI. The dental search for a common denominator in craniocervical pain and dysfunction. *JAOA.* July 1979:78.

65. Myofascial Trigger Points

AN INTRODUCTION

MICHAEL L. KUCHERA AND JOHN M. McPARTLAND

Key Concepts

- **Difference between tender points and trigger points**

- **Descriptions of significant or complete overlap between two types of myofascial points**

- **Physiologic mechanisms that have been described as causes of referred pain from trigger points**

- **Role of posture in forming trigger points**

Myofascial structures make up the largest organ system in the body, constituting approximately half of the body's mass. Somatic dysfunction affecting this system has far-reaching implications in the diagnosis and treatment of:

Pain syndromes
Disability
Disrupted visceral homeostasis
Reduced muscle functions

Myofascial points are only one manifestation of somatic dysfunction in this system, but they provide significant osteopathic insights. Knowing how to diagnose, interpret, and treat myofascial points as a form of somatic dysfunction provides a better understanding of the osteopathic perspective. It expands our interpretation of structure–function relationships and offers possible mechanisms for treatment of other somatic tissues. It also enhances our clinical diagnostic and treatment skills. In return, osteopathic medicine continues to contribute greatly to the documentation, interpretation, and treatment of myofascial tender points and trigger points.

TENDER POINTS VERSUS TRIGGER POINTS

Myofascial points have certain common clinical characteristics. All are subjectively tender[1(p.24)] with moderate to deep palpation, and all are characterized and recognized as palpably small, circumscribed, hypersensitive myofascial thickenings. Often they are associated with local or referred autonomic disturbances.[1(p.25), 2] They may exhibit localized tenderness alone, or they may also have a referred pain pattern to a reference zone that may or may not have a neurologic distribution. The term "trigger point"[1(p.4)] as described by Janet Travell is usually reserved for any myofascial point that refers pain in a certain predictable distribution. The system described by Lawrence Jones, associated with locally tender myofascial points that do not refer pain beyond the location being pressed, is described in Chapter 58. Simons[3] describes a significant overlap in location between tender points and trigger points. Chaitow[4] believes their distinction is arbitrary. He notes that tender points can develop referral capabilities by the simple introduction of a chill or strain to the affected muscle. Similarly, Bennett[5] suggests that tender points become trigger points as a result of enhanced pain perception in patients.

Mapping

Throughout the history of medicine, tender points have been observed and mapped in the myofascial tissues. In addition to their prominence in ancient eastern systems such as Chinese acupuncture and southeast Asian Ayurveda,[6] various western physicians have also correlated palpable myofascial points with patient histories and their accompanying symptoms and have described a number of modern myofascial point systems. Unfortunately, this has made the medical literature extremely confusing. Only recently has there been a serious attempt to agree on consistent terminology. Generally accepted definitions of commonly used terms have been coined and/or redefined since 1975. These include:

Fibrositis
Fibromyalgia
Overuse syndrome
Chronic fatigue syndrome
Repetitive strain injury

When reading different authors on these subjects, one must take care to heed publication dates, definitions, and authors' perspectives to interpreting information.

While many of these myofascial terms and systems have overlapping characteristics, they also have unique factors[1(p.21)] related to the perspective and philosophy of the physician mapping them. Some clinicians have correlated tender points and trigger points with visceral pathology. Head[7] and Mackenzie,[8] both in 1893, associated dermal and myofascial tender points with internal pathology. Twenty years later, Fitzgerald[9] described a series of points on the extremities reflecting activity elsewhere in the body. Owens[10] recorded a number of points now referred to as Chapman's viscerosomatic reflexes (see

Chapter 67) in recognition of the osteopathic physician, Frank Chapman, who first delineated them in the 1920s. Dicke[11] correlated visceral or systemic diseases with altered skin tissue, which occurs in "zones" rather than points.

Treatment

Myofascial points have been treated in a number of ways. Chinese physicians have addressed these points with acupuncture for thousands of years. Needles unearthed from Stone Age dwellings were made of sharp rocks; now they are made of stainless steel and are disposable. Many western clinicians are impressed with acupuncture as a modality. Some osteopathic physicians use acupuncture as a way of achieving osteopathic goals. A less invasive Chinese technique, acupressure, uses digital pressure over points instead of needles. This technique resembles Chapman's treatment of reflex points. It also resembles manual inhibition and the massage techniques advocated by Travell to treat trigger points. The Japanese honed this to a fine art, calling it shiatsu.

Several European allopathic physicians who now practice in the United States have adopted osteopathic techniques and given them new names. Lewit, a Czech physiatrist, renamed muscle energy technique as "post-isometric relaxation." Although Lewit freely acknowledges his debt to osteopathic physicians,[12] Travell, Simons, and many others refer to this technique as "Lewit technique," ignoring its osteopathic heritage. "Gaymans-Lewit technique" is another European variation, owing its name to Gaymans, a Dutch physician who studied under osteopathic physicians in New York.[13]

CAUSATION

Central Nervous System

The central nervous system plays an integrating role in the causation and maintenance of the myofascial point phenomenon. This view is consistent with Korr's observations[14] that the spine can be viewed as an "organizer" of disease and dysfunctional processes. Many direct stimuli are capable of initiating trigger points with distinct pain reference zones. Initiation is even more likely when indirect stimuli "facilitate"

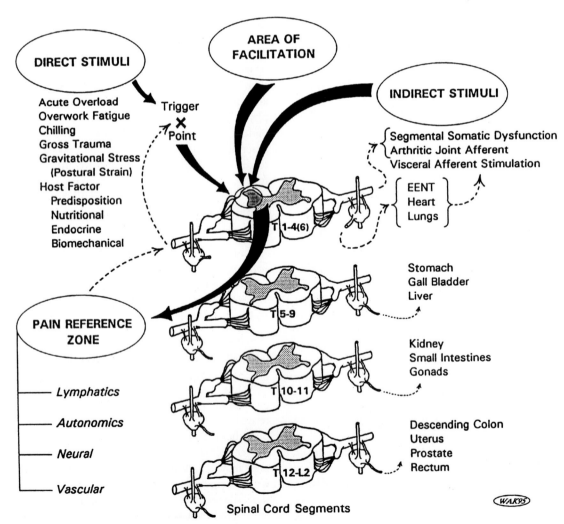

Figure 65.1. Spinal cord as "neurologic lens" for variety of stressors to initiate somatic and/or visceral symptoms.

segmentally related levels. Conversely, trigger points are capable of facilitating the cord with somatic afferent stimuli. Resultant neural, lymphatic, and vascular changes affect segmentally related viscera and are a source of somatic palpatory clues. The central integration of afferent data with predictable modification of efferent responses is one neurologic model used to explain somatic dysfunction, myofascial points, referred pain, and a number of reflexes between the soma, the viscera, and the sympathetic systems. Regardless of the specific model, however, there is agreement that the spinal cord behaves as a "neurologic lens" for a variety of stressors to initiate somatic and/or visceral symptoms (Fig. 65.1).

A role for the central nervous system is also included in the explanation of trigger points proposed by Travell and Simons.[15(pp.1,15)] Several physiologic mechanisms[16,17(pp.1,31)] related to central nervous system integration have been postulated to explain these myofascial points and their relationship to dysfunction and/or pain referred elsewhere in the body. The most frequent explanations for referral from trigger points are:

1. Convergence–projection
2. Convergence–facilitation
3. Activity of the sympathetic nervous system
4. Convergence or image projection at the supraspinal level
5. Axon branching in a subpopulation of primary afferent nociceptive nerves

The first and fifth mechanisms relate to the structure of the nervous system, while the others relate to functional factors. The fifth mechanism is peripheral; the others are central.

Physiologic Mechanisms

Local conditions resulting from, or accompanying, the development of myofascial points have been studied.[18] A summary of these factors is proposed in Figure 65.2. Both sympathetic and biochemical processes enter into the physiology of the tissues in the region of a myofascial point, altering somatic and other parameters. Palpatory findings in the area of a myofascial point include an alteration of cutaneous temperature and humidity. There is a small nodular or spindle-shaped thickening of the tissues representing the myofascial point itself. The point is extremely tender to the patient and usually invokes a generalized jump sign or some other patent response of discomfort. In the case of myofascial trigger points, there is a local twitch of the taut muscle band containing the point when the muscle is palpated perpendicular to its long axis. There may be localized goose flesh or trophic changes at the site. Physiologically, there appears to be local metabolic crisis in the presence of impaired circulation, a factor that leads to tissue texture abnormalities. These aid in finding the point by palpation.

Studies further suggest that palpatory tenderness is increased by intrinsic tissue sensitizing substances, including[18]:

Bradykinins
Serotonin
Histamine
Potassium

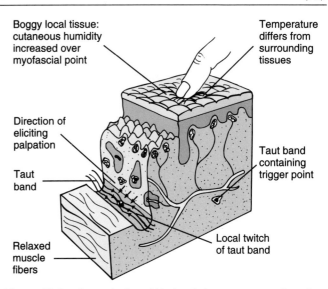

Figure 65.2. Sympathetic and biochemical processes enter into physiology of tissues in region of myofascial point, altering somatic and other parameters.

Prostaglandins
Substance-P
Leukotrienes

Branching axon subpopulations, as well as local microtrauma and/or macrotrauma, lead to a more widespread release of these substances. They are important factors in the causation of myofascial points. Somatic dysfunction, which alters the local biochemical milieu and prevents removal of these sensitizing substances, is also significant. The sympathetics have recently been shown to play a major role in maintenance of trigger points.[19]

Regardless of the exact mechanism or mechanisms involved, afferent information to the central nervous system from both somatic and visceral structures figures prominently in the proposed origin of myofascial points. In the Travell system, overuse of somatic structures, especially chilled muscle, is most often implicated in myofascial point development,[1(p.52–53)] while primary visceral dysfunction related to facilitated segments is more frequently associated with Chapman's reflex points.[20] Travell and Simons also note the association of segmentally related visceral dysfunction in the initiation and/or perpetuation of trigger points.[1(p.15)] Proponents of Chapman's points recognize the importance of segmentally related somatic dysfunction[21] in the interpretation and treatment of that myofascial point system. Jones relates tender points to a hypertonic state of a strained muscle's antagonist, and to segmentally related visceral dysfunction.

Posture

Posture is also prominently implicated in the formation of both Chapman's reflexes and Travell's trigger points. Jones relates strained muscles and their tender points to abnormal postures. Myofascial structures are constantly working to maintain postural homeostasis within the pervasive influence of gravity.

Continuous postural strain has been charged by numerous authors[1,22–26] with precipitating and/or perpetuating myofascial points and other manifestations of somatic dysfunction. Furthermore, patients with crossover points secondary to postural factors have a higher propensity to develop somatic dysfunction, facilitated segments, and related visceral dysfunction.[27] A crossover commonly occurs at sites where postural curves, convex on one side, cross the gravitational line and continue on the opposite side, reversing direction. Proponents of myofascial systems rely on an understanding of functional anatomy in the diagnostic prediction and clinical treatment of myofascial point sites. All emphasize the need for structural stability of posture to achieve lasting therapeutic relief.

CONCLUSION

An analysis of the systems of myofascial pain and dysfunction pioneered by Chapman, Travell, Jones, and others provides additional insight into the system conceived by Andrew Taylor Still. They reinforce the clinical utility of careful observation and palpation of the musculoskeletal system when looking for clues to a differential diagnosis. Each views the body as an interconnected unit with all parts and systems working together. Each expresses a common goal: the identification and treatment of somatic elements to reestablish normal functional characteristics that promote beneficial changes in body homeostasis.

The following chapters seek to examine the unique and common elements associated with two of these clinically useful myofascial point systems, Travell myofascial trigger points and Chapman's reflexes, and examine myofascial points from an osteopathic perspective.

REFERENCES

1. Travell JG, Simons DG. *Myofascial Pain and Dysfunction: The Trigger Point Manual.* Vol. I. Baltimore, Md: Williams & Wilkins; 1983. (For this reference only, page numbers are given in the body of the text with the note number.)
2. Hubbard DR, Berkoff GM: Myofascial trigger points show spontaneous needle EMG activity. *Spine.* 1993;18(13):1803–1807.
3. Simons DG. Muscle pain syndromes. *J Man Med.* 1991;6:3–23.
4. Chaitow L. *Soft Tissue Manipulation.* Ellington, Great Britain: Thorston Publ; 1987.
5. Bennett RM. Myofascial pain syndrome and the fibromyalgia syndrome: a comparative analysis. *J Man Med.* 1991;6:34–45.
6. McPartland JM. Manual medicine at the Nepali interface. *J Manual Med.* 1989;4:25–27.
7. Head H. On disturbance of sensation with especial reference to the pain of visceral disease. *Brain* 1893;16:1–133.
8. Mackenzie J. Some points bearing on the association of sensory disorders and visceral disease. *Brain* 1893;16:321–354.
9. Fitzgerald WH. *Key to Zone Therapy or Relieving Pain and Disease.* Columbus, Ohio: IW Long Publ; 1918.
10. Owens C. *An Endocrine Interpretation of Chapman's Reflexes.* 2nd ed. Chattanooga, Tenn: Chattanooga Printing & Engraving Co; 1937.
11. Dicke E. *Meine Bindegewebsmassage.* Stuttgart: Hippokrates; 1953.
12. Lewit K. Postisometrische Relaxation in Kombination mit anderen Mes muskularer Fazilitation und Inhibition. *Manuelle Medizin.* 1986;24:30–34.
13. Greenman PE. In memoriam: FHC Gaymans. *J Man Med.* 1988;3:158.
14. Korr IM. The spinal cord as organizer of disease processes. In: Peterson B, ed. *The Collected Papers of Irvin M. Korr.* Newark, Ohio: American Academy of Osteopathy; 1979:207–221.
15. Simons DG. Muscle pain syndromes. *J Man Med.* 1991;6:3–23.
16. vanBuskirk RL. Nociceptive reflexes and the somatic dysfunction: a model. *JAOA.* 1990;90(9):792–809.
17. Simons DG. Muscle pain syndromes. *J Man Med.* 1991;6:3–23.
18. Simons DG. *Myofascial Pain Syndrome Due to Trigger Points (International Rehabilitation Medicine Association Monograph Series Number 1).* Cleveland, Ohio: Rademaker Printing; 1987.
19. Hubbard DR, Berkoff GM. Myofascial trigger points show spontaneous needle EMG activity. *Spine.* 1993;18(13):1803–1807.
20. Kuchera ML, Kuchera WA. *Osteopathic Considerations in Systemic Dysfunction.* 2nd ed. rev. Columbus, Ohio: Greyden Press; 1994:200–201.
21. Kuchera ML, Kuchera WA. *Osteopathic Considerations in Systemic Dysfunction.* 2nd ed. rev. Columbus, Ohio: Greyden Press; 1994:79–84.
22. Jungmann M. *Backaches, Postural Decline, Aging and Gravity Strain.* Lewiston, Me: Penmor Lithographers; 1988.
23. Kuchera ML. Gravitational stress, musculoligamentous strain, and postural alignment. *Spine State Art Rev.* 1995;9(2):463–490.
24. Irwin R. Reduction of lumbar scoliosis by use of heel lift to level the sacral base. *JAOA.* 1991;91(1):34, 37–44.
25. Hench PK. Myofascial pain syndromes in clinical insights into musculoskeletal problems. *Myology.* 1980;5(1):5.
26. Janda V. Muscles, central nervous motor regulation, and back problems. In: Korr IM, ed. *The Neurobiologic Mechanisms in Manipulative Therapy.* New York, NY: Plenum Press; 1978:27–41.
27. Korr IM, Wright HM, Chace JA. Cutaneous patterns of sympathetic activity in clinical abnormalities of the musculoskeletal system (1964). In: Peterson B, ed. *The Collected Papers of I.M. Korr.* Newark, Ohio: American Academy of Osteopathy; 1979:66–72.

66. Travell and Simons' Myofascial Trigger Points

MICHAEL L. KUCHERA

Key Concepts

- **Definition of a trigger point in the Travell system**

- **Difference between active and latent trigger points**

- **Incidence rate of trigger points in the healthy population and in those seeking medical care**

- **Contributing and perpetuating factors for trigger points**

- **Palpatory techniques for diagnosing trigger points**

- **Techniques for treatment of trigger points, including soft tissue techniques, cooling with stretch, deep massage, injection, and others**

- **Commonalities between Travell myofascial points and traditional osteopathic descriptions of somatic dysfunction, including somatovisceral and viscerosomatic reflexes**

- **Effects of Travell myofascial points on somatic function, venous and lymphatic drainage, and autonomic function**

The Travell myofascial point system was developed by Janet Travell, M.D., who devoted her career to the understanding of myofascial pain and dysfunction and the clinical application of the trigger point system for their treatment. Her prominence in using this system in the care of President John F. Kennedy, and her excellent two-volume text, *Myofascial Pain and Dysfunction: The Trigger Point Manual*,[1,2] coauthored with David Simons, M.D., have brought recognition to the use of this form of somatic dysfunction. Without the efforts of Travell and Simons, this particular myofascial system may have been overlooked. Diagrammatic summaries of trigger point maps affecting different regions are shown in Figure 66.1. When a patient complains of pain in a particular region, examine these points.

A myofascial trigger point (TP) is defined in the Travell system as *"a hyperirritable spot, usually within a taut band of skeletal muscle or in the muscle's fascia, that is painful on compression and that can give rise to characteristic referred pain, ten-*derness, and autonomic phenomena."[1(p.3)] TPs are classified as "active" or "latent" depending on their ability to refer pain into the characteristic distribution empirically mapped for each point. Active points refer pain at rest, with muscular activity, or with palpation. Latent points usually produce pain only when probed with more steady pressure. Unless a skilled palpatory examination is conducted, latent trigger points are often overlooked. The true cause of a patient's dysfunction may be misdiagnosed.

INCIDENCE

The incidence of latent TPs has been reported[1(p.13)] as 54 and 45%, respectively, in asymptomatic 19-year-old female and male Air Force recruits. Trigger points are most likely to develop in the upper trapezius muscle.[1(pp.183–184)] Overall, however, trigger points in the quadratus lumborum muscle are reported to be the most common and are the most commonly overlooked cause of myogenic low back pain.[3] Different centers have reported the incidence of primary myofascial syndromes: 85% of 283 consecutive admissions for chronic pain,[4] and 55% of 296 patients admitted for chronic head and neck pain.[5] Of 61 consecutive patients presenting to an internal medicine practice,[6] 10% with general medical symptoms and 31% presenting with the chief complaint of pain had TPs as the primary cause.

TPs are both more likely to occur and, once present, are more likely to remain in patients with perpetuating factors. Postural and other mechanical disorders, including articular somatic dysfunction,[2,7,8] are reported to be some of the most pervasive perpetuating factors. An osteopathic structural analysis is warranted in any patient with myofascial TPs. Other contributing factors include:

Hypothyroidism, anemia, and various endocrine dysfunctions[1(pp.143–148)]
Nutritional deficiencies[1(pp.114–143)]
Chronic infections[1(pp.151–153)]
Psychologic stressors[1(pp.148–151),9]

Systemic perpetuating factors may include any structural or functional disorder that compromises homeostasis of the local energy supply to the involved muscle(s).

DIAGNOSIS

Laboratory, imaging, and neuroelectrodiagnostic tests are not diagnostic for primary myofascial TPs, nor for most other forms of somatic dysfunction. They may prove useful, how-

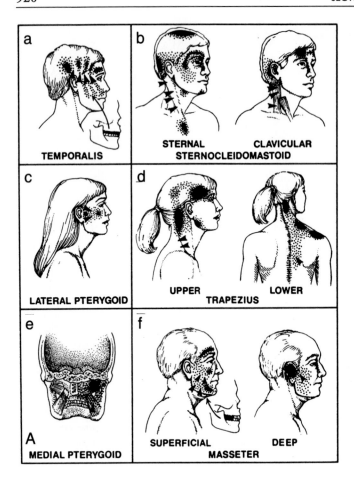

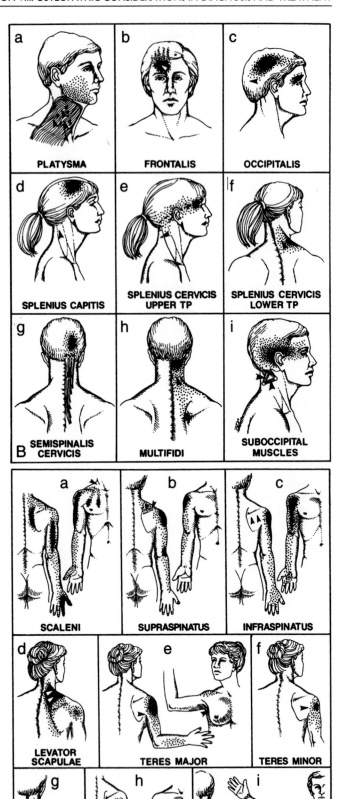

Figure 66.1. Regional depiction of myofascial Travell trigger points; referred pain patterns (*black stippled area*) and location of trigger points (*arrows*): A. Masticatory and two neck muscles. B. Several head and neck muscles. C. Neck muscles (scaleni) that refer pain in the upper extremity and for many shoulder girdle muscles. D. Arm and a number of forearm muscles. E. Forearm and intrinsic hand muscles. F. Shoulder girdle, chest, and iliocostalis paraspinal muscle. G. Superficial paraspinal, several deep paraspinal, quadratus lumborum back muscles, and two abdominal wall muscles. H. Pelvic girdle muscles and three parts (vastus medialis, rectus femoris, and vastus intermedius) of quadriceps femoris muscle. I. Vastus lateralis of quadriceps femoris, several muscles of leg, and selected intrinsic foot muscles. (From Wall PD, Melzack R, eds. *Textbook of Pain.* 2nd ed. Edinburgh: Churchill Livingstone; 1989:368–385.)

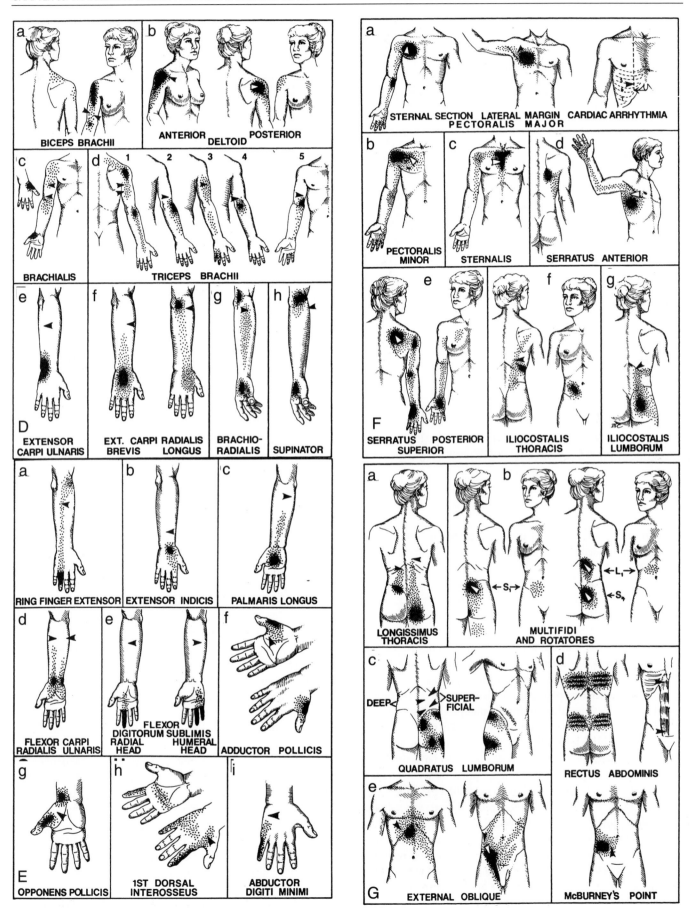

a BICEPS BRACHII

b ANTERIOR DELTOID POSTERIOR

c BRACHIALIS

d 1 2 3 4 5 TRICEPS BRACHII

D **e** EXTENSOR CARPI ULNARIS **f** EXT. CARPI RADIALIS BREVIS LONGUS **g** BRACHIO-RADIALIS **h** SUPINATOR

a RING FINGER EXTENSOR **b** EXTENSOR INDICIS **c** PALMARIS LONGUS

d FLEXOR CARPI RADIALIS ULNARIS **e** FLEXOR DIGITORUM SUBLIMIS RADIAL HEAD HUMERAL HEAD **f** ADDUCTOR POLLICIS

E **g** OPPONENS POLLICIS **h** 1ST DORSAL INTEROSSEUS **i** ABDUCTOR DIGITI MINIMI

a STERNAL SECTION LATERAL MARGIN CARDIAC ARRHYTHMIA PECTORALIS MAJOR

b PECTORALIS MINOR **c** STERNALIS **d** SERRATUS ANTERIOR

F **e** SERRATUS POSTERIOR SUPERIOR **f** ILIOCOSTALIS THORACIS **g** ILIOCOSTALIS LUMBORUM

a LONGISSIMUS THORACIS **b** MULTIFIDI AND ROTATORES S_1 L_1 S_4

c DEEP SUPER-FICIAL QUADRATUS LUMBORUM **d** RECTUS ABDOMINIS

G **e** EXTERNAL OBLIQUE McBURNEY'S POINT

Figure 66.1—*continued*

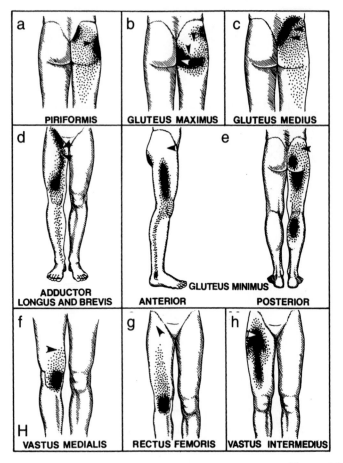

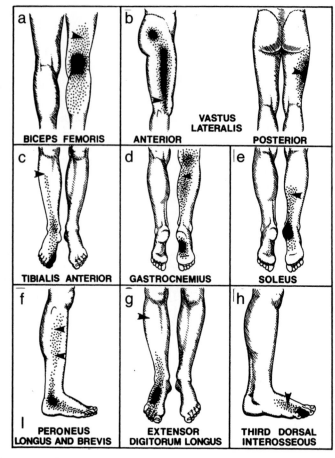

Figure 66.1—*continued*

ever, in identifying factors that perpetuate trigger points or in ruling out a variety of clinical conditions from which secondary myofascial TPs may arise.

Diagnosis of myofascial TPs depends on distinctive palpatory findings, distribution of the pain pattern, and the patient's history. Joints controlled by muscles with myofascial TPs may show restricted ranges of motion in the direction of stretch, and the muscles are painful with either active or passive stretching. Patchy weakness during muscle testing may result from a conscious or unconscious desire to avoid pain. If present, attention to the precise pain patterns is extremely important in the diagnosis, because the empirically mapped patterns for each given muscle are fairly consistent among patients (Fig. 66.1). Histories of activities leading to the onset of pain and dysfunction, or detailed descriptions of the muscular activities no longer comfortable for the patient, are often sufficient to identify specific muscles that need to be examined for TPs.

Myofascial TPs are locally very tender. They are palpated as small nodular or spindle-shaped thickenings within a taut band of tissue. Depending on the muscle examined, use either flat palpation or palpation with a pincer type grip (Fig. 66.2). The most appropriate palpation for a myofascial trigger point is that which permits pressure to be applied perpendicular to the long axis of the muscle suspected of harboring the point.

Seek a local twitch sign as well as determination of a triggered pain. Precise localization is required for accurate TP diagnosis as well as in accomplishing many of the specific treatments. In large flat muscles like the quadratus lumborum, fingertips can be drawn across the muscle perpendicular to its fibers. Some muscles, like the trapezius or those in the axillary folds, are better palpated with a pincer grip.

Each suspicious muscle is examined. A muscle contains a myofascial TP when fingertip pressure across the long axis of the muscle produces a generalized jump sign by the patient and a local twitch of the taut band. This latter finding is clinically significant because it is usually absent in the fibromyalgia syndrome but present in myofascial pain syndromes due to TPs.[1(p.62)]

Dysfunction in a given muscle places additional demand on others in the functional myotatic unit. A myotatic unit is made up of muscles sharing the same functional responsibilities. Functional overuse may result in associated TPs in a given myotatic unit. Satellite trigger points, on the other hand, may develop in muscles covered by the referred pain pattern of another myofascial TP. They may be apparently unrelated to functional considerations. Successful treatment depends on removing the primary myofascial TP, its associated and satellite TPs, and any underlying or perpetuating factors. Failure to

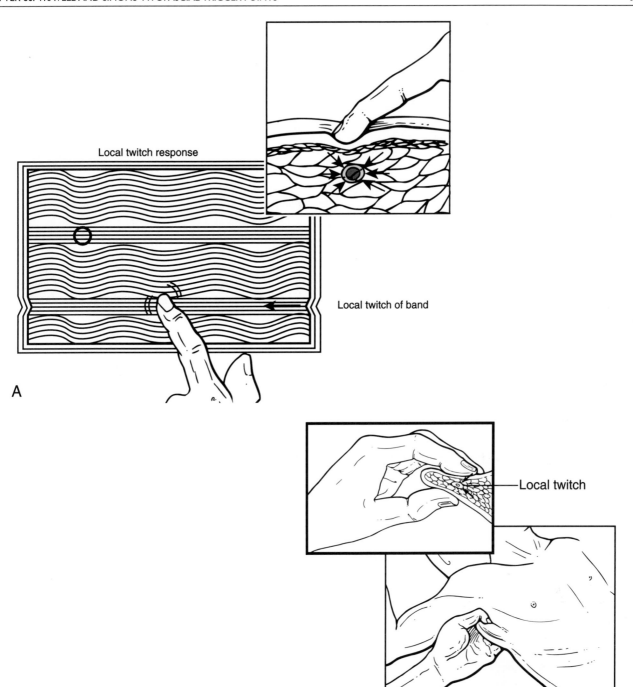

Figure 66.2. Palpation for myofascial trigger points. **A.** Draw finger-tips across large flat muscles. **B.** Use pincer grip for muscles like trapezius or those in axillary folds. (Modified from Travell JG, Simons DG. *Myo-fascial Pain and Dysfunction: The Trigger Point Manual. The Upper Extremities.* Vol I. Baltimore, Md: Williams & Wilkins; 1983:60, 61, 398.)

address all of these elements usually results in the full return of the dysfunctional myofascial situation.

TREATMENT

Treatment is directed toward inactivation of the trigger points in the involved muscles and toward identification and resolu-tion of contributing and perpetuating factors. Lasting success depends on:

Correction of associated somatic dysfunction
Patient education to prevent recurrences
Appropriate self-stretch exercise programs
Correction of underlying perpetuating and facilitating factors

Specific treatment of myofascial TPs can be accomplished with:

Inhibition soft tissue technique
Vapocoolant spray or other intermittent cooling with stretch
Deep massage
Injection
Jones' counterstrain
Isometric muscle energy techniques
Myofascial release
Other osteopathic manipulative treatment[2(pp.9–11),10]

Successful TP treatment addresses the central nervous system's response to nociceptive information or modifies peripheral input. These techniques may be ineffective if the patient is unable to relax and involuntary tensing takes place. If the operator releases the pressure too soon or too quickly, or if perpetuating factors are not addressed, there may also be reoccurrence or incomplete resolution of the TPs.

Cooling with Stretching

Intermittent cooling with a vapocoolant spray followed by myofascial stretch ("spray with stretch") is probably the most commonly used method to inactivate TPs. Stroking with plastic-covered ice followed by passive stretching is also effective, however. These techniques will restore the muscle to its normal resting length with full range of motion without causing pain or reflex spasm. Spray-with-stretch technique is believed to act through the gate theory of Wall and Melzack[1(p.73)] (Fig. 66.3).

The cooling activates Kraus receptors, which report centrally through fast fibers. The afferent volley of neural impulses conveyed through these fast fibers reflexly blocks the TP nociceptive impulses conveyed by slow fibers at the substantia gelatinosa. Blocking this neurologic reflex prevents the pain–spasm–pain cycle that results from stretching a muscle harboring a trigger point. This allows the operator to stretch the muscle containing the TP without producing reflex muscle spasm. The common adage is that "spray is the distraction, stretch is the action."[1(p.64)]

Vapocoolant spray with Fluori-Methane spray is best applied to the skin at an angle of 30° from a distance of about 18 inches and at a rate of approximately 4 inches per second. The rate and distance for Fluori-Methane spray are advised to stimulate cold receptors in the skin without chilling the underlying muscle. Adjust these parameters for other cooling sources. For example, apply the "colder" ethyl chloride spray at a more rapid rate and/or from a greater distance. Apply cooling in unidirectional parallel sweeps over the entire length of the muscle in the direction of its fibers, being sure to pass over the TP. Gently stretch the muscle. Subsequent passes of the spray should include similar application continuing over the TPs reference zone. Again follow this by a gentle stretch of the muscle. Care should be taken to activate the cold receptors of the skin while carefully avoiding chilling the muscle. Chilling of the underlying muscle will often activate a TP and prevent the effective muscle stretch needed to eliminate that TP. After intermittent cooling with stretch, warm the area with

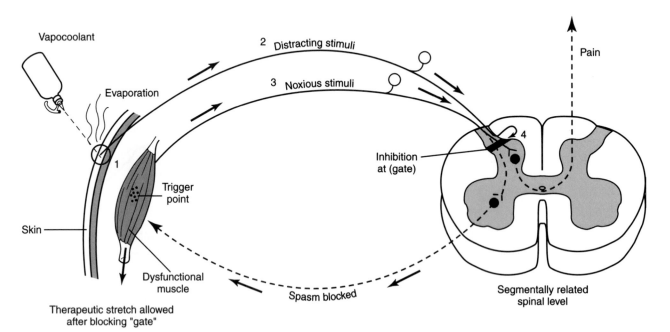

Figure 66.3. Spray-with-stretch technique. Cooling (1) must occur at rate that significantly activates Kraus (cold) receptors in skin but avoids chilling underlying muscle. Cold is conveyed centrally by fast afferents (2) that "block" noxious afferent information (3) from dysfunctional muscle at substantia gelatinosa (4) or "gate." (Modified from Travell JG, Simons DG. *Myofascial Pain and Dysfunction: The Trigger Point Manual. The Upper Extremities.* Vol. I. Baltimore, Md: Williams & Wilkins; 1983:72.)

moist heat and take the muscle through its full active range of motion.

Injection

Injection is sometimes necessary to inactivate a TP. While dry needling of the TP has been reported to be successful by some operators, most inject procaine. Some mix the procaine with a steroid preparation. Aspirate before injecting. The needle should be placed directly into the TP (Fig. 66.4) to be most effective. This will be intensely uncomfortable and will reduplicate the patient's pain pattern. Warn the patient of this. Successful penetration of the TP will create a local twitch response that correlates highly with a successful injection. Injection of a TP may fail if:

Primary or secondary trigger points are missed by the needle
The injected solution causes irritation of the tissues
Local bleeding acts as an irritant to reinitiate a trigger point
Perpetuating factors are not addressed

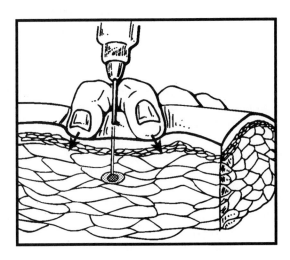

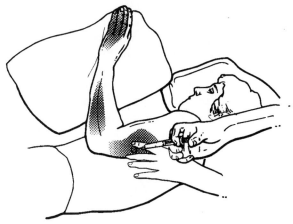

Figure 66.4. Triceps TP$_3$ and injection precipitated pain pattern. (Modified from Travell JG, Simons DG. *Myofascial Pain and Dysfunction: The Trigger Point Manual. The Upper Extremities.* Vol. I. Baltimore, Md: Williams & Wilkins; 1983:83, 473.)

If injection of a TP with a radicular or peripheral nerve distribution is attempted, omit steroids to avoid accidental injection into the nerve itself.

OSTEOPATHIC APPROACH

Somatic dysfunction is present when there is *"impaired or altered function of the somatic system and its related neural, lymphatic, and circulatory elements."*[11] Travell and Simons' description of myofascial dysfunction also includes:

Neural entrapment
Arterial entrapment
Venous entrapment
Lymphatic entrapment
Autonomic sequelae
Viscerosomatic–somatovisceral reflex phenomena resulting from myofascial dysfunction

Travell myofascial points can easily be integrated into the diagnostic and treatment considerations of an osteopathic physician as a subset of somatic dysfunction. Unfortunately, this osteopathic perspective has not been widely applied. Simons reports that *"the interface between (myofascial pain syndromes) and somatic dysfunction is one of the greatest voids in our knowledge."*[12]

Travell Myofascial Points Affecting Somatic Functions

Travell myofascial points typically result in weakness and/or dysfunction of the muscle harboring them. Overuse in the myotatic unit because of this primary myofascial point may cause secondary associated myofascial points, resulting in further weakness and reduced function. If the point is latent,[1(p.2)] it may be clinically silent unless it is palpated directly or the muscle harboring it is functionally stressed. If the point is active,[1(p.1)] it weakens and prevents full lengthening of the muscle. It may produce referred pain and/or autonomic phenomena in a predictable "trigger or reference zone." These zones are characteristic for each muscle and have been empirically mapped and documented.[1,2]

Altered somatic functions that have been noted include[1]:

Disturbed motor coordination[1(p.15)]
Temporomandibular joint dysfunction[1(pp.224,240,264)]
Depressed deep tendon reflexes[1(p.15)]
Muscular stiffness and weakness[1(p.16)]
Diminished ranges of motion[1(pp.56–57)]

The patient often complains of these symptoms as well as dysesthesia, paresthesia, and pain. The pain is described as steady, deep, and achy in nature. Symptoms are often aggravated by:

Use of the muscle
Chilling
Psychogenic stress

Viral infection
Prolonged shortening of the muscle

Chronic pain may lead to secondary depression, sleep disturbance, and chronic pain behavior.[1(p.53)]

Diminished range of motion caused by myofascial TPs should be differentiated from structural limitations of the joints, such as occur in osteoarthritis, and functional arthrodial limitations, such as occur in other forms of somatic dysfunction. In particular, Travell myofascial points should be distinguished from fibromyalgia syndrome[13] and other rheumatologic disorders.[14] Appropriate recognition and treatment of Travell points have provided dramatic restoration of function in numerous patients previously misdiagnosed as having these other conditions.

Similarly, as a component element of somatic dysfunction, myofascial TPs must sometimes be specifically addressed to allow complete resolution of the joint dysfunction. Clinically, this is often the case in recurrent exhalation somatic dysfunction of rib 12 related to quadratus lumborum TPs. The presence of trigger points must be considered when the usual treatment for shoulder dysfunction fails to respond fully to manipulative techniques such as the Seven Stages of Spencer (see Chapter 55). Table 66.1 delineates these trigger points associated with Spencer technique.

Many clinical diagnoses have associated myofascial trigger points in which the dysfunctional trigger zone overlaps with the structural symptoms profile. While a cause-and-effect relationship has not been demonstrated, treatment of those myofascial elements contributes significantly to patient management and symptom reduction.

Two common clinical diagnoses illustrate this point very well. In lateral epicondylitis, or tennis elbow syndrome, myofascial trigger points in the supinator, wrist and finger extensor muscles, anconeus, and triceps are all capable of referring symptoms to the lateral epicondyle.[1(pp.510–521)] Conversely, all become significantly stressed with the altered biomechanics adopted in a true inflammatory process of the lateral epicondyle.

In carpal tunnel syndrome (CTS), myofascial trigger points are found in the pronator teres, and wrist, finger, and thumb flexors.[15] Here also, triggered referral zones from the myofascial points overlap with the wrist pain, finger and thumb paresthesias, grip weakness, and referred forearm pain perception common to patients with carpal tunnel syndrome. Forearm muscles also become significantly stressed with the altered extremity mechanics adopted by patients with CTS.

Failure to address the trigger points in patients with lateral epicondylitis results in failure to help a significant number of patients.[1(pp.510–521)] Osteopathic treatment protocols that specifically address treatment of these myofascial structures, in addition to traditional conservative care, have been more effective than wrist splints and medication alone in CTS.[16] The stretch component addressing each of these conditions is pictured in Figure 66.5. Note in Figure 66.5A that the same general position is modified to localize in turn the supinator, wrist, and finger extensors, with a separate positioning of the anconeus and triceps. In Figure 66.5B, general positioning with slight localization modifications during the stretch component effectively, and in a time-efficient manner, addresses the ventral forearm muscles most commonly involved in patients with CTS or its symptoms.

Myofascial points also result from and contribute to postural disorders.[7,8,17] Travell and Simons[1(pp.103–113)] cite postural disorders as one of the primary perpetuating factors of myofascial trigger points. Active TPs are most often seen in postural muscles.[1(p.13)] They even go so far as to state that *postural training should be one of the first parts, if not the first part, of the treatment program.*[2(p.548)] Patterns of recurrent TPs in various combinations should alert the clinician to an underlying postural disorder. Figure 66.6 depicts muscles most commonly contributing to postural patterns.

The so-called "short leg syndrome" has been implicated in causing multiple TPs, including those in the paraspinal,[1(p.651)] sternocleidomastoid,[1(p.207)] and quadratus lumborum[1(p.104),2(pp.41–63)] muscles. Quadratus lumborum TPs have already been implicated as an extremely common primary cause of myogenic low back pain.[3(p.85)] Conversely, trigger points in this muscle are capable of producing a false short-leg syndrome caused by muscular attachments to the iliac crest.[2(pp.42–63)] This situation is likely to result in compensatory postural charges, recurrent somatic dysfunction, and TPs in local and distant areas. It also may lead to lift therapy being incorrectly or inappropriately instituted.

Impairment of Venous and Lymphatic Drainage

Optimal venous and lymphatic drainage depends on unobstructed myofascial pathways through which these circulatory vessels pass and on respiratory–circulatory mechanisms efficiently creating pressure differentials. Zink stated the relevance of this perspective to the osteopathic clinician.[18,19] Travell and

Table 66.1
Limitation of Shoulder Range of Motion (ROM)

Motion Restricted[a]	Myofascial Point Found
Flexion	Triceps
Abduction	Subscapularis
	Infraspinatus
	Supraspinatus
	Teres major (levator scapulae)
Internal rotation	Teres minor
	Infraspinatus
External rotation	Subscapularis
	Pectoralis minor

[a]Stage of Spencer that is restricted. Note: The majority of muscles are rotator cuff muscles.

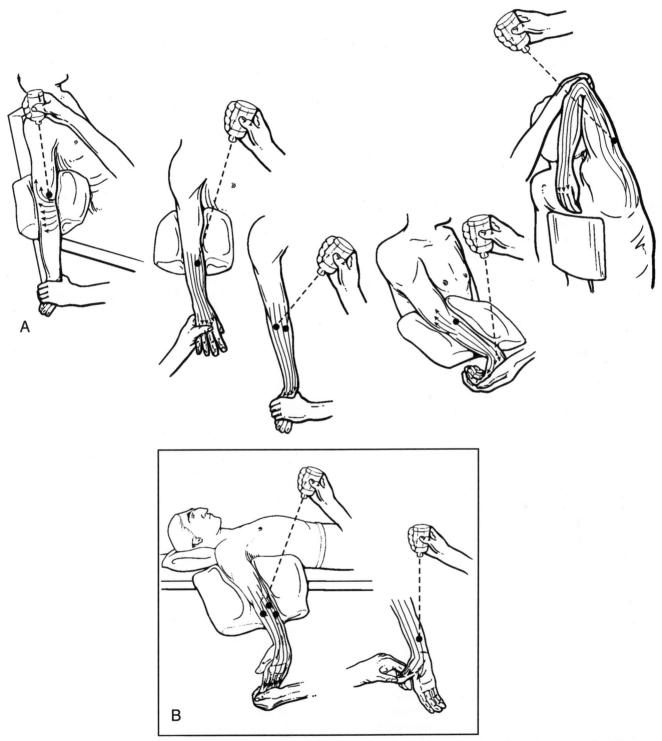

Figure 66.5. A. Spray and stretch of the "SWEAT" muscles most commonly found in tennis elbow syndrome. **B.** Spray and stretch in carpal tunnel syndrome. (Modified from Travell JG, Simons DG. *Myofascial Pain and Dysfunction: The Trigger Point Manual. The Upper Extremities.* Vol. I. Baltimore, Md: Williams & Wilkins; 1983:471, 492, 504, 517, 544.)

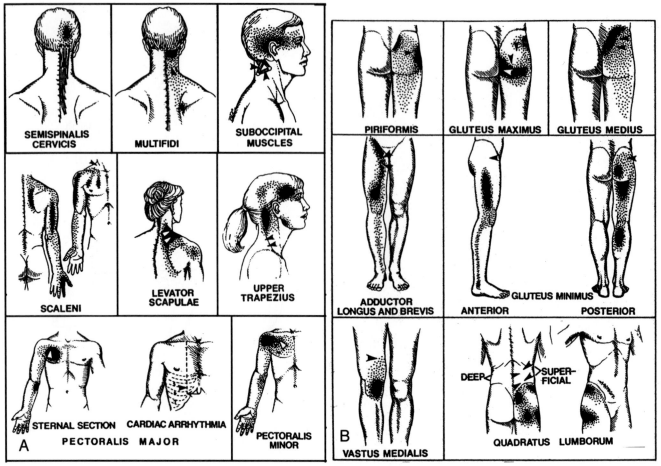

Figure 66.6. Trigger points commonly precipitated by poor posture. *black stippled area,* referred pain patterns; *arrows,* location of trigger points. (Modified from Wall PD, Melzack R, eds. *Textbook of Pain.* 2nd ed. Edinburgh: Churchill Livingstone; 1989:371, 372, 376, 377.)

Simons have also documented the effect of certain myofascial points in creating lymphatic dysfunction and have reported improvement of congestive sequelae by removing this type of somatic dysfunction. The osteopathic profession and Travell emphasize the importance of proper and effective respiration and attention to the somatic factors involved.

The scalene muscles are often referred to as "the entrappers"[1(p.344)] because of their clinical tendency to entrap structures passing through the superior thoracic aperture (thoracic inlet). The subclavian lymphatic trunk and the subclavian vein are particularly susceptible to muscular compression caused by TPs in the anterior scalene muscles (Fig. 66.7). This compression is further aggravated by elevation of the first rib, which may result from a variety of dysfunctional phenomena, including TPs in the anterior or middle scalene muscles. Somatic dysfunction of the first rib and other parts of the functional superior thoracic inlet should also be treated because of their effect on this region. Scalene TP activity has been implicated[1(p.357)] in reflex suppression of lymphatic duct peristaltic contractions in the affected extremity.

Palpation of the posterior and anterior axillary folds for ev-

idence of myofascial dysfunction is clinically important in assessing the degree of lymphatic dysfunction affecting the upper extremities and/or breasts. The posterior axillary fold is the location of palpable myofascial points in the subscapularis, teres major, and latissimus dorsi muscles. It is also the site of terminal lymphatic drainage dysfunction for the upper extremities (Fig. 66.8). Zink et al.[20] discuss diagnosis and treatment of this region to relieve lymphatic congestion in the upper extremity. Those findings closely parallel the palpatory and clinical findings described independently by Travell and Simons, using myofascial points located in the posterior axillary fold.[1(pp.393–424)] Figure 66.8*B* shows that points higher in the posterior axillary fold correlate predominantly with shoulder referral, while lower points refer distally. Zink and Travell report that treatment of myofascial dysfunction in this area results in reduction of swelling, joint dysfunction, and dysesthesia (Fig. 66.9). Likewise, appropriate treatment of anterior axillary fold dysfunction results in reduction of breast tenderness and congestive changes attributed to entrapment of breast lymphatics traveling around and through the pectoralis muscle toward the subclavicular lymph nodes.[1(p.587)]

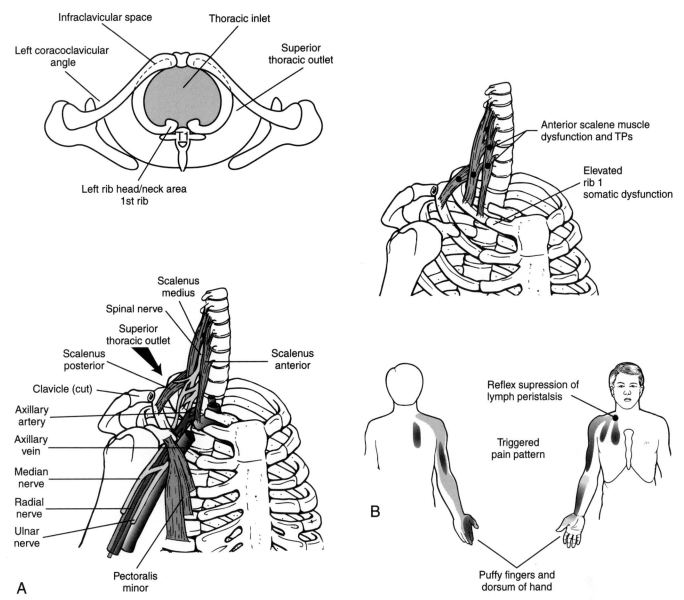

Figure 66.7. **A.** Entrapment of vascular and lymphatic structures in thoracic inlet. **B.** Anterior scalene muscle referred pain and lymphaticovenous congestion in affected extremity. (Modified from Travell JG, Simons DG. *Myofascial Pain and Dysfunction: The Trigger Point Manual. The Upper Extremities.* Vol. I. Baltimore, Md: Williams & Wilkins; 1983:345, 356; A, top illustration by W.A. Kuchera.)

Autonomic Effects of Travell Myofascial Points

Clinically, autonomic effects of myofascial dysfunction are common.[1(p.25),13] Travell's term, *"referred autonomic phenomena,"* refers to the *"vasoconstriction (blanching), coldness, sweating, pilomotor response, ptosis, and/or hypersecretion that is caused by activity of a trigger point in a region separate from the trigger point. The phenomena usually appear in the same area as the pain referral for that trigger point."*[1(p.3)] Korr[21] and Travell and Simons[1(p.69)] have postulated an organizing role for the spinal cord by relating somatic and visceral input to palpatory and symptomatic findings in both systems (Fig. 66.10). Afferent input to the spinal cord may facilitate the segment at the spinal level it enters. Efferent consequences include sympathetic changes to somatic and visceral tissues at the same spinal level, and palpable somatic dysfunction including tissue texture changes. A series of reflexes and referred symptoms result. Trigger zones for each muscle have been mapped by Travell and Simons.[1] Viscerosomatic reflexes have been documented by Chapman (see Chapter 67). The autonomic effects produced in both somatic and visceral systems should be recognized in the patient and elicited in the history. Furthermore, the asso-

Figure 66.8. **A.** Zink's posterior axillary fold technique. **B.** Location and overlapping patterns of Travell and Simons' trigger points located in posterior axillary fold. *1*, subscapularis; *2*, teres major; *3*, latissimus dorsi; *4*, serratus anterior. Overlapping patterns between *1* and *2* and between *3* and *4* are shown in *black*. (Modified from Travell JG, Simons DG. *Myofascial Pain and Dysfunction: The Trigger Point Manual. The Upper Extremities.* Vol. I. Baltimore, Md: Williams & Wilkins; 1983:398.)

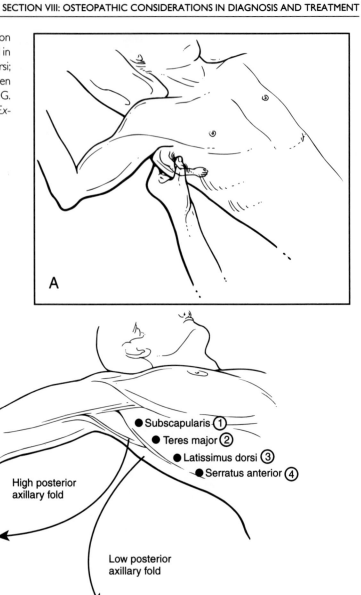

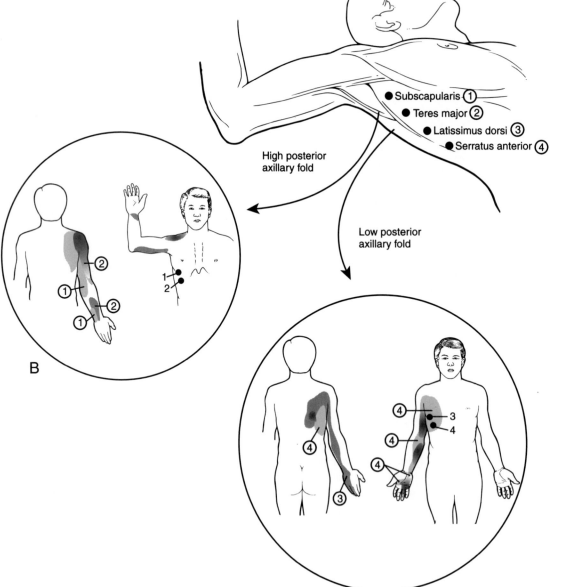

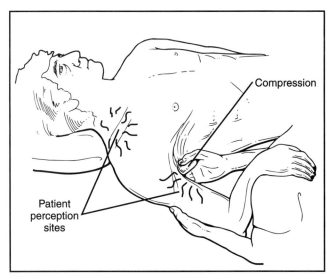

Figure 66.9. Compression of posterior axillary fold at palpatory site of each thickened tender point. (Modified from Travell JG, Simons DG. *Myofascial Pain and Dysfunction: The Trigger Point Manual. The Upper Extremities.* Vol. I. Baltimore, Md: Williams & Wilkins; 1983:418.)

Pectoralis TPs may result in cardiac dysfunction, a demonstrable somatovisceral reflex. Supraventricular tachyarrhythmias have been documented to arise from TPs located in the right pectoralis major muscle between the fifth and sixth ribs, midway between the sternal margin and the nipple line (Fig. 66.11). Pectoralis trigger points are common in patients with a slumped posture and rounded shoulders. They also occur as a viscerosomatic reflex in over 60% of patients with cardiac disease. A trigger point in the right pectoralis muscle (at the level of the fifth intercostal space) can produce a somatovisceral reflex, causing a supraventricular tachyarrhythmia. Treatment involves both removing the trigger point and correcting the underlying postural problem if present. Correction of this somatic dysfunction results in immediate return of normal cardiac function.[1(p.585)]

Pectoralis TPs may also arise as a consequence of coronary artery insufficiency. This example of a viscerosomatic reflex has a significant prevalence as demonstrated by one study of 72 patients. Chest muscle TPs were reported in 61% of patients with cardiac disease.[1(p.586)] Treatment of these TPs is an im-

ciated tissue texture changes should be actively sought throughout the physical examination to enhance the differential diagnosis process.

Clinical symptoms attributed to the autonomic sequelae of myofascial dysfunction include:[1]

Diarrhea and dysmenorrhea due to autonomic control changes in the activity of smooth muscle[1(p.672)]

Diminished gastric motility and aggravation of duodenal ulcer activity[1(p.677)]

Vasoconstriction with headache[1(p.238)]

Dermatographia[1(p.17)]

Proprioceptive disturbances and dizziness[1(p.204)]

Excessive secretion from the maxillary sinus[1(p.263)]

Localized sweating[1(p.204)]

Cardiac arrhythmias[1(p.577)]

Goose flesh[1(p.189)]

Ptosis, excessive lacrimation, conjunctival reddening[1(pp.203,286)]

Association with Viscerosomatic and Somatovisceral Reflexes

When considering the interaction between somatic and visceral systems, recognizing somatovisceral and viscerosomatic reflexes is important for arriving at a differential diagnosis. Travell and Simons' two-volume *Myofascial Pain and Dysfunction: The Trigger Point Manual*[1,2] adds to the literature documenting these reflexes. TPs in the pectoralis major muscle provide an example of each phenomenon. They illustrate the clinical concern that should be raised by the discovery of this important somatic clue.

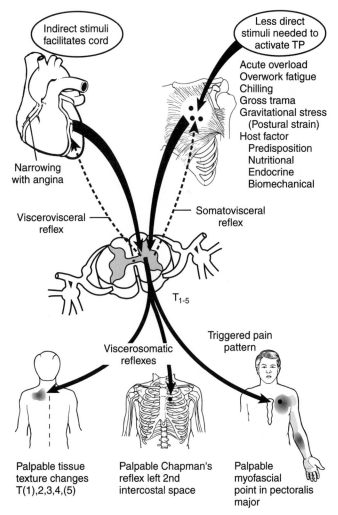

Figure 66.10. Spinal cord as organizer of disease processes.

portant factor in reducing reflex coronary artery spasm,[1(p.591)] but reduction of chest pain in this particular situation may inadvertently present an associated clinical dilemma. Symptomatic relief provided by treatment of somatic findings does not eliminate the need clinically to assess and treat a specific underlying primary visceral cause.

In the case of somatic findings resulting from viscerosomatic reflexes, healing of the primary visceral component does not mean that the secondary somatic dysfunction will spontaneously resolve. Pectoralis TPs originating in this manner have been shown to be self-perpetuating and a source of referred chest/arm pain even after recovery from or successful treatment for the initial visceral event.[1(p.586)] Precipitated by cold or overuse of the pectoralis muscles, these somatically referred symptoms may unfortunately promote unnecessary emotional distress and disability in a cardiac patient until identified and removed. Similar myofascial points occur in patients with a variety of visceral disorders, including duodenal ulcer[1(p.673)] (Fig. 66.12) and postcholecystectomy syndrome.[22]

CONCLUSION

An analysis of the system of myofascial pain and dysfunction pioneered by Travell and Simons provides additional insight into the system conceived by Andrew Taylor Still, M.D., a century earlier. Both systems reinforce the clinical utility of

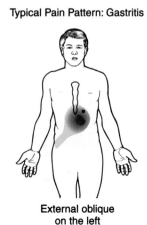

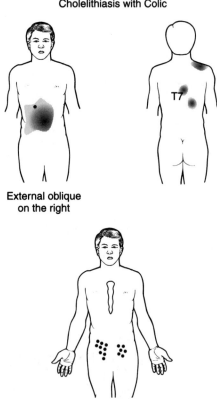

Figure 66.12. Myofascial trigger points associated with viscerosomatic reflexes. (See also Fig. 66.11.) (Modified from Travell JG, Simons DG. *Myofascial Pain and Dysfunction: The Trigger Point Manual. The Upper Extremities.* Vol. I. Baltimore, Md: Williams & Wilkins; 1983:662.)

Figure 66.11. Pectoralis trigger points and associated reflexes. *SA,* sinoatrial node of the heart.

careful musculoskeletal palpation when looking for clues to a differential diagnosis. Each views the body as an interconnected unit with all parts and systems working together. Each expresses a common goal, the identification and treatment of somatic elements to reestablish normal functional characteristics. This promotes, enhances, and restores body homeostasis.

Travell myofascial points can be viewed by osteopathic physicians as a particular subset of somatic dysfunction. They represent impaired or altered function of the myofascial system and its related neural, lymphatic, and circulatory elements. Several points have been linked to viscerosomatic and somatovisceral reflexes; others are known to entrap circulatory and/or neural structures. Many have autonomic sequelae, and most involve pain and/or musculoskeletal dysfunction. All require careful and skilled palpation for diagnosis and an understanding of the underlying anatomy and physiology for successful treatment.

Travell points, as a form of somatic dysfunction, respond to a balanced osteopathic approach integrating postural, psychoemotional, and nutritional factors with manual techniques and modalities. These reestablish the homeostatic relationship between the musculoskeletal system and the central nervous system.

The general impact resulting from somatic dysfunction in patients from any osteopathic practice is consistent with the potential for the myofascial points to:

Contribute to a wide range of clinical conditions
Impair homeostatic mechanisms
Evoke depression and sleep disturbances
Cause pain, weakness, dysesthesia, and restricted range of motion

Recognition of somatic dysfunction as an aid in the differential diagnosis and treatment of patients with both musculoskeletal and visceral disturbances has been greatly enhanced by the work of Travell, Simons, and other students of myofascial trigger points.

REFERENCES

1. Travell JG, Simons DG. *Myofascial Pain and Dysfunction: The Trigger Point Manual: The Upper Extremities.* Vol. I. Baltimore, Md: Williams & Wilkins; 1983.
2. Travell JG, Simons DG. *Myofascial Pain and Dysfunction: The Trigger Point Manual: The Lower Extremities.* Vol. II. Baltimore, Md: Williams & Wilkins; 1992:547.
3. Simons DG, Travell JG. Low back pain, Part 2: torso muscles. *Post Grad Med.* 1983;73(2):81–92.
4. Fishbain DA, Goldberg M, Meahger BR, et al. Male and female chronic pain patients categorized by DSM-III psychiatric diagnostic criteria. *Pain.* 1986;26:181–197.
5. Fricton JR, Kroening R, Haley D, et al. Myofascial pain syndrome of the head and neck: a review of clinical characteristics of 164 patients. *Oral Surg.* 1985;6:615–623.
6. Simons DG. Myofascial pain syndrome due to trigger points. *International Rehabilitation Medicine Association Monograph Series Number 1.* Cleveland, Ohio; Rademaker Press; 1987:4.
7. Kuchera ML. Gravitational stress, musculoligamentous strain and postural alignment. *Spine State Art Rev.* May 1995;9(2):463–490.
8. Kuchera ML. Gravitational strain pathophysiology, Parts I and II. In: Vleeming A, ed. *Low Back Pain: The Integrated Function of the Lumbar Spine and Sacroiliac Joints.* Proceedings of the 2nd Interdisciplinary World Congress, November 1995.
9. McNulty WH, Gevirtz RN, Hubbard DR, Berkoff GM. Needle electromyographic evaluation of trigger point response to a psychological stressor. *Psychophysiology.* 1994;31:313–316.
10. Greenman PE. *Principles of Manual Medicine.* Baltimore, Md: Williams & Wilkins; 1989:106–122.
11. The Glossary Review Committee of the Educational Council on Osteopathic Principles. In: Allen TW, ed. Glossary of osteopathic terminology. *AOA Yearbook and Directory of Osteopathic Physicians.* Chicago, Ill: American Osteopathic Association; 1991:678–690.
12. Simons DG. Muscle pain syndromes. *J Man Med.* 1991;6:18.
13. Bennett RM. Myofascial pain syndromes and the fibromyalgia syndrome: a comparative analysis. *J Man Med.* 1991;6(1):34–45.
14. Wolfe F, Smythe HA, Yunus MB, et al. American College of Rheumatology 1990 criteria for the classification of fibromyalgia: Report of the Multicenter Criteria Committee. *Arthritis Rheum.* 1990;33:160–172.
15. Melchior DE et al. A study of the components of somatic dysfunction in relationship to the carpal tunnel syndrome. Residency paper accepted by the Osteopathic Manipulative Medicine Department, Kirksville College of Medicine, Kirksville, Mo, 1990.
16. Strait B, Kuchera ML. Osteopathic manipulation for patients with confirmed mild, modest, and moderate carpal tunnel syndrome. *JAOA.* 1994;94(8):673.
17. Janda V. Muscles, central nervous motor regulation, and back problems. In: Korr IM, ed. *The Neurobiologic Mechanisms in Manipulative Therapy.* New York, NY: Plenum Press; 1978:27–41.
18. Zink JG. Respiratory and circulatory care: the conceptual model. *Osteopath Ann.* 1977;5(3):108–112.
19. Zink JG, Lawson WB. An osteopathic structural examination and functional interpretation of the soma. *Osteopath Ann.* 1979;7(12):433–440.
20. Zink JG, Fetchik WD, Lawson WB. The posterior axillary folds: a gateway for osteopathic treatment of the upper extremities. *Osteopath Ann.* 1981;9(3):81–88.
21. Korr IM. The spinal cord as an organizer of disease processes. In: Peterson B, ed. *The Collected Papers of Irvin M. Korr.* Newark, Ohio: American Academy of Osteopathy; 1979:207–221.
22. Kuchera ML, Kuchera WA. *Osteopathic Considerations in Systemic Dysfunction.* 2nd ed. rev. Columbus, Ohio: Greyden Press; 1994:87.

67. Chapman's Reflexes

DAVID A. PATRIQUIN

Key Concepts

- **General uses of anterior and posterior Chapman's reflex points, and the relationship between them**

- **Distinguishing characteristic of Chapman's reflex points**

- **Importance of treating whole person when using technique**

- **Importance of resolving pelvic dysfunction before beginning Chapman's reflex points treatment**

- **Locations and uses of Chapman's reflex points**

- **How to treat Chapman's reflex points**

Most physicians and basic scientists have never heard of Chapman's reflexes, yet these particular viscerosomatic reflexes are an osteopathic entity dating from the 1920s. They are a viscerosomatic reflex mechanism that has diagnostic and therapeutic importance.

Frank Chapman, DO, described the reflex as a "gangliform contraction" that blocks lymphatic drainage, causing inflammation in tissues distal to the blockage. Current thinking ties it into the sympathetic nervous system. Regardless of the mechanism, both somatic and visceral tissues suffer from the presence of this reflex. Chapman did not write about his reflex system, but his brother-in-law, Charles Owens, DO, and Chapman's wife, Ada Hinckley Chapman, DO, published the only reference text on this subject. Owens' book[1] discusses using the anterior points for diagnosis and as an evaluation of successful treatment, and using the posterior points for soft tissue treatment to affect an organ. Today, physicians tend to use these reflexes as another clue to visceral disease and as an indicator of which organ is most likely to be dysfunctional.

In current clinical practice, Chapman's reflex points are used more for diagnosis than for treatment. Treatment of these somatic representations of visceral dysfunction is a part of a complete osteopathic health management plan. Many posterior Chapman's reflexes are located in the paraspinal areas near the thoracic transverse processes. Those reflexes may be treated incidentally as soft tissue treatment is applied to the area. Chapman's reflexes may thus be treated by design or inadvertently.

Treatment of these somatic points still remains a way of enlisting the patient's body in its own recovery from dysfunction.

PALPATORY CHARACTERISTICS

On palpation, Chapman's reflexes are located deep to the skin and subcutaneous areolar tissue, most often lying on the deep fascia or periosteum. For the most part, they are found paired on both the dorsal and ventral surfaces of the body. For example, an anterior point found next to the sternum at the 5th intercostal space has a corresponding posterior point between the transverse processes of T5 and T6, adjacent to the costotransverse junction. Both reflex points represent the same viscus (Fig. 67.1).

A Chapman's reflex point is fixed in its anatomic location. It may have a characteristic palpatory quality that makes its identification positive. When an anterior Chapman point is gently compressed, the patient's response is one of greater pain than expected. Attempts to describe the reflex change microscopically have failed; biopsy attempts have provided no information concerning the tissue involved or altered in the reflex change. Still, Chapman's reflexes have good interexaminer reliability and correlate well with final hospital diagnoses.[2]

Distinguishing Characteristics

What are the distinguishing characteristics of a Chapman's reflex? They are nodules that are:

Small
Smooth
Firm
Discretely palpable
Approximately 2–3 mm in diameter

Sometimes they are described as feeling like small pearls of tapioca lying, partially fixed, on the deep aponeurosis or fascia. The masses are dense but not hard. One gets the impression of a circumscribed area of rather firm edema. They move slightly but are otherwise firmly moored in place and cannot be displaced. Occasionally, they are somewhat confluent and thought to represent longstanding visceral reflexes of greater magnitude, or chronicity, than those palpable as a single, discrete mass.

Once a Chapman's reflex point is identified and isolated by the examiner's fingertip, gentle but firm pressure usually causes a deep, disagreeable pain response in the patient. The pain is characteristically:

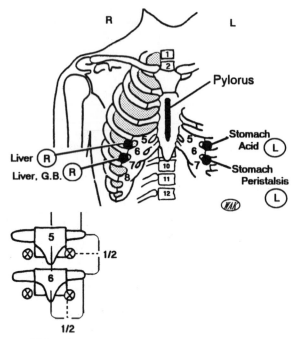

Figure 67.1. Often, anterior Chapman's reflex points have corresponding posterior points. (Reprinted with permission from Kuchera ML, Kuchera WA. *Osteopathic Considerations in Systemic Dysfunction.* rev. 2nd ed. Columbus, Ohio: Greyden Press; 1994.)

Pinpoint
Located under the finger
Nonradiating
Sharp
Exquisitely distressing

Patients invariably wince or complain while stating that they didn't know they had such a sore spot. Equivalent deep pressure on any adjacent "normal" tissue will produce only vague, local distress.

Locating Reflexes

How are these reflexes found? Owens' personal commentary on Chapman's work suggests that the novice practitioner should refer to the book early and often. When a differential diagnostic dilemma exists, look in the book for the location of reflexes related to the items on the differential diagnostic list. Then find the reflex locations identified on the chart as relating to the organs to be considered. The subsequent identification of a reflex can help to reduce the number of diagnostic items on the list.

HISTORY AND PHILOSOPHY

This systematized method of diagnosis and treatment is an empirical system developed from the observations recorded by Chapman, an osteopathic physician who practiced in Chattanooga, Tennessee. Ada Hinckley Chapman, DO, Charles

Owens, DO, and W.F. Link, DO, collected his notes, arranged them, and, in 1932, published the only reference text material on the subject.[1] Owens notes in a later edition of the book that he became convinced of the efficacy of the reflex system by using it in his practice only after Chapman's death.

Osteopathic physicians who use Chapman's reflexes select from the many reflex points they have frequently found to be helpful to them in their practice. They refer to Chapman's charts if they wish to search for a less common point. For example, one pathologist palpated the tip of the right twelfth rib to identify the typical appendix reflex. Some physicians learn the location of the Chapman's reflex for the appendix during their internship. The presence of this particular reflex point for the appendix helps to direct the differential diagnosis of lower right quadrant abdominal pain in children or in women of childbearing age more toward acute appendicitis rather than toward acute mesenteric lymphadenitis, acute right salpingitis, ruptured right ectopic pregnancy, or chronic appendicitis. This sort of focal push-button diagnosis has great appeal to any physician faced with the dilemma of undiagnosed abdominal pain. This noninvasive examination is performed quickly and without altering the position of the patient.

The whole person approach is critical in the application of Chapman's system and is a basic principle of all osteopathic treatment. His description of the pelvic-thyroid-adrenal syndrome (PTAS) confirms his dedication to the concept of the interconnectedness and interrelatedness of all parts of the body. He insisted that treatment of reflex points should not begin until the pelvis is made to function properly. This requires an accurate diagnosis of pelvic function or dysfunction with proper and successful pelvic treatment before the local reflex treatment is initiated. Chapman emphasized the important relatedness of the endocrine components—the thyroid and adrenals—by including them in his acronym for treatment of neuroendocrine dysfunction. A physician using Chapman's reflex treatments finds that a much enhanced response follows a complete Chapman's reflex treatment, especially when all pelvic dysfunctions are successfully resolved as the initiating step of the treatment protocol (see Chapter 49, "Pelvis and Sacrum").

CURRENT CLINICAL USE

Today, Chapman's reflexes are more likely to be used as an integral part of an osteopathic physical examination than as a specific therapeutic intervention. They are more likely to contribute to the differential diagnosis and implicate dysfunction of an organ system rather than be the basis of a specific pathophysiologic diagnosis. They are more likely to be used selectively than as a complete systematized diagnostic process.

Specific Reflexes to Seek and Treat

What specific reflexes might be sought and treated frequently or advantageously in practice? The reflex for appendicitis can be valuable in the differential diagnosis of lower abdominal pain. We need all the help we can find when we are faced with the lower right quadrant dilemma. The presence of Chapman's reflex for appendiceal involvement helps in differential diagnosis of this vexing complaint.

The presence of colon reflexes aids in the clinical identification of chronic constipation of irritable bowel syndrome (IBS). Such reflexes are easily identified by palpatory examination along the anterior aspect of the iliotibial fascial tract from the trochanter to within one inch of the patella on one or both legs. Those reflexes lie just superficial to the deep fascia and are slightly adherent to it. The reflex gangliform masses may be single, multiple, or, in chronic or severe cases, coalescent mats or even "strings of pearls." Owens suggests that the anatomic location of the Chapman's reflexes on the iliotibial tracts correlates with specific portions of the colon (Fig. 67.2):

Starting with the trochanter on the right side, a gangliform contraction in the tissues of the upper fifth shows that there is an inflammation within the mucous membrane of the cecum or that there is a spastic state of the circular fibers of the cecum.

The next succeeding three-fifths will show a similar state of the ascending colon, while the last fifth will have the same indication for the first two-fifths of the transverse colon.

Starting on the left thigh just above the knee, the first fifth corresponds to the last three-fifths of the transverse colon, indicating the same condition as has been explained before regarding the right side.

The middle three-fifths shows a similar state of the descending colon and the last fifth corresponds with the sigmoid, and more especially, the extreme upper end of the trochanter on the left side, effects the junction of the sigmoid with the rectum, which will often cause a stricture to form, almost closing the lumen of the bowel.[1]

The reflexes for the colon are distributed along the lateral thigh, lateral to the shaft of the femurs. It is as if the upper portions of the large bowel were removed from the abdomen and rotated ventrally around a transverse axis through the cecum and low sigmoid regions so that the transverse colon lies on the ventral surfaces of the two legs extended side by side. The ascending colon then lies over the proximal and midportion of the right femur; the hepatic flexure and right half of the transverse colon lie over the distal right femur. The left half of the transverse colon and the splenic flexure lie in relation to the distal left femur. The descending colon lies along the midshaft of the left femur and the sigmoid and rectum are represented on the proximal left femur in order (Fig. 67.2).

The palpatory finding of tissue texture changes consistent with Chapman's reflexes alerts the practitioner to screen the lower gastrointestinal system even more carefully. It also leads to correlating any history, abdominal and rectal examination findings, and other musculoskeletal reflex clues with the Chapman's findings. Because of the proximity of this reflex to those associated with the prostate or broad ligament, clinicians should carefully screen these viscera as well.

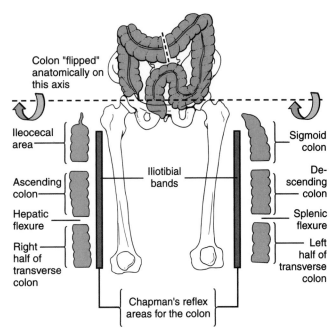

Figure 67.2. Anterior Chapman's reflexes for colon.

Other reflex points that are clinically useful in a general practice include those in the upper respiratory system (sinus, pharynx, middle ear), the upper gastrointestinal system (stomach, gallbladder), and the genitourinary system (kidney, gonads, prostate/broad ligament). Figures 67.3 and 67.4 show anterior and posterior Chapman's points summarized by the College of Osteopathic Medicine from Chapman's book.[3]

Use of Chapman's Reflexes

How do we use Chapman's reflexes? In some clinical situations, the differential diagnosis hinges on whether the cause is visceral dysfunction or primary musculoskeletal dysfunction. Palpating for Chapman's reflexes provides clinical evidence of the presence or absence of visceral disease. It suggests to the physician the possible cause of abdominal pain. The clinical ability to better differentiate a pathologic condition in the urinary bladder from that in the uterus or prostate can be critical. Chapman's reflex diagnosis is highly efficient in these days of expensive diagnostic, medical, and surgical care. Imagine how useful it is to have evidence that a patient's abdominal pain more likely arises from the colon than from the ovary.

Chapman's reflexes can also be clinically manipulated to specifically reduce adverse sympathetic influence on a particular organ or visceral system. Improved function of the disturbed organ often follows treatment of its corresponding Chapman's point. For example, patients with frequent bowel movements from the effects of irritable bowel syndrome report that they have normal or near normal bowel movements for days to months after soft tissue treatment over the iliotibial bands and/or the lumbosacral paraspinal tissues and associated Chapman's reflexes.

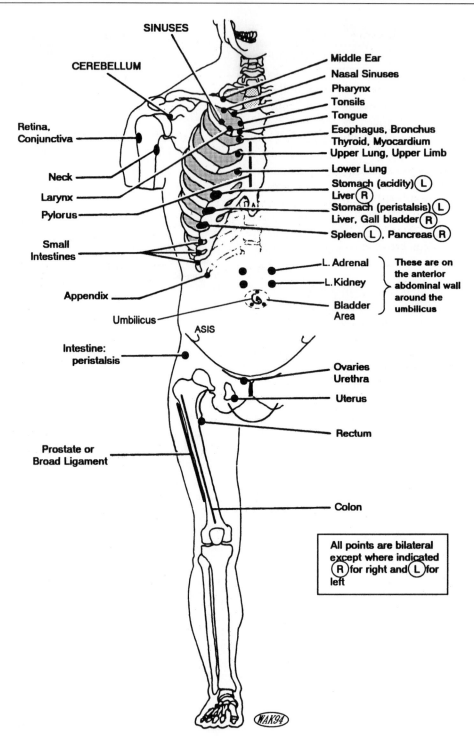

Figure 67.3. Chapman's reflexes: anterior points. (Reprinted with permission from Kuchera ML, Kuchera WA. *Osteopathic Considerations* *in Systemic Dysfunction.* rev. 2nd ed. Columbus, Ohio: Greyden Press; 1994.)

Research into the efficacy of Chapman's reflex treatment has been limited. One study of hypertensive patients in which posterior points to the adrenals were treated reported a blood pressure drop of 15 mm Hg systolic and 8 mm Hg diastolic pressure, and decreased serum aldosterone levels, 36 hours after Chapman's treatment.[4]

Treatment

How does one treat Chapman's reflexes? Treat these reflex points with firm pressure on the volar-distal finger pad of one finger. Assuming that the pelvis has been normalized first, apply somewhat heavy and even uncomfortable pressure to the gangliform mass. Slowly move the tip of the finger in a circular

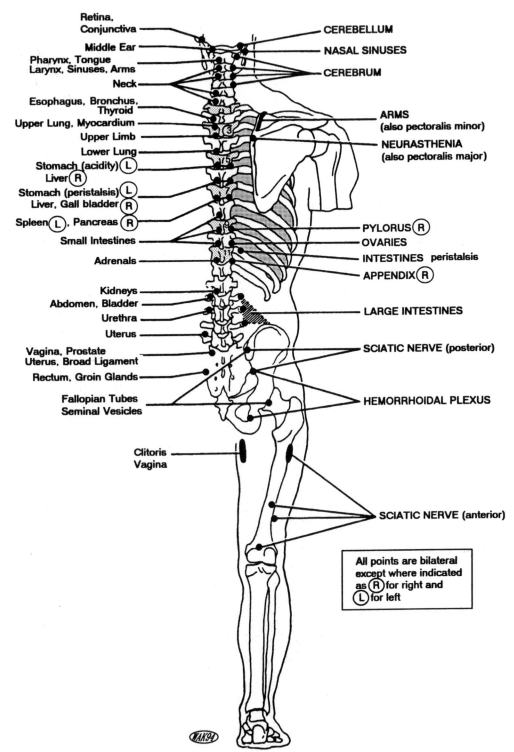

Figure 67.4. Chapman's reflexes: posterior points. (Reprinted with permission from Kuchera ML, Kuchera WA. *Osteopathic Considerations in Systemic Dysfunction.* rev. 2nd ed. Columbus, Ohio: Greyden Press; 1994.)

fashion, attempting to work (flatten) the mass as if to mobilize a localized fluid accumulation. Continue the moving pressure for 10–30 seconds. Cease treatment when the mass disappears or the patient or physician can no longer tolerate the procedure.

CONCLUSION

Chapman's reflexes have particular value in the differential diagnosis of visceral disease and should be integrated with historical and other physical examination findings. The reflex itself is described as a neurolymphatic gangliform structure. The few histopathologic studies of biopsies of Chapman's reflexes have identified nothing. While its cellular structure has yet to be described, the anatomic location of a Chapman's reflex is predictable and consistent. These anatomic sites are typically viscerosomatic representations in or on somatic structures. This suggests that the sympathetic nervous system may play an important role in the generation and maintenance of the reflexes. It further suggests that treatment of the reflexes may alter sympathetic influences on any related viscus. Most of these reflexes are found loosely attached to the deep fascia near the costotransverse structures posteriorly and in the intercostal spaces near the sternum anteriorly. Other important reflex sites include the iliotibial tracts overlying the femora and in several locations related to the pubic symphysis.

A Chapman's reflex treatment includes general and specific components. The general component deals with management of postural factors as well as the care of short-term and long-term pelvic dysfunctions. Specific treatment consists of deep rotary finger pressure applied to one or a series of Chapman's reflexes. The combination of general and specific treatment supports and assists the self-regulating and self-healing capabilities of the patient.

REFERENCES

1. Owens C. *An Endocrine Interpretation of Chapman's Reflexes.* Carmel, Calif: Reprinted by the American Academy of Osteopathy; 1932.
2. Byrnes TR, Kuchera ML, Guffey JM, Steele KM, Beatty DR, Haman JL, Lockwood MD. Correlation of palpatory findings with visceral diagnoses. *JAOA.* September 1992;92(9):1177.
3. Kuchera ML, Kuchera WA. *Osteopathic Considerations in Systemic Dysfunction.* rev. 2nd ed. Columbus, Ohio: Greyden Press; 1994:65, 90–92, 119, 124, 200–201, 231, 233.
4. Mannino JR. The application of neurologic reflexes to the treatment of hypertension. *JAOA.* December 1979;79(10):607–608.

ADDITIONAL READINGS

Brown EA. Clinical aspects of the Chapman's reflexes. In: Northup TL, ed. *Academy of Applied Osteopathy Yearbooks, 1949.* Ann Arbor, Michigan: Edwards Brothers, Inc; 1949:212–214. (Brown discusses the possible physiologic basis of the reflexes with more attention paid to patterns of reflexes and their possible mechanism of action.)

Patriquin DA. Viscerosomatic reflexes. In: Patterson MM, Howel JN, eds. *The Central Connection: Somatovisceral—Viscerosomatic Interactions.* 1989 International Symposium. Athens Ohio: University Classics, Ltd; 1992:4–18. (Patriquin introduces Chapman's reflexes as a model of osteopathic diagnosis and treatment of visceral dysfunction. He suggests that the somatic changes termed Chapman's reflexes, which clinicians find by palpation, represent specific visceral dysfunction and that the sympathetic nervous system is most likely the connecting link.)

Soden CH. Lecture notes on Chapman's reflexes. In: Northup TL, ed. *Academy of Applied Osteopathy Yearbooks, 1949.* Ann Arbor, Michigan: Edwards Brothers, Inc; 1949:201–211. (Soden reviews Chapman's work from a theoretical and practical perspective. Several pages contain labeled diagrams much like those found in Owens' book.)

Young MD. Osteopathy unlimited. In: Northup TL, ed. *Academy of Applied Osteopathy Yearbooks, 1947.* Ann Arbor, Michigan: Edwards Brothers, Inc; 1947:34–35. (Dr. Young presents Chapman's reflexes integrated into osteopathic practice.)

68. Lymphatic System

LYMPHATIC MANIPULATIVE TECHNIQUES

ELAINE WALLACE, JOHN M. McPARTLAND, JOHN M. JONES III, WILLIAM A. KUCHERA, AND BOYD R. BUSER

We strike at the source of life and death when we go to the lymphatics.

—A.T. STILL[1]

Key Concepts

- **Anatomy of the lymphatic system**

- **Physiology and pathophysiology of the lymphatic system**

- **Theories of treatment**

- **Diagnostic techniques and treatment approaches to lymph-related problems**

- **Techniques to remove impediments to lymphatic drainage**

The lymphatic system is known as the second circulatory system of the body and as the great integrator for all body fluids. If this system were to stop functioning, the patient would be dead within 24 hours as a result of massive edema and the effects from retention of toxic metabolic wastes. The lymphatic system is a passive system whose functioning can be greatly influenced and altered by extrinsic forces. Of all the systems of the body, osteopathic manipulative treatment (OMT) can exert perhaps its greatest influence on lymphatic function.

This chapter reviews the anatomy, physiology, pathophysiology, and theories of treatment of the lymphatic system. Diagnostic techniques as well as treatment approaches and techniques are presented.

When Harvey solved the circulation of the blood, he only reached the banks of the rivers of life.
—A.T. STILL[1]

EMBRYOLOGIC DEVELOPMENT

The lymphatic system and the immune system both begin developing at approximately 20 weeks of fetal age. The lymphatic system is immature at the time of birth and continues to undergo changes until approximately puberty. In infancy, lymphoid tissue is plentiful and actually increases in amount until approximately 6–9 years of age. At that time, a regression in the system begins, and by the age of 15 or 16, stable adult levels of lymphoid tissue remain.

COMPONENTS

The lymphatic system comprises approximately 3% of the total body weight.[2] It can be divided into three distinct components:

Organized lymph tissues
Collecting ducts
Lymph fluid

Organized Lymph Tissues

Organized lymph tissues consist of the spleen, the thymus, the tonsils, the vermiform appendix, the visceral lymphoid tissues located in the gastrointestinal and pulmonary systems, and the liver. There are structures of lymphoid material that are not located along the course of the lymph ducts and that do not directly function in the filtration of lymph. Each organ serves a specialized and ancillary function in the immune system.

The spleen is the largest single mass of lymphoid tissue in the body. Located deep to ribs 9, 10, and 11 on the left side of the thorax, the superior surface of the spleen abuts the abdominal surface of the diaphragm, and its inferior surface extends to the area just cephalad to the left costal margin. In the normal physiologic state, the spleen is approximately 12 cm long and 7 cm wide and is generally nonpalpable. The spleen serves important ancillary services for the lymphatic system by destroying deformed or damaged red blood cells and synthesizing immunoglobulins. The spleen is also a clearance site for particulate antigens, microorganisms, and poorly organized bacteria; well-organized bacteria are cleared by the liver. This is why the liver is also sometimes considered an organ of the lymphatic system.

The thymus is located in the superior mediastinum, anterior to the great vessels of the heart and extending upward into the neck. In infancy, the thymus is a relatively large structure that continues to develop, reaching its greatest size at the age of 2 years. The thymus provides immunologically potent cells that appear to be essential to the development of mature immune functions. It is the preprocessing site for the T-lymphocyte immune cells. After puberty, the thymus undergoes involution, and by adulthood, most of the gland has been replaced by fatty tissue. It is presently believed that the minimal tissue that does remain serves little or no function in the adult.

The tonsils are an aggregate of lymphoid tissue lying in a ring formation at the posterior oropharynx. The palatine tonsils line the lateral aspects of the pharynx at the base of the tongue and are continuous with the lingual tonsils, which cover the posterior one-third of the tongue. When enlarged, the pharyngeal tonsils—known as the adenoids—lie in the mucosa at the nasopharyngeal border of the tonsillar ring. The tonsils, like the thymus, provide cells that appear to influence and build immunity early in life but appear to be nonessential contributors to adult immunologic function.

The vermiform appendix is a long tapered structure, 2–20 cm in length at the medial surface of the cecum. Although the exact function of the appendix is unknown, it is richly imbued with lymphoid tissue and presumably offers support to the immune system. However, like the thymus and the tonsils, we know that this support is nonessential to the adult patient.

Visceral lymphoid tissue is also located in the respiratory and gastrointestinal systems. The lymphoid tissue of the respiratory system aids filtration of toxins from the lungs. The lymphoid tissues located in the mucosa of the small intestine are the most highly organized of all visceral tissues. In the small intestines, both Peyer's patches and lacteals can be identified. Peyer's patches are nonencapsulated areas of lymphoid tissue that are most highly concentrated in the distal ileum. Lacteals are small lymphatic capillaries located centrally in each small intestinal villus. These capillaries converge to form a lymphatic capillary plexus in the submucosal layer. Both Peyer's patches and the lacteals are the structures by which fats in the digestive system enter the circulatory system. These tissues drain into the superior and inferior mesenteric lymphatic trunks and ultimately into the thoracic duct.

Lymph nodes are perhaps the most highly organized of all lymphoid tissues. Lymph nodes differ from other organized lymphoid tissues in that they are dispersed along the course of the lymph vessels and are involved primarily in the filtration of lymph. The nodes can be divided into two categories: the superficial nodes, located in the subcutaneous connective tissues accompanying the superficial veins, and the deep nodes that lie beneath the fascia and muscle layers and are adjacent to the deep veins. A normal young adult body contains some 400–450 lymph nodes.[3] Aggregates of lymphocytes, interme-

shed with lymphatic sinuses, are supported in a framework of reticular tissue and encased in a connective tissue capsule. These structures vary in size from a few millimeters to a few inches in diameter. They serve a dual function of filtration and synthesis (production). Afferent lymph vessels deliver lymph to the node wherein reticuloendothelial cells phagocytize bacteria, particulate matter, and fragments of cells. In the germinal centers of the nodes, lymphocytes are manufactured and enter into the lymph as it passes through the node.

The superficial lymph nodes receive lymph from the skin as well as from the deeper tissues of the upper extremities, lower extremities, head, and neck. Superficial nodes drain into three main groups of nodes located in the cervical, axillary, and inguinal regions. The cervical nodes receive lymph from the head and areas superior to the clavicle and send it on to the jugular nodes. Lymph from the superficial areas between the clavicle and the umbilicus drain into the axillary nodes that drain into the deeper subclavian nodes; superficial areas caudal to the umbilicus drain into the inguinal nodes and eventually into the right and left lumbar nodes in the deep tissues. Deep nodes drain into a system of collecting channels.

Lymph Channels

The second component of the lymphatic system are lymph channels. These channels perfuse all tissues of the body with the exception of the central nervous system (brain and spinal cord), the epidermis (including the hair and the nails), the endomysium of muscles and cartilage, the bone marrow, and selected portions of the peripheral nerves. These tissues, although devoid of lymph channels, are perfused by minute interstitial conduits or by direct diffusion.

The anatomic arrangement of the lymph channels mirrors that of the lymph nodes in that there are both superficial and deep vessels. The superficial lymph vessels follow the course of the superficial veins and the superficial nodes. The deep lymphatic vessels, as in the case of the deep nodes, follow the course of the deep veins and drain the deep structures of the thorax, the abdomen, the pelvis, and the perineum. Deep lymph channels lie around all major organs of the body.

The structure of the lymphatic system differs significantly from all other fluid flow systems in the body. It begins in the tissues as lymphatic capillaries or blind endothelial tubes composed of a single layer of leaky squamous epithelium (Fig. 68.1). These thinly walled capillaries are supported by anchoring filaments that are attached to the endothelial cells and extend into the surrounding interstitium. These filaments bind the endothelial tubes to the proteinaceous fibers in the interstitial matrix. They also function to open spaces between the endothelial cells as fluid accumulates and prevent collapse of the thinly walled lymph capillaries.

At the level of the arterial capillaries, filtration of intravascular fluid occurs, allowing for the passage of fluid, proteins, and particles from the vascular system directly into the interstitium. This fluid then diffuses along the connective tissue fibers and the anchoring filaments in the interstitium, where

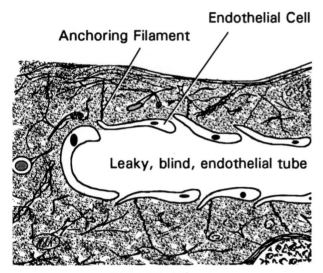

Anchoring Filament   **Endothelial Cell**

Leaky, blind, endothelial tube

Figure 68.1. *Beginnings of lymphatic system. (Illustration by W.A. Kuchera.).*

it actively mixes with extracellular fluids. More fluid gets into the interstitial spaces than is removed by the capillaries, even when all is normal. Because the simple squamous epithelium of the lymphatic capillaries contains no basement membrane, it possesses a greater permeability than do the blood capillaries. This promotes ready passage of the excess transudate from the interstitium back into the closed circuit of the lymphatic system.

Peripheral lymphatic capillaries join to form capillary plexus that in turn form larger trunks. In the superior portion of the body, the chest wall and the pleural spaces are drained by the intercostal trunks. The mediastinal trunks drain the thoracic viscera. The internal jugular trunk drains the left side of the head and neck, and the subclavian trunk drains the left arm and shoulder. The pelvis is drained by the internal iliac trunk, while the lower extremities are drained by the external iliac trunk. The lumbar trunk drains the lumbar area; the small intestine trunk drains the small intestine, the lacteals, and Peyer's patches. The colon and the mesentery are drained by the superior and inferior mesenteric trunks. The gastric trunk receives drainage from the liver, spleen, stomach, and pancreas. All of these trunks eventually drain into two main trunks that empty into the venous system in the cervicothoracic area, either the right lymphatic duct (RLD) or the thoracic duct, also called the left lymphatic duct (LLD).

The trunks of the abdomen, pelvis, and lower limbs drain into the cisterna chyli, a saccular dilation of the thoracic duct that lies on the anterior right side of the Ll and L2 vertebral bodies, at the level of the renal vessels. The cisterna chyli lies behind the right crus of the diaphragm next to the abdominal aorta and represents the distal portion of the thoracic duct. In some cases, the lumbar trunks unite above the level of the L2 vertebra, forming a plexus of vessels that drain directly into the thoracic duct, in which case the cisterna chyli is absent.

All of the aforementioned trunks (from the left side of the

head and neck, the left arm and thorax, left and right portions of the lower body, and the thoracic viscera) drain into the LLD. Only the right side of the head, the right side of the neck, the right arm, and the right chest (inclusive of the heart and portions of the lungs) drain into a separate main duct, the RLD. Sodeman and Sodeman state that sometimes the posterior portion of the left upper lobe of the lung drains into the thoracic duct.[4]

The thoracic duct is the largest lymph vessel in the body, typically measuring 36–45 cm in total length. The thoracic duct lies directly against the vertebral column as it courses cephalically. It passes through the aortic hiatus of the diaphragm and traverses the posterior mediastinum between the aorta and the azygos vein, passing in front of the phrenic nerve and behind the vagus nerve. At the level of the sternal angle (T4), it inclines to the left of midline and enters the superior aperture of the thorax behind the aortic arch and to the left of the esophagus. At this juncture, it passes laterally across the carotid sheath and then arches caudally and anteriorly to the subclavian artery. The thoracic duct terminates at its junction with the venous system. It empties into the venous circulation in the region of the junction between the left subclavian and left brachiocephalic vein.

The RLD is formed by a merger in the right jugular trunk, the right subclavian trunk, and the right transverse cervical trunks. This short duct courses the medial border of the anterior scalene muscle and terminates in the jugulosubclavian junction in the anterior neck. A distinct RLD, approximately 1 cm in length, is present in only 20% of patients.[4(p841)] Usually, the three main contributing trunks of the duct empty separately via two or three separate openings.

The terminal points of both main trunks are protected by valves that prevent the back flow of blood into the lymphatic system. These are one-way valves under sympathetic autonomic control. In addition, the lymph vessels possess a series of one-way valves situated in the vessels every few millimeters that prevent regression of lymph as it returns to the central lymphatic collection sites. All lymph moves unidirectionally. Each segment between valves acts independently, filling and emptying on fluid demand. The larger lymph vessels contain smooth muscle, which is also innervated by the sympathetic nervous system. The extent of sympathetic innervation suggests that response to stress may hinder optimal decongestion of tissues via the lymphatic system.

Lymph

Lymph is the final component of the lymphatic system. Lymph is the substance that leaks out of the arterial capillaries, into the interstitium, and into the single-cell lymphatic vessels. Lymph is usually clear in color and contains proteins (2–6 gm%)[5] and salts. After a meal, the lymph in the thoracic duct becomes richly laden with emulsified water-soluble fats, and its color may actually change to yellow. The primary cells of lymph are lymphocytes. Lymphocytes have been found in quantities of 2000–20,000/mm%[6] in the thoracic duct.

Lymph also contains clotting factors; it clots on standing. Finally, large particles such as bacteria and smaller viruses are found in the peripheral lymph before filtration through a lymph node or one of the organized lymphoid tissues. These larger particles are brought into close contact with lymphatic cells having immune functions.

PHYSIOLOGY

Let the lymphatics always receive and discharge naturally, if so we have no substance detained long enough to produce fermentation, fever, sickness, and death.
　　—A.T. STILL[1]

Function

The lymphatic system has four basic functions:

　　Maintaining fluid balance in the body
　　Purification and cleansing of tissues
　　Defense
　　Nutrition

Fluid Balance

One of the most important functions performed by the lymphatic system is that of fluid balance. At least 50% of all plasma proteins that diffuse out of the vascular system within a 24-hour period return to the body by way of the lymphatic system.[2] On a daily basis, approximately 30 liters of fluid filters out of the capillaries and into the interstitial spaces.[6] Of this 30 liters, approximately 90% (27 liters) drains back into the blood capillaries, but the remaining 10% (3 liters) drains into the lymphatic channels. In addition to absorption of this 3-liter volume, the system has a capacity to absorb a limited amount of excess fluid from the cavities of the pleura, the peritoneum, the pericardium, and the joints. Although 10% is a proportionately small amount of fluid that is returned to the circulation by way of the lymphatics, this lymph flow is vital because proteins and other substances of high molecular weights, unable to pass easily into the pores of the vascular capillaries because of their large size, are able to enter the lymphatic capillaries with relative ease. In the case of significant fluid overload, it is the lymphatic system that provides the homeostatic reserve to resist or forestall damage.[6]

PURIFICATION AND CLEANSING

The lymphatic system serves important functions in cleansing the body, both within the structure of the lymphatic conduits and without. Because lymph forms as a filtrate from the arterial capillaries into the extracellular spaces, lymph actually bathes all of the organs of the body. Before passing into the capillaries of the lymphatic system, it cleanses the extracellular spaces of particulate matter, exudates, and bacteria. Once inside of the lymphatic system, it readily delivers all of these substances to the lymph nodes, which act as purifying filters for removal of this waste matter from the circulation.

DEFENSE

Intimately associated with the cleansing and purification functions of lymph are the defensive properties of the lymphatic system. Because of the pervasive quantities and locations of lymphoid tissues in the body, lymph comes in fairly immediate contact with any toxins, bacteria, and viruses entering the system. The lymphatic system provides the first line of defense against this invasion. Acquired immunity does not develop until the body has first exposure to these invading antigens. All of these substances contain proteins, polysaccharides, or lipoprotein complexes, and these are the essential substrates by which the body is able to develop acquired (adaptive) immunity. The lymphatic system's importance is underlined by the fact that any individual who genetically lacks lymphoid tissue or who has had chemical or radiation obliteration of the body's lymphoid tissue cannot defend against antigenic invasion and will die. The lymphatic defense system is broken down into two separate divisions, both embryologically derived from lymphocytic stem cells in the bone marrow. The T-lymphatic division contains those sensitized lymphocytes that have been processed through the thymus gland and function to provide cellular immunity. The majority of this preprocessing occurs before birth of the infant, and the remainder shortly thereafter. Cellular immunity, also known as lymphocytic immunity, is the capability of the sensitized lymphocyte to attach to a foreign substance and to destroy it.

The B-lymphocytic division is named for the bursa of Fabricius, a structure not found in mammals but found in birds, where B-lymphocytes were first identified. These B-lymphocytes are believed to be processed in the liver or the spleen in humans (although the exact location is unknown) and give rise to humoral immunity. Humoral immunity is the capability of the body to produce globulin molecules known as antibodies, which possess the specific capability of attacking the invading antigens.

Not only is the lymphatic system responsible for the production and maintenance of these two essential defensive armies, but also the free flow of lymph is vital for direct contact of the invading agents with the defense factors. Whenever injury occurs, the subsequent inflammation brings increased vascular perfusion, increased capillary filtration, and increased lymph production to the area. This is the body's obvious mechanism for increasing contact between antigens and antibodies as well as phagocytes. The greater the lymphatic flow through the body, the greater the contact of body defenses with all toxins, particulate matter, and other foreign substances.

NUTRITION

As stated earlier, 50% or more of all plasma proteins are carried by the lymphatic system back to the vascular system after their efflux from the arterial capillaries into the extracellular spaces.

Many of these proteins are capable of binding nutrients that the cells need. Long chain fats, chylomicrons, and cholesterol are absorbed in large quantities from the lacteals in the villi of the small intestine. After a large and fatty meal, the thoracic duct may contain up to 2% fat. With fat absorption, the lymph of the gastrointestinal tract changes from its normal clear appearance to a yellow or milky color. This particular kind of lymph is called chyle.

Mechanisms of Flow

Several factors determine the rate of lymph flow in the body. Interstitial fluid pressure is one important factor. Normally, interstitial fluid pressure is maintained at −6.3 mm Hg. Any increase in this pressure increases the absorption of lymph into lymph capillaries. An increase, from −6 or −7 mm Hg to O mm Hg, increases lymphatic flow approximately 20 times its normal rate of 120 ml/hr.[6]

At O mm Hg, a ceiling of efficiency is reached. Above that level, interstitial fluid pressure becomes greater than the pressure inside of the lymph channels, causing them to collapse, obstructing the pathways; drainage ceases.

Several elements increase interstitial pressure:

Increased arterial capillary pressure (such as in systemic hypertension)

Decreased plasma colloid osmotic pressure (as in cirrhosis of the liver, in which there is a decrease of plasma protein synthesis)

Increased interstitial fluid protein (as in plasma hypoalbuminemia associated with starvation)

Increased capillary permeability (associated with toxins such as rattlesnake poisoning)

A second element affecting lymph flow is the intrinsic lymphatic pump. As stated earlier, each section between the valves of the lymph channels functions as an independent unit. When lymph enters into a segment of the lymph vessel, distension of that individual section occurs. In the larger vessels, this distension causes contraction of the smooth muscle within the walls of the lymph channel and effectively pumps the lymph to the next independent segment, where the dilation and pumping process is repeated. A similar process occurs in the lymph capillaries. Although there is no smooth muscle in the lymph capillary, the endothelial cells contain contractile fibers (myoendothelial fibers) that respond to fluid distension in the same way. This lymphatic pumping at the capillary level also creates a slight degree of suction as the capillary passes from relaxed to distended to relaxed states, and it is this suction that helps pull fluids from the interstitium in the face of the −6 mm Hg interstitial fluid pressure.

Finally, in the same way that lymph flow is pumped by intrinsic mechanisms, extrinsic pressures on the lymph channel also promote passive filling of lymphatic segments with subsequent pumping effect.

Direct external pressure on a lymph channel increases the flow of lymph. Internally, wherever pressure is exerted over the lymph vessel, flow increases. Wherever arteries with their rhythmic contractions cross lymph channels, flow increases.

The diaphragm is considered by many to be an extremely important extrinsic pump for the lymphatic system. Movements of the diaphragmatic crura exert a pumping influence on the cisterna chyli. All movements of internal organs, such as respiration and abdominal peristalsis, as well as movements of the extremities, exert an effective external pump. Not only does the diaphragm directly massage the lymphatics, but respiration produces pressure gradients between the chest and the abdomen. These pressure gradients, along with the one-way valves, help to pull lymph toward the venous circulation. If a person breathes 12 breaths per minute, this produces 17,280 pressure changes per day. Rate and depth of breathing can therefore increase or decrease lymphatic flow.

The overall effect of the extrinsic pump is best underlined by the fact that vigorous exercise, with its movement of extremities, organs, and the diaphragm, may increase lymph flow 15–20 times the normal resting flow amount.

Other functional diaphragms, such as the pelvic diaphragm, normally work in synchrony with the abdominal diaphragm. When this happens, there is optimal movement of interstitial fluids from the pelvis and optimal pressure gradients from abdominal diaphragmatic contractions. The pelvic organs predominantly rest on the soft tissues of the perineal floor, in contrast to the abdominal contents that rest against the large iliac fossae. The soft tissues that form the urogenital diaphragm, pelvic diaphragm, and other perineal ligaments and tissues close the pelvic outlet. They form a solid yet elastic floor that also allows for periodic opening to occur for excretion and, in females, for childbirth.

The abdominal viscera constitute a dynamic column that rests on the iliac fossa and the edge of the ischiopubic rami. In spite of these supports, some pressure is still exerted on the pelvic inlet from above. The pelvic organs themselves add their weight and, along with the effects of gravity, add to the load that must be supported by the perineal floor.

To completely fulfill its function, the pelvic floor needs to provide elasticity in addition to its supportive function. If the floor were rigid, thoracic inhalation would compress the pelvic organs from above. Compensation by the pelvic floor must dissipate or alleviate the permanent, cyclic respiratory pressure and also the transient or temporary increased pressures produced by coughing, sneezing, hiccups, pregnancy, and so on. This synchronized contraction of the abdominal diaphragm and descent of the relaxed pelvic diaphragm, and the reciprocal motions with exhalation, produces a mechanical pump for the lymphatic vessels and venous sinuses in the pelvis and around the rectum and perineum.

Within the perineal floor are openings for the urogenital tract and rectum. These orifices are anatomic weak points, and because of the number and size in women, the female perineum is much more fragile than the male perineum. Structurally, these orifices provide a weakness that may allow herniations or ptosis in the adult. Because of these weak areas where the urinary and vaginal tracts exit, the body has developed a second layer of reinforcement distal to the shelf of the levator ani muscles. This is called the urogenital diaphragm.

The pelvic diaphragm needs to acts as a support and yet remain elastic. Distension of the pelvic diaphragm must be in phase with the continual movements of the thoracic diaphragm and also with the transient changes in intrapelvic pressure. This helps assure that the pelvic organs escape undue pressure and that there is a free flow of fluids within the vascular and lymphatic channels of the pelvic region.

PATHOPHYSIOLOGY

The consequence of a poorly functioning lymphatic system is congestion or frank edema from the buildup of interstitial fluids. Edema is the result of too much fluid getting into the interstitium or too little fluid getting out. Its presence signifies that the body's compensatory mechanisms have already failed. Conditions that overload the interstitium produce congestion and edema by overriding the absorptive capabilities of the lymphatic system. Excessive interstitial fluid produces excessive interstitial pressure, which in turn is associated with collapse of the lymph capillaries, resulting in further interstitial congestion and edema. Edema has a second deleterious effect of dilating the lymphatic capillaries. With dilation, the endothelial cells separate and the flap valves of the capillaries become nonfunctional. This is associated with a shutdown of the intrinsic lymphatic pumping of the capillaries.

Conditions of high venous pressure are associated with increased capillary filtration rates and have an increased tendency to produce edema. These conditions include congestive heart failure, incompetent heart valves, venous obstruction, and the effects of gravity. Arteriolar dilation and venous constriction are also associated with increased capillary permeability, as are the effects of substances such as kinins and histamines.

Conditions of starvation and cirrhosis of the liver, as well as other states of abnormal protein metabolism, affect interstitial fluid gradients by altering the osmotic effect of plasma protein levels. Decreased osmotic pressure gradients across the capillary, which occur with decreased plasma protein level or the accumulation of osmotically active substances in the interstitium, promote increased accumulation of fluid in the extracellular spaces with all the ramifications that go along with the edematous state.

Inadequate drainage also results in the development of edema because of the relative imbalance created in pressure gradients, even in the face of normal capillary filtration. Posttraumatic or postsurgical scarring may cause mechanical obstructions to absorptive flow and mechanical blockages, such as those produced by filariasis or intraluminal carcinoma, creating absorptive insufficiency that will eventually lead to edema.

The results of edema are pervasive and profound to all surrounding tissues. Edema causes compression not only on the lymphatic channels but also on the nearby vascular and neurologic structures, thus potentially diminishing their function-

ing. Edema is associated with increased tissue congestion. Stasis of interstitial fluids promotes changes in the pH of tissues and organs, further compromising function. This promotes inflammation that in turn produces greater edema and continuation of the cycle. It also is associated with infiltration of fibroblasts, which can lead to fibrosis and contracture of tissues. Edema also affects the delivery of nutrients to the affected sites and is associated with even greater changes in tissue function and healing abilities. Finally, edema affects bioavailability of drugs and hormones, hampering not only medical management of the primary fluid buildup but also, because of tissue congestion, decreasing the efficacy of any pharmacologic treatment.

PRINCIPLES OF TREATMENT

Goals

The goal for treatment of the lymphatic system is to have a balanced, well-functioning system in which no edema occurs. The fact that the lymphatic system is a passive system underlines the importance of motion and adequate drainage of lymph. OMT has long provided an extra measure of movement that promotes proper fluid dynamics. Manipulation is associated with:

Increased resorption of fluids
Increased circulation and respiration
Decreased proteins in the interstitium
Facilitation from a more beneficial pH balance

FASCIAL PATTERN DIAGNOSIS (ZINK)

Although there was previous talk about the fascias of the body having rotatory preferences, J. Gordon Zink, DO, was the first to provide a written, understandable, and clinically useful explanation for treatment, with a method of diagnosing and manipulative methods of treating the fascial patterns of the body. Fascias form the pathways for lymphatic vessels as well as for arteries, veins, and nerves. Torsion of these pathways can hinder the flow of lymph through the lymphatic vessels. Zink identified four areas of the body as crossover sites where fascial tension could occur[7]:

Occipitoatlantal (OA)
Cervicothoracic (CT)
Thoracolumbar (TL)
Lumbosacral (LS)

He tested the fascial preference for rotation and side-bending of those regions of the body. Zink had observed that almost all people who thought they were well and healthy had alternating patterns of rotatory preference at the key sites. When testing rotation from the OA to the LS regions, he found that approximately 80% of these people had the body pattern of L/R/L/R, and the other 20% had R/L/R/L, so he named the former pattern the common compensatory pattern (CCP). Zink reasoned that, ideally, there should be equal motion to the right or to the left in all of these reference zones, but apparently the stress of gravity and living produced the alternative patterns.

People in the hospital tend to have patterns that do not alternate; this is also true for people who are easily stressed, who get sick easily, and who have low levels of wellness. When reference zones do not indicate equal or alternating patterns of rotational preference among the four regions of the body, Dr. Zink called these uncompensated fascial patterns. These need OMT. The goal of treatment for these people is to return their fascial patterns to ideal so that their bodies can establish more efficient fascial patterns, usually of the compensated form. Since fascia attaches to bone, direct (thrust or muscle energy) or indirect methods of OMT can be performed to normalize the fascial preferences. Dr. Zink's diagnostics and treatment for the fascial regions of the body improved the pathway for lymph flow.

Types of Treatment

Lymphatic treatments are essentially divided into two broad categories: those techniques that remove restrictive impediments to lymphatic flow and those that promote and augment the flow of lymph. A thorough treatment regime usually includes techniques from both categories, in that sequence. A sequence for a basic lymphatic treatment program includes:

1. Rib raise and/or use paraspinal inhibition (T1-L2). This is designed to reduce hypersympathetic activity to the lymphatic vessels in the area of concern and around the major lymphatic duct that anatomically drains that area or region. Mobilizing the ribs also enhances respiration.
2. Diagnose and treat any thoracic inlet somatic dysfunction. The thoracic inlet is the common obstruction to lymphatic flow from anywhere in the body.
3. Dome (relax) the abdominal diaphragm. This improves the ability of this major fibromuscular diaphragm to produce effective pressure gradients between the thoracic and abdominal cavities.
4. Apply some additional form of lymphatic pump and/or techniques to further promote lymphatic flow. This may be optional in a basic plan but would further enhance lymphatic flow.

More than one type of treatment affects the lymphatic system. For instance, use of high-velocity low-amplitude treatment alters muscle tone and neural reflexes that affect structures such as the diaphragm, adding to the efficiency of the system. Muscle energy, deep articulatory, or other direct techniques do the same thing. An example of a deep articulatory technique is rib raising in a repetitive fashion, freeing the ribs and diaphragm to have a more relaxed, efficient performance and normalizing sympathetic autonomic activity from the thoracolumbar sympathetic chain ganglia. Myofascial release techniques, conversely, are particularly effective in eliminating inappropriate tension in tissues surrounding lymphatic channels

that tend to be constrictive in nature. Cranial techniques are thought to have a balancing effect on the sympathetic/parasympathetic nervous system, leading to deeper diaphragmatic breathing as well as promoting appropriate cranial venous fluid return.

TREATMENT PLAN (ONE EXAMPLE)

Treatment of the lymphatic system should begin with the removal of all restrictions resulting from tissue hypertonicity that may be affecting lymph flow. Release of the central lymphatic system should be accomplished first, followed by release of the periphery. This decreases the likelihood of exceeding the system's innate 7 mm Hg maximum increase in capability of handling increased flow.

Treatment begins by releasing the central lymphatic system: the area of the thoracic inlet, then the abdominothoracic diaphragm and the pelvic diaphragm. Release of the peripheral lymphatic systems should include drainage techniques of the head and neck as well as the extremities (in each case beginning centrally and progressing peripherally). Lymphatic treatment should be accompanied by a release of all respiratory restrictions (rib or clavicular somatic dysfunctions) as well as restrictions of the muscles, joints, and the abdomen. Rib raising and treatment of any spinal somatic dysfunction are also prudent to optimize autonomic activity. Attention should also be given to dysfunctions of the cranium, including the temporals, the occiput, and the sphenoid, to promote optimal functioning of the cranial nerves, particularly the vagus nerve (cranial nerve X).

CONTRAINDICATIONS OF LYMPHATIC TREATMENTS

Contraindications of individual treatments are included along with the following individual techniques. Relative contraindications for lymphatic treatment techniques include osseous fracture, bacterial infections with a temperature over 102° F (in which case antibiotic control should first be implemented to reduce the chance of seeding and encouraging a generalized body infection), and certain stages of carcinoma.

LYMPHATIC MANIPULATIVE TECHNIQUES

Even under normal conditions, more blood gets to the tissues than can be removed by the venous system. This amount is even greater when there is dysfunction or inflammation. An important principle in the efficient care of patients with dysfunction or disease is to be sure that the lymphatic drainage is as efficient as possible. This can be performed by diagnosing impediments to flow and then designing osteopathic manipulative techniques to remove those impediments, improve the pumps, and directly promote decongestion of an organ or region of the body. The lymphatic system has no intrinsic pump and must heavily rely on the production of efficient pressure gradients between the thoracic and abdominal regions, produced by the efficient action of a well-domed abdominal dia-

Figure 68.2. Thoracic inlet: static landmarks. (Illustration from W.A. Kuchera.)

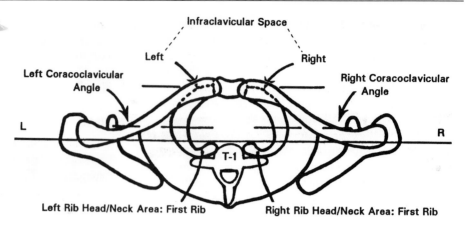

phragm. Recent studies reveal that there are sympathetic fibers innervating muscle fibers in the larger lymphatic vessels, implying that sympathicotonia may reduce the amount of lymph that the lymphatic vessels can carry.

TECHNIQUES TO REMOVE IMPEDIMENTS

Open Thoracic Inlet Fascia

The thoracic inlet (Fig. 68.2) is anatomically the first ribs, the first thoracic vertebra, and the manubrium. Clinically the thoracic inlet is the first two ribs, the first four thoracic vertebrae, and the manubrium of the sternum. Fascia from the scalenus and the longus coli muscles join together to produce a functional fascial diaphragm for the superior thoracic inlet. Lymphatic fluid returning from any site outside the thorax must pass through this diaphragm.

The thoracic fascial inlet is a common diaphragm for both the right and the left lymphatic ducts. The left lymphatic duct (thoracic duct) passes through this diaphragm twice. The tissues of the thoracic inlet are frequently subjected to the stresses associated with carriage of the head on the shoulders as well as the muscular pull of the shoulders themselves. Some physicians evaluate the thoracic inlet fascias by examining first rib motion during respiration and then determining the direction of fascial ease or restriction to the application of traction in all directions at the cervicothoracic junction. This is an organized method of determining preference of the tissues at the cervicothoracic junction:

1. The patient may be supine or seated, and the physician may approach the patient from either the anterior or the posterior position.
2. Place the fingertips at the superior aspect of the shoulders in the region of the first rib (Table 68.1).

The fascias at the inlet tend to pull the cervicothoracic region into side-bending and rotation to the same side. Opening the thoracic inlet relieves obstruction to lymphatic flow at this level.

Table 68.1
Thoracic Inlet Diagnosis: Static and Motion Test Findings

	Inlet Fascia Rotated and Side-bent Left	Inlet Fascia Rotated and Side-bent Right
First rib	Left rib ↓ /right rib ↑	Left rib ↑ /right rib ↓
Infraclavicular space	Left deep	Right deep
Coracoclavicular angle	Left posterior	Right posterior
Spring upper ribs	Left spring/right resist	Right spring/left resist

THORACIC INLET—TWO-STEP WITH MUSCLE ENERGY ACTIVATION

Patient Position

Supine.

Physician Position

Sitting or standing at the head of the table (to treat side-bending restriction).

Procedure

1. Side-bend the neck to the side of restricted side-bending, using IP joints of the index finger of one hand as a fulcrum at the cervicothoracic junction on that side (Fig. 68.3).
2. Rotate the patient's head to the opposite side to lock out the cervical spine above the cervicothoracic junction.
3. Ask the patient to attempt side-bending the head to the side opposite the fulcrum hand as you isometrically resist the effort.
4. Ask the patient to completely relax and repeat step 3 three or four times.
5. Place the head and neck back to neutral position; now, rotate the head to the restrictive barrier of rotation (without side-bending) using your hand on the side of the head and the fingers of the IP joints of the index finger of that hand at the cervicothoracic junction (the fulcrum) (Fig. 68.4).

6. Ask the patient to attempt to rotate the head and neck toward your fulcrum hand as you isometrically resist the effort.
7. Ask the patient to completely relax, and repeat Step 6 three or four times.
8. Recheck the fascial preference at the thoracic inlet.

THORACIC INLET—DIRECT MYOFASCIAL RELEASE

Patient Position

Supine with arm abducted 90° from the body.

Physician Position

Seated at the side of the patient.

Procedure

1. Use your knee to support the patient's elbow and cephalad hand to support the patient's wrist.
2. With caudal fingers placed on the superior aspect of the supraclavicular fossa, apply downward pressure to the patient's wrist (Fig. 68.5). The caudal fingers apply gentle anterior pressure against the clavicle.
3. Then move the patient's wrist superior. The caudal hand follows the rotation of the clavicle posteriorly until tension develops. Hold this until some relaxation is noted.
4. Repeat this two or three times.

NOTE: This technique can be uncomfortable to those who need it the most. Please be aware of your whole patient and not just the clavicle.

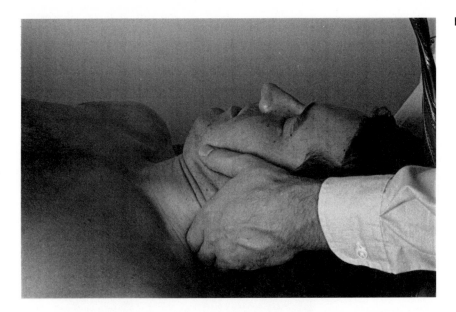

Figure 68.3. Thoracic inlet: side-bending.

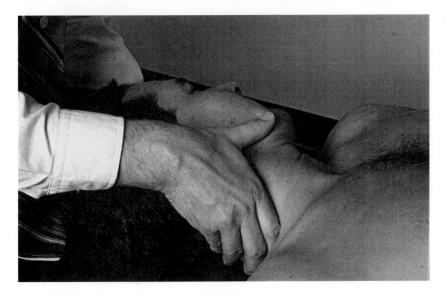

Figure 68.4. Thoracic inlet: rotation.

Figure 68.5. Thoracic inlet: direct myofascial release.

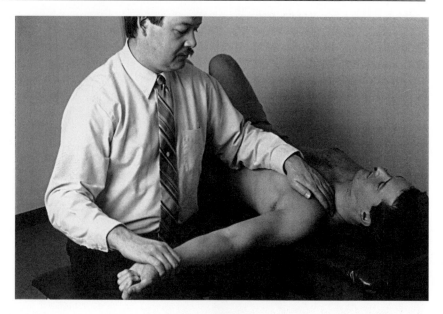

Normalize Sympathetic Activity

Treatment by rib raising reduces constriction of larger lymphatic vessels. Rib raising that raises the rib heads also stimulates the thoracic sympathetic chain ganglia. This initially stimulates regional sympathetic efferent activity to organs related to that spinal level of sympathetic innervation, but in the long run, rib raising results in a prolonged reduction in sympathetic outflow from the area treated. By freeing rib motion, the excursion of the rib cage during respiration is also freed. By freeing the rib heads, the excursion of the chest during breathing is increased and lymphatic flow is improved.

RIB RAISING—SEATED

Patient Position

Seated on table.

Physician Position

Standing at the side of the table, facing the patient

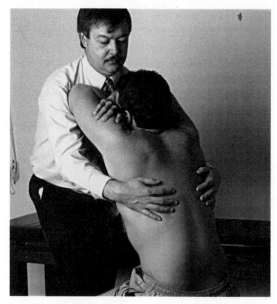

Figure 68.6. Rib raising: seated.

Procedure

1. Have the patient cross his or her arms and grasp the deltoid muscles.
2. Have the patient lean toward you resting his or her crossed arms on your chest. (A variation: patient's arms raised overhead, draped on your shoulders instead of crossed.)
3. Grasp the posterior, inferior rib angles bilaterally in the area you are treating (Fig. 68.6). (Begin cephalad, move caudad, return to cephalad.)
4. Apply a lateral traction bilaterally at the rib angle while pulling the patient toward you.
5. Have the patient breathe deeply to aid the mobilization of the entire rib cage.

RIB RAISING—SUPINE

Patient Position

Supine.

Physician Position

Standing or seated at the patient's side.

Procedure

1. Place your hands (palms) under the patient's thorax, contacting the rib angles with the pads of your fingers (Fig. 68.7).
2. Flex your fingers to achieve contact with the rib angle and the patient's posterior thorax.

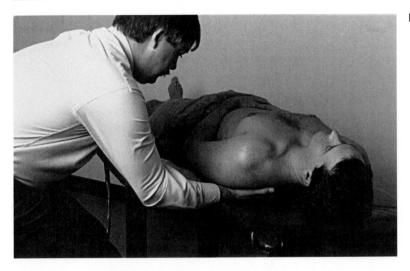

Figure 68.7. Rib raising: supine.

3. Apply traction on the rib angle.
4. While maintaining traction, bend your knees and lower your trunk, which raises the ribs by moving your hands upward. This is a fulcrum/lever action. Do *not* bend your wrists. (Particularly if the patient is in a hospital bed, it is easier to move your hands upward if you reciprocally push your forearms down.)
5. Move your hands to subsequent rib angles until all ribs are treated.
6. Treat the opposite side of the rib cage in the same manner.

NOTE: If you have an assistant, a two-person technique can be used treating both sides of the rib cage at once. Care must be taken to treat both sides of the rib cage with equal traction, and motions of the operators must be synchronous.

Improve Extrinsic Lymphatic Pump

Osteopathic manipulative techniques affect diaphragms so that they can more efficiently create alternating pressure gradients. This can usually be done most time-efficiently if the abdominal diaphragm's muscular attachments are first treated for maximal structure–function; cervical somatic dysfunction should also be treated because this is the region associated with the diaphragm's innervation. The thoracoabdominal diaphragm is a strong muscular structure innervated by the phrenic nerve (C3-C5). Tension in this structure produces substantial alterations in the lymphatic flow.

The body is constructed in such a fashion that lymph flow predominately runs in a longitudinal plane. At several significant regions, however, horizontal tissues transect this pattern. Should these horizontal tissues be placed on tension for any reason, lymph flow could be significantly impeded. Osteopathic physicians have long considered that there are four of these regions:

Abdominal diaphragm: placed between the abdomen and the chest cavity, it is muscular and tendinous in nature, forming a continuous sheet interrupted only by the aorta, esophagus, inferior vena cava, and accompanying blood vessels, lymphatics, and nerves.

Pelvic diaphragm: this is a group of muscles and fascia that span the perineum and form a lower border to the abdominal contents.

Thoracic inlet or outlet: these are located in the cervicothoracic region.

Tentorium cerebelli: this diaphragm affects venous return from the brain because the brain has no lymphatic system and relies on the veins to perform both functions.

Dome Abdominal Diaphragm

"Doming the diaphragm" is a term used to refer to relaxing the resting state of the abdominal diaphragm (or the pelvic diaphragm). If the diaphragm can be completely relaxed and well-domed, its contraction and relaxation produce greater pressure gradients between the thoracic and abdominal cavities, along with the one-way valves, and promotes better lymphatic drainage back into the venous circulation. The pressure gradients act as an extrinsic pump for the lymphatic system. The doming techniques may also directly engage the inferior surface of the diaphragm and augment its excursion during expiration.

Thoracoabdominal Diaphragm

DIAGNOSIS OF FASCIAL RESTRICTION AT THORACOABDOMINAL DIAPHRAGM

Procedure

1. Place the palmar surfaces of your hands on the right and left side of the lower rib cage of the patient, with the fingers pointing toward the table (Fig. 68.8).
2. Rotate the tissues of the thoracoabdominal cylinder to the right and then to the left about a vertical axis, to test the ease of or restriction to rotatory motion.

Figure 68.8.   Diagnosis of thoracoabdominal restriction.

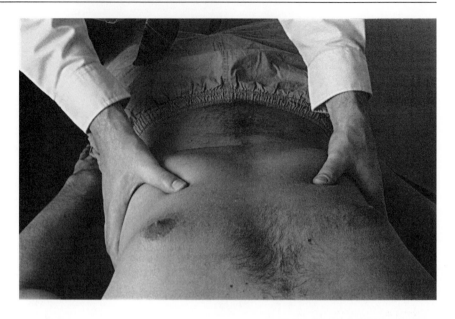

Figure 68.9.   Direct fascial release of thoracic diaphragm.

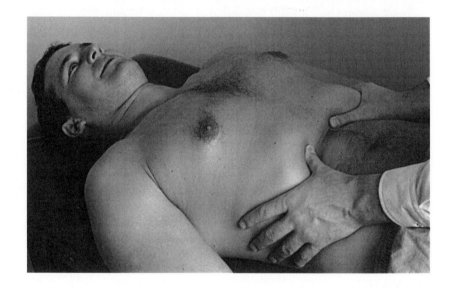

3. This region can then also be tested for side-bending preference by inducing translation of the region in each direction.

Treatment examples for thoracic diaphragm dysfunction point out a problem: fascias at the thoracoabdominal diaphragm prefer to rotate to the left side.

THORACIC DIAPHRAGMATIC FASCIAL RELEASE—DIRECT METHOD

Patient Position

Supine on the table.

Physician Position

Standing beside the table.

Procedure

1. Rotate the tissues of the thoracoabdominal region (tube) in the direction of their restriction; rotate to the restrictive barrier (Fig. 68.9).
2. Hold there and ask the patient to "take a deep breath in and out through the mouth." Notice the side of greatest movement and the side of least movement.
3. Maintain the rotation but adjust tension through your hands to produce a vertical shearing force on the thoracoabdominal tube, and ask the patient to repeat the big breath in and out through the mouth.
4. Adjust the tensions through your hands until there is equal excursion produced by the right and the left side of the thoracoabdominal diaphragm.

5. Hold those vectors while the patient breathes deeply two or three times.
6. Return the patient to neutral and retest rotational preference of the tissues of the thoracoabdominal region.

THORACIC DIAPHRAGMATIC FASCIAL RELEASE—MYOFASCIAL

Patient Position

Seated, erect and not slumped; the patient may relax but not collapse.

Physician Position

Standing behind the patient.

Procedure

1. Pass your hands around the thoracic cage (under the patient's arms) and gently but firmly introduce your fingers underneath the costal margin.
2. Test for motion by passively rotating the thorax to the left and to the right. Determine (in one cycle of motion testing) in which direction there is greater freedom/ease of motion.
3. Treatment phase: with the fingers on the diaphragm, i.e., underneath the costal margin, carry the thorax in the direction toward which it moves more freely. Hold it in that position. Follow it as it goes through its fascial release (unwinds) and continue until it finally settles down into a free, gentle, rhythmic, vertical motion.
4. Retest the range of motion and evaluate treatment effectiveness.

DOME ABDOMINAL DIAPHRAGM—DIRECT MECHANICAL

Patient Position

Supine.

Physician Position

Standing at the patient's side.

Procedure

1. Place fingers on the outer aspect of the inferior border of the ribs with thumbs pointed toward each other medially and positioned directly caudad to the xiphoid process of the sternum.
2. On the first respiration, gently press downward with thumbs toward the table as the patient exhales; follow the diaphragm motion.
3. Hold this end position (barrier); the patient inhales again. (NOTE: There will be a sensation of resistance to respiration by the thumbs.)
4. On the second exhalation, press in further downward toward the table, following the diaphragm.
5. Repeat step #3.
6. On the third exhalation, press the thumbs cephalad following the superior course of the diaphragm.

Dome Pelvic Diaphragm

The pelvic diaphragm is a muscular sling located on the bony floor of the true pelvis that provides support for the pelvic organs. It is composed of two main muscles, the coccygeus muscle and the levator ani muscle. The coccygeus muscle attaches to the ischial spine and then to the sacrum and coccyx. The levator ani muscle is subdivided into two main parts according to its attachments to the innominate bone. The various muscles are as follows:

Iliococcygeus muscle: attaches to the iliac bone and the tendinous arch of the obturator internus to the coccyx and the anococcygeal ligament
Pubococcygeus muscle: attaches to the pubic bone and then to the coccyx and the midline structures of the perineum; it can be divided into three attachments according to attachments to the midline structures:

Pubococcygeus proper muscle: pubic bone to the coccyx and anococcygeal ligament
Puborectalis muscle: pubic bone to rectum forming a muscular sling behind the rectum near the anorectal junction
Pubovaginalis or puboprostatic muscle: pubic bone to one of these structures in the midline

Diagnosis of Pelvic Diaphragm Somatic Dysfunction

PROCEDURE

1. To approach the pelvic diaphragm, position the patient supine and sit at the side of the pelvis to be treated. Face toward the patient's head.
2. Flex the patient's knee and hip on this side. Identify the ischial tuberosity with your outside hand. Introduce the fingers of the other hand medial to the ischial tuberosity, letting the pads of the fingers keep contact with the medial surface of the ischium. Your fingers are now pressing into the ischiorectal fossa, the inclined roof of which is the pelvic diaphragm (Fig. 68.10). (See also Chapter 54, "Muscle Energy Treatment Techniques for Specific Areas.")
3. As the patient inhales, the pelvic diaphragm should press down on your fingertips. With exhalation, the pelvic diaphragm should move cephalically.
4. If the pelvic diaphragm is unable to descend, it is in an exhalation somatic dysfunction and is restricted in its inhalation phase. If it does not ascend well, it is in an inhalation somatic dysfunction and is restricted in its exhalation phase.

DOME EXHALATION PELVIC DIAPHRAGM: INDIRECT METHOD

Diagnosis

The pelvic diaphragm is in a cephalad position and does not descend during inhalation.

Patient Position

Supine, with knee and hip flexed on the side to be treated.

Figure 68.10. Dome pelvic diaphragm.

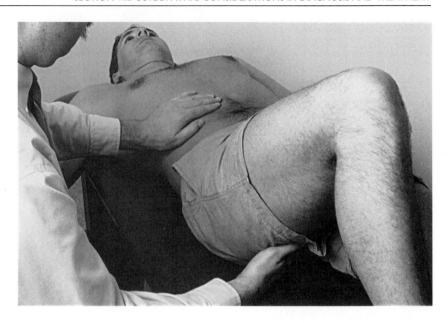

Physician Position

Sitting by the table on the side of the pelvis to be treated.

Procedure

1. With the hand closest to the patient, introduce the fingers as described above into the ischiorectal fossa. Place the other hand just below the costal margin on the same side to monitor movement of the thoracic diaphragm.
2. Ask the patient to take a deep inhalation, then exhale to the limit and hold the exhalation until forced to breathe. Repeat this procedure two or three times.
3. Recheck pelvic diaphragmatic tension.
4. Repeat treatment until both the thoracic and pelvic diaphragm come into phase with good amplitude (i.e., descend and ascend together).

DOME INHALATION PELVIC DIAPHRAGM—INDIRECT METHOD

Diagnosis

The pelvic diaphragm is in an inferior position and does not ascend in exhalation.

Patient Position

Supine, with knee and hip flexed on the side to be treated.

Physician Position

Sitting by the table on the side of the pelvis to be treated.

Procedure

1. Instruct the patient to hold his or her breath to the limit in inhalation. The pelvic diaphragm begins to ascend a moment before forced exhalation occurs.
2. The procedure may need to be repeated two or three times.

DOME INHALATION PELVIC DIAPHRAGM—DIRECT METHOD

Diagnosis

The pelvic diaphragm has descended and is restricted in moving superiorly into an inhalation position.

Patient Position

Supine, with knee and hip flexed on the side to be treated.

Physician Position

Sitting by the table on the side of the pelvis to be treated.

Procedure

1. Use the same hand placements as above.
2. Have the patient inhale, then exhale. With exhalation, encourage the diaphragm to move superiorly into its exhalation phase by providing fingertip pressure in a cephalic direction.
3. Maintain this position. Ask the patient to inhale. Be sure to hold ground, not allowing the pelvic diaphragm to descend.
4. As the patient exhales a second time, follow the diaphragm cephalically even more.
5. Repeat the treatment until both the thoracic and pelvic diaphragm come into phase with good amplitude (i.e., descend and ascend together).

TECHNIQUES TO PROMOTE LYMPHATIC FLOW

Pump Techniques

Lymphatic pump techniques are techniques designed to augment the pressure gradients that develop between the thoracic and abdominal regions during normal respirations. Some techniques are rhythmic; some are continuous. Some of the techniques influence the negative intrathoracic pressure of the thorax and some affect the abdominal pressure gradient.

PECTORAL TRACTION

Pectoral traction influences lymph flow by means of influencing the pectoralis minor muscle. By exerting a cephalic traction on the pectoralis minor, the range of motion of the first six ribs is augmented during inhalation, thereby increasing the negative pressure in the thorax as well as the volume of the chest. It is estimated that a 1-cm increase in the diameter of the chest increases the intake of air by 200–400 cc.[8] This is an efficacious technique that can be used with relative ease with patients with brittle bones, with patients in the intensive care unit where multiple tubes and monitoring devices may be in place, and with postsurgical patients.

PECTORAL TRACTION TECHNIQUE

Patient Position

Supine.

Physician Position

Standing at the head of the patient.

Procedure

1. Gently grasp the inferior border of the pectoralis muscles of each anterior axilla in a meat hook fashion, taking care not to gouge with fingertips (Fig. 68.11).
2. With your arms fully extended, apply a bilateral cephalad traction. (Lean back, using your body to produce the traction.)
3. While maintaining traction, have the patient breathe deeply. The combination of traction and respiratory motion releases the upper thoracic muscle tension.

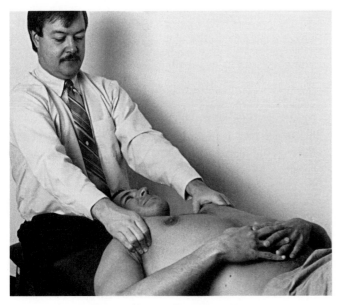

Figure 68.11. Pectoral traction.

THORACIC PUMP

Thoracic pump techniques, like pectoral traction, affect the intrathoracic pressure gradients by augmenting the thoracic range of motion and also by increasing expiratory efficacy. These techniques are indicated as initial treatments for clearing the thoracic duct region and are also especially effective for patients with chronic obstructive pulmonary disease (COPD), upper and lower respiratory infections, mastitis, or swollen upper extremities, and for postsurgical reduction of respiratory volume. Preliminary studies and a long history of clinical efficacy suggest that lymphatic pump techniques enhance immune function.[9]

Contraindications to these (and rib raising) techniques include:

1. Thoracic cage bony derangements:
   Fractures
   Dislocations
   Osteoporosis (relative contraindication)
2. Malignancy of lymphatic system
3. Be cautious with patients with a decreased cough reflex

REPETITIVE (CLASSIC) THORACIC PUMP

Patient Position

Supine. Caution: be sure that the patient does not have any food, gum, or foreign body (loose dentures, etc.) in the mouth.

Physician Position

Standing at the head of the table.

Procedure

1. Place your hands on the patient's thoracic wall with the thenar eminence of each hand over the pectoralis muscles, just distal to the respective clavicle; fingers are spread and angled toward the sides of the patient's body. The heels of the hands are on ribs 2–4 (Fig. 68.12). (With females it is important not to apply heavy pressure to the breast, but gentle pressure can assist in lymphatic drainage of congested breasts.)
2. A rhythmic pumping action is induced by alternating pressure and release through the operator's hands at a rate of approximately 110–120 times/minute. The motion is generated through a slight extension/flexion of the operator's elbows, with forearm, wrist, and hand acting as a fixed lever.
3. The rate of pumping action should be in sync with the natural response of the patient's body tissues; during this rhythmic treatment, the patient continues to breathe as usual.

THORACIC PUMP VARIATION OF ACTIVATION

Patient Position

Supine. Be sure that the patient does not have any food, gum, or foreign body (loose dentures, etc.) in the mouth.

Figure 68.12. Thoracic pump.

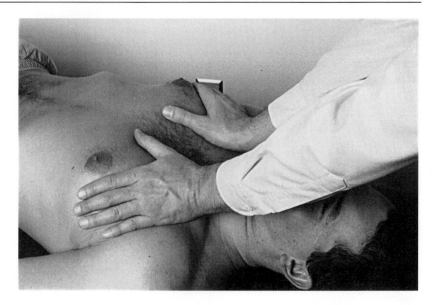

Physician Position

Standing at the head of the table.

Procedure

1. Position hands the same as in the first step of the classic pump technique.
2. Have the patient breathe in deeply with the mouth open. As the patient exhales, and with your elbows straight, follow the exhalation motion downward and maintain the endpoint. This applies a compressive force. With each subsequent breath, follow the exhalation motion downward, increasing the intrathoracic pressure with each exhalation.
3. One-third of the way through the fourth or fifth inhalation, as the patient's inhalation is creating a negative intrathoracic pressure within the thoracic cavity, briskly remove your hands. This will suddenly release the pressure from the chest, and you will hear a suction or vacuum release as air rushes into the lungs.
4. The rate of pumping action should be in sync with the natural response of the patient's body tissues.

Abdominal and Pedal Pumps

The abdominal pump and the pedal pump both work by intermittently pushing the abdominal contents up against the diaphragm, therefore indirectly affecting intrathoracic/abdominal pressure gradients. These techniques also indirectly massage the thoracic duct at its origin in the cisterna chyli.

INDICATIONS

1. Congestive heart failure (CHF)
2. Infective processes (in these patients it may increase immune competence)
3. Upper respiratory tract infection, asthma, and COPD

4. Restricted mobility of lumbar spine and thoracic cage
5. Hiatal hernia
6. Upper and lower GI dysfunctions

CONTRAINDICATIONS

1. Thoracic cage mechanical derangements:
    Fracture
    Dislocation
2. Traumatic disruption of liver, spleen, or adjacent organs
3. Recent surgery to gallbladder or other adjacent organs
4. A full stomach (postprandial)

ABDOMINAL PUMP

Patient Position

Supine.

Physician Position

Standing or kneeling at patient's side (on table).

Procedure

1. Place your palms on the patient's abdomen with fingers pointing to the patient's head, thumbs side by side (Fig. 68.13). (For small patients, or for greater control, you may place your hands on top of one another.)
2. Keep your arms extended and elbows locked.
3. Pump in a rhythmic manner. (Pumping motion is similar to the pedal or thoracic pump.) The rate should be 20–30 times/minute.

PEDAL PUMP (DALRYMPLE PUMP)

Patient Position

Supine (or prone).

Physician Position

Standing at the patient's feet.

Procedure

1. Grasp the patient's feet and dorsiflex (Fig. 68.14).
2. Introduce a force that hyperdorsiflexes the feet. Continue the force along the longitudinal axis of the body. The force should send a wave of motion cephalad, which will followed by a rebound wave moving caudally. (NOTE: Use an umbilicus, osseous landmark, or dermal lesion to appreciate the wave motion.)
3. As the rebound wave returns to the feet, reapply the dorsiflexion force, thereby creating a oscillatory pump.
4. The above technique may also be combined with the application of force through the plantarflexed feet (Fig. 68.15), thereby stretching the anterior body wall fascial structures.

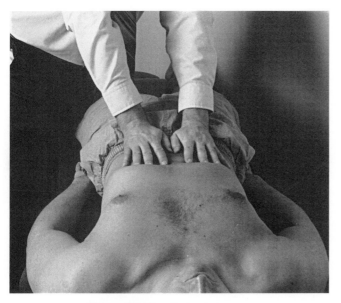

Figure 68.13. Abdominal pump.

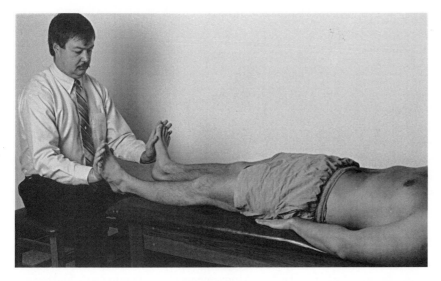

Liver and Spleen Pump Techniques

Both the liver and spleen are pressure-sensitive organs in the sense that they respond quickly to intermittently changing pressure gradients. The liver has a rich bed of lymphatic vessels, and its decongestion is postulated to aid in detoxification and in relief of visceral congestion.[9(p219)] The spleen stores red and white blood cells and screens the blood of damaged cells; the spleen pump is most commonly used for patients with systemic infections and for selected anemic patients with low resistance to infection. The proximity of these organs to the diaphragm and their pressure-sensitive nature suggest that this attribute may be important in the homeostatic functional mechanisms associated with these structures. Although other lymphatic pump techniques and diaphragm techniques indirectly or secondarily enhance pressure gradients affecting the liver and spleen, these pumps have long been available in the osteopathic armamentarium and are specifically designed for the liver and spleen.

INDICATIONS

1. Passive congestion of liver or spleen
2. Congestive heart failure (especially right-sided failure)
3. Consider in patients with infective processes (may increase immune competence)
4. Consider in patients with parenchymal disease of liver or spleen (may affect disease process by modulating blood and lymph fluid dynamics)

CONTRAINDICATIONS

1. Thoracic cage mechanical derangements:
   Fracture
   Dislocation
2. Lymphatic system malignancy
3. Traumatic disruption of liver, spleen, or adjacent organs
4. Acute hepatitis
5. Friable hepatomegaly as in infectious mononucleosis

Figure 68.14. Pedal pump: dorsiflexion.

Figure 68.15. Pedal pump: plantar flexion.

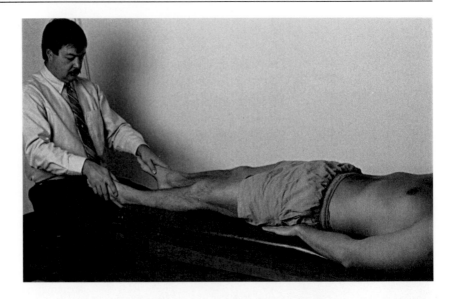

Figure 68.16. Liver drainage.

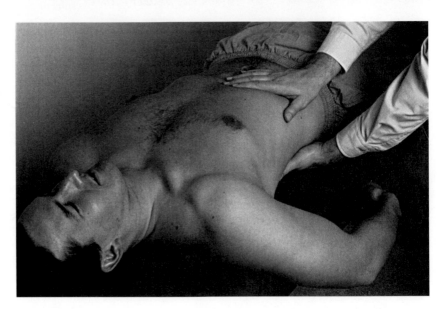

LYMPHATIC DRAINAGE OF THE LIVER ("LIVER QUIVER")

Stand on the right side of the supine patient, beside the lower thorax and facing the head (Fig. 68.16). Pass the left hand underneath the lower ribs and the right hand on the abdominal wall immediately below the costal margin. Request the patient to take a deep breath and identify the inferior border of the liver with the tips of the fingers of the right hand. As the exhalation occurs, the fingers penetrate over the liver and underneath the thoracic cage. Again, a deep breath; this time, as the breath goes out, use a vibratory motion of the right hand on the liver. This may be done three or four times; each time penetrate a little deeper into the area underneath the costal margin in relation to the liver.

LIVER/SPLEEN PUMP

An alternative technique for the liver pump is performed with the patient lying on the left side with the hips and knees flexed

to stabilize the body (Fig. 68.17). Sit on the table behind the thorax, facing toward the patient's feet. Have the patient places the right hand on the back of your right shoulder. Place both your hands on the lower thoracic cage, the left hand anteriorly, the right posteriorly, and the thumbs meeting in the axillary line. As you lean slightly backward, open up the rib cage while increasing abduction on the arm, and the patient takes a deep breath. As the patient exhales, lean on the thoracic cage with a vibratory motion to apply the pumping action to the liver. A similar technique can be used for the splenic area with the patient lying on the right side while you sit behind the patient on the left side of the table.

Direct Pressure Techniques to Move Lymph

Direct pressure techniques exert their influence by extrinsically increasing pressure on the lymphatic vessels. This extrinsic pressure facilitates movements of lymph into segmental regions

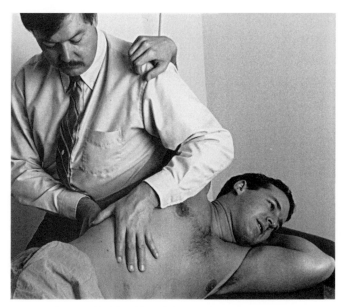

Figure 68.17. Liver drainage: alternative method.

of the lymphatic channel that, in turn, dilates the lymph vessel and invokes the intrinsic pressure of the lymphatic conduit via contraction of the smooth muscle within the lymph channel and the myoendothelial fibers within the lymph capillaries. This is especially effective for locally decongesting tissues.

Effleurage is defined in the *Glossary of Osteopathic Terminology* as "light or deep stroking of the skin toward the heart from any place in the body to force fluids through lymphatic vessels." Pétrissage is defined as "deep kneading or squeezing action to express swelling."

HEAD EFFLEURAGE

MANDIBULAR TECHNIQUE (GALBRAITH'S TECHNIQUE)[8(p17),10]

Patient Position

Supine (Fig. 68.18).

Physician Position

Standing beside the patient.

Procedure

1. Rotate the patient's head to face you.
2. With your right hand, place your fingers at the temporomandibular joint and your thenar eminence along the ramus of the mandible as shown in Figure 68.18.
3. Apply a repetitive downward traction on the mandible. Anterior and medial motion should be done slowly.

SUBMANDIBULAR TECHNIQUE

Patient Position

Seated.

Physician Position

Standing.

Procedure

1. Start at the angle of the jaw (Fig. 68.19).
2. Use the palmar aspect of the fingertips and walk your fingers medially on the inferior mandibular line until you reach the chin.
3. The fingertips make contact with the submandibular nodes using a gentle vertical karate-chop motion.

PREAURICULAR AND POSTAURICULAR NODE

Patient Position

Seated.

Physician Position

Standing behind patient (may be performed in front of patient).

Procedure

1. The preauricular and postauricular nodes are situated in front of and behind the ear.
2. Spreads your fingers and contact the lateral side of the head such that the index fingers contact the postauricular node and the third fingers contact the preauricular node.
3. Apply a rotary motion both in clockwise and counterclockwise directions over the ear.

Cervical Soft Tissue

INDICATIONS

1. As an initial central lymphatic treatment to be followed by peripheral lymphatic treatments

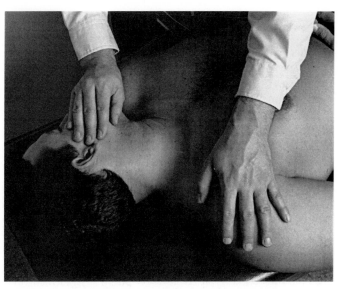

Figure 68.18. Mandibular technique: supine.

Figure 68.19. Mandibular drainage: seated.

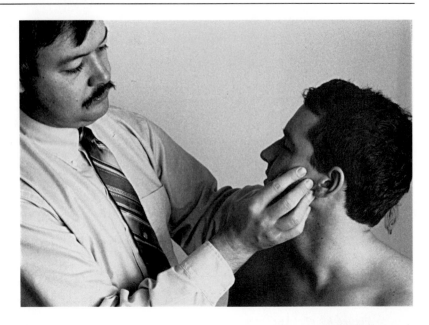

Figure 68.20. Cervical stroking.

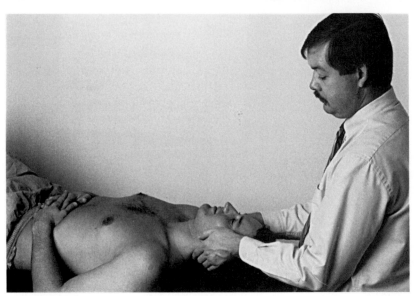

2. As an integrated treatment for an upper respiratory tract infection
3. Swollen upper extremities
4. Mastitis
5. Infections of HEENT system

CONTRAINDICATIONS

1. Structural derangement, bony abnormalities, or fractures in the area to be treated
2. Cervical ribs
3. Malignancy

CERVICAL STROKING

Cervical stroking is a method of stretching the muscle groups surrounding the cervical vertebrae.

Patient Position

Supine.

Physician Position

Standing or seated at the head of the table.

Procedure

1. Place your hands along the paravertebral muscles (Fig. 68.20).
2. Slowly stroke these muscles in a cephalic direction, not letting the muscles slip, but giving the muscles a good stretch.

ANTERIOR CERVICAL TRACTION

Patient Position

Supine.

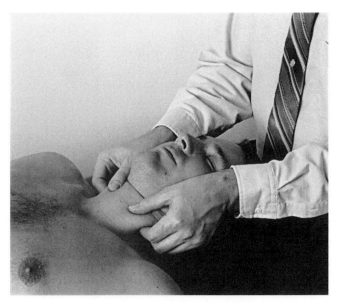

Figure 68.21. Anterior cervical traction.

Physician Position

Standing or seated at the head of the patient.

Procedure

1. Locate the anterior and posterior border of the inferior portion of the sternocleidomastoid muscle (SCM). Place your thumb along the anterior margin, and second through fifth digits along the posterior margin (Fig. 68.21).
2. Beginning in the lower portion of the SCM and anterior cervical fascia, gently lift anteriorly and laterally until you note relaxation.
3. Move superiorly to middle portion, and repeat again on superior portion. This procedure may be repeated up to three times.

SUPRAHYOID AND INFRAHYOID NODE TECHNIQUE

Patient Position

Prone (must allow the hyoid to fall forward off the nodes, which are located superior and inferior to the hyoid bone).

Physician Position

Standing.

Procedure

1. Place your fingers on the lateral aspect of the hyoid bone (Fig. 68.22).
2. Gently move the hyoid bone from side to side four or five times.

3. If notable restriction continues, gently position the hyoid by translating it to the soft tissue barrier and ask the patient to swallow as you maintain the resistance.

ANTERIOR TRACHEAL TECHNIQUE

Patient Position

Seated or supine.

Physician Position

Standing in front of the patient.

Procedure

1. Place your fingers along the lateral borders of the trachea. Move the trachea from side to side (Fig. 68.23).
2. Move lymph in the cervical region in a downward fashion toward the thorax.

Thoracic Soft Tissue

See Chapter 55, "Articulatory Techniques," on rib raising.

Abdominal

Manipulative techniques can be used in the abdominopelvic region to reduce congestion and improve circulation to the abdominal and/or pelvic viscera. Mesenteric lift techniques involve careful hand positioning to apply direct pressures in directions that take stress off of the mesenteries and/or ligaments supporting that organ. Jean-Pierre Barral, DO,[11] describes release techniques for each abdominopelvic organ; see this reference for further insights and applications of these techniques. Visceroptosis, most commonly resulting from upright postural

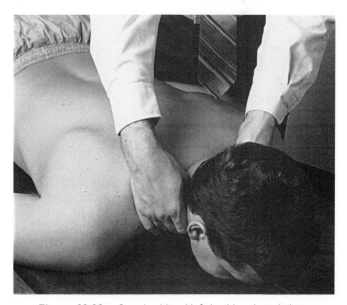

Figure 68.22. Suprahyoid and infrahyoid node technique.

Figure 68.23. Anterior tracheal technique.

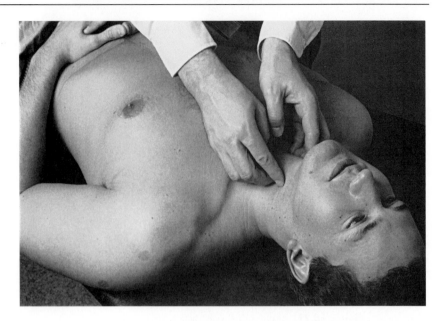

problems, is a major cause of congestion in the abdominopelvic organs. Treatment improves organ function and can decrease many functional visceral symptoms, including bloating, constipation, and pelvic or abdominal pain.

Application of this principle can be seen with the following mesenteric lift techniques.[9(pp22,89)] The small intestines have an interesting anatomic relationship to its mesentery (Fig. 68.24). The small intestines hang from a 6-inch mesenteric attachment located under a line approximately from a point 1 inch to the left and 1 inch above the umbilicus to the lower right quadrant of the abdomen just anterior to the right sacroiliac joint and the cecum.

MESENTERIC LIFT—SMALL INTESTINES

Patient Position

Supine.

Physician Position

At patient's right side.

Procedure

1. To relax the abdomen, bend the patient's knees with his or her feet placed on the table or bed.
2. Gently apply your fingers from the middle interphalangeal joints to the finger pads into the left lower quadrant of the abdomen.
3. Gently scoop the abdominal wall and underlying loops of small intestine toward their mesenteric attachment (Fig. 68.25*A*). Do not force tissues or cause pain (Fig. 68.25*B*).
4. It is often helpful to gently turn the tissues in slight clockwise or counterclockwise directions for maximal tissue freedom.
5. Hold the tissues until a sense of relaxation is palpated, or hold

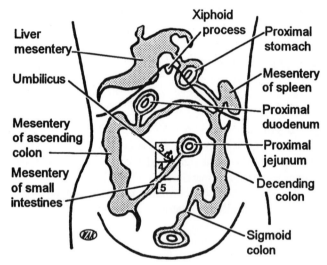

Figure 68.24. Mesenteric attachments. (Illustration from W.A. Kuchera.)

for approximately 90 seconds to allow time for visceral tissues to decongest.

MESENTERIC LIFT—CECUM

Patient Position

Supine.

Physician Position

At patient's right side.

Procedure

1. To relax the abdomen, bend the patient's right knee with that foot placed on the table or bed.

2. Gently apply the heel of your right hand to the inferior portion of the right lower quadrant of the abdomen.
3. Gently lift the cecum superiorly away from any pelvic entrapment by pushing toward the hepatic flexure of the colon (Fig. 68.26).
4. Hold the tissues until a sense of relaxation is palpated, or hold for approximately 90 seconds to allow time for visceral tissues to decongest.

PÉTRISSAGE WITH COUGH ACTIVATION—ABDOMINAL SCARS

Throughout the body, pétrissage and deep friction soft tissue techniques can also be used to break down connective tissue impediments to lymphatic drainage and free movement between adjacent fascias (Fig. 68.27). In the case of an abdominal scar where superficial tissues restrict complete motion between the region of the scar and deeper fascial layers, the fascias associated with the scar can be treated with gentle pétrissage and a cough activation to improve mobility in the region and to subsequently improve lymphatic flow. This technique should be used only in well-healed scars where restriction of motion between fascial layers is noted. This can be evaluated by gently attempting to move the scar in various directions on the abdomen and either sensing restriction or observing fascial dimpling/retraction adjacent to the scar at the end of motion testing.

Patient Position

Supine.

Physician Position

At the patient's side.

Procedure

1. Gently grasp the abdominal scar between the thumb(s) and fingers. Include some of the nearby adjacent superficial tissue.
2. Lift the scar and superficial tissues perpendicularly away from the abdomen to tissue tension (Fig. 68.28).
3. Now take the scar and superficial tissues in the direction of restricted motion to tissue tension.
4. Ask the patient to cough deeply enough to feel the deeper fascia of the abdominal wall pull into the scar that you are holding, but not so deep that you cause discomfort.
5. Recheck and repeat in any other direction where restriction is palpated.
6. This technique can be taught to the patient to perform at home.

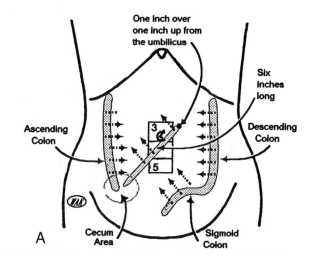

Figure 68.25A. Direction for tissue treatment of intestinal mesenteries. (Illustration from W.A. Kuchera.)

Figure 68.25B. Mesenteric lift: small intestine.

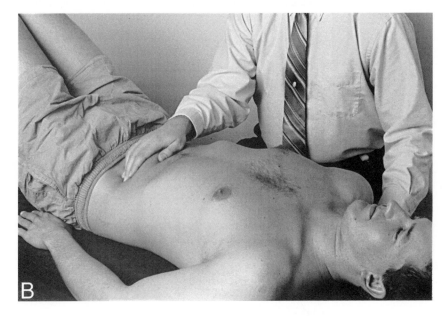

Figure 68.26.   Mesenteric lift: cecum.

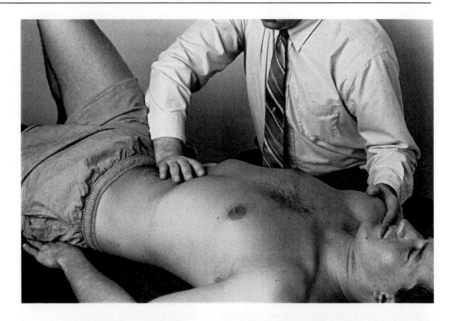

Figure 68.27.   Abdominal scar: identification.

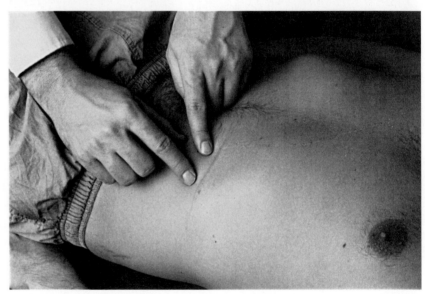

Extremities

INDICATIONS

1. Edema
2. Infection
3. Lymphatic stripping (especially postmastectomy)

CONTRAINDICATIONS

1. Fracture
2. Friable skin or stasis ulcers (for example, from diabetes)
3. Malignancy

POSTERIOR AXILLARY FOLD TECHNIQUE

This technique is related to ipsilateral upper extremity congestion.

Diagnosis

Thick, tender, and congested right axillary fold.

Patient Position

Supine.

Physician Position

Seated at the right side of the patient, facing the patient's head.

Procedure

1. Place the extended fingers of your right hand high up under the posterior surface of the posterior axillary fold with the in-

dex finger next to the patient's chest cage. Place your right thumb over the axillary fold high in the axillary cavity and also next to the patient's chest wall (Fig. 68.29).

2. Bring the thumb and fingers toward each other along their longitudinal surfaces chest wall, creating tension between the extended thumb and fingers. The fingers of your right hand can be strengthened by the fingers of your left hand.

3. Hold the compression until the tissues relax.

4. Move the grip inferiorly to a new area and repeat the inhibition if signs of congestion are found. Continue caudally until the border of the latissimus muscle disappears over the back as it progresses medially toward the spine.

EFFLEURAGE AND PÉTRISSAGE—UPPER EXTREMITY

Diagnosis

Signs and symptoms of a congested right upper extremity.

Patient Position

Supine.

Physician Position

Seated at the right side of the patient, facing the patient's head.

Figure 68.28. Abdominal scar: treatment.

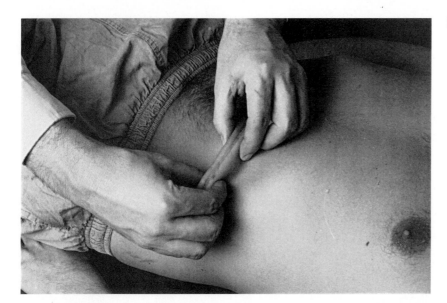

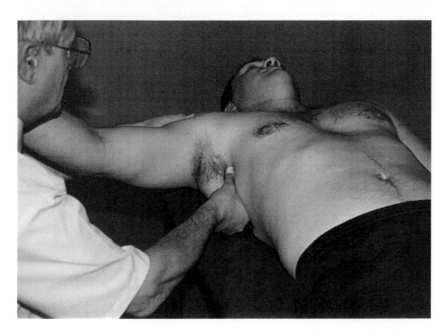

Figure 68.29. Posterior axillary fold technique.

Figure 68.30. Effleurage and pétrissage: upper extremity.

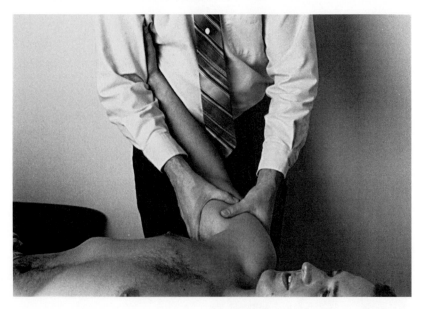

Procedure

1. Tuck the patient's right hand into your right axilla and hold it there.
2. Grasp the upper arm close to the shoulder, and with a hand on either side of the limb, apply a wringing motion, moving from proximal to distal (Fig. 68.30).
3. When the second step is completed, start closer to the elbow with the wringing motion, and again move distally.
4. Continue this process of lymphatic movement an additional three or four times or until adequate drainage has been achieved in the arm.
5. When step 4 is completed, go to the forearm, placing your thumbs on the ventral surface between the flexor and extensor muscle masses and the rest of your digits around the other side. Squeeze the muscle masses simultaneously, then relax.
6. Repeat this process again, moving from proximal to digital.

EFFLEURAGE AND PÉTRISSAGE—LOWER EXTREMITY

Diagnosis

Signs and symptoms of a congested right lower extremity.

Patient Position

Supine; the right knee is flexed to a right angle; the lower leg is horizontal, parallel with the table; the thigh is flexed at a right angle with the body.

Physician Position

Seated on the table facing the patient's head.

Procedure

1. Balance the patient's right leg on your shoulder.
2. Place the palmar surface of both hands on opposing sides of

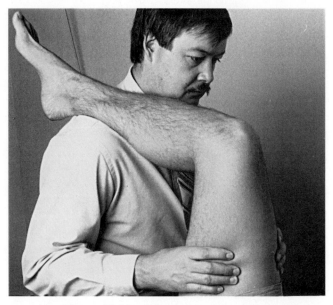

Figure 68.31. Effleurage: lower extremity.

the proximal end of the thigh, and perform a rotatory wringing-out type of movement in a clockwise direction.
3. As tissue change takes place, move distally down the thigh toward the knee, one hand's width at a time.
4. Repeat the sequence of motions, going back again to the inguinal area and progressively moving toward the knee.
5. When the tissues have softened and there is less congestion in the thigh, move below the knee.
6. Place the hand on either side of the lower leg; with the thumbs press deeply between and into the calf muscles, squeezing out the muscles, progressing down from the knee toward the ankle.

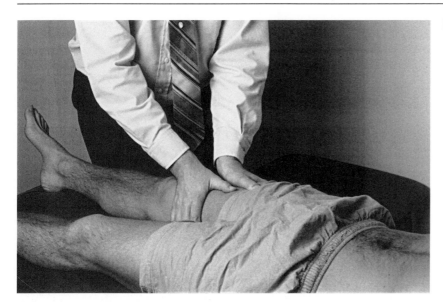

Figure 68.32. Pétrissage: lower extremity.

7. During each squeezing motion, rock your body forward and backward using your body weight to flex and extend the knee and hip in a rhythmic fashion.

EFFLEURAGE—ARMS AND LEGS

Effleurage is the stroking of appendages from distal to proximal. This facilitates the flow of lymph to the axilla and the thorax from the upper limb and facilitates the flow of lymph to the abdomen from the lower limb.

Patient Position

Supine.

Physician Position

At the patient's side.

Procedure

With effleurage you stroke the appendages from distal to proximal (Fig. 68.31) using a milking motion.

PÉTRISSAGE—ARMS AND LEGS

Pétrissage is a method of draining lymph from the extremities into the thoracic duct.

Patient Position

Supine.

Physician Position

At the patient's side.

Procedure

Knead the extremity, starting distally (Fig. 68.32) and proceeding toward the trunk.

CONCLUSION

Because lymphatic function can be critically influenced and altered by extrinsic forces, osteopathic diagnosis, and manipulative treatment, using the techniques outlined in this chapter can greatly influence lymphatic function.

REFERENCES

1. Still AT. *Philosophy of Osteopathy.* Kirksville, Mo: A.T. Still; 1809:108.
2. Gangong W. Review of Medical Physiology, *Lange Medical Physiology.*
3. Williams PL, Warwick R, Dyson M, Bannister LH. *Gray's Anatomy.* 37th ed. Edinburgh: Churchill Livingstone; 1989:841.
4. Sodeman WA Jr, Sodeman TM. Protective mechanism of the lungs; pulmonary disease; pleural disease. *Pathologic Physiology: Mechanism of Disease.* 6th ed. Philadelphia, Penn: WB Saunders Company; 1979:452.
5. Guyton A. *Textbook of Medical Physiology.* Philadelphia, Penn: WB Saunders Company; 1976.
6. Woodburne R. *Essentials of Human Anatomy.* 8th ed. New York, NY: Oxford University Press; 1988.
7. Zink G, Lawson WB. An osteopathic structural examination and functional interpretation of the soma. *Osteopath Ann.* December 1979;7:12–19 (433–440).
8. Kuchera ML, Kuchera WA. *Considerations in Systemic Dysfunction.* Columbus, Ohio: Greyden Press; 1994:43.
9. Measel JW Jr. The effect of the lymphatic pump on the immune response: preliminary studies on the antibody response to pneumonococcal polysaccharide assayed by bacterial agglutination and passive hemagglutination. *JAOA.* September 1982;82(1):28–31 (59–62).
10. Cathie A. Sino-bronchial syndrome. In: Barnes MW, ed. *AAO Yearbook.* Indianapolis, Ind: American Academy of Osteopathy; 1974:180–181.
11. Barral JP, Mercier P. *Visceral Manipulation.* Seattle, Wash: Eastland Press; 1988.

69. General Postural Considerations

MICHAEL L. KUCHERA AND WILLIAM A. KUCHERA

If we regard posture as the result of the dynamic interaction of two groups of forces—the environmental force of gravity on one hand, and the strength of the individual on the other—then posture is but the formal expression of the balance of power existing at any time between these two groups of forces. Thus, any deterioration of posture indicates that the individual is losing ground in his contest with the environmental force of gravity.[1]

Key Concepts

- **What constitutes optimal posture**
- **Four factors that produce postural decompensation**
- **Mechanism of compensation and spinal patterning**
- **Role of central nervous system in maintaining posture**
- **Possible treatments for postural decompensation**

Analysis of a patient's posture provides an enormous amount of information about the body. The endurance of antigravity (postural) muscles, the capability of the musculoskeletal system to adjust homeostatically to physical stressors, and the locations of postural spinal crossovers all offer insight into structure–function relationships on a physical level. Observation of posture may also offer the clinician the first clues to the emotional, spiritual, and psychological elements of a patient's health.

Treatment of posture has wide implications in the general health status of each patient. It especially involves reduction or elimination of a constant precipitating and perpetuating factor of group curves and recurrent somatic dysfunction. Postural treatment can also play a significant role in the treatment of certain conditions associated with postural decompensation, such as scoliosis and spondylolisthesis.

ASPECTS OF POSTURE

Base of Support

Posture is the distribution of body mass in relation to gravity over a base of support. The base of support includes all structures from the feet to the base of the skull. The effect of the lower extremities, pelvis, and base of the skull are especially important. Distribution of weight over the base of support depends on the following:

Energy requirements for homeostasis
Integrity of musculoligamentous structures
Compensation that structures at or below the base of the skull have on the visual and/or balance functions of the body

Optimal Posture

Optimal posture is a balanced configuration of the body with respect to gravity. It depends on normal arches of the feet, vertical alignment of the ankles, and horizontal orientation (in the coronal plane) of the sacral base. The presence of an optimum posture suggests that there is a perfect distribution of the body mass around the center of gravity. The compressive force on spinal disks is balanced by ligamentous tension; there is minimal energy expenditure from postural muscles.[2,3] Structural or functional stressors on the body, however, may prevent achievement of optimum posture. In this case, homeostatic mechanisms provide for "compensation" in an effort to provide maximum postural function within the existing structure of the individual. Compensation is the counterbalancing of any defect of structure or function.[4]

Compensated Posture

A compensated posture is the result of the patient's homeostatic mechanisms working through the entire body unit to maximize function. Postural compensation in the musculoskeletal system occurs in all three planes of body motion to keep the body balanced and the eyes level. The central nervous system (CNS) places a high priority on visual and vestibular (balance) functions. Spinal compensation involves CNS correlation of proprioceptive information from tendons and muscles as well as vestibular information from the semicircular canals. The CNS also integrates this proprioceptive information with information received from the eyes.

Postural homeostatic lessons are learned gradually by the central nervous system from visual and proprioceptive input as the individual grows and develops. The process has implications for treatment that includes postural reeducation; this should be progressive and consistent if it is to succeed. Structural compensation allows a person to function despite musculoskeletal imbalances. Because of an accumulated history of genetic, traumatic, and habitual processes requiring compensation, few patients have ideal posture.

Posture is both static (structural) and dynamic (functional). It is static in its alignment of body mass with respect to gravity. It is dynamic because this alignment constantly adjusts to the individual's changing postural demands.

Over time, individual static postural alignment conforms to inherent connective tissue structure. It also responds to the cumulative functional demand placed upon it by static and dynamic postural conditions. Both static and dynamic posture are influenced by and influence soft tissue functions. Examination includes analysis of static postural alignment in the upright weight-bearing position. It also includes osteopathic examination of the selective tensions of the soft tissues. Palpatory examination of dynamic posture and segmental motion testing is vital to understanding structure–function interrelationships. This combination of examinations provides clinical clues about the inherent capability of the patient's neuromusculoskeletal system to balance and maintain biomechanical alignment. Radiographic analysis of bony relationships can further add to this understanding.

Compensatory changes of the spine are often named according to the group curve with the most prominent postural feature (Fig. 69.1). Compensatory curves in the sagittal plane are called kyphotic or lordotic curves. Compensatory curves primarily in the coronal plane are called scoliotic curves, and compensation in the horizontal plane is called rotation. Scoliotic curves are sometimes referred to as rotoscoliotic curves because rotation and side-bending are inseparable. A curve may be called a kyphorotoscoliotic curve if all three planes are significantly involved.

POSTURAL DECOMPENSATION

Gravitational strain acts universally to affect upright posture. Decompensation occurs when an individual's homeostatic mechanisms are overwhelmed.[5] Host factors can be overwhelmed by several conditions.

Traumatic decompensation occurs when macrotrauma or recurrent microtrauma disrupts ligamentous stability of the spine. Fractures of the spine, pelvis, or lower extremity may produce sacral base unleveling or the need for other compensatory changes above the area of the trauma.

Congenital or acquired structural changes create chronic postural strain. Unleveling of the sacral base or a deformed vertebra due to fracture or congenital deformation leads to compensatory curvatures of the spine. Occasionally an unlevel sacral base is observed in an x-ray image with a straight spine above it. This requires muscular effort, resulting in spinal musculoligamentous strain. As the person grows older and the muscular compensation becomes inadequate, functional scoliosis manifests and structural scoliosis eventually develops. Spondylolisthesis likewise initiates stress with spinal changes occurring predominantly in the sagittal plane.

Personal conditions, inactivity, and aging potentially predispose people to decompensation of the spine. Changes of body habits that accompany pregnancy, obesity, muscular weakness of aging, and poor sitting or standing habits produce postural stress and can initiate decompensation. Work environments or recreational activities requiring strenuous posturing may also result in postural decompensation.

Abnormal gait may initiate the need for compensation or precipitate decompensation. Examples include the gait produced from unilateral pes planus (flat foot), wearing shoes with high or worn heels, and dysfunctional gaits following ankle sprains or strains. These conditions affect the base of support and therefore stimulate compensatory changes in posture. If continued indefinitely, these changes could progress to decompensation with rotation, scoliosis, lordosis, and/or kyphosis.

Postural progression from a healthy state to a dysfunctional state leads to symptoms and a structural pathological state. The body first tries to compensate for imbalance by altering motion characteristics and tissues in its spinal structure. The result is a functional scoliosis in the coronal plane. If this remains too long, it develops a fixed component and becomes a structural scoliosis.

Other symptoms occur in a person with spinal decompensation. These usually originate at the areas of crossover where the spinal curve crosses from right to left or anterior to posterior across the weight-bearing line (Fig. 69.2). These crossover points may be the site of local subjective joint and tissue symptoms. They could also result in facilitated segments and somatovisceral reflexes, producing inappropriate increases in sympathetic activity and related organ dysfunction.

PATTERNING

Spinal Patterning

The nature of postural compensation is to react to a disturbance of posture with change throughout the remaining somatic tissues. These changes tend to overcorrect slightly for postural disturbances. They alternate from one body region to

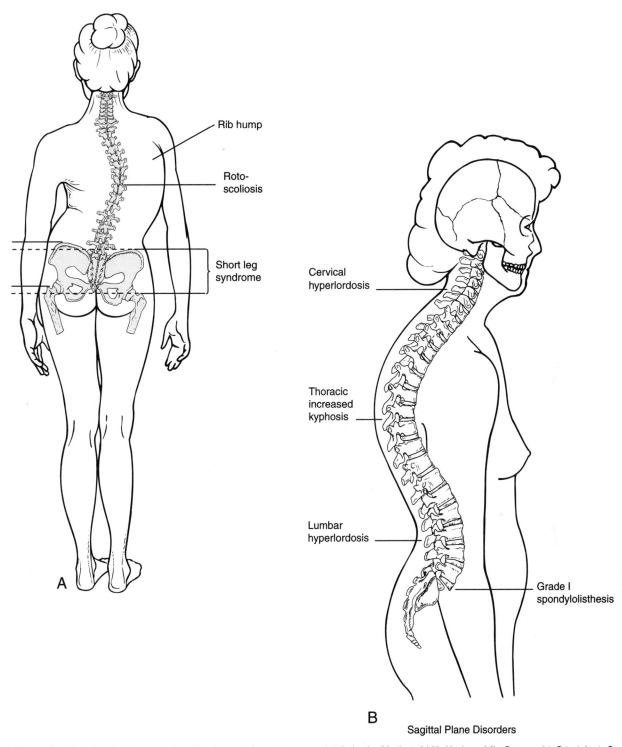

Figure 69.1. **A.** Disorders in the coronal and horizontal plane: short leg syndrome and rotoscoliosis. **B.** Disorders in the sagittal plane: lumbar and cervical hyperlordosis, thoracic kyphosis, and L5-S1 isthmic spon- dylolisthesis. (Kuchera WA, Kuchera ML. *Osteopathic Principles in Practice.* 2nd ed. rev. Columbus, Ohio: Greyden Press; 1994:47.)

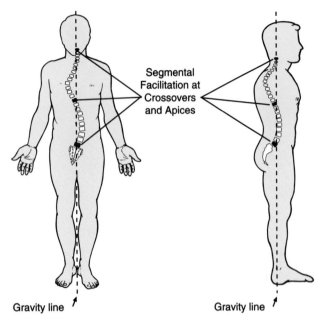

Segmental
Facilitation at
Crossovers
and Apices

Gravity line

Gravity line

Figure 69.2. Gravitational strain pathophysiology. Crossover sites are found where center of gravity line crosses bony posture. These sites have a high incidence of segmental facilitation. (Kuchera WA, Kuchera ML. *Osteopathic Principles in Practice.* 2nd ed. rev. Columbus, Ohio: Greyden Press; 1994:47.)

the next and tend to occur in regions above and below the initial change. Most commonly these changes occur at the so-called "transition zones," areas where anatomical structure changes create the potential for the greatest functional change (Fig. 69.3). Describing these regional changes in a patient can lead to recognition of patterns. Patterning provides a convenient way of summarizing common prototypes of compensation. Postural patterns or patterning refer to classifiable combinations of regional compensatory change.

Compensation involves all three cardinal planes because spinal motions are biomechanically linked.[6] Scoliotic, rotational, lordotic, or kyphotic curves can therefore develop as compensation for postural stressors. The curve in a given plane often occurs in one direction in one region and in the opposite direction in the next spinal region so that the body can maintain some type of postural balance.

Postural patterns can be classified by whether they can be reduced by specific functional maneuvers. If a lateral curve can be reduced by some spinal motion such as side-bending, it is known as a functional or secondary scoliotic curve. If it is unable to be reduced, it is known as a structural, fixed, or primary scoliosis. Functional scoliosis is reversible. Structural scoliosis is fixed. Because structure and function are interrelated, many scoliotic curves are a mixture of these two classifications. This phenomenon is also seen with postural patterns in the other planes.

Fascial Patterning of Zink

Postural patterning influences and is influenced by the fascias and related structures. J. Gordon Zink described patterns[6] that

are clinically relevant to the diagnosis and treatment of fascial compensation and decompensation. Based on the palpatory fascial preference to motion (see Chapter 68, "Lymphatic System"), these fascial patterns can be classified as ideal, compensated, or uncompensated (Fig. 69.4). The postural influence on fascial patterning is important for understanding the effect that postural management has in improving the respiratory–circulatory model.[7] Conversely, fascial preference influences tissues and skeletal structures of each region producing the dynamic postural characteristics of that body region.

Musculoligamentous Patterning

Musculoligamentous structure and function are also significantly influenced by, and responsible for, static and dynamic postural alignment. Gravitational stress placed on these structures to maintain a patient's posture is a constant and greatly underestimated stressor. In a patient with less than ideal postural alignment, gravitational stresses are amplified. When the viscoelastic deformation properties of muscle are unable to resist the stress imposed, predictable pathophysiologic changes occur. These changes are both functional and structural. The elastic component represents the transient functional change in connective tissue length occurring in response to stress. The viscous component, on the other hand, is responsible for the more permanent deformation of connective tissue that occurs with static postural change.

Musculoligamentous structures are affected early in patients with gravitational strain and can be easily recognized. The symptoms arising from the resultant pathophysiological condition have certain associated palpable characteristics, including the following:

Muscle spasm
Edema or bogginess
Myofascial trigger points
Subtle weakness to muscle testing

Not missing such palpable changes or postural pattern clues is important. Myofascial structures undergo sustained changes in length; studies[8] suggest that deleterious change is most pronounced in shortened muscles. New collagen, with a half-life of 10–12 months, realigns the connective tissues in response to vectors of stress, perpetuating postural problems and maintaining the biomechanical amplification of gravitational stress. Postural patterns that are compensated can decompensate.

The structure of the muscle and its function are related. Structure and function play a major role in the muscle patterns commonly seen in posturally initiated pain and dysfunction. Postural stress on muscles leads to chronic, recurrent trigger points,[9] consistent myotomal and sclerotomal pain patterns, and predictable functional changes. Postural muscles are structurally adapted to resist fatigue and function in the presence of prolonged gravitational exposure. When their capacity to resist stress is overwhelmed, these postural muscles become irritable, tight, and shortened.[10] Many muscles, antagonists to these postural muscles, react when stressed by becoming weak or pseudoparetic. Therefore, gravitational strain patterns reveal

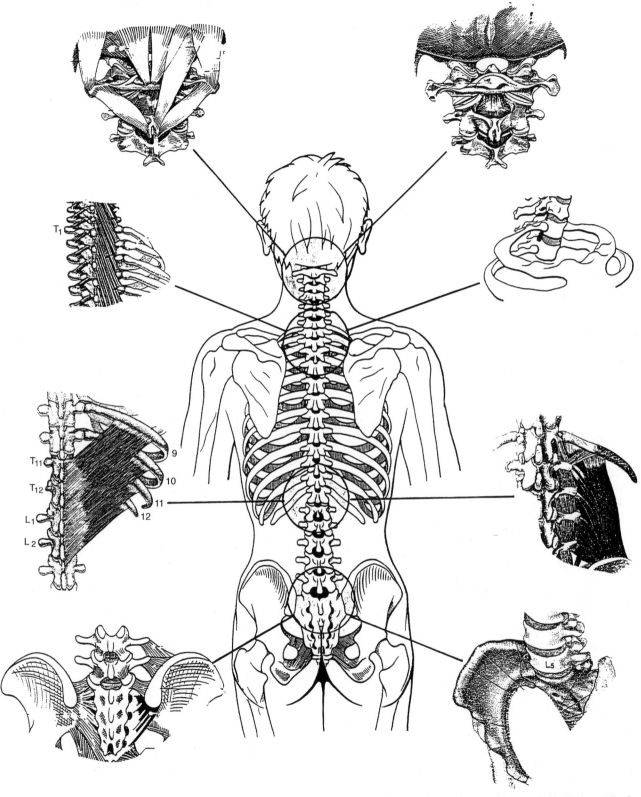

Figure 69.3. Transition zones are anatomically defined and their function is affected by skeletal, arthrodial, and myofascial anatomy. Transition zones occur at occipitocervical junction, cervicothoracic junction, thoracolumbar junction, and lumbosacral junction. Between each transition zone lies definable region of spine. (Kuchera WA, Kuchera ML. *Osteopathic Principles in Practice*. 2nd ed. rev. Columbus, Ohio: Greyden Press; 1994:47.)

Figure 69.4. Fascial patterns that alternate in direction from region to region are typically compensated patterns. Those that do not are uncompensated and usually traumatically induced. *OA*, occipitoatlantal; *CT*, cervicothoracic; *TL*, thoracolumbar; *LS*, lumbosacral. (Kuchera WA, Kuchera ML. *Osteopathic Principles in Practice.* 2nd ed. rev. Columbus, Ohio: Greyden Press; 1994:47.)

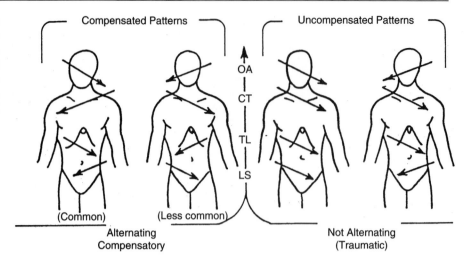

a dysfunctional pattern of tight and weak muscles in a postural pattern (Fig. 69.5). Involvement of a number of the muscles in Tables 69.1 and 69.2 should alert the osteopathic physician to this underlying cause. In these patients, treatment of the dysfunctional postural alignment yields more lasting results than treatment of the recurrent myofascial trigger points or muscle imbalances in isolation.

TREATMENT

Treating a patient with postural decompensation requires appropriate diagnosis of the functional capabilities of that individual's structure. The treatment goals may depend on how long the imbalance has been present and how much decompensation has already occurred. Structural treatment goals are directed at establishing the optimal function the existing structure is capable of achieving. Functional treatment goals promote free motion within an optimally balanced posture.

Treatment of postural problems emphasizes compliance, especially in the initial phases of the reeducation program. Compliance by the patient is essential and can be enhanced if the patient understands the rationale behind the treatment procedures and requirements.

The choice of treatment modalities to achieve these goals also depends on the degree of decompensation present in the patient and an estimate of the patient's homeostatic reserves. The physician may choose a combination of the modalities described in the following sections.

Osteopathic Manipulative Treatment

Manipulation plays an intimate role in the formulation of any postural treatment protocol. Manipulation is defined as the use of the hands in a patient management process using instructions and maneuvers to achieve maximum painless movement of the musculoskeletal (motor) system in postural balance.

Osteopathic manipulative treatment (OMT) helps prepare muscles, joints, ligaments, and other supportive soft tissue to better accept positive postural change. Unaddressed tension in these structures often prevents optimal compensatory re-

sponses. Additionally, hypomobility often creates pain or ache in the sites seeking to change under the forces of homeostasis.

Education

Educating and modifying a patient's perspective are often required in addition to the treatment of the myofascial system. Teenage girls, for example, may slump severely because they are embarrassed about the development of their breasts. They may also not want to look taller than teenage boys who mature later chronologically. This personal attitude toward their body must be changed by education about normal growth and development. Other patients need treatment of their primary psychologic depression that results in a secondary postural "slump." Proper postural education for the work site and other activities of daily living is also beneficial.

Exercise

Exercise programs (see Chapter 76, "Exercises and Recovery") must be carefully prescribed. Exercise of a muscle that is under continued stress only weakens and strains associated soft tissues further. Rest and reduction of postural stressors with adjunctive postural orthoses and/or manipulation may be required before prescribing a directed exercise program. Pelvic coil exercises[11] are often beneficial for sagittal plane postural problems. In patients with coronal plane postural decompensation, the Konstancin[12,13] exercise program has been statistically shown to improve postural alignment. Effective postural exercise protocols optimally include the goal of proprioceptive reeducation. Promotion of flexibility for realignment and selective strengthening for stability in hypomobile areas are goals for postural exercise.

Bracing

Static structural bracing has both positive and negative aspects. Although such devices support the structure and initially reduce ligamentous and muscular stress, the muscles soon become dependent on the support provided. The longer the brace

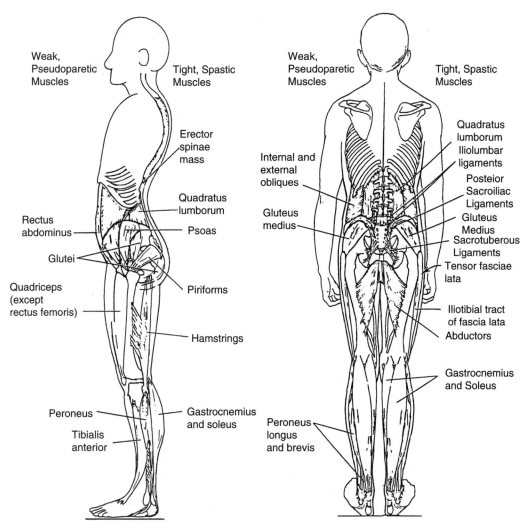

Figure 69.5. Coronal and horizontal postural patterns usually alternate from side-to-side in adjacent regions with stressed muscle group typically on convex side of each postural curve. Sagittal plane postural patterns involve postural muscles and their antagonists as listed in Table 69.1. (Kuchera WA, Kuchera ML. *Osteopathic Principles in Practice.* 2nd ed. rev. Columbus, Ohio: Greyden Press; 1994:47.)

is worn, the weaker the patient's own muscles become. It is therefore imperative that the physician link the patient's brace treatment with an ongoing exercise program. Static braces are better for providing rest in an acute condition than for treating a chronic one. Ideally a physician should not introduce a static brace without having a plan to replace it.[14]

Orthotics

Functional orthotics serve to direct, guide, and/or reeducate the body, as opposed to directly taking over support. They are capable of influencing physiologic parameters and reducing associated low back pain. With respect to postural realignment, this class of treatment modalities includes several specific orthotics. The Levitor orthotic, which was biomechanically designed specifically to reduce gravity-induced musculoligamentous stress, has its greatest effect within the sagittal plane. Foot orthotics incorporating heel lifts have their effect primarily within the coronal plane. Anterior sole lifts maximally affect

the horizontal plane. All three of these examples, however, affect posture in all cardinal planes simultaneously,[15] and each ultimately has systemic effects. Functional orthotics in conjunction with an osteopathic approach have been documented to reduce or reverse lordosis, kyphosis, and scoliosis, decrease low back pain and other musculoskeletal symptoms, improve respiratory–circulatory functions, and decrease segmental facilitation. Flexible foot orthoses and the Levitor do not replace normal muscular function. Therefore, their use does not weaken associated muscles.

Electrical Stimulation

Electrical stimulation of paraspinal muscles has been used in some centers. Electrodes are placed in the muscles on the side of the spinal convexity. The electrodes are connected to a direct current from a control box. An electrical current causes contraction of the muscles on the side of the convexity and is postulated to help reduce scoliotic curvature. This can be used

Table 69.1
Spastic Muscle Symptoms

Structure	Symptoms
Iliopsoas muscle	Inability to stand straight (psoas posturing); knees flexed; recurrent L1–2 somatic dysfunction; pain referral to back and anterior groin; positive Thomas test
Quadratus lumborum muscle	Low back pain referred to the groin and hip; exhalation 12th rib somatic dysfunction; diaphragm restriction
Hamstring muscles	Pain sitting or walking; pain disturbs sleep; pain referral to posterior thighs; straight leg raising limited mechanically
Piriformis muscle	Pain down posterior thigh; may entrap peroneal portion of sciatic nerve; perpetuated by sacroiliac dysfunction; associated with pelvic floor dysfunction, dyspareunia, and prostatodynia
Thigh adductor muscles (short)	Pain referral to the inguinal ligament, inner thigh, and upper medial knee
Gastrocnemius–soleus complex	Nocturnal leg cramps; pain referral to upper posterior calf, instep, and heel

Table 69.2
Inhibited Muscle Symptoms

Structure	Symptoms
Gluteus minimus muscle	Pain characteristic when arising from chair; pain referral to buttock, lateral and posterior thigh; "pseudosciatica"; antalgic gait; positive Trendelenburg test
Gluteus medius muscle	Pain aggravated by walking; pain referral to posterior iliac crest and sacroiliac joint; positive Trendelenburg test
Gluteus maximus muscle	Restlessness; pain sitting or walking up hill; antalgic gait
Vastus muscles	Buckling knee; weakness going up stairs; thigh and knee pain; chondromalacia patellae
Rectus abdominis muscle	Increased lordosis; constipation
Tibialis anterior muscle	Pain referred to great toe and anteromedial ankle; may drag foot or trip when tired

only in the thoracic area and is used only when the patient is asleep. Opinions on its efficacy vary.

Prolotherapy

Prolotherapy (sclerotherapy) is injection of a proliferant solution into a ligament. When postural strain biomechanically overwhelms structural integrity, ligamentous laxity can result. Injection of a proliferant solution into the ligament at its fibro-osseous insertion can increase stability. Coupled with exercise, OMT, and postural realignment to prevent return of ligamentous strain, this protocol can be an effective conservative alternative to surgical intervention.

Surgery

When an insurmountable problem is primarily structural, its treatment is primarily structural. In unstable situations, or in situations that have not responded to conservative care, surgery may be performed. In the case of severe scoliosis or highly symptomatic spondylolisthesis, this could consist of fusing vertebrae. Surgical implantation of orthopaedic rods or other stabilizing apparatuses may also be required.

CONCLUSION

Postural diagnosis and treatment are perfectly consistent with the tenets of the osteopathic philosophy. Careful exploration of the homeostatic response of the body unit as reflected in the structure and function of that individual's posture permits specific treatment design for total patient management.

Posture is not just a stack of spinal curves with musculoligamentous connectors. Posture is influenced by the patient's emotional–spiritual–psychological self. It has been astutely observed that *"posture to a large degree is also a somatic depiction of the inner emotions. There is no doubt that posture can be considered a somatization of the psyche."*[16] Postural realignment requires reintegration of peripheral and central factors that are physiologically, psychologically, and biomechanically linked.

Several modalities are available to the osteopathic physician to aid in the realignment process. These include osteopathic manipulative treatment, functional orthotics and orthopaedic braces, exercise protocols, and patient education. There is an intimate relationship between osteopathic manipulative treatment and postural balance. The osteopathic physician seeks to achieve maximum function of the neuromusculoskeletal system in postural balance and to prepare the patient's neuromusculoskeletal system to respond to postural realignment. Postural treatment generally supports the patient's homeostasis.

Postural gravitational stress should be considered a factor in the general health status of each and every patient. It should not be reserved only for consideration in cases of recurrent somatic dysfunction, myofascial trigger point syndromes, scoliosis, or spondylolisthesis.

REFERENCES

1. Jungmann M, McClure CW. Backaches, postural decline, aging and gravity-strain. Abstract delivered at the New York Academy of General Practice, New York City, October 17, 1963.
2. Kappler RE. Postural balance and motion patterns. In: Peterson B, ed. *Postural Balance and Imbalance (1983 AAO Yearbook)*. Newark, Ohio: American Academy of Osteopathy; 1983:6–12.
3. Kuchera ML, Kuchera WA. Postural decompensation. In: *Osteo-

pathic Principles in Practice. 2nd ed. rev. Columbus, Ohio: Greyden Press; 1994.

4. *Dorland's Medical Dictionary.* Philadelphia, Pa: WB Saunders; 1989.

5. Denslow JS, Chase JA. Mechanical stresses in the human lumbar spine and pelvis. In: Peterson B, ed. *Postural Balance and Imbalance (1983 AAO Yearbook).* Newark, Ohio: American Academy of Osteopathy; 1983:76–82.

6. Zink JG, Lawson WB. An osteopathic structural examination and functional interpretation of the soma. *Osteopath Ann.* December 1979;7:12–19.

7. Zink JG. Respiratory and circulatory care: the conceptual model. *Osteopath Ann.* 1977;5(3):108–112.

8. Gossman MR, Sahrmann SA, Rose SJ. Review of length-associated changes in muscle. *Phys Ther.* 1982;62(12):1799–1807.

9. Travell JG, Simons DG. *Myofascial Pain and Dysfunction: A Trigger Point Manual.* Vol II. Baltimore, Md: Williams & Wilkins, 1992:547.

10. Janda V. Muscle weakness and inhibition (pseudoparesis) in back pain syndromes. In: Grieve GP, ed. *Modern Medicine Therapy of the Vertebral Column.* Edinburgh: Churchill Livingstone; 1986:197–200.

11. Travell JG, Simons DG. *Myofascial Pain and Dysfunction: The Trigger Point Manual.* Vol I. Baltimore, Md: Williams & Wilkins; 1983:680.

12. Kuchera WA, Kuchera ML. Postural decompensation. In: *Osteopathic Principles in Practice.* 2nd ed. rev. Columbus, Ohio: Greyden Press; 1994.

13. Kuchera WA, Kuchera ML. *Osteopathic Principles in Practice.* 2nd ed. rev. Columbus, Ohio: Greyden Press; 1994:385–389.

14. Grieve GP. Lumbar instability. *Physiotherapy.* 1982;68(1):2–9.

15. Kuchera ML, Irvin RE. Biomechanical considerations in postural realignment. *JAOA.* 1987;87(11):781–782.

16. Calliet R. *Low Back Syndrome.* 3rd ed. Philadelphia, Pa: FA Davis; 1981:24.

70. Management of Group Curves

ROBERT E. KAPPLER

Key Concepts

- **Group curves, and planes of motion involved**
- **Major causes of group curves**
- **Physical findings that occur with group curves, and their clinical significance**
- **Basis for management of group curves**
- **Direct treatment techniques, including epigastric thrust, patient astride table technique, muscle energy technique**

A group curve is a spinal curve that involves several segments. The motion pattern in these curves follows the first principle of physiologic motion of the spine. When the spine is in neutral position, that is, with an absence of marked flexion or extension, and side-bending is introduced, the vertebrae rotate into the produced convexity.[1] In these curves, rotation is to the opposite side of side-bending. Lateral curves that exceed 5° as measured by the Cobb method are called scoliosis.

CAUSES

Spinal joints are designed to provide motion; spinal motion is necessary in most of our ordinary activity. Most spinal motion involves a group of vertebral segments. This motion follows the first principle of physiologic motion of the spine and is necessary to allow for positional changes of the body. Every time a person side-bends, a lateral curve is produced. This sometimes leads to restriction of motion. Lateral curves become a problem when restriction occurs and the spine no longer straightens.

Spinal curves may be produced by unilateral muscle contraction. This muscle pull creates a concavity, resulting in a curve. The vertebrae rotate into the convexity. This type of lateral curve disappears when the muscle hypotonicity is gone.

Another type of lateral curve involves long-term anatomic adaptation. For example, the spine is initially in a curved position to compensate for an anatomic short leg, structural deformity, postural balance, or even a long-term positional change that becomes a pattern. Over time, the tissues associated with this curve change. Tissues on the convex side become lengthened. Tissues on the concave side become shortened. Deformity of a vertebral body with lateral wedging results in a spinal curve. Long-standing curves with anatomic adaptation resist change. Over time the curved position becomes the neutral position.

DIAGNOSIS

The patient has humping of a paravertebral region on the convex side of a coronal plane curve as a result of stretched muscles or deformation of ribs brought about by rotation of the vertebrae in the curve. Stretched muscles may be tender to palpation. Side-bending is toward the concavity, and rotation occurs into the convexity with maximal rotation occurring at the apex of the curve.

Consider kyphoscoliosis. Anteroposterior (AP) curves may be increased at the apex. AP curves flatten at the crossover. The crossover is a point where an S curve crosses the midline to the other side. Scoliotic curves are named for their convex side. For example, rotoscoliosis right means a curve that is convex to the right by being side-bent to the left.

CLINICAL SIGNIFICANCE

Lateral curves contribute to postural imbalance by producing positional asymmetry that may lead to back pain. They may involve a loss of energy because of the increased active muscle contraction needed to counteract gravity. Not all anatomic asymmetries can be corrected. In searching for an answer to the significance of a lateral curve in a patient, consider both structure and function. Although the physician often tries to improve the structure, reducing asymmetry does not necessarily improve the function of the patient. The objective of treatment is to maintain or improve function of the patient within the existing structure.

Group curves (type I, neutral) involve multiple segments. Often the longer outer muscles are involved rather than the short, deep segmental muscles. Multiple segments lack segmental specificity in terms of altered neural activity. By contrast, type II nonneutral dysfunction involves single segments. Segmental dysfunction is more likely to be associated with changes in spinal cord function, which osteopathic physicians associate with somatic dysfunction.

Osteopathic physicians differ regarding the significance of group curves. Some physicians focus on nonneutral type II single segmental dysfunction, while others emphasize treating group curves as well. The approach should depend on the individual patient: what is the functional significance of a group curve for the patient? If the group curve contributes to dysfunction of the patient, it should be treated.

TREATMENT

Several principles govern the management of group curves.

First, identify and treat the cause of the curve. If a patient has an anatomic short leg with sacral base unleveling, treat the short leg to level the sacral base and decrease the curve. As a patient adjusts to treatment for postural rebalancing, the spine must remain mobile to compensate for the change; this is where osteopathic manipulation is useful. Long-term anatomic change, however, does not disappear with manipulation.

Second, if a focal muscle hypertonicity has produced a curve, the muscle hypotonicity that produces the curve must be found. When this is removed, the curve disappears. Causes of muscle hypertonicity are varied. Segmental dysfunction may be the cause. The dysfunction may be the result of a viscero-somatic reflex. Myofascial triggers may be involved. Kimberly[2] looked for nonneutral dysfunction within a neutral curve. A nonneutral segment involves rotation into the concavity. This might be a segment that is out of step with the rest of the segments forming the group curve.

The concavity of a curve is the tight or restricted side, while the convexity is the unstable side. Exercises or manipulation involve stretching or mobilizing the concavity while strengthening the convex side. If a curve has been present for some time, treatment of the curve improves motion within the curve. However, the curve itself or some asymmetry within the spine may remain.

DIRECT TECHNIQUES

Epigastric Thrust

FINDINGS

The patient has group curve (type I, neutral) convex right, apex at T7. The curve is rotated right, side-bent left. There is restriction of right side-bending and left rotation.

PROCEDURE (Fig. 70.1)

1. Stand behind your seated patient.
2. Patient's hands are behind his or her neck.
3. Place a towel or small pillow over apex (T7 right side).
4. Place your arms under axilla and over patient's wrists.
5. Contact pillow (T7 right side) with your epigastrium.
6. Side-bend right, translate T7 left to engage barrier.
7. Final corrective force is a thrust with your epigastrium over the apex, combined with gentle upward traction force through the patient's axilla/arms.
8. Recheck.

Patient Astride Table

FINDINGS

The patient has group curve (type I, neutral) convex left, apex at L1. The curve is rotated left, side-bent right. There is restriction of left side-bending and right rotation.

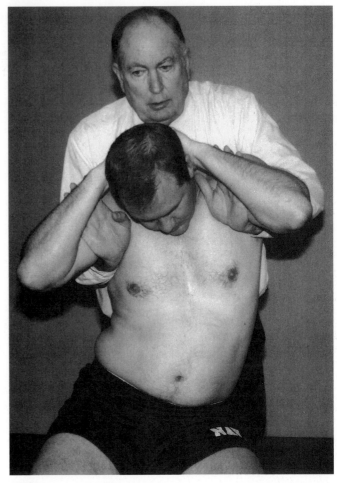

Figure 70.1. Epigastric thrust for group curve convex right. Treatment position reverses side-bending.

PROCEDURE (Fig. 70.2)

1. Stand behind your patient seated astride the end of the table.
2. Patient places hands behind the neck, interlacing fingers.
3. Place your right arm in front of patient's thorax and contact patient's left arm.
4. Contact apex (L1 left side) with your hand, adding forward or backward bending to localize the sagittal plane barrier.
5. Side-bend the patient to the left, to barrier.
6. Rotate the apex (L1) right, engaging the barrier.
7. Apply a high-velocity, low-amplitude final force, increasing the rotation to the right.
8. Recheck.

Muscle Energy

FINDINGS

The patient has group curve (type I, neutral) convex right, apex at T9. The curve is rotated right, side-bent left. There is restriction of right side-bending and left rotation.

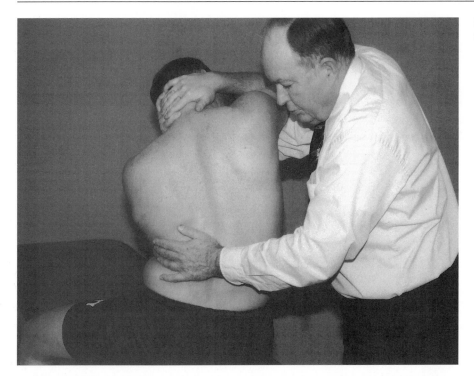

Figure 70.2. Patient astride table for treatment of group curve convex left.

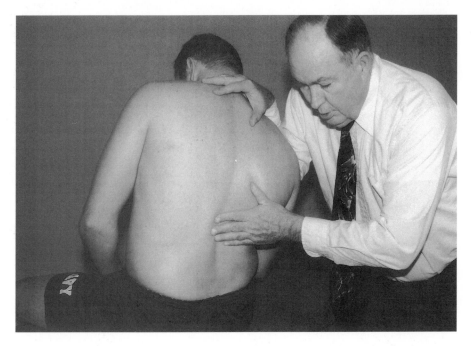

Figure 70.3. Treatment with muscle energy, with emphasis on side-bending.

PROCEDURE (Fig. 70.3)

1. Stand behind your seated patient.
2. Drape your right arm over patient's right shoulder.
3. Place your left hand over apex (T9 on right), adding forward or backward bending to localize to that level.
4. Side-bend right by depressing patient's right shoulder.
5. Translate apex (T9) to the left.
6. Engage side-bending barrier. Hold.
7. Patient attempts to raise right shoulder for 3–5 seconds.
8. Wait, then engage new barrier.
9. Repeat several times.
10. Recheck.

CONCLUSION

Spinal joints are designed to provide motion; spinal motion is necessary in most of our ordinary activity. Most spinal motion involves a group of vertebral segments. This motion follows the first principle of physiologic motion of the spine and is necessary to allow for positional changes of the body. Curves become a problem when restriction occurs and the spine no longer straightens. If the group curve contributes to dysfunction of the patient, it should be treated. Exercises or manipulation should involve stretching or mobilizing the concavity while strengthening the convex side. If a curve has been present for some time, treatment of the curve improves motion within the curve.

Though the physician often tries to improve the structure, it must be remembered that reducing asymmetry does not necessarily improve the function of the patient. The objective of treatment is to maintain or improve function of the patient within the existing structure.

REFERENCES

1. Fryette HH. Physiologic movements of the spine. *JAOA.* September 1918;18:1–2.
2. Kimberly P. *Outline of Osteopathic Manipulative Procedures.* 3rd ed. Kirksville, Mo: KCOM Press; 1980:16.

71. Postural Considerations in Coronal and Horizontal Planes

MICHAEL L. KUCHERA AND WILLIAM A. KUCHERA

Be sure the foundation is level and all will be well.

—A.T. STILL

Key Concepts

- **"Short leg syndrome" as a misnomer**
- **Biomechanical changes that contribute to short leg syndrome, and application of these as principles used for treatment rationale**
- **Role of osteopathic manipulative treatment in treatment of short leg syndrome**
- **Rationalization of treatment modalities for pelvic rotation**
- **Major criteria for classification of scoliosis**
- **Treatment goals for scoliosis, and implications of each treatment modality as it relates to patient's lifestyle and activities**

References to the existence of leg length inequality in 90% of the population have appeared in the medical literature since the latter half of the 1800s.[1-3] Lift therapy as a treatment for this problem was specifically mentioned by John Hilton in 1863:

Thus I have seen many patients wearing spinal supports, in order to correct a lateral curvature when the deformity might have and has been subsequently, corrected by placing within the shoe or boot a piece of cork thick enough to compensate for the shortness of the less well developed limb.[4]

The osteopathic profession began studies on the diagnosis and treatment of coronal plane asymmetry in 1921, when Hoskins and Schwab introduced the standing postural x-ray view.[5-6] A compilation of many of the classic osteopathic articles discussing diagnosis, clinical impact, and treatment of this subject can be found in the *1983 Yearbook of the American Academy of Osteopathy, Postural Balance and Imbalance.*[7]

SHORT LEG SYNDROME

Within the profession, the term "short leg syndrome" is recognized as a misnomer. This text refers to short leg syndrome because of historical precedence. The actual cause of the condition, however, may not be related to the actual length of the legs at all. It is called a syndrome because it is associated with a variety of biomechanical findings and symptoms. An unlevel sacral base is the clinically relevant element in this so-called short leg syndrome. Because a short lower extremity usually results in an unlevel sacral base, the spine compensates by changing its spinal curvatures. Subsequently, the person often must stand and walk differently. If the sacral base is unlevel for any reason, the innominates often rotate to compensate. This creates the appearance of a functionally short lower extremity. In either case, the most common spinal response is development of a rotoscoliosis with side-bending toward the side opposite the low sacral base, or short leg. Atypical patterns do occur, however, providing clinically challenging cases (Fig. 71.1).

A number of studies[7] indicate that sacral base unleveling and leg length inequality are fairly common. Approximately half of an unselected population has radiographic leg length inequality of more than 3/16 inch. Short leg syndrome is suspected with certain constellations of asymmetry, recurrent somatic dysfunction, and tissue texture change. When this syndrome is caused by leg length inequality, often the standing trochanteric plane, the plane of the posterior superior iliac spine (PSIS), and the iliac crests are depressed on the side of the unlevel sacral base. Usually the more cephalad horizontal planes (shoulders, occipital) are also depressed to compensate for the sacral base unlevelness (Fig. 71.2).[8] The number of curves between the pelvis and the upper body determine on which side the more cephalad horizontal planes are depressed. To find these planes, stand behind the patient and assess the levels of the following:

983

Mastoid processes
Acromioclavicular joints
Inferior scapula
Iliac crests
Greater trochanters

These static landmarks are helpful in predicting underlying spinal response to coronal plane postural asymmetry.

Early compensation in the short leg syndrome (with an unlevel sacral base) is associated with the development of a single long scoliotic curve. In this C-shaped curve, the cephalad horizontal planes are typically depressed on the side opposite the pelvic horizontal planes. Later, the compensatory mechanisms redistribute postural responsibilities over several lateral curves. In an S-shaped scoliotic curve, the shoulders and the greater trochanteric planes are typically depressed on the same side. Long-term radiographic postural studies demonstrate that the pattern of spinal curvature changes and evolves in one-third of a maturing population.[9] The likelihood of several lateral curves evolving is higher when the leg length inequality is greater than 10 mm.[8(p47)]

Pelvic rotation occurs concomitantly with the short leg syndrome[10] and can present a therapeutic challenge when preyscribing foot orthotics in an attempt to level the sacral base. There is often approximately equal declination of femoral head, sacral base (extrapolated laterally to femoral head line), and iliac crest. Postural adaptations rarely occur purely in one plane or in one region, however. The lumbar spine side-bends away from and rotate toward the short leg. The biomechanics of the typical spinopelvic response to sacral base unleveling is shown in Figure 71.3. As a curve forms in one spinal area, curves in all spinal areas change.

Each person with short leg syndrome progressively compensates in a different way. Certain guiding principles apply,

however. Postural changes take place throughout the musculoskeletal system in an attempt to coordinate visual, vestibular, and kinesthetic input while distributing the stresses. Typically, the changes occur more predictably in the lumbopelvic region because of its proximity to both the problem and the center of gravity.

The remainder of the changes involved depend on compensatory responses. In general, the pelvis side-shifts and rotates toward the long leg side. The innominate typically rotates anteriorly on the side of the apparent short leg to lengthen that extremity relative to the other. The innominate on the side of the apparent long leg may rotate posteriorly to relatively shorten that extremity. Often, on the long leg side, the foot assumes a pronated position, and the lower extremity medially rotates. There is an increase of 2–3° in the lumbosacral angle. The increased lumbosacral angle and pelvic rotation frequently mask the presence of an unlevel sacral base.[11] The vertebrae of the most caudal scoliotic curve usually side-bend away from and rotate toward the apparent short leg side. Often degener-

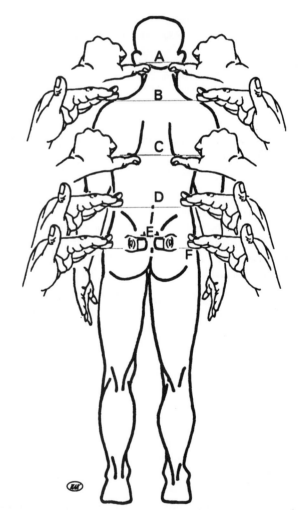

Figure 71.2. Levelness of horizontal planes. A, Occipital plane; B, Shoulder plane; C, Scapular plane (inferior); D, Iliac crest plane; E, PSIS plane; F, Greater trochanteric plane.

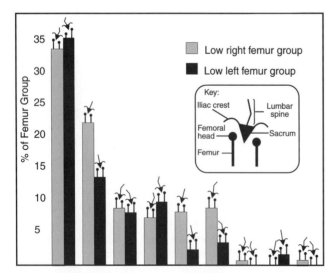

Figure 71.1. Frequency distribution of lumbosacral relationships to unlevel femoral head heights. n = 738. (Reprinted with permission from Kirksville College of Osteopathic Medicine).

ative arthritis of the hip joint develops on the long leg side,[12] accompanied by tenderness over that greater trochanter.

Diagnosis

Compensatory measures are sometimes so good that any single landmark measurement may fail to provide a true and accurate diagnosis. Neither alignment of spinous processes nor level of iliac crests are good indicators of sacral base unleveling or short leg syndrome. Anterior superior iliac spine (ASIS) or hip-to-ankle measurements using a tape measure are also inaccurate.[13–14] Comparison of the levels of the medial malleoli in the supine position is similarly inaccurate or incorrect.[15] The greater trochanters in the standing position are somewhat more helpful clinically but can be in error when unilateral coxa varus or coxa valgus is present.[16] Diagnosis based on clinical findings alone, then, is difficult and not always accurate. In one study of standing patients with known radiographic leg length inequality, the wrong extremity was identified as short in 13% of clinical observations; more than half of the 196 clinical estimates of leg length were incorrect by more than 3/16 inch.[17]

Recurrent somatic dysfunction of the pelvis, spine, cranium, or myofascial structures may be a clue that the sacral base is unlevel or that a short leg is present. Soft tissue involvement with respect to the compensation occurring in the short leg syndrome is particularly common and a cause of many patient complaints. Tissues on the concavity shorten and demonstrate increased electromyographic activity.[18–19] Tissues on the convex side lengthen. Patients with coronal plane postural imbalance develop tight abductors on one side and tight thigh adductors on the contralateral side. Associated horizontal plane imbalance often results in tight hamstrings on one side and tight rectus femoris on the other thigh. The iliolumbar ligament on the side of the convexity of the lumbopelvic curve is often the first structure to react to added stress in the lumbosacral area. The iliolumbar ligament is pain-sensitive. The point of maximal tenderness to palpation is typically located over the attachments of the iliolumbar ligament at the ilial or L4 or L5 transverse processes. When stressed, it often refers pain around the ipsilateral side to the groin, and sometimes into the testicle or the labia and the upper medial thigh (Fig. 71.4).[20] The pain may be mistaken for arthritis of the hip, greater trochanteric bursitis, or even an inguinal hernia.

The sacroiliac ligaments on the side of the convexity may also become stressed and tender to palpation and may refer pain down the lateral side of the leg. Unilateral sciatica and hip pain, as well as pain over the greater trochanter, are more frequently expressed on the long leg side, however. Numerous postural muscles are strained, and significant physiologic changes related to segmental facilitation have been documented. There may subsequently be visceral dysfunction related to increased sympathetic hyperactivity coming from spinal crossover areas located between T1 and L2.

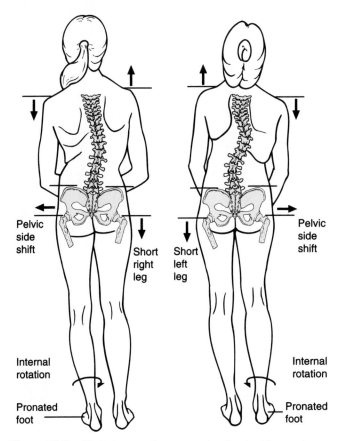

Figure 71.3. Typical postural compensation for short leg syndrome.

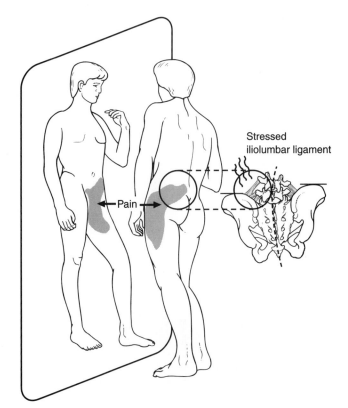

Figure 71.4. Iliolumbar ligament pain pattern from postural imbalance.

Before definitive diagnosis of a patient's posture, a thorough osteopathic manipulative treatment (OMT) should be directed to all somatic dysfunction. It is extremely important not to overlook sacral or innominate shear somatic dysfunctions. After OMT, the presence of a positive standing flexion test coexisting with a negative seated flexion test should raise the suspicion that lower extremity influences, such as a short lower extremity, are affecting the function of the sacroiliac joint and the patient's posture.[21]

When the spine is as mobile as possible and any nonphysiologic (shear) somatic dysfunctions have been removed, a standard standing postural x-ray series may be taken. After first manipulating the patient, this x-ray series primarily portrays structural data indicating the best homeostatic compensation possible by the patient at the time. These standard standing postural x-ray images can then be used to measure coronal plane values accurately, including the following:

Iliac crest heights
Femoral head heights
Sacral base unleveling
Degree and type of scoliotic compensatory curvatures

When reading the x-ray image (Fig. 71.5), remember that there is still potentially a 2-mm human error in measurement. This can occur even with flawless technique by the radiologic technician and perfect patient cooperation. There can also be up to a 25% bony magnification (distortion).[22] Compensatory changes such as innominate rotations, pelvic rotation, and changes in the LS angle may alter the x-ray appearance. This can misrepresent the extent of the patient's actual problem. For these reasons, a leg length difference of less than 5 mm may not be treated unless the patient has other clinically relevant factors. Conversely, the desire to attain peak physical performance may be an indication for treating the patient in

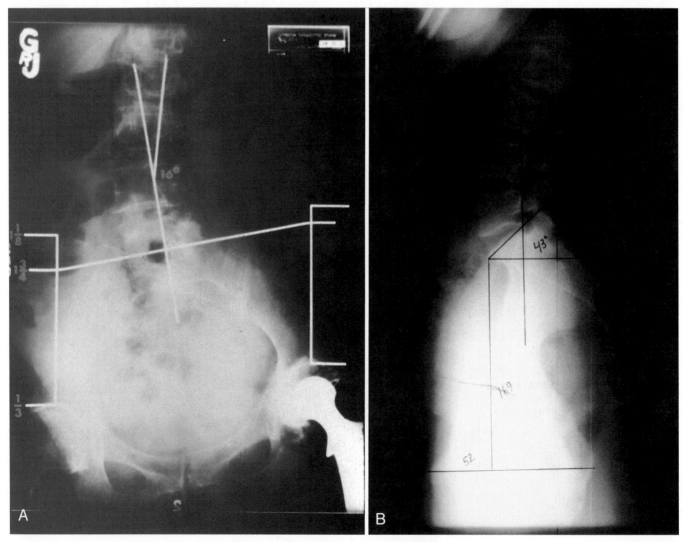

Figure 71.5. X-ray image marked for coronal (**A**) and horizontal (**B**)plane measurements. Ideal values would be no side-to-side unleveling of any of these landmarks and no pelvic rotation.

this case. Patterns of imbalance recorded along the spine may be caused by as little as ¹⁄₁₆ of an inch (1.5 mm) difference in leg length. Clinical symptoms can occur in these cases, including low back pain.[8(p37–63),23]

Treatment

Typically, treatment of the short leg syndrome involves lifting the heel of the leg on the side of the depressed sacral base. This is especially true if there is a compensatory curvature that side-bends to the side opposite the short leg. In the less common situation where the curve has its concavity toward the side of the short leg, it is usually necessary to lift the side of the long leg. This first effects a change in the lumbar scoliosis and also relieves some of the pelvic and lumbar strain.[24(p26–38)] Reduce the lift on the long leg side later to begin to lift the unlevel sacral base.

Heel lift treatment within the osteopathic profession is always combined with OMT and is usually not attempted until after an appropriate trial of OMT. The rationale for both was clearly implied by Harrison Fryette:

In the average case I do not attempt a correction until I have mobilized the lumbar joints and established rotation in them; furthermore, if this region cannot be rotated toward the midline, the lift will not do what it is intended of it, for the correction will not take place in the lumbar region—the spine higher up will compensate by increasing its curve and only more trouble will result.[25]

OMT may alleviate a functional condition that presents as an apparent short leg syndrome. In the situation in which lift therapy is indicated, OMT prepares the somatic tissues to accept the realignment needed in response to the newly established sacral base level.

Whenever lift therapy is initiated, osteopathic physicians consider the implications of postural realignment and "reeducation," which must take place throughout the entire body. For many reasons, the initial amount of lift selected is rarely the full amount needed. In most cases, compensation and decompensation have occurred over a period of time, leading to shortening and fibrosis of soft tissues, bony remodeling, and regional somatic dysfunction. The easiest but least sensitive guideline used by clinicians is to select an initial lift that is one-third to one-half of the measured sacral base difference.

Attempts to formulate specific guidelines to better quantify the amount of lift are best appreciated by studying the writings of David Heilig.[26] Heilig found that one-third to one-half the measured sacral base unleveling was too much initial lift in selected clinical situations. He developed a formula[26] (Table 71.1) that considered the amount of lift to be directly proportional to the measured sacral base unleveling and inversely proportional to host factors such as the age, duration of the condition, and amount of compensation or adaptation acquired by the body.

Heilig offered examples of patients who all had ½-inch sa-

cral base unleveling but who, based on the formula, would receive different initial lifts (Table 71.2).

One of the safest protocols taught at many of the colleges of osteopathic medicine is less complicated than the Heilig formula yet sensitive to individual host factors. It employs conservative rules of thumb that can later be modified with clinical experience and judgment. This protocol is designed to avoid any unexpected flare-ups of pain or somatic dysfunction that can occur if lift therapy is introduced too rapidly or if it exceeds the capability of the body to realign in response to the changes being made in the sacral base level.

The following are guidelines only and must be adapted to each individual patient's evaluation and response.[27(p343–350)]

If lift therapy is required and if the patient is considered to be a "fragile" patient (arthritic, osteoporotic, aged, having significant acute pain, etc.), begin with ¹⁄₁₆-inch lift and lift no faster than ¹⁄₁₆ of an inch every 2 weeks.

If the spine is flexible and no more than mild to moderate strain is noted in the myofascial system, begin with ⅛-inch lift and lift at a rate no faster than ¹⁄₁₆ of an inch per week, or ⅛ of an inch every 2 weeks.

If there was a recent sudden loss of leg length on one side, as might occur following fracture or a recent hip prosthesis, and the patient had a level sacral base before the fracture or surgery, lift the full fractional amount that was lost.

Table 71.1
The Heilig Formula

The Heilig formula suggests that the initial lift can be calculated as follows:

$$L < [SBU]/[D + C]$$

L = Lift required; SBU = Sacral base unleveling; D = Duration; C = Compensation.
Duration allotted as (1) = 0–10 years; (2) = 10–30 years; (3) = 30+ years.
Compensation allotted as (0) = none observed; (1) = rotation of lumbar vertebrae into convexity of compensatory side-bending; (2) = wedging of the vertebrae, altered size of facets, horizontal osseous developments from endplates, and/or spurring.

Table 71.2
Patients with Same Sacral Base Leveling but Receiving Different Lifts

Case 1: Following fracture, minimal duration, no compensatory changes
   L = [SBU]/[D + C] = ½″/[0 + 1] = ½″
Case 2: Patient age 35, injured in early youth, minimal compensation
   L = [SBU]/[D + C] = ½″/[2 + 1] = ½″/3 = ⅙″
Case 3: Patient age 75, injured in youth, spurring, horizontal endplate development, rotation is marked
   L = [SBU]/[D + C] = ½″/[3 + 2] = ½″/5 = ¹⁄₁₀″
Case 4: Patient age 26, polio affecting right leg in youth, minimal compensatory change
   L = [SBU]/[D + C] = ½″/[2 + 0] = ½″/2 = ¼″

Regardless of the method used to select the amount of the initial lift, certain other guidelines should be followed for optimum clinical results.

Because of magnification, measurement error, and compensatory changes, the final lift height in a chronic short leg syndrome may only be one-half to three-fourths of the shortness in that leg measured by the standard standing x-ray method.

When a proper lift has eventually been reached and there are no pelvic or lower extremity somatic dysfunctions, the standing flexion test should become negative. If a repeat x-ray image is desired, it should be taken using the same radiographic protocol and parameters but with the shoes on and the lift in place.

Guidelines used in lift treatment are not absolute rules. One aspect of the art of medicine is an appreciation of the concerns that patients have about cost, cosmetic appearance, and convenience. Ideally, the shoe is rebuilt with every increment of lift to prevent alteration of foot mechanics and introduction of unwanted pelvic rotation. Few patients, however, would agree with this approach. The following guidelines emphasizing clinical tolerances can be pragmatically used in lift treatment. If problems arise, reducing the tolerances or insisting on the ideal may be necessary.

The true height of a lift is measured from the bottom of the lift to a point where the calcaneal bone strikes the lift; it is not measured from the bottom of the lift to the most posterior part of the lift.

Up to and including one-fourth of replaceable lift can be used inside of the shoe before the foot no longer fits well.

Up to and including a total of ½-inch lift can be placed between the heel of the patient's foot and the floor before foot mechanics are significantly disturbed.

If only the heel is lifted, a tendency toward pelvic rotation, muscle imbalance, and alteration of foot mechanics is progressively introduced.

Application of these principles to change the relative leg length by ½-inch may result in:

¼-inch lift being placed inside the shoe and ¼ inch added to the heel of that shoe
½ inch added to the heel of one shoe
¼ inch added to one sole and ¼ inch removed from the opposite side[26,28]

Many other combinations exist within these general guidelines, permitting the osteopathic practitioner the latitude to balance nonphysical factors (such as vanity and cost) with those related to posture.

Any increase beyond the ½-inch heel lift must be added to the heel and also to the half-sole of the shoe (Fig. 71.6). This principle preserves the relationship of the heel to the forefoot by maintaining a certain normal angle.

Studies[23] indicate that an 80% reduction in pain and other posturally related symptoms could be expected as a result of

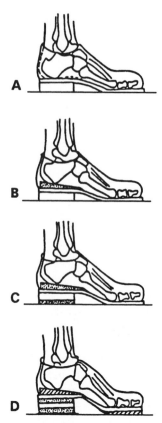

Figure 71.6. Principles of lift therapy. Heel lift measurements made at midcalcaneal line. *A*, Foot in typical shoe. *B*, Heel lift in place. Maximum in shoe is ¼ inch. *C*, If more lift needed, add to outside heel. *D*, If more than ½ inch is required, or to create minimal disturbance of foot mechanics, entire sole can be lifted.

properly balancing the sacral base with lift therapy to within 1 mm of levelness.

Try to balance the weight of both shoes, especially if large lifts are required.

If a big lift is needed, cork material between the shoe and the heel may be necessary to reduce the weight being added to one side. In some cases, small lead weights may be added to the other shoe to maintain balance.

OMT helps the patient's spine to compensate better for the new posture that results from treatment for a short leg.

Compressive force makes bone grow faster. A lift under a growing child's short leg may be expected to stimulate faster growth in that leg.

The physician must closely monitor leg lengths when using lift therapy for a child. The height of the lift must be adjusted according to clinical responses and the results observed on follow-up x-ray studies. In growing athletes, alternating lower extremity growth parameters have been reported.[26] This has prompted the clinical recommendation to check the pelvic and extremity levels at regular intervals. Fryette went as far as to remark, "In the last 15 years I have added lifts to the short side in many cases under the age of fourteen and in every case that I have kept under my observation for some time I have been astonished to find that the legs grew to the same length."[29]

ANTERIOR LIFT TREATMENT OF PELVIC ROTATION

The clinical use of anterior sole lifts (in distinction from heel lifts) or the combination of an anterior lift in one shoe and/or a heel lift in the opposite shoe to affect posture in the horizontal plane has largely been explored by Ross Pope and James Carlson.[30] An increase in the sole height of a shoe encourages rotation of the pelvis toward that same side. A unilateral heel lift rotates the pelvis to a lesser degree and rotates it away from the lifted side.[27(p351-356)] Because this method is new, few clinical trials have been performed. The predominance of clinical experience, however, suggests the following guidelines, which are adapted to each individual patient's evaluation and response.

Anterior lift therapy rotates the pelvis toward the same side; heel lifts may rotate the pelvis away from the lift side. Treatment of both planes simultaneously is often warranted, as side-bending and rotation are biomechanically linked motions (Fig. 71.7).

Behind the axis of motion, heel lifts push that side of pelvis anteriorly in the horizontal plane. Anterior sole lifts are in front of the axis and rotate that side of the pelvis posteriorly in a horizontal plane.

In the treatment of pelvic rotation assuming coexistent sacral base unleveling, follow these principles:

For pelvic rotation less than 5 mm: Usually it is not necessary to treat a pelvic rotation less than 5 mm. Treat the sacral base unleveling with heel lifts according to coronal plane postural balancing principles. Recheck to determine if any unwanted pelvic rotation has occurred secondary to heel lift therapy.

For pelvic rotation of 5–10 mm: For pelvic rotation of 5–10 mm, treat both sacral base (coronal plane) and rotational (horizontal plane) components simultaneously. Begin with appropriate ⅛ inch anterior and heel lifts, progressively increasing in ⅛-inch increments every 2 weeks.

For pelvic rotation greater than 10 mm: For pelvic rotations more than 10 mm, first treat with an anterior lift of ¼ inch, and then recheck the postural study before attempting heel lifts. Thereafter, treat sacral base unleveling and pelvic rotation simultaneously with ⅛-inch incremental changes in anterior and heel lifts every 2 weeks.

ANTERIOR AND HEEL LIFTS

Lift therapy is initiated to help the body return to better structural alignment and function. Properly managed, the patient's postural mechanisms are "reeducated" toward the ideal posture. Balancing mechanisms are known to become more precise as evidenced by graphic center-of-gravity plots before and after appropriate lift therapy. Paraspinal muscle tension and various spinal physiologic parameters become more symmet-

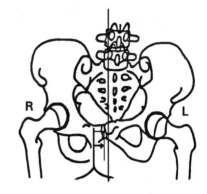

With lifts in the heel or in the opposite half-sole, the pelvis can be derotated.

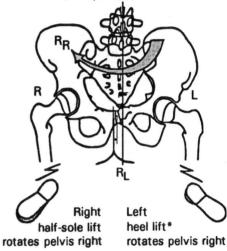

Right half-sole lift rotates pelvis right   Left heel lift* rotates pelvis right

Figure 71.7. Left half-sole lift and right heel lift rotating pelvis left.

rically normalized, and patient symptoms throughout the body are dramatically reduced.

SCOLIOSIS (ROTOSCOLIOSIS)

Ten in every two hundred children (10:200) develop scoliosis by the age of 10–15 years; one in every 200 (1:200) has clinical symptoms related to the curvatures. Boys and girls are equally affected, but the curvatures in girls are three to five times more likely to progress and produce subjective symptoms. Most cases (75–90%) of scoliosis in children are discovered between the ages of 10 and 15 because of widespread screening programs and because this is the time of most rapid bone growth. Curvatures are more likely to progress during times of rapid bone growth.

Scoliosis primarily affects the coronal plane. It is officially named according to the direction of the convexity of the curve. A curve that is side-bent to the left is called a right scoliosis because the convexity of the curve is toward the right.

Diagnosis

Scoliosis may be classified by its reversibility, severity, cause, or location.

REVERSIBILITY

Scoliosis can be functional or structural. A simple physical examination technique to assess the proportion of functional to structural scoliosis can be accomplished by standing behind a patient (Fig. 71.8). The patient is forward-bent until maximal rib hump appears on horizon. With that much forward-bending, the patient swings the upper body first left, then right, while the operator observes the functional ability of rib hump to reduce. The amount of rib hump remaining is associated with the structural component. Functional scoliotic curves go away with side-bending, rotation, or forward-bending. If they remain in the body too long, they may become structural.[31] Structural scoliotic curves are fixed curves that do not reduce with side-bending or rotation.

SEVERITY

There are four degrees of severity. The normal case shows no scoliosis. Mild scoliosis shows a thoracic curve of 5–15° (Fig. 71.9). Moderate scoliosis curves from 20 to 45°. Severe scoliosis has a curve of more than 50°. Severe scoliosis affects structure and systemic function. A thoracic curve of more than 50°

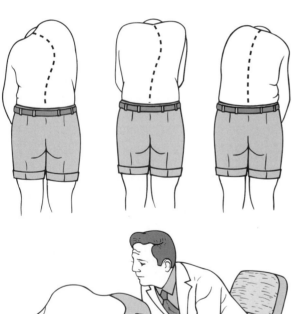

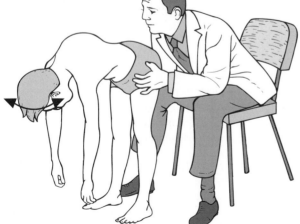

Figure 71.8. Assessment of structural or functional scoliosis.

compromises respiratory function. A curve of more than 75° compromises cardiovascular function.

CAUSE

The following causes are listed according to decreasing frequency.

Idiopathic

This diagnosis accounts for 70–90% of the scoliotic curves. By definition, this term implies that there is no known reason for this type of scoliosis to occur. Osteopathic physicians feel that some of these may be explained as compensatory curves for unlevel sacral[23] or cranial bases.[32] In those cases where such a biomechanical basis exists for the development of scoliosis, the idiopathic classification is inappropriate. Other clinicians have implicated sagittal plane biomechanics in the genesis and progression of different types of idiopathic scoliotic patterns.[33] Better understanding of scoliosis may further reduce the number of cases classified as idiopathic.

Congenital

Of congenital cases, 75% are progressive. This classification is the second most common type according to cause.

Acquired

Acquired scoliosis may arise from causes such as the following:

Osteomalacia
Response to inflammation or irradiation
Sciatic irritability
Psoas syndrome
Healed leg fracture
Following a hip prosthesis

Obviously, if a short leg syndrome is documented as the reason for the patient's scoliosis, this should be reclassified as an acquired scoliosis.

LOCATION

Various locations of scoliosis are listed below according to decreasing frequency (Fig. 71.10). Regions involved in scoliosis may be balanced or not. Unbalanced curves are more likely to decompensate, while balanced curves are subject to degeneration at crossovers.

Double Major Scoliosis

These are balanced curves but they are subject to degeneration at the crossovers. This is the most common scoliosis, with a thoracic and lumbar combination being the most frequent.

Single Thoracic Scoliosis

Cosmetically, this curve is rather noticeable. It is usually side-bent right. If this type of curve should progress, it could com-

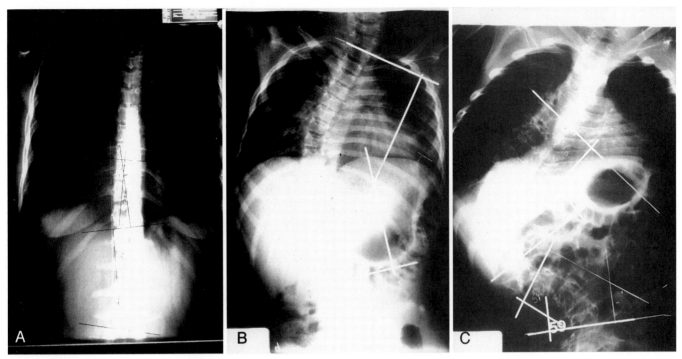

Figure 71.9. Curve patterns in idiopathic scoliosis. **A**, mild (14° + 15°); **B**, moderate (38°); **C**, severe (59° and 85°). Assessment of scoliotic severity defined by Cobb angle measurements (see Fig. 71.11) for each portion of coronal plane curve. Classification system quoted allows 5° gray zone between severity classes.

promise the function of the heart or lungs. It is the second most common scoliosis.

Single Lumbar Scoliosis

This curve is associated with arthritic change. It is the third most common scoliosis.

Junctional Thoracolumbar Scoliosis

This scoliosis often results in structural (arthritic) change because such long curves functionally overstress the spine. It is not a common scoliosis.

Junctional Cervicothoracic Scoliosis

This scoliosis is very uncommon.

Screening

Children with scoliosis are usually asymptomatic, yet scoliosis is most often seen between 10 and 15 years of age. For this reason, school children should be routinely screened for scoliosis. Physicians casually looking for scoliosis may miss a curve of up to 35°.[27(p351–356)] Careful screening with physical examination alone should pick up all scolioses less than 10°.

In the standing position, analyze the space around the patient's body, especially in the arm and waist area. Does one hand hang by the side and the other hand lay on or over the thigh? Look at the levelness of the occipital, shoulder, iliac crest, PSIS, and trochanteric planes. Run your fingers along the spinous processes from top to bottom. Have the patient forward-bend and observe for an asymmetric hump along the horizon of vision. Its presence would indicate rotoscoliotic deformity with rotation to that side and side-bending of the spine to the side opposite the hump.

If spinal curvature is found, have the patient bend over to that area of the spine and determine if it goes away with side-bending toward the side of the rib hump (Fig. 71.8). Check the patient for conditions that could give the appearance of a short leg, such as sacral shear somatic dysfunction on that side. If you find somatic dysfunction, correct it with manipulation and then recheck for the short leg. If there is continued recurrence of a scoliotic curve, provide OMT until there is good mobilization of the spine and then get a standing postural x-ray image. The x-ray image provides the quantitative data to determine:

Any bony pathology
Type and severity of the curvatures
Amount of sacral base unleveling
Femoral head and iliac crest levelness

Scoliotic curvatures are measured from the radiographs by the Cobb method (Fig. 71.11). The same vertebrae defining the top and the bottom of the curve are used for future Cobb measurements to see if the curve is progressing. Scoliosis often increases rapidly during the growth spurt of adolescence. Take an x-ray image of the hands and epiphyses and obtain a bone

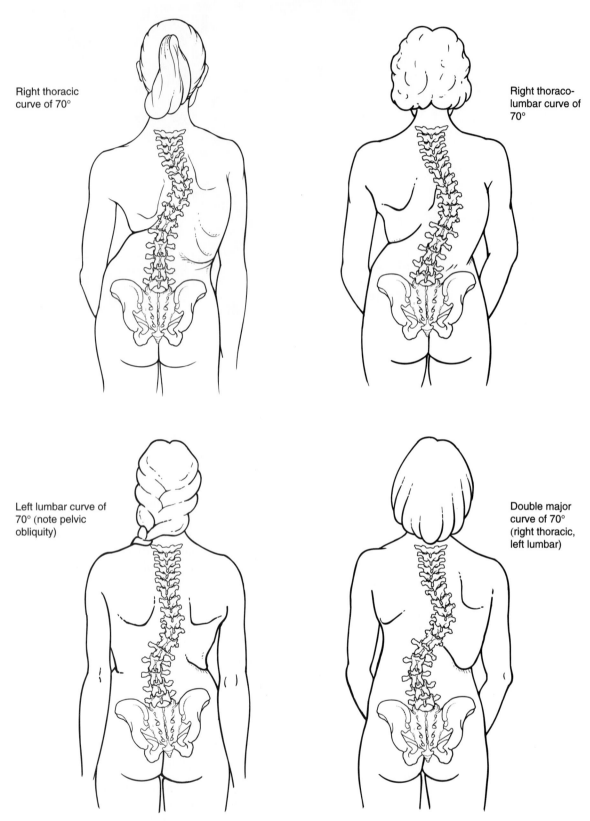

Right thoracic
curve of 70°

Right thoraco-
lumbar curve of
70°

Left lumbar curve of
70° (note pelvic
obliquity)

Double major
curve of 70°
(right thoracic,
left lumbar)

Figure 71.10.   Curve patterns in idiopathic scolioses classified by location.

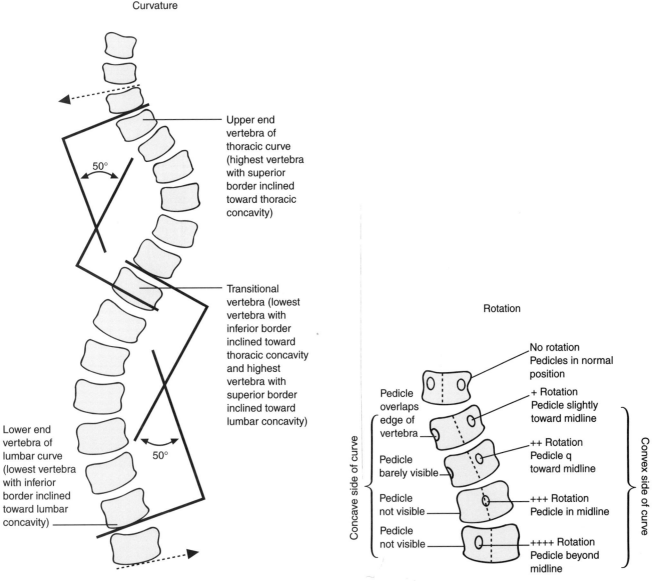

Curvature

50°

Upper end vertebra of thoracic curve (highest vertebra with superior border inclined toward thoracic concavity)

Transitional vertebra (lowest vertebra with inferior border inclined toward thoracic concavity and highest vertebra with superior border inclined toward lumbar concavity)

Lower end vertebra of lumbar curve (lowest vertebra with inferior border inclined toward lumbar concavity)

50°

Rotation

Concave side of curve

Pedicle overlaps edge of vertebra

Pedicle barely visible

Pedicle not visible

Pedicle not visible

No rotation
Pedicles in normal position

+ Rotation
Pedicle slightly toward midline

++ Rotation
Pedicle q toward midline

+++ Rotation
Pedicle in midline

++++ Rotation
Pedicle beyond midline

Convex side of curve

Figure 71.11. Measurement of curvature and rotation by Cobb method. In Cobb method, identification of top and bottom of each curve is most important.

age for those patients with significant scoliotic progression. For females, the scoliosis is more likely to undergo a more rapid progression. Significant progression of the curve is considered to be occurring if there is a 5° or greater increase in the curvature between an initial and a follow-up x-ray image taken within 5 months. The Cobb method is used to classify scoliosis by severity (Fig. 71.9).

Symptoms of Rotoscoliosis

Scoliosis is also often asymptomatic in the adolescent and therefore would be overlooked unless screening was performed. The patient may have only noticed that clothing does not fit properly. As the person gets older, several symptoms bring the scoliotic patient to the physician. These include:

Arthritic symptoms
Backaches

Chest pains
Neck aches
Headaches
Symptoms of organ dysfunction

Treatment

Appropriate treatment protocols are based on classification of the scoliosis, taking into consideration factors affecting potential compliance. The treatment for scoliosis according to its severity follows the following general guidelines.[27(p351–356)]

For mild scoliosis, use:

OMT
Konstancin exercises
Functional orthotics
Patient and family education

Figure 71.12. Milwaukee brace.

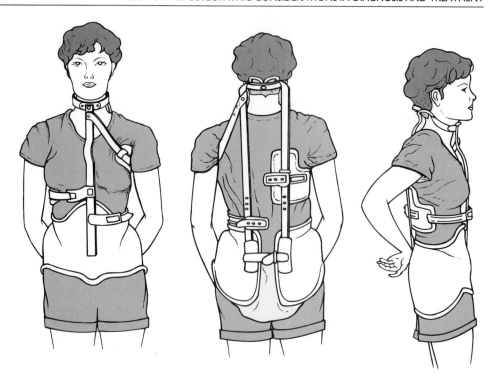

Figure 71.13. Boston brace.

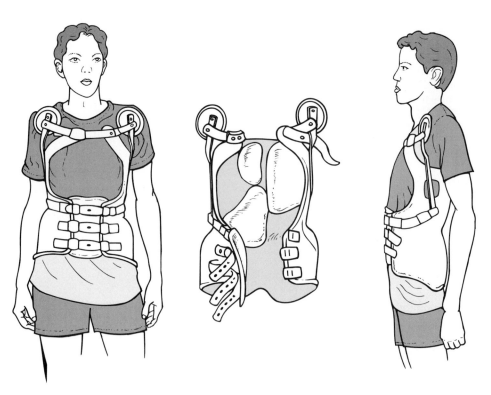

For moderate scoliosis, use:

OMT
Konstancin exercises
Patient and family education
Bracing
Electrical stimulation

For severe scoliosis, use surgery and adjunctive measures, including those listed for moderate scoliosis.

Anyone with scoliosis of more than 15–20°, with progression of curvature, or with intractable low back pain in spite of adequate conservative treatment measures, should have a specialist's consultation.

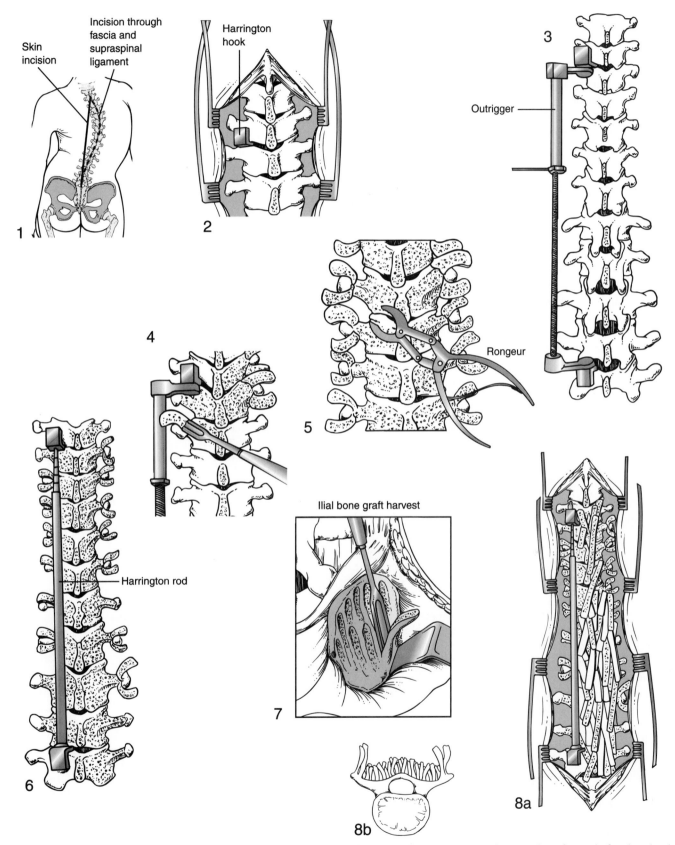

Figure 71.14. Surgical fusion with Harrington rod implantation. This extensive surgery is reserved for patients with curves greater than 45°. Clinical goal is to stop structural progression of curve before it seriously compromises cardiopulmonary function.

The goals of treatment are to obtain flexibility and improved balance of the spine. Decide what can be improved and then correct the primary cause or at least prevent the scoliosis from progressing. Postpone fusions as long as possible without endangering function or the patient's life. Osteopathic manipulation is a definite part of the management of a patient with scoliosis. The person with scoliosis must be able to compensate for the new posture introduced by the treatment methods used to prevent progression or reduce the severity of the curvatures.

OMT

When structural scoliosis is present, direct manipulation to optimize the function of the existing structure. It is not primarily intended to straighten the curvatures. Treatment should remove joint somatic dysfunction but should also include improvement of the general range of body motion through soft tissue, fascial releases, and indirect treatments. Stretch the lumbosacral tissues and institute exercises to reduce the lumbosacral angle and strengthen the psoas and abdominal muscles. After structural strains are allowed to heal, introduce Konstancin exercises.

Orthopaedic appliances, orthotics, braces, and electrical stimulation may also be used in the management program. These adjunctive modalities support, align, or prevent deformity and may stabilize function of a hypermobile part of the body. Braces are more effective if the scoliosis is moderate, if the spine is mobile, and if the spine still has not fully matured.

BRACES

The Milwaukee brace (Fig. 71.12) was introduced in 1945 and has been the standard for scoliotic bracing for many years. It is individually fitted and easy to prescribe, but it is also hard to wear and costly. It is worn 23 hours/day with only 1 hour out of the brace to allow for skin care. This brace is used in a growing patient with 20–40° curves. It works to control the scoliotic (lateral) curves until the spine matures (generally around age 21).

It is necessary to exercise supported muscles when static braces or appliances are used. Studies suggest that even for patients with a good reduction in the Cobb measurements, after a few years their curves return to approximately the extent present at the time that the brace was introduced.

An alternative brace is possible for some patients with scoliosis. The Boston brace (Fig. 71.13) is made of plastic and is designed to work on deformities such as lordosis and rotation as well as scoliosis. This brace can be used only if the apex of the curve is below T10. It is helpful in addressing postural curves in all three cardinal planes.

ELECTRICAL STIMULATION

Electrical stimulation was introduced in the l970s. It is applied to the convexity of the curve and is usually considered when the curve is 10–40°, the spine is flexible, and the curve is in the thoracic area. Electrical stimulation applied to a lumbar curve increases the lumbar lordosis. This concept enjoyed some degree of popularity but is not often used today.

SURGERY

Surgical fusion is performed only in 1 in 1000 cases of scoliosis; the curve must usually be greater than 45°. The placement of stainless steel Harrington rods (Fig. 71.14) and spinal fusion is an extensive surgery. The mechanical power of the body is dramatically demonstrated by the propensity of the rods to become stressed and break, requiring another extensive surgery to replace them. Surgery is considered for progressing scoliotic curves at 45–50° to prevent the heart and lung complications that accompany greater curvatures.

CONCLUSION

Patients' philosophies toward illness, their ways of life, and the environments in which they function may affect their compliance, in turn affecting the outcome of the treatment program. OMT helps the patient's spine compensate better for the new posture that results from treatment for a short leg or scoliosis.

REFERENCES

1. Hunt W. Inequality to length of the lower limbs, with a report of an important suit for malpractice; and also a claim for priority. *Am J Med Sci.* 1879;77:102–107.
2. Cox WC. On the want of symmetry in the length of opposite sides of persons who have never been the subject of disease or injury to their lower extremities. *Am J Med Sci.* April 1875;69:438–439.
3. Garson JG. Inequality in length of lower limbs. *J Anat Physiol.* July 1879;13:502–507.
4. Hilton J. *Rest and Pain.* 6th ed. Philadelphia, Penn: JB Lippincott Co; 1950:404.
5. Schwab WA. Principles of manipulative treatment: II. Low back problem. *JAOA.* February 1932;31:216–220.
6. Beilke MC. Roentgenological spinal analysis and the technic for taking standing x-ray plates. *JAOA.* May 1936;35:414–418.
7. Peterson B, ed. Postural balance and imbalance. In: *1983 AAO Yearbook.* Newark, Ohio: American Academy of Osteopathy; 1983.
8. Travell JG, Simons DG. *Myofascial Pain and Dysfunction: A Trigger Point Manual.* Vol. II. Baltimore, Md: Williams & Wilkins; 1992:47.
9. Hagen DP. A continuing roentgenographic study of rural school children over a 15-year period. *JAOA.* 1964;63:546–557.
10. Denslow JS, Chase JA, Gardner DL, Banner KB. Mechanical stresses in the human lumbar spine and pelvis. *JAOA.* 1962;61:705–712.
11. Kuchera ML, Irvin RE. Biomechanical considerations in postural realignment. *JAOA.* November 1987;87(11):781–782.
12. Gofton JP, Trueman GE. Studies in osteoarthritis of the hip: part II. Osteoarthritis of the hip and leg-length disparity. *Can Med Assoc J.* 1971;104:791–799.
13. Nichols PJR, Bailey NTJ. The accuracy of measuring leg-length differences. *Br Med J.* 1955;2:1247–1248.
14. Clarke GR. Unequal leg length: an accurate method of detection and some clinical results. *Rheum Phys Med.* 1972;11:385–390.
15. Beal MC. The short-leg problem. *JAOA.* 1950;50:109–121.

16. Hoskins ER. The development of posture and its importance: III. Short leg. *JAOA*. 1934;34:125–126.

17. Friberg O, Nurminen M, Korhonen K, et al. Accuracy and precision of clinical estimation of leg length inequality and lumbar scoliosis: comparison of clinical and radiological measurements. *International Disability Studies*. 1988;10:49–53.

18. Strong R, Thomas PE. Patterns of muscle activity in the leg, hip, and torso associated with anomalous fifth lumbar conditions. *JAOA*. 1968;67:1039–1041.

19. Strong R, Thomas PE, Earl WD. Patterns of muscle activity in the leg, hip, and torso during quiet standing. *JAOA*. 1967;66:1035–1038.

20. Hackett GS. *Ligament and Tendon Relaxation Treated by Prolotherapy*. 3rd ed. Springfield, Ill: CC Thomas; 1958:27.

21. Sutton SE. Postural imbalance: Examination and treatment utilizing flexion tests. In: Peterson B, ed. *Postural Balance and Imbalance (1983 AAO Yearbook)*. Newark, Ohio: American Academy of Osteopathy; 1983:102–112.

22. Denslow JS, Chace JA, Gutensohn OR, Kumm MG. Methods in taking and interpreting weight-bearing x-ray films. In: Beal MC, ed. *Selected Papers of John Stedmen Denslow (1993 AAO Yearbook)*. Indianapolis, Ind: American Academy of Osteopathy; 1993:109–120.

23. Irvin RE. Reduction of lumbar scoliosis by use of a heel lift to level the sacral base. *JAOA*. January 1991;91(1):34–44.

24. Beal MC. A review of the short-leg problem. In Peterson B (ed) *Postural Balance and Imbalance (1983 AAO Yearbook)*. Newark OH, American Academy of Osteopathy, 1983, pp. 26–38.

25. Fryette HH. Some reasons why sacroiliac lesions recur. *JAOA*. November 1936;36:119–122.

26. Heilig D. Principles of lift therapy. In: Peterson B, ed. *Postural Balance and Imbalance (1983 AAO Yearbook)*. Newark, Ohio: American Academy of Osteopathy; 1983:113–118.

27. Kuchera WA, Kuchera ML. Postural decompensation. In: *Osteopathic Principles in Practice*. rev. 2nd ed. Columbus, Ohio: Greyden Press; 1994:343–356.

28. Greenman PE. Lift therapy: Use and abuse. In: Peterson B, ed. *Postural Balance and Imbalance (1983 AAO Yearbook)*. Newark, Ohio: American Academy of Osteopathy; 1983:123–134.

29. Patriquin DA. Lift therapy: A study of results. In: Peterson B, ed. *Postural Balance and Imbalance (1983 AAO Yearbook)*. Newark, Ohio: American Academy of Osteopathy; 1983:119–122.

30. Carlson JA, Carlson JM, Earl DT. Three-dimensional counterstrain lifts (3-DCL)—theoretical concept and applications. *AAOJ*. Summer 1995;5(2):23–27.

31. Giles LGF, Taylor JR. Lumbar spine structural changes associated with leg length inequality. *Spine*. 1982;7:159–162.

32. Magoun HI. Idiopathic adolescent spinal scoliosis: A reasonable etiology. In: Peterson B, ed. *Postural Balance and Imbalance (1983 AAO Yearbook)*. Newark, Ohio: American Academy of Osteopathy; 1983:94–100.

33. Cruickshank JL, Koike M, Dickson RA. Curve patterns in idiopathic scoliosis: a clinical and radiographic study. *J Bone Joint Surg*. 1989;71B(2):259–263.

72. Postural Considerations in the Sagittal Plane

MICHAEL L. KUCHERA

Key Concepts

- **Anatomic landmarks that ideal postural weightbearing line passes through, and implications of failure to meet this ideal center of gravity**

- **Modalities useful in treating postural decompensation and spondylolisthesis**

- **General structural condition of spondylolisthesis, and role of radiology in evaluating patients for postural decompensation**

- **Evaluation of spinal x-ray films, and grading severity of spondylolisthesis using Meyerding system**

- **Clinical presentation of spondylolisthesis and different age-related manifestations**

- **Reasons why palpatory findings are more diagnostic than x-ray images for instability and valuable for spondylolisthesis**

- **Role of orthotics in managing spondylolisthesis, and types of devices used in treating postural insufficiencies**

- **Two basic rules of exercise and importance of patient compliance**

- **Osteopathic manipulations used to treat postural problems in musculoskeletal system**

GRAVITATIONAL STRAIN

Gravity is one of the major disrupters of sagittal plane postural homeostasis.[1] Although gravity is a constant force on everyone, some individuals appear less capable of resisting its stress than do others. These individuals often have weakened structure,[2] increased functional demand in the sagittal plane,[3] or biomechanical risk factors that augment the gravitational stress challenging their homeostatic resources.

The homeostatic response to gravity in the sagittal plane begins as soon as the individual assumes an upright position (Fig. 72.1) and continues throughout life. Two secondary lordotic curves, in the cervical and lumbar regions, develop to counterbalance the primary thoracic curve present at birth. These three spinal curves resist gravity much better than one

long one. They allow a person to function in an upright position but they also result in some uniquely human problems affecting both structure and function.

Ideal postural alignment depends on balancing the cervical, lumbar, and thoracic sagittal curves against the effects of gravity. Failure to do so results in lordosis or kyphosis and numerous symptoms associated with postural decompensation in the sagittal plane. Recent literature implicates lordosis as a key destabilizing factor in the development and progression of scoliosis.[4]

Ideal postural alignment in the sagittal plane (Fig. 72.2) has a center of gravity or weightbearing line that passes through the following anatomic landmarks:

External auditory meatus
Humeral head
Middle of the body of the L3 vertebra
Anterior third of the sacral base
Femoral head
Just behind the midknee
Just anterior to the lateral malleolus

Failure of the body to maintain this center of gravity results in additional functional demands on soft tissues and joint facet structures that are not designed for weightbearing. Structural change and pain results from decompensation in the postural sagittal plane.[5]

Biomechanical Principles

The biomechanical principles of gravity's effect on the pelvis are specific. Because the gravitational line falls anterior to the middle transverse sacral axis and behind the femoral axis, gravity encourages the sacral base to rotate anteriorly and encourages innominates to rotate posteriorly (Fig. 72.3).[6] Homeostatic mechanisms to resist this counterrotation are provided by muscular tone as well by as pelvic and lumbosacral ligaments.

The iliolumbar ligaments are usually the first structures to be involved with postural decompensation because they are affected by both sacral and innominate rotations (Fig. 72.4). When stressed, these ligaments' attachments are bilaterally tender to palpation. Calcification may be seen in one or both of these ligaments when there has been long-standing postural strain; calcium is laid down along lines of stress (Wolff's law).[7] Functional changes include tenderness, edema, and pain referred to the lower extremity; these findings disappear with treatment.

Gravity stresses a number of other somatic structures in-

Figure 72.1. Changes in sagittal plane spinal curves from day 1 through age 10 years. (Reprinted with permission from Kapandji IA. *The Physiology of the Joints.* Vol 3. New York, NY: Churchill Livingstone; 1974:17.)

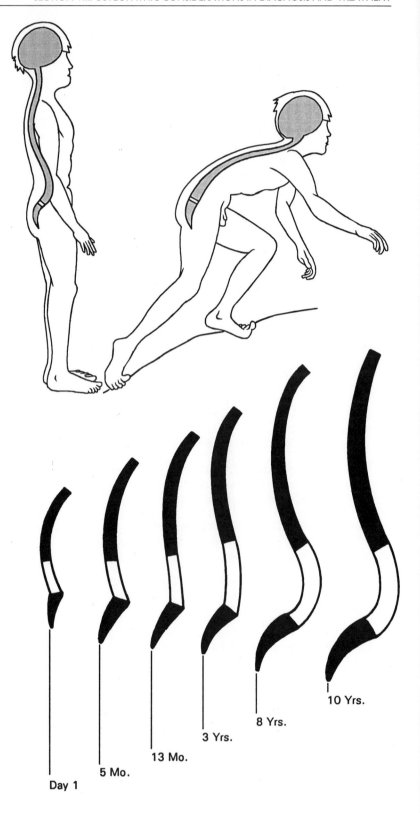

Day 1   5 Mo.   13 Mo.   3 Yrs.   8 Yrs.   10 Yrs.

volved in homeostasis. Each of these structures alone responds predictably when stressed. For example, postural muscles that are structurally adapted for prolonged stress typically respond when strained by becoming tight and spastic. Postural antagonists (phasic muscles) typically become pseudoparetic and are somewhat weak when tested (Table 72.1).[8] In combination, a pattern of postural decompensation can be recognized.[9] Patients with increased sagittal plane curves often have trigger points in a number of the muscles listed in Table 72.1. Such patterns of involvement should alert the osteopathic clinician

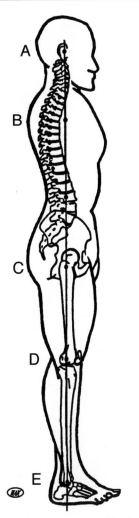

Figure 72.2. "Ideal" postural alignment of body in relation to gravitational line. *A*, external auditory meatus; *B*, shoulders; *C*, center of the body of L3; *D*, through the knee; *E*, just anterior to the distal.

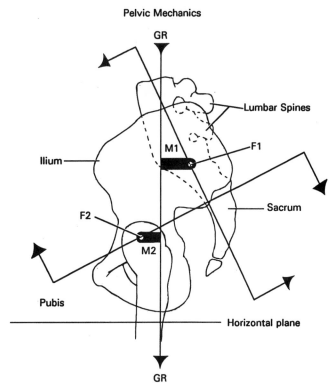

Figure 72.3. Pelvic mechanics. Intrapelvic rotations occur biomechanically about their axes of rotation in relation to gravitational line (*GR*).[6,43] Sacrum rotates anteriorly because weightbearing falls anterior to its S2 axis (*F1*). Innominates rotate posteriorly because weightbearing is posterior to femoral axes (*F2*). (Reprinted with permission from Jungmann M. *The Jungmann Concept and Technique of Antigravity Leverage.* Rangely, Me: Institute for Gravitational Strain Pathology, Inc; 1982.)

to consider a postural diagnosis and can often be traced biomechanically to gravitational stress on these muscles.

Diagnosis

RADIOGRAPHIC

Posture is both static (structural) and dynamic (functional). X-ray images primarily visualize the static or structural aspect of posture. These static postural measurements can be viewed as biomechanical risk factors. Using a standard protocol,[10] radiographic measurements outside the normative range suggest a biomechanical disadvantage that increases functional demand. As the number of biomechanical risk factors increases, homeostatic maintenance of posture is more likely to fail. These factors not only strain musculoligamentous structures but also may predispose the patient to develop spondylolysis or spondylolisthesis.[11]

Radiographic x-ray series are extremely valuable in measuring sagittal plane posture. They also aid in identifying congen-

ital anomalies and other structural deficiencies that enable gravitational and other functional strain to overcome the body's homeostatic mechanisms. Key radiographic measurements (Fig. 72.5) used to evaluate a patient for postural management of sagittal plane problems are the weightbearing line from L3 (N = anterior one-third to one-half of the sacral base) and the modified lumbosacral angle of Fergusson (N = 30–40°).

Another clinically relevant radiographic measurement is Jungmann's pelvic index (N = age-dependent). This pelvic index (PI) is the ratio of measurements representing the position of the sacrum relative to the innominates. The index appears to rise as gravity overcomes the individual's homeostatic ability to resist it. The index is higher for patients with chronic low back pain[12] and for those with other elevated sagittal plane postural measurements.[13] It is also elevated for athletes with high functional demand in the sagittal plane.[3] The highest measurements of pelvic index are seen in people with isthmic (L5-SI) spondylolisthesis.[14] For this reason, if the PI is very high and spondylolisthesis is not visualized on routine lumbopelvic x-ray views, the clinician may order oblique films of the lumbosacral area to detect a defect at the pars interarticularis (Fig. 72.6). This condition is called spondylolysis. Spondylolysis may progress to spondylolisthesis and is sometimes called prespondylolisthesis.

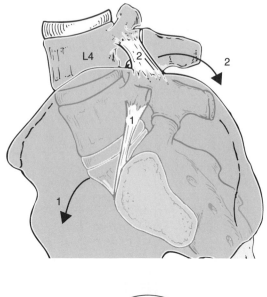
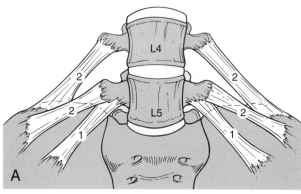
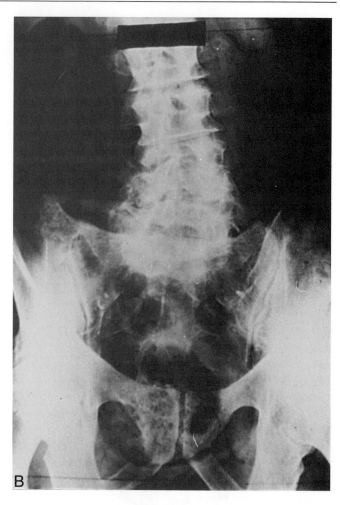

Figure 72.4. A, Anterior rotation of sacrum bilaterally stresses fibers labeled 1. Posterior rotation of innominates bilaterally stress fibers labeled 2. **B**, Calcification of iliolumbar ligament is an excellent example of structural change resulting from excessive functional demand. (Radiograph reprinted with permission from the Institute for Gravitational Strain Pathology, Inc.)

Many other radiographic measurements are possible. Mitchell's angle, for example, is a true lumbosacral angle. Lumbolumbar or lumbosacral lordotic angles are objective measurements of lordosis.[15] The observation of hyperlordosis is significant in the evaluation of patients with sagittal plane postural problems. Some of these measurements may eventually prove to be relevant, whereas others may never add any clinical relevance. Current research at the Kirksville College of Osteopathic Medicine is delineating these and other postural measurements that may add to the understanding of postural decompensation.

PALPATORY

Palpation of the spine and pelvis is essential when evaluating the dynamic or functional component of posture. Observation and palpation of postural muscles, their antagonists, and sagittal plane spinal curves should be performed with the patient in the upright position.

With the patient supine, determine whether the lumbar curve can relax and be flat against the table, especially when

Table 72.1
Postural Antagonists

Postural Muscles	Phasic Muscles
Cervical and upper thoracic muscles	
Upper trapezius muscle	Latissimus dorsi muscle
Levator scapulae muscle	Mid/lower trapezius muscles
Pectoralis major (upper part)	Rhomboid muscles
Pectoralis minor muscle	Anterior cervical muscles
Cervical erector spinae muscles	
Scalenus muscles	
Lumbar and lumbopelvic muscles	
Tensor fasciae latae muscle	Quadriceps muscles
Hamstring muscles	Dorsiflexor muscles
Hip adductor muscles (short adductors)	Abdominalis muscles
Gastrocnemius/soleus muscles	Gluteus maximus muscle
Piriformis muscle	
Iliopsoas muscles	

Reprinted with permission from Kuchera M. Gravitational stress, musculoligamentous strain and postural alignment. In: Dorman T, ed. *Spine: State of the Art Reviews on Prolotherapy.* Philadelphia, Pa: Hanley and Belfus; 1995:463–490.

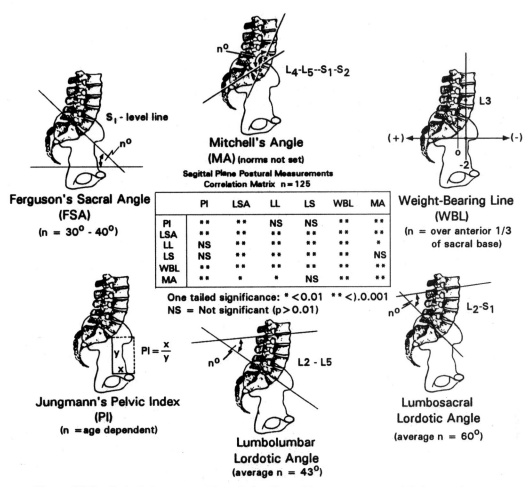

Figure 72.5. Sagittal plane postural (standing) radiographic measurements and their normal ranges.

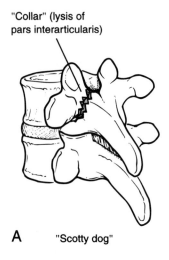

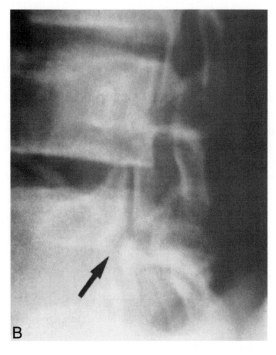

Figure 72.6. Spondylolysis. 45° oblique radiographic view best visualizes pars interarticularis. (Radiograph (**B**) reprinted with permission from

Roy S, Irvin R. *Sports Medicine: Prevention, Evaluation, Management, and Rehabilitation.* Englewood Cliffs, NJ: Prentice-Hall; 1983:280.)

the knees are bent (Fig. 72.7). In functional lumbar lordosis, bending the knees as shown should permit the lumbar region to flatten onto the table (or floor). Inability to flatten this curve actively or passively represents the structural component. Be sure to palpate the lumbar spine when evaluating this element, as other soft tissues in the adjacent flanks may mask the lordotic curve.

Alternatively, or additionally, objective measurements can be ascertained using varying computerized measurement instruments. Some of these instruments can measure intersegmental as well as regional motions and are used to reinforce the palpatory determination of areas requiring manipulative treatment (hypomobile areas) and those that need strengthening exercise, prolotherapy, or extrinsic stabilization (hypermobile areas).

Sagittal plane decompensation is often associated with palpation of extension mechanics in the craniosacral mechanism, along with an anterior sacral base and hyperlordosis. The extension phase is often accompanied by loss of energy and psychological depression. These patients may have problems in many activities of daily living as well as poor compliance with the postural treatment program.

Treatment

The principles used to prescribe a treatment plan for patients with sagittal plane postural decompensation do not vary significantly from the process used to treat postural problems in the coronal and horizontal planes. Rational treatment depends on accurate diagnosis and the recognition that every postural curve has both a structural and a functional component. These components must be evaluated with respect to their relative contributions to the whole. The chief tools for evaluation continue to be observation and palpation. Radiographic and computerized range-of-motion analyses provide additional or supportive information.

Identification of functional factors, such as muscle imbalance and joint somatic dysfunction, provides strategies for reducing postural stress and reversing the process of postural decompensation. Identification of structural involvement provides insight into the patient's prognosis.

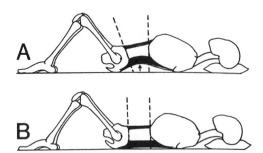

Figure 72.7. Lumbar lordosis, with patient actively attempting to flatten spine to table. **A**, Structural component; **B**, No structural component. (Reprinted with permission from Travell JG, Simons DG. *Myofascial Pain and Dysfunction: The Trigger Point Manual.* Vol I, The Upper Extremities. Baltimore, Md: Williams & Wilkins; 1983.)

If compensatory mechanisms are overwhelmed, treatment of sagittal plane postural decompensation should include some combination of the following:

1. Sound biomechanical and ergonomic education emphasizing appropriate footwear. This includes the reduction of high heels, proper lifting technique, and dietary counseling when necessary for appropriate weight distribution.
2. A functional orthosis such as the Levitor to reverse the mechanics involved in decompensation.
3. Specific exercise designed first to rest and then to functionally replace ineffective ligamentous structures.
4. Injection techniques using proliferative medication (prolotherapy) for ligamentous laxity if other conservative modalities alone fail to restore stability.
5. Osteopathic manipulative treatment (OMT) to allow postural compensation associated with treatment intervention and to address the somatic dysfunction that consistently and recurrently accompanies postural problems.

Treatment of postural problems emphasizes compliance, especially in the initial phases of the program of reeducation. Compliance by the patient is essential and can be enhanced if the patient understands the rationale behind the treatment procedures and requirements.

Exercise is a frequently misunderstood and misused activity. Clinically, the patient needs a precise prescription for the goal, the dose, the frequency, and the duration of physical activities. In this manner, exercise prescription can help the patient achieve rest, flexibility, strength, and endurance, depending on the desired goal. Further tissue damage may also be prevented.

Exercise prescriptions should always consider the muscles' present status and their ability to respond to the desired goal. In general, a person with decompensated posture requires a period of rest before exercise and compensation are effective. The bioenergic cycle (Fig. 72.8) espoused by Jungmann[16] describes the requirement of resting the body until it is physiologically capable of resuming its postural fight against gravity. Energy expenditure throughout each day is cyclic, with sequencing important for the efficacy of the process. Postural strain increases the load in the early stages of the cycle and delays or even subverts later stages. On lying down at night, patients whose homeostatic reserves have been exceeded often experience a 30-minute (or more) delay before relaxation is possible in the erector spinae and quadratus lumborum muscles.

The appropriate exercise prescription for a patient with postural decompensation may be to decrease activities of daily living. The exercise prescription should promote healing of strained and injured tissues before striving to accomplish any other postural goal. Monitor reduction in iliolumbar ligament tenderness and edema to indicate when active postural exercises may be introduced to achieve strength, stability, and proprioceptive reeducation.

Select OMT to improve structure–function relationships with a minimum of side effects for patients with posturally induced pathophysiologic change. Indirect method OMT is particularly useful for treating somatic dysfunction in hypermobile areas. Recognize that hypermobile areas may represent either primary traumatized tissue or secondary compensation for areas of restricted motion. Use direct methods, physical modalities, and stretching exercises in regions of hypomobility. The percussion hammer technique, as taught by Robert Fulford, DO, is particularly helpful in treatment of some chronic postural problems.

Static braces are often helpful adjunctive therapy, promoting rest and healing in an acute strain. Chronic postural strain, however, is a situation in which functional orthotics or elimination of biomechanical risk factors are required to support homeostasis. The chronicity of the situation precludes replacing function and mandates that functions be modified. Use of static bracing in chronic situations requires careful and continuous exercise as well as care to prevent muscle atrophy and dependence on the static brace.

A functional orthosis such as the Levitor is a more appropriate choice than a static brace for patients with chronic postural decompensation. This orthosis has been used in the United States since 1939 and is a prescription custom-fitted device. It weighs 6 ounces and is made of a high-test aluminum alloy that transfers pressure to air-filled cushioned pads, one over the superior portion of the pubic symphysis and the other below the S2 middle transverse axis on the posterior part of the sacral apex. This orthosis was specifically designed to resist the counterrotation of the sacrum and innominates (Fig. 72.9) occurring under the influence of gravity strain. It aids but does not replace the function of postural muscles, thus avoiding the dependency side effects of static bracing. A functional orthosis is added to a patient care treatment regimen to enhance homeostatic postural mechanisms. This enables the osteopathic approach to function even more effectively.

A functional orthosis is indicated in those chronic or recurrent conditions resulting from, or aggravated by, postural strain or decompensation. Its use can realistically be expected to im-

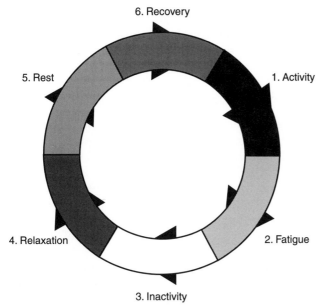

Figure 72.8. Bioenergic model. (Modified from Jungmann M. *The Jungmann Concept and Technique of Antigravity Leverage.* Rangely, Me: Institute for Gravitational Strain Pathology, Inc; 1982.)

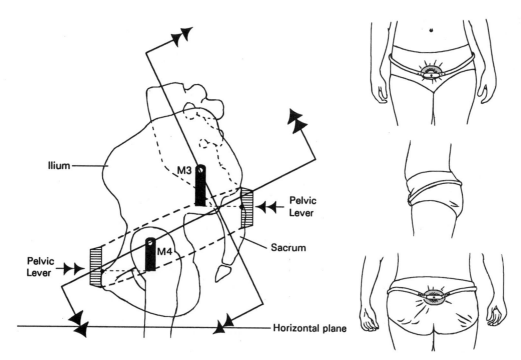

Figure 72.9. Pelvic lever action and Levitor. (Reprinted with permission from Jungmann M. *The Jungmann Concept and Technique of Antigravity Leverage.* Rangely, Me: Institute for Gravitational Strain Pathology, Inc; 1982.)

prove the body's ability to resist strain and decompensation by altering biomechanical alignment or assisting soft tissue structures. Concomitant symptoms such as back pain, headache, fatigue, muscle imbalance, and functional visceral complaints may be relieved in a program that incorporates a functional postural orthosis, OMT, and patient education. These symptoms alone in the absence of the underlying postural cause are not a sufficient indication. Functional orthotics may be especially indicated for patients who have had failed back surgery for chronic back pain, chronic disk disease, spondylolisthesis, or who have had failed medical treatment for low back arthritic conditions. All of these structural conditions make it more difficult for the patient to functionally resist gravity.

A functional orthosis should not to be used alone. It requires systemic OMT and carefully prescribed exercise to be maximally effective. Conversely, OMT and exercise may greatly benefit from the addition of an orthotic device. Adjunctive use of the Levitor, for example, has been demonstrated to improve measurable sagittal plane risk factors and to reduce posturally related low back pain.[17–18] In a 1985 study[18] of 109 patients with recalcitrant chronic low back pain, 33% of patients were found to improve with manipulation and postural exercise alone. When a functional orthosis (Levitor) was added to this program, 76% improved. The likelihood of improved results is achieved by decreasing functional demand on postural structures, modifying biomechanical risk factors, and allowing postural homeostatic mechanisms to operate under more optimal conditions.

In summary, numerous modalities are used to assist the body's postural response to gravity. An individually designed program includes a carefully selected combination of patient education, OMT, exercise, and functional orthotics. All of these are aimed at modifying the structure–function relationship and enhancing the body's ability to self-heal. Postural balancing therefore requires an understanding of the biomechanical nature and functional anatomy of each patient and a full understanding of osteopathic philosophy.

SPONDYLOLISTHESIS

The biomechanical principles of diagnosis and treatment of patients with sagittal plane postural problems can be directly applied to the management of patients with spondylolisthesis. The generic term "spondylolisthesis" is derived from Greek roots roughly meaning "vertebra sliding down a slippery path." It is a generic term for a group of spinal disorders having this phenomenon in common. It identifies a group of spinal disorders in which there is a forward displacement of one vertebra over another, usually the fifth lumbar over the body of the first sacral segment.

Classification

With the advent of radiology and more definition, the study of spondylolisthesis began, including its true incidence, location, classification, and significance. The classification

of spondylolisthesis subsequently evolved into the currently accepted causal categories delineated by Wiltse, Newman, and MacNab[19] as shown in Table 72.2.

Causes

Regardless of specific hereditary and developmental factors, spondylolisthesis refers to a group of disorders having a particular mechanical consequence in common. The mechanical perspective permits better understanding of the general symptoms complex. Applying mechanical treatment protocols provide the rational basis of osteopathic conservative management of patients diagnosed as having spondylolisthesis.

HEREDITARY PREDISPOSITION

Two observations argue against a direct inheritance of spondylolisthesis. First, although there is an increased incidence of spondylolisthesis within family groups,[20–22] a significant number of these family members exhibit different types of spondylolisthesis. Second, infants are rarely reported to have spondylolysis, called prespondylolisthesis. The incidence increases after children assume an active upright position up until age 20, when it matches the 5% incidence of the general population.[23]

The genetic link appears more likely to involve those factors that predispose the region to instability. Posterior defects such as spina bifida occulta and open sacrum are inherited almost invariably in dysplastic spondylolisthesis and in a third of patients with the isthmic type.[24] This lack of posterior support may concentrate postural weightbearing forces in the area, resulting in forward subluxation of the entire L5 unit in dysplastic spondylolisthesis. It could predispose a patient to stress fracture of the pars interarticularis and then sliding of the anterior elements of L5 on S1 in isthmic spondylolisthesis.[24] Conversely, degenerative spondylolisthesis, (formally called pseudospondylolisthesis) occurs two to three times more frequently in African-Americans, who are also known to have greater L5-S1 stability.[25] In general, patients with degenerative spondylolisthesis have a low pelvic index for age[26] and a higher incidence of sacralization of L5 and block-shaped L5 vertebra. They also have a much lower incidence of posterior defects[25] than seen in the general population. The increased stability established at L5 lends itself to instability higher in the lumbar spine.

DEVELOPMENTAL FACTORS

Certain developmental factors, statistically and/or logically, have been implicated in spondylolisthesis. Foremost among these factors are posture and microtrauma.[14,27–31]

Posture is strongly implicated in the development of spondylolisthesis and spondylolysis (prespondylolisthesis). Spondylolysis does not develop prior to the assumption of the standing posture. In one study of 125 institutionalized patients who had never assumed a standing position, none demonstrated a pars defect.[27] No other primate has fully adopted human up-

Table 72.2
Classification of Spondylolisthesis

Diagnosis	Type	%	Criteria	Comments
Type I Dysplastic spondylolisthesis 	Dysplastic	21	Congenital deficiencyof neural arch of L5 or upper sacrum. Insufficiency of superior sacral facets.	2 girls: 1 boy is the ratio; almost exclusively L5; lumbosacral facets also approach horizontal
Type II A Isthmic spondylolisthesis Type IIB 	Isthmic Subtype A Subtype B Subtype C	51	Pars interarticularis defect A. Lytic-fatigue fracture of pars B. Elongated but intact pars C. Acutely fractured pars	Almost exclusively L5 A. Most common type below age 50 years B. Probably due to repeated micro-fractures healing elongated fashion as slippage occurs C. History of severe trauma may heal with immobilization
Type III Degenerative spondylolisthesis 	Degenerative	25	Degenerative changes at apophyseal joints due to long-standing intersegmental instability	4 female: 1 male; 3 black: 1 white; 6–9 times more common at L4; sacralization 4× general population; not seen before age 40; rare between 40–50; slippage 30% maximum
Type IV Traumatic spondylolisthesis 	Traumatic	1	Due to fractures in other areas of the bony hook than the pars	Heals with immobilization
Type V	Pathologic	2	Generalized or localized bone disease	Neoplasm, osteogenesis imperfecta, Paget's disease, arthrogryposis, iatrogenic postlumbar fusion; Kuskokwim disease

Reprinted with permission from Kuchera WQ, Kuchera ML. *Osteopathic Principles in Practice.* Columbus, Ohio: Greyden Press; 1994.

right posture, nor does any other primate develop a lytic type of spondylolisthesis.

Postural decompensation as measured by Jungmann's pelvic index is substantially higher in patients with L5-S1 spondylolisthesis[14] than in the general population. Increasing pelvic index and increasing lumbosacral instability may, in part, address Wiltse's observation that so many patients develop lesions in the pars at approximately age 6 and then have no problems with it until their mid-30s.

Hyperlordosis in particular has been the postural fault most implicated.[29,30–32] Increased lordosis transfers weightbearing from the vertebral bodies onto the articular facets in joint capsules.[33] These structures are ill-designed to carry the body's weight continuously. An anterior weightbearing line is also known to create similar mechanics and should be evaluated. Certain activities such as gymnastics further increase backward bending demands in the lumbar spine. Subsequently, many young gymnasts permanently adopt an exaggerated lordotic posture. Not surprisingly, female gymnasts demonstrate spondylolysis with an incidence four times that of the general female population.[34]

Other groups are specifically subject to increased stress in the lumbopelvic area. Among these, weight lifters, soldiers carrying backpacks, and college football linemen have all been shown to have an increased incidence of spondylolysis. Repetitive lumbosacral motion is a common characteristic in all except traumatic spondylolisthesis. Frequent stress in posturally or congenitally unstable areas (especially during the adolescent growth spurt) is thus implicated in the development of fatigue fracture, the proposed basic lesion in isthmic spondylolisthesis.[19]

Diagnosis

Of the estimated 5% of the population with spondylolisthesis, approximately half are asymptomatic.[35] Those who become symptomatic do so commonly after the age of 20. Preventive care depends on early and accurate diagnosis. Diagnostic testing should include the following:

Radiography
Pelvic index measurement
History
Physical examination
Spinal palpation
Neurologic testing

RADIOGRAPHIC

Radiology has greatly enhanced our ability to diagnose spondylolisthesis even in totally asymptomatic patients; it provides a prognostic modality.[14,36] There are significant differences between weightbearing and non-weightbearing films.[36–37] From a pragmatic point of view, the postural standing film offers structural information in functional context and is preferred. Radiographically, gross spondylolisthesis can be seen and quantified in the lateral view (Fig. 72.10). However, 45° oblique films may be necessary to see a subtle or unilateral spondylolysis. In this view, the pars interarticularis in isthmic type II-B

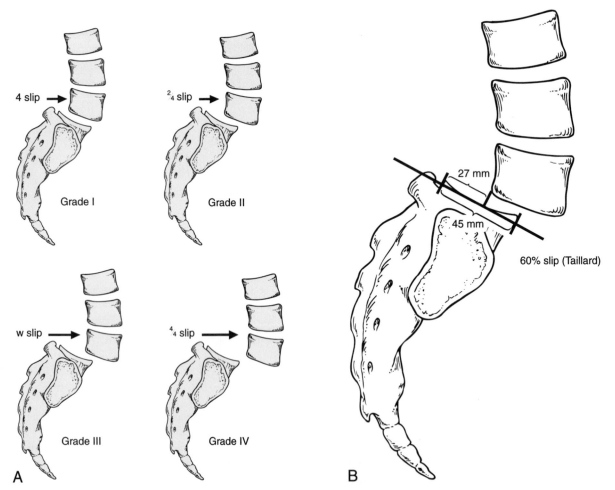

Figure 72.10. **A**, Classification of spondylolisthesis using Meyerding system. **B**, Taillard method of classifying spondylolisthesis.

spondylolisthesis has been described as the "greyhound of Hensinger."[38]

Meyerding[39] provided the simplest system of grading by assigning I, II, III, or IV, respectively, for each quarter of the upper vertebra displaced off the vertebra below. The more precise displacement measurement of Taillard[40] can detect minor progression but it is rarely needed clinically. The Meyerding system is more commonly used, more quickly applied, and is clinically relevant.

The fastest progression of isthmic spondylolisthesis is seen between ages 9 and 15. Less often, there is progression in the Meyerding grading over the age of 20,[27] especially in the presence of a sclerotic buttress on the anterior lip of the sacrum.[41] Other signs of instability or its effects in the area can be seen with radiographic analysis, including:

Angle of slip
Osteophytes
Calcified ligaments (especially iliolumbar)
Increased pelvic index[12,14,42–43]
Anterior weightbearing mechanics
Increased lordosis or lumbosacral angle
Disk narrowing[32]

Whenever possible, radiographic typing of the spondylolisthesis should be performed because it may affect treatment or prognosis.

CLINICAL

The age of the symptomatic patient determines the clinical presentation. While spondylolisthesis is perhaps the most common cause of persistent low back pain and sciatica in children and adolescents,[44] most in this age group do not have pain. These individuals are often identified when a school official or parent notes a change in gait or posture.[44] If any pain is expressed, it is described as a dull ache in the buttock or posterior thigh. Rarely are there symptoms expressed below the knee.[38] Tight hamstrings,[36,45] probably resulting from postural stress and an attempt to stabilize the unstable lumbosacral junction (and not from root impingement), are found in 80% of young people with symptomatic spondylolysis or spondylolisthesis and to a lesser extent in nonsymptomatic patients. Inability to bend over to touch one's toes reveals this deficit. It can also be used to uncover the nonfixed scoliosis[27,46] that exists in approximately 30% of these patients secondary to lumbar irritation and paraspinal spasm. Furthermore, as a result of having tight hamstrings, those with greater than Meyerding grade II spondylolisthesis have a pathognomonic stiff-legged, short-stride, waddling gait[45,47] in which the pelvis rotates with each step. Distortion of the pelvis and trunk appears in patients having a Meyerding grade II-III[45,47] with flared ilia in the back and an abdomen that is thrust forward. These young people have a short waist, a transverse abdominal crease at the level of the umbilicus, and flattened heart-shaped buttocks. Only 2% of young people demonstrate any objective neurologic

change[33] requiring extensive electromyographic or myelographic workup.

One of the most consistent physical findings in patients younger than 30 years of age with dysplastic or isthmic spondylolisthesis is tight hamstrings restricting forward flexion of the trunk. In contrast, the most constant physical finding in patients older than 50 years of age with degenerative spondylolisthesis is the ease with which they are able to touch their toes without bending their knees or obliterating their lumbar lordosis.

The flexibility of the patient with degenerative spondylolisthesis is thought to result from laxity of the pelvitrochanteric and hamstring muscles. This patient is also likely to have neurologic symptoms arising from the unstable spondylolisthetic joint manifesting in L5 root symptoms. He or she is more likely to complain of somatovisceral complaints of a hypersympathetic nature, such as constipation and irregular menses.[1] Symptoms of pelvic congestion and vague complaints in the lower extremity are also common in adults with spondylolisthesis. These result from poor thoracic abdominal diaphragmatic function initiated by the hyperlordosis and visceroptosis[1,24,48–49] that accompanies spondylolisthesis.

Adult patients are more likely to complain of pain. Their pain is usually aggravated by moderate activity or prolonged standing and relieved by rest or limited activity. Because of chronic overt instability of the lumbosacral region, these patients have poorly responsive soft tissues,[50] somatic dysfunction, and multiple myofascial points that, when stressed, react out of proportion to the initiating event and produce palpable spasm and low back pain. Pain can thus be caused by several structures in the area other than the spondylolisthetic segment. These structures are also subject to the instability of the region and the mechanical disadvantage placed there. It is, therefore, difficult to sort out when the pain is caused by the spondylolisthesis, when it is the result of somatic dysfunction of muscular, ligamentous, or joint structures, or when it is of diskogenic origin.

Wiltse[27p276–288] proposes that for patients older than 20 years of age with spondylolisthesis of less than 33%, pain is probably caused by one of three mechanisms:

Disk degeneration at the level of the defect
Root impingement by fibrocartilaginous buildup
Referral from stressed posterior ligaments and soft tissues

In our clinical experience, pain in these patients is most commonly referred from trigger points in the quadratus lumborum, glutei, and piriformis muscles, and from iliolumbar and posterior sacroiliac ligaments. This best supports Wiltse's third mechanism.

With more than a 50% slip in patients with isthmic spondylolisthesis, the cauda equina[27p276–288] is physically involved. In this case, low back pain is attributable directly to the spondylolisthesis itself. Because the dysplastic type carries the posterior arch forward, no more than 25% slippage is necessary to manifest a cauda equina syndrome.[22] Degenerative spondylolisthesis, by nature of its mechanism, does not progress beyond a 30% slip.[22,27,32] The instability of this joint (usually L4-L5), coupled with physical continuity with the posterior arch, usually results in L5 root impingement. Myelograms performed on these patients generally show hourglass constriction[32] at that level. Differential diagnosis of back pain in a patient with spondylolisthesis therefore requires careful palpatory and neurologic physical diagnosis in addition to the radiographic and historical findings just outlined.

PALPATORY

Increased intersegmental motion in the lumbosacral region is usually a sign of instability and severe degeneration. This increased motion is grossly apparent even on x-ray films, but palpatory evidence[50] by those trained to palpate segmental motion is generally considered to have twice the diagnostic yield for instability (28.6%) than that of x-ray studies (15%).

Palpatory findings in patients with spondylolisthesis reveal an anteriorly located spinous process (Fig. 72.11) or "drop-off" sign. This is the spinous process of the vertebra that has slipped forward in dysplastic and degenerative spondylolisthesis. It is the adjacent vertebra above the slipped segment in isthmic spondylolisthesis. Sacral base motion is excessively lax when it is rocked anteriorly around the middle transverse axis; this may also cause subjective buttock or posterior thigh discomfort. If testing sacral base motion causes neurologic symptoms, particular care should be taken in designing a treatment protocol.

Paraspinal tissues vary in palpatory quality depending on the degree of symptoms present. Often they display multiple myofascial tender points. Even in the asymptomatic state, they are slow to relax and are somewhat boggy (congested) to palpation. Any muscle strength testing of the low back muscles would demonstrate nearly full flexibility but decreased strength and endurance.

The iliolumbar ligament should be palpated bilaterally in every patient with symptomatic spondylolisthesis. Attached to the transverse processes of L5, the anterior sacroiliac joint, and the iliac crest, the iliolumbar ligament is anatomically positioned to resist any forward slip of L5 on the sacrum. Palpatory tension and subjective tenderness over its attachments bilaterally are often noted. The patient may experience lateral thigh and/or groin referral. Palpation of this ligament is a valuable and sensitive indicator of the success of conservative management programs designed to reduce mechanical stress in symptomatic spondylolisthesis patients.

NEUROLOGIC

The physical examination of each patient should include a neurologic evaluation including deep tendon reflexes, muscle strength testing, and straight leg raising. Electromyographic testing (EMG) and/or myelography is indicated if radicular symptoms are present. It is especially important to assess

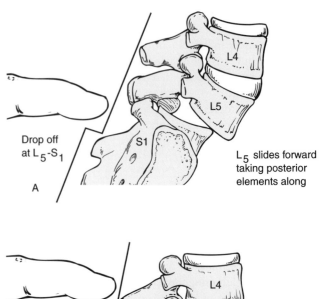
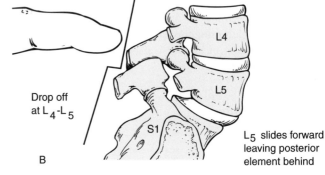
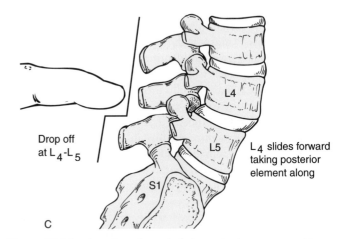

Figure 72.11. Location of anteriorly located spinous process (drop-off sign) depends on underlying mechanism of spondylolisthesis. **A,** In dysplastic spondylolisthesis, L5-S1 horizontal facets allow entire spine to glide forward creating drop-off between L5 and S1. **B,** In isthmic spondylolisthesis, pars defect between L5 and S1 allows anterior elements of L5 to slide forward along with rest of spine. Posterior elements of L5 remain behind with sacrum creating drop-off between L4 and L5. **C,** Degenerative spondylolisthesis at L4-L5 does not affect anterior and posterior elements of vertebral unit and therefore drop-off sign is located between L4 and L5.

the condition of the L4 disk[27] when surgical fusion is contemplated.

Treatment

Conservative management is 85–90% successful in degenerative spondylolisthesis.[27,32] It is successful in only 50% of the minority of children who are symptomatic.[27,38] Conservative management is probably not indicated without extensive bracing or surgical fusion for immature patients with Meyerding grade III-IV spondylolisthesis, with progressive subluxation, or for spondylolisthesis secondary to acute fractures. This third group responds best to immediate immobilization.[27] For those patients requiring surgery (or bracing), conservative management should be added afterward because the conditions that led to the instability preoperatively are still present postoperatively. In all cases, conservative management should attempt to maximize structure–function relationships.

PATIENT EDUCATION

Education is a key element in conservative management[35,51–52] of the patient with either asymptomatic or symptomatic spondylolisthesis. Goals center on decreasing stress in the unstable lumbosacral region through application of back mechanics, proper exercise and nutrition, and improvement of posture. Back schools offering 3–6 hours of instruction in teaching back mechanics and appropriate choices for optimum back care are effective.[51] These approaches increase patient compliance immensely. In the absence of a back school, the individual practitioner should use a minimum of one patient visit (more if necessary) to explain lumbosacral mechanics. Teach all patients to avoid improper lifting, especially over the head, as this increases lumbar lordosis. Advocate proper footwear because high heels also increase lumbar lordosis.[33] Advise patients on correct sleeping, sitting, and standing postures; also counsel them on weight loss, if necessary. This minimal investment of time reduces the frequency of reinjury or the failure of an otherwise well-conceived conservative program.

Pregnancy significantly affects posture by shifting the weightbearing line anteriorly and accentuating the lumbar lordotic curve. Unfortunately, this postural stress occurs at a time when the hormonal changes of pregnancy reduce soft tissue stabilization. Women with spondylolisthesis who contemplate pregnancy should prepare their posture and muscle tone in advance, if possible. They should also strictly adhere to their obstetrician's weight gain limits. Often the addition of a Levitor is extremely beneficial, even if it is only for the duration of the pregnancy.

For asymptomatic young people with less than a Meyerding grade I spondylolisthesis, avoid creating a "back cripple" with excessive restrictions. It is wise to direct these individuals toward a vocation not requiring heavy lifting or strenuous activity.[21] In asymptomatic young people with more than grade I spondylolisthesis, the same vocational goals are upheld but they should also avoid contact sports. Inform young patients and

their parents of the concerns and uncertainties involved; stress the need for close follow-up.

EXERCISE

The response to exercise does not depend on the type of spondylolisthesis (I, II, or III).[52] The goals of exercise should be eventually to stabilize the lumbosacral region and diminish the lumbar lordosis.[48,52] Weight loss for an overweight patient can also be facilitated by exercise. As with any exercise program, overly stressed or strained muscles cannot effectively be exercised until they have first recovered.[53] Thus, rest, medication, indirect OMT, and certain physical modalities may be necessary before beginning an individually designed exercise program.

Exercise should be of a flexion type only, rather than flexion-extension combination programs.[52] Excellent results with the flexion program were reported by Gramse. The variables examined included relief of pain, need for back supports, return to work status, and "recovery." Combination flexion-extension exercise significantly reduced the effectiveness in all of the variables. Pelvic narrow and coil exercise[54–56] with the knees bent in the supine position is extremely effective, although flattening the back against the wall while standing, or bringing the chest to the thigh while sitting in a chair, can also be beneficial.

The patient must be able to demonstrate his or her ability to maintain a reduced lordosis before abdominal strengthening exercises such as bent-knee sit-ups are considered. Good abdominal strength adjunctively supports weightbearing and "unloads" the spine. Gymnastics, diving, and the contact sports are not encouraged. Swimming, however, is considered an excellent activity to cultivate. Strongly advocate two basic rules of exercise[33]:

1. Avoid exercising to the point of fatigue
2. Discontinue any exercise causing pain until a reason for the pain is discovered by the physician

MANIPULATION

Several authors report a benefit[1,33,43,57] from the manipulative management of patients with spondylolisthesis. Manipulative treatment of the patient with spondylolisthesis is extremely helpful in attempting to redress some of the postural decompensation that has occurred over time and to alleviate segmental limitation of motion known to upset the forces resisting spondylolisthesis.[32]

The goals[1,43,57–58] are reduction of lumbar lordosis and somatic dysfunction. This transfers weightbearing from the posterior elements and tissues back to the vertebral bodies. It specifically relaxes strained irritable lumbar paraspinal tissues, permitting them to better resist stresses of the activities of daily living. It also reduces the patient's somatic pain and somatovisceral symptomatology. These goals seek gradual reestablishment of fascial and muscular balance to promote maximal functional weightbearing posture. The manipulative program is not just directed to the lordosis and specific somatic dysfunctions, but to all support structures as well. Because of the instability and injury in the lumbosacral junction, avoid high-velocity techniques in that area.

In correcting lordosis, often the first concern is balancing the pelvis horizontally.[33,59–60] An undiagnosed or uncorrected unilateral sacral shear somatic dysfunction thwarts the most expert manipulator in achieving this goal and renders functional orthoses such as the Levitor ineffective. Treat this and other nonphysiologic somatic dysfunctions promptly and effectively with OMT.

An unlevel sacral base needs gradual heel lift orthotics before instability and recurrent somatic dysfunction can be effectively addressed. A minimal heel lift, when indicated, can reduce the lumbosacral angle by 2–4 degrees and may move an anterior weightbearing line as much as an inch posterior.[61] Correction of a short leg is also extremely helpful in reducing long-term strain on the iliolumbar ligament. It eliminates somatosomatic referral of groin pain from this structure as well as reduces low back pain and instability in the lumbosacral junction.[58,62] A heel lift may also be helpful to the one-third of spondylolisthetic young people having concomitant scoliotic change and the long-term somatovisceral changes resulting from it.

Remove any intrapelvic somatic dysfunction; the sacroiliac articulations should be freely mobile. Gently stretch tight hamstring muscles with isometric muscle energy technique. Fascial unwinding of the lower extremities is well-received by patients and eliminates many of the vague congestive complaints in this area (JG Zink, personal communication, 1978).

Next address the thoracic spine and thoracolumbar junction. Schwab[57] reported improvement of compensatory lumbar lordotic stresses with mobilization of increased thoracic kyphosis. Fryette[33] emphasized that somatic dysfunction in this area must be corrected before any effective changes could be maintained in the lower lumbosacral junction. Additional consideration of the diaphragm and quadratus lumborum has proven particularly successful in helping to promote lymphatic drainage.[24] The quadratus lumborum and the iliolumbar ligament are functionally and structurally related and both should be treated.[62]

Lastly, approach the lower lumbar region in a general manner with soft tissue, counterstrain, myofascial release, and fascial unwinding techniques. Address any specific somatic dysfunction with indirect technique. A clinically useful endpoint is achieved when the intrinsic rhythm of the craniosacral mechanism is easily palpated between hands monitoring both the thoracolumbar junction and sacrum.

ORTHOTICS, BRACES, AND CASTS

Orthotics play a significant role in the conservative management of patients with spondylolisthesis. The benefits of a heel lift orthotic in helping to lend stability to the lumbosacral region have already been discussed, and the heel lift orthotic is potentially a permanent part of the patient's treatment program. A corsetlike lumbosacral support, conversely, should

only be considered for short-term stability.[35,50] Grieve[50] goes as far as to say, *"a support should, however, never be supplied without a plan to eliminate it."* Most lumbosacral supports worn for prolonged periods weaken the patient's own supportive mechanisms,[35] thereby increasing long-range instability and promoting dependence on the support. For short-term management of lumbar strain, however, these supports can be invaluable in reducing pain and preparing the tissues for a subsequent exercise program.

For spondylolisthesis resulting from an acute fracture, the types of immobilization, ranging from knee to nipple casting to ordinary body casts to corsets, have been studied.[38] The latter two types of immobilization suppress the extremes of bending but do a poor job of diminishing lumbosacral motion with walking.[41]

The Levitor has proven extremely effective as an adjunct in the long-term management of symptomatic isthmic spondylolisthesis.[1,43] Exerting pressure between the pubic symphysis and the base of the sacrum, the Levitor effectively[18] aids in decreasing postural decompensation as measured by pelvic index, in reducing lumbosacral angle, and in transferring weightbearing off the posterior tissues and forward to the vertebral bodies. By reducing the chronic strain on these tissues, symptomatic relief from low back pain is accomplished in days to weeks, and implementation of an exercise program can begin shortly thereafter.

MEDICATION

Antiinflammatories, analgesics, muscle relaxants, and bowel softeners all have a limited role in the symptomatic relief of various common symptoms experienced by patients with spondylolisthesis. Because spondylolisthesis is a chronic problem, narcotics have no place in symptom management of these patients. Vapocoolant spray-and-stretch technique[63] and trigger point injection with local anesthetics[63] may be helpful in relieving the secondary myofascial points that occur. Injections of proliferative agents are also useful for cases of ligamentous laxity uncorrected by conservative means.[64]

CONCLUSION

Rational, conservative management of a patient with spondylolisthesis presupposes early and accurate diagnosis and a thorough understanding of the mechanics involved. While the cause is important for prognosis, treatment addressing the underlying instability, spinal mechanics, and patient homeostasis provides optimum benefit. Postural decompensation in the sagittal plane is particularly prominent in patients with isthmic spondylolisthesis and must be treated to maximize both patient homeostasis and body mechanics.

REFERENCES

1. Kuchera ML. Diagnosis and treatment of gravitational strain pathophysiology: Research and clinical correlates (parts I & II). In: Vleeming A, ed. *Low Back Pain: The Integrated Function of the Lumbar*

Spine and Sacroiliac Joints. Proceedings of the 2nd Interdisciplinary World Congress, University of California (San Diego), Nov 9–11, 1995, pp. 659–693.

2. Cathie AG. The applied anatomy of some postural changes. In: Peterson B, ed. *Postural Balance and Imbalance (1983 AAO Yearbook).* Newark, Ohio: American Academy of Osteopathy; 1983:44–46.

3. Kuchera ML, Bemben MG, Kuchera WA, Piper F. Athletic functional demand and posture. *JAOA.* September 1990;90(9):843–844.

4. Cruickshank JL, Koike M, Dickson RA. Curve patterns in idiopathic scoliosis: a clinical and radiographic study. *J Bone Joint Surg.* March 1989;71B(2):259–263.

5. Kuchera ML. Gravitational stress, musculoligamentous strain and postural alignment. In Dorman T, ed. *Spine: State of the Art Reviews.* May 1995;9(2):463–490.

6. Beal MC. The sacroiliac problem: review of anatomy, mechanics, and diagnosis. *JAOA.* June 1982;81(10):667–679

7. Educational Council on Osteopathic Principles: Glossary of osteopathic terminology. In: *AOA Directory and Yearbook.* Chicago, Ill: American Osteopathic Association; 1994.

8. Janda V. Muscle weakness and inhibition (pseudoparesis) in back pain syndromes. In: Grieve GP, ed. *Modern Manual Therapy of the Vertebral Column.* Edinburgh: Churchill Livingstone; 1986:197–210.

9. Kuchera ML. Gravitational strain pathophysiology and "Unterkreuz" syndrome. *Manuelle Medizin.* April 1995;33(2):56.

10. Willman MK. Radiographic technical aspects of the postural study. *JAOA.* July 1977;76:739–744.

11. Kuchera ML. Conservative management of symptomatic spondylolisthesis. On file with the American Academy of Osteopathy in partial fulfillment of FAAO, 1987.

12. Kuchera ML. Aging, postural decompensation and low back pain. *JAOA.* October 1986;86(10):74.

13. Kuchera ML, Barton J. Sagittal plane postural measurements. *JAOA.* October 1990;90(10):932.

14. Kuchera ML. Postural decompensation in isthmic spondylolisthesis. *JAOA.* November 1987;87(1l):781.

15. Fernand R, Fox DE. Evaluation of lumbar lordosis: a prospective and retrospective study. *Spine.* November 1985;10(9):799–803.

16. Gallant R, ed. *The Jungmann Concept and Technique of Anti-Gravity Leverage: A Clinical Handbook.* rev. 2nd ed. Rangeley, Me: Institute for Gravitational Strain Pathology, Inc; 1992:4–6.

17. Kuchera ML. Alteration of intrapelvic spatial relationships utilizing an external pelvic orthosis in patients with low back pain. *Proceedings of the International Society for Prosthetics and Orthotics.* June 1992:291. (Also see *JAOA.* September 1992;92(9):1182.)

18. Kuchera ML, Jungmann M. Inclusion of Levitor Orthotic Device in the management of refractive low back pain patients. *JAOA.* October 1986;86(10):673.

19. Wiltse LL, Newman PH, MacNab I. Classification of spondylolysis [sic] and spondylolisthesis. *Clin Orthop.* 1976;117:23–29.

20. Friberg S. Studies on spondylolisthesis. *Acta Chir Scand.* 1939; 82(suppl 55):1440.

21. Wiltse LL. The etiology of spondylolisthesis. *J Bone Joint Surg.* 1962; 44A:536–569.

22. Wiltse LL, Widell EH, Jackson DW. Fatigue fracture: the basic lesion in isthmic spondylolisthesis. *J Bone Joint Surg.* 1975;57A:17–22.

23. Wiltse LL. Spondylolisthesis in children. *Clin Orthop.* 1961;21:156–163.

24. Zink JG, Lawson WB. An osteopathic structural examination and functional interpretation. *Osteopath Ann.* 1987;7(12):12–19.

25. Rosenberg NJ. Degenerative spondylolisthesis—predisposing factors. *J Bone Joint Surg Am Vol.* June 1975;57(4):467–474.

26. Kuchera ML, Miller K. Postural measurements in L4 degenerative spondylolisthesis. *JAOA.* August 1995;95(8):496.

27. Finneson BE. *Low Back Pain.* Philadelphia, Penn: J.B. Lippincott Co; 1973:276–288.

28. Krauss H. Effect of lordosis on the stress in the lumbar spine. *Clin Orthop.* 1976;117:56–58.

29. Newman PH. The etiology of spondylolisthesis. *J Bone Joint Surg.* 1963;45B:39–59.

30. Troup DG. Mechanical factors in spondylolisthesis and spondylolysis. *Clin Orthop.* 1976;117:59–67.

31. Wynne-Davies R, Scott JHS. Inheritance and spondylolisthesis: a radiographic family survey. *J Bone Joint Surg.* 1979;61B:301–305.

32. Farfan HF, Osteria V, Lamy C. The mechanical etiology of spondylolysis and spondylolisthesis. *Clin Orthop.* 1976;177:40–55.

33. Luibel GJ. Lordosis. *JAOA.* 1954;54(3):126–130.

34. Jackson DW, Wiltse LL, Cirincione RJ. Spondylolysis in the female gymnast. *Clin Orthop.* 1976;117:68–73.

35. Magora A. Conservative treatment in spondylolisthesis. *Clin Orthop.* 1976;117:74 –79.

36. Boxall D, Bradford DS, Winter RB, Moe JH. Management of severe spondylolisthesis in children and adolescents. *J Bone Joint Surg.* 1979;61A:479–495.

37. Lowe RW, Hayes TD, Kaye J, Bogg RJ, Luekens CA. Standing roentgenograms in spondylolisthesis. *Clin Orthop.* 1976;117:80–91.

38. Hensinger RN, Lang JR, MacEwen GD. Surgical management of spondylolisthesis in children and adolescents. *Spine.* 1976;1:207–216.

39. Meyerding HW. Spondylolisthesis. *Surg Gynecol Obstet.* 1932; 54:371–377.

40. Taillard WF. Le spondylolisthesis chez l'enfant et l'adolescent. *Acta Orthop Scand.* 1955;24:115–144.

41. Eisenstein S. Spondylolysis: a skeletal investigation of two population groups. *J Bone Joint Surg Br Vol.* 1978;60:488–494.

42. Hoyt H, Bard D, Shaffer F. Experience with an antigravity leverage device for chronic low back pain: a clinical study. *JAOA.* March 1981;80(7):474–479.

43. Jungmann M. *The Jungmann Concept and Technique of Antigravity Leverage.* Rangeley, Me: Institute for Gravitational Strain Pathology, Inc; 1982.

44. Laurent LE, Oskman K. Operative treatment of spondylolisthesis in young patients. *Clin Orthop.* 1976;117:85–91.

45. Phalen GS, Dickenson JA. Spondylolisthesis and tight hamstrings. *J Bone Joint Surg.* 1961;43A:505–512.

46. Fisk JR, Noe JH, Winter RB. Scoliosis, spondylolysis, and spondylolisthesis. *Spine.* 1978;3(3):234–245.

47. Newman PH. A clinical syndrome associated with severe lumbosacral subluxation. *J Bone Joint Surg.* 1965;47B(3):472–481.

48. Freeman JT. Posture in the aging and aged body. *JAMA.* 1957; 165(7):843–846.

49. Kimberly P. Visceroptosis: an osteopathic explanation of cause and symptoms. *JAOA.* 1944;43(6):270–273.

50. Grieve G. Lumbar instability. *Physiotherapy.* 1982;68(1):2–9.

51. Fisk JR, DiMonte P, Courington SM. Back schools—past, present and future. *Clin Orthop.* 1983;179:18–21.

52. Gramse RR, Sinaki M, Ilstrup DM. Lumbar spondylolisthesis—a rational approach to conservative treatment. *Mayo Clin Prac.* 1980; 55:681–686.

53. Semon RL, Spengler D. Significance of lumbar spondylolysis in college football players. *Spine.* 1981;6(2):172–174.

54. Cochran A. From handout distributed at Kirksville College of Osteopathic Medicine (1983) entitled "Useful exercises for pelvis and spine," derived from "Physio-synthesis" by Amy Cochran, DO.

55. Lay EM. Personal communication; Lectures delivered annually while teaching at Kirksville College of Osteopathic Medicine, 1976–1982.

56. Pheasant HC. Practical posture building. *Clin Orthop.* 1962;25:83–91.

57. Schwab WA. Principles of manipulative treatment—low back problem. In: Barnes MK, ed. *1965 AAO Yearbook.* Carmel, Calif: Applied Academy of Osteopathy; 1965:90–94.

58. Cathie AG. Structural mechanics of the lumbar spine and pelvis. In: Barnes MW, ed. *1965 AAO Yearbook.* Carmel, Calif: Applied Academy of Osteopathy; 1965:14–20.

59. Friberg O. Clinical symptoms and biomechanics of lumbar spine and hip joint in leg length inequality. *Spine.* 1983;8(6):643–651.

60. Kuchera ML, Irvin RE. Biomechanical considerations in postural realignment. *JAOA.* November 1987;87(11):781–782.

61. Magoun HI Sr. Mechanics of chronic spinal lesion. *JAOA.* 1943; 42:489–500.

62. Luk KDK. The iliolumbar ligament. *J Bone Joint Surg.* 1986; 68B:197–200.

63. Travell JG, Simons DG. *Myofascial Pain and Dysfunction: The Trigger Point Manual.* Vol I. Baltimore, Md: Williams & Wilkins; 1983.

64. Dorman T, Ravin T. *Diagnosis and Injection Techniques in Orthopedic Medicine.* Baltimore, Md: Williams & Wilkins; 1991:34–35.

73. Efficacy and Complications

EILEEN L. DiGIOVANNA, MICHAEL L. KUCHERA, AND PHILIP E. GREENMAN

Key Concepts

- Current state of research on efficacy of osteopathic manipulation, and problems in current studies

- Difficulties of research trials studying effectiveness of osteopathic manipulation on low back pain, and success rates

- Effectiveness of manipulation on systemic disease

- Osteopathic practice guidelines, and reasons osteopathic physicians cannot follow existing written guidelines

- Difference between symptom exacerbation and true complication

- Incidence of complications, difference between physician-related and patient-related complications, and best ways to avoid complications

- Cervical spine manipulation as source of most manipulation complications

- Difficulty in listing absolute contraindications to osteopathic manipulation

- Complications most likely to result from high-velocity low-amplitude manipulation

- Discomfort or complications associated with muscle energy, counterstrain, and craniosacral treatments

Manipulation has enjoyed wide usage for many centuries of medical practice in most cultures. In most cases, it has been applied empirically, based on clinical observations. As with many forms of medical treatment, ongoing clinical successes have contributed to its continuous and expanding use.

Osteopathic manipulation uses palpatory diagnosis and manipulative treatment methods as integrated components of a patient encounter. It is an important element of an osteopathic approach to total patient care. Osteopathic manipulation is prescribed not only as care for a variety of musculoskeletal and systemic pathophysiologic problems but also as part of general health maintenance and enhancement strategies. It is directed toward optimizing structure–function relationships and assisting the patient's homeostatic mechanisms. Its processes help to strengthen physician–patient relationships, allowing better diagnostic insights and treatment for all aspects of human problems.

Osteopathic manipulative techniques are among the safest medical treatments a physician can provide. Whenever manipulative treatment is carried out, however, certain risks are present, along with potential side effects ranging from mild to severe, including death, when particularly aggressive maneuvers are used. Such risks also occur with pharmaceutical, surgical, and a variety of other mechanical treatments.

Even though osteopathic manipulation has a very low risk-to-benefit ratio, it is necessary that the operator be aware of inherent risks and avoid untoward occurrences while weighing anticipated benefits against the risk of treating or not treating.

EFFICACY OF MANIPULATION

Despite years of successful use of osteopathic and other forms of manipulation, the orthodox medical community continued to be critical of its use, often referring to its practitioners as cultists. The reasons are both cultural and scientific. The latter problem arises because of a lack of adequate scientific methods to explore not only clinical efficacy but also basic mechanisms. Researchers with a directed osteopathic focus, such as Louisa Burns, DO, Irvin M. Korr, PhD, J. Stedman Denslow, DO, and Wilbur V. Cole, DO, have been few. Clinically, when osteopathic models were originally proposed, double-blind research methods were yet to emerge. When they were developed, they were more readily applied to pharmacologic and surgical practices. More ambiguously defined clinical processes, such as osteopathic manipulation, remain difficult to evaluate. Progress is occurring, however.

In 1975, the first of several international seminars brought together a group of international basic scientists and clinicians to examine the scientific basis for the use of manipulation.[1] The National Institute of Communicative Diseases and Stroke held this conference in Bethesda, Maryland. Attendees were drawn from the osteopathic, allopathic, and chiropractic professions. The goal was to define the current state of research and identify areas for future study; several areas of agreement were reached.

In 1977, a second international conference was held at Michigan State University (MSU). The conference focused on neurobiologic mechanisms thought to underlie the effects of manipulative treatment.[2] Again, basic scientists and clinicians from the osteopathic, allopathic, and chiropractic professions discussed areas of mutual interest and concern, particularly in areas of neuroscience. Impulse and non–impulse-based neural control mechanisms were discussed in a context that uses manipulative treatments for a wide range of conditions.

In 1980, another international conference was held at MSU. This conference dealt with various models and mechanisms for the use of manipulation.[3] Conferees examined the effects of a variety of manipulative models considered to be beyond neurally mediated factors. These included:

Respiratory-circulatory models
Biomechanical models of postural and structural techniques
Inherent force concepts arising from the craniosacral treatment system

In 1983, a third international conference, again at MSU, examined an increasing number of outcome-based clinical trials, particularly in relation to low back pain.[4] Attendees also looked at issues necessary for development of future clinical trials. Many discussants were invited from the available clinical trials, along with a number of others with expertise in areas such as epidemiology. Their role was to discuss specific research methodologies, particularly in relation to the following:

The specific diagnosis; i.e., the entity treated by the manipulation
Inclusion and exclusion criteria
Type of manipulation performed
Outcome measures to identify efficacy, including statistical methods and data interpretation

From the outset, it was clear that a variety of manipulative methods are used; procedures are seldom identical. In many procedures, definition of the specific problem to be manipulated was limited and unclear. Most patients were treated for generic "low back pain" with or without radiation to the lower extremity. Despite the lack of specificity in these areas (such as lack of diagnostic and treatment specificity, small sample sizes, and differences in follow-up and outcome measures), the conference concluded that the trials demonstrated efficacy for the use of manipulative procedures when dealing with acute and acute recurrent mechanical low back pain. None of the trials dealt with chronic low back pain. By the end of the conference, generic issues surrounding the design and implementation of clinical trials were identified. They continue to be germane.

In 1989 and 1991, the American Academy of Osteopathy presented international symposia to discuss the scientific underpinnings of osteopathic principles and the role that osteopathic treatment of somatic dysfunction plays in applying the osteopathic philosophy to patient care. The Academy asked a leading group of international basic scientists and clinical researchers to explore relevant research and to draw clinical corollaries.

The 1989 conference entitled, "The Central Connection: Somatovisceral/Viscerosomatic Interaction"[5] focused on structure–function relationships. Discussants examined central and peripheral reflex mechanisms, including the perpetuation of altered reflex patterns in the somatic and visceral systems. They also discussed effects of manipulative treatment, exploring its relevance to the practice of osteopathic medicine.

The 1991 conference was entitled, "Nociception and the Neuroendocrine-Immune Connection."[6] It was inspired by the osteopathic concept of body unity. The roles of somatic dysfunction and other somatic stressors were examined in relation to both psychological and immune functioning.

Each of the above conferences published its proceedings. Other Academy symposia are planned.

Low Back Pain

Manipulation of all types is widely used to treat musculoskeletal pain and dysfunction. It is considered beneficial by millions of patients receiving care from a wide variety of practitioners, including:

Osteopathic physicians
Allopathic physicians
Chiropractors
Physical therapists
Lay persons

Textbooks from the professional groups discuss indications and contraindications for manipulation, without clear scientific evidence that the recommendations are appropriate and useful. Empirical recommendations dominate. Considering the empirical effectiveness of manipulation in a wide range of neuromusculoskeletal disorders, it is surprising that most current studies focus nearly exclusively on low back pain. Only a few studies have examined the benefits of cervical manipulation[7–8] or other musculoskeletal complaints.

Over 70 studies have been published dealing with low back pain with and without radiation to the lower extremities.[9,10] Some recent studies have dealt with chronic back pain[11] in addition to acute and acute recurrent populations. It is not always possible to identify the training of the individual(s) who performed the manipulations. In most cases in which training could be identified, the work was performed by chiropractors and physical therapists. Two studies describe manipulation performed by osteopathic practitioners trained in the British system.[12–13]

In 1984, Stiles reported a 24% reduction in the length of hospital stay for patients admitted for low back pain when an osteopathic manipulative medicine consultation and treatment program was added to the patient's traditional medical care.[14]

In 1995, a subacute low back pain project was completed by the Rush-Anchor HMO network. It was a double-blind, matched random sample patient study begun in 1992, comparing osteopathic care (which included manipulation) with so-called standard care. Sponsored by the Bureau of Research of the American Osteopathic Association (AOA), the study was directed by Gunnar B. Andersson, MD, PhD, an internationally renowned orthopedic surgeon and researcher. Approximately 300 patients who met inclusion criteria were randomly assigned to either a standard care group, staffed by MDs, or an osteopathic care group, staffed by DO manipulation specialists from the Midwestern University Chicago College of Osteopathic Medicine. The study proposed to assess any differences in osteopathic care, including manipulative treatment and standard care. As of this writing, the data have been gathered and analyzed in a preliminary way, but the first paper has yet to appear.

Despite the many variations in trial design, implementation, and evaluation, all published studies suggest that manipulation is useful for syndromes of acute low back pain.[3] This is demonstrated by reports of:

Pain reduction
Earlier return to work
Generally shortened disability and impairment

Analysis of clinical trial reports reveals that manipulative methods most used were:

Soft tissue kneading
Mobilization without impulse (articulatory procedures)
Mobilization with impulse (high-velocity low-amplitude thrust procedures)

High-velocity low-amplitude thrusting maneuvers were most common, with rotary thrusting to the lumbar area with the patient in a lateral recumbent position. A few studies identify muscle energy procedures.[15] None describe use of the following procedures:

Indirect
Functional
Counterstrain
Myofascial/fascial release
Craniosacral

With the exception of the AOA/Rush-Anchor HMO protocol, other research protocols have not accurately integrated the total patient approach characteristic of osteopathically oriented manipulative interventions.

Systemic Disease

Controlled trials for manipulation in conditions other than low back and cervical pain are few. Most studies represent pilot observations by experienced osteopathic clinicians. Stiles[14] reported reduction in hospital length of stay when osteopathic manipulative care was used for patients with the following:

Asthma: 14%
Pneumonia: 10%
Cholecystectomy: 7%
Hysterectomy: 12%

Stiles also reported a reduction in shock, dysrhythmias, and mortality when osteopathically-oriented manipulative care was integrated into the care of a group of patients with myocardial infarction (Fig. 73.1).

There are a greater number of studies in the osteopathic literature documenting the incidence of somatic dysfunction findings in certain systemic diseases. Kelso[16] reported on a

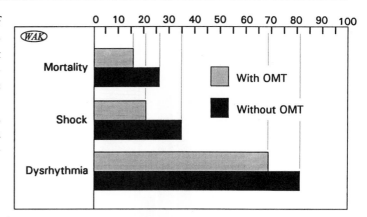

Figure 73.1. Response of 50 patients with myocardial infarction. (Adapted from work by Ed Stiles, DO)

double-blind clinical study of osteopathic findings in hospital patients. Student examiners were compared with experienced osteopathic clinicians. In 5174 separate examinations, somatic findings were significantly more frequent in acute visceral disease than in controls.

Nicholas[17] reported a pilot study that examined 286 hospitalized patients with 73 different diseases. Again, a variety of identifiable somatic patterns were identified with different disease entities. The study focused on somatically identified cervical and thoracic spine pattern differences associated with respiratory, gastrointestinal, and genitourinary diseases.

Other osteopathically based observational studies assessed somatic correlations with gastrointestinal diseases. Their findings closely mirror pain pattern findings recorded by Mayo Clinic surgeons.[18]

Several well-controlled studies have identified common somatic dysfunction patterns in patients with coronary artery disease and myocardial infarction.[19–21] Somatic findings are primarily located in the left upper thoracic area (Fig. 73.2). There was also evidence of upper cervical (C2) dysfunction in patients with acute visceral diseases. It is hypothesized that these findings correlate with the anatomy of the proximal vagus nerve in relation to the second cervical vertebra.

Beal and Kleiber evaluated 70 patients prior to angiography. Specificity for both positive and negative cervicothoracic palpatory findings in patients with and without coronary artery diseases was 79%.[20]

Many other authors have reported on the efficacy of manipulation in managing coronary heart disease, but no controlled studies have been performed.[22–26] Nevertheless, these authors have identified similar clinical findings and results associated with the addition of manipulative treatment to an overall management plan.

Similar studies have been done for spinal levels of somatic findings associated with pulmonary diseases.[27–28] Authors report a strong dominance of problems located in the upper thoracic and C2 region of the spine. Many of these authors report beneficial outcomes associated with osteopathic manipulative treatment (OMT).

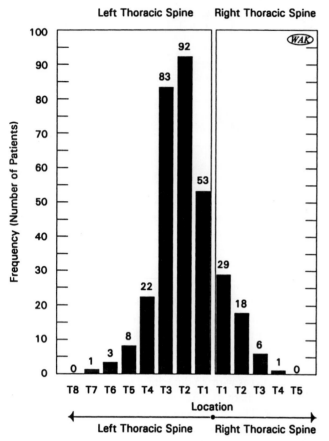

Figure 73.2. Location and incidence of thoracic somatic dysfunction in 94 cardiac patients. (Reprinted with permission from Kuchera ML, Kuchera WA. *Osteopathic Considerations in Systemic Function.* rev. 2nd ed. Columbus, Ohio: Greyden Press; 1994.)

Howell et al.[29] reported on the efficacy of OMT in 17 patients who showed improvement in the severity score over a 1-year time frame. Miller[30] reported on a study of 23 patients with chronic obstructive lung disease, randomly assigned to a treatment or control group. With the exception of OMT, the treatment received by all patients was the same. Although there was a small change in the mean vital capacity of the treated versus the untreated group, this parameter was not considered statistically significant. What did prove to be clinically significant was a clear improvement in functional capacity of the treated group with reduction of cough, increased walking capacity, less dyspnea, and fewer respiratory tract infections.

Numerous other observational studies and pilot projects suggest the value of continuing use of manipulative treatment to enhance self-healing mechanisms in patients with systemic illnesses. For example, two pilot studies suggest that preoperative and postoperative OMT reduce the incidence of atelectasis[31] and ileus, respectively.[32]

Some reports suggest that OMT can be effective in decreasing blood pressure and aldosterone levels in hypertensive patients.[33–35] Other OMT research reports suggest that fibromyalgia-related tender points can be decreased, with improved quality of life measures.[36–38]

Travell and Simons document[39] improved visceral functions when related somatic components are corrected with manipulative treatment and other manual neuromuscular release techniques. Problems that improved include:

Supraventricular tachyarrhythmia
Gastrointestinal functioning
Reduced recurrences of peptic ulcer disease

Korr, drawing from his and others' published research, has hypothesized about neurophysiologic factors, such as segmental facilitation and sympathetic nervous system factors that contribute to these phenomena.[40]

COMPLICATIONS AND CONTRAINDICATIONS

Although manual treatment methods have been used for centuries, little has been recorded regarding morbidity and mortality arising from their use. The earliest documentations were recorded as case histories in various journals.

Complications associated with various procedures have been reported only recently. Most center on impulsed thrust manipulations and focus on isolated case reports of manipulation of the upper cervical spine. Greater interest in the gathering of data regarding these problems began in the 1980s. Attempts were made to identify the actual incidence, nature, and causes of the injuries.

Any discussion of complications must make a clear distinction between symptom exacerbation and true complication. Even though uncomfortable, symptom exacerbations following manipulative treatments are often normal, temporary outcomes of the treatment process. This is particularly true following changes associated with long-term, chronic tissue texture abnormalities and a resulting short-term acute inflammatory response.

True complications are those that worsen the patient's pathologic condition or result in development of new injury or disorder as a direct result of the manipulative treatment.

When describing manipulative treatment contraindications, one must also differentiate between absolute and relative factors. There are few absolute contraindications, but many are relative. If the condition being treated risks worsening when activating forces of a particular technique are apt to create harm, it constitutes a relative contraindication. Other manipulative techniques that use different activating forces may be appropriate and useful, however.

Incidence

A true incidence of complications is difficult to identify. Most studies arrive at similar conclusions: major, serious, or significant complications range from 1 in 400,000 to 1 in 1,000,000 (Table 73.1).[41–52]

Dvorak and Orelli[53] surveyed members of the Swiss Manual Medicine Society in 1981. The survey reports a serious incidence of 1 in 400,000 procedures, most of which were mobilization with impulse (high-velocity low-amplitude) with considerable accompanying rotation. Of 1408 reported com-

Table 73.1
Possible Serious Consequences of Manipulation Reported in the World Literature[a]

Sequelae	Preexisting Condition	Incidence

Vertebrobasilar artery sequelae
  Locked-in syndrome
  Wallenberg syndrome
  Vertigo/dizziness/posterior
    headache
  Aneurysm/dissection
  Subintimal tears
  Intraluminal clot
  TIA/stroke
  Death
	Unilateral atresia of vertebral
	  artery
	Prior neck trauma including
	  prior traumatic cervical
	  manipulation
		1:400,000 to
		1:1,000,000

Cervical cord compression	Agenesis of odontoid process
	Odontoideum
	Down's syndrome with:
	  agenesis of transverse axial
	    ligament
	  odontoid developmental
	    variation
	Ligamentous laxity in:
	  severe rheumatoid arthritis
	  other rheumatologic disorders
	Posterior osteophytes
		1:1,000,000

Exacerbation of disk
  disease[41,42]
  sequestration and acute
  radiculopathy
	Disk disease	Rare

Thrombosis anterior spinal artery		Very rare
Dissecting hematoma of int. carotid[43]		Very rare
Paralysis of diaphragm[44]		Very rare
Hearing loss		Very rare
Horner's syndrome[45]		Very rare
Herniation of thoracic disk[46]		Very rare
Rib fracture	Osteoporosis/metastasis	1:1,000,000
Spinal meningeal hematoma[47]	Concurrent anticoagulation	Very rare
Thoracic spine fracture/diskitis	Alcoholic patient	Very rare
Cauda equina syndrome[48–52]	Disk herniation	1:1,000,000

[a]NOTE: In a survey of the literature, only approximately 5% of these rare sequelae have occurred as a result of osteopathic physicians using osteopathic manipulative techniques.

plications, 1255 were associated with cervical procedures. Most were minor complications such as vertigo. More serious complications included 10 patients with altered consciousness, 12 with loss of consciousness for as long as 5 minutes, and 11 with an undefined neurologic disturbance. Four underwent surgery. The Swiss survey reported less frequent complications relating to the lumbar spine, with most being an increase in subjective pain reports.

Although the Swiss survey did not involve American osteopathic techniques, it was among one of the first careful reports on manipulative treatment-related morbidity. It also highlights the low risk involved with these procedures. In addition, in a 1991 lecture to students at Michigan State University College of Osteopathic Medicine, Dvorak[54] reported a zero incidence of manipulative treatment complications in the decade of the 1980s when cervical manipulations were modified to principally use muscle energy/postisometric relaxation procedures.

Patijn[55] identified 93 papers yielding 129 cases of significant

manipulation-related complications. He notes that of the reports:

67% (85 cases) involved chiropractors
5% involved physical therapists
5% involved European osteopathic practitioners
2% were unknown
2% were self-induced
2% were performed by unqualified persons
18% (23 cases) were unspecified

The most frequent significant complication (65%) involved vertebral artery injury. Other complications included:

Cauda equina syndrome (12%)
Ruptured lumbar disk (6%)
Cervical fracture and/or dislocation (5%)
Thoracic disk rupture (2%)
Other occurrences (<1% each)

All appeared to involve high-velocity low-amplitude activations. Vertebral artery complications occurred in a younger group than might be anticipated, with a mean age of 35–40 years. Male and female distributions were equal. Despite these occurrences, spontaneous vertebral artery dissection is more likely to occur during normal daily activities, such as looking backward over one's shoulder.

Koss[56] reports on the higher incidence of side effects from medications when compared with manipulative procedures. He notes that 5% of hospital admissions result from adverse drug reactions and that 36% of patients on an internal medicine service had an adverse reaction to a drug or diagnostic or therapeutic procedure.

Choice of Osteopathic Technique

Because a wide variety of mild to assertive impulsed manipulative techniques are available to American-educated osteopathic physicians, it is difficult to list or generalize absolute contraindications for the procedures. Rather than rely on one method, one should tailor treatment to the individual patient's circumstances. An essential key is the practitioner's familiarity with the approaches discussed in this text.

Kleynhans and Terrett[57] divide causes of manipulative complications into two categories: physician-related and patient-related. Physician-related problems include:

Diagnostic errors
Lack of manual skills
Lack of interdisciplinary communication and consultation with those who are specially skilled in manipulative techniques

Kleynhans and Terrett report that patient-related problems arise from physical intolerance to the procedures as well as pathologic and structural factors. Other factors are often pertinent:

Personal expectations of both physician and patient
Previous experiences with other practitioners

Subjective pain responses
Other psychological and behavioral factors
Congenital abnormalities
Osteophytes
Atheromatous plaques
Active arthritis
Joint instabilities

Physician examination and diagnostic errors can lead to improper or inappropriate use of manipulation, with complications potentially occurring. For example, using manipulation in the absence of an appropriate physician encounter runs the risk of delayed diagnosis of potentially life-threatening diseases such as cancer and heart disease. Anecdotal reports of such problems are common. Properly performed history, physical, and testing procedures avoid this pitfall.

Lack of diagnostic and manipulative treatment skills can result in:

Poor choice of manipulative procedures
Use of manipulation in a contraindicated situation
Improper soft tissue preparation
Incorrect patient positioning
Poorly applied techniques that use excessive force

Finally, trauma severe enough to raise the suspicion of fracture, dislocation, or neurovascular insult requires that imaging procedures be performed before manipulation is undertaken.

High-Velocity Low-Amplitude Thrusting

High-velocity low-amplitude thrusting (mobilization with impulse, or HVLA) techniques reportedly cause the most serious complications, occurring in 1 of 400,000 procedures to 1 in 1,000,000 procedures. They are designed to apply low-amplitude planar and rotational forces along planes of both single and multiple joint systems. The most frequent of the severe complications are neurovascular accidents following manipulations of the upper cervical spine. These include:

Occipitobasilar strokes (Wallenberg syndrome)
Vertebral artery compression with thrombosis
Arterial dissections
Cerebellar infarctions

Vascular complications occur primarily with the use of cervical rotational forces with the head extended on the neck. The risk increases when the neck is moved away from the midline. Injuries at C1 and C2 are more prone to create vascular complications than are other cervical regions. Several living and cadaveric studies have shown that during rotation, the extracranial portion of the vertebral arteries can be occluded on the side opposite to the rotation; i.e., rotation right can occlude the left vertebral.[58] Fortunately, decreased blood flow to the brain as a result of cervical rotation is a rare complication arising only in the presence of a significant preexisting compromise of the other vertebral artery. Basmajian states, furthermore, *"The cervical spine is, without doubt, quite resistant, and the atheromatous vertebral arteries are quite tolerant."*[59]

Patients with rheumatoid arthritis and Down's syndrome are at particular risk to cervical direct method manipulation because the odontoid ligament is likely to be weakened and susceptible to rupture.

Complications are less frequent in the lumbar and thoracic spine. Increased pain reports are most common in this group. Complications also may include fractures in patients with the following underlying conditions:

Osteoporosis
Metastatic bone disease
Bone infections
Vertebral tuberculosis

Cauda equina syndromes have occasionally been reported in conjunction with the use of HVLA procedures.

Muscle Energy

When indicated, muscle energy/postisometric relaxation (MET) procedures are effective alternatives for HVLA. MET is most effective when a specific joint or muscle is involved and when patient cooperation and operator forces can be well controlled. Posttreatment discomfort and complications are uncommon. The most frequent complications are temporary increases of pain. MET is not effective for someone if muscle contracting increases pain or if proper patient positioning cannot be achieved.

Absolute MET contraindications are fractures and severe neuromuscular injuries involving potential treatment sites.

Counterstrain

Counterstrain technique is a gentle, nontraumatic, indirect manipulative treatment. Posttreatment pain can occur several hours after the procedure, particularly in antagonist muscles, but this is usually well-accepted by patients who have been informed of this possibility. Take care to avoid combined upper cervical hyperrotation and hyperextension. Stop treatment immediately if the patient reports any unusual neurologic sensations. Anecdotally, one documented case of counterstrain-related stroke has been reported in Europe during formal course teaching. A 38-year-old physical therapist, with unknown vascular disease but with many risk factors including smoking, sustained an internal carotid artery stroke after multiple classroom procedures. The complication was documented by angiography. It had not been previously reported (R. Ward, personal communication, 1993).

Avoid positioning that fails to relieve pain and discomfort, as well as positions that produce dizziness or radicular pain. Osteoporotic patients should avoid positions that require extreme forward bending of the thoracolumbar spine.

Craniosacral

Osteopathically based cranial manipulations, with their potential for providing valuable help in a wide variety of cases, also can create problems when used by the unskilled. For example, unanticipated lassitude and temporary emotional reactions ranging from tears to laughter occur at times. Uncomfortable side effects include:

Nausea
Vertigo
Lightheadedness
Headache
Loss of appetite
Sleep problems

Most are temporary and respond to rest. If problems occur in the clinic, the gentle use of CV4 techniques usually calms the reaction.

In the hands of nonprofessionals, serious complications have occurred. One author (E.L.D.) reports the case of a young man who developed hypopituitarism following an unskilled and forceful cranial treatment. After several months of hormone treatment and osteopathic treatment for the cranial dysfunctions, he had a favorable recovery.

Prevention of Complications

Proper diagnosis and treatment of any kind, including manipulative procedures, occur when one links the patient's background and presenting story with present circumstances. This includes:

Mechanism of injury
Medication use and abuse
Exercise levels
Lifestyle factors
Mental and emotional well-being

A well-performed history and physical, including a careful, osteopathically oriented history and physical examination, complete this essential process. The application of osteopathic principles associated with functional anatomy, biomechanics, and manipulative skills reduce the potential for complications.

Histories of trauma, joint and soft tissue diseases, infectious diseases, and cancer are major considerations. When appropriate, include blood work and imaging studies.

Another line of defense is the appropriate choice of manipulative procedure. Indirect and neuromuscular-activating methods are typically safe and effective. If HVLA procedures are considered, consider the risk-to-benefit ratio. Most complications have occurred with HVLA maneuvers in the upper cervical spine during combined extension and rotation. Statistically, there is less chance of injury if cervical flexion and side-bending maneuvers are used. Take care to keep the neck in the midline, remembering the basic rule of spinal motion: modification of motion in one plane limits motion in all other planes.

Finally, the broader the manipulative armamentarium possessed by the clinician, the better the chances for safe and effective outcomes.

OSTEOPATHIC PRACTICE GUIDELINES

Disease and dysfunction-based allopathically designed medical practice guidelines have been developed and are under contin-

ued development for a wide variety of diagnoses. For example, the American Association of Family Physicians established a guideline for depression after more than a year in development and at a cost of more than $1,000,000. Such MD-oriented guidelines are often difficult to implement for osteopathically oriented physicians because they do not allow for the wide range of patient responses (i.e.,the host). As a "parallel but distinctive" health care system,[60] osteopathic medicine is ill-served by directly adopting another group's standard of practice as anything more than partial "guidelines" in the strictest sense of that word.

In general, osteopathically oriented guidelines consider both the host and the etiologic factors. They should include an appropriate osteopathic diagnosis that includes palpatory diagnosis and potential manipulative treatment relatively early in the evaluation and treatment process, respectively. Goals of manipulation within an osteopathic practice guideline may include:

Resolution of primary somatic dysfunction
Resolution of secondary somatic dysfunction
Improvement of homeostatic mechanisms (e.g., respiratory, circulatory, immune, etc.)
Reduction of inappropriate afferent neural stimuli

Significant somatic dysfunction is that which reduces the body's ability to recover, compensate, and repair itself. Psychologically, it is the somatic component that causes the patient discomfort and concern. It is also the somatic component of a problem that prevents the patient from functioning with a high level of efficiency. This is of particular importance for patients such as high-level athletes and ballet dancers.

Functional disorders of other systems affected by a primary disorder need to be a part of osteopathically oriented practice guidelines. The strategy is to reduce or remove identifiable lingering elements of somatic dysfunction to improve the body's ability to:

Compensate
Repair
Recover
Improve health

Finally, osteopathically oriented practice guidelines include all related elements relating to the diagnosis, treatment, and long-term health enhancing strategies embodied in the application of osteopathic principles.

CONCLUSION

Osteopathic manipulative treatment has the potential for complications and side effects, but the risk is low. Properly selected and applied osteopathic procedures are beneficial for a wide variety of human ailments and health-enhancing activities. Palpatory diagnosis and manipulative treatment enlists the patient's cooperation in the process of maintaining health and overcoming the detrimental effects of somatic dysfunction. In general, the benefits far outweigh the rare and usually minor risks. Serious complications have occurred with the work of some practitioners but are only anecdotally documented in the practice of American-trained osteopathic physicians. Osteopathically based manipulative treatment is tailored to the individual patient's needs in a context of total health care that is in the patient's best interests. When osteopathic treatment is appropriate, it should be performed with gentleness, care, and skill.

REFERENCES

1. Goldstein M, ed. *The Research Status of Spinal Manipulative Therapy.* Bethesda, Md: DHEW publication number (NIH) 76-998, 1975.

2. Korr IM. *The Neurobiologic Mechanisms in Manipulative Therapy.* New York, London: Plenum Press; 1978.

3. Greenman PE, ed. *Concepts and Mechanisms of Neuromuscular Functions.* Berlin: Springer-Verlag; 1984.

4. Beurger AA, Greenman PE, eds. *Empirical Approaches to the Validation of Spinal Manipulation.* Springfield, Ill: Charles Thomas; 1985.

5. Patterson MM, Howell JN. *The Central Connection: Somatovisceral/Viscerosomatic Interaction.* Proceedings of the 1989 American Academy of Osteopathy International Symposium. Athens, Ohio: University Classics, Ltd; 1989.

6. Willard FH, Patterson MM. *Nociception and the Neuroendocrine-Immune Connection.* Proceedings of the 1991 American Academy of Osteopathy International Symposium. Athens, Ohio: University Classics, Ltd; 1991.

7. Parker GB, Tupling H, Pryor DS. A controlled trial of cervical manipulation for migraine. *Aust NAJ Med.* 1978;8:589–593.

8. Sloop PR, Smith DS, Goldenberg E, et al. Manipulation for chronic neck pain: a double-blinded controlled study. *Spine.* 1982;7:532–535.

9. Shekelle PA, Adams AH, Chassin MR, et al. Spinal manipulation for low back pain. *Ann Int Med.* 1992:117:590–598.

10. Koes BW, Assendelft WJJ, von der Heijden GJMG, et al. Spinal manipulation and mobilisation for back and neck pain: a blinded review. *Br Med J.* 1991;303:1298–1303.

11. Waagen GN, Haldeman S, Cook G, et al. Short-term trial of chiropractic adjustments for the relief of chronic low back pain. *Man Med.* 1986;2:63–67.

12. Gibson T, Grahame R, Harkness J, et al. Controlled-wave diathermy treatment comparison of short wave with osteopathic treatment in non-specific low back pain. *Lancet.* 1985:1258–1261.

13. Dyer C. Osteopathic vs medical manipulation in clinical trials. *Br Osteopath J.* 1983;15:65–67.

14. Fitzgerald M, Stiles E. Osteopathic hospitals' solution to DRG's may be OMT. *The DO.* November 1984:97–101.

15. Brodin H. Inhibition-facilitation technique of lumbar pain treatment. *Man Med.* 1987;3:24–26.

16. Kelso AF. A double-blind clinical study of osteopathic findings in hospitalized patients: progress report. *JAOA.* 1970;70:570–592.

17. Nicholas N. Correlation of somatic dysfunction with visceral disease. *JAOA.* 1975;75:426–428.

18. Smith LA, et al. *An Atlas of Pain Patterns: Sites and Behavior of Pain in Certain Common Disease of the Upper Abdomen.* Springfield, Ill: CC Thomas; 1961.

19. Nicholas AS, DeBias DA, Ehrenfeuchter W, et al. A somatic component to myocardial infarction. *Br Med J.* 1985;291:13–17.

20. Beal MC. Palpatory testing for somatic dysfunction in patients with cardiovascular disease. *JAOA.* 1983;82:73–82.

21. Cox JM, Gorbis S, Dick LM, et al. Palpable musculoskeletal findings in coronary artery disease: results of a double-blind study. *JAOA.* 1983;82:832–836

22. Rogers JT, Rogers RC. The role of osteopathic manipulative therapy in the treatment of coronary heart disease. *JAOA.* 1976;76:23–31.

23. Robuck SV. *Osteopathic Manipulative Therapy in Organic Heart Disease: Yearbook.* Indianapolis, Ind: American Academy of Osteopathy; 1956:11–25.

24. Patriquin DH. *Osteopathic Management of Coronary Disease: Yearbook.* Indianapolis, Ind: American Academy of Osteopathy; 1956:75–79.

25. Koch RS. A somatic component in heart disease. *JAOA.* 1961; 60:92–97.

26. Stookey JR. OMT for angina. *Osteopathic Symposium.* May 1975:16–18.

27. Beal MC, Morlock JW. Somatic dysfunction associated with pulmonary disease. *JAOA.* 1984;84:179–183.

28. Koch RS. *Structural Patterns and Principles of Treatment in the Asthmatic Patient: Yearbook.* Indianapolis, Ind: American Academy of Osteopathy; 1957:71–72.

29. Howell RK, Allen TW, Kappler RE. The influence of osteopathic manipulative therapy in the management of patients with chronic lung disease. *JAOA.* 1975;74:757–760.

30. Miller WD. Treatment of visceral disorders by manipulative treatment. In: *The Research Status of Spinal Manipulative Therapy.* Bethesda, Md: US Dept of Health, Education, and Welfare; 1975:295–301.

31. Henshaw RE. Manipulative and postoperative pulmonary complications. *The DO.* September 1963;4(1):132–133.

32. Hermann E. Postoperative adynamic ileus: its prevention and treatment by osteopathic manipulation. *The DO.* October 1965; 6(2):163–164.

33. Northup TL. Manipulative Management of hypertension. *JAOA.* 1961;60:973–978.

34. Mannino JR. The application of neurologic reflexes to the treatment of hypertension. *JAOA.* 1979;10:607–608.

35. Mannino JR. The application of neurological reflexes to the treatment of hypertension. *JAOA.* 1979;12:225–231.

36. Lo KS, Kuchera ML, Preston SC, Jackson RW. Osteopathic manipulative treatment in fibromyalgia syndrome. *JAOA.* 1992l;9:1177.

37. Rubin BR, Gamber RG, Cortez CA, et al. Treatment options in fibromyalgia syndrome. *JAOA.* 1990;90:844.

38. Rubin BR, Gamber RG, Shores J, et al. The effect of treatment options on perceived pain in fibromyalgia syndrome. *JAOA.* 1991; 91:1032.

39. Travell JG, Simons DG. *Myofascial Pain and Dysfunction: A Trigger Point Manual.* Baltimore, Md: Williams & Wilkins; 1983.

40. Korr IM. The spinal cord as organizer of disease processes: III. Hyperactivity of sympathetic innervation as a common factor in disease. *JAOA.* December 1979;79(4):232–237.

41. Wolff HD. Akute Wurzelkeompression durch zervikalen Bandscheibensequester nach gezielter Handgrifftherapie. *Manuelle Medizine.* 1989;27:14–15.

42. Hooper J. Low back pain and manipulation. *Med J Aust.* 1973; 1:549–557.

43. Beatty RA. Dissecting hematoma of the internal carotid artery following chiropractic cervical manipulation. *J Trauma.* 1977;17:248–249.

44. Heffner JE. Diaphragmatic paralysis following chiropractic manipulation of the cervical spine. *Intern Med.* 1985;145:562–564.

45. Grayson MF. Horner's syndrome after manipulation of the neck. *Br Med J.* 1987;295:1381–1382.
46. Lanska DJ, Lanska MJ, Fenstermaker R, et al. Thoracic disk herniation associated with chiropractic spinal manipulation. *Arch Neurol.* 1987;44:996–997.
47. Darbert O, Freeinna DG, Weis AJ. Spinal meningeal hematoma, warfarin therapy and chiropractic adjustment. *JAMA.* 1970; 214:2058.
48. Dan NG, Saccasan PA. Serious complications of lumbar spinal manipulation. *Med J Aust.* 1983;2:672–673.
49. Richard J. Disk rupture with cauda equina syndrome after chiropractic adjustment. *NYJ Med.* September 1967:2496–2498.
50. Malmivaara A, Pohjola R. Cauda equina syndrome caused by chiropraxis on a patient previously free of lumbar spine symptoms. *Lancet.* October 30, 1982:986–987.
51. Schvartzman P, Abelson A. Complications of chiropractic treatment for back pain. *Post Grad Med.* 1988;83:57–61.
52. Quon JA, Cassidy JD, O'Conner SM, et al. Lumbar intervertebral disc herniation: treatment by rotational manipulation. *J Manip Physical Ther.* 1989;12:220–227.
53. Dvorak J, Orelli FV. How dangerous is manipulation to the cervical spine? Case report and results of a survey. *Man Med.* 1985;2:1–4.
54. Deleted in proof.
55. Patijn J. Complications of manual medicine: a review of the literature. *Man Med.* 1991;6:89–92.
56. Koss RW. Quality assurance monitoring of osteopathic manipulative treatment. *JAOA.* May 1990;90(5):427–434.
57. Kleynhans AM. Complications of and contraindications to spinal manipulative therapy. In: Haldeman S, ed. *Modern Developments in the Principles and Practice of Chiropractic.* New York, NY: Appleton-Century-Crofts; 1980;359–384.
58. Heinking K, Kappler R, et al. Vertebral artery blood flow during cervical extension and rotation as assessed by color flow duplex ultrasound. *JAOA.* September 1995;95(9):548.
59. Basmajian JV. *Grant's Method of Anatomy.* 8th ed. Baltimore, Md: Williams & Wilkins; 1983.
60. Gevitz N. Parallel and distinctive. The philosophic pathway for reform in osteopathic medical education. *JAOA.* 1994;94:328–332.

74. Radiographic Technical Aspects of the Postural Study

MICHAEL K. WILLMAN, MICHAEL L. KUCHERA, AND WILLIAM A. KUCHERA

Key Concepts

- **Use of postural study x-ray series**
- **Importance of standardization of postural x-ray series**
- **Equipment used in performing postural study**
- **Essential views for complete postural x-ray series**
- **Methods for obtaining postural x-ray series and reasons for following these procedures**
- **Explanations of concepts related to radiographic image analysis:**
  - **Vertebral rotation**
  - **Vertebral side-bending**
  - **Cobb angles**
  - **Sacral base unleveling**
  - **Pelvic rotation**
  - **Angle of sacral base**
  - **L3 weight-bearing line**
  - **Pelvic index**
  - **Lumbosacral lordotic angle**
  - **Lumbolumbar lordotic angle**

Osteopathic physicians have used radiographs for many years to better understand structure and function of the spine and pelvis. The roentgen ray was discovered in 1895; by 1898 the American School of Osteopathy in Kirksville, Missouri, had acquired the second machine west of the Mississippi. In 1898, this equipment provided the earliest roentgenologic studies of circulation.[1] Hoskins and Schwab introduced the standing postural x-ray series in 1921, opening the field for clinical interpretation and integration. Martin Beilke in 1936 acknowledged the value of the technique by observing:

The osteopathic profession can lay claim to these contributions as being strictly original and especially applicable to our approach in finding etiological factors in a given pathological process and in applying corrective measures.[2]

For many years, lack of standardization for a postural x-ray procedure prevented the profession from combining important multicenter data. It also prevented universal clinical interpretation of postural studies. J. Stedman Denslow and his co-workers called for standardization in 1955,[3] although even today relatively few academic institutions have adopted that recommendation. A standard protocol would provide accurate, reproducible methods to research measurable discrepancies related to structural examination. Standardized postural x-ray views do *"show repeatable findings when the state of the patient is unchanged and provide valid information concerning improvements or regressions in skeletal structure which are associated with changes in the patient's condition."*[3] Postural x-ray views taken according to a standardized protocol can be accurately and consistently measured for postural information by radiologists or attending nonradiologist physicians.[4]

Many radiologists are not trained to do postural studies specifically for osteopathic analysis but will do them for primary care physicians if given an appropriate protocol. This chapter provides a method[5] for evaluating the pelvis and spine. The advantages of this method are that it is:

Practical
Reproducible
Inexpensive
Accurate
Standardized

The measurements obtained through the use of this protocol can be interpreted clinically in the context described in other chapters of this text.

MATERIALS

The following equipment is needed to employ this standardized protocol:

1. Vertical Bucky diaphragm
2. Adjustable holder for plumbed wire
3. Piano wire
4. Plumb bob
5. Level metal base plate or level floor

The vertical Bucky diaphragm is wall-mounted for best results (Fig. 74.1). The adjustable holder (Fig. 74.2) is designed to move the plumbed wire exactly over the desired point on the base plate. Piano wire, 0.020 inch in diameter, is ideal for this system. It is pliable and durable for adjusting to the desired shape, and it is readily identified on the exposed film because of its density. A plumb bob (Fig. 74.3) of any size or configuration is attached to the wire. These items are relatively inexpensive and available from hardware stores.

The level, rectangular metal base plate (Fig. 74.4) is made from 1/4-inch gauge steel and measures 70 by 50 cm. It is

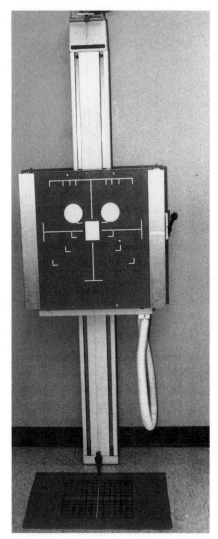

Figure 74.1.   Vertical Bucky diaphragm and piano wire reference.

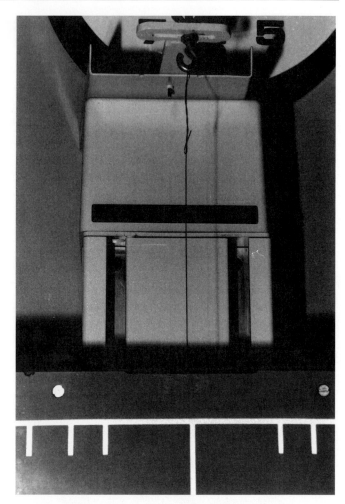

Figure 74.2.   Adjustable film cassette holder.

leveled and cemented or fixed to the floor. This ensures a level plane for the patient to stand on (unlevel floors may accentuate or hide a short leg). The floor may be used instead of the metal plate if it is level in two planes. Paint a modified cross-hatched grid on the surface of the plate or on the floor to ensure accurate alignment of the patient's feet.

Attach the piano wire to the adjustable holder and pass it behind the protective covering on the Bucky diaphragm (Fig. 74.1). Attach the plumb bob to the wire to establish a vertical reference line. Adjust it to lie directly over two main cross-sectional base lines perpendicular to each other (Fig. 74.4). The posterior line (Fig. 74.4, *1*) lies in a plane parallel to the film and the coronal plane of the body. The midheel line (Fig. 74.4, *2*) and the plumbed wire lie in the sagittal plane of the body and perpendicular to the posterior line. This plane is equidistant from both heels for the anteroposterior view. It is just anterior to the lateral malleolus for the lateral view.

In the anteroposterior (AP) view, the reference line is known as the midheel line. In the lateral view, the reference line is known as the postural or weight-bearing line (Fig. 74.4).

PROCEDURE

Postural films of the pelvis or any section of the spine are exposed at a film-tube distance of 40 inches. Record all information, including radiographic factors and the position of the feet, on a separate form that is filed with the patient's radiographic records. Future examinations are then performed using the same technical factors. This ensures a uniform, acceptable, and reproducible method.

The patient prepares for the anteroposterior (AP) x-ray view by removing all clothing and putting on a gown. He or she stands on the adjustable metal base plate with the back facing, but not touching, the Bucky diaphragm (Fig. 74.5). The feet are positioned equidistant from and parallel to the midheel base line (Fig. 74.6), far enough apart so that they are directly under the femoral heads. Record this distance by noting the distance from the base line to the medial aspect of the feet, as indicated by the markings on the base plate. The heels are placed equidistant from the posterior line (Fig. 74.4, *1*), with the patient standing as close to the film as possible, in a relaxed posture. This method ensures a reproducible, standard position for the feet (the base for support of posture). Ask the patient to extend the knees in a locked but comfortable position, with arms re-

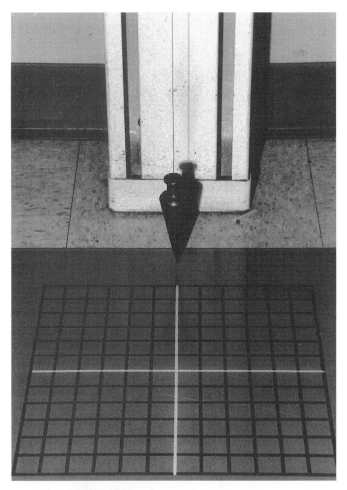

Figure 74.3. Plumb bob and piano wire.

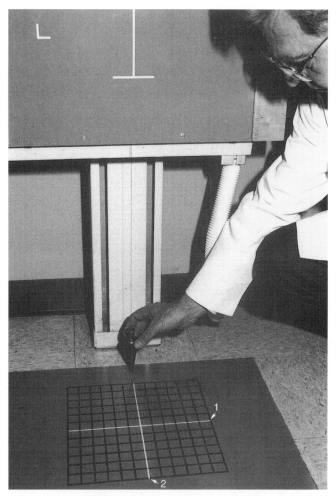

Figure 74.4. Rectangular metal base plate with reference lines. *1*, posterior line; *2*, midheel line.

laxed to the sides and the head forward with the eyes straight ahead (Fig. 74.5).

Adjust the x-ray tube to position the central ray at the level of the iliac crest for pelvic and lumbar spine radiographs. Adjustment of the Bucky diaphragm to the desired height assures that the AP pelvic film includes the femoral heads, the pubic symphysis, and most of the lumbar vertebrae. Center the central beam for a postural study of the thoracic spine at the xiphoid process or at about the T9 level.

The piano wire, behind the patient but in front of the Bucky diaphragm and film, is recorded in an undistorted fashion on the film. It becomes the reference line in the midsagittal plane of the patient. Measurements are obtained from this reference line.

Obtain the lateral view by having the patient turn to the standing lateral position with the lateral malleolus of the innermost ankle (closest to the wire) placed in a position where the wire lies just anterior to the lateral malleolus (Fig. 74.7). This positioning is very important, because it places the piano wire in the plane of the patient's lateral weight-bearing line. In a patient with an ideal posture, the lateral weight-bearing line should pass through a point just anterior to the lateral malleolus, and through the greater trochanter, the center of the L3

vertebral body, and the external auditory canal.[6] The other foot is positioned parallel to the contralateral foot and apart the same distance as determined in the AP view. The patient's arms are crossed in front of the body to obtain an unobstructed view of the spine. The knees are locked and the normal posture maintained as for the AP view (Fig. 74.8). Again, by adjusting the Bucky diaphragm, the lateral x-ray view may be obtained of the pelvis and spine using the landmarks described for the AP view. The film must contain the lumbar vertebrae, lumbosacral junction, sacrum, and pubic bone. Both of these films are exposed immediately after positioning the patient to eliminate movement from fatigue.

All of these procedures are performed with the patient's shoes off to determine postural discrepancies. At times, films may also be obtained with the patient wearing lift therapy shoes to determine the amount of sacral base unleveling that still remains to be corrected. Oblique views may be obtained in the standing posture, although this has not proved helpful in evaluating the spine structurally. Sometimes right and left oblique views are necessary to evaluate the neural arches and intervertebral foramina.

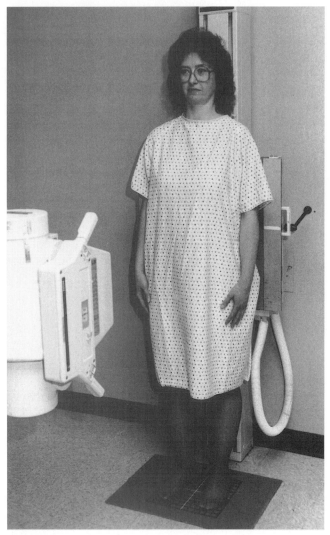

Figure 74.5. Patient positioned for anteroposterior postural x-ray view.

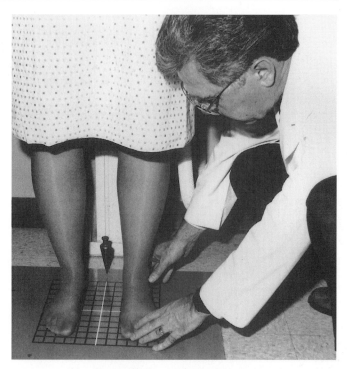

Figure 74.6. Midheel positioning.

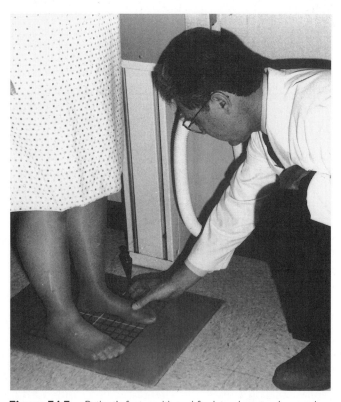

Figure 74.7. Patient's feet positioned for lateral postural x-ray view.

RESULTS

The x-ray method described is amenable to rapid adjustment and placement, making it useful in a busy department. It also positions the patient in a reproducible posture and records an independent reference line on the film (see Fig. 74.10, *RL*) that is used for accurate measurements. The reference line is unrelated to the position of the cassette, yet it is perpendicular to the line of the horizon. Measurements taken from the edge of the film may produce undesirable results. This is due to the unavoidable inability to place the cassette, and thus the film, in a square position relative to the patient. This rotational component of the cassette in its holder can accentuate or reduce the measurable difference in leg lengths, iliac crests, etc.

The postural x-ray series may provide other clinically relevant findings including:

Facet tropism
Sacralization

Lumbarization
Spondylolisthesis
Spondylosis, scoliosis
Facet arthritis
Fracture

Anteroposterior Film of Thoracolumbar Region

The anteroposterior film of the thoracolumbar region shows coronal and horizontal plane postural data in two areas.

Vertebral rotation can be qualitatively assessed by noting the relative positions of the two pedicles and the spinous process. In the absence of vertebral rotation, the spinous process is located equidistant from each pedicle. With right vertebral rotation (named in relation to the direction of movement of a reference point on the anterior portion of the vertebral body), the spinous process visualized on the x-ray film appears closer to the left pedicle. With left vertebral rotation, the spinous process appears closer to the right pedicle on the x-ray film.

Vertebral side-bending is also easily observed on this radio-

graphic view and can be qualitatively reported. Quantitative measurement of group curves is often more formally reported using scoliosis nomenclature. Scoliosis, by convention, is usually reported in reference to the convexity of the curve. A right scoliosis is side-bent left (convex right). The Cobb method is used to measure scoliotic curves (Fig. 74.9). Lines are constructed across the top of the superior vertebral segment and across the bottom of the inferior vertebral segment of a spinal scoliotic curve. Perpendicular lines are then constructed from these lines. These perpendicular lines intersect to form an angle, the Cobb angle measurement.

Anteroposterior Film of Pelvis

The anteroposterior film of the pelvis shows coronal and horizontal plane postural data. This film is especially important in evaluating the degree of sacral base unleveling as well as determining structural leg lengths and pelvic rotation with the patient in a weight-bearing position (Fig. 74.10A).

Lines are drawn from the most superior aspect of the femoral heads (D), perpendicular to the reference line, and discrepancies are measured in millimeters.

Similar lines are drawn from the superior margins of the iliac crests (E), perpendicular to the reference line, to determine the relative iliac crest heights.

The junction of the articular pillars and the sacral ala are marked with small dots (a), and a straight line (7) connecting these dots is extended to intersect a perpendicular line extending from the superior margins of each femoral head. A line that is perpendicular to the reference line is then drawn from where the line through a and the perpendicular lines from the femurs meet (C). The difference between the level of these lines indicates the amount of sacral base unleveling (Fig. 74.10A, 1–9). Dots b in Figure 74.10 mark the sites where the sacral ala and the iliac crests cross each other on the x-ray film, and they

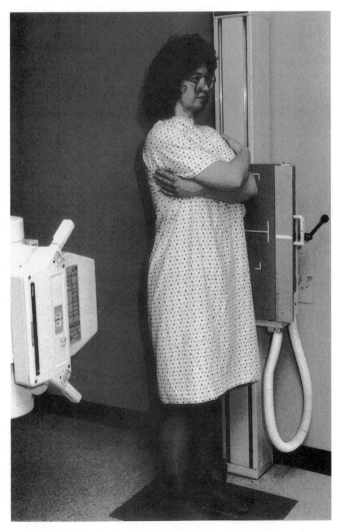

Figure 74.8. Patient positioned for lateral postural x-ray view.

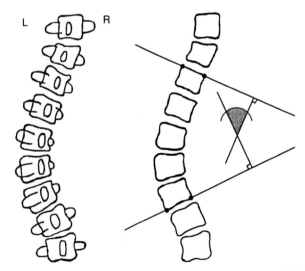

Figure 74.9. Measurement of scoliotic curve: Cobb method. This left scoliosis is functionally $S_R R_L$. (Illustration by W.A. Kuchera.)

Figure 74.10. Measurements for postural x-ray view. *Diagram A,* anteroposterior postural measurements. *Diagram B,* lateral postural measurements. (From Kuchera WA, Kuchera ML. *Osteopathic Principles in Practice.* 2nd ed. rev. Columbus, Ohio: Greyden Press; 1994:63.)

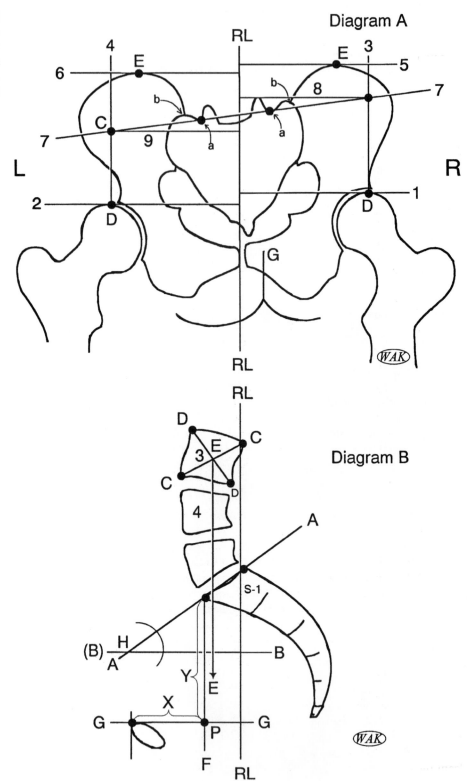

may be used as alternatives for reference points *a* when calculating sacral base unleveling. The final measurement will be the same either way. This alternative may be used in instances in which this set of reference points is more easily and accurately identified.

The physician is more interested in leveling a sacral base than making the leg lengths equal, that is, the sacral base unleveling is usually of more clinical significance than comparison of leg lengths. In the presence of sacral base unleveling, the direction of the lumbar side-bending component is clinically relevant. Roughening of the iliac crest where the iliolumbar ligament attaches or calcification of the iliolumbar ligament should be noted, as these are markers for postural stress.

Pelvic rotation is determined by measuring the distance between the pubic symphysis and either the dark line representing the air in the gluteal fold or the median sacral crest.[7] The pelvis is said to rotate in the direction in which the anterior portion of the pelvis (pubic symphysis) moves. Pelvic rotation is also recognized qualitatively by asymmetry of the obturator foramina.

Lateral Film of Pelvis

The lateral film of the pelvis and its sagittal plane postural data show the determinations of the angle of the sacral base, the weight-bearing line from L3 to the sacral base, and the pelvic index (Fig. 74.10*B*). (See Chapter 72, "Postural Considerations in the Sagittal Plane.")

The angle of the sacral base, also known as Ferguson's angle, or the lumbosacral angle, is calculated by drawing a line (*A*) across the sacral base. Another line (*B*) is constructed to cross line *A* and to be perpendicular to the reference line (Fig. 74.10*B*, *lines A and B*).

The line of weight bearing, previously described as running just anterior to the lateral malleolus, is represented by the lucent line produced by the reference wire's image on the x-ray film. This reference line (*RL*) can be used to evaluate the position of the third lumbar vertebra relative to the lateral malleolus of the ankle, the sacral base, and the femoral heads. To do this, calculate the center of the third lumbar vertebra by marking the four corners of the vertebral body and then connecting the dots. A line constructed from the center of L3, down past the sacral base and parallel to the weight-bearing line, is the L3 weight bearing. The weight-bearing line should fall through the anterior one-third of the sacral base. If the weight-bearing line falls posterior to the sacral base, the lumbar facets are under increased load. Examine the facets on the radiograph for arthritic change, which is seen as increased density (eburnation) of these articulations (Fig. 74.10*B, C–E*).

The pelvic index is calculated from measurements obtained from the lateral postural x-ray view. The sacral promontory is marked with a small dot. A line parallel to the reference line is constructed downward past where a horizontal line from the pubic symphysis would be drawn. The most superior and anterior part of the pubic symphysis is then marked with a dot, and a second line is constructed that is perpendicular to the

reference line. These two constructed lines will cross forming a reference point (*P*). The measurement of distance in millimeters from the pubic symphysis to the reference is called *x*. The measurement of distance in millimeters from the sacral promontory to the reference point is called *y*. Pelvic index (PI) is a calculation of the ratio of *x/y* (Fig. 74.10*B*, *letters F, G, X, and Y*). The PI indicates the relative position of the innominates to the sacrum (Fig. 74.11). Normal values are age-related and are typically less than 1. As posture "ages," the ratio approaches and exceeds the value of 1.0. The PI is known to be increased in some patient populations, including those with chronic low back pain and those with isthmic spondylolisthesis.

Lumbar lordosis can be qualitatively assessed as normal, increased, or decreased; it can be quantified by measuring the angle created by lines along the top of L2 and S1 (Fig. 74.12) or the top of L2 and the bottom of L5 (Fig. 74.13).[8] These angles average 60 and 43°, respectively.[9]

EXERCISE IN MEASUREMENT

Two exercises follow, using Figure 74.10, illustrating how to measure postural x-ray films taken with the method described in this chapter.

AP Postural View of Pelvis

Refer to Figure 74.10*A*.

1. Identify the midheel reference line (*RL*) on the x-ray film. This represents a line that is perpendicular to the horizon.
2. Put a dot (*D*) at the most superior border of each femoral head.
3. Draw line *1* perpendicular to the reference line (*RL*) from point *D* on one of the femoral heads.

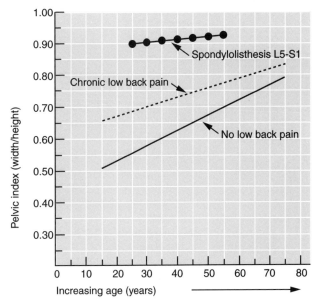

Figure 74.11. Pelvic index. (Illustration by W.A. Kuchera.)

Figure 74.12. Lumbosacral lordotic angle using L2 and S1 (average 60°). (Illustration by W.A. Kuchera.)

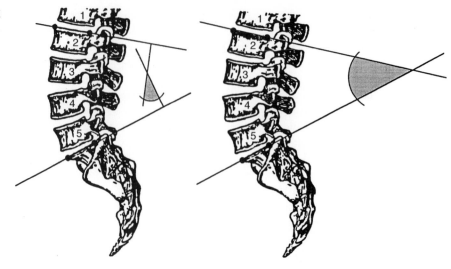

Figure 74.13. Lumbolumbar lordotic angle using L2 and the bottom of L5 (average 43°). (Illustration by W.A. Kuchera.)

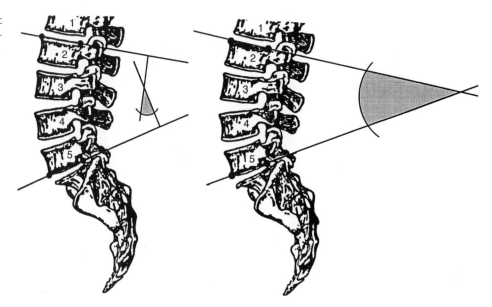

4. Draw line *2* by repeating step 3 on the other side of the body. Step 3 and 4 indicate if there is any inequality in the femoral head heights.

5. From point *D* on one of the femoral heads, draw line *3*, parallel to the reference line (*RL*) and perpendicular to line *1*.

6. Draw line *4* by repeating step 5 from dot *D* on the other femoral head.

7. Place a dot (*E*) at the most superior edge of each iliac crest.

8. Draw line *5*, perpendicular to the reference line (*RL*) from point *E* on one of the iliac crests.

9. Draw line *6* by repeating step 8 on the other side of the body. Steps 8 and 9 indicate any inequality of the iliac crests.

10. Mark two points (indicated as *a* on the diagrammed example), which are located at the junction of the articular pillars with the sacral ala **or** two points (indicated as *b* on the example), which are at the superior junction of the sacroiliac joints. Draw a line *7*, which passes through two of the matching points, either *a*'s or *b*'s. Extend that line past lines *3* and *4* drawn in steps 5 and 6 above. Place a dot, *C*, where these lines cross on the right and the left sides.

11. Now construct line *8* perpendicular to the reference line (*RL*) from point *C*.

12. Draw line *9* by repeating step 11 on the other side of the body. Steps 11 and 12 will indicate unlevelness of the sacral base.

13. Find the soft tissue shadow on the x-ray view that indicates the position of the natal crease or gluteal crease (*G* in the diagrammed example).

14. At the reference line (*RL*) report the following in millimeters:

    a. Horizontal distance between the natal crease shadow (*G*) and middle of the shadow of the pubic symphysis (= amount of pelvic rotation and symphyseal direction)

b. Difference between lines *1* and *2* (= femoral head unleveling)

c. Difference between lines *5* and *6* (= iliac crest inequality)

d. Difference between lines *8* and *9* (= sacral base unleveling)

Lateral Postural View of Pelvis

Refer to Figure 74.10*B*.

1. Identify the reference line (*RL*) on the lateral x-ray view.
2. Place a dot at the most anterior and the most posterior border on the superior surface of the body of the first sacral vertebra.
3. Draw line *A* through these two points and extend it far enough anterior on the film (at least 2 inches anterior to the sacral promontory) to allow easy measurement of its angle.
4. Near the anterior end of line *A* construct line *B*, perpendicular to the reference line (*RL*) and crossing line *A*. (*H* indicates the point of crossing of lines *A* and *B* on the diagrammed example.)
5. Now identify L3 vertebra and find its center by constructing two diagonal lines, *C* and *D*, from corner to corner, like a big "X."
6. Construct line *E*, passing through the midpoint of the L3 vertebra and parallel to the reference line (*RL*). It must pass at least past the level of the sacral base (indicated by line *A* on the diagrammed example.) This is the weight-bearing line.
7. Draw line *F*, parallel to the reference line and extending caudally from the sacral promontory past the horizontal level of the pubic bone.
8. Draw line *G*, perpendicular to the reference line from the most anterior and superior aspect of the pubic bone. Lines *F* and *G* will cross (designated as point *P* on the diagrammed example.)
9. Measure the following:
   a. Measure the angle *AHB* (= the lumbosacral angle)
   b. Does the weight-bearing line (step 6 above) pass through the anterior, middle, or posterior third of the sacral base? Or does it pass anterior or posterior? (How many millimeters?)
   c. Measure *X* and *Y* and determine the PI:
      1. *X* is the mm or distance from the most superior and anterior point on the pubes to *P*, the intersection of lines *G* and *F*
      2. *Y* is the mm of distance from the sacral promontory to *P*, the intersection of lines *G* and *F*
      3. The PI is *X/Y*

CONCLUSION

This protocol provides a simple and inexpensive way to obtain accurate structural measurements for either research or clinical interpretation (Table 74.1). These requirements can be shared with the radiologist to whom the osteopathic primary care practitioner is referring patients. Anteroposterior views of the pelvis, lumbar, and thoracic spines are obtained, as well as lateral views of the pelvis and lumbar spine. Consistent reference lines produced on the radiographs are available for proper eval-

Table 74.1
Sample Analysis Report on Weight Bearing Postural X-ray Series

Subject _____ Examiner _____ Date _____
Other Examiners: _____
Height of Femur Heads:
  (Indicate side of shortness by R or L; measure in millimeters.)
Height of Iliac Crests:
  (Repeat process used above.)
Sacral Base:
  (Is it level or is it depressed? How many millimeters on R or L side? How does this finding relate to the plane of the femoral heads?)
Lumbar Rotation:
  (Indicate R or L and which ones.)
Lumbar Lateral Flexion:
  (Indicate side-bending, right or left, and vertebrae involved.)
Pelvic Rotation:
  (R or L; measure millimeter difference.)
Pelvic Tilt:
  (R or L)
Lateral Disalignment of Trunk:
  (At L5; R or L)
Lumbosacral Angle:
  (Degrees)
Relation of L3 to the Sacral Base:
  (Where is the weight-bearing line in relation to the sacrum?)
Lordosis:
  (Qualitative: Normal, decreased, or increased? Quantitative: Measurement of lumbosacral or lumbolumbar lordotic angle.)
Pelvic Index:
  X = _____ mm
  Y = _____ mm
  PI = X/Y =
Anomalies:
  (Bat-wing, sacralization, lumbarization, facet asymmetry, spina bifida, etc.)
Summary:
  (Comment concerning disalignment and related disturbances. This includes changes in the density of both osseous and soft tissues such as muscles and ligaments.)

uation of the patient when lift therapy is being applied. This method lends itself to an accurate evaluation.

These static (structural) findings can be effectively correlated with dynamic (functional) physical findings for a more complete and accurate assessment of a patient.

REFERENCES

1. Smith W. Skiagraphy and the circulation. *J Osteopathy*. January 1899; 3:356–378.
2. Beilke M. Roentgenological spinal analysis and the technic for taking standing X-ray plates. *JAOA*. May 1936;35:414–418.
3. Denslow JS, Chace JA, Gutensohn OR, Kumm MG. Methods in taking and interpreting weight-bearing films. *JAOA*. July 1955; 54:663–670.
4. Kuchera ML, Bemben MG, Kuchera WA, Willman MK. Comparison of manual and computerized methods of assessing postural radiographs. *JAOA*. August 1990;90(8):714–715.
5. Willman MK. Radiographic technical aspects of the postural study. *JAOA*. June 1977;76:739–744.

6. The Glossary Review Committee of the Educational Council on Osteopathic Principles. Glossary of osteopathic terminology. In: Allen TW, ed. *AOA Yearbook and Directory of Osteopathic Physicians.* Chicago, Ill: American Osteopathic Association; 1995.

7. Denslow JS, Chace JA. Mechanical stresses in the human lumbar spine and pelvis. Postural balance and imbalance. In: Peterson B, ed. *1983 AAO Yearbook.* Newark, Ohio: American Academy of Osteopathy; 1983:76–82.

8. Fernand R, Fox DE. Evaluation of lumbar lordosis: a prospective and retrospective study. *Spine.* 1985;10(9):799–803.

9. Kuchera ML, Gitlin R, Frey-Gitlin K. Aging, lumbar lordosis and low back pain. *JAOA.* 1992;92(9):1182.

Osteopathic Considerations in Health Restoration

75. Treatment of the Acutely Ill Hospitalized Patient

KAREN M. STEELE

Key Concepts

- **Osteopathic examination of acutely ill hospitalized patients, including history and physical examination**

- **Treatment of hospitalized patients, including special cases**

- **Recording diagnosis and treatment on hospital charts**

- **Follow-up evaluation and treatment**

- **Osteopathic consults in the hospital**

The dynamic interaction between anatomy and physiology in the development of illness was summarized by Dr. Andrew Taylor Still in the following statement: *"Disease is the result of anatomical abnormalities followed by physiological discord."*[1] By using manipulative treatment, the osteopathic physician can alter this interaction in the medically compromised, hospitalized patient. This is accomplished by treatment of somatic dysfunction to:

Alter visceral and somatic function
Normalize neurologic control
Improve arterial circulation
Improve venous and lymphatic drainage

The correlation between dysfunction of the musculoskeletal system and visceral disease has been well-documented by many.[2–18] Osteopathic manipulative diagnosis and treatment offer a practical mechanism by which the somatovisceral and viscerosomatic reflexes can be reduced, thus facilitating recovery. An afferent impulse from a dysfunctional viscera may manifest itself in facilitation of its related motor and autonomic spinal cord segments, producing contraction, spasm, and trophic changes at the segmental area involved. This afferent input with resulting facilitation is the basis for a viscerosomatic reflex. The reflex may also manifest itself as hyperalgesia of the myofascial tissues or skin at the corresponding vertebral segments. Pottenger describes this in his second law:

Every important internal viscus is so connected in the central nervous system that it is able to produce reflexes through afferent sympathetic and efferent spinal nerves, with definite skeletal structures; and if acutely inflamed, trophic changes. Therefore, spasm

of muscles, altered cutaneous sensation and degeneration of muscles, subcutaneous tissue and skin, in areas having definite limited segmental innervation become important diagnostic phenomena.[19]

These alterations in cutaneous sensation, subcutaneous tissue, skin, and spasm of muscles have been termed "tissue texture changes" by Larson.[8] The level at which these changes are clinically palpated generally correspond to a spinal level. This is the level of the cell bodies that originate in the sympathetic efferents of the diseased viscus. The levels of this association have been reviewed by Beal[20] and are an important part of the osteopathic palpatory examination and treatment.

OSTEOPATHIC EXAMINATION OF THE HOSPITALIZED PATIENT

History

Begin the osteopathic history of the hospitalized patient with a review of the medical record, paying close attention to factors affecting or affected by the neuromusculoskeletal system. Next, take the patient's history. If the patient is unable to give the history because of age, neurologic damage, intubation, or other causes, ask a family member to provide the history. The history for the neuromusculoskeletal evaluation includes the routine medical history, in addition to questioning the patient or family member about previous injuries and structural abnormalities. Typically, the following are included in the patient's history:

Head trauma
Motor vehicle accidents
Pratfalls
Fractures
Episodes of loss of consciousness
Presence of known short leg
Scoliosis
Previous experience with osteopathic manipulative treatment (OMT)
Previous experience with other manual medicine modalities
Response to previous treatments

The historical data assists in deciding which musculoskeletal areas might contain primary somatic dysfunction and/or which might contain secondary somatic dysfunction produced by somatovisceral reflexes from related visceral dysfunction. The history also assists in deciding which manipulative techniques are most appropriate.

Figure 75.1.   ASIS compression test.

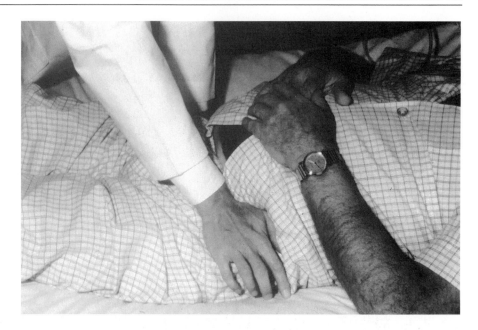

Physical Examination

Begin the examination with a review of the patient's original radiographs. This is extremely important because bony and fascial abnormalities significant to the patient's disease process may not have been mentioned in the radiology report. Only after review of the chart, review of the original radiographs, and recording of an integrated history is the physician prepared to perform a physical examination of the patient. As with the history, integrate the osteopathic palpatory examination into the routine medical examination of the patient. The history and chief complaint dictate that some areas of the body must be more thoroughly investigated than others. It is generally easier to use a standard approach to the patient that can be modified slightly to fit each individual patient's needs. Follow routine body fluid contamination procedures during the examination of all patients.

The following protocol is suggested, although alterations are necessary depending on the patient's needs and the physician's preference. This protocol is based primarily on the respiratory, circulatory, and neurologic models of osteopathic evaluation and treatment.[21–22] Emphasize the major diaphragms of the body that impede normal fluid flow, and the bony and fascial attachments of those diaphragms. Emphasize rib function because of its relationship both to fluid movement within the body and to reflexes mediated by the sympathetic nervous system via the chain ganglia that lie anterior to the rib heads. Emphasize the paraspinal myofascial elements of the suboccipital, sacral, and thoracolumbar areas because of their involvement with autonomic reflexes that manifest in these areas.

If the patient is ambulatory, the musculoskeletal examination is not significantly different from an outpatient structural evaluation. However, the routine outpatient musculoskeletal examination is not appropriate for acutely ill patients. A bedside osteopathic evaluation in the supine position is necessary.

The examination begins with bilateral compression of the anterior superior iliac spines (ASIS), an ASIS compression test. This test indicates restrictions in iliosacral mobility that interfere with sacral and pubic motion, and pelvic diaphragm tension (Fig. 75.1).

Evaluate and treat the sacrum and lumbar areas from the patient's side. Generally, the patient is lying on an absorbent pad over a draw-sheet and fitted mattress sheet. The sacrum and lumbar areas are easily approached by slipping the hands under the patient, palms up, between the draw-sheet and the fitted mattress sheet. This is made easier by loosening the draw-sheet from under the mattress and rolling it up parallel to the patient on either side of the bed (Fig. 75.2). This rolled-up draw-sheet serves as a sling with which the patient can be gently lifted and rolled away, enabling the physician to place a hand under the pelvic or lumbar area without any effort required by the patient. Although this treatment procedure requires palpating and treating through the thickness of the absorbent pad and draw-sheet, it becomes easy with practice. This approach also protects the patient's modesty, and the physician is less likely to come into contact with any discharge, drainage, urine, or feces in the bed.

Next, place the fingertips of one hand at the inferolateral angle of the sacrum and the fingertips of the other hand at the ipsilateral sacral base (Fig. 75.3). Exert alternate pressure in an anterior direction with the fingertips, ascertaining the ability of the sacrum to "rock" on its L-shaped articulation. This procedure reveals sacral motion restrictions.

Next, place one or both hands under the patient's lumbar spine, and assess the tissue texture changes and motion restrictions of the lumbar spine according to the protocol suggested by Larson.[8] This is carried out by pressing anteriorly on the paraspinal elements. First note tissue texture changes, then note any ease in rotatory motion induced by using an alternating

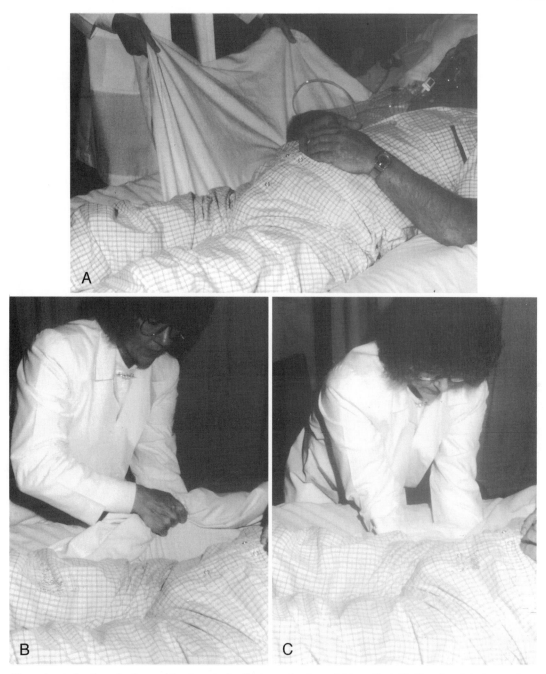

Figure 75.2. Draw-sheet sling for palpation and treatment of patient posteriorly. **A,** Loosen draw-sheet from under mattress. **B,** Roll draw-sheet parallel to patient. **C,** Place hands between draw-sheet and mattress to contact lumbar areas.

anterior pressure on the transverse processes. The characteristic texture changes resulting from viscerosomatic referral are most easily discerned with the patient supine, and with the examiner executing anterior palpatory pressure. With the patient relaxed as much as possible, estimate the degree of lumbar lordosis.

If the patient is not in the immediate postoperative period after abdominal or pelvic surgery, palpate the abdomen for visceral dysfunction. Assess restrictions of the thoracoabdominal diaphragm by placing one hand under the patient at the T10-L2 area posteriorly, and the other hand anteriorly, just

inferior to the xiphoid process. One hand gently twists the underlying fascia clockwise while the other hand twists counterclockwise; then, reverse the direction of testing. The abdominal diaphragm dysfunction is named according to the direction of preferred fascial movement sensed by the abdominal hand.

Assess the excursion of the lower and upper ribs by having the patient breathe deeply. Lightly palpate the rib cage at the midaxillary line for the lower ribs. Palpate over the midclavicular line lateral to the sternum for the upper ribs. If the patient

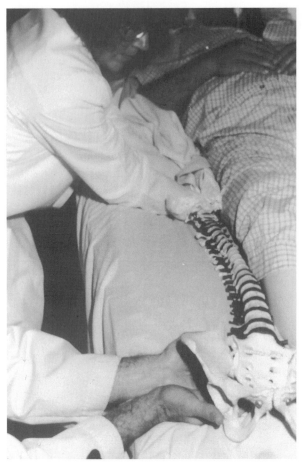

Figure 75.3. Sacral rocking.

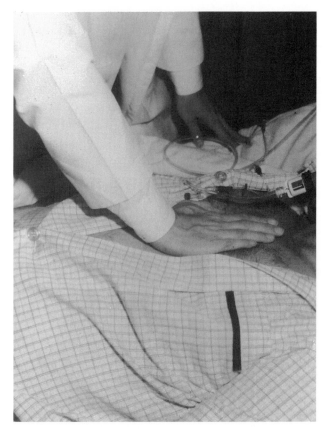

Figure 75.4. Sternal palpation.

has a chest tube in place or is on a respirator, follow the motion present by lightly resting hands on the rib cage. Gently rest the palpating hand on the sternum and follow its motion, noting any fascial pulls and any costosternal articular restrictions (Fig. 75.4). Perform a screen of the anterior Chapman's[23] and Jones points[24] in the thoracic and abdominal areas. Note any specific rib restrictions so that they can be treated later. Note the symmetry of the thorax and tension of the accessory muscles of respiration.

Adjust the bed to place the patient in the Fowler's position (approximately 15° head elevation), elevating the mattress until it is even with the top of the headboard. Move to the head of the bed and remove the patient's pillow. This positioning allows treatment with minimal stooping, and without removing the headboard. If the Fowler's position is contraindicated, the entire bed may be elevated. The bed may need to be pushed away from the wall to permit access to the head of the bed. Be careful not to disturb peripheral and central lines, suction tubing, urinary catheters, etc. Follow this same procedure in the intensive care unit as well. If the patient is on a respirator, treat him or her in the position dictated by the life support systems.

Standing and leaning over the head of the bed, place a hand on each side of the patient's head, palms facing upward, and glide them between the draw-sheet and the bed, or between

the bed sheet and the mattress, down to the T12-L2 area of the patient's back (Fig. 75.5). With elbows leaning on the head of the bed for support, place the fingertips over the transverse processes. Push anteriorly with the fingertips of both hands, assessing first the tissue texture changes. Then, push alternately to assess the rotatory motion of the paraspinal elements. This is the same assessment used for the lumbar area. Move the hands more cephalad and repeat the process until the entire thoracic spine has been evaluated. Also note fascial restrictions of the thorax, and further define rib somatic dysfunction noted on the rib motion screening examination. Place the fingertips of the anterior hand against the costochondral junction, and those of the posterior hand at the rib head of the same rib (Fig. 75.6).

Next, evaluate the thoracic inlet for fascial restrictions (Fig. 75.7). If the patient has any central venous lines, the hand on that side must be placed more laterally, near the acromioclavicular joint. The presence of these lines does not contraindicate evaluating and treating this area but makes it even more imperative that it be evaluated. Evaluate the cervical area for the presence of somatic dysfunction.

Assess the suboccipital area for condylar compression and occipitoatlantal (OA) and atlantoaxial (AA) somatic dysfunction (Fig. 75.8). Gently cradle the head and upper cervical area with the fingertips and hands. If craniosacral diagnosis is to be performed, the cranium is now palpated for somatic dysfunction. The cranium can be evaluated with many hand positions. In one position(Fig. 75.9), the palms and fingertips gently rest on the head with thumbs at the vertex or off the head, index fingers at the area of the great wing of the sphenoid bone, middle and ring fingers on either side of the ear, and little fingers on the occiput. The bed is in Fowler's position, and the physician is resting his or her elbows on the head of the bed for support.

At this point, the neuromusculoskeletal system of the patient has been assessed, including:

1. *Sympathetic nervous system:* evidence of somatic dysfunction associated with the sympathetic nervous system is indicated by

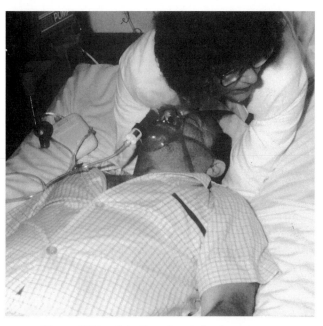

Figure 75.5. Palpation of posterior thoracic area.

palpation of the thoracic and upper lumbar area (spinal levels of origin of the sympathetic nervous system) for viscerosomatic and articular restrictions, and of the rib cage for restrictions affecting or being affected by the sympathetic chain ganglia.

2. *Parasympathetic nervous system:* evidence of somatic dysfunction associated with the parasympathetic nervous system is indicated by palpation of the sacral, suboccipital, and cranial areas (its central nervous system site of origin).

3. *Lymphatic system:* evidence of dysfunction affecting lymphatic flow is indicated by assessing the four major diaphragms of the body (pelvic, thoracoabdominal, thoracic inlet, and foramen magnum) and rib motion.

4. *Visceral dysfunction:* visceral dysfunction is reflected by positive anterior Chapman's points, visceral palpation (when possible), and spinal somatic dysfunction that may be related to facilitated segments.

5. *Structural component:* asymmetries and abnormalities of the cervical, thoracic, rib, and pelvic areas affect optimal functioning of the autonomic and lymphatic systems.

TREATMENT OF THE HOSPITALIZED PATIENT

General Considerations

When treating the hospitalized patient, remember that the patient is acutely ill. The treatment goal is to promote homeostasis and the body's ability to heal itself. Each intervention performed requires energy from that patient to incorporate the changes induced into that person's body by the manipulation. Therefore, treat only those dysfunctions that impede the homeostatic processes. Leave long-standing or unrelated problems for outpatient care. Norman Larson put it this way: *"The acutely ill patient can only take so much of a dose, don't waste your manipulative effects on areas of the body that do not require your immediate attention"* (Larson N. Personal communication from WA Kuchera to K Steele). For example, a short leg and mild functional scoliosis may not need to be addressed during

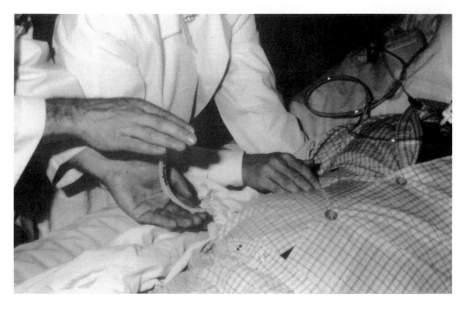

Figure 75.6. Individual rib evaluation and treatment position.

Figure 75.7. Thoracic inlet evaluation and treatment position.

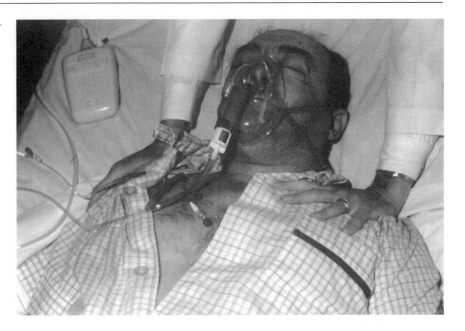

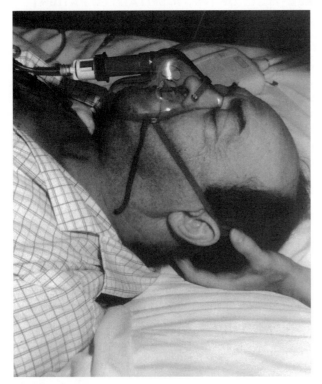

Figure 75.8. Suboccipital evaluation and treatment position.

a hospitalization for pneumonia unless they contribute to impaired homeostasis during the acute illness. The short leg, though it may be a contributing factor in lowering the patient's resistance to infections and trauma, can usually be evaluated after recovery from the acute incident.

Alterations in tissue texture changes are helpful in following the patient's medical progress. The presence of new tissue texture changes at a given level alerts a physician to possible early organ dysfunction. Likewise, resolution of the viscerosomatic reflex indicates improved health in that area. One notable exception occurs when treating extremely compromised patients. The severely ill patient whose vital resources or immune system has been exhausted will fail to show tissue texture changes that should, in fact, be present considering the site of the organ dysfunction. In these patients, the presence of new tissue texture change in areas that are appropriate for that patient's illness may be a favorable sign.

When formulating a manipulative prescription[25] for an inpatient osteopathic treatment, determine the duration. As a rule, the sicker the patient, the shorter the treatment should be. A patient in the intensive care unit can generally tolerate only 5–15 minutes of osteopathic treatment. Treat only those areas most likely to impair the recovery process, considering both lymphatic flow and autonomic balance.

Treatment frequency also varies according to the patient's condition. Generally, the sicker the patient, the more often the physician should provide OMT. This usually means once daily, although some literature suggests more frequent application.[26–28] As the patient improves, the interval between treatments and the treatment duration may be lengthened if needed. When a hospitalized patient can tolerate 3 or 4 days between treatments, the manipulative treatments may essentially be provided on an intensive outpatient schedule. Psychiatric inpatients and those in drug and alcohol inpatient treatment programs may require a different schedule, and are discussed separately.

If the patient is unfamiliar with osteopathic treatments, especially those given at the bedside, briefly explain the philosophy and reason for the OMT. A simple explanation seems to work best, such as: "There are nerves from your spine that go to both the back muscles and the organs inside. When an internal organ is sick, a reflex is created that causes your back muscles to get tense. By treating your back, the reflex is calmed so that the organs can heal faster." Or you might say, "When you have pneumonia (or congestive heart failure, etc.), the fluids in your body pool in your lungs, making your illness worse. Your ribs don't move normally either, making it more difficult to get rid of this fluid. The osteopathic treatment will help your ribs work more normally, and help pump the fluids out of your lungs."

Further answers may be provided if the patient expresses an interest. Usually, however, the patient simply relaxes with the physician's soothing touch, and no further explanations are needed.

For any medically ill, hospitalized patient, the presence of somatic dysfunction in areas that impede normal autonomic or lymphatic functioning can and should be treated. The patient's disease process dictates the areas to treat and the techniques to use. This discussion uses the generalizations in Table 75.1 concerning levels of autonomic innervation.[29–30]

Treatment Protocol

Decide which areas most impair the patient's homeostatic balance, which techniques are best suited for the patient, and how much of a treatment the patient can tolerate. In other words, make a manipulative prescription.[22] A general rule of thumb is to select three or four principle areas for treatment that are most relevant to the patient's recovery. Additional areas may be added, depending on the response of the patient. In this way, the patient is not overtreated, and no important areas are missed. Hospital patients typically respond to a limited dose of osteopathic treatment, but they also need to be treated more often. As they recover, they become more like outpatients in their tolerance for the treatment and the duration of the treatment response.

Table 75.2 outlines a means of deciding which areas to treat

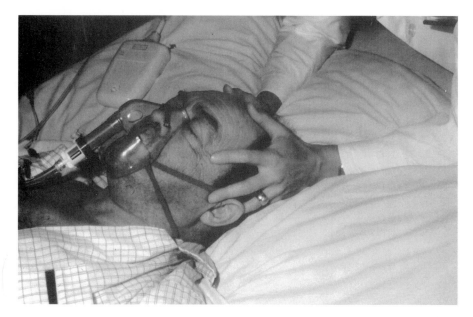

Figure 75.9. Cranial evaluation with vault hold position.

Table 75.1
Summary of Autonomic Innervations

Nerve	Area Treated	Body Area Affected
Parasympathetic		
III, VII, IX, X	Cranial	Head and neck, thorax, right half of GI tract
Vagus X, IX	OA, AA, C2, occipitomastoid suture	Head, neck (parotid, tongue, pharynx), thorax; hepatic flexure or midtransverse colon
S2–S4	Sacrum, innominate	Left half of colon and pelvis
Sympathetic		
Cord and sympathetic chain	T1–T5	Head, neck, thorax
	T2–T8	Upper extremity
	T5–T9	Upper GI, digestive organs
	T10–T11	Small intestines, gonads, and adrenals
	T10–L2	Kidney, lower extremity
	T12–L2	Left colon, pelvic organs, and lower extremity

in three typical types of inpatients: postsurgical or trauma, medical illness, and newborn feeding disorder or colic. Select one or two techniques to affect each of the following areas:

Sympathetic
Parasympathetic
Lymphatic
Visceral or structural

This method of selecting techniques yields six to eight techniques per treatment session. By following this table, important autonomic, lymphatic, visceral, and structural components relevant to the patient's recovery are evaluated and treated. The process can then be extrapolated to any type of patient, remembering to consider the autonomic, lymphatic, visceral, and structural components of each patient's disease process and recovery.

Some manipulative techniques appropriate in one situation may not be appropriate in another. For example, for a patient with fractures, avoid any treatment positioning that could destabilize the fracture site. A patient in the intensive care unit with a myocardial infarction generally should not receive techniques using isometric patient contractions. The decision of where and why to treat the patient lies with the physician and is part of the medical decision-making process.

Special Considerations

ACQUIRED IMMUNE DEFICIENCY SYNDROME PATIENTS

Persons with acquired immune deficiency syndrome (AIDS) who are hospitalized should be treated manipulatively with the same rational and systemic approach as all hospitalized patients. The nature of the disease process for which they have been hospitalized dictates which areas should be treated manipulatively and the intensity, duration, and frequency of the treatment. Routine body fluid precautions should be taken, as with all patients. If the patient is in isolation, special precautions are necessary, as discussed below.

Table 75.2
Protocol for Treatment of Patients after Surgery or Trauma[a]

Type of Patient	Area	Technique
Postsurgical/trauma patient		
Thoracic (i.e., thoracotomy, rib fracture, chest drainage tube, etc.)		
Sympathetic	T1–T5	PI, CS, DA
Parasympathetic	OA, cranium	Suboccipital ST, cranial,[b] CS, DA
Lymphatic	TI, abd. diaphragm	MR, RR, DA (no vigorous lymphatic pumps)
Other	Viscera	Visceral[c]
Abdominal surgery (i.e., cholecystectomy, bowel resection, etc.)		
Sympathetic	T1–T5	PI (to decrease respiratory complications), RR, CS, DA
	T5–T9	PI (if upper GI surgery), RR, CS, DA
	T10–L2	PI (to decrease ileus), RR, CS, DA
Parasympathetic	OA, cranium	Suboccipital ST, cranial,[b] CS, DA
	Sacrum	Sacral rocking (see Fig. 75.11), CS, DA
Lymphatic	TI–T12	RR, CS, DA
	Thoracic inlet, abd. diaphragm	MR, DA
Other	Viscera	Visceral[c]
Medical patient (i.e., MI, pneumonia, peritonitis, etc.)		
Sympathetic	T1–T5	PI, CS, DA
Parasympathetic	OA, cranium	Suboccipital ST, cranial,[b] CS, DA
Lymphatic	TI–T12	RR
	Thoracic inlet, abd. diaphragm	MR, lymphatic pump, DA
Other	a. respiratory muscles, rib; b. abdomen	a. ST, MR, CS, DA; b. ST, mesenteric release (to decrease sluggish bowel function), visceral[c]
Newborn infant feeding disorder/colic		
	Suboccipital area	ST, condylar decompression (to improve sucking and swallowing), reduce irritability[b]

PI, paraspinal inhibition; CS, counterstrain; DA, direct action (muscle energy, articular, etc.); OA, occipitoatlantal; ST, soft tissue; TI, thoracic inlet; abd. diaphragm, abdominal diaphragm; MR, myofascial release; RR, rib raising.

[a]This table is organized to encourage a thoughtful approach to treatment. It is time-efficient and does not miss treatment of critical areas. The protocol is organized under the headings of Sympathetic, Parasympathetic, Lymphatic, and Other for each area. The physician is encouraged to pick one or two techniques for each of the three functions to be assisted with OMT, yielding 3–6 techniques for each treatment encounter.

[b]For recommendations of appropriate cranial techniques indicated for patients with various medical illnesses, refer to *Osteopathy in the Cranial Field*,[33] *Craniosacral Therapy*,[38] or other texts on cranial technique.

[c]For recommendations of appropriate visceral techniques, see Barral JP, Mercier P. *Visceral Manipulation*. Seattle, Wash: Eastland Press; 1988.

DRUG AND ALCOHOL DETOXIFICATION AND REHABILITATION PATIENTS

During drug or alcohol detoxification, the patient is not usually responsive to OMT. After the detoxification has been completed, OMT is helpful in aiding the recovery process. Most patients undergoing drug or alcohol treatment have a long history of trauma and/or abuse. OMT should address the lasting effects of that trauma on the musculoskeletal, emotional, and cranial systems. These patients are usually treated one or two times in the first week, and then weekly as needed. Any medical or surgical conditions are treated according to the protocol for the condition as described earlier (Table 75.2).

OMT in the inpatient psychiatric or drug/alcohol treatment setting is generally more effective than treatment of the same patient as an outpatient. Presumably, the intensive setting, where nutrition, medication, exercise, peer support, situation control, and counseling are structured into the patient's existence, allows an increased recovery rate in the entire person (mind, body, and spirit). OMT is extremely effective in this optimal setting.[18]

INTENSIVE CARE UNIT AND RESPIRATOR PATIENTS

Request assistance when moving a patient in the bed or changing the bed position so as not to endanger the stability of any drainage, intravenous, arterial, endotracheal, or feeding tubes. Patients on respirators can and should be treated manipulatively. Avoid techniques that interfere with the respiratory rate, such as the pedal pump or classic lymphatic pump.

ISOLATION PATIENTS

If the patient has been placed in some form of isolation, requirements for gloves, gown, and mask must be followed. Palpatory examination and OMT with gloves are not ideal, but protection is necessary. For patients with profuse secretions, it is wise to use gloves even if there are no isolation protocols ordered. During the treatment, position yourself and the patient in a manner that will reduce your chances of becoming infected.

PEDIATRIC PATIENTS

Newborns occasionally need treatment in the nursery for cranial entrapment neuropathies resulting in colic and feeding disorders.[31] These conditions can often be relieved by simple, gentle, condylar decompression.

Treatment of pediatric patients for medical illnesses such as pneumonia and OMT for infants postoperatively involve the same processes used for treating adults. The techniques recommended, however, are usually articular or myofascial approaches. One treatment for children described by Max Gutensohn (personal communication) enables the physician to articulate vertebral levels and encourage lymphatic flow simultaneously, while seemingly playing a game with the child. This is especially nice for assisting recovery from respiratory disease.

The child is held in the air with the physician's hands encircling the child's chest under the axillae. The legs are then gently swung in a circle, thereby mobilizing the area just distal to the hands on the torso. To articulate other areas, hold the child higher or lower on the torso.

POSTOPERATIVE OR POSTTRAUMA PATIENTS

When treating postoperative patients who are in the hospital, avoid excessive jiggling and overhead arm techniques. Techniques such as the lymphatic pump with arms overhead or vigorous pedal pump may endanger the stability of the operative site or injury.

PSYCHIATRIC PATIENTS

The osteopathic premise states that the body is a unit, with mind, body, and spirit as interwoven parts of one being. This supports the concept of treating a patient with psychiatric illness to improve functioning of the rest of the body. If the psychiatric patient is hospitalized for a medical or surgical condition, he or she is treated for that condition following the protocols described earlier (Table 75.2). Patients who are hospitalized for their psychiatric disease also deserve an osteopathic structural evaluation and manipulative treatment if indicated.

The structural examination should closely evaluate the cranial sacral mechanism and the upper thoracic regions, looking for evidence of somatic dysfunctions that could be produced by autonomic reflexes. Older literature makes a strong case for dysautonomia as a significant factor in psychiatric disease, based in part on clinical observations at the Still-Hildreth Osteopathic Hospital. Dunn discusses the association of autonomic dysfunction with psychiatric disease, and supports this association with data from 1000 psychiatric patients. More than 50% of these patients demonstrated palpable somatic dysfunction at C2 and T4-T6 paravertebral regions of the spine.[32] In 2288 examinations, Woods demonstrated an altered rate of the cranial rhythmic impulse in various psychiatric diseases, as compared with controls.[33]

In addition to calming autonomic reflexes, the calming effect of manipulation also helps in the treatment of the psychiatric patient. Psychiatric patients generally do not tolerate high-velocity low-amplitude techniques well. Use a soothing treatment approach and a slow, gentle touch.[34] When psychiatric patients are receiving electroconvulsive shock treatments (ECTs), OMT within 24 hours of a treatment event is not generally productive. Providing OMT on the day following ECT, however, is often extremely effective. Osteopathic treatment of the cranial and pelvic areas is especially important for these patients.[35]

OMT may be contraindicated for some psychiatric patients. A paranoid schizophrenic patient may interpret a hands-on treatment modality as threatening and usually does not tolerate it well. Touch may be misinterpreted by patients having difficulty differentiating fantasy from reality. For patients with a history of abuse, the manipulative treatment may be seen as a sexual advance or assault. In rare cases, the physician may decide against the manipulative treatment because of concerns of personal safety.

As with all patients, the benefits of osteopathic treatment for psychiatric patients must be weighed against its potential adverse outcomes. Most psychiatric patients tolerate the treatment extremely well and respond to treatment quickly in inpatient settings.

Recording Osteopathic Diagnosis and Treatment on the Hospital Chart

Following a session with a patient, the following must be recorded in the hospital chart:

History
Physical examination (including the osteopathic diagnoses)
Treatment plan
Treatment provided

A protocol for adequately recording an osteopathic structural examination is outlined by the American Osteopathic Association in the Accreditation Requirements for Acute Care Hospitals[36] and is used in hospital credentialing. Each hospital may also have individual guidelines for the recording of osteopathic structural examinations.

In general, the following should be included in the recorded neuromusculoskeletal examination:

Position(s) in which the patient was examined
Notation of asymmetries of the spine, ribs, head, shoulders, and extremities noted by visual examination or palpation
Results of screening the range of motion of the spine and extremities
Location of tissue texture changes
Any other relevant positive or negative findings from the neuromusculoskeletal examination, as described above
Correlation of the musculoskeletal examination with the chief complaint(s)

FOLLOW-UP EVALUATION AND TREATMENT

Begin the follow-up examination with a review of any new radiographs, followed by a review of the medical record since the last evaluation. Take an interval history. Perform the physical examination following the protocol described above, noting any changes in response to the previous treatment or in the disease process.

The areas to be treated may change at every visit and are determined by the interval history and physical examination. The tolerance for a longer treatment generally increases as the patient improves. The intervals between treatments are also usually increased as the patient improves.

OSTEOPATHIC CONSULT

All osteopathic physicians are trained to provide osteopathic diagnosis and treatment for their patients. Some osteopathic physicians, with additional training and skill, elect to provide this service on a consultation basis for other physicians. In this case, the physician becomes a consultant in osteopathic manipulative medicine (OMM) to the patient's attending physician. Most hospitals require that physicians serving as consultants go through a credentialing process and be granted privileges in their area of specialty. This credentialing also applies to OMM.

The Consult

The OMM consultant becomes involved with a patient's care when the attending physician writes an order requesting an OMM consult. The order should state the reason for the consult, specifying either the specific patient complaint (e.g., headache) or the organ system or disease to be evaluated. This order may be written as a consultation only, or as an order to consult and treat manipulatively as indicated ("Consult regarding left lower lobe pneumonia with OMT as indicated"). If the order does not also specify for the consultant to "treat the patient if indicated," the consultant provides only an examination and recommendations for treatment. In most cases, the attending physician also specifies that treatment is requested. The attending physician may sometimes specify a certain number of treatments, essentially dictating part of the manipulative prescription. However, the consultant is the one performing the procedure (OMT); the burden of actually formulating the manipulative prescription rests on that physician's shoulders.

As in the process described earlier, the OMM consult begins with a review of the patient's radiographs and medical record, with special notation of findings that relate to the neuromusculoskeletal, fascial, and visceral systems. The osteopathic physician then evaluates the patient for the presence of somatic dysfunction of the neuromusculoskeletal, fascial, and visceral systems, and determines its relevance to the disease process for which the patient has been hospitalized. If the attending physician does not request treatment, the consultant is ready to write the consultation. If the attending physician also orders "treatment if indicated," the consultant is obliged to determine if treatment is indicated. If so, the consultant proceeds with the OMT of the patient, following the treatment protocol described earlier.

After the examination and treatment (if ordered and indicated) are completed, a consult is written in the medical record. Usually, a specially designated sheet is provided for the consultant's written summary, which includes impressions and recommendations. A summary is written so that it can be immediately used by the attending physician; the full report is then dictated. A written note should also be made in the progress note section stating that a consult was completed, including the date and time. If the results of the examination or treatment indicate a clinical need for immediate information, the consultant should also contact the attending physician directly and discuss the patient's case.

The dictated OMM consultation should contain the following:

1. Date and time of the consult.
2. Name of the attending physician, reason for consult request, and whether the patient's chart and x-rays were reviewed.
3. Statement that a history was taken from the patient (or family member), and a written summary of findings.
4. Statement of the positions in which the patient was examined ("was examined in the sitting, supine, and lateral recumbent position," or "examined in the supine position only due to presence of an endotracheal tube"), and the results of the patient's physical examination.
5. Impressions. Generally, the consultant limits his or her diagnoses to somatic dysfunctions. Also include any other diagnoses that are directly related to the somatic dysfunction and the disease process, and the viscerosomatic and somatovisceral reflexes. The consultant is functioning as an OMM specialist, not assuming other parts of the patient's medical management.
6. Recommendations. This includes the manipulative prescription if OMT is indicated, and recommendations for x-rays, further evaluations, and treatment modalities relevant to the consult.
7. Treatment given, if any. Areas treated, techniques used, and the patient's response to treatment are recorded here. Use standard nomenclature as defined in the Glossary of Osteopathic Terminology.
8. Follow-up recommendations.
9. "Thank you" to the requesting physician for the consult.
10. Request that the original consult be placed in the medical chart and that photocopies of the consult be sent to the attending and consulting physicians.

Follow-up

Follow-up consultations are performed at the request of the attending physician or if the consultant feels that a reevaluation is indicated. The protocol is essentially the same as the initial consultation, with the exception that radiograph and chart reviews are only necessary from the date of the initial consultation.

Follow-up treatment is provided at the consultant's discretion if he or she has been asked to participate in the patient's care. In this case, the consultant is then seeing the patient as an established patient and no longer as a consultant. The protocol for follow-up treatment is described in the section "Follow-Up Evaluation and Treatment."

CONCLUSION

Osteopathic manipulative treatment has been shown clinically to effectively improve vegetative functioning, leading to an enhanced rate of healing in acutely ill patients. With the advent of sophisticated medicines for the treatment of specific diseases, the appreciation of osteopathic manipulative treatment as a treatment modality for visceral disease waned. However, appreciation of its efficacy has experienced a resurgence as patients are demanding both "high tech and high touch." The

osteopathic physician is uniquely able to assist in all of these demands, to the benefit of the acutely ill hospitalized patient.

ACKNOWLEDGMENTS

Appreciation is expressed to Mr. Lowell Jackson for allowing photography of an actual inpatient osteopathic treatment for educational purposes, and to Richard Koss, DO, for assisting in the treatment and photography. Appreciation is also expressed to Ross Carlson, DO, for his assistance in the research and writing of this chapter, and to William A. Kuchera, DO, FAAO, for his development of the three-part approach to the osteopathic evaluation and treatment of patients with medical illness (i.e., sympathetic, parasympathetic, and lymphatic areas) and for his invaluable critique of this chapter.

REFERENCES

1. Still AT. *Research and Practice.* Republished by American Academy of Osteopathy; 1910:15.
2. Burns L. Spinal lesions and their effects on viscera. *The Western Osteopath.* October 1927:13–20.
3. MacFarlane Tilley RM, Young GS, Eble JN. *Practical Aspects of Viscera Somatic Reflex Interchange with Special Reference to Surgery.* Carmel, Calif: Academy of Applied Osteopathy; 1959:9–19.
4. Koch RS. A somatic component in heart disease. *JAOA.* May 1961; 60:735–740.
5. Henshaw RE. Manipulation and postoperative pulmonary complications. *The D.O. Precepts & Practice.* September 1963:132–133.
6. Nicholas NS. Correlation of somatic dysfunction with visceral disease. *JAOA.* December 1975:119–122 (75:425–428).
7. English W. The somatic component of colon disease. *Osteopath Ann.* April 1976:13–22.
8. Larson N. Summary of site and occurrence of paraspinal soft tissue changes in the intensive care unit. *JAOA.* May 1976:117–119 (75:840–842).
9. Larson N. Manipulative care before and after surgery. *Osteopath Med.* January 1977:41–49.
10. Stiles EG. Somatic dysfunction in hospital practice. *Osteopath Ann.* January 1979:35–38.
11. Stiles EG. Fitzgerald M, staff writer. Indiana convention report: osteopathic hospitals' solutions to DRGs may be OMT. *DO.* November 1984:97–101.
12. TePorten BA. Insight osteopathic management: spinal palpatory diagnosis of visceral disease. *Osteopath Med.* August 1979:52–53.
13. Beal MC. Palpatory testing for somatic dysfunction in patients with cardiovascular disease. *JAOA.* July 1983:73–82 (82:822–831).
14. Cox JM, Gorbis S, Dick LM, Rogers JC, Rogers FJ. Palpable musculoskeletal findings in coronary artery disease. Results of double-blind study. *JAOA.* July 1983:86–90 (82:832–836).
15. Rogers F, Glassman J, Kavieff R. Osteopathic techniques: effects of osteopathic manipulative treatment on autonomic nervous systems function in patients with congestive heart failure. *JAOA.* September 1986:122 (86:605).
16. Nicholas AS, England RW, Greene CH, Heilig D, Kirschbaum M. A somatic component to myocardial infarction. *JAOA.* February 1987:62–68 (87:123–129).
17. Sato A. Reflex modulation of visceral functions by somatic afferent activity. In: Patterson MM, Howell JN, eds. *The Central Connection: Somatovisceral/Viscerosomatic Interaction, 1989 International Symposium.* Athens, Ohio: University Classics Ltd; 1992:53–72. Published by the American Academy of Osteopathy.

18. de Groat WC. Viscerosomatic interactions and neuroplasticity in the reflex pathways controlling lower urinary tract function. In: Patterson MM, Howell JN, eds. *The Central Connection: Somatovisceral/Viscerosomatic Interaction: 1989 International Symposium.* Athens, Ohio: University Classics, LTD; 1992:91–110.

19. Pottenger FM. *Symptoms of Visceral Disease: A Study of the Vegetative Nervous System in Its Relationship to Clinical Medicine.* 6th ed. St. Louis, Mo: CV Mosby; 1944:193.

20. Beal MC. Viscerosomatic reflexes: a review. *JAOA.* December 1985; 85(12):53–68.

21. Hruby RJ. Pathophysiologic models: aids to the selection of manipulative techniques. *JAAO.* 1991;1(3):8–10.

22. Zink JG. Respiratory and circulatory care: the conceptual model. *Osteopath Ann.* 1987;10:108–111.

23. Owens C. *An Endocrine Interpretation of Chapman's Reflexes.* Carmel, Calif: American Academy of Osteopathy; 1963.

24. Jones L. *Strain Counterstrain.* Newark, Ohio: American Academy of Osteopathy; 1981.

25. Kuchera WA, Kuchera ML. *Osteopathic Principles in Practice.* rev. 2nd ed. Columbus, Ohio: Greyden Press; 1994:297–302.

26. Herrmann EP. Postoperative adynamic ileus: its prevention and treatment by osteopathic manipulation. *The DO. Precepts & Practice.* October 1965:163–164.

27. Young GS. *Post-operative Osteopathic Manipulation.* Colorado Springs, Colo: Academy of Applied Osteopathy Yearbook; 1970:77–82.

28. Rumney IC. Osteopathic manipulative treatment of infectious disease. *Osteopath Ann.* July 1974:29–33.

29. Beal MC. Viscerosomatic reflexes: a review. *JAOA.* December 1985; 85(12):53–68.

30. Kuchera WA, Kuchera ML. *Osteopathic Principles in Practice.* rev 2nd ed. Columbus, Ohio: Greyden Press; 1994:68–70.

31. Magoun HI. *Osteopathy in the Cranial Field.* 2nd ed. (completely rewritten) Kirksville, Mo: Journal Printing Co; 1966:234, 263.

32. Dunn FE. Osteopathic concepts in psychiatry. *JAOA.* March 1950; 49(7):354–357.

33. Woods JM, Woods RH. A physical finding related to psychiatric disorders. *JAOA.* August 1961;60:988–993.

34. Bradford, SG. Role of osteopathic manipulative therapy in emotional disorders—a physiologic hypothesis. *JAOA.* January 1965:64–73 (64:484–493).

35. Upledger JE, Vredevoogd JD. *Craniosacral Therapy.* Seattle, Wash: Eastland Press; 1983:268.

36. *Accreditation Requirements, Acute Care Hospitals.* Chicago, Ill: American Osteopathic Association; 1992:75–76.

76. Exercises and Recovery

ROBERT E. KAPPLER

Key Concepts

- **Detrimental and beneficial effects of exercise**

- **Different types of exercise and their purposes**

- **Difference between warm-up and stretching, and when each one is appropriate**

- **Different types of stretching**

- **How exercise can benefit a person with spinal somatic dysfunction problems**

- **How to perform the exercises described in this chapter**

- **Principles and terms used to write an exercise prescription, and how to write an exercise prescription**

This chapter presents information about exercises that is especially useful to primary care osteopathic physicians. To write meaningful and effective exercise prescriptions, it is necessary to:

Understand the terminology of exercise
Be familiar with various types of exercise
Understand the principles involved and objectives to be accomplished by the exercises prescribed

Some common exercises for back problems are presented in this chapter, along with a practical approach to exercises for other back pain patients. Important information on tailoring exercises to fit the patient's needs is also presented. This information enables a greater level of success in the management of patients with musculoskeletal problems.

ASPECTS OF EXERCISE

Beneficial Aspects

The following aspects of exercise are beneficial to the patient:

1. Exercise enhances joint stability and mobility.
2. Exercise maintains bone density and lean body weight.
3. Exercise is useful for decreasing anxiety and releasing tension.
4. Exercise is useful for reducing depression.
5. Exercise reverses the harmful effects of disuse syndrome and deconditioning.
6. Exercise is helpful in any weight loss program. Losing weight during a time when the patient cannot exercise is difficult.
7. Exercise elevates the level of functional capacity by enhancing physical conditioning and the quality of life. Exercise also improves self-esteem.

Detrimental Aspects

There are possible detrimental aspects to exercise, including the following:

1. Exercise may produce an endorphin high, leading to compulsive exercise behavior and physical side effects such as overuse syndromes.
2. In those addicted to an endorphin high, inability to exercise will cause depression.
3. In strain and overuse syndromes, improper exercise may cause or perpetuate musculoskeletal imbalance or dysfunction and may activate myofascial triggers.
4. Improper equipment, inadequate warm-up, unrealistic expectations, or frequent jarring may lead to musculoskeletal or visceral injury.
5. Excessive exercise may lead to amenorrhea in women who have associated very low body fat levels and poor body image.

Terms Associated with Exercise

Several important terms are used in the following discussions and prescriptions of exercise:

Agonist: a muscle that contracts to achieve a particular motion (prime mover)
Antagonist: a muscle that counteracts the action of another muscle, its agonist
Concentric contraction: the muscle shortens while developing tension (contracting)
Eccentric contraction: the muscle lengthens while developing tension (contracting)
Endurance: ability of muscles to contract repetitively without fatigue
Fatigue: weakening and loss of strength resulting from depletion of substrates and accumulation of byproducts
Isokinetic: a term used to describe exercises performed using equipment, which produces variable resistance and maintains a constant contraction velocity throughout the range of motion of a joint

Isotonic: a contraction that produces joint movement without a change in muscle tension (e.g., lifting weights)

Speed: primarily the result of fast-twitch muscle contractions

Strength or power: the amount of force generated by a muscle contraction over a given amount of time

Tonic muscle: a muscle that holds some continuous contraction to maintain posture or to oppose gravity (e.g., red slow-twitch muscles of the hamstrings or erector spinae that function aerobically)

TYPES OF EXERCISE

Flexibility/Stretching

Flexibility or stretching exercises are used to relax and lengthen or to reduce tension in tight muscles and fascia. Increased range of motion or increased freedom of motion are the goals.

Aerobic Exercise

Aerobic exercise develops, trains, and improves the cardiopulmonary system. Examples include running, cycling, and swimming. Oxygen is consumed at the same rate that the patient is ventilating; any muscle can act as an oxygen consumer. An effective exercise program for the average patient is to exercise for 20 minutes three times a week, which produces a significant increase of pulse rate during each exercise session.

The old formula for maximal heart rate with exercise was 220 minus age; 85% of this target rate was considered the appropriate maximum. Treadmill testing, especially for patients who are deconditioned or at risk, is used to identify a maximal heart rate for the patient being tested. Eighty-five percent of this maximum determined by treadmill testing is the proper level for increase of heart rate during exercise.

Recent studies show that 30 minutes per day of cumulative exercise is appropriate.[1] An example of cumulative exercise is two 10-minute and two 5-minute periods of exercise totaling 30 minutes.

Recently, there has been increasing interest in the application of prescribed aerobic exercise for the promotion and maintenance of general health. The benefits of exercise are supported by a large body of scientific information. The United States Public Health Service declared, *"Physical fitness and exercise is one of five priority areas in which improvement is expected to lead to substantial reduction in premature morbidity and mortality."*[2]

Most members of western industrialized societies remain sedentary at work and in their leisure time. Primary care providers are in a good position to encourage patients to become more active. It is important to educate patients about the benefits of aerobic activity and an active lifestyle. Exercise is essential in the prevention and treatment of coronary artery disease. Cross-sectional studies appear to support the hypothesis that individuals demonstrating increased levels of physical fitness have a more desirable cardiac risk profile and appear to be healthier.

The amount of exercise necessary is still under study. There are considerable data on the benefits of vigorous activity such as running, swimming, and cross-country skiing.[3–6] Public education has led many potential exercise patients to conclude that there is no training effect or benefit unless they can do a vigorous aerobic workout for at least 20 minutes per day. However, lower levels of activity do appear to offer a beneficial effect.[7]

There are risks involved when sedentary individuals and high-risk individuals suddenly start an exercise program. The American College of Sports Medicine (ACSM) has developed a system to classify risk factors for individuals based on age and underlying cardiac condition.[8] The three categories are:

1. "Apparently healthy individuals" without known cardiac risk factors or evidence of underlying disease
2. "Higher risk individuals" with one or more coronary risk factors
3. "Individuals with disease" who have known active cardiopulmonary or metabolic diseases or who have symptoms suggestive of underlying disease that have not yet been evaluated[9]

Chisholm et al.[9] have developed a self-administered set of seven questions known as the Physical Activity Readiness Questionnaire. On this questionnaire, individuals responding "yes" to any question should consult a physician before implementing an exercise program. Individuals classified as "higher risk" or "individuals with disease" in the sports medicine categories should be evaluated by a physician before beginning exercise.

The preexercise evaluation should include a focused history and a physical examination. The examination should attempt to identify abnormalities in the following systems:

Cardiopulmonary
Peripheral vascular
Musculoskeletal
Metabolic or endocrine

Although resting electrocardiograms are considered of no value, cardiac stress testing is necessary to evaluate the function of coronary arteries. Protocols for the evaluation of patients at risk are beyond the scope of this chapter but should not be ignored. The reader is referred to the ACSM guidelines for exercise testing and prescription.[10]

Musculoskeletal problems may prevent the patient from doing the aerobic exercise necessary to achieve the benefits. These factors may appear during the physical examination, or they may become apparent when the patient starts exercising. The osteopathic physician is in a unique position to evaluate and treat musculoskeletal complications so that the patient can realize the benefits of aerobic exercise.

Many patients are unable to tolerate an initial vigorous aerobic exercise program because of musculoskeletal problems and general deconditioning. Low-impact aerobics are preferable to high-impact activity. Water exercises offer an exercise opportunity for the patient whose musculoskeletal system is too compromised to deal with the effects of gravity as well as exercise activity. A therapeutically directed Tai Chi program is useful before proceeding to heavy exercise.

Recent information evaluating exercise methods used in cardiac rehabilitation suggests that resistance exercises and circuit weight training are of value.[11] Previously, exercises had been limited to aerobic activity and resistance exercises were avoided.

Anaerobic Exercise

Anaerobic exercises (e.g., power lifting) are resistance exercises that can provide trophic stimulus for strengthening all involved tissues. Muscles can metabolize glucose to lactic acid without oxygen. Oxygen and adenosine triphosphate (ATP) are necessary to complete the metabolic process. Some strengthening exercises may involve short-term anaerobic activity.

Strengthening Exercises

This type of exercise requires muscle contractions under load to strengthen the muscles.

Exercises to Stabilize Weak or Unstable Joints

Exercises to stabilize joints strengthen the muscles and connective tissue that support a weak or unstable joint. The challenge is to find ways to contract muscles actively without straining or injuring the weak or unstable joint.

Toning Exercises

Toning exercises are designed to "firm" muscles. Mild muscle contractions at 30–40% of capacity are performed with 15–25 repetitions per set.

Kinesthetic Balance

Certain types of exercises can be designed to improve kinesthetic balance, e.g., walking on a balance beam or standing on a board balanced on a cylinder.

EXERCISE PREPARATION

A period of warm-up exercises should precede any prescribed exercise program. Warm-up requires mild muscle contractions to promote circulation. These exercises literally warm up the muscles by stimulating arterial dilation. Warm-up prior to activity is not synonymous with stretching, discussed below.

Warm-up

Warm-up exercises for a runner would involve walking first and then running slowly. For a tennis player, walking, slow running, and "lobbing" the ball warm up the muscles.

Stretching

PRINCIPLES OF STRETCHING

Stretching is used to prepare the body for vigorous activity. Stretching increases range of motion and general freedom of motion by decreasing muscle hypertonicity and fascial tension. Stretching is capable of moving the physiologic barrier to provide a greater range of active motion.

Observe these precautions when stretching:

1. Muscles must be stretched slowly.
2. Avoid stimulating the Golgi tendon receptors, which causes the muscle to contract and "fight" against the stretching force.
3. Stretch slowly (approximately 30 seconds per stretch). Stretching requires type B behavior. Type A behavior is inappropriate for effective stretching.[12]
4. Avoid high-velocity stretching maneuvers.
5. Avoid a terminal bounce (sudden quick increase of force).

In addition to muscle, collagen fibers are also subjected to the stretching force. The viscoelastic properties of collagen dictate that stretching requires time. Collagen has properties of fluids and of solids, termed viscoelastic properties. The fluid component of collagen requires time for the collagen to flow as it is lengthened. Collagen must be stretched slowly.

If stretching is overdone or done improperly, it can lead to adverse side effects. Collagen can be overstretched to a point at which it is permanently deformed and will not return to its original length, the same way a spring can be overstretched so that it is permanently deformed. This overstretching is called plastic deformation. Joint instability is the usual consequence of plastic deformation of tissues. It is possible to overstretch a strong low back and produce a weak, unstable, painful low back. Stretching provides no trophic stimulus and so does not strengthen muscles. Active muscle contraction produces increased muscle strength.

Stretching after warm-up exercises and after exercising is appropriate.

TYPES OF STRETCHING

Stretching is usually performed by applying a force to tissues. This applied force is called active stretching. Force applied by another person (therapist, trainer, partner) to stretch is called passive stretching. It is also possible for individuals to stretch their own muscle(s) by applying the stretching force using a different part of their body. An example of the stretching force being self-applied would be to stretch the right wrist and hand by applying a stretching force with the left hand. This type of stretching is similar to passive stretching done by a trainer or therapist, except that the patient or athlete has complete control of the force being applied. There are alternative forms of stretching, such as using a table, chair, or counter surface as a stabilizer.

A muscle can be stretched by actively contracting the antagonist muscle. This type of stretching takes advantage of a neurophysiologic phenomenon called reciprocal inhibition. When the antagonist muscle contracts, nerve impulses to the agonist muscle are inhibited, allowing the agonist muscle to lengthen. An example of the use of reciprocal inhibition would be stretching the psoas major muscle (a hip flexor) by having the prone patient raise the involved leg off the table and actively extend the hip.

Another type of stretching involves an isometric muscle energy technique that probably uses the Golgi tendon body reflex. The muscle to be stretched is lengthened to engage the restrictive barrier, held in that position, and then actively contracted against some isometric holding force. The hamstrings may be stretched using this muscle energy approach. The person stands on one leg, places the heel of the other leg (leg straight and knee locked) on a chair or stool, and positions the body to "load" the hamstrings. While maintaining this position, the heel is pushed against the stool by actively contracting the tight hamstring. The muscle stretch is repositioned to engage a new restrictive barrier, and the process is repeated. Isometric muscle contraction away from the restrictive barrier not only stretches the muscle but also provides a circulatory benefit with movement of fluids. This muscle contraction is believed to reduce the gamma tone to the tight muscle.

POSTEXERCISE MUSCLE SORENESS

Clinicians have studied soreness after exercise by examining muscle biopsies under the electron microscope. Microscopic study reveals abnormalities involving disruption of the Z bands of the muscles. Muscle soreness is not entirely a lactic acid phenomenon. Eccentric muscle contractions are most commonly associated with postexercise muscle soreness. Soreness is uncommon in well-conditioned athletes but is common in poorly conditioned individuals who engage in vigorous exercise. Fortunately, the problem is self-limiting, and the muscles return to normal after several days.

SPECIFIC PROBLEM AREAS OF SPINAL DYSFUNCTION

Extended Somatic Dysfunctions of the Spine

The motion restriction is flexion (forward-bending) with increased freedom of extension. Extension exercises are essential for treatment of extended somatic dysfunction of the spine. This dysfunction is maintained by flexed areas (extension restriction) above and below the extended dysfunction. Extension exercises address the flexed areas that maintain the segment with extended dysfunction. Hyperextension, however, is painful for these patients. If the upper thoracic interscapular area is involved and the patient must perform a prone spinal extension exercise, excess extension can be controlled by limiting extension of the head and neck. This is accomplished by keeping the patient's chin toward the chest.

Neck Pain

Neck pain is often associated with instability of some of the cervical joints. Active exercises are necessary to strengthen and stabilize those weakened segments of the cervical spine. First, find a dose of strengthening exercises that will work without causing pain. Mild isometric exercises with the neck in a comfortable neutral position often fit this starting point. The "circumduction" neck exercises (neck rolls) that were often recommended by physicians in the past have been found to localize the forces to the unstable area and compound the instability that is present.

Lumbosacral Pain

L5 is the most mobile of the lumbar segments, and it is often unstable. Patients with backache need extension exercises to strengthen paraspinal extensor muscles, yet it is common to find L5 extended (backward bent) while the upper lumbar region is flexed. In this position, extension movement of L5 will produce subjective pain. The extension exercises can be performed comfortably if you position your patient prone on the table and place a pillow or pillows under the pelvis to flex L5. This positioning tends to restrict extreme hyperextension of L5 so that the patient can tolerate the spinal extension exercises.

Lumbar Disk

Lumbar disk problems usually will not tolerate a flexion load of the lumbar spine. Flexion exercises are, however, usually indicated in these patients. If the patient's head is elevated to reduce the gravitational load and a slant board is used for sit-up or "curl" abdominal exercise, lumbar exercises are much easier for the patient to tolerate. Be sure to stop short of pain.

ILLUSTRATED EXERCISES FOR PATIENTS

CONSTANT REST POSITION

Purpose

The purpose of the constant rest position is to reduce lumbar and cervical lordotic curves and relax paraspinal and psoas muscles. This position reduces lumbar intradisk pressure.

Instructions

1. Place your lower legs on a chair or on a similar device.
2. Position your torso so that your thighs are perpendicular to the floor or even at a 45° angle with the abdomen (Fig. 76.1).
3. Place a pillow under your head. Remain in this position 15–20 minutes.

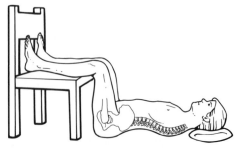

Figure 76.1. Constant rest position.

Strengthening Exercises

PELVIC TILT

Purpose

The purpose of the pelvic tilt is to strengthen lower abdominal muscles and reciprocally inhibit lower lumbar paraspinal muscles.

Instructions

1. Start from the constant rest position or, alternatively, lie with your thighs flexed and feet on the floor.
2. Attempt to curl your buttocks off the ground, flattening the lumbar curve to the floor (Fig. 76.2).
3. Hold for a few seconds, then return slowly.

TORSO CURL ("CRUNCHES")

Purpose

The purpose of the torso curl is to strengthen the upper abdominal muscles and inhibit the paraspinal muscles.

Instructions

1. Start from the constant rest position or supine with thighs flexed. The psoas muscles must be relaxed and not used in the exercise.
2. Place fingers on abdominal muscles.
3. Tuck chin down and in.
4. Slowly curl head and then shoulders off the floor (Fig. 76.3).

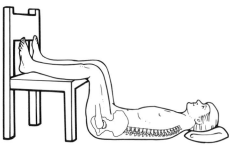

Figure 76.2.   Pelvic tilt.

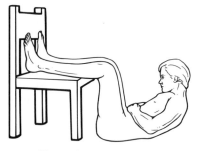

Figure 76.3.   Torso curl.

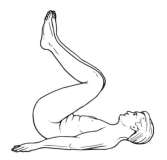

Figure 76.4.   Reverse torso curl.

5. Continue to ascend upward, with each vertebra moving off the floor individually rather than as a group.
6. Hold top position.
7. Return slowly to starting position. The slow approach can be accomplished with a count of four-four-four: four counts up, hold for four counts, four counts down.

REVERSE TORSO CURL

Purpose

The purpose of the reverse torso curl is to strengthen the lower abdominal muscles. This exercise is a progression from the pelvic tilt.

Instructions

1. Lie supine on the floor.
2. Rest your hands at your sides or grasp the end of the table over your head.
3. Draw your knees to your chest, flexing knees and hips as far as possible.
4. Using your lower abdominal muscles, slowly curl buttocks off the ground to the approximate level of T12 (Fig. 76.4).
5. Hold this position for a few seconds, then return slowly. Use the four-four-four count.

TORSO (BACK) EXTENSION

Purpose

The purpose of the torso extension is to strengthen the paraspinal muscles.

Precaution: This exercise can increase low back pain, especially in the acute state. Hyperextension of L5 can be painful in some patients. The patient must adhere to the rule Stop Short of Pain. If back pain is worsened by doing this exercise, even if it doesn't hurt at the time, it should be stopped or the dosage decreased. Sometimes placing one or more large pillows under the pelvis will flex L5 and allow the exercise to be done without pain.

Instructions

1. Lie prone on the floor.
2. Place your hands at your sides, supinating your forearms (thumbs pointing out).

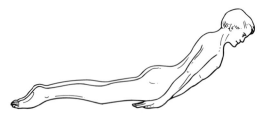

Figure 76.5. Torso (back) extension.

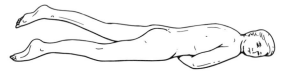

Figure 76.6. Hip hyperextensions (psoas resets).

3. Keep your chin tucked in, maintaining your head in line with your torso.
4. Slowly raise your head and torso off the floor (Fig. 76.5).
5. Hold the position; return slowly to the floor. Use the four-four-four count.

HIP HYPEREXTENSIONS (PSOAS RESETS)

Purpose

The purpose of hip extensions is to stretch (lengthen) and reciprocally inhibit the psoas muscle.

Instructions

1. Lie prone on the floor, hands under the anterior superior iliac spine (ASIS).
2. Keep your chin tucked in.
3. Slowly raise one leg, keeping the knee locked and the ASIS pressed into the hand (Fig. 76.6). Note: Once hip extension is maximized, additional movement of the thigh (upward) is achieved by rotating the pelvis, which is not desired. By keeping the ASIS pushed into the hand, pelvic rotation is avoided.
4. Hold the position for a few seconds; return slowly to the floor.
5. Do both sides.

ANGRY CAT

Purpose

The angry cat exercise is designed to relax the low back muscles and to relieve the spasm or cramp that causes pain in the lower lumbar region. This exercise alone eases tired backs and minor aches and pains caused by bad posture. It will help a person stand erect without pain, even after a tough day.

Instructions

1. Get on all fours on the floor.
2. Keep knees and hands apart.
3. Arch the back and lift up the chin (Fig. 76.7A).

4. Arch as much as you can. Lift the chin as high as you can.
5. Raise your back and tuck in your chin (Fig. 76.7B).
6. Raise your back as high as you can.
7. Tuck in your chin as close as you can.
8. Combine numbers 3 and 5 into one smooth exercise; do not pause. Do both parts of this exercise smoothly.

CERVICAL ISOMETRICS

Purpose

The purpose of cervical isometrics is to strengthen the neck by performing isometric exercises.

Instructions

1. Flexion: place the hand on the forehead, push the forehead into the hand, but do not allow the head to move (Fig. 76.8).

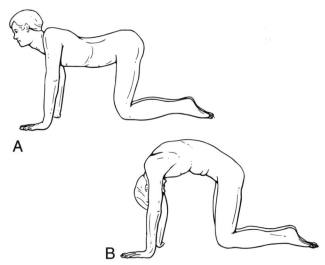

Figure 76.7. **A**, Angry cat (raise chin and sway back). **B**, Angry cat (tuck chin and arch or raise back).

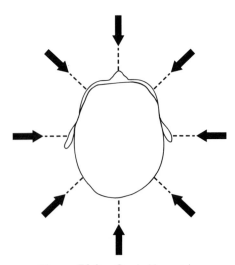

Figure 76.8. Cervical isometrics.

2. Extension: place the hand on the back of the head.
3. Side-bending: place the hand on the side of the head.
4. Rotation: place the hand on the side of the head, slightly more anteriorly than when doing the side-bending exercise.
5. Amount of force: start with a mild amount (3–5 pounds), and increase as needed.

WRITING THE EXERCISE PRESCRIPTION

Elements

A complete exercise prescription should contain the following elements:

1. Goals of the exercise: What is to be accomplished? Assess initial strength, endurance, and mobility.
2. Mode of exercise: flexibility, strength training, etc. Examples include weight lifting, games, swimming.
3. Intensity: How much load or resistance? How fast or slow?
4. Duration: How many repetitions? How long do they last?
5. Frequency: number of sets, times per day, times per week.
6. Progression: incremental increase of intensity, duration, and/or frequency.

Principles and Terms

Exercises should involve the patient's cerebral cortex controlling the muscle activity. Ballistic or uncontrolled motions must be avoided. Keep the cortex attached to the muscle. The following principles of exercise are illustrated by examples shown in Figures 76.1–76.8. To be effective, these exercises must be performed slowly so that the intersegmental muscles of each segment are required to participate. Fast exercises will actually skip over the stiff areas, and the objective of the exercises will not be achieved.

1. Position to obtain relief: the constant rest position (Fig. 76.1) or bringing the thighs toward the chest to reduce a lumbosacral hyperextension.
2. Passive stretching: the physician stretches the muscle.
3. Active stretching: the patient stretches the psoas by extending the hip.
4. Use motion to promote circulation of tight, congested muscles: getting out of bed and walking around the room.
5. Use exercises to mobilize tight, stiff, restricted areas: active muscle contraction to provide shoulder rolls and mobilize the shoulder girdle area.
6. Use exercises to strengthen weak areas: curls or sit-ups strengthen abdominal muscles.
7. Use exercises to improve spinal motion so that all segments of the spine contribute to total motion. The objective is to provide for smooth, coordinated spinal motion: core exercises focusing on the trunk include torso curl, reverse torso curl, and torso (back) extension.
8. Use exercise to provide stability, strength, and endurance throughout the range of motion. This type of exercise requires multiple repetitions with a moderate significant resistance.

9. There is a continuum within the spectrum of exercise. Establish an acceptable range of motion first. This involves eliminating specific restrictions as well as achieving an overall range of motion. Strength, stability, and endurance follow. The trophic stimulus of active exercise strengthens all tissues involved (bone, connective tissue), not just muscle.
10. Group activity has a much higher compliance rate than does individual effort.

The body is no stronger than its weakest link. Many well-conditioned patients have a back or musculoskeletal problem that severely limits their function. Direct treatment to strengthen the weak link. The proper dosage of exercise may be minimal. An overdose will cause harm and worsen the condition. Physically active patients instinctively look for an exercise program tailored to the strong parts of their body without regard for the "weak link." Pursuing exercises with type A aggressive behavior will usually make a condition worse, not better. It is impossible to know what exercises are right for any given patient without the patient actually trying them.

Exercises must stop short of pain. Pain is an indication that the joint is being stressed or overloaded. The object is to find ways to strengthen the muscle and tissues without causing more injury or stress to the joint. Discomfort, as with stretching muscles, is acceptable. Avoiding injury or stress to joints often requires an exercise program specifically tailored for the patient. For compulsive exercise patients, the exercise prescription may decrease their activity level from excessive to appropriate. Giving a paper handout containing a series of exercises to well people is acceptable, but this is not suitable for patients with problems.

The dose of exercise may vary from day to day. One day, a patient may be able to do the exercise easily. On another day, the exercise may cause pain, and the patient cannot tolerate the exercise. Patients should be instructed to back off when appropriate, and told always to stop short of pain.

Flexion and extension should be performed in the same exercise session. Flexion and extension exercises for the spine must precede exercises involving rotation and side-bending. This order comes from the following biomechanical concept: flexion and extension are pure and uncoupled motions. If free flexion and extension motion can be obtained, rotation and/or side-bending will introduce group motion rather than single segmental motion. Most spinal motion involves neutral or type I mechanics. This type of motion is group motion, when a number of contiguous spinal segments contribute to an overall positional change. By contrast, local spinal dysfunctions often produce nonneutral mechanics (type II). This effect localizes force to a single segment.

A strong, functional extremity must be attached to a strong trunk. A strong limb is no better than the trunk to which it is attached. Programs to strengthen extremities should therefore include the trunk.

Osteopathic diagnosis and osteopathic manipulative treatment (OMT) to relieve somatic dysfunction or fascial tension of the spine and/or extremities may be the key to a successful exercise program for the patient. OMT can provide improved motion of the spine, making it possible for the body to compensate, mobilize, and strengthen.

Patients frequently ask if it is acceptable to perform certain exercise activities. If it doesn't hurt, the activity is probably acceptable. If the patient develops discomfort later, such as the next day, the dose of activity should be reduced.

There is a proper time for rest following injury, but bed rest and inactivity do not increase muscle strength. The rehabilitation phase requires active work on the patient's part. Continued inactivity will only lead to a progressive cycle that includes weakness, reduced resistance, and increasingly severe clinical consequences resulting from minor stresses. These patients are said to be "going downhill." Get involved with your patients. Be prepared to help them fully recover or rehabilitate by instructing them and monitoring a good exercise program for them. Seek health with your patients.

CONCLUSION

There are many exercise programs for back pain patients. Some physicians prescribe exercise programs in stages that depend on the patient's fitness level. Others use handouts listing specific exercises for injury rehabilitation. These programs are common but are likely to fail because they are focused on having the patient complete a process.

Physician and patient energies should be focused on the objectives to be accomplished. Categorizing exercises with objectives in mind makes it easier to prescribe appropriate exercises for the patient.

Osteopathic physicians are especially trained in understanding the relationship of the musculoskeletal system to a patient's somatic and visceral problems. Osteopathic diagnosis and manipulative treatment to relieve somatic dysfunction or fascial tension of the spine and/or extremities may be the key to a successful exercise program for the patient. You must be able to demonstrate and write an exercise prescription that will meet the specific needs of patients with back pain, postural imbalance, or musculoskeletal decompensation. The exercises enhance the benefits of treatment as well as continue the process of functional restoration between treatments.

REFERENCES

1. Pate RR, Pratt M, Blair SN, et. al. Physical activity and public health. *JAMA.* February 1, 1995;273(5):402–407.
2. Friewaid WT. Physical activity research and coronary heart disease. *Public Health Rep.* 1985;100:115–117.
3. Paffenbarger RS Jr, Wing AL, Hyde RT, Jung DL. Physical activity and incidence of hypertension in college alumni. *Am J Epidemiol.* 1985;117:245–257.
4. Sobolski J, Komitzer M, DeBacker G, et al. Protection against ischemic heart disease in the Belgian Physical Fitness Study: physical fitness rather than physical activity? *Am J Epidemiol.* 1987;125:601–610.
5. Paffenbarger RS Jr, Hyde RT, Wing AL, Hsieh CC. Physical activity, all-cause mortality, and longevity of college alumni. *N Engl J Med.* 1986;314:605–613.
6. Leon AS, Connett J, Jacobs DR, Rauramaa R. Leisure time physical activity levels and risk of coronary heart disease and death. *JAMA.* 1987;258:2388–2395.
7. Rippe JM, Ward A, Porcari JP. Walking for health and fitness. *JAMA.* 1988;259:2720–2724.
8. American College of Sports Medicine. *Guidelines for Exercise Testing and Prescription.* 3rd ed. Philadelphia, Penn: Lea & Febiger; 1986.
9. Chisholm DM, Collis ML, Kulak LL, Davenport W, Gruber N. Physical activity readiness. *Br Columbia Med J.* 1975;17:375–378.
10. American College of Sports Medicine. *Guidelines for Exercise Testing and Prescription.* 4th ed. Philadelphia, Penn: Lea & Febiger; 1991.
11. 1993 AOA Research Conference—presentation by Felix Rogers, DO, at the 1993 AOA Research Conference; October 10–14, 1993; Boston, Mass. *D.O.* January 1994:98–102.
12. Kaplan HI, Saddock BJ. *Comprehensive Textbook of Psychiatry.* 5th ed. Baltimore, Md: Williams & Wilkins; 1989:1193.

Applications of Basic and Clinical Research for Osteopathic Theory and Practice

INTRODUCTION

Albert F. Kelso

The foundation for osteopathic medicine is supported by research in many fields. The search to advance osteopathic medicine includes the fields of philosophy, science, education, and management. Information in each field appears in the world literature, while specific information on the osteopathic component of health care is available from the profession's publications. Osteopathic philosophy[1] associates patient health with the status of the somatic system. Other histories provide a background on the profession's scientific efforts.[2–3] The histories in this section identify ideas and their development and contribution to osteopathic concepts and practice.

RESEARCH ON MEDICAL PRACTICE AND KNOWLEDGE

Research in Medical Educational and Health Care Management

Research in education and health care management ensures that the delivery of health care by osteopathic institutions and its clinicians meets public expectations. Patients, communities, and the public trust their health to the hands of individuals qualified by education, training, experience, and licensure to provide quality health care. Educational research adapts physician education programs to advances in knowledge and technology, to the needs for personal and community health, and to regulations affecting the practice of medicine. Management research examines the processes used in the health care system by measuring the impact of process on health outcomes.[4] Research in these fields provides a competitive edge for clinicians and for the health care institutions in which they practice.

Advancing Medicine by Scientific Investigation

Scientific investigation furnishes the evidence to answer questions and test hypotheses about health, disabilities, illness, and health care.[5–7] Evaluating the research evidence determines whether it supports or refutes the idea that initiated the question. Recognized and accepted research designs provide controls for variables and reduce bias. Current and future research must advance the knowledge and practice of osteopathic medicine and rely on established research designs, models, and methods. Innovations are limited to changes in designs and methods required to meet unique situations encountered when answering questions in unexplored fields. Even innovative changes must have scientific validity and reliability established.

Epidemiologic Investigation of Patients and Populations

The evidence supplied by clinical and epidemiologic research is used for specific purposes in two different fields: in patient care and in the protection and promotion of public health. Advances in osteopathic patient health care focus on processes that alter a patient's health or the course of health with or without an intervention to change the course. For example, research on the effects of somatic dysfunction and manipulative treatment investigates their influences during illness, disability, recovery, or health. Advances in public health depend on detecting influences that place persons at risk, the causes and control of risk, and the resources needed to restore and maintain public health. For example, research on the health and cost-effectiveness of treating somatic dysfunction is conducted as a survey of osteopathic medical practice. Survey data are aggregated to identify the:

Prevalence of somatic dysfunction
Frequency of use of manipulative treatment
Patients' satisfaction with this aspect of care
Health and cost-effectiveness of manipulative treatment for somatic dysfunction

Sources and Use of Medical Research Data

Clinical research is published in peer-reviewed scientific journals as a contribution to medical knowledge. Epidemiologic research is reported internally to governmental agencies. These agencies use the data to evaluate:

Quality of public health
Public health care needs
Resources to provide needed care
Budgets for developing and maintaining public health

External reporting appears in agency publications or is obtained by requesting the internal reports. In the field of patient care, the unit of investigation is the patient; in the field of public health, the unit of investigation is a large sample or an entire population. The patient's medical record is an important source document for both patient and epidemiologic research.

Value of Established Research Design

Most accepted research designs have been used for several decades and tested in many investigations. These designs provide controls that minimize the influence of the many variables in a patient's health or illness and environments. The designs also provide methods that reduce the effects of bias on the experimental results and conclusions.

A major variable relates to the differences in clinicians' education, training, and experience. Special efforts are required to reduce interclinician and intraclinician variability.[8] This section emphasizes clinical and epidemiologic research; clinical practice must be advanced to the current frontiers of medicine and knowledge. Basic research is equally important; its use provides a sound foundation for osteopathic theory. Research relies on current references for planning, proposing, and conducting investigation. Basic research designs provide definitive evidence to support or reject researchable ideas in established fields. Collaboration with established investigators is recommended to increase the quality of research.

Public and Governmental Expectations on Improving Health Care

The public expects clinical research to identify needed, safe, effective, and efficient procedures for health care.[9] Research on interventions or modes of therapy used in practice, other than Food and Drug Administration-approved medications and devices, requires modified medical research designs and methods to meet the public's expectations. Research on the quality of health care requires experienced research team members. Competent teams include expertise in:

Clinical diagnosis and management
Clinical research designs
Statistical analysis
Research management

The team approach produces better results than those provided by a single investigator. Giving clinical research a high priority in the immediate future ensures perfection in the clinical investigation that basic research achieved over the last century.

HISTORY

Roots of Osteopathic Medicine

The milestones in osteopathic medicine's foundation for clinical practice up to 1975 are presented here as background for current and future research. Nineteen seventy-five is a benchmark in manual medicine, a date that represents a challenge to the use of manual procedures in health care. At the request of the U.S. Senate in 1975, the National Institute of Neurologic Diseases and Stroke convened a workshop in which international representatives reviewed the scientific status of manual medicine. The review and analysis of the Workshop on Research Status of Spinal Manipulative Therapy are summarized as follows:

"...specific conclusions cannot be derived from the scientific literature for or against either the efficacy of spinal manipulative therapy or the pathophysiologic foundations from which it is derived."[10]

Scientific investigation is expected to support practice and to establish a credible biologic basis for its effects. The researcher is reminded that we stand on the shoulders of the practitioners, clinicians, scientists, and scholars who have preceded us. Their efforts developed our knowledge base from humble beginnings and expanded the base with evidence from all fields of knowledge. Continued efforts to investigate all contributions to osteopathic theory and practice will help meet the public's expectations for quality health care.

Models for Medical Practice

Medicine has its roots in practice espoused by leading physicians who provide the model for current practice. These leaders rely heavily on medical procedures that they perceive to be sound and that provide benefits to patients. The history of medicine and healers includes transitions from one leader or model to another. Transition occurs when a new model appears to be better than the previous one or when there are misconceptions or failures in the leader's model. A.T. Still's dissatisfaction with results of 19th century medicine is an example of a failure leading to a different model for practice. Each AOA Yearbook and Directory[11] sketches the important events in osteopathic history that followed Still's introduction of a new model.

Clinical Responses to Osteopathic Manipulative Treatment

Research in osteopathic medicine began with clinical observations by A.T. Still and other early osteopathic physicians. Their treatments provided patients with relief from discomfort and disability caused by injury and illness. These patient benefits, plus the physician's experience in palpatory examination and manipulative treatment, created theories about the role of the neuromusculoskeletal system in health and illness. They identified somatic dysfunction (called Still or osteopathic lesions in that era) as a specific response of the musculoskeletal system to bodily disturbances. This focus guided a philosophy for practice, established principles for patient care, and stimulated speculations on their clinical observations.

From Speculation to Hypotheses

The formulation of theories derived from speculation on the nature of somatic dysfunction and from patient responses to manipulative treatment is the first milestone in the evolution of osteopathic medicine. These speculations survived the test of time and had a sound basis in the known science and medicine of that day. The pioneers in osteopathic research recognized that observation and formulations of plausible explanations alone are not sufficient. Public, academic, and medical acceptance requires the formulation of testable hypotheses on theory and practice that are then investigated in basic and clinical research. It is evident from history that, as knowledge in medicine and science advance, the theoretical models must be rethought and restated. A balance must exist between retaining viable knowledge and discarding or revising outdated models, theories, and procedures.

Early Years

Clinicians and faculty members of the early osteopathic colleges speculated on the nature of somatic dysfunction. Their explanations for its clinical, structural, and functional nature stimulated the creation of the Memorial Institute.[12] Local and remote effects of somatic dysfunction on health and its response to manipulative treatment were attributed to structural relations and functional mechanisms present in all individuals. *Osteopathic Research: Growth and Development*[13] and *The D.O.'s*[14] present a historical perspective on the development of a theoretical and scientific basis for osteopathic medicine.

Role of Osteopathic Practitioners

Answers were sought in the organization of the body to these questions:

What is the origin of somatic dysfunction?
How is it associated with the local physical findings?
What are the remote effects of somatic dysfunctions and response to treatment?
How does manipulative treatment change the local condition, provide relief, and restore health?

These questions, augmented now to include cellular and molecular mechanisms, continue to guide osteopathic research. Osteopathic researchers report their research at annual research conferences.[15] These reports are published in the *Journal of the American Osteopathic Association* (JAOA). The conference proceedings include related research seminars and lectures.

Structural and Functional Changes Associated with Somatic Dysfunction

Pioneer basic science researchers reached a second milestone when they demonstrated mechanisms in animal models that supported their theories. In the early 20th century, Deason, McConnell, and Burns conducted research in laboratories supported by the American Osteopathic Association (AOA).[16] They demonstrated structural and functional aspects of somatic dysfunction and its effects in animal models. Such demonstration provided insight into fundamental processes. However, lack of similarity to currently used experimental procedures precluded widespread recognition. Publications from the A.T. Still Memorial Institute appear in separate reports published in the *JAOA*[17], Yearbooks, and in publications of the American Academy of Osteopathy[18] and are archived in osteopathic college libraries.

Role of the American Osteopathic Association

The AOA initiated and has continued to provide a stimulus for the conduct of basic research and to encourage clinical research. In 1938, the AOA[19] established the Bureau of Research to increase funding for research and to formalize the profession's methods for supporting osteopathic research. It has funded pilot studies in basic and clinical research. The Bureau also supports the annual AOA Research Conferences, programs to recognize research and researchers, and assists in the publication of osteopathic research, theory, and practice. The Bureau has been assisted by the Burroughs Wellcome Foundation and the Smith Kline and French Laboratories in recognizing researchers. Recipients of the Gutensohn-Denslow award, selected by the AOA Bureau of Research, present an honorary Louisa Burns Memorial Lecture. Students receive the Burnett Osteopathic Student Research Award for independently writing an outstanding paper on osteopathic medicine.

Clinical and Basic Research on Somatic Dysfunction

The third milestone, evolution of osteopathic clinical and basic research studies on the role of structure, received less attention than did the research on function. Extending from the late 19th century to the present, basic and clinical research has supported structural theory. Research by Smith (1898) used the Skiagraph, a forerunner of x-ray machines, to image bony structure and circulation.[20] Such research continues in the present.

Clinical Evidence to Support Structural Components of Somatic Dysfunction

Clinicians accepted the structural theories and applied them to practice. They used evidence from postural analysis and x-ray studies to guide decisions on selection of manipulative treatments, exercise, and use of prosthetic devices. This phase of osteopathic clinical research has gained the recognition of radiologists and introduced new procedures for imaging and analysis of structural components. In Chapter 77, Heath identifies currently available imaging systems and some other measurement techniques used in osteopathic research.

Functional Role of Somatic System

The fourth milestone, basic research on osteopathic theory, is exemplified in the basic research by Denslow and colleagues at the Kirksville College of Osteopathic Medicine (KCOM).[21–24] Denslow's pioneering efforts were preceded by consultation with leading scientists of his day. His initial research provided evidence that reflex thresholds were lowered in regions of somatic dysfunction, thereby supporting a role for reflexes in the origin of somatic dysfunction.

Investigation of Somatic Dysfunction

Within a few years, Korr, Thomas, Wright, Hix, and Eble joined the Kirksville research effort. This group of scientists continued to expand in number and productivity. Their investigations not only supported the somatosomatic and viscerosomatic reflex role of somatic dysfunction but also identified remote effects in the body mediated by somatovisceral and somatosomatic reflexes. Basic research that tested osteopathic theory was published in scientific journals beginning with Denslow's research in the early 1940s. Research chronicled in the JAOA has been summarized through 1975.[25]

Frontiers of Science and Medicine

The most recent advance in osteopathic theory, "learning" in the spinal cord, resulted from neurophysiologic research by Patterson. His research is at the forefront of neuroscience. His and other published neuroscience research support some components of learning as occurring in the spinal cord. This advance in theory provides plausible explanations for long-term maintenance of somatic dysfunction and for the creation of a common set of characteristics, whether originating from structural stresses, or somatosomatic or viscerosomatic reflexes. Patterson's and other osteopathic researchers' contributions to medical knowledge appear in peer-reviewed scientific and clinical journals. Patterson, with support from the American Academy of Osteopathy and world leaders in science, organized international symposia on the body's integrative mechanisms in health and disease.[26–27]

Interactions between Nerves and Muscles

KCOM researchers Korr, Wilkenson, and Chornock conducted basic research on non–impulse-mediated interactions between nerve and muscles. They identified the delivery of substances from nerves into muscle. This process, axoplasmic flow, is a slow process requiring days for delivery from its origin in the neuronal cell body into muscle or the antegrade transport from muscle to the neural cell body. Korr and Appeltauer subsequently identified delivery of substances by antegrade axonal transport at much faster rates. Related research on antegrade and retrograde neuronal transport discovered a communication system across the synaptic membrane that connects the neuron with the environment.[28] This communication provides information for control mechanisms in both neurons and innervated cells. The substances involved in axonal transport have biologic and clinical significance that need further investigation.

Facilitated Synaptic Transmission

Korr and his KCOM colleagues advanced osteopathic theory by introducing the concept of segmental facilitated nerve impulse transmission in spinal cord regions related to somatic dysfunction. Denslow and Korr have published on the basic research conducted at Kirksville, on the implications for osteopathic medicine, and on its contributions to the advancement of osteopathic theory. Korr's collected writings are published in an American Academy of Osteopathy Yearbook[29] commemorating his contributions to osteopathic medicine.

The experiments by Deason and Burns, cited earlier, sought histologic evidence of tissue changes in regions of somatic dysfunction. Cole continued the investigation of tissue changes and included extensive study of motor endplates in affected somatic muscles. Cole's research is presented in a Louisa Burns Memorial Lecture and appears with selected papers in an American

Academy of Osteopathy publication.[30] Burns' research continued throughout her career and is summarized in the 1994 yearbook of the American Academy of Osteopathy.[31]

FORCES ADVANCING OSTEOPATHIC MEDICINE

The recognition of osteopathic medicine was accelerated by basic research conducted in well-equipped laboratories, testing theories on the nature of somatic dysfunction and on developing other theories based on research results. The application of current medical, scientific, and technical knowledge to this research will keep osteopathic basic research at the frontiers of science. The historian or researcher interested in the background for basic osteopathic research will find investigations that qualify as basic research before 1942.

Early Challenges

The major difference from earlier investigations was the establishment by KCOM, after 1942, of a continuing research effort that lasted for more than a quarter of a century. The KCOM president, Morris Thompson, and Board of Trustees not only supported the development of osteopathic research but also made it one of their highest priorities. Investigation occurred in a favorable environment supported by the KCOM administration, the osteopathic profession, and grants from the National Institutes of Health. A cadre of qualified researchers joined Denslow and Korr in team research; their research efforts made important contributions to knowledge and osteopathic medicine.

Present and Future Challenges

The fifth milestone in evolution of osteopathic research—evidence of the safety, efficacy, and effectiveness of treating somatic dysfunction with manipulation—had not been reached by the year 1975.[32–33] This milestone represents basic and clinical research that produces evidence to support osteopathic theory and practice by use of current research methodology. A paradigm for obtaining evidence to evaluate manual medicine, osteopathic diagnosis and treatment, and other non–medicine-based interventions has not been established. Modified or new research designs and methods are needed to support the clinical efficacy and effectiveness of physical interventions used in health care. Efficacy is the effectiveness observed under the controlled experimental conditions of a clinical trial. Effectiveness is the outcome observed in practice.

AUTHORS AND THEMES

In the following chapters, the authors introduce methods that will assist osteopathic researchers in selection of designs and methods. Reading the background for contributions of selected procedures identifies facts, methods, and contributions relevant to the proposed project. Also, published research identifies current research procedures that have been accepted by peer-reviewed publications. Historical and methodological information is essential in a sound research plan, proposal, report, or publication. Each author introduces research methods that are applicable to advancing osteopathic theory and practice. The details on models, designs, methods, and analysis change frequently; current information and knowledgeable consultants assist the researcher.

Six chapters in this section are devoted to clinical investigation. Heath introduces the role of somatic dysfunction in osteopathic research. Friedman addresses recording and reporting osteopathic examination, findings, and assessment of somatic dysfunction. Glassman suggests the advantages of and identifies the problems in population studies and epidemiologic research. Kelso indicates the applications of descriptive, analytic, and intervention strategies for investigating the natural history of somatic dysfunction and the benefits obtained in treating the dysfunction.

These four clinical chapters have increased importance in an era of cost-containment that simultaneously seeks to maintain quality health care. Reliable research data obtained from medical records are essential for both clinical and epidemiologic research; medical records are the only original source to document what occurs in practice.

Sheldon introduces clinical trials and research that evolved in medical research during the past half century and set the standard for medical research. A similar standard must be established for research on osteopathic diagnosis and treatment. In a subsequent chapter, Kelso and Heath suggest adaptation of outcome research design to continuous improvement in quality health care.

The last two chapters in this section indicate the designs, methods, and future goals to be achieved by research in the laboratory and clinic. Willard explains the basic scientist's approach to investigating the theoretical basis for osteopathic medicine. Patterson predicts future developments that will advance osteopathic theory and practice. His experience in the Kirksville College research program and in introducing the profession to developments in worldwide research provides a basis for defining the future.

CONCLUSION

Through the efforts of its national and state organizations, colleges, and affiliates, the osteopathic profession from its very inception has advanced the role of osteopathic medicine in the nation's health care system. Osteopathic physicians are graduates of accredited colleges of medicine, licensed for the full practice of medicine, and rely on all modes of therapy used in medical practice. Osteopathic medicine differs from allopathic medicine in the attention given to the role of the somatic system in health and disease. The use of manipulative treatment for somatic dysfunctions and the consequences on total body function are a unique concern. The most reliable source of information on this topic must be provided with the assistance of the profession.

All modes of therapy used in medical practice are subject to regulation. Medical practice is also influenced by social and economic forces, by the health care traditions of cultures and families, and by individual preferences. These influences require scientific and clinical evidence on individual and community health needs and on the benefits obtained from health care. Basic, clinical, and outcome research studies provide acceptable evidence to address these requirements. Such research involves investigation of all aspects of the health care system. These investigations are shared by all persons involved in health care. The osteopathic practicing physician, staff and faculty members of teaching institutions, and researchers, basic and clinical, share the burden and opportunity to investigate the unique aspects of osteopathic practice.

Research on osteopathic medical practice, including osteopathic evaluation and manipulative treatment, must be reviewed by an Institutional Review Board (IRB) and acted on before any research is conducted.[34] The IRB requires monitoring research in progress and reporting incidents that may represent an unpredicted consequence. Clinical researchers should be familiar with these requirements and comply with them.[22]

Many forces will modify clinical practice and research in the future. Those interested in osteopathic research are advised to use currently accepted research designs and information from the literature and from consultants to keep a current perspective while reading or planning research. Duplication in some of these chapters results from the intent to provide three views on research, from:

Established investigators
Younger generation of DO graduates
Basic scientists

Their suggestions help future researchers to locate usable research designs, methods, and ideas. The protocols developed with current resources for investigating osteopathic theory and practice aid in planning sound research protocols. Research collaboration between clinicians, scientists, and patients continues to advance osteopathic medicine.

REFERENCES

The following references identify useful fields of information. Multiple fields contribute research planning. Osteopathic clinician-researchers use specific details to develop their research protocols.

1. Northup GW. *Osteopathic Medicine: An American Reformation.* Chicago, Ill: American Osteopathic Association; 1979.

2. Northup GW, ed. *Osteopathic Research: Growth and Development.* Chicago, Ill: American Osteopathic Association; 1987.

3. Gevitz N. *The D.O.'s: Osteopathic Medicine in America.* Baltimore, Md: The Johns Hopkins University Press; 1982.

4. Couch JB, ed. *Health Care Quality Management for the 21st Century.* Tampa, Fla: Hillsborro Printing Co; 1991.

5. Hulley SB, Cummings SR, eds. *Designing Clinical Research.* Baltimore, Md: Williams & Wilkins; 1988.

6. Friedman LW, Fuchsias CD, DeMets DL. *Fundamentals of Clinical Trials.* 2nd ed. Littleton, Mass: PSG Publishing Company, Inc; 1985.

7. Payton OD. *Research: The Validation of Clinical Practice.* 2nd ed. Philadelphia, Penn: F.A. Davis Company; 1988.

8. Johnston WL, Friedman HD. *Functional Methods.* Indianapolis, Ind: American Academy of Osteopathy; 1994.

9. Brecher C. The government's role in health care. In: Kovner AL, ed. *Jonas's Health Care Delivery in the United States.* 5th ed. New York, NY: Springer Publishing Company; 1995.

10. Goldstein M, ed. Introduction, Summary and analysis. In: *The Research Status of Spinal Manipulative Therapy.* Bethesda, Md: US Department of Health, Education and Welfare; 1975. DHEW publication number (NIH) 76-988.

11. Annual AOA Yearbook and Directory, published annually. Chicago, Ill: American Osteopathic Association. (Section titles vary. Section contents contain: organization and roster of the AOA; directory of osteopathic physicians; AOA documents and data; component societies; osteopathic licensing summary; predoctoral and postdoctoral education; osteopathic hospitals; osteopathic postdoctoral training programs; requirements for specialty certification; osteopathic research; general information—policies, conferences, and programs; handbook and instructions for research grant applications and processing; review process for applications, awards, and fellowships.)

12. AOA Yearbook and Directory, published annually. Chicago, Ill: American Osteopathic Association. (See AOA History: dates, events, and people, in documents and data section.)

13. Meck ME. Foreword; Northup GW. Introduction. In: Northup GW, ed. *Osteopathic Research: Growth and Development.* Chicago, Ill: American Osteopathic Association; 1987.

14. Gevitz N. Andrew Taylor Still; The Missouri Mecca; Structure and Function. In: *The D.O.'s: Osteopathic Medicine in America.* Baltimore, Md: The Johns Hopkins University Press; 1982.

15. *Journal of the American Osteopathic Association, 1901– .* Chicago, Ill: American Osteopathic Association. (See Annual Research Conferences in each annual's index.)

16. Cole WV. Historical basis for osteopathic theory and practice. In: Northup GW, ed. *Osteopathic Research: Growth and Development.* Chicago, Ill: American Osteopathic Association; 1987.

17. Denslow JS. *The Early Years at the Kirksville College of Osteopathic Medicine.* Kirksville, Mo: Kirksville College of Medicine Press; 1982.

18. American Academy of Osteopathy Publications, Indianapolis. Yearbooks, Reviews, and Symposia on osteopathic medical practice and research. (The publications listed in the Bibliography provide specific support for the citation.)

19. AOA Yearbook and Directory, published annually. Chicago, Ill: American Osteopathic Association. (See AOA Bureau of Research Programs in Osteopathic Research section.)

20. Cole WV. Historical basis for osteopathic theory and practice. In: Northup GW, ed. *Osteopathic Research: Growth and Development.* Chicago, Ill: American Osteopathic Association; 1987.

21. Beal MC, ed. *1993 Year Book: The Collected Papers of John Stedman Denslow.* Indianapolis, Ind: American Academy of Osteopathy; 1993.

22. Kugelmass IN, ed. *The Physiologic Basis of Osteopathic Medicine.* New York, NY: The Postgraduate Institute of Osteopathic Medicine and Surgery; 1970.

23. Kelso AF. Physiology. In: Northup GW, ed. *Osteopathic Research: Growth and Development.* Chicago, Ill: American Osteopathic Association; 1987.

24. Patterson MM. A model mechanism for spinal segmental facilitation. *JAOA.* 1976;76:62–72. (See also: Patterson MM. Louisa Burns Memorial Lecture. *JAOA.* 1980;80:106–112.)

25. Northup GW. *Osteopathic Medicine: An American Reformation.* Chicago, Ill: American Osteopathic Association; 1979.

26. Patterson MM, Howell JN, eds. *1989 International Symposium: The Central Connection: Somatovisceral/Viscerosomatic Interaction.* Indianapolis, Ind: American Academy of Osteopathy; 1989.

27. Patterson MM, Willard FH. *1992 International Symposium. Nociception and the Neuro–Immune Connection.*

28. Cole WV. Anatomical and histopathologic evidence. In: Northup GW, ed. *Osteopathic Research: Growth and Development.* Chicago, Ill: American Osteopathic Association; 1987.

29. Patterson B, ed. *The Collected Papers of Irvin M. Korr.* Indianapolis, Ind: American Academy of Osteopathy; 1979.

30. Beal MC, ed. *The Cole Book.* Indianapolis, Ind: American Academy of Osteopathy; 1989.

31. Beal MC, ed. *1994 Year Book: Louisa Burns, D.O. Memorial.* Indianapolis, Ind: American Academy of Osteopathy; 1994.

32. Goldstein M, ed. *The Research Status of Spinal Manipulative Therapy.* Bethesda, Md: US Department of Health, Education and Welfare; 1975. DWEH publication number (NIH) 76-988.

33. Rodwin AR. Comparative health systems. In: Kovnar AR, ed, with contributors. *Jonas's Health Care Delivery in the United States.* 5th ed. New York, NY: Springer Publishing Company; 1995.

34. Greenwald RA, Ryan MK, Mulvihill JE, eds. *Human Subjects Research: A Handbook for Institutional Review Boards*. New York, NY: Plenum Press; 1982.

BIBLIOGRAPHY

The Collected Papers of Irvin M. Korr, edited by Peterson B, 1979.

1989 International Symposium—The Central Connection: Somatovisceral/Somatosomatic Interaction, edited by Patterson MM, Howell JN.

1992 International Symposium—Nociception and the Neuroendocrine-immune Connection.

1993 Year Book: Selected Papers of John Stedman Denslow, DO.

1994 Year Book: Louisa Burns Memorial, edited by Beal MC.

The Cole Book, edited by Beal MC.

77. **Somatic Dysfunction**

EFFECTS OF MANIPULATIVE TREATMENT AND IMPACT ON HEALTH STATUS

DEBORAH M. HEATH

Key Concepts

- **Purpose and methods for investigating the role of the somatic system in health, disability, and illness**

- **Importance of describing somatic dysfunction, the effects of its treatment, and health outcomes**

- **Measurements that indicate changes in somatic dysfunction and their use in clinical research**

- **Value of instrumental measurements that verify clinical observations obtained in osteopathic examination**

Clinical research advances medical theory and incorporates new knowledge into practice ultimately for the patient's benefit. Historically, clinical research has been performed mostly by physicians associated with an academic institution or hospital. Recent trends reveal a shift with an ever-increasing patient population utilizing ambulatory care settings. Simultaneously, there is a growing emphasis on the quality of patient care delivered at all levels. Research on osteopathic examination and manipulative treatment adapts readily to the office-based practice with careful recording of all data in the patient's medical record. The medical records of health care in private practice are the only information source for verifying[1]:

Requests
Claims
Surveys
Reports on practices
Physician network research data

RESEARCH ON AMBULATORY CARE PRACTICE

Forces driving research into routine practice include public concerns about the delivery of cost-effective quality health care.[2] Concerns are also prompted by factors such as diverse practice patterns and lack of uniformity in health service. These factors increase the scrutiny of both inpatient and outpatient medical records and the use of stringent criteria in judging the medical decision-making process.[3]

Justifying Management Decisions

Justification of patient management decisions includes analysis of the cost–benefit equation. The meaning of benefit has expanded from solely addressing patient's complaints, problems, and diagnoses to assessing the patient's health outcomes and functional status. Attention is given to the patients' environment and to the physician's practice profile, accessibility, and patients' satisfaction with the care provided. These factors and health outcomes are important measures in clinical research.

Monitoring and Improving Health Care

Predictable and measurable value of health care services provided is important. The objective is to achieve the highest quality at the lowest possible cost.[4] The 2-year Medical Outcome Study (MOS) is an example of a multidisciplinary, multi-institutional study that used advanced methodology and verified the validity of health status measures.[5] The goal of these studies and of similar research is to monitor and improve medical practice. The scope of clinical assessment includes estimates and measurements of response to treatment as evidence of the health status benefit. This new emphasis increases the need to document the health benefits associated with osteopathic manipulative treatment (OMT) of somatic dysfunction.

CLINICAL RESEARCH

Developments in clinical research methodology are adaptable to routine patient encounters but are still cumbersome and need refinement and further validation. Scientists and physicians need to collaborate to develop methods and measurement tools to assess a patient's health status and response to therapeutic interventions. The clinician collaborating in research acquires an additional role, that of a clinician-researcher. In this role, the physician becomes familiar with ways to reliably and systematically collect the original data and enter it in the medical record. Any derived reports and records from the medical record must be monitored for accuracy. The physician requires training to become adept in research skills while adapting practice to rapidly changing demands in medical care.

Quantitative Measures

As information managers, physicians must often cope with an overload of patient and test data, with assessment of this data, and with their incorporation into a formal treatment plan.

Quantitative data are already included in the medical record; data such as rate of progress or reduction of symptoms—sometimes called soft data—have been mostly ignored. Methods to measure and report clinical observations have not been standardized. The science of clinometrics deals with physical signs and symptoms that have been relegated to the category of soft data.[6]

SCALES AND INDICES AS MEASURES

Rating scales of soft data combined into an index fulfills the need for quantitative measures in the patient's medical record. Indices or some other type of data reduction condense clinical observations to standard formats used in transferring medical record data, enabling office staff to complete the task without having to interpret the data. Physical signs of somatic dysfunction identified by palpatory diagnosis can accommodate a quantitative value. This value, recorded in the medical record and in reports, summarizes a process used in health care. The strategy ensures concise reports while retaining a direct relation to the original data in the medical record. The index or quantitative assessment in reports and records represents the evaluation and decision process recorded in the medical record as findings and an assessment summed as the same value that appears in the report. This strategy ensures concise reports while original data in the medical record is available for verification.

INDEX VALUES FOR SOMATIC DYSFUNCTION

Index values obtained from uniform records of services are likely to accurately reflect the palpatory findings and their assessment. These values also reflect the treatment prescription and its administration, and responses to the interventions prescribed. Clinical services such as osteopathic evaluation and manipulative treatment (OEMT) must include more than segmental levels or locations of somatic dysfunction. Information provided for each component of service provides complete information on the patient encounter. The components include:

Interview
Examination
Health assessment
Decisions on management
Report on outcomes
Patient perceptions

These data are essential in seeking the associations between somatic dysfunction, its changes, and health outcomes. Korr[7] suggests that the clinician-researcher use this paradigm to study the in vivo process of osteopathic medical management.

Statistical Analysis

Physical signs of somatic dysfunction identified by palpatory diagnosis are suited to the assignment of a quantitative value. Scale items for each component of asymmetry, restricted motion, and tissue texture change (ART) are converted to indices. The value assigned for each scale affects the sensitivity and

reliability of the scale value. Scales of presence or absence of somatic dysfunction rarely assist the researcher in detecting changes related to OMT. Scales with many values are time-consuming and less reliable.

RATING SCALE

Clinical experience suggests that the numerical scale used in a standard neurologic rating of reflexes, 0–4/4, is feasible and familiar to most physicians. The same scale for the components of ART provides a convenient and familiar method for rating:

Zero is no response
1–2 is mildly responsive
3 is moderate
4 is more exaggerated or very pronounced

In describing the motion restriction component of somatic dysfunction:

0 represents no restriction
1–2 represents mild restriction
3 represents moderate restriction
4 represents pronounced or severe restriction to a specific motion test and test direction

The rating scale is used for each test of motion, tissue texture, and asymmetry. Other suitable systems are feasible; many experienced osteopathic physicians have developed their own system in practice. Modifying these independently developed systems to fit a uniform system for research will accelerate the advance of osteopathic medicine.

Clinical and Research Analysis

Characterizing the components of regional or segmental palpatory examination findings with a quantitative value translates qualitative clinical assessment into specific data for analysis. This methodology enables the clinician-researcher to evaluate the usefulness of the scales and indices for reproducible and sensitive measurements. Scales that increase interexaminer reliability and correlations with instrumental measurements are valued in clinical research. Research on practice is feasible when scales reliably detect changes during research in a hospital stay or in a series of outpatient visits. The introduction of scales and indices to measure somatic dysfunction also increases the credibility of research that suggests OMT improves health and healing.

Numerical Ratings

Numerical rating of components allows an analysis of the course of somatic dysfunction and the influences on it. Rating somatic dysfunction aids the clinician-researcher in interpreting the process of development and resolution of the condition. Certain components are more time-dependent and responsive than others and can be studied separately. For example, motion restriction responds almost immediately to manipulation, whereas tissue texture usually requires more time. These factors, identified and isolated, are useful in research.

Analysis of Factors Affecting Somatic Dysfunction

The analysis assists in separating mechanical from segmental and central nervous control of effector systems. Clinical experience shows that some palpatory tests are less reliable for short-term, visit-by-visit assessment in interexaminer agreement as compared with long-term follow-up. Beal discusses this time factor and Johnston describes its application.[8] He states that the physician must be able not only to pinpoint the specific location of a lesioned area but alto "to record the elements of . . . motion . . . for comparison in time."[9]

ANALYSIS OF CHANGE

A uniform system provides sufficient data to characterize the components of a regional or segmental examination for somatic dysfunction. Uniformity allows clinical estimates to be converted to analyzable specific and sensitive quantitative data. These measurements provide the researcher with an accurate assessment at each visit. The differences between indices obtained for different examinations (or scales if needed to verify where the change occurred) evaluate the influences that cause change in somatic dysfunction and indicate other responses to manipulative treatment. Total correction of somatic dysfunction is unlikely to occur in chronic or even long-standing acute conditions. Changes in the scale values or indices are available for study when the dysfunction is still present. The use of numerical values in research replaces previous attempts to describe the phenomenon or just evaluate it as an "all-or-none" assessment.

Clinometrics

The potential for developing a prognosis from severity of the somatic dysfunction is another useful application of clinometrics. Location and patterns of segmental dysfunctions are already in use as indicators of disease processes.[10] Clinically, osteopathic physicians have used severity of somatic dysfunction to estimate the intensity of reflex inputs to somatic dysfunction. Quantitative values are needed to test this observation and its value in predicting whether an individual will become symptomatic. Clinometric indices improve observer predictions and increase interexaminer reliability. Further research in the application of quantitative descriptions of somatic dysfunction contributes to developing these potential advantages. This research should include instrumental measures of somatic dysfunction components to support clinical evidence obtained by palpatory examination.

EFFECTS OF INTERVENTION

Documenting outcomes of osteopathic management is a final task in developing a complete record of health care. A number of scales and indices are established as outcome measures and used to assess treatment of low back pain. The pain scales provide a model for rating somatic dysfunction, given that pain is not always perceived by the patient or elicited in examination. The Comprehensive Pain and Rehabilitation Center at the University of Miami Medical School[11] uses four categories to measure effectiveness of therapeutic intervention:

1. Self-reported pain level (0–10 scale)
2. Static strength of back extensors
3. Lumbar paraspinal muscle activity
4. Range of motion (primarily lumbar)

All of these measures qualify for development of four scales and a clinometric index. The measures include:

Rating scale
Clinical test
Palpatory findings
Inclinometer measurement

Similar criteria to quantify effectiveness of manipulative treatment for low back pain provide an outcome index. The value of well-planned and verified scales and indices is its versatility. These semiquantitative measures are equally applicable as measures of the condition being treated and the changes associated with treatment.

Other Scores, Scales, and Indices

Other scales in research on somatic dysfunction and its treatment include ratings for disability or impairment. The Oswestry Disability Score and the Waddell Physical Impairment and Disability Rating are reported in a study of low back pain.[12] Ottenbacher has discussed qualitative methods to increase measurement precision.[13] Ottenbacher evaluated effectiveness of manipulative treatment with ratings for:

1. Pain
2. Flexibility
3. Physical activity

Improvements associated with manipulation and mobilization were observed in short-term studies; longitudinal studies are needed. Long-term follow-up studies require reliable and accurate measures made at baseline and exit examinations. The advantages of clinometric indices and similar measures are apparent in longitudinal studies.[14]

International Assessment of Health Outcomes

The World Organization of National Colleges and Associations has studied standardized summary measurements of clinical health in its efforts to encourage a uniform method for worldwide reporting. WONCA assesses nine major areas[15]:

1. Physical condition
2. Emotional condition
3. Daily work
4. Social activities
5. Pain
6. Change in condition
7. Overall condition
8. Social support
9. Quality of life

These functional measures combine objective with subjective measures and increase reliability of the measurement while the researcher conducts longitudinal studies. Use of WONCA standards for clinical investigation of somatic dysfunction and its treatment increases communication with the entire field of manual medicine. The goal of WONCA is to establish a gold standard for assessment of functional status.[16-17] Instruments to measure functional status on a daily basis in primary care should satisfy five criteria. These measurements must be[18]:

1. Person-oriented
2. Reliable and valid
3. Useful
4. Sensitive
5. Internationally acceptable

Some disease states may require more than one functional measurement.[19]

Patient Diaries

Patient diaries of the activities of daily living and of health problems have advantages and disadvantages. Daily assessments are subject to emotional and mental states that vary greatly among individuals. Other individuals have positive feedback from the activity, much like a Hawthorne effect. The diary is one method of following day-to-day trends that are usually unavailable for study. The record of daily activities may not reflect the effects of all somatic dysfunctions; somatic dysfunction that creates disability or impaired mobility is less likely to be affected than dysfunctions that alter the presence of pain to affect activities. Many aspects of the patient's life experience can be recorded to study the effects and usefulness of manipulation.

PATIENT'S EXPECTATIONS

A patient's perception of the experience of osteopathic management is an important outcome measure in treating somatic dysfunction. This perception is obtained as a written report that provides data on quality of care.[20] Quality is customer (patient) satisfaction with the services received. Patient expectations for care are collected by a clinic receptionist and included in the patient's packet for review before the encounter with the physician. These expectations, discussed with the physician, result in mutual understanding of realistic expectations. The physician gains insight into the patient's perceptions of the expected benefit; the patient is apprised of the limitations and resources available at this encounter that may affect outcomes.

After the visit, the patient evaluates the encounter for satisfaction with care. Subsequent follow-up evaluation by telephone or during repeat visits is evaluated in the same manner. The information is treated confidentially to avoid bias.[21] Collated responses reported on physician performance as perceived by patients provide feedback on quality of care and on potential sources of differences in perceptions. Confirmation of differences in patients' perceptions and actual progression in re-sponse to OMT helps the physician. Improvement in palpatory findings may precede the patient's subjective experience and the level of satisfaction. An explanation of this phenomenon helps the patient understand the expected course of somatic dysfunction and the role of treatment in healing. Patient interactions with the physician increase reliability of the patient's satisfaction index and improve the process of health care.

Patient Perceptions of Quality Care

Scales are devised for the:

1. Patient's report of expectations
2. Agreed on expectations
3. Rating of the encounter and progress

These scales are used to score the patient's pre- and postencounter reports and are entered in the clinician-researcher's records. The patient's written evaluation is coded; this avoids use of the patient's name and maintains a paper trail to the original research data. The insight gained from reviewing the patient's and physician's experiences helps improve practice.

The important factor in all research on somatic dysfunction as a clinical entity is a quantitative measure for each component. The outcomes related to the presence of somatic dysfunction and the response to treatment also need quantification. Scales, indices, or instrumental measurements should be used in osteopathic clinical research to support treatment assessments and outcomes.[22-23]

CHARACTERISTICS OF SOMATIC DYSFUNCTION FOR RESEARCH

The science of palpatory description is ongoing for use in documenting osteopathic health care. Precise descriptions indicate what is to be palpated, measured, and recorded. These procedures increase interexaminer agreement on the same research subject or patient.

Locating Somatic Dysfunction

One of the most precise methods of describing palpatory examination is outlined in a series of articles by Johnston. He isolates the central segmental location of a somatic dysfunction, in part by defining compensatory restrictions immediately above and below the central location of the lesion complex. The adjacent areas behave opposite to the central segment for all motions introduced:

Side-bending
Rotation
Flexion or extension
Translation
Respiration

Adjacent areas contribute to a specific definition of the segmental complex of somatic dysfunction.[8,24-25] Johnston notes, *"It is possible to record these findings with considerable precision."* Repeatability is an essential aspect in defining characteristics of somatic dysfunction. Interexaminer and intra-examiner reliability have been extensively studied.[26-27] Beal notes that, from a research standpoint, recording assessment of somatic dysfunction with good agreement between examiners requires:

1. Specific agreement before examinations on the exact test to be used
2. Preselection of examiners who share the same testing methods and concepts
3. Study design that includes control patients (blinded to the examiners) who are not receiving treatment or who do not have chronic conditions. These controls are expected to have minimal change in their findings during multiple examinations.
4. Tests used should be appropriate to the patients' clinical condition

Responses to Treatment

A continuum of responses occurs when controlled stimuli such as manipulative treatments are used as an intervention, creating a desired therapeutic effect. This continuum involves local palpable tissue responses that guide decisions during treatment. These tissue responses determine the direction and localization of forces with the appropriate degree of force needed for proper execution of a particular procedure. Dynamic interaction to a stimulus results in some instantaneous tissue responses. Subsequent effects may take place over longer periods (seconds, minutes, weeks, or months). Changes initiated by OMT may act locally while other responses occur at a distant site or may occur as global systemic effects. These effects are the result of OMT directed toward particular palpatory findings defining a regional or segmental dysfunction. The effects of OMT include:

Alleviating symptoms of pain
Modifying illness and disability
Assisting recovery of health
Creating a feeling of well-being

These effects support the principle that restoring somatic function assists the body in its ability to heal itself (within physiologic limits). OMT facilitates recovery in ways that are predictable and often measurable with various instrumental measures, clinometric scales, and indices.

MECHANICAL AND FUNCTIONAL MECHANISMS

In clinical research, a distinction exists between neurophysiologically and mechanically induced changes following manipulative treatment. This distinction identifies the source of change and clarifies the processes that are observed as health outcome changes. In clinical research designed to advance theory and practice, response of the somatic dysfunction and outcomes of treatment must be identified and defined.

ATTENTION TO CHANGES

There are research questions about the assessment of desired tissue changes and the local and systemic effects associated with OMT. The parameters involve characteristics of somatic dysfunction, health status, and functional changes following treatments. The decision on the research method and measurements depends on practical considerations, availability, and costs. Available equipment and measurement tools, personnel time available for research, and the research tasks determine feasible research studies using instrumental measurements.

Pretreatment, Reevaluation, and Discharge Research

After the characteristics of somatic dysfunction are defined, pretreatment, reevaluation, and reexamination are scheduled to determine how these characteristics change during and after treatment. Often, the measurements are based on clinical scales and indices and on findings and instrumental measurements (when available). Schedules for testing are planned to obtain data on instantaneous and obvious changes such as motion while other, slower, and more subtle response measures are scheduled after several hours, days, or years. Reevaluation over longer periods of time reveals long-term effects, including some that were not anticipated. Delayed evaluations require reproducing baseline methods and measurements to obtain valid estimates of change.

Some methods seem more appropriate for clinical research in the office setting because of the ease of measuring the variables in osteopathic examination and evaluation, health outcomes, and patient satisfaction. The factors presented earlier should be considered and included when feasible. Also, research records and the medical record used for research purposes should include characteristics of:

1. Patients, their health status and problems, knowledge, and experience with osteopathic health care
2. Osteopathic physician's profile
3. Purpose of the study

Any of a number of manipulative techniques and decisions may achieve the desired outcome. For research and future medical records, the prescription and its administration are important. Outcomes are assessed to obtain data on immediate, short-term, or long-term responses. The data for the longer term responses must rely on reliable and reproducible methods and measurements of the specific local and systemic changes. The ideal contribution from clinician-researchers is feedback on practice and the production of reliable information for use in surveys, reports, and databases.

INSTRUMENTAL MEASUREMENTS

Measured Components

Advancement of osteopathic medical research requires quantitative data to support osteopathic theory and practice. Evaluation of health outcomes and other changes following manipulative treatment of somatic dysfunction needs the support of instrumental data. These measurements must meet scientific requirements for validity, reliability, and accuracy for research.[28] Health status, like somatic dysfunction, has many components to be measured[29]:

Physical functioning
Psychological well-being or distress
Cognitive functioning
Perceptions of distress or relief
Social functioning
Role functioning in personal, family, community, and work settings.

CLINICALLY SIGNIFICANT COMPONENTS

Research on somatic dysfunction requires selecting a clinically significant component of somatic dysfunction and a related instrumental measurement to support the clinical evaluation of the component. Appropriate measures provide numerical data on a component of somatic dysfunction that is identified by clinical examination. Using a clinical characteristic allows correlation between the instrumental and clinical measures. The characteristic must be one that the clinician relies on to assess the presence, location, and severity of somatic dysfunction for instrumental measurement.

Research on outcomes of an intervention used in practice, such as improved health and functioning, requires selecting measurements that are sensitive to changes following manipulative treatments. Research identifies association between instrumental and clinical measures supporting or refuting the osteopathic principle that the body has the capacity to restore and maintain health (within physiologic limits). Measurements of renal function by Hix[30] and respiratory capacity by Slezynski[31] supported the hypothesis that somatovisceral reflexes mediated the visceral responses. The research by Hix used an animal model and a basic research design. The research by Slezynski used incentive spirometry, a clinically accepted treatment to prevent postoperative atelectasis, as a standard for comparison with the effects of the thoracic pump, a manipulative treatment.

BENEFITS OF INSTRUMENTAL MEASUREMENT

Desirable instrumental measures are minimally subject to errors (reading, transcribing, and bias) and sufficiently sensitive to detect the amount of change that occurs between two measurements of a patient's status. Reduction in errors requires written test protocols that are carefully followed. Further improvement in accuracy also requires training the examiner and subject. Reduction depends on monitoring test data for possible instrumental error, malingering, and extraneous influences on the clinical and instrumental measurements.

Measuring Variables

Instruments are selected after the characteristic is chosen. It is important to select a measurement that correlates with a significant variable used in osteopathic evaluation of somatic dysfunction and changes in somatic dysfunction, health, and functional status. Strong correlation supports research conclusions. Support for speculation and hypothetical associations is established only through experimental research.

INSTRUMENTAL MEASUREMENTS FOR RESEARCH

Often, several instruments are suitable for measuring significant variables. For example, quality of life (QOL) questionnaires are used in clinical trials[32] to detect the changes in health status during testing of a drug for safety and efficacy. Similar questionnaires on activities of daily living (ADL) provide information on outpatients who are participating in clinical research.[33] Either QOL or ADL might be used; QOL is appropriate in clinical trials because most researchers are familiar with it. Reading the background literature on instrumental measurements and their application helps the researcher make an appropriate selection.

Osteopathic Approach

Diagnosis and treatment of somatic dysfunction are unique characteristics of osteopathic medicine. They are distinctive features that differentiate osteopathic physicians from:

Orthopedists
Physiatrists
Chiropractors
Naturopaths
Physical therapists
Others who use manipulative treatment

Disturbances in structure and nervous control of motor functions accompany regional somatic dysfunction. The disturbances are prominent in identifying spinal segments to be treated. Information for selecting established instrumental measurements exists in the fields of physical medicine, sports medicine, and radiology, and for functional measurements in cardiology, gastroenterology, neurology, obstetrics and gynecology, and sports and rehabilitation medicine. Literature sources identify research models, protocols for use of instruments, and methods of measurement.

Preparation

New technology often requires the development of technical specifications as well as normative and standardized data. Upper and lower limits of normal must be established. For instance, skeletal motion analysis with the Metrecom yields numerical data in digital readouts on degrees of motion between vertebral segments. However, no criteria for normal ranges are available for evaluating the influence of somatic dysfunction on mobility. The researcher expends considerable time and effort in establishing the needed reference data. Researchers omit or overlook the tasks that establish credibility for instrumental data by using published and peer-reviewed methods. This information includes calibration standards and protocols for instrument and application uses. When such information is lacking, the researcher is advised to complete the tasks of calibration and to develop protocols before submitting grant proposals. Most overruns in research schedules and costs occur because of instrumental difficulties.

Standard for Quality

It is important that the osteopathic evaluation and manipulative treatment be equal to the quality attained in practice by an experienced osteopathic physician. The method for assessing the presence of somatic dysfunction should be referenced or accompanied by a detailed description of examination procedures and the criteria for decisions. Correlating patient response to manipulative treatment with changes in health status and functions requires descriptions of changes in somatic dysfunction. A reference should be cited or descriptions provided on how measurements were made and how differences were calculated.

Information on instrumental measurement suitable for research appears in at least two fields of literature: medicine and bioengineering. Names may differ; for example, biomechanics and bioengineering include theory and practice of physical measurements. Clinical publications on therapeutic outcomes provide information on instrumental and clinical measurements. Specific information from the literature or consultation should confirm the researcher's choices of instrumentation and plans to correlate the data with outcomes of osteopathic health care.

MANUAL MEDICINE IN AMBULATORY CARE

Osteopathic principles of practice and philosophy are available but provide little insight into planning clinical research protocols that include quantitative measurements. The resource information can be organized as background information on ambulatory care research, instrumental measurements of structure, movement, and health status. Textbooks and references on medical physiology supply needed information on functional measurements. Computerized laboratories are available for detailed and accurate analysis of motion. Arrangements to collaborate with researchers who have access to these facilities provides mutual benefits to the researcher and is a cost-effective use of expensive facilities.

Data on Medical Practice

Questions on ambulatory care and its health and cost-effectiveness alerted clinical researchers to the lack of reliable data on outpatient care. Their publications provide information for developing protocols and insight into ambulatory care research. Specific information is needed on investigations by individuals or physician networks, or in a multicentered clinical trial. *Osteopathic Research: Growth and Development* includes clinical and basic research information from the late 1890s to 1975.[34] *Research: The Validation of Clinical Practice* emphasizes measurements and improving health care in the fields of occupational and physical therapy.[35] *Research Methods for General Practitioners* is an English textbook that is a practical guide and training manual for research on practice.[36] Helpful hints are provided for a clinical researcher and for a team of general practitioners. *Epidemiology in General Practice* recognizes the potential for epidemiologic research by general practitioners.[1(p142–149)] Morrell introduces this aspect of the scientific method and the methods available for research in outpatient settings. *Research Methods in Primary Care* consists of six short volumes that address topics of interest to clinician-researchers.[37] The volumes include *Primary Care Research, Tools for Research, Strategies for Qualitative Research, Assessing Interventions, Implementing Research in the Primary Care Setting,* and *Disseminating Research Findings.* The goal of these six monographs is to evaluate and improve primary care by supporting the processes and interventions used in practice with evidence from clinical research.

RESOURCES FOR RESEARCH

The osteopathic history of structural examination and the clinical experience with structural problems are summarized by Cole and Beal in several chapters of *Osteopathic Research: Growth and Development.*[38–41] Recent additions to the investigation of structure and movement are included in publications by Schwabb[42] and Irvin.[43] Greenman's text, *Principles of Manual Medicine,* emphasizes osteopathic manipulation with inclusion of some aspects of other approaches to manual medicine.[44] Its research value is in the principles and clinical descriptions of manual procedures and techniques. Johnston[45] quantified range of motion and correlated this loss with presence of somatic dysfunction. Inclinometers are accepted as standard methods for measuring range of motion.[14] Other devices for measuring range of motion include:

Electrogoniometers
Spinoscopes[46]
X-ray studies[47]
Soft tissue compliance meter[48]
Three-dimensional CT scan images[49]
MRI[50]
MRI with positron-emission tomography (PET)[51]

INSTRUMENTAL MEASUREMENTS OF BODY FUNCTIONS

Functional measurements are of interest to clinical researchers. Electromyograms (EMGs) obtained by needle electrodes or surface electrodes provide records of muscle activity.[52] Under standardized conditions, the activity corresponds to static and dynamic muscle activity.[53] Thermography and sweating are noninvasive methods for accurate measurement of skin temperature and sympathetic control.[54–55] Thermographic changes in cutaneous areas reflexly related to the kidney have been observed.[56] Under controlled conditions, the measurements aid diagnosis of peripheral nerve anomalies or damage as reported by Wexler[57] and aid evaluation of sympathetic control of cutaneous circulation as reported by Schnitzlein,[58] Heath,[59] Einstein and Einstein,[60] Sucher,[61] and Clark and Edholm.[62] Other uses of thermography are proposed but require development of a theoretical bias and clinical documentation for use in pain syndromes and somatic dysfunction.[63]

CONCLUSION

Osteopathic diagnosis and manipulative treatment of somatic dysfunction are among many interventions used by osteopathic physicians in providing health care. The role of the somatic system in health and in recovery from illness, disability, and disease is not well-understood. Clinical investigation expands the knowledge base, supports osteopathic theories and principles of practice, and tests speculations and hypotheses on the effects of somatic dysfunction and its treatment. The research requires investigation of patients' health benefits, satisfaction with their care, and effective health outcomes. Investigation in outpatient settings requires the clinician to assume the additional roles of researcher and information manager to ensure the quality of clinical and research data. Clinicians must obtain quantitative data with instrumental measurements that support clinical observations. Another task is to monitor the medical records for complete documentation of patient characteristics, the services provided, and health outcomes. An additional task is to develop summary indices for:

Somatic dysfunction
Health status
Patient satisfaction
Health benefits and outcomes

These indices, or their equivalent, in the patient's medical record are transferred to reports, surveys, and third-party claims without the need for office personnel to interpret the medical record. The development of physician networks and a cadre of clinical researchers will advance osteopathic medicine and will increase knowledge about the unique aspect of osteopathic medical practice and the effects of somatic dysfunction on the somatic system's role in health.

ACKNOWLEDGMENTS

An osteopathic research fellowship was awarded by The Center for Osteopathic Research and Education and assisted by funding from The Burroughs Wellcome Foundation. The direction by Albert F. Kelso, PhD, Robert E. Kappler, DO, and John H. Sloan, DO, supported my interest in clinical research. Benjamin M. Sucher provided valuable assistance with information on instrumental measurements.

REFERENCES

1. Morrell D, ed. *Epidemiology in General Practice.* New York, NY: Oxford University Press; 1988:vii–viii.

2. Couch JB, ed. *Health Care Quality Management for the 21st Century.* Tampa, Fla: The American College of Physician Executives; 1991:iv.

3. Feinstein AR. *Clinical Epidemiology: The Study of the Outcome of Illness.* New York, NY: Oxford University Press; 1986:3–32.

4. Jennison K. Total quality management—Fad or paradigmatic shift? In: Couch JB, ed. *Health Care Quality Management for the 21st Century.* Tampa, Fla: The American College of Physician Executives; 1991:431–443.

5. Greenfield S. The use of outcomes in medical practice applications of the Medical Outcome Study. In: Couch JB, ed. *Health Care Quality Management for the 21st Century.* Tampa, Fla: The American College of Physician Executives; 1991:431–442.

6. Feinstein A. *Clinical Epidemiology: The Architecture of Clinical Research.* Philadelphia, Penn: WB Saunders; 1985:69–86.

7. Korr IM. Osteopathic research: the needed paradigm shift. *JAOA.* 1991;91:156–163.

8. Johnston WL. Segmental definition: I. A focal point for diagnosis of somatic dysfunction. *JAOA.* 1988;88:99–105.

9. Johnston W. Segmental behavior during motion: III. Extending behavioral boundaries. *JAOA.* 1973;88:211–217.

10. Johnston W, Kelso AF, Babcock HG. Changes in the presence of a segmental dysfunction pattern associated with hypertension, I. A short-term longitudinal study. *JAOA.* 1995;95(4):243–260.

11. Kahlil TM, Asfour SS, Martinez LM, et al. Stretching in the rehabilitation of low-back pain patients. *Spine.* 1992;17:311–317.

12. Greenough CG, Fraser RD. Assessment of outcome in patients with low back pain. *Spine.* 1992;17:36–41.

13. Ottenbacher K, Difabio RP. Efficacy of spinal manipulation/mobilization therapy. *Spine.* 1985;10:833–837.

14. Johnston W, Kelso AF. Changes in the presence of a segmental dysfunction pattern associated with hypertension, II. A long-term longitudinal study. *JAOA.* 1995;95(5):315–318.

15. Froom J. Preface. In: S Greenfield, *Functional Status Measurement in Primary Care.* New York, NY: Springer-Verlag; 1990:ix–x.3.

16. Greenfield S, Preface. In: WONCA Classification Committee. *Functional Status Measurement in Primary Care.* New York, NY: Springer-Verlag; 1990.

17. Lamberts H. The use of functional status assessment within the framework of the international classification of primary care. In Froom J, Preface in S Greenfield, *Functional Status Measurement in Primary Care.* New York, NY: Springer-Verlag; 1990:45–56.

18. Bensten BG. The history of health status assessment from the point of view of the general practitioner. In Froom J, Preface in S Greenfield, *Functional Status Measurement in Primary Care.* New York, NY: Springer-Verlag; 1990:57–65.

19. Froom J. Disease-specific functional status assessment. In Froom J, Preface in S Greenfield, *Functional Status Measurement in Primary Care.* New York, NY: Springer-Verlag; 1990:66–71.

20. Macintyre K, Kleman CC. Measuring customer satisfaction. In: McLaughlin CP, Kaluzny AD, eds. *Continuous Quality Improvement in Health Care.* Gaithersburg, Md: Aspen Publishers, Inc; 1994:102–121.

21. Internal Customers—the patient. In: McLaughlin CP, Kaluzny AD, eds. *Continuous Quality Improvement in Health Care.* Gaithersburg, Md: Aspen Publishers, Inc; 1994:115–117.

22. Pocock SJ. A perspective on the role of quality-of-life assessment in clinical trials. *Controlled Clinical Trials.* 1991;12:257–265S.

23. Chapman CG, Syrjala K. Measurement of pain. In: Bonica J, ed. *The Management of Pain.* Philadelphia, Penn: Lea & Febiger; 1990:580–594.

24. Johnston WL. Segmental definition: III. Definite basis for distinguishing somatic findings of visceral reflex origin. *JAOA.* 1988; 88:347–353.

25. Johnston W. Segmental behavior during motion: II. Somatic dysfunction—the clinical distortion. *JAOA.* 1972;72:53–57.

26. Johnston W, Allan BR, Hendra JL, et al. Interexaminer study of palpation in detecting location of spinal segmental dysfunction. *JAOA.* 1983;82:839–845.

27. Beal MC, Goodridge JP, Johnston WL, et al. Interexaminer agreement on patient improvement after negotiated selection of tests. *JAOA.* 1979;79:432–440.

28. Dunn EV. Basic studies for analytic studies in primary care research. In: Norton PG, Stewart M, Todiver JF, et al., eds. *Primary Care Research.* London, England: Sage Publications; 1991:78–96.

29. Stewart AL. The Medical Outcomes Study Framework of Health Indicators. Stewart AL, Ware JE Jr, eds. In: *Measuring Functioning and Well-Being.* 1993:15.

30. Kelso AF. Physiology. In: *Osteopathic Research: Growth and Development.* Chicago, Ill: American Osteopathic Association; 1987:65.

31. Slezynski SL, Kelso AF. Comparison of thoracic manipulation with incentive spirometry in preventing postoperative atelectasis. *JAOA.* 1993;93(8):834–845.

32. Spilker B, ed. Introduction. In: *Quality of Life Assessments in Clinical Trials.* New York, NY: Raven Press; 1990:3–5.

33. Stewart AL, Ware JE Jr. Questionnaires, design, and administration. In: Stewart AL, Ware JE Jr, eds. *Measuring Functioning and Well-Being.* 1993:67–272.

34. Northup GW, ed. In: *Osteopathic Research: Growth and Development.* American Osteopathic Association; 1987.

35. Payton OD. *Research: The Validation of Clinical Practice.* 2nd ed. 1988.

36. Armstrong D, Calnan M, Grace J. In: *Research Methods for General Practitioners.* New York, NY: Oxford University Press; 1990.

37. *Primary Care Research: Traditional and Innovative Approaches,* series editors, PG Norton, M Stewart, F Tudiver, et al., Chicago, Ill: American Osteopathic Association; 1991.

38. Cole WV. Historical basis for osteopathic theory and practice. In: Northup GW, ed. *Osteopathic Research: Growth and Development.* Chicago, Ill: American Osteopathic Association; 1987:3–22.

39. Cole WV. Osteopathic research: Anatomical and histopathological evidence. In: Northup GW, ed. *Osteopathic Research: Growth and Development.* American Osteopathic Association; 1987:27–34.

40. Beal MC. Biomechanics: A foundation for osteopathic theory and practice. In: Northup GW, ed. *Osteopathic Research: Growth and Development.* Chicago, Ill: American Osteopathic Association; 1987:37–54.

41. Beal MC. Clinical research. In: Armstrong D, Calnan M, Grace J, eds. *Research Methods for General Practitioners.* New York, NY: Oxford University Press; 1990:73–87.

42. Schwabb WA, Strachan WF. The human mechanism as it is affected by unequal leg lengths. In: Peterson B, ed. *Postural Balance and Imbalance.* Indianapolis, Ind: The American Academy of Osteopathy; 1983.

43. Irvin RE. Reduction of lumbar scoliosis by use of a heel lift to level the sacral base. *JAOA.* 1991;91:474–479.

44. Greenman PE. *Principles of Manual Medicine.* Baltimore, Md: Williams & Wilkins; 1989.

45. Johnston WL, Voro J, Hubbard RP. Clinical/biomechanical correlates for cervical function: I. A kinematic study. *JAOA.* 1985; 85:429–437.

46. Smythe HA. Control and "fibrositic" tenderness comparison of two dolorimeters. *J Rheumatol.* 1992;19:768–771.

47. Hagberg C. General musculoskeletal complaints in a group of patients with craniomandibular disorders (CMD). A case control study. *Swed Dent J.* 1991;15:179–185.

48. Fisher AA. Tissue compliance meter for objective, quantitative documentation of soft tissue consistency and pathology. *Arch Phys Med Rehabil.* 1987:122–125.

49. Kojima T, Kurokawa T. Quantitation of three-dimensional deformity of idiopathic scoliosis. *Spine.* 1992;17:S22–S29.

50. Kamin M. Headache. In: *Textbook of Family Practice.* 4th ed. Philadelphia, Penn: WB Saunders Company; 1995:1430.

51. Hall S. *Mapping the Next Millennium.* New York, NY: Random House; 1992.

52. Denslow JS, Clough HG. Reflex activity in the spinal extensors. *J Neurophysiol.* 1941;5:393–402.

53. Voro J, Johnston WL. Clinical biomechanic correlates for cervical function: II. A myoelectic study. *JAOA.* 1987;87:353–367.

54. Wright HM, Korr IM, Thomas PE. Local and regional variations in cutaneous vasomotor tone of the human trunk. *J Neural Transm.* 1960;22:3,34–52.

55. Thomas PE, Korr IM. Relationship between sweat gland activity and electrical resistance of skin. *J Neural Transm.* 1957;17:77–96.

56. Kelso AF. Physiology. In: Northup GW, ed. *Osteopathic Research: Growth and Development.* Chicago, Ill: American Osteopathic Association; 1987:65.

57. Wexler CE. An overview of liquid crystal and electronic lumbar, thoracic and cervical thermography. In: Abernathy M, Uematsu S. *Medical Thermology.* Hanover, Me: Sheridan Press; 1986:198–209.

58. Schnitzlein HN, King PS. Review of sympathetic regulation of cutaneous vasculature. *Mod Med.* September 1987(special supplement):8–12.

59. Heath DM, Sloan JH, Kelso AF, et al. A prospective clinical study on the efficacy of osteopathic manipulative treatment in managing ischemic rest pain in the lower extremities. *JAOA.* 1986;86:603–604.

60. Einstein SA, Einstein G. Computerized electronic thermography in evaluation of muscle pain. In: *Journal Academy Neuromuscular Thermography, Clinical Thermography, Scripta Medica and Technica.* South Orange, NJ: 1989:38–48.

61. Sucher JM. Thermographic documentation of dysfunction in repetitive strain syndrome. *J Am Acad Thermol.* 1991;3:281.

62. Clark RP, Edholm OG. *Man and His Thermal Environment.* London, England: Edward Arnold Ltd; 1985.

63. Hales JRS, ed. In: *Thermal Physiology.* New York, NY: Raven Press; 1984.

78. Medical Records in Clinical Research

HARRY D. FRIEDMAN

Key Concepts

- **Components of the medical record that identify services provided to patients during osteopathic evaluation and treatment**

- **Importance of the medical record in providing information about the outcomes of osteopathic health care**

- **Use of medical record data for clinical research**

- **Use of medical record data for abstracts, reports, reimbursement requests, and research on osteopathic practice**

Other chapters in this text explore the philosophy and practice of osteopathic medicine and define somatic dysfunction as a clinical entity reflecting important changes in the body. Several questions about somatic dysfunction remain:

What do we know about its most basic features?
Who has it?
Who is likely to get it?
What circumstances promote its occurrence?
Once present, how long does it persist?
Does it change over time?
With what clinical syndromes is it associated?
What is its role in the natural history of health, disability, and illness?

Our answers are incomplete; changes in environment, knowledge, and patients may alter the existing answers.

We need to characterize the basic epidemiologic features of somatic dysfunctions. Additionally, we are interested in studying the course and character of health status during osteopathic manipulative treatment (OMT) to address further questions:

What changes in the patient's somatic system and health identify the benefits of manipulative treatment?
What is the time course of the changes and benefits?
How many and what type of treatments are necessary to resolve a somatic dysfunction, influence the response to health stresses, and support the healing process?
What other factors influence response to manipulative treatment?

THE MEDICAL RECORD

The nature of somatic dysfunction, its response to treatment, and the influence of the nature and response alter the outcomes of health care. Such changes, associated with somatic dysfunction, are not easily identified by classical medical research. The medical records of patients who have had continuing health care that included manipulative treatment provide clues that suggest these associations. An accurate and complete medical record increases effectiveness of patient health care and ensures the value of the records for communication and information retrieval.[1] Records also contain essential information about patients, about their health status and problems, and about their care and its effectiveness. This information contributes to clinical research.[2]

An accurate and reliable medical record is needed to advance osteopathic knowledge and practice in multiple settings. Especially important is the use of procedures that have been carefully standardized, which ensures uniformity in records and improves their communication value. This standardization enables the use of research designs that rely on medical record data for analysis.[3–7] Standardized formats for record keeping make it possible not only to communicate medical information but also to collect, abstract, and analyze data to advance medical knowledge.[8]

The answers to questions raised in medical practice require continual research because the answers may change with advances in knowledge and technology. Medical progress adds new dimensions to the questions. In some instances, personal or environmental factors influencing health care also change and modify the previously established answers. Medical knowledge is modified by research that produces new information on health and illness, on technological advances, and on changes in health care needs. Evaluating these sources of change provides a basis for updating current practice.

Functions of the Medical Record

The medical record serves many important functions. First, it stores information pertaining to the patient's medical care and as such is the common point of reference for all problem-solving and communication activities within that medical care. Stored information in the medical record greatly enhances the quality of patient care in the health care system. The medical record also serves as a document[9] in which scientific, ethical, and quality care issues are met, maintained, and advanced. The standards of science, the tenets of philosophy, and the principles of practice can be formulated, evaluated, and reformulated to effectively manage the complex and ever-changing nature of the health care system. Recognition of and compliance with these influences ensures quality data for osteopathic research.

Medical Records in Clinical Research

There are rational problem-solving approaches to[10–12]:

- Medical history-taking
- Physical examination
- Formulating a differential diagnosis
- Arriving at a definitive diagnosis on which to implement and follow a plan of medical management

This medical problem-solving model is reflected in the medical record. The quality of the record to a great extent determines the quality and the impact of research when medical record data is used for research. Advancement in knowledge that results from research improves osteopathic medical practice.

Medical Records in Hospital and Ambulatory Care

Practice in hospital and ambulatory care settings requires similar medical record formats. In private and group practice, the initial history, physical record, and follow-up notes are similar to the hospital inpatient record. The ambulatory osteopathic structural examination can be much more detailed and inclusive of all body regions. A definitive record is obtained because the patient's function and mobility are improved in the outpatient setting.

EXPANDING MEDICAL RECORD INFORMATION

The global, health restoration, and maintenance nature of outpatient medical services stimulates a complete osteopathic evaluation and ongoing comprehensive osteopathic care. The patient's medical record in the office setting reflects a more detailed examination, including screening, scanning, and segmental examination findings. Osteopathic examination is combined with assessment and selection of treatment. For this reason, the osteopathic structural evaluation form may be more detailed and may vary from clinician to clinician, as styles dictate and as requirements change. This individuality in methods and records should not interfere with providing uniform information on osteopathic evaluation and manipulative treatment or with reporting the health status during osteopathic health care.

RECORDING DIAGNOSIS OF SOMATIC DYSFUNCTION

In the ambulatory record, the same basic parameters are needed to fulfill the criteria for a diagnosis of somatic dysfunction. Gross structure and motion as well as tissue texture findings are recorded region by region using one of the standard formats. Reliability of findings is increased by testing segmental characteristics and by using specific criteria for location and positive findings, characteristics or acuteness or chronicity and severity, and response to OMT.

FOLLOWING RESPONSES TO OMT IN LONG-TERM PATIENT CARE

Following long-term patient responses to OMT is possible in the ambulatory care setting. Reexamination of a patient at subsequent visits using the same procedures, criteria for positive findings, and recording methods identifies trends in the patient's somatic dysfunctions and health status. Using the same procedures ensures that palpatory findings, accompanying symptoms, and health status can be evaluated for persistence or change. Research protocols for use in office settings can be implemented with patients who are examined at regular intervals. Accurate medical records used for a retrospective study identify the long-term health outcomes associated with osteopathic health care.

Standardized Record Forms

There are standardized record forms for screening, scanning, and segmental examinations.[7,13–16] These forms and associated sets of procedures provide reliable information on somatic dysfunction. The screening and scanning examination for somatic dysfunction can be completed in a few minutes. The number of segmental examinations varies according to the information needed on verification of the location, on the acute/chronic and severity characteristics of somatic dysfunction, and on the basis for planning manipulative treatment. Limiting segmental examinations to locating sites of new or exacerbated somatic dysfunctions reduces the need for segmental examinations outside of the areas of somatic dysfunction. The immediate and follow-up assessment of somatic dysfunction response to OMT is important, but there is no standard format for recording such changes. Changes are measured by the differences between the initial and reexamination records. Differences from accurate data obtained with the same tests and criteria that were used originally identify changes in somatic dysfunction and other measures of patient health status and outcomes.

Standardized Format

A standardized record format is essential for multisite data collection, for collecting data for public health care statistics, and for osteopathic research. A standardized format ensures consistency at multiple data collection sites and facilitates the task of abstracting, analyzing, and reporting medical record data. A standardized record format appears in Figure 78.1. This format was used in the Care-a-Van project commemorating the 100th anniversary of the founding of the Kirksville College of Osteopathic Medicine. With this standardized format, data analysis from medical records collected across the country is facilitated, and important questions can be answered on the incidence of somatic dysfunction in a cross-sectional population study.

Medical Records Provided in Different Settings

While the medical record is the key element in hospital, clinic, and office record systems, equally important is an organized

Regional exam: Musculoskeletal system

Required: The essential record of a screen for dysfunction during physical exam is formatted in the upper left table.

Patient _____

	ALTERED		SOMATIC DYSFUNCTION
	Tiss, Tex >2 sp.segs	Structure or Motion	
Head/face			
Cervical			
Thoracic			
Lumbar			
Sacro Pelvic			
Costal cage			
Extrems: up			
lower			

COMMENTS: _____
_____
_____
_____
_____
_____
_____
_____
_____
_____
_____

(+) Presence of altered findings

(-) Absence of altered findings

(0) Omitted

Somatic dysfunction = alted tissue texture and/or alted motion

MAKE USE OF the Comments section above, and the Diagram below, to facilitate description of the dysfunction when indicated:

Gross visual asymmetry

1. Levels (high ↑, low ↓)

2. Cures

Palpable

1. Tissue texture change (x)

2. Altered motion (→I)

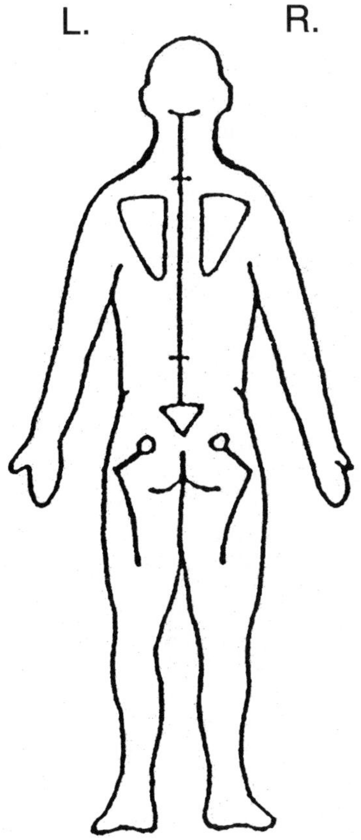

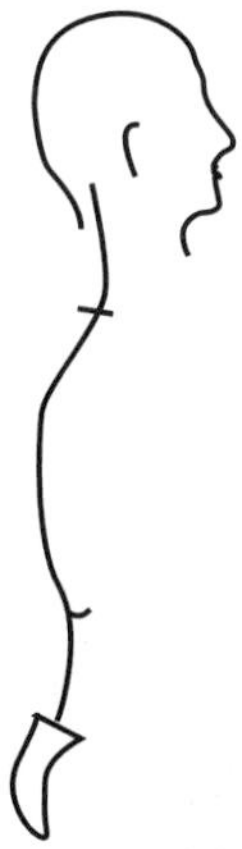

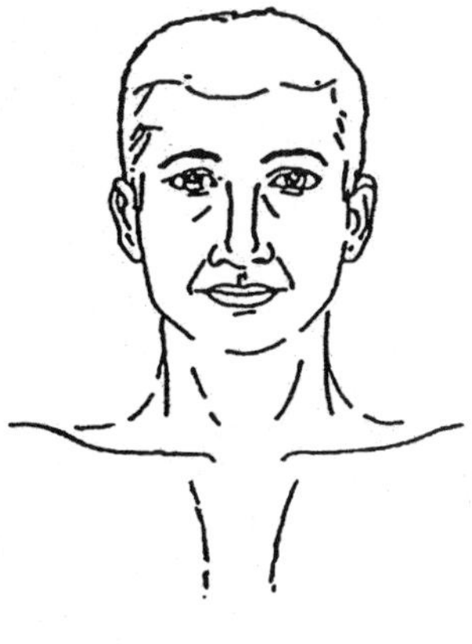

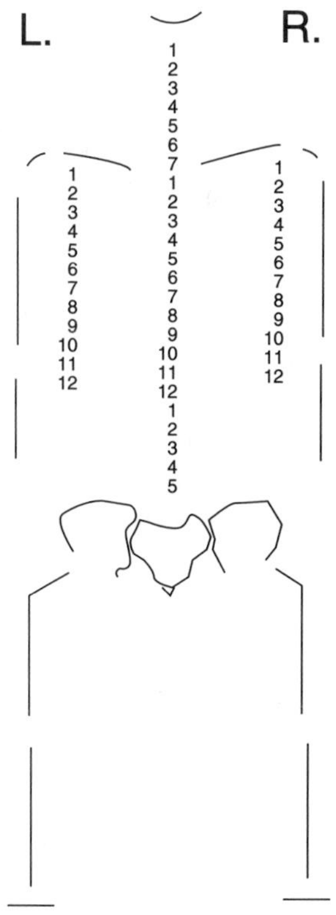

Signature

Figure 78.1. Example form used for regional examination of musculoskeletal system.

system for management of patient encounters, required services, and records in patient health care. Management defines tasks, establishes training programs, and monitors performance of assistants and allied health and administrative personnel, who are involved in data entry, filing, retrieval of records, and reporting the information on what health services have been provided.

Including OMT in Problem-Oriented Medical Records

Reorganization of the source-oriented medical record, in which the data was filed according to its origin, occurred with the introduction of the Problem-Oriented Medical Record (POMR).[1] The POMR begins with a problem list, identifying patient problems whether included in the current management of the patient or not. The list provides an index, the number assigned to the problem that is used in the Subjective Objective Assessment Plan (SOAP) notes to track the decisions, management, and course related to the health care and attention given individual problems.

POMR FORMS FOR AMBULATORY CARE

The POMR is currently accepted for use in most health care settings. Soon after its acceptance, a set of forms was designed for managing private and group practice.[4] The Bjorn and Cross system for managing ambulatory care included the POMR and other records that ensure the ability to track information on patient, physician, and office performance. Such records are a valuable source of information to plan health care improvements.

SOAP NOTES

Progress notes based on a SOAP format are entered into the medical record during the course of care. This format provides information on the patient's subjective (S) and physician's objective (O) data about the patient's problem and response to treatment. SOAP notes include the physician's initial and continuing assessment of findings (A) and the physician's decisions that establish or modify the management plan (P). Decisions are (or should be) based on previous record entries:

Findings
Progress relative to the expected course
Current health status
Outcomes that have occurred

This evaluation of changes associated with care is feasible for short-term, e.g., during a hospital stay or a series or encounters for a specific problem. Accurate records that were based on using the same procedures, observations, and tests with the same criteria for findings, assessment, and decisions also provide the basis for detecting long-term changes in somatic dysfunction, in patient progress, and in health.

OSTEOPATHIC COMPONENTS IN THE MEDICAL RECORD

A medical record should include:

Osteopathic findings
Diagnosed somatic dysfunctions
Decisions (plan or modifications of the plan during care) on treating somatic dysfunctions
Administration of OMT
Observed responses to OMT

This information identifies the need for osteopathic care and benefits. This is essential information about patient care. Reports based on the patient's medical record also provide data for the profession. The information helps community and public health agencies assess health care needs, available services, and planning (including budgets) to meet unmet and anticipated needs.

Health Care Research Team

A team approach to medical record keeping improves the record for health care and makes it feasible to conduct research. Members of the team are the:

Leader (the physician-researcher)
Patient
Allied health personnel
Staff

A hospital manual indicates the tasks for all personnel. An office manual provides the same information. The office manual should be more detailed because of the varied background and multiple tasks performed by office personnel. It is important that the leader ensures that personnel are trained[17]; they must know what and how the data should be entered in the medical record. Research in the hospital or office setting can be a routine part of all personnel tasks. Adding the research tasks to the manuals and training personnel in these tasks improves the conduct of health care research and the accuracy of data in the medical record. A research technician or assistant performs tasks similar to that of a medical assistant and improves the quality of research.

Quality Control

Quality of care and research records are a special concern. In the hospital setting, quality assurance is established by review of medical records to ensure that the content meets established standards. Quality control personnel review records for content and accuracy. Hospitals and clinics that conduct research routinely use research assistants or technicians who are responsible for many tasks, including the completeness and accuracy of medical and research data.

CONTROLLING QUALITY OF MULTISITE RESEARCH DATA

Using the team approach makes it feasible to conduct research during health care. Producing quality data for reports, surveys, and use in databases can be accomplished with little increase in time or effort. Participating in planned, network office-based studies can be accomplished within the normal operation of the office.[18] The task of controlling data collection for quality and completeness, and for tabulating, analyzing, and reporting data belongs to the research leader or organizer. Without the participating physician-researcher's cooperation, the credibility and quality of network data is questionable.

MEDICAL RECORDS KEPT BY CLINICIAN-RESEARCHERS

Though medical researchers have their own scientific and personnel agenda, their use of a medical record reflects its important role: to enhance the delivery and quality of patient care. To researchers, the medical record provides the data for answering clinical questions and for advancing medical theory and practice. The physician-researcher role is unique and must be preserved and encouraged amidst the many demands, some with high priorities, for performing in the health care system.

Recording Osteopathic Procedures and Outcomes

The remainder of this chapter emphasizes recording osteopathic procedures and outcomes of care in both the hospital and ambulatory setting. Such records not only improve patient health care but also provide a data source for reporting to the patient, community, and public on the effectiveness of osteopathic health care. Chapter 77, "Somatic Dysfunction," identifies the data components of osteopathic examination and testing. These data are entered into the medical record and used in the physician's decisions on patient care. The data on decisions, services provided, and outcomes of care recorded in the medical record are used in:

　　Discharge summaries
　　Face sheets
　　Periodic ambulatory care reviews[16]
　　Abstracts (transfer notes, summaries)
　　Surveys
　　Databases

The reliability and credibility of these derived documents is only as good as the accuracy of the data in the medical record and its reproduction in the records and reports.

Summary of Data

Table 78.1 shows the information necessary for the record; the information is easily obtained from hospital and ambulatory care records. Information from walk-in ambulatory care and emergency care may not be relevant to a research design that requires baseline information or an initial workup, or that anticipates follow-up care. The care for an industrial patient may or may not be relevant, depending on whether such records have a bearing on the purpose of the research under consideration and whether the medical records are available for verifying the data. Similarly, student examinations usually lack sufficient baseline data and are not easily followed up.

Table 78.1
Information Included in Medical Records and Reports

Information to be included in the medical record
　　Admitting note (H)
　　Initial history on hospital admission (H)
　　Discharge summary and plan (H)
　　Hospital medical record face sheet (H)
　　Complaint(s)/purpose of encounter (AC)
　　Initial history and periodic histories (AC)
　　Admitting (H) or periodic physical examination (AC)
　　Laboratory data (B)
　　SOAP notes (B)
　　Transfer note of patient's health care (B)
Information to be included in medical reports
　　Surveys
　　Questionnaires
　　Third-party billing
Reports for inclusion in a professional database should abstract data from
　　the medical record on these components
　　Osteopathic diagnosis
　　Treatment
　　Changes in somatic dysfunction
　　Patient's health risk/benefit
　　Health status and outcomes

H, hospital medical record; AC, ambulatory care medical record; B, hospital and ambulatory care record.

NOTE: The periodic examination in general or family practice benefits the patient who is receiving continuing care by ensuring a periodic review and evaluation by the provider for needs met and the effectiveness of care. It provides a means for identifying the patient's health risks and current health status and is a potential method for following somatic dysfunction as a risk indicator and associated changes in health.

Planning Research in Different Health Care Settings

Health care is provided in a number of different settings and for many purposes. Unless specific research is planned for these settings, only carefully recorded data in the medical record is suitable. This is particularly true of data needed in longitudinal studies because changes in patients are being studied.

FLAGGING MEDICAL RESEARCH RECORDS

Many persons use the medical record to find instructions for patient care and to record their services. Flagging medical records of patients who are participating in approved research facilitates research data entries and alerts other users to research in progress. Researchers rely on the medical record for health-related information and may keep additional information in their research record. In this case, an entry could be made in the medical record: "a research encounter occurred on this date." This additional information ensures that the physician responsible for the patient's care can contact the researcher if information is needed.

Contributions of Medical Record to Quality Health Care

Increased use of medical record data, in both hospital and ambulatory care records, accompanies the emphasis on health care, manages patients with health risks, and provides access to efficacious, quality health care. Many persons can contribute to this research effort by completing records of their services and ensuring the accuracy of such entries.

Medical Record Data Source for Information

Physicians writing discharge summaries should use the medical record as a source for information in the osteopathic component of health care: what was provided and what were the outcomes. Medical librarians complete the face sheet for the medical record, and the osteopathic component of health care should be included: diagnosis of somatic dysfunction and its treatment and benefits. Surveys and databases on the osteopathic component of health care rely on medical record data:

Diagnosis of somatic dysfunction
Characteristics of somatic dysfunction
Administration of OMT for specific somatic dysfunction
Response of the somatic dysfunction to treatment
Accompanying changes in health and healing

Requests for reimbursement from third-party payers and inpatient billing must be supported with information in the medical record that includes osteopathic diagnoses, the care provided, and changes in health status. The persons providing services related to osteopathic health care need to ensure that the information needed for reporting the community and public benefits of osteopathic care are entered into the medical record.

Physician Data in Medical Records

Data on the osteopathic components of patient health care obtained by the osteopathic physician include:

1. Elucidating the somatic component of the patient's chief complaint and the general health status for entry into the patient's problem list
2. Performing specific visual and palpatory tests of the somatic system that can be repeated during the patient's health care management to identify changes in somatic dysfunction that accompany altered health status or progression of illness
3. Arriving at the diagnosis of somatic dysfunction and determining its relationship to the patient's chief complaint and the problem list
4. Planning diagnostic testing, consultations, and treatments to be included in the patient's management
5. Assessing the patient's response to treatment and implementing management modifications
6. Writing a discharge summary of assessments and treatment outcomes, including documentation to support all of the above
7. Including the observed benefits of osteopathic care in the patient's medical record, abstract, and reports to third-party payers and to community and public health agencies

Recording Osteopathic Findings, Assessments, and Diagnoses

Somatic dysfunctions are recorded during the physical examination as somatic dysfunction by region. A similar record is made during each encounter and examination for somatic dysfunction. Data on the nature of the somatic dysfunction needed for research purposes is included and indexed by the problem number in the problem list.

EVALUATING FOR CHANGES IN SOMATIC DYSFUNCTION

Somatic dysfunction changes with time, disease, and interventions. The only records of somatic dysfunction that can be used to identify these changes must have a uniform base. For valid retests of somatic (segmental) dysfunction, there are several requirements:

The original methods of examination and testing; criteria for positive findings, assessment, and diagnosis; and recording of somatic dysfunction must be the same on reexamination to make a comparison.
The same methods of examination and testing, and the criteria for positive findings, assessment, decisions, and recordings must be used for retesting or identifying progress or changes in the patient's other problems, health risks, and health.

The comparison of information in the two records provides information on any changes.

SEGREGATING POSITIVE FINDINGS

Positive findings from a group of tests, each for a specific characteristic, are aggregated for assessment to provide a reliable and repeatable measurement. This method, in addition to standardizing the research protocol and verification of internal consistency, improves the precision of testing.[2] Johnston has reported 27 specific tests for segmental motions in a central vertebral segment and the two adjacent ones, which provides a statistically significant basis for assessing segmental motion dysfunction.[19] Sets, groups, or aggregated data usually provide more information than can be obtained from individual data. Statistical significance is increased by pooling results from different studies or by increasing numbers of subjects.

COMBINED EXAMINATION AND TREATMENT

During health care encounters, a physician may combine segmental examination and treatment. It is difficult to record osteopathic findings when examinations are made during treatment. A voice-activated recorder used during examination and treatment ensures that all the information is recorded. (It should be transcribed and validated soon after the treatments are completed).

QUANTITATIVE MEASUREMENTS

Records of instrumental measurements provide evidence to support the diagnosis of somatic dysfunction. Sources of instrumental data include:

Imaging and image analysis
Video recording
Thermography
Computerized records of movement
Electrophysiologic monitoring of movement

The procedures for obtaining valid information from such measurements should be included in either the instrument record or the progress note. Information on measurements should include technical procedures such as calibration and controls for accuracy. They also include procedural controls such as patient positioning and activities, and others such as environment conditions, which should be in the technician's record and report.

Orders for Osteopathic Manipulative Treatment

The plan for including OMT in the patient's health care is developed after:

1. Considering the somatic dysfunctions in the problem list with other information for planning patient management
2. Examining and treating somatic dysfunctions during a patient care encounter

Diagnoses of somatic dysfunctions aid in the decisions on which patient problems are selected and when OMT is involved in the management of the patient's health care. The findings, assessment, and plan should be completed and entered into the medical record regardless of whether planning or providing manipulative treatment during an encounter because they represent decisions on patient care.

Orders should be written or described when the physician provides the treatment. The order or description should contain:

Region of somatic dysfunction
Contraindications in the choice of treatment
Intensity, duration, and frequency of treatment
Request for assessment of the patient's response to treatment

The treating physician should be alert for other changes in patient behavior or conditions that represent possible response to OMT. Knowing possible responses in advance ensures observation; a prepared mind is a key to awareness.

Recording Changes in Somatic Dysfunction

The specific tests used in segmental examinations should also be used for assessing changes in somatic dysfunctions. A diagnosis of somatic dysfunction is based on the findings of structural asymmetry, gross motion disturbance, and tissue texture abnormalities observed during a screening and scanning examination. These findings are gathered using many different testing procedures that have been reported in the literature.[20–21] These procedures provide data to answer the following questions:

Is there a problem in the musculoskeletal system that relates to this patient's chief complaint, health problems, and risks? Are there benefits evident in other systems related to administering OMT?

Specific tests and criteria for positive findings in segmental examinations allow precise description of the location and characteristics of somatic dysfunction. Recording the segmental tests, criteria, and positive findings in the SOAP note provides a reference for evaluating changes in somatic dysfunctions following treatment or later in the course of patient health care. Recording similar tests, criteria, and findings on other characteristics, for example, the status of a problem or the patient's health, provides a comparison reference for evaluating concomitant changes in somatic dysfunction and in other health conditions. Using specific tests and standard criteria for positive findings and assessments ensures that changes can be detected. The recording of changes following OMT obtained without the use of specific tests are subject to faults in memory.

RATE OF HEALING AND HEALTH STATUS

The benefits of interventions used in health care include providing relief, aiding recovery, and maintaining health. The benefits are presently estimated by many methods. Investigations of better methods to establish health status and to evaluate the patient's subjective perceptions are ongoing.[1,5,22] The newer measurements of health, pain, perceptions, or changes in a problem should be used (see Chapter 77, "Somatic Dysfunction"). The measurement procedure for obtaining subjective data and the steps taken to reduce variability in the data and the results should be recorded. The reliability of these measurements is subject to the errors introduced by variable testing procedures. Data obtained by using different tests or modified procedures may not be comparable. Using standardized tests, procedures, and controls ensures a basis for comparison.

CHANGES FOLLOWING TREATMENT

Research on the association of somatic dysfunction and its response to OMT as a beneficial intervention in health care requires the use of accurate measures of change in somatic dysfunction. The most reliable data, to date, are obtained by using specific segmental tests for motion asymmetry or tissue changes with specific criteria for positive findings and results. Variability in the methods used to assess changes in somatic dysfunction requires establishment of criteria for comparison between different measurements. Similarly, the data on health, healing, and response to risk require identical measurements if data from different encounters, hospitalizations, and periodic examinations are compared.[2] The strategy for ensuring the quality of future research is to establish procedures for obtaining, recording, and reporting information in osteopathic practice. The expectation is that the plan will produce accurate data for use in research.

Accuracy of Osteopathic Medical Data

The accuracy of the osteopathic component in medical record data determines its research credibility. Established research designs or newer designs developed to study ambulatory care benefit from osteopathic physicians' and their health care teams' efforts to provide information.

Obtaining Evidence from Experience of Physicians

Clinicians who practice osteopathic manipulative medicine have considerable experience in providing total health care that includes diagnosis and treatment of somatic dysfunction. Their experience also provides the insight needed to answer questions concerning medical practice. The collective experiences of osteopathic physicians form the body of knowledge that supports osteopathic practice and theory. Valid and reliable recording supports the practice of osteopathic medicine by identification of patient, community, and public health benefits. Records must include osteopathic health care:

Procedures
Findings
Assessments
Plan
Treatment
Outcomes

CONCLUSION

Attention should be given to epidemiologic research on the characteristics of somatic dysfunction:

Nature
Occurrence
Relation to health status
Influence of its treatment

The benefits of osteopathic diagnosis and OMT as medical intervention also needs further research. These benefits can be identified using research designs that identify associations or cause–effect relationships between somatic dysfunction and changes in health problems or status.

Benefits from osteopathic health care can also be researched by osteopathic professional, community, and public health agencies using routinely reported data, surveys, or analysis of information stored in databases. This latter type of research includes ambulatory care data and is an addition to previously conducted osteopathic research. Newer and older types of research provide a response to the American and World Health Organization initiatives to provide access to health and cost-effective health care.

In all types of research, accurately recorded osteopathic components of health care in the patient's medical record is essential. The statistical reliability of epidemiologic and inter-

vention research is limited by variability in the research data. Reducing this variability improves the inferences that can be drawn from the data.

Surveys and databases obtain data from medical records and are limited by the accuracy of the recorded information. Increasing accuracy in the original record and its transcription to other records and reports ensures that the use of aggregated data from these medical records provides reliable information. Professional regulation of osteopathic practice and education depends on such information. Community and public planning and budgeting to meet health care needs, maintain adequate health care services and facilities, and support the health care infrastructure also rely on aggregate data or specialized surveys. The use of specialized surveys to obtain such information is expensive and still subject to errors and inaccuracies.

REFERENCES

1. Rakel RE, ed. In: *Textbook of Family Practice.* Philadelphia, Penn: WB Saunders Company; 1990:209–217, 401–416, 1693–1719.
2. Hulley SB, Cummings SR, eds. In: *Designing Clinical Research.* Baltimore, Md: Williams & Wilkins; 1988:34–36, 159–163.
3. Acheson ED. *Record Linkage in Medicine.* Baltimore, Md: Williams & Wilkins; 1969.
4. Bjorn JC, Cross HD. *Problem-Oriented Private Practice of Medicine.* Chicago, Ill: Hospital Press, McGraw-Hill; 1977.
5. Feinstein AR. *Clinimetrics.* New Haven, Conn: Yale University Press; 1987.
6. Friedman LM, Furberg CD, DeMets DL. *Fundamentals of Clinical Trials.* 2nd ed. Littleton, Mass: PSG Publishing Company; 1985:137–140, 272–273.
7. Friedman HD, Johnston WL, Kelso AF, Schwartz FN. Effects of an educational intervention on quality and frequency of osteopathic structural documentation on hospital admitting examination. *JAOA.* 1990;90:840. Abstract.
8. Hill AB. *Principles of Medical Statistics.* 8th ed. New York, NY: Oxford University Press; 1966.
9. Report of the Secretary's Advisory Committee on Automated Personal Data Systems. *Records, Computers, and the Rights of Citizens.* Washington, DC: US Government Printing Office; 1973. US Dept of Health, Education, and Welfare publication DHEW (OS) 73–97.
10. DeGowin EL, DeGowin RL. *Bedside Diagnosis and Examination.* New York, NY: MacMillan Publishing Co; 1981.
11. Isselbacher TR, Braunwald E, Wilson J, eds. *Harrison's Principles of Internal Medicine.* 13th ed. New York, NY: McGraw-Hill; 1994.
12. Melasanos L. *Health Assessment.* 2nd ed. St. Louis, Mo: CV Mosby Co; 1981.
13. Seffinger MA, Johnston WL. Relationship between musculoskeletal findings and somatic dysfunction. *JAOA.* 1990;90(7):656. Abstract.
14. Beal MC. Palpatory testing for somatic dysfunction in patients with cardiovascular disease. *JAOA.* 1983;82:822–831.
15. Johnston WL. Passive gross motion testing, I. *JAOA.* 1982;81:298–303.
16. Kelso AF. Records to assist osteopathic physicians. *JAOA.* 1975; 74(4):751–755.
17. Kinn ME. *The Administrative Medical Assistant.* 2nd ed. Philadelphia, Penn: WB Saunders Co; 1988.
18. Michigan State University/College of Osteopathic Medicine: De-

velopment of a Michigan Osteopathic Network for the training of clinician-researchers and conduct of epidemiologic and outcome studies on osteopathic practice. Prepared and distributed in the Michigan State University, College of Osteopathic Medicine, by the Primary Medicine Initiative, Research Work-Group; MSU/COM; Director, Martin J. Hogan.

19. Johnston WL, Hill JL, Elkiss ML, Marino RV. Identification of stable somatic findings in hypertensive subjects by trained examiners using palpatory examination. *JAOA.* 1982;81:830–836.

20. Dinar U, Beal MC, Goodridge JP, et al. Description of fifty diag-nostic tests used with osteopathic manipulation. *JAOA.* 1982; 81:314–321. Reprinted in Beal MC, ed. *The Principles of Palpatory Diagnosis and Manipulative Technique.* Indianapolis, ind: American Academy of Osteopathy; 1992.

21. Johnston WL. Louisa Burns Memorial Lecture: inter-examiner re-liability studies spanning a gap in medical research. *JAOA.* 1982; 81:819–829.

22. Spector WD. Functional disability scales. In: Spilker AS, ed. *Quality of Life Assessments in clinical trials.* New York, NY: Raven Press; 1990:115–127.

79. Use of Data on Osteopathic Aspects of Health Care

JEREL H. GLASSMAN

Key Concepts

- **Use of observation in population studies to understand relationships between causes and effects on health**

- **Need for valid, reliable, and consistent medical records of patient health care**

- **Statistical basis for drawing inferences about the associations**

- **Importance of medical records as a source document for population studies**

- **Utilization of population studies for protecting and promoting public health**

- **Application of public health data in planning, financing, and maintaining health care resources**

Federal, state, and local governments need information on citizens' health, disabilities, and illnesses. Governments use this information to promote and protect community health. They also use it to evaluate needs for health care and to plan the development, maintenance, and budgeting of health care services. Public health surveys, statistics, and special projects collect some information. A great deal of information comes from medical practice reports. The original medical records are rarely reviewed. Medical record data appears in:

Medical abstracts
Statistics on health care
Requests for reimbursement
Required reports

Staff personnel, rather than physicians, translate information from medical records that was transcribed from dictation or copied from other sources of this patient's data. Omissions in the medical record and errors in transcription decrease the value of the medical record as a source of data. Population studies, as compared with patient studies, require a valid source of data for public health research.

The strength of population studies is that pooling large bodies of information allows inferences to be made. Common events are significantly associated with diseased states. Somatic dysfunction, the hallmark of structural diagnosis performed by

osteopathically trained physicians, is such a commonly occurring event.

ASSOCIATION OF DYSFUNCTIONS WITH HEALING

A.T. Still proposed the controversial association between anatomic alteration and illness. In recent years, clinical trials have begun to clarify the association of certain somatic dysfunctions with conditions of pain and immobility.[1] Many groups have attempted to associate specific somatic dysfunction with alterations in autonomic-mediated processes such as cardiac or pulmonary function.[2–3] These studies have focused on small groups and have generally not been of a random design.

Cause–Effect Relationships

In cases where a strong cause–effect relationship exists between a pathologic agent, process, or illness, such as with exposure to influenza virus or with extreme cholesterol levels, relatively small groups are needed to show cause and effect. Using basic approaches of epidemiologic research, such as cross-sectional, case-control, or prospective study designs, associations suggest cause and effect for risk factors.

Similarity or Difference in Effects

Somatic dysfunction rarely exists as a solitary finding. More often, discrete somatic dysfunctions are found within each region of the body. It is left to the clinician to identify and treat the most problematic of these findings. In some cases, a cause–effect relationship seems likely; in other cases, somatic dysfunction either is a contributory factor or is present as a response to stress placed on the system. Study designs such as case reports and small control trials are helpful in situations where the specific cause–effect relationships are suspected. In cases where multiple factors result in higher probability of disease, simple study designs do not suffice.

Large-Scale Study Populations

To establish subtle associations between risk factors and diseased states, large-scale study populations are needed. Many of the conditions to which somatic dysfunction contributes appear multifactorial. For example, with coronary artery disease, large data tests were necessary to establish the relationship of multiple factors such as blood pressure, race, exercise, and cholesterol levels in the cause of the disease. Before the subtle contributions of somatic dysfunction to lumbar disk disease, ligamentous strain, and various nonmusculoskeletal conditions can be inferred, a method of amassing large study populations is necessary. Screening methods and systems of recording findings enable statistical power. Some researchers seek a link between osteopathically oriented structural diagnosis and treatment. Investigators now have a method of demonstrating associations between diagnosis and disease and between treatment and control of disease.

MEDICAL RECORD DATA

The study of somatic dysfunction presents special challenges for investigators researching osteopathic diagnosis and treatment. An osteopathically trained evaluator can identify somatic dysfunction in an individual. Researchers in this field have to quantify the persistence or dynamic quality of these structural findings over time. The identification of somatic dysfunction has traditionally been a palpatory process. Questions exist regarding the reliability, consistency, and validity of this diagnostic process.

Sensitivity and Specificity

Two indices are used to evaluate the accuracy of a test: sensitivity and specificity.[4] These indices are usually determined by administering a test to one group of persons who have a disease and to another group who do not and then comparing the results. This process has been difficult in osteopathic research. Osteopathic researchers have not agreed on a universally objective measure of somatic dysfunction. This problem exists, however, in all areas of medical research; it arises from the inherent difficulty in providing accuracy and continuity for systems that may be changing throughout their natural history.

Examiners Reduce Errors

Yerushamy initially clarified the problem of variability in his studies of the interpretation of chest x-ray films in the diagnosis of tuberculosis.[5] He found that both interrater and intrarater errors existed. Much of the variability was the result of differences in training and experience of the different examiners. Johnston and Beal have similarly shown this to be true in the analysis of osteopathic structural findings.[6–7]

Costs and Contributions

In setting a test level to identify those individuals with a specific condition and to omit those individuals without it, the research plan must justify the relative costs of classifying persons as false–negatives and false–positives. The prevalence of the condition in a community and the cost of additional examinations that may be necessary must be considered.[8]

Data Collection

Medicine is in a transitional stage in that the skills of diagnosis in some areas have been augmented by advances in technology. However, the accuracy of a diagnostic technology, such as ultrasonic evaluation of cardiac function, has not led to the abandonment of the stethoscope. So too, advances in technology may assist in the diagnosis of somatic dysfunction but are unlikely to eliminate the need for palpation in observation of the patient.

Surveys and Interviews

Information acquired through surveys and questionnaires can greatly assist researchers in linking somatic dysfunction to behaviors or activities that occur within the community at large. Some question the accuracy of information obtained by interview.[9] For example, if the prevalence of somatic dysfunction was thought to be associated with a sedentary lifestyle, the possibility exists that interviewed persons might overestimate their activity levels. Information obtained by interview might need to be validated with past medical or other types of records.

Research Protocols

Additional methods of data collection exist. An individual or team can collect information directly from observation of patients. Designing and carrying out specific projects of this type is extremely costly. All study personnel must be paid; test subjects may have to receive free care. To adhere to controlled trial design, the control group must be identical in every way to the test group; thereby doubling costs. The osteopathic profession could create a professional database by standardizing procedures and record keeping. Developing the procedures and database enables the conduct of multicenter research and retrospective studies. Both database and observational studies contribute valuable information at reduced costs. Large-scale studies offer a way for manual medicine data to impact public health policy and planning.

PUBLIC HEALTH UTILIZATION OF MEDICAL DATA

If efforts are made to successfully and reliably collect information on osteopathically oriented medical care, how could these data be used in the development of health care planning?

Interventions Affect Rationing Decisions

There must first be a need for intervention. A medical need is defined as: "Some disturbance in health and well-being which requires medical care services."[10] One of the first orders of business in establishing an osteopathic basis for health care policy is to define the need for osteopathic treatment. To do this, some approximation of the prevalence and incidence of osteopathically defined structural findings should be undertaken. How large is the problem of somatic dysfunction, or is it a problem at all? Epidemiologists and others who study populations frequently find that a far larger proportion of disease is hidden from view than is evident to administrators, physicians, or the general public. Somatic dysfunction is likely to have a greater role in health and disease than we now suspect; it has to be documented.

Availability, Quality, and Appropriateness

A corollary to the apparent need for intervention is the availability of services to meet a need. Some attempts should be made to quantify the supply and demand of osteopathic services. Such services are more likely to occur in areas for which osteopathic services have been developed to meet a perceived need. It is not enough to identify a need if the resources to meet that need are unknown. Policy formation should be rooted in the capacity to address needs and not just identify them.

Projecting and Planning

What are the resources of information that can allow us to quantify needs and services available? These resources include[10]:

    Large national and statewide databases
    Smaller employee, educational, and hospital-based collections
    Individual physician and clinic services

If the need to include osteopathically relevant information in data sets is clear, then multiple hypotheses can be tested for the cause, consequences, and treatment of somatic dysfunction. Until such a national policy exists, osteopathic researchers must link their findings with data sets to generalize to the population at large.

Questions that need to be addressed include stability and natural history of somatic dysfunction, and the incidence and prevalence in various population groups sorted by age, sex, vocational and recreational activities, and so on. Once these data are in the medical database, associations with general health and disease processes could be made.[11]

PHYSICIAN'S ROLE

No national effort is underway to establish the identification and treatment of somatic dysfunction as a national priority. Once osteopathically trained physicians and therapists can begin to add to the health care database, valuable information can lead to answering questions concerning the nature of somatic dysfunction.

Epidemiologic Studies of Somatic Dysfunction

John Snow, a physician in 19th century London, is considered as the originator of intervention-oriented epidemiology. Although many theories of cholera transmission existed in his day, Snow systematically charted the occurrence of cases. He was able to account for findings and boldly stop the epidemic by removing the pump handle on the offending well that was the source of the infectious agent.[8(pp4–12,40)] Although somatic dysfunction does not represent a lethal risk to the general community, its identification and control is likely to reduce mor-

bidity of many conditions. Investigating somatic dysfunction requires bold effort to quantify the effects of somatic dysfunction, as well as successful approaches to its control in the population.

Data Collection

Osteopathically oriented physicians and therapists are at the front lines of patient care and must assume a leading role in collection efforts towards a national database. It is these individuals who see, touch, and interview patients. Attempts to create consistent, reliable data gathering and abstracting methods are most important. Once data on somatic dysfunction are recorded in the medical record, data sources can be linked. This is a simple concept. Because the potential for pooling information is powerful, linking somatic dysfunction to health risks and its treatment to health benefits can lead to changes in regional and national planning for health care resources. Without documentation, the valuable contribution of osteopathically oriented health care may never be fully appreciated.

Population and Impact on Health Care

In summary, the prevalence and incidence of somatic dysfunction must be established. This effort can be greatly enhanced by organizing the efforts of osteopathically trained physicians and therapists. As noted in Chapter 78, "Medical Records in Clinical Research," on the recording of palpatory diagnosis, a mechanism is being developed to accomplish this task. Concerned practitioners and researchers must insist that these palpatory findings be recorded in the public record.

With consistent recording of somatic dysfunction, efforts can be made to link these databases via regular abstraction and sampling techniques. It is not the purpose of this text to discuss specific sampling methods; great sophistication has been developed that permits inferences from carefully selected data.

Physicians' Records

To ensure reliable, consistent data collection, an effort must be made to standardize data collection in recording methods. These methods must meet certain criteria. They must be reliable and simple to use and record; they must permit linkage with other data sets. This effort is enhanced by emphasizing a consistent method of gathering data on somatic dysfunction. To achieve this goal, we need the leadership of the Educational Counsel on Osteopathic Principles (ECOP) and the American Academy of Osteopathy (AAO). These organizations are affiliates of the American Osteopathic Association. ECOP membership includes faculty members of family medicine and manual medicine departments. AAO members include family and general practice physicians; the Academy promotes the use of manual medicine. A commitment must be made by the AOA for the programs of its organizations and services of graduates from osteopathic medical education to emphasize the role of the somatic system in health and disease.

CONCLUSION

Health care policy can be influenced by those providing services, but not if it is assumed that the community will always want and need these services. In an era of limited resources, osteopathically trained health care providers have to prove the value of their unique services. A national database of somatic dysfunction is the key to demonstrating the value of managing somatic dysfunction in patient care.

REFERENCES

1. Buerger AA. A control trial of rotational manipulation in low back pain. *Manuelle Medizin.* 1980;2:1726.
2. Beal M, Morlock JW. Somatic dysfunction associated with pulmonary disease. *JAOA.* 1984;84:179.
3. Cox J, Rogers F, Gorbiss S, et al. Palpatory musculoskeletal findings in coronary artery disease: results of a double-blind study. *JAOA.* 1983;82:832.
4. Moynihan C. Perspectives on quality in American health care. In: *Quantifying Quality.* New York, NY: McGraw-Hill Book Co; 1988;2.
5. Yerushamy J. Statistical problems in assessing methods of medical diagnosis, with special reference to x-ray techniques. *Pub Health Reps.* 1947;62:1432.
6. Beal M, Go JP, Johnston WL, McConnell DG. Interexaminer agreement on long-term patient improvement: an exercise in research design. *JAOA.* 1982:322–328.
7. Johnston WL, Allen BR, Hendra JL, et al. Interexaminer study of palpation in detecting location of spinal segmental dysfunction. *JAOA.* 1983;82:842.
8. Hennekens CH, Buring JE. *Epidemiology in Medicine.* Boston, Mass: Little Brown & Co; 1982:327–347.
9. Feinstein A. *Clinical Epidemiology.* Boston, Mass: Little Brown & Co; 1985:403–406.
10. Donabedian A. *Aspects of Medical Care Administration: Specifying Requirements for Health Care.* Cambridge, Mass: Harvard Press; 1973.
11. Feinstein A. *Clinimetrics.* New Haven, Conn: Yale University Press; 1987:vii–ix.

80. Clinical Research and Clinical Trials

STEPHEN H. SHELDON

Key Concepts

- **Research designs used to develop clinical protocols that provide scientific support for medical theory and practice**

- **Sources for information used to plan and evaluate clinical research protocols**

- **General references on clinical research and clinical trials**

A standard definition of research is an "investigation or experimentation aimed at the discovery and interpretation of facts, revision of accepted theories or laws in light of new facts, or practical application of such new or revised theories or laws."[1] The goal of research is to discover truth. Scientific method requires that truth to one should be truth to all.

BASIC RESEARCH

In basic research, a question is refined, a hypothesis developed, and an experiment designed to test the hypothesis. To test the hypothesis, the investigator develops a specific protocol that permits manipulation of one variable while all other variables are controlled (kept constant). In this way, outcomes of the manipulation can be observed and recorded. Results of the experiment are then statistically analyzed to decide the likelihood that the observation could have occurred by chance. Scientific method requires, however, that results of experimentation are universal truth only if they are reproducible by others using the same methods and protocol.

Applied or clinical research differs from basic research in several important aspects. In contrast to the basic science laboratory, the clinical laboratory is often difficult to define. It may range from an entire geographic region to an individual hospital or physician's office. Humans are the subject of clinical investigations. Control of all human variables is beyond the scope of any single experiment. Often it is impossible to study an entire population. Therefore, a small number of subjects are chosen as population representatives.

There is always a possibility that subjects selected do not represent the population of interest. When the characteristic to be investigated occurs infrequently, many subjects are required. Therefore, selection of individuals and grouping of subjects into cohorts (subjects with similar characteristics) require rigorous attention to detail to reduce representation bias. Con-

clusions based on results from small segments of the population require internal validity. When these results are generalized to the entire population, external validity is essential.

Adherence to the scientific method requires that the results of clinical research be reproducible. Difficulties may be encountered because of variations among:

Individual subjects
Geographic locations
Societal norms
Genetic differences
Cultural influences

ELEMENTS OF CLINICAL RESEARCH

Hulley, Newman, and Cummings have eloquently described the anatomy and physiology of clinical research.[2] Anatomy of clinical research refers to the tangible elements of the study plan:

Research question
Research design
Subjects
Measurements
Sample size calculation

Physiology of clinical research refers to how research works. The usefulness of clinical investigations depends on internal and external validity. Internal validity is concerned with the correctness of conclusions based on events that occurred within the study sample. External validity relates to the ability to generalize observed events in the cohort to people outside the study sample. The investigator's goal is to reduce errors that may threaten the soundness of conclusions based on these data.

Research Question

Clinical research begins with the development of a clear, concise research question.[3] Doubt or reservations about something that begs resolution develop in the investigator's mind. Uncertainty may be based on:

Problems encountered during prior observations
New approach to old problems
New technologies
Healthy skepticism about current knowledge and beliefs

Statement of this uncertainty forms the basis of the research question.

Good research questions possess certain characteristics. They must be ethical as well as clear, concise, focused, and testable. Research of an unclear, nebulous question is generally considered a fishing expedition, results in unreliable data, and lacks internal and external validity. Questions must:

Be feasible
Be relevant
Be interesting to the researcher
Confirm or refute previous findings
Extend previous information
Provide new knowledge

According to Cummings and coworkers, the question must pass the "so what?" test.[3]

Research Protocol

A protocol is a written plan of the study. It describes methods and promotes a logical, efficient, focused approach that may be replicated by other investigators. The significance and rationale of the study are stated, and the design of the investigation is described. Subjects who represent the target population are identified. Variables are defined, and a sample size is calculated. Statistical issues are addressed. During the development of the protocol, the investigator must make several important decisions regarding the study design. Determinations of study design are typically based on the research question and on the variables to be observed during the study.

INVESTIGATIONAL DESIGNS

Clinical research generally occurs in three phases.[4] In the first phase, an observation or descriptive study is undertaken to provide background information, to characterize the disease process being studied, and to describe the population affected. This initial phase furnishes a general picture from which to begin. In the second phase, investigators analyze correlations and clarify cause-and-effect associations. Finally, the investigators may design an experiment to test the efficacy of an intervention on the disease process.

OBSERVATIONAL STUDIES

This design requires the investigator to step back from the events taking place within the study population and record observations.[4(pp10–11)] Populations observed at a single point in time and data recorded on a single occasion represent a cross-sectional study. Observations over an extended period with data recorded on multiple occasions are longitudinal studies. Retrospective observational studies focus only on past or recent events. In contrast, prospective studies monitor populations for events that have not yet happened. Data collected may be descriptive of the study population or it may be analytical, assessing first association or cause–effect relationships.

Types of Observation

Three basic observational designs are the[4(pp4–8)]:

Cohort study
Cross-sectional study
Case-control study

These types of clinical investigations are designed to analyze a predictor variable that may have influenced outcome; they may be conducted prospectively or retrospectively. Cohort studies follow a group of subjects over time. Cross-sectional studies are similar, except measurements are generally made only once. Cross-sectional studies are useful in describing population and distribution variables. In contrast, case-control studies are generally retrospective. Groups of individuals with a specific disease or condition (cases) and individuals without the disease or condition (controls) are identified and matched according to certain characteristics such as age or sex. The investigator then looks backward to find differences in a predictor variable that might explain why the cases acquired the disease or condition and why the controls did not.

No design is superior to another. Investigators' judgment and experience are required to choose the study design best suited to reliably answer the initial research question.

EXPERIMENTAL STUDIES

Experimental studies require some manipulation of a variable followed by measurement of the effect of this change.[5] A variable may change naturally (e.g., the presence or absence of disease). A variable changed by the researcher might involve the administration of a medication, a surgical procedure, or modified behavior. Change occurs in the predictor variable; observation identifies changes in an outcome variable. Causal inference is based on comparing the outcomes observed in two or more groups of subjects receiving different interventions, a between-group design. Outcomes observed in a single group before and after the intervention use a within-group design or self-controlled design.

Controlling for Bias

Bias can render observations meaningless and destroy the ability to make causal inferences from an experiment.[4(pp98–101)] All clinical investigations are potentially subject to bias that may affect outcome and conclusions. Inherent differences among individual subjects and groups and preconceived notions of the investigators may significantly prejudice data. In addition, if the sample size (number of subjects in the study) is too small, internal and external validity may be profoundly affected.

Minimizing Differences

The randomized clinical trial has become the method of choice for evaluation of safety and for determining treatment efficacy under controlled conditions. Clinical trials are randomized, double-blinded, and controlled. Random allocation of subjects to control and experimental groups guards against any systematic association of treatment assignment with prognosis or outcome.[5(pp76–77,97)] Outcomes, therefore, probably result from the manipulation of the predictor variable rather than from differences between groups.

Randomization

Randomization begins with an appropriate selection of the cohort.[4(pp37–38,80–84,93–94)] Inclusion criteria are established that are appropriate and specific to the research questions; subjects must meet these characteristics to be considered for participation. After baseline data are gathered, some potential subjects are excluded from the study sample. Exclusion criteria help in eliminating subjects who possess extraneous features that might affect the outcome or results. Once the sample is identified, demographic and clinical measurements are made. These measurements identify the population represented by the sample. Strong predictors of outcome are identified and baseline measurements are made to assure that the outcome has not already occurred. During randomization, subjects are assigned to two or more study groups. Subjects may be assigned to a group according to a simple random number table or by computer-generated randomization.

Two important features of randomization must be assured. First, there must be a true random allocation of subjects; second, the process must be tamper-proof. Once the plan for randomization is established, it must be irreversible. All methods share a common goal of eliminating the bias of one group being significantly different from the other. The randomization process eliminates patients', physicians', and researchers' influences on choice of assignment.

Interventions are administered according to the procedures described in the written protocol. The manner of administration is the same for all groups. In drug therapy, this procedure prevents the research subjects, their physicians, and the researchers from knowing whether different drugs or placebos are administered. Outcome variables are measured as described in the protocol and in the same manner for all subjects. The choice of variable to be measured and the way it is measured enhances the power of the study. For example, assessment of a continuous variable (such as hemoglobin concentration) is more powerful than measurement of a dichotomous variable (such as normal versus abnormal hemoglobin concentration).

Blinding

Investigator and subject bias is reduced during clinical experiments by blinding. The importance of blinding cannot be emphasized enough. Outcome variables must be measured without knowledge of which group the subject is assigned to. Double-blinding eliminates the subject's and investigator's bias and is used when the assessment of an outcome requires judgment by the observer. It prevents ascertainment prejudice from affecting groups differently. A triple-blind design requires that the subjects, the person manipulating the predictor variable and administering the intervention, and the person measuring the outcome are unaware of the group assignment and the type of intervention being administered. In a triple-blind study, the

measurements are protected against investigators or subjects influencing the outcome and creating unreliable results.

Using Subjects as Own Controls

Crossover designs are employed in some studies on medications to enhance internal validity. For example, subjects may be randomly assigned to two groups and blinded to the intervention. One group receives a medication and the other a placebo. The investigator is blinded to the group assignment. Outcomes after administration are monitored in the two groups, assessed, and recorded. In a crossover design, the intervention for the two groups is exchanged and responses are observed over a second period. Researchers allow time between crossover to avoid carryover effects. They also obtain interim histories to detect changes in subjects' health status.

Sample Size

Sample size is the number of subjects needed for statistically significant results.[4(pp21–26)] The number of subjects required for internal and external validity of the study should be determined early in the development of the protocol. Sample size calculation estimates the influence of change in the outcome variable on the statistical significance of results. Small degrees of change in the outcome variable require larger sample sizes.

When a large sample size is required for a clinical trial, multiple medical centers or research sites provide a sufficient number of subjects. Training and monitoring performance at each site with periodic follow-up on data collection for accuracy and completeness assures compliance with the protocol and quality of the data. Accurate and complete data collection reduces errors during multicenter trials but increases responsibilities for administering the protocol. Data collection, central randomization, frequent audits of research records, and site visits are added burdens planned and accepted by the clinical trial investigators. Clearly, even minor deviations from the protocol confound data from one or more centers and decrease reliability of results.

Data Analysis

Plans for analysis of data should be decided at the outset of the study, not after data have been collected.[6] The research question and outcome variables are the basis for the method of statistical analysis. The research question is stated originally and refined into a specific, clear, concise, and testable hypothesis. Hypotheses too broad in scope become fishing expeditions and rarely provide reliable or reproducible data. The research question is then refined into a null hypothesis. Statistical analysis reduces the chance of making unsupportable statements.[6(pp105–129)] Statistics test a null hypothesis that there is no real difference between an observed sample value and the absolute value for a population that the sample represents. Statistical tests evaluate an acceptable probability level that the hypothesis is not true and, therefore, should be rejected. The null hypothesis used in statistical tests should be focused and testable. Nonspecific hypotheses cause unreliable conclusions.

The null hypothesis may be tested using a variety of statistical analyses. The type of statistical test employed depends on the type of outcome variable being measured. Typically, the statistical analysis searches for truth by testing the degree to which the measurements could have occurred by chance alone. Choosing the level of significance reduces two sources of errors. Type I errors involve concluding the null hypothesis is true when it is false (beta or power). Type II errors conclude that the null hypothesis is false when it is true (alpha). The levels of confidence (alpha and beta) are chosen arbitrarily by the investigator. They are generally set at a beta of 0.2 and an alpha of 0.05. An alpha of 0.05 typically means that there is a 5% chance of concluding that the null hypothesis is false when it is true. If there is a difference seen in outcome variables at a p value (significance) of 0.05, there is a 5% likelihood that the results occurred by chance alone.

CONCLUSION

The goal of clinical research is to seek truth using the most appropriate and acceptable tools available. Truth to one should be truth to all.

Principles and practices of osteopathic medicine have been documented in anecdotes, observational studies, and descriptive statistics. Unfortunately, few studies have been published that have subjected these principles and practices to the rigors of scientific methodology. Clinical investigation of osteopathic principles and practices is difficult because of problems encountered in the design of experiments and the control of predictor and outcome variables.

The art of osteopathic medicine is sound. Clinical application of principles and techniques has been highly successful for many years. Documentation of the clinical science of osteopathic medicine, however, has been dramatically hampered by the subjective nature of diagnostic findings. Difficulties include reducing ascertainment bias that results from manipulating the

predictor variable and measuring outcomes consistently. Available technology provides scientific support for clinical observations; however, only limited aspects of observation are supported. This situation requires the researcher to select variables for measurement. Selecting the best predictive and reliable measurement provides the needed scientific support.

Providing a scientific basis for osteopathic principles and practices is possible. Rigorous analysis of the question with insight, creativity, and attention to details is required. Demanding precision for both clinical and technical measures provides answers to questions. Remain focused on the question, however, and do not get lost in the mire of methodology.

This chapter has briefly overviewed the structure and function of clinical research and the complexities of clinical investigation. Successful clinical researchers:

Understand the clinical and research processes
Can critically evaluate published research reports
Find imaginative and creative approaches to pursue the discovery of truth

REFERENCES

1. Woolf HB. *Webster's New Collegiate Dictionary.* Springfield, Mass: Merriam Company; 1979.
2. Hulley SB, Newman TB, Cummings SR. Getting started: The anatomy and physiology of research. In: Hulley SB, Cummings SR, (with major contributors), eds. *Designing Clinical Research.* Baltimore, Md: Williams & Wilkins; 1988:1–11.
3. Cummings SR, Browner WS, Hulley SB. Conceiving the research question. In: Hulley SB, Cummings SR, (with major contributors), eds. *Designing Clinical Research.* Baltimore, Md: Williams & Wilkins; 1988:12–17.
4. Kelsey JL, Thompson WE, Evans AS. *Methods in Observational Epidemiology.* New York, NY: Oxford University Press; 1986:3–18.
5. Payton OD. *Research: The Validation of Clinical Practice.* 2nd ed. Philadelphia, Penn: FA Davis Company; 1988:49–53.
6. Shott S. *Statistics for Health Professionals.* Philadelphia, Penn: WB Saunders Co; 1990.

81. Epidemiology

APPLICATION TO CLINICAL RESEARCH

ALBERT F. KELSO AND FREDERIC N. SCHWARTZ

Key Concepts

- **Types of epidemiologic studies and their purposes**

- **Epidemiologic sources of data used by governments to regulate public health and plan health care resources**

- **How epidemiologic investigation of somatic dysfunction and its treatment advances osteopathic medical theory and practice**

Epidemiology originated as a research design to study the causes of infectious disease in human populations or subgroups within a population.[1] A recent addition to the field includes studying causes of noninfectious conditions that influence health. Research with this additional focus is often called clinical epidemiology[2-3] because identical strategies are used for investigating causes of infectious disease and illness.

ROLE IN PUBLIC HEALTH

Multiple uses of epidemiologic research attest to its importance in protecting public health. Epidemiology provides data on factors affecting citizens' health and information for planning budgets for health care resources and services. Many federal, state, and local agencies collect vital statistics, conduct surveys, and analyze reports on health care. These sources of information allow agencies and departments to follow trends in disease, disability, and illness. This data is analyzed and used in developing education programs and regulations to protect citizen and community health.[4] Similar use of epidemiologic investigations by the medical and allied health professions advances theories and suggests further investigation of the practice of medicine. Emphasis in this chapter is on the use of clinical epidemiologic research; there is a continuous need for investigation of osteopathic medicine. New or modified theories about the somatic system's roles in health, healing, disability, and illness are required to meet advances in medical knowledge and practice and to meet governmental regulations. These studies also contribute scientific support for use of osteopathic manipulative treatment (OMT) in medical practice.

CLASSICAL AND CLINICAL EPIDEMIOLOGY

Clinical epidemiologic investigation identifies potential causes of disease and illness in human populations.[1(pp12–13)] Epidemiology of infectious disease identifies the source of exposure involving persons, place, or time, and the course from exposure to disease. In clinical epidemiology, putative sources that lead to citizens' noninfectious health problems are investigated to develop recommendations for individual health and regulations to protect public health. For example, clinical epidemiology identified cancer risks associated with cigarette smoking, the effects of personal lifestyles, and environmental influences through a series of epidemiologic studies.[5] Particularly in slowly developing conditions, unknown influences confound the inferences of single studies; many causes are suspected with only a few supported by further investigation.[5(pp168–169)] This contrasts with epidemiologists' successes in highly infections conditions such as AIDS and Legionnaire's disease, which were quickly identified and their causes confirmed. The need to confirm putative sources of illness by further investigation suggests that researchers, the media, and the public must be aware of differences in inferences drawn early in clinical investigation and conclusions confirmed by further research.

Large Cohort Studies of Osteopathic Practice

Epidemiologic strategies and research designs are introduced in the next section. The details of planning research protocols are beyond the scope of this chapter but are readily available in other texts.[1,2,4,6–7] Team planning and investigation are suggested for developing protocols for epidemiologic investigations of somatic dysfunction. First, somatic dysfunction should be investigated as a condition initiated by somatosomatic and viscerosomatic reflexes. Second, treating somatic dysfunction is investigated as an influence on patients' health and healing. Collaboration is recommended between experienced epidemiologists and osteopathic physicians who emphasize osteopathic evaluation and treatment of somatic dysfunction in their practices. Joint efforts are essential to reach conclusions that advance osteopathic theory and practice.

HISTORY

Modern epidemiology has its origins in England.[1(pp5–13)] Recognition of the value of routinely collected data on human diseases and the basis for modern epidemiology is attributed to John Gault. Beginning in 1662, his weekly publication of births, deaths, and disease gave an analysis of how patterns of disease in London related to specific types of infections. Later, in 1839, England established a medical statistics record bank under William Farr.

Hypothesis Formulation

Application of these vital statistics in 1854 by an English physician, John Snow, helped differentiate cholera death rates in separate areas within London. He suspected cholera was transmitted by exposure to contaminated water. This hypothesis was tested with data he collected on persons using water supplied from a sewage-contaminated section of the Thames. He compared these data with information from persons using a clean water supply. A high death rate in the area supplied by contaminated water compared with a low death rate in the area with a clean water supply supported his hypothesis.

Development of Public Health Programs

Application of Snow's studies eventually led to public health regulations to protect citizens' health. Today, federal, state, and local public health departments and other governmental agencies continue epidemiologic studies, provide educational information, and enforce regulations to protect citizens' health.[4(pp263–310)] Regulations now include:

Housing
Accident prevention
Nutrition
Food
Drugs
Cosmetics
Quarantine
Environment risks
Seasonal influences
Medical interventions used in health care

Epidemiology of noninfectious disease is more complex than epidemiology of infectious disease, and is influenced by more variables.

PROBLEMS

Researching the influence of illness, work-related factors, and environmental health risks requires additional controls. Sometimes two or more populations are represented in a study. For example, employees as a population often come from different socioeconomic environments, or exposed individuals attending a convention may reside in many different areas.

The number of variables involved in these complex studies limits the confidence in conclusions unless the results and details of analysis are included in the published discussion. A discussion of variables considered in planning research allows a reader to account for some aspects of bias and confounding that may alter any conclusions. Confirmation by subsequent

studies should provide needed support for the initial inferences. It is worth noting that, in spite of scientific weakness, epidemiologic studies and the application of findings to public health programs have steadily modified mortality patterns. Since 1900, in the United States, chronic disease and accidents replaced infectious diseases as the major threat to life and extended life expectancy toward its theoretical limits.[1(p9)]

BENEFITS

Epidemiologic investigations of the conditions that change patterns of illness and contribute to improved well-being and health now include attention to health risks as an important strategy to reduce health care costs.[5(p166),8] In the 1990s, increased attention is being given to the quality of health care and to the effectiveness of interventions (modes of therapy, alternative medicine) used in practice.[9] Health and cost-effectiveness focuses attention on interventions used in health care. The next development of federal regulations to protect citizens from undue health risks is likely to establish requirements for all interventions used in medical practice.

These regulations will require a scientific basis for therapies that have evolved during the history of medicine. Patients' experiences with cultural medicine available through practitioners often determines their preferences for health care. Some of their experiences may have major influence on their response to this type of health care. Many of these modes of therapy, unsupported except by experience, have been in use for centuries. Scientific support for these experiential modes of therapy can be obtained from epidemiologic and medical outcome studies[2(pp321–325)] as described in Chapter 77, "Somatic Dysfunction."

FUNDAMENTALS OF EPIDEMIOLOGIC INVESTIGATION

Epidemiology, with the exception of studying interventions, uses documented observations as a source of data and statistical analysis to support inferences and hypotheses. Three strategies, descriptive, analytic, and experimental, organize the epidemiologic research designs for data collection and analysis.[1(pp16–28)]

Descriptive Strategy

Descriptive observations involve[1(pp21–26)]:

Case reports
Case-series
Correlational study designs
Cross-sectional surveys

The strength of these designs in classical epidemiology relates exposure and development of disease, or in clinical epidemiology identifies influences that alter development of health problems or promote health. The weakness of the designs is incomplete data for analysis because exposure, influence, and related variables are difficult to document completely. Also, unknown variables contribute to false–positive or false–negative conclusions.

Analytic Strategy

Analytic strategy uses an experimental group (known to have the disease or condition being studied) and a control group (known not to have the disease or influences being studied) within the same population.[1(pp26–27)] An hypothesis is developed from descriptive studies, experience, or theoretical considerations and is tested with an analytic study design. Differences in frequency of occurrence between experimental and control groups are compared and analyzed statistically for significance. The statistical analysis supports or refutes the hypotheses on association. The weakness in these studies is in the potential differences between the experimental and control groups' mix of uncontrolled variables. Small samples are prone to this type of error. Large samples of a population, randomly assigned as experimental or control cases, are needed to ensure a uniform mix. Also, selection bias, occurring unintentionally or in poorly planned studies, may alter the distribution of unknown variables in the two groups.

Experimental Strategy

Experimental strategy for clinical trials relies on knowing and measuring the cause and effect being studied.[10] Clinical trials often have theoretical support for the interactions occurring between cause and effect.[1(pp178–208)] The theories represent previous research seeking mechanisms that are involved in cause-and-effect relationships. For example, basic research in osteopathic medicine established somatosomatic and viscerosomatic reflexes[11] as mechanisms associated with somatic dysfunction. Basic research complemented by observation in clinical practice strongly suggests that somatosomatic and somatovisceral reflexes are involved in the clinical response to OMT.[12] The scientific support for effects on healing and health status remains to be documented in ambulatory care practice and supported by analytic, clinical, and basic research. The rates of healing observed in hospital care units by Stiles,[12] in coronary care units by Larson,[13] and in several postoperative studies are small—approximately a 15% difference between experimental and control groups. Continued research is needed to substantiate these initial observations and rule out chance variations.

Comparison of Strategies

Descriptive and analytic strategies rely on the natural course of events that takes place between exposure and the development of disease or health problems. Intervention studies, also known as clinical trials, are based on experimental study designs and are accepted as the "gold standard" for testing the safety and efficacy of interventions under controlled conditions (see Chapter 80, "Clinical Research and Clinical Trials"). Clinical trial strength lies in randomizing subjects to control and experimental groups, blinding researchers and subjects to group assignment, and paying rigorous attention to measurement of both cause and effects during investigation. Further investigation of these effects is needed to support their effectiveness in ambulatory care practice. Theories on the proposed effectiveness of OMT provide additional scientific support.

EPIDEMIOLOGIC STUDIES OF SOMATIC DYSFUNCTION

Epidemiologic research designs offer answers to questions about reflex influences in the development of dysfunctional motor control. Descriptive research studies on humans provide clinical information on the question of when somatosomatic and viscerosomatic reflexes develop into somatic dysfunctions. Analytic research design provides a method for testing hypotheses developed from observations in descriptive research.

Development of Somatic Dysfunction

Reflexes,[14] somatosomatic and somatovisceral (also called somatosympathetic reflexes in medical publications[15]), are theoretical mechanisms associated with changes observed in somatic dysfunction. No evidence is available to indicate when normal motor controls become dysfunctional. It is essential to establish when this happens and how the change can be detected. These questions and available information to answer them are included as background in proposed epidemiologic study protocols or grant applications. The following should be discussed in research protocols, applications, and publications:

Evidence that motor controls in regions or segments of somatic dysfunctions are dysfunctional

Measurements used to identify status and changes in somatic dysfunction

Response of Somatic Dysfunction to Treatment

Descriptive research designs used to develop protocols for longitudinal clinical studies seek information on what influences motor control in the presence of somatic dysfunction. The methods section includes the observations and analysis for when and how the modification occurs. The identified modifiers and the sequence for their effects are verified using analytic or basic research studies. The planned studies in the clinical arena provide information for planning basic research in biologic models. The combined approach of clinical and basic research supports or refutes hypotheses about mechanisms that alter motor control. Epidemiologic studies document important observations used in clinical decisions; basic research provides details on changes in functional motor control.

A similar plan is feasible for establishing scientific support for the health benefits provided by manipulative treatment of somatic dysfunction. However, clinical trials are the preferred design for investigating the effects of OMT on health status and systemic functions in human populations. Epidemiologic studies document clinicians' observations made in practice.

CLINICAL EXPERIENCE

Clinical experience over the last 100 years established and continues to support a principle of practice: the treatment of somatic dysfunction improves a patient's capacity for healing and helps maintain health. Epidemiologic research to support the principle requires:

Evidence that improvements of health status and rate of healing are associated with OMT of somatic dysfunction

Measuring the status of somatic dysfunction before and after manipulative treatment to document changes in somatic dysfunction as an influence on health and healing

Measuring health and/or functional status before and after treatment to document the health benefit of treatment

Retrospective cohort studies on information obtained from practice are feasible and are the quickest source of information. Many osteopathic physicians provide manipulative treatments for a stable group of patients. A pilot study conducted at CCOM by Karrat, Grujanac, and Kelso in 1993 investigated the effects of treating somatic dysfunction and performance of corrective exercises. Subjects rated their somatic pain and reported their feeling of well-being and ability to function in daily tasks. Their experience was that they were either pain-free or had reduced pain, felt better, and were better able to perform their daily tasks.

VERIFICATION OF ASSOCIATIONS

Planned research to verify the initial observations tests the osteopathic principle of practice that treating somatic dysfunction improves patients' health and healing. Background for research protocols includes:

Statement of the principle

Summary of clinical experience that established the principle

Data from clinical observations, preferably as a descriptive study

Methods for assessing change in somatic dysfunctions

Estimating health benefits of manipulative treatment

Hypothesis being tested: the treatment of somatic dysfunction improves healing and maintenance of health

Analytic strategy, case control, and cohort research designs provide evidence to support or refute the hypothesis. The documented clinical benefits from epidemiologic studies furnish the basis for planning a clinical trial.

DISCUSSION

Epidemiologic studies are planned and conducted using protocols based on established designs. A written protocol for a planned investigation specifies the purpose, problem, or hypothesis of the investigation, the background information, and the details for data collection and analyses. An excellent discussion of this with suggestions for writing protocols appears in Spilker.[16] Although written for clinical trials, protocols are applicable to most planned research. Planners select a design based on its relevance to the investigators' goals and the availability of resources required by the plan.

Descriptive epidemiologic strategy provides evidence from observations on the natural history or relationship between exposure and effects. The researcher chooses case-series studies,[1(pp20,106–108)] correlational studies,[1(pp17–28,102–106,343)] or cross-sectional surveys[1(pp20–21,108–112)] and develops a research protocol. Case and case-series studies document a suspected exposure or health risk. Additional cases with the same characteristics verify the initial observations. Correlational studies are similar to case-series studies; the data collection is from population samples, usually small, rather than from individuals. Cross-sectional surveys of physicians' practices use their patients as a population for presenting osteopathic health care outcomes. The detailed data on patients, their characteristics and environments, and the physicians' practice profile with the modes of therapy used and outcomes obtained suggest researchable questions for analytic or other scientific studies.

The small numbers of subjects for these studies and the lack of controls limit inferences from the data and are the basis for challenges to the credibility of conclusions. They are, however, important sources of clues for designing rigorous protocols for further research. Including a discussion of strengths, weaknesses, confounding influences, and biases in the published reports is recommended to decrease the likelihood of misinterpretation of the studies and challenges.

Analytic strategies to test hypotheses use case-control, cohort, and intervention (clinical trial) designs for planning research protocols. The descriptive studies, literature, experience, and theoretical considerations are used to develop a hypothesis and select a design for the protocol. Either case-control or cohort research designs provide analytic methods to test for association. Case-control experimental subjects have a diagnosed disease or known health problem; a selected group of subjects from the same population without the condition form the control group. The proportions of exposed subjects in each group are compared to evaluate support for assuming an association between the exposure and the condition.

Cohort studies are retrospective when both the exposure and the condition of interest exist at the time of the study. They are prospective when the exposure is known but the presence of the condition of interest has not been determined when the study is initiated. The prospective cohort study may require years of observation to determine occurrence of the condition. For example, some of the Framingham risk factor studies have lasted more than 10 years,[17] and the Nurses Health Studies are rarely shorter than 5 years.[18] The inferences drawn from analytic research studies are still open to question. Case-control and cohort studies provide evidence of strong statistical differences. Rigorous analytic research in primary care is possible. It requires both understanding and maintaining the standards that are appropriate to the study being undertaken.

Intervention studies discussed as clinical trials in Chapters 80 and 82 are similar to basic research. Food and Drug Administration approval for prescription drugs requires clinical trials and strong statistical evidence that a drug is safe and efficacious (effective under controlled research conditions). The measurements of drug administration and its effects are valid, reliable, and accurate in phase II and III FDA studies; there is little doubt about either drug administration or its effects. Many FDA studies require extensive laboratory testing in phase I investigation that provides a theoretical basis for drug effects. A theoretical basis for an intervention's effects in a clinical trial increases the likelihood that clinical trial conclusions can be accepted.

Preliminary research to justify the massive expenditure of resources (time, personnel, and funds) for a clinical trial of osteopathic practice is suggested in Chapter 82, "Planning Research on Health Care. Clinical trials on the role of somatic dysfunction and its effects on health, disability, and illness will have greater acceptance when there is a research basis for the relationship between dysfunction and reported health outcome.

CONCLUSION

Clinical epidemiology provides an initial base for development and an accepted sequence of studies to support or refute the suggestions evolving from clinical experience. Epidemiologic, clinical, and basic research designs provide information for designing research protocols and conducting research. Epidemiologic descriptive, analytic, and clinical trial studies convert observations in practice to documented and supported associations. Accepted descriptions of clinical phenomenon are an initial step that often saves time when the researcher is tempted to proceed directly to clinical trials on safety and efficacy of interventions or basic research to develop theory and mechanisms for the association.

REFERENCES

1. Hennekens CH, Buring JE. *Epidemiology in Medicine.* Boston, Mass: Little, Brown and Company; 1987:5.
2. Feinstein AR. *Clinical Epidemiology.* Philadelphia, Penn: WB Saunders Company; 1985.
3. Weiss NS. *Clinical Epidemiology: The Study of the Outcomes of Illness.* New York, NY: Oxford University Press; 1986:v.
4. Raffel MW, Raffel NK. *The U.S. Health System: Origins and Functions.* 3rd ed. Albany, NY: Delmar Publishers, Inc; 1989:263–312.
5. Taubes G. Special new report: epidemiology faces its limits. *Science.* 1995;269(14 July):165.
6. Kelsey JL, Thompson WD, Evans AS. *Methods in Observational Epidemiology.* New York, NY: Oxford University Press; 1986.
7. Spilker B. *Guide to Clinical Studies and Developing Protocols.* New York, NY: Raven Press; 1984.
8. Morse RM, Heffron WA. Preventive health care. In: Rakel RE, ed. *Textbook of Family Practice.* 5th ed. Philadelphia, Penn: WB Saunders Company; 1995:192–212.
9. Mission: a forum for sharing information concerning the practical use of alternative therapies in preventing and treating disease, healing illness, and promoting health. *J Alternative Ther Health & Med.* 1995;1(1):4.
10. Friedman LM, Furberg CD, DeMets DL. *Fundamentals of Clinical Trials.* 2nd ed. PSG Publishing Company, Inc; 1985:3–4.
11. Guyton AC, Hall JE. *Textbook of Physiology.* 9th ed. Philadelphia, Penn: WB Saunders Company; 1995:690–691, 777.
12. Stiles EG. Osteopathic manipulation in the hospital environment. *JAOA.* 1976;76(4):243–258.
13. Larson NL. Summary of site and occurrence of paraspinal soft tissue changes of patients in the intensive care unit. *JAOA.* 1976;75:840–842.
14. Kelso AF. Physiology. In: Northup GW, ed. *Osteopathic Research: Growth and Development.* Chicago, Ill: American Osteopathic Association; 1987:59–70.
15. Sato A. Reflex modulation of visceral functions by somatic afferent activity. In: Paterson MM, Howell JN, eds. *The Central Connection: Somatovisceral/ Viscerosomatic Interaction.* 1989 International Symposium. Indianapolis, Ind: American Academy of Osteopathy; 1989:53–69.
16. Spilker B. *Guide to Clinical Studies and Developing Protocols.* New York, NY: Raven Press; 1984:154–184.
17. Hennekens CH, Buring JE; Mayrent SL, ed. *Epidemiology in Medicine.* Boston, Mass: Little, Brown and Company; 1989:5.
18. Dunn EV. Basic standards for analytic studies in primary care research. In: Norton PG, Stewart M, Tudiver F, et al., eds. *Primary Care Research: Traditional and Innovative Approaches.* Newbury Park, Calif: Sage Publications; 1991:95.

82. Planning Research on Health Care

ACCESS TO SAFE, QUALITY HEALTH CARE

ALBERT F. KELSO AND DEBORAH M. HEATH

Key Concepts

- **Public, professional, and governmental roles in changing medical practice**

- **Regulations that provide access to high-quality, safe, healthy, and cost-effective care**

- **Use of clinical trial, outcome, and survey research to supply data on safety and health effectiveness of manipulative treatment in osteopathic practice**

- **Purpose and methods used in research with each design**

- **Planning research to evaluate osteopathic practice and manipulative treatment**

Clinical, basic, and management research supply essential information for the osteopathic profession and physicians. Researchers plan research using clinical trial,[1] epidemiologic,[2] outcome,[3–4] and research survey[5–6] designs. These designs adapted for use in manual medicine provide specific information to support osteopathic practice and osteopathic manipulative treatment (OMT). The challenge to the profession and to physicians in practice is to provide evidence that treating somatic dysfunctions or using any other intervention improves health benefits for patients and is a valuable asset in health care.

Meeting this challenge with evidence from research includes initial descriptive studies of osteopathic practice followed by studies of clinical trials that establish the safety and efficacy of OMT. The response also requires continual epidemiologic and outcome research[7] as changes in knowledge, technology, medicine, and society provide opportunities for new applications or reduce the need for medical interventions. These forces change medical practice and alter available medical resources for intervening in health and illness. These forces are sources for governmental regulations designed to protect citizens' health and welfare.

INVESTIGATING INTERVENTIONS

Federal Agencies

Federal agencies approve interventions for use in health care.[8] Before 1980, the Food and Drug Administration (FDA) re-

quired only medicines, prosthetic devices, and laboratory procedures to obtain approval before use in health care. The FDA was established in 1906 to control food purity. In 1938, responsibility for drug purity and efficacy was added to the FDA's authority. The term "safety" in regulations means an acceptable risk and is not the total absence of undesirable side effects, morbidity, or mortality. Efficacy is an intervention's effectiveness established under controlled experimental conditions.

Health Care Financing Administration

Regulation of practice and interventions is shifting to the Health Care Financing Administration (HCFA) and other agencies.[9] Increased use of resources led to requiring quality assurance for reimbursement from Medicare funds. Other aspects of cost containment also threaten the health care system. Expensive interventions developed from new technology threaten to deplete financial resources. This drain results in government seeking to curtail the use of some interventions in practice.

Osteopathic Interventions

OMT and osteopathic practice are important elements in the health care system. A failure to anticipate future needs for approved interventions, however, will change osteopathic medicine's image and physicians' medical practice. Clinical trials of the interventions used in osteopathic practice should be pursued vigorously, now and in the future. Osteopathic and allopathic medicine face the alternatives of passive or active roles in regulating medical practice. Physicians must decide which interventions and what type of practice will occur in the 21st century. Research, particularly outcome research, supplies information for decisions on changes to the health care system. Targeted clinical research to support medical decisions is the only method available to plan regulations or contest decisions that change the practice of medicine.

Equal Access

Equal access to health care changed the delivery and pressures for health care. A major change was the medical and cost burdens created by free access to health care. These burdens and increased use of resources led to limiting practice and requiring quality assurance for reimbursement from Medicare funds. Other aspects of cost containment also threatened the health care system and research into methods of cost control. Expensive interventions have threatened available resources.[10] Cost containment now focuses on high-tech and high-volume interventions that need support from clinical trials. The authority for approving applications for untested interventions, including manual medicines, is assigned to the Office of Alternative Medicine (OAM).[10–11] Theoretically, all remedies, proprietary and unsupported interventions require a clinical trial or similar research to obtain approval for use.

Variability in Health Outcomes

Variability in health outcomes representing differences in medical practice is another force altering medical practice. Monitoring variations in population studies or comparison between practices should identify sources of variation. The HCFA review[12] and the National Health Interview Surveys by the Centers for Disease Control and Prevention (CDC) monitor health care and outcomes.[13] Variability in health outcomes, related to the same or similar processes for providing health care, is the target of monitoring. Important variable influences include:

Patient demographics
Health history
Health status
Family and socioeconomic background

Health outcomes also depend on local and regional resources for health care. Large variations occur in ability to diagnose, stage, or detect severity of disease. Little attention is given to health for its influence. The physician's contribution to variation in outcomes is an important influence. However, available facilities influence their effectiveness in practice. An important factor that should decrease variation is physicians' evaluation of monitor reports and opportunity to change causes of the reported variation.[14]

Federal efforts contribute to an increased life expectancy and quality of living.[15] Similar improvements should accompany approval for manual medicine and other unsupported interventions in the near future.

RESEARCH SUPPORT FOR OSTEOPATHIC CARE

Improving the quality of ambulatory care in the 21st century depends on clinician-researchers' contributions (see Chapter 80, "Clinical Research and Clinical Trials"). This is a role for dedicated physicians who receive training in obtaining quality research data from practice. Clinician-researchers represent a new cadre of researchers who supplement the efforts of basic and clinical researchers. The clinician-researcher is a team member who participates in planning and conducting research in the office setting.

Consortium

A consortium or network of cooperating clinician-researchers provides another method for reducing variation in practice (WL Johnston, personal communication, 1993–1994). A physician network established to collaborate with the Department of Family Medicine at Michigan State University is training physicians for ambulatory care research. Obtaining information on osteopathic evaluation of somatic dysfunction in noninstitutional settings is the first objective. Clinician-researchers in solo, small group, and managed care practice collect data in accordance with a research manual. Office and medical records are the major source of data; special data may be needed for some cooperative projects. Research data unrelated to the patient's health care are kept in separate files. Office assistants are trained to obtain reliable data from records and create the research reports. The clinician-researcher verifies the data before it is forwarded to the research coordinator. Data collection from practices in a network or cooperative study is similar to that of multicenter clinical trial research. In the clinician-research cooperative studies, the research coordinator tabulates, analyzes, and reports on the data, decreasing the research burden on practice and increasing research efficiency.

Analysis

Analysis is required to create specific research hypotheses or clinical questions. The components of need, quality, treatment, and criteria used in decisions on practice are variables to be controlled or measured during research:

Is the need related to a patient's concern for health, well-being, distress, or medical problem?

Does patient satisfaction, change in health status, improvement in performance, restoration of function, and expected benefit provide a complete list for measuring quality of care?

Where is the somatic dysfunction located and what are its characteristics (such as acuteness or chronicity, severity or stage of development, responsiveness to movement)?

Does the treatment modify or remove the somatic dysfunction? Does treatment provide relief, improve feeling of well-being, alter the course of illness or the clinical problem?

Is OMT used as primary care in managing acute self-limiting health problems, in chronic disease, or as an adjunct treatment that improves a patient's response to primary treatment, health status, and feeling of well-being?

Are patients satisfied with use of OMT, and is it an appropriate intervention to be used in their health care?

What is its relative value (health cost–benefit) compared with other available interventions for managing the patient's complaint, problem, illness, or preventive care?

Answers to these questions not only characterize the use of OMT as an intervention but also identify variables to be measured or controlled. In addition, the answers aid researchers in evaluating proposed changes in the use of OMT. The answers also assist the profession in evaluating government regulations of practice and responding to questions raised in managed care.

INVESTIGATING OSTEOPATHIC PRACTICE AND OMT

Research Designs

There is an advantage in using established research designs. The delays, frustrations, and difficulties in gaining acceptance for some new research design outweigh the small advantage gained by developing the design. Clinical trial, epidemiologic, and medical outcome research designs are established models suitable for planning research on osteopathic practice and OMT. A major problem encountered in trials of manual medicine not present in drug studies is blinding patients, physicians, and researchers to the administration of alternative interventions. There are also ethical constraints in requiring physicians to deny treatments for patients when these treatments had been previously accepted for routine use in practice. These issues are addressed and resolved during planning clinical trial, epidemiologic, and outcome research and surveys to investigate osteopathic practice.

ESTABLISHED RESEARCH DESIGNS

Reliance on established research designs to guide planning decreases the likelihood that faulty design will invalidate the research. Planned research purpose, methods, and analysis are clearly defined and stated for researchers who participate in targeted research on osteopathic practice. The purpose of a clinical trial is to investigate the safety and efficacy of OMT as an intervention used in providing health care.[16] The design requires a description of entrance criteria, measurement of variables, and the organization of research teams and administrators. Adaptations modify methods and analysis for testing a specific hypothesis but do not change the basic design. The discussion section of research proposals and publications explains these adaptations and the rationale.

SAFETY AND EFFICACY

Requests for approval of interventions submitted to the FDA are required to use a clinical trial design to test for safety and efficacy. This section of an application is the major source of evidence to support the application. Similar design, methods, and analysis are anticipated if the HCFA, the Agency for Health Care Policy and Research (AHCP&R), or the OAM develops regulations for investigating unsupported interventions.[17] Modifications are frequently made to the basic clinical trial design. These include changes based on previous experience and on advances in the theoretical and statistical basis for design and analysis. Modification of clinical trial designs is identified by reading the current literature and by consulting with authorities. Important modifications include additional methods for measuring outcome variables.

ADDITIONS TO MEASUREMENTS

Recent additions to measurements used in clinical trials include quality of life (QOL)[18] and activities of daily living (ADL).[19] These measurements provide evidence that the intervention not only addresses the patient's problem but also maintains or improves the quality of life. QOL is a concern when interventions such as radiation or chemotherapy decrease the patient's capacity to function or increase the burden of illness. ADL is a valuable tool for short-term and long-term studies. There are self-administered questionnaires designed to obtain reliable information on the patient's perceived capacity to function in personal, family, and community roles. Indices developed from physical, mental, and socioeconomic scales are sensitive and specific for health status changes in these parameters.

RESEARCH PLAN

The intervention being investigated is described in the literature. There may be variations in administration, particularly in manual medicine. The research plan should address patient selection, diagnostic criteria for selecting the intervention for improving health or recovery from illness, administration, and the specific outcomes. The plan should describe each of these research methods in detail.

OTHER VARIABLES

Other variables may be important in clinical outcome research. The value of added measurements depends on their specificity and sensitivity.[20] Sensitive measures provide information on change in the variable. This allows changes during the treatment or during the course of the condition to be followed. Specific and sensitive predictors of patients' health status are available for investigating OMT. However, similar predictors for the course of somatic dysfunction have not been addressed. The available standardized examination for somatic dysfunction has been validated as a useful method to answer questions on the course of somatic dysfunction.[21]

Outcome Studies

Outcome studies are planned to include a large number of subjects because so many uncontrolled or unknown variables are present. An exception to the need for many research subjects occurs if the changes between encounters are large. A single investigator's small patient base requires collecting data from cooperating investigators at multiple sites to increase the number of subjects. This aspect of a clinical trial requires committed collaboration from all researchers. Data collected by uniform procedures, assessed by the same criteria, and accurately recorded contribute to reliable investigation. A research team of experts plans the trial with practicing physicians' input on feasibility. Resources to conduct the research may be deficient at some sites, requiring development or use of regional facilities. Training the site research teams for their tasks is required to reduce variability in data. Deficiencies in other resources must be identified during planning and corrected before starting the trial. The management team provides training, monitors research in progress, and receives data for analysis. The tasks of the management team ensure blind controls, completeness of data, analysis, and reports on the results.

DISCUSSION

Reform

Reform in health care and change in medical practice is inevitable. The history of medicine has recorded continuous changes that evolved because different forces present at that time or place influenced healing systems.[22] In the Middle Ages, physicians practiced on the basis of health benefits that they and their patients believed resulted from interventions. Medical authorities were replaced when doubt developed or stronger beliefs were established. Today, the art of practice still exists but is rapidly being replaced by scientifically supported medical practice.

Research

Research provides information on the present status of medicine, detects trends that forecast change, and monitors the forces for change. Planned research, targeted and prioritized when appropriate, is more efficient than independently conceived research. However, both planned and independent forms of research are important. The emphasis on one or the other shifts with pressures to meet different demands for information.

Challenges to Osteopathic Medicine

Public, governmental, and scientific challenges to osteopathic medicine establish the use, safety, and efficacy of OMT. In the near future, health and the cost effectiveness of medical practice will be challenged. Epidemiologic and outcome population studies are a source of information to evaluate changes required to protect citizens' health and welfare. Outcome case and medical practice studies provide information on health effectiveness and the characteristics of interventions used in practice. Clinical trials are used to obtain scientific support for medical interventions.

Changing Clinical Trial Design

A clinical trial to obtain approval for an intervention is time-consuming. Researchers have revised the original clinical trial design based on experience and theoretical advances. Frequent revisions occurred in the past 50 years; further modifications are likely to occur. Adapting clinical trial design to physical interventions requires time and resources. Creating a new procedure to obtain approval requires its recognition, acceptance, and adoption for use. Establishing either the clinical trial or the alternative procedure is a lengthy process. New research designs are unpredictable, whereas modifying existing designs avoids the uncertainties of gaining recognition and acceptance. OMT and osteopathic medicine are important elements in the health care system; failure to anticipate future needs for approved interventions will change osteopathic medicine's image. Clinical trials of the interventions used in osteopathic practice should be pursued vigorously, now and in the future.

SURVEYS

Surveys provide semiquantitative measures and are tools for research by the medical professions. Cross-sectional data contributes information on the current practice of graduates and the contributions made to patient, family, and community health. Data from reliable cross-sectional studies entered into a computerized database create the basis for longitudinal studies. Such studies detect trends associated with environmental influences on health and practice as well as preferences and perceived value for interventions.

Research Plan

Use a research plan based on established research designs. Different research designs fit specific purposes; proper application provides reliable data, analysis, and conclusions. Each era contains forces that lead to health care reform and modification of medical practice. These forces create a need for continuing research in medicine. Research conducted or sponsored by the osteopathic profession provides information for the profession's self-direction and evaluation of external forces that threaten health care reform and change in medicine.

APPLIED DESIGNS

Research on and treatment with applied clinical trial and outcome research designs should be targeted, rather than individual initiatives. Professional standards for medical practice and guidelines for decisions are needed to expedite continuous quality improvement in osteopathic medicine. Targeted research evaluates current forces that are changing practice while advancing osteopathic theory and practice. Documenting osteopathic evaluation and manipulative treatment used in practice and including data on full medical practice supports or refutes the principle that maintaining the structure and function of the somatic system influences health and healing. Such research emphasizes the general contributions of OMT in patient care and identifies its values in treating disabled, distressed and diseased patients.

Research Manual

Create a research manual. It is a valuable asset. An overview of planned research provides quick access to the goal, procedures, tasks, and responsibilities. Including schedules and location of contact persons improves communication. The details for data collection on hypotheses, methods, assessment or process, and outcomes are available as a quick reference that helps researchers and staff in preparing for and conducting their tasks. Similar information helps the researcher with tabulation, data reduction, and analysis. Manuals that include information for participating organizational sections and departments expedite their assistance and cooperation. Preparing a manual as part of planning is as valuable for a single institution as it is in multicenter trials. The manual is indispensable in multicenter trials.

CHECKLIST

Include a checklist in the manual for monitoring progress during research and to increase efficiency. A checklist of important events improves the quality of research. The plan specifies scheduling different events, such as recruiting subjects and obtaining clearances. List missed appointments and data collections for follow-up to ensure completeness of data. Including periodic verification of data in the checklist increases the quality of the research.

SCHEDULE

List completion dates in a schedule. Placing these dates in a prominent place in the manual keeps the study from extending past the expected completion date. Prompt completion reduces expenses caused by an extension and improves the image of the researchers. Listing schedules recognizes the value of time and decreases waiting time for subjects, clinicians, and staff. Respect for persons' time increases commitment to the research and decreases lost data and dropouts. Monitoring decreases errors and initiates corrections at an appropriate time. Follow-up on missed data collection; ask questions on data or schedules to obtain timely answers that are difficult to obtain at a later date.

Steering Committee

To maximize effectiveness in conducting clinical research, create a steering committee to bridge the gap between planning and executing research. Appoint key members of the planning committee as a steering committee to interpret, safeguard the plan, and provide a means for dealing with problems. A participating research physician should be a member. A meeting of the committee or a member handles interpretations of the plan or questions on responsibilities, tasks, data collection, and analysis. Include a cost analysis of practice and the interventions used in managing a patients' health care; this provides a health cost–benefit measure. It allows evaluation of the current value and trends in the values to be analyzed for a competitive edge in health care.

Human Research Subjects

The protection of human research subjects is an important but often delaying factor in conducting research.[23–24] The research subject is a volunteer participant who is essential to the research. Respect for his or her contribution and rights is as important as obtaining approval for informed consent. Institutional Review Boards (IRB) have weighty tasks in evaluating scientific merit, risks to patients, and reasonable risk/benefit associated with volunteering to participate.[25] The IRB requires time for deliberation and possible research on their concerns with a study. Requests for IRB approval should be submitted as early as possible to avoid this source of delay. Its decisions require deliberation and deserve respect and compliance.

CONCLUSION

Clinical research today occurs in all aspects of the health care system. Inclusion of physician input in management outcome research and management's input in medical outcome research integrates the organization's efforts to provide quality and cost-effective health care. Analysis of the interaction between business and medicine is expedited. In business outcome studies,

emphasis is on the management or delivery components. Emphasis on health outcomes uses the financial data in efforts to continuously improve the quality of health care.

Continuous quality improvement in health care with advancement in osteopathic theory and practice is feasible. The resources for a program to achieve these goals need to be identified and developed. The program benefits osteopathic education from a database on what physicians need to know for medical practice. The program benefits patients of osteopathic physicians with evidence to support expected health outcomes. The program develops the resources to meet challenges to the profession, including the most recent ones occurring in managed care.

REFERENCES

1. Friedman L, Furberg CD, DeMets DL. *Fundamentals of Clinical Trials.* 2nd ed. Littleton, Mass: PSG Publishing Company; 1985.
2. Feinstein A. *Clinical Epidemiology.* Philadelphia, Penn: WB Saunders; 1985.
3. McLaughlin CP, Kaluzny AD. *Continuous Quality Improvement in Health Care: Theory, Implementation, and Applications.* Gaithersburg, Md: Aspen Publishers, Inc; 1994:3–69.
4. Couch JB, ed. *Health Care Quality Management for the 21st Century.* Tampa, Fla: American College of Physician Executives; 1991:1–136.
5. Macintyre K, Kleman CC. Measuring customer satisfaction. In: Feinstein A, ed. *Clinical Epidemiology.* Philadelphia, Penn: WB Saunders; 1985:110–115.
6. Barry SH. Methods of collecting data. In: Stewart AL, Ware JE Jr, eds. *Measuring Functioning and Well-being.* Durham, NC: Duke University Press; 1992:48–64.
7. Simpson KN, McLaughlin CP. Strategic decision-making, economic analysis, and TQM. In: Feinstein A, ed. *Clinical Epidemiology.* Philadelphia, Penn: WB Saunders; 1985:148–166.
8. Granatar T. Quality and community accountability: A view of the American Hospital Association. In: Kazandjian VA, ed, with Sternberg EA. *The Epidemiology of Quality.* Gaithersburg, Md: Aspen Publishers, Inc; 1995:253–268.
9. Shoemaker D, Burke G, Dorr A, Temple R, Friedman MA. A regulatory perspective. In: Spilker B, ed. *Quality of Life Assessments in Clinical Trials.* New York, NY: Raven Press, Ltd; 1990:3–204.
10. Epstein AA. The outcomes movement: Will it get us where we want to go? In: Graham NO, ed. *Quality in Health Care: Theory, Application, and Evolution.* Gaithersburg, Md: Aspen Publishers, Inc; 1995:188–197.
11. Moran J. Making alternative therapies everyone's issue. *Alternative Therapies.* September 1995;1:79.
12. Brown SW, Nelson A-M, Bronkesh SJ, Wood SD. *Patient Satisfaction Pays: Quality Service for Practice Success.* Gaithersburg, Md: Aspen Publishers, Inc; 1993.
13. Counte MA, Kjerulff KH. Survey methods for quality improvement. In: Kazandjian VA, ed, with Sternberg EA. *The Epidemiology of Quality.* Gaithersburg, Md: Aspen Publishers, Inc; 1995:38–54.
14. James BC. Implementing practice guidelines through clinical quality improvement. In: Graham NO, ed. *Quality in Health Care: Theory, Application, and Evolution.* Gaithersburg, Md: Aspen Publishers, Inc; 1995:162–165.
15. Raffel MW, Raffel NK. Public health. In: *The U.S. Health System:*

Origin and Functions. 3rd ed. Albany, NY: Delmar Publishers, Inc; 1989:292.

16. Friedman L, Furberg CD, DeMets DL. *Fundamentals of Clinical Trials.* 2nd ed. Littleton, Mass: PSG Publishing Company; 1985:1–10, 51–81.

17. Jencks SF, Wilensky GR. Appendix B: The health care quality improvement initiative: A new approach to quality assurance in Medicare. In: Graham NO, ed. *Quality in Health Care: Theory, Application, and Evolution.* Gaithersburg, Md: Aspen Publishers, Inc; 1995:341–354.

18. Jaeschke HG, Guyatt. How to develop and validate a new quality of life instrument. In: Spilker B, ed. *Clinical Trials.* New York, NY: Raven Press, Ltd; 1990:47–57.

19. Stewart AL, Sherbourne CD, Hays RD, et al. Summary and discussion of MOS measures. In: Stewart AL, Ware JE Jr, eds. *Measuring Functioning and Well-being.* Durham, NH: Duke University Press; 1992:345–371.

20. McWhinney IR. Clinical problem-solving in family medicine. In: *Textbook of Family Practice.* 5th ed. Philadelphia, Penn: WB Saunders; 1995:309–314.

21. Johnston WL, Friedman HD. *Functional Methods.* Indianapolis, Ind: American Academy of Osteopathy; 1994.

22. Lyons AS, Petrucelli RJ. *Medicine: An Illustrated History.* New York, NY: Harry N Abrams, Inc; 1987 edition.

23. Katz J. *Experimentation with Human Beings.* New York, NY: Russell Sage Foundation; 1972.

24. Report of the Secretary's Advisory Committee on Automated Personal Data Systems. *Records, Computers and the Rights of Citizens.* US Dept of Health, Education and Welfare; 1973. DHEW publication (OS) 73–97.

25. Greenwald RA, Ryan MK, Mulvihill JE, eds. *Human Research Subjects: A Handbook for Institutional Review Boards.* New York, NY: Plenum Press; 1982.

83. Basic Research and Osteopathic Medicine

FRANK H. WILLARD AND BARBARA SWARTZLANDER

Key Concepts

- **Philosophy and science of basic research**
- **Assumptions of principles of basic research**
- **Steps of scientific method**
- **Mechanics of experimental design and data collection**
- **Interpretation and evaluation of data**
- **Future of basic research in osteopathic medicine**

Basic research is founded on the principles of the scientific method and has had a long and intimate history with clinical medicine.

The principles used in basic research represent a philosophy as well as a science. As a philosophy, basic research provides a framework in which to organize observations, sharpen critical thoughts, and develop carefully formulated definitions and meanings. As a science, it represents a systematic attempt to organize, catalogue, and integrate the materials and phenomena of the surrounding world. In essence, it is a way through which we may come to understand the phenomena of the body and the mind, their interactions, and our relationship to the surrounding universe.

HISTORY

Basic research and clinical medicine have a long and interwoven history. Many individuals critical in the development of basic science knowledge were initially trained in clinical medicine. Medicine was traditionally considered a necessary precursor to the study of science.[1] British medicine was the first to shift away from a purely philosophic approach to medical knowledge when it used the basic research field of anatomy to make observations on disease processes. Anatomy was followed by experimental research in microbiology such as developed in French and German schools.[2] The experimental approach has precipitated many advances in understanding the physiology and biochemistry of disease processes.

BASIC VERSUS CLINICAL RESEARCH

There are no concrete boundaries between basic and clinical research, the latter essentially being a continuation of the for-

mer. Both approaches use intuitive logic and the scientific method to derive their underlying principles. The distinction, to the extent that it can be made, lies more in their range of topics and techniques and not in their fundamental philosophies. In general, the topics investigated in basic research have a much broader range, extending across the whole range of science and, as such, provide the necessary background for interpretation of the more focused area of clinical research. Basic research has the benefit of carefully constructed control situations along with statistical methods, whereas clinical research frequently has to rely on elaborate statistical methods in place of control populations for ethical reasons.

There are several fundamental assumptions when applying the principles of basic research to any field of Western medicine. The routines used in medicine can be explained in light of scientific principles. These principles can be induced and studied through the scientific method. Based on tested medical principles, additional or improved treatments in medicine can be deduced and tested. This is not to imply that all aspects of the practice of medicine are reducible to the principles of the scientific method. Although aspects of the patient–physician relationship can be analyzed with scientific principles, there remains the humane element that arises from the intrinsic desire to help a fellow human being who is ill.

Knowledge of body homeostasis and its response to external, internal, and emotional stimuli is expanding. It is imperative for the future growth and development of the osteopathic medical profession, as well as for improved awareness of its past, that it embrace the principles of basic research and that it encourage its students and clinicians to become involved in medical science research. To this end, this chapter first describes the fundamental steps used when applying the scientific method in basic research, followed by the mechanics of experimental design and the processes involved in data collection. Guidelines used to distinguish between the research data collected in a study and its subsequent interpretation are then discussed. Finally, this chapter underscores not only the need but the necessity for future basic research in osteopathic medicine.

SCIENTIFIC METHOD

The scientific method is based on a series of logical steps proceeding from observation through hypothesis to testing and interpretation.

The scientific method has been used to develop conceptual schemes for the organization of phenomena of the universe. The scientific method has elements closely related to common sense reasoning.[3] It is based on a logical progression or hierarchy of principles, each principle related to its predecessor through causal demonstrations. Many first principles are underived, such as the existence of points on a number line, the value of the unit in mathematics, and the progression of time, and as such are simply accepted as true. All other principles are largely derived in logical progression from the first principles.[4] The distinctive features of the scientific method involve the logical achievement of systematic classification of the known phenomena in this universe.[3]

The medical field also uses the scientific method of analysis—involving induction and deduction first articulated by Aristotle[5]—in both its research and its teaching programs (Fig. 83.1). In the inductive process, one observes a series of particular events (observations) from which a general or universal proposition is then induced.[4] Knowledge expands from particulars to generalizations in the inductive process. The scientific method is based primarily on induction.[6] Researchers collect numerous specific observations from which a generalized theory is induced. Conversely, in the deductive process, one progresses from a general proposition to deduce that specific situations may occur. Medical education is based primarily on the deductive method.[6] Rules, induced from medical research, are described for handling the generalized patient, from which the student can deduce the specific course of action for an individual patient.

The progress of knowledge from particulars to general rules used to predict new particulars is called an inductive-deductive couple. An example of the inductive-deductive couple in medical practice is as follows. Studies have demonstrated that individual patients with the signs of Parkinson's disease such as tremor and bradykinesia experience some amelioration of these signs when given the drug levodopa. From these observations, the generalization that patients with Parkinson's disease should be given levodopa has been induced and disseminated to the physician population.[7] A physician who recognizes tremor and bradykinesia in a specific patient, recalls his or her medical instruction, and prescribes levodopa, is using a deductive process of reasoning, going from general principles to specific cases.

The scientific method of basic research involves six cardinal steps (Fig. 83.2). Although these are separate steps, they may overlap in time. Research begins with observations that may

be of clinical or nonclinical phenomena and should be augmented by extensive background literature reviews. Through inductive reasoning, the observations lead to generalizations concerning the phenomena, and from these generalizations an overall hypothesis is formulated. The hypothesis is essentially a well thought out question to be investigated. From a carefully constructed hypothesis, predictions are made that can be turned into tests or experiments, ultimately producing research data. Replication of the tests as well as modification of the test procedures then produces additional data from which the consistency of the initial results can be judged. As data are accumulated, the validity of the hypothesis can be determined by inspection and statistical testing, and conceptual schemes (called working models) may be developed to fit the results into the overall knowledge of science. As additional studies demonstrate support for the conceptual scheme, research will advance the level of theory. Ultimately, theories that cannot be refuted progress to laws of science.

Research Studies

Research studies can be prospective or retrospective. In either case, they should begin with a carefully articulated hypothesis and a search of the background literature.

Before beginning the process of research, one has to identify the problem to be investigated. Two general approaches to problem identification have been used. The first, the prospec-

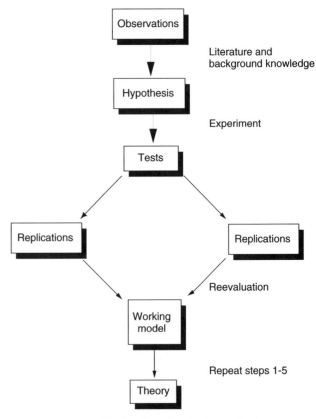

Literature and background knowledge

Experiment

Reevaluation

Repeat steps 1-5

Figure 83.2. Steps in scientific method.

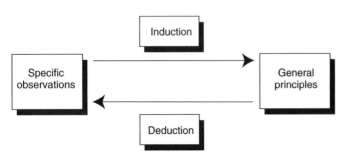

Figure 83.1. Relationship between induction and deduction in scientific method.

tive study, has taken basic research findings and derived useful clinical practices by forward thinking: "Here's what I've got, and here's what I want to have, now what do I have to do to get there?" Examples of prospective study are the quest for an antiviral agent to be employed against the AIDS virus and the development of pharmaceuticals targeting specific subtypes of neurotransmitter receptors involved in the class of neurologic diseases called movement disorders. In both cases, specific needs have been identified, and answers are being sought by medical research.

The second approach, the retrospective study, occurs when a clinical observation is investigated to gain an understanding of its underlying mechanism: "This technique appears to work well, but we need to examine why." Examples of retrospective studies are research into the mechanism of clinically effective pharmaceuticals and the investigations into the mechanisms of specific manipulative techniques. In both cases, the effectiveness of the therapy may be known through years of use in clinical practice, but the mechanism through which it works is not understood and represents the object of the quest.

Steps

The sequence of steps taken in the scientific method is similar for both prospective and retrospective studies. In the initial step, observations of a phenomena are accrued and the problem articulated. The observations and the problem statement should be carefully recorded. This description states what is known about the problem as well as what needs to be known and why. Continual review of the thesis statement is extremely helpful in fine-tuning the arguments. This step, if properly done, saves considerable time as the study progresses.

Although the scientific method begins with observations, a critical next step in the development of a hypothesis is a review of the existing information. Literature reviews represent an organized method of approaching the established body of scientific knowledge. Such reviews provide the background on which the initial phase of the proposed study can be evaluated. In addition, the literature can also provide information on whether a specific or a closely related study has been done previously, saving time and embarrassment in the future.

LITERATURE REVIEW

A good literature review requires thorough investigation through multiple information channels. Several methods exist for conducting such reviews. Initially, general information can be obtained by examining the bibliographies in the secondary literature, such as review articles in the field of interest. As an initial step, a quick perusal of current primary research papers in the field usually locates several references to pertinent review articles. The bibliographies of these review articles are an excellent source of reference citations. As with the review articles, the introductory sections and bibliographies of primary articles also form a good introduction to the problem area and source of references.

Numerous bibliographic databases, such as MEDLINE or BIOSIS, can provide a more thorough and systematic approach to the literature (a more detailed list of sources is included in Table 83.1). These resources require a knowledge of specific keywords and/or authors and are best approached after gaining initial familiarity with the characteristic of the discipline. Searches of these large databases can usually be accomplished with Boolean logic allowing the use of AND, OR, or NOT as operators between terms. Some knowledge of the discipline coupled with clever use of these logical operators can focus a search toward just the articles you desire.

Storing information once it has been collected from the literature is also a critical problem in research. The amount of information available far exceeds the human capacity for storage and retrieval. Older methods often involved use of index cards and file catalogs to organize and store reference citations and notes. These techniques for indexing material provided only limited methods for retrieval, making information searches difficult and cumbersome. The construction of personalized computer databases has allowed much better indexing of information, facilitating its retrieval. Several good personal database programs are currently available: Ref-11 or Reference Manager, for example. These databases are empty when purchased and can be used to hold thousands of references you encounter in your study. Each entry into the database can be conceived of as an index card. Multiple indices or keywords can be placed on the entry; this allows the computer to locate the information during a search. There are several things to look for in choosing a personal database for storing research article citations and information:

1. The program should be interactive with commercial reference services such that pretyped references can be transferred (downloaded) from these commercially available sources (Table 83.1).
2. With each entry, the program should be capable of storing large quantities of notes or an abstract of the article.
3. The program should be able to produce bibliography files or note files that are compatible with popular word processors programs, facilitating rapid transfer of information between these programs.
4. There should be a mechanism, intrinsic to the program, for quickly generating a list of references from citations placed in a text of a manuscript written on a word processor.

Scientific papers are a specialized form of technical writing. As such, it is far too extensive a job for an individual to read every paper of interest in its entirety. Use shortcuts to obtain information from a research paper. There are several techniques for rapidly reading and extracting information from research articles. Read the abstract alone to gain the main points of the article; this is all that is necessary for many papers. File and index in a database for future use any information obtained from the article, along with the reference citation. Storing the information without the reference citation is useless when it comes time to writing an article because the bibliography must be referred to in a written paper. The introduction of the article can also help place the specific information in context with previously established information; it also may be a good source of additional references, including review articles.

Examine critically the methods used for data collection of any scientific paper that is to be used as a key point in research. This requires critical reading of the materials and methods section as well as the results section. Keep the following questions in mind:

1. Are the methods used appropriate for the study?
2. Are the methods performed correctly?

3. Do the authors' conclusions fit with their findings?
4. Do the authors fit their observations into existing information in the field?

DEVELOPING A TESTABLE HYPOTHESIS

The construction of a testable hypothesis requires a considerable understanding of the problem and the background literature as well as the limitations of the investigative techniques available. Write this stage of the planning down in detail, as it

Table 83.1
Major Reference Sources for the Medical and Life Sciences.[a]

Print	CD-ROM	Online

Index Medicus (1879+)	Medline (1966+)
	  OVID
	  Cambridge Scientific Abstract
	  DIALOG
	  SilverPlatter
		Medline (1966+)
		  OVID
		  NLM
		  DIALOG
		  DataStar

Excerpta Medica (1946+)	EMBASE (1974+)
	  OVID
	  SilverPlatter
		EMBASE (1974+)
		  OVID
		  DIALOG

Biological Abstracts (1926+)	Biological Abstracts (1985+)
	  OVID
	  SilverPlatter
		BIOSIS Previews (1969+)
		  OVID
		  DIALOG
		  DataStar

Cumulative Index to Nursing
  & Allied Health (1960+)
	CINAHL (1983+)
	  OVID
	  SilverPlatter
	  Cambridge Scientific Abstracts
		CINAHL (1983+)
		  OVID
		  DataStar

Chemical Abstracts (1907+)		CA Search (1967+)
		  OVID
		  DIALOG
		  DataStar
		  ORBIT

Science Citation Index (1961+)	SCISEARCH
	  Institute for Scientific Information (ISI)
		SCISEARCH (1974+)
		  DIALOG
		  DataStar

Hospital Literature Index
  (1945+)
	Health Planning and Administration
	  OVID
		Healthline (1975+)
		  NLM
		Health Planning and Administration (1975+)
		  OVID
		  DIALOG

Current Contents-Clinical
  Medicine (1973+)
Current Contents-Life Sciences
  (1958+)
	Current Contents on Diskette
	  Institute for Scientific Information (ISI)
		Current Contents
		  OVID
		  DIALOG

Psychological Abstracts
  (1894+)
	PsycLIT (1974+)
	  OVID
	  SilverPlatter
		PsycINFO (1967+)
		  OVID
		  DIALOG

Nutrition Abstracts (1931+)	CAB Abstracts
	  SilverPlatter
		CAB Abstracts (1972+)
		  OVID
		  DIALOG

		CHIROLARS (1900+) OVID

Physician's Desk Reference
  (PDR)
Merck Manual
	Physician's Desk Reference
	Medical Economics with or without
	  Merck Manual	

Table 83.1—*continued*

Print	CD-ROM	Online

Martindale: The Extrapharmacopoeia	Martindale CD-ROM Microindex	Martindale Online
		  DIALOG
		  DataStar

		Comprehensive Core Medical Library (CCML) (1982+) OVID (full text)

		National Library of Medicine (NLM)
		  MEDLINE
		  AIDSLINE
		  AIDSDRUGS
		  AIDSTRIALS
		  BIOETHICSLINE
		  CATLINE
		  AVLINE
		  CHEMLINE
		  HEALTH
		  CANCERLIT
		  TOXLINE
		  TOXLIT
		  DIRLINE
		  SERLINE
		  HSTAR
		  SPACELINE
		  PDQ

*The underlined terms represent specific databases; nonunderlined terms represent the vendors carrying the databases.

MEDLINE, produced by the U.S. National Library of Medicine (NLM), is one of the premier sources of biomedical literature. MEDLINE corresponds to three print indexes: Index Medicus, Index to Dental Literature, and International Nursing Index. More than 3700 journals are indexed and more than 70% of the records contain author abstracts.

EMBASE, the Excerpta Medica database, is a leading source for biomedical and pharmaceutical literature. It contains citations and abstracts to more than 3500 international journals.

BIOSIS Previews is one of the world's most comprehensive databases in the life sciences. More than 6500 serials, 2000 international meetings, as well as books and monographs are monitored for inclusion.

CINAHL provides bibliographic access to important nursing and allied health journals in the fields of cardiopulmonary technology, emergency services, laboratory technology, medical assistants, occupational therapy, physical therapy, physician's assistants, radiologic technology, respiratory therapy, and surgical technology.

CA SEARCH database includes more than 10 million citations to the literature of chemistry and its applications.

SCISEARCH is a multidisciplinary index to the literature of science and technology prepared by the Institute for Scientific Information (ISI). Cited reference searches are possible in this database.

Health Planning and Administration contains references to nonclinical literature on all aspects of health care planning and facilities, health insurance, the aspects of financial management, personnel administration, manpower planning, and licensure and accreditation that apply to the delivery of health care.

Current contents is a weekly service that reproduces the tables of contents from current issues of leading journals in clinical medicine and life sciences and five other subsets.

PsycINFO database provides access to the international literature in psychology and related behavioral and social sciences, including psychiatry, sociology, anthropology, education, pharmacology, and linguistics.

CAB Abstracts is a comprehensive file of agricultural and biological information and contains all records in the 26 main abstract journals published by CAB International.

CHIROLARS is a health care database that emphasizes health promotion, prevention, and conservation care. More than 700 periodicals are included from medical, osteopathic, physical therapy, chiropractic, and other disciplines.

National Library of Medicine computer files contain approximately 15 million records covering its holdings of books, journal articles, and more. With GRATEFUL MED software, health professionals from even the most rural areas can access the files listed in this table.

is often easier to spot inconsistencies in written arguments than in verbal ones. Seek outside consultation, especially that of peer review, as the test protocol matures to eliminate errors in design.

Differentiating between a testable and an untestable hypothesis is not always easy. A hypothesis can be untestable either because it asks for a subjective or value judgment or because the techniques are not yet developed to collect the data. For example: "Do neurons in lamina I of the spinal cord process nociception better than those in lamina V?" requires a value judgment on what "better" means. "Do laminae I neurons in the dorsal horn of the spinal cord have a shorter response latency than lamina V neurons to C fiber, primary nociceptive inputs?" is a more testable hypothesis because the latencies for small-caliber, primary afferent fibers to definable stimuli can be reproduced, quantified, and compared.

A testable hypothesis has to have a variable that can be critically defined for observation or quantification. For example, the hypothesis "Depressed people are more anxious than are nondepressed people" is difficult to test because quantifiable definitions for depression and anxiety are not available. "People with above average blood cortisol levels have elevated blood catecholamine levels" is a more testable hypothesis because, under controlled conditions, both of these substances can be quantified, baselines determined, data compared, and the hypothesis judged true or false. If the techniques have not been developed to observe or measure the variable, the hypothesis remains untestable, awaiting future technical developments. "People with above average blood cortisol levels have elevated activity of the locus ceruleus" is not very testable as of this writing because methods for accessing locus ceruleus activity in the human brain are not well-developed. To make the hypothesis more testable with current methods, one might assay indirect components of the activity on the locus ceruleus, such as the metabolic byproducts of ceruleus neurons, or use animal models to record neural activity in the locus ceruleus and extrapolate the data to humans.

Once a hypothesis has been formulated, develop specific experimental paradigms for testing. For each experiment, write explicit outlines; have them carefully peer reviewed for flaws. This review process can save enormous amounts of time at later stages in the study when data from the experimental design is being analyzed.

IDENTIFYING VARIABLES

Each of the variables in the study, where possible, should be identified along with its controlling factors. In the actual testing process, as many variables as possible should be fixed in value while the specific variable in question is run through a range of values. Such a study results in a range of data points. Statistical methods assist in determining how well these points support the hypothesis.

There are certain variables that cannot be controlled in any experiment. Having uncontrolled variables in an experiment does not automatically negate the study; if it did, almost all studies would be eliminated. However, uncontrolled variables can increase the range of values over which the data fluctuate. Sometimes this range of values is so large that the data are rendered useless. A knowledge of as many as possible of the uncontrolled variables present in the experiment is important for evaluating the results. The uncontrolled variables must also become a significant part of the written discussion when the study is finalized.

ANALYSIS AND EVALUATION

Once data have been collected, the process of analysis and evaluation can begin. Data analysis is in large part a search for meaningful patterns in the study results.[8]

How is one variable related to another in the study?
Does weakness and reduced size in a paravertebral muscle group relate to low back pain?
Can manual treatment of low back structures shorten the time spent away from work?

To evaluate such relationships, statistical methods must be used because it is not possible to observe all conceivable events in any given study paradigm. Although these methods cannot prove a hypothesis, they can be used to assist in eliminating incorrect assumptions when reasoning from specific to general situations.[9] A description of the numerous statistical tests available and their usage is beyond the scope of this chapter. Numerous packaged computer programs are available to perform statistical calculations. Examples of statistical programs are SYS STAT, SIGMA STAT, and SAS.

The values collected in the study represent raw data and may contain a range of variation. Transformations may be necessary to prepare the data for interpretation.[10] Statistical methods can assist the observer with the interpretations by demonstrating that, within a certain range of probability, the phenomena tested are compatible with the hypothesis. A review of statistical methods related to medicine can be found in Bailar and Mosteller,[10] and a more detailed treatment of statistical theory is present in Box et al.[11]

Having formulated a problem and collected the data, the interpretative phase follows. After examining the data accrued in the current studies as well as that found in the literature and supported by the statistics, the observer determines whether the hypothesis is valid. This step is an interpretation. It is not data or fact but is based on statistical probabilities. It is extremely important to distinguish between the experimental data and its interpretation. The data, if properly collected, should not change in the future. Data should grow in quantity as additional experiments are performed and reported, but the basic data values of each study do not change. It is expected that the interpretation of the data will change as additional data points are accrued and the hypothesis is more completely developed.

Continual criticism of the interpretation by the observers and other experimenters is necessary to refine the hypothesis. Seek alternative interpretations of the hypothesis as each new batch of data is added to the collection. When alternative explanations for the data are found, the simplest interpretation rules, a phenomena called Occam's razor (see entry in *Compton's Interactive Encyclopedia*, Compton's NewMedia Inc., 1994). The discovery that an interpretation is false does not necessarily mean that the data are wrong; it simply means that a new interpretation is required.

Out of the critical phase of data evaluation may come modification of the original hypothesis. Keep in mind that critical thinking dictates that one is attempting to disprove the original hypothesis. Observations not in agreement with the hypothesis or statistical results that do not support the hypothesis do not necessarily mean that all is wrong. Modification of the original hypothesis, based on the experimental results, can lead to new predictions and other testable hypotheses.

APPLICATION OF BASIC RESEARCH TO OSTEOPATHIC MEDICINE

The application of basic research methods to further understand osteopathic practices reaps many benefits.

The definition of osteopathic philosophy emphasizes the self-regulatory mechanisms of the body and their role in preventing disease processes.[12] The physician's role is to assist these mechanisms in the repair of the body. It follows from these statements that osteopathy as a profession requires a powerful knowledge of the body and its function, regardless of whether this knowledge involves renal function and electrolyte balance, or the processing of nociception in the neural circuits of the spinal cord. Based on the principles of osteopathic philosophy, the more one understands body functions, the more one is able to assist these functions in regaining their normalcy in the face of pathologic processes.

Basic biomedical research, which in part represents a quest to understand the body and its compensatory mechanisms, increases our general fund of knowledge and facilitates osteopathic practices. Other benefits derived from strong basic research programs linked to osteopathic medicine are:

1. The development and testing of new models regarding specific osteopathic techniques
2. Better explanations of existing osteopathic techniques thus facilitating patient education as well as the presentation of osteopathic practices and principles to the surrounding medical community

Future directions for basic research in osteopathy should target anatomy, neural sciences, endocrinology, and immunology.

Anatomy

The continued study of anatomy is a necessary avenue to further knowledge of human structural variation. The following suggestions mark areas of particular concern for the practitioner. A few references have been included to act as seed crystals. Exploration into the general organization and innervation of the paravertebral muscles and associated joints of the back[13–14] brings greater understanding of lumbar mechanisms and techniques. Particularly, examination of the innervation of the pelvic basin and its surrounding ligamentous structures[15] helps us understand the pain presentation syndromes in the thoracolumbar area. Exciting research in the advanced imaging of muscle groups and fluid surrounding facilitated segments could provide methods for clinical studies using osteopathic manipulative treatment.[16]

Research into the innervation of the cranial vault and the movement of fluids in the surrounding tissue may provide further insight into the mechanisms underlying the practice of osteopathy in the cranial field.[17] In addition, investigations into the tonic muscle contractions of paravertebral musculature attached to the base of the vault may shed light on the association of movements between the cranial vault and the sacral base.

Neural Sciences

The study of neural sciences is extremely important for explanations of osteopathic techniques. The interactive and highly integrated network of regulating substances released by sensory nerve endings and immune cells in the vicinity of an inflammatory process[18–19] leads to a better understanding of the processes underlying the palpable lesion in somatic dysfunction. The neurophysiology of spinal cord segments exposed to elevated nociceptive input such as neurogenic inflammatory processes[20–21] is a necessary step to understanding what factors can influence or control these facilitated segments. Anatomic and biochemical studies of the changes in gene expression in interneurons in the spinal cord gray matter consequent to prolonged exposure to nociception[22–23] lead to an understanding of spinal cord facilitation. Investigation of the convergence of somatic and visceral input in the gray matter of the spinal cord is of great benefit in the understanding of viscerosomatic and somatovisceral reflexes.[24–26] Little is known with regard to the output of the autonomic nervous system to the vasculature of the body; even less is known concerning the interaction between autonomic efferent fibers and their parallel afferent neurons (somatosympathetic neurons).[15,27] Much can be gained from these studies in the understanding of facilitated segments. The types of sensory information derived from the spindle organs in the paravertebral muscles and the vestibular apparatus are of extreme importance with respect to its influence on posture, locomotion, and pain perception.[28–29]

Endocrinology and Immunology

The response of the body to dysfunction is an important concept in osteopathy. Recent studies have opened new venues of basic research into the function of the neuroendocrine-immune system[30–33] and revealed the key role that this network plays in the maintenance of homeostasis and the initiation of a general adaptive response to stressors.[19,34] Future work describing the response of this system to somatic and visceral nociception, neural control of the endocrine and immune systems, as well as the immune and endocrine control of neural function, will be rewarding for osteopathic medicine.

CONCLUSION

In all of these approaches, the future of osteopathic medicine lies in our ability to understand and teach its principles. To this end, basic research can provide the solid foundation on which the house is constructed.

REFERENCES

1. Shryock RH. *The Development of Modern Medicine: An Interpretation of the Social and Scientific Factors Involved.* Madison, Wis: University of Wisconsin Press; 1974.
2. Howell TD. The history of medicine. In: Kelley WG, ed. *Textbook of Internal Medicine.* Philadelphia, Penn: JB Lippincott; 1989:6–8.
3. Nagel E. *The Structure of Science: Problems in the Logic of Scientific Explanation.* New York, NY: Harcourt, Brace, & World, Inc; 1961.
4. Smith VE. *The Science of Nature: An Introduction.* Milwaukee, Wis: The Bruce Publishing Company; 1966.
5. Losee J. *A Historical Introduction to the Philosophy of Science.* London, England: Oxford University Press; 1972.
6. Elston RC, Johnson MS. *Essentials of Biostatistics,* Philadelphia, Penn: FA Davis Company; 1987.

7. Tsui JKC, Calne DB. Approach to the patient with abnormal movements and posture, including cerebellar ataxia. In: Kelly WN, ed. *Textbook of Internal Medicine.* New York, NY: JB Lippincott; 1992:2321–2323.

8. Godfrey K. Simple linear regression in medical practice. *N Engl J Med.* 1985;313:1629–1636.

9. Steel RGD, Torrie JH. *Principles and Procedures of Statistics with Special Reference to Biological Science.* New York, NY: McGraw-Hill Book Company, Inc; 1960.

10. Bailar JC, Mosteller F. *Medical Uses of Statistics.* Boston, Mass: NEJM Books; 1992.

11. Box GEP, Hunter WG, Hunter JS. *Statistics for Experimenters: An Introduction to Design, Data Analysis, and Model Building.* New York, NY: John Wiley & Sons; 1978.

12. The Glossary Review Committee. In: Allen TW, ed. *Glossary of Osteopathic Terminology. 1995 Yearbook and Directory of Osteopathic Physicians.* Chicago, Ill: American Osteopathic Association; 1995; 86:692–703.

13. Bogduk N, Wilson AS, Tynan W. The human lumbar dorsal rami. *J Anat.* 1982;134:383–397.

14. Groen GJ, Baljet B, Drukker J. Nerves and nerve plexuses of the human vertebral column. *Am J Anat.* 1990;188:282–296.

15. Jinkins JR, Whittermore AR, Bradley WG. The anatomic basis of vertebrogenic pain and the autonomic syndrome associated with lumbar disk extrusion. *Am J Radiol.* 1989;152:1277–1289.

16. Parke WW. The significance of venous return impairment in ischemic radiculopathy and myelopathy. *Orthop Clin North Am.* 1991; 22:213–221.

17. Norton JM. A tissue pressure model for palpatory perception of the cranial rhythmic impulse. *JAOA.* 1991;91:975–994.

18. Payan DG. The role of neuropeptides in inflammation. In: Gallin JI, Goldstein IM, Snyderman R, eds. *Inflammation: Basic Principles and Clinical Correlations.* New York, NY: Raven Press; 1992.

19. Willard FH. Neuroendocrine-immune network, nociceptive stress, and the general adaptive response. In: Everett T, Dennis M, Ricketts E, eds. *Physiotherapy in Mental Health: A Practical Approach.* Oxford, England: Butterworth, Heinemann; 1995:102–126.

20. Grigg P, Schaible H-G, Schmidt RF. Mechanical sensitivity of group III and IV afferents from posterior articular nerve in normal and inflamed cat knee. *J. Neurophysiol.* 1986;55:635–643.

21. Zimmermann M. Pain mechanisms and mediators in osteoarthritis. *Semin Arthritis Rheum.* 1989;18:22–29.

22. Dubner R, Ruda MA. Activity-dependent neuronal plasticity following tissue injury and inflammation. *Trends Neurosci.* 1992;15:96–103.

23. Coderre TJ, Katz J, Vaccarina AL, Melzack R. Contribution of central neuroplasticity to pathological pain: review of clinical and experimental evidence. *Pain.* 1993;52:259–285.

24. Sato A, Swenson RS. Sympathetic nervous system response to mechanical stress of the spinal column in rats. *J Manipulative Physiol Ther.* 1984;7:141–147.

25. Sato A, Schmidt RF. Somatosympathetic reflexes: afferent fibers, central pathways, discharge characteristics. *Physiol Rev.* 1973; 53:916–947.

26. Patterson MM, Howell JN. *The Central Connection: Somatovisceral/Viscerosomatic Interaction.* Athens, Ohio: University Classics, Ltd; 1992.

27. Prechtl JC, Powley TL. B-afferents: a fundamental division of the nervous system mediating homeostasis? *Behav Brain Sci.* 1990; 13:289–331.

28. Yates BJ, Kasper J, Wilson VJ. Effects of muscle and cutaneous hindlimb afferents on L4 neurons whose activity is modulated by neck rotation. *Exp Brain Res.* 1989;77:48–56.

29. Suzuki I, Timerick SJB, Wilson VJ. Body position with respect to head or body position in space is coded by lumbar interneurons. *J Neurophysiol.* 1985;54:123–133.

30. Gold PW, Goodwin FK, Chrousos GP. Clinical and biochemical manifestations of depression: relation to the neurobiology of stress: I. *N Engl J Med.* 1988;319:348–353.

31. Johnson EO, Kamilaris TC, Chrousos GP, Gold PW. Mechanisms of stress: a dynamic overview of hormonal and behavioral homeostasis. *Neurosci Biobehav Rev.* 1992;16:115–130.

32. Gold PW, Goodwin FK, Chrousos GP. Clinical and biochemical manifestations of depression: relation to the neurobiology of stress: II. *N Engl J Med.* 1988;319:413–420.

33. Maier SF, Watkins LR, Fleshner M. Psychoneuroimmunology. The interface between behavior, brain, and immunity. *Am Psychol.* 1994; 49:1004–1017. Review.

34. Willard FH, Patterson MM. *Nociception and the Neuroendocrine-Immune Connection.* Athens, Ohio: University Classics, Ltd; 1994.

84. Osteopathic Research

THE FUTURE

MICHAEL M. PATTERSON

Key Concepts

- **The issues that challenge osteopathic theory and practice, and sources of knowledge to meet the challenge**

- **Research models constructed and used for investigating osteopathic manipulative treatment and the associated health benefits**

- **Differences among speculation, theory, statistical support obtained from research, and knowledge accepted as support for osteopathic principles and practice**

The osteopathic profession faces a future filled with unknown and unpredictable forces that will shape the profession and challenge it in many ways. The osteopathic profession is challenged more and more strongly to show that the claims it makes for its unique philosophy and practice are beneficial to the patients it serves. The existence of osteopathy as a unique and separate profession rests on its ability to continually demonstrate that its practices are efficacious and its theories sound. Government and third-party insurance carriers mandate that the outcomes of health care be used as evidence of the quality of service. Meeting this challenge is not a simple task or one to be taken for granted. To achieve this goal, all components of the profession are required to take an active role. This includes:

Educational institutions
Hospitals
Affiliated societies
Individual physicians in practice

In addition, those active in research and teaching must make special efforts to use new information from research performed outside the profession to buttress and support osteopathy's unique ideas and insights.

It is not that no data exist to show that the osteopathic profession has made unique contributions to health care and that its philosophy is sound. The research from the Kirksville group in the 1940s and 1950s, data from the Chicago College and other osteopathic schools, and papers published in the *Journal of the American Osteopathic Association* over the years show that the osteopathic contribution to health care is sub-

stantial. Showing the unique contributions and emerging quality of osteopathic care requires new and innovative ways to measure health care and outcomes and the development of new and innovative research techniques. The art of clinical research is a fairly new endeavor; necessary new techniques and understandings must be developed.

This chapter looks at some of the issues facing the profession for meeting this challenging future, and at some of the research models that might be considered for future research efforts designed to demonstrate the unique aspects of osteopathic philosophy and practice.

TYPES OF RESEARCH IN OSTEOPATHIC MEDICINE

Basic Science

Within the purview of osteopathic research there are several valid types of studies. Perhaps the most basic is that outlined by Willard in Chapter 83, "Basic Research and Osteopathic Medicine," which flows from basic science studies. This research includes studies designed to define the basic functions of the body and mind and explain how they interact with the environment. These studies are mainstream biomedical research. An increased understanding of the human organism and its function should help validate osteopathic practice. The osteopathic profession therefore must nurture the basic sciences.

BASIC RESEARCH IN OTHER INSTITUTIONS AND PROFESSIONS

Basic science has been performed for many years in most biomedical facilities and research institutes. Most basic research relevant to the osteopathic profession is done not in the educational institutions of the profession but in other biomedical settings. The amount of research that can be supported directly by the profession is small compared with the amount of such research performed around the world. The total amount of funding available from within the osteopathic profession for support of its research programs is less per year than the annual budgets of many individual laboratories outside the profession. This suggests two things. First, maximal use must be made of data from laboratories outside the profession. Osteopathic researchers and clinicians must cultivate interactions with biochemical researchers at other institutions who can supply data and interpretations.

Second, the limited resources of the profession must be put into research endeavors that provide the greatest return in ex-

1115

plaining osteopathic experience and theory. The funding agencies of the profession must insist that their funds go to efforts that have direct bearing on the questions the profession deems important. This requires that investigators within the osteopathic profession understand the unique and defining concepts of osteopathy within which to interpret their findings. Without this understanding, the investigator is unable to interpret the findings in ways that are useful to the profession, and a large part of the investment is lost.

RECRUITING AND ORIENTING BASIC SCIENTISTS

Cultivating basic scientists who understand the clinical tenets of the profession and training basic scientists to gain such understanding pays off in increased theory building and data interpretation. One excellent way to begin the process of understanding osteopathic principles and practice is to ask PhD faculty to attend osteopathic manipulative treatment (OMT) courses. Experience in learning and receiving manipulative treatment is an enlightening experience. A cadre of investigators must be developed who understand the principles and clinical experiences of osteopathy so that they can frame their research questions in the light of osteopathic clinical experience and theory. Without this understanding, data will not be examined from the perspective of osteopathic treatment and insight.

A good example of this is the lack of scientific interest in viscerosomatic and somatovisceral reflexes in the general neuroscientific community until recently. Although these reflex connections are vital in osteopathic theory, they were not generally deemed important in general medical research. Only when the National Institutes of Health recognized the importance of these interactions and set aside funds for research did research interest increase. Had the insights from osteopathic theory and practice been well-known in the neurophysiologic community, the importance of these reflex connections may have been recognized much earlier. However, even in areas that are well-recognized as important, such as the role of the muscle proprioceptors in regulating muscle tone, the experiences of the osteopathic profession often allow the data to be examined in another light, exposing different potential roles.[1]

INTERFACE BETWEEN RESEARCHERS AND OSTEOPATHIC PROFESSION

It is the role of the researcher to be the interface between data and relevant osteopathic philosophy. The osteopathic profession must provide the means by which the investigator can become familiar with the clinical and theoretical aspects of the profession. This makes it possible for researchers to interpret their data and insights. To facilitate this interaction and to assure the profession of the best return on its investment, the funding agencies of the profession must think of themselves as agencies with specific missions and must direct their funds to investigators willing to meet those missions and willing to learn about the profession and its goals.

Integrative Model Building

INTEGRATING BASIC SCIENCE AND CLINICAL OBSERVATION

A second type of research activity necessary within the profession is the integration of basic science knowledge and clinical observation. This endeavor is extremely valuable and potentially dangerous. A recent article by Van Buskirk[2] illustrates such research. In this article, Van Buskirk builds a theoretical model of somatic dysfunction based on nociceptive inputs. He marshals an impressive array of basic science data and synthesizes it in a unique way from his clinical understandings and observations. The result is a well-grounded look at one of the central concepts of the osteopathic philosophy of health and disease. This is the valuable aspect of the article.

The dangerous part is that the model will be taken as fact. Van Buskirk goes to great lengths to point out that the model seems to be explanatory but still needs to be subjected to rigorous research verification and clinical observation before it can be accepted as proven. Unfortunately, the pioneering models that came out of the research of Korr and Denslow[3-4] suffered from being taken as factual explanation rather than as models in need of experimental verification. Once a model has been accepted as truth, the perceived need for further research or theory is impeded or stopped and the model becomes accepted truth. This can be disastrous if the model is then shown to be erroneous because there are no alternatives to take its place. Integrative model building provides much needed directions for both basic and clinical research but must not be taken at face value without verification and experimental testing.

CHALLENGES IN ACCEPTING CLINICAL EXPERIENCE

The osteopathic profession must continually examine its theories and subject its explanations to close scrutiny. The vast body of clinical evidence demonstrates that the precepts of the osteopathic profession are sound; often the profession embraces explanations that are not solidly research-based. The result is theory taken for fact; further exploration of alternative theory or factual basis is stymied.

Research on Manipulation

As one of the key elements of osteopathic care, manipulative treatment should be the subject of increasing amounts of research in the profession. In research aimed at investigating the usefulness of manipulative treatment, there is much confusion about proper research methodology. The researcher approaching osteopathic manipulation as an independent variable must decide if a technique is to be evaluated, if OMT is to be tested, or if osteopathic health care is to be the subject of the study so that the appropriate research design can be employed.

MANIPULATIVE TECHNIQUES

The most carefully performed study of manipulative technique is the Irvine study, performed by Buerger and colleagues at the

School of Medicine at the University of California, Irvine, in the late 1970s and early 1980s.[5–6] They wished to determine the effects of a single lateral recumbent roll (high-velocity, low-amplitude thrust) on low back pain. The study was elegantly designed and executed, with a result that showed an immediate effect of the lateral recumbent roll on certain measured variables; simply positioning the patient for a lateral recumbent roll and omitting the thrust did not provide the same changes. After a few weeks, however, no differences between the experimental and control groups remained, probably the result of the nature of the presenting complaint, which has a natural history of relief in a few weeks. Nonetheless, an immediate effect of the thrust was seen. The point missed by many readers was that the investigation was not of OMT but of a treatment technique.

THE IRVINE STUDY COMPARED WITH CLINICAL TRIALS OF MEDICAL INTERVENTIONS

In many ways, the Irvine study was similar to drug studies. In the typical drug trial, the specific effects of a certain chemical compound on the course of a specific set of symptoms are studied. The design of the study controls for any other factors that might cause a change in the outcome. This is a legitimate model for the study of a specific technique within manipulative treatment. If the intent of the study is to determine the effect of a specific and repeatable manipulation, the research design should emulate the design of a drug trial, including attempts to blind the patient to whether the technique was delivered. Such studies are useful in instances where there may be reason to suspect that a specific manipulative technique would change a particular condition. Great care must be taken to control for:

The actual presenting complaint
Whether the patient has knowledge of manipulation
The actual delivery of the technique to make certain that it is
    given in the same way to each patient

Such studies can be useful as long as it is recognized that the study's purpose is to evaluate the effect of a specific, single, or small group of physical manipulations on a specific condition.

MANIPULATIVE TREATMENT DESIGNS

This research design is used to study the effects of OMT on one or more measurable patient parameters. The research design and the goals are somewhat different from those used in technique designs. Korr[7] has elegantly reviewed these differences. Osteopathic theory and practice holds that the full treatment of an individual by an osteopathic physician entails an interaction between the physician and the patient that is not static but dynamic, changing from treatment to treatment and instant to instant as the treatment progresses. The physician responds to the dynamic changes in the patient's function; the patient responds to the attitudes and touch of the physician. The treatment is not a prearranged set of movements and thrusts but an ongoing stimulus–response synergism between

the physician and patient, with the patient's response guiding the actions of the physician.

In this case, the manipulation cannot be predetermined or prescribed by the research protocol but must go with the flow in response to the reactions of both participants. The manipulative treatment is properly a black box. The physician–patient interaction determines what manipulative treatment is performed. The physician is free to do what is deemed best for the interaction. Because one of the basic axioms of osteopathy is that each person responds differently to stress and treatment, this freedom of interaction cannot be removed from the physician without reducing the research to an investigation of the technique. To investigate manipulative treatment rather than technique, manipulative treatment must be used.

TECHNIQUE VERSUS MANIPULATIVE TREATMENT

Once the difference between the two basic types of research on manipulation is realized, many of the other problems associated with investigating manipulation can be much more easily resolved. Both types of research are valuable and valid. Research on techniques gives information on specific techniques; research on treatment gives information on what the osteopathic physician does in practice. Both are necessary and essential for the future of the profession. Their differences must be recognized and appreciated for appropriate studies to be designed.

SUBTYPES OF MANIPULATIVE TREATMENT DESIGNS

Within the general design of research on manipulative treatment, there can be several subtypes. One aims at the effect of manipulative treatment in general on some aspect of a disease or on body function. This could be called the nonspecific design. It is done to improve body function without specific somatic dysfunction in patients with some clinical presenting complaint. The treating physician provides a general manipulative treatment without specifying areas of somatic dysfunction or specific areas to be addressed. By contrast, in specific treatment designs, the physician applies manipulative treatment to specific somatic dysfunction as defined by palpatory diagnosis and documented with signs such as asymmetric motion, tissue texture changes, and so forth. This type of treatment is designed to restore function or ameliorate functional difficulties and may or may not be related to actual presenting complaints (the patient may not be aware of some somatic dysfunctions). In each of these study types, appropriate data on what is done must be collected and specific measures of outcome must be made.

EFFECTIVENESS STUDY

A third type of study incorporates either of the first two: the effectiveness study, in which manipulative treatment is given to alleviate a specific presenting complaint. The patient is selected for a particular complaint, such as low back pain; the treating physician gives appropriate manipulative treatment. The effect of the treatment on the complaint (e.g., low back pain) is measured. This study type may or may not require the delineation of somatic dysfunction during treatment. Efficacy studies are the most usual in the literature because the measure of results is the most straightforward.

FUNCTIONAL OUTCOMES OF MANIPULATIVE TREATMENT

In the fourth design subtype, the functional outcome design, the general effect of manipulative treatment on general physiologic function is assessed. In the philosophy of the osteopathic profession, the origin of disease is believed to be some loss of normal function in the body which then allows for the development of clinical symptoms. This type of study is accomplished on clinically disease-free subjects with somatic dysfunction who are addressed with specific treatment. Measures of outcome are such things as:

Immune system function
Tolerance to stress
General activities of daily living assessments (in older subjects)
Other measures of normal function that assess general health and function

Presumably, such studies would find increases in the functional ability or capacity of treated subjects.

Total Osteopathic Care

Another general study design takes into account the total care given by the osteopathic physician; it is not limited to manipulative treatment. This study type assesses the health status of patients given care by osteopathic physicians and presumably, but not necessarily, includes manipulative treatment over the course of care. Such studies are longitudinal or cross-sectional in nature and include as data such things as disease episodes and measures of total body function and activities of daily living. If the osteopathic philosophy of health is taken seriously by a physician, there is a heavy component of preventive care that includes periodic manipulative treatment to correct somatic dysfunction as it occurs and that should prevent a least some of the acute disease episodes seen in nonmanipulated subjects. Such a study is expensive and long-term and may be approached in various ways. These approaches include such procedures as meta-analysis and research designs evolving in the study of organization to determine which factors lead to outstanding results in leadership and management.[9] Research of this type could show whether the application of osteopathic principles to health care are differentiated from disease care. Practitioners applying total osteopathic care to their patients would be carefully selected. Obviously, there would be many potentially confounding factors that would have to be analyzed. Interesting results, such as cost–benefit ratios, quality of life issues, and others, could be addressed. Other study types such as epidemiologic studies are discussed in other chapters in this text.

Other Designs

The research designs reviewed above include mainly those that use planned comparisons between experimental and control groups, or long-term determinations of health status that are then compared with the general population. Another group of study types should receive careful attention when the effects of manipulative techniques or treatment are studied. These designs are single subject designs; they essentially use the same subject as both the control and experimental group. Keating et al.[9] have summarized this type of design in some detail.

The single subject study usually involves following a patient for a period of time to determine the baseline symptoms and whether they are fairly stable or changing in some fairly predictable fashion. After some period of baseline measurement, treatment is introduced and the measurements continued. The measured variables can be compared before and after treatment to see if the treatment had an effect. The baseline measurement period will vary among several subjects, allowing the treatment to be introduced at different times, assuring that there was no peculiar effect of time on treatment intervention. This is known as the variable baseline study design. In a variation of this design, one group of subjects would receive the treatment immediately while another group would have no treatment for a time, then the treatment would be discontinued for the first group and introduced in the second.

Such crossover and variable baseline studies are not especially effective if the measurements and symptoms are not somewhat stable for a period of time that can be used as the control condition. In addition, there is some problem with establishing whether the manipulative intervention actually did cause any change in the symptoms being measured. However, this type of design allows the use of treatment for every subject in the study, whereas the control group does not receive treatment in traditional experimental and control group studies.

RESEARCH DESIGNS TO FIT PURPOSE OF RESEARCH

An understanding of the type of research being undertaken is important in the design, record keeping, and analysis of the study. By carefully thinking through the various aspects of any project and determining the correct study type to be applied, the investigator can better plan the conduct of the study and be more confident of the outcomes and their acceptance. Other issues must also be addressed in planning any research project.

INTERPRETING MANIPULATIVE STUDIES

Shams and Placebos

One of the most interesting issues facing the design of research in osteopathic manipulative treatment or techniques is whether to use placebos or sham procedures and, if so, what to use. The use of placebos is well-known and documented in clinical research literature, as is the use of sham controls.[10] The placebo treatment was initially developed for research on the effectiveness of drugs; the treatment entails the delivery of a substance that is, from the standpoint of the patient and physician, indistinguishable from the drug being tested. Such a placebo is often in the form of a capsule that is the same color, size, and weight as the capsule containing the drug, but the placebo contains only inert substances. The patient is given either the drug-containing capsule or the inert-substance capsule, not knowing which is being given. The sham procedure is given to the patient but has been shown or is thought to have no effect on the symptoms being treated. With both placebos and shams, the intent is to keep the patient from knowing whether he or she is receiving an active or inactive drug or procedure. This should keep the expectations of both the experimental and control groups equal and thus allow the effect of the active ingredient or procedure to be seen, independent of patient expectations.

Issues in Clinical Trial Designs

In the case of drug tests or for specific procedures, such as ultrasound, placebo and sham controls are entirely appropriate. The intent of such studies is to ascertain the effect of the active ingredient alone. They look at the effect of either a certain molecule (or, more precisely, many millions of molecules) on the natural course of something like a bacterial invasion of the body, or of a particular procedure (such as ultrasound) on the restoration of muscle function. The patient's expectations and conscious processes are not at issue. The use of placebo or sham procedures as control groups against which the drug or procedure groups can be compared gives the researcher a measure of the effectiveness of the drug or technique alone.

CONTROLS IN CLINICAL TRIALS

In the design of manipulative technique research, it seems entirely appropriate to use sham treatment control groups. Here, the rationale is to test the effectiveness of a certain specific technique, which is administered in the same way to each patient for presumably the same symptom or symptoms. The treating physician has no leeway in how the maneuver is accomplished, and the patients are screened closely so that the symptoms are much the same from patient to patient.

This was the approach used in the Irvine study.[5-6] Low back pain patients were carefully screened to ensure that only a certain type of low back pain patient was admitted to the study and that the patients had not previously experienced manipulative treatment. The only manipulation was a lateral recumbent roll, with both groups receiving the positioning but only the experimental group receiving the final thrust. The two groups were identical following the study in their reports of whether they thought manipulation had been done. The active ingredient in this study was the thrust. The sham was positioning. The researchers had reason to believe that the thrust would be beneficial over and above the positioning, which they postulated to have no effect. That may be an erroneous assumption, since no group receiving either thrust or positioning

was used. However, an immediate effect of the thrust was seen on some of the measures being taken, when compared with the sham control.

BLINDING AND HAWTHORNE EFFECT

A second issue closely related to that of shams and placebos is that of blinding. Shams and placebos are given to equate patient expectations. The patients are thus blinded to the treatment. In a similar vein, it is often essential to blind the attending physician to the treatment the patient is receiving. In such studies, the physician is also unaware of whether the patient is being given an active or control treatment. This procedure is instituted to keep the physician from treating the groups differently. Studies in which both the patient and physician are unaware of the treatment condition are known as double-blind studies. Again, the intent is to equate the expectations and actions of the study participants. In research with manipulative techniques or manipulative treatment, the physician delivering the technique or treatment cannot be blind to the treatment. In research on specific techniques, the patient may be blind to whether the technique is or is not being delivered, at least under some circumstances.

Blinding Outcome Observer

Under circumstances in which blinding the physician or the patient is not possible, it is important that measures of treatment outcome be recorded by a blind observer. A blind observer is one who does not know whether the patient received treatment. In this way, the reporting of alterations in the patient's function or symptoms is not influenced by the expectations of the reporter. This is probably one of the most difficult requirements to meet in many office studies. In a small practice, there if often no one available to assess the results of treatment who does not have any knowledge of whether a treatment has been given. Unfortunately, the measurement of treatment results by an individual who knows the patient's treatment history is almost always a reason for being suspicious of the data. Even the best of researchers can introduce errors into the data if they know the patient's treatment. Expectations can have real influences not only on the patient's behavior but also on the observer's behavior.

Hawthorne Effect

Another influence on the outcome of experiments is called the Hawthorne effect, named after a study done at the Hawthorne Company of the Western Electric Company in the late 1920s and early 1930s.[11] In this study, investigators wanted to evaluate the effects of lighting intensity on productivity. As the study progressed, they found that no matter how they changed the lighting, productivity went up. Apparently, just the knowledge that they were in a study was sufficient to make the workers more active and feel less tired. The message here is that the fact of being in a study may make patients feel different than they would if they were under regular treatment. This, like the placebo effect, is another reason for the judicious use of control groups of the appropriate sort.

Validity and Reliability

The issues of validity and reliability of data are complex for studies of manipulative treatment. In experimental design, validity is either internal or external. Internal validity refers to the extent to which any changes in the measures being taken (dependent variables) are the result of the influences of the experimental variables (independent variables). In other words, a study is internally valid if the differences observed between the experimental and control groups are the result of the variable given to the experimental group but not the control group. Internal validity is suspect if there are other, uncontrolled variables operating that the investigator does not recognize and that influence the results.

EXTERNAL VALIDITY OF MANUAL MEDICAL RESEARCH

In the case of the Irvine study, the independent variable was the high-velocity, low-amplitude thrust. It apparently was the cause of the differences between the two groups; the study was internally valid. External validity is how far results can be generalized from the study groups to the general population. If any experimenter wanted to have an externally valid study of the effects of a manipulative technique on asthma in the general population, the study group would be chosen not from a hospitalized population but from the whole group of people with asthma. If the asthma study patients were all hospitalized, the effects of a manipulative technique may be different than if the technique were performed on patients with a less severe form of the disease. The study would not be externally valid because it would not be generalizable to the whole population of asthma sufferers. Of course, if the intent of the study were to study the effects of manipulative interventions on asthma in hospitalized patients, it would be externally valid. Many things can affect validity, including[12]:

Lack of proper control procedures
Improper selection of patients
Simple length of time the patient is in the study (symptoms may change over time even without treatment)
Other factors

RELIABILITY OF DATA

Reliability is the concept that the measurements taken in a study are repeatable. The more carefully the measures of a study are taken, the more reliable it is likely to be because the measures can be accurately repeated. However, a study with good reliability may not have good validity because the measures may not be generalizable or may not be measuring the results of the experimental procedure.

IMPROVING RELIABILITY WITH EXPERIENCED CLINICIAN-RESEARCHERS

Studies of manipulative techniques or manipulative treatment require delivery by a skilled physician who can enter fully into the interaction with the patient. Although this requirement is not so great when testing the effects of a technique, the technique must be given in a skilled manner and in a way consistent with others using the technique. The use of such skilled physicians in any study increases the reliability of the study (because it decreases the variability of the data), while the use of several such physicians in any one study may also increase our confidence that the results are generalizable to other physician–patient interactions. The use of more than one manipulator also provides an opportunity to test for differences between manipulators in producing the outcomes being measured. External validity of the results of studies of manipulation (techniques and treatment) can be increased by making sure that the characteristics of the patients studied are known, so that it is possible to make statements about who would benefit from the treatment. Internal validity of technique studies is increased by using sham controls and making sure that the subjects are treated equally and selected carefully. In studies of manipulative treatment, the use of untreated controls or the provision of standard medical therapy as a control increases internal validity, while the use of inappropriate controls decreases that validity. In either study type, the use of blind observers to measure the results is an absolute necessity for internal validity of the data.

How to Evaluate Manipulative Treatment

VALID AND RELIABLE RESEARCH STUDIES

When one wishes to evaluate the effectiveness of a specific manipulative technique, the use of an appropriate sham control and a blind evaluator seem to be the minimal control conditions. The evaluation of OMT presents another set of considerations. Korr[12] has set out many of these considerations.

INFLUENCE OF TOTAL BODY RESPONSE

At the heart of osteopathic philosophy is the premise that treatment should be aimed at normalization of function by removing the barriers to the body's ability to normalize its function. Once these barriers are removed, the body can regain its optimal function and return to or maintain health. To think that this is purely a physiologic function and has nothing to do with conscious processes or the mind (i.e., the patient's expectations, desires, beliefs, and will) is to return to a belief in mind–body dualism such that the mind has nothing to do with physiologic function, and vice versa. It is to deny the most vital part of the whole equation of health and disease, the patients themselves. In addition, the treating physician is a part of the equation. Both the skill and the manner of the treating physician affect the results of the treatment, because both the patient's tactile and mental perceptions of the physician influence how the patient responds to the treatment. Indeed, Gribbin[13] has argued that many patients could effectively be treated by placebos alone, that the effect of the knowledge of treatment is a powerful factor in treatment outcome.

PLANNING AND EVALUATING PLACEBO EFFECT

In OMT, the treatment is an interaction between patient and physician, each responding to the other throughout the treatment. The osteopathic physician relies on the very effect that is labeled placebo or expectation in the testing of a drug to help with the alteration he or she is attempting to produce, that of normalized function. The patient's expectation is an important and vital factor in OMT; it must not be cast off as some spurious side effect. It is also a real and unusually safe therapeutic tool. There are few deleterious side effects to positive expectations. Expectations can influence such far-flung body systems as the immune system.[14]

In addition, the use of a sham treatment group in which the patient is exposed to a treatment considered ineffective presents another real problem for the evaluation of OMT (again, as contrasted to the evaluation of a particular technique). It is assumed that in the sham control group, the treatment of a body area distant from a particular somatic dysfunction does not influence the resolution of a diagnosed dysfunction being treated in the experimental group. Much data available shows that the simple act of touching and moving an individual produces real changes in function and response. The act of manipulative treatment involves touching and moving the patient as an integral part of the process. To compare a manipulation group with some sham group that has also received touch and movement leads to an underestimation of the effects of manipulative treatment, unless it can be shown that the sham treatment had no effect on total mind and body function of the patient.

COMPARISON STUDIES EVALUATE EFFECTIVENESS

Initial attempts to evaluate the true effectiveness of manipulative treatment on either the progression of symptoms or on total body function requires the use of a control group that either receives some standard medical therapy not requiring manipulation or the use of a totally untreated control group that would simply undergo the natural course of the malfunction being studied. This could be done by simply requiring control subjects to come to the physician's office for diagnostic measurements. To try to factor out the mental process involved in manipulative treatment is to deny much of the actual treatment. It is akin to studying the effectiveness of a drug by giving only a partial dose.

To study the effects of osteopathic manipulation, one must study osteopathic manipulation as it is given, as an interaction between physician and patient, with all components intact and functioning. To factor out any particular component, such as the so-called hands-on effect, and call it an artifact is to underestimate the effect of manipulative treatment and deny that

the natural power of the person's cognitive and recuperative processes are factors in the effects of OMT.

ASSOCIATION OR CAUSAL EFFECTS

Once the total effects of manipulative treatment have been established, studies can be designed to tease apart the various components of the treatment, including the effects of touching the patient and so forth. However, to try to do such studies in the absence of demonstrated effects is both inefficient and impractical. The study of OMT must flow from the philosophy of osteopathy and not from some other philosophic orientation.

CONTROL SUBJECTS FOR MANUAL MEDICAL RESEARCH

The investigator designing studies of OMT must determine which type of research is to be done so that the appropriate contrast control can be used. Using the incorrect control results in dramatic underestimation of the effect of manipulative treatment, although the same control may well be the appropriate one for evaluation of a manipulative technique. The decision rests on whether the total response of the individual to the interaction between patient and physician is being evaluated or whether manipulative technique is being studied as a procedure.

Selecting Appropriate Measures

It is often difficult to determine the best measures to determine if the manipulation had an effect. These measures are known as the dependent variables because their values are supposedly dependent on the experimental treatment. In studies of the efficacy of a manipulative technique or a manipulative treatment on the outcome of a specific disease process, the measures are presumably some aspect of the disease process or of the natural course of the symptoms. In assessing the contributions of manipulative treatment to resolution of somatic dysfunction or to the maintenance of health, the task of defining sensitive dependent variables becomes more difficult. Some dependent measures include:

Measures of immune system function
Studies of the activities of daily living
Episodes of loss of health (for long-term studies)
Other measures of body function, including reports of feelings of well-being and comfort

Whatever the dependent variable or variables, the measures of manipulative treatment results should include an evaluation of whether the treating physician determined that the treatment given actually did what it was designed to do. Sometimes the manipulation fails to accomplish the desired immediate outcome in restoring range of motion or proper muscle relaxation. These facts must be recorded and used in analysis of the outcome of the treatment so that unsuccessful treatments can be looked at separately from those judged to achieve the desired endpoints. This will help reduce the variability in the data collected.

FUNDING AND ENVIRONMENT FOR RESEARCH

In setting up any research program or project, the investigator must take into account the research environment.

Are there sufficient patients to assure adequate numbers for the study?

Is there knowledgeable support personnel with time to do the study?

What provisions are made for data recording and analysis?

These are not trivial matters, and they must be addressed prior to the initiation of a project. Included are the issues of funding for the research and whether there is an appropriate Institutional Review Board to oversee the design and execution of the study, if one is required. The official bodies of the American Osteopathic Association can help in the areas pertaining to administrative issues and funding. Most clinical research studies that require more than routine record keeping and tabulation are expensive. The profession must support clinical research efforts, as well as the efforts of basic scientists who are willing to apply their data to the osteopathic concepts and philosophy. In addition, the educational institutions of the profession must take some responsibility to promote such research in their clinics and hospitals. Members of the profession in their practices can participate in some types of research if the central organization is provided to receive and tabulate data. These tasks are daunting but manageable. They are also important for the long-term health of the profession.

Models for Future Research

Many avenues exist for research into the effects of osteopathic manipulation and osteopathic health care. From the application of basic science data to the concepts of the profession and theory building through long-term studies of the health status of individuals given osteopathic care, the possible types of research are many and varied. As has been pointed out in an earlier chapter, the epidemiology of somatic dysfunction is an important area for study. Cost–benefit analyses of the application of preventive manipulative treatment are especially appealing to those supporting the cost of health care, as is the evaluation of manipulative treatment used in chronic pain problems and disability claims. The possibilities are vast, but the techniques for each type of study must be evaluated carefully to ensure that the proper type of design is used and that the use of manipulative technique is not confused with the use of OMT. It must be remembered that the osteopathic philosophy includes the response of the individual in the total measure of effectiveness of treatment and that manipulative treatment includes all manipulative procedures that the treating physician deems necessary in the restoration of function. With these concepts in mind, research designs will be found to study the many and varied aspects of OMT and the osteopathic philosophy in relation to health care.

Academic Role for Osteopathic Researchers

Another important aspect of research designs for the future is the aspect of where this research should be carried out. The osteopathic profession must increase dramatically its contact with basic science research centers and scientists outside the profession. It must also cultivate a cadre of basic scientists at the profession's educational institutions, both schools and hospitals, who are intimately familiar with osteopathic theory and practice and who can perform basic research important to the profession and assist in designing and carrying out clinical studies. Training programs for DO-PhD researchers must be strongly encouraged.

Research Outside of Osteopathic Institutions

Recent developments in clinical research stimulated by the AIDS epidemic are useful models for the osteopathic profession to follow. In the past, there has been little clinical research performed outside major research centers. In response to increasing pressure for clinical data on the AIDS epidemic, there has been an increasing use of smaller neighborhood clinics and solo practitioners to collect data on the disease (M. Goldstein, personal communication, 1992). It is becoming evident that there is an important role for the practicing physician in collecting data for clinical studies. Studies using this important resource for data collection must be designed to take advantage of the practice of medicine in the office setting so as not to disrupt the daily flow of the practice. However, it is here that the real practice of osteopathic medicine takes place. It is here that there is the best chance to ask such questions as:

What is the incidence of somatic dysfunction?

What is its natural course?

What is the effectiveness of manipulative treatment on it?

The questions of real life in osteopathic medicine can be approached at the office level. Such research must be encouraged. That such research can be accomplished is seen in the recent report from the office of Dr. Viola Frymann[15] on the effects of osteopathic care on neurologic development in children. Other office-based studies that include many practitioners would provide much important data on the basis for and efficacy of osteopathic care.

FUTURE OF OSTEOPATHIC RESEARCH

Forces Affecting Practice of Medicine

The introduction to this chapter pointed out that there are many unknown and unpredictable forces that will challenge and shape the profession in the future. One such force is the need for research in the profession. It is only with a strong and continuing commitment to research that the osteopathic profession will continue to thrive and to achieve its potential to alter medical thought and practice, which was the prime motivation of the profession's founder, A.T. Still. How can research be encouraged in the profession to achieve these ends? What are the most important questions emerging from our changing understanding of human health and disease and from osteopathic clinical experience?

Role of Osteopathic Philosophy in Future Research

Basic to the philosophy and theory of osteopathy is the idea that the body is an integrated functional unit. This unit includes the physical, cognitive, and spiritual aspects of the individual. How these elements interact within the total individual and with the external environment determine the long-term health status of the person. From the beginning of osteopathy, osteopathic practitioners have held that there was some entity that would adversely affect a person's health status. This entity, which could be palpated and specifically treated with manipulation, was first known as the osteopathic lesion and then, more recently, as the somatic dysfunction. In the 1940s and 1950s, Denslow and Korr and their colleagues postulated that a major component of the osteopathic lesion was the facilitated segment.[16] The facilitated segment concept arose from the data gathered by these researchers, which showed that in most individuals, there was no uniform excitability throughout the spinal cord. The areas of hyperexcitability were shown to react more strongly to afferent input, exposing innervated structures, both visceral and somatic, to increased activation. This break in body unity was postulated to lead over time to early breakdown and malfunction; in short, to disease. Clinical disease was, then, a consequence of earlier body dysfunction. Indeed, this was a data-based theory that truly embodied one of Still's basic insights; that clinical disease was simply a manifestation of body malfunction rather than a primary event.

DETERIORATION OF NORMAL FUNCTION AS CENTRAL CONCEPT

That clinical disease is a result of earlier deterioration of normal function is central to osteopathic philosophy. It is perhaps best manifest in the treatment of somatic dysfunction, an entity not recognized by most medical practitioners as a clinical entity at all. Why treat it? Because it is the beginning of disease, the start of body breakdown. To treat the root of disease would seem to be more cost-effective than waiting until the final breakdown of clinical disease has occurred before beginning treatment.

OTHER ROLES FOR SOMATIC DYSFUNCTION

Given this view, the research of the profession should be aimed at elucidating the relationships between disturbances of body function and health status:

How does the presence of somatic dysfunction predict the health status of the individual?

What is the incidence of serious somatic dysfunction and its natural history?

What are the predictors of somatic dysfunction?

What environmental and lifestyle attributes seem to contribute to the incidence of somatic dysfunction?

How does lifestyle contribute to the incidence of somatic dysfunction in old age?

Flowing from these questions are even larger questions that should be at the forefront of osteopathic thinking:

What is the contribution of early lifestyle or events that happen to a the person to the health status of the individual in old age?

What regime of manipulative treatment in early life will contribute most to deterring the deterioration of health usually associated with old age?

More simply, why are some very old people vital and healthy and others completely overtaken by deterioration and disease?

What role do long-lasting somatic dysfunctions play in the presence or absence of vitality in old age?

These questions are complex and not easily answered. The critical point is that the research of the profession should take as its starting point body unity and that the start of disease is the deterioration of that functional unity, not a bacterial or viral invasion.

INTEGRATION AND SELF-REGULATION IN HEALTH

These questions suggest several important areas of research for the osteopathic profession. In the basic sciences, increasing attention must be paid to understanding the integration of body systems and what can cause the fine-tuned integration of body function to deteriorate. The capacity of the body to self-regulate (homeostasis) and the limits of that capacity in both the short-term and long-term must be better understood. Research aimed at elucidating the fine control and adaptation of body function would be especially useful. Integration of basic science data with data from studies of cognitive function gives a greater understanding of the role of the physician in the health maintenance process. A greater understanding of the effects of afferent inputs and cognitive function on the immune system, and how manipulative treatment can affect this system, would be useful. The profession should encourage basic scientists toward an increased understanding of the basis of osteopathy. These researchers can then design their studies and interpret their data in light of this understanding.

HEALTH BENEFITS OF MANIPULATIVE TREATMENT

Within the clinical research areas there must be studies of the efficacy of manipulative techniques and manipulative treatment. Measurements of the effects of manipulation on specific disease entities need to be carried out as demonstrations that manipulation can be used to great effect in treating specific disease processes. To rely on such demonstration studies to show the most significant benefits of manipulation would, however, be unwise. The most beneficial and lasting effects of manipulation and, indeed, of osteopathic care should be searched for in the effects on total functional capacity of individuals and in their long-term health status. The current health care system is preoccupied with the treatment of disease, especially in the chronic degenerations of old age. It is by no means clear that the chronic diseases commonly associated with old age are inevitable. What are the enabling or protective roles of early and continued normal body function in the aging process? Osteopathy is ideally suited by its philosophy and clinical experience to look at the effects of early disruptions of body unity on the deteriorations of old age. This is a golden opportunity for osteopathic research.

TOTAL NATURE OF SOMATIC DYSFUNCTION

Clinical research should continue to look at the effects of manipulation on specific disease processes. Such studies can be effectiveness studies such as the use of manipulative treatment in low back and chronic pain syndromes. These studies could have fairly quick and valuable outcomes for the profession. Other less specific studies, such as the effects of manipulation on sympathetic tone, vasomotor reactivity, and muscle spasticity, contribute to an understanding of the more general effects of manipulation on body function. Studies of the effects of somatic dysfunction, its etiology, prevalence, and contributions to the long-term health of the individual form a solid base for a greater understanding of the fundamental dynamics of health and disease. Investigation of the effects of manipulation on somatic dysfunction and of osteopathic care on old age health status is probably the most important area of study to which the profession can aspire.

CONCLUSION

By following closely the basic philosophy of osteopathy and the insights from its years of clinical experience, the research efforts of the profession can truly add to the most beneficial aspects of health care—that to which osteopathy is fundamentally dedicated—the maintenance of health and optimal function of the total person throughout life.

REFERENCES

1. Korr IM. Proprioceptors and somatic dysfunction. *JAOA*. 1975; 74:638–650.
2. Van Buskirk RL. Nociceptive reflexes and the somatic dysfunction: a model. *JAOA*. 1990;90(9):792–809.
3. Denslow JS, Korr IM, Kremms AD. Quantitative studies of chronic facilitation in human motoneuron pools. *Am J Physiol*. 1947; 150:229–238.
4. Korr IM. The neural basis of the osteopathic lesion. *JAOA*. 1847; 47:191–198.
5. Buerger AA. A controlled trial of rotational manipulation in low back pain. *Man Med*. 1980;2:17–26.
6. Hoehler FK, Tobis JS, Buerger AA. Spinal manipulation for low back pain. *JAMA*. 1981;245(18):1835–1838.
7. Korr IM. Osteopathic medicine: the profession's role in society. *JAOA*. 1990;90(9):824–837.
8. Bateman TS, Ferris GR, eds. *Methods and Analysis in Organizational Research*. Reston, Va: Reston Publishing Co; 1984.
9. Keating JC, Seveille J, Meeker WC, et al. Intrasubject experimental designs in osteopathic medicine: applications in clinical practice. *JAOA*. 1985;85(3):192–203.
10. Pocock SJ. *Clinical Trials: A Practical Approach*. Somerset, NJ: John Wiley & Sons; 1983.
11. Payton OD. *Research: The Validation of Clinical Practice*. Philadelphia, Penn: FA Davis Co; 1979:128–129.
12. Korr IM. Osteopathic research: the needed paradigm shift. *JAOA*. 1991;91(2):156–171.
13. Gribbon M. Placebos: the cheapest medicine in the world. *New Science*. 1981;89:64–65.
14. Kiecolt-Glasser JK, Glaser R. Stress and immune function. In: Ader R, ed. *Psychoimmunology*. 2nd ed. San Diego, Calif: Academic Press; 1991.
15. Frymann VM, Carney RE, Springall P. Effect of osteopathic medical management on neurologic development in children. *JAOA*. 1992; 92(6):729–744.
16. Peterson B, ed. *The Collected Papers of Irvin M. Korr*. Indianapolis, Ind: American Academy of Osteopathy; 1979.

Glossary

INTRODUCTION

William A. Kuchera

The Glossary of Osteopathic Terminology was created by the Educational Council on Osteopathic Principles (ECOP). This committee was established in 1969 as an independent group and shortly after became a part of the American Association of Colleges of Osteopathic Medicine (AACOM). Two areas emerged for their prime consideration:

Lack of standardized osteopathic terminology
Lack of standardization of Osteopathic Principles and Practice (OPP)

ECOP spent the next fifteen years addressing these two issues. The first edition of a "Glossary of Osteopathic Terminology" was published In 1981. It has been updated many times since then.

The Core Curriculum Document, "Teaching Standards for Osteopathic Principles and Practice," was completed in 1989. This present AOA-sponsored osteopathic principles textbook, *Foundations for Osteopathic Medicine*, is the consensus by Colleges and Universities of Osteopathic Medicine, which have worked together through the years to standardize the OPP curriculum in osteopathic medical training.

The process of developing the glossary involved obtaining financial support from Colleges of Osteopathic Medicine to fund the Project on Osteopathic Principles. Robert Ward, D.O., was the Principal Investigator, and Sarah Sprafka, Ph.D., the Project Director. Criteria for inclusion and exclusion of words were developed:

Words to be included must have special significance to the osteopathic profession.
Words must be a part of our language or appear in osteopathic literature
Terms that were defined in medical dictionaries were excluded, unless they had a special significance to osteopathic physicians.

A large number of potential terms were assembled. ECOP members worked in small groups writing the definition or description of each term. The work of the small groups was then reviewed by the total group, and consensus was achieved on terms and definitions to be included and excluded.

The glossary has had a major impact on standardizing terminology used in the osteopathic profession. The National Board of Osteopathic Medical Examiners has approved the Glossary of Osteopathic Terminology for use in their examinations. Terms appearing in test items must be in conformity with the glossary. Since it is a published reference, if anyone wishes to use a different definition of a term, that person has the obligation to identify to the students that his or her use of a term is contrary to the glossary definition.

"Words should be employed as the means, not as the end; language is the instrument, conviction is the work" (Sir J. Reynolds).

Glossary of Osteopathic Terminology

Prepared by The Glossary Review Committee. Sponsored by The Educational Council on Osteopathic Principles of the AACOM

Revised September 30, 1995

The Glossary of Osteopathic Terminology and its revisions are a continuing function of the Educational Council on Osteopathic Principles, Chairman, John M. Jones 111, D.O. Forward any comments or suggestions to the Chairman of the Glossary Review Committee, William Kuchera, D.O., F.A.A.O., Kirksville College of Osteopathic Medicine, 800 W. Jefferson, Kirksville, MO 63501. The glossary first appeared in the JAOA 80:552-67 in April of 1981. It is now printed yearly in the AOA Yearbook and Directory of Osteopathic Physicians.

The most recent glossary review was performed by William Kuchera, D.O., F.A.A.O., Michael L. Kuchera, D.O., F.A.A.O., John M. Jones 111, D.O., Robert Kappler, D.O., F.A.A.O., Walter Ehrenfeuchter, D.O., F.A.A.O., John Glover, D.O., David Vick, D.O., F.A.A.O., Raymond Hruby, D.O., F.A.A.O., Guy DeFeo, D.O., Tom Shaver, D.O., Eileen DiGiovanna, D.O., F.A.A.O., John G. Hohner, D.O., David L. Eland, D.O., Donald D. Downing, D.O., F.A.A.O., Donald V. Hampton 11, D.O., and David Hyler-Both, D.O., Jane E. Carreiro, D.O., Ann Habenicht, D.O.

The purpose of this osteopathic glossary is to present important and often used words, terms and phrases of the osteopathic profession. It is not meant to replace a dictionary. The glossary offers the consensus of a large segment of the osteopathic profession and is to serve to standardize terminology.

We also expect this glossary to be useful to the student of osteopathic medicine and to be helpful to authors and other professionals in understanding and making proper use of osteo-pathic vocabulary.

Dictionary definitions are included from:
Dorland's Medical Dictionary, 28th edition, W.B. Saunders Company, Philadelphia, PA.1994.
Stedman's Medical Dictionary, 26th ed-ition, The William & Wilkins Company, Baltimore, MD,1995.

abbreviations: types of osteopathic manipulative treatment.
ART: articulatory treatment
BLT: balanced ligamentous tension treatment/ligamentous articular strain treatment
CR: cranial treatment/osteopathy in the cranial field/ cranial osteopathy
CS: counterstrain treatment
D: direct treatment
DIR: direct treatment
FPR: facilitated positional release treatment

HVLA: high velocity/low amplitude treatment
I: indirect treatment
IND: indirect treatment
LAS: ligamentous articular strain treatment/balanced ligamentous tension treatment
ME: muscle energy treatment
MFR: myofascial release treatment
OCF: osteopathy in the cranial field/cranial treatment
OMT: osteopathic manipulative treatment
ST: soft tissue treatment
VIS: visceral manipulative treatment

acceleration: the instantaneous change in rate of motion (also applies to deceleration).

accessory movements: movements used to potentiate, accentuate, or compensate for an impairment in a physiologic motion (e.g., the accessory activities in an asthmatic's breathing or compensatory movements needed to move a paralyzed limb).

accommodation: a self-reversing and non-persistent adaptation

active motion: see *motion: active motion*

acute somatic dysfunction: see *somatic dysfunction*

anatomical barrier: see *barrier (motion barrier).*

angle, lumbosacral: represents the angle of the lumbosacral junction as measured by the inclination of the superior surface of the first sacral vertebra to the horizontal (this is actually a sacral angle); usually measured from standing lateral x-ray films; also known as Ferguson's angle. (Fig. 1)

angle of Ferguson: see *angle, lumbosacral.*

anterior component: a positional descriptor used to identify the side of reference when rotation of a vertebra has occurred; in a condition of right rotation, the left side is the anterior component; usually refers to the less prominent transverse process; see also *posterior component.*

anterior iliac rotation: see *ilium, somatic dysfunctions of: anterior (forward) innominate (iliac) rotation.*

A.R.T.: see *T.A.R.T.*

articular pillar: refers to the columnar arrangement of the articular portions of the cervical vertebrae.

articulation: 1. the place of union or junction between two or more bones of the skeleton; 2. the

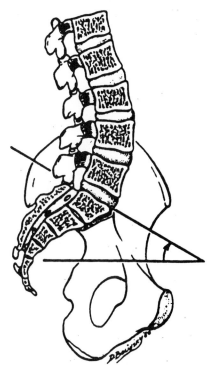

Figure I. Lumbosacral angle

active or passive progress of moving a joint through its permitted anatomic range of motion; see also *osteopathic manipulative treatment: articulatory treatment.*

articulatory pop: refers to a characteristic popping sound made by a joint.

articulatory technique: see *technique.* see also *osteopathic manipulative treatment: articulatory treatment.*

asymmetry: absence of symmetry of position or motion; dissimilarity in corresponding parts or organs on opposite sides of the body which are normally alike; of particular use when describing position or motion alteration resulting from somatic dysfunction.

axis: 1. an imaginary line about which motion occurs; 2. the second cervical vertebra; 3. one component of an axis system.

axis of rib motion: an imaginary line through the costotransverse and the costovertebral articulations of the rib.
anteroposterior rib axis: (Fig. 2); see *bucket handle rib motion definition;* see also (Fig. 3).

1127

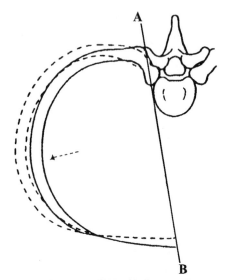

Figure 2. The functional anterior-posterior rib axis about which bucket handle motion of a rib occurs. The interrupted lines indicate the position of the rib in inhalation (see Fig. 3)
(Modified by *Gray's Anatomy*, 35th edition, p. 421 @ 1973 by Churchill Livingston)

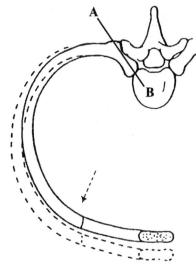

Figure 4. The functional transverse rib axis of a vertebrosternal rib about which pump handle rib motion occurs. The interrupted lines indicate the position of the rib in inhalation. (see also fig. 5)
(Modified by *Gray's Anatomy*, 35th edition, p. 421 @ 1973 by Churchill Livingston)

Anteroposterior Axes

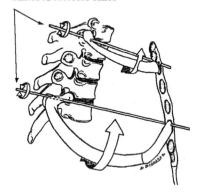

Figure 3. Bucket handle rib motion

"Transverse Axes"

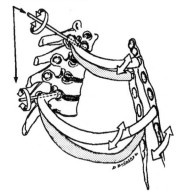

Figure 5. Pump handle rib motion

transverse rib axis: (Fig. 4); see *pump handle rib motion definition;* see also (Fig. 5).

axis of sacral motion: see *sacral motion, axis of.*

axoplasmic flow: see *axoplasmic transport.*

axoplasmic transport: the antegrade movement of substances from the nerve cell along the axon toward the terminals, and the retrograde movement from the terminals toward the nerve cell.

backward bending: opposite of forward bending; see *extension.*

balanced ligamentous tension technique: see *osteopathic manipulative treatment: ligamentous articular strain.*

barrier (motion barrier): the limit to motion; in defining barriers, the palpatory end-feel characteristics are useful.
anatomic barrier: the limit of motion imposed by anatomic structure; the limit of passive motion.
elastic barrier: the range between the physiologic and anatomic barrier of motion in which passive ligamentous stretching occurs before tissue disruption.
physiologic barrier: The limit of active motion; can be altered to increase range of active motion by warm-up activity.
restrictive barrier: a functional limit within the anatomic range of motion, which abnormally diminishes the normal physiologic range.
pathologic barrier: 1. restrictive barrier; 2. permanent restriction of joint motion associated with pathologic change of tissues (example: contracture, osteophytes).

batwing deformity: see *transitional segment: sacralization.*

bind: relative palpable resistance to motion of an articulation or tissue. Synonym: resistance; antonyms: ease, compliance, resilience.

biomechanics: mechanical principles applied to the study of biological functions; the application of mechanical laws to living structures; *the study and knowledge of biological function from an application of mechanical principles.*

bogginess: a tissue texture abnormality characterized principally by a palpable sense of sponginess in the tissue, interpreted as resulting from congestion due to increased fluid content.

bucket handle rib motion: movement of the ribs during respiration such that with inhalation the lateral aspect of the rib moves cephalad resulting in an increase of transverse diameter of the thorax; this type of rib motion is predominantly found in lower ribs (*Fig. 3*), increasing from the upper to the lower ribs; see *axis of rib motion;* see also *pump handle rib motion.*

caliper rib motion: rib motion of ribs 11 and 12 characterized by single joint motion; analogous to internal and external rotation.

caudad: toward the tail or inferiorly.

caught in inhalation: see *inhalation rib*

caught in exhalation: see *exhalation rib*

cephalad: toward the head.

cephalad pubic dysfunction: see *pubes, somatic dysfunctions of.*

cerebrospinal fluid, fluctuation of: a description of the hypothesized action of cerebrospinal fluid with regard to the craniosacral mechanism.

Chapman's reflex: a system of reflex points originally used by Frank Chapman, D.O. were described by Charles Owens, D.O. These reflexes present as predictable anterior and posterior fascial tissue texture abnormalities assumed to be reflections of visceral dysfunction or pathology (viscerosomatic reflexes). A given reflex is consistently associated with the same viscus; Chapman's reflexes are manifested by palpatory findings of plaque-like changes of stringiness of the involved tissues.

chronic somatic dysfunction: see *somatic dysfunction.*

circumduction: the active or passive circular movement of a limb; the rotary movement by which a structure or part is made to describe a cone, the apex of the cone being a fixed point (e.g., the circular movement of a ball and socket joint).

combined technique: see *osteopathic manipulative treatment: combined treatment.*

compensatory fascial patterns: see *fascial patterns.*

conditioned reflex: see *reflex.*

contraction: shortening and/or development of tension in muscle.
concentric contraction: contraction of muscle resulting in approximation of attachments.
eccentric contraction: lengthening of muscle during contraction due to an external force.
isolytic contraction: 1. contraction of a muscle against resistance while forcing the muscle to lengthen; 2. operator force greater than patient force.
isometric contraction: 1. change in the tension of a muscle without approximation of muscle origin and insertion; 2. operator force equal to patient force.
isotonic contraction: 1. approximation of the muscle origin and insertion without change in its tension; 2. operator force less than patient force.

contracture: a condition of fixed high resistance to passive stretch of a muscle, resulting from fibrosis of the tissues supporting the muscles or the joints, or from disorders of the muscle fibers.
Dupuytren's contracture: shortening, thickening and fibrosis of the palmar fascia, producing a flexion deformity of a finger (Dorland).

contractured muscle: as contrasted to contracted muscle; contracted muscle is regarded as the physiologic function of neuromuscular excitation-response, whereas contractured muscle is due to histologic change substituting non-contractile tissue for muscle tissue which prevents the muscle from reaching normal relaxed length.

coronal plane: see *plane.*

counternutation: posterior movement of the sacral base around a transverse axis in relation to the ilia (*Fig.* 8); see also *nutation.*

counterstrain technique: see *osteopathic manipulative treatment: counterstrain.*

cranial concept: see *primary respiratory mechanism.*

cranial rhythmic impulse: a palpable, rhythmic fluctuation believed to be synchronous with the primary respiratory mechanism. (Term coined by Drs. John and Rachel Woods.)

cranial technique: see *primary respiratory mechanism*; see also *osteopathy in the cranial field.*

craniosacral mechanism: a term used to refer to the anatomical connection between the occiput and the sacrum by the spinal dura mater, as used by William G. Sutherland, D.O.; it was not used by Dr. Sutherland in any other sense.

decompensation: a dysfunctional, persistent pattern, in some cases reversible, resulting when homeostatic mechanisms are partially or totally overwhelmed.

diagnostic palpation: see *palpatory diagnosis.*

diagonal axis: see *sacral motion, axis of: diagonal (oblique).*

direct method (technique): see *osteopathic manipulative treatment: direct treatment.*

drag: see *skin drag.*

ease: relative palpable freedom of motion of an articulation or tissue. synonyms: compliance, resilience; antonyms: bind, resistance.

easy normal: see *neutral.*

-ed: a suffix describing status, position, or condition (e.g., extended, flexed, rotated, restricted).

effleurage: stroking movement in massage used to move lymphatic fluids (Dorland).

elastic deformation: any recoverable deformation; see also *plastic deformation.*

elasticity: ability of a strained body or tissue to recover its shape after deformation; see *plasticity; viscosity.*

end feel: perceived quality of motion as an anatomic or physiologic restrictive barrier is approached.

enthesitis: traumatic disease occurring at the insertion of muscles where recurring concentration of muscle stress provokes inflammation with a strong tendency toward fibrosis and calcification (Stedman); inflammation of the muscular or tendinous attachment to bone (Dorland).

ERS: a descriptor of spinal somatic dysfunction used to denote a combination extended (E), rotated (R), and sidebent (S) vertebral position.

exaggeration technique: see *osteopathic manipulative treatment: exaggeration treatment.*

exhalation rib: 1. a somatic dysfunction usually characterized by a rib being held in a position of exhalation such that motion toward exhalation is more free and motion toward inhalation is restricted; synonyms: inhalation restriction of rib(s), exhalation strain, depressed rib; 2. an anterior tender point in strain-counterstrain.

extension: 1. accepted universal term for backward motion in a sagittal plane of the spine about a transverse axis; in a vertebral unit when the superior part moves backward (*Fig.* 6); 2. *in extremities,* it is the straightening of a curve or angle (biomechanics). 3. separation of the ends of a curve in a spinal region; see *extension, regional.*.
extension, craniosacral: motion occurring during the cranial rhythmic impulse, when the sacrum nutates and the sphenobasilar symphysis descends (*Fig.* 7); see *nutation.*

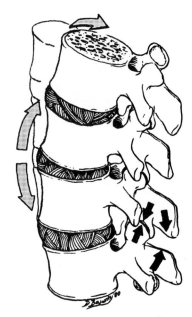

Figure 6. Extension

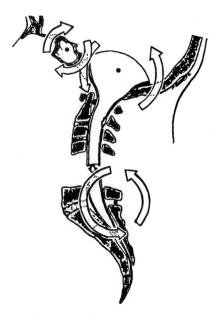

Figure 7. Craniosacral extension

extension, regional: historically, is the straightening of the sagittal plane in a spinal region; also called Fryette's regional extension; see *extension.* (*Fig.* 6)
extension, sacral: [fm] posterior movement of the base of the sacrum in relation to the ilia (*Fig.* 8); see also *flexion, sacral.*

extension lesion of the sacrum: see *sacrum, somatic dysfunctions of.*

extrinsic corrective forces: treatment forces, the sources of which are external to the patient; they may include operator effort, effect of gravity, mechanical tables, etc; see also *intrinsic corrective forces.*

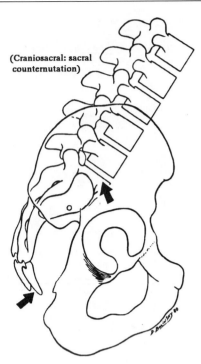

(Craniosacral: sacral counternutation)

Figure 8. Sacral extension

facet asymmetry: vertebral structure in which the orientation of the facets is not anatomically bilaterally comparable; see *facet symmetry; tropism, facet.*

facet symmetry: describes the structure of a vertebra in which the facets are anatomically bilaterally comparable; see *facet asymmetry; symmetry.*

facilitated segment: see *facilitation.*

facilitated segmental release technique: see *osteopathic manipulative treatment , facilitated positional release.*

facilitation: 1. the maintenance of a pool of neurons (e.g., premotor neurons, motoneurons or preganglionic sympathetic neurons in one or more segments of the spinal cord) in a state of partial or subthreshold excitation; in this state, less afferent stimulation is required to trigger the discharge of impulses; 2. a theory regarding the neurophysiological mechanisms underlying the neuronal activity associated with somatic dysfunction; 3. facilitation may be due to sustained increase in afferent input, aberrant patterns of afferent input, or changes within the affected neurons themselves or their chemical environment. Once established facilitation can be sustained by normal central nervous system (CNS) activity.

fascial patterns: systems for classifying and/or recording the preferred directions of fascial motion throughout the body in classifiable combinations of regional compensatory change. Major systems of fascial patterns include the observations of W. Neidner, D.O. and J. Gordon Zink, D.O.

compensatory pattern of Zink: fascial patterns which alternate at transitional regions of the body (occipitocervical, cervicothoracic or superior thoracic inlet, thoracolumbar, and lumbopelvic).

fascial release technique: see *osteopathic manipulative treatment: fascial release treatment.*

Ferguson's angle: see *angle, lumbosacral.*

flexion: 1. accepted universal term for forward motion in a sagittal plane of the spine about a transverse axis (*Fig. 9*); in a vertebral unit when the superior part moves forward; see *forward bending;* 2. *in the extremities,* is approximation of a curve or angle (biomechanics); 3. approximation of the ends of a curve in a spinal region; see *flexion, regional.*

flexion, craniosacral: motion occurring during the cranial rhythmic impulse, when the sacrum counternutates and the sphenobasilar symphysis ascends (*Fig. 10*); see *counternutation*

flexion, regional: historically, is the approximation of the ends of a curve in the sagittal plane of the spine; also called Fryette's regional flexion; see *flexion (Fig. 9).*

flexion, sacral: anterior movement of sacral base in relation to the ilia; see also *extension, sacral.* (*Fig. 11*)

flexion somatic dysfunction of the sacrum: see *sacrum, somatic dysfunctions of.*

forward bending: reciprocal of backward bending; see *flexion.*

FRS: a descriptor of spinal somatic dysfunction used to denote a combination flexed (F), rotated (R), and sidebent (S) vertebral position.

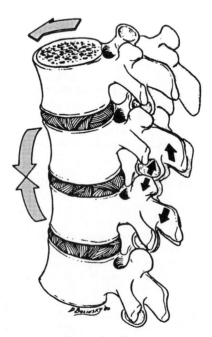

Figure 9. Flexion

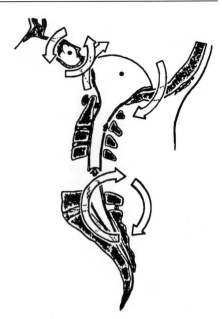

Figure 10. Craniosacral flexion

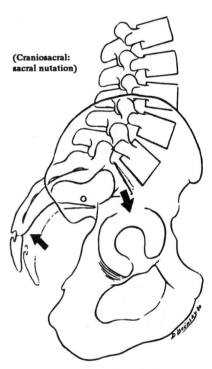

(Craniosacral: sacral nutation)

Figure 11. Sacral flexion

Fryette's laws or principles: see *physiologic motion of the spine.*

functional technique: see *osteopathic manipulative treatment: functional treatment.*

Galbraith treatment: see *mandibular drainage.*

gravitational line: viewing the patient from the side, an imaginary line in a coronal plane which, in the theoretical ideal posture, starts slightly anterior to the lateral malleolus, passes across the lateral condyle of the knee, the greater trochanter, through the lateral head of the humerus at the tip of the shoulder to the external auditory meatus; if this were a plane through the body, it would intersect the middle of the third lumbar vertebra and the anterior one third of the sacrum; it is used to evaluate the AP curves of the spine; see also *midmalleolar line. (Fig. 12)*

guiding: gentle movement by the operator following the path of least resistance in the movement of a body part within its normal range.

habituation: decreased response to repeated stimulation; hypothetically, a short-term (minutes or hours) decremental central nervous system (CNS) process; it interacts with the incremental CNS process of sensitization and yields a final behavioral outcome.

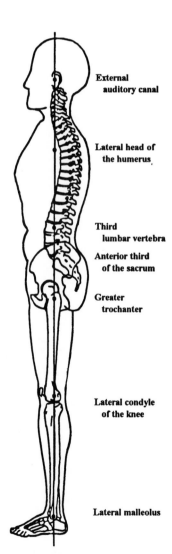

Gravitational Line

Figure 12. Gravitational line

External auditory canal

Lateral head of the humerus

Third lumbar vertebra

Anterior third of the sacrum

Greater trochanter

Lateral condyle of the knee

Lateral malleolus

health: adaptive and optimal attainment of physical, mental, emotional, spiritual, and environmental well-being.

hip bone: the os coxae; a large, irregular shaped bone which consists of three parts: ilium, ischium, and pubis which meet at the acetabulum, the cup-shaped cavity for the head of the femur; the pelvis is made up of the right and left hip bones, the sacrum, and the coccyx; see *pelvic bone.*

homeostasis: 1. maintenance of static or constant conditions in the internal environment; 2. the level of well-being of an individual maintained by internal physiologic harmony; it is the result of a relatively stable state or equilibrium among the interdependent body functions.

hypertonicity: a condition of excessive tone of the skeletal muscles; increased resistance of muscle to passive stretching.

iliosacral motion: motion of the ilia on an inferior transverse axis through the sacrum, as occurs in walking; considered to be primarily influenced by the attachments and movements of the pelvis, hips, and lower extremities.

ilium, somatic dysfunctions of:
anterior (forward) innominate (iliac) rotation: a somatic dysfunction in which the anterior superior iliac spine (ASIS) is anterior and inferior to the contralateral landmark; the ilium moves more freely in an anterior inferior direction, and is restricted in posterior superior motion.
inferior innominate (iliac) shear: a somatic dysfunction (qv) in which the anterior superior iliac spine (ASIS) and posterior superior iliac spines (PSIS) are inferior to the contralateral landmarks; the ilium (innominate pelvic bone) moves more freely in an inferior direction and is restricted in superior motion.
inflare: (of the ilium i.e. innominate) a somatic dysfunction of the ilium resulting in medial positioning of the anterior ileum (ASIS); the ilium moves more freely in a medial direction, restriction is in lateral direction.
outflare: (of the ilium, i.e. innominate) a somatic dysfunction of the ilium resulting in lateral positioning of the anterior ilium (ASIS); the ilium moves more freely in a lateral direction, restriction is in medial direction.
posterior (backward) innominate (iliac) rotation: a somatic dysfunction in which the anterior superior iliac spine (ASIS) are posterior and superior to the contralateral landmarks; the ilium moves more fully in a posterior superior direction and is restricted in an anterior inferior motion.
superior innominate (iliac) shear: a somatic dysfunction in which the anterior superior iliac spine (ASIS) and posterior superior iliac spines (PSIS) are superior to the contralateral landmarks; the ilium (innominate pelvic bone) moves more freely in a superior direction and is restricted in inferior motion.

inferior ilium: see *ilium, somatic dysfunctions of.*

inferior lateral angle (ILA) of the sacrum: the point on the lateral surface of the sacrum where it curves medially to the body of the fifth sacral vertebrae. (Gray's Anatomy)

inferior pubis: see *pubes, somatic dysfunctions of.*

inhalation rib: a somatic dysfunction usually characterized by a rib being held in a position of inhalation such that motion toward inhalation is more free and motion toward exhalation is restricted; synonyms: inhaled rib, anterior rib, inhalation strain, elevated rib, exhalation restriction.

inhibition, reflex: 1. in osteopathic usage, a term that describes the application of steady pressure to soft tissues to effect relaxation and normalize reflex activity, 2. effect on antagonist muscles due to reciprocal innervation when the agonist is stimulated; see *laws, Sherrington's; osteopathic manipulative treatment: inhibitory pressure treatment.*

innominate bone: now called hip bone, pelvic bone, or os coxae; The pelvis is made up of the two innominate bones, the sacrum and coccyx; see *hip bone;* see *ilium, somatic dysfunction of.*

intersegmental motion: designates relative motion taking place between two adjacent vertebral segments or within a vertebral unit; described as the upper vertebral segment moving on the lower.

intrinsic corrective forces: voluntary or involuntary forces from within the patient that assist in the manipulative treatment process. (For comparison, see *extrinsic corrective forces.*)

-ion: a suffix describing a process or movement (e.g., extension, flexion, rotation, restriction).

isokinetic exercise: exercise using a constant speed of movement of the body part.

isolytic contraction: see *contraction: isolytic contraction.*

isometric contraction: see *contraction: isometric contraction.*

isotonic contraction: see *contraction: isotonic contraction.*

junctional region: see *transitional region.*

kinesthesia: the sense by which muscular motion, weight, position, etc. are perceived.

kinesthetic: pertaining to kinesthesia.

kinetics: the body of knowledge that deals with the effects of forces that produce or modify body motion.

klapping: striking the skin with cupped palms to produce vibrations with the intention of loosening material in the lumen of hollow tubes or sacs within the body, particularly the lungs.

kneading: a soft tissue technique which utilizes an intermittent force applied perpendicular to the long axis of the muscle.

kyphoscoliosis: a spinal curve pattern combining kyphosis and scoliosis; see also *kyphosis; scoliosis.*

kyphosis: 1. the exaggerated (pathologic) AP curve of the thoracic spine with concavity anteriorly; 2. abnormally increased convexity in the curvature of the thoracic spine as viewed from the side (Dorland).

kyphotic: pertaining to or characterized by kyphosis.

lateral flexed: a term used to describe a position of a vertebral body; defined as the movement of a point on the anterior-superior aspect of the vertebral body about an anteroposterior axis in a coronal plane.

lateral flexion: also called lateroflexion; see *sidebending.*

lateral masses (of the atlas): the most bulky and solid parts of the atlas; they support of the weight of the head.

law, Head's: when a painful stimulus is applied to a body part of low sensitivity (e.g., viscus) that is in close central connection with a point of higher sensitivity (e.g., soma), the pain is felt at the point of higher sensitivity rather than at the point where the stimulus was applied.

law, Wolff's: every change in form and function of a bone, or in its function alone, is followed by certain definite changes in its internal architecture, and secondary alterations in its external conformations (Stedman's, 25th ed.); e.g., bone is laid down along lines of stress.

laws of motion, Fryette's (principles of motion): see *physiologic motion of the spine.*

laws, Sherrington's: 1. every posterior spinal nerve root supplies a specific region of the skin, although fibers from adjacent spinal segments may invade such a region; 2. when a muscle receives a nerve impulse to contract, its antagonist receives, simultaneously, an impulse to relax. (These are only two of Sherrington's contributions to neurophysiology; these are the ones most relevant to osteopathic principles.)

lesioned components: see *osteopathic lesion; somatic dysfunction.*

lesion (osteopathic): see *osteopathic lesion.*

ligamentous articular strain technique: see *osteopathic manipulative treatment: ligamentous articular strain.*

ligamentous strain: motion and/or positional asymmetry associated with elastic deformation of connective tissue (fascia, ligament, membrane); see *strain.*

line of gravity: see *gravitational line.*

localization: 1. in manipulative technique, the precise positioning of the patient and vector application of forces required to produce a desired result; 2. the reference of a sense impression to a particular locality in the body.

lordosis: 1. the anterior convexity in the curvature of the lumbar and cervical spine as viewed from the side; the term is used to refer to abnormally increased curvature (hollow back, saddle back, sway back) and to the normal curvature (normal lordosis). cf. kyphosis and scoliosis; (Dorland) 2. hollow back or saddle back; an abnormal extension deformity; anteroposterior curvature of the spine, generally lumbar with the convexity looking anteriorly (Stedman).

lordotic: pertaining to or characterized by lordosis.

lumbolumbar lordotic angle: an objective radiographic measurement of lumbar lordosis determined by measuring the angle between the superior surface of the second lumbar vertebra and the inferior surface of the fifth lumbar; best measured from a standing lateral x-ray film.

lumbosacral angle: see *angle, lumbosacral.*

lumbosacral lordotic angle: an objective radiographic measurement of lumbar lordosis determined by measuring the angle between the superior surface of the second lumbar vertebra and the superior surface of the first sacral segment; best measured from a standing lateral x-ray film.

lymph pumps: see *osteopathic manipulative treatment: pedal pump or thoracic pump.*

mandibular drainage: soft tissue manipulative technique using passively induced jaw motion to effect increased drainage of middle ear structures via the eustachian tube and lymphatics; see *Galbraith treatment.*

manipulation: therapeutic application of manual force; see also *technique.*

manual medicine: the use of the hands to diagnose and treat disorders of the somatic system.

massage: therapeutic friction, stroking, and kneading of the body; see also *osteopathic manipulative treatment: soft tissue treatment.*

mechanoreceptor: a receptor excited by mechanical pressures or distortions, as those responding to touch and muscular contractions. (Dorland).

middle transverse axis: see *sacral motion, axis of: middle (postural) transverse axis.*

mid-heel line: a vertical line used as a reference in standing anteroposterior (AP) x-rays and postural evaluation, passing equidistant between the heels.

mid-malleolar line: a vertical line passing through the lateral malleolus, used as a point of reference in standing lateral x-rays and postural evaluation.

motion: 1. a change of position (rotation, and/or translation) with respect to a fixed system; 2. an act or process of a body changing position in terms of direction, course and velocity.
active motion: movement produced voluntarily by the patient.
inherent motion: that spontaneous motion of every cell, organ, system, and their component units within the body.
passive motion: motion induced by the physician while the patient remains passive or relaxed.
physiologic motion: changes in position of body structures within the normal range; see *physiologic motion of the spine.*
translatory motion: motion of a body part along an axis; see *translation.*

motion barrier: see *barrier (motion barrier).*

muscle energy technique: see *osteopathic manipulative treatment: muscle energy treat-ment.*

myofascial release technique: see *osteopathic manipulative treatment: myofascial release treatment.*

myofascial technique: see *osteopathic manipulative treatment: myofascial treatment.*

myofascial trigger point: see *trigger point.*

Neidner, W: see *fascial patterns.*

neurotrophicity: see *neurotrophy.*

neurotrophy: the nutrition and maintenance of tissues as regulated by direct innervation.

neutral: 1. the range of sagittal plane spinal positioning in which the first principle of physiologic motion of the spine applies (Fig. 13); 2. the point of balance of an articular surface from which all the motions physiologic to that articulation may take place.

nociceptor: a peripheral nerve organ or mechanism for the appreciation and transmission of painful or injurious stimuli. (Stedman).

non-neutral: the range of sagittal plane spinal positioning in which the second principle of physiologic motion of the spine applies.

normalization: the therapeutic use of anatomic and physiologic mechanisms to facilitate the body's response toward homeostasis and improved health.

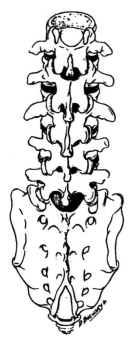

Figure 13. Neutral spinal position

NSR: a descriptor of spinal somatic dysfunction used to denote a combination neutral (N), sidebent (S), and rotated (R) vertebral position; similar descriptors may involve flexed (F) and extended (E) position; examples of combinations are FRS, ERS.

nutation: nodding forward; anterior movement of the sacral base around a transverse axis in relation to the ilia, occurring during sphenobasilar extension of the craniosacral mechanism (Fig. 7); see also *counternutation*.

oblique axes of the sacrum: see *sacral motion, axis of: diagonal (oblique)*.

OMM: 1. osteopathic manipulative medicine; 2. primary care specialty emphasizing in-depth application of osteopathic philosophy and special proficiency in osteopathic diagnosis and treatment.

OMT: see *osteopathic manipulative treatment*.

OP&P: osteopathic principles and practice.

-osis: word element [GR], disease; morbid state; abnormal increase.

osteopathic lesion (osteopathic lesion complex): term originally used to identify what is currently defined as somatic dysfunction; see *somatic dysfunction*.

osteopathic manipulative treatment (OMT): the therapeutic application of manually guided forces by an osteopathic physician to improve physiologic function and/or support homeostasis; this is accomplished by a variety of techniques:

active treatment: technique in which the person voluntarily performs a physician directed motion.

articulatory treatment (ART): a low velocity/moderate to high amplitude technique where a joint is carried through its full motion with the therapeutic goal of increased freedom range of movement.

balanced ligamentous tension (BLT/LAS): see *ligamentous articular strain*.

combined treatment: 1. a term coined by Paul Kimberly, D.O., to describe a technique where the initial movements are indirect; as the technique is completed the movements change to direct forces; 2. a manipulative sequence involving two or more different techniques (e.g. Spencer technique combined with muscle energy technique).

counterstrain (CS): a system of diagnosis and treatment developed by Lawrence Jones, D.O. that considers the dysfunction to be a continuing, inappropriate strain reflex, which is inhibited by applying a position of mild strain in the direction exactly opposite to that of the false strain reflex; this is accomplished by use of the specific point of tenderness related to this dysfunction followed by specific directed positioning to achieve the desired therapeutic response.

cranial treatment (CR): see *primary respiratory mechanism*; see also *osteopathy in the cranial field*.

Dalrymple treatment: see *pedal pump*.

direct treatment (D/DIR): any technique engaging the restrictive barrier and then carrying the dysfunctional component into the restrictive barrier.

exaggeration treatment: 1. operator movement of the dysfunctional component away from the restrictive barrier through and beyond the range of voluntary motion to a point of palpably increased tension; 2. an indirect procedure that involves carrying the dysfunction part away from the restrictive barrier, then applying a high velocity/low amplitude force in the same direction.

facilitated positional release (FPR): a system of indirect myofascial release treatment developed by Stanley Schiowitz, D.O. The component region of the body is placed into a neutral position, diminishing tissue and joint tension, in all planes, and an activating force (compression or torsion) is added.

fascial release treatment: see *myofascial release treatment*.

functional treatment: an indirect treatment method in which the physician guides the manipulative procedure while the dysfunctional area is being palpated in order to obtain a continuous feedback of the physiologic response to induced motion; the physician guides the dysfunctional part so as to create a decreasing sense of tissue resistance (increased compliance).

Galbraith treatment: see *mandibular drainage*.

indirect treatment (I/IND): a manipulative technique where the restrictive barrier is disengaged; the dysfunctional body part is moved away from the restrictive barrier until tissue tension is equal in one or all planes and directions.

inhibitory pressure treatment: the application of steady pressure to soft tissues to reduce reflex activity and produce relaxation.

ligamentous articular strain (LAS/BLT): a set of myofascial release techniques described by Howard Lippincott, D.O. and Rebecca Lippincott, D.O.

lymphatic pump: a term coined by C. Earl Miller, D.O., to describe the impact of intrathoracic pressure changes on lymphatic flow; this was the name originally given to the thoracic pump technique before the more extensive physiologic effects of the technique were recognized.

mandibular drainage: a technique used to effect increased drainage of middle ear structures via the eustachian tube and lymphatics.

muscle energy treatment: a term first used by Fred L. Mitchell, Sr, D.O., to describe the form of osteopathic manipulative treatment in which the patient voluntarily moves the body as specifically directed by the physician; this directed patient action is from a precisely controlled position, against a defined resistance by the physician.

myofascial treatment: any technique directed at the muscles and fascia; see also *soft tissue treatment*.

myofascial release treatment (MFR): treatment form first described by Andrew Taylor Still and his early students, which engages continual palpatory feedback to achieve release of myofascial tissues.

direct MFR: a restrictive barrier is engaged for the myofascial tissues; the tissue is loaded with a constant force until tissue release occurs.

indirect MFR: the dysfunctional tissues are guided along the path of least resistance until free movement is achieved.

passive treatment: technique in which the patient refrains from voluntary muscle contraction.

pedal pump: a venous and lymphatic drainage technique applied through the lower extremities; also called the pedal fascial pump or pedal pump; also known as *Dalrymple treatment*.

positional treatment: a direct segmental technique in which a combination of leverage, patient ventilatory movements and a fulcrum are used to achieve mobilization of the dysfunctional segment; may be combined with springing or thrust technique.

range of motion treatment: active or passive movement of a body part to its physiologic or anatomic limit in any or all planes of motion.

soft tissue treatment (ST): procedure directed toward tissues other than skeletal or arthrodial elements; a direct technique which usually involves lateral stretching, linear stretching, deep pressure, traction and/or separation of muscle origin and insertion while monitoring tissue response and motion changes by palpation; also called myofascial treatment.

Spencer technique: a series of direct manipulative procedures to prevent or decrease soft tissue restrictions about the shoulder.

springing treatment: a low velocity/moderate amplitude technique where the restrictive barrier is engaged repeatedly to produce an increased freedom of motion.

thoracic pump: a technique developed by C. Earl Miller, D.O., which consists of intermittent compression of the thoracic cage.

thrust treatment (HVLA): a direct technique which uses high velocity/low amplitude forces; also called mobilization with impulse treatment.

traction treatment: a procedure of high or low amplitude in which the parts are stretched or separated along a longitudinal axis with continuous or intermittent force.

ventral techniques: see *osteopathic manipulative treatment, visceral manipulation.*

visceral manipulation (VIS): manual techniques directed to the viscera to improve physiologic function; typically the viscera are moved toward their fascial attachments to a point of fascial balance; also *called ventral techniques.*

osteopathic philosophy: osteopathic medicine is a philosophy of health care and a distinctive art, supported by expanding scientific knowledge; its philosophy embraces the concept of the unity of the living organism's structure (anatomy) and function (physiology). Its art is the application of the philosophy in the practice of medicine and surgery in all its branches and specialties. Its science includes the behavioral, chemical, physical, spiritual and biological knowledge related to the establishment and maintenance of health as well as the prevention and alleviation of disease. Osteopathic concepts emphasize the following principles: 1. The human being is a dynamic unit of function; 2. The body possesses self-regulatory mechanisms which are self-healing in nature; 3. Structure and function are interrelated at all levels; 4. Rational treatment is based on these principles.

osteopathic postural examination: the part of the osteopathic musculoskeletal examination that focuses on the static and dynamic responses of the body to gravity while in the erect position.

osteopathic structural examination: the examination of a patient by an osteopathic physician with emphasis on the neuromusculo-skeletal system including palpatory diagnosis for somatic dysfunction and viscerosomatic change, in the context of total patient care. The examination is concerned with range of motion of all parts of the body, performed with the patient in multiple positions to provide static and dynamic evaluation.

osteopathy (osteopathic medicine): A system of medical care with a philosophy that combines the needs of the patient with current practice of medicine, surgery and obstetrics, and emphasis on the interrelationships between structure and function, and an appreciation of the body's ability to heal itself; see *osteopathic philosophy.*

osteopathy in the cranial field (OCF): diagnosis and treatment by an osteopathic physician using the primary respiratory mechanism; see *primary respiratory mechanism.* 1. refers to the work of William G. Sutherland, D.O., in applying the philosophy and principles of osteopathy to the whole body, 2. title of reference work by Harold Magoun, Sr, D.O., see *primary respiratory mechanism.*

palpation: the application of the fingers to the surface of the skin or other tissues, using varying amounts of pressure, to selectively determine the condition of the parts beneath.

palpatory diagnosis: a term used by osteopathic physicians to denote the process of palpating the patient to evaluate the neuromusculoskeletal and visceral systems.

palpatory skills: sensory skills used in performing palpatory diagnosis and osteopathic manipulative treatment.

passive motion: see *motion: passive motion.*

patient cooperation: voluntary movement by the patient (on instruction from the operator) to assist in the palpatory diagnosis and treatment process.

pedal pump: see *osteopathic manipulative treatment: pedal pump.*

pelvic bone: preferred current term replacing the term innominate bone. The two pelvic bones with the sacrum and coccyx is referred to as the pelvis; see *hip bone;* see *innominate;* see *ilium, somatic dysfunction of.*

pelvic declination (pelvic unleveling): pelvic rotation about an A-P axis.

pelvic index: an objective radiographic measurement representing the relative positions of the sacrum and innominates; normal values are age-related and increase in subjects with sagittal plane postural decompensation.

pelvic rotation: movement of the entire pelvis in a relatively horizontal plane about a vertical (longitudinal) axis.

pelvic sideshift: deviation of the pelvis to the right or left of the central vertical axis as translation along the horizontal (z) axis, usually observed in the standing position.

pelvic tilt: pelvic rotation about a transverse (horizontal) axis (forward or backward tilt) or about an anterior-posterior axis (right or left side tilt).

pétrissage: deep kneading or squeezing action to express swelling.

physiologic barrier: see *barrier: physiologic barrier.*

physiologic motion: see *motion: physiologic motion.*

physiologic motion of the spine: Principles I and II of thoracic and lumbar spinal motion described by Harrison H. Fryette, D.O. (1918). Principle III was proposed by C.R. Nelson, D.O. (1948); see *rotation and rotation of vertebra.* The three major **principles** are:

I When the thoracic and lumbar spine is in a neutral position [Fig. 13] (easy normal), the coupled motions of sidebending and rotation for a group of vertebrae are such that sidebending and rotation occur in opposite directions (with rotation occurring toward the convexity); [Fig. 14]; see *somatic dysfunction, type I.*

II When the thoracic and lumbar spine is sufficiently forward or backward bent (non-neutral), the coupled motions of sidebending and rotation in a single vertebral unit occur in the same direction. [Fig. 15]; see *somatic dysfunction, type II.*

III Initiating motion of a vertebral segment in any plane of motion will modify the movement of that segment in other planes of motion.

plagiocephaly: an asymmetric condition of the head.

plane: a flat surface determined by the position of three points in space; any of a number of imaginary surfaces passing through the body and dividing it into segments. (Fig. 16)

coronal plane: frontal plane.

frontal plane: a plane passing longitudinally through the body from one side to the other, and dividing the body into anterior and posterior portions.

sagittal plane: a plane passing longitudinally through the body from front to back and dividing it into right and left portions; the median or midsagittal plane divides the body into approximately equal right and left portions.

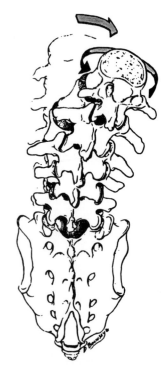

Figure 14. Physiologic motion of the spine (Type I) Sidebending and rotation from neutral

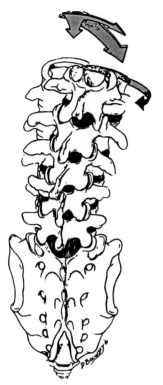

Figure 15. Physiologic motion of the spine (Type II) Forward bending and sidebending from a non-neutral position

transverse plane: a plane passing horizontally through the body perpendicular to the sagittal and frontal planes, dividing the body into upper and lower portions.

plastic deformation: a non-recoverable deformation; see also *elastic deformation.*

plasticity: ability to retain a shape attained by deformation; see also *elasticity; viscosity.*

posterior component: a positional descriptor used to identify the side of reference when rotation of a vertebral segment has occurred; in a condition of right rotation, the right side is the posterior component; usually refers to a prominent transverse process; see also *anterior component.*

posterior ilium: see *ilium, somatic dysfunctions of: posterior (backward) innominate rotation.*

postural balance: a condition of optimal distribution of body mass in relation to gravity.

postural decompensation: distribution of body mass away from ideal when postural homeostatic mechanisms are overwhelmed; occurs in all cardinal planes but is classified by the major plane(s) affected. (Fig. 16)

coronal plane postural decompensation: scoliotic changes

horizontal plane postural decompensation: rotational changes

sagittal plane postural decompensation: kyphotic and/or lordotic changes

posture: position of the body; the distribution of body mass in relation to gravity.

primary machinery of life: the neuromusculoskeletal system; a term used by I.M. Korr, Ph.D., to denote that body parts "act together to transmit and modify force and motion through which man acts out his life"; this integration is achieved via the central nervous system acting in response to continued sensory input from the internal and external environment.

primary respiratory mechanism: a model proposed by William G. Sutherland, D.O., to describe the interdependent functions among five body components as follows: 1. the inherent motility of the brain and spinal cord; 2. fluctuation of the cerebrospinal fluid; 3. mobility of the intracranial and intraspinal membranes; 4. articular mobility of the cranial bones; 5. the involuntary mobility of the sacrum between the ilia (pelvic bones).

primary: refers to the internal tissue respiratory process.

respiratory: refers to the process of internal respiration, i.e., the exchange of respiratory gases between tissue cells and their internal environment consisting of the fluids bathing the cells.

mechanism: refers to the interdependent movement of tissue and fluid with a specific purpose.

prime mover: a muscle primarily responsible for causing a specific joint action.

pronation: in relation to the anatomical position, as applied to the hand, rotation of the forearm in such a way that the palmar surface turns backward (internal rotation) in relationship to the anatomical position; applied to the foot, a combination of eversion and abduction movements taking place in the tarsal and metatarsal joints, resulting in lowering of the medial margin of the foot; see also *supination.*

prone: lying face downward (Dorland).

proprioception: the sensing of motion and position of the body.

proprioceptor: sensory nerve terminals found in muscles, tendons and joint capsules which give information concerning movements and position of the body (Dorland).

pubes, somatic dysfunctions of:

inferior pubic shear (inferior pubis): a somatic dysfunction in which one side of the pubic symphysis is inferior to the contralateral side as the result of a shearing in the sagittal plane.

superior pubic shear (superior pubis): reciprocal of inferior pubis.

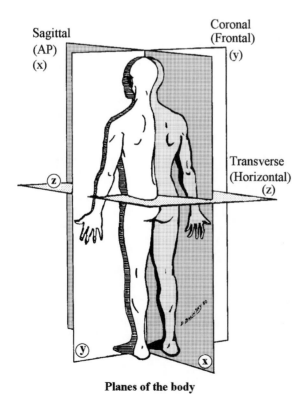

Planes of the body
(Fig. 16)

Figure 16. Planes of the body

pubic symphysis, somatic dysfunctions of: see *pubes, somatic dysfunctions of.*

pump handle rib motion: movement of the ribs during respiration such that with inhalation the anterior aspect of the rib moves cephalad and causes an increase in the anteroposterior diameter of the thorax; this type of rib motion is found predominantly in the upper ribs (Fig. 5), decreasing from the upper to the lower ribs; see *axis of rib motion;* see also *bucket handle rib motion.*

reciprocal inhibition: the inhibition of antagonist muscles when the agonist is stimulated; see also *laws, Sherrington's.*

reciprocal tension membrane: the intracranial and spinal dural membrane including the falx cerebri, falx cerebelli, tentorium and spinal dura.

reflex: an involuntary nervous system response to a sensory input; the sum total of any particular involuntary activity; see also *Chapman's reflexes.*

conditioned reflex: one that does not occur naturally in the organism or system but that is developed by regular association of some physiological function with an unrelated outside event; soon the physiological function starts whenever the outside event occurs; see also *somatic dysfunction; facilitation.*

red reflex: 1. the erythematous biochemical reaction (reactive hyperemia) of the skin in an area that has been stimulated mechanically by friction; the reflex is greater in degree and duration in an area of acute somatic dysfunction as compared to an area of chronic somatic dysfunction; it is a reflection of the segmentally related sympathicotonia commonly observed in the paraspinal area; 2. a red glow reflected from the fundus of the eye when a light is cast upon the retina.

somato-somatic reflex: localized somatic stimuli producing patterns of reflex response in segmentally related somatic structures.

somato-visceral reflex: localized somatic stimulation producing patterns of reflex response in segmentally related visceral structures.

viscero-somatic reflex: localized visceral stimuli producing patterns of reflex response in segmentally related somatic structures.

viscero-visceral reflex: localized visceral stimuli producing patterns of reflex response in segmentally related visceral structures.

region: see *transitional region.*

resilience: property of returning to the former shape or size after mechanical distortion; see also *elasticity; plasticity.*

respiratory axis of the sacrum: see *sacral motion, axis of: superior transverse axis.*

respiratory cooperation: a physician-directed inhalation and/or exhalation by the patient to assist the manipulative treatment process.

restriction: a resistance or impediment to movement; for joint restriction see *barrier (motion barrier).*

retrolisthesis: posterior displacement of one vertebra relative to the one immediately below.

rib dysfunction (rib lesion): a somatic dysfunction in which movement or position of one or several ribs is altered or disrupted; for example, an elevated rib is one held in a position of inhalation such that motion toward inhalation is freer, and motion toward exhalation is restricted; a depressed rib is one held in a position of exhalation such that motion toward exhalation is freer, and there is a restriction in inhalation; see also *inhalation rib; exhalation rib.*

rib motion: see *axis of rib motion; bucket handle rib motion; pump handle rib motion, caliper rib motion.*

ropiness: a tissue texture abnormality characterized by a cord-like feeling; see *tissue texture abnormality.*

rotation: motion about an axis.

rotation dysfunction of the sacrum: see *sacrum, somatic dysfunctions of.*

rotation of sacrum: movement of the sacrum about a vertical (y) axis (usually in relation to the innominate bones).

rotation of vertebra: movement about the anatomical vertical axis (y axis) of a vertebra; named by the motion of a midpoint on the anterior superior surface of the vertebral body. (Fig. 17)

sacral base unleveling (declination): with the patient in a standing or seated position, any devia-

tion of the sacral base from the horizontal in a coronal plane; generally, the rotation of the sacral base around an anterior-posterior axis.

sacral motion, axis of: motion of the sacrum about any of its hypothetical axes. (Fig. 18)

anterior-posterior (x) axis: axis formed at the line of intersection of a sagittal and transverse plane.

oblique axis (diagonal): a hypothetical functional axis proposed by Fred Mitchell, Sr, D.O., that is from the superior area of a sacroiliac articulation to the contralateral inferior sacroiliac articulation; it is designated as right or left relevant to its superior point of origin.

longitudinal axis: the hypothetical axis formed at the line of intersection of the midsagittal plane and a coronal plane, see *vertical axis.*

postural axis: see *middle (postural) transverse axis.*

superior transverse axis: see *superior (respiratory) axis.* (Fig. 19)

transverse (z) axes: axes formed by intersection of the coronal and transverse planes about which flexion/extension occurs. (Fig. 19)

inferior transverse axis (innominate axis): the hypothetical functional axis of sacral motion proposed by Fred Mitchell, Sr, D.O., that passes from side to side on a line through the inferior auricular surface of the sacrum, and represents the axis for movement of the ilia on the sacrum. (Fig. 19)

middle transverse axis (postural axis): the hypothetical functional axis of sacral flexion/extension

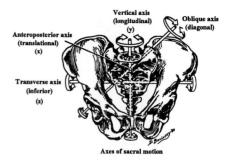

Figure 18. Axes of sacral motion

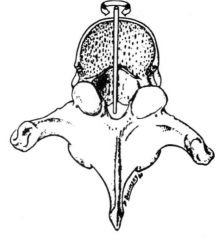

Anatomical vertical axis (y)

Figure 17. Rotation of a vertebra (thoracic)

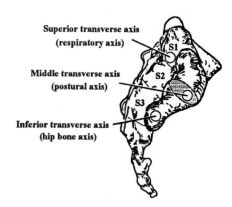

Figure 19. Sacral transverse axes

in the standing position proposed by Fred Mitchell, Sr, D.O., passing from side to side through the anterior aspect of the sacrum at the level of the second sacral segment. (Fig. 19)

superior transverse axis (respiratory axis): the hypothetical transverse axis about which the sacrum moves during the respiratory cycle proposed by Fred Mitchell, Sr, D.O.; it passes from side to side through the articular processes posterior to the point of attachment of the dura at the level of the second sacral segment; involuntary sacral motion occurring as a part of the craniosacral mechanism is believed to occur about this axis. (Fig. 19)

respiratory axis: see transverse axes: *superior transverse axis. (Fig. 19)*

vertical (y) axis (longitudinal): the axis formed by the intersection of the sagittal and coronal planes. (Fig. 18)

sacral somatic dysfunction: ee *sacrum, somatic dysfunctions of.*

sacral torsion: a somatic dysfunction in which a torque occurs between the sacrum and the lumbar spine; see *sacrum, somatic dysfunctions of.*

sacral sulcus: a depression just medial to the PSIS as a result of the spatial relationship of the PSIS to the dorsal aspect of the sacrum.

sacrum, somatic dysfunctions of (sacral somatic dysfunction): any of a group of somatic dysfunctions involving primarily the sacrum.

anterior sacrum: a positional term referring to sacral somatic dysfunction in which one side of the sacral base relative to the pelvic bones has rotated *forward* and sidebent to the side opposite the rotation about a diagonal axis; the dysfunction is named for the side on which the forward rotation occurs; anterior sacrum right describes a condition in which the sacrum is rotated left and sidebent to the right, such that rotation left and sidebending right are freer motions and rotation right and sidebending left are restricted; the use of the term anterior (or posterior) to describe dysfunctions of the sacrum uses the pelvic bones for reference.

extension dysfunction of the sacrum (sacral base posterior): a sacral somatic dysfunction that involves rotation of the sacrum about a middle transverse axis such that the sacral base has moved posteriorly relative to the pelvic bones; backward movement of the sacral base is freer and forward movement is restricted; this is the reciprocal of flexion sacrum.

flexion dysfunction of the sacrum (sacral base anterior): 1. a sacral somatic dysfunction that involves rotation of the sacrum about a middle transverse axis such that the sacral base has moved anteriorly between the pelvic bones; forward movement of the sacral base is freer and backward movement is restricted; 2. reciprocal of an extension sacrum.

left on left (forward) sacral torsion: see *sacral torsions. left on right (backward) torsion:* see *sacral torsions.*

posterior sacrum: a positional term referring to a sacral somatic dysfunction in which the sacral base has rotated *backward* and sidebent to the side opposite the rotation; the dysfunction is named for the side on which the backward rotation occurs; for example, a posterior sacrum left describes a condition in which the sacrum is rotated left and sidebent to the right, such that rotation left and sidebending right are freer motions and rotation right and sidebending left are restricted.

right on left (backward) torsion: see *sacral torsions. right on right (forward) torsion:* see *sacral torsions. rotated dysfunction of the sacrum:* a sacral somatic dysfunction in which the sacrum has rotated about an axis approximating the longitudinal (y) axis; motion is freer in the direction that rotation has occurred, and is restricted in the opposite direction.

sacral shear (unilateral sacral flexion): a non-physiologic sacral somatic dysfunction which is usually traumatically induced; characterized by a deep sacral sulcus and ipsilateral inferior-posterior inferolateral angle of the sacrum.

sacral torsions: rotational motion about an oblique or diagonal sacral axis; primarily a term used to designate somatic dysfunction that results in torsion at the L/S junction. One of the dysfunctions described by Fred Mitchell, Sr, D.O., based on the motion cycle of walking. *Forward torsions* (neutral torsions) occur when the lumbar spine is in *neutral* and sidebending; for example, to the left engages the left oblique axis (L/L). The sacrum then rotates left about the left oblique axis. The lumbar spine in neutral rotates right with left sidebending. The term torsion originates from the fact that the sacrum has rotated in a direction opposite to the supported vertebra (sacrum rotates left, the lumbar spine rotates right). A left rotation about a left oblique axis produces a right anterior sacral base with a deep right sacral sulcus, a more posterior left inferolateral angle and a decrease in the tension of the right sacrotuberous ligament. A *backward torsion* (non-neutral) occurs when the lumbar spine is in *non-neutral* and the sacral base then rotates posteriorly about an oblique axis. Backward or non-neutral torsions are identified for convenience by "right on left" or "left on right." *The use of the term torsions describes sacral dysfunctions in relationship to the axial spine.*

translated sacrum: a non-physiological sacral somatic dysfunction as a result of trauma in which the entire sacrum has moved forward between the pelvic bones (an anterior translated sacrum), or backward between the pelvic bones (posterior translated sacrum).

anterior translated sacrum: a sacral somatic dysfunction in which the entire sacrum has moved forward between the ilia; anterior motion is freer, and there is a restriction to posterior motion; (Fig. 20)

posterior translated sacrum: a sacral somatic dysfunction in which the entire sacrum has moved backward between the ilia; posterior motion is

freer, and there is a restriction to anterior motion. (Fig. 21)

scan: an intermediate detailed examination of specific body regions which have been identified by findings emerging from the initial screen; the scan focuses on segmental areas for further definition or diagnosis.

scoliosis: 1. pathological or functional lateral curvature of the spine; 2. an appreciable lateral deviation in the normally straight vertical line of the spine (Dorland). (Fig. 22)

screen: the initial general somatic examination to determine signs of somatic dysfunction in various regions of the body; see also *scan.*

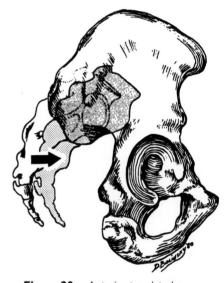

Figure 20. Anterior translated sacrum

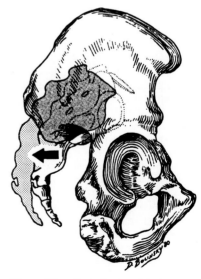

Figure 21. Posterior translated sacrum

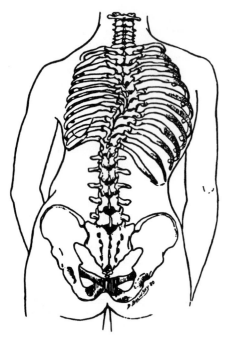

Figure 22. Scoliosis

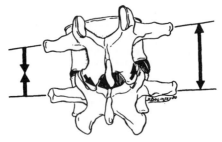

Figure 23. Sidebent

secondary joint motion: involuntary or passive motion of a joint; also called accessory joint motion.

segment: a portion of a larger body or structure set off by natural or arbitrarily established boundaries; often equated with spinal segment, i.e., 1. to describe a single vertebrae, viz. a vertebral segment, 2. a portion of the spinal cord corresponding to the sites of origin of rootlets of individual spinal nerves.

segmental diagnosis: the final stage of the spinal somatic examination in which the nature of the somatic problem is detailed at a segmental level; see also *scan; screen.*

segmental motion: movement within a vertebral unit described by displacement of a point at the anterior-superior aspect of the superior vertebral body.

sensitization: hypothetically, a short-lived (minutes or hours) increase in central nervous system (CNS) response to repeated sensory stimulation that generally follows habituation (qv)

shear: an action or force causing or tending to cause two contiguous parts of an articulation to slide relative to each other in a direction parallel to their plane of contact [e.g., pubic shear (qv); sacral shear, innominate shear].

Sherrington's laws: see *laws, Sherrington's.*

sidebending: movement in a coronal (frontal) plane about an anterior-posterior (x) axis; also called lateral flexion, lateroflexion or flexion right (or left).

sidebent: the position of any one or several vertebral bodies after sidebending has occurred. (Fig. 23)

skin drag: sense of resistance to light traction applied to the skin; related to the degree of moisture and degree of sympathetic nervous system activity.

soft tissue technique: see *osteopathic manipulative treatment: soft tissue treatment.*

somatic dysfunction: impaired or altered function of related components of the somatic (body framework) system: skeletal, arthrodial, and myofascial structures, and related vascular, lymphatic, and neural elements. Somatic dysfunction is treatable using osteopathic manipulative treatment. The positional and motion aspects of somatic dysfunction are best described using at least one of three parameters: 1. the position of a body part as determined by palpation and referenced to its adjacent defined structure, 2. the directions in which motion is freer, and 3. the directions in which motion is restricted. see also *osteopathic lesion (osteopathic lesion complex).*

somatic dysfunction, acute: immediate or short-term impairment or altered function of related components of the somatic (body framework) system; characterized in early stages by vasodilation, edema, tenderness, pain and contraction; identified by T.A.R.T. (qv); palpatorily diagnosed by assessment of tenderness, asymmetry of motion and relative position, restriction of motion and tissue texture change (T.A.R.T.). see *T.A.R.T.*

somatic dysfunction, chronic: impairment or altered function of related components of the somatic (body framework) system, characterized by tenderness, itching, fibrosis, paresthesias, contracture; identified by T.A.R.T. (qv). see *T.A.R.T.*

somatic dysfunction, secondary: somatic dysfunction (qv) arising subsequent to or as a consequence of other etiologies.

somatic dysfunction, type I: a group of thoracic and/or lumbar vertebrae in which the freedoms of motion are in neutral with sidebending and rotation in opposite directions (rotation occurs toward the convexity of the curve).

somatic dysfunction, type II: thoracic or lumbar somatic dysfunction of a single vertebral unit in which the vertebra is flexed or extended with sidebending and rotation in the same direction (rotation occurs into the concavity of the curve).

somatogenic: that which is produced by activity, reaction, and change originating in the musculoskeletal system.

somato-somatic reflex: see *reflex: somato-somatic reflex.*

somato-visceral reflex: see *reflex: somato-visceral reflex.*

spasm: (compare with hypertonicity) a sudden, violent, involuntary contraction of a muscle or group of muscles, attended by pain and interference with function, producing involuntary movement and distortion (Dorland).

Spencer techniques: see *osteopathic treatment, Spencer techniques*

spondyl-, spondylo-: combining form denoting relationship to a vertebra, or to the spinal column (Dorland).

spondylitis: inflammation of vertebrae. (Dorland)

spondylolisthesis: anterior displacement of one vertebra relative to one immediately below (usually L-5 over the body of the sacrum or L-4 over L-5).

spondylolysis: dissolution of a vertebra, aplasia of the vertebral arch, and separation at the pars interarticularis; platyspondylia, pre-spondylolisthesis.

spondylosis: 1. ankylosis of adjacent vertebral bodies; 2. degeneration of the intervertebral disk.

sprain: stretching injuries of ligamentous tissue (compare with strain). Grade 0: plastic deformation of the ligament without any tissue tearing; first degree: microtrauma; second degree: partial tear; third degree: complete disruption.

springing technique: see *osteopathic manipulative treatment: springing treatment.*

static contraction: see *contraction, isometric contraction.*

Still, M.D., Andrew Taylor: founder of osteopathy; 1828-1917; first announced the tenets of osteopathy on June 22, 1874, established the American School of Osteopathy in 1892 at Kirksville, MO.

still point: a term used by William G. Sutherland, D.O., to identify and describe the brief cessation of rhythm attributed to the fluctuation of cerebrospinal fluid (a component of the primary respiratory mechanism (qv) observed by palpation during osteopathic manipulative treatment when a point of balanced membranous tension (or balanced ligamentous tension) is achieved.

strain: 1. stretching injuries of muscle tissue; 2. distortion with deformation of tissue; see *ligamentous strain.*

stretching: separation of the origin and insertion of a muscle and/or attachments of fascia and ligaments.

stringiness: a palpable tissue texture abnormality characterized by fine or stringlike myofascial structures.

structural examination: see *osteopathic structural examination.*

subluxation: 1. a partial or incomplete dislocation; 2. a term describing an abnormal anatomical position of a joint which exceeds the normal physiologic limit but does not exceed the joint's anatomical limit.

superior ilium (upslipped innominate): see *ilium, somatic dysfunctions of: superior innominate shear.*

superior pubis: see *pubes, somatic dysfunctions of.*

superior transverse axis: see *sacral motion, axis of: superior (respiratory) axis and transverse (z) axis.*

supination: 1. beginning in anatomical position, applied to the hand, the act of turning the palm forward (anteriorly) or upward, performed by lateral external rotation of the forearm; 2. applied to the foot, it generally applies to movements (adduction and inversion) resulting in raising of the medial margin of the foot, hence of the longitudinal arch; a compound motion of plantar flexion, adduction and inversion; see also *pronation.*

supine: lying with the face upward (Dorland).

symmetry: the similar arrangement in form and relationships of parts around a common axis, or on each side of a plane of the body (Dorland).

symphyseal shear: the resultant of an action or force causing or tending to cause the two parts of the symphysis to slide relative to each other in a direction parallel to their plane of contact; it is usually found in an inferior/superior direction but is occasionally found to be in an anterior/posterior direction. (Fig. 24)

tapotement: striking the belly of a muscle with the hypothenar edge of the open hand in rapid succession in an attempt to increase its tone and arterial perfusion.

T.A.R.T.: a mnemonic for the four diagnostic criteria of somatic dysfunction—tissue texture abnormality, asymmetry, restriction of motion and tenderness—any one of which must be present for the diagnosis.

technic: see *technique.*

technique: methods, procedures and details of a mechanical process or surgical operation. [. . . method, treatment, maneuver . . .] (Dorland); see also *osteopathic manipulative treatment.*

tenderness: 1. discomfort or pain elicited by the physician through palpation; 2. a state of unusual sensitivity to touch or pressure (Dorland).

tender points: 1. system of points originally described by Lawrence Jones, D.O., F.A.A.O., in strain/counterstrain diagnosis and treatment; see *osteopathic manipulative treatment: counterstrain;* 2. small, hypersensitive points in the myofascial tissues of the body used as diagnostic criteria and treatment monitors.

terminal barrier: see *barrier: physiologic barrier.*

thoracic aperture (superior): see *thoracic inlet.*

thoracic inlet: 1. *the functional thoracic inlet* consists of T1-4 vertebrae, ribs 1 and 2 plus their costicartilages, and the manubrium of the sternum; see *fascial patterns;* 2. *the anatomical thoracic inlet* consists of T1 vertebra, the first ribs and their costal cartilages, and the superior end of the manubrium (Moore); see *thoracic aperture, superior.*

thoracic pump: see *osteopathic manipulative treatment: thoracic pump.*

thrust: see *osteopathic manipulative treatment: thrust treatment.*

tissue texture abnormality (TTA): a palpable change in tissues from skin to periarticular structures that represents any combination of the following signs: vasodilation, edema, flaccidity, hypertonicity, contracture, fibrosis; and the following symptoms: itching, pain, tenderness,

paresthesias; types of TTA's include: bogginess (qv), thickening, stringiness (qv), ropiness (qv), firmness (hardening), increased/decreased temperature, increased/decreased moisture.

tonus: the slight continuous contraction of muscle which, in skeletal muscles, aids in the maintenance of posture and in the return of blood to the heart (Dorland).

myogenic tonus: 1. tonic contraction of muscle dependent on some property of the muscle itself or of its intrinsic nerve cells. 2. Contraction of a muscle caused by intrinsic properties of the muscle or by its intrinsic innervatrion (Stedman).

torsion: 1. a motion or state where one end of a part is twisted about a longitudinal axis while the opposite end is held fast or turned in the opposite direction; 2. motion of the sacrum about an oblique axis, with sacral rotation opposite to rotation of L5; 3. an unphysiologic motion pattern about an anteroposterior axis of the sphenobasilar symphysis/synchondrosis; see *sacrum, somatic dysfunctions of: sacral torsions.*

traction: a linear force acting to draw structures apart.

transitional region: areas of the axial skeleton where structure changes significantly leading to functional change; transitional areas commonly include the following:

occipitocervical region (OA): typically the OA-AA-C2 region is described

cervicothoracic region (CT): typically C7-T1

thoracolumbar region (TL): typically T10-L1

lumbosacral region (LS): typically L5-S1

transitional segment (transitional vertebral segment): a congenital anomaly of a vertebra in which it develops characteristic(s) of the adjoining structure or region; e.g., lumbosacral, cervicothoracic; the clinical significance of this lies in its aberrant motion characteristics; gross postural effects on the super incumbent spinal column, or pseudoarthrosis between the enlarged transverse processes and either the sacrum or ilia.

batwing: see *transitional segment: sacralization.*

lumbarization: a transitional segment in which the first sacral segment becomes like an additional lumbar vertebra articulating with the second sacral segment.

sacralization: 1. incomplete separation and differentiation of the fifth lumbar vertebra (L5) such that it takes on characteristics of a sacral vertebra; 2. when transverse processes of the fifth lumbar (L5) are atypically large, causing pseudoarthrosis with the sacrum and/or ilia(um), referred to as batwing deformity, if bilateral.

translation: motion along an axis.

translatory motion: see *motion: translatory motion.*

transverse axis of sacrum: see *sacral motion, axis of: transverse (z) axis.* (Fig. 19)

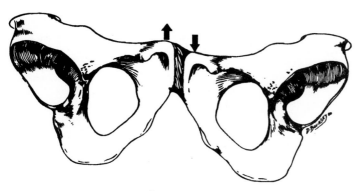

Figure 24. Symphyseal shear

treatment, osteopathic manipulative techniques: see *osteopathic manipulative treatment.*

trigger point (myofascial trigger point): a small hypersensitive site that, when stimulated, consistently produces a reflex mechanism that gives rise to referred pain or other manifestations in a constant reference zone, and consistent from person to person. This system of points was most commonly documented by Janet Travell, M.D. and David Simons, M.D.

trophic: of or pertaining to nutrition, especially in the cellular environment; example: trophic function - a nutritional function.

trophicity: 1. a nutritional function or relation, 2. the natural tendency to replenish the body stores that have been depleted.

trophotropic: concerned with or pertaining to the natural tendency for maintenance and/or restoration of nutritional stores.

-tropic: a word termination denoting turning toward, changing, or tendency to change.

tropism, facet: unequal size and/or facing of the zygapophyseal joints of a vertebra; see also *facet asymmetry.*

type I somatic dysfunction: see *somatic dysfunction, type I.*

type II somatic dysfunction: see *somatic dysfunction, type II.*

uncompensated fascial patterning: historic

velocity: the instantaneous rate of motion in a given direction.

ventral technique: see *osteopathic manipulative treatment: visceral manipulation.*

vertebral unit: two adjacent vertebrae with their associated intervertebral disk, arthrodial, ligamentous, muscular, vascular, lymphatic and neural elements (Fig. 25).

visceral manipulation: see *osteopathic manipulative treatment: visceral manipulation:*

viscero-somatic reflex: see *reflex: viscero-somatic reflex.*

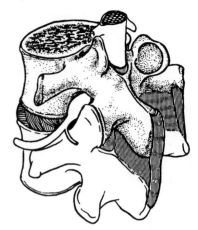

Figure 25. Vertebral unit

viscosity: 1. a measurement of the rate of deformation of any material under load; 2. the capability possessed by a solid of yielding continually under stress; see also *elasticity; plasticity.*

weight-bearing line of L3: see *gravitational line.* (Fig. 12)

Index

Abdominal region (*see also* Lumbar and
    abdominal region)
  innervation of organs in, 68–80
  lymphatic pump, 956
  oblique muscles, 603
  rectus abdominis muscle, 603
    inhibited, symptoms of, 976
  surgery, 388–389
  techniques to promote lymphatic flow,
    961–964
  transverse muscle, 603
Abdominopelvic plexus of nerves, 68–69, 77–79
Abducens nerve, 529–530
Abscess, tubo-ovarian, 368
Absorption, intestinal, 380
  disorders of, 380–381
Acanthosis nigricans in malignancies, 421
Accessory nerve, 530
Acetabular notch, 646, 656
Acetabulum, 601
Acetylcholine secretion by parasympathetic
    nervous system, 57
Achalasia of esophagus, 377
Achilles tendon
  bursitis, 657
  reflex, 506, 643
Acid, gastric
  in gastroesophageal reflux disease, 375–376
  in peptic ulcer, 378–379
Acromioclavicular joint, 548
  motion tests, 553
Acromion drop test, 493
ACTH, 84, 115, 122
  ectopic, and Cushing's syndrome in
    malignancies, 422
  secretion related to photoperiod, 89
  in stress response, 100
Activities of daily living
  assessment in geriatric patients, 277–278
  measurements in clinical trials, 1103
Acupressure, 916
Acupuncture, 916
  in pain syndromes, 432
Acute phase proteins, 104
Adaptations, regulatory, 99–105
  and general adaptation response, 100, 127–129
Addison's disease, 91, 123
  cortisol deficiency in, 91–92
Adductor muscles of hip, 645, 646
Adenohypophysis
  affecting neural activity, 88–89
  hormones of, 84
Adenoids, 295, 942
Adenomyosis, 367
Adhesive capsulitis, 560–561
Adolescence, 193

Adrenal hormones, 84
  cortical, 115–116, 122
Adrenergic axons in peripheral vasculature, 61–62
β-Adrenergic blocking agents in hypertension,
    324
Adrenocorticotrophic hormone (*see* ACTH)
Adson's test, 558
Adulthood as life phase, 193–194
Aerobic exercise, 1050–1051
Aging (*see* Geriatrics)
AIDS
  diarrhea in, 381–382
  in hospitalized patients, 1044
Alcohol intake, 161
  stress-induced, 211–212
Aldosterone, 84
Allen's test, 559
Allergic rhinitis, 292–293
Aluminum toxicity, bone disease in, 394, 395
Alveolar macrophages, 111
Alzheimer's disease, 279–280
Ambulatory outpatients, musculoskeletal
    examination for, 501–504
American Academy of Osteopathy, symposia
    presented by, 1016
American Association of Colleges of Osteopathic
    Medicine, 18
American Association of Orthopaedic Medicine,
    329
American College of Osteopathic Family Practice,
    249
American College of Osteopathic Pediatricians,
    261, 267
American College of Osteopathic Surgeons,
    387
American Medical Association, conflict with, 16
American Osteopathic Academy of Sports
    Medicine, 285
American Osteopathic Association, 16, 18–19
  research supported by, 1061
American Society of Osteopathic Internists, 257
Amine type hormones, 84
Anaerobic exercise, 1051
Anal canal, external, 604
Anal triangle, 369
Analgesic drugs, 180–181
  adjuvants with, 181
  excessive intake of, 181
  tolerance for, 181
Anatomy, 24–25, 27–43
  cartilage and bone, 30
  connective tissue, 29–30
  and embryologic development, 27–29
  microscopic features of, 29–31
  and myofascial continuity, 41–43
  research applied to osteopathic practice, 1113

  rules of, 25, 45–51
    connectedness, 49–50
    difference, 51
    drainage, 48
    function, 46
    pain, 48–49
    proximity, 45–46
    supply, 47–48
  segmental organization of systems in, 36–39
  skeletal muscle, 30–31
  and somatic dysfunction, 512
  upper and lower limbs, 39–41
Androgens affecting reproductive function, 91
Anemia in renal failure, 357
Aneurysms
  abdominal, 588
  cerebral, headache in, 406
Angina pectoris, 304–305
  grading of, 305
  treatment of, 307
  unstable, 305
Angiogenesis and remodeling in atherosclerosis,
    302–303
Angiotensin, 84
  converting enzyme inhibitors
    in heart failure, 310–311
    in hypertension, 324
Angle of anteversion, 626
Angle of inclination, 626
Ankle, 633–635
  deltoid ligament, 637–638
  dorsiflexion, 634
    muscle energy technique in, 755–766
    thrust technique in, 689
  muscle energy techniques, 755–756
  muscles of, 648
  myofascial and integrated neuromusculoskeletal
    release, 887
  plantar flexion, 634
    muscle energy technique in, 756
    thrust technique in, 689–690
  sprains, 636–637
  stabilizing ligaments, 636–637
  subtalar joint, 633, 634–635
  talocrural joint, 633–634
Ankle tug, 689
Anococcygeal nerve, 606
Antagonist muscles, 36, 1000, 1002
Anterior component, 1127
Anteversion, angle of, 626
Antibiotics, diarrhea from, 382
Antidiuretic hormone, 84
  inappropriate secretion in malignancies, 422
Anxiety
  exercise therapy in, 200–201
  measurement of, 210

Anxiety—continued
    stress-induced, 209–211
    treatments of, 210–211
Aorta
    abdominal, 586–587, 588
        innervation of, 68
    thoracic, 586
        innervation of, 67–68
Aortic bodies as chemoreceptors, 448
Apley scratch test, 552, 559
Apneustic center in pons, 447
Appendix, 942
    viscerosomatic reference sites for, 450
Apprehension test for shoulder dislocation,
        559
Arachidonic acid inhibition, 122
Arch of foot, 639
    relaxation of muscles in, 794
Arm (see Upper extremities)
Arteries (see Vasculature)
Arteriovenous malformations, cerebral, 537
Arteritis, temporal, 537–538
Arthritis, 459–466
    crystal-induced, 463
    gonococcal, 463
    infectious, 463
    inflammatory, 460–463
    osteoarthritis, 463–464. (see also Osteoarthritis)
    rheumatoid, 461–463
        juvenile, 463
Articulation, 1127
Articulatory techniques, 763–780, 1122
    cervical, 766–767
    cervicothoracic, 767–768
    contraindications, 764, 765
    costal, 764–765, 769–771
    indications for, 763–764, 765
    lumbar, 771–775
    pelvic, 775–777
    Spencer shoulder treatment, 552, 765,
        777–780, 1133
    thoracic, 768–769
Asthma, osteopathic treatment of, 455–456
Astrocytes, 112
Asymmetry, 1127
Atelectasis, postoperative prevention of, 388, 389,
        456
Atherosclerosis, coronary artery disease in,
        300–303
Athletes, and sports medicine, 285–287
Atlantoaxial joint
    muscle energy techniques, 700–702
    thrust technique, 667–668
Atlas, 541
    anterior, 544
    motion test, 544
Auerbach's plexus, 67, 72
Auras in migraine headaches, 405
Auscultation, abdominal, 593
Automobile safety measures, 161
Autonomic nervous system, 25, 53–80, 402
    afferent fibers of, 61
    divisions of, 57–61

innervation of various regions, 61–80, 1043
    abdominopelvic organs, 68–80
    cardiac, 141–143
    connective tissue, 62
    head and neck organs, 62–63
    sweat glands, 62
    thoracic organs, 63–68
    vasculature, 61–62
interactions with somatic system, 26
modulation of immune system, 119–121
myofascial trigger points affecting, 929–931
parasympathetic division, 60–61 (see also
        Parasympathetic nervous system)
peripheral distribution of, 54–57 (see also
        Peripheral nervous system)
reflexes in ganglia, 144
sympathetic division, 58–60. (see also
        Sympathetic nervous system)
Axillary artery, 548
Axillary folds
    myofascial trigger points in, 928
    posterior technique to promote lymphatic flow,
        964–965
    relaxation technique, 791
Axillary lymph nodes, 549–550
Axillary vein, 549
Axis
    cervical spine, 541
    of rib motion, 1127
    of sacral motion, 1136
Axons, 54
    myelinated, 55
    postganglionic, 55, 56, 57, 61
    preganglionic, 55, 56, 57, 60
    unmyelinated, 55
Axoplasmic transport, 1128
    two-way communication of, 149

B-lymphocytes, 111, 295, 944
Back pain, 337–345, 591–592
    causes of, 338
    differential diagnosis of, 343–345
    efficacy of manipulation in, 1016–1017
    exercises for, 1052
    history and physical examination, 339
    in malignancies, 423
    management of, 345
    in metastatic disease, 420
    neuromuscular symptoms in, 369
    pathophysiology of, 339–343
    in postfracture or postoperative ileus, 597–598
    postpartum, 359
    in postural stress, 596–597
    in pregnancy, 350–351
    in psoas syndrome, 597
    from quadratus lumborum myofascial triggers,
        598–599
    in radiculopathy, 598
    in spondylolisthesis, 1009
Backward bending test, 616
Baker's cyst, 657, 659
Ballottement test for effusions in knee, 657, 659
Barlow test for hip reduction, 625

Baroreceptor reflexes, somatic afferents affecting,
        133
Barr-Lieou syndrome, 522, 524
Barrett's esophagus, 376
Barriers to motion, 484, 1128
Basal ganglia, 401
Basic research, 1091, 1107–1113
Basophils, 111
Batson's venous plexus, 423, 589
Bayes' theorem, and analysis of ECG, 240–241
Behavioral sciences, 154–215
    health maintenance in, 187–194
    lifestyles and health habits, 157–166
    pain management, 171–185
    psychoneuroimmunology, 167–169
Bell's palsy, 530
Bending tests (see also Side-bending)
    backward, 616
    seated, 499
    standing, 496–497
Biceps femoris, 646, 647
Biceps reflex, 551
Bicipital tendinitis, 559
Bigelow's Y-ligament, 625
Biliary system, innervation of, 70
Biofeedback
    in pain management, 183
    in stress management, 214
Bladder innervation, 76–77
Blood-brain barrier, and effects of drugs, 96
Blood pressure
    and baroreceptor activity, 144
    drugs affecting, 321
    elevated (see Hypertension)
    measurements of, 321–322
Blood supply, and health maintenance, 47 (see
        also Vasculature)
Blush sign after blanching in thoracolumbar
        release, 851
Body unity (see Unity of body)
Bogginess, 1128
Bombesin, ectopic production of, 419
Bone (see also Skeletal anatomy)
    exercise affecting, 200
    metastases to, 420
    microscopic appearance of, 30
    muscle attachment to, 35, 41–42
    in renal osteodystrophy, 394–396
Bone marrow, efferent innervation of, 120
Braces
    in sagittal plane postural decompensation, 1005
    in scoliosis, 994, 996
    in spondylolisthesis, 1012
Brachial artery, 548
Brachial nerve entrapment, 411
Brachial plexus, 38, 550, 3941
Brachial pulse, 551
Brachiocephalic vein, 549
Brachioradialis reflex, 551
Bracing in postural decompensation, 974–975
Brain, 401
    blood supply of, 517, 521, 525
    fourth ventricle, 530–531

inherent motility of, 903
tumors of, 421
headache in, 537
Bronchi, innervation of, 66
Bronchiolitis, osteopathic treatment of, 455
Bucky diaphragm, 1025–1026
Bulge test for effusions in knee, 657, 659
Bunions, 642
Bursae of lower extremity, 658
Bursitis, 464
Achilles tendon, 657
lower extremity, 655–658
patellar, 656–657
trochanteric, 656
Buttocks, nerve supply in, 646

Cachectin (*see* Tumor necrosis factor)
Calcaneal heel spur, 639
Calcaneocuboid joint, 639
Calcaneofibular ligament, 637
Calcaneonavicular ligament, 639
Calcitonin, 84
Calcium
channel blockers in hypertension, 325
hypercalcemia in malignancies, 422
serum levels in renal osteodystrophy, 395
Calcium pyrophosphate deposition disease, 463
Caloric intake, recommendations for, 159
Cancer (*see* Oncology)
Capsulitis, adhesive, 560–561
Carbon dioxide
hypercapnia, 447
respiratory exchange with oxygen, 441
Carcinoma (*see* Oncology)
Cardiac plexus of nerves, 65
Cardiovascular system, 299–313
coronary artery disease, 299–307
endocrine system interaction with, 87–88
heart failure, 307–313
innervation of, 64, 65–66
in renal failure, 397–398
Carotid arteries
dissections causing headache, 406
internal, 517
Carotid bodies as chemoreceptors, 448
Carotid nerve, internal, 63
Carotidynia in cluster headaches, 407
Carpal tunnel
myofascial and integrated neuromuscoskeletal
release, 899
syndrome, 411–412
management of, 412, 559–560
myofascial trigger points in, 926
postpartum, 358
tests for, 559
Carpometacarpal joints, 548
somatic dysfunction of, 558
Cartilage
articular, 32
microscopic appearance of, 30
Cartilaginous joints, 34
Casts in spondylolisthesis, 1012
Catecholamines in stress response, 100

Cauda equina syndrome, 342, 583
in spondylolisthesis, 1009
Celiac artery, 70, 587
Celiac ganglion, 56, 70
Central nervous system, 401–402 (*see also*
Neurology)
in malignancies, 421–422
organization of, 54
role in myofascial trigger points, 916–917
in ventilatory control, 447–448
Cerebellum, 401, 517
subacute degeneration, 421
Cerebrospinal fluid fluctuation, 903
Cerebrovascular disease, headache in, 537
Cerebrum, 517
aneurysm of, headache in, 406
cortex of, 401
fourth ventricle of, 530–531
vasculature innervation, 63
Cervical lymph nodes, 522
Cervical plexus, 38, 39
Cervical region
anterior traction to promote lymphatic flow,
960–961
counterstrain techniques, 814
facilitated positional release, 833–834
fascial-ligamentous release, 826
functional technique, 802–803
isometric exercise, 1054
pain in, exercises for, 1052
soft tissue techniques, 781–783
effleurage to promote lymphatic flow,
959–961
Cervical spine, 541–546
articulatory techniques, 766–767
extension of, 542, 543
flexion of, 542, 543
functional anatomy of, 541–542
motion biomechanics, 542
muscle energy techniques, 698–704
myofascial and integrated neuromuscoskeletal
release, 874–880
palpation of, 543
skeletal anatomy of, 541
symptoms of problems in, 545–546
thrust techniques, 667–669
treatment of problems in, 546
Cervicothoracic articulatory technique, 767–768
Cervix uteri innervation, 79
Chapman's reflexes, 353–355, 371, 915–916,
935–940, 1128
anterior points, 938
palpation of, 593, 595
for colon, 937
palpatory characteristics of, 935–936
posterior points, 939
Chemoreceptors in ventilatory control, 448
Chest wall surgery, 388–389
Childhood (*see* Pediatrics)
Cholesterol, and steroid hormone biosynthesis,
85–86
Cholinergic axons in peripheral vasculature,
61–62

Cholinergic preganglionic neurons
in craniosacral system, 57
in thoracolumbar system, 57
Chondroblasts, 29
Chopart's joint, 639
Chromaffin cells, 112
Chyle, 945
Circulation
in pregnancy, 351–352
pulmonary, 444–446
Circumduction, 1128
Cisterna chyli, 587, 943
innervation of, 68
Clinical problem solving, 219–241
data gathering and synthesis in, 220–226
decision analysis in, 225–226
hypothetico-deductive method in, 222–224
illustrative cases, 219–220, 227–238
for osteopathic physicians, 226–239
pattern recognition in, 220–222
problem-oriented perspective in, 224–225
Clinical research and trials, 1091–1094
activity of daily living measurements in, 1103
bias in, 1092
blinding in, 1093, 1119
compared to basic research, 1107
crossover designs in, 1092
data analysis in, 1093–1094
epidemiology applied to, 1095–1099
established designs used in, 1102–1103, 1104
experimental studies in, 1092
Hawthorne effect in, 1119–1120
investigating osteopathic practice, 1102–1105
outcome studies in, 1103
protocol in, 1092
quality of life measurements in, 1103
questions in, 1091–1092
randomization in, 1093
sample size in, 1092
validity and reliability of data in, 1120
Clitoris, innervation of, 79
Clostridium difficile infection, diarrhea in, 382
Cluster headaches, 406–407, 536
Cobb measurements in scoliosis, 993, 1029
Coccygeal nerve plexus, 606
Coccygeus muscles, 602
Coccyx, 602
Cochlear nerve, 530
Cognition disorders, geriatric, 279–280
Cognitive behavioral factors in depression, 208
Cold, therapeutic, 432
COLDER mnemonic for pain studies, 609
Colds, common, 532
Colitis, ulcerative, 382–383
Collagen in connective tissue, 29
Collateral ligaments of knee, 630
Colles' fascia, 50
Colloid, thyroid, 86
Colon, innervation of, 71
Communication in doctor–patient relationship,
164
Compartment syndromes, lower leg, 650, 655,
657

Compliance
  in respiratory system, 442
  with treatment, factors affecting, 245
Complications from manipulations, 1018–1021
  in counterstrain techniques, 1020
  in cranial treatments, 1020–1021
  and guidelines for osteopathic practice, 1021
  incidence of, 1018–1019
  in muscle energy techniques, 1020
  patient-related causes of, 1019–1020
  physician-related causes of, 1019
  prevention of, 1021
  in thrust techniques, 1020
Compression test, 799–800
Conditioned reflex, 1136
Confusion, geriatric, 279–280
Connectedness of body regions and systems, 24,
    49–50
  autonomic nervous system in, 53–80
Connective tissue, 50
  dense, 29, 35
  diseases, 464–465
  of head, 517
  innervation of, 62
  loose, 29, 35
  microscopic appearance of, 29–30
  thoracic, 370
Constipation alternating with diarrhea, 383
Consultants in osteopathic manipulative
    medicine, 1046–1047
Contraction, 1129
  of skeletal muscles, 36
Control, and mitigation of stress, 213
Conus medullaris, 583
Cooling with stretching, in myofascial trigger
    points, 924, 927
Coronal plane of body, 1134, 1135
Coronary artery disease, 299–307
  analysis of ECG in, 239–241
  and angina pectoris, 304–305
  diagnosis of, 303–384
  and myocardial infarction, 305
  osteopathic approach to, 305–307
  pathophysiology and natural history of,
    299–303
  treatment of, 304
Corticosteroids, 84, 115–116, 122–123
  affecting neural activity, 88
Corticotropin (ACTH), 84, 115, 122
  releasing factor, 84, 115, 117–118, 122
    in stress response, 100
Cortisol, 84, 91, 115
  deficiency of, 91–92
  in stress response, 100
Costosternal joint of first rib, motion tests, 553
Costovertebral joints, 564
  motion tests, 553
Counseling in pain management, 183
Counternutation, 1129
  sacral, 607–608, 851
Counterstrain techniques, 809–818, 820, 1133
  cervical, 814
  complications from, 1020
  location of tender points in, 810–811

lumbar, 816–817
pelvic, 817–818
position of comfort in, 809, 811–813
in postoperative disorders, 390
posttreatment reaction in, 812
rechecking of tender points in, 813–814
and returning patient to neutral, 813
ribs, 815–816
therapeutic pulse in, 812–813
thoracic, 814–815
Coupled motions of spine, 513
  lumbar, 591
  thoracic, 572
Coxa valga, 626
Coxa vara, 626
Cranial dura mater, 34
Cranial field, 901–913, 1134
  articular mobility of bones in, 903
  evaluation in hospitalized patients, 1041, 1043
  motion assessment, 539–540
    palpation in, 904–905
    still point in, 913, 1138
  primary respiratory mechanisms in, 902–904,
    1135 (see also Primary respiratory
    mechanisms)
Cranial nerves, 60, 63, 371, 524–530
  entrapment, 411
  neuropathies, 413
Craniosacral extension, 1129
Craniosacral flexion, 1130
Craniosacral mechanism, 1129
Cranium, 515, 901–913 (see also Head)
Cremasteric reflex, 506
Crepitus in knee joint, 628
Cretinism, 88
Crohn's disease, 382–383
Cruciate ligaments, 631
Crystal-induced arthritis, 463
Cuboid bone
  Hiss plantar whip for displacement, 690
  somatic dysfunction of, 640
Cuneiform bones
  Hiss plantar whip for displacement, 690
  somatic dysfunction of, 640
Cushing's disease, 123
Cushing's syndrome from ectopic ACTH in
    malignancies, 422
Cyst, Baker's, 657, 658
Cytokines
  characteristics of, 101
  in inflammation, 101
  proinflammatory, 123

Dalrymple pump, 956–957, 1133
Dartos fascia, 50
Death, leading causes of, 157
Decompensation, 1129
  postural, 970, 1135
Deep tendon reflex
  Achilles, 643
  patellar, 642
Defense reactions, inflammatory mediators in,
    101–103
Definition of osteopathic medicine, 11–12

Delirium diagnosis, criteria for, 279–280
Deltoid ligament, 637–638
Dementia diagnosis, criteria for, 279–280
Dental problems, primary respiratory mechanisms
    in, 911
Depression
  cognitive behavioral factors in, 208–209
  drug-induced, 209
  exercise therapy in, 201
  geriatric, 279
  hypothalamic-pituitary-adrenal axis in, 120,
    123
  measurement of, 208
  and physical illness, 168
  stress-induced, 207–209
De Quervain's tenosynovitis, postpartum, 358
Dermatomes, 37, 39, 41
  lower extremity, 643
  lumbar, 582, 589
  thoracic, anterior, 611
Dermatomyositis, 464–465
  in malignancies, 421
Desensitization, systematic, in stress management,
    213–214
Detrusor muscle, 76
Development (see Life phases)
Diabetes mellitus
  exercise in, 199
  hypertension in, 325
  insulin deficiency in, 91–92
Diagnostic problem solving, 219–241
Diaphragm
  pelvic, 369, 602–603, 945–946
    dysfunction diagnosis and treatment,
      953–954
    muscle energy treatment for myofascial
      tension, 760–761
  thoracoabdominal, 568, 569, 585–586, 588
    affecting lymph flow, 945
    doming of, to improve lymphatic flow,
      951–953
    evaluation of, 578
    fascial restriction diagnosis and treatment,
      951–953
    muscle energy techniques, 756–760
    myofascial and integrated
      neuromusculoskeletal release, 870–874
    neuroregulation of, 448
  urogenital, 370, 603, 945–946
Diaries by patients, on health problems, 1070
Diarrhea, 381–382
  alternating with constipation, 383
  antibiotic-induced, 382
  from endocrine-producing tumors, 382
  invading organisms in, 381
  osmotic, 381
  secretory, 381
  toxigenic, 381
Diet (see Nutrition)
Digestion disorders, 380–381
Digitorum longus muscles of foot
  extensor, 648, 649
  flexor, 649
Dihydrotestosterone, 84

Diltiazem in hypertension, 325
Disease, and body-mind-spirit triad, 246–247
Disks, intervertebral
   degeneration of, 342, 408
   lumbar, 583, 622
   thoracic, 564
Diuretics in hypertension, 323–324
Diverticular disease, 383–384
   bleeding in, 384
Diverticulitis, 384
Diverticulosis coli, 384
Doctor–patient relationship, 164–165
Drainage pathways for blood and lymph, 48
Drawer tests of cruciate ligaments, 631, 633
Drop arm test, 558–559
Drop of foot, 643
Drop-off sign, spinal, in spondylolisthesis, 1010
Drop test of hip, 492, 497–498, 593–594
Drug therapy (see Pharmacology)
Drug-induced conditions
   blood pressure alterations, 321
   depression, 209
   in elderly persons, 282
Duodenum
   innervation of, 70
   peptic ulcer, 378–379
Dura mater, 517, 524
   cranial, 34
      innervation of, 63
      meningeal layer of, 34, 43
      periosteal layer of, 34
   mobility of, 903
   spinal, 34, 43
Dwarfism, 91
Dynamic motion, sacral, 608
Dynorphin, 148
Dysmenorrhea, 365–366

Ears, 293–295, 532
   anatomy and physiology of, 293
   osteopathic approach to, 296
   otitis media, 294–295
   pathophysiology of, 293–294
Eaton-Lambert syndrome in malignancies, 423
Ecology, pediatric, 269–270
Edema, 946
   drainage pathways in, 48
Education
   in osteopathic medicine
      history of, 15–18
      and state licensure, 17–18
   for patients
      in postural decompensation, 974
      in spondylolisthesis, 1011
Efficacy of manipulation, 1015–1018
   in low back pain, 1016–1017
   research studies, 1117–1118
   in systemic disease, 1017–1018
Effleurage, 1129
   lower extremity, 966–967
   to promote lymphatic flow, 959–967
   upper extremity, 965–966
Effusions in knee, tests for, 657, 659
Elastic cartilage, 30

Elastic recoil, pulmonary, 442
Elbow joint, 548, 553–556
   muscle energy techniques, 740–742
   muscles of, 550
   myofascial and integrated neuromusculoskeletal
      release, 891–899
   somatic dysfunction of, 555–556
   tennis, 559, 925
   thrust technique for restriction, 685–686
Elderly persons (see Geriatrics)
Electrical nerve stimulation, transcutaneous, 182,
      432, 435
   in angina pectoris, 307
   in postural decompensation, 975–976
   in scoliosis, 996
Electrocardiography
   analysis in diagnostic problem solving, 239–241
   in coronary artery disease, 303–384
Electromyography, 436
Embryology of neuromusculoskeletal system,
      27–29
   limb development in, 39–41
Emotional stimuli affecting neuroendocrine-
      immune network, 128
Emphysema, pulmonary, 442
   osteopathic treatment of, 455–456
Encephalitis, headache in, 406
Encephalopathy, uremic, 396
Endocrine system, 25, 83–92 (see also
      Neuroendocrine-immune system)
   biosynthesis of hormones in, 85–86 (see also
      Hormones)
      regulation of, 89–90
   cardiovascular system interaction with, 87–88
   cellular processing in, 85–86
   chemical structure of hormones in, 84, 85
   modulation of immune system, 122–126
   nervous system interaction with, 88–89,
      116–119
   processes regulated by hormones, 90–92
   research applied to osteopathic practice,
      1113
   stress affecting, 99–100
   structure and function of, 85–87
Endocytosis, and thyroid hormone release, 86
Endometrial cells, 112
Endometriosis, 367–368
Endorphins, 123, 125–126
Endothelial cells, 112
Endothelial-derived relaxing factor, 302
Endurance exercise, 436
Enteric nervous system, 69, 72
Enterochromaffin cells, 112
Enthesitis, 1129
Entrapment neuropathies, 411–413
   of central nervous system, 910
Eosinophils, 111
Epidemiology, 1095–1099
   analytic strategy in, 1097
   descriptive strategy in, 1096–1097
   experimental strategy in, 1097
   studies of somatic dysfunction, 1097–1099
Epididymis, innervation of, 78
Epidural stimulation in angina pectoris, 307

Epinephrine, 84
Erector spinae muscles, 569, 581
Esophagus, 375–377
   achalasia, 377
   cancer, 377
   diffuse spasm, 376–377
   innervation, 64, 67
   reflux disease, 375–376
Estrogens, 84
   and reproductive function, 91
Ethmoid sinus, 290, 532
Ethyl chloride in pain management, 182
Eustachian tube, 293, 532
Exaggeration treatment, 1133
Exercise, 158–159, 1049–1055
   aerobic, 1050–1051
   anaerobic, 1051
   angry cat, 1054
   in anxiety disorders, 200–201
   beneficial aspects of, 1049
   in cardiac rehabilitation, 304
   cervical isometrics, 1054–1055
   constant rest position, 1052
   in depression, 201
   detrimental aspects of, 1049
   to develop sense of touch, 479–482
   in diabetes mellitus, 199
   dose of, 1055
   dynamic, physiologic adaptations to, 197–198
   flexibility or stretching, 1050
   and health, 197–201
   and heart disease prevention, 198–199
   hip hyperextensions, 1054
   and hypertension prevention, 199
   illustrated for patients, 1052–1055
   isokinetic, 434
   isotonic, 434
   for kinesthetic balance, 1051
   lipoprotein levels in, 199
   muscle soreness from, 1052
   in obesity, 199–200
   and osteoarthritis, 464
   in osteoporosis, 200
   pelvic tilt, 1053
   in postural decompensation, 974
      in sagittal plane, 1004
   in pregnancy, 353
   preparation for, 1051–1052
   program with myofascial and integrated
      neuromusculoskeletal release, 849
   and psychological health, 200–201
   for spinal areas, 1052
   in spondylolisthesis, 1011
   and sports medicine, 285–287
   to stabilize joints, 1051
   strengthening, 1051, 1053
   stretching, 1051–1052
   therapeutic, 432–436
   toning, 1051
   torso curl, 1053
      reverse, 1053
   torso extension, 1053–1054
   warm-up, 1051
   writing prescription for, 1055–1056

Exocytosis, and hormone release, 85
Extension, 1129
  cervical spine, 542, 543
    test for C2-7 motion, 544–545
  craniosacral, 1129
  hip, 625
    hyperextension, 1054
  knee, 630
  lumbar spine, 591
    testing of, 595
  sacral, 607, 1130
    bilateral, 621
    unilateral, 621
  thoracic spine, 572
    testing of, 576
  wrist, 557
Eye muscles and nerves, 532

FABERE test of hip, 627
Face
  arterial supply, 517
  bones of, 515
  muscles of expression, 43
Facial nerve, 63, 522, 530, 571
  paralysis of, 530
Facilitated positional release, 831–832, 1133
  cervical, 833–834
  gluteal and hip, 840–841
  in intervertebral motion restrictions, 832
  lumbar, 836–840
    in diskogenic pain syndrome, 839–840
    in extension dysfunction, 836–838
    in flexion dysfunction, 838–839
    soft tissue treatment, 836
  sacroiliac, 840
  thoracic, 834–836
  in tissue texture changes, 832
Facilitation, 1130
  neuromuscular proprioceptive, in pain
      management, 183
  segmental, 402–403
  in upper thoracic cord segments, 522
Falls, in geriatric patients, 281–282
Falx cerebelli, 517
Family life, 162–163
Family practice, osteopathic, 249–254
  basics of, 250–251
  case studies of, 250, 251–252
  foundations of, 249–250
  and gatekeeper role of physician, 254
  office diagnosis and treatment procedures in,
      253
  palpatory diagnosis and manipulative care in,
      252
  pharmacotherapeutics in, 252–253
  preventive medicine and health maintenance in,
      254
  psychosocial considerations in, 253
Fascia, 35, 819–820
  as connector, 50
  deep, 35
    connective tissue in, 29
  innervation of, 62
  in intermuscular septa, 35

lata, 603
  relaxation techniques, 792–793
  lumbar, 584–585
  myofascial continuity, 41–43
  in neurovascular bundle, 35
  patterns of rotatory preference, 946–947, 972,
      974, 1130
  restrictions of pelvis, 616–617
  superficial, 35
  thoracic, 570
Fascial-ligamentous release, 819–829
  axillary, 826
  basilar axes of skull, 829
  cervical area, 826
  clavicular and glenohumeral, 827–828
  diagnostic touch in, 821
  liver, 823
  lower extremity, 823–825
  lumbar, 822
  observation and palpation in, 821
  occipitoatlantal articulation, 829
  pelvis and sacrum, 821–822
  ribs, 825
  scapulofascial, 826
  supine treatment, 821
  thoracic aperture expansion
    inferior, 827
    superior, 828
  thoracic region, 825–826
  treatment considerations in, 820–821
  wrist and hand, 828
Feedback mechanisms in hormone secretion
      regulation, 89–90
Femoral artery, 646, 650
Femoral nerve, 588
  entrapment of, 411
  lateral cutaneous, 588, 611
  posterior cutaneous, 605, 611
Femoral triangle, 650, 656
Femoroacetabular joint (see Hip)
Femorotibial joint (see Knee)
Femur, 626
  angle of inclination, 626
  longitudinal axis, 626–627
Ferguson lumbosacral angle, 1001, 1031,
      1127
Fibroblasts, 29, 112
Fibroids, uterine, 367
Fibromyalgia, 464
  manipulative therapy in, 465
Fibrous cartilage, 30
Fibrous joints, 33
Fibula
  head dysfunction, 631, 633
  motions of, 631, 633
  thrust techniques
    anterior head, 687
    posterior head, 686–687
Filum terminale, 583
Fixator muscles, 36
Flares, innominate, 617–618
Flexion, 1130
  cervical spine, 542, 543
    test for C2-7 motion, 544–545

craniosacral, 1130
hip, 625–626
lumbar spine, 591
  testing of, 595
plantar, 634
sacral, 607, 1130
  bilateral, 620–621
  unilateral, 621
in sacroiliac dysfunction
  seated test, 613
  standing test, 612–613
seated tests, 498, 613
standing tests, 496, 612–613
thoracic spine, 572
  testing of, 576
wrist, 557
Follicle-stimulating hormone, 84, 91
Food and Drug Administration (FDA), 1101
Foot, 635–642
  arches of, 639
  drop, 643
  fascial-ligamentous release, 824–825
  motion of, 635–636
  muscles of, 649
  myofascial and integrated neuromusculoskeletal
      release, 887
  nerve supply, 646
  plantar ligaments, 639
  soft tissue techniques, 793–794
  somatic dysfunction of, 640–642
  transverse tarsal joint, 639–640
Foramen magnum, 34, 43
Forearm
  interosseous membrane of, 553–554, 555
    relaxation technique, 791
  myofascial and integrated neuromusculoskeletal
      release, 891–899
  palpation of motions in, 555
  pronation of, 554, 555
  somatic dysfunction of, 556
  supination of, 554, 556
Fowler's position for examination of hospitalized
      patient, 1040
Frankenhäuser plexus of nerves, 79
Frontal plane of body, 1134, 1135
Frontal sinus, 290, 531–532
Frozen shoulder, 560–561
Functional assessment of geriatric patients,
      277–278
Functional technique, 795–808, 829
  cervical, 802–803
  compression test in, 799–800
  guidelines for, 800
  history of, 795–799
  innominate, 803–804
  knee, 805
  positional concepts in, 800–801
  ribs, 805–808
  in thoracic, lumbar, and sacral regions,
      801–802

Gait
  examination of, 491, 494
  training in pain management, 183

Galbreath mandibular drainage
    in otitis media, 294, 296
    to promote lymphatic flow, 959, 1132, 1133
Gallbladder
    innervation of, 70
    viscerosomatic reference sites for, 450
Ganglia, autonomic, 54, 56–57
    paravertebral, 56, 57, 58–59
    prevertebral, 56, 57, 58–59
Gas exchange, respiratory, 441–442, 446–447
Gastritis, 378
Gastrocnemius muscle, 647, 648
Gastroesophageal reflux disease, 375–376
Gastrointestinal system, 375–385
    diarrheal illnesses, 381–385
    esophageal disorders, 375–377
    gastric inflammatory disease, 378–379
    innervation of, 69–74
    lymphoid tissue in, 942
    small intestine and colon disorders, 380–381
    stomach disorders, 377–378
Gate-control theory of pain, 173–174
Gemellus muscles, 603
General adaptation response, 100, 127–129
General internists, osteopathic, 257–259
Genetic factors in spondylolisthesis, 1006
Genitalia, external, lymphatic drainage of,
        604
Genitofemoral nerve, 364, 588
Genu
    recurvatum, 630
    valgum, 627
    varum, 337, 627
Geriatrics, 273–283
    clinical impact of physiology of aging, 275–276
    comprehensive assessment in, 274–279
        functional, 277–278
        medical, 276–277
        psychological, 278–279
        social, 279
    falls in, 281–282
    hip fracture in, 334–335
    iatrogenic disorders in, 282–283
    laboratory values in, 278
    neuroendocrine-immune system in, 129–130
    and osteopathic medicine, 283
    structural changes in, 51
    theories of aging, 273–274
    urinary incontinence in, 280–281
Giantism, 91
Glaucoma, headache in, 406
Glenohumeral joint, 548
    motion tests, 552
    muscle energy techniques, 735–738
    muscles of, 549
Glomerular filtration rate, estimation of, 393
Glossary of osteopathic terminology, 1126–1140
Glossopharyngeal nerve, 63, 530, 571
Glucagon, 84
    in stress response, 100
Glucocorticoid hormones, 115–116, 122
Glutamate as neuroregulator, 109–110
Gluteus muscles, 603, 645, 646
    facilitated positional release, 840–841

inhibited, symptoms of, 976
Gonadal plexus of nerves, 78
Gonadotropin-releasing hormone, 91
    inhibition of, 125
Gonococcal arthritis, 463
Gout, 463
Gracilis muscle, 603, 647
Gravitational line, 1001, 1130–1131
Gravitational stress, postural, 970, 999–1001
Growth and development, hormones affecting,
        91
Growth hormone, 84, 91, 124
    inhibiting hormone, 84, 124
    releasing hormone, 84
    secretion in sleep, 89
    in stress response, 100
Guidelines for osteopathic practice, 1021
Gynecology, 363–371
    pelvic floor dysfunction, 369–371
    pelvic pain, 363–369

Habits
    health, 157–166
    sleep, 215
Habituation, 1131
    in reflexes, 147
Hallucis longus muscles, 649
Hallux valgus, 640
Hammer toes, 642
Hamstring muscles, 645, 646
    spastic, symptoms of, 976
    test of, 613–614
    unequal length of, 618
Hand, somatic dysfunction of, 557–558 (see also
        Upper extremities)
Hawthorne effect in clinical trials, 1119–1120
Head, 515–540, 901–913
    arterial supply, 517, 521, 525
    in common cold, 532
    complications from manipulations of,
        1020–1021
    connective tissue of, 517
    cranial motion assessment, 539–540 (see also
        Cranial field)
    cranial nerves, 524–530
    ear structures, 532
    effleurage to promote lymphatic flow, 959
    eye muscles and nerves, 532, 533
    innervation of, 62–63
        parasympathetic, 522, 528
        sympathetic, 522, 524, 528
    lymphatic drainage, 521–522, 527
    muscles of, 515–517
    paranasal sinuses, 531–532
    primary respiratory mechanism in, 902–904
    skeletal structure of, 515
    strains of sphenobasilar synchondrosis, 906–907
    venous drainage, 521, 525
Headache, 403–408, 532–539
    classification of, 403
    cluster, 406–407, 536
    in cranial neuralgias, 538–539
    migraine, 404–406, 535–536
    in systemic or neurologic disorders, 406

in temporomandibular joint dysfunction,
        538–539
    tension, 403, 536–537
    traction and inflammatory, 537–538
    treatment of, 408
    in trigeminal neuralgia, 538
    vascular, 535–536
Head's law, 1132
Healing and repair at microscopic level, 31
Health
    criteria for, 246
    exercise and fitness in, 197–201
    habits of, 157–166
    in life phases, 191–194
    maintenance of, 187–194
        in family practice, 254
        innovative program for, 188–189
        in internal medicine, 258–259
        patient's role in, 187
        and physician as patient, 189
        physician's role in, 188
        planning research on, 1101–1105
Health Care Financing Administration (HCFA),
        1101
Health-oriented care, 7
    as national strategy, 11
    and self-regulation principle, 5, 10
Heart
    disease prevention with exercise, 198–199
    innervation of, 64, 65–66
        afferent nerves in, 66
        efferent nerves in, 65
        parasympathetic, 143
        sympathetic, 141–143
    ischemic disease, 299–307
    in renal failure, 398
    viscerosomatic reference sites for, 450
    viscerosomatic reflexes, 143
Heart failure, 307–313
    diagnosis of, 310
    natural history of, 309–310
    osteopathic approach to, 311–313
    pathophysiology of, 308–309
    treatment of, 310–311
Heartburn, 375–376
Heat, therapeutic, 431–432
    and hot packs for pain management, 182
Heel
    lifts for
        in short leg syndrome, 987–989
        in spondylolisthesis, 1012
    mid-heel line, 1132
Heilig formula for lifts in short leg syndrome,
        987
Helicobacter pylori infection, 378
    treatment of, 379
Hemorrhage
    and diverticular bleeding, 384
    intracranial, headache in, 536
Hepatocytes, 112
Hering-Breuer inflation reflex, 448
Hernia, hiatal, 376
Herpes zoster, headache in, 406
Hiatal hernia, 376

High-velocity low-amplitude forces
   in sacroiliac dysfunction, 618–619
   in thrust techniques, (see Thrust techniques)
Hip, 601, 625–627, 1131
   anteriorly rotated technique, 683–684
   Barlow test for reduction, 625
   coxa valga, 626
   coxa vara, 626
   developmental dysplasia of, 331–334
   drop test, 492, 497–498, 593–594
   extension of, 625
   facilitated positional release, 840–841
   flares, 617–618
   flexion of, 625–626
   fracture in elderly persons, 334–335
   functional technique, 803–804
   hyperextension exercise, 1054
   ligaments of, 625
   motion of, 606–607
   muscle energy techniques, 720–722, 746–753
   muscles of, 643, 645–646
   myofascial and integrated neuromusculoskeletal
      release, 866–869
   Ortolani test for dislocation, 331, 624, 625
   pain referred from, 643
   posteriorly rotated technique, 684
   rotations, 617
   sheared, 617
   somatic dysfunctions of ilium, 1131
   superior shear technique, 684–685
   trochanteric bursitis, 656
   upslipped technique, 684–685
Hiss plantar whip, 690
Histaminergic axons in peripheral vasculature,
      61–62
History of osteopathic medicine, 3–4, 15–21
   activities of American Osteopathic Association,
      18–19
   conflict with American Medical Association, 16
   first school chartered, 15–16
   hospitals established, 7, 20
   professional education, 15–18
      curriculum in, 16–17
   recognition by federal government, 19
   specialties developed, 19–20
HIV infection
   diarrhea in, 381–382
   in hospitalized patients, 1044
Home safety measures, 162
Homeostasis, 1131
   drugs affecting, 94
   endocrine physiology in, 89–91
   and internal personal health care system, 5, 10
      as guide to medical practice, 11
   neuroendocrine and immune systems in,
      107–132
   stressors affecting, 103
Hormones
   in adaptive response to stress, 115–116
   biosynthesis of, 85–86
   changes in pregnancy, 352
   chemical structure of, 83, 84 (see also Endocrine
      system)
   counterregulatory, 100

in defense of internal environment, 91
   and energy metabolism, 91–92
   in growth and development, 91
   hydrophilic, 87
   hypophysiotropic, 89, 117
   interactions with receptors, 87
   lipophilic, 87
   mechanism of action, 86–87
   processes regulated by, 90–92
   and reproductive function, 91
   role in body unity, 87–89
   secretion regulation, 89–90
      control mechanisms in, 89–90
      temporal patterns in, 90
   transport and metabolism of, 86
Horner syndrome, 522
   in cluster headache, 536
Hospice care, 426–427
Hospitalized patients, 1037–1047
   AIDS in, 1044
   for drug and alcohol detoxification, 1045
   elderly, 282–283
   follow-up evaluation and treatment, 1046
   history-taking procedure, 1037
   in isolation, 1045
   musculoskeletal examination for, 501, 505–506
   osteopathic consultations for, 1046–1047
   pediatric, 1045
   physical examination of, 1038–1041
      recording of, 1046
   postoperative or posttrauma, 1045
   psychiatric, 1045–1046
   on respirators or in intensive care unit, 1045
   treatment of, 1041–1047
      protocol for, 1043–1044
Hot packs for pain management, 182
Humeroulnar joint (see Elbow joint)
Hyaline cartilage, 30
   in synovial joints, 32
Hydrocephalus, headache in, 406, 537
Hydrocollator packs, 431
Hydrophilic hormones, 87
Hydrotherapy, 431
Hypercalcemia in malignancies, 422
Hypercapnia, 447
Hyperextension
   hip exercise, 1054
   lumbopelvic, 725
Hypermobile joints, unstable, thrust technique
      affecting, 664–665
Hypertension, 319–326
   accelerated, 319
   clinical trials in, 320–321
   in diabetes mellitus, 325
   diagnosis of, 321–322
   diastolic, 319
   drug-induced, 321
   drug therapy in, 96–97
   essential or secondary, 319–320
   etiology of, 96
   exercise for prevention of, 199
   headache in, 406, 537
   heart failure in, 308
   intracranial, headache in, 406

labile, 319
   laboratory tests in, 322
   left ventricular hypertrophy with, 325
   osteopathic approach to, 326
   physical examination in, 321–322
   pulmonary, 446
   in renal failure, 397–398
   resistant, 325
   systolic, isolated, 319
   treatment of, 322–325
Hypogastric ganglia, 56, 57
Hypogastric plexus
   inferior, 60, 68, 76, 79, 606
   superior, 68
Hypoglossal nerve, 530
Hypothalamic-pituitary-adrenal axis, hormones
      of, 122–123
Hypothalamic-pituitary-thyroid axis, hormones
      of, 123–124
Hypothalamus, 53, 116–119
   hormones of, 84
   neuroendocrine cells in, 99
Hypothetico-deductive method in clinical
      problem solving, 222–224
Hypothyroidism, congenital, 88
Hypoxemia, 447

Ice, in pain management, 182
Ileum, innervation of, 70
Ileus
   adynamic, 390
   postfracture, 597–598
   postoperative, 389–390, 597–598
Iliac arteries, 604
Iliac crest levelness test, 612
Iliac spines
   anterior superior (ASIS)
      compression test, 616, 1038
      levelness test, 614
   posterior superior (PSIS), levelness test, 482,
      491, 612, 614
Iliacus muscle, 582, 585
Iliococcygeus muscle, 369
Iliocostalis muscles, 567, 585
Iliofemoral ligament, 625
Iliohypogastric nerve, 588
Ilioinguinal nerve, 588
   entrapment of, 411
Iliolumbar ligaments, 584, 602
   pain from postural imbalance, 985
   pain referral from, 603
   in postural decompensation, 999
   in spondylolisthesis, 1010
Iliopsoas muscles, 582, 603, 645
   referred pain pattern, 592
   spastic, symptoms of, 976
   tender points, 595
   unequal length of, 618
Iliosacral dysfunction, 617–618
Ilium, 601 (see also Hip)
Immobilization of elderly persons, problems with,
      282
Immune system
   afferent innervation of glands in, 121

autonomic nervous system affecting, 119–121
cell types in, 111
cellular immunity, 944
efferent innervation of glands in, 119–121
endocrine modulation of, 122–126
humoral immunity, 944
interaction with neuroendocrine system, 103
  and aging, 129–130
  factors affecting, 126–129
  and psychoneuroimmunology, 167–169
  signal coding in, 108–116
in malignancies, 427
modulation by central nervous system, 116–119
research applied to osteopathic practice, 1113
stress affecting, 168
thoracic lymphatic pump affecting, 453–454
Immunoregulators, 111–115
Inclination, angle of, 626
Incontinence, urinary, 370–371
geriatric, 280–281
Indirect or functional technique, 795–808
Infancy, 192
Infarction, myocardial, 305 (*see also* Coronary
  artery disease)
circadian pattern of onset, 301
Infectious arthritis, 463
Inflammation, 101–103
mediators of, 122
Inflammatory disease
arthritis, 460–463
bowel, 382–383
gastric, 378
headache, 537–538
pelvic, 368
Infrahyoid node technique to promote lymphatic
  flow, 961
Inguinal ligament, 603
Inherent motion
of brain and spinal cord, 903
cranial, palpation of, 904–905
monitoring of, 846
sacral, 607–608
  palpation of, 610
Inhibited muscle symptoms, 976
Inhibition in soft tissue techniques, 781, 1131
Injections in myofascial trigger points, 925
in spondylolisthesis, 1012
Innominate bones (*see* Hip)
Insomnia, psychological management of,
  214–215
Insulin, 84, 91
deficiency of, 91–92
in stress response, 100
Integrated neuromusculoskeletal release (*See*
  Myofascial and integrated
  neuromusculoskeletal release)
Integration of body regions and systems, 24,
  49–50
autonomic nervous system in, 53–80
Intercarpal joints, 548
somatic dysfunction of, 557–558
Intercostal muscles, 566
Intercostal nerve entrapment, 411
Interferons, 114–115

Interleukins, 101–102
IL-1, 112–113, 123
  biologic effects of, 102
IL-2, 113
IL-6, 113–114, 123
Intermuscular septa, 35
Internal medicine, osteopathic, 257–259
diagnosis and treatment in, 258
preventive medicine and health maintenance in,
  258–259
Interneurons, 55
in pulmonary plexus, 66
Interosseous membrane of forearm, 553–554,
  555
relaxation technique, 791
strains of, 555
Interphalangeal joints of hand, 548
somatic dysfunction of, 558
Interspinales muscles, 568, 584
Interstitial fluids affected by primary respiratory
  mechanisms, 910
Intertransversarii muscles, 568, 585
Intervertebral disks
degeneration of, 342, 408
lumbar, 583
thoracic, 564
Intestines, 380–385
colorectal neoplasms, 384–385
diarrhea, 381–382
diverticular disease, 383–384
inflammatory bowel disease, 382–383
innervation of, 70–74
  large bowel, 71
  small bowel, 70
irritable bowel syndrome, 383
malabsorption, 380–381
postoperative ileus, 389–390
Irritable bowel syndrome, 383
Irvine study of manipulative treatment,
  1116–1117
Ischemia
myocardial (*see* Coronary artery disease)
transient attacks of, headaches in, 537
Ischiococcygeus muscle, 369
Ischiorectal fossa, landmarks of, 760
Isokinetic exercise, 434
Isolytic contraction, 693
Isometric contraction, 36, 693
and postisometric relaxation, 694
Isotonic contraction, 36
concentric, 693
eccentric, 693
Isotonic exercise, 434

Jejunum, innervation of, 70
Joints
cartilaginous, 34
dysfunction of, 35
fibrous, 33
in malignancies, 420–421
nonsynovial, 33–34
play of, 35
synovial, 31–33
Jones tender points, 810

Jugular veins, internal, 521
Jungmann pelvic index, 1001, 1031

Kegel's exercises, 371
Kidneys, 393–398
acute failure, 393
  causes of, 396
chronic failure, 393–394
  anemia in, 397
  basic management of, 395
  encephalopathy in, 396
  hypertension in, 397–398
  musculoskeletal manifestations of, 39
  myocardial function in, 398
  neuropathies in, 396–397
  osteodystrophy in, 394–396
end-stage disease, 393
innervation of, 74–75
renal cell cancer, 418
Kinesthesia, 1131
Kinetics, 1131
Kirksville Krunch, 671
Klapping, 1132
Kneading of soft tissue, 781, 1132
Knee, 33, 627–631
extension of, 630
functional technique, 805
gliding of, 630
ligaments and cartilage, 630–631
muscle energy techniques, 753
muscles of, 647
osteoarthritis of, 335–337
patella, 627–630
  bursitis of, 656–657
in Q-angle, 627
tests for effusions in, 657, 659
vascular supply of, 650
Kupffer cells, 111
Kyphoscoliosis, 1132
Kyphosis, 1132
Kyphotic curves, thoracic, 563, 970, 972

Labor, 356–358
Laboratory values, age affecting, 278
Lachman test of cruciate ligaments, 631, 633
Lacteals, 942
Laryngopharynx, 295
Lateral translation test
for C2-7 motion, 545
for occipital motion, 544
Latissimus dorsi muscle, 565, 581
Learning
observational, and coping with stress, 213
patterns in depression, 208–209
Leg (*see* Lower extremities)
Leiomyomas, uterine, 367
Leptomeningeal carcinomatosis, 420
Lesion, osteopathic, (*see* Somatic dysfunction)
Levator ani, 369, 602
Levator scapulae, 541, 565
Levatores costarum, 566
Levitor orthotic, 975
in sagittal plane postural decompensation, 1005
in spondylolisthesis, 1012

Lhermitte's sign, 410
Licensure, state laws for, 17–18
Life expectancy, 157
Life phases, 191–194
    adolescence, 193
    adulthood, 193–194
    continuities and discontinuities in, 191
    elders, 194
    infancy, 192
    one-to-five-year olds, 192
    prenatal period, 101–192
    school-age children, 192–193
Lifestyles, and health habits, 157–166
Lift therapy
    anterior, for pelvic rotation, 989
    in short leg syndrome, 987–989
        in childhood, 988
        Heilig formula for, 987
    in spondylolisthesis, 1012
Ligaments (see also Fascial-ligamentous release)
    cervical spine, 542
    connective tissue in, 29
    hip, 625
    knee, 630–631
    lumbar, 584
    pelvis and sacrum, 602
    of synovial joints
        accessory, 32
        capsular, 32
Limbic system, 53, 128
    bridge with hypothalamus, 118
Lipophilic hormones, 87
Lipoprotein levels, exercise affecting, 199
Liver
    fascial-ligamentous release, 823
    innervation of, 70, 74
    lymphatic pump, 957–958
Longissimus muscle, 567, 584
Lordosis, 1132
    in lumbosacral spring test, 615–616
    in spondylolisthesis, 1007–1008
        correction of, 1011–1012
Lordotic curves, lumbar, 584, 970, 972
Lower extremities, 623–660
    anatomy, 39–41
    ankle, 633–635
    compartment syndromes, 650, 655, 657
    effleurage and pétrissage, 966–967
    fascial-ligamentous release, 823–824
    foot, 635–642
    functional technique, 805
    hip, 625–627
    knee, 627–631
    muscle energy techniques, 746–756
    muscles of, 646, 647–649, 651–654
    nerve supply, 646, 655
    neuromuscular structures and function,
        642–649
    referred pain, 643
    screening examination, 493, 500
    skeletal and ligamentous structures and
        function, 623–642
    soft tissue techniques, 792–794

    somatic dysfunction
        muscular, 643–646
        skeletal, 640–642
    thrust techniques, 686–690
    vascular and lymphatic structures and function,
        646–660
Lumbar and abdominal region, 581 (see also
        Abdominal region)
    articulatory techniques, 771–775
    counterstrain techniques, 816–817
    diagnosis of problems in, 592–596
    exercises for disk problems, 1052
    facilitated positional release, 836–840
    fascial-ligamentous release, 822
    functional anatomy of, 582–591
    functional technique in, 801–802
    ligaments, muscles, and fascia, 584–586
    motion of, 591
        testing of, 593–595
    muscle energy techniques, 716–720
    myofascial and integrated neuromusculoskeletal
        release, 851–858
    nerves of, 588–591
    pain referred from, 643
    palpation of, 593
    reflexes and muscle strength tests, 506
    soft tissue techniques, 787–790
    treatment of problems in, 596–599
    vasculature and lymphatics, 587–588
Lumbar plexus, 38, 39, 581, 588, 605
Lumbopelvic hyperextension, 725
Lumbosacral angle, 1031, 1127
    measurement of, 1001, 1002
Lumbosacral pain, exercises for, 1052
Lumbosacral spring test, 615–616
Lungs, 441
    carcinoma, 418–419
        and paraneoplastic syndromes, 418–419, 421,
            422
    chronic obstructive disease, osteopathic
        treatment of, 455–456
    circulation in, 444–446
    in emphysema, 442
    fibrosis of, 442
    function measurements, 444
    gas exchange in, 446–447
    innervation of, 66
    osteopathic manipulations affecting, 452–453
    prevention of postoperative complications, 456
    viscerosomatic reference sites for, 450
Lupus erythematosus, 464–465
    manipulative therapy in, 465
Luschka's joints, uncinate, 541
Luteinizing hormone, 84, 91
Lymph, 943–944
    flow mechanisms, 945–946
Lymph nodes, 942
    efferent innervation of, 121
    enlargement of, 48
Lymphatic drainage
    rectal, 604–605
Lymphatic system, 48, 941–967
    anatomy of, 941–944

    channels in, 942–943
    in cleansing of tissues, 944
    defensive properties of, 944
    direct pressure techniques, 958–966
        abdominal, 961–964
        head effleurage, 959–961
        lower extremity, 966–967
        rib raising, 950–951
        upper extremity, 964–966
    drainage from head, 521–522, 527
    ducts in, 943
    efferent innervation of, 120–121
    embryology of, 941
    in fluid balance maintenance, 944
    lower extremity, 650
    lumbar and abdominal region, 587–588
    manipulative techniques, 947–967
        doming of diaphragm, 951–954
        effleurage and pétrissage, 959–967
        to open thoracic fascial inlet, 948–949
        to promote lymphatic flow, 954–967
        to remove impediments to flow, 948–954
        rib raising in, 950–951
    myofascial trigger points affecting, 926–928
    in nutrition, 944–945
    organized tissues in, 941–942
    pathophysiology of, 946
    pectoral traction affecting, 955
    pelvis and sacrum, 604–605
    physiology of, 944–946
    pump techniques, 954–958, 1133
        abdominal, 956
        cervical, 542
        contraindicated in malignancies, 428
        liver, 957–958
        in lower extremity dysfunction, 658
        pedal, 956–957
        spleen, 957–958
        thoracic, 389, 453–454, 955–956, 1134
    thoracic, 452, 569–570
    types of treatment for, 947
    upper extremity, 549–550
Lymphocytes
    B cells, 111, 295, 944
    T cells, 111, 295, 944

Macrophages, 111
Malabsorption, intestinal, 380–381
Malignancies (see Oncology)
Malleoli
    lateral, thrust techniques, 688–689
    medial, levelness test, 613
    mid-malleolar line, 1132
Mandibular drainage technique of Galbreath,
        959, 1132, 1133
    in otitis media, 294, 296
Mandibular nerve, 528–529
Manipulative treatments, 1133 (see also
        Osteopathic treatment)
Manual medicine, 1132
Massage, 1132
Mast cells, 111
Maxillary nerve, 526, 528

Maxillary sinus, 290, 532
McMurray meniscal tests, 631, 632
Mechanoreceptor, 1132
Median nerve entrapment, 411
    in carpal tunnel syndrome, 559–560
Medical assessment of geriatric patients, 276–277
Medical records, 1077–1084
    in clinical research, 1078
    functions of, 1077–1078
    in hospital and ambulatory care, 1078
    information included in, 1081
    osteopathic components in, 1046, 1080–1084
        changes after treatment recorded, 1083–1084
        orders for manipulative treatment, 1083
    problem-oriented (POMR), 224, 1080
    public health utilization of data in, 1087–1090
    quality control in, 1080–1081
    standardized format in, 1078
    standardized forms in, 1078
    and subjective objective assessment plan
        (SOAP), 1080
    team approach to, 1080
Medical therapy (see Pharmacology)
Meissner's plexus, 67, 72
Melanocyte-stimulating hormone, 84
Melatonin, circadian cycle of, 126
Meningeal layer of cranial dura mater, 34
Meningitis, headache in, 406
Meniscus, ligament attachments to, 630
Menstruation
    dysmenorrhea, 365–366
    and premenstrual syndrome, 366
Mental examination in geriatric patients,
    278–279
Mesangial cells, 112
Mesenchyme in limb development, 39
Mesenteric arteries, 70, 587
Mesenteric ganglia, 56
    inferior, 70–71
    superior, 70
Mesenteric lifts, 596
    to promote lymphatic flow, 962–963
Mesenteric plexus, 68
Mesentery, 586
    palpation of, 589–590
Metabolism
    disorders of, exercise in, 199–200
    hormonal regulation of, 91–92
    in stress response, 99–100
Metacarpophalangeal joints, 548
    somatic dysfunction of, 558
Metastases of tumors, 419–424
Metatarsophalangeal joints, 640
Microglia, 111
Microscopic anatomy of musculoskeletal system,
    29–31
Migraine headaches, 404–406, 535–536
    auras in, 405
    management of, 405–406
Mitchell lumbosacral angle, 1002
Monocytes, 111
Monosynaptic reflex, 55
Mood disorders, psychoimmunology in, 168

Morley reflex, somatic pain from, 590–591
Mortality rates, 157
Morton's foot, 640, 642
Motion, 1132
    ankle, 633–635
    barriers to, 484, 1128
    cervical spine biomechanics, 542
    cranial, assessment of, 539–540
    external rotation, 631
    fibular, 631, 633
    foot, 635–636
    gliding, 633
    in joint play, 35
    loss with somatic dysfunction, 662–663
    lumbar spine, 591
    in muscle, 35–36
    pelvis and sacrum, 606–608
    of ribs, 573–574
    spinal, palpation of, 481–482
    in synovial joints, 33
    test pattern of passive gross motions, 797–798
    thoracic spine, 572–573
    upper extremity, 548
    in walk cycle, 608
    wrist joint, 557
Motion testing
    cervical spine, 543–545
    costal region, 577–578
    in functional technique, 799
    lumbar, 593–595
    pelvis and sacrum, 611–617
    thoracic spine, 576–577
    upper extremity, 552–553
Motor neurons, 55
Motor strength tests, upper extremity, 552
Mucociliary clearance, 290
Multifidi muscles, 568, 584
    referred pain pattern, 592
Muscle
    antagonist, 36, 1000, 1002
    attachment to bone, 35, 41–42
    cervical spinal, 542
    energy in sacroiliac dysfunction, 618–619
    of facial expression, 43
    fixator, 36
    hip, 643, 645–646
    inhibited, symptoms of, 976
    intermuscular septa, 35
    isometric contractions, 36
    isotonic contractions, 36
    lumbar, testing of strength in, 596
    metastases to, 421
    microscopic appearance of, 30–31
    motor unit in, 35–36
    movements of, 35–36
    myofascial continuity, 41–43
    pelvic floor, 369–370
    in pelvis and sacrum region, 602–604
        assessment of, 611
    polymyositis, 464
    postural
        antagonists, 1000, 1002
        palpation of, 1002–1003

    prime movers, 36
    shortened, lengthening of, 694, 697–698
    spastic, symptoms of, 976
    synergist, 36
    in thigh and leg, 646, 647–649, 651–654
    in thoracic region and rib cage, 564–569
    in upper extremities, 548, 549
Muscle energy techniques, 691–696, 1133
    activating forces in, 694
    in acute torticollis, 545
    cervical, 698–704
        atlantoaxial joint, 700–702
        occipitoatlantal joint, 698–700
        oculocephalogyric reflex in, 700, 701, 703
    complications from, 1020
    and diagnostic assessment of movements, 692
    efficacy factors in, 695–696
    history of, 691–692
    isolytic contraction in, 693
    isometric contraction in, 693
    isotonic contraction in
        concentric, 693
        eccentric, 693
    to lengthen shortened muscles, 694, 697–698
    lower extremity, 746–756
        ankle joint, 755–756
        hip joint, 746–753
        knee joint, 753
        proximal tibiofibular joint, 753–755
    lumbar region, 716–720
        multiple plane, 717–720
        single plane, 716–717
    in nonarticular dysfunction, 756–761
    and palpatory exercise in diagnosis, 692–693
    pelvis and sacrum, 720–734
        innominate bone, 720–722
        pubic bone, 722–724
        sacral torsion, 724–734
    physiologic principles in, 694
    postisometric relaxation in, 694
    reciprocal inhibition in, 694
    ribs, 710–716
        anterior rib, 712–713
        in exhalation, 711–712
        first rib, 713
        in inhalation, 710–711
        ribs 11 and 12, 713–716
    in sacral torsion, 724–734
        backward, 731–734
        forward, 725–731
    sequential steps in, 695
    for spinal group curves, 980–981
    technical principles in, 693
    in temporomandibular joint dysfunction, 539
    thoracic spine, 704–710
        lower, 706–710
        upper, 704–706
    thoracoabdominal diaphragm, 756–760
    upper extremity, 734–746
        elbow, 740–742
        glenohumeral joint, 735–738
        sternoclavicular joint, 738–740
        wrist, 742–746

Musculoskeletal examination, 489–508
  for ambulatory outpatients, 501–504
  general appearance and gait in, 491
  for hospitalized patients, 501, 505–506
  information needed in, 522
  in neurologic disorders, 411
  for outpatient and hospitalized patients,
      500–501
  primary, 490–494
  recording of findings in, 506–508
  in seated position, 492–493
    motion tests in, 492–493, 498–499
    spinal palpation in, 493, 499
    static findings in, 492
    upper extremity testing in, 493, 499–500
  secondary, 491–500
  in standing position, 491–492
    motion findings in, 491–492, 496–498
    static findings in, 491, 494–495
  in supine position for lower extremity and ribs,
      493, 500
Musculoskeletal system, 26
  changes in pregnancy, 349–351
  functional concepts of, 31–35
  metastases to, 420–421
  patterns in problems of, 221
  in pediatric patients, 269
  in renal failure, 398
  response to injury, 31
  in rheumatology, 459–466
  role in total health care, 8–10
    as guide to medical practice, 11
  segmental organization of, 36–39
Musculotendinous junction, 35
Myasthenic syndrome in malignancies, 423
Myelinated axons, 55
Myeloma, multiple, 419
  metastasis to bone, 343
Myenteric plexus, 67, 72
Myofascial and integrated neuromusculoskeletal
      release, 843–849, 1133
  anterior pelvic-innominate, 864–866
  carpal and palmar tunnel, 899
  combined sacroiliac, sacral base, and
      lumbopelvic, 851–858
  craniocervical spine, 874–880
  exercise program with, 849
  focused prone sacral base, 858
  forearm, elbow, and wrist, 891–899
  identification of tethering effects in, 846
  inherent tissue motions in, 846
  lower extremity, 880–887
  lumbosacral spine and pelvis, 848–851
  maneuvers in, 848
    unwinding, 882–887
  mechanics and forces in, 844–846
  palpation in, 845–846
  passive and active patterns in, 844–845
  posttreatment discomfort in, 848
  pubic symphysis, 861–864
  sacroiliac, 866–869
  sacrotuberous ligament, 859–860
  thoracic cage, spine, and diaphragm, 870–874
  thoracolumbar, 851

  three-dimensional patterns in, 847–848
  tight-loose concept in, 844, 847
  upper limb and shoulder, 887–891
Myofascial continuity, 41–43
Myofascial pain syndromes, 464
  headache in, 406
Myofascial tender points, 810, 915–916
Myofascial tension of pelvic diaphragm, 760–761
Myofascial trigger points, 810, 915–918, 1140
  and associated reflexes, 931–932
  autonomic effects of, 929–931
  in axillary folds, 928
  causes of, 916–918
  central nervous system role in, 916–917
  diagnosis of, 919–923
  incidence of, 919
  injection of
    in pain syndromes, 432, 925
    in spondylolisthesis, 1012
  and lower extremity pain, 643
  osteopathic approach to, 925–933
  and pain in head and neck, 515–517
  and pain in lumbar region, 591
  physiologic mechanisms in, 917
  posture in, 917–918, 928
  in quadratus lumborum, 598–599
  regional depiction of, 920–922
  in scalene muscles, 928
  in somatic dysfunctions, 925–926
  treatment of, 916, 923
    cooling with stretching, 924–925, 927
    injections, 432, 925
    in spondylolisthesis, 1012
    in venous and lymphatic drainage impairment,
        926–928
Myotomal pain patterns, 643

Naffziger sign, 409
Nasopharynx, 295
Natural killer cells, 111
  in mood disorders, 168
NAVEL mnemonic for femoral triangle
      structures, 650
Navicular bone
  Hiss plantar whip for displacement, 690
  somatic dysfunction of, 640
Neck (see Cervical region)
Nephrology, 393–398 (see also Kidneys)
Nerves
  autonomic innervations, 61–80, 1043
  blocks in pain management, 181–182
  in buttock and thigh, 646
  conduction studies, 436
  cranial, 524–530
  electrical stimulation of, transcutaneous, 182,
      432, 435
    in angina pectoris, 307
    in postural decompensation, 975–976
    in scoliosis, 996
  in head and neck, 522, 524, 528
  in lumbar and abdominal region, 588–591
  in pelvis and sacrum, 605–606
  spinal cord, 541–542
  supply to organs, 47–48

  in thigh, leg, and foot, 646, 655
  in thoracic region, 570–572
  in upper extremities, 550
  in uterus and perineum, 363–364
Nervous system
  autonomic, 25, 53–80, 402, 1043
  central, 401–402 (see also Neurology)
    autonomic components of, 54
    interaction with endocrine and immune
        systems, 88–89, 116–119
  enteric, 69, 72
  parasympathetic, 60–61, 402, 1043
  peripheral, 54–57, 402
    in malignancies, 422–424
    in renal failure, 396–397
  segmental organization of, 36–39
  sympathetic, 58–60, 402, 560, 570–571, 1043
Neuralgia, trigeminal, 529, 538
Neuroendocrine cells in hypothalamic-pituitary
      complex, 88
Neuroendocrine-immune system, 26, 53, 103
  and aging, 129–130
  factors affecting, 126–129
  and psychoneuroimmunology, 167–169
  signal coding in, 108–116
  in stress responses, 100
Neurohypophysis, hormones of, 84
Neurologic examination of pelvic region, 611
Neurology, 401–414
  and embryology of neuromusculoskeletal
      system, 27–29
  entrapment neuropathies, 411–413
  headaches, 403–408
  musculoskeletal examination in, 411
  research applied to osteopathic practice, 1113
  spinal disorders, 408–410
Neuromuscular junction, transmission in, 55
Neurons
  hypophysiotropic, 88
  motor, 55
  sensory, 55
Neuropathies
  carcinomatous, 422–424
  entrapment, 411–413
  uremic, 396–397
Neuropeptides
  in cardiac nerves, 66
  in cerebrovascular nerves, 63
  in enteric neurons, 72
  in respiratory tract, 66, 67
  in ureters, 76
  in vascular nerves, 61, 62
Neurophysiology, 137–150
  integrative function of, 137–145
    alteration of, 145–150
    non–impulse-based, 148–149
Neuroregulators, 109–111
Neurotransmitters in enteric neurons, 72
Neurotrophy, 1132
Neurovascular bundle, 35
Neutral spinal position, 514, 1133
Neutrophils, 111
Nitric oxide, and neurotransmission in enteric
      nervous system, 72

Nociception, 175–176
  in abdominopelvic organs, 73–74
  cardiac, 66
  and reflex excitability, 146–148
Nociceptors, 175, 1132
Noncognitive stimuli, 121
Norepinephrine, 84
  as neuroregulator, 110
  secretion by sympathetic nervous system, 57
Normalization, 1133
Nose
  allergic rhinitis, 292–293
  anatomy and physiology of, 289–290
  osteopathic approach to, 296
  pathophysiology of, 290–291
Nutation, 1133
  sacral, 607–608, 851
Nutrition, 157–158
  food guide pyramid in, 158
  lymphatic system in, 944–945
  in malignancies, 426

Obesity, 159–160
  exercise in, 199–200
Obliquus abdominis muscles, 603
Obliquus capitis inferior muscle, 568
Obstetrics, 349–359 (see also Pregnancy)
Obturator muscles
  externus, 603
  internus, 646
Obturator nerve, 588
Occipital lymph nodes, 522
Occipitoatlantal joint
  fascial-ligamentous release, 829
  muscle energy techniques, 698–700
  thrust technique with side-bending force, 667
Occiput
  motion testing, 544
  movement of, 542
Oculocephalogyric reflex in muscle energy techniques
  for atlantoaxial joint, 701
  for cervical spine segments, 703
  for occipitoatlantal joint, 700
Oculomotor nerve, 63, 522, 525–526, 571
O'Donaghue triad, 631
Olfactory nerve, 524
Oligodendrocytes, 112
Oncology, 417–429
  brain tumors, headache in, 537
  central nervous system symptoms in, 421–422
  colorectal tumors, 384–385
  diagnostic and treatment options presented to patient, 424–425
  esophageal cancer, 377
  fibroids of uterus, 367
  gastric cancer, 379
  index tumors, 418–424
  lung carcinoma, 418–419
  metastases, 419–424
  modulators of biologic response in, 427–428
  musculoskeletal symptoms in, 420–421
  osteopathic approach to, 428–429
  paraneoplastic syndromes, 418–419

  peripheral nervous system symptoms in, 422–424
  philosophic principles in patient care, 427
  plasma cell tumors, 419
  renal cell cancer, 418
  spinal tumors, 343–344
  supportive care for patients, 425–427
  viscerosomatic-type responses in, 424
Ophthalmic nerve, 526
Opioid peptides, 125–126
Optic nerve, 524–525
  neuritis of, headache in, 406
Oropharynx, 295
Orthopaedics, 329–346
  developmental dysplasia of hip, 331–334
  fracture of hip in elderly persons, 334–335
  low back pain, 337–345
  osteoarthritis of knee, 335–337
  osteopathic approach to, 329–331
Orthotics, 436
  in Morton's foot, 640, 642
  in postural decompensation, 975
    sagittal plane, 1005–1006
  in spondylolisthesis, 1012
Ortolani test for hip dislocation, 331, 624, 625
Osteoarthritis, 463–464
  of knee, 335–337
  manipulative therapy in, 465
  of vertebral body, 408
Osteoarthropathy, hypertrophic pulmonary, 421
Osteoblasts, 29
Osteocytes, 30, 112
Osteodystrophy, renal, 394–396
  diagnosis of, 395
  treatment of, 395–396
Osteomyelitis, headache in, 406
Osteopathic treatment
  approach in, 484–485
  and art of medicine, 470–471
  consideration of entire person in, 469–470
  definition of, 244
  direct or indirect techniques in, 486–487
  dose and frequency in, 496
  evaluation and management in, 473–508
  exercises to develop sense of touch in, 479–482
  forms of, 468
  knowledge of anatomy in, 471–472
  methods of, 485
  models of, 468–469
  musculoskeletal examination in, 489–508
  philosophy of, 3–12, 1134
  plan of intervention in, 487
  and primary care, 245–247
  regional examination and treatment, 511–660
  selection of technique in, 469
  sequence of, 485–496
Osteoporosis, 464
  exercise in, 200
Otitis media, 294–295
Ovarian plexus, 78
Ovaries
  hormones of, 84
  innervation of, 78

  pain in, 368–369
  viscerosomatic reference sites for, 450
Oxygen
  hypoxemia, 447
  respiratory exchange for carbon dioxide, 441
Oxytocin, 84

Pacemaker, gastric, 377
Pain, 48–49
  acute, 174
  in back, 337–345, 591–592 (see also Back pain)
  central control processes in, 176
  in chest, 304–305
    palpatory examination in, 306–307
  chronic, 174–175
    biomechanical deficiencies in, 413–414
  in headaches, 403–404, 534–535
  information processing in, 176–179
  management of, 179–185
    acupuncture in, 432
    analgesics in, 180–181
    in cancer, 426
    cold therapy in, 432
    counterirritants in, 182
    electrical stimulation in (see Electrical nerve stimulation, transcutaneous)
    heat therapy in, 431–432
    individualization of, 180
    medications in, 179–182
    nerve blocks in, 181–182
    osteopathic approach in, 182–184
    osteopathic manipulations in, 432
    patient-controlled analgesia in, 180
    placebos in, 180–181
    trigger point injections in, 432, 925, 1012
  in myofascial syndromes, 464
  myotomal, 643
  nociception in, 175–176
    in abdominopelvic organs, 73–74
    cardiac, 66
    and reflex excitability, 146–148
  ovarian, 368–369
  pattern appraisal in, 178–179
  pattern recognition in, 177–178
  pelvic, 363–369
    COLDER mnemonic for, 609
    contributory factors in, 610
    posterior, in pregnancy, 351
    PQRST mnemonic for, 609
  pelvic floor, 362
  perceptual field in, 177
  referred, 49, 140, 582
    from esophagus, 67
    from gonadal tissues, 78
    from heart, 66
    from hiatal hernia, 73
    from iliolumbar ligament, 603
    from kidneys, 75
    from liver and biliary tree, 74
    in lower extremity, 643
    from lumbar and abdominal region, 589–590
    from lungs and bronchi, 67
    from myofascial trigger points, 591, 915
    from thoracic aorta, 67

Pain, referred—*continued*
   from ureters, 76
   from uterus, 79
   visceral, 582
   response execution in, 179
   sclerotomal, 589, 593, 643
   somatic, from reflex of Morley, 590–591
   in spinal disorders, 409
   in spondylolisthesis, 1009
   theories of, 171–174
   uterine, 366–367
   visceral, 590
      from lumbar and abdominal region, 589–590
      referred, 582
   viscerosomatic, 590
Pain drawings, use of, 345
Palmar tunnel, myofascial and integrated
      neuromusculoskeletal release, 899
Palpation, 473–477, 1134
   of anterior Chapman's points, 593, 595
   of cervical spine, 543
   of Chapman's reflexes, 935–936
   of cranial motion, 904–905
   dominant eye in, 474
   dominant hand in, 474
   and exercises to develop sense of touch,
         479–482
      forearm of partner palpated in, 480
      inanimate objects palpated in, 479
      layer palpation in, 479–480
      for somatic dysfunction diagnosis, 481–482
   of forearm motions, 555
   of hospitalized patients, 1038
   learning of technique in, 474–475
   of lumbar spine, 593
   of mesentery, 589–590
   motion perception in, 475
   of pelvis and sacrum, 609–611
   postural muscles in, 1002–1004
   in somatic dysfunction diagnosis, 475–476,
         483–484
      in cervical area, 481
      in lumbar area, 482
      in sacroiliac area, 482
      TART mnemonic for, 475
      in thoracic area, 481
   for spinal motion and paravertebral tissue
         texture in, 480–481, 491–492
   in spondylolisthesis, 1010
   of thoracic spine and rib cage, 575
   of upper extremity, 551
Pancreas
   hormones of, 84
   innervation of, 70, 74
Paraneoplastic syndromes, 418–419
   central nervous system in, 421–422
Parasympathetic nerves, 60–61, 402, 1043
   cardiac, 143
   cranial system, 60
   of head, 522, 528
   lumbar and abdominal region, 581
   sacral system, 60
   thoracic region, 571

Parathyroid hormone, 84
   in renal osteodystrophy, 395
Paraventricular nucleus of hypothalamus, 117,
      122
Paravertebral ganglia, 56, 57, 58–59
Parietal peritoneum, 586
Parotid lymph nodes, superficial, 522
Patella, 627–630
   bursitis, 656–657
   deep tendon reflex, 642
Patellofemoral joint dysfunction, 627–628
Patrick FABERE test of hip, 627
Pattern recognition in clinical problem solving,
      220–222
   for established patients, 221
   musculoskeletal patterns in, 221
   seasonal and environmental patterns in,
         220–221
   visual patterns in, 220
Pavlik harness, 332
Pectineus muscle, 645
Pectoral traction technique, 791
   to promote lymphatic flow, 955
Pectoralis muscles
   major, 565
   minor, 565
Pedal lymphatic pump, 956–957, 1133
Pediatrics
   development in childhood, 192–193
   hospitalized patients, 1045
   lift therapy for short leg syndrome, 988
   neonatal dysfunction of primary respiratory
         mechanisms, 909–910
   osteopathic approach in, 261–262, 267–271
      and concept of child ecology, 269–270
      diagnosis in, 270–271
      guiding principles in, 267–269
      musculoskeletal system in, 269
      and primary care, 271
   screening for scoliosis, 991–993
Pelvic bones, 1134
Pelvic diaphragm, 369, 602–603, 945–946
   muscle energy treatment for myofascial tension,
         760–761
Pelvic floor dysfunction, 369–371
   anatomy in, 369–370
   incontinence in, 370–371
   pain in, 362
Pelvic index, 1001, 1031, 1134
Pelvic ligaments, 602
Pelvic plexus (*see* Hypogastric plexus, inferior)
Pelvic tilt exercise, 1053
Pelvis and sacrum region, 601–622
   anatomic landmarks in, 611
   articulatory techniques, 775–777
   congestion syndrome, 366–367
   counterstrain techniques, 817–818
   diagnosis of problems in, 609–611
   dysfunctions, 608
      pelvic, 617–618
      sacroiliac, 618–622
   fascial-ligamentous release, 821–822
   fascial restrictions of, 616

   functional anatomy of, 601–606
   functional techniques, 803–804
   inflammatory disease, 368
   motion of, 606–608
   motion testing, 611–621
      in iliosacral dysfunction, 617–618
      prone, 614–616
      in sacroiliac dysfunction, 612–617
      seated, 613
      side shift, 492, 498
      standing, 612–613
      supine, 613–614
   muscle energy techniques, 720–734
   myofascial and integrated neuromusculoskeletal
         release, 851–858
   pain in, 363–369
      anatomy in, 363–364
      causes of, 365
      differential diagnosis of, 365–369
      in dysmenorrhea, 365–366
      in endometriosis, 367–368
      history and physical examination in, 364–365
      in inflammatory disease, 368
      ovarian, 368–369
      posterior, in pregnancy, 351
      in premenstrual syndrome, 366
      uterine, 366–367
   palpation of, 609–611
   physical examination of, 609
   rotation in anterior lift therapy, 989
   thrust techniques, 682–685
      anterior sacrum, right, 682
      anteriorly rotated ilium, 683–684
      posterior sacrum, left, 682–683
      posteriorly rotated ilium, 684
      superior ilial shear, 684–685
   types of, 356–357
Penis, innervation of, 79
Peptic ulcer, 378–379
Peptides
   hormones, 84
      affecting CNS activity, 88
      biosynthesis of, 85
      opioid, 125–126
Percussion hammer technique in postural
      problems, 1005
Perineal muscle, deep transverse, 76
Perineum, nerves of, 363
Periosteal layer of cranial dura mater,
      34
Periosteum
   of bones in face and cranial vault, 43
   connective tissue in, 29
   in synovial joints, 21
   tendon attachment to, 35, 41–42
Peripheral nervous system, 54–57, 402
   ganglia in, 54, 56–57
   in malignancies, 422–424
   somatic reflex arc in, 55
   visceral reflex arc in, 55–56
Peritoneum
   parietal, 586
   visceral, distension of, 589

Peroneal nerve, 646
  entrapment of, 411
Peroneus muscles, 648, 649
Pes cavus, 635
Pes planus, 635
Pétrissage, 959, 1134
  with cough activation, to release abdominal
    scars, 963–964
  lower extremity, 966–967
  upper extremity, 965–966
Peyer's patches, 942
Phalen test, 559
  in carpal tunnel syndrome, 412
Pharmaceutics, 94–95
Pharmacodynamics, 95
Pharmacokinetics, 95
Pharmacology, 93–97
  drug therapy opposed by Still, 4, 7, 16–17
  factors affecting responses to drugs, 94
  in family practice, 252–253
  in hypertension therapy, 96–97, 323–325
  and individualization of therapy, 93–94
  and osteopathic principles, 96
  in pain relief, 179–182
  processes in, 94–95
  rational use of drugs in, 25–26
  receptors for drugs in, 95
Pharyngitis, 296
Pharynx, 295–296
  anatomy and physiology of, 295
  osteopathic approach to, 296
  pathophysiology of, 295–296
Philosophy of osteopathic medicine, 3–12, 1134
  in areas of basic science, 24–26
  body unity in, 4–5
    and person as a whole, 8
  evolution of, 4
  key principles in, 4–7
    explication of, 7–12
    as guides to medical practice, 10–12
  rational treatment in, 6–7
  role of drugs and surgery in, 7
  self-regulation in, 5
    as guide to medical practice, 11
    and internal personal health care systems, 10
  structure and function interdependence in, 5–6
    as guide to medical practice, 11
    and role of musculoskeletal system, 8–10
Photoperiod, and ACTH secretion, 89
Phrenic nerves, 448, 570
Physiatry (see Physical medicine and
    rehabilitation)
Physical activity (see Exercise)
Physical examination
  in back pain, 339
  of geriatric patients, 276–277
  of hospitalized patients, 1038–1041
  in hypertension, 321–322
  in pelvic pain, 364–365
  in rheumatic diseases, 459–460
Physical medicine and rehabilitation, 431–439
  case histories in, 436–439
  cold in, 432

electrical stimulation in, 432, 435
electromyography and nerve conduction in, 436
exercise in, 432–436
heat in, 431–432
in malignancies, 426
orthotics and prosthetics in, 436
osteopathic manipulations in, 432
therapeutic modalities in, 431–436
trigger point injections and acupuncture in, 432
Pierce, Charles S., 3–4
Pineal gland, circadian control of, 126
Pinocytosis, reverse, 85
Piriformis muscle, 603, 645
  location of tender point in, 793
  referred pain pattern, 592
  structure–function relationships, 646, 650
Pituitary gland
  anterior
    affecting neural activity, 88–89
    hormone production and release, 117–118
    hypothalamic-pituitary-adrenal axis, 122–123
    hypothalamic-pituitary-thyroid axis, 123–124
    neuroendocrine cells in, 88
    posterior, hormones of, 84
Pituitary hormones, 84, 117–118
Placebos
  in pain management, 180–181
  in research on osteopathic medicine,
    1118–1119
Planes of body, 1134–1135
Plantar fascia, relaxation and stretching of, 793
Plantar flexion of talus, 634
  muscle energy technique in, 756
  thrust technique in, 689–690
Plantar ligaments, 639
Plasma cell neoplasms, 419
Pleura, innervation of, 67
Pneumonia, osteopathic treatment of, 454–455
Pneumotaxic center in pons, 447
Polymyositis, 464
  in malignancies, 421
Polypeptide hormones, biosynthesis of, 84
Polyps, adenomatous, and colorectal cancer, 384
Polysynaptic reflexes, 55
Popliteus muscle, 647
Position of comfort, 809, 811–813
Positional treatment, 1133
Postauricular lymph nodes, effleurage to promote
    lymphatic flow, 959
Posterior component, 1135
Posttreatment reaction
  in counterstrain techniques, 812
  in myofascial and integrated
    neuromusculoskeletal release, 848
Postural motion, sacral, 607
Posture, 969–976
  base of support in, 969
  compensated, 970
  decompensated, 970, 1135
    back pain in, 596–597
    bracing in, 974–975
    in coronal and horizontal planes, 983–997
    electrical stimulation in, 975–976

exercise in, 974
manipulative treatment of, 974
orthotics in, 975
patient education in, 974
in sagittal plane, 999–1014
sclerotherapy in, 976
surgery in, 976
dynamic, 970, 1001
gravitational stress affecting, 970, 999–1001
and management of group curves, 979–982
muscles in
  antagonists of, 1000, 1002
  palpation of, 1002–1003
  and myofascial trigger points, 917–918, 926,
    928
optimal, 969
patterning of, 970–974
  fascial, 972, 974
  musculoligamentous, 972–974
  spinal, 970–972
radiographic studies, 1025–1033
sagittal plane decompensation, 999–1012
  radiographic measurements in, 1001–1002,
    1003
  treatment of, 1004–1006
in scoliosis, 989–996
in short leg syndrome, 983–989
in spondylolisthesis, 1001, 1006–1012
static, 970, 1001
PQRST mnemonic for pain studies, 609
Preauricular lymph nodes, effleurage to promote
    lymphatic flow, 959
Pregnancy, 349–359
  body fluid and circulation changes in, 351–352
  first trimester, 353
  hormonal changes in, 352
  labor and birth, 356–358
  lightening in, 351
  low back pain in, 350–351
  musculoskeletal changes in, 349–351
  osteopathic care in, 262
  osteopathic manipulations in, 356
  postpartum period, 358–359
  second trimester, 355–356
  spondylolisthesis in, 1011
  third trimester, 356
Premenstrual syndrome, 366
Prenatal development, 191–192
Presacral nerve, 68
Prespondylolisthesis, 1001, 1006
Preventive medicine
  in family practice, 254
  by general internists, 258–259
Prevertebral ganglia, 56, 57, 58–59
Primary care
  and family practice, 249–254
  geriatric, 273–283
  and internal medicine, 257–259
  managed care concepts in, 247
  osteopathic considerations in, 245–247
  in pediatric practice, 261–262, 271
  stress management in, 204–215
  and team for health promotion, 165

Primary care—*continued*
   treatment strategies in, 247
   and understanding of health and disease,
      246–247
Primary respiratory mechanisms, 902–904, 1135
   articular mobility of cranial bones in, 903
   brain and spinal cord motility in, 903
   cerebrospinal fluid fluctuation in, 903
   dura mater mobility in, 903
   dysfunctions
      in dental problems, 911
      diagnosis of, 907–909
      neonatal, 909–910
      in trauma, 911
      treatment of, 911–913
      vascular supply affecting, 910
   and sacral mobility between ilia, 903–904
Problem-oriented medical record (POMR), 224,
      1080
Problem solving (*see* Clinical problem solving)
Procaine injections in myofascial trigger points,
      925
   in spondylolisthesis, 1012
Progesterone, 84
Progestogens, and reproductive function, 91
Prolactin, 84, 91, 124–125
Prolotherapy in postural decompensation, 976
Pronation, 1135
   foot, 636
   forearm, 554, 555
Pro-opiomelanocortin, 123–125
Proprioception, 1135
   and neuromuscular facilitation in pain
      management, 183
Prostaglandins, 122
Prosthetics, 436
Protein hormones, 84
   biosynthesis of, 85
Proteins, acute phase, 104
Pseudogout, 463
Psoas muscles, 581–582, 585
   fascial-ligamentous release, 823
   shortened, 594
   syndrome of, 593, 597
   tension test, 621
   unequal length of, 618
Psychiatric patients, hospitalized, 1045–1046
Psychoimmunology
   alternative treatments in, 168
   in mood disorders, 168
   research in, 167–168
Psychological health
   affecting neuroendocrine-immune network, 128
   assessment in geriatric patients, 278–279
   exercise affecting, 200–201
   problems in, 245
   stressors affecting, 99
Psychoneuroimmunology, 167–169
Psychosocial considerations in family practice,
      253
Pubic symphysis, 601
   compressions, 618
   levelness test, 614

   motion of, 607
   muscle energy techniques, 722–724
   myofascial and integrated neuromusculoskeletal
      release, 861–864
   shears of, 618, 1135, 1139
Pubococcygeus muscle, 369
Pudendal nerve, 77
Pulmonary conditions (*see* Lungs)
Pulmonary plexus, 66
Pulse
   brachial, 551
   radial, 551
   recording of amplitude, 551
Pump techniques, lymphatic, 954–958
Purinergic axons in peripheral vasculature, 61–62
Pyrosis, 375–376

Q-angle, 627
Quadratus lumborum muscle, 566, 585, 603
   myofascial trigger points, 598–599
   referred pain pattern, 592
   spastic, symptoms of, 976
Quadriceps angle, 627
Quadriceps femoris muscle, 603, 647
Quality of life, measurements in clinical trials,
      1103

Radial nerve entrapment, 411
Radial pulse, 551
Radiculopathy, 409
   lumbar, 584
      management of, 598
   in malignancies, 423
   reflexes in, 642–643
Radiocarpal joint, 548, 553, 554, 557 (*see also*
      Wrist joint)
Radiography
   in postural studies, 1025–1033
      anteroposterior films in, 1029–1031
      and Cobb measurements in scoliosis, 991,
         993, 1029
      exercises for measurements in, 1031–1033
      Ferguson lumbosacral angle in, 1001, 1031
      lateral film of pelvis in, 1031
      materials used in, 1025–1026
      pelvic index in, 1001, 1031
      procedure in, 1026–1027
      results of, 1028–1031
      sagittal plane measurements in, 1001–1002,
         1003, 1031
      sample analysis report in, 1033
   in rheumatic diseases, 460
   in short leg syndrome, 986
   in spondylolisthesis diagnosis, 1008–1009
Radioulnar joint, 548
Radius
   head of, posterior thrust technique, 685
   reciprocal motion of, 554
Range of motion
   active, 434
   lower extremity, testing of, 493
   myofascial trigger points affecting, 926
   passive, 434

   in somatic dysfunction, 484
   spinal, 341
      tests for, 491–493
   in treatment, 1133
   upper extremity, testing of, 493, 499–500
Rational treatment as principle in osteopathic
      medicine, 6–7
Receptors, drugs interacting with, 95
Reciprocal inhibition reflex, 694, 1136
Reciprocal motion of radius, 554
Reciprocal tension membrane, craniosacral, 903,
      1136
Rectal venous plexus, 604
Rectum
   innervation of, 71
   lymphatic drainage of, 604–605
Rectus abdominis muscle, 603
   inhibited, symptoms of, 976
Rectus femoris muscle, 645
Red reflex, 575, 1136
Reflex arc
   somatic, 55
   visceral, 55–56
Reflex sympathetic dystrophy, 560
Reflexes, 138–139
   alterations in, 145–148
   association with myofascial trigger points,
      931–932
   in autonomic ganglia, 144
   biceps, 551
   brachioradialis, 551
   changes in excitability, 146
   Chapman, 354–355, 935–940
   habituation in, 147
   high-excitability areas in, 145
   interactions of, 139–145
      in cardiac control, 141–144
      neural basis for, 140–144
   low-threshold areas in, 145–146
   monosynaptic, 55
   of Morley, somatic pain from, 590–591
   nociceptive stimuli affecting, 146–148
   polysynaptic, 55
   recording of amplitude, 552
   somatosomatic, 139
   somatovisceral, 140, 141, 1136
   structure of, 138–139
   triceps, 551
   viscerosomatic, 61, 139–140, 141, 1136 (*see
      also* Viscerosomatic reflexes)
   viscero-visceral, 139, 1136
   wind-up or sensitization in, 144–145, 147
Reflux, gastroesophageal, 375–376
Regulatory adaptations, 99–105
Rehabilitative care (*see* Physical medicine and
      rehabilitation)
Relaxation, progressive, in stress management,
      213
Relaxin levels in pregnancy, 352
Renal arteries, 587
Renal disorders, 393–398 (*see also* Kidneys)
Repetitive strain syndrome, 464
Reproduction, hormones affecting, 91

Reproductive tract, innervation of, 77–80
Research, 1058–1064
  basic research, 1091, 1107–1113
    analysis and evaluation in, 1112
    applied to osteopathic practice, 1112–1113
    hypothesis construction in, 1110–1112
    literature review in, 1109–1110
    in osteopathic medicine, 1115–1116
    prospective studies in, 1108–1109
    retrospective studies in, 1109
    scientific method in, 1107–1108
    sequence of steps in, 1109–1112
    variables identified in, 1112
  challenges in, 1063
  clinical research and trials, 1091–1094 (see also
      Clinical research and trials)
  on history of osteopathy, 1059–1063
  on medical practice and knowledge, 1058–1059
  medical records in, 1077–1084
  in osteopathic medicine, 1102–1105,
      1115–1124
    appropriate measures in, 1121
    basic science in, 1115–1116
    clinical trial designs in, 1119–1121
    funding and environment for, 1122
    integrative model building in, 1116
    manipulative treatment evaluation in,
        1116–1118, 1120–1121
    placebos and sham procedures in, 1118–1119
    total care in, 1118
  in pediatric care, 262
  on somatic dysfunction, 1061–1062,
      1067–1075
    instrumental measurements in, 1071–1073
    measured components in, 1071–1072
    patient diaries in, 1070
    quantitative measures in, 1067–1068
    reevaluation and outcome studies in, 1071
    reference data in, 1072
    resources for, 1073
    responses to treatment in, 1071
    scores and scales in, 1069–1070
    standard for quality in, 1073
    statistical analysis of, 1068–1069
    tests used in, 1070–1071
    variables in, 1072, 1103
Respiration, 441–444
  control of, 447–448
  primary respiratory mechanisms, 902–904
  sacral motion in, 607
Respiratory distress in newborn, osteopathic
    treatment of, 456
Respiratory system, 441–456
  control of respiration in, 447–448
  gas exchange in, 446–447
  innervation of, 66–67
    afferent fibers in, 67
    efferent fibers in, 66
  lymphoid tissue in, 942
  osteopathic approach to, 448–456
    in chronic obstructive pulmonary disease,
        455–456
    in pneumonia, 454–455

    in prevention of postoperative pulmonary
        complications, 456
    thoracic lymphatic pump in, 453–454
    pulmonary circulation in, 444–446
    ventilation in, 441–444
Restrictive barriers to motion, 484, 1128
Reticular cells, 112
Retroauricular lymph nodes, 522
Rexed layers of spinal cord, 140
Rheumatism, soft-tissue, 464
Rheumatoid arthritis, 461–463
  juvenile, 463
Rheumatology, 459–466
  arthritis
    inflammatory, 460–463
    noninflammatory, 463–464
  connective tissue diseases, 464–465
  history-taking in, 459
  laboratory studies in, 460
  manipulative therapy in, 465
  medications in, 465
  physical examination in, 459–460
Rhinitis, allergic, 292–293
Rhomboid muscles, 566
  relaxation technique, 792
Rib raising to improve lymphatic flow, 950–951
Ribs, 564
  articulatory techniques, 764–765, 769–771
  bucket-handle motion, 573, 574, 710,
      1128
  counterstrain techniques, 815–816
  evaluation of, 577–578
    in hospitalized patients, 1041
  exhalation, 1129
  facilitated positional release, 836
  fascial-ligamentous release, 825
  functional techniques, 805–808
  inhalation, 1131
  mechanics of, 573–574
  muscle energy techniques, 710–716
  myofascial and integrated neuromusculoskeletal
      release, 870–874
  pump-handle motion, 573–574, 710, 1128
    and thrust technique, 677
  screening examination, 493, 500
  thrust technique, 674–679
Risk perception, stress in, 213
Romberg sign, 410
Ropiness, 1136
Rotation
  cervical spine, 542
    testing of, 545
  innominate, 617
  lumbar spine, 591
    testing of, 593–595
  test for occipital motion, 544
  thoracic spine, testing of, 576
Rotator muscle of hip, 646
Rotatores muscles, thoracolumbar, 568,
    584
  referred pain pattern, 592
Rotoscoliosis, 970, 971, 989–996 (See also
    Scoliosis)

Sacral hiatus, 601–602
Sacral plexus, 38, 39, 605
Sacral promontory, 601
Sacral sulcus, 602
Sacroiliac joint, 602
  dysfunction
    diagnosis of, 618–622
    motion tests in, 612–617
  facilitated positional release, 840
Sacroiliac ligaments, 602
  pain from postural imbalance, 985
Sacrospinous ligaments, 602
Sacrotuberous ligaments, 602
  myofascial and integrated neuromusculoskeletal
      release, 859–861
Sacrum
  anterior, 619
  axes of motion, 1136–1137
  in backward bending test, 616
  extension of, 1130
    bilateral, 621
    unilateral, 621
  fascial-ligamentous release, 821–822
  flexion of, 1130
    bilateral, 620–621
    unilateral, 621
  functional techniques in, 801–802
  inferolateral angles of, 614–615
  lumbosacral spring test, 615–616
  mobility between ilia, 903–904
  motion of, 607–608
    test about oblique axis, 615
    test about transverse axis, 615
  muscle energy techniques in torsion, 724–734
  myofascial and integrated neuromusculoskeletal
      release, 851–858
  posterior, 619
  rocking of, 1038, 1040
  sheared, 621, 1137
  soft tissue techniques, 790
  test for base position, 614
    posterior, 615
  thrust techniques, 682–683
  torsions, 620, 1137
  translated, 1137
  transverse axes, 1138
Safety measures, 161–162
  in automobiles, 161
  in homes, 162
Sagittal plane of body, 1134, 1135
Salpingo-oophoritis, 368
Sartorius muscle, 603, 645, 647
Scalene muscles, 541
  myofascial trigger points in, 928
Scalp, arterial supply of, 517
Scapulothoracic joint, 547
  motion tests, 553
  muscles of, 550
Scarpa's fascia, 50, 603
Sciatic nerve, 605, 646
  entrapment of, 411
Scleroderma, 464
Sclerotherapy in postural decompensation, 976

Sclerotomal pain, 589, 593, 643
Scoliosis, 989–996, 1137, 1138
  braces in, 994, 996
  causes of, 990
  Cobb measurements in, 993, 1029
  curve patterns in, 970, 972, 991, 992
  diagnosis of, 989–991
  electrical stimulation in, 996
  locations of, 990–991
  manipulative treatment in, 993–996
  reversibility of, 990
  screening for, 991–993
  severity of, 990
  surgery in, 995, 996
  symptoms of, 993
  treatment of, 993–996
Screening for scoliosis, 991–993
Second messenger in hormone-receptor
        interaction, 87
Segmental motion, 1138
Self-regulation as principle in osteopathic
        medicine, 5
  and guide to medical practice, 11
  and internal personal health care systems,
        10
Semimembranosus muscle, 603, 647
Semispinalis muscle, 567
Semitendinosus muscle, 603, 647
Sensation testing
  in pelvic region, 611
  in upper extremity, 552
Sensitization, 1138
  in reflexes, 144–145, 147
Sensory neurons, 55
  in A-afferent system, 55
  in B-afferent system, 55
Sensory-motor polyneuropathy, mixed, in
        malignancies, 423
Serratus muscles
  anterior, 566
  posterior, 566
Sex act, viscerosomatic reflexes in, 79–80
Sexual behavior, 162
Sham procedures in research on osteopathic
        medicine, 1118–1119
Sharpey's fibers, 41
Shears, 1138
  innominate, 617
  pubic, 618, 1135, 1139
  sacral, 621
Sherrington's laws, 1132
Shiatsu, 916
Shin splints, 655
Short leg syndrome, 621, 983–989
  diagnosis of, 985–987
  lift therapy in, 987–989
    for children, 988
    Heilig formula for, 987
  myofascial trigger points in, 926
  patellar tracking in, 630
  spinal compensatory changes in, 971
  treatment of, 987–989
Shoulder
  frozen, 560–561

motion testing, 552
muscles of, 549
myofascial and integrated neuromusculoskeletal
        release, 887–891
Spencer articulatory techniques, 552, 765,
        777–780, 1133
Side-bending, 1138
  cervical spine, 542
  lumbar spine, 591
    testing of, 593–595
  thoracic spine, 572
    testing of, 576
Signal transduction in hormone-receptor
        interaction, 87
Sinuses, paranasal, 531–532
  anatomy and physiology of, 289–290
  osteopathic approach to, 296
  pathophysiology of, 290–291
  sinusitis, 291–292
Sinusitis, 291–292
  headache in, 406
Skeletal anatomy
  cervical, 541
  lower extremity, 623–642
  lumbar region, 582–584
  pelvis and sacrum, 601–602
  thoracic region and rib cage, 563–564
  upper extremity, 547–548
Skull, 515
  frontal view of, 516
  inferior view of, 521
  interior view of, 520
  lateral view of, 518–519
  orbital view of, 517
  sutures of, 33, 34
Sleep
  good habits of, 215
  and growth hormone secretion, 89
  psychological management of insomnia,
        214–215
Smoking, 160–161
Social considerations
  assessment in geriatric patients, 279
  psychosocial factors in family practice, 253
  in readjustment scale, 164
  in support for stress management, 212
Soft-tissue rheumatism, 464
Soft-tissue techniques, 781–794, 1133
  cervical, 781–783
  lower extremity, 792–794
  lumbar, 787–790
  sacrum, 790
  thoracic, 783–787
  upper extremity, 791–792
Soleus muscle, 648
Somatic afferents affecting baroreceptor reflexes,
        144
Somatic and autonomic systems, interactions of,
        26
Somatic component of disease, 572
Somatic dysfunction, 1138
  anatomy in, 512
  as central concept of disease, 1123
  classification of, 476

diagnosis with palpation, 475–476, 483–484
  exercises for, 481–482
epidemiologic studies of, 1097–1099
musculoskeletal examination for, 489–508
range of motion in, 484
research on, 1061–1062, 1067–1075
total nature of, 1124
Somatic reflex arc, 55
Somatic stimuli affecting neuroendocrine-
        immune network, 127
Somatogenics, 1138
Somatomammotrophs, 124–125
Somatomedins, 91, 124
Somatosomatic reflexes, 139, 1136
Somatostatin, 84, 124
Somatotropin, 84
Somatovisceral reflexes, 140, 141, 1136
  association with myofascial trigger points,
        931–932
  wind-up phenomenon in, 144–145
Spasm, 1138
  diffuse esophageal, 376–377
  muscle symptoms, 976
Spencer shoulder techniques, 552, 765, 777–780,
        1133
Spermatic plexus, 78
Sphenobasilar synchondrosis, strains of, 906–907
Sphenoid sinus, 290, 532
Sphenopalatine ganglion, 522, 528
Sphincter urethrae muscle, 7677
Sphinx test in sacral torsion, 725
Spina bifida occulta, 583
Spinal canal stenosis, lumbar, 583
Spinal cord, 38, 402, 570–571
  cervical, 541–542
  compression by malignancies, 423–424
  inherent motility of, 903
  lumbar, 582–583
  Rexed layers of, 140
  somatic and visceral afferents in, 141
  in sympathetic innervation of heart, 142–143
  syndromes of, 408–409
  viscerotropic map in lateral horns, 74
Spinal nerves, 570–571
  disorders of, 408
  lumbar, 581–582, 588–589
Spinalis muscle, 567
Spine, 408–410
  cervical, 541–546
  changes in pregnancy, 351
  compensatory changes in, 970, 971
  curvature affecting respiration, 453
  disorders causing back pain, 342
  drop-off sign in spondylolisthesis, 1010
  dura mater of, 34, 43
  exercises for problem areas, 1052
  facilitated segments at crossover sites, 970,
        972
  functional spinal units, 339–341
  group curves, 979–982
    causes of, 979
    diagnosis of, 979
    significance of, 979
    treatment of, 980–981

intervertebral disks
  degeneration of, 342, 408
    lumbar, 583, 622
    thoracic, 564
  lumbar, 582–584
  motion of
    compound, 513
    coupled, 513
    lumbar, 591
    neutral, 514
    nonneutral, 514
    physiologic, 1134–1135
    range of motion in, 341
    simple, 513
    thoracic, 572–573
  motion tests
    seated, 492–493, 498–499
    standing, 491–492, 496–498
  neutral position, 514, 1133
  palpation of motion and paravertebral tissue
      texture, 480–481, 491–492
    in cervical area, 481
    in lumbar area, 482
    in sacroiliac area, 482
    in thoracic area, 481
  patterning, 970–972
  side-bent vertebra, 1138
  thoracic, 563–564
    movements of, 572–573
    neutral and nonneutral dysfunctions,
        572–573
  transition zones in, 972, 973
  tumors of, 343–344
  vertebral rotation, 1136
  vertebral unit in, 1140
Spinothalamic system, 175–176
Spiritual support in stress management, 212–213
Splanchnic nerves, 571, 581
  lumbar, 59
  pelvic and sacral, 59, 60, 71–72, 606
  thoracic, 59
    in abdominopelvic plexus, 68
    afferent axons to liver and pancreas, 74
Spleen, 941
  innervation of, 70
    efferent, 120
  lymphatic pump, 957–958
Splenius muscle, 566
Spondylitis, 1138
  ankylosing, 343
Spondyloarthopathies, seronegative, 461–463
Spondylolisthesis, 1001, 1006–1012, 1138
  causes of, 1006–1008
  classification of, 1006, 1007, 1008
  diagnosis of, 1008–1011
  exercise in, 1011
  manipulation in, 1011–1012
  patient education in, 1011
  in pregnancy, 1011
  treatment of, 1011–1012
Spondylolysis, 343, 1001, 1003, 1006, 1138
Spondylosis, 1138
Sports medicine, 285–287
  goals of physicians in, 286

  needs of athletes in, 286
  osteopathic approach to, 286–287
Sprains
  ankle, 636–637
  ligamentous, 623–624
Spray-and-stretch techniques
  for myofascial trigger points, 924, 927
  in spondylolisthesis, 1012
Spring ligament in foot, 639
Spring test in sacral torsion, 724
Springing technique, articulatory, 763, 1133
Steatorrhea, 380
Sternal angle, 564, 575
Sternal notch, 564, 575
Sternoclavicular joint, 33, 548
  motion tests, 553
  muscle energy techniques, 738–740
Sternocleidomastoid muscle, 541
Sternomanubrial joint, 564
  motion testing, 578
Sternum, 564
  evaluation of, 578
  palpation of, 1040
Steroid hormones, 84
  adrenal cortical, 84, 115–116, 122–123
    affecting neural activity, 88
  biosynthesis of, 85–86
  gonadal, affecting neural activity, 88
Still, Andrew Taylor, 3–4, 15, 137
Still point, 913, 1138
Stomach, 377–379
  cancer, 379
  inflammatory disease, 378
  innervation, 70
  motility disorders, 377–378
  peptic ulcer, 378–379
  viscerosomatic reference sites, 450
Strain and counterstrain, 809–818, 820 (see also
    Counterstrain techniques)
Strains, 1138
  of interosseous membrane in forearm, 555
  repetitive strain syndrome, 464
  of sphenobasilar synchondrosis, 906–907
Strength
  dynamic, 434
  static, 434
Strengthening exercises, 1053
  in pain management, 182
Stress, 205–215
  adaptation to, 163
  alcohol use and dependence in, 211–212
  anxiety from, 209–211
  approaches to
    changing responses to, 207
    changing stressors in, 207
  biofeedback in, 214
  and biologic response to illness, 427
  and body-mind-spirit triad, 246–247
  definitions of, 205
  depression from, 207–209
  effects on health and disease, 167
  and general adaptive response, 100, 127–129
  immune system in, 168
  insomnia management in, 214–215

  management techniques, 212–215
  observational learning in, 213
  perceptions of risk in, 213
  physiologic responses to, 205–206
  postural, lumbar pain from, 596–597
  progressive relaxation in, 213
  responses to, 99–105
    molecular basis of, 104
  sense of control in, 213
  and social readjustment scale, 164
  support systems in, 163
    social, 212
    spiritual, 212–213
  systematic desensitization in, 213–214
  theories of, 206
Stretching, 1138
  exercise with, 1051–1052
  in pain management, 182
  in soft tissue techniques, 781
  and spray-with-stretch technique
    for myofascial trigger points, 924, 927
  in spondylolisthesis, 1012
Stringiness, 1139
Structure
  interdependence with function, 137
    in endocrine system, 85–92
    as guide to medical practice, 11
    in pharmacology, 94
    as principle in osteopathic medicine, 5–6
    and role of musculoskeletal system, 8–10
    and rules of anatomy, 25, 45–51
  in somatic dysfunction, 512–513
  variations in, 51
Subclavian arteries, 548
Subclavian muscle, 568
Subclavian vein, 549
Subcostal muscles, 566
Subluxation, 1139
Submandibular effleurage to promote lymphatic
    flow, 959
Submandibular lymph nodes, 521
Suboccipital region, evaluation in hospitalized
    patients, 1040, 1042
Substance abuse, 160–161
Substance P as neuroregulator, 110–111
Subtalar joint, 633, 634–635
Summation
  and somatovisceral reflexes, 144–145
  in theories of pain, 173
Supination, 1139
  foot, 636
  forearm, 554, 556
Support systems for patients, 163
  for cancer patients, 163
  in pain management, 183–184
Suprahyoid node technique to promote lymphatic
    flow, 961
Supraoptic nucleus, 117
Surgery, 387–391
  abdominal and chest wall, 388
    postoperative complications of, 388–389
  alimentary tract, 389–390
  osteopathic approach to, 387–388
  in scoliosis, 995, 996

Sutherland, William G., 901–902
Sutures of skull, 33, 34
Sweat glands, innervation of, 62
Symmetry, 1139
Sympathetic dystrophy, reflex, 560
Sympathetic nervous system, 58–60, 402, 570–571, 1043
    cardiac, 141–143
    of head, 522, 524, 528
    organization of, 59
    in upper extremities, 550
    vascular component, 58
    visceral component, 58
Symphysis pubis (see Pubic symphysis)
Synapses, 55
Synergist muscles, 36
Synovial fluid, 32
Synovial joints, 31–33
    disks or menisci in, 33
    motions of, 33
    specialized types of, 33
    structure of, 31–33
Synovial membrane, 32
Synoviocytes, 111
Systemic illness
    and body-mind-spirit triad, 246–247
    efficacy of manipulation in, 1017–1018
    and treatment of hospitalized patients, 1037–1047

T-lymphocytes, 111, 119, 295, 944
Talocalcaneal joint, 633
Talocrural joint, 633–634
Talofibular ligaments, 637
Talonavicular joint, 639
Talotibial joint, thrust technique for, 689
Talus, inverted, thrust technique for, 689–690
Tapotement, 1139
Tarsal bones, somatic dysfunction of, 640
Tarsal joint, transverse, 639–640
TART findings in somatic dysfunction, 475, 491, 610, 1139
    in lumbar region, 590
Temporal arteritis, 537–538
Temporomandibular joint, 33
    dysfunction of, 538–539
        muscle energy treatment of, 539
Tender points, myofascial, 810, 1139
    location of, 810–811, 915
Tendinitis, 464
    bicipital, 559
Tendons
    attachment to bone, 35, 41–42
    connective tissue in, 29
    deep reflexes, 506
    tap reflex, 138
Tennis elbow, 559
    myofascial trigger points in, 926
Tenosynovitis, de Quervain's, postpartum, 358
Tension headaches, 403, 536–537
Teres muscles
    major, 565
    minor, 565

Testes
    hormones of, 84
    innervation of, 78
Testosterone, 84
Tethering, sources of, 846
Thiazide diuretics in hypertension, 323–324
Thigh
    fascia lata relaxation, 792–793
    muscles of, 646, 647–649, 651–654
        symptoms of spastic adductor muscles, 976
    nerve supply in, 646
Thoracic duct, 569–570, 587, 943
    innervation of, 68
Thoracic inlet, 1139
    evaluation in hospitalized patients, 1040, 1042
    lymphatic drainage in, 527
    opening to improve lymphatic flow, 948–949
Thoracic lymphatic pump, 389, 955–956
    and immune function, 453–454
Thoracic outlet syndrome, 413, 542, 561
Thoracic region, 563–579
    anatomy and physiology of, 563–572
    articulatory techniques, 768
    connective tissue and fascia in, 570
    counterstrain techniques, 814–815
    evaluation of, 574–575
    facilitated positional release, 834–836
    fascial-ligamentous release, 825–826
    functional techniques in, 801–802
    innervation of organs in, 63–68
    lymphatics of, 452, 569–570
    mobility reduction in, 448–449
    motion testing, 575–578
    movements of, 572–574
    muscle energy techniques, 704–710
        lower spine, 706–710
        upper spine, 704–706
    muscles of, 564–569
    myofascial and integrated neuromusculoskeletal release, 870–874
    neural connections of, 570–572
    palpation of, 575
        posterior, in hospitalized patients, 1041
    pump actions of, 448
    skeleton of, 563–564 (see also Ribs)
    soft tissue techniques, 783–787
    thrust technique, 669–674
    treatment of problems in, 578–579
Thoracolumbar region
    aponeurosis in, 584–585
    thrust technique, 679–682
Throat, 295–296
Thrombosis, coronary, 300–301
Thrust techniques, 661–665, 1134
    cervical, 667–669
        atlantoaxial, 667–668
        occipitoatlantal, 667
        rotational focus in, 669
        side-bending focus in, 668–669
    complications from, 1020
    direct method, 663–664
    dose of, 665
    epigastric, for spinal group curves, 980

    guidelines for safety, 665
    Hiss plantar whip, 690
    history of, 661
    indications for, 661–662
    lower extremity, 686–690
        ankle tug, 689–690
        anterior fibular head, 687
        anterior tibia on talus, 689
        lateral malleoli, 688–689
        posterior fibular head, 686–687
    mechanism of action, 664
    in motion loss with somatic dysfunction, 662–663
    pop or click in, 664
    precautions and contraindications, 665
        in malignancies, 428
    ribs, 674–679
        crossed hand, 677–678
        inhalation and exhalation in, 677
        prone, 674–675, 677–679
        seated, 676–677
        supine, 675–676, 677
    thoracic, 669–674
        crossed hand, 672–673
        extension, 670, 671–672, 674
        flexion, 669–670, 671, 673
        hand as fulcrum in, 670
        multiple plane, 670–674
        pillow fulcrum in, 673–674
        prone, 672–673
        seated, 673–674
        single plane, 669–670
        supine, 669–671
    thoracolumbar, 679–682
        extension, 680–681
        flexion, 681–682
        lateral recumbent, 679–682
        posterior transverse process down, 679, 680–683
        posterior transverse process up, 679–680
    unstable hypermobile joints in, 664–665
    upper extremity, 685–686
        abducted elbow, 685–686
        posterior radial head, 685
        wrist, 686
Thymocytes, 111, 119
Thymosins, 116
Thymulin, 116
Thymus, 942
    efferent innervation of, 119–120
    hormones of, 116
Thyroglobulin, 86
Thyroid colloid, 86
Thyroid hormones, 84, 123–124
    affecting neural activity, 88
Thyroid-stimulating hormone (see Thyrotropin)
Thyrotropin, 84, 123
    releasing hormone, 84, 118, 123
Thyroxine, 84, 123
Tibia
    anterior on talus, thrust technique in, 689
    posterior on talus, thrust technique in, 689
Tibial nerve, 646
    entrapment of, 411

Tibialis anterior muscle, 648, 649
  inhibited, symptoms of, 976
Tibiofibular joint, 631
  proximal, muscle energy techniques, 753–755
Tibiotalar joint, 633
Tic douloureux, 528
Tinel's sign, 559
  in carpal tunnel syndrome, 412
Tissue repair, activities in, 102–103
Tissue texture abnormality, 1139
  facilitated positional release in, 832
  paravertebral, palpation of, 480–481, 491–492
Tobacco use, 160–161
Toeing out and toeing in, 634
Tonsillitis, 296
Tonsils, 295, 942
Tonus, 1139
Torsion, 1139
  sacral, 620
Torso curl exercise, 1053
  reverse, 1053
Torso extension exercise, 1053–1054
Torticollis, 530
  acute, muscle energy technique in, 545
Touching, as communication with cancer
      patients, 427
Traction headache, 537
Traction therapy, 1134
  cervical, anterior, to promote lymphatic flow,
      960–961
  pectoral, 791
    to promote lymphatic flow, 955
  in soft tissue techniques, 781
Transcutaneous nerve stimulation (see Electrical
      nerve stimulation, transcutaneous)
Transfusions for cancer patients, 426
Transitional regions, 1139
  in postural changes, 972, 973
Transitional vertebral segment, 1139
Translation
  lateral translation test
    for C2-7 motion, 545
    for occipital motion, 544
  sacral, 1137
Transverse abdominis muscle, 603
Transverse plane of body, 1135
Trapezius muscle, 541, 565
Trauma
  ankle sprains, 636–637
  from falls in geriatric patients, 281–282
  hip fractures in elderly persons, 334–335
  ligamentous sprains, 623–624
  of primary respiratory mechanisms, 911
Travell and Simons myofascial trigger points,
      810, 915, 919–933 (see also Myofascial
      trigger points)
Travell tender points, 595
Trendelenburg test, 612
Triceps reflex, 551
Trigeminal nerve, 63, 526, 528–529
  entrapment of, 411
  neuralgia, 529, 538
    headache in, 406
Trigger points (see Myofascial trigger points)

Trigone muscle, 76
Triiodothyronine, 84, 123
Trochlear nerve, 526
Trophicity, 1140
Trunk bending tests
  seated, 499
  standing, 496–498
Tubo-ovarian abscess, 368
Tumor(s) (see Oncology)
Tumor necrosis factor, 114, 123, 424
  in stress response, 104
Turbinates, nasal, 290
Tympanic membrane, 293

Ulcer, peptic, 378–379
Ulcerative colitis, 382–383
Ulna, abduction and adduction of, 553, 554
Ulnar nerve entrapment, 411
Ulnohumeral joint, 548, 553
Ulnomeniscotriquetral joint, 33
Umbilicus, 588
  tender points near, 595
Uncovertebral joints of Luschka, 541
Unity of body
  connectedness in, 49–50
  and endocrine system, 83–92
  as guide to medical practice, 10–11
  and person as a whole, 8
  as principle in osteopathic medicine, 4–5
  role of hormones in, 87–89
Unstable hypermobile joints, thrust technique
      affecting, 664–665
Unwinding maneuvers in myofascial and
      integrated neuromusculoskeletal release,
      882–887
Upper extremities, 547–561
  adhesive capsulitis, 560–561
  anatomy, 39–41
  articulatory techniques, 777–780
  axillary fold technique, posterior, 964–965
  carpal tunnel syndrome, 559–560
  Chapman's points (see Chapman reflexes)
  diagnosis of problems in, 551–553
  effleurage and pétrissage, 965–966
  fascial-ligamentous release, 826–828
  functional anatomy of, 547–550
  glenohumeral joint and shoulder muscles,
      549
  motion testing, 499–500, 552–553
  motor strength tests, 552
  muscle energy techniques, 742–746
  myofascial and integrated neuromusculoskeletal
      release, 887–899
  palpation of, 551
  pulses in, 551
  reflex sympathetic dystrophy, 560
  reflexes in, 551–552
  sensation testing in, 552
  soft tissue techniques, 791–792
  special tests for, 558–559
  thrust techniques, 685–686
  thumb joint motions, 549
  treatment of problems in, 559–561
  trigger points (see Myofascial trigger points)

Uremia
  encephalopathy in, 396
  neuropathies in, 395–397
Ureter, innervation of, 75–76
Urethral sphincters, 76, 77, 370
Urinary incontinence, 370–371
  geriatric, 280–281
Urine voiding mechanisms, 77
Urogenital diaphragm, 603, 945–946
Urogenital triangle, 369
Uterus
  innervation of, 78–79, 363
  pain in, 366–367
  viscerosomatic reference sites for, 450

Vagina, innervation of, 79
Vagus nerve, 60, 371, 530, 581
  afferent and efferent fibers of, 63
  afferent axons to liver and pancreas, 74
  axons in abdominal cavity, 71
  in cardiac innervation, 65, 66
  in esophageal innervation, 67
  pulmonary branches of, 66
Valgus stress testing of knee, 630
Varus stress testing of knee, 630–631
Vas deferens, innervation of, 78
Vasculature
  blood supply affecting health, 47
  of brain, affecting primary respiratory
      mechanisms, 910
  of head and neck, 517, 521, 542
  innervation of, 61–62
  lower extremity, 646, 650, 655
  lumbar and abdominal region, 586–587
  pelvis and sacrum, 604
  pulmonary, 445
  segmental organization of, 36–39
  upper extremity, 548–549
  venous drainage, 48
Vasculitis, 464
Vasomotor nerve fibers, 61–62
Vasopressin, 84
Vastus muscles, inhibited, symptoms of, 976
Venous drainage, 48
  of head, 521, 525
  of lumbar and abdominal region, 588
  myofascial trigger points affecting, 926–928
  of upper extremity, 549
Ventilation, 441–444
  control of, 447–448
  inequality with perfusion, 447
  obstructive and restrictive patterns of, 444
Ventricles
  fourth, cerebral, 530–531
  of heart
    dysfunction in heart failure, 308
    hypertrophy with hypertension, 325
Verapamil in hypertension, 325
Vertebrae (see Spine)
Vertebral arteries, 517, 521
  dissections causing headache, 406
Vertebral unit, 1140
Vertigo, cervical, 542
Vesical plexus, 76, 79

Vestibulocochlear nerve, 530
Vibration in pain management, 182
Viscera
    innervation of, 571
    manipulation of, 1134
    pain in, 590
        from lumbar and abdominal region, 583,
            589–590
        peritoneum of, distended, 589
    reflex arc, 55–56
    stimuli affecting neuroendocrine-immune
        network, 127–128
Viscerosomatic pain, 590
Viscerosomatic reflexes, 61, 139–140, 141, 1136
    association with myofascial trigger points,
        931–932
    cardiac, 143
    and lung disease, 449–452

in nausea and vomiting of pregnancy, 353
    in pelvic pain, 364
    postoperative, 389
    sacroiliac, 622
    in sex act, 79
    somatic component of, 389
Viscero-visceral reflexes, 139, 1136
Viscosity, 1140
Voiding of urine, mechanisms in, 77

Waldeyer's ring, 295
Walk cycle, normal motion of, 608
Weight problems in obesity, 159–160
    exercise in, 199–200
Wolff's law, 572, 999, 1132
Work situations, satisfaction with, 163
Wrist joint, 548, 553, 557
    motion of, 557

muscle energy techniques, 742–746
myofascial and integrated neuromusculoskeletal
    release, 891–899
somatic dysfunction of, 557
thrust technique for restriction, 686

Xiphisternal joint, 564
    motion testing, 578
X-ray studies (see Radiography)
D-Xylose test in malabsorption, 380

Y-ligament of Bigelow, 625
Yergason test, 558

Zink, J. Gordon
    fascial patterning of, 946–947, 972, 974
    treatment of axillary fold dysfunction, 928, 930
Zygapophyseal tropism, 584